FOURTH EDITION

Veterinary Pharmacology and Therapeutics

FOURTH EDITION

Veterinary Pharmacology and Therapeutics

EDITED BY L. Meyer Jones
Nicholas H. Booth
Leslie E. McDonald

AMES: The Iowa State University Press

TO OUR TEACHERS

whose promptings and examples have guided so well

L. Meyer Jones taught veterinary pharmacology and therapeutics at Iowa State University for 25 years. He wrote the first edition of this textbook in 1954. He revised and enlarged the text as edition two for publication in 1957. Dr. Jones was coauthor and editor of edition three that appeared in 1965. He is a member of the American Society of Pharmacology and Experimental Therapeutics and of the Society of Toxicology. Dr. Jones served as the first Director of Scientific Activities of the American Veterinary Medical Association. Subsequently, he was Dean of the School of Veterinary Medicine at the University of Georgia and later was Dean of the College of Veterinary Medicine, University of Illinois. Dr. Jones was awarded the A.B. degree by DePauw University, the D.V.M. and M.S. degrees by Iowa State University, and the Ph.D. degree by the University of Minnesota.

Nicholas H. Booth taught pharmacology to veterinary medical students at Colorado State University for 18 years. He later served as Dean of the College of Veterinary Medicine and Biomedical Sciences in Colorado and then as Director of the Division of Veterinary Medical Research of the U.S. Food and Drug Administration. Dr. Booth is a Fellow of the American College of Veterinary Toxicology and is currently Professor of Physiology and Pharmacology within the College of Veterinary Medicine at the University of Georgia. He received the D.V.M. degree from Michigan State University, the M.S. degree from Colorado State University, and the Ph.D. degree from the University of Colorado School of Medicine.

Leslie E. McDonald, Professor of Physiology and Pharmacology at the University of Georgia, has specialized in veterinary endocrinology and reproduction. He has held teaching, research, and administrative posts at the University of Illinois, Oklahoma State University, Ohio State University, and the University of Georgia. He is also the author of *Veterinary Endocrinology and Reproduction,* a widely used textbook in colleges of veterinary medicine. Dr. McDonald holds the B.S. and D.V.M. degrees from Michigan State University and the M.S. and Ph.D. degrees from the University of Wisconsin.

Composed and printed by
The Iowa State University Press

Fourth edition, 1977

Library of Congress Cataloging in Publication Data
Jones, Leo Meyer, 1913–
Veterinary pharmacology and therapeutics.

Includes bibliographies.
1. Veterinary pharmacology. I. Booth, Nicholas H., 1923– joint author. II. McDonald, Leslie Ernest, 1923– joint author. III. Title. [DNLM: 1. Pharmacology. 2. Drug therapy—Veterinary. 3. Poisoning—Veterinary. SF915 V587]
SF915.J67 1977 636.089'51 76-44946
ISBN 0-8138-1740-4

Contents

Contributors

ADAMS, H. RICHARD, D.V.M., Ph.D. Associate Professor of Pharmacology, Southwestern Medical School, University of Texas, Dallas, Texas

BAGGOT, J. DESMOND, M.V.B., Ph.D. School of Veterinary Studies, Murdoch University, Murdoch, Western Australia

BEVILL, RICHARD F., D.V.M., Ph.D. Associate Professor of Physiology and Pharmacology, College of Veterinary Medicine, University of Illinois, Urbana, Illinois

BOOTH, NICHOLAS H., D.V.M., Ph.D. Professor of Physiology and Pharmacology, College of Veterinary Medicine, University of Georgia, Athens, Georgia

CLARK, DONALD R., D.V.M., Ph.D. Professor of Physiology and Pharmacology, College of Veterinary Medicine, Texas A & M University, College Station, Texas

DETWEILER, DAVID K., V.M.D. Professor of Physiology, School of Veterinary Medicine, University of Pennsylvania, Philadelphia, Pennsylvania

GROSS, DAVID R., D.V.M., Ph.D. Associate Professor of Physiology and Pharmacology, College of Veterinary Medicine, Texas A & M University, College Station, Texas

HATCH, ROGER C., D.V.M., Ph.D. Associate Professor of Pharmacology and Toxicology, College of Veterinary Medicine, University of Georgia, Athens, Georgia

HUBER, WILLIAM G., D.V.M., Ph.D. Professor of Comparative Pharmacology, College of Veterinary Medicine, Washington State University, Pullman, Washington

JONES, L. MEYER, D.V.M., Ph.D. Professor of Anatomy, Physiology, and Pharmacology, College of Veterinary Medicine, University of Illinois, Urbana, Illinois

LEWIS, LON D., D.V.M., Ph.D. Assistant Professor of Clinical Sciences, College of Veterinary Medicine and Biomedical Sciences, Colorado State University, Fort Collins, Colorado

McCRADY, J. D., D.V.M., Ph.D. Professor of Physiology and Pharmacology, College of Veterinary Medicine, Texas A & M University, College Station, Texas

McDONALD, LESLIE E., D.V.M., Ph.D. Professor of Physiology and Pharmacology, College of Veterinary Medicine, University of Georgia, Athens, Georgia

NOLAN, MAXCY P., Ph.D. Extension Entomologist, Cooperative Extension Service, University of Georgia, Athens, Georgia

PHILLIPS, ROBERT W., D.V.M., Ph.D. Professor of Physiology and Biophysics, College of Veterinary Medicine and Biomedical Sciences, Colorado State University, Fort Collins, Colorado

ROBERSON, EDWARD L., D.V.M., Ph.D. Assistant Professor of Parasitology, College of Veterinary Medicine, University of Georgia, Athens, Georgia

SZABUNIEWICZ, MICHAEL, D.V.M., D.V.Sc. Professor Emeritus of Physiology and Pharmacology, College of Veterinary Medicine, Texas A & M University, College Station, Texas

Preface

WHEN Dr. L. Meyer Jones asked us to take the major editorial responsibility for the revision of this textbook, we were pleased to accept the challenges and tasks of this important endeavor. As in previous editions, the main thrust of the book has been directed to the professional student in veterinary medicine. In addition, it is anticipated that the book will continue to serve as a valuable reference for the practicing veterinarian and those engaged in specialized disciplines such as laboratory animal medicine.

More space has been devoted in this edition to the important discipline of veterinary toxicology. Also, more in-depth information has been introduced that was not covered in previous editions such as molecular pharmacology and drug residues in food products derived from animals. The benefits versus the public health risks of using drugs in food-producing animals in the prevention, control, and treatment of animal diseases have been discussed. Information has been included on many veterinary drugs, most of which have been approved for use in animals by the U.S. Food and Drug Administration (FDA) as well as the drugs regulated by the U.S. Drug Enforcement Agency under the Controlled Substances Act of 1970. Although its coverage is not comprehensive in all species, this edition has been expanded to include the use of pharmacologic agents in the exotic species and those of importance in laboratory animal medicine.

Since the last edition, a number of new drugs and

drug combinations have been introduced for veterinary medical use. The pharmacologic, therapeutic, and toxicologic activities of many of these new preparations have been discussed throughout the textbook. Some of the "old drugs" have been omitted because they have been withdrawn from use by the FDA or have been replaced by superior products. Additionally, there are some drugs that are discussed only briefly because their use is limited.

Most of the pharmacologic agents in the book are identified by their generic and/or proprietary names. However, reference to a specific drug by proprietary name does not constitute endorsement of the product by the authors to the exclusion of similar products. It is virtually impossible to list all proprietary names.

The first three editions of *Veterinary Pharmacology and Therapeutics* have enjoyed widespread acceptance in the United States and internationally. Translations into several languages have extended usage of the book. To enable the continued success of future editions, every effort will be made to keep pace with the important advances in knowledge through frequent revisions. Although the span of time between this and the last edition was inordinately long, it is anticipated that subsequent editions will be more prompt.

In conclusion, the authors wish to acknowledge the encouragement and support of their wives and colleagues during the preparation of this edition.

N. H. Booth and L. E. McDonald

SECTION 1

Introduction

CHAPTER 1

VETERINARY PHARMACOLOGY—PAST, PRESENT, AND FUTURE

L. MEYER JONES

HISTORY OF PHARMACOLOGY

Ancient Era

The origin of medical knowledge and the use of drugs were entwined with the differing mythology of each group of ancient peoples. Among the Greeks, the first efforts to control disease were associated with Apollo, the god of healing. The son of Apollo was Asclepius, whose priest-physician followers founded temples of healing where diseased people were treated by prayer, mineral spring baths, and massage. In addition, plants and animals or their products were used in sacrifices to appease a wrathful god or applied to patients to eliminate the disease agent or evil spirit.

The *Papyros Ebers,* written about 1550 B.C. in Egypt, is a collection of folklore dating from dynasties of various countries five to twenty centuries earlier. The *Papyros* is composed mainly of prescriptions, which specified ailments, and the substances and procedures to be used for treatment. It contains 811 prescriptions in the form of salves, plasters, poultices, snuffs, inhalations, gargles, draughts, confections, pills, fumigations, suppositories, and clysters.

The Greek philosopher-physicians of around 500 B.C. proposed and then taught the concept that health was maintained by a balance of body "humors," which were influenced by heat and cold, moisture and dryness, and acidity and sweetness, and that disease was due to an imbalance of these qualities. Elements of the earth were associated with these characteristics, i.e., fire was hot and dry; water was cold and moist; air was hot and moist; the earth was cold and dry; and certain minerals and other substances were acid and some were sweet (as were vinegar and honey). The Greek philosopher-physicians associated elements of the universe with the four body humors: yellow bile was hot and dry; blood was hot and moist; phlegm was cold and moist; and black bile was cold and dry.

Hippocrates (460–370 B.C.) is purported to have originated the theory that disease is due to the imbalance of the body humors (humoral pathology). As a result of his bedside method of observation, the keeping of clinical records, and his belief in the healing power of nature and in simple remedies, Hippocrates stands as a monument in the early recorded history of medicine and is called the Father of Medicine. Hippocrates raised medicine from the art of philosophy to a systematic clinical science by the art of observation of the patient's symptoms. He attributed the causes of disease to an imbalance of body humors rather than to gods or demons. His treatments included massage, hydrotherapy, and bloodletting, which was practiced until recent decades in an empirical effort to correct an imbalance of body humors or fluids.

About A.D. 77, Dioscorides, a pupil of Aristotle, wrote the first materia medica (materials of medicine), which was principally a qualitative classification of medicinal herbs but included minerals and a few products of animal origin. Information regarding these materials and their uses was gathered by Dioscorides while he served as a surgeon in the Roman armies and traveled around the Mediterranean Sea. His materia medica was probably the more authoritative guide to drugs until the seventeenth century, although it was not as widely used as were the later writings of Galen. The latter's materia medica have been called galenical preparations. Thereafter, and leading to the Renaissance, the knowledge of medicine degenerated to a state of ignorance through use of complex, irrational prescriptions consisting of a vast number of ingredients with apparently no beneficial effect in the control or successful treatment of disease.

The Renaissance

The spirit of inquiry is exemplified best by Paracelsus (1493–1541) who wrote, "Reading never made a physician. Medicine is an art and requires practical experience." Paracelsus rejected medical theorists and traditional practitioners because, as he said, ". . . nothing resulted from their practice but killing, laming, and distorting. . . . They administered scarcely anything but syrups, laxatives, purgatives and oatmeal gruel with everlasting clysters. . . ." Paracelsus induced medical practitioners to use laudanum (an opium preparation), sulfur, iron, copper sulfate and potassium sulfate, mercurials, and tinctures or fluid extracts of various plants for the treatment of disease.

In 1628 William Harvey (1578–1657) discovered the phenomenon of circulation. This observation was followed by the injection of water, colored fluids, ink, and wax into the blood vessels of animals. In 1656 Sir Christopher Wren and assistants made the first intravenous injection of drugs (opium and *Crocus metallorum*), using a dog as the subject.

During this same period, members of the Order of Jesuits brought the bark of the cinchona tree from South America for use in treatment of malaria in human beings. This treatment was relatively effective against malaria and was used to differentiate other febrile conditions from malaria. More significantly, this discovery brought recognition that specific therapy was possible and started a never-ending search in pharmacology for a specific drug to use in treating a specific disease condition.

In 1783 William Withering, an English physician, reported on his experience in the use of crude digitalis (the foxglove plant) for the treatment of "dropsy" (generalized edema generally from cardiac malfunction). Later, the experimental investigation of digitalis by Claude Bernard (1813–1873), and subsequently by Schmiedeberg, revealed that the primary pharmacological action of the drug was exerted on the heart. These investigations employing experimental techniques of drug study established the philosophy and *modus operandi* of modern pharmacology and, therefore, the foundation of the discipline. Such comments about Bernard and Schmiedeberg are not intended to detract from the major contribution of Withering, who was indeed an astute practitioner and clinical observer. In an age still tainted with witchcraft, quackery, and secret remedies, Withering stands out above the early physicians in England.

It is interesting to note that in the eighteenth century the English physician was truly a family doctor. He was paid an annual stipend and it was his responsibility to keep the family free from disease insofar as possible. One is reminded also of the earlier Chinese custom of paying a physician to keep the family free from disease but not paying him when members of the family were sick. These earlier customs show an appreciation of the value of preventive medicine that frequently is not fully exploited in modern medicine.

During the nineteenth century, the tree of experimental sciences grew vigorously. Magendie (1783–1855), a French physiologist-pharmacologist, published many experimental observations on the effects of intravenous injection of ipecac, morphine, hydrocyanic acid, strychnine, iodine, potassium, veratrine, quinine, and many other drugs. He published a "formulary" in which he discussed the action and preparation of a large number of drugs, many of which he introduced into medical practice.

A systematic investigation of poisonous substances was undertaken by M. J. B. Orfila, who published the results of many experiments in 1813 under the title of *Toxicologie Générale*. Orfila (1787–1853), a chemist and physician, is regarded as the founder of the science of toxicology. Taylor of England, Casper of Germany, and Christison of Scotland made many contributions toward identification of toxic agents, quantitative chemical tests, and the examination of dead bodies for legal purposes when poisoning was suspected.

Origin of General Pharmacology

It is hard to recognize the beginnings of medicine, but even more so the beginning of the discipline of pharmacology. The term "Pharmakologie" was applied to the science of materia medica by S. Dale in London as early as 1692; however, the formal birthplace of modern pharmacology is claimed to be the city of Dorpat on the Baltic Sea where Rudolph Buchheim, primarily a biochemist, established in 1846 the first laboratory devoted exclusively to experimental pharmacology at the University of Dorpat. The term "Father of Pharmacology" is applied to Buchheim, a professor at Dorpat University. Buchheim felt it insufficient to merely describe drugs and list their indications. He considered it necessary to explain actions of drugs upon the organs and cells of the body. Such information gathered from these experiments resulted in 118 publications about a variety of drugs and their activities. Using these data and other information, Buchheim published in 1856 his textbook of materia medica in which he arranged drugs in an unprecedented method of classification determined by their pharmacological action upon living tissue. He discarded many remedies then current because a rational scientific action or explanation could not be demonstrated in his laboratories; thus was the era of critical pharmacology initiated.

Oswald Schmiedeberg (1838–1921) was the most outstanding student of Buchheim while the latter was at Dorpat University. Schmiedeberg succeeded Buchheim as professor at Dorpat when the latter moved to the University of Geissen. In 1872 Schmiedeberg moved to the University of Strasbourg where he became Professor of Pharmacology and did most of his research work, writings, and training of students who became famous pharmacologists at many universities around the world.

Professor Schmiedeberg's goal was to establish pharmacology as an independent scientific discipline based upon exact experimental methodology. In his textbook, he defined pharmacology as "an experimental science which has for its purposes the study of the changes brought about in living organisms by chemically acting substances (with the exception of food, whether used for therapeutic purposes or not)." One of his students, John J. Abel, said, ". . . more than any other man . . . Schmiedeberg turned the ages-old materia medica and therapeutics of our medical schools into the modern and fundamental science of pharmacology" (Abel 1926). Schmiedeberg and his students carried out vast numbers of superb investigations demonstrating the effect of drugs upon living tissues of the body. When Schmiedeberg collected the results of these investigations into a textbook, he followed the classification of drug actions generated by Buchheim and entitled the book *Grundriss der Ärzneimittellehre.* This title was chosen to indicate that these drugs provided a groundwork for therapy and were selected because their therapeutic value had been established by scientific experimentation. Later editions substituted the word "Pharmakologie" to indicate the wider scope of the textbook, i.e., a study of the effects of drugs on the living organism without confining attention to therapeutics. He felt that the discipline of pharmacology should guide the clinicians to practice rational therapeutics. Among the many pupils of Schmiedeberg were several men whose contributions formed the foundation of modern pharmacology and who were prominent in the development of pharmacology in the United States: Abel, Cushney, Sollmann, Meyer, Cash, and Heubner. In addition, Schmiedeberg founded the first pharmacological journal, *Archiv für Experimentelle Pathologie und Pharmakologie.*

The title "Father of American Pharmacology" has been conferred on Professor John Jacob Abel, Ph.D., M.D. Abel (1857–1938) was born in Ohio and educated at the Universities of Michigan and Pennsylvania before going to Strasbourg to study with the great Schmiedeberg. Abel returned to the University of Michigan School of Medicine to accept the first full-time professorship in the United States devoted to the new discipline of pharmacology. The spirit of Magendie, Buchheim, and Schmiedeberg was brought to the United States by Abel, who probably was more effective than anyone else in the United States in promoting the growth and recognition of pharmacology as a discipline of medical science. Abel's teachings in pharmacology dealt with the dynamic action of drugs on the living tissues of human beings and animals. His teachings, research, and philosophy contributed much to the demise of materia medica as a discipline, which described and otherwise emphasized the physical characteristics of medical materials, i.e., mostly crude plant drugs and minerals. Materia medica devoted little or no attention to the actions of drugs within and upon the living cells of the body.

After 2 years at Michigan, Abel accepted a chair of pharmacology at Johns Hopkins Medical School, where he remained the rest of his life. Abel was noted for his originality, keenness of observation, breadth of knowledge, thoroughness, and productivity in his research on a variety of important drugs. His major fields of investigation encompassed the isolation of active endocrine substances, metabolism and pharmacokinetics of drugs, clinical pharmacology, chemotherapy, and the identification of certain diagnostic agents. Abel shared his laboratory with various investigators and trained many young scientists who became prominent pharmacologists.

In 1905 Abel, with C. A. Herter, founded the *Journal of Biological Chemistry.* In 1909 Abel founded the *Journal of Pharmacology and Experimental Therapeutics.* He was also instrumental in the formation of the respective sponsoring organizations, the American Society of Biological Chemistry and the American Society of Pharmacology and Experimental Therapeutics.

Origin of Veterinary Pharmacology

Although archaeologists have unearthed the ruins in India of an army hospital only for horses and elephants dating back to about 5000 B.C., the oldest of the present veterinary colleges and hospitals were established in the 1760s in western Europe. Earlier in that century, great epizootics (viz., rinderpest) decimated the animal population in western Europe, especially cattle. In response to public demand, five veterinary colleges were established in France and other colleges were started in Austria, Germany, and the Netherlands. In 1791 a veterinary college was started in London, England, and soon thereafter another began in Edinburgh, Scotland.

In the United States, one so-called college was started in Philadelphia (1852) and another in Boston (1854), but these were short-lived apprenticeship programs appended to existing private practices. During the next half century, thirty or more privately owned and generally successful veterinary colleges educated veterinarians in the United States. Although the educational curricula and teaching varied widely, the graduates of such programs appeared to meet the social needs for animal health care that existed in those times. With advancements in scientific knowledge, higher standards of training were required in all medical science education by various agencies of the U.S. federal and state governments acting in behalf of the public. The newly established educational requirements for teaching and licensing of the veterinarian and also for employment in government positions led to the demise of the privately owned colleges of veterinary medicine, mostly in the 1920s. At present in the United States, public tax monies support all colleges of veterinary medicine (although Cornell, Pennsylvania, and Tuskegee receive substantial private funding), awarding degrees to students that qualify them to write licensing examinations in the various states.

The early schools of veterinary medicine were established in conjunction with schools of medicine and the faculties were intermingled. In London, England, the first faculty members of the Royal College of Veterinary Surgeons taught jointly in the medical and veterinary schools. The same was true at the Royal (Dick) Veterinary College in Edinburgh. This tradition was carried to the American colonies when the first schools of veterinary medicine were established. The first professor of therapeutics at the School of Veterinary Medicine at Iowa State College was D. S. Fairchild, M.D., according to the college catalog of 1881. Dr. Kenelm Winslow, assistant professor of Materia Medica and Therapeutics and author of a textbook published while at the School of Veterinary Medicine, Harvard University, had degrees both in veterinary medicine and medicine. The professions of medicine and veterinary medicine were one and the same in the Western world until about a century ago when the two professions and their schools went their separate ways.

The origin and development of veterinary pharmacology as a discipline in the veterinary medical profession need to be more clearly defined. In earlier centuries, teaching was by lecture, demonstration, and/or performance under supervision by the apprenticeship system. Originally no books on veterinary drugs were available for student use. Later books were available but expensive and scarce. An examination of textbooks generally gives the reader an indication of the state of knowledge taught to students.

TEXTBOOKS

The early veterinary textbooks discussing drugs and their uses dealt with the physical characteristics of medicinal materials and their sources, incompatibilities, and compounding (preparing the medicine in a dosage form). The books also discussed the toxic or poisonous effects of certain medicines, plants, and minerals. Instruction in therapeutics consisted principally in listing disease conditions for which certain drugs were empirically and traditionally used. The problem faced by the student was to memorize and prescribe the traditional drug in the proper dosage and form of administration to match the indication, i.e., diagnosed ailment.

An early veterinary textbook in English dealing with drugs was *The Veterinarians' Vade Mecum* by John Gamgee, which was published in England in its second edition in 1868. No discussion of drug activities or mechanisms of effect on tissues appears in this textbook. About 20% of the page space was devoted to a listing of materia medica used by the veterinarian, about 26% to formulas for compounding prescriptions, and about 54% to descriptive toxicology involving minerals and plants mostly. Such space allocation was typical of other books.

A *Manual of Veterinary Therapeutics and Pharmacology,* written by Professor E. Wallis Hoare of the Royal College of Veterinary Surgeons in London, went through many editions. In the United States, several early books dealt with posology (dosages and prescriptions). Prominent among these were *Synopsis of Veterinary Materia Medica, Therapeutics and Toxicology* by E. L. Quitman, Professor of Materia Medica, Therapeutics and Toxicology at the Chicago Veterinary College, published in the third edition in 1907; the *Book of Veterinary Dosages: Therapeutic Terms and Prescription Writing,* published in the third edition in 1908 by P. A. Fish, Professor of Veterinary Physiology, New York State Veterinary College, Cornell University; and the *Book of Veterinary Posology and Prescriptions,* published in 1924 by O. V. Brumley, Professor of Small Animal Medicine, Ohio State University.

A prominent textbook in the United States entitled *Veterinary Materia Medica and Therapeutics* was that written by Kenelm Winslow, Assistant Professor of Materia Medica and Therapeutics, School of Veterinary Medicine, Harvard University. The eighth edition, published in 1919, devoted about 7% of its space to the general actions of drugs, 9% to pharmacy and prescription writing, 2% to posology, 24% to general therapeutic measures, and about 58% to materia medica; however, Winslow's discussions of materia medica emphasized the action of drugs on living tissues more than did other veterinary authors of his generation. Winslow was much influenced by newer knowledge of the physiology of organs and the publications in the new discipline of pharmacology, which revealed the activities of drugs on living tissue.

A more widely used textbook, *Practical Veterinary Pharmacology and Therapeutics,* was published by H. J. Milks, Professor of Therapeutics and Director of Small Animal Clinic, New York State Veterinary College, Cornell University. The 1917 edition devoted about 13% of its space to pharmacy and prescription writing and the remaining 87% to a consideration of materia medica and the clinical uses of drugs. The sixth edition, appearing in 1949, was entitled *Practical Veterinary Pharmacology, Materia Medica and Therapeutics* and, although much more current, this prominent textbook still emphasized the materia medica and the clinical use of drugs for the treatment of disease. It was a very reliable text for drug dosages for common species of animals treated by veterinarians.

This textbook, *Veterinary Pharmacology and Therapeutics* by L. Meyer Jones, Nicholas H. Booth, and Leslie E. McDonald, authorized first in 1954 by Jones, attempted to introduce more information regarding the actions of drugs on living tissues. It has been translated into five foreign languages. Among the books in the German language, the most influential were those written at the turn of the century by Eugen Fröhner of the Veterinary College at Berlin, Germany, and by Professor Carl Steinmetzer of the School of Veterinary Medicine in Vienna, Austria, at the close of World War II. The latter clearly emphasized pharmacodynamics as the basis for the selection and use of drugs for the treatment and control of disease in animals.

EARLY PROGRAMS AND PERSONALITIES IN THE UNITED STATES

The following discussion deals with three colleges of veterinary medicine that in early years developed strong programs in veterinary pharmacology with different characteristics arising out of the local needs, situations, and personalities involved. Iowa State University had a strong program of veterinary pharmacology in the Department of Veterinary Physiology and Pharmacology. Cornell University developed a strong program in veterinary materia medica and therapeutics in the Small Animal Clinic. Texas Agricultural and Mechanical University developed a strong program in veterinary toxicology in the Department of Veterinary Physiology and Pharmacology.

At Iowa State University, instruction about drugs used in veterinary medicine has received a great deal of attention throughout the history of the College of Veterinary Medicine. Among the documents in the substantial collection of veterinary literature in the archives of the library at Iowa State University is a catalog for the School of Veterinary Science of the Iowa Agricultural College for 1881. The veterinary curriculum covered 2 years with the subject of materia medica taught throughout the first year and therapeutics taught throughout the second; one-half year of toxicology was taught also during the second year. Later, the curriculum was extended to 4 years, and during the 1920s, the instruction about drugs took on the character of pharmacology and therapeutics with the offerings concentrated in the second curricular year plus a brief course in therapeutics taught in the fourth year.

Around the turn of the century, George Judisch, a pharmacist, gave much of the early instruction at Iowa State on the materia medica and compounding of veterinary drugs. About 1913, Henry D. Bergmann, a veterinarian, assumed responsibility for the instruction in pharmacology and therapeutics for the next 33 years and introduced much information on the actions of drugs on body tissues. Bergmann was considered by many to be the leading veterinary pharmacologist in the United States. He was ably supported by physiologists H. H. Dukes and E. A. Hewitt, who emphasized the experimental methodology in the laboratories of the Department of Physiology and Pharmacology. Although a course in therapeutics was taught in that department, according to the catalog, it is obvious that instructors in clinical courses discussed therapeutic measures employed in treatment of specific disease conditions.

The New York State Veterinary College at Cornell University was a contrast to Iowa State University in the type and emphasis of instruction regarding veterinary drugs. Fish apparently taught posology to veterinary students, because he published a small book that appeared in 1908 in its third edition. He was primarily a physiologist and, at least in later years, most of the information about the selection and administration of drugs was taught by Milks. Milks was the author of a widely used textbook and was a prominent and highly respected teacher of materia medica and therapeutics, especially in eastern United States. Hadley Stephenson, also in the Small Animal Veterinary Clinic, assisted Milks extensively. In later years, H. H. Dukes, who moved to Cornell as Head of the Department of Veterinary Physiology, taught some pharmacokinetics of drug activities in his laboratories in physiology, although this was never an assigned and formal responsibility.

The College of Veterinary Medicine at Texas A & M University established a Department of Veterinary Physiology and Pharmacology in 1916 and taught a course in toxicology for veterinary students separate from other courses in pharmacology and physiology. The total responsibility and nearly all the instruction in toxicology for 40 years (1926–1966) was contributed by P. W. Burns. Also during some of these years R. D. Radeleff and J. W. Dollahite were active in research and diagnostic toxicology. Among the veterinary colleges, only Texas maintained formal programs of instruction and research in veterinary toxicology. The contamination of the environment with chemicals and drugs has prompted recognition in recent years of the importance of toxicology by other universities.

RECENT TRENDS IN VETERINARY PHARMACOLOGY

During the first 35 years of the twentieth century, the respect of practitioners for materia medica and the efficacy of drug therapy declined and few young veterinarians were attracted to a study of drugs. There were many reasons for this, including the introduction and use of new vaccines and antisera for the control of specific diseases.

Starting in 1935 there were reports about the phenomenally specific action of an azo dye compound, Prontosil, introduced by Gerhard Domagk, for control of streptococcal bacterial infections in human beings and animals. The active agent soon was shown to be sulfanilamide, so many related sulfonamides were immediately synthesized. This discovery created a new era of chemotherapy, the doctrine introduced in 1910 by Paul Erhlich by the synthesis and use of arsphenamine to treat syphilis and trypanosomiasis. The chemotherapeutic uses of sulfonamides, antibiotics, and various antiparasitics reawakened interest in the discipline of pharmacology. The basis for experimental therapeutics, established by Buchheim, Schmiedeberg, Abel, and later pharmacologists, provided the necessary foundation for phenomenal growth in general pharmacology and specifically in veterinary pharmacology during the next four decades.

The age of miracle drugs started at the outbreak of World War II and offered great promise for the control of bacterial diseases. For several years following World War II, new drugs were introduced into the general drug market at the unprecedented rate of fifty to ninety per year. Prominent among these were the alkylating agents and antimetabolites for treatment for neoplasms; adrenergic and ganglionic blocking drugs for essential hypertension; thiazide and carbonic anhydrase as diuretics; antipsychotic, antianxiety, and antidepressant agents; and corticosteroids and oral antidiabetic drugs as substitutes for natural hormones.

At the present time, the rate of introduction of new drugs has been curtailed by increasingly restrictive regulations of the U.S. Food and Drug Administration at the direction of the U.S. Congress, so that by the mid-1970s only a dozen or so drugs have been introduced annually.

There are fewer veterinary schools with fewer veterinary pharmacologists than schools of human medicine and pharmacologists. Developments in veterinary pharmacology tend to parallel or follow those in medical pharmacology. The following discussion of recent trends in medicine and medical pharmacology will be helpful to the reader in identifying patterns in veterinary pharmacology.

Marketing reports on drugs used in human beings indicate that most physicians are acquainted with and prescribe a limited number of drugs. In a 1971 study, 30 drugs accounted for 75% of the dollar value of drugs marketed in the United States. These 30 drugs were covered in about one-tenth of the total course time devoted to pharmacology instruction in medical schools. These data led a teacher and author of a current textbook (Aviado 1972) to select 100 prototypes for detailed consideration as most representative of drugs likely to be used in the treatment of diseases in human beings. These 100 drug prototypes included digoxin, ephedrine, and chloroquin and 47 others used from before 1948 plus 50 other drugs introduced after 1963.

Following World War II, change characterized the teaching pattern and the amount of research done in the health science institutions. The number of teaching personnel in medical pharmacology increased about fourfold, but these scientists also devoted an increasing amount of time to research. Both the teaching and research of a given individual generally have become narrower in scope and more specialized. During the same period, the number of clock hours allotted to teaching pharmacology in the medical curriculum has been reduced to about one-half of what it was 25 years ago. This decrease must have originated chiefly from fewer clock hours of laboratory instruction because 25% of 74 medical schools surveyed eliminated pharmacology laboratories during the period 1961–62 to 1971–72 (Visscher 1973). The same survey showed that the total hours of instruction in physiology decreased an average of 31% in all schools, and as much as 70% in one school. In some schools, pharmacology is taught in conjunction with other disciplines by integration in organ systems or diseases; this mechanism seems to create greater problems for the pharmacologist than the physiologist or anatomist.

A general trend exists in medical schools, and to a lesser extent in veterinary schools, to decrease the hours of instruction in preclinical courses and to increase the time in clinical instruction. This trend has gained support from two sources: (1) the Carnegie Commission on Higher Education (1970), which based its report and recommendations for revision of medical education on data collected by educational psychologists who claim that specific, testable knowledge of medical students is learned in a fraction of the time and cost by reading as compared to laboratory experience, although long-term retention of such knowledge was not checked; and (2) the Congress and general public, who criticized the insufficient and maldistributed health services in the United States. Improving delivery of health services depends on many factors (viz., attracting practitioners to rural and ghetto areas, promoting student interest in general practice instead of specialization, etc.) and not alone on the unsupported assumption that the solution rests with increased clinical instruction in the professional curriculum accompanied by a coincident decrease in the time devoted to instruction in pharmacology and the basic sciences.

In 1910 the Carnegie Foundation supported a study by Abraham Flexner that severely chastized the U.S. health science schools for their failure to instruct students adequately in the basic sciences with laboratory experience, and for devoting too much curricular time to clinical instruction. The recommendations of the Flexner report were adopted by the health science colleges of the United States. During the next 60 years, the U.S. health science schools became the preeminent educational institutions of the world. The present anti-Flexnerian movement in health sciences education may be extremely dangerous to the welfare of veterinary pharmacology and all preclinical sciences and generally to the caliber of health science education. This anti-Flexnerian trend is also dangerous for the public at large, because the diagnosis and management of disease are today more complexly scientific and dependent on a thorough understanding of science than ever before. This is a poor time to decrease the training in the basic sciences for the future practitioners who will serve the public.

Although programs, personnel, and budgets in veterinary pharmacology are still comparatively small, a comparison of the present situation to that of 40 years ago shows that impressive gains have been made in veterinary pharmacology. There is, however, one prominent and serious deficiency characterizing veterinary pharmacology today, i.e., a lack of graduate degree training opportunities in veterinary colleges, especially for the new veterinarian but also for the new science graduate. This deficiency is not new and explains why there are so few trained veterinary pharmacologists available at present. Thirty to 35 years ago, several veterinarians obtained Ph.D. degrees in pharmacology at a medical school and returned to veterinary faculties. During the past 10 to 15 years, few such specialists have returned to veterinary colleges due to a lack of understanding, vision, and funding of the discipline of pharmacology. Therefore, it is important to attract those still young, well-trained, experienced veterinary pharmacologists currently employed on medical school faculties back to key positions on veterinary college faculties.

PROJECTIONS FOR VETERINARY PHARMACOLOGY

To project the future of veterinary pharmacology is an uncertain undertaking; however, substantial justification exists for the following personalized assertions that are accompanied by specific recommendations for constructive actions necessary for proper development of the discipline of veterinary pharmacology.

Status as a Discipline

Veterinary pharmacology will continue to exist as a discipline composed of the three subdisciplines of (1) pharmacokinetics, (2) clinical veterinary pharmacology, and (3) veterinary toxicology.

There should be increasing interdisciplinary activities in clinical veterinary pharmacology by a team of teachers and researchers composed of pharmacologists with knowledge of experimental therapeutics and interest in clinical medicine and of clinicians with knowledge in clinical medicine and an interest in experimental pharmacology. There is a clear need for more research in problems in clinical pharmacology. The teaching of clinical pharmacology in some veterinary and medical schools appears to have significantly augmented the knowledge and competence of a student to use drugs upon completion of his curriculum. The specific administration of drugs in the control and treatment of animal diseases will continue to be the responsibility of the clinicians.

Funding

The discipline of veterinary pharmacology has been grossly underfunded in educational institutions in the United States. The same assertion can be made in varying degrees of many disciplines of veterinary medical education and research.

The need for advice, supervision, and research by veterinary pharmacologists in the agricultural sector of our economy is indicated by noting that in the United States the sales of drugs used in animal health during 1974 totaled nearly $1 million. It has been loosely estimated that the total sales of drugs used in animal health approaches $8 million currently and by 1980 may reach $15 million in the world at large.

Manpower

Manpower is lacking in the disciplinary area of veterinary pharmacology. A survey of the faculties of veterinary schools in Canada and the United States in 1974–75 showed a total of 44 pharmacologists among 18 colleges (Davis 1975). This provides an average of 1 pharmacologist per 163 veterinary students. Excluded from this calculation is Michigan State University, which has a Department of Pharmacology with 15 faculty members that teach students in all 6 health professions on that campus.

The same survey identified only 36 toxicologists on the veterinary faculties of 18 colleges. Four of these schools had no toxicologist. This is a very serious and grim situation, especially in view of the increased use of chemicals and drugs in rations of food-producing animals because of the danger that human beings will consume the tissues containing drug residues. Furthermore, the extensive addition of various chemicals (fertilizers, pesticides, herbicides, and industrial effluents) to the environment of food-producing animals identifies a hazardous and ever-worsening situation.

Veterinary pharmacologists and toxicologists in education are so few in number and so overloaded with teaching duties that insufficient time remains for research and supervision of graduate student training. This shortage leads to the less obvious but perhaps more critical problem that available personnel by necessity tend to be scientific generalists for lack of time and funding to specialize in narrow areas and to conduct research in significant depth for advancement of the discipline of veterinary pharmacology.

Manpower deficiencies exist in industry and in the state and federal governments where veterinary pharmacologists are in great demand and command relatively high salaries. Meeting future manpower needs is dependent upon the development of larger graduate training programs in veterinary pharmacology. A survey of the veterinary colleges of Canada and the United States by the American Society of Veterinary Physiologists and Pharmacologists for 1974–75 indicated that in 10 schools only 23 students were studying toward a Ph.D. degree in pharmacology and 21 were studying toward the M.S. degree. The same survey revealed that in 6 veterinary colleges 8 students were studying toward a Ph.D. degree in toxicology and 11 students were studying toward the M.S. degree (Tumbleson 1975).

Evaluation of the Present Status

A Subcommittee on Pre- and Postdoctoral Training of Pharmacologists of the American Society of Pharmacology and Experimental Therapeutics has identified a dire shortage of professionally trained pharmacologists in the field of "agricultural pharmacology," which includes veterinary medicine. A preliminary report of this subcommittee found that "a serious deficiency of high-quality pharmacologic education, advice, training, and research (exists) in the whole area of animal production. . . ." (Subcommittee Report 1975).

Recommendations

Worthy recommendations made to the above subcommittee aimed at improving the status of veterinary pharmacology in North America (Davis 1975) include the following: (1) veterinary colleges should enlarge the existing pharmacology faculty by hiring Ph.D. pharmacologists trained outside the veterinary colleges to provide reasonable numbers of personnel for teaching and research. These non-D.V.M. pharmacologists should receive postdoctoral training to orient them to animal health problems. (2) A special effort should be made by veterinary college administrators to recruit veterinarians with special training in pharmacology who are now employed outside the veterinary profession and principally in medical schools. (3) A larger number of appointments for graduate training of young veterinarians in pharmacology should be funded on recurring dollars by our veterinary colleges. Some of these appointments should be for training veterinarians in clinical pharmacology. When trained, such clinical pharmacologists should be retained on veterinary faculties on joint appointments between clinics and pharmacology, but with their salaries coming from the pharmacology budget. (4) Continuing education programs to update veterinary practitioners in pharmacology, toxicology, and therapeutics deserve greater emphasis. (5) Members of existing pharmacology faculties should make special efforts to obtain funding for research and graduate training programs in the general area of comparative pharmacology.

SCOPE OF PHARMACOLOGY

Pharmacology is an experimental science that studies the changes produced in living organisms by drugs. Traditionally, pharmacology has included a study of the sources of drugs (pharmacognosy), their action and fate in the animal body (pharmacodynamics), their use in the treatment of disease (therapeutics), and their poisonous action (toxicology). The word "drug" has been defined by the U.S. Food, Drug and Cosmetic Act to refer to all medicines and preparations recognized in the *United States Pharmacopeia* (U.S.P.) and the *National Formulary* (N.F.) for internal or external use, and to substances or mixtures of substances intended to be used for the successful treatment, mitigation, or prevention of disease of either human beings or other animals. As defined, the word "drug" includes all chemical substances except foods that are used to promote or safeguard the health of human beings or animals.

Pharmacology, which studies the effects of drugs in living organisms, emphasizes the study of pharmacodynamics and pharmacotherapy. *Pharmacodynamics* investigates the response of living organisms to drugs in the absence of disease. *Pharmacotherapy* studies the response of the living organisms to drugs in the presence of disease. More specifically, pharmacotherapy deals with the clinical application of pharmacodynamics in the treatment of disease in the sick animal.

Recently, two new terms have been used by pharmacologists, i.e., pharmacokinetics and clinical pharmacology. Many new research techniques have been applied on a quantitative and time basis to reveal how a drug may be absorbed, distributed, absorbed selectively by tissues, transformed, and excreted by the body. This type of kinetic study is called *pharmacokinetics* and is defined briefly as a study of the actions of a drug in the body over a defined period of time. As a more specific and expressive term, pharmacokinetics is likely to supplant pharmacodynamics. Another term that has come into favor is *clinical pharmacology,* which, because of its simplicity, may easily replace its synonym, pharmacotherapy. It was these current trends that led to the statement earlier in this chapter that pharmacology is composed of three discrete subdisciplines, i.e., pharmacokinetics, clinical pharmacology, and toxicology.

Chemotherapy is the use of a pure chemical compound in the specific treatment of a certain pathogen. In addition to clinical effects, chemotherapy is concerned with the relationship between chemical constitution and the antiinfective activity of drugs on both the host and the pathogen.

Toxicology is a study of poisoning. Toxicology is concerned with the effects of therapeutic agents administered in excess and of substances having only a toxic action. In addition, toxicology is concerned with environmental health that may require investigation of the toxic properties of water containing industrial or sewage wastes and of toxic vapors from industrial plants and numerous other things hazardous to life.

Posology is a study of dosage of medicine. The dosage varies with the species of animal, with the intended effect of the drug, and with individual tolerance or susceptibility. In general, the dose of a drug is that amount necessary to elicit the desired therapeutic response in the patient.

Metrology is a study of weights and measures as applied to the preparation and administration of drugs.

Pharmacy is an additional field sometimes included in pharmacology, but which actually entails a parallel, though closely related, study of drugs. *Pharmacy* is concerned with the collection, preparation, standardization, and dispensing of drugs. Although the preparation of drugs for use in treatment of disease is the responsibility of pharmacists, the pharmacologist must be conversant in this field of drug activity. *Pharmacognosy* is concerned with the sources and the physical and chemical properties of drugs of vegetable and animal origin. It is a purely descriptive science. The importance of pharmacognosy has decreased in recent years as many of the vegetable drugs have been replaced by synthetic organic chemicals.

Materia medica is an older term that encompassed the entire field of pharmacy and pharmacology. It constituted a didactic descriptive study of pharmacognosy, pharmacy, posology, and indications for the use of drugs with therapeutic intent. In this sense, the term "materia medica" is obsolete.

Pharmacology is the youngest of the medical sciences. Its contribution to the treatment and control of disease is unquestioned. Pharmacology has become especially well established during the last four decades through its part in the development of many widely used therapeutic agents. Pharmacology integrates its studies with the fields of clinical medicine, physiology, and biological chemistry in particular. Pharmacology also must correlate its study with other fields of medical science, such as pathology and microbiology.

Pharmacology may be viewed as both a preclinical and a clinical subject because it includes pharmacodynamics and pharmacotherapy. Pharmacology has an added responsibility in bridging the gap in the medical curriculum between the basic medical sciences and the clinical sciences.

It is obvious that the scope of pharmacology is broad and that it ramifies throughout the entire field of basic and clinical medicine.

REFERENCES

Abel, J. J. 1926. Arthur Robinson Cushney and pharmacology. J Pharmacol Exp Ther 27:266.

Aviado, D. M. 1972. Pharmacologic Principles of Medical Practice, 8th ed., p. 9. Baltimore: Williams & Wilkins.

Carnegie Commission on Higher Education. 1970. A special report and recommendations on Higher Education and the Nation's Health: Policies for Medical and Dental Education. New York: McGraw-Hill.

Davis, L. E. 1975. Pharmacology training in schools of veterinary medicine. Proc Am Soc Exp Pharmacol Ther (Fall Meet).

Subcommittee on Pre- and Post-doctoral Training. 1975. Report of the Committee on

Education and Professional Affairs, American Society of Pharmacology and Experimental Therapeutics. Pharmacology 17:63.

Tumbleson, M. 1975. Survey of faculty and graduate students in pharmacology and toxicology in Canada and U.S.A. in 1974–75. Am Soc Vet Physiol Pharmacol (Bus Meet July).

Visscher, M. B. 1973. The decline and emphasis on basic medical sciences in the medical school curriculum. Physiologist 16:43.

DRUG STANDARDS AND REGULATIONS

L. MEYER JONES

The preparation and sale of medicines for administration to human beings and animals are particularly vital to the health of the nation. In the United States these processes are regulated by special laws intended to establish and maintain standards of quality, purity, and uniformity of all drugs. The laws are made by the Congress of the United States to control interstate commerce in drugs. The interpretation and enforcement of these laws are the responsibility of the Food and Drug Administration (FDA) of the Department of Health, Education and Welfare. Each state of the United States in a more or less parallel fashion controls drug commerce confined to the limits of the state.

DRUG STANDARDS

The FDA is responsible for enforcement of the Food, Drug and Cosmetic Act and its amendments, including the 1972 amendment pertaining to animal drugs. This act, which was made law by the Congress of the United States, contains standards and regulations established and recommended by members of the professions of medicine, pharmacy, dentistry, and veterinary medicine. The standards are found in the *United States Pharmacopeia* (U.S.P.) and the *National Formulary* (N.F.), both of which are officially and legally accepted compendia in the legal courts of the United States.

In addition to requiring that all drugs meet the official standards of purity, quality, and uniformity required by the U.S.P. and the N.F., the FDA has certain other requirements that must be met in the marketing of drugs. The container must be correctly and completely labeled; it must bear the identity of the manufacturer or distributor; and it must give adequate directions for use. All advertisements and all information accompanying drugs, either on the labels or on enclosed package inserts, must be true and correct statements regarding the indication, toxicity, and general usage of the drug. Only preparations conforming to the requirements of the *United States Pharmacopeia* or the *National Formulary* can be labeled as U.S.P. or N.F. preparations. Preparations of nonofficial drugs must give certain specified information about the ingredients upon the label. No drug may be distributed for sale to the public until an application establishing its safety and efficacy by adequate testing data has been submitted to and approved by the FDA.

THE *United States Pharmacopeia*

This publication is the most eminent and recognized legal drug standard for the United States. It is revised and published periodically by a committee of the U.S. Pharmacopeial Convention. The convention is formed of delegates from all the major organizations of health and medical science in the United States. The first U.S.P. was published in 1820 and revised approximately every decade until recently, when revisions have been made every 5 years. At present the *Pharmacopeia* is in the nineteenth edition, which became official on July 1, 1975. The *Pharmacopeia* contains a description of the source, appearance, properties, standards of purity, and other requirements of the most important pure drugs. Any drug meeting these standards may be labeled U.S.P. The comparable authority for the United Kingdom is the *British Pharmacopoeia* (B.P.).

THE *National Formulary*

This publication was written and published by pharmacists because they needed some standards for certain pure drugs that were not important or widely enough used in the United States as a whole to be in the U.S.P. and yet were frequently used in some localities. In addition, the *National Formulary* contains standards for many medicinal mixtures in common use. It is published and revised by the American Pharmaceutical Association simultaneously with the U.S.P. It is now in the thirteenth edition, which became official September 1, 1970. The N.F. is a recognized legal standard. All drugs or mixtures of drugs listed in the U.S.P. or N.F. are called "official drugs" by the Food, Drug and Cosmetic Act.

AMA Drug Evaluations (AMA-DE)

This volume, published in its second edition in 1973, is a collection of monographs of drugs generally introduced within the last 10 years. The discussion of each drug is based on an evaluation of available laboratory and clinical data by the consultants and staff of the Department of Drugs, American Medical Association (AMA). Products not approved by the Drug Efficacy Study of the National Academy of Sciences–National Research Council are not included. This book, published first in 1965, was an outgrowth of the former *New and Non-Official Drugs* published by the AMA. The AMA-DE is intended to meet the specific needs of the practicing physician for a source of up-to-date, authoritative, unbiased information on recently introduced drugs.

THE *United States Dispensatory*

This encyclopedic volume contains general information on all drugs, both old and new, found throughout the world. It is a nonofficial publication. The twenty-seventh edition was published in 1973.

FOREIGN PHARMACOPEIAS

The most prominent of the foreign pharmacopeias are the *French Codex,* the *British Pharmacopoeia,* the *German Pharmacopeia,* and the Spanish edition of the *United States Pharmacopeia.* The Council of the Pharmaceutical Society of Great Britain has a publication comparable to the N.F. that is designated as the *British Pharmaceutical Codex* (B.P.C.). This same agency, in conjunction with the National Veterinary Association, published the *British Veterinary Codex* (B.V.C.) in 1953.

DRUG ASSAY STANDARDS

In the therapeutic administration of drugs, it is essential that the amount of active ingredient be known in any given dose of drug. In dealing with pure chemical substances, the careful measurement of active principle is a good indication of expected drug activity, assuming that no deterioration has occurred.

Many important drugs are mixtures or chemically impure preparations that must be measured by biological assay. The method of biological assay assumes that a given quantity of drug will produce an average response in the average animal of given species. The biological standard is determined by measuring the reaction of a large number of animals under test conditions to calculated dosages of drug. When properly performed with consideration for variants such as age, sex, and weight, the method of biological assay can determine the approximate dose that the clinician should employ. The reaction of the patient to this average dose is not always predictable because there are individual variations involving the condition of the animal, its idiosyncrasies, and other uncontrollable factors. Herein lies the opportunity and the need for expression of the art in addition to the science of therapeutics by the clinician.

Some drugs are extremely difficult to assay biologically for uniformity. For these cases a given quantity of drug, known as a Reference Standard, is maintained and distributed to research laboratories and pharmaceutical manufacturers in the United States by the U.S. pharmacopeial authorities. In the United Kingdom, the National Institute for Medical Research performs the same service. International drug standards were originally established and maintained by the League of Nations and are available from its successor, the United Nations.

SPECIFIC LEGISLATION REGULATING DRUGS

Only the general aspects of the more important drug regulatory measures can be mentioned here. The U.S. Congress passed the original version of the Food, Drug and Cosmetic Act in 1906. This legislation was an achievement by name rather than by effect because it did not provide the FDA with significant enforcement power. In 1938 the Food, Drug and Cosmetic Act was amended, giving the federal government authority to control the manufacture, sale, and use of "dangerous" drugs for human beings or animals. Under this legislation the FDA was also authorized to regulate and police labeling, instructions for use, and advertising employed in the sale of foods, drugs, and cosmetics.

Following World War II, an increasing number of chemicals was produced for use in, on, or by human beings and animals as drugs, cosmetics, food additives, or pesticides. These developments necessitated increased protection for the public, which was provided by a series of amendments to the Food, Drug and Cosmetic Act. For example, the amendment in 1972, Section 512 on "New Animal Drugs," requires the manufacturer of a drug to demonstrate that the drug is safe for animal use and possesses the therapeutic efficacy claimed on the label. The manufacturer also must provide a satisfactory analytical method for detection of drug residues in edible animal products. He also must establish an acceptable drug withdrawal period following the last administration of the drug to a food-producing animal to assure the consuming public that the foodstuff is wholesome and safe.

To the veterinary practitioner, an important aspect of the above regulations and of his professional responsibility is the fact that a variety of therapeutic agents, administered by many routes to a food-producing animal, could be present in a food product (milk, butter, eggs, meat, fat) intended for human consumption. A practitioner must be particularly careful to provide explicit instructions (preferably in writing) to the owner regarding the sale of edible products from livestock to avoid subsequent complications arising from drug residues in edible foods of animal origin.

The U.S. Congress has enacted over 50 pieces of legislation regulating narcotic and other drugs since the Harrison Act of 1914. The Controlled Substances Act of 1970, officially designated as the Comprehensive Drug Abuse Prevention and Control Act, collected most of these diverse laws into one piece of legislation. A "controlled substance" is defined under the law and includes opiates, barbiturates, hallucinogens, methadone, stimulants such as amphetamines, and other addictive or habituating drugs. This Act of 1970 regulates the manufacturing, distribution, and dispensing of controlled substances by providing for a "closed" system of legitimate handlers (drug manufacturers and distributors, pharmacists, and licensed practitioners) of these drugs, which is designed to reduce illicit marketing. The veterinarian licensed to practice by a state and wishing to use or prescribe controlled substances must register annually under the Controlled Substances Act with the Drug Enforcement Administration (DEA) of the U.S. Department of Justice (Registration Branch, Drug Enforcement Administration, Department of Justice, P.O. Box 28083, Central Station, Washington, D.C. 20005). The controlled drugs and drug products are categorized in five "schedules" and the applicant requests certification for those schedules or categories of drugs that he expects to purchase, store, dispense, and use. The registered practitioner or hospital is given a DEA certificate for display, a registration number, and official forms for ordering the controlled substances from a drug distributor. The registration number must be used on all prescriptions and supply order forms. The registered practitioner and other authorized handlers must keep careful records of orders, receipts, uses, and thefts of controlled substances for 2 years following each transaction. The registrant is expected to keep and to file every 2 years with the DEA an inventory of controlled substances on hand and to file a revised form if his location changes. All such records and activities are subject to inspection at anytime by DEA personnel.

The manufacturer and distributor are required to identify a controlled substance on a label of the original container by a symbol corresponding to the "schedules" specified by DEA for each controlled substance, i.e., a capital letter "C" containing the Roman numeral of the schedule or the letter "C" followed by the schedule number (C-II). This designation is used also in catalogs of distributors selling schedule II drugs so that the registered practitioner will be reminded to submit the special DEA form with the distributor's conventional order form.

Both the veterinarian and/or the pharmacist filling a prescription are legally responsible for the proper prescribing and dispensing of drugs covered by the Controlled Substances Act. Controlled substances must be stored in a locked cabinet or preferably in a safe attached to a concrete floor.

There may be differing federal, state, and municipal regulations to control purity, manufacture, sale, and dispensing of drugs. The most stringent regulation takes precedence but generally the practitioner should follow the federal regulations of the Controlled Substances Act. This act classifies controlled substances into five schedules as follows:

Schedule I. Drugs in this schedule have a high abuse potential and are not currently accepted in the United States for treatment of any practice situation. They may be obtained for research or instructional use by application to the DEA. Examples are heroin, LSD, peyote, mescaline, dihydromorphine, morphine methylsulfonate, tetrahydrocannibinols, and marihuana.

Schedule II. Drugs in this schedule have a high abuse potential that in human beings produces severe psychic or physical dependence. These drugs apparently have similar effects in animals. These are the former class-A narcotic drugs plus certain stimulant drugs. Examples are opium, morphine, hydromorphone (Dilaudid), codeine, methadone (Dolophine), meperidine (Demerol), and cocaine; phenmetrazine (Preludin), methylphenidate (Ritalin), and methaqualone (Quaalude, Parest, Somnafac, and Sopor) and its salts; and amobarbital (Amytal), pentobarbital (Nembutal), and secobarbital (Seconal) and their salts alone, in combination with each other, or in combination with other controlled substances. The amphetamines are no longer available under schedule II for veterinary use.

Schedule III. These drugs have less abuse potential than those listed in schedules I and II. Abusive use of schedule III drugs leads to moderate or low physical dependence and high psychological dependence in human beings. Drugs in this schedule were formerly known as class-B narcotics (any preparation containing limited amounts of opium, morphine, ethylmorphine, codeine, dihydrocodeine, or hydrocodone) and some nonnarcotic drugs such as glutethimide (Doriden), nalorphine, phencyclidine, benzphetamine, paregoric, and barbiturates (except those in another schedule).

Schedule IV. Drugs in this schedule have a low abuse potential that leads to limited physical or psychological dependence in human beings. Included here are barbital, phenobarbital, methylphenobarbital, chloral hydrate, ethinamate (Valmid), meprobamate (Miltown, Equanil), chlordiazepoxide (Librium), and diazepam (Valium).

Schedule V. These drugs have a lesser abuse potential and include those preparations formerly known as "exempt" narcotics, except for paregoric.

CHAPTER 3

PRESCRIPTION WRITING

L. MEYER JONES

A *prescription* is an order to a pharmacist written by a licensed veterinarian, physician, or dentist to prepare the prescribed medicine, to affix the directions, and to sell the preparation to the client or patient. The prescription is a legally recognized document and the writer is held responsible for its accuracy.

FORM OF THE PRESCRIPTION

The essential parts of a "classical" prescription consist of the following:

1. The *date* of writing the prescription.

2. The *identity* and *address* of the owner and the patient.

3. The *superscription,* ℞, is an abbreviation of the Latin word recipe meaning "take thou of." This superscription is the symbol of the Roman god Jupiter and is a relic of the times when all prescriptions were begun with a prayer to Jupiter asking his help in making the prescription effective in the cure of disease.

4. The inscription lists the names and amounts of the drugs to be incorporated in the prescription. The names of the drugs should be written in English and the total amounts required should be written in the metric system—the procedure preferred and official in the U.S.P. and the N.F. Previously the apothecaries' system of measurement and Latin terminology were preferred for prescription writing. The tendency in therapeutics is to employ as few drugs as possible and to strive for specific therapy. The complicated and useless mixtures ("shot-gun" prescriptions) of earlier decades have been discarded in favor of single drugs or simple combinations of drugs. Most of the drugs needed by the practitioner are listed in the U.S.P. and the N.F.

5. The *subscription* gives the instructions to the pharmacist. These instructions may be entirely in English or with Latin abbreviations. Prescriptions are seldom written entirely in Latin.

6. The *signa* (Sig. or S.) consists of instructions for administration of the medicine, which the pharmacist is to write on the label.

7. The *name* of the practitioner must be signed to the prescription.

The modern prescription is written as simply as possible. It consists of a minimum number of drugs, is written in English, employs the metric system and may use several abbreviations.

ABBREVIATIONS

It is unwise to abbreviate the names of drugs to be used in the prescription. These names should be written out in full to avoid error. Chemical formulae, even short ones, should not be used in prescription writing because of the increased probability of error.

Several abbreviations of Latin words are commonly used to advantage in writing a prescription because they save time. The more common abbreviations are:

ā	(ante)	before
$\overline{\text{aa}}$	(ana)	of each
ad lib.	(ad libitum)	freely as wanted
aq.	(aqua)	water
b.i.d.	(bis in die)	twice a day
C.	(congius)	gallon
$\bar{\text{c}}$	(cum)	with
cap.	(capula)	capsule
div.	(divide)	divide
dos.	(dosis)	dose
eq. pts.	(equalis partes)	equal parts
ft.	(fiat)	make
h.	(hora)	hour
haust.	(haustus)	drench
M.	(misce)	mix
no.	(numero)	number
n.r.	(non repetatur)	not to be renewed
O.	(octarius)	pint
o.d.	(omnie die)	daily
pil.	(pilula)	pill
p.r.n.	(pro re nata)	according to circumstances
pv.	(pulvis)	powder
q.i.d.	(quater in die)	4 times a day
q.s.	(quantum sufficit)	as much as needed
q. 3 h.	(quaque 3 hora)	every 3 hours
s.i.d.	(semel in die)	once a day
Sig. or S.	(signa)	write on the label
sol.	(solutio)	solution
s.o.s.	(si opus sit)	if necessary
$\bar{\text{s}}$	(sine)	without
$\overline{\text{ss}}$	(semisse)	half
stat.	(statim)	immediately
tab.	(tabella)	tablet
t.i.d.	(ter in die)	3 times a day

METROLOGY

Metrology is the study of weights and measures used in prescription writing. The metric system is preferred to the apothecaries' system, but since the latter is still used occasionally, both systems with conversion values should be learned.

In the United States the weight/volume method (w/v) of measuring solids and liquids is employed; i.e., the solids are weighed and the liquids are measured. The weight/weight method (w/w) is employed in Continental Europe; i.e., both liquids and solids are weighed in prescription compounding. The completely gravimetric method is more accurate because it compensates for differences in specific gravity of liquids. However, for most purposes the weight by volume method employed in this country proves satisfactory.

The use of different or mixed systems of metrology is extremely confusing. Although there is no simple solution to this problem, Table 3.1 should provide some graphic help in common conversions.

The metric system uses Arabic numerals to indicate the quantities of drug required. The Arabic numeral is followed by the unit of measurement. A single ver-

TABLE 3.1. Conversion factors for obtaining approximate equivalents

To Convert	To	Multiply by
grains/lb	mg/lb	64.8
grains/lb	mg/kg	143.0
mg/lb	grains/lb	0.015
mg/lb	mg/kg	2.2
mg/kg	grains/lb	0.007
mg/kg	mg/lb	0.454

THE METRIC SYSTEM

Weight		
	1 picogram	= 10^{-12} gram
	1,000 picograms (pg)	= 1 nanogram (ng) or 10^{-9} gram
	1,000 nanograms	= 1 microgram (μg) or 10^{-6} gram
	1,000 micrograms	= 1 milligram (mg) or 10^{-3} gram
	1,000 milligrams	= 1 gram (g)
	1,000 grams	= 1 kilogram (kg)
Volume		
	1,000 milliliters (ml)	= 1 liter (L)

THE APOTHECARIES' SYSTEM

Weight		
	20 grains (gr)	= 1 scruple (℈)
	3 scruples	= 1 dram (ʒ) = 60 grains
	8 drams	= 1 ounce (℥) = 480 grains
Volume		
	60 minims (m)	= 1 fluid dram (ʒ)
	8 fluid drams	= 1 fluid ounce (℥)
	16 fluid ounces	= 1 pint (O.)

CONVERSION EQUIVALENTS

	Exact	*Approximate*
1 milligram	=1/65 grain	(1/60)
1 gram	= 15.432 grains	(15)
1 kilogram	= 2.2 pounds (avoirdupois)	
1 milliliter	= 16.23 minims	(15)
1 liter	=1.06 quarts or 33.8 fluid ounces	
1 grain	= 65 milligrams	(60)
1 dram	= 3.88 grams	(4)
1 ounce	= 31.1 grams	(30)
1 avoirdupois pound	= 454 grams	
1 minim	= 0.062 milliliter	(0.06)
1 fluid dram	= 3.7 milliliters	(4)
1 fluid ounce	= 29.57 milliliters	(30)
1 pint	= 473 milliliters	(500)
1 quart	= 946 milliliters	(1,000)
1 drop	=	1 minim
1 teaspoonful	=	5 milliliters
1 dessertspoonful	=	8 milliliters
1 tablespoonful	=	15 milliliters

tical line may be substituted for a series of decimal points placed on successive lines. The figures to the left of the line are whole numbers, while those to the right are decimal fractions. In the metric system the quantities automatically indicate grams (g) for solids and milliliters (ml) for liquids without specific designation.

In modern prescription writing, the apothecaries' system should no longer be used. However, the veterinarian must be familiar with these basic units in the United States for conversion to the metric system because a number of dosage forms are still provided in the apothecaries' system of weights and measures.

In commerce the avoirdupois pound, which contains 16 ounces, is employed, but this system is not used in fine measure of drugs. The avoirdupois system of weight allows only 437.5 grains per ounce, whereas the apothecaries' ounce contains 480 grains.

WRITING THE PRESCRIPTION

Several examples of prescription writing are given in this section. Oftentimes the prescription is very simple and requires

Telephone (999)123–4567

Date ______________

JAMES J. SMITH, D.V.M.

2511 Broad Street — Columbus, Ohio

Client's name *Mr. Ross Barnes* Address *Rt. 3, Columbus, Ohio*

Patient *horse (Standardbred)* Age *2 yrs.* Sex *Female*

℞ g or ml

Calamine liniment *480*

M.

Label: Apply daily to skin lesions

D.V.M.

DEA No. XX1234 Refills

FIG. 3.1. A sample prescription form.

little writing and calculation. In the prescription given in Fig. 3.1, dosage is not important because the liniment would be applied by the owner in quantity sufficient to cover the lesions on the skin. The amount of 480 ml of liniment was chosen for dispensing because this volume exactly fills a 16-oz. prescription bottle. The veterinarian should know that prescription bottles are available in the following volumes in ounces: 1, 2, 3, 4, 6, 8, 12, 16, and 32. Bottles are also available that are calibrated in the metric system, i.e., ml. The veterinarian should prescribe volumes that will fill a given size bottle because the client is better satisfied when paying for a full bottle.

Some drugs are not soluble in the common solvents and must be administered as solids.

Powders may be administered as such when sprinkled on the solid feed of the animal. Many powders are distasteful and must be masked by some flavoring agent or administered in a more palatable form. A very common way of administering powders is by packing into a hard gelatin capsule. The capsule is tasteless, readily swallowed, and disintegrates rapidly in the stomach. Hard gelatin capsules are available in two series of sizes. The smallest capsule is known as No. 5. In order of increasing size, the capsules are numbered as follows: 5, 4, 3, 2, 1, 0, 00, 000. Another numbering scheme is used for the next series of hard gelatin capsules, which increase in size from the last mentioned. In succession they are 13, 12, 11, and 10. In addition, there are the infrequently used sizes 9, 8, and 7. The weight of drug contained in a capsule varies too widely with the ingredient to be of significance, but the No.

10 gelatin capsule is commonly referred to as the 1-oz size, the No. 11 as the ½-oz, the No. 12 as the ¼-oz, and the No. 13 as the ⅛-oz capsule.

It may be desirable for the owner to administer tablets to a dog at home. The following prescription directs the pharmacist to dispense 15 tablets, each containing 30 mg of phenobarbital sodium. It is the pharmacist's responsibility to write the directions for the owner *(signa)* on the label of the dispensing bottle.

℞
Phenobarbital Sodium Tablets, U.S.P., 30 mg
Dispense 15
Sig. Give one tablet each morning.

Codeine phosphate may be prescribed for a dog suffering from a chronic cough. The intended dose is 15 mg administered every 3 hours for 4 doses each day to a total of 6 days. The veterinarian should assume the responsibility of calculating and stating the total amount of ingredients needed. This problem could be calculated as follows:

4 doses × 6 days = 24 doses
24 doses × 15 mg = 360 mg of codeine phosphate needed.

The next step has to do with measurement of the dose. Any household would have a teaspoon to administer medicine to a dog. The teaspoon holds 5 ml. Any other convenient form of household measurement could be employed by adjusting the volume of the vehicle.

24 doses × 5 ml = 120 ml of vehicle needed

℞
Codeine Phosphate, U.S.P. 360
Syrup of cherry q.s. 120
ft.sol.
Sig. One teaspoonful every 3 hours for 4 doses daily.

Many modern prescriptions stipulate proprietary pharmaceutical preparations. There is no objection to their use if there is no parallel preparation in the U.S.P. or N.F. The use of a proprietary rather than an official preparation increases the cost of the medicine considerably, because official preparations are more commonly and widely produced in a competitive market. When a proprietary preparation is stipulated in a prescription, the ingredient is identified by the name of the manufacturer and the copyright name of the preparation.

If a veterinarian writes a prescription to be filled by a pharmacist, it cannot be refilled unless authorized by the prescriber. The latter should indicate on the prescription the number of times it may be refilled. Prescriptions containing drugs regulated by the Controlled Substances Act of 1970 must have appended the registration number obtained by the veterinarian from the Drug Enforcement Administration (DEA) of the U.S. Department of Justice. The full name and address of both the veterinarian and the owner, as well as the identity of the animal patient, must be on all such prescription forms along with the permit number issued to the practitioner. Prescriptions for controlled substances in schedule II must be typewritten or written in ink or indelible pencil and signed by the registered practitioner. Prescription orders for schedule II drugs must be limited to a 34-day supply and cannot be refilled. Prescription orders for schedule III or IV drugs may be issued orally or in writing by a practitioner and may be refilled, when authorized, but not more than 5 times and not later than 6 months after the date of writing the prescription. Thereafter a new prescription authorization must be issued. Drugs in schedule V can be prescribed like those of schedules III and IV, and some may be sold over the counter by a pharmacist under specified conditions.

The label on the container of any controlled substance in schedules II, III, or IV when dispensed for animal use must contain the following warning: "Caution: Federal law prohibits the transfer of this drug to any person other than the (client and) patient for whom it was prescribed."

PRESCRIPTION INCOMPATIBILITY

Prescription incompatibilities are unnecessary and arise only from the carelessness or ignorance of the prescriber. An incompatibility nullifies the desired therapeutic effect of the prescription. Prescription incompatibilities are therapeutic, chemical, or pharmaceutic in nature.

Therapeutic incompatibility arises from prescribing drugs having an antagonistic action as would occur from simultaneous administration of physostigmine to constrict the iris of the eye and atropine to dilate it. A medical scientist must know the pharmacologic activities of individual drugs thoroughly to avoid simultaneous use of drugs acting antagonistically. Likewise, it is advantageous for the medical scientist to know which drugs have a synergistic or additive action; for example, the preanesthetic action of morphine to a patient decreases proportionately the anesthetic dose of pentobarbital sodium and facilitates induction of anesthesia.

Chemical incompatibility arises from the interaction of compounds during or following their compounding in a prescription. Such chemical reaction could result in the production of a toxic substance (chloral hydrate plus alkali gives chloroform) or an inert substance having no therapeutic value whatever (mercuric iodide plus tannic acid gives a tannate). Occasionally a prescription may call for a combination of materials intended to produce a chemical interaction that results in the formation of a substance that is unstable under other circumstances. An example of the latter is the preparation of a lotion of zinc acetate by the combination of lead acetate and zinc sulfate.

Pharmaceutical incompatibility generally arises from a lack of miscibility, i.e., the ingredients are not mutually soluble (oil in water). The practitioner can best avoid pharmaceutical incompatibility by prescribing official preparations of the U.S.P. or N.F.

The following materials should be prescribed alone because they are frequently incompatible with other substances: alkaloids, arsenic iodide, iron salts, mercury salts, methenamine, permanganates, salicylates, silver salts, strong alkalis, strong acids, and tannic acid.

SAFETY PACKAGING FOR DISPENSING

The U.S. Congress passed the Poison Prevention Packaging Act in 1970, which allocated responsibility to the FDA to require special packaging for drugs that may be dangerous to small children. Broadly, the required special packaging is a container that cannot be readily opened by children but all adults under 45 years of age should be able to open and reclose the packages easily. These rather stringent requirements arose from recognition by the National Clearing House for Poison Control Centers in its 1970 report of an excessive number of hospitalizations of children under 5 years of age from ingestion of amphetamines, barbiturates, meprobamate, and methadone, which are among the more toxic agents ingested. At present, the regulations apply only to the drug manufacturers and pharmacists and not to veterinarians; nevertheless, veterinarians should be guided by these regulations for the protection of their clients and to protect themselves against legal actions. Some of the drugs covered by these regulations include drugs prescribed for human beings in all dosage forms, all "controlled" drugs (viz., opiates, hallucinogens, barbiturates), aspirin, methyl alcohol, methylsalicylate, and strong alkalies.

The veterinarian must use great care to dispense drugs in safe containers with proper labeling that includes the date, veterinarian's name and address, the name of the drug, the amount or quantity dispensed, and directions for use. The veterinarian must be careful not to knowingly create the possibility of human use of the drug. Grounds for malpractice action by a client against a veterinarian may exist for several reasons, including the following: failure to adequately inform the client, failure to test for allergy when such is indicated, improper storage of the drug causing it to become defective, failure to get the client's consent when a drug that may have adverse reactions is used, employing an improper dosage for the animal, using the wrong drug, and using a defective drug. Damage may occur to drugs while being transported in a practice vehicle because of overheating or excessive agitation.

It is quite clear that a veterinary practitioner has a professional responsibility arising from the acquisition, storage, dispensing, and record keeping of drugs used in his practice.

S E C T I O N 2

Pharmacodynamics

CHAPTER 4

MECHANISMS OF DRUG ACTION

J. DESMOND BAGGOT

INTRODUCTION

Pharmacodynamics is the study of the biochemical and physiological effects of drugs and their mechanisms of action. A drug may be defined as a chemical substance that acts in a biological system to preferentially give a beneficial pharmacological or chemotherapeutic effect. The action of a drug is the process by which the drug brings about a change in some preexisting physiological function or biochemical process of the living organism. The part of the body in which a drug acts and thereby initiates the series of biochemical and physiological changes that are characteristic of the drug is known as the *site of action*. The means by which a drug initiates the series of events, measured or observed as an effect, is its *mechanism of action*. The mechanism of action of most drugs is believed to involve a chemical interaction between the drug and a functionally important tissue component, called a *receptor*, in the living organism. The hypothetical receptor is regarded as a macromolecular tissue constituent with which a drug interacts to produce its characteristic biological effect (Ariens and Simonis 1964; Albert 1968). Only the initial consequence of the drug-receptor combination is correctly termed the action of the drug; the succeeding events are properly called drug effects. The effects produced by a drug can be measured and expressed only in terms of an alteration of some known function or process that maintains the existence of the organism; effects of drugs are quantitative, never qualitative. It is axiomatic that no drug can cause a tissue to exert any response of which it is not naturally capable.

DRUG-RECEPTOR INTERACTION AND STRUCTURE-ACTIVITY RELATIONSHIPS

The binding force that holds a drug in combination with its receptor arises from the concerted operation of several bond types. The drug-receptor combination usually involves ionic bonds, hydrogen bonds, and van der Waals forces; a reversible interaction is established, which obeys the law of mass action (Clark 1937). Consider the combination of acetylcholine with a hypothetical receptor. The chemical formula of acetylcholine and its postulated interaction with a receptor are shown in Fig. 4.1. The quaternary nitrogen atom of acetylcholine has a strong positive charge and is thought to be ionically bonded to a negatively charged group of the receptor. This electrostatic attraction may be sufficient to draw acetylcholine close to

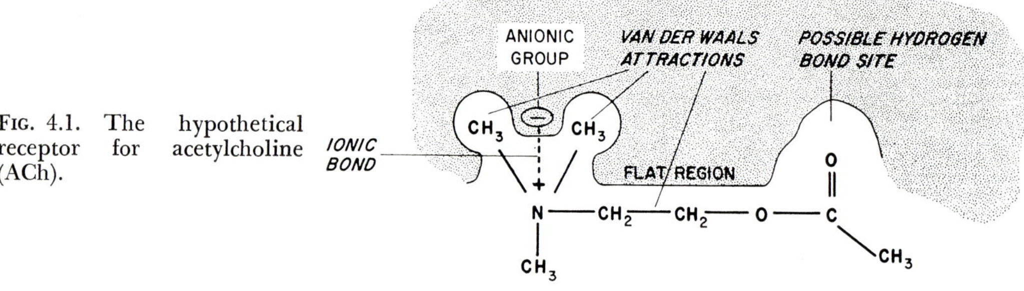

FIG. 4.1. The hypothetical receptor for acetylcholine (ACh).

the receptor. The assumption is made that two of the methyl (—CH_3) groups help to stabilize the acetylcholine-receptor complex through van der Waals forces by fitting into the cavity in which the charged (anionic) site of the receptor is embedded. It is likely that the carbon chain between the nitrogen and oxygen atoms lies in close proximity to a flat portion of the receptor surface, contributing further van der Waals attractions to the overall binding. The carbonyl oxygen atom might well participate in hydrogen bond formation with an appropriate receptor group (e.g., the —NH of a peptide bond), thus further stabilizing the interaction. Although this concept of a receptor is entirely hypothetical, the inferences concerning individual points of binding are based on the results of structure-activity relationship studies reported by Waser (1960).

The narcotic analgesics act upon pain pathways in the central nervous system (CNS) by a similar mechanism and constitute a series of drugs with different potencies. Structurally, morphine was thought of as a substituted phenanthrene derivative, as indeed it is (Fig. 4.2); but eventually it was realized that although the phenanthrene nucleus could be modified or even eliminated without loss of analgesic activity, the piperidine ring is essential. The nitrogen atom of this ring is about 80% cationic at physiological pH, so it is postulated that one important element of the drug-receptor interaction may be ionic binding to an anionic site on the receptor surface. The narcotic analgesics are best thought of as *N*-methylpiperidine compounds with bulky ring substituents. Receptor attachment (Beckett and Casy 1954) and analgesic activity (Gero 1954) are related to the γ-phenyl-*N*-methylpiperidine moiety of these molecules. Substitution of allyl (—$CH_2CH = CH_2$) for methyl (—CH_3) on the nitrogen atom produces a remarkable change in activity. Such compounds (e.g., nalorphine) behave as specific competitive antagonists of analgesia (and other effects) produced by the narcotics (Martin 1967). It is assumed, therefore, that they interact with the same receptors.

The covalent binding of drugs to receptors, unlike most drug-receptor interactions, results in stable persistent complexes. An example of drug-receptor interaction through formation of a covalent

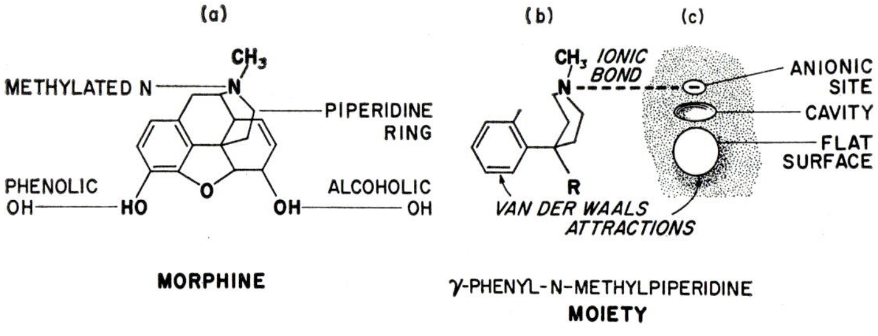

FIG. 4.2. *(a)* Structure of morphine; *(b)* active portion of morphine molecule; *(c)* hypothetical receptor surface for narcotic analgesics.

bond is the long-lasting inhibition of the cholinesterase enzymes by organic phosphates and carbamates. The specificity and selectivity of drug-receptor interactions arise not just from the nature of the bonds formed but also from the spatial configuration of the sites for bond formation on the receptor surface.

Acetylcholine (ACh) is a neurotransmitter that is released from cholinergic neurons at many locations in the body. It acts upon receptors (cholinoceptive sites) in skeletal muscle end-plates, in smooth muscles, in cells of secretory glands, in ganglion cells of the autonomic nervous system, and probably in certain nerve cells of the CNS. This molecule has the appropriate structure and relative flexibility to interact with two different kinds of receptor sites: the nicotinic site at somatic neuromuscular junctions and autonomic ganglia; and the muscarinic site at parasympathetic neuroeffector junctions in smooth muscle, the heart, and secretory glands. Many drugs combine specifically with one or the other site. Acetyl-β-methylcholine (methacholine) and carbamylmethylcholine (bethanechol) exert mainly muscarinic actions. Carbamylcholine (carbachol) acts rather selectively on the smooth muscle of the gastro-intestinal tract and urinary bladder but it also displays nicotinic activity, particularly on autonomic ganglia, which is due, at least in part, to release of endogenous ACh from the terminals of cholinergic fibers (Koelle 1970). Atropine is a highly selective antagonist of ACh and congeners that act at muscarinic sites. It competitively occupies the cholinoceptive sites on autonomic effector cells and the secondary muscarinic receptors of autonomic ganglion cells. Blockade of the muscarinic receptor by atropine can be reversed by drugs that allow ACh to accumulate and compete for receptor sites, i.e., reversible cholinesterase inhibitors (e.g., neostigmine, physostigmine, edrophonium). The nicotinic receptors of autonomic ganglia and skeletal muscle are not identical, since they respond differently to certain stimulating (dimethylphenylpiperazinium [DMPP], phenyltrimethylammonium [PTMA]) and blocking (hexamethonium, decamethonium) agents. The essential difference between the ganglionic and muscle end-plate receptors is presumed to be in the distance between anionic sites on the nicotinic receptors. Succinylcholine, a depolarizing agent, interacts specifically with the muscle end-plate receptor to produce neuromuscular block; the blocking effect is preceded by activation (depolarization). There is a wide variation in sensitivity to the neuromuscular blocking action of succinylcholine among the various species of domestic animals. A competitive neuromuscular blocking agent, *d*-tubocurarine, effectively interrupts transmission of the nerve impulse by combining with cholinoceptive sites at both motor end-plates and autonomic ganglia, although it acts predominantly at the former site. The reversible cholinesterase inhibitors hasten recovery from competitive neuromuscular blocking agents (*d*-tubocurarine and gallamine) but augment the effects of depolarizing agents (succinylcholine). Respiratory paralysis, caused by overdosage with neuromuscular blocking agents of both types, should be treated by the application of positive-pressure artificial respiration.

The active center of acetylcholinesterase (AChE) has two main subsites (Fig. 4.3). The first is an anionic site that attracts the positive charge in ACh and the second, about 5 Å distant, is an esteratic site that binds the carbonyl carbon atom of ACh. The overall hydrolytic reaction can be written as follows:

$$\text{Enzyme} + \text{ACh} \rightleftharpoons \text{Enzyme} \cdot \text{ACh complex} \rightarrow \text{Acetylenzyme} + \text{Choline}$$

$$\text{Acetylenzyme} \xrightarrow{H_2O} \text{Enzyme} + \text{Acetic Acid}$$

The very rapid rate of hydrolysis of ACh by both AChE and butyrocholinesterase (also called pseudocholinesterase) limits therapeutic value of this endogenous substance. Information on the architecture of the active center of AChE has been de-

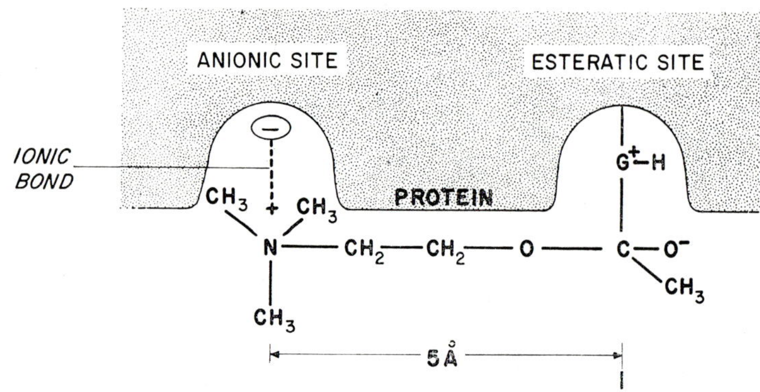

FIG. 4.3. Active center of acetylcholinesterase (AChE). The enzyme-substrate complex (shown in diagram) is formed by electrostatic attraction between the N^+ atom of the choline moiety and anionic site of the enzyme and the electrophilic C atom of the carboxyl group of ACh and a protonated acidic group (:G-H) of the esteratic site of AChE.

rived not only from kinetic studies using model compounds but from anticholinesterase compounds. The anticholinesterases are classified as reversible (carbamates) and irreversible (organic phosphates) inhibitors of the enzyme. The effects of cholinesterase inhibitors are manifestations of ACh activity. While the acetyl- and carbamyl-enzyme bonds undergo spontaneous hydrolysis, the phosphoryl-enzyme bond is hydrolyzed spontaneously at a negligible rate. The spontaneous recovery of enzyme activity in organic phosphate toxicity is governed by the generation of new enzyme protein, a process taking several days. To hasten recovery, pralidoxime (*N*-methylpyridinium 2-aldoxime, formerly known as 2-PAM), which is a nucleophilic reactivating agent for phosphorylated cholinesterase, is an effective antidote to organic phosphate toxicity when administered in conjugation with atropine. The oxime functions as an antidotal agent by displacing the phosphorus from the enzyme (Loomis 1968). Pralidoxime, with its quaternary ammonium group, does not penetrate the blood-brain barrier well enough to overcome central actions of the anticholinesterase. Atropine, at high dosage, does exert activity in the CNS. The same principles apply in treating overdosage with the reversible inhibitors of ACh (e.g., neostigmine, physostigmine). These inhibitors form carbamylated enzymes analogous to the phosphorylated enzymes, except that their rates of spontaneous hydrolysis are much faster (Wilson et al. 1961). Consequently, atropine and supportive therapy suffice.

QUANTITATIVE ASPECTS OF DRUG-RECEPTOR INTERACTION

One of the most fundamental principles of pharmacology states that the intensity of response elicited by a drug is a function of the dose administered. This relationship between dose and response may be interpreted in two ways: (1) as the dose of a drug is increased, the magnitude (or intensity) of the response is also increased; or (2) as the dose is increased, the number or proportion of animals exhibiting a particular, stated response is also increased. These two fundamental relationships between dose and response have been termed graded and quantal, respectively.

Graded Dose-Response Relationship

A pharmacological effect is considered to be the consequence of a reversible combination of drug molecules with receptors. The product of this reaction becomes the stimulus for the events leading to the effect:

$$\text{Drug} + \text{Receptor} \rightleftarrows \begin{matrix}\text{Drug-receptor}\\ \text{complex}\end{matrix} \xrightarrow{\text{Stimulus}} \text{Effect}$$

A. J. Clark (1885–1941) was largely responsible for applying the law of mass action to the dose-response relationship. The magnitude of a response (pharmacological effect) elicited by a drug was postulated to be directly proportional to the number of receptors occupied by drug molecules, with a maximal response corresponding to occupancy of all the receptors.

In the drug-receptor interaction, the reacting substances are the drug and the unoccupied receptors and the product is the drug-receptor complex:

$$\underset{C_X}{\text{Drug}} + \underset{(100 - Y)}{\text{Free receptor}} \underset{k_2}{\overset{k_1}{\rightleftarrows}} \underset{Y}{\text{Drug-receptor complex}}$$

where C_X is the concentration of the drug at the site of action and Y is the percentage of the total number of receptors occupied by the drug. To apply the law of mass action to the dose-response phenomenon, two important assumptions must be made. First, the drug response is directly proportional to the percentage of the total receptors occupied by the drug. Second, a negligible fraction of the total drug is combined with receptors. At equilibrum,

$$k_1 \cdot C_X(100 - Y) = k_2 \cdot Y$$

$$\text{i.e., } C_X = \frac{k_2 Y}{k_1(100 - Y)}$$

and substituting K_X, the equilibrium constant of the reaction, for k_1/k_2,

$$C_X = \frac{Y}{K_X(100 - Y)}$$

Since the drug concentration remains essentially unchanged during the reaction, the ratio of the percentage of occupied receptors to that of unoccupied receptors is proportional to the dose of the drug administered. The mathematical expression of the relationship between the dose and the response is the equation for a hyperbola. The increments in response to equal increases in the dose become progressively smaller as a maximum value is approached, until further increases in the dose produce no perceptively greater effect; a maximum response would be equivalent to 100% occupancy of receptors.

The graphic representation of the typical relationship between the graded response and the dose takes the form of a hyperbola with concavity downward when the effect (the dependent variable) and the dose (the independent variable) are expressed in arithmetic units. In pharmacology, it is conventional to plot the independent variable (dose) on a logarithmic scale. Such a transformation converts the hyperbola into a sigmoid curve with a central segment that is practically linear (Fig. 4.4). The log dose-response curve is symmetrical about the point at which 50% of the maximum response is elicited, and its maximum slope and point of inflection occur at this midpoint. Drugs that produce

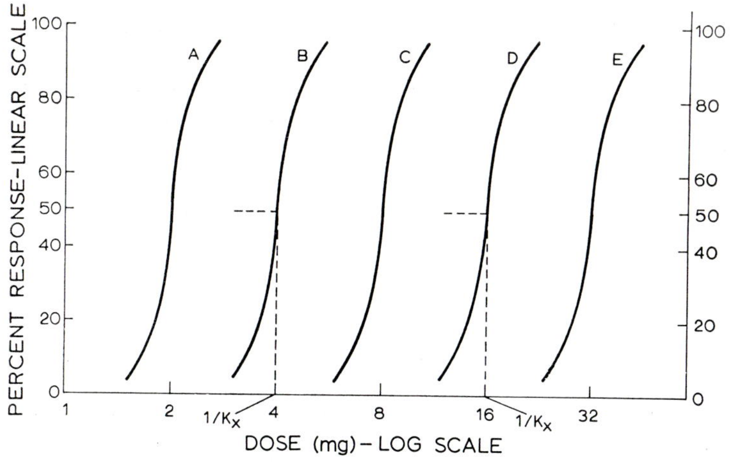

FIG. 4.4. Log dose-response (LDR) curves for drugs that produce similar effects by the same mechanism of action but differ in potency. Drug *B* is four times more potent than drug *D*. In terms of affinity for the receptor, drug *A* has the greatest and drug *E* the least affinity for the same receptor site.

similar effects by the same mechanism of action but differ in potency generally have similarly shaped log dose-response (LDR) curves with the same maximum; their linear segments are usually parallel. Another practical advantage of the logarithmic dosage scale is that a wide range of doses can be presented readily in a single graph.

The intensity of effect produced by a drug is directly proportional to the percentage of total receptors that are occupied by the drug. Receptor occupancy is a function both of drug concentration and its ability to combine with its receptor. The ability (or tendency) of a drug to combine with a particular receptor is a constant, which is known as the affinity constant. The affinity of a drug for its receptor is reflected by the position of its LDR curve on the abscissa. The abscissal intersection of a perpendicular line, drawn from the point of 50% maximal response on an LDR curve, is the drug concentration that is equal to the reciprocal of affinity, i.e., $1/K_X$. One would expect a series of congeneric drugs that interact with the same receptor (i.e., have a similar mechanism of action) to yield a set of parallel log dose-response curves; the curve for the drug with greatest affinity for the receptor (acts at lowest concentration) will lie closest to the ordinate, i.e., the greater the affinity, the farther the curve will lie to the left (Fig. 4.4). Although the receptors for most drugs have not been characterized and the estimated values of the affinity of a drug for its receptor are approximations, there is little doubt that drug receptor combinations obeying mass law kinetics are involved in drug action.

Potency is the dose of a drug required to produce a particular effect of given intensity. The positions of the log dose-response curves of several drugs along the abscissa (dose axis) provide an expression of the relative potencies of the drugs. Like affinity, potency varies inversely with the magnitude of the dose required to produce the effect; the closer the LDR curve is to the ordinate the more potent the drug. Only drugs that act at the same group of receptors (i.e., same mechanism of action) and that are capable of eliciting the same maximal response can be compared with respect to potency, e.g., narcotic analgesics for analgesic effect, glucocorticoids for antiinflammatory effect, and benzothiadiazides for diuretic effect. Potency, unlike affinity, is a comparative rather than an absolute expression of drug activity. The relative potencies of narcotic analgesics in human beings are found by comparing the doses, administered by the same route (e.g., subcutaneously) and required to relieve pain induced by the same stimulus, with 10 mg of morphine. For example, it has been found that 1.5 mg of hydromorphone (Dilaudid) or 120 mg of codeine have similar analgesic activity to 10 mg of morphine; one can say that morphine is about seven times less potent than hydromorphone, but about twelve times more potent than codeine. Potency embodies the conceptual aspects of drug-receptor interactions; it is influenced by the drug's affinity for its receptor and by factors regulating the drug concentration in the biophase (immediate vicinity of the receptor), i.e., absorption, distribution, biotransformation, and excretion. The potency of a drug is not related to its efficacy or safety, and there is no justification for the view that the most potent drug among agents with similar actions is clinically superior. The appropriate dosage of drugs having similar mechanisms of action (i.e., interact with the same receptor site) should be based on their relative potencies.

A drug whose interaction with a receptor initiates an action-effects sequence is known as an agonist and is endowed with two independent properties: affinity and efficacy, or intrinsic activity (Ariens 1954). Affinity describes the tendency of a drug to form a stable complex with a receptor. Efficacy describes the biological effectiveness of the drug-receptor complex. The efficacy of a drug is reflected as a plateau in the LDR curve, and it is a measure of the maximum effect of a drug relative to that of a standard whose intrinsic activity is assigned the arbitrary number 1. Since aspirin and morphine (or codeine) act at different sites and produce their analgesic effects by different mechanisms, it is inappropriate to express the relative activities of the salicylate and opiate in terms of potency. Morphine has the potential to relieve pain of nearly all intensities, whereas aspirin is effective against mild-to-moderate pain only, so that these drugs differ in maximum analgesic effect.

Drug Antagonism

Whenever the conjoint effect of two drugs is less than the sum of the effects of the drugs acting separately, the phenomenon is called drug antagonism. Drugs that interact with a receptor but do not initiate the sequence of events leading to an effect are known as antagonists. The antagonism is competitive when the two molecular species, agonist and antagonist, compete for the same receptors. Competitive antagonism is completely reversible; an increase in the concentration of agonist will overcome the effect of the antagonist and vice versa. The degree of antagonism produced depends on the concentration of the antagonist and its affinity constant. The antagonist effect is seen as a reduction in the apparent affinity of the agonist for its receptor. In competitive antagonism, the efficacy of the agonist is unchanged. The antagonism is noncompetitive when its effects cannot be reversed by increasing concentrations of the agonist. The noncompetitive antagonist may produce its effect by combining either with the same sites as the active drug or with different sites in a manner that alters the capacity of the agonist to combine with its own receptor sites. In noncompetitive antagonism, the effects upon receptors may be reversible or irreversible; the essential point is that the agonist has no influence upon the degree of antagonism or its reversibility.

The quantitative aspects of drug antagonism are readily analyzed from LDR curves (Fig. 4.5). In the presence of a competitive antagonist, the LDR curve for the agonist will be shifted to the right, but neither the slope nor the maximum response is altered. This indicates that the competitive antagonist simply alters the effective affinity of the agonist for its receptor. The influence of a noncompetitive antagonist upon the LDR curve is quite different from that of a competitive antagonist. The agonist curve will again be shifted to the right, but the slope will be reduced and the maximum response will diminish, in relation to the degree of noncompetitive blockade established. Another method of analyzing drug antagonisms, particularly enzyme inhibitions, is by means of the double-reciprocal (or Lineweaver-Burk) plot (Webb 1963). A graph of the reciprocal of intensity of effect (response magnitude) versus reciprocal of

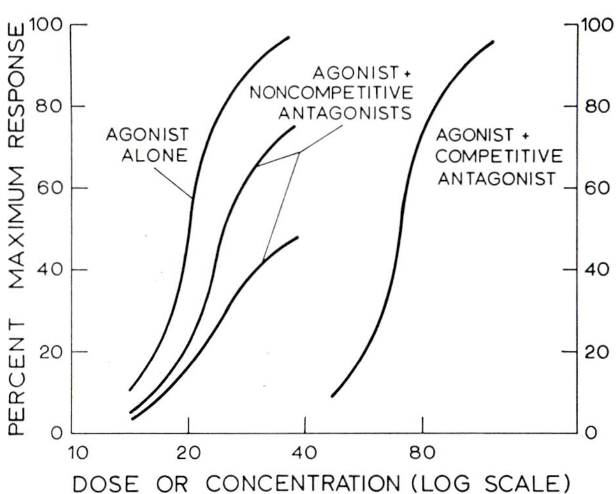

Fig. 4.5. LDR curves in analysis of drug antagonism.

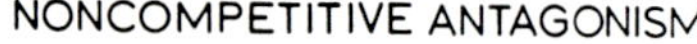

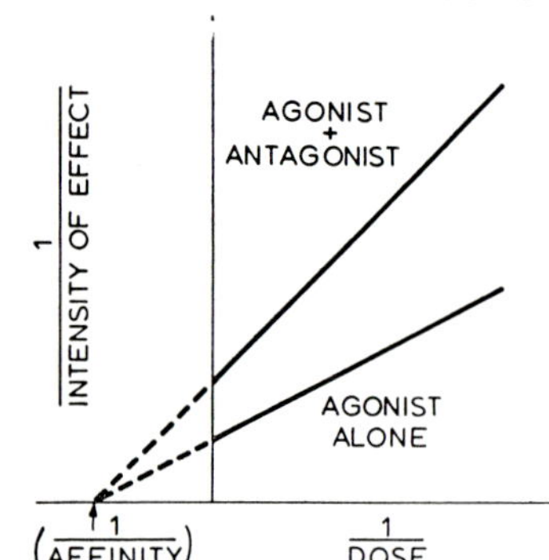

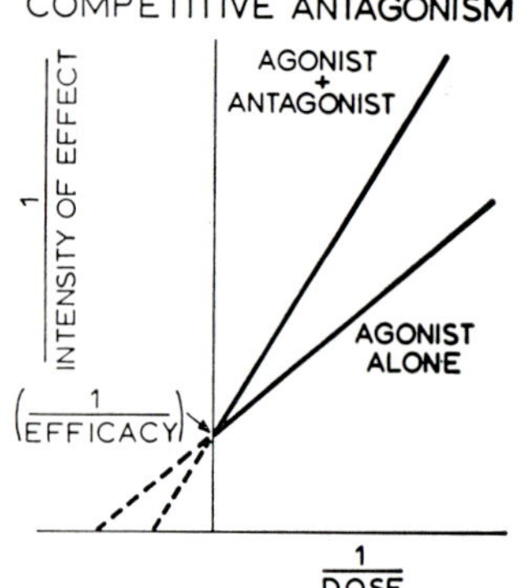

FIG. 4.6. Analysis of antagonisms by double-reciprocal plots.

dose gives a straight line for any drug; the intercept on the *Y*-axis gives the reciprocal of efficacy, and the *X*-axis intercept is the negative reciprocal of affinity (Fig. 4.6). If the dose-response range is first explored with an agonist alone and then in the presence of a fixed dose (or concentration) of a noncompetitive antagonist, the system will behave as though the total number of available receptor sites had been reduced. Nevertheless, whatever receptors remain should display unchanged affinity for the agonist. In the double-reciprocal plot, since the maximum response is reduced proportionately to the decrease in free receptors, the *Y* intercept will increase. On the other hand, the *X* intercept will remain unchanged. In competitive antagonism, the maximum response (efficacy) of the agonist is not altered. In the double-reciprocal plot, therefore, the *Y* intercept remains unchanged, but the affinity (*X* intercept) is reduced.

The type of drug antagonism that has been discussed is known as pharmacological antagonism, since the antagonist interferes with the mechanism by which most pharmacological effects are produced. Physiological antagonism is observed when two agonists, acting at different sites, counterbalance each other by producing opposite effects on the same physiological function. Biochemical antagonism occurs whenever one drug indirectly decreases the concentration of a second drug at its site of action. The usual mode of action of a biochemical antagonist is to increase the elimination from the body of an agonist, e.g., by inducing hepatic microsomal enzyme activity. A fourth type of antagonism, chemical antagonism, is simply a chemical inactivation (or neutralization) effect, e.g., antacids. Combination of certain chemotherapeutic agents, especially one with bacteriostatic and another with bactericidal action, may be detrimental in antibacterial therapy owing to their opposite effects (Jawetz 1968).

QUANTAL DOSE-RESPONSE RELATIONSHIP

The graded dose-effect curve provides information about the dose required to provide a specified intensity of effect in an individual. In the graded type of dose-effect relationship, it is assumed that the response of an individual biological unit increases measurably with increasing concentration of drug. Quantal effects, in contrast to graded effects, are all-or-none responses. Each individual is categorized as responding or not responding, according to whatever criterion of response has been adopted. The quantal dose-effect relationship relates dose to an expression of the frequency with which any dose of a drug evokes a stated, all-or-none pharmacological effect. Biological variation imposes variable sensitivity to a drug in animals within a species, and even breed or strain. As a rule, the sensitivity of animals to different doses of a drug is distributed normally with respect to the logarithm of the dose (Barlow 1964). If log dose is plotted on the *X*-axis and the relative frequency of

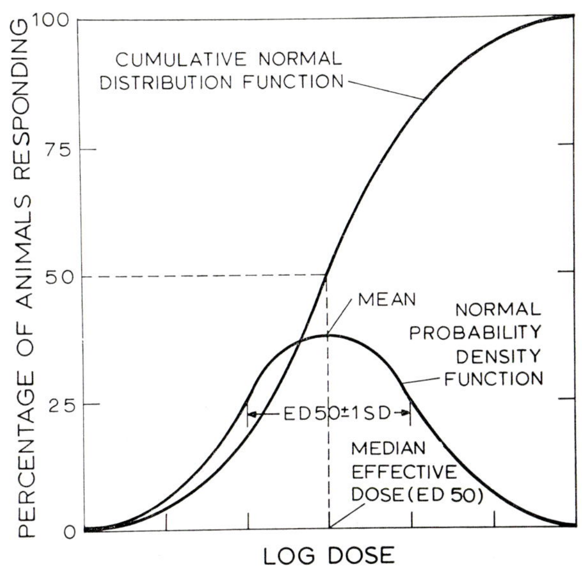

FIG. 4.7. Statistical distribution of receptor sensitivities.

animals sensitive to the various doses is plotted on the *Y*-axis, a gaussian (normal) distribution is usually approximated (Fig. 4.7). The median (also mean) of the quantal curve is the dose at which 50% of the animals manifests the predetermined effect. Hence, the term "median effective dose" (ED50) or "median lethal dose" (LD50) is used to express the smallest dose required to produce the stated or lethal effect, respectively, in 50% of the population. The most useful measure of variability of the normal distribution curve is the standard deviation. Unlike the median, which is calculated only from the number of individuals in the sample, the standard deviation takes into account all the individual values, even those at the extremes, since its calculation is based on the difference of each observation from the mean value. The cumulative (integral) form of the normal distribution curve is a more useful form of graphic presentation of the data and relates the dose of the drug to the cumulative percentage of animals showing the response. The cumulative quantal dose-effect curve is sigmoid in shape, and at any dose the cumulative curve gives the percentage of animals responding to that dose and to all lower doses.

Long before the birth of modern pharmacology, Paracelsus (1493–1541) observed that "all things are poisons, for there is nothing without poisonous qualities. It is only the dose which makes a thing a poison." There is no single dose-response relationship that can adequately characterize a drug in terms of its full spectrum of activity. Every drug has at least two quantal dose-response curves, one for the desired therapeutic effect and one for a toxic effect (Fig. 4.8). The margin of safety is the dosage range between the dose producing a lethal effect and the dose producing the desired effect. This margin of safety is referred to as the therapeutic index, which is obtained from the ratio of the median lethal dose to the median effective dose (ie., LD50/ED50). The essential attribute we seek in a drug is efficacy at a safe dose; this implies a large value of the therapeutic index. However, this index alone is not sufficient for a true assessment of drug safety, since median doses tell nothing about the slopes of the dose-response curves for therapeutic and toxic effects. Since there is no fixed dose or concentration of a chemical that can be relied upon to produce a given biological effect in a population and the aim of drug therapy is to achieve a therapeutic effect

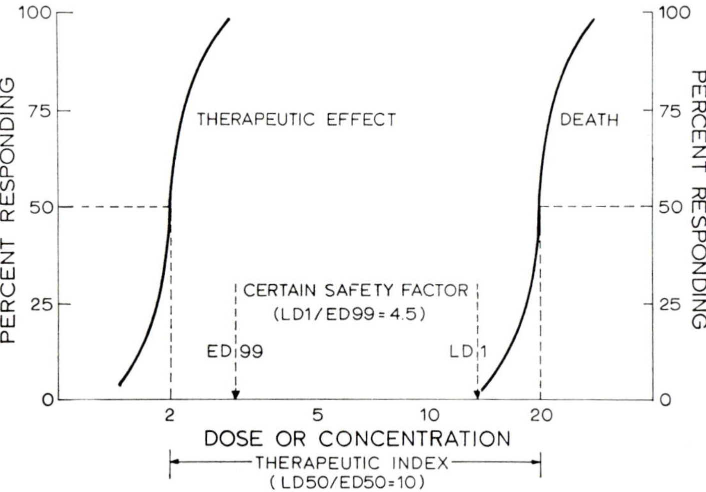

FIG. 4.8. Quantal dose-response curves representing the cumulative number of animals responding as the dose is increased. The margin of safety of a drug is a dose ratio obtained from these curves.

in all individuals, drug safety can be better assessed by using a ratio derived from the extremes of the respective quantal curves, such as LD1/ED99. This ratio is known as the *certain safety factor*. If all quantal LDR curves had the same slopes, it would make no difference what ratio were chosen; the ratio LD1/ED99, for example, would always be a fixed fraction of the therapeutic index.

Selectivity of Drug Action

A drug is usually described by its most prominent effect or by the action thought to be the basis of this effect. However, such descriptions should not obscure the fact that most drugs produce many effects and have many dose-response curves. The varied effects of a drug with a specific action (e.g., atropine, propranolol, acetazolamide) are the consequence of a single mechanism of action taking place at a multiplicity of sites. If the effects are due to several mechanisms of action, the drug is nonspecific, e.g., diphenhydramine (antihistaminic). A drug's selectivity depends on its capacity to preferentially produce one particular effect, i.e., the characteristic effect of the drug is the effect produced at lower doses than those required to elicit other responses. It follows that a comparison of the dose-response curves for the desired and undesired (side) effects of a single drug determines its selectivity. The selectivity of drug action is measured by the therapeutic index or certain safety factor, in which the relationship between two effects is expressed, e.g., intensity of analgesia and degree of respiratory depression produced by morphine. Differences in physiochemical properties influencing distribution among agents that have a similar mechanism of action may confer selectivity on a member of the group by virtue of its unique ability to attain an effective concentration at a particular site of action (usually the CNS). For therapeutic applications, selectivity of a drug is clearly one of its more important characteristics.

DRUG ACTIONS NOT MEDIATED DIRECTLY BY RECEPTORS

Certain mechanisms of drug action do not entail the formation of a drug-receptor complex. The actions of some of the drugs used in veterinary medicine fall into this category.

The biological effect may be a nonspecific consequence of physical or chemical properties of a drug. The osmotic diuretics (e.g., urea, mannitol) produce their effects by increasing the osmolarity of tubular urine and thereby slowing reabsorption of water. The saline cathartics or purgatives (e.g., magnesium sulfate, sodium sulfate) when given orally retain an osmotic equivalent of water within the lumen of the gut. Neither Mg^{2+} nor SO_4^{2-} ions traverse the gastrointestinal mucosa. Certain drugs owe their actions entirely to their acidic or basic properties, e.g., antacids (aluminum hydroxide, sodium bicarbonate) and urinary acidifiers (ammonium chloride). The most notable among those drugs whose actions do not involve receptors are the volatile general anesthetic agents. Substances as unrelated as diethyl ether, cyclopropane, halothane, and nitrous oxide produce very similar effects on the brain. It has long been recognized that the usual drug-receptor models would not accommodate these drugs. Theories of narcosis either have related the phenomenon of anesthesia to similarities in some physicochemical properties (e.g., lipid-to-water partition coefficient) of anesthetic agents or have described biochemical or physiological phenomena that occur during anesthesia. The ability of the volatile anesthetics to stabilize water clathrates has been made the basis of a theory of anesthesia (Pauling 1964), the validity of which, however, has been questioned (Miller et al. 1972). While the various observations have provided valuable information, a fundamental, experimentally proved theory of narcosis is lacking at the present time. Anesthesia could be the result of a composite change in the total lipoprotein cell membrane and in the adjacent water phase (DiFazio et al. 1972) or it may also occur from biomembrane expansion (Seeman 1972); see the discussion in Chapter 10 on the mode of action of general anesthetics.

The biological effect may be a consequence of direct chemical interaction between the drug and a small molecule or ion. The therapeutically useful chelating agents provide the best examples of this mechanism of action. Chelation is the formation of coordination complexes through ring systems, often 5- or 6-membered rings. Chelate complexes vary greatly in stability (i.e., in the tendency to dissociate), depending upon the nature of the chelating agent and of the complexed atom. Stability is expressed quantitatively by the stability constant (K_c) in the mass law equation for the equilibrium relationship between free and complexed reactants:

$$\text{metal cation} + \text{chelating agent} \underset{k_2}{\overset{k_1}{\rightleftarrows}} \text{coordination complex}$$

$$\frac{[\text{complex}]}{[\text{metal}] \times [\text{chelating agent}]} = \frac{k_1}{k_2} = K_c$$

For any given chelating agent, the magnitude of the stability constants is determined largely by the atomic structures of the various metals, e.g., the values of K_c for metal-EDTA complexes increase in the order $Na^+ < Ca^{2+} < Pb^{2+}$. A metal with a higher stability constant would effectively compete for the chelating agent with a metal of lower stability and, given sufficient time, would displace the less tightly bound metal from complexes already formed (Martell and Calvin 1952; Loomis 1968).

Calcium disodium edetate, a salt of EDTA, is a specific antidote in lead poisoning. The drug removes free lead ions from blood and other tissues and renders it inert by complexing Pb^{2+} very tightly. Since the attractive force between the drug and Pb^{2+}, its affinity for lead, is many orders of magnitude (10^7-fold) greater than that between the drug and Ca^{2+}, the lead effectively displaces calcium from EDTA. Eventually the soluble lead chelate is eliminated from the body by renal excretion. Disodium edetate is a satisfactory *in vitro* anticoagulant, the EDTA exchanges Na^+ for Ca^{2+} of blood. Penicillamine is a relatively safe and orally effective copper-binding chelating agent. Desferrioxamine (Deferoxamine) is a useful chelating agent for the systemic treatment of iron toxicity. It binds the iron from transferrin and ferritin but does not remove iron from hemoglobin or the cytochromes, to which the metal is bound even more tightly. Thus the chelate stability constant is of a magnitude suitable for the removal of excessive iron without disrupting the biologically indispensable iron compounds. The principle of mercaptide formation is applied in the use of dimercaprol (British anti-lewisite, BAL). This drug is a simple glycerol derivative containing two vicinal sulfhydryl groups capable of forming a very stable mercaptide ring. Certain heavy metals, notably mercury and arsenic, owe their toxicity primarily to their ability to react with and inhibit sulfhydryl enzyme systems involved in several vital processes in the body, such as those involved in the production of cellular energy. BAL is capable of forming metal complexes of greater stability than the enzyme-metal complex. By virtue of its free hydroxyl group, dimercaprol remains soluble even after it has chelated a metal atom. Thus various heavy metals (mercury, arsenic, antimony), whether present as free ions or in organic complexes, may be removed from the tissues and body fluids, rendered nontoxic by combination with dimercaprol, and then excreted in the urine. Dimercaprol must be administered parenterally (intramuscularly) and is itself potentially toxic.

REFERENCES

Albert, A. 1968. Selective Toxicity, 4th ed., p. 68. London: Methuen.

Ariens, E. J. 1954. Affinity and intrinsic activity in theory of competitive inhibition: Problems and theory. Arch Int Pharmacodyn Ther 99:32.

Ariens, E. J., and Simonis, A. M. 1964. A molecular basis for drug action. J Pharm Pharmacol 16:137.

Barlow, R. B. 1964. Introduction to Chemical Pharmacology, 2nd ed., p. 27. London: Methuen.

Beckett, A. H., and Casy, A. F. 1954. Synthetic analgesics: Stereochemical considerations. J Pharm Pharmacol 6:986.

Clark, A. J. 1937. Handbuch der Experimentellen Pharmakologie. Begrundet von A. Heffter. Erganzungswerk 4, p. 63. Berlin: Springer-Verlag.

DiFazio, C. A.; Brown, R. E.; Ball, C. G.; Heckel, C. G.; and Kennedy, S. S. 1972. Additive effects of anesthetics and theories of anesthesia. Anesthesiology 36:57.

Gero, A. 1954. Steric considerations on the chemical structure and physiological activity of methadone and related compounds. Science 119:112.

Jawetz, E. 1968. The use of combinations of antimicrobial drugs. Annu Rev Pharmacol 8:151.

Koelle, G. B. 1970. Drugs acting at synaptic and neuroeffector junctional sites. In L. S. Goodman and A. Gilman, eds. The Pharmacological Basis of Therapeutics, 4th ed., p. 402. New York: Macmillan.

Loomis, T. A. 1968. Essentials of Toxicology, p. 131. Philadelphia: Lea & Febiger.

Martell, A. E., and Calvin, M. 1952. Chemistry of the Metal Chelate Compounds, pp. 184, 191. New York: Prentice-Hall.

Martin, W. R. 1967. Opioid antagonists. Pharmacol Rev 19:463.

Miller, K. W.; Paton, W. D. M.; Smith, E. B.; and Smith, R. A. 1972. Physicochemical approaches to the mode of action of general anesthetics. Anesthesiology 36:339.

Pauling, L. 1964. The hydrate microcrystal theory of general anesthesia. Anesth Analg 43:1.

Seeman, P. 1972. The membrane actions of anesthetics and tranquilizers. Pharmacol Rev 24:583.

Waser, P. G. 1960. The cholinergic receptor. J Pharm Pharmacol 12:577.

Webb, J. L. 1963. Enzyme and Metabolic Inhibitors, vol. 1, p. 149. New York: Academic Press.

Wilson, I. B.; Harrison, M. A.; and Ginsburg, S. 1961. Carbamyl derivatives of acetylcholinesterase. J Biol Chem 236:1498.

CHAPTER 5

DISPOSITION AND FATE OF DRUGS IN THE BODY

J. DESMOND BAGGOT

TRANSPORT OF DRUGS ACROSS BIOLOGICAL MEMBRANES

Pharmacodynamics not only describes the mechanisms of drug action but also deals with the factors determining the intensity and temporal course of drug action. The processes of absorption and distribution influence the accessibility of a drug to its site of action, while biotransformation and excretion are responsible for terminating the action of a drug in the body (Fig. 5.1). The duration of action, which is related to the concentration at the site of action, depends in a complex way upon

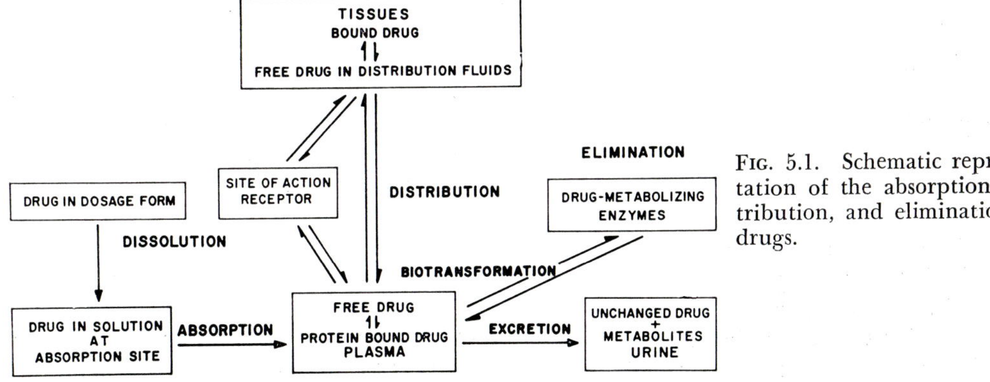

FIG. 5.1. Schematic representation of the absorption, distribution, and elimination of drugs.

the relative rates of the various translocation and drug-metabolizing processes. Either directly or indirectly, all these processes involve passage of drugs across membranes. It is essential, therefore, to consider the nature of biological membranes and how they are penetrated by drugs.

Nature of Biological Membranes

Biological membranes may be viewed as mosaics of functional units composed of lipoprotein complexes (Dowben 1969). The characteristic feature of cell membranes appears to be a bimolecular layer of phospholipid molecules, oriented perpendicular to the plane of the membrane, with polar head groups aligned at both surfaces and long hydrocarbon chains extending inward (Davson and Danielli 1952). It was thought that sheets of unfolded protein covered the inner and outer membrane surfaces and that an additional layer of globular proteins (e.g., enzymes) was localized at the inner surface. Recent advances in electron microscopy and analytical data on membrane proteins have led to a different concept, the "fluid mosaic" model (Singer and Nicolson 1972). In this model, the proteins that are integral to the membrane are a heterogeneous set of globular molecules, each arranged in an amphipathic structure, that is, with the ionic and highly polar groups protruding from the membrane into the aqueous phase and the nonpolar groups largely buried in the hydrophobic interior of the membrane. These globular molecules are partially embedded in a matrix of phospholipid. The bulk of the phospholipid is organized as a discontinuous, fluid bilayer, although a small fraction of the lipid may interact specifically with the membrane proteins.

Passage of Drugs across Membranes

Drug molecules pass across membranes either by passive transfer processes or by specialized transport processes (Schanker 1964). In passive transfer processes, the membrane behaves as an inert lipoid-pore boundary and solutes traverse this barrier either by diffusing through the lipoprotein region or by filtering through the postulated aqueous pores (or channels). The rate of transmembrane movement of lipid-soluble compounds is directly proportional to the concentration gradient across the membrane and the lipid-to-water partition coefficient (i.e., lipid solubility) of the drug. Passive diffusion is characterized by the movement of drug molecules down a concentration gradient without cellular expenditure of energy.

Many drugs are weak organic acids or bases and exist in solution as both the nonionized and ionized forms. The nonionized molecules are usually lipid soluble and can readily diffuse across the cell membrane. In contrast, the ionized fraction is often unable to penetrate the lipoidal barrier because of its low degree of lipid solubility and is too large to pass through the aqueous channels. Passage of an organic electrolyte across a biological membrane is therefore dependent upon the pH of the environment and the dissociation constant of the drug, since according to the Henderson-Hasselbalch equation:

for an acid,

$$\mathrm{pH} - \mathrm{p}K_a = \log \frac{\text{(conc. of ionized acid)}}{\text{(conc. of nonionized acid)}} \quad (5.1)$$

and for a base,

$$\mathrm{pH} - \mathrm{p}K_a = \log \frac{\text{(conc. of nonionized base)}}{\text{(conc. of ionized base)}} \quad (5.2)$$

In these equations, the dissociation constant of both acids and bases is expressed as $\mathrm{p}K_a$, which is the negative logarithm of the acidic dissociation constant. From the equations it can be seen that, when the pH and $\mathrm{p}K_a$ values are equal, 50% of the drug is in either form. The majority of drugs used in medicine have $\mathrm{p}K_a$ values between 3 and 11 and exist accordingly in both nonionized and ionized forms within the range of physiological pH

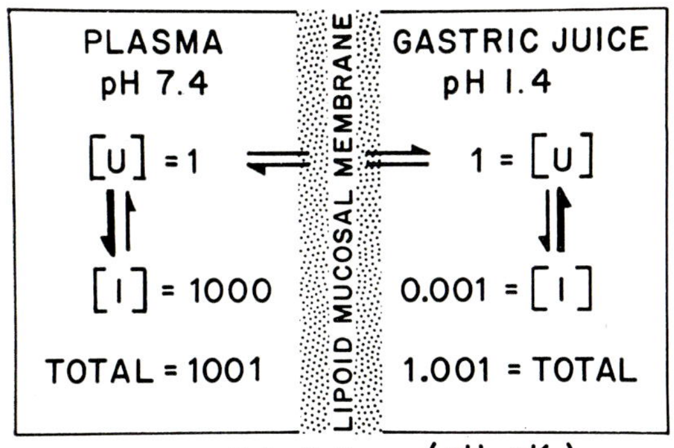

FIG. 5.2. The effect of the pH gradient on the distribution of a weak organic acid ($pK_a = 4.4$) between blood plasma ($pH = 7.4$) and gastric juice ($pH = 1.4$). In this figure, $[I]$ and $[U]$ represent the concentrations of the ionized and nonionized fractions of the drug, respectively.

values. The quaternary ammonium compounds are an exception and exist in biological fluids only in cationic form.

Equilibrium is achieved when the concentrations of nonionized drug are equal on both sides of the membrane. The rate of equilibration of the nonionized moiety is directly related to its lipid solubility. When a pH differential exists across the membrane, the concentrations (nonionized plus ionized) of drug on either side of the membrane are unequal; at equilibrium, there will be more total drug on the side where the degree of ionization is greater (Fig. 5.2). This mechanism is known as ion trapping. Acidic drugs (e.g., salicylates, sulfonamides, barbiturates) are found in higher concentrations in the more alkaline fluids. Basic drugs (e.g., narcotic analgesics, antihistamines, phenothiazines) accumulate in the more acidic fluids (including intracellular). Weak organic acids are rapidly absorbed from the stomachs of dogs and cats. Likewise, the acidic urinary reaction in carnivorous species promotes passive reabsorption of acidic drugs from the distal portion of the nephron. Weak bases, administered parenterally, diffuse into the rumen of cattle and sheep where they become trapped by ionization and exposed to the action of ruminal microorganisms. Studies of the penetration of chemotherapeutic agents from the systemic circulation into milk indicate that the mammary gland epithelium behaves as a lipoidal membrane that separates blood of pH 7.4 from milk of a somewhat lower pH value (normal range is 6.5–6.8). It has been shown that only the lipid-soluble, nonionized moiety of an organic electrolyte in the water phase of blood plasma diffuses into milk (Rasmussen 1966). Weak acids give milk ultrafiltrate-to-plasma ultrafiltrate concentration ratios of less than or equal to 1; weak bases, in general, attain concentration ratios ($R_{\text{milk/plasma}}$) of greater than or equal to 1 (Table 5.1). The choice of chemotherapeutic agent for systemic therapy of mastitis should be based both upon the susceptibility of the infecting microorganisms to the drug and its diffusibility into milk. At equilibrium, the theoretical concentration ratio of a drug ($R_{x/y}$) on opposite sides of a biological membrane may be calculated, on the basis of the degree of ionization of the drug, according to the following equations:

for an acid,

$$R_{x/y} = \frac{1 + 10^{(\text{pH}_x - \text{p}K_a)}}{1 + 10^{(\text{pH}_y - \text{p}K_a)}} \tag{5.3}$$

and for a base,

$$R_{x/y} = \frac{1 + 10^{(\text{p}K_a - \text{pH}_x)}}{1 + 10^{(\text{p}K_a - \text{pH}_y)}} \tag{5.4}$$

One should be aware that, while the "pH partition hypothesis" usually provides a good approximation of the distribution of a weak organic electrolyte between the water phase of blood plasma (or serum)

TABLE 5.1. Passage of chemotherapeutic agents from the systemic circulation into milk

Drug	pK_a	Milk pH	Concentration Ratio (milk ultr:plasma ultr) Theoretical	Experimental	Reference
Organic acids					
Benzyl penicillin (G)	2.7	6.8	0.20	0.13–0.26	Ziv et al. 1973
Cloxacillin	. . .	6.8	0.20	0.25–0.30	Ziv et al. 1973
Ampicillin	. . .	6.8	0.26	0.24–0.30	Ziv et al. 1973
Cephaloridine	3.4	6.8	0.25	0.24–0.28	Ziv et al. 1973
Sulfadimethoxine	6.0	6.6	0.19	0.23	Stowe and Sisodia 1963
Sulfamethazine	7.4	6.6	0.55	0.59	Rasmussen 1958
Organic bases					
Tylosin	7.1	6.8	3.0	3.5	Ziv and Sulman 1973a
Lincomycin	7.6	6.8	2.83	2.50–3.60	Ziv and Sulman 1973b
Trimethoprim	7.6	6.5–6.8	2.8–5.3	2.90–4.90	Rasmussen 1970
Erythromycin	8.8	6.8	. . .	8.7	Rasmussen 1959
Kanamycin	(7.8)	6.5–6.9	. . .	0.60–0.80	Ziv and Sulman 1974

Note: Individual references should be consulted for the design of each experiment. It is important to know the method of drug administration, because after a single intravenous injection equilibrium will never be established.

and another biological fluid, it cannot be considered so seriously as to postulate that biological barriers are generally impermeable to ions and to attribute observed deviations from its predictions to thermodynamically untenable mechanisms that invoke a virtual pH (Smolen 1973). In many instances, equilibrium is not achieved, either because the drug diffuses from a small volume into a much larger volume or because the drug is rapidly removed by elimination; the diffusion process is then unidirectional.

Specialized transport processes appear to be responsible for the rapid cellular transfer of certain foreign organic ions and polar molecules as well as many natural substrates such as sugars, amino acids, and pyrimidines. Specialized transport is generally thought to be mediated by carriers, i.e., membrane components that form a reversible complex with the substance to be transported. Two types of carrier-mediated transport can be distinguished, namely, facilitated diffusion and active transport (Wilbrandt and Rosenberg 1961; Stein 1967). Specialized transport processes differ from passive transfer in that the former exhibits relative selectivity and saturability, and active transport requires the direct expenditure of energy. Competitive inhibition is characteristic of carrier-mediated transport. Facilitated diffusion is responsible for the rapid transfer of glucose and amino acids across membranes of various cells. Active transport processes are involved in renal and biliary excretion of certain unchanged drug molecules as well as polar metabolites of the majority of drugs, in the removal of some drugs from the CNS at the choroid plexus and ciliary body and, to a lesser extent, in the intestinal absorption of compounds structurally related to normal dietary constituents.

Pinocytosis is a transport mechanism also requiring an expenditure of cellular energy. It differs from active transport in that the transfer of the solute is not mediated by combination with a carrier but by the local invagination of the cell membrane and subsequent budding off of a vesicle containing the solute (Lewis 1931; Fawcett 1965). The capacity of the newborn calf to absorb soluble protein molecules from colostrum is attributed to pinocytosis. Pinocytotic activity may be responsible for transcapillary passage of macromolecules and uptake of solutes by pulmonary alveolar epithelial cells.

Water and small-sized lipid insoluble molecules may traverse aqueous channels, but ultrafiltration and bulk flow are important processes for the translocation of drugs only at sites where the plasma membrane has been specially modified to accommodate these processes (e.g., renal glomerulus, arachnoid villi).

Cell membrane permeability of various tissues is influenced quite selectively by certain hormones. For example, the cells of the distal and collecting tubules of the nephron respond to vasopressin (antidiuretic hormone, ADH) by a great increase in permeability to water, probably the result of an increase in diameter of the aqueous channels.

Membrane Potentials

Cell membranes are electrically polarized; a potential difference exists across the membrane of most living cells, which is due to the relative distribution of the intracellular and extracellular ions. The extracellur fluid is particularly rich in sodium and relatively low in potassium. Inside the cell, the cytoplasm is relatively high in potassium content and very low in sodium. While the cell membrane permits potassium ions to diffuse freely in either direction, it appears to resist the movement of sodium ions from the extracellular fluid to the inside of the cell. With radioisotope experiments it has been established that a certain amount of sodium leaks into the resting cell from outside. An active transport process, colloquially known as the "sodium pump," continuously maintains the low intracellular sodium concentration. This pump mechanism ejects sodium from the inside of the cell against the high concentration and electrical gradients attracting it to within. However, the pump does not handle sodium exclusively but requires the presence of extracellular potassium, so that when a sodium ion is ejected from the cell, a potassium ion is incorporated into the cell. The pump is dependent upon metabolic energy and can be blocked by several metabolic poisons such as dinitrophenol and the rapidly acting cardiac glycoside, ouabain. The excitability of nerve cells arises from the unique ability of their membranes to become depolarized quite suddenly by the inrush of sodium ions. Local anesthetics appear to act by blocking activation of the sodium conductance preventing depolarization.

ABSORPTION OF DRUGS

The purpose of drug administration is to obtain a desired clinical response that will most likely be produced by establishing and maintaining, for a certain time, an effective concentration of drug at its site of action. To act and produce effects, unless it acts topically at the site of application, a drug must be absorbed into the blood. Drug absorption is governed by the route of administration, the dosage form, and certain physicochemical properties of the drug. Administration of a drug by any route other than directly into the bloodstream (i.e., intravenous injection) presents a potential bioavailability problem.

Bioavailability is a term used to indicate the rate and relative amount of the administered drug reaching the general (or systemic) circulation intact. In the context of this definition, general circulation refers primarily to venous blood (excepting the hepatic portal blood during the absorptive phase) and arterial blood carrying the drug to the tissues. The systemic availability of a drug contained in a drug product is determined relative to a reference dosage form, which may be a single intravenous injection of an equivalent dose of the same drug. Bioavailability is the first of many factors that determine the relation between drug dosage and intensity of action. There is often marked individual variation in the rate of drug absorption, and slow or incomplete absorption is probably a common but rarely recognized cause of therapeutic failure in clinical practice.

Absorption from the Alimentary Canal

While the entire length of the alimentary canal has absorptive capacity, the stomach and small intestine are the most important sites of absorption of drugs and nutrients excluding water. The gastrointestinal mucosa has the properties of a lipoidal barrier endowed with aqueous pores and has, in addition, a large number of enzyme or carrier systems responsible for the transport of water-soluble nutrient molecules. The theory of nonionic diffusion, also known as the "pH partition hypothesis" (Jacobs 1940) states that the absorption of drugs from the alimentary canal can be explained by passive diffusion of the nonionized, lipid-soluble molecules across a lipid membrane. The physicochemical properties of each drug determine the extent and principal site of absorption (Brodie and Hogben 1957). Low degree of ionization and high lipid-to-water partition coefficient of the nonionized form of organic electrolytes, and small atomic or molecular radius of water-soluble substances, are properties favorable for rapid absorption. Polar molecules, whether neutral (mannitol) or ionized (aminoglycoside antibiotics), are either absorbed poorly or not at all, unless they are sufficiently small to pass through the pores of the membrane (urea). Certain quaternary amines may be absorbed in part in the form of chemical complexes (Levine and Pelikan 1964). Ionic iron is absorbed as an amino acid complex, at a rate usually determined by the body's need for iron (Bothwell 1968). Sodium ion is probably transported actively across the intestinal wall. Magnesium ion is very poorly absorbed and, when administered orally as a salt (e.g., magnesium sulfate), will act as a cathartic, retaining an osmotic equivalent of water as it passes along the intestinal tract. Sulfate ion is also very slowly absorbed; sodium sulfate solution, given by stomach tube, is the saline purgative of choice for the horse (Alexander 1969).

Passive diffusion is the most important mechanism of absorption and depends essentially on the movement of the drug across the mucosa to the circulation down a concentration gradient. Absorption of a drug from the gastrointestinal tract involves release of the drug from its dosage form, unless the latter is a solution, and access to and transfer across the mucosal barrier into the hepatic portal venous blood. The term "dosage form" includes the chemical nature (salt or simple derivative), physical state (amorphous or crystalline, solvated or nonsolvated, etc.), and the particle size distribution and surface area of the drug itself in the dosage form. Drug release from a tablet involves both disintegration and dissolution. When drugs are administered as tablets, suspensions, or in capsules, release from the dosage form, reflected by the rate at which the drug dissolves in gastrointestinal fluids, is frequently rate limiting in the overall absorption process and may determine the rate and extent of absorption (Levy 1968). Occasionally the dissolution rate of sparingly soluble drugs is so protracted that dissolution controls not only the absorption process but also the overall rate of elimination of the drug from the body; the drug may be present in blood for a prolonged period after a single dose. Dissolution may be enhanced by using the salt form of a drug (e.g., potassium phenoxymethyl penicillin, diphenylhydantoin sodium, morphine sulfate, promazine hydrochloride) or by decreasing the particle size (e.g., spironolactone, griseofulvin), thereby increasing bioavailability of the therapeutic agent. Absorption of a drug from a suspension is usually more rapid than from a tablet. A drug in solution will probably be well absorbed if it is lipid soluble, not completely ionized, and stable (i.e., neither chemically nor enzymically inactivated) in the gastrointestinal contents. Penicillin G and erythromycin are unstable in the acidic contents of the stomach; chloramphenicol is inactivated by ruminal microorganisms. Antibacterial drugs that are not inactivated and have low systemic availability when administered orally may be used in treatment of enteric infections and for preoperative sterilization of the gut. Aminoglycoside antibiotics (e.g., streptomycin, kanamycin) and succinylsulfathiazole, a pro-drug that is hydrolyzed by microorganisms in the large intestine to sulfathiazole, are poorly absorbed when given by mouth.

The presence of food in the stomach can impair the absorption of drugs given by the oral route. Because the absorptive capacity of the small intestine is much greater than that of the stomach, gastric emptying time is a critical determinant of the overall absorption rate of drugs, particularly when the drugs are in solution (Hunt and Knox 1968). Information on the steady-state distribution of drugs indicates that the reaction of intestinal contents (pH 6.6) might not be the same as the effective pH at the site of absorption. An effective pH of 5.3 in the microenvironment of the absorbing surface of the intestinal epithelial barrier appears to determine the degree of ionization and extent of absorption of organic electrolytes. Detailed studies with a large number of drugs in unbuffered solutions revealed that in the normal intestine acids with a pK_a above 3 and bases with a pK_a less than 7.8 were very well absorbed; outside these limits the absorption of acids and bases, respectively, fell off rapidly (Hogben et al. 1959). While most drugs and other foreign compounds appear to cross the intestinal barrier by simple diffusion, there is evidence that a drug can be absorbed by a specialized transport process if its chemical structure closely resembles a nutrient that is actively absorbed.

During the process of absorption, drug molecules are exposed to enzymes in the intestinal mucosa, and molecules absorbed from the stomach and small intestine are conveyed to the liver, which is the principal site of drug biotransformation, before they are distributed throughout the body. Biotransformation by enzymes in the gut mucosa and/or liver may significantly reduce bioavailability of an orally administered drug, particularly if the drug is extensively metabolized, e.g., lidocaine (Boyes et al. 1970). The effect of biotransformation preceding entry into the general circulation (first-pass effect) would be similar to, and could be misinterpreted as, incomplete absorption. The amount of drug lost depends on the rate of absorption, the hepatic extraction ratio, and the portal blood flow. The quantitative assessment of availability from a given drug product can be determined by comparing the total area under the plasma or serum concentration of the drug versus the time curve after giving the drug orally with the area obtained following intravenous administration of an equivalent dose of the same drug. The area is measured by an appropriate numerical integration procedure and is expressed as the product of concentration and time (i.e., mg/L $\times$ hours). For best correlation of the area under the curve with completeness of absorption, plasma drug concentrations must be determined over a period that is many times longer than the usual absorption half-time of the drug. Since a formulation that releases a drug slowly over an extended time could have the same quantitative availability as a formulation with a more rapid rate of absorption, it is important to consider both extent and rate of absorption as criteria for assessing therapeutic equivalency. Drug solutions injected intraperitoneally (i.p.) are absorbed primarily into the portal venous circulation and, therefore, pass through the liver before entering the general circulation (Lukas et al. 1971).

Comparative Aspects of Drug Absorption

The domestic animals may be divided, on the basis of dietary habit, into herbivorous (horse, ox, sheep, and goat), omnivorous (pig), and carnivorous (dog and cat) species. The physiology of digestion and drug absorption processes are, in general, similar in the dog, cat, and pig and are not unlike those in human beings. The gastric juice is highly acid (pH 1–2) in these species, whereas the intestinal contents are nearly neutral, actually slightly acid, in reaction. The stomach is a significant site of absorption for many acidic and neutral compounds. Only the weakest bases ($pK_a < 1.5$, e.g., caffeine) are absorbed to any appreciable extent at normal gastric pH values. Because of its extensive surface area and rich blood supply, the upper small intestine is the major site of absorption for all drugs. The rate of gastric emptying therefore markedly influences the rate at which drugs are absorbed, regardless of whether they are weak acids, weak bases, or neutral compounds (Levine 1970). Buccal absorption of drugs has not been investigated and is probably insignificant in domestic animals, at least in monogastric species. It is difficult to appreciate the functions of the stomach of the adult horse. Under normal conditions of feeding, this organ is never empty and the reaction has been observed to vary from pH 1.13 to 6.8 (Schwarz et al. 1926). Evidence exists that substantial amounts of lactic acid are produced in the stomach as a result of bacterial fermentation and most of this acid appears to be absorbed in the small intestine, thus contributing to the nutrition of the horse (Alexander 1972). Another distinguishing feature of the equine digestive tract is the adaptation of the large intestine for microbial digestion of polysaccharides.

The anatomical structure of the anterior portion of the alimentary canal characterizes the ruminant animal. The rumen, reticulum, and omasum, collectively called the forestomachs, are lined with a stratified squamous epithelium, keratinized in its outer layer. The approximate capacities of the adult reticulorumen are 100–225 L in cattle and 6–20 L in sheep and goats. Ruminal contents are of a semisolid consistency and have an acidic reaction, pH 5.5–6.5 (Annison and Lewis 1959). Despite the stratified squamous nature of its epithelial lining, the rumen has been shown to have considerable absorptive capacity (Phillipson and McAnally 1942; Danielli et al. 1945; Gray 1948; Masson and Phillipson 1951; Sperber and Hyden 1952). The principal feature of digestive physiology in the ruminant is that fermentative digestion occurs on a massive scale in the first two parts of the stomach. The ruminal microflora may inactivate certain drugs by metabolic transformations of a hydrolytic or reductive nature. Drugs administered by the oral route enter ruminal fluid, and weak organic electrolytes in the water phase of blood plasma may diffuse into the rumen. Nonionic diffusion and subsequent trapping by ionization in ruminal fluid is an important aspect of drug distribution in ruminant animals. Further, organic acids in particular may enter the rumen by way of alkaline saliva (pH 8.0–8.4). The flow of mixed saliva for cows fed in different ways was estimated to be 98–190 L during 24 hours (Bailey 1961). The mucosa of the abomasum has similar histological features to those of the stomach in the monogastric animal; the abomasum is the only part of the ruminant stomach that secretes digestive juices. The reaction of abomasal contents does not vary much and usually remains close to pH 3 (Masson and Phillipson 1952).

For the purposes of most bioavailability studies it is sufficient to determine three indices: the maximum plasma drug concentration (peak of plasma concentration-time curve), the time of maximum drug concentration, and the area under the plasma drug concentration-time curve (Fig. 5.3). The time at which the plasma drug concentration reaches its maximum is closely related to the rate of drug absorption. The peak plasma level increases with both the completeness and the rate of absorption. The area under the plasma concentration-time curve is useful as a measure of occupancy, the time during which a given volume of plasma is occupied by a drug, which is the antithesis of plasma clearance (Orr et al. 1969). Variation among species in absorption of chloramphenicol was observed after oral administration of the drug (Davis et al. 1972). Maximum (peak) concentrations of chloramphenicol in plasma were attained at 2 hours in dogs and swine and at 3 hours in ponies and cats (Fig. 5.4). Systemic availability of chloramphenicol from the proprietary product, i.e., chloromycetin capsules, was highest in cats. Chloramphenicol was not detectable in the plasma of goats and sheep after oral and intraruminal administration of the drug, respectively. Theodorides et al. (1968)

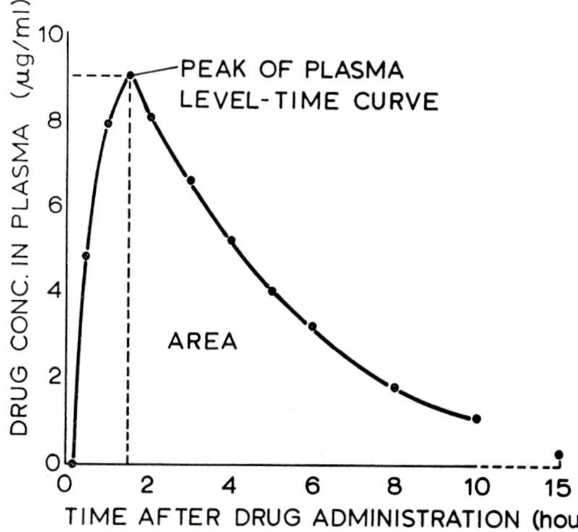

FIG. 5.3. Drug concentration in plasma versus time curve after oral administration of a single dose of a hypothetical drug. The plasma drug concentration reached a maximum level (9 µg/ml) at 1.5 hours after administration.

showed that the drug was rapidly degraded to bacterially inactive products by the strong reducing environment in the rumen of sheep. In a comparative study of salicylate absorption (Davis and Westfall 1972), peak concentrations of salicylate in plasma were highest in swine and dogs and considerably lower in the herbivorous animals (ponies and goats). The limited data on systemic availability of orally administered drug products suggest that absorption is fast and relatively complete in the dog, cat, and pig; highly variable in the equine species; and slow in ruminant animals. Absorption is usually more rapid than elimination in monogastric species but may control the rate of elimination and prolong the action of some drugs in ruminant species. In any species, individual variation in response to a given dose of a drug is likely to be more marked when the route of administration is oral rather than parenteral.

PARENTERAL ADMINISTRATION OF DRUGS

Parenteral administration implies that the gastrointestinal tract is bypassed. Parenteral routes include intravenous (i.v.), intramuscular (i.m.), and subcutaneous (s.c.) injections when a systemic effect is desired, and tissue infiltration, intra-articular, or epidural injection when a localized action is sought. Parenteral therapy necessitates that strict asepsis be maintained. Some drugs may be inhaled as gases (e.g., gaseous and volatile liquid anesthetics) and enter the general circulation by diffusing across the alveolar membranes. Topical application and intramammary infusion are routes of drug ad-

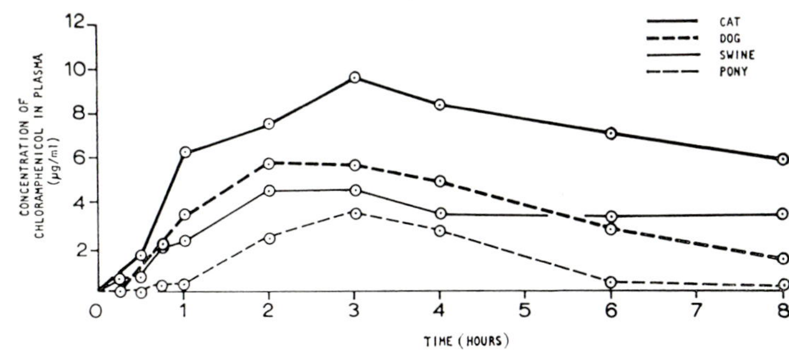

FIG. 5.4. Serum concentrations of chloramphenicol in domestic animals after oral administration of chloramphenicol capsules (22 mg/kg). The drug was undetectable in serum of goats. Each point represents the mean drug concentration determined in 4 cats or dogs, and 8 swine, ponies, or goats. (Reproduced from Am J Vet Res 33 (Nov. 1972):2259, with permission of the editor.)

ministration employed when local effects are sought; a variable degree of absorption, which depends on physicochemical properties of drug and vehicle, takes place from these sites of application.

Intravenous Injection

Injection of a drug directly into the bloodstream gives a predictable concentration of the drug in plasma and produces an extremely rapid pharmacological response. Another advantage of the intravascular route is control over the rate of introduction of a drug into the general circulation. Intravenous infusion is a satisfactory method of maintaining therapeutic plasma concentrations of drugs that have short (biological) half-lives and relatively narrow margins of safety. While the intravenous route has many advantages, it is potentially the most dangerous route of drug administration and great care must be exercised in computing the total dose to be administered and with the rate of injection. A drug should never be introduced directly into the bloodstream unless specifically indicated. Complete bioavailability of a drug is assured only when the intravascular route of administration is employed.

Absorption from Intramuscular and Subcutaneous Sites

Intramuscular and subcutaneous administration of drugs can result in absorption rates very different from those after oral administration. The absorption rate of drugs from aqueous solutions depends mainly on the vascularity of the injection site, the degree of ionization and lipid solubility of the drug, and the area over which the injected solution has spread (Schou 1961; Sund and Schou 1964). Absorption of most drugs from aqueous solutions injected intramuscularly or subcutaneously is relatively rapid; the peak concentration in serum is usually reached within 30 minutes. A drug may affect its own rate of absorption and uptake of another drug administered simultaneously if it alters the blood supply or capillary permeability at the site of absorption. Addition of epinephrine, 1 part in 200,000 (Scott et al. 1972), or other vasoconstrictor (e.g., vasopressin) to a solution of local anesthetic (e.g., procaine) will extend the duration of local analgesia beyond that produced by the anesthetic alone. It has generally been assumed that drugs injected intramuscularly and subcutaneously are completely bioavailable. This assumption has been found invalid for intramuscularly administered diazepam (Gamble et al. 1973), digoxin (Greenblatt et al. 1973), and diphenylhydantoin (Wilkensky and Lowden 1973). Drugs that are insoluble at tissue pH, or that are in an oily vehicle, form a depot in the muscle tissue, from which absorption proceeds very slowly. Certain drug solutions cause severe pain when injected subcutaneously, owing to a pH reaction outside that within the physiological range of values. These irritant solutions may be administered by slow intravenous injection.

DRUG DISPOSITION

Drug disposition is a term used to describe the simultaneous effects of distribution and elimination. After intravenous injection, drug levels in plasma are initially high and rapidly decline biphasically or, in some cases, polyphasically. The early phases are associated mainly with distribution of the drug into tissues, and the last phase is associated with elimination of the drug after the distribution phases have been completed. Pharmacokinetics is defined as the mathematical description of concentration changes of drugs within the organism. Plasma concentration-time curves are important largely because they provide the only relevant information that can be measured for most drugs.

Distribution of Drugs

For an active drug molecule to be therapeutically effective it must reach the site of its intended pharmacological activity within the body at a sufficient rate and in sufficient amounts so that an effective concentration can be achieved. After a drug is injected or absorbed into the blood there are various cellular barriers that must be traversed before it reaches its site of action. The distribution of a drug is influenced by blood flow to tissues, the propensity of the drug for binding to plasma albumin and tissue proteins, and physicochemical properties governing diffusion, such as degree of ionization and lipid solubility of organic electrolytes. Differences in perfusion may account for variation in the rate of equilibration of drug concentrations in different tissues. In the kidney, liver, heart, and brain, which are richly perfused, equilibrium is established rapidly if the drug readily crosses membranes. Drugs enter muscle and viscera more slowly than they enter the very highly perfused organs; however, because of their considerable mass, these tissues can significantly affect overall distribution of the drug. Fat-soluble compounds partition slowly into the poorly perfused adipose tissue. In time, however, substantial amounts of lipophilic drugs (e.g., DDT, the thiobarbiturates) can accumulate in body fat, which then acts as a reservoir for the drug. The amount of any drug in the tissues where it acts is usually a very small fraction of the bioavailable dose. Most of the drug remains in various body fluids in solution, or is localized in tissues other than the site of action. At some time after drug administration, an apparent distribution equilibrium is attained between the tissue compartment and the plasma. Thereafter, it is assumed that the drug is removed from the tissues containing the receptor sites and cleared from the plasma in a parallel fashion.

Pharmacokinetic Concepts

The purpose of pharmacokinetics is to study the time courses of drug and metabolite concentrations and amounts in various body fluids, tissues, and excreta, and thereby develop mathematical models to describe and interpret absorption, distribution, biotransformation, and excretion processes (Wagner 1968a). A common approach to studying the pharmacokinetic behavior of drugs is to depict the body as a system of compartments. In many instances these compartments, which are mathematical entities, have no physiological meaning but are useful in describing the disposition kinetics of a drug.

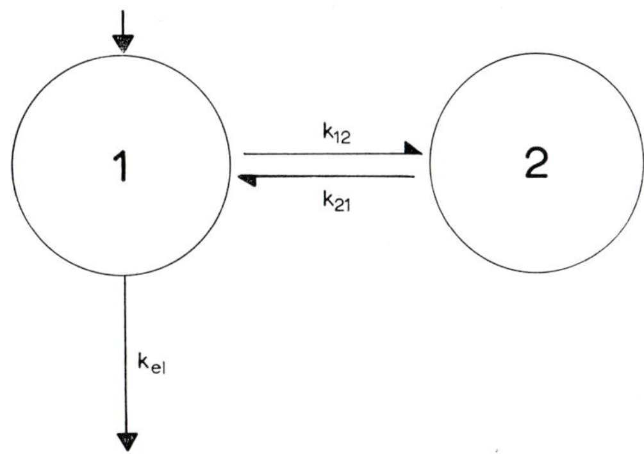

Fig. 5.5. When a drug is introduced into the bloodstream, it distributes between *(1)* the central and (2) the peripheral compartments. The individual rate constants k_{12} and k_{21} reflect the rate of distribution into and out of the peripheral compartment; k_{el} reflects the rate of drug elimination from the central compartment. Elimination (i.e., biotransformation and excretion) takes place exclusively from the central compartment.

A single model (Fig. 5.5) can be used to represent both one- and two-compartment systems. A one-compartment system is arbitrarily defined as one in which the drug entering the body is distributed instantaneously into the available space. The one-compartment model is particularly useful for describing the time course of most drugs in the plasma (or urine) after oral or intramuscular administration. However, it may or may not adequately describe the time course of a drug in the body after intravenous administration. The adequacy of the model depends upon the rate of attainment of apparent distribution equilibrium. When distribution between the central and peripheral compartments is slow relative to elimination, Fig. 5.5 represents a two-compartment model. The two-compartment open model accurately describes the pharmacokinetics of most drugs after intravenous administration. The model assumes that a drug entering the body distributes instantaneously and homogeneously into a space termed the central compartment, which consists of the blood and other readily accessible tissues and fluids. Distribution into the rest of the available body space, or peripheral compartment, is somewhat slower. The term "central compartment" can be frequently applied to such physiological systems as the extracellular fluid, which consists of the circulating blood plasma and interstitial fluid, and well-perfused organs such as the kidney and liver. The peripheral or tissue compartment may be considered to consist of less perfused organs and tissues such as muscle and fat. The distribution and elimination processes associated with the model are assumed to follow first-order kinetics, where the rate of a given process is proportional to the amount or concentration of the drug. An important feature of the model is that drug elimination (i.e., biotransformation and excretion) is assumed to take place exclusively from the central compartment.

A biexponential expression frequently describes the drug concentration in plasma versus time profile after intravenous administration of a drug. The concentration of a drug in the plasma (C_p) as a function of time (t) is given by the equation

$$C_p = Ae^{-\alpha t} + Be^{-\beta t} \qquad (5.5)$$

where A and B are the zero-time plasma concentration intercepts, and α and β are the distribution and elimination rate constants, respectively, and their values are related to the slopes of the drug disposition curve. The above mathematical expression may be described graphically by a semilogarithmic plot of drug concentration in plasma versus time (Fig. 5.6). The linear portion of the curve has a slope that may be defined as $-\beta/2.303$ and an extrapolated zero-time intercept of B (in units of concentration). Resolving the curve into its two components by the method of residuals yields a second linear

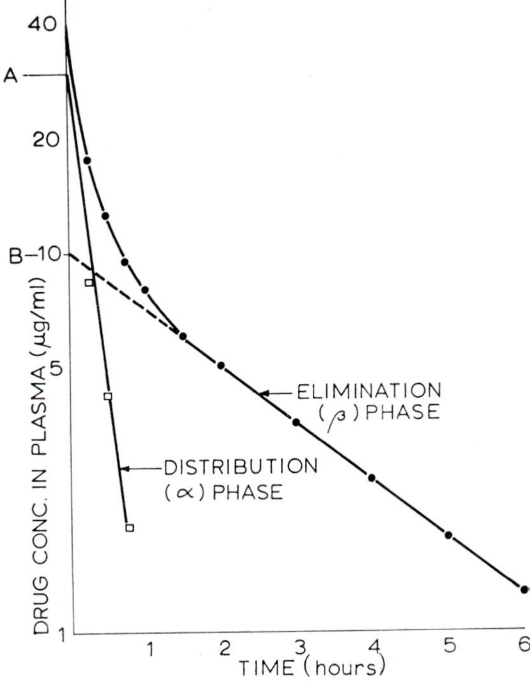

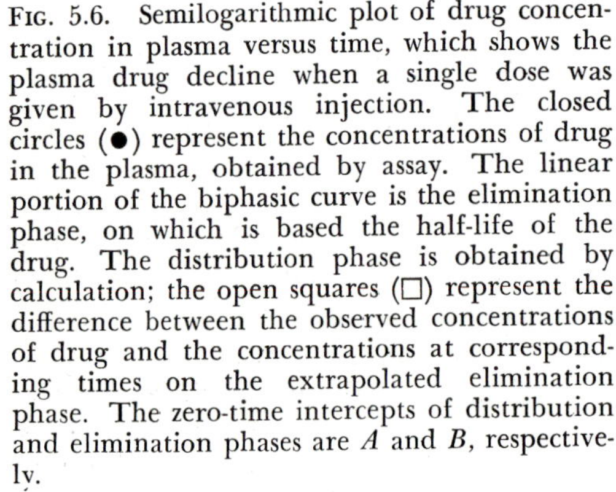

FIG. 5.6. Semilogarithmic plot of drug concentration in plasma versus time, which shows the plasma drug decline when a single dose was given by intravenous injection. The closed circles (●) represent the concentrations of drug in the plasma, obtained by assay. The linear portion of the biphasic curve is the elimination phase, on which is based the half-life of the drug. The distribution phase is obtained by calculation; the open squares (□) represent the difference between the observed concentrations of drug and the concentrations at corresponding times on the extrapolated elimination phase. The zero-time intercepts of distribution and elimination phases are A and B, respectively.

segment with a slope of $-\alpha/2.303$ and a zero-time intercept of A (Gibaldi et al. 1969). If the ordinate of the semilogarithmic plot is in natural logarithms, the slopes are simply $-\alpha$ and $-\beta$. Accordingly, it is a simple procedure to obtain values for A, B, α, and β from a semilogarithmic plot of C_p versus time; these terms, however, are hybrid parameters and mathematically complex (Nelson 1961; Notari 1971).

While a biexponential expression accurately describes the plasma concentration-time course of most drugs after their intravenous injection, a monoexponential expression may adequately approximate disappearance of some drugs from plasma. If the rate of drug equilibration between the central and peripheral compartments is very rapid relative to the rate of elimination (i.e., $k_{12} + k_{21} >> k_{e1}$), the drug concentration in plasma as a function of time may be described mathematically by

$$C_p = Be^{-\beta t} \tag{5.6}$$

where B is the extrapolated zero-time intercept of the monoexponential curve and β is the apparent overall elimination rate constant. The value of B is an estimate of the initial drug concentration in plasma based on instantaneous attainment of distribution equilibrium. The relationship described by Equation 5.6 also applies to the decline in plasma drug levels with time for the postabsorptive phase after oral or intramuscular administration.

Of prime importance in determining the duration of drug action in the body is the (biological) half-life of the drug. The (biological) half-life, $t_{1/2}$, may be defined as the time required for the body to eliminate one-half the drug that it contains. The half-life value of a drug may be calculated from the expression:

$$t_{1/2} = \frac{0.693}{\beta} \tag{5.7}$$

where β represents the negative value of the slope of the first-order curve for a one-compartment model or the slope of the terminal portion of the curve for a two-compartment model. It is assumed that the ratio of drug in the peripheral to central compartments remains constant during the elimination phase. Iterative least squares regression methods should be used to find the terminal exponential portion of the drug plasma concentration-time profile, as it may be difficult to be sure when distribution equilibrium has been reached. Drug elimination may involve several processes, which include various metabolic pathways and routes of excretion, operating in parallel. Overall elimination of the majority of drugs in human beings and domestic animals obeys first-order kinetics. The half-life of a first-order process is independent of the route of administration and the dose. This means that doubling the dose does not double the duration of action of a drug but increases it only by one biological half-life. When a zero-order process is involved in the elimination of a drug, e.g., phenylbutazone in the horse (Piperno et al. 1968) and dog (Dayton et al. 1967) and salicylate in the cat (Yeary and Swanson 1973), the time to eliminate 50% of the drug becomes progressively longer as the dose increases. Significant differences in half-life values of several drugs, in particular those extensively metabolized, have been found among the species of domestic animals (Table 5.2).

An estimate of the half-life value of a drug may be obtained graphically from a semilogarithmic plot of drug concentration in plasma versus time after intravenous administration of the drug (Fig. 5.7). The half-life is found by measuring the time required for a given plasma level of drug to decline by one-half during the terminal exponential (β-) phase of the curve. Knowledge of the half-life of a drug can be extremely useful in a predictive sense, particularly with respect to the design of rational dosage regimens. Assuming first-order kinetics, the fraction of the original amount of drug remaining in the body is easily estimated from the (bio-

TABLE 5.2. The half-life values (in hours) of drugs eliminated mainly by metabolism

Drug	Pony	Cow (Goat)	Pig	Dog	Cat	Reference
Salicylate	1.0	0.54* (0.78)	5.9	8.6	37.6†	Davis and Westfall 1972
Chloramphenicol	0.9	(2.0)	1.3	4.2	5.1	Davis et al. 1972
Trimethoprim	3.8‡	(0.5)§	2.0§	3.0‖	. . .	
Sulfadimethoxine	11.3#	12.5**	15.5††	13.2*	10.2*	
Amphetamine	1.4	(0.6)	1.1	4.5	6.5	Baggot and Davis 1973a
Quinidine	4.4	(0.85)	5.4	5.6	1.9	Neff et al 1972

* Baggot 1975.
† Half-life of salicylate in the cat is dose-dependent.
‡ Alexander and Collett 1974b.
§ Nielsen and Rasmussen 1972.
‖ Kaplan et al. 1970.
\# Tschudi 1972.
** Boxenbaum 1974.
†† Tschudi 1973.

logical) half-life (Table 5.3). Considerably more information can be obtained from a nomogram for graphical determination of the time necessary to eliminate a certain percentage of a drug, knowing either the overall elimination rate constant or the (biological) half-life of the drug (Wagner 1968b).

Within any species of animal many factors can alter the half-life value of a given drug, e.g., age of animal, impaired liver or renal function, interaction with (or influence of) another drug, and dose administered if overall elimination is zero-order (i.e., constant rate). Some important types of drug interaction are interference with carrier-mediated transport mechanisms, displacement from binding sites on plasma proteins, and stimulation or depression of hepatic microsomal drug-

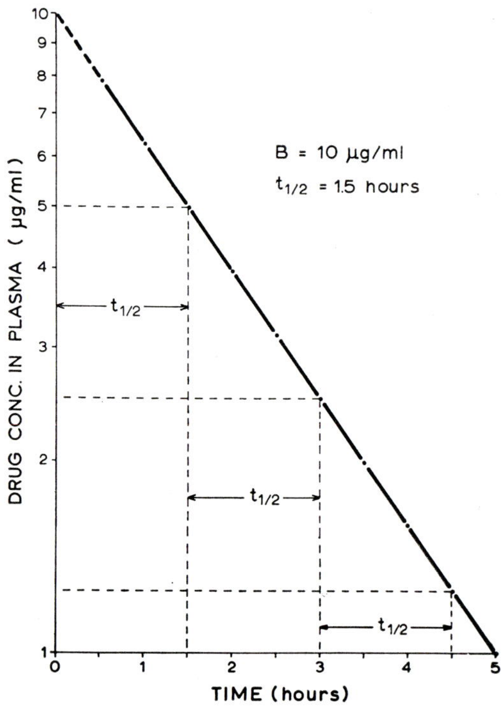

FIG. 5.7. Semilogarithmic plot of drug concentration in plasma versus time. The monoexponential drug decline (solid line) shown in this figure represents first-order elimination. The half-life value (i.e., half-time of elimination) is constant (1.5 hours) and independent of the plasma-drug concentration. The value of B(10 μg/ml) is the zero-time intercept of the extrapolated "elimination" phase of drug decline in plasma.

TABLE 5.3. Estimation of fraction of drug remaining in the body from the biological half-life, assuming first-order kinetics

Portion of Original Amount Remaining:		Cumulation of
Fraction	Percent	Half-Life
1/2	50	1
1/4	25	2
1/8	12.5	3
1/16	6.25	4
1/32	3.125	5
1/64	1.5625	6
1/256	0.3906	8
1/1024	0.097	10

metabolizing enzyme systems. Alteration of the urinary pH reaction will influence the overall rate of elimination of organic acids and bases whose pK_a values lie within certain ranges, provided renal excretion constitutes a major mechanism of their elimination. The urinary pH may be appropriately adjusted to favor ionization of the weak organic electrolyte and, thereby, inhibit reabsorption from distal tubular urine.

Another useful pharmacokinetic parameter is the apparent volume of distribution of the drug. It can be defined as that volume of fluid required to contain the amount of drug in the body if it were uniformly distributed at a concentration equal to that in the plasma. The assumption is made that the body acts as a single homogeneous compartment with respect to the drug. The apparent volume of distribution, V_d, does not represent an actual volume but serves as a proportionality constant relating the concentration of drug in plasma at any time after distribution equilibrium has been attained to the amount present in the body, i.e.,

$$C_p \cdot V_d = A_{B(t)} \tag{5.8}$$

where C_p and A_B are the plasma concentration and amount of drug in the body, respectively, at time t. The apparent volume of distribution parameter is frequently obtained from the terminal exponential (elimination) phase of drug decline in plasma after intravenous injection of a known amount of the drug. Extrapolation of the straight line in Fig. 5.7 to time zero gives the initial concentration of drug in the plasma (B), assuming instantaneous distribution. A value of V_d can be calculated from the expression:

$$V_d\ (\text{L}) = \frac{\text{Dose (mg)}}{B\ (\text{mg/L})} \tag{5.9}$$

The extrapolation method provides an estimate of the apparent volume of distribution by neglecting the distributive or α-phase of drug disposition. This method of calculating V_d should be used only for drugs injected intravenously and whose disposition kinetics can be adequately described by a one-compartment open model. The kinetics of drugs that are extensively metabolized or excreted during the distribution phase are best represented by the two-compartment open model. The volume of distribution obtained by the extrapolation method overestimates the value of V_d for these drugs. The area equation provides a more satisfactory method of calculating the volume of distribution parameter:

$$V_{d(\text{area})} = \frac{\text{Dose}}{(\text{Area}) \cdot \beta} \tag{5.10}$$

where (Area) is the total area under the linear drug concentration in plasma versus time curve from $t = 0$ to $t = \infty$, in units of mg • min/L. This equation may be employed to calculate V_d after administration of a drug by any route, provided the dose is completely available systemically.

In general, many acidic drugs, including sulfonamides, phenylbutazone, salicylates, and penicillins, are highly protein bound or too hydrophilic to diffuse across cell membranes and enter cellular water and adipose tissue in significant amounts. These drugs have low volumes of distribution, approximately 0.2–0.4 L/kg of body weight in monogastric animals. Basic drugs (e.g., narcotic analgesics, amphetamine, quinidine, lidocaine, chloramphenicol) are widely distributed. Plasma concentrations of bases are usually low, and the volumes of distribution exceed the volume of the total body fluids. Organic bases may have particularly large apparent volumes of distribution in ruminant animals, as these drugs diffuse into the rumen and become trapped by ionization in ruminal liquor.

The clearance of a drug is defined as the volume of blood plasma cleared of drug by metabolism and excretion per unit time. By definition, this is also the number of ml of V_d cleared per unit time and therefore equal to $\beta \cdot V_d$. Appropriately, $\beta \cdot V_d$ is termed the (total) body clearance:

$$Cl_B = \beta \cdot V_d \qquad (5.11)$$

The half-life and body clearance of pentobarbital in the pony can be calculated from values of the overall elimination rate constant ($\beta = 0.46$ hour^{-1}) and the apparent specific volume of distribution ($V^1_d = 0.8$ L/kg) in the following manner:

$$t_{1/2} = \frac{0.693}{0.46} = 1.5 \text{ hours},$$
$$Cl_B = 0.46 \times 0.8 = 0.368 \text{ L/kg/hour.}$$

The clearance of certain substances can be used to quantitatively assess renal function (inulin, para-aminohippurate [PAH]) or hepatic function (bromsulphthalein). Renal clearance values of inulin, creatinine, and either para-aminohippurate or Diodrast in normal adult animals of different species are tabulated (Table 5.4). From a pharmacological viewpoint, the much lower value of the renal clearance of inulin in the horse and cow as compared with that in the dog is the most important feature of the species variation in renal function. For clinical evaluation of renal function, body clearances of ^{125}I-iothalamate (Glofil-125) and ^{131}I-iodohippurate (Hipputope), which are indices of glomerular filtration rate (GFR) and effective renal plasma flow (ERPF), respectively, are easily performed and are satisfactory. The clearance values of these radioisotopes can be obtained by giving a single intravenous injection, calculating the slopes (β) and intercept values (B) from the monoexponential curves that describe their elimination from the blood plasma, and substituting the values of β and V_d in the equation. Using this technique, renal function was measured in Beagle dogs (Table 5.5).

TABLE 5.4. Renal clearance values in adult animals of different species

Animal	Substance Cleared	Clearance Value (ml/kg/min)	Reference
Horse	Inulin	1.66 (1.00–2.32)	Knudsen 1959
	Creatinine	1.46 (1.02–1.90)	
	Diodrast	6.91 (5.29–8.53)	
Cow	Inulin	1.84 (1.30–2.20)	Poulsen 1957
	Creatinine	1.68 (1.32–2.23)	
	Diodrast	9.11 (5.82–12.60)	
Pig	Inulin	2.1 (1.8–2.5)	Gyrd-Hansen 1968
	Creatinine	2.2 (1.5–3.4)	
	PAH	6.4 (5.2–8.4)	
Dog	Inulin	3.77 (1.74–5.86)	Asheim et al. 1961
	Creatinine	4.3 (2.2–8.3)	
	PAH	12.88 (6.30–21.18)	

Protein Binding

The binding of a drug to plasma and tissue proteins can influence the distribution of the drug, the intensity of its pharmacological effect, and its elimination rate. Drugs of diverse chemical structures interact reversibly and to a variable extent with proteins. Ionic, van der Waals, hydrogen, and hydrophobic binding forces contribute in varying degrees to protein binding.

TABLE 5.5. Measurement of renal function in Beagle dogs ($n = 11$) by determining body clearance of labeled compounds

Compound Cleared	Half-Life (min) Mean ± S.E.M.	Body Clearance (ml/kg/min) Mean ± S.E.M.	Renal Clearance Process
^{125}I-Iothalamate	36.1 ± 2.0	4.5 ± 0.6	GFR
^{131}I-Iodohippurate	16.3 ± 0.9	12.9 ± 0.5	ERPF

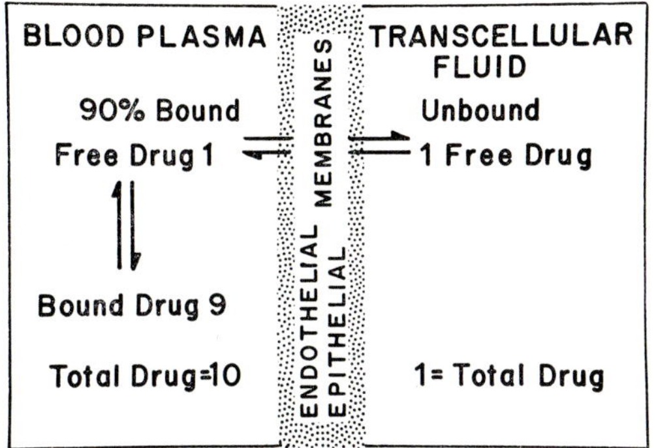

FIG. 5.8. The effect of protein binding on distribution of a drug between blood plasma and transcellular fluid (relatively protein-free), for example, cerebrospinal and synovial fluids.

Plasma albumin is most frequently involved in drug binding, but the globulins were shown to have a high affinity for certain compounds, notably the corticosteroids (Gala and Westphal 1965).

Protein binding may influence a drug's therapeutic efficacy, since only the unbound molecules are diffusible and pharmacologically active. Extensive binding to plasma proteins reduces the proportion of the plasma level of a drug that is available to enter transcellular fluids and milk (Fig. 5.8). Only the lipid-soluble, nonionized moiety of a weak organic electrolyte in the water phase of blood plasma can enter these fluids. When designing a dosage regimen for a chemotherapeutic agent, both serum binding and minimum inhibitory concentration of susceptible microorganisms must be taken into consideration. The clinical efficacy of similar antibiotics (e.g., penicillin analogues or tetracycline derivatives) may be quite different despite equivalent total concentrations in serum (Kunin 1974). High serum concentrations of one penicillin analogue may be due to its high binding affinity to albumin (e.g., cloxacillin) and of another to high concentrations of free drug (e.g., ampicillin). Protein binding does not retard carrier-mediated transport processes, e.g., renal tubular excretion of penicillins. Removal of unbound drug from blood plasma instantly causes dissociation of the drug-protein complex so that equilibrium is maintained.

Species variations, which are of statistical significance, in the binding of drugs to plasma proteins are frequently found (Table 5.6) and may be attributed not only to differences in the total concentrations and relative proportions of the various plasma proteins but also to the composition and conformation of albumins. In general, human beings tend to bind acidic drugs more extensively to their plasma proteins than do other mammals. Variation in drug-protein binding among species may play a role in determining differences

TABLE 5.6. Extent of binding of drugs to plasma (or serum) proteins at therapeutic concentrations

Drug	Concentration (μg/ml)	Percentage Bound Man	Ruminant		Dog	Reference
Salicylate	200	85	62	(goat)	60	Davis and Westfall 1972
Sulfadiazine	100	33	24	(cow)	17	Anton 1960
Sulfisoxazole	100	84	76	(cow)	68	Anton 1960
Chloramphenicol	20	46	30	(goat)	39.5	Davis et al. 1972
Cloxacillin	20	95.2*	71.3	(cow)†	64.5‡	
Benzylpenicillin	10	64.6*	48.3	(cow)§	. . .	
Diphenylhydantoin	10	87	82.5	(cow)	81	Baggot and Davis 1973d
Lincomycin	5	72‖	34.2	(ewe)†	. . .	
Kanamycin	5	2.8#	4.0	(ewe)†	. . .	
Morphine	1	34**	23.6	(cow)	12.1	Baggot and Davis 1973b
Digitoxin	0.05	92.3	86.6	(cow)	88.8	Baggot and Davis 1973c

* Kunin 1967.
† Ziv and Sulman 1972.
‡ Acred et al. 1970.
§ Keen 1965.
‖ Gordon et al. 1973.
Gordon et al. 1972.
** Olsen 1975.

in tissue levels of the drug, in relative toxicity, and in overall disposition kinetics particularly when the extent of binding is high (>80%).

Important clinical situations that may influence the drug-protein interaction include certain disease states (e.g., uremia, hypoproteinemia) and competition between drugs for binding sites on plasma albumin. For extensively bound drugs, a small decrease in binding can elevate significantly the concentration of free drug in plasma and may result in a more intense pharmacological response and a shorter duration of action. Salicylate appears to produce substantial changes in the plasma protein binding of a variety of anionic substances (Anton 1961; Dawkins et al. 1970; Judis 1972). The antibacterial activity of sulfonamides, particularly the long-acting agents that are more highly protein bound (inactive) can be enhanced by several other acidic, highly protein-bound drugs (Anton 1960, 1968).

MECHANISMS OF DRUG ELIMINATION

As soon as drug molecules enter the bloodstream, a portion may bind reversibly to plasma proteins, usually albumin, and the remainder undergo simultaneous distribution and elimination. Drug elimination refers to all the processes that operate to reduce the effective concentration in the body fluids. Hepatic metabolism and renal excretion are the principal mechanisms of drug elimination. Less important mechanisms include biliary and salivary excretion, loss in milk, sweat, and via the lungs. Extensive binding of a drug to tissue components reduces the fraction of the amount in the body that is contained in plasma and available for elimination. Similarly, the uptake of lipophilic compounds by fat reduces their rate of elimination. Lipid solubility limits the excretion of drugs by the kidney, since lipid-soluble compounds are readily absorbed from renal tubular fluid by passive diffusion. Lipid-soluble compounds undergo metabolic transformations in the body (i.e., biotransformation) to more polar, less lipid-soluble products that often have diminished or no pharmacological activity. While the halogenated hydrocarbon anesthetics (e.g., halothane, methoxyflurane) are metabolized to some degree (ca. 10%) by the liver, they are eliminated mainly unchanged by pulmonary excretion.

DRUG METABOLISM (BIOTRANSFORMATION)

The basic pattern of drug metabolism is usually biphasic, the initial phase of the process consisting of reactions classified as oxidations, reductions, and hydrolyses, and the second phase as syntheses or conjugations (Williams 1967). Very often a drug is subjected to several competing pathways simultaneously, and the amounts of the metabolites formed depend on the relative rates of the various metabolic processes. In addition, phase I metabolites frequently react with endogenous substrates (acetate, glycine, sulfate, or glucuronic acid) to yield conjugated products. Drug conjugates are pharmacologically inactive, water-soluble, and rapidly cleared from the body, mainly by renal excretion.

The liver is the principal site of drug biotransformation. Drug-metabolizing enzymes are associated mainly with the smooth-surfaced endoplasmic reticulum (microsomal fraction) of hepatic cells, but the soluble and mitochondrial fractions of mammalian liver, the blood plasma, kidney, placenta, intestinal mucosa, and gut microflora are also capable of drug metabolism. Numerous factors may influence the metabolism, and consequently the pharmacological activity, of a chemical compound. These factors include dose and frequency of administration of the drug; route of administration; species of animal; diet; nutritional status; liver and kidney function of the individual animal; and chronic and concurrent administration of, or exposure to, certain chemical agents that inhibit or induce important metabolic pathways. Biotransformation is a reflection of the drug-metabolizing enzyme systems of various animal species and for many therapeutic substances is the most important single factor in the regulation of drug levels in plasma. Wide interspecies variations exist in the rates of drug biotransformation. Species differences in biotransformation are due to quantitative differences in activity of drug-metabolizing enzymes and the presence of certain capacity-limited metabolic pathways in some species, e.g., glucuronide formation in the cat. Variations in the nature and rate of formation of phase I metabolites may have considerable significance, as a metabolite formed in one species might be pharmacologically more active than the metabolite(s) in other species. Divergence between plasma levels and effects of a drug suggests the possibility of active metabolites being formed from the administered compound. Knowledge of the metabolic pathways and rates of formation of metabolites of a drug is important in the proper understanding and use of data, derived from animal experimentation, in further drug development. It is imprudent to disregard a metabolite merely because it is generated in very small amounts. The rate of formation of conjugates (phase II) is the metabolic process determining the biological half-life and, indirectly, the length of the dosing interval for many drugs administered repeatedly on a multiple dosage regimen. Irrespective of the conjugating agent, the product formed is usually pharmacologically inactive and rapidly excreted. Species differences in conjugation reactions are determined by the availability of the conjugating agent and the amount and activity of the transferring enzyme involved in the final stage of the conjugation process.

Chemical Pathways of Drug Biotransformation

PHASE I (NONSYNTHETIC) REACTIONS

Oxidation is the most general metabolic reaction of foreign compounds in domestic animals. The microsomal fraction of liver, and to a much lesser extent lung and kidney, contains enzymes that oxidize a wide variety of lipid-soluble drugs. These enzymes have a requirement for reduced nicotinamide adenine dinucleotide phosphate (NADPH) and molecular oxygen and have been classified as mixed function oxidases (Mason 1957). The ability of the microsomal drug-metabolizing system to mediate a wide variety of oxidation reactions may be ascribed to a common mechanism, hydroxylation (Brodie et al. 1958; Gillette 1963, 1966). The mixed function oxidase mechanism requires that NADPH reduce a component, cytochrome P-450, in microsomes. The reduced cytochrome P-450 reacts with molecular oxygen to form "active" oxygen, which is then transferred to a drug or steroid substrate (Fig. 5.9). The overall reaction involves the oxidation of NADPH and the hydroxylation of the drug substrate. Oxidation reactions associated with hepatic microsomes (Table 5.7) include

$$\text{NADPH} + \text{A} + \text{H}^+ \rightarrow \text{AH}_2 + \text{NADP}^+$$

$$\text{AH}_2 + \text{O}_2 \rightarrow \text{"active oxygen complex"}$$

$$\text{"active oxygen complex"} + \text{drug} \rightarrow \text{oxidized drug} + \text{A} + \text{H}_2\text{O}$$

This oxidative mechanism requires that equivalent amounts of NADPH, oxygen, and drug substrate be utilized in the reaction. A represents the oxidized form and AH_2 is the reduced form of cytochrome P-450.

FIG. 5.9. Hepatic microsomal drug-oxidizing system.

TABLE 5.7. Some oxidative transformations catalyzed by the liver microsomal enzyme system

Oxidation Reaction	Substrate	Metabolite
Aromatic hydroxylation	Amphetamine*	*p*-Hydroxyamphetamine
	Phenylbutazone*	Oxyphenbutazone*
	Phenobarbital*	Hydroxyphenobarbital
	Acetanilid*	Acetaminophen*
Aliphatic hydroxylation	Pentobarbital*	Pentobarbital alcohol
O-Dealkylation	Phenacetin*	Acetaminophen*
	Codeine*	Morphine*
N-Dealkylation	Imipramine*	Desmethylimipramine*
Deamination	Amphetamine*	Phenylacetone
Desulfuration	Parathion	Paraoxon*
S-Oxidation	Chlorpromazine*	Chlorpromazine sulfoxide

* Therapeutically active compound.

aromatic hydroxylation, oxidation of alkyl chains (aliphatic hydroxylation), *O*- and N-dealkylation, oxidative deamination, desulfuration, *N*-oxidation, and *S*-oxidation (sulfoxide formation).

All mammalian species can probably oxidize most foreign organic compounds, though the rates and relative importance of various routes of oxidation may differ from one species to another. Amphetamine could be metabolized along two pathways, either by hydroxylation of the aromatic ring or by deamination of the side chain. These two pathways have been shown to occur and their relative extent appears to vary with species (Axelrod 1954; Ellison et al. 1966; Dring et al. 1970; Baggot and Davis 1973a). The known metabolites of amphetamine in urine, apart from the unchanged drug itself, were *p*-hydroxyamphetamine and benzoic acid and their conjugates. Clindamycin is eliminated by a combination of metabolism and excretion, biliary and renal (Sun 1973). Based on the metabolic products found in urine, sulfoxidation and *N*-demethylation were the predominant metabolic pathways in the rat, while conjugation with glucuronic acid and sulfoxidation were the major routes in the dog. However, since the major excretion route of clindamycin in both species is the feces (60%–70%), the urinary excretion products may not reflect the overall metabolic pattern of this antibiotic. Species differences in duration of action of many lipid-soluble drugs can be attributed to differences in their rates of biotransformation, e.g., hexobarbital (Quinn et al. 1958), meperidine (Burns et al. 1955; Alexander and Collett 1974a), antipyrine, and phenylbutazone (Burns 1968). A rate-limiting step in the mechanism of drug oxidation by liver microsomal enzymes may be the reduction of cytochrome P-450, and species differences in P-450 reductase activity have been shown to parallel differences in rates of drug oxidation (Davies et al. 1969). Remarkable differences in effective dosage between human beings and experimental animals do not primarily reflect differences in sensitivity of the target organs to the drug. They may depend upon different rates and patterns of drug metabolism (Brodie 1964; Williams 1969).

In addition to catalyzing the oxidation of drugs, the NADPH-dependent enzymes in microsomes also reduce azo- and nitro-compounds. A wide variety of azo dyes are cleared reductively to primary aromatic amines; nitro-compounds are reduced to primary amines. Nitroreductase is active only under anaerobic conditions. Ruminal microflorae were shown to reduce the nitro (NO_2) group of chloramphenicol. The reduced product is inactive so that the oral route of administration is unsuitable for systemic therapy with chloramphenicol in ruminant animals (Davis et al. 1972). The monoglucuronide derivative is the principal metabolite of chloramphenicol in various species (Glazko et al. 1950). In cats and in newborn infants, which have in common a low activity of the glucuronide conjugating mechanism, a small amount of a dehalogenated product is also formed (Dill et al. 1960).

Foreign compounds may be metabolized by nonmicrosomal enzyme systems (Parke 1968). These reactions include deamination of amines, oxidation of alcohols and aldehydes, reduction of aldehydes and ketones, hydrolysis of esters and amides, and certain types of synthetic or conjugation reactions (sulfate and glycine conjugation, acetylation). Monoamine oxidase is a mitochondrial enzyme found especially in liver, kidney, intestine, and nervous tissue. This enzyme (MAO) catalyzes deamination of several naturally occurring amines, including catecholamines, as well as some drugs (e.g., isoproterenol). Compounds that inhibit the action of monoamine oxidase (e.g., isocarboxazid, phenelzine, tranylcypromine) and thereby cause elevations in the norepinephrine and serotonin levels in the CNS were developed for the treatment of severe depression. Alcohol dehydrogenase and aldehyde dehydrogenase, which catalyze several important oxidative transformations, are rather nonspecific enzymes found in the soluble fraction of liver. The substrates include some compounds normally found in the body, e.g., the alcohol vitamin A and the aldehyde retinine. Alcohol dehydrogenase functions as a reductase when it catalyzes the conversion of the (hypnotic) drug chloral hydrate to the pharmacologically active metabolite trichloroethanol (Friedman and Cooper 1960; Mackay and Cooper 1962). Intravenously administered chloral hydrate was rapidly and quantitatively converted to trichloroethanol in the dog, with an apparent half-life of 3 minutes (Garrett and Lambert 1973). The major route of trichloroethanol metabolism in dogs was glucuronidation; the conjugate was rapidly excreted in the urine by glomerular filtration and tubular excretion.

Drug metabolism by hydrolysis is confined to compounds with an ester linkage ($-\overset{\overset{\displaystyle O}{\|}}{C}-O-$) or an amide linkage ($-\overset{\overset{\displaystyle O}{\|}}{C}-NH-$). Nevertheless, hydrolysis is an important reaction in the inactivation and quite often the activation of drugs. Ester linkages occur in widely different types of drugs such as local anesthetics (procaine, cocaine), narcotic analgesics (meperidine, heroin), insecticides (parathion, malathion), the esters of choline (acetylcholine, neostigmine), atropine, and aspirin. A low esterase activity in insects as compared with that in mammals is the basis of the selectively toxic action of organic phosphate insecticides (Loomis 1968). The esterases are found in blood plasma and many other tissues, including the liver. The amidases are also nonmicrosomal enzymes and are found principally in the liver. In human beings it has been shown that there are large individual differences in the ability to hydrolyze succinylcholine by pseudocholinesterase (Kalow 1962). It was found that there are two types of pseudocholinesterase in human plasma that are determined by two allelic genes. While succinylcholine is normally inactivated by rapid hydrolysis, the presence of an "atypical esterase" in plasma of some individuals causes a prolonged action of the muscle relaxant due to a very low affinity of the atypical enzyme for succinylcholine. In domestic animals there is a wide species variation in the dose of succinylcholine required to produce neuromuscular block. Relatively small doses of the drug produce blockade in dogs, sheep, and cattle, but much higher doses are required in the cat, pig, and horse (Tavernor 1971).

A number of amides (e.g., lidocaine, procainamide) are hydrolyzed in the animal body, but the rate of hydrolysis is considerably slower than for esters. The local anesthetic procaine is an ester that is rapidly metabolized by plasma and liver esterases. In contrast, procainamide is slowly hydrolyzed and can be used as an antiarrhythmic agent.

PHASE II (SYNTHETIC) REACTIONS

A synthetic or conjugation reaction may take place when a drug contains a group such as hydroxyl (—OH), carboxyl

(—COOH), amino (—NH_2), or sulfhydryl (—SH) that is suitable for combining with a compound provided by the body. If the drug does not have any of these chemical groups, it may acquire one through a phase I reaction, i.e., by oxidation, reduction, or hydrolysis. The endogenous conjugating agents are derived from carbohydrate, protein, or fat metabolism and include glucuronic acid, glycine (or ornithine), glutathione, methionine, sulfate and acetic acid. Almost without exception, conjugation reactions convert drugs and normal metabolites into products that are, respectively, pharmacologically and biologically inactive. Moreover, the conjugated products are invariably less lipid soluble or more polar than the parent compounds. Consequently, this metabolic pathway not only causes inactivation of drugs but also facilitates their excretion.

Conjugation reactions can be considered to take place in two steps. In the first step, either the drug or the conjugating agent forms part of an "activated" nucleotide. In the second step, the nucleotide reacts with the other component of the conjugation system, under the influence of a transferring enzyme. The synthesis of glucuronides is an extremely important pathway in the metabolism of drugs. Glucuronides are synthesized mainly in the liver but also in the kidney, gastrointestinal tract, and skin (Dutton 1962). The functional chemical groups for glucuronide conjugation are an amino, a sulfhydryl, a carboxyl, or a hydroxyl, which can be either an aliphatic or an aromatic radical. The conjugating agent is glucuronic acid, which is derived from glucose. Uridine diphosphate glucuronic acid, the "activated" form of glucuronic acid, is synthesized by enzymes in the soluble fraction of the cell. The synthesis of the glucuronide proceeds by way of transfer of glucuronic acid from the "activated" nucleotide, uridine diphosphoglucuronic acid (UDPGA), to an acceptor molecule; the transfer reaction is catalyzed by the microsomal enzyme, glucuronyl transferase (Isselbacher et al. 1962). The microsomal enzymes involved in glucuronide syntheses are unique in that this is the only conjugation reaction associated with microsomal enzymes, and a wide range of endogenous compounds (e.g., steroid hormones, thyroxine, bilirubin) as well as drugs are utilized as substrates. Morphine, acetaminophen, salicylic acid, meprobamate, and chloramphenicol are metabolized by this pathway. Some drugs, such as chloral hydrate, phenobarbital, phenacetin, diazepam, and nortriptyline, are also excreted as glucuronides, but only after they have acquired a functional chemical group by a nonsynthetic reaction. The glucuronides are rapidly excreted by the kidney by a combination of glomerular filtration and tubular excretion processes. In certain species, notably the rat, dog, and hen, the biliary route of excretion may predominate for glucuronide conjugates with molecular weights exceeding 400, e.g., bilirubin glucuronide, diethylstilbestrol glucuronide, morphine glucuronide (m.w. 461), sulfadimethoxine N^1-glucuronide (m.w. 487), and chloramphenicol glucuronide (m.w. 500). Compounds of molecular weights above 500 (e.g., indomethacin glucuronide, bromsulphthalein, iopanoic acid) are excreted in bile of all mammalian species. Following passage of glucuronide conjugates into the gut, they may undergo hydrolysis mediated by intestinal β-glucuronidase with liberation of the aglycone, and, if the latter is lipid soluble, it will be reabsorbed (Smith and Williams 1966). The presence of an enterohepatic cycle will prolong the persistence of the drug in the body.

The domestic cat appears to have a defect in glucuronide synthesis, as the rate of formation of glucuronide conjugates is extremely slow in the cat as compared with other species of animals. It has been demonstrated that the cat can synthesize UDPGA but has a deficiency of glucuronyl transferases (Dutton 1966). The limited capacity of this metabolic pathway may increase the pharmacological response or potential toxicity and lengthen the duration of action of lipid-soluble drugs in cats (e.g., salicylate). In insects, glucuronide formation is replaced by β-glucoside conjugation, the activated conjugating agent is uridine diphosphate glucose, and glucosyl transferases mediate transfer of the sugar moiety to a foreign compound (Parke 1968). Among fish, goldfish and perch do not appear to form glucuronides (Brodie and Maickel 1962), but conjugation of aminobenzoic acids with glucuronic acid has been reported to occur in some other breeds (Adamson 1967).

Phenolic or, to a much lesser extent, alcoholic groups of drugs may be conjugated with sulfate to form sulfate esters, called ethereal sulfates. *N*-sulfates, or sulfamates, may be formed by reaction of amino groups of aromatic amines with activated sulfate. In the first stage of the conjugation reaction, sulfate is activated by reaction with ATP to form 3¹-phosphoadenosine-5¹-phosphosulfate (PAPS), catalyzed by enzymes in the soluble fraction of liver cells (Robbins and Lipmann 1957). Relatively specific sulfokinases, also present in the soluble fraction, mediate the second stage of the conjugation process, which is the reaction between PAPS and a phenolic drug to form the ethereal sulfate (Nose and Lipmann 1958). The ethereal sulfates appear to be more water soluble than their parent compounds and are readily excreted in the urine. Phenolic and alcoholic compounds metabolized along this pathway include phenol, acetaminophen, morphine, chloramphenicol, isoproterenol, *p*-hydroxyamphetamine, 3-hydroxycoumarin, estrone, polysaccharides, and ethanol to a small extent. Formation of the sulfate esters of phenolic compounds is widely distributed among species (Smith 1968). The pig, however, does not readily synthesize ethereal sulfates (Stekol 1936). The sulfate pool in the body is easily exhausted so that conjugation with glucuronic acid usually predominates over sulfate conjugation.

The acetylation of OH and SH groups has been shown to occur *in vivo* for natural compounds (e.g., choline), but NH_2 is the only important functional group of drugs that undergoes this type of synthetic reaction. At least five types of amino groups that can be acetylated are distinguishable, and this may indicate the existence of several *N*-acetylases (Williams 1967). The active conjugating agent is acetyl-CoA, which reacts with free amino groups on the drug to form an amide bond, catalyzed by transacetylases. Acetylation of amino groups takes place in reticuloendothelial cells, rather than parenchymal cells, of the liver, spleen, lungs, and gastrointestinal mucosa (Govier 1965). Most mammalian species, except the dog and fox, can acetylate the various types of amino groups (Fig. 5.10). The dog and fox were the only species unable to acetylate the aromatic amino group ($Ar \cdot NH_2$) of sulfanilamide, whereas the sulfamoyl group ($Ar \cdot SO_2NH_2$) was acety-

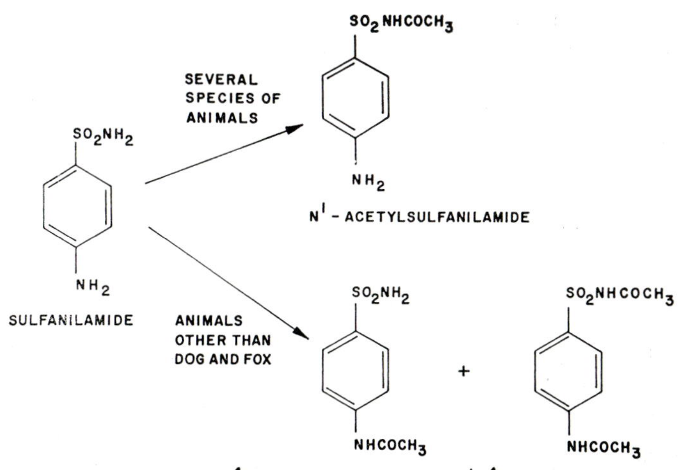

FIG. 5.10. Acetylation of sulfanilamide in various species.

lated in all the several species studied (Williams 1967). Decreased lipid solubility of a drug metabolite does not necessarily mean increased water solubility. The sulfonamides are metabolized to more polar, less lipid-soluble acetyl derivatives, but some of these are less water soluble than their parent compounds (e.g., sulfathiazole). As a result of the decrease in aqueous solubility, the acetylated derivatives have an increased tendency to precipitate in the renal tubules (crystalluria). Acetylation of sulfapyrimidines (e.g., sulfamethazine) increases their solubilities in water, so that conjugation of these sulfonamides decreases their potential toxicity. The sulfonamides are more soluble and are excreted more rapidly and in larger amounts unchanged in alkaline than in acid urine.

METABOLIC INTERACTIONS AMONG ENVIRONMENTAL CHEMICALS AND DRUGS

Metabolic interactions can occur among drugs, insecticides, food additives, carcinogenic hydrocarbons, and a wide variety of environmental chemicals (Conney and Burns 1972). A common denominator governing these effects is the versatile nature of the liver microsomal enzymes that metabolize chemicals with diverse structures and biological activities and the fact that these enzymes can be stimulated or inhibited by other chemicals administered simultaneously. Increased activity, or induction, of liver microsomal enzymes leads to an accelerated biotransformation and alteration, usually decrease, in the intensity and duration of the pharmacological effects of the inducing agent or of other concurrently administered drugs. Enzyme induction is also of physiological significance as endogenous lipid-soluble compounds, such as cortisol, bilirubin, and the sex steroids, are substrates for inducible drug-metabolizing enzymes (Conney 1967). Foreign chemicals stimulate metabolism by increasing the amount of drug-metabolizing enzymes in liver microsomes. Phenobarbital is the most widely recognized and one of the most potent of the inducing agents, but chronic use of other barbiturates, diphenylhydantoin, phenylbutazone, griseofulvin, and DDT can also induce the microsomal enzymes. Induction usually develops over a period of several days or weeks and persists for a similar period following withdrawal of the inducing agent. The effects of chlorinated hydrocarbon insecticides, such as DDT, are more persistent since they are stored in body fat and have a very long biological half-life. Enzyme inducers have been used for lowering insecticide residues in cattle. Treatment with phenobarbital stimulates hepatic drug-metabolizing enzymes in the cow, sheep, goat, calf, and pig (Cook and Wilson 1970), and chronic administration of low doses of phenobarbital to dairy cows given DDT for 2 months resulted in a significant decrease in the content of DDT-related substances in the milk (Alary et al. 1971). Stimulation of the metabolism of coumarin anticoagulants (e.g., warfarin) by barbiturates and other hypnotics is one of the most important induction interactions in human beings. This effect requires that the dosage of coumarins be raised to obtain an adequate anticoagulant response; serious toxicity can result when the inducing agent is withdrawn and the anticoagulant is continued without an appropriate decrease in dose.

Drug metabolites usually have little or no pharmacological activity, and in such circumstances drug effects are reduced by enzyme-inducing drugs. This may explain the development of tolerance to some drugs. Tolerance to narcotics such as morphine and meperidine does not result from accelerated biotransformation. Microsomal enzyme induction may result in enhanced drug effects when metabolites are more active than the parent compound. For example, the metabolite (i.e., paraoxon) is more toxic than the pesticide or parent compound (i.e., parathion).

Inhibition of drug metabolism may result in exaggerated and prolonged response with an increased risk of toxicity. Many interactions of this type involve liver microsomal enzymes, and mechanisms include substrate competition, interference with drug transport, depletion of hepatic glycogen, and functional impairment of enzyme activity due to hepatotoxicity. Environmental chemicals that inhibit microsomal function in animals include organophosphorus insecticides, pesticide synergists of the methylenedioxyphenyl type (e.g., piperonyl butoxide), quinidine, carbon tetrachloride, and chloramphenicol. Compounds that inhibit drug-metabolizing enzymes in liver microsomes also inhibit steroid metabolism and augment the action of steroids in animals.

Some interactions arise through inhibition of nonmicrosomal enzymes that inactivate drugs. Plasma pseudocholinesterase is irreversibly inhibited by organophosphorus insecticides. The drugs, 6-mercaptopurine and azathioprine, are metabolized to uric acid analogues by xanthine oxidase. The xanthine oxidase inhibitor, allopurinol, greatly enhances the toxicity of these drugs so that their dosage must be reduced in patients receiving allopurinol. Inhibition of monoamine oxidase, a mitochondrial enzyme, increases the sensitivity (hypertensive effect) of an individual to catecholamine-releasing drugs (e.g., sympathomimetic agents such as amphetamine, ephedrine, and metaraminol) and natural products rich in tyramine.

EXCRETION OF DRUGS

Renal

The principal route of excretion of polar drugs and the majority of drug metabolites is in the urine. The primary role of the kidney is to regulate the composition and volume of the internal fluid environment, and in performing this task polar foreign compounds are cleared from blood plasma by renal excretion. Drugs that are eliminated mainly unchanged in urine include many antibiotics (e.g., penicillin G, ampicillin, kanamycin, gentamicin, oxytetracycline); most diuretics, with the notable exception of ethacrynic acid; the competitive neuromuscular blocking agents (e.g., *d*-tubocurarine, gallamine); and digoxin. Renal excretion of drugs is complex and involves the processes of glomerular filtration, carrier-mediated excretion in the proximal convoluted tubules, and passive reabsorption, by diffusion, in the distal portion of the nephron. Foreign compounds having low lipid solubility or a high degree of ionization will be excreted, while highly lipid-soluble compounds may be reabsorbed from tubular urine into the blood. The renal excretion mechanisms generally have the net effect of removing a constant fraction of the drug presented to the kidneys by the renal arterial blood, i.e., excretion is usually a first-order process. The relationship between glomerular filtration rate and the overall rate of elimination of a drug that is excreted unchanged and is not transported by a specialized process is influenced by the degree of binding to plasma proteins and extent of reabsorption from glomerular filtrate.

Drug molecules that are free in blood plasma will be filtered through the porous glomerular capillary membrane into the tubular lumen. Since the drug concentration increases progressively as water is reabsorbed from the glomerular filtrate, a concentration gradient favoring drug reabsorption is established as the filtrate moves along the nephron. The tubular epithelium is permeable only to the lipid-soluble nonionized form of a drug. Accordingly, the extent of reabsorption of weak organic electrolytes is determined by the pH reaction of tubular fluid and the pK_a value of the drug (Milne et al. 1958). The normal urinary reaction of carnivores, such as the dog and cat, is acid while that of horses, cattle, and sheep is alkaline. In any species, however, urinary pH is dependent upon the diet. The significance of urinary pH changes in altering the elimination rate of a weak organic electrolyte is determined by the pK_a of the drug and the contribution of renal excretion to overall clearance of the drug from the body. Alkalinization of urine increases the excretion of weak organic acids, e.g., salicylate (pK_a 3.0) and phenobarbital (pK_a 7.2), while urinary acidification hastens excretion of organic bases, e.g., amphetamine (pK_a 9.9). Induction of an alkaline diuresis may successfully combat intoxication, which was caused by overdosage, with a lipid-soluble weak organic acid.

Certain drugs (e.g., penicillins, *p*-aminohippurate, procainamide) and many drug metabolites, in particular conjugates (i.e., phase II metabolic products), are excreted into renal tubular fluid by carrier-mediated transport processes (Weiner and Mudge 1964). While the transport systems responsible for excretion of organic anions and cations are independent, both have similar characteristics and are located in the proximal portion of the nephron. The tubular excretion processes require an energy source and carrier substances, which are rather nonspecific and handle either organic anions or cations. The transport system is susceptible to interference by metabolic or competitive inhibitors, rapidly removes certain foreign organic compounds and metabolites from blood, but has a maximum capacity. Concurrent administration of either acidic or basic drugs that are substrates for carrier-mediated excretion processes will prolong persistence in the body of the less readily transported compound. Probenecid and phenylbutazone reduce renal tubular excretion of penicillin and thereby decrease the rate of elimination of the antibiotic (Kampmann et al. 1972). Even though some drugs enter tubular fluid by glomerular filtration and carrier-mediated excretion, their renal clearance is low because they are substantially reabsorbed in the distal portion of the nephron. The handling of salicylate by renal mechanisms in dogs and cats exemplifies this point.

Biliary

Certain drugs and their metabolites are actively excreted by hepatic parenchymal cells into bile and are then conveyed in this fluid into the gallbladder and small intestine. The metabolites, both of drugs and endogenous substances, that enter bile are frequently formed in liver cells. Glucuronide conjugation in particular seems to produce compounds with suitable properties for the carrier-mediated hepatic transfer system. Generally, polar compounds of molecular weight above 300 are likely to be excreted in bile in significant amounts, e.g., chlortetracyline, erythromycin, steroid hormones, bile acids, bromsulphthalein (BSP), iopanoic acid, and glucuronides of chloramphenicol, morphine, bilirubin, and stilbestrol (Smith 1966). The BSP clearance is widely used to assess hepatic function in domestic animals (Cornelius 1970). The major portion of BSP is conjugated in the liver with glutathione and excreted in bile (Grodsky et al. 1959).

Compounds excreted in bile may be passively reabsorbed from the small intestine if they are sufficiently lipid soluble, and an enterohepatic cycle will be established (Fig. 5.11). Glucuronide conjugates may be hydrolyzed by enzymes in the gut with liberation of parent drug. The pharmacological significance of enterohepatic cycling depends on the fraction of the dose excreted in bile. When the quantity is substantial, the effects of a single dose will be prolonged (e.g., digitoxin). The main importance of biliary excretion as a mechanism of drug elimination is for clearance of organic anions and cations that are highly ionized and have low lipid solubility. A drug with these physicochemical properties can only be poorly absorbed from the intestine by passive diffusion.

SOME ASPECTS OF DRUG DOSAGE

Therapeutic Range of Plasma Drug Concentrations

Dose is a quantitative term estimating the amount of drug that must be administered to produce a particular biological response, i.e., to establish a certain effective concentration of drug in the body fluids. For most therapeutic substances, there exists a range of plasma drug concentrations that relates to an effect of desirable intensity (Table 5.8). Plasma levels of drugs whose action is not rapidly reversible reveal little about their therapeutic activity (e.g., reserpine). Species differences in response to many drugs, particularly lipid-soluble compounds, may be attributed to differences in bioavailability and disposition rather than differences in sensitivity. Consequently, it is probable that a drug has the same effective range of concentrations in different mammalian species.

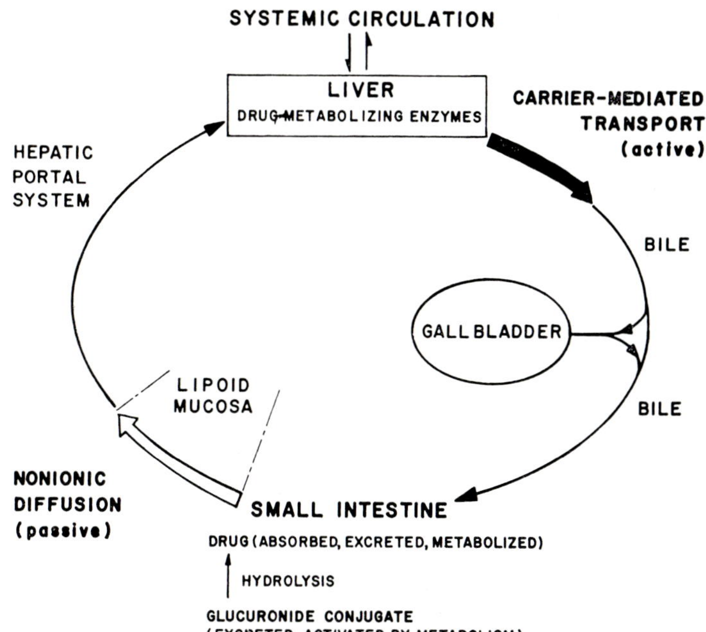

FIG. 5.11. The enterohepatic cycle for a lipid-soluble drug. All species of domestic animals, except the horse, have gallbladders and may intermittently release bile containing unchanged drug and the glucuronide conjugate (inactive), which are conveyed into the small intestine. When the physicochemical properties of the drug in the intestinal environment are suitable for diffusion across the lipoid mucosa, absorption will take place.

When the pharmacological activity is associated with a metabolite and not the parent compound, comparison of metabolite levels only is relevant. Since wide variation exists among species in absorption, distribution, and elimination of the majority of drugs, it is not surprising that appropriate dosage regimens cannot be derived by extrapolation of information from one species to another. However, knowledge of the pharmacological effects, bioavailability, and disposition kinetics of a drug in two species of animals, preferably the dog and a ruminant species, is a useful guideline for dosage of drugs in domestic animals. Among monogastric animals, the cat is the species in which the response to lipid-soluble drugs is least predictable. When conjugation (glucuronide formation) is an important process of elimination, the poten-

TABLE 5.8. Relationship between plasma drug concentrations and therapeutic effect

Drug	Usual Range of Therapeutic Plasma Concentrations (μg/ml)	Principal Pharmacological Effect
Salicylate	50–100	Analgesia
	200–350	Antiarthritic
Acetaminophen	10–20	Analgesia
Diphenylhydantoin	10–20	Anticonvulsive
Chloral hydrate	5–10	Hypnosis
Quinidine	2–5	Antiarrhythmic
Propranolol	0.025–0.100	β-Adrenergic blockade
Digoxin	0.001–0.003	Stabilize sinus; rhythm and antiarrhythmic; antimicrobial effect
Sulfonamides	50–150	Bacteriostatic
Chloramphenicol	5–15	Bacteriostatic
Tetracyclines	1.5–4	Bacteriostatic
Kanamycin	4–32	Bactericidal
Gentamicin	4–16	Bactericidal
Tylosin	1–8	Bactericidal
Penicillin	0.1–25	Bactericidal

Note: The minimum effective serum level of antimicrobial agents depends upon susceptibility of the microorganisms.

tial toxicity may be increased and the duration of action is usually prolonged. Bioavailability of orally administered drug products is unpredictable in the equine species. Some pharmacodynamic features of ruminant animals include slow absorption from the reticulorumen and possibly inactivation by ruminal microorganisms, diffusion from the systemic circulation into ruminal liquor, and extremely efficient hepatic biotransformation mechanisms. It is evident that comprehensive appreciation of what occurs following drug administration is possible only when pharmacokinetic analyses complement pharmacodynamic studies. Drugs are potentially toxic chemical agents that, after correct diagnosis and given in proper dosage only, are likely to produce beneficial effects.

Therapy with Antimicrobial Agents

Antimicrobial agents behave similarly to other drugs, but their efficacy depends on their ability to act on invading microorganisms rather than on tissue receptors of the host animal. The effective range of levels of a chemotherapeutic agent in serum is determined by the susceptibility of the invading microorganisms to the particular antibiotic, its degree of penetration (by passive diffusion) to the site of infection, and the margin between the effective and toxic serum levels. Ideally with bacteriostatic agents, the serum level of free (not bound to serum proteins) drug should not fall below the minimum effective concentration during the course of treatment. The minimum effective concentration of drug in serum (or plasma) is a multiple of the minimum inhibitory concentration for the particular microorganism; the latter is determined *in vitro*.

Since most antibiotics, with the notable exceptions of chloramphenicol and clindamycin, are eliminated unchanged, one would not expect wide species variations in the serum half-lives of many antibiotics. The apparent specific volume of distribution, however, may vary considerably among species, particularly between monogastric and ruminant animals when diffusion into ruminal fluid is a feature of distribution. Consequently, variation among species may exist in the body clearance of antibiotics, particularly those that are bases.

Dosage Regimen

By dosage regimen is meant the systematized dosage schedule. A dosage regimen entails two variables: the magnitude of each dose and the frequency with which the dose is repeated, usually expressed as a dosing interval. The regimen that, in theory, should be most effective can be designed for any drug, provided that a desirable body content of the drug can be clinically defined. When circumstances necessitate drug therapy, it is usually desirable to establish an effective concentration of drug in the body fluids as soon as possible and to maintain this concentration for an adequate period of time. To achieve this objective, the dosage regimen often consists of an initial priming or loading dose followed by lower maintenance doses, which are administered at fixed time intervals. Inappropriate choice of the maintenance dose or the dosing interval leads to inadequate therapy or to accumulation of drug with attendant signs of toxicity. Cumulation is not a property of the drug itself but rather a consequence of the dosage regimen (Dettli 1970).

The priming dose is intended to establish a therapeutic amount of drug in the body and thereby produce an almost immediate effect (Fig. 5.12). Drug levels are maintained within the therapeutic range, $C_{P(\text{ther})} = C_P{}^{\infty}{}_{(\text{max})}$ to $C_P{}^{\infty}{}_{(\text{min})}$, by administering appropriate maintenance doses at fixed time intervals. The dosing interval is normally chosen among the values 4, 6, 8, 12, and 24 hours. The same steady state concentrations of a drug can be achieved gradually by accumulation and without a priming dose. Accumulation of drug by administering a fixed dose at constant time intervals will eventually produce a therapeutic amount in the body. When the steady state level of drug has been achieved, each maintenance dose replaces the amount lost during the preceding interval. A properly designed and carefully exe-

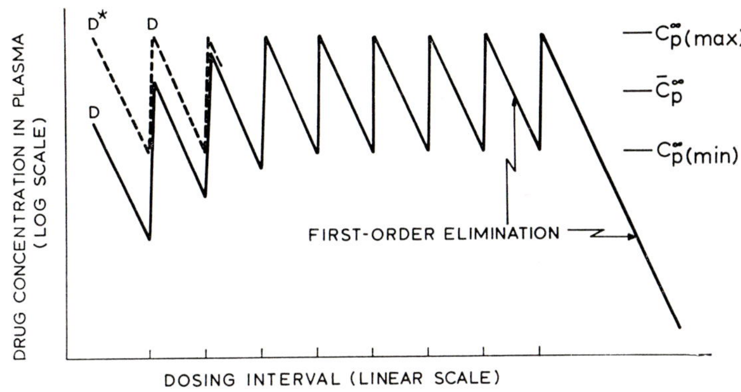

FIG. 5.12. Drug concentration in plasma time curves depicting the ideal profiles for a multiple dosage regimen. Both priming (D^*) and maintenance (D) doses are administered intravenously (or by a route giving rapid absorption). At the steady state, each maintenance dose replaces the amount of drug eliminated during the preceding dosing interval.

cuted multiple dose schedule ensures effective drug levels and gives the greatest degree of control throughout the course of treatment. To be relevant clinically, however, dosage regimens based on drug levels require that a well-defined relationship exists between plasma (or serum) levels of drug and pharmacological or antimicrobial effects.

The dosage regimen for a drug is determined by its (biological) half-life and the range of plasma levels that is considered therapeutic. Initiation of therapy with a priming dose and careful selection of the dosing interval are particularly important for drugs with long half-life values (e.g., cardiac glycosides) and for chemotherapeutic agents with a bacteriostatic action (e.g., the tetracyclines, the sulfonamides). Using a priming dose twice the maintenance dose, which is given at intervals equal to the half-life of the drug (assuming the absorption rate to be much greater than the elimination rate), constitutes a suitable dosage regimen for most bacteriostatic drugs (Kruger-Thiemer 1960; Kruger-Thiemer and Bunger 1965/66). The duration of therapy with bacteriostatic drugs is unrelated to their properties, unless toxicity is imminent, and depends on the relationship of the bacteria to the defense mechanisms of the body. The only significant indication of a therapeutic effect is a favorable clinical response.

When the maintenance dose is given at intervals equal to the biological half-life of a drug, 50% fluctuation (or oscillation) is obtained in plasma levels during the steady state. The greater the extent of fluctuation, or range of plasma levels, that is acceptable for a drug, the longer the time that may elapse between successive doses (Table 5.9). Penicillin analogues can be

TABLE 5.9. Relationship between length of the dosing interval and half-life of drugs with variable extent of fluctuation

		Percent Fluctuation (f_{el})				
$t_{1/2}(h)$	$\beta(h^{-1})$	$\tau(h)$:4	6	8	12	24
2	0.3465	75	87.5	93.75	98.4	. . .
6	0.116	37	50	60	75	93.75
12	0.058	20	30	37	50	75

given at intervals of up to eight times their half-life values as an extremely wide range of therapeutic concentrations is feasible against most susceptible microorganisms. When a drug has a relatively narrow margin of safety and a short (biological) half-life (e.g., gentamicin), a dosing interval of several times the half-life value cannot be used, as a potentially toxic plasma drug concentration would be produced by the necessarily large maintenance dose. For a first-order elimination, the duration of a therapeutically effective drug concentration increases as the logarithm of the amount of drug in the body fluids (i.e., the dose). Administration of a priming dose is unnecessary for drugs with short half-lives (e.g., penicillins and cephalosporins, kanamycin, gentamicin).

Prediction of Steady State Levels

When a fixed dose of a drug is administered repeatedly at fixed time intervals, a steady state will eventually be established in which the plasma level-time curves will be the same during successive dosing intervals (Wagner et al. 1965). This concept enables one to predict the average steady state plasma concentration of a drug ($\overline{C}_P^{\infty}$) after long-term administration of a fixed dose at fixed time intervals:

$$\overline{C}_P^{\infty} = \frac{(1.44)\ t_{1/2} \cdot FD}{V_d \cdot \gamma} \qquad (5.12)$$

here F is the fraction of each dose (D) which is absorbed, γ is the dosing interval, $t_{1/2}$ and V_d are the half-life and apparent volume of distribution, respectively, of the drug. When the dose is injected intravenously, $F = 1$. In the case of oral or intramuscular administration, the more rapid the rate of absorption, the greater the oscillation of plasma levels about the average steady state concentration. The equation holds true for any route of administration and kinetic model, provided that absorption, distribution, and elimination can be described by a set of linear differential equations. A dosing interval of 1.44 times the half-life of a drug is equivalent to the time for the amount of drug in the body to be reduced from some value to 36.8% of that value, assuming that absorption is complete at the time the observation is made (Wagner 1967). Dosing at intervals of approximately 1.5 times the half-life value provides a satisfactory regimen for many drugs with half-lives between 4 and 16 hours and simplifies the equation that predicts average steady state plasma levels.

Prediction of the average steady state plasma concentration of a drug, under a variety of dosage regimens, may be made by using quantitative information ($t_{1/2}$, V_d, F) obtained from single-dose studies (Wagner and Metzler 1969). While there are several possible sources of error in such predictions, the increased accuracy of dosage that would be achieved should enable the drug to exert its optimum therapeutic effect.

Special Dosage Forms

If the maintenance dose rate (D/γ) of a drug is either impractical or is likely to cause toxicity, the drug should be administered either by constant infusion or as a special dosage form. The constant infusion of a drug that has a short half-life and narrow therapeutic index eliminates fluctuation in steady state levels and provides for the greatest degree of control over the intensity of pharmacological response. Both sustained-release dosage forms and prolonged-action preparations (special dosage forms) of drugs that have short half-lives provide an extended response (i.e., a longer duration of action) and overcome the necessity for dosing at short intervals or administering unduly large doses of the usual drug products. Sustained-release dosage forms, in theory, provide an initial therapeutic dose that is available upon administration of the product followed by a gradual release of drug over a prolonged period of time. Variability in drug absorption is a feature of the sustained-release dosage form (Crosland-Taylor et al. 1965). Prolonged-action preparations release the drug at a rate that will provide a significantly longer duration of action than the usual single dose. The half-life of penicillin G in the cow is 0.7 hour (Ziv et al. 1973). A dose (6 million units, injected intramuscularly) of procaine penicillin G in aqueous solution was shown to provide a serum level of penicillin above 0.05 unit/ml for at least 24 hours in the cow (Schipper et al. 1971). Dissolution rather than absorption is the rate-limiting step determining entry of drugs into the systemic circulation from prolonged-release dosage forms, whether they are intended for oral or parenteral administration.

An effective way of achieving extremely slow absorption is to incorporate a drug into a compressed pellet, which can be implanted subcutaneously. The drug must be relatively insoluble (e.g., certain steroid hormones) and the pellet resistant to disintegration in the subcutaneous fluid environment. It has been predicted that the ideal shape of a pellet for achieving a constant rate of absorption is a flat disk. The principal disadvantage of controlled release formulations is probably the loss of flexibility in dosage of a drug.

GLOSSARY OF PHARMACOKINETIC TERMS

Pharmacokinetic variables associated with a two-compartment open model:

C_P—drug concentration in plasma at any time, t

C_T—drug concentration in distribution fluids (tissues) at time t

$A_{B(t)}$—amount of a drug in the body at time t

Pharmacokinetic evaluation of plasma level data after intravenous administration of a drug yield A, B, α, and β directly, and k_{12}, k_{21}, and k_{el} by calculation.

A, B—zero-time plasma concentration intercepts

α, β-hybrid rate constants dependent on all three specific rate constants of the model. Values of α and β are obtained from the slopes of distribution and elimination phases, respectively, of biexponential drug concentration in plasma versus time profile. β is the first-order rate constant for overall elimination of a drug by the body and is obtained from the terminal exponential phase.

C_P°—extrapolated zero-time plasma concentration of a drug ($C_P^\circ = A + B$)

k_{12}, k_{21}—first-order rate constants of distribution between the central and peripheral compartments

k_{el}—first-order elimination rate constant for loss of a drug from the central compartment

All rate constants are in units of reciprocal time (i.e., $time^{-1}$)

$t_{1/2}(\alpha)$—drug distribution half-time

$t_{1/2(\beta)} = t_{1/2}$—drug elimination half-time. This value is the (biological) half-life of the drug. As defined the terms biological and serum half-life are synonymous.

Volume terms:

V_c—volume of central compartment

V_d—apparent volume of distribution

$V_{d(B)}$—apparent volume of distribution obtained by neglecting the α- or distributive phase of drug disposition (extrapolation method)

$V_{d(area)}$—apparent volume of distribution based on total area under linear plasma concentration-time curve after administration of a drug by any route

Area—total area under the linear drug concentration in plasma versus time curve from $t = 0$ to $t = \infty$ after administration of a single dose

The dimensions of clearance are volume/unit of time (usually ml/min)

Cl_B—(total) body clearance, which is the sum of all clearance processes in the body

Cl_R—renal clearance

Cl_{cr}—endogenous creatinine clearance

GFR—glomerular filtration rate

ERPF—effective renal plasma flow

Terms associated with a dosage regimen (i.e., multiple dose schedule):

$C_{P(ther)}$—therapeutically effective range of drug concentrations in plasma (or serum)

$C_P{}^\infty{}_{(max)}$, $\bar{C}_P{}^\infty$, $C_P{}^\infty{}_{(min)}$—maximum desirable, average, and minimum effective concentrations of a drug in plasma during a dosing interval once the steady state (equilibrium) has been achieved

$\bar{A}_B{}^\infty$—average steady state amount of a drug in the body

D^*, D—priming (or loading) dose and maintenance dose of a drug, respectively, used in dosage regimens

τ—length of a dosing interval

D/τ—maintenance dose rate

f_{el}—fraction eliminated during a dosing interval. This represents the extent of fluctuation in steady state levels of a drug that occurs between successive doses.

F—fraction of a dose that is absorbed. This term is the systemic availability of a drug (i.e., the fraction of the dose reaching the systemic circulation unchanged).

REFERENCES

Acred, P.; Brown, D. M.; Clark, B. F.; and Mizen, L. 1970. The distribution of antibacterial agents between plasma and lymph in the dog. Br J Pharmacol 39:439.

Adamson, R. H. 1967. Drug metabolism in marine vertebrates. Fed Proc 26:1047.

Alary, J. G.; Guay, P.; and Brodeur, J. 1971. Effect of phenobarbital pretreatment on the metabolism of DDT in the rat and the bovine. Toxicol Appl Pharmacol 18:457.

Alexander, F. 1969. An Introduction to Veterinary Pharmacology, 2nd ed., p. 170. Edinburgh: Livingstone.

———. 1972. Certain aspects of the physiology and pharmacology of the horse's digestive tract. Equine Vet J 4:166.

Alexander, F., and Collett, R. A. 1974a. Pethidine in the horse. Res Vet Sci 17:136.

———. 1974b. Some observations on the pharmacokinetics of trimethoprim in the horse. Br J Pharmacol 52:142.

Annison, E. F., and Lewis, D. 1959. Metabolism in the Rumen, p. 124. London: Methuen.

Anton, A. H. 1960. The relation between the binding of sulfonamides to albumin and their antibacterial efficacy. J Pharmacol Exp Ther 129:282.

———. 1961. A drug-induced change in the distribution and renal excretion of sulfonamides. J Pharmacol Exp Ther 134: 291.

———. 1968. The effect of disease, drugs, and dilution on the binding of sulfonamides in human plasma. Clin Pharmacol Ther 9:561.

Asheim, A.; Persson, F.; and Persson, S. 1961. Renal clearance in dogs with regard to variations according to age and sex. Acta Physiol Scand 51:150.

Axelrod, J. 1954. Studies on sympathomimetic amines. II. The biotransformation and physiological disposition of *d*-amphetamine, *d-p*-hydroxyamphetamine and *d*-methamphetamine. J Pharmacol Exp Ther 110:315.

Baggot, J. D. 1975. To be published.

Baggot, J. D., and Davis, L. E. 1973a. A comparative study of the pharmacokinetics of amphetamine. Res Vet Sci 14:207.

———. 1973b. Species differences in plasma protein binding of morphine and codeine. Am J Vet Res 34:571.

———. 1973c. Plasma protein binding of digitoxin and digoxin in several mammalian species. Res Vet Sci 15:81.

———. 1973d. Comparative study of plasma protein binding of diphenylhydantoin. Comp Gen Pharmacol 4:399.

Bailey, C. B. 1961. Saliva secretion and its relation to feeding in cattle. III. The rate of secretion of mixed saliva in the cow during eating, with an estimate of the magnitude of the total daily secretion of mixed saliva. Br J Nutr 15:443.

Bothwell, T. H. 1968. The control of iron absorption. Br J Haematol 14:453.

Boxenbaum, H. 1974. Research Division, Hoffmann-LaRoche, Inc., Nutley, N.J. Personal communication.

Boyes, R. N.; Adams, H. J.; and Duce, B. R. 1970. Oral absorption and disposition kinetics of lidocaine hydrochloride in dogs. J Pharmacol Exp Ther 174:1.

Brodie, B. B. 1964. Of mice, microsomes and man. Pharmacologist 6:12.

Brodie, B. B., and Hogben, C. A. M. 1957. Some physicochemical factors in drug action. J Pharm Pharmacol 9:345.

Brodie, B. B., and Maickel, R. P. 1962. Comparative biochemistry of drug metabolism. In B. B. Brodie and E. G. Erdös, eds. Metabolic Factors Controlling Duration of Drug Action, vol. 6, p. 299. Oxford, Eng.: Pergamon Press.

Brodie, B. B.; Gillette, J. R.; and LaDu, B. N. 1958. Enzymatic metabolism of drugs and other foreign compounds. Annu Rev Biochem 27:427.

Burns, J. J. 1968. Variation of drug metabolism in animals and the prediction of drug action in man. Ann NY Acad Sci 151:959.

Burns, J. J.; Berger, B. L.; Lief, P. A.; Wollack, A.; Papper, E. M.; and Brodie, B. B. 1955. The physiological disposition and fate of meperidine (Demerol) in man and a method for its estimation in plasma. J Pharmacol Exp Ther 114:289.

Conney, A. H. 1967. Pharmacological implications of microsomal enzyme induction. Pharmacol Rev 19:317.

Conney, A. H., and Burns, J. J. 1972. Metabolic interactions among environmental chemicals and drugs. Science 178:576.

Cook, R. M., and Wilson, K. A. 1970. Metabolism of xenobiotics in ruminants. Phenobarbital induction of liver microsomal nitrogen demethylase. J Agric Food Chem 18:441.

Cornelius, C. E. 1970. Liver function. In J. J. Kaneko and C. E. Cornelius, eds. Clinical Biochemistry of Domestic Animals, 2nd ed,. vol. 1, p. 161. New York: Academic Press.

Crosland-Taylor, P.; Keeling, D. H.; and Cromie, B. W. 1965. A trial of slow-release tablets of ferrous sulphate. Curr Ther Res 7:244.

Danielli, J. F.; Hitchcock, M. W. S.; Marshall, R. A.; and Phillipson, A. T. 1945. The mechanism of absorption from the rumen as exemplified by the behaviour of acetic, propionic and butyric acids. J Exp Biol 22:75.

Davies, D. S.; Gigon, P. L.; and Gillette, J. R. 1969. Species and sex differences in electron transport systems in liver microsomes and their relationship to ethylmorphine demethylation. Life Sci 8(2):85.

Davis, L. E., and Westfall, B. A. 1972. Species differences in biotransformation and excretion of salicylate. Am J Vet Res 33:1253.

Davis, L. E.; Neff, C. A.; Baggot, J. D.; and Powers, T. E. 1972. Pharmacokinetics of chloramphenicol in domesticated animals. Am J Vet Res 33:2259.

Davson, H., and Danielli, J. F. 1952. The Permeability of Natural Membranes, 2nd ed., p. 57. London: Cambridge Univ. Press.

Dawkins, P. D.; McArthur, J. N.; and Smith, M. J. H. 1970. The effect of sodium salicylate on the binding of long-chain fatty acids to plasma proteins. J Pharm Pharmacol 22:405.

Dayton, P. G.; Cucinell, S. A.; Weiss, M.; and Perel, J. M. 1967. Dose dependence of drug plasma level decline in dogs. J Pharmacol Exp Ther 158:305.

Dettli, L. 1970. Multiple dose elimination kinetics and drug accumulation in patients with normal and with impaired kidney function. In G. Raspé, ed. Advances in the Biosciences, vol. 5, p. 39. Oxford, Eng.: Pergamon Press.

Dill, W. A.; Thompson, E. M.; Fisken, R. A.; and Glazko, A. J. 1960. A new metabolite of chloramphenicol. Nature 185:535.

Dowben, R. M. 1969. Composition and structure of membranes. In R. M. Dowben, ed. Biological Membranes, p. 1. Boston: Little, Brown.

Dring, L. G.; Smith, R. L.; and Williams, R. T. 1970. The metabolic fate of amphetamine in man and other species. Biochem J 116: 425.

Dutton, G. J. 1962. Glucuronide conjugation. In B. B. Brodie and E. G. Erdös, eds. Metabolic Factors Controlling Duration of Drug Action, vol. 6, p. 39. Oxford, Eng.: Pergamon Press.

Dutton, G. J., ed. 1966. The biosynthesis of glucuronides. Glucuronic Acid, Free and Combined. Chemistry, Biochemistry, Pharmacology and Medicine, p. 185. New York: Academic Press.

Ellison, T.; Gutzait, L.; and Van Loon, E. J. 1966. The comparative metabolism of *d*-amphetamine-^{14}C in the rat, dog and monkey. J Pharmacol Exp Ther 152:383.

Fawcett, D. W. 1965. Surface specializations of absorbing cells. J Histochem Cytochem 13:75.

Friedman, P. J., and Cooper, J. R. 1960. The role of alcohol dehydrogenase in the metabolism of chloral hydrate. J Pharmacol Exp Ther 129:373.

Gala, R. R., and Westphal, U. 1965. Corticosteroid-binding globulin in the rat: Studies on the sex difference. Endocrinology 77:841.

Gamble, J. A. S.; Mackay, J. S.; and Dundee, J. W. 1973. Plasma levels of diazepam. Br J Anaesth 45:1085.

Garrett, E. R., and Lambert, H. J. 1973. Pharmacokinetics of trichloroethanol and metabolites and interconversions among variously referenced pharmacokinetic parameters. J Pharm Sci 62:550.

Gibaldi, M.; Nagashima, R.; and Levy, G. 1969. Relationship between drug concentration in plasma or serum and amount of drug in the body. J Pharm Sci 58:193.

Gillette, J. R. 1963. Metabolism of drugs and other foreign compounds by enzymatic mechanisms. Prog Drug Res 6:13.

———. 1966. Biochemistry of drug oxidation and reduction by enzymes in hepatic endoplasmic reticulum. Adv Pharmacol 4:219.

Glazko, A. J.; Dill, W. A.; and Rebstock, M. C. 1950. Biochemical studies on chloramphenicol (Chloromycetin). III. Isolation and identification of metabolic products in urine. J Biol Chem 183:679.

Gordon, R. C.; Regamey, C.; and Kirby, W. M. M. 1972. Serum protein binding of the aminoglycoside antibiotics. Antimicrob Agents Chemother 2:214.

———. 1973. Serum protein binding of erythromycin, lincomycin, and clindamycin. J Pharm Sci 62:1074.

Govier, W. C. 1965. Reticuloendothelial cells as the site of sulfanilamide acetylation in the rabbit. J. Pharmacol Exp Ther 150: 305.

Gray, F. V. 1948. The absorption of volatile fatty acids from the rumen: The influence of pH on absorption. J Exp Biol 25:135.

Greenblatt, D. J.; Duhme, D. W.; Koch-Weser, J.; and Smith, T. W. 1973. Evaluation of digoxin bioavailability in single-dose studies. N Engl J Med 289:651.

Grodsky, G. M.; Carbone, J. V.; and Fanska,

R. 1959. Identification of metabolites of sulfobromophthalein. J Clin Invest 38: 1981.

Gyrd-Hansen, N. 1968. Renal clearances in pigs. Inulin, endogenous creatinine, urea, para-aminohippuric acid, sodium, potassium, and chloride. Acta Vet Scand 9:183.

Hogben, C. A. M.; Tocco, D. J.; Brodie, B. B.; and Schanker, L. S. 1959. On the mechanism of the intestinal absorption of drugs. J Pharmacol Exp Ther 125:275.

Hunt, J. N., and Knox, M. T. 1968. Control of gastric emptying. Am J Dig Dis 13:372.

Isselbacher, K. J.; Chrabas, M. F.; and Quinn, R. C. 1962. The solubilization and partial purification of a glucuronyl transferase from rabbit liver microsomes. J Biol Chem 237:3033.

Jacobs, M. H. 1940. Some aspects of cell permeability to weak electrolytes. Cold Spring Harbor Symp Quant Biol 8:30.

Judis, J. 1972. Binding of sulfonylureas to serum proteins. J Pharm Sci 61:89.

Kalow, W. 1962. Esterase action. In B. B. Brodie and E. G. Erdös, eds. Metabolic Factors Controlling Duration of Drug Action, vol. 6, p. 137. Oxford, Eng.: Pergamon Press.

Kampmann, J.; Molholm Hansen, J.; Siersboek-Nielsen, K.; and Laursen, H. 1972. Effect of some drugs on penicillin half-life in blood. Clin Pharmacol Ther 13:516.

Kaplan, S. A.; Weinfeld, R. E.; Cotler, S.; Abruzzo, C. W.; and Alexander, K. 1970. Pharmacokinetic profile of trimethoprim in dog and man. J Pharm Sci 59:358.

Keen, P. M. 1965. The binding of three penicillins in the plasma of several mammalian species as studied by ultrafiltration at body temperature. Br J Pharmacol 25:507.

Knudsen, E. 1959. Renal clearance studies on the horse. I. Inulin, endogenous creatinine and urea. Acta Vet Scand 1:52.

Krüger-Thiemer, E. 1960. Dosage schedule and pharmacokinetics in chemotherapy. J Am Pharm Assoc [Sci Ed] 49:311.

Krüger-Thiemer, E., and Bunger, P. 1965–66. The role of the therapeutic regimen in dosage design. Chemotherapia 10:61.

Kunin, C. M. 1967. Clinical significance of protein binding of the penicillins. Ann NY Acad Sci 145:282.

———. 1974. Blood level measurements and antimicrobial agents. Clin Pharmacol Ther 16:251.

Levine, R. R. 1970. Factors affecting gastrointestinal absorption of drugs. Am J Dig Dis 15:171.

Levine, R. R., and Pelikan, E. W. 1964. Mechanisms of drug absorption and excretion. Passage of drugs out of and into the gastrointestinal tract. Annu Rev Pharmacol 4:69.

Levy, G. 1968. Kinetics and implications of dissolution rate limited gastrointestinal absorption of drugs. In E. J. Ariens, ed. Physicochemical Aspects of Drug Action, vol. 7, p. 33. Oxford, Eng.: Pergamon Press.

Lewis, W. H. 1931. Pinocytosis. Johns Hopkins Hosp Bull 49:17.

Loomis, T. A. 1968. Essentials of Toxicology, p. 116. Philadelphia: Lea & Febiger.

Lukas, G.; Brindle, S. D.; and Greengard, P. 1971. The route of absorption of intraperitoneally administered compounds. J Pharmacol Exp Ther 178:562.

Mackay, F. J., and Cooper, J. R. 1962. A study on the hypnotic activity of chloral hydrate. J Pharmacol Exp Ther 135:271.

Mason, H. S. 1957. Mechanisms of oxygen metabolism. Science 125:1185.

Masson, M. J., and Phillipson, A. T. 1951. The absorption of acetate, propionate and butyrate from the rumen of sheep. J Physiol (Lond) 113:189.

———. 1952. The composition of the digesta leaving the abomasum of sheep. J Physiol (Lond) 116:98.

Milne, M. D.; Scribner, B. H.; and Crawford, M. A. 1958. Nonionic diffusion and the excretion of weak acids and bases. Am J Med 24:709.

Neff, C. A.; Davis, L. E.; and Baggot, J. D. 1972. A comparative study of the pharmacokinetics of quinidine. Am J Vet Res 33: 1521.

Nelson, E. 1961. Kinetics of drug absorption, distribution, metabolism, and excretion. J Pharm Sci 50:181.

Nielsen, P., and Rasmussen, F. 1972. Elimination of trimethoprim in pigs and goats. Acta Pharmacol Toxicol [Suppl 1] (Kbh) 31:94.

Nose, Y., and Lipmann, F. 1958. Separation of steroid sulfokinases. J Biol Chem 233: 1348.

Notari, R. E. 1971. Biopharmaceutics and Pharmacokinetics: An Introduction, p. 126. New York: Dekker.

Olsen, G. D. 1975. Morphine binding to human plasma proteins. Clin Pharmacol Ther 17:31.

Orr, J. S.; Shimmins, J.; and Speirs, C. F. 1969. Method for estimating individual drug dosage regimens. An application of the occupancy principle. Lancet 11(Oct. 11):771.

Parke, D .V. 1968. The Biochemistry of Foreign Compounds. Oxford, Eng.: Pergamon Press.

Phillipson, A. T., and McAnally, R. A. 1942. Studies on the fate of carbohydrates in the rumen of sheep. J Exp Biol 19:199.

Piperno, E.; Ellis, D. J.; Getty, S. M.; and Brody, T. M. 1968. Plasma and urine levels of phenylbutazone in the horse. J Am Vet Med Assoc 153:195.

Poulsen, E. 1957. Year Book, p. 97. Copenhagen: R Vet Agric College.

Quinn, G. P.; Axelrod, J.; and Brodie, B. B. 1958. Species, strain and sex differences in metabolism of hexobarbitone, amidopyrine, antipyrine, and aniline. Biochem Pharmacol 1:152.

Rasmussen, F. 1958. Mammary excretion of sulphonamides. Acta Pharmacol Toxicol (Kbh) 15:139.

———. 1959. Mammary excretion of benzylpenicillin, erythromycin, and penethamate hydroiodide. Acta Pharmacol Toxicol (Kbh) 16:194.

———. 1966. Studies on the Mammary Excretion and Absorption of Drugs. Copenhagen: Carl Fr. Mortensen.

———. 1970. Renal and mammary excretion of trimethoprim in goats. Vet Rec 87:14.

Robbins, P. W., and Lipmann, F. 1957. Isolation and identification of active sulfate. J Biol Chem 229:837.

Schanker, L. S. 1964. Physiological transport of drugs. In N. J. Harper and A. B. Simmonds, eds. Advances in Drug Research, vol. 1, p. 71. New York: Academic Press.

Schipper, I. A.; Filipovs, D.; Ebeltoft, H.; and Schermeister, L. J. 1971. Blood serum concentrations of various benzyl penicillins after their intramuscular administration to cattle. J Am Vet Med Assoc 158:494.

Schou, J. 1961. Absorption of drugs from subcutaneous connective tissue. Pharmacol Rev 13:441.

Schwarz, C.; Steinmetzer, K.; and Caithaml, K. 1926. Arch Ges Physiol 213:595. Cited by H. H. Dukes. 1955. The Physiology of Domestic Animals, 7th ed., p. 330. Ithaca, N.Y.: Comstock.

Scott, D. B.; Jebson, P. J. R.; Braid, D. P.; Ortengren, B.; and Frisch, P. 1972. Factors affecting plasma levels of lignocaine and prilocaine. Br J Anaesth 44:1040.

Singer, S. J., and Nicolson, G. L. 1972. The fluid mosaic model of the structure of cell membranes. Science 175:720.

Smith, J. N. 1968. Comparative metabolism of xenobiotics. In O. E. Lowenstein, ed. Advances in Comparative Physiology and Biochemistry, vol. 3, p. 173. New York: Academic Press.

Smith, R. L. 1966. The biliary excretion and enterohepatic circulation of drugs and other organic compounds. Prog Drug Res 9:299.

Smith, R. L., and Williams, R. T. 1966. Implication of the conjugation of drugs and other exogenous compounds. In G. J. Dutton, ed. Glucuronic Acid, Free and Combined. Chemistry, Biochemistry, Pharmacology and Medicine, p. 457. New York: Academic Press.

Smolen, V. F. 1973. Misconceptions and thermodynamic untenability of deviations from pH-partition hypothesis. J Pharm Sci 62: 77.

Sperber, I., and Hyden, S. 1952. Transport of chloride through the ruminal mucosa. Nature 169:587.

Stein, W. D. 1967. The Movement of Molecules Across Cell Membranes, p. 1. New York: Academic Press.

Stekol, J. A. 1936. Comparative studies in the sulfur metabolism of the dog and pig. J Biol Chem 113:675.

Stowe, C. M., and Sisodia, C. S. 1963. The pharmacologic properties of sulfadimethoxine in dairy cattle. Am J Vet Res 24: 525.

Sun, F. F. 1973. Metabolism of clindamycin. II. Urinary excretion products of clindamycin in rat and dog. J Pharm Sci 62: 1657.

Sund, R. B., and Schou, J. 1964. The determination of absorption rates from rat muscles: An experimental approach to kinetic descriptions. Acta Pharmacol Toxicol (Kbh) 21:313.

Tavernor, W. D. 1971. Muscle relaxants. In L. R. Soma, ed. Textbook of Veterinary Anesthesia, p. 114. Baltimore: Williams & Wilkins.

Theodorides, V. J.; Dicuollo, C. J.; Guarini, J. R.; and Pagano, J. F. 1968. Serum concentrations of chloramphenicol after intraruminal and intra-abomasal administration in sheep. Am J Vet Res 29:643.

Tschudi, P. 1972. Eliminierung, Plasmaproteinbindung und Dosierung einiger Sulfonamide. I. Pferd. Zentralbl Veterinaermed [A] 19:851.

———. 1973. Elimination, Plasmaproteinbindung and Dosierung einiger Sulfonamide. III. Untersuchungen beim Schwein. Zentralbl Veterinaermed [A] 20:155.

Wagner, J. G. 1967. Drug accumulation. J Clin Pharmacol 7:84.

———. 1968a. Pharmacokinetics. Annu Rev Pharmacol 8:67.

———. 1968b. Pharmacokinetics. III. Half-life and volume of distribution. Drug Intell 2:126.

Wagner, J. G., and Metzler, C. M. 1969. Prediction of blood levels after multiple doses from single-dose blood level data: Data generated with two-compartment open model analyzed according to the one-compartment open model. J Pharm Sci 58:87.

Wagner, J. G.; Northam, J. I.; Alway, C. D.; and Carpenter, O. S. 1965. Blood levels of drug at the equilibrium state after multiple dosing. Nature 207:1301.

Weiner, I. M., and Mudge, G. H. 1964. Renal tubular mechanisms for excretion of organic acids and bases. Am J Med 36:743.

Wilbrandt, W., and Rosenberg, T. 1961. The concept of carrier transport and its corollaries in pharmacology. Pharmacol Rev 13:109.

Wilensky, A. J., and Lowden, J. A. 1973. Inadequate serum levels after intramuscular administration of diphenylhydantoin. Neurology 23:318.

Williams, R. T. 1967. Comparative patterns of drug metabolism. Fed Proc 26:1029.

———. 1969. The fate of foreign compounds in man and animals. Pure Appl Chem 18:129.

Yeary, R. A., and Swanson, W. 1973. Aspirin dosages for the cat. J Am Vet Med Assoc 163:1177.

Ziv, G., and Sulman, F. G. 1972. Binding of antibiotics to bovine and ovine serum. Antimicrob Agents Chemother 2:206.

———. 1973a. Serum and milk concentrations of spectinomycin and tylosin in cows and ewes. Am J Vet Res 34:329.

———. 1973b. Penetration of lincomycin and clindamycin into milk in ewes. Br Vet J 129:83.

———. 1974. Distribution of aminoglycoside antibiotics in blood and milk. Res Vet Sci 17:68.

Ziv, G.; Shani, J.; and Sulman, F. G. 1973. Pharmacokinetic evaluation of penicillin and cephalosporin derivatives in serum and milk of lactating cows and ewes. Am J Vet Res 34:1561.

SECTION 3

Drugs Acting on the Autonomic and Somatic Nervous Systems

CHAPTER 6

INTRODUCTION TO THE AUTONOMIC NERVOUS SYSTEM

H. RICHARD ADAMS

INTRODUCTION

The autonomic nervous system is a peripheral complex of efferent and afferent nerves, plexuses, and ganglia that modulate the involuntary activity of secretory glands, smooth muscles, and visceral organs. Historically, this system also has been termed the visceral, involuntary, or vegetative nervous system. The autonomic nervous system reacts to maintain respiration, heart rate, blood pressure, gastrointestinal motility and secretion, urinary output, and virtually all other visceral functions within well-defined physiologic limits. In addition, autonomic activity to various organs can rapidly increase or decrease in response to sudden changes in the environment. Thus the autonomic nervous system functions to sustain homeostatic conditions within an organism during periods of reduced physical and emotional activity and, just as importantly, to assist in internal bodily reactions to stressful circumstances.

The autonomic nervous system occupies a rather unique position in the clinical interrelationships of disease, pathophysiology, and pharmacotherapeutics in that diseases of the autonomic nervous system per se are infrequently encountered in lower animals; and yet drugs that alter autonomic function are commonly used in the clinical practice of veterinary medicine. This is because the physiologic functions of diseased organs can still be influenced by their relatively intact nervous supply and, therefore, may respond to drugs that simulate autonomic effects. Also, autonomic drugs are routinely used during anesthetic and surgical procedures to prevent inadvertent stimulation or depression of autonomic influence on visceral functions.

It is, therefore, apparent that a comprehensive examination of pharmacologic characteristics of the autonomic nervous system is required for a practical understanding of the therapeutic management of various clinical disorders in animals.

ORGANIZATION OF THE AUTONOMIC NERVOUS SYSTEM

The most important components of the autonomic nervous system, in relation to clinical pharmacology, are the outflow (efferent) nerve tracts. Efferent autonomic nerves supply motor innervation to visceral structures. The *efferent* segment of the autonomic nervous system is divided into two principal components: (1) the *sympathetic nervous system* and (2) the *parasympathetic nervous system*. A schematic representation of the sympathetic and parasympathetic outflows is shown in Fig. 6.1.

Sympathetic and parasympathetic outflow tracts comprise (1) *preganglionic neurons* and (2) *postganglionic neurons* (Fig. 6.1). The cell body of a preganglionic neuron is located within the central nervous system (CNS). The synapse (junction) of a preganglionic axon with a postganglionic neuronal body occurs outside the CNS within an autonomic ganglion. Autonomic ganglia are specialized nodular structures comprising numerous ($>$ 100,000) neuronal bodies. An axon of a postganglionic cell passes peripherally and innervates its effector organ or organ substructure. The junction of a postganglionic axonal terminal with its effector organ is termed a *neuroeffector junction*.

Sympathetic Nervous System

The sympathetic nervous system is often synonymously referred to as the *thoracolumbar outflow* due to the anatomic origin of this system (Fig. 6.1). Sympathetic preganglionic fibers (axons) originate from cell bodies that are localized within the intermediolateral columns of the thoracic and lumbar regions of the spinal cord. These fibers are myelinated; they exit the spinal cord with the ventral (anterior) nerve roots and then form bundles (white rami communicantes) before entry into the paravertebral chain of sympathetic ganglia. The gray rami communicantes are composed of nonmyelinated post-ganglionic fibers that exit the sympathetic chain and reenter spinal nerve roots to be distributed to target structures (sweat glands, blood vessels, and hair follicles) within the limbs and body trunk.

The paravertebral (or vertebral) ganglia are located bilaterally to the ventral aspects of the vertebral column. The ganglia on each side are interconnected by nerve fibers to form the *sympathetic ganglionic chain*. This chain extends into the cervical and sacral regions; however, ganglia in these areas receive fibers only from the thoracolumbar spinal cord.

Upon entering the sympathetic ganglionic chain, a preganglionic fiber may terminate in one of several manners. It may synapse with a neuronal body that is located within the immediately adjacent ganglion; it may ascend or descend the sympathetic chain and synapse with a neuron of a distant ganglion; or it may pass through the chain and synapse in a prevertebral ganglion rather than in the vertebral chain. Prevertebral ganglia are located more peripherally than the vertebral chain. Prevertebral ganglia include the celiac, cranial (anterior) mesenteric, and caudal (posterior) mesenteric ganglia. They supply fibers to abdominal and pelvic viscera. Sympathetic control to the head and neck arises from the cranial (anterior, or superior), middle, and caudal (posterior, or inferior) cervical ganglia. Fibers from

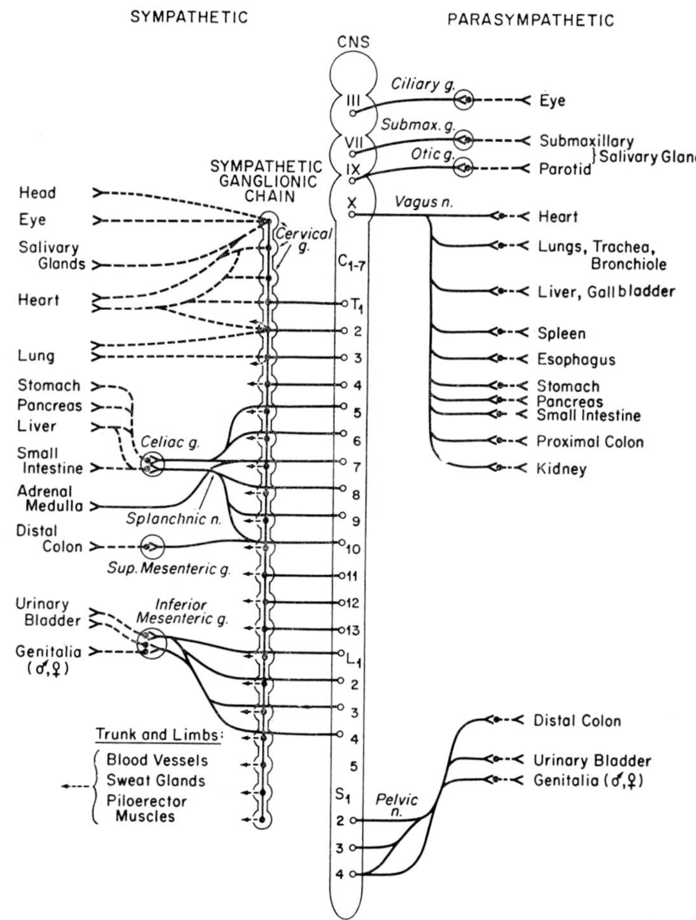

FIG 6.1. Schematic representation of sympathetic and parasympathetic motor innervation of various body organs. Sympathetic fibers and the left sympathetic ganglionic chain are depicted on the left side of the drawing. Parasympathetic fibers are shown on the right side of the drawing. Central nervous system (CNS) preganglionic cell bodies are represented as open circles (o). Ganglionic cell bodies are represented as closed circles (●). Preganglionic fibers are solid lines; postganglionic fibers are dashed lines. The small arrows (←) represent postganglionic sympathetic fibers to blood vessels, sweat glands (cholinergic), and piloerector muscles of the trunk and limbs; these fibers pass peripherally with spinal nerves. g = ganglion. n = nerve.

the cervical ganglia and fibers from the anterior thoracic ganglia innervate the thoracic organs.

Sympathetic postganglionic fibers are as a rule relatively long since most sympathetic ganglia are located in close proximity to the spinal cord. Sympathetic preganglionic fibers may ramify, form plexuses and subsequently synapse with numerous different postganglionic cell bodies. Furthermore, one sympathetic ganglionic neuron may be innervated by preganglionic fibers that originate from several different nerve bodies. Sympathetic discharge may, therefore, affect several different target organs and organ substructures.

The *adrenal medulla* is an extremely important component of the sympathetic nervous system. It is embryologically and functionally homologous to a sympathetic ganglion but does not contain postsynaptic neuronal cells. Instead, secretory *chromaffin cells* are present. They are innervated by typical preganglionic fibers that issue from the midthoracic spinal cord. Adrenal chromaffin cells contain epinephrine and norepinephrine; these hormonal substances are released from the adrenal gland into the circulatory system.

Parasympathetic Nervous System

Parasympathetic outflow tracts originate from the midbrain, the medulla oblongata, and the sacral spinal cord (Fig. 6.1). The parasympathetic component of the autonomic nervous system is, therefore, often referred to anatomically as the *craniosacral outflow.*

The vagus nerve is the tenth cranial nerve, and it is considered to be the most important parasympathetic nerve trunk. It arises from the medulla oblongata and sends efferent fibers to all thoracic and abdominal viscera from the caudal pharyngeal region to the cranial portions of the large colon. Fibers from the spinal accessory nerve (eleventh cranial nerve) may also join the vagus trunk. The facial (seventh cranial nerve) and glossopharyngeal (ninth cranial nerve) nerves arise from the medulla oblongata and carry parasympathetic fibers to various glands and smooth muscles within the head. The third cranial nerve (oculomotor) carries preganglionic efferent fibers from the Edinger-Westphal nucleus of the midbrain to the ciliary ganglion that then supplies postganglionic autonomic motor fibers to ocular structures.

The sacral portion of the parasympathetic system comprises nerve fibers arising from the sacral spinal cord. These fibers form the pelvic nerves; they terminate in ganglion cells located in the colon, bladder, and sex organs.

Parasympathetic ganglia are invariably localized more peripherally than sympathetic ganglia and usually they are close to innervated structures. In many cases, parasympathetic ganglia are actually located within innervated organs. Accordingly, postganglionic parasympathetic fibers are usually quite short. Parasympathetic discharge is usually discrete and may affect specific effector systems individually.

GENERAL CONCEPTS OF AUTONOMIC FUNCTION

Autonomic Interrelationships

Virtually all visceral organs are innervated by nerves from both the parasympathetic and sympathetic divisions (see Fig. 6.1); however, each division produces contrasting effects on the same structure. For example, parasympathetic fibers of the vagus nerve elicit a decrease in heart rate and a diminution of myocardial contractile force. Sympathetic cardiac nerves, on the other hand, accelerate heart rate and increase the strength of myocardial contraction. Such reciprocating relationships allow varying degrees of qualitative as well as quantitative changes in organ function, depending upon the relative needs of the organism. Principal organ responses that are mediated by sympathetic and parasympathetic discharge are summarized in Table 6.1.

If parasympathetic outflow traffic is momentarily hypoactive, sympathetic influence on a particular structure will dominate. The converse is also true. An important example of this type of relationship involves the autonomic control of the digestive tract. Gastrointestinal functions are normally under parasympathetic dominance. Enhanced activity of this division elicits a pronounced increase in gastrointestinal secretion and smooth muscle motility. However, sympathetic nerve traffic causes an inhibition of smooth muscle activity and secretory processes in the gastrointestinal tract. Abolishment of parasympathetic control initially produces a quiescent hypoactive gastrointestinal tract that is characterized by sympathetic dominance. Destruction of sympathetic control to the gastrointestinal tract accentuates parasympathetic activity. However, since the gastrointestinal system is already functioning under slight parasympathetic dominance, removal of sympathetic activity produces a relatively smaller demonstrable change in normal function.

It should be remembered that autonomic nerves modulate organ activity and in many structures do not exert absolute control. In the denervated heart, for example, intrinsic regulatory processes will continue to sustain heart beat and cardiac output, although within less-defined physiologic limits. Similarly, gastrointestinal smooth muscle exhibits rhythmic contractile movements in the absence of autonomic innervation. The fact remains, however, that autonomic nerves mediate

TABLE 6.1. Responses of effector organs to sympathetic and parasympathetic nerve impulses

Effector Organs	Sympathetic-mediated Responses*	Parasympathetic-mediated Responses†
Heart	General excitation	General depression
S-A node	β_1-Increase heart rate	Decrease heart rate
Atria	β_1-Increase contractile force and conduction velocity	Decrease contractile force
A-V node	β_1-Increase conduction velocity	Decrease conduction velocity; A-V block
Ventricles	β_1-Increase contractile force Increase irritability‡	Decrease contractile force§
Blood vessels		
Coronary	β_2-Dilatation;∥ α-constriction	Dilatation
Cutaneous, mucosal	α-Constriction	Dilatation#
Skeletal muscle	β_2-Dilatation;** α-constriction	Dilatation#
Splanchnic	α-Constriction	Dilatation#
Renal	α-Constriction	Dilatation#
Gastrointestinal tract	General inhibition	General excitation
Smooth muscle	α-Relaxation; β-relaxation	Contraction
Sphincters	α-Contraction	Relaxation
Secretions	Decrease	Increase
Bronchial muscle	β_2-Relaxation	Contraction
Kidney renin release	α-Decrease; β-increase	...
Eye		
Pupil	α-Dilatation	Constriction
Radial muscle of iris	α-Contraction	...
Sphincter muscle of iris	...	Contraction
Urinary bladder		
Fundus	β-Relaxation	Contraction
Trigone, sphincter	α-Contraction	Relaxation
Splenic capsule	α-Contraction	...
Salivary glands	α-Thick, viscous secretion	Profuse, watery secretion
Sweat glands	Secretion (cholinergic)†† α-secretion (horse)	...
Piloerector muscles	α-Contraction	...
Adrenal medula	Secretion of epinephrine > norepinephrine (cholinergic)	...
Autonomic ganglia	Ganglionic discharge (cholinergic)	Ganglionic discharge
Liver	β-Glycogenolysis (α in some species?)	...

* Alpha (α) and beta (β) designate the basic type of adrenergic receptor present in a particular tissue. β_1 or β_2 designates, when known, the tentative classification of β receptor subtypes.

† All listed parasympathetic responses are associated with muscarinic receptors except ganglia where nicotinic receptors are predominant. All autonomic ganglia (sympathetic and parasympathetic) are innervated by cholinergic nerve fibers.

‡ Catecholamine-induced irritability of the myocardium may be associated with β_1 and/or α receptors.

§ Although muscarinic receptors are demonstrable in isolated ventricular muscle, the significance is not definitely known. *In vivo,* atrial effects are predominant.

∥ In coronary arteries, β receptors are believed to be predominant and/or to be more sensitive than α receptors to agonists.

Arterial beds are not innervated by the parasympathetic nervous system; thus cholinergic receptors in vascular smooth muscle are not associated with parasympathetic nerve terminals. In certain areas (e.g., blood vessels of skeletal muscles, facial skin), sympathetic cholinergic vasodilator fibers may be present; their physiologic significance is poorly understood.

** In skeletal muscle blood vessels, β receptors are more sensitive than α receptors; thus vasodilatation occurs at low doses of epinephrine, but vasoconstriction occurs with high doses.

†† Sweat glands are innervated "atypically" by postganglionic sympathetic fibers that release acetylcholine rather than norepinephrine. In the horse, however, sweat glands seem to be innervated by adrenergic fibers.

very specific changes that are integrated into the entire nervous system of the organism. A denervated organ thus rarely functions well when sudden changes are required to sustain homeostasis.

Organ Responses to Autonomic Discharge

The sympathetic outflow tract and the closely associated adrenal medulla are often referred to as the sympathoadrenal (or sympathoadrenomedullary) axis. This axis is extremely reactive, and activity varies discretely on a moment-to-moment basis consistent with the needs of the organism. Thus small changes required for homeostasis are readily accomplished. The sympathoadrenal axis may also discharge in a mass or unit action affecting virtually all sympathetically innervated structures. Such a unitary sympathoadrenal discharge occurs in response to severe fear or rage and readies the organism for either "fight or flight." Accordingly, cardiovascular activity is accelerated; an increase in heart rate, myocardial contractile strength, cardiac output, and blood pressure is observed. Also, blood is redistributed from splanchnic and cutaneous beds to voluntary skeletal muscles; bronchiolar pathways dilate and respiration increases; pupils enlarge; and blood glucose concentration increases. The organism is now better prepared to effectively react to the stimulus that instigated the sympathetically mediated fight-or-flight reaction.

The parasympathetic nervous system, on the other hand, functions mainly to regulate localized organ changes and is not organized for mass action. Whereas sympathetic activation results in expenditure of energy, the parasympathetic system reacts to generate and maintain biological energy. Perhaps parasympathetic activity could, therefore, be referred to as a "live-and-let-live" type of response. Digestive breakdown of nutrients, for example, is enhanced by increased parasympathetic activity to the gastrointestinal system. Myocardial oxygen consumption and energy utilization are decreased by vagal-mediated decreases in heart rate and contractile strength of the heart.

How an individual organ will respond to sympathetic or parasympathetic impulse traffic may be foreseen by considering if a particular response would benefit the fight-or-flight response (sympathetic) or the live-and-let-live response (parasympathetic). For example, it is logical that an increase in cardiac output and an increase in skeletal muscle blood flow would be required for an effective reaction to fear or rage. Thus activation of the heart and concurrent relaxation of skeletal muscle blood vessels would be due to sympathetic discharge. Under the same circumstances, less blood would be needed in cutaneous and splanchnic beds; thus vasoconstriction in these areas would also be due to sympathetic discharge.

On the other hand, digestion of foodstuff obviously would not be required for an immediate sympathetic reaction to stressful environmental changes. Thus sympathetic discharge inhibits gastrointestinal activity whereas parasympathetic (live-and-let-live) discharge enhances gastrointestinal function. One apparently contradictory aspect, however, is quite familiar to veterinarians. Occasionally, some animals (e.g., dogs, nonhuman primates) that experience profound fright will exhibit signs of increased intestinal and urinary bladder activity, i.e., defecation and micturition. However, it should be appreciated that in severe incidences of fear it is likely that parasympathetic centers in the brain may be activated by "overspill" of central sympathetic impulses that originate from emotional centers. Thus sympathetic inhibition of intestinal and urinary bladder activity may momentarily be overridden by parasympathetic discharge.

Information Transmission

Information is communicated from nerve to nerve and from nerve to effector organ by a process termed *neurohumoral transmission*. This process involves the release from a nerve terminal of a chemical (neurotransmitter substance), which then reacts with specialized receptor areas on the innervated cell. Interaction of the neurotransmitter with the receptor instigates characteristic physiologic responses in the effector cell. The neurotransmitter at all autonomic (parasympathetic and sympathetic) ganglia and all parasympathetic neuroeffector junctions is acetylcholine. Norepinephrine (noradrenalin) is released at the majority of sympathetic neuroeffector junctions and is considered to be "the" sympathetic neurotransmitter. (At a few sympathetic neuroeffector junctions, e.g., sweat glands, acetylcholine is the transmitter.) Nerves that release acetylcholine are referred to as *cholinergic* nerves. Nerves that release norepinephrine are referred to as *adrenergic* nerves.

The preganglionic and postganglionic relationships of sympathetic and parasympathetic efferent fibers are shown schematically in Fig. 6.2. This figure should be thoroughly studied. Often, difficulty is encountered in correlating classifications of sympathetic and parasympathetic nerves and adrenergic and cholinergic nerves. It should be remembered that an adrenergic nerve is a sympathetic postganglionic nerve. A cholinergic nerve, on the other hand, can be (1) a parasympathetic preganglionic nerve, (2) a parasympathetic postganglionic nerve, and also (3) a sympathetic preganglionic nerve.

Central Integration of Autonomic Activity

Most attention is usually directed toward the efferent adrenergic and cholinergic pathways of the autonomic nervous system. However, the afferent fibers and the brain nucleii that influence peripheral motor function are equally important when physiologic interactions of the autonomic nervous system are considered. For example, afferent fibers transmit information concerning visceral pain, cardiovascular activity, respiration, and numerous other organ functions from peripheral receptive areas to the CNS.

Afferent fibers are usually nonmyelinated and pass into the CNS along autonomic nerve trunks such as the vagus, pelvic, and splanchnic nerves. Sensory fibers, in fact, often make up a considerable portion of autonomic nerve trunks (Paintal 1963). The nerve bodies of sensory afferent fibers are believed to be located in the dorsal root ganglia of spinal nerves and in specialized sensory ganglia of autonomic nerve trunks.

An *autonomic reflex arch* involves (1) the passage of information along an afferent pathway, (2) the reaction of CNS sites to the received impulse, and (3) the resulting change in efferent discharge. Well-known examples involve the baroreceptor (pressure sensitive) areas localized in the

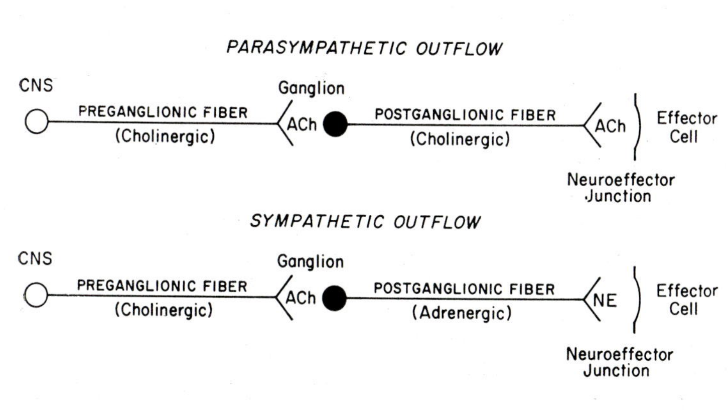

Fig. 6.2. Schematic representation of the preganglionic and postganglonic relationships of sympathetic and parasympathetic outflow tracts. CNS preganglionic nerve bodies are represented as open circles (o). Ganglionic cell bodies are shown as closed circles (●). Acetylcholine (Ach) is the neurotransmitter released at sympathetic and parasympathetic ganglia and at parasympathetic neuroeffector junctions. Norepinephrine (NE) is the neurotransmitter released at adrenergic sympathetic neuroeffector junctions. Cholinergic fibers release ACh. Adrenergic fibers release NE.

aortic arch and carotid sinus, and the chemoreceptive cells localized within the aortic arch and carotid bodies. Information concerning blood pressure, blood O_2 and CO_2, and respiration is relayed from these sites via afferent fibers to CNS areas. Depending upon receipt of afferent impulses, central nuclei alter the discharge of efferent activity accordingly.

Some drugs exert their pharmacologic action principally by altering afferent receptor areas and afferent impulse traffic. The *veratrum alkaloids,* for example, increase impulse traffic along those afferent vagal fibers that arise from the sensory areas in the left ventricle of the heart and the carotid and coronary sinuses (Benforado 1967). A veratrum-induced increase in afferent impulse traffic will misinform the brain that blood pressure and heart rate are greater than normal. Vagal parasympathetic efferent traffic emitting from brain centers are reflexly increased, with bradycardia and hypotension resulting. Efferent impulses along cardiac sympathetic nerves and sympathetic vasoconstrictor fibers are decreased.

Other drugs may also influence afferent autonomic fibers and sensory areas. However, most commonly used autonomic drugs exhibit pharmacologic profiles that can best be explained by changes exerted primarily at peripheral efferent or CNS nerve pathways.

The *hypothalamus* is the principal supraspinal site involved in modulation of both sympathetic and parasympathetic outflow traffic. Posterior and lateral hypothalamic nuclei are primarily sympathetic, whereas medial and anterior nerve bodies are believed to be associated with parasympathetic functions. Autonomic participation in regulation of blood pressure, body temperature, carbohydrate metabolism, water-electrolyte balance, sexual responses, emotions, and sleep is mediated through hypothalamic pathways. The medulla oblongata contains nuclei that integrate blood pressure and the expiratory-inspiratory respiratory phases, often interacting with hypothalamic regions.

Cerebral cortical foci may also influence autonomic activity. The Pavlovian experiments are classic examples of conscious and emotional brain centers affecting peripheral autonomic activity. In these experiments, a dog was repeatedly fed only after the ringing of a bell. Eventually, ringing a bell would evoke an increase in secretory activity of the gastrointestinal tract in anticipation of a meal. Such basic experiments have led numerous research workers to subsequently propose that certain disorders of body viscera may actually represent psychic influence on central autonomic sites rather than organic disease. Central influences on peripheral autonomic function were reviewed by Chase and Clemente (1968).

Numerous drugs have very pronounced effects on central autonomic control centers. The pharmacologic activity of certain drugs, in fact, is characterized by dominant CNS effects rather than peripheral-mediated responses. Amphetamine, for example, affects peripheral adrenergic neuroeffector junctions; however, the overall response to amphetamine in an intact animal is characterized by CNS stimulation. Just the opposite, some drugs that are used for their CNS effects (e.g., tranquilizers) may also have profound peripheral autonomic actions. The promazine family of tranquilizers, for example, may depress blood pressure rather markedly (Popovic et al. 1972) by blocking the interaction of norepinephrine with adrenergic receptor sites in blood vessels. Such peripheral and central interactions should always be kept in mind when the total pharmacologic profile of a drug is evaluated prior to its clinical use.

NEUROHUMORAL TRANSMISSION

Virtually every autonomic drug that is clinically used exerts its primary pharmacologic activities by altering some essential step(s) in the neurohumoral transmission process. In the remaining portions of this chapter, the physiologic steps involved in neurohumoral transmission will be discussed. In subsequent chapters, autonomic drugs that affect the neurohumoral transmission process in the parasympathetic and sympathetic nervous systems will be examined.

General Concepts

The discovery and subsequent characterization of events involved in communication of information from nerve to nerve and from nerve to effector organ represent major scientific achievements. Although numerous investigators have provided various relevant information, the first definitive evidence of chemical neurotransmission seems to have been obtained by Loewi and coworkers (1921, 1926). In these experiments, Loewi electrically stimulated the vagus nerve of an isolated perfused frog heart. The perfusate leaving this preparation was reperfused through another frog heart. Upon stimulation of the vagus nerve to the first heart, Loewi observed that this heart was immediately depressed. Within a few seconds, the second heart was also depressed. Certainly, the most logical explanation for this finding was that stimulation of the vagus nerve liberated a chemical "myocardial inhibitory" substance that was carried in the perfusate to the second heart. This substance, referred to as *Vagusstoff* (vagus-substance), was later identified as acetylcholine.

Similar experiments showed that stimulation of the cardiac accelerator nerves released a myocardial stimulatory substance that was similar in action to the adrenal hormone, epinephrine (adrenalin). Subsequent studies identified the epinephrinelike "adrenergic" transmitter as norepinephrine (noradrenalin), the immediate precursor of epinephrine.

The basic techniques proved by Loewi have been modified and utilized by numerous investigators to map other adrenergic and cholinergic pathways. As previously mentioned, acetylcholine was found to be the chemical released from all (parasympathetic and sympathetic) autonomic preganglionic fibers and from all postganglionic parasympathetic fibers. Norepinephrine is the neurotransmitter released at the majority of sympathetic neuroeffector junctions (see Fig. 6.2).

Several criteria should be met before a chemical can be accepted as a neurotransmitter: (1) stimulation of a nerve should markedly increase the concentration of the active substance in the effluent; (2) the proposed mediator should be chemically and pharmacologically identified and characterized; (3) exogenous administration of the chemical should identically simulate nerve stimulation; (4) other drugs should have basically similar effects on responses to nerve stimulation and the proposed transmitter substance; and (5) cellular mechanisms that are capable of manufacturing, storing in an inactive form, and inactivating the neurotransmitter should be demonstrable. These basic criteria have been challenged as being too rigorous and, in some cases, not necessary (Werman 1966). Currently, however, these stipulations seem to be generally accepted.

Several recent textbooks have presented explicit and finite details of neurohumoral transmission. The reader is referred to these references for critical examinations of proposed neurotransmitter concepts (Bennett 1972; Mandell 1973; Usdin and Snyder 1973; Bennett 1974).

Physiologic Events

Events involved in neurohumoral transmission at ganglionic synapses and at neuroeffector junctions may, for ease of examination, be subdivided into (1) axonal conduction, (2) release of neurotransmitter, (3) receptor events, and (4) catabolism of the neurotransmitter.

axonal conduction

Axonal conduction refers to the passage of an impulse along a nerve fiber. It is dependent upon selective changes in the permeability of the axonal membrane to electrolytes. At rest, membrane potential within mammalian axons is approximately a minus 70 mV. This negative intracellular potential is maintained at rest basically because the axonal membrane is relatively more permeable to K^+ than to Na^+. Sodium ions are in higher concentrations in the extracellular than in the intracellular fluid, whereas potassium ions are in greater concentration in the intracellular than in the extracellular fluid. Thus the relatively small amounts of K^+ that do leak into the interstitial space in conjunction with the large amounts of Na^+ that are extracellular result in a net positive charge outside the cell and, accordingly, a net negative charge within the axon (Curtis and Cole 1942; Bullock and Hagiwara 1957).

An action potential represents a reversal of the polarization state that is present at rest and is, therefore, a depolarization process. Functionally, an action potential represents the permeability changes that occur at the axonal surface as an impulse is propagated along a nerve fiber. A suprathreshold stimulus initiates a localized change in the permeability of the axonal membrane. Suddenly, the permeability of the fiber to Na^+ is greatly increased in relation to K^+; Na^+ moves inward and K^+ moves outward in the direction of their respective concentration gradients. Electrically, this electrolyte movement is detected by an instantaneous change in the membrane potential in a positive direction. The positive charged sodium ions increase in concentration within the axon; the membrane potential moves from a minus 70 mV toward zero and then overshoots to the extent that momentarily the inside of the fiber is positive in relation to the exterior of the cell.

Repolarization of the membrane occurs rapidly as the selective membrane permeability characteristics of the axonal membrane are quickly reestablished after the passage of an action potential. The axon once again becomes relatively impermeable to Na^+ and relatively more permeable to K^+, and the negativity of the interior of the cell is quickly reestablished. A schematic representation of axonal conductance and resulting neurohumoral transmission events is presented in Fig. 6.3.

Although the localized permeability changes associated with an action potential are extremely short-lived, these changes elicit similar alterations in membrane function in immediately adjacent quiescent areas of the axon. Thus the action potential is self-propagating and in this manner an action potential is conducted along an axonal fiber. Over long periods, the absolute concentration gradients of electrolytes are maintained by energy-utilizing transport systems such as the sodium pump. The axonal membrane is refractory for a brief interval after the passage of an action potential, thereby preventing antidromic and excess impulse trafffic.

Axonal conduction is insensitive to most drugs. Even the local anesthetics must be used in high concentrations in immediate contact with the nerve before ex-

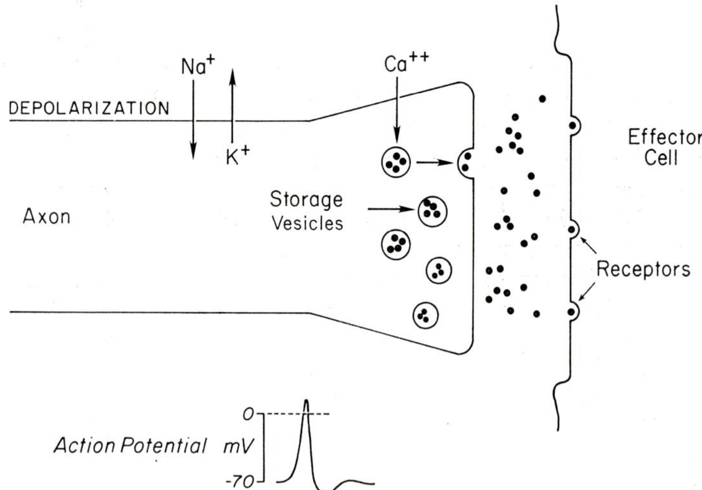

FIG. 6.3. Schematic representation of neurohumoral transmission. The axonal action potential represents a self-propagating depolarization of the axon that is characterized by an influx of Na^+ and an efflux of K^+. As the action potential arrives at the nerve terminal, it facilitates an inward movement of Ca^{++}. Ca^{++} triggers the discharge of neurotransmitter (●) from storage vesicles into the junctional cleft. Neurotransmitter reacts with specialized receptor areas on the postjunctional membrane and initiates a physiologic response in the effector cell.

citability is blocked. However, subsequent events in neurohumoral transmission are quite susceptible to drug actions. Physiologic and pharmacologic aspects of axonal conductance have been reviewed (Katz 1966; Cole 1968).

NEUROTRANSMITTER RELEASE

Release of neurotransmitter substance is triggered by the arrival of the axonal action potential at the nerve terminal (Fig. 6.3) where neurotransmitters are stored in vesicular structures (Klein 1973; Winkler and Hörtnagl 1973). Upon arrival of an action potential, the nerve terminal suddenly releases large quantities of transmitter. The actual mechanism(s) of transmitter release is not completely known; however, the imperative participation of calcium ions (Ca^{++}) in the excitation-secretion coupling process is established beyond a doubt (Douglas and Rubin 1961; Burn and Gibbons 1965). Calcium ions act to link or couple the excitation of the membrane (action potential) with the discharge of neurotransmitter from the nerve terminal. The sources of these Ca^{++} are believed to be the interstitial space and/or superficial membrane binding sites at the axonal terminal. The action potential initiates an inward movement of Ca^{++} into the nerve terminal from these sites. The inward movement of Ca^{++} somehow triggers the discharge of neurotransmitter from the vesicles into the junctional cleft (Hubbard 1971; Bogdanski 1973).

RECEPTOR EVENTS

The processes involved in association of transmitter with autonomic receptor areas are poorly understood. After rapid migration of neurotransmitter across the cleft, the mediator substance forms some type of bond with receptive areas on the postsynaptic membrane. Receptors may be considered simply as those portions of the cell that a neurotransmitter interacts with to elicit a response. Receptors are usually envisioned as specialized macromolecular structures; however, receptors have yet to be satisfactorily isolated.

Receptor events that are caused by interaction of transmitter substance with the receptor may be of two general types: *excitatory* or *inhibitory*. If the neurotransmitter initiates an excitatory response in the cell, receptor activation triggers a general increase in permeability of the postsynaptic membrane to all ions. Thus, in a manner analogous to the axonal action potential, there is a sudden depolarization of the postsynaptic membrane that is characterized by a net inward movement of Na^{+} and an efflux of K^{+} along their respective concentration gradients. Electrically, these changes are characterized as an excitatory postsynaptic potential (EPSP). The EPSP then propagates localized permeability changes in adjacent portions of the cell membrane and an action potential is conducted along the remainder of the innervated cell.

An inhibitory postsynaptic potential (IPSP), on the other hand, occurs when the neurotransmitter initiates a selective increase in permeability of the postsynaptic membrane to only smaller ions (e.g., K^{+}, Cl^{-}). Thus outward movement of K^{+} and inward movement of Cl^{-} along their respective concentration gradients increase the net negative charge within the cell and actually hyperpolarize the postsynaptic membrane. The resulting hyperpolarization of the membrane increases the threshold to stimuli and, in effect, elicits an inhibitory response in the cell.

CATABOLISM OF NEUROTRANSMITTER

Termination of the duration of action of released neurotransmitter substances involves different mechanisms. The adrenergic neurotransmitter, norepinephrine, is metabolized by both intraneuronal and extraneuronal enzymes. However, the uptake of norepinephrine back into the adrenergic nerve terminal and the diffusion of norepinephrine away from receptor sites are probably more important pathways for termination of norepinephrine activity. Extraneuronal acetylcholine is rapidly hydrolyzed by acetylcholinesterase, a quite specific enzyme that is localized in close proximity to the synaptic cleft.

ADRENERGIC NEUROHUMORAL TRANSMISSION

Physiologic and pharmacologic aspects of adrenergic neurohumoral transmission processes are intensely investigated by laboratories located throughout the world. For critical examination of adrenergic mechanisms, the interested reader is referred to the lengthy and detailed volume edited by Usdin and Snyder (1973).

CATECHOLAMINES

Norepinephrine, epinephrine, and dopamine are endogenous catecholamines; they are the sympathetic neural and humoral transmitter substances in most mammalian species. Norepinephrine and dopamine are believed to transmit impulse information in specific areas within the CNS; norepinephrine is also the neurotransmitter at most peripheral sympathetic neuroeffector junctions. Perhaps epinephrine should be thought of as a hormone rather than a neurohumoral transmitter; it is the major hormone released from the adrenal medulla. Catecholamines are stored in an inactive form within granular structures in adrenergic nerve terminals and chromaffin cells (Hokfelt 1973).

SYNTHESIS

It should be emphasized that although the names of the enzymes involved in catecholamine synthesis often imply specificity, these enzymes are usually nonspecific and will catalyze similar types of reactions with other similarly structured substrates (Usdin and Snyder 1973). Norepinephrine is synthesized from the amino acid phenylalanine in a stepwise process as summarized in Fig. 6.4. The aromatic ring of phenylalanine is hydroxylated by the action of an enzyme, phenylalanine hydroxylase; this reaction yields tyrosine. Tyrosine is converted to dihydroxyphenylalanine (DOPA) by the enzyme, tyrosine hydroxylase. This reaction involves additional hydroxylation of the benzene ring, and it is believed to represent the rate-limiting step in catecholamine synthesis.

Dopa is decarboxylated by the enzyme L-aromatic amino acid decarboxylase (dopa

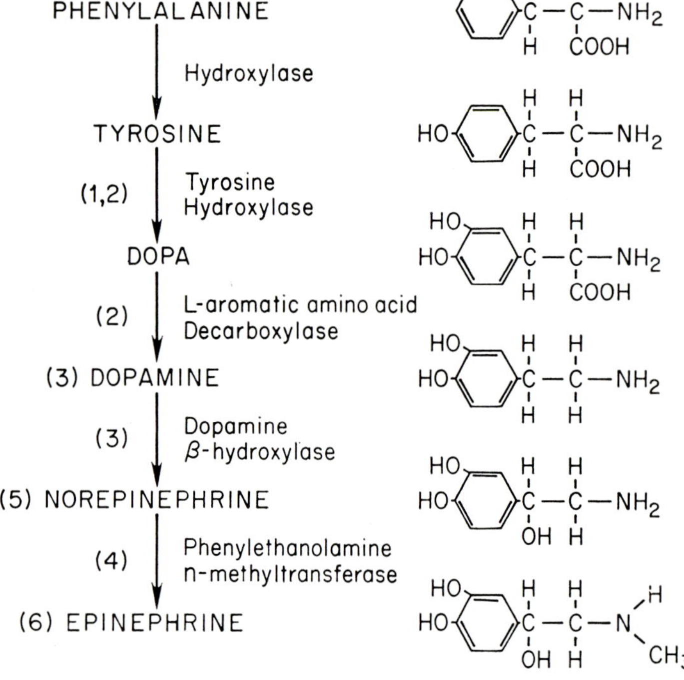

FIG. 6.4. The biosynthetic pathway of norepinephrine and epinephrine. *(1)* = the rate-limiting step; *(2)* = occurs within axoplasm; *(3)* = occurs within amine storage granule; *(4)* = occurs primarily within cytoplasm of adrenal medullary chromaffin cells; *(5)* = stored primarily within amine storage granule of adrenergic neurons; (6) = stored within amine storage granule of chromaffin cells.

decarboxylase) to dihydroxyphenylethylamine (dopamine). The conversion of tyrosine to dopa to dopamine is believed to occur within the cytoplasm. Dopamine is taken up into the storage granule. In some central anatomic sites (e.g., mammalian extrapyramidal system), dopamine seems to act as the primary neurotransmitter rather than its metabolites, norepinephrine and epinephrine (Aghajanian and Bunney 1973; Bartholini et al. 1973).

In peripheral adrenergic neurons and adrenal medullary chromaffin cells, intragranular dopamine is hydroxylated in the β position of the aliphatic side chain by dopamine-β-hydroxylase to form norepinephrine. In the adrenal medulla, norepinephrine is released from the granules of chromaffin cells and is *N*-methylated within the cytoplasm by phenylethanolamine *N*-methyltransferase to form epinephrine. Epinephrine is subsequently localized in what seems to be another type of intracellular storage granule prior to its release from the adrenal medulla.

STORAGE, RELEASE, REUPTAKE, AND METABOLISM

The physiologic events involved in adrenergic neurotransmission and the susceptibility of these events to pharmacologic agents are outlined schematically in Fig. 6.5. Storage within the granular vesicles is accomplished by complexation of the catecholamines with adenosine triphosphate (ATP) and a specific protein, chromogranin. This complexation renders the amines inactive until their release (Shore 1972).

According to many researchers, the amine storage process represents a net result of several subtle functional interrelationships. For example, the intragranular pool of norephinephrine consists of (1) a tightly bound fraction (ATP-protein complex) that acts as a reservoir and (2) a more mobile pool. The mobile intragranular pool may represent amine that is in transit to or from complexation with the ATP-specific protein system; it may also represent "newly synthesized" norepinephrine. Catecholamines are taken up from the cytoplasm into the granules by an active transport system that is ATP and Mg^{++} dependent. The intragranular pool of norepinephrine is believed to be the principal source of neurotransmitter that is released upon nerve stimulation.

The cytoplasmic amine pool is not bound. It is probably made up of amine that has leaked from the granules or that has been taken up from the extracellular space. Amines within the cytoplasm may be taken up by the granules for storage or they may be inactivated by a deaminating enzyme, monoamine oxidase (MAO), that is located in the neuronal mitochrondria. Intracytoplasmic dopamine may also be deaminated by MAO.

A very active amine uptake system is present in the axonal membrane of postganglionic sympathetic nerve terminals. This transport system is Na^+ and energy dependent and it functions to recapture or reuptake catecholamines that have been released from the nerve. Furthermore, exogenously administered norepinephrine and epinephrine are taken up into sympathetic nerve endings by this uptake process (Bogdanski 1973; Iversen 1973). Conservation of catecholamine neurotransmitters by reuptake represents one of the first examples of "recycling" used products.

All the physiologic events necessary for release of adrenergic neurohormones have not been completely defined. In the adrenal chromaffin cells, acetylcholine released from the preganglionic axon acts on specific receptors resulting in depolarization of the membrane. Membrane depolarization of the chromaffin cell enhances the influx of Ca^{++}, which then instigates the discharge of granular constituents into the interstitial fluid to be carried into the circulation (Douglas and Rubin 1961).

Excitation-secretion coupling and release of norepinephrine from adrenergic nerve terminals are similarly dependent upon an inward movement of Ca^{++} (Burn and Gibbons 1965; Bogdanski 1973). Released norepinephrine migrates across the synaptic cleft and interacts with specific

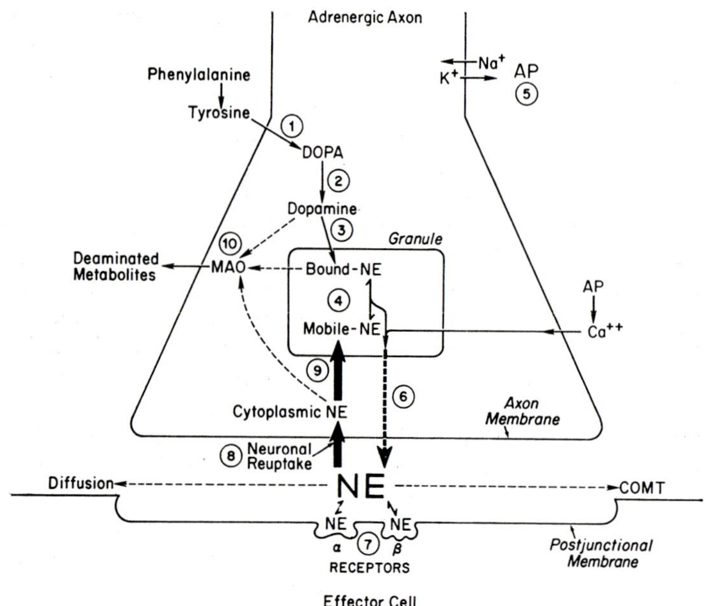

FIG. 6.5. Neurohumoral transmission at the adrenergic neuroeffector junction: proposed physiologic pathways and sites of action susceptible to modification by pharmacologic agents. *1.* Tyrosine is hydroxylated to dopa. This reaction, considered to be the rate-limiting step in catecholamine synthesis, is inhibited by α-methyl-*p*-tyrosine. *2.* Dopa is decarboxylated to dopamine. Dopa decarboxylase inhibitors (e.g., α-methyldopa) inhibit this step. *3.* Dopamine is taken up into the storage granules and is oxidized to norepinephrine (NE). α-Methyldopamine inhibits conversion of dopamine to NE and is converted to α-methylnorepinephrine. α-Methyl NE is then stored in the granule and upon nerve stimulation may be released as a "false neurotransmitter." *4.* Norepinephrine is stored in the granule in a bound and free (mobile) form. Tyraminelike drugs release NE from adrenergic neurons. *5.* The axonal action potential (AP) is a self-propagating depolarization process that upon reaching the nerve terminal increases influx of Ca^{++}, which then triggers the discharge of NE from the nerve terminal. Bretylium inhibits this step. *6.* Norepinephrine is released from the neuron via exocytotic emptying of the contents of the storage granules into the junctional cleft. Newly synthesized NE may be preferentially released. *7.* Released NE reacts with receptor sites on the postjunctional membrane of the effector cell. This step is blocked by adrenergic blocking agents (e.g., α-phentolamine, β-propranolol). Receptive areas (that modify NE release) may also be located on the prejunctional membrane of the nerve terminal (see Fig. 6.7). *8.* Extraneuronal NE can be taken back up into the nerve terminal by an active Na^+-dependent uptake process. This step is inhibited by cocaine and imipraminelike drugs. Extraneuronal NE may also diffuse from the junction or be catabolized by catechol-O-methyltransferase (COMT). *9.* Cytoplasmic NE may be taken up into the granule by a Mg^{++}-ATP–dependent uptake process. Reserpinelike drugs inhibit this step. *10.* Monoamine oxidase (MAO) can deaminate cytoplasmic norepinephrine and dopamine. MAO inhibitors (e.g., pargyline) suppress this step.

The bold dashed line represents release of NE from the granular pool into the junctional cleft. Small dashed lines denote catabolic pathways. Bold solid lines indicate uptake processes. Double-headed arrows indicate reversible pathways.

adrenergic receptor sites on the postsynaptic membrane. The duration of action of norepinephrine may be terminated by (in descending order of importance) (1) active reuptake into the nerve across the axoplasmic membrane (the amine reuptake pump), (2) diffusion from the cleft space via the extracellular fluid, or (3) metabolic breakdown by an extraneuronal enzyme, catechol-O-methyltransferase (COMT). The activity of COMT involves methylation of one of the ring hydroxyl groups (3-OH).

Norepinephrine that has been taken back into the nerve may be restored in granules, or it may be deaminated by MAO. Deamination of norepinephrine or epinephrine by MAO initially yields the corresponding aldehyde, which in turn is further oxidized to 3,4-dihydroxymandelic acid. Alternatively, the 3-hydroxyl group of norepinephrine and epinephrine can first be methylated by COMT to yield normetanephrine and metanephrine, respectively. The O-methylated or deaminated metabolites can then be acted upon by the other enzyme to yield 3-methoxy-4-hydroxymandelic acid. The deaminated O-methylated metabolites can then be conjugated with sulfate or glucuronide prior to excretion by the kidneys. The structural steps involved in catabolism of norepinephrine and epinephrine have been summarized by Goth (1974).

PHARMACOLOGIC CONSIDERATIONS

Many drugs exert their pharmacologic activity by altering the synthesis, storage, and release mechanisms of the catecholamines (Usdin and Snyder 1973). Most of these agents are used in human beings to control hypertension or to affect central autonomic centers (e.g., tranquilization, antidepression, antiparkinsonism). Few of these drugs are commonly employed in clinical veterinary medicine. It seems important to briefly mention some of these drugs, however, since they are often used as "model" drugs in research to characterize the mechanism of action of new drugs that are intended for clinical veterinary use.

Certain drugs act as false substrates for the catecholamine synthesizing enzymes. Alpha-methyl-para-tyrosine, for example, inhibits tyrosine hydroxylase, the rate-limiting step in norepinephrine formation. Thus norephinephrine stores are not replenished by newly synthesized norepinephrine. Alpha-methyldopa may be converted to α-methyldopamine to α-methylnorepinephrine by dopa decarboxylase and dopamine-β-hydroxylase, respectively. The α-methylnorepinephrine may be stored in granules, replace granular stores of norepinephrine, and be released upon nerve stimulation. However, the α-methyl derivative seems to be a less effective agonist than norepinephrine. It may, therefore, act as a "false transmitter" (Kopin 1968).

Reserpinelike drugs block the granular uptake process (Shore 1972). Catecholamine stores are depleted and adrenergic functions are markedly altered by prolonged treatment with even small doses of reserpine (Adams et al. 1971, 1972). Guanethidine may slowly deplete norepinephrine and interfere with its release. Bretylium blocks the neuronal release of neurotransmitter. The new experimental drug, 6-hydroxydopamine, produces a functional peripheral sympathectomy apparently by destroying adrenergic nerve terminals (Gauthier et al. 1974).

Other drugs (e.g., cocaine, imipramine) inhibit the neuronal reuptake process so that released norepinephrine is available for a longer period for reaction with receptor sites. Inhibition of MAO by drugs may result in accumulation of catecholamines. Drugs like tyramine and amphetamine release intraneuronal stores of catecholamines.

Most adrenergic drugs that are important to clinical veterinary medicine act by activating or blocking the postsynaptic adrenergic receptors.

ADRENERGIC RECEPTORS

The interaction of neurohormone with an adrenergic receptor (i.e., adrenoceptor) may elicit either an excitatory or inhibitory response in different sympathetically innervated structures. Following the isolation and identification of norepinephrine as the adrenergic neurotransmitter at these sites, attention was directed to differences in postsynaptic events that might explain such contrasting results. Based on the relative potencies of a series of catecholamines in producing excitatory and inhibitory effects, Ahlquist (1948) proposed that there were two basic types of adrenergic receptors: α and β. In most tissues α-receptor activation elicits an excitatory response, and β receptors mediate an inhibitory response. Major exceptions to this rule include the heart, where β adrenoceptors mediate excitatory responses, and the intestinal smooth muscle, where α receptors instigate relaxation. Epinephrine is the most potent α-receptor stimulant, norepinephrine is intermediate, and isoproterenol is the least active. On the other hand, isoproterenol is the most potent β-receptor agonist, epinephrine is intermediate, and norepinephrine is least active. Epinephrine is, therefore, classified as a mixed α-β agonist, whereas isoproterenol is virtually a pure β agonist with little if any α-receptor effects. Norepinephrine is primarily an α agonist; however, norepinephrine does activate the excitatory β receptors in the heart.

The concept of dissimilar adrenoceptors has been strongly supported by observations that certain adrenergic antagonists block only the α or β receptors (Moran 1973). Furthermore, recent studies with selective antagonists and agonists have demonstrated that β receptors may be divided into subtypes. Confusion over the classification of β receptors was clarified somewhat by the tentative subclassification of β receptors as β_1 or β_2 (Lands et al. 1967). β_1 receptors are located in the heart, and they are associated with excitatory responses. Isoproterenol, epinephrine, and norepinephrine activate β_1 adrenoceptors. β_2 receptors are localized in vascular smooth muscle and bronchiolar smooth muscle; they instigate inhibitory (relaxant) effects. Norepinephrine has little effect on β_2 receptors, whereas epinephrine and isoproterenol are very active at β_2 receptor sites.

Summarization of the presence of α, β_1, and β_2 receptors in different sympathetically innervated organs, where known, is presented in Table 6.1. The designation of receptors as α or β is now accepted. However, subclassification of β receptors into a β_1 or β_2 subtype should be considered as a "working" hypothesis at the present time.

CHOLINERGIC NEUROTRANSMISSION

Acetylcholine is the neurotransmitter substance at parasympathetic neuroeffector junctions, autonomic ganglia, the adrenal medulla, somatic myoneural junctions, and probably certain CNS regions. Brimblecombe (1974) recently reviewed peripheral and central aspects of cholinergic mechanisms. Neurohumoral transmission processes seem to be basically quite similar at all cholinergic junctions. Autonomic ganglionic and somatic myoneural transmission will be discussed in greater detail in subsequent chapters.

SYNTHESIS, STORAGE, RELEASE, AND CATABOLISM OF ACETYLCHOLINE

Acetylcholine is synthesized within cholinergic nerves by the enzymatic transfer of an acetyl group from acetylcoenzyme A to choline. This reaction is catalyzed by the enzyme cholineacetylase (also referred to as choline acetyltransferase), which is summarized in Fig. 6.6. The acetylcoenzyme A is formed by the action of an enzyme, acetyl kinase, which mediates the transfer of an acetyl group from adenyl-

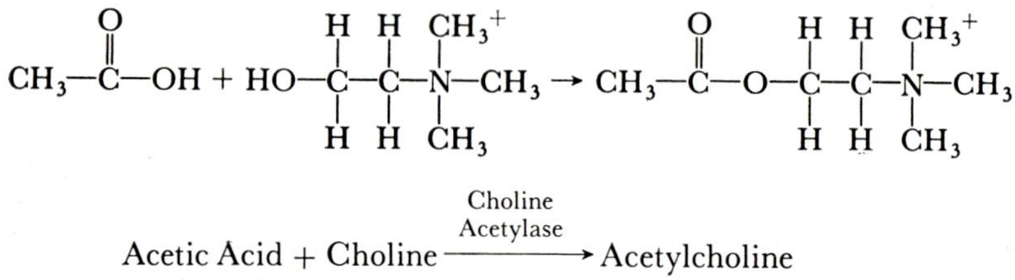

$$CH_3{-}\overset{O}{\overset{\|}{C}}{-}OH + HO{-}\underset{H}{\overset{H}{\overset{|}{\underset{|}{C}}}}{-}\underset{H}{\overset{H}{\overset{|}{\underset{|}{C}}}}{-}\underset{CH_3}{\overset{CH_3^+}{\overset{|}{\underset{|}{N}}}}{-}CH_3 \rightarrow CH_3{-}\overset{O}{\overset{\|}{C}}{-}O{-}\underset{H}{\overset{H}{\overset{|}{\underset{|}{C}}}}{-}\underset{H}{\overset{H}{\overset{|}{\underset{|}{C}}}}{-}\underset{CH_3}{\overset{CH_3^+}{\overset{|}{\underset{|}{N}}}}{-}CH_3$$

$$\text{Acetic Acid} + \text{Choline} \xrightarrow{\text{Choline Acetylase}} \text{Acetylcholine}$$

FIG. 6.6. Formation of acetylcholine involving choline acetylase, choline, and acetic acid.

acetate (formed from acetate and ATP) to the coenzyme A molecule. Choline is transported from the extracellular fluid into the cholinergic nerve by an energy-requiring axoplasmic uptake process. Acetylcholine is stored within axonal vesicular structures in either a concentrated solution or bound to membranes, or both. Intraneuronal stores of acetylcholine have been functionally classified as "more readily releasable" and "less readily releasable." These terms may relate to the free and bound pools, respectively.

Acetylcholine is released from the nerve terminal upon arrival of an axonal action potential. Depolarization of the nerve terminal membrane instigates Ca^{++} influx, which triggers the release of large quanta of acetylcholine from storage sites (Katz and Miledi 1965).

Acetylcholine that is within the junctional space is rapidly inactivated by hydrolysis by a specific enzyme, acetylcholinesterase. Acetylcholinesterase is present in cholinergic nerves, autonomic ganglia, and neuromuscular and neuroeffector junctions. A somewhat similar enzyme, pseudocholinesterase (butyrocholinesterase), is present in various body tissues.

CHOLINERGIC RECEPTORS

There are two basic types of cholinergic receptors within the peripheral efferent autonomic nerve tracts: nicotinic and muscarinic. Early studies demonstrated that small doses of nicotine mimicked certain actions of acetylcholine, and large doses inhibited the same acetylcholine responses. The nicotinic responsive sites were found to be present in autonomic ganglia, adrenal medullary chromaffin cells, and also the neuromuscular junction of the somatic nervous system. Accordingly, these sites have been referred to as *nicotinic cholinergic receptors.*

Nicotine does not, however, simulate or block the action of acetylcholine at the parasympathetic neuroeffector junctions in heart muscle, smooth muscle, and secretory glands. The plant alkaloid muscarine was found to simulate the activity of acetylcholine at these sites but not at the previously described nicotinic receptors. *Muscarinic receptors,* therefore, designate the type of receptor present at cholinergic neuroeffector junctions.

A nicotinic response usually denotes an excitatory response, whereas muscarinic receptor activation may elicit an excitatory (e.g., in gastrointestinal tract) or inhibitory (e.g., in heart muscle) response. As previously discussed, this seems to be related to either a general increase in permeability to all ions (depolarization-excitatory) or to a selective increase in permeability to small ions like K^+ (hyperpolarization-inhibitory), respectively.

Pharmacologic Considerations

A wide variety of chemical and biological agents affect cholinergic neurotransmission. The synthesis of acetylcholine is inhibited by hemicholinium, which blocks the entrance of choline into the cholinergic nerve. Botulinum toxin interferes with the release of acetylcholine. The plant alkaloids nicotine and muscarine have been mentioned in the preceding paragraph. Atropine and related alkaloids block muscarinic receptors, whereas curare blocks nicotonic receptor sites. The activity of endogenous and exogenous acetylcholine is markedly augmented by many chemicals that act as cholinesterase inhibitors (anticholinesterase agents). The therapeutic importance of cholinergic and anticholinergic agents will be discussed in a subsequent chapter.

CHOLINERGIC LINK IN ADRENERGIC NEUROTRANSMISSION

Several investigators have proposed that acetylcholine may also participate in adrenergic neurotransmission. This theory, originally proposed by Burn and Rand (1959, 1965), states that the axonal action potential releases acetylcholine from intraneuronal vesicles of the *sympathetic nerve terminal.* The released acetylcholine is not in sufficient quantity to activate nearby postsynaptic cholinergic receptors. However, it does affect the axonal terminal via activation of nicotinic-type receptors resulting in a release of norepinephrine. The released norepinephrine then acts on postsynaptic adrenergic receptors. Available evidence in support of this theory has been obtained by several different laboratories; however, this concept has not received worldwide acceptance at this time.

AUTONOMIC RECEPTOR SITES ON NERVE TERMINALS

Several studies have presented evidence that immediately released acetylcholine from the cholinergic nerve may not exert its primary action on postsynaptic sites (Koelle 1962). It has been proposed that the nerve action potential mediates the release of only a small amount of acetylcholine that by itself is inadequate to activate postsynaptic receptors. Instead, this initial release of acetylcholine may primarily act to depolarize the cholinergic nerve terminal. Acetylcholine-mediated depolarization of the nerve terminal would lead to additional release of greater quanta of acetylcholine, which would then activate the postsynaptic receptors (Volle and Koelle 1961). This theory is supported, in part, by the finding that in some tissues acetylcholinesterase is primarily located at the axoplasmic membrane of the axonal terminals (Koelle and Koelle 1969). The presynaptic scheme of acetylcholine-mediated release of neurotransmitter is also viewed as being operative in the proposed cholinergic link in adrenergic neurotransmission. Indeed, evidence is continuing to be obtained that indicates the presence of several different receptor sites on autonomic nerve terminals.

As mentioned, Burn and Rand (1959, 1965) proposed the existence of nicotinic-type cholinergic receptors at adrenergic nerve terminals that act to release norepinephrine. Several laboratories have now reported the presence of muscarinic cholinergic receptors at adrenergic nerve terminals as well as the nicotinic sites (Muscholl 1973). Muscarinic receptor activation, however, actually results in inhibition of the release of norepinephrine. Recently, prostaglandin has been shown to decrease the release of norepinephrine from adrenergic nerves; these results were interpreted as evidence for an inhibitory presynaptic prostaglandin receptor (Horton 1973).

In addition, it now seems that there are α-adrenoceptive sites on adrenergic nerve terminals as well as the cholinergic (nicotinic and muscarinic) and prostaglandin receptors (Rand et al. 1973; Starke 1973). The prejunctional α receptors, when activated, cause a decrease in the amount of norepinephrine that is released upon nerve stimulation. The function of these α sites has been envisioned as a local feedback control mechanism through which norepinephrine may inhibit its own release once a threshold concentration has been been obtained in the junctional space (Langer 1973). A schematic representation of proposed prejunctional receptors and their effects in adrenergic nerves is presented in Fig. 6.7.

It is very tempting to speculate on the physiologic significance and implications of such local inhibitory feedback mechanisms. However, although these extremely complex interrelationships most likely exist, neither the complete physiologic nor pharmacologic significance of presynaptic receptors has been definitely established at this time.

PUTATIVE NEUROHUMORAL SUBSTANCES

Biological substances other than acetylcholine and the catecholamines have been proposed as probable (putative) neurotransmitter substances (Koelle 1970). Histamine, for example, has been suggested as a potential neurotransmitter at certain peripheral and CNS sites; however, the existence of peripheral histaminergic nerves has not been definitely established. On the other hand, histamine is known to be concentrated in certain autonomic centers within the brain (e.g., hypothalamus). Also, histamine-synthesizing and histamine-metabolizing enzymes are present within the

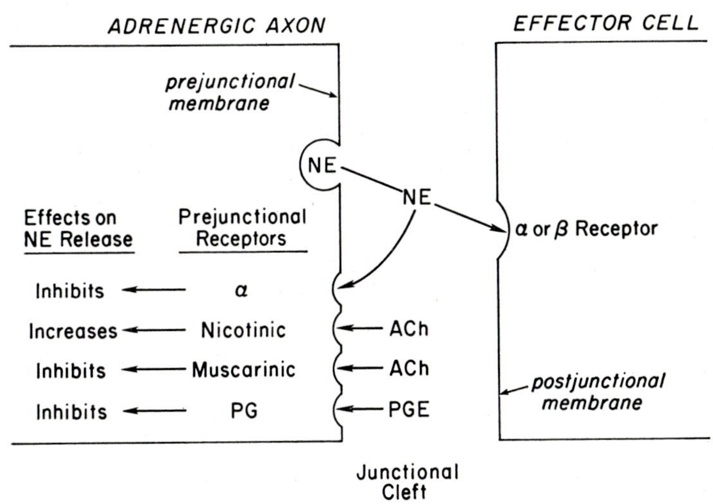

FIG. 6.7. Proposed prejunctional receptor areas on the adrenergic nerve terminal. Release of norepinephrine (NE) from adrenergic nerves may be influenced by receptors that are located on the nerve terminal. Acetylcholine (ACh) may act on nicotinic cholinergic receptors to facilitate NE release (i.e., Burn and Rand theory). ACh may also act at muscarinic cholinergic receptors to inhibit release of NE. Prostaglandin (PGE) may act on prostaglandin (PG) receptive areas to inhibit release of NE. Norepinephrine itself may act on prejunctional α receptors to inhibit (in a local feedback mechanism?) the subsequent release of additional amounts of NE.

CNS. It seems likely that histamine in some way acts as a neurotransmitter in certain specific neural pathways; however, this thesis remains to be conclusively proved.

Considerable evidence has suggested that serotonin (5-hydroxytryptamine) acts as a neurotransmitter in specific brain centers and perhaps in some peripheral nerves. The functional consequences of tryptaminergic transmission have not been completely defined, but it is very likely that 5-hydroxytryptamine participates in thermoregulation, sleep cycles, and extrapyramidal influences on motor control of skeletal muscles. Gamma aminobutyric acid (GABA) has been proposed as an inhibitory neurotransmitter at certain CNS sites. Recently, the presence of noncholinergic and nonadrenergic inhibitory innervation to the gut was proposed (Burnstock 1972). These fibers, referred to as purinergic nerves, are believed to release substances that are structurally related to adenosine triphosphate (ATP).

Although several putative neurotransmitter substances are believed to be involved in information transfer in the central and peripheral nervous systems, the fact remains that the pharmacologic activity of most autonomic drugs and numerous centrally acting agents can best be explained by actions on cholinergic or adrenergic pathways. However, it now seems almost certain that transmitters other than acetylcholine and the catecholamines play important roles that remain to be clearly elucidated in nervous system function.

INVOLVEMENT OF CYCLIC AMP IN AUTONOMIC FUNCTION

Physiologic events involved in neurohumoral transmission have been well characterized, as previously outlined. Until recent times, relatively little has been known concerning the linkage of receptor activation with the resultant physiologic responses of the cell. Considerable evidence has now accumulated indicating that adenosine 3,5-monophosphate (cyclic AMP), a cyclic nucleotide, may act as a "second messenger" to link certain agonist-receptor interactions with cellular responses (Sutherland and Rall 1960a,b; Robison et al. 1967, 1971).

Cyclic AMP is formed from adenosine triphosphate (ATP) by the catalytic action of the enzyme adenylate cyclase. Cyclic AMP is broken down to 5′-adenosinemonophosphate by another enzyme, phosphodiesterase. Adenylate cyclase is believed to be localized in the cell membrane in those mammalian cells that contain the cyclic AMP system. It has been strongly suggested that adenylate cyclase itself may actually be the β-adrenergic receptor. Alternatively, it has been proposed that adenylate cyclase represents at least a portion of the β receptor and may also be very closely related to numerous hormonal receptor sites. This theory has been challenged and currently it remains equivocal. The fact remains, however, that changes in the intracellular concentration of cyclic AMP can often be correlated with the activity of autonomic drugs and hormones.

It is known, for example, that the adrenergic drugs norepinephrine, epinephrine, and isoproterenol increase the concentration of cyclic AMP in the liver. This effect is mediated through an activation or acceleration of the activity of adenylate cyclase. Isoproterenol, primarily a β agonist, has the greatest effect, whereas norepinephrine, primarily an α agonist, has the least potent action. These relationships correspond closely with catecholamine-mediated glycogenolysis in the hepatocytes, which has now been attributed to cyclic AMP-mediated increase in phosphorylase activity.

Alteration of adenylate cyclase and resultant change in cyclic AMP by various adrenergic drugs have been demonstrated in numerous other mammalian tissues including spleen; kidney; brain; adipose cells; and cardiac, skeletal, and smooth muscles. An increase in the tissue concentration of cyclic AMP is generally associated with β-receptor activation, whereas a decrease in cyclic AMP seems to be mediated by a α receptors. Numerous endocrine hormones may also act via alteration of tissue levels of cyclic AMP (see Section 8).

The interrelationship of β adrenoceptors and cyclic AMP has been intensely studied in heart muscle. Catecholamines increase the concentration of cyclic AMP in the myocardium by activating adenylate cyclase. Increases in cyclic AMP correspond with an increase in heart rate and contractile strength. Thus it has been suggested that the effects of catecholamines in the heart are carried out by the formation of cyclic AMP. The temporal relationship of these events seems established; however, the absolute role of cyclic AMP as the link has been challenged by several investigators (Benfey et al. 1974). Considerable research effort in different laboratories is being directed toward solving this and related problems.

Several groups of drugs have been known to elicit autonomiclike activity in various tissues, but attempts to associate these effects with change in neurohumoral transmission have historically failed. It now seems that certain of these drugs bypass receptor sites and act on the same cyclic AMP system as do the catecholamines. The *methylxanthines* (caffeine, theobromine, theophylline), for instance, elicit changes in heart function that are reminiscent of β-receptor activation in that they elicit positive inotropic and chronotropic responses. However, β blockers have no effect on the cardiac actions of the methylxanthines. It now seems that these drugs are *phosphodiesterase inhibitors.* By inhibiting the phosphodiesterase enzyme, the catabolism of cyclic AMP is impaired and the cellular concentration of this nucleotide increases. Furthermore, under certain conditions, the methylxanthines potentiate the effect of catecholamines and other drugs that activate adenylate cyclase (Amer and Kreighbaum 1975).

It must be emphasized that the role of cyclic AMP as a universal second messenger has not at this time been completely proved. Several problems remain to be resolved. For example, β-receptor–mediated responses in cardiac muscle increase the level of cyclic AMP and cause increased contractile strength. In most smooth muscles, however, increased levels of cyclic AMP resulting from β-receptor activation cause relaxation rather than contraction. Furthermore, research with some tissues has suggested a temporal or parallel relationship rather than a causal or series relationship of cyclic AMP and β-receptor–mediated cellular responses. Recently, other studies have indicated that another

TABLE 6.2. Classification of autonomic drugs

Classification	Other Terms	Pharmacologic Effects	Mechanisms and Examples
Sympathomimetic	Adrenergic* Adrenomimetic*	Resemble effects caused by stimulation of adrenergic neurons Simulate effects of epinephrine and norepinephrine	Direct acting—α,β adrenergic receptor agonists (α-phenylephrine; β-isoproterenol; α,β-epinephrine) Indirect acting—release endogenous stores of catecholamines (tyramine and amphetamine) (Increase sympathetic discharge—nicotinic cholinergic agonists)†
Sympatholytic			
Receptor blocking effects	Adrenergic blocking drugs	Inhibit effects of sympathomimetic drugs, and inhibit responses caused by stimulation of adrenergic neurons	Block α or β receptors (α blocker—phentolamine; β blocker—propranolol)
Neuronal blocking effects	Adrenolytic	Inhibit responses caused by stimulation of adrenergic neurons	Deplete endogenous catecholamines (reserpine) Inhibit release of norepinephrine from nerve terminals (bretylium)
Parasympathomimetic	Cholinergic‡ Cholinomimetic‡	Resemble effects caused by stimulation of postganglionic parasympathetic neurons Simulate effects of acetylcholine	Direct acting—cholinergic receptor agonists (acetylcholine, carbachol) Indirect acting—cholinesterase inhibitors (neostigmine, organophosphates)
Parasympatholytic			
Receptor blocking effects	Cholinergic‡ blocking drugs	Inhibit effects of acetylcholine; inhibit responses caused by stimulation of postganglionic parasympathetic neurons	Block nicotinic‡ or muscarinic receptors (muscarinic blocker—atropine; nicotinic blocker—hexamethonium)
Neuronal blocking effects	Anticholinergic‡	Inhibit responses caused by stimulation of postganglionic parasympathetic neurons	Inhibit release of acetylcholine from nerve terminals (botulinum toxin)

* These terms refer specifically to activities at adrenergic synapses, adrenergic neuroeffector junctions, and adrenergic receptors.

† Sympathomimetic effects may be produced by nicotinic *cholinergic* agents by their excitatory action on sympathetic ganglia, the adrenal medulla, and adrenergic nerve terminals causing sympathetic discharge and release of epinephrine and norepinephrine. However, these activities should be considered as secondary when broad-based classifications of autonomic drugs are considered.

‡ These terms also refer to nonautonomic sites (e.g., somatic neuromuscular junction, CNS). Thus the terms parasympathomimetic and parasympatholytic are reserved to describe activities at the parasympathetic neuroeffector junction (i.e., in relation to muscarinic receptors; see text).

related nucleotide, cyclic guanine monophosphate (GMP), may be of greater importance as a second messenger in some cell types (Robison et al. 1971).

Certainly, future investigations of the involvement of cyclic AMP and cyclic GMP in the mediation of drug-induced changes will prove to be extremely important contributions not only to autonomic function but also to basic cellular processes (Rall 1972).

AUTONOMIC DRUGS

Drugs that exert pharmacologic effects that simulate activation, intensification, or inhibition of either the sympathetic or parasympathetic nervous system have been historically referred to as autonomic drugs. As a rule, autonomic drugs are classified according to the physiologic activity that they mimic. Table 6.2 summarizes the classification of the basic types of autonomic drugs that will be discussed in subsequent chapters.

REFERENCES

Adams, H. R.; Smookler, H. H.; Clarke, D. E.; Jandhyala, B. S.; Dixit, B. N.; Ertel, R. J.; and Buckley, J. P. 1971. Clinicopathologic effects of chronic reserpine administration in mongrel dogs. J Pharm Sci 60:1134.

Adams, H. R.; Dixit, B. N.; Smookler, H. H.; and Buckley, J. P. 1972. Clinical and biochemical effects of chronic reserpine administration in mongrel dogs. Am J Vet Res 33:699.

Aghajanian, G. K., and Bunney, B. S. 1973. Central dopaminergic neurons: Neurophysiological identification and responses to drugs. In E. Usdin and S. Snyder, eds. Frontiers in Catecholamine Research, p. 643. Elmsford, N.Y.: Pergamon Press.

Ahlquist, R. P. 1948. A study of the adrenotropic receptors. Am J Physiol 153:586.

Amer, M. S., and Kreighbaum, W. E. 1975. Cyclic nucleotide phosphodiesterases: Properties, activators, inhibitors, structure-activity relationships, and possible role in drug development. J Pharm Sci 64:1.

Bartholini, G.; Stadler, H.; and Lloyd, K. G. 1973. Cholinergic-dopaminergic relation in different brain structures. In E. Usdin and S. Snyder, eds. Frontiers in Catecholamine Research, p. 471. Elmsford, N.Y.: Pergamon Press.

Benfey, B. G.; Kunos, G.; and Nickerson, M. 1974. Dissociation of cardiac inotropic and adenylate cyclase activating adrenoceptors. Br J Pharmacol 51:253.

Benforado, J. M. 1967. The veratrum alkaloids. In W. S. Root and F. G. Hofmann, eds. Physiological Pharmacology. Vol. 4, The Nervous System. Part D: Autonomic Nervous System Drugs, p. 331. New York: Academic Press.

Bennett, M. R. 1972. Autonomic Neuromuscular Transmission. London: Cambridge Univ. Press.

Bennett, M. V. L., ed. 1974. Synaptic Transmission and Neuronal Interaction. Society of General Physiologists Series, vol. 28. New York: Raven Press.

Bogdanski, D. F. 1973. Effect of electrolytes on amine transport and release mechanisms in nerve endings. In E. Usdin and S. Snyder, eds. Frontiers in Catecholamine Research, p. 427. Elmsford, N.Y.: Pergamon Press.

Brimblecome, R. W. 1974. Drug Actions on Cholinergic Systems. Baltimore: University Park Press.

Bullock, T. H., and Hagiwara, S. 1957. Intracellular recording from the giant synapse of the squid. J Gen Physiol 40:565.

Burn, J. H., and Gibbons, W. R. 1965. The release of noradrenaline from sympathetic fibres in relation to calcium concentrations. J Physiol (Lond) 181:214.

Burn, J. H., and Rand, M. J. 1959. Sympathetic postganglionic mechanism. Nature 184:163.

———. 1965. Acetylcholine in adrenergic transmission. Annu Rev Pharmacol 5:163.

Burnstock, G. 1972. Purinergic nerves. Pharmacol Rev 24:509.

Chase, M. H., and Clemente, C. D. 1968. Central neural components of the autonomic nervous system. Anesthesiology 29:625.

Cole, K. S. 1968. Membranes, Ions, and Impulses: A Chapter of Classical Biophysics. Berkeley: Univ. of California Press.

Curtis, H. J., and Cole, K. S. 1942. Membrane resting and action potentials from the squid giant axon. J Cell Comp Physiol 19:135.

Douglas, W. W., and Rubin, R. P. 1961. The role of calcium in the secretory response of the adrenal medulla to acetylcholine. J Physiol (Lond) 159:40.

Gauthier, P.; Nadeau, R. A.; and de Champlain, J. 1974. Cardiovascular reactivity in the dog after chemical sympathectomy with 6-hydroxydopamine. Can J Physiol Pharmacol 52:590.

Goth, A. 1974. Medical Pharmacology, 7th ed. St. Louis: C. V. Mosby.

Hokfelt, T. 1973. Neuronal catecholamine storage vesicles. In E. Usdin and S. Snyder, eds. Frontiers in Catecholamine Research, p. 439. Elmsford, N.Y.: Pergamon Press.

Horton, E. W. 1973. Prostaglandins at adrenergic nerve-endings. Br Med Bull 29(2): 148.

Hubbard, J. I. 1971. Mechanism of transmitter release from nerve terminals. Ann NY Acad Sci 183:131.

Iversen, L. L. 1972. Neuronal and extraneuronal catecholamine uptake mechanisms. In E. Usdin and S. Snyder, eds. Frontiers in Catecholamine Research, p. 403. Elmsford, N.Y.: Pergamon Press.

Katz, B. 1966. Nerve, Muscle, and Synapse. New York: McGraw-Hill.

Katz, B., and Miledi, R. 1965. The effect of calcium on acetylcholine release from motor nerve terminals. Proc R Soc Lond [Biol] 161:496.

Klein, R. L. 1973. A large second pool of norepinephrine in the highly purified vesicle fraction from bovine splenic nerve. In E. Usdin and S. Snyder, eds. Frontiers in Catecholamine Research, p. 423. Elmsford, N.Y.: Pergamon Press.

Koelle, G. B. 1962. A new general concept of the neurohumoral function of acetylcholine and acetylcholinesterase. J Pharm Pharmacol 14:65.

———. 1970. Neurohumoral transmission and the autonomic nervous system. In L. S. Goodman and A. Gilman, eds. The Pharmacological Basis of Therapeutics, 4th ed., p. 402. New York: Macmillan.

Koelle, W. A., and Koelle, G. B. 1959. The localization of external or functional acetylcholinesterase at the synapses of autonomic ganglia. J Pharmacol Exp Ther 126:1.

Kopin, I. J. 1968. False adrenergic transmitters. Annu Rev Pharmacol 8:377.

Lands, A. M.; Arnold, A.; McAuliff, J. P.; Luduena, F. P.; and Brown, T. G., Jr. 1967. Differentiation of receptor systems activated by sympathomimetic amines. Nature 214:597.

Langer, S. Z. 1973. The regulation of transmitter release elicited by nerve stimulation through a presynaptic feed-back mechanism. In E. Usdin and S. Snyder, eds. Frontiers in Catecholamine Research, p. 543. Elmsford, N.Y.: Pergamon Press.

Loewi, O. 1921. Über humorale übertragbarkeit der herznervenwirkung. Pfluegers Arch Ges Physiol 189:239.

Loewi, O., and Navratil, E. 1926. Über humorale übertragbarkeit der herznervenwirkung. X. Mitteilung. Über das schicksal des vagusstoffs. Pfluegers Arch Ges Physiol 214:678.

Mandell, A. J., ed. 1973. New Concepts in Neurotransmitter Regulation. New York: Plenum Press.

Moran, N. C. 1973. The classification of adrenergic receptors. In E. Usdin and S. Snyder, eds. Frontiers in Catecholamine Research, p. 291. Elmsford, N.Y.: Pergamon Press.

Muscholl, E. 1973. Regulation of catecholamine release: The muscarinic inhibitory mechanism. In E. Usdin and S. Snyder, eds. Frontiers in Catecholamine Research, p. 537. Elmsford, N.Y.: Pergamon Press.

Paintal, A. S. 1963. Vagal afferent fibres. Ergeb Physiol 52:74.

Popovic, N. A.; Mullane, J. F.; and Yhap, E. O. 1972. Effects of acetylpromazine maleate on certain cardiorespiratory responses in dogs. Am J Vet Res 33:1819.

Rall, T. W. 1972. Role of adenosine 3′,5′-monophosphate (cyclic AMP) in actions of catecholamines. Pharmacol Rev 24:399.

Rand, M. J.; Story, D. F.; Allen, G. S.; Glover, A. B.; and McCulloch, M. W. 1973. Pulse-to-pulse modulation of noradrenaline release through a prejunctional α-receptor auto-inhibitory mechanism. In E. Usdin and S. Snyder, eds. Frontiers in Catecholamine Research, p. 579. Elmsford, N.Y.: Pergamon Press.

Robison, G. A.; Butcher, R. W.; and Sutherland, E. W. 1967. Adenyl cyclase as an adrenergic receptor. Ann NY Acad Sci 139:703.

———. 1971. Cyclic AMP. New York: Academic Press.

Shore, P. A. 1972. Transport and storage of biogenic amines. Annu Rev Pharmacol 12:209.

Starke, K. 1973. Regulation of catecholamine release: α-Receptor mediated feedback control in peripheral and central neurones. In E. Usdin and S. Snyder, eds. Frontiers in Catecholamine Research, p. 561. Elmsford, N.Y.: Pergamon Press.

Sutherland, E. W., and Rall, T. W. 1960a. The relation of adenosine-3′,5′-phosphate and phosphorylase to the actions of catecholamines and other hormones. Pharmacol Rev 12:265.

———. 1960b. The relation of adenosine-3′,5′-phosphate to the action of catecholamines. In J. R. Vane; G. E. W. Wolstenholme; and M. O'Connor, eds. Adrenergic Mechanisms (a Ciba Foundation symposium), p. 295. Boston: Little, Brown; London: J. & A. Churchill.

Usdin, E., and Snyder, S., eds. 1973. Frontiers in Catecholamine Research. Elmsford, N.Y.: Pergamon Press.

Volle, R. L., and Koelle, G. B. 1961. The physiological role of acetylcholinesterase (AChE) in sympathetic ganglia. J Pharmacol Exp Ther 133:223.

Werman, R. 1966. Criteria for the identification of a central nervous system transmitter. Comp Biochem Physiol 18:745.

Winkler, H., and Hörtnagl, H. 1973. Composition and molecular organization of chromaffin granules. In E. Usdin and S. Snyder, eds. Frontiers in Catecholamine Research, p. 415. Elmsford, N.Y.: Pergamon Press.

CHAPTER 7

ADRENERGIC AND ANTIADRENERGIC DRUGS

H. RICHARD ADAMS

Amine substances that cause physiologic responses similar to those evoked by the endogenous adrenergic mediators, epinephrine and norepinephrine, are known as *adrenergic drugs.* They are commonly referred to as *sympathomimetic* agents in reference to their mimic of sympathetic nervous system activity. Sympatholytic, adrenolytic, and adrenergic blocking drugs exert pharmacologic effects that, in general, simulate a decrease in adrenergic nerve activity. These terms are not synonymous, however, and they have been used to describe different types of antiadrenergic actions, as will be discussed later in this chapter.

ADRENERGIC (SYMPATHOMIMETIC) DRUGS

Pharmacologic effects of sympathomimetic amines are mediated by activation of adrenergic receptors of effector cells innervated by the sympathetic nervous system. Ahlquist (1948) proposed the existence of two types of adrenergic receptors, α and β, to explain dissimilar effects of sympathomimetic agents in different tissues. This classification was based on the relative potencies of several adrenergic drugs to elicit excitatory and inhibitory effects in different organs, as discussed in Chapter 6.

Epinephrine is the most potent α agonist; it is 2–10 times more active than norepinephrine and 100 times more potent than isoproterenol. Just the opposite sequence was found at the β receptors; isoproterenol is the most potent β agonist; it is 2–10 times more active than epinephrine and over 100 times more active than norepinephrine. However, norepinephrine is quite active at the cardiac β receptors. Lands et al. (1967) subclassified the β receptors of the myocardium as β_1, and the β receptors of blood vessels and bronchial smooth muscle as β_2. Distribution of adrenergic receptors in different body organs and associated physiologic effects are presented in Table 6.1.

The validity of designating adrenergic receptors as α or β has been substantiated by the discovery of different drugs that selectively block either the α or β responses. These agents, termed *adrenergic blocking drugs,* are so selective in their action that they are now routinely used in determining the α and β agonistic characteristics of adrenergic drugs. For example, a drug is considered to be an α agonist if its activity is blocked by a known "alpha blocker" such as phentolamine but unaffected by a "beta blocking agent" such as propranolol. Conversely, if propranolol blocks the effect of a drug that is unaffected by phentolamine, this effect is considered to be mediated by β receptors.

Structure-Activity Relationships

Several factors have complicated determination of optimal structural requirements for adrenergic drugs. Many studies of structure-activity relationships were based on blood pressure responses. Pressor effects in intact animals, however, are influenced by indirect factors such as, for example, reflexogenic changes. Also, most adrenergic drugs affect both α and β receptors, and the ratio of α and β activity varies tremendously between drugs. Therefore, to determine the potency of a particular agent at one receptor, the other type of receptor must be blocked. In addition, some sympathomimetic amines are taken up into the adrenergic nerve, whereas others are not subjected to this pathway. Inactivation by neuronal uptake of some but not all drugs examined in a study may yield inaccurate estimates of potency at the receptor and simply reflect differences in susceptibility to the amine uptake pump. Furthermore, except for the catecholamines, many adrenergic agents cause some indirect effects mediated by release of endogenous norepinephrine. Despite these various and often conflicting interrelationships, some general and some rather specific aspects of the structure-activity relationship of sympathomimetic amines have been determined, as described below.

The basis for the sympatheticlike activity of various drugs depends upon the similarity of their chemical structure to that of the endogenous adrenergic mediators, norepinephrine and epinephrine. The nucleus of this chemical structure, β-phenylethylamine, is a benzene ring and an ethylamine side chain. Substitution may be made on the aromatic ring, on the α and β carbons of the side chain, and on the amine moiety. (The α and β nomenclature of the carbon atoms represents organic chemical terminology and has no relationship to the α- and β- receptor classification.)

The chemical structures and related pharmacologic characteristics of several adrenergic drugs are summarized in Table 7.1. Epinephrine, norepinephrine, dopamine, and isoproterenol have a hydroxyl group on both the 3 and 4 positions of the benzene ring. Since 3,4-dihydroxybenzene is also known as "catechol," sympathomimetic amines containing this nucleus are termed *catecholamines.* In general, the catechol nucleus is required for maximum α and β potencies. Removal of one or both hydroxyl groups from the aromatic ring especially reduces β activity. Phenylephrine, for instance, is identical in structure to epinephrine except for the lack of one hydroxyl group on the ring (Table 7.1). Phenylephrine is almost exclusively an α agonist, whereas epinephrine is a mixed α–β agonist. Substitution of a ring hydroxyl group similarly reduces potency and may actually yield an antagonist (i.e., an adrenergic blocking drug such as the β blocker, dichloroisoproterenol).

Substitution on the β-carbon atom of the side chain results in less active central actions in relation to peripheral effects. Substitution on the α-carbon atom yields a compound that is not susceptible to oxidation by monoamine oxidase (MAO). Thus α-substituted amines may influence other agents that are normally inactivated by MAO. For example, α-methylnorepinephrine is not metabolized by MAO but it is stored in the amine granule. Endogenous norepinephrine is displaced from storage granules, metabolized by MAO,

TABLE 7.1. Chemical structures and related pharmacologic activities of some commonly used sympathomimetic amines.

Drug	Ring (positions 1–6)	β CH	α CH	NH	Activity	Clinical Use
β-Phenylethylamine	...	H	H	H	...	...
β-Phenylethanolamine	...	OH	H	H	...	...
Catecholamines						
Dopamine*	3-OH,4-OH	H	H	H	α,$β_1$,D	P,C,K
Norepinephrine	3-OH,4-OH	OH	H	H	α,$β_1$	P,C
Epinephrine	3-OH,4-OH	OH	H	CH_3	α,β	P,C,A,B
Isoproterenol	3-OH,4-OH	OH	H	$CH(CH_3)_2$	β	C,B
Noncatecholamines						
Metaraminol	3-OH	OH	CH_3	H	α	P
Phenylephrine	3-OH	OH	H	CH_3	α	P,Rb*
Tyramine	4-OH	H	H	H	I	...
Hydroxyamphetamine	4-OH	H	CH_3	H	I	CNS
Amphetamine	...	H	CH_3	H	I	CNS
Methamphetamine	...	H	CH_3	CH_3	I	CNS
Ephedrine	...	OH	CH_3	CH_3	I,α,β	P,C,CNS

Note: α = α receptor; β = β receptor; A = allergic reactions; B = bronchodilator ($β_2$ receptor); C = cardiac stimulation ($β_1$ receptor); CNS = central nervous system excitation; D = dopamine may interact with α, $β_1$, and "dopaminergic" receptors; I = indirect-acting, causes release of endogenous norepinephrine which acts on α and β receptors; K = renal vasodilatation (dopaminergic receptors); P = pressor activity; Rb = reflex bradycardia due to pressor activation of baroreceptor-vagal reflex.

* Clinical use in human beings, experimental studies in animals

and replaced by α-methylnorepinephrine (i.e., false transmitter concept).

Alkyl substitutions on the amino moiety affect the ratio of α and β agonistic properties. Within limits, increasing the size of the aliphatic substitution increases β activity. Epinephrine (*N*-methylnorepinephrine) is a more potent β agonist than norepinephrine. Isoproterenol (*N*-isopropylnorepinephrine) is a more potent β agonist than epinephrine or norepinephrine. Naturally occurring norepinephrine and epinephrine are in the levo configuration at the β-carbon atom. Dextrorotatory substitution on the β carbon yields the many times less potent *d* isomers.

Pharmacologic Relationships

All adrenergic drugs do not necessarily produce identical effects. Their pharmacologic profiles may vary depending upon their basic chemical structure and resulting activities as α, β, or mixed α-β agonists. Nevertheless, such differences usually cause only quantitative dissimilarities in intact patients, and sympathomimetic amines exhibit similar and characteristic properties. Therefore, only representative adrenergic drugs will be examined in detail; other agents will be compared in relation to differences that they may exhibit in agonistic properties (i.e., activity at α or β receptors) and in mechanisms of action (i.e., direct- or indirect-acting sympathomimetic activity).

CATECHOLAMINES

These agents are direct-acting sympathomimetic amines. They activate receptors of effector cells; therefore, adrenergic nerves are not required for their effects.

Epinephrine, Norepinephrine, and Isoproterenol

Epinephrine (adrenaline) and norepinephrine (noradrenaline, levarterenol, arterenol) are endogenous biogenic amines; isoproterenol (isopropylarterenol) is not found in the body but is chemically synthesized. The subtle differences in the pharmacologic effects of structurally related adrenergic drugs can be demonstrated by comparing the cardiovascular effects of these three agents, as shown schematically in Fig. 7.1.

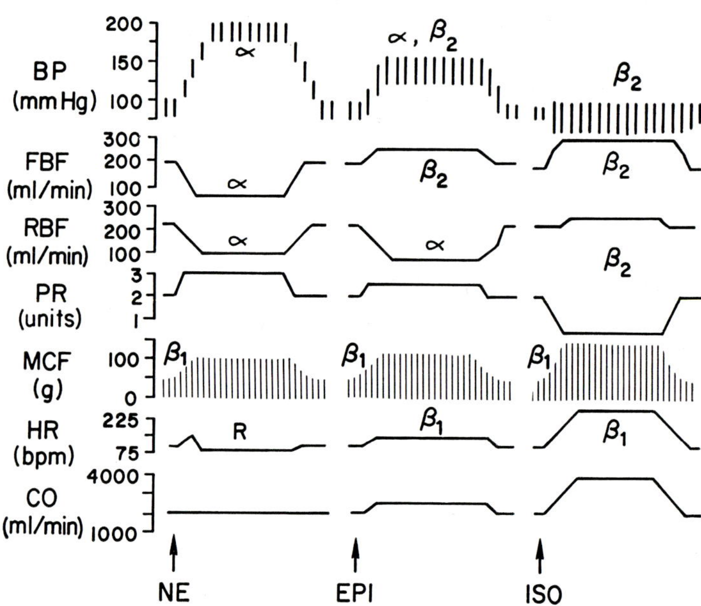

FIG. 7.1. Cardiovascular effects of intravenously administered norepinephrine (NE), epinephrine (Epi), and isoproterenol (ISO) in a dog. Schematic representations of effects of "equivalent" doses of these amines on blood pressure (BP), femoral blood flow (FBF), renal blood flow (RBF), peripheral vascular resistance (PR), myocardial contractile force (MCF), heart rate (HR), and cardiac output (CO). α = response mediated primarily by α-adrenergic receptor; β = response mediated primarily by β-adrenergic receptor (β_1 or β_2 subtype); R = reflex mediated. Characteristics of cardiovascular excitation evoked by these agents are due to differences in their α-β agonistic properties (Table 7.2). See text for explanation of each response.

The different cardiovascular responses seen with epinephrine, norepinephrine, and isoproterenol in Fig. 7.1 are due to differences in the ratios of their α and β agonistic properties. Classification of adrenergic receptors in the heart and blood vessels, related effects, and the order of potency of epinephrine, norepinephrine, and isoproterenol are shown in Table 7.2.

Norepinephrine, primarily an α agonist, activates the α vascular receptors resulting in intense vasoconstriction; peripheral resistance increases and femoral and renal blood flow decrease (Fig. 7.1).

Although epinephrine is a potent α stimulant, it also is very active at β receptors. Beta receptors in blood vessels subserve vasodilatation. In response to epinephrine, vasoconstriction occurs in those vascular beds that have predominantly α receptors (e.g., abdominal viscera); however, vasodilatation can occur in those beds that contain β receptors (e.g., skeletal muscle). Blood flow increases in areas in response to regional vasodilatation (e.g., femoral flow) but decreases if vasoconstriction dominates (e.g., renal flow) (Fig. 7.1).

Since isoproterenol is a selective β agonist, it causes vasodilatation, a fall in diastolic blood pressure, a decrease in peripheral resistance, and an increase in blood flow to those areas containing β receptors (e.g., femoral blood flow). The renal vasculature has few β receptors and is, therefore, little affected by isoproterenol (Fig. 7.1).

As also seen in Fig. 7.1, the heart is activated by epinephrine, norepinephrine,

TABLE 7.2. Adrenergic receptor activation by catecholamines

Receptor Type	Tissue	Response	Potency of Agonists
α	Blood vessels	Vasconstriction	Epinephrine>norepinephrine>>>isoproterenol
β_1	Heart	Positive inotropic and chronotropic effects	Isoproterenol>epinephrine≧norepinephrine
β_2	Blood vessels*	Vasodilatation	Isoproterenol>epinephrine>>>norepinephrine

Note: > = greater than; ≧ = greater than or equal; >>> = many times greater.
* Receptor of coronary arteries may be β_1.

and isoproterenol. Isoproterenol is the most potent of the three and causes a relatively greater increase in myocardial contractile force, heart rate, and cardiac output than does the similarly acting epinephrine. Norepinephrine also increases myocardial contractile force, but bradycardia occurs at the peak pressor effect of this amine. This is due to an increase in vagal tone reflexly instigated by the pronounced norepinephrine-induced increase in mean blood pressure. Norepinephrine-mediated peripheral vasoconstriction may decrease venous return so that cardiac output does not increase although the heart is activated.

These examples demonstrate differences in selective cardiovascular effects of these closely related catecholamines. Nevertheless, it should be apparent that all three agents elicit the same basic result: a net increase in cardiovascular activity.

PHARMACOLOGIC EFFECTS

Blood Pressure. Norepinephrine administered intravenously either by slow infusion or bolus injection causes a dose-related increase in systolic and diastolic blood pressures due to bodywide vasoconstriction. Mean blood pressure increases accordingly; little change is seen in pulse pressure.

Slow intravenous infusion of small amounts of epinephrine usually causes a fall in diastolic blood pressure that may or may not be accompained by a slight increase in systolic pressure. This response is due to regional vasodilatation (β-receptor–mediated) causing a decrease in peripheral resistance. However, a bolus intravenous injection of a large amount of epinephrine (e.g., 1–3 $\mu g/kg$) causes a pronounced increase in blood pressure that is as remarkable as that produced by norepinephrine. It should be appreciated that epinephrine is an extremely potent pressor agent. This pressor response depends upon vasoconstriction, myocardial stimulation, and tachycardia. Vasoconstriction is the most important, however. Bradycardia can occur at the peak pressor response due to reflex vagal activity. A depressor effect may be observed after the pressor response to a large dose of epinephrine. This secondary response is related to residual activation of β receptors in some blood vessels.

Following a single bolus injection of norepinephrine or epinephrine, the pressor response lasts for several minutes then gradually decreases and returns to normal within 5–10 minutes. Repeated injections continue to elicit similar effects in contrast to repeated administration of drugs like tyramine that act by releasing endogenous stores of norepinephrine. Isoproterenol increases pulse pressure predominantly by lowering diastolic pressure. This effect is due to β-receptor–mediated vasodilatation.

Vascular Smooth Muscle. Epinephrine and norepinephrine are very potent constrictors of cutaneous and mucosal blood vessels in mammalian species. Adrenergic receptors in these vessels are almost exclusively α. Intense vasoconstriction, increased vascular resistance, and decreased blood flow occur in these regions in response to norepinephrine and epinephrine. This is often seen as a "blanching" type response in skin or mucosal membranes.

Since epinephrine is a more potent α agonist than norepinephrine, it is 2–10 times more active than norepinephrine in constricting cutaneous and mucosal vessels. Smaller arterioles and precapillary sphincters are particularly responsive to the vasoconstrictor catecholamines. They are active regardless of whether they are applied topically to blood vessels, sprayed upon mucosal surfaces, injected perivascularly, or administered systemically. Isoproterenol has little, if any, effect on cutaneous and mucosal vessels, due to the lack of β receptors in these tissues.

The renal vasculature has predominantly α receptors. Epinephrine and norepinephrine cause vasoconstriction in the kidney and a generalized increase in vascular resistance in this organ. Renal blood flow is decreased even in the presence of an elevated systemic blood pressure (Fig. 7.1). Large doses of α-agonistic catecholamines may actually induce a functional renal shutdown, due to decreased perfusion of the kidney. During this period, urinary output is substantially decreased, due to lowered glomerular filtration rate. During exposure to moderate concentrations of norepinephrine or epinephrine, urinary output, electrolyte excretion, urine pH, and other renal parameters vary considerably. Local regulatory processes in the renal arteriolar segments probably act to modulate flow in the presence of α-receptor–mediated vasoconstriction.

Isoproterenol has little effect on renal arteries, due to the small number of β receptors in the vasculature of the kidney. However, direct injection of the drug into the renal artery increases renal blood flow (McNay and Goldberg 1966). In addition, there is some evidence of β receptors in the kidney that upon activation cause a release of renin into the circulation for angiotensin formation.

Mesenteric arteries are constricted by norepinephrine and epinephrine, due to activation of α receptors. Mesenteric arterial resistance is markedly increased and splanchnic blood flow decreases proportionately. In some circumstances, i.e., with small doses, epinephrine may cause slight vasodilatation of splanchnic arteries, due reportedly to the presence of β receptors (Greenway and Lawson 1966).

Skeletal muscle blood vessels have both α and β receptors. Vasoconstriction or vasodilatation can be induced, depending upon the α- and β-agonistic profiles of a vasostimulatory amine. Norepinephrine, due to its relative lack of effect on β vascular receptors, elicits vasoconstriction in skeletal muscles, due to activation of α receptors. Vascular resistance increases and blood flow decreases proportionately.

Beta receptors in skeletal muscle blood vessels are more sensitive to epinephrine than are the α recptors. Therefore, small amounts of epinephrine actually cause a decrease in vascular resistance and an increase in blood flow to voluntary muscles due to vasodilatation. This effect is blocked by a β blocking agent such as propranolol. However, large doses of epinephrine cause vasoconstriction in skeletal muscles due to α-receptor–mediated contraction overriding β-mediated relaxation. If α receptors are blocked, the response to epinephrine is converted to vasodilatation, due to "unmasking" of the β sites. If a β blocker is used, the α-mediated constrictor effects of epinephrine are accentuated.

Isoproterenol causes relaxation of skeletal muscle blood vessels, increased blood flow to voluntary muscle masses, and decreased vascular resistance in these structures due to activation of the vascular β receptors. Since isoproterenol has little effect on α receptors, β blockade abolishes the vasodilator effect of isoproterenol but does not convert the response to vasoconstriction.

The coronary arteries dilate after exposure to catecholamines (isoproterenol > epinephrine > norepinephrine). Portions of this response are metabolic effects that are secondary to changes in the heart muscle (Schaper 1967). Alpha receptors that mediate vasoconstriction seem to be present in the coronary vasculature; however, they are believed to be less sensitive than the β sites. Beta receptors seem to dominate, causing vasodilatation, decreased resistance, and increased coronary flow. Recent studies in kittens, dogs, and pigs indicate that coronary β receptors may respond more like β_1 than like β_2 receptors (Cornish and Miller 1975). If established, this is in contrast to other vascular beds that have been characterized as β_2.

Vascular Mechanisms. Mechanical function of a vascular smooth muscle cell depends upon the availability of free intracellular Ca^{++} in the vicinity of the contractile proteins. Norepinephrine and epinephrine have been found to alter Ca^{++}-related events in the vascular smooth muscle fiber.

Isolated arterial strips from mammalian species contract in the presence of appropriate amounts of norepinephrine or epinephrine. Usually, this contractile response is biphasic and is composed of an initial fast component and a slow prolonged component. Only the initial rapid component of contraction is observed if an arterial strip is immersed for a short period of time in a Ca^{++}-free (but otherwise physiological) salt solution. If the tissue is maintained in a zero Ca^{++} solution for a prolonged period of time, however, the vascular strip fails to contract. These findings indicate that norepinephrine and epinephrine produce vascular contraction by initially causing release of an intracellular (sequestered) source of Ca^{++} to the contractile proteins; this Ca^{++} is not readily depleted by placing the tissue in a zero Ca^{++} solution. The slow, sustained phase of a norepinephrine response seems to be dependent upon mobilization of a superficial Ca^{++} source that is more readily depleted by incubating the artery in a low Ca^{++} environment (Goodman and Weiss 1971).

Although it is known that these Ca^{++}-dependent responses depend upon a preceding activation of an α-adrenergic receptor, the molecular mechanisms and intermediate steps are only poorly understood. Cyclic AMP may be involved. In some cases, α-receptor–mediated effects in blood vessels have been associated with a decrease in cyclic AMP, whereas β effects have often been associated with an increase in cyclic AMP. Such interrelations of drugs with biological systems exemplify the complexities involved in physiologic expression of the action of a pharmacologic agent. Further, they demonstrate quite clearly that receptor-agonist classifications are simply useful descriptive terms and they do not identify cellular mechanisms.

Myocardial Effects. Isoproterenol, epinephrine, and norepinephrine are potent myocardial stimulants. They increase the strength of myocardial contractile force and acelerate the heart rate. These changes represent direct effects that are not dependent upon changes in venous return (pre-load), after load, or other hemodynamic variables. Contractile and rate effects of catecholamines are mediated via direct activation of β receptors of the myocardial and pacemaker cells. Myocardial β receptors are subtyped as β_1. Isoproterenol is 10–20 times more active in the heart than epinephrine; norepinephrine is somewhat less potent than epinephrine.

The increase in myocardial contractility (positive inotropic effect) seen with each of the three agents is produced in both atrial and ventricular muscles. The positive inotropism in the whole heart is characterized by a more rapid and forcible systolic ejection. The rate of pressure changes in the ventricular chambers (i.e., dP/dt, which is expressed as mm Hg per second) is increased. In isolated heart muscle, the positive first derivative of contractile force (dF/dt) is increased during exposure to the catecholamines, indicating that the rate at which contraction takes place is accelerated. The systolic interval (time to peak tension) is shortened. Negative dF/dt (rate of relaxation) of heart muscle is also increased by catecholamines, indicating that diastolic relaxation takes place more quickly. However, oxygen consumption is accelerated to a relatively greater extent when the heart work is increased. Therefore, cardiac efficiency is sacrificed in expense of the absolute increase in myocardial contractility produced by the catecholamines.

Acceleration of heart rate (positive chronotropism) induced by epinephrine, norepinephrine, and isoproterenol is due to changes in the excitability of the pacemaker cells. The depolarization process in the S-A node cells is accelerated; the velocity of the action potential is enhanced in these and other conduction system cells. Purkinje fibers are similarly affected by epinephrine and norepinephrine. Latent or normally inactive pacemaker cells seem to be activated by these agents. In essence, their threshold is reset so that they become more excitable and fire more easily or even spontaneously. By similar mechanisms, epinephrine antagonizes the A-V block produced by other drugs or by vagal stimulation.

Norepinephrine and epinephrine also increase myocardial irritability resulting, with large doses, in serious arrhythmias. Some investigators have shown that this can be partially blocked by an α blocker (Nickerson and Nomaguchi 1949). However, pure α agonists such as phenylephrine and methoxamine are very weak arrhythmogenic agents. Also, a β blocker such as propranolol is much more active than an α blocker in decreasing the arrhythmias evoked by epinephrine and norepinephrine. Certain halogenated anesthetics (e.g., halothane, chloroform) increase the sensitivity of the heart to the cardiac rhythm irregularities induced by epinephrine and norepinephrine (Katz and Katz 1966).

Bradycardia often occurs during the peak pressor response seen after administration of epinephrine or norepinephrine to intact animals. This can be blocked by vagotomy or atropine; it is dependent upon the hypertensive response causing an increase in vagal discharge via the baroreceptor reflex mechanisms. It is usually more pronounced with norepinephrine than with epinephrine, due to the relatively greater increase in mean blood pressure seen with the former drug. A tachycardia is invariably produced by isoproterenol.

The positive inotropic and chronotropic effects of norepinephrine, epinephrine, and isoproterenol can best be demonstrated in isolated heart muscle. Such preparations are free from the influence of peripheral circulatory and reflex nervous mechanisms. The right atrium of the guinea pig heart beats spontaneously due to the presence of S-A cells. As seen in tracings obtained from guinea pig right atria in Fig. 7.2, norepinephrine, isoproterenol, and epinephrine cause concentration-related increases in contractile force and heart rate. Heart rate is seen to increase from about 160 beats/minute to 240 beats/minute. The inotropic response is characterized by (1) an increase in contractile force (developed tension) generated by the heart muscle, (2) an increase in the rate of systolic contraction ($+dF/dt$, expressed in g/second), and (3) an increase in the rate of diastolic relaxation ($-dF/dt$) (Fig. 7.2). Notice that isoproterenol is considerably more potent than epinephrine or norepinephrine in both inotropic and chronotropic activities. When the concentrations used in these experiments (i.e., 1.6×10^{-10} to 1×10^{-8} g/ml) are considered, the exceptional potencies of these agents on myocardial function are striking.

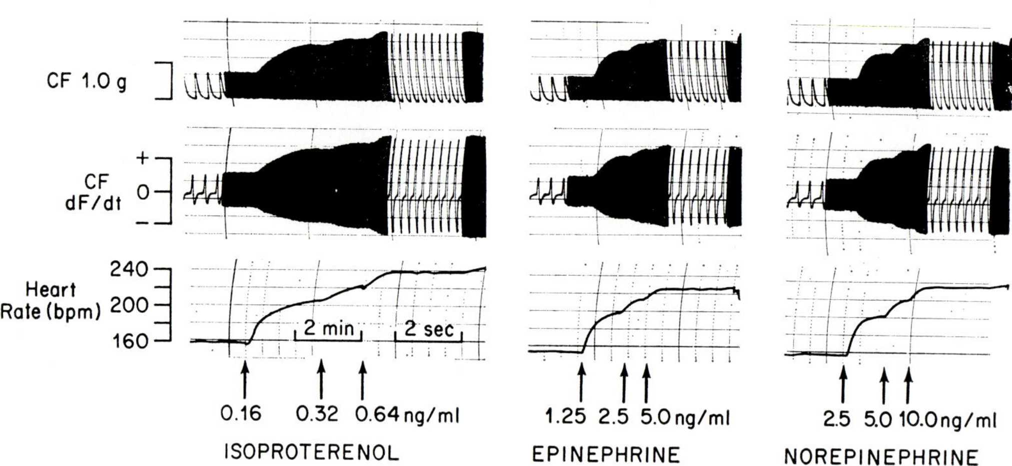

FIG. 7.2. Positive inotropic and chronotropic effects of isoproterenol, epinephrine, and norepinephrine in isolated spontaneously beating right atria of guinea pigs. CF = contractile force (developed tension); dF/dt = the rate of increase (+) or decrease (—) in CF; bpm = beats per minute. Concentrations refer to cumulative amounts; amine added at designated arrows.

Myocardial Mechanisms. In a heart muscle cell, contractile Ca^{++} is believed to originate in part from superficial sarcolemmal sites. Calcium bound at these sites is in rapid equilibrium with the Ca^{++} within the extracellular space (Langer 1974). It is believed that Ca^{++} influx from superficial sites links membrane excitation (i.e., the cardiac action potential) to the contraction of the myofibers. Catecholamines enhance the influx of Ca^{++} into the myocardial cell. Drugs that have no direct influence on adrenergic mechanisms can alter inotropic responses to catecholamines by interfering with Ca^{++}-dependent contractile events (Adams 1975). It has been proposed that catecholamine-mediated influx of Ca^{++} into the myocardial cell is due to increased intracellular concentrations of cyclic AMP.

As previously outlined (Chapter 6), activation of the cardiac β receptor by epinephrine, norepinephrine, and isoproterenol increases the activity of adenylate cyclase, an enzyme localized in the cell membrane (Robison et al. 1967, 1971). This enzyme catalyzes the conversion of ATP to cyclic AMP. Cyclic AMP has been reported to cause an increased Ca^{++} influx through the "slow Ca^{++} channels" of the sarcolemma, resulting in increased availability of Ca^{++} at the contractile proteins (Watanabe and Besch 1974). Further, cyclic AMP activates phosphorylase, resulting in glycogenolysis and increased energy availability.

A schematic representation of the proposed involvement of cyclic AMP in the inotropic activity of catecholamines in heart muscle is shown in Fig. 7.3. This model is not universally accepted, however, and many investigators have obtained results that do not support the mediation of cardiac effects of catecholamines by cyclic AMP (Benfey et al. 1974). The importance of the involvement of cyclic AMP in activating phosphorylase in heart muscle has been particularly challenged (Young and McNeill 1974). Other energy-yielding reactions seem to be more important.

Several drugs alter the cyclic AMP system in complementary manners. For example, the methylxanthines inhibit the enzyme (phosphodiesterase) that inactivates cyclic AMP (Fig. 7.3). These drugs, termed phosphodiesterase inhibitors, cause an increase in cyclic AMP concentrations and a positive inotropic effect in heart muscle. They potentiate the inotropic activity of the catecholamines.

It now seems likely that the effects of some inotropic drugs and hormones (e.g., catecholamines, glucagon, histamine) may be mediated by, or at least be associated with, fluctuations in cyclic AMP concentrations in the myocardial cell. However, the definitive interrelationships remain equivocal at the present time.

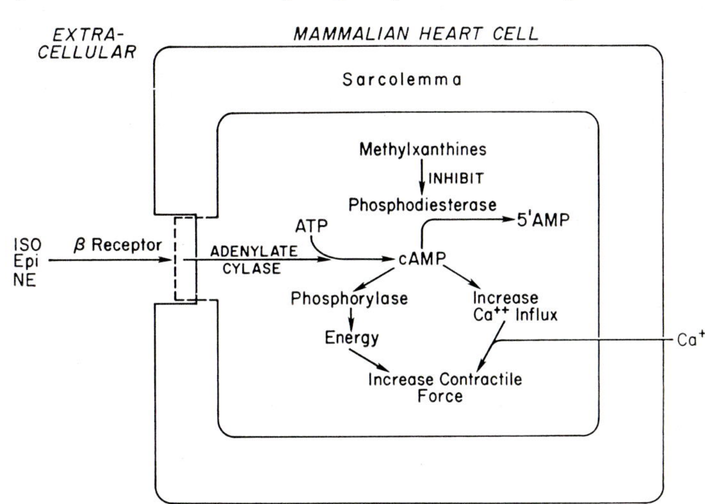

Fig. 7.3. Representation of the proposed involvement of cyclic adenosine monophosphate (cAMP) in the myocardial effects of catecholamines. ISO = isoproterenol; Epi = epinephrine; NE = norepinephrine; ATP = adenosine triphosphate; 5′ AMP = 5-adenosine monophosphate. *Phosphorylase* represents this and/or other energy-yielding biochemical reactions that may be influenced by cAMP (see text).

Respiratory Effects. Effects of catecholamines on respiration are not striking, and these agents have no practical application as analeptics. In fact, dyspnea and even temporary apnea can occur during the peak pressor responses to injection of epinephrine or norepinephrine. These respiratory changes are primarily mediated by reflex inhibition of medullary respiratory centers.

Epinephrine is a potent bronchodilator due to relaxation of bronchial smooth muscle. This effect is particularly pronounced if bronchial muscle is contracted by other drugs (e.g., acetylcholine, histamine) or by anaphylactoid or asthmatic conditions. Adrenergic receptors in bronchiolar muscle are of the β_2 type. Isoproterenol is, therefore, a potent bronchiolar dilator, whereas norepinephrine has relatively less effect. Epinephrine and isoproterenol are often used clinically to dilate bronchiolar passageways during episodes of allergic reactions.

Gastrointestinal System. Adrenergic drugs inhibit gastrointestinal (GI) activity in a manner similar to that seen upon stimulation of the sympathetic nerves. The frequency and amplitude of peristaltic contractions in the gut are decreased due to relaxation of the intestinal smooth muscle. These effects are due to activation of adrenergic receptors of the smooth muscle cells. Adrenergic drugs may also inhibit the function of the parasympathetic nerves of the Auerbach's and Meissner's plexuses. Such an effect would contribute further to GI quiescence.

Problems were encountered during original attempts to classify adrenergic receptors in the gut. Epinephrine was found to relax intestinal muscle; however, this effect was not completely blocked by either an α or β blocking agent. Subsequent studies showed that both α and β blocking agents were required to abolish the relaxant effects of epinephrine. Thus the presence of α and β receptors that both subserve inhibitory (relaxant) effects in the gut was established. Isoproterenol, due to β effects, exerts a rather potent inhibitory effect on GI smooth muscle. GI sphincters are in general contracted by α-sympathomimetic agents. This is in basic agreement with the overall "slowing down" of GI activity produced by sympathetic nerve stimulation.

Secretion of digestive juices is also decreased by α-sympathetic agents. Although salivary glands are activated in response to sympathetic activity, the saliva produced is scant and viscous. This is in contrast to the profuse and watery salivation seen with parasympathetic activity.

Adrenergic drugs have no application as GI inhibitory agents in clinical situations. Cardiovascular effects are usually concurrently produced by those dosages required to inhibit GI function. In addition, parasympathetic activity in the GI system can quickly override the depressant effects exhibited by most sympathomimetic drugs.

Uterine Muscle. Both α and β receptors seem to be present in the uterus; epinephrine, norepinephrine, and isoproterenol affect motor activity. Responses of uterine smooth muscle to catecholamines are quite variable, depending on species and stage of the estrous and gestational cycles. In the cat, for example, epinephrine relaxes the nongravid uterus but contracts the uterus during late pregnancy. In the rabbit, epinephrine contracts the gravid and nongravid uterus. In human beings, epinephrine contracts the pregnant or nonpregnant uterus when examined *in vitro* in isolated uterine muscle strips. *In situ,* however, the responses vary; and epinephrine may cause relaxation of the uterus during late pregnancy. Isoproterenol usually exerts relaxant effects in uterine muscle, even in the presence of epinephrine-induced contraction. It seems likely that the presence of circulating hormones such as estrogen and progesterone modify and may even reverse responses of the uterus to other agents. There is little clinical application of catecholamines as effectors of uterine motility.

Spleen. The smooth muscle of the splenic capsule is contracted by epinephrine and norepinephrine. The size of the spleen decreases and blood is discharged into the circulation. This response is probably functional in physiologic states such as acute hypoxia, severe fear or rage, hemorrhage, or other conditions that elicit a generalized activation of the sympathoadrenal axis.

The splenic effects of catecholamines are easily and decisively demonstrable in dogs anesthetized with pentobarbital. Under these circumstances, the spleen is enlarged and engorged with blood. Injection of small amounts of norepinephrine or epinephrine into the splenic artery causes a pronounced contraction of the spleen and a remarkable diminution of its size. Injection of these agents directly under the splenic capsule causes intense localized contraction of the capsule. These effects are associated with α receptors.

Pilomotor Effects. Norepinephrine and epinephrine cause contraction of piloerector muscles; hairs become erect. This effect is mediated by α receptors; it is often seen in animals, particularly carnivores, during severe reaction to fear or rage.

Ocular Effects. Mydriasis occurs in response to stimulation of the sympathetic innervation to the eye. Intravenous administration or topical application of epinephrine or norepinephrine causes pupillary dilation. Parasympathetic activity easily overrides adrenergic activity in the eye, however, and responses to adrenergic drugs may vary considerably. The nictitating membrane, or third eyelid, is contracted by norepinephrine and epinephrine; conjunctival and scleral blood vessels are constricted. Intraocular pressure may decrease slightly upon local instillation of epinephrine; this effect is too insignificant to be useful in treating glaucoma.

Central Nervous System Effects. Catecholamines are not believed to readily cross the blood-brain barrier. Therefore, epinephrine and norepinephrine have little effect on the CNS. With large doses, anxiety and apprehension have been reported in human beings, but this effect may be due to awareness of cardiovascular disturbances produced by large dosages. Although the CNS may be slightly affected by norepinephrine or epinephrine, this effect is of little importance in most situations in animals. This is in contrast to certain noncatecholamine adrenergic agents, like amphetamine, that readily cross the blood-brain barrier and elicit very pronounced stimulation of the CNS.

Metabolic Effects. Catecholamines exert several rather striking effects on anabolic and catabolic activities in different organs and tissues. In mammals, there is an overall calorogenic effect (increase in general metabolism) associated with a 20%–30% increase in oxygen consumption. Glycogenolysis occurs in the liver and in skeletal and cardiac muscle following exposure to epinephrine, norepinephrine, or isoproterenol. In addition, there is an acceleration of fatty acid mobilization and lactic acid formation. Accordingly, the concentrations in the blood of glucose, free fatty acids, and lactic acid are increased. The order of potency of the catecholamines in eliciting these metabolic changes varies in different tissues and species. In general, the glycogenolysis effect in muscles and liver follows the potency order of that associated with the β receptors.

The metabolic activities of the catecholamines have been associated with alterations of tissue concentration of cyclic AMP. In hepatic and muscle tissue, for example, adenylate cyclase activity is increased by the catecholamines resulting in an accelerated conversion of ATP to cyclic AMP. Cyclic AMP, in turn, accelerates the conversion of the inactive phosphorylase enzyme (phosphorylase b) to an active form (phosphorylase a), which then catalyzes the catabolism of glycogen to glucose. Similarly, the catecholamines have been associated with changes in the relative activities of tissue lipases and phosphofructokinases, purportedly by increases in cyclic AMP formation. The direct causal relationship of catecholamines and cyclic AMP in relation to all the metabolic effects remains to be definitively established.

Epinephrine causes a leukocytosis with concurrent eosinopenia. The effects on circulating eosinophils have mistakenly been attributed to changes in the ACTH-adrenal cortex relationship. However, the effects seem to be direct since eosinopenia occurs in adrenalectomized animals.

ABSORPTION AND BIOTRANSFORMATION

Epinephrine and norepinephrine are not absorbed to any appreciable extent following oral administration, due to destruction within the gastrointestinal tract. The liver rapidly inactivates by oxidative deamination and conjugation any norepinephrine or epinephrine that may be absorbed into the portal system. Isoproterenol is absorbed following oral or sublingual administration but often in such an erratic manner as to be therapeutically nonuseful. Catecholamines are readily absorbed from aerosolized sprays or after parenteral administration. Subcutaneous dosages are more slowly absorbed than are intramuscular injections.

Injected norepinephrine and epinephrine are metabolized by both MAO and COMT (catechol-O-methyltransferase) enzymes; the inactive metabolites are excreted in the urine. A portion of the O-methylated and deaminated metabolites are conjugated prior to excretion. MAO and COMT are present in many tissues; breakdown of catecholamines does not depend entirely upon the liver or kidney. It should be remembered that uptake of norepinephrine and epinephrine into adrenergic neurons away from their active receptor sites is an important pathway for termination of their pharmacologic activities (see Chapter 6). This is demonstrated by injecting a drug that blocks the amine uptake pump, e.g., cocaine; cocaine potentiates the pressor response to norepinephrine and epinephrine. Inhibition of MAO and COMT has little effect on responses to single injections of catecholamines.

PREPARATIONS

Epinephrine, U.S.P. The free base, it is obtained from adrenal medullary extracts of domestic farm animals or is chemically synthesized. It is a white or light brown crystalline powder that is relatively insoluble in water but readily forms the water-soluble salt, epinephrine hydrochloride, upon addition to dilute hydrochloric acid. Solutions are unstable in alkaline mediums or upon exposure to light or heat and discolor to pink and eventually brown. Discoloration indicates oxidation of epinephrine to an inactive form; such solutions should be discarded.

Epinephrine Injection, U.S.P., and *Epinephrine Solution,* U.S.P., are aqueous solutions of epinephrine hydrochloride (adrenaline hydrochloride) prepared in a 1:1000 (1 mg/ml; 0.1%) solution; they are probably the most commonly used preparations of epinephrine. The former solution is sterile. Addition of small amounts of sodium bisulfite retards the oxidative breakdown of epinephrine.

Sterile Epinephrine Suspension, U.S.P., is a sterile suspension of epinephrine, usually 2 mg/ml, in sesame or peanut oil for intramuscular injection only. This product is used when prolonged activity is desired.

Epinephrine Bitartrate, U.S.P., is available in aerosol and ophthalmic solutions.

Levarterenol (Norepinephrine) Bitartrate, U.S.P., l-norepinephrine bitartrate is a white crystalline powder (monohydrate salt) that readily dissolves in water. Solutions turn pink upon exposure to light, heat, or air and should be discarded if discoloration occurs.

Levarterenol (Norepinephrine) Bitartrate Injection, U.S.P., is a sterile aqueous solution usually containing 0.2% (2 mg/ml) of the salt (equivalent to 0.1% or 1 mg/ml of norepinephrine base). Bisulfite is included to delay oxidation.

Isoproterenol Hydrochloride, U.S.P., (Isuprel hydrochloride) is the water-soluble hydrochloride salt. Solutions of this compound also oxidize when exposed to light or air.

Isoproterenol Hydrochloride Injection, U.S.P., is a sterile aqueous solution of isoproterenol hydrochloride for parenteral injection. Preparations available usually contain 0.2 mg/ml (0.02%).

Isoproterenol Hydrochloride Tablets, U.S.P., are available in 10-mg and 15-mg tablets.

CLINICAL USE

With Local Anesthetics. Epinephrine is commonly used in concentrations of 1:100,000 to 1:20,000 in local anesthetic solutions. It causes pronounced local vasoconstriction and thereby localizes the action and delays the absorption of the infilterable anesthetic. Since norepinephrine is a less potent α agonist than epinephrine, it is infrequently used in local anesthetic solutions.

Local Hemostatic. Vasoconstrictor effects of epinephrine (1:100,000 to 1:20,000 solution) may be utilized to control superficial bleeding of mucosal and subcutaneous surfaces by application of moistened gauze sponges or by aerosol sprayed directly onto the damaged region. Epinephrine solutions have been used topically during ophthalmic surgery to control hemorrhage. Epistaxis and dental extractions are other indications. Epinephrine is effective only against hemorrhage from capillaries and arterioles and should not be used in attempts to control bleeding from larger vessels. Although smooth muscle of large vessels contract in response to amines, this effect is by no means sufficient to occlude the lumen. During surgery, topical application of epinephrine should be considered only as a temporary aid for controlling bleeding to assist in visualization of the operative field. Serious bleeding may well recur subsequent to termination of activity of this catecholamine if routine ligation of blood vessels is disregarded.

Hypotension. Pressor amines are often used to maintain blood pressure during spinal surgery, and epinephrine is quite effective in treating hypotension associated with anaphylactic shock. The peripheral vasoconstrictor effects of norepinephrine, epinephrine, and other adrenergic drugs have also been used in attempts to treat and prevent hypotension occurring during other shock syndromes. It should be recognized, however, that blood pressure elevation due to peripheral vasoconstriction is not an adequate substitution for correcting serious underlying problems such as hypovolemia, undetected hemorrhage, and electrolyte and fluid imbalances. In fact, some shock states are characterized by peripheral vasoconstriction secondary to a generalized sympathoadrenal discharge. Under such circumstances, administration of epinephrine or norepinephrine may serve to compound the problem by causing further intensification of vasoconstriction in vital areas, e.g., splanchnic and renal vascular beds. In some cases, the exact opposite effect, i.e., blockade of α-adrenerigc receptors, has been proposed as a treatment in shock. These factors should always be considered when the use of sympathomimetic amines during shock therapy is considered. Treatment of shock is discussed in Chapter 29.

In those shock cases that are characterized by a loss of vascular tone, the use of pressor amines has been suggested. Also, reestablishment of normal blood volume in some shock patients does not seem to correct the vascular complications, and blood pressure remains seriously depressed. Pressor agents may be of some use. Norepinephrine has been utilized under these circumstances. Usually, a 4-ml vial of 0.2% norepinephrine bitartrate (0.1% of free norepinephrine base; 1 mg/ml) is added to 1 L of sterile isotonic saline solution or 5% dextrose solution, which gives a final concentration of norepinephrine base of 4 μg/ml of solution. This solution is slowly infused intravenously until blood pressure is maintained somewhat lower than normal. Usually, an infusion rate of 0.1–0.2 μg/kg/minute proves effective; however, administration should be to effect. The pressor response to norepinephrine can be readily controlled since it disappears within 1 or 2 minutes after stopping the infusion. Blood pressure should be closely monitored during the infusion process. An attempt should always be made to closely monitor cardiovascular function during treatment with any of the catecholamines. Isoproterenol has been used in some low cardiac output stages of stock. Soma et al. (1974) recommend a slow intravenous infusion of a 0.1–0.2 μg/ml solution of isoproterenol.

Cardiac Effects. Catecholamines are indicated in the treatment of certain cardiac disorders: cardiac arrest, partial or complete atrioventricular (A-V) block, and Stokes-Adams syndrome. With cardiac arrest, an attempt is first made to restore heartbeat by mechanical means such as a precordial blow, electrical shock, or external cardiac massage. If the heart starts contracting, isoproterenol or epinephrine can be given by slow intravenous drip to maintain heart rate and cardiac output after circulation is restored. Care should be taken with intravenous infusion since epinephrine may precipitate ventricular fibrillation if prefibrillatory rhythm is presented.

If asystole persists, norepinephrine, epinephrine (0.5–1.0 ml of a 1:10,000 solution; i.e., 50–100 μg), or isoproterenol (20–40 μg) may be administered directly into the left ventricular chamber in an attempt to restore contraction. Larger doses may be required in some instances. The heart should then be massaged to insure circulation of the catecholamine through the coronary vasculature. Peripheral circulation should be maintained by cardiac massage until myocardial contraction is restored.

Isoproterenol is the drug of choice for treating heart block. Complete A-V heart block in a dog was treated with 0.05 mg (approximately 3.5 μg/kg) of isoproterenol administered intravenously; the heart rate increased almost immediately from 44 beats/minute to 68 beats/minute (Buchanan et al. 1968). Due to its potency, isoproterenol should be administered by slow intravenous infusion rather than by rapid bolus injection. Slow intravenous drip of a dilute solution can be instituted until the heart rate is maintained at 80–100 beats/minute. Thereafter, intramuscular injections of 0.1–0.2 mg of isoproterenol every 4 hours may prove effective. Isoproterenol tablets (15–30 mg) have been given every 4 hours; however, patients should be closely monitored since absorption after oral administration is erratic. Buchanan et al. (1968) found that orally administered isoproterenol (30 mg twice daily) was ineffective in treating complete A-V block in a dog. In treating A-V block in dogs, Ettinger (1969) infused isoproterenol hydrochloride (5 μg/ml in dextrose and water) intravenously at a rate (usually 1 ml/minute) sufficient to maintain the ventricular rate at 80/minute. With this procedure, all premature ventricular contractions were suppressed. Isoproterenol was then administered subcutaneously every 6 hours at the dose of 0.2 mg. Oral administration of an isoproterenol tablet (30 mg) every 6 hours was prescribed for several weeks. Catecholamines should not be used in the presence of acute or chronic heart failure. These agents decrease efficiency of myocardial contraction by increasing oxygen demands of the heart muscle and compound the heart failure syndrome.

Anaphylactic and Allergic Reactions. Epinephrine is extremely effective and often lifesaving in the treatment of acute anaphylactic shock. It quickly reverses the precipitous fall in blood pressure and the cardiac irregularities associated with this type of syndrome. Histaminelike constriction of bronchiolar smooth muscles occurs during anaphylaxis; these effects are rapidly antagonized by epinephrine. Bronchiolar passageways are dilated by epinephrine due to relaxation of the smooth muscle, and dyspnea is quickly counteracted.

Epinephrine is beneficial in reversing many types of allergic responses. Acute anaphylactoid reactions to biological vaccination products respond quite well to epinephrine administration. Care should be taken that allergic signs do not recur after epinephrine activity has terminated.

Bronchial Asthma. Isoproterenol and epinephrine are particularly valuable for providing immediate relief from bronchial asthma. These agents activate the β receptors of the bronchial smooth muscle cells, causing relaxation and prompt relief by dilating the airways. Norepinephrine is ineffective in dilating passageways even though it may transiently decrease mucosal congestion by constricting mucosal blood vessels. For systemic relief from allergic and anaphylactoid reactions, epinephrine can be administered subcutaneously or intramuscularly, since with these routes effective blood levels are quickly achieved. However, if a patient is presented in late stages of anaphylactic shock or other similar life-threatening situations, intravenous administration may be required.

In large domestic animals, e.g., cattle and horses, 4–8 mg of epinephrine can be given intramuscularly or subcutaneously by injection of 4–8 ml of a 1:1000 dilution of epinephrine hydrochloride solution. Sheep and swine may be administered 1–3 ml of the 1:1000 dilution. Dogs and cats are usually given 1–5 ml of a 1:10,000 (0.1 mg/ml) dilution. Based on a body weight range of approximately 5–25 kg, this represents a dosage schedule of approximately 20 μg/kg of body weight. A dose this large should be administered only by intramuscular or subcutaneous injection. Response of animals to adrenergic drugs may vary considerably. Therefore, repeat injections or somewhat larger doses may be required in some cases. If intravenous administration is necessary, one should proceed cautiously and give no more than 0.25–0.5 μg/kg. In experimental animals, 1–2 μg/kg of epinephrine or norepinephrine administered by intravenous bolus injection causes a pronounced increase in cardiovascular activity, and even slightly larger doses may well lead to serious arrhythmias.

TOXICITY

As implied in the preceding discussion, toxicity of the catecholamines is usually characterized by untoward cardiovascular responses. In particular, cardiac dysrhythmias such as tachycardia and even fatal ventricular fibrillation may occur following inadvertent overdosage. Hyperthyroid conditions, thyroid therapy, digitalis therapy, halogenated hydrocarbon anesthetics, and thiobarbiturates predispose a patient to the myocardial toxicity of catecholamines. The influence of anesthetics on the arrhythmogenicity of catecholamines is believed to be due to "sensitization" of the heart muscle. Myocardial sensitization to catecholamines is evoked by trichlorethylene, ethyl chloride, cyclopropane, halothane, chloroform, methoxyflurane, and fluroxene (listed in order of decreasing effect) (Katz and Katz 1966). The thiobarbiturates thiamylal and thiopental have been reported to increase the incidence of epinephrine- and norepinephrine-induced arrhythmias in chloroform-anesthetized dogs (Claborn and Szabuniewicz 1973; Wiersig et al. 1974).

Hypertensive crises occur from norepinephrine or epinephrine overdosage; cerebral vascular accidents and ruptured aneurysms may result. The latter represents a potential problem in horses due to a fairly common incidence of undiagnosed verminous aneurysms. Large or repeated dosages of epinephrine and isoproterenol have been associated with myocardial ischemia and necrosis; these effects are prevented by β blocking agents. Local necrosis and sloughing of tissue may occur at injection sites due to intensive vasoconstriction and resulting ischemia. Subcutaneous administration is particularly likely to present this complication.

In short, the catecholamines are extremely potent agents. Under no circumstances should they be considered as innocuous agents. Therapeutic use of these drugs should always be carefully monitored by a trained individual familiar with their indications, limitations, and toxicities.

Dopamine

Until relatively recent times, dopamine (3,4-dihydroxyphenylethylamine) was thought to be important only as the immediate precursor to norepinephrine. However, dopamine itself is now believed to have some physiologic functions in mammalian species and is receiving attention in certain clinical circumstances in human beings. Parkinson's disease, for example, has been related to decreased concentrations of dopamine in the basal ganglia, and treatment with L-dopa has proved effective in controlling motor disorders in some Parkinsonism patients. L-Dopa crosses the blood-brain barrier (dopamine does not in significant quantities) and is decarboxylated to dopamine.

Experimental hemodynamic studies indicate that dopamine may have some use as a selective cardiovascular agent. In anesthetized dogs, intravenous injection of 1–9 μg/kg of dopamine caused a slight depressor response associated with a decrease in total peripheral resistance, a decrease in renal vascular resistance, an increase in renal blood flow, and an increase in cardiac output. Large amounts, 9–81 μg/kg, produced pressor responses and a more pronounced increase in myocardial contractile force (Setler et al. 1975). The cardiovascular effects of dopamine seem to depend on activation of different types of catecholaminergic receptors. The pressor response is blocked by an α blocker (e.g., phenoxybenzamine), and the cardiac stimulatory effects are blocked by a β blocker (e.g., propranolol). Part of the myocardial effects of dopamine are thought to be indirect and to be mediated by release of norepinephrine from cardiac sympathetic nerves.

The depressor effects of dopamine are not blocked by a β blocker, but they are blocked by haloperidol and bulbocapnine. Since these drugs are dopamine antagonists in the brain, it has been proposed that there are specific "dopaminergic" receptors in certain vascular beds (Goldberg 1972, 1975). Dopamine-responsive receptors in blood vessels subserve relaxation of vascular smooth muscle and evoke vasodilation. They appear to be particularly prevalent in the renal and splanchnic circulation. Dopamine causes decreased vascular resistance and increased blood flow to the kidneys and mesenteric circulation concurrent with myocardial stimulation. This particular aspect may be an advantage over conventional catecholamines in the treatment of shock since norepinephrine and epinephrine markedly constrict renal and mesenteric arteries due to α-receptor effects and since isoproterenol has little effect on resistance in these regions, due to a relative lack of β vascular receptors in these tissues.

Selective vasodilation of renal and splanchnic beds by dopamine has prompted the use of this agent in clinical cases of cardiovascular dysfunction in human beings and during experimental shock in lower animals. In some cases, dopamine has been found to be effective in maintaining cardiovascular function in human patients that were nonresponsive to other catecholamines. Dopamine is now approved for use in human beings for treatment of certain cardiovascular disorders. Although it has not received clinical use in lower animals, extension of the use of dopamine into clinical veterinary medicine seems likely in the future.

NONCATECHOLAMINES

Although the 3,4-dihydroxybenzene structure yields maximum potency, many drugs lacking the catechol nucleus have proved to be clinically useful in many situations. As with the catecholamines, the end effects of these drugs are mediated by the adrenergic receptors of effector cells. However, the mechanism of obtaining receptor activation varies considerably from one drug to another. For example, it has been known for some time that surgical sympathetic denervation abolishes or markedly reduces the effects of some agents, like tyramine (an experimental sympathomimetic amine), but does not reduce the effects of epinephrine. Reserpine causes a "functional" sympathectomy by depleting adrenergic neurons of their stores of norepinephrine. Pretreatment with reserpine markedly decreases the response to tyramine but does not decrease the effects of epinephrine. Bretylium blocks the release of norepinephrine from nerves; it decreases the effects of tyramine but does not reduce responses to epinephrine or norepinephrine. An α blocking agent, however, prevents the effects of tyramine, epinephrine, and norepinephrine. These findings indicate that tyramine acts presynaptically to cause a release of endogenous norepinephrine from the nerve, which in turn acts on postjunctional receptors. Based on these types of findings, adrenergic drugs can be classified into three groups: (1) direct-acting (effects not decreased by denervation), (2) mixed-action (effects partially reduced by denervation), and (3) indirect-acting (effects markedly reduced by denervation). Prototypes for each class are norepinephrine (direct-acting), ephedrine (mixed-acting), and tyramine (indirect-acting).

The catecholamines are direct-acting agents. In general, drugs with only the 3-OH group have predominantly direct effects, while those with 4-OH act primarily by indirect means. However, most of the noncatecholamine adrenergic drugs have been found to have both direct and indirect effects, and the ratio of these effects may even vary from one tissue to another. Ephedrine, for example, releases norepinephrine as part of its action but seems to act directly on β receptors of bronchial smooth muscle, an effect that is not seen with norepinephrine. Agents with a methyl substitution on the α-carbon atom effectively cross the blood-brain barrier and exert marked CNS stimulation in addition to peripheral actions.

Despite these very complex interrelationships, the peripheral effects of adrenergic drugs can invariably be explained by an activation, whether direct or indirect, of the α and/or β receptors. Therefore, the effects of these drugs are similar to and can be compared with the previously discussed pharmacologic effects of the direct-acting agents, norepinephrine, epinephrine, and isoproterenol.

Ephedrine

Ephedrine was originally isolated from the Chinese shrub, *Ma huang (Ephedia* genus), but is now chemically synthesized. The natural product has been used in oriental medicine for centuries and was introduced into modern therapeutics during the 1920s (Chen and Schmidt 1930). The structure of ephedrine and related pharmacologic effects are shown in Table 7.1. The levo isomer is the most active form of this component. Ephedrine exerts its sympathomimetic effects both by direct activation of adrenergic receptors and by release of endogenous norepinephrine.

PHARMACOLOGIC EFFECTS

Cardiovascular. Intravenous administration of ephedrine produces hemodynamic changes similar to those caused by bolus injection of epinephrine. Systolic and diastolic blood pressures increase, myocardial contractile force increases, heart rate increases if vagal reflexes are blocked, and cardiac output increases if venous return is adequate. Vasoconstriction occurs in the kidney, mesenteric, and cutaneous circulation; blood flow to these regions decreases. Blood flow may increase, however, through coronary, cerebral, and skeletal muscle vascular beds. Ephedrine is many times less potent a pressor agent than epinephrine, but its effects last 7–10 times longer. Cardiovascular effects are obtained after oral administration of ephedrine, whereas epinephrine is inactive if given by mouth.

In contrast to epinephrine and norepinephrine, repeated injections of ephedrine evoke progressively smaller pressor responses in intact animals. This condition, termed *tachyphylaxis,* is probably dependent upon different factors. First, since ephedrine causes a release of endogenous amines, stores of norepinephrine may eventually be depleted so less and less is available for release. The long duration of action of ephedrine may also contribute to development of tachyphylaxis. During long courses of cardiovascular stimulation, reflex mechanisms attempt to return hemodynamic function toward normal. Blood pressure may return to somewhat normal values, although ephedrine, due to its delayed elimination, is still present at receptor sites. Repeated injections, therefore, prove less effective if a relative blockade of the receptors by prior administration of ephedrine still exists.

Central Nervous System. Ephedrine is a CNS stimulant. It stimulates corticomedullary regions and, in large doses, causes excitement, apparent anxiety, and muscular tremors. Respiratory centers of the medulla oblongata are activated by appropriate doses of ephedrine. This effect has been used clinically to reverse respiratory depression, particularly if respiratory problems are associated with barbiturate overdosage. Ephedrine is infrequently used for this purpose now since other central stimulants have proved more effective or more reliable. Other adrenergic drugs, such as amphetamine, stimulate the CNS to a greater extent than ephedrine.

Ocular. Mydriasis occurs after local or systemic administration of ephedrine due to active stimulation of the radial muscle of the iris. A 10% solution has been used to enlarge the pupillary space to facilitate ophthalmic examination.

Bronchial Smooth Muscle. Ephedrine is effective in causing relaxation of bronchial smooth muscle and increasing the diameter of bronchiolar passageways; these effects are believed to be due to direct activation of β receptors.

CLINICAL USE

Ephedrine has not been used extensively in veterinary medicine. It offers no particular advantage over epinephrine except that its duration of action is longer and it is effective when given by the oral route. Indications for use of an adrenergic drug in veterinary medicine usually require an immediate response, which can often best be obtained with injection of epinephrine.

The prolonged duration of the pressor effect of ephedrine may be of some benefit in maintaining blood pressure without having to resort to repeated injection or constant perfusion with a catecholamine. The use of 10–20 mg of ephedrine administered by intravenous or intramuscular injection has been advocated for pressor effects in dogs (Soma et al. 1974).

Ephedrine solution, 1%–1.5%, can be applied topically onto congested mucosal membranes to evoke vasoconstriction and decongestion. Ephedrine is effective in reducing allergic responses, but the onset of action is slower than with epinephrine. Ephedrine is sometimes included in cough suppressant preparations for relief from bronchiolar congestion and vascular constriction. It is stable in solution and has a longer duration of relaxant effect on bronchial muscle than epinephrine.

AMPHETAMINE

Amphetamine, or β-phenylisopropylamine, induces pronounced stimulation of the CNS as well as causes marked peripheral α and β effects. A considerable portion of the pharmacologic effects of amphetamine is due to release of endogenous norepinephrine. Cardiovascular effects of amphetamine are somewhat similar to those produced by ephedrine. An increase of systolic and diastolic blood pressures is observed. Heart rate is reflexly slowed and cardiac output is not affected to any appreciable extent. Cardiovascular effects are observed after the drug is given by the oral route. The *l*-isomer is a somewhat more active pressor agent than the *d*-isomer. The chemical structure of amphetamine is shown in Table 7.1.

Topical application of amphetamine to mucosal membranes evokes vasoconstriction and decreased secretions and shrinks the membranes. It causes pupillary dilatation but has less effect on bronchiolar muscle than ephedrine. Gastrointestinal activity is inhibited.

Amphetamine and its analogues, methamphetamine and hydroxyamphetamine, have been used primarily as CNS stimulants. Of the three, amphetamine (benzedrine) has been used most frequently in veterinary medicine. Amphetamine is no longer available for use in veterinary medicine and is now subject to strict control under the 1970 Controlled Substances Act. It is active if given by mouth; CNS effects persist for several hours. The entire CNS is affected, but effects on the cerebrum are most evident in human beings: increased alertness, loss of fatigue, euphoria, and a sense of exhilaration. The performance of athletes is improved; this is attributed to improvement of those activities requiring mental and physical coordination. After the effects of amphetamine have dissipated, pronounced depression may occur. In human beings amphetamine is most often used in the treatment of neuropsychiatric disorders such as mild but chronic depression, narcolepsy, alcoholism, and in some cases of hyperkinesis in children.

Prior to the strict control of amphetamine by the Controlled Substances Act it was used almost exclusively in veterinary therapeutics for its stimulatory effects on the respiratory centers in the medulla oblongata. The entire cerebrospinal axis is affected, but particularly the brain stem and cortex. The *d*-isomer, dextro-amphetamine (Dexedrine), is the most centrally active isomer. Its analeptic potency is similar to that of pentamethylenetetrazol (Metrazol). Amphetamine increases both the rate and depth of inspiration in anesthetized animals. It was often used intravenously (4–4.5 mg/kg) in the dog to overcome the respiratory depressant effects of barbiturate overdosage.

Phenylephrine

Phenylephrine is similar in structure to epinephrine except that it lacks the 4-OH group on the benzene ring; the chemical structure and pharmacologic characteristics of phenylephrine are shown in Table 7.1. Phenylephrine is primarily a direct-acting sympathomimetic amine at α receptors and does not depend upon release of endogenous norepinephrine for its effects. Similar to norepinephrine, phenylephrine causes peripheral vasoconstriction due to direct activation of α receptors of blood vessels. However, dissimilar to norepinephrine, it has very little effect at cardiac β receptors. Systolic and diastolic blood pressures are increased by phenylephrine; reflex bradycardia usually occurs. In fact, the predictable reflex-mediated slowing of the heart rate by phenylephrine has led to the use of this agent in human patients to control episodes of paroxysmal atrial tachycardia.

Phenylephrine is a less potent pressor agent than norepinephrine but has a longer duration of action. The intravenous dose for dogs is 0.088 mg/kg; approximately twice this amount should be given if administered by the subcutaneous or intramuscular route.

Methoxamine and Metaraminol

The chemical structure of methoxamine is β-hydroxy-β-(2,5-dimethoxyphenyl)-isopropylamine. The chemical structure and related pharmacologic effects of metaraminol are included in Table 7.1. Like phenylephrine, these drugs act almost exclusively as direct-acting sympathomimetic amines at peripheral α receptors. They have minimal detectable myocardial stimulatory properties. Their pressor effects on systolic and diastolic blood pressures can be explained by peripheral vasoconstriction and increased peripheral resistance. Reflex bradycardia usually results. These drugs are used as pressor agents. After intravenous injection, the pressor response to methoxamine occurs rapidly and may persist for 1 hour. With intramuscular administration, 15 minutes is usually required for the pressor response to take effect and it usually lasts 1–1.5 hours.

ANTIADRENERGIC DRUGS

Numerous agents have been discovered that prevent either the pharmacologic effects of sympathomimetic drugs or the physiologic responses evoked by stimulation of adrenergic nerves, or both. The terms adrenolytic and sympatholytic have been used in the past to describe such activities; however, more precise terminology is presently in use. *Adrenergic blocking drug* is a term used in reference to a very explicit mechanism of action. These drugs interact with adrenergic receptors of effector cells and by occupying these sites do not allow an adrenergic agonist access to the receptor. *Adrenergic neuron blocking drugs,* on the other hand, do not block the postsynaptic receptor. Instead, they act presynaptically at the nerve terminal to cause a decreased release of the endogenous neurotransmitter, norepinephrine.

Adrenergic Blocking Drugs

Immediately after the beginning of this century, Dale (1906) reported that pretreatment of cats with ergot alkaloids prevented some of the hemodynamic effects of epinephrine. These studies presented the first evidence of the drug action now commonly referred to as *adrenergic blockade.* Adrenergic blocking drugs exert their pharmacologic effects by interlocking with and occupying adrenergic receptors of effector cells. In this manner, adrenergic agonists are prevented from affixing to the receptor site; effects of the agonist are abolished or markedly decreased.

The adrenergic blocking effects of ergot alkaloids (and some drugs like phentolamine that were subsequently synthesized) were identified as being present only at those adrenergic receptors designated by Ahlquist (1948) as *alpha.* In fact, for over 50 years the only adrenergic blocking agents identified inhibited α-receptor–mediated effects. This problem delayed full acceptance of Ahlquist's (1948) differentiation of α- and β-receptor sites. However, in 1958, Powell and Slater and Moran and Perkins demonstrated that the 3,4-dichlorophenyl analog of isoproterenol selectively inhibited those responses ascribed by Ahlquist (1948) to be mediated by *beta* receptors. This drug, dichloroisoproterenol, blocked the vasodilatation, cardiac stimulation, and bronchial smooth muscle relaxing effects of catecholamines but had no effect on α-mediated effects. Dichloroisoproterenol is not used clinically, since it causes a transient stimulation of the β receptors prior to blockade, i.e., it is a *partial agonist.* Propranolol was subsequently identified as a β blocking agent that did not have agonistic properties.

Pharmacologic Considerations of α and β Blocking Drugs

Receptor Blockade

The selective α or β inhibitory effects of representative adrenergic blocking drugs (e.g., α blockade with phentolamine and β blockade with propranolol) on the blood pressure and myocardial effects of sympathomimetic drugs are shown in Fig. 7.4. Alpha blockade abolishes the pressor response to norepinephrine. Epinephrine is a mixed α-β agonist; α blockade by phentolamine not only prevents the pressor response to epinephrine, it actually converts it to a depressor response. This is called *epinephrine reversal.* Since the α receptors are occupied by phentolamine, only the vasodilator-related β receptors are available for interaction with epinephrine. Thus epinephrine causes a fall in blood pressure. Alpha blockade does not affect the β-receptor–mediated depressor effect of isoproterenol nor does it affect the cardiac stimulant effects of the catecholamines.

Propranolol, a β blocker, inhibits the cardiac stimulant effects of isoproterenol, epinephrine, and norepinephrine (Fig. 7.4). It also blocks the depressor response to isoproterenol but does not prevent the α-receptor–mediated pressor response to norepinephrine. The secondary depressor effect of epinephrine seen in the control situation is due to residual β-receptor–mediated vasodilation; this is abolished by propranolol.

Some β blocking agents are considerably more active at either the β_1 myocardial receptors (e.g., practolol) or the β_2 vascular receptors (e.g., butoxamine) (Moran 1973). Recent studies have provided preliminary evidence indicating that, in addition to α and β receptors, there may also exist a dopamine receptor subserving vasodilatation in certain arterial beds (i.e., renal, mesenteric) (Goldberg 1975). Table 7.3 summarizes characteristics of catecholaminergic receptors in relation to agonists and antagonists.

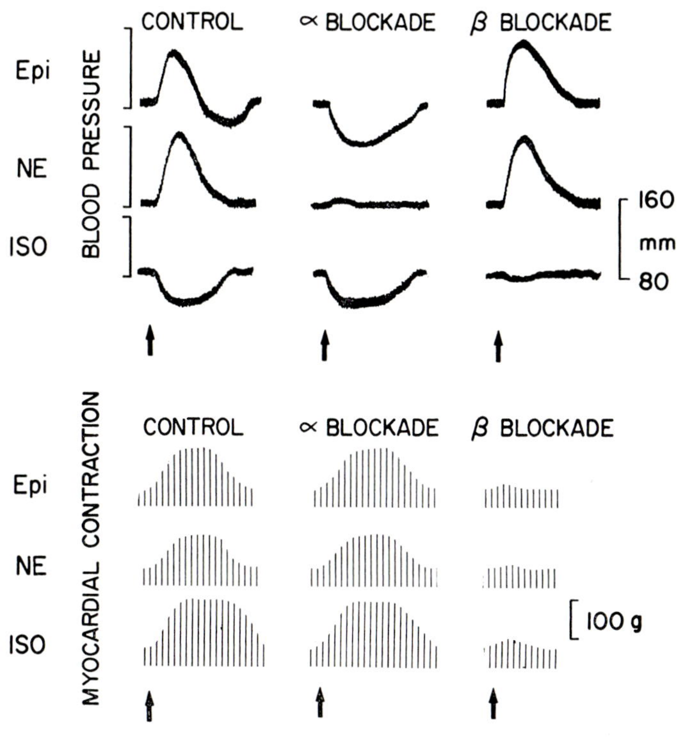

FIG. 7.4. Effects of α- and β-adrenergic blockade on the blood pressure and myocardial effects of epinephrine (Epi), norepinephrine (NE), and isoproterenol (ISO) in a dog. Control = effects of the amines in the absence of an adrenergic blocking drug. α Blockade = effects of the amines after administration of an α blocker (e.g., phentolamine). β Blockade = effects of the amines after administration of a β blocker (e.g., propranolol). Epi, NE, or ISO was injected intravenously at arrow. α Blockade (1) inhibits the pressor response to NE, (2) does not affect the depressor effect of ISO, (3) converts the pressor effect of Epi to a depressor effect ("epi reversal"), and (4) does not affect the cardiac stimulant effects of the amines. β Blockade (1) does not affect pressor responses to NE, (2) inhibits the depressor effects of isoproterenol, (3) inhibits the secondary depressor effect of Epi, and (4) inhibits the myocardial stimulant effects of all three amines (see text for details).

TABLE 7.3. Classification and characteristics of catecholaminergic receptors

Characteristics	Receptor Types			
	α	β_1	β_2	Dopamine
Potency of agonists	E>NE>D>I	I>E≧NE>D	I>E>NE>D	D>E,NE,I
Antagonists				
α blockers (PHEN)	Block	No	No	No
β blockers				
General (PROP)	No	Block	Block	No
β_1 (PRACT)	No	Block	Weak block	No
β_2 (BUT)	No	Weak block	Block	No
Dopamine antagonist (HAL)	No	No	No	Block

Source: Modified from Moran 1973.

Note: E = epinephrine; NE = norepinephrine; D = dopamine; I = isoproterenol; PHEN = phentolamine; No = no blocking effect; PROP = propranolol; PRACT = practolol; BUT = butoxamine; HAL = haloperidol.

PHARMACOLOGIC EFFECTS

The degree of autonomic nervous system activity at any one time plays an important role in determining the extent of pharmacologic effects that will be produced by an adrenergic blocking agent. For example, administration of a β blocking drug to a trained quiescent patient does not cause profound cardiovascular effects. This is because at rest the heart is not under pronounced sympathetic influence. Upon physical exertion, however, an increase in heart rate and cardiac output is produced, due to increased sympathetic nervous system activity. If the patient is required to exercise during treatment with propranolol, these characteristic cardiac responses are not obtained since the β-adrenergic receptors of the heart are blocked by this drug.

Effects of an α blocking agent are similarly influenced by the existing state of autonomic nervous system activity. If the cardiovascular system is under pronounced sympathetic dominance (e.g., during fright or severe hypovolemia), an α blocking drug will cause a decrease in blood pressure. This occurs because the α receptors of blood vessels are occupied by the α blocking agent and are no longer available to norepinephrine or to circulating epinephrine.

The pharmacologic effects of adrenergic blocking agents can be reliably predicted by considering the distribution of α and β receptors in the body and the respective physiologic functions that they subserve. The distribution of α and β receptors in various organs and tissues and their functional characteristics are summarized in Tables 6.1 and 7.2. Distinctive and specific inhibitory effects of α or β blockade similar to those shown in Fig. 7.4 are demonstrable with adrenergic responses that have been definitely associated with either α or β receptors.

ALPHA-ADRENERGIC BLOCKING AGENTS

Ergot Alkaloids. Ergot alkaloids are not used clinically in human beings or in lower animals for α blocking effects. In fact, they affect a variety of organs at concentrations less than those required for α blockade. Therefore, they are not truly prototypical α blockers; however, they were the first adrenergic blocking agents identified (Dale 1906).

Ergot is a fungus *(Claviceps purpurea)* that parasitizes rye and other grains. Ingestion of contaminated grain products has caused outbreaks of ergotism in human beings and domestic animals throughout the world. This problem is infrequently encountered in modern times.

Ergot is a mixture of different types of alkaloids that have biological effects. The ergonovine group lacks a polypeptide side chain; this group does not cause adrenergic blockade but has potent oxytocic activity. The ergotamine group causes adrenergic blockade but has little effect on nonvascular smooth muscle. See Chapter 60 for information on the toxic activity of ergot as well as procedures for its prevention, control, and treatment.

Cardiovascular Effects. The predominant vascular effect of ergot is not α blockade but is related to intense peripheral vasoconstriction. These compounds cause a direct stimulation of smooth muscle, including that of peripheral blood vessels. Due to peripheral vasoconstriction, ergot initially causes a pressor response that may persist for a fairly long time. Larger doses eventually block the α-adrenergic recptors; α-receptor–mediated effects of norepinephrine, epinephrine, and other agonists are inhibited. Beta receptors are not affected.

Due to α blocking effects, ergot produces epinephrine reversal, as previously described (Fig. 7.4). In ergot-treated animals, vasodilation and hypotension occur after administration of epinephrine (or other mixed α-β agonists) due to β-receptor dominance in the presence of α blockade. Although this is not the most prominent effect of ergot, it is the most interesting, since it led to identification of other more selective α blockers. Large doses of ergot cause serious circulatory disturbances, due to intense and persistent vasoconstriction of peripheral vessels. This is characterized by stasis of blood in the capillaries and arterioles, thrombosis, and eventually obliterative endarteritis, leading to gangrene of the extremities. Sloughing of portions of the feet, hooves, tails, ears, and tongues have occurred in ergot-poisoned animals.

Other Effects. Ergot initially causes a slight stimulation of the CNS, followed by depression. Vasomotor and respiratory centers are depressed; medullary centers seem less responsive to reflexogenic signals. Gastrointestinal motility is increased. Emesis is induced by ergot, due to stimulation of the chemoreceptor trigger zone of the medulla oblongata. Smooth muscle of the uterus is stimulated to contract by ergot. The most common use of ergot, in fact, is for motor stimulation of the postparturient uterus.

Synthetic Alpha Blocking Agents. The synthetic α blockers fall into several classes of structurally unrelated chemical compounds; structure-activity relationships have not been clarified. There are several groups of α blockers, such as the haloalkylamine derivatives (phenoxybenzamine, dibenamine), the imidazoline derivatives (phentolamine, tolazoline), the benzodioxans (piperoxan, dibozane), and the dibenzazepine derivatives (azapetine); see Fig. 7.5 for the chemical structures of these compounds.

Members of the phenothiazine derivative tranquilizers also have α-adrenergic blocking properties. These drugs are discussed in detail in relation to their CNS effects (Chapter 17); their peripheral vascular actions are also of interest. Chlorpromazine and several other related compounds cause a characteristic blockade of α receptors, shown on examination of *in vitro* preparations. *In vivo* responses are not as clearly defined. These agents alter pressor effects of catecholamines (they can cause epinephrine reversal) but it seems likely that the total cardiovascular effects are due to a variety of factors such as concomitant antihistaminic, antiserotonergic, and anticholinergic effects.

Inhibition of pressor responses to catecholamines by the other synthetic α blockers, however, can be ascribed almost entirely to α-receptor blockade. Phentolamine and phenoxybenzamine are the most frequently used α blocking drugs. Their site of action is the α receptor of effector cells; β responses are not blocked. Phenoxybenzamine and other related haloalkylamines such as dibenamine produce a noncompetitive block; increasing the dosage of an α agonist will not overcome the α blockade produced by phenoxybenzamine. This characteristic seems to be due to the drug binding in a very stable manner to the receptor or nearby structures in a persistent manner. Phentolamine and tolazoline, however, cause a competitive blockade of α receptors that can usually be antagonized by increasing the availability of agonist.

Cardiovascular Effects. Slow intravenous infusion of phenoxybenzamine or phentolamine to a normal patient usually does not cause a remarkable change in blood pressure. Occasionally, a slight fall in diastolic pressure occurs. However, these drugs will cause a marked hypotensive response if a patient's cardiovascular system is under pronounced sympathetic tone. This is particularly evident during hypovolemia since in this state sympathetic discharge increases to maintain adequate blood pressure in the presence of low circulating blood volume.

If phenoxybenzamine or other potent α blockers are given by rapid intravenous injection, severe hypotension and other adverse cardiovascular effects are seen; however, these effects probably involve factors other than α blockade.

In human beings, α blockade evokes little change in blood pressure if the patient is supine, but pronounced hypotension occurs when the patient stands. This response is called *postural hypotension*. It is due to blockade of the vascular α receptors that are normally active in the efferent limb of reflex blood pressure pathways.

Other reflexogenic changes are also altered. Reflex hypertension caused by anoxia is prevented by α blockade, as is the pressor response to occlusion of the carotid

HALOAKLYAMINE DERIVATIVES

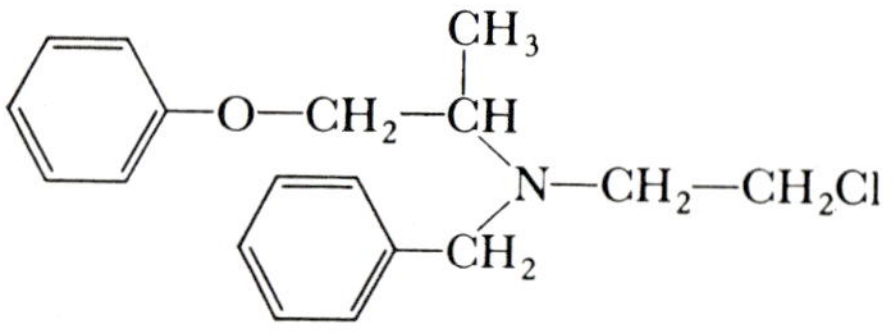

Phenoxybenzamine

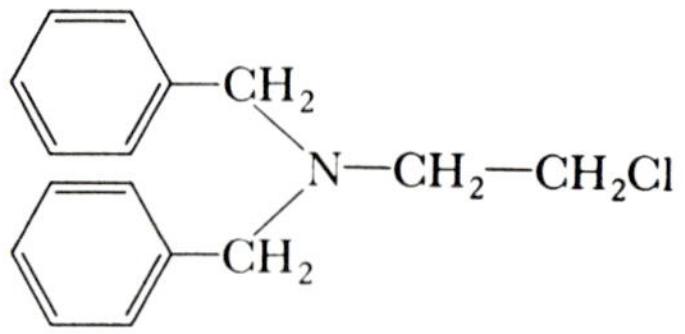

Dibenamine

IMIDAZOLINE DERIVATIVES

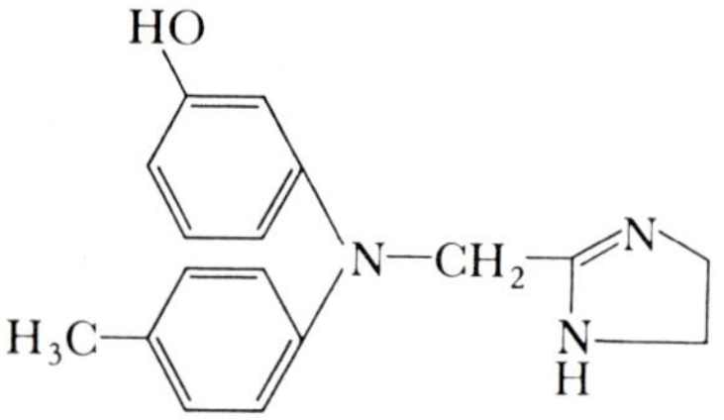

Phentolamine

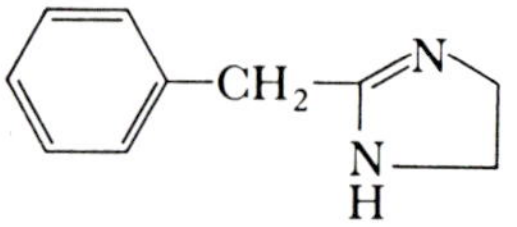

Tolazoline

BENZODIOXAN DERIVATIVES

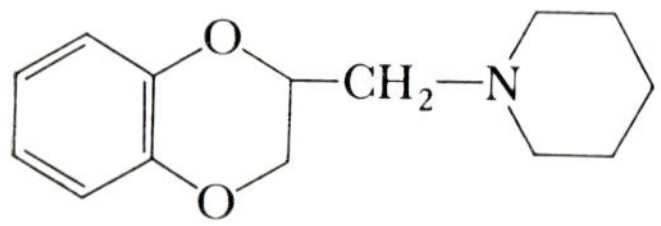

Piperoxan

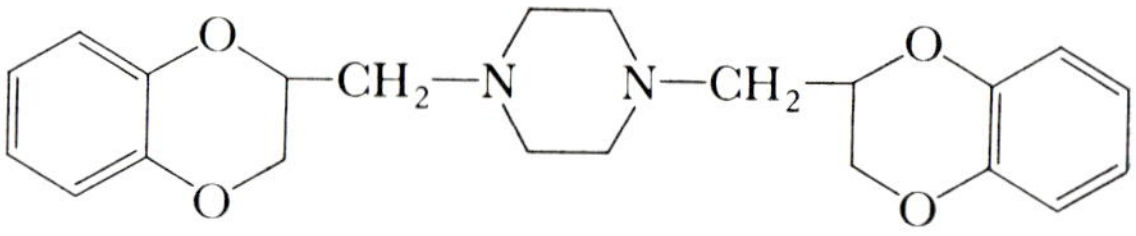

Dibozane

DIBENZAZEPINE DERIVATIVE

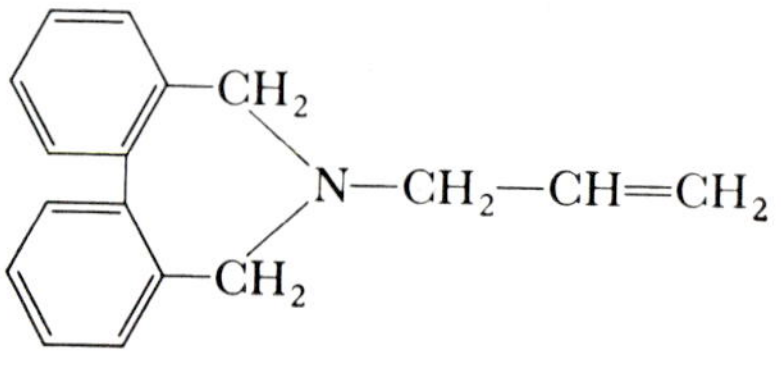

Azapetine

FIG. 7.5. Chemical structures of α-adrenergic blocking drugs.

arteries (the bilateral carotid artery occlusion reflex depends upon increased sympathetic vasoconstrictor tone and increased release of epinephrine from the adrenal gland). Due to their occupation of α receptors, α blocking agents prevent the transmission of the nerve impulse to the α receptors of the blood vessel cells and also block the interaction of circulating epinephrine with α receptors. In this manner, reflexogenic pressor responses are inhibited. Alpha blocking agents increase blood flow through capillaries and arterioles due to α-receptor blockade and perhaps due to some direct relaxing effect on vascular smooth muscle.

The positive inotropic and chronotropic effects of catecholamines in heart muscle are not prevented by phentolamine or by phenoxybenzamine. However, studies have shown that drugs having α blocking effects decrease the arrhythmias caused by catecholamines (Claborn and Szabuniewicz 1973; Wiersig et al. 1974). This has been demonstrated in nonanesthetized subjects and after sensitization of the myocardium by halogenated hydrocarbon anesthetics. It is not known if this is mediated entirely by α blockade. The haloalkylamines have a slight direct depressant effect on the heart that may be involved. Also, inhibition of the pressor effects of the catecholamines (which is known to contribute to sensitization of the myocardium to arrhythmias) may also contribute (Katz and Katz 1966).

It should also be mentioned that within the past few years experimental studies have demonstrated that, under certain conditions, α blocking agents partially decrease the inotropic effects of catecholamines in isolated heart muscle (Wagner et al. 1974). This response varies from species to species, however, and in some cases it is demonstrable only during abnormally low temperatures. Until these results have been clarified and verified *in vivo,* the inotropic and chronotropic effects of catecholamines in heart muscle should be considered only as β-receptor–mediated events.

Other Effects. Phentolamine and phenoxybenzamine cause relaxation of the nictitating membrane (3rd eyelid); contractile responses caused by stimulation of sympathetic nerves or by administration of an α agonist are blocked in this structure. The ocular effects of epinephrine and norepinephrine are inhibited by α blockers, as are the pilomotor effects. The gastrointestinal tract is variably influenced by α blockers, due in part to the presence of β receptors in this system that also subserve relaxation. Effects of α blocking agents on the CNS have not been clarified.

Pharmacokinetics. The haloalkylamines and the imidazolines are effective whether administered by mouth or by injection. However, the former group is absorbed inefficiently after oral administration; only 20%–30% of the drug is absorbed in active form from the gastrointestinal tract. The onset of action of phenoxybenzamine and dibenamine is prolonged even after intravenous administration. These drugs may be converted to active intermediates, which then exert α blocking effects. Their local irritating properties restrict their clinical use to oral or intravenous administration. Effective blood levels of tolazoline may not be obtained after oral administration, since it is slowly absorbed from the gastrointestinal tract and since it is rapidly excreted by the kidneys. Phentolamine is less than 30% as active when given by mouth as when injected. Biotransformation pathways of the α-adrenergic blocking agents have not been clarified. Several of these drugs may localize in body adipose tissue due to their relatively high fat solubility.

Clinical Use. Alpha-adrenergic blocking agents are not used extensively in clinical medicine in animals. In human beings these drugs have been used to control vasospasms in peripheral vascular disease such as Raynaud's syndrome, to reduce cold damage to extremities, as an aid in diagnosis of pheochromocytoma, and unsuccessfully in treating hypertension.

Certain types or stages of shock syndromes have been reported to respond favorably to an α blocking agent. This is believed to be due to antagonism of catecholamine-induced peripheral vasoconstriction in vital visceral regions (e.g., renal and splanchnic circulation). Phenoxybenzamine (0.44–2.2 mg/kg diluted in 500 ml of isotonic saline or glucose) administered by slow intravenous infusion has been suggested as a treatment procedure for preventing ischemia of the microcirculation during shock in animals (Sattler 1968). If hypotension occurs upon administration of an α blocking agent during shock, adequate fluid replacement has not been achieved. It is essential that additional administration of blood or plasma expanders should be instituted prior to continuing the infusion of the α blocking agent.

Chlorpromazine (2 mg/kg) and acepromazine (1 mg/kg) administered intravenously have been shown to prevent anesthetic-induced sensitization of the myocardium to catecholamines and to decrease the incidence of ventricular fibrillation induced by administration of epinephrine and norepinephrine during anesthesia in dogs (Claborn and Szabuniewicz 1973; Wiersig et al. 1974). This may be related to mechanisms other than the α blocking effects of these phenothiazine-derivative tranquilizers.

BETA-ADRENERGIC BLOCKING AGENTS

Dichloroisoproterenol was the first drug demonstrated to cause a specific blockade of β-adrenergic receptors. Since it also caused an initial stimulation of the same receptors, subsequent studies were directed to identification of other β blocking agents that lacked agonistic properties. *Pronethalol* was found to produce less β-receptor stimulant effects; however, it was subsequently associated with thymic tumors in mice and was withdrawn from clinical use. *Propranolol* is structurally related to its precursors; it is many times more potent than pronethalol and has very minimal agonistic effects. Other β blocking agents have been identified and are now being investigated.

Propranolol blocks all β receptors; it is available for clinical use; and it is considered a prototypical β-adrenergic blocking agent. Propranolol and related β antagonists are somewhat similar in structure to the β agonist isoproterenol, as seen in Fig. 7.6. All these compounds have an isopropyl-substituted secondary amine on the carbon side chain; this moiety appears to be essential for effective interaction with the β receptor. The levo-configuration of the asymmetrical carbon atom on the side chain of propranolol yields the many times more potent β blocking isomer than does the *d*-configuration.

Pharmacologic Effects. *Cardiovascular.* Propranolol causes minimal depression of heart rate, myocardial contractile force, and cardiac output during normal conditions, since at rest the heart is not under pronounced sympathetic tone. However, if the heart is functioning under sympathetic nervous system dominance (e.g., during exercise), a relative bradycardia and a rather pronounced decrease in myocardial contraction and cardiac output will be produced. This drug prevents the positive inotropic and chronotropic effects of catecholamines in the heart due to β-receptor blockade.

Under most physiological conditions, β vascular receptors participate only in a limited manner to homeostatic regulation. Thus β blocking agents affect blood pressure primarily through their effects on cardiac output rather than by peripheral vascular effects. Vasodilation produced by isoproterenol or epinephrine is blocked by propranolol, however, and the vasoconstrictor response to epinephrine (α response) may be somewhat accentuated. The vasoconstrictor effects of norepinephrine or other α agonists are not blocked by propranolol.

Bronchiolar airways seem to be under slight sympathetic dominance resulting in

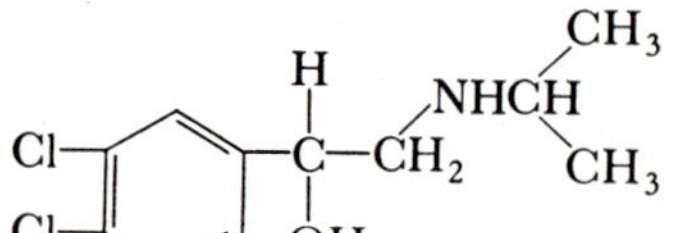

Dichloroisoproterenol

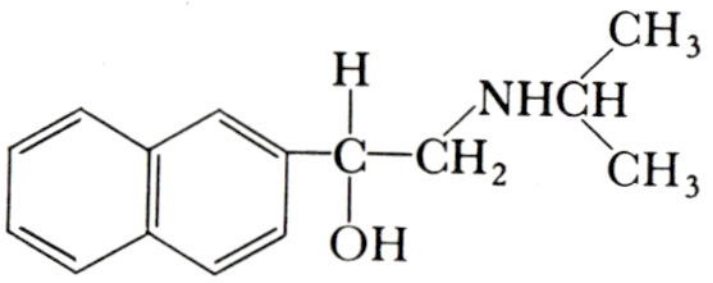

Pronethalol

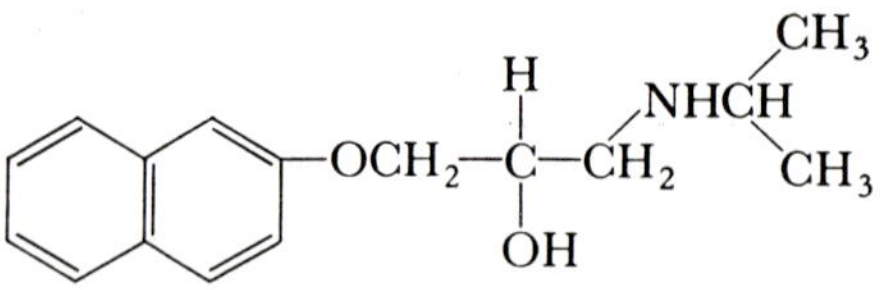

Propranolol

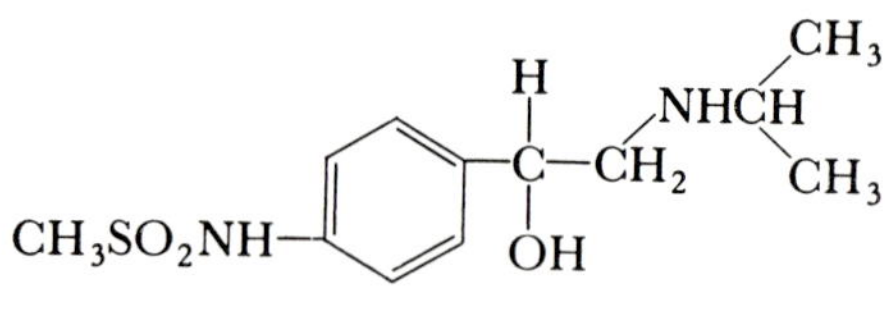

Sotalol

FIG. 7.6. Chemical structures of β-adrenergic blocking drugs.

an active state of relaxation of the bronchiolar smooth muscle. By blocking β receptors, propranolol inhibits sympathetic bronchiodilator activity and causes bronchiolar constriction. This effect is especially prominent during episodes of allergic reactions and bronchiolar asthma; β blocking drugs are contraindicated in these and related conditions.

Propranolol and pronethalol exert antiarrhythmic effects in the heart due primarily to β-receptor blockade (Fitzgerald and Wale 1971). However, this effect may partially be related to a non–β-dependent mechanism. Propranolol causes a direct stabilization of cell membranes that somewhat resembles effects caused by local anesthetics. This has been called a "quinidinelike" effect. Racemic (*d-l*) propranolol and the non–β-blocking *d*-isomer of propranolol exert these effects as does the β-blocking *l*-isomer. Propranolol causes a prolongation of A-V conduction time and decreases upstroke velocity and overshoot of the cardiac action potential without affecting resting membrane potential. The membrane stabilizing effects are probably only minimally important clinically.

Pharmacodynamics. Effective blood concentrations of propranolol are obtained after oral administration, but a large dose is required when given by this route. Biotransformation takes place primarily within the liver, and several active metabolites have been identified. In some species, 4-hydroxypropranolol is as active a β-adrenergic blocking agent as is the parent compound. Propranolol causes a competitive blockade of β receptors. Therefore, large doses of β agonists can overcome the β blocking effects of this drug.

Clinical Use. Recently, antihypertensive therapy in human beings has involved the use of vasodilator drugs that act specifically upon the arterial smooth muscle cell, in combination with a β blocking drug to prevent the reflex tachycardia caused by the decrease of peripheral vascular resistance.

Propranolol and other β blockers have also been used to control angina attacks since the oxygen-consuming effects of norepinephrine in the myocardium are decreased by β-receptor blockade.

Beta blocking agents have been used to protect the heart from arrhythmias induced by adrenergic agents. Wiersig et al. (1974) reported that 1 mg/kg of racemic propranolol administered intravenously to dogs markedly decreased the incidence of ventricular fibrillation induced by epinephrine and norepinephrine during halothane and thiobarbiturate anesthesia. In this respect, propranolol was more effective than chlorpromazine or acepromazine. Adrenergic antagonists should be infused very slowly when given by the intravenous route, since cardiovascular depression may occur if they are administered by bolus intravenous injection.

Beta blocking drugs are frequently effective in increasing the degree of A-V block in patients with digitalis-resistant atrial fibrillation and atrial flutter. Propranolol has been shown to be effective in controlling atrial and ventricular arrhythmias induced by digitalis excess and in treating paroxysmal arrhythmias that prove resistant to digitalis and quinidine. In dogs, slow intravenous infusion of propranolol (1–3 mg) has been proposed for treatment of digitalis-induced supraventricular tachycardia, idiopathic sinus tachycardia, and supraventricular tachycardia of noncardiac origin. The oral dosage is 10–40 mg every 8 hours (Bolton 1974).

Adrenergic Neuron Blocking Drugs and Catecholamine Depleting Agents

These drugs act presynaptically at the adrenergic nerve terminal and prevent the release of norepinephrine; they do not block the postsynaptic adrenergic receptor. Therefore, responses to direct-acting sympathomimetic amines are not prevented. However, effects of indirect-acting sympathomimetic amines (agents that cause release of endogenous norepinephrine) are attenuated by neuronal blocking and amine depleting drugs since the latter agents affect neuronal mechanisms that are active in the norepinephrine release process. For example, reserpine is a catecholamine depleting agent that causes a severe reduction in the neuronal stores of norepinephrine. Therefore, less is available for release by an indirect-acting amine such as tyramine. Pressor effects of tyramine are thereby attenuated. Fig. 7.7 demonstrates the differential effects of an adrenergic blocking agent and an agent that affects adrenergic neurons on the pressor responses produced by sympathetic nerve stimulation, injection of a direct-acting amine (norepinephrine) and injection of an indirect-acting amine (tyramine).

Adrenergic neuron blocking and amine depleting drugs have not been used in clinical veterinary medicine to any appreciable extent. Following early experiments in animals, it was suggested that reserpine would have a wide and extensive application in the veterinary field (Earl 1956). However, this has not been substantiated. The onset of action of reserpine is very long (24–48 hours after oral administration and several hours after intravenous injection), and the drug has found little application in clinical veterinary medicine. Some of the clinical uses of reserpine are discussed in Chapter 17.

Reserpine has been used for treating psychic disorders in human beings and is extensively used in research as a "pharmacologic tool" to deplete endogenous catecholamines from peripheral and CNS adrenergic pathways. Chronic daily treatment of dogs with reserpine (approximately 26 μg/kg, administered orally) caused a marked decrease in the concentration of norepinephrine in the hypothalamus, pons-medulla oblongata, and heart (Adams et al. 1971, 1972). Pronounced disturbances in peripheral and central sympathetic functions were observed, and myocardial damage was suspected.

The mechanism of action of reserpine is related to an impairment of the Mg^{++}- and ATP-dependent capacity of intraneuronal vesicles to accumulate and store catecholamines. After treatment with reserpine, amines are released from granular storage sites into the neuronal cytoplasm where they are metabolized by MAO (Shore 1972).

Guanethidine is another agent that depletes catecholamines from adrenergic nerves. However, responses to adrenergic nerve stimulation are inhibited by guanethidine before detectable amine depletion occurs. A local anestheticlike effect at the

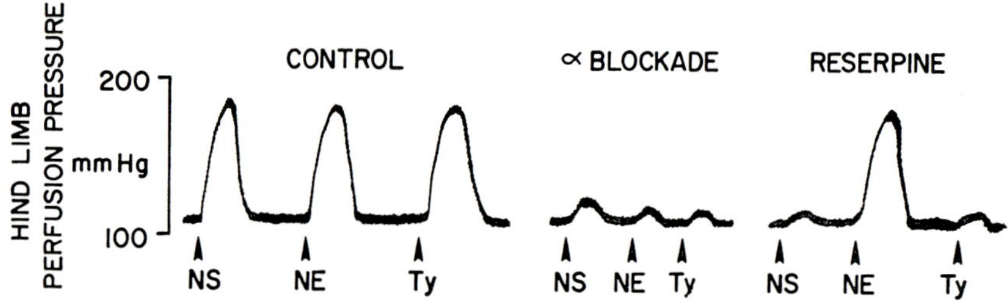

FIG. 7.7. Effects of an adrenergic blocking drug and a catecholamine depleting agent on the pressor responses caused by stimulation of sympathetic nerves (NS), administration of a direct-acting sympathomimetic amine (norepinephrine, NE), and administration of an indirect-acting sympathomimetic amine (tyramine, Ty). Simulated effects obtained from a constant flow-rate perfused hind limb of the dog. NS = electrical stimulation of the lumbar sympathetic chain; NE and Ty = injection of NE or tyramine, respectively, into the femoral artery supplying the perfused hind limb. α Blockade = effects observed after administration of phentolamine; reserpine = effects observed after pretreatment with reserpine. α Blockade inhibits responses to NS, NE, and Ty. Reserpine depletes endogenous norepinephrine from adrenergic nerves; thus effects of NS and Ty are inhibited. NE acts directly on the receptor of the effector cell and its effects are not inhibited by reserpine. (Atropine was also administered to block vasodilation resulting from stimulation of sympathetic cholinergic innervation to the blood vessels of skeletal muscles.)

adrenergic nerve terminal is thought to be involved. Guanethidine does not effectively pass the blood-brain barrier and has relatively less effect on central adrenergic pathways than does reserpine. Guanethidine is used in antihypertensive therapy in human beings; propranolol is sometimes given concurrently to block the reflex tachycardia resulting from guanethidine-induced hypotension.

Bretylium is an adrenergic neuron blocking drug that was originally used in attempts to control hypertension. Side effects such as postural hypotension precluded the extensive use of this drug in clinical situations. Bretylium is often used in research to prevent the release of norepinephrine from adrenergic nerves. This drug does not deplete adrenergic neurons of their catecholamine stores; in this respect, it is dissimilar to reserpine and guanethidine. Bretylium seems to exert a local anestheticlike effect at the adrenergic nerve terminal, and, by this mechanism, decreases the amount of norepinephrine discharged from the nerve.

Miscellaneous Agents

A chemical sympathectomy is produced by 6-hydroxydopamine. This compound is taken up into adrenergic nerves and causes anatomic destruction of the nerve terminal. Several weeks are required for regeneration of these structures after treatment with 6-hydroxydopamine.

Alpha-methyldopa is taken up into the adrenergic nerves where it is biotransformed by the catecholamine synthesizing enzymes into α-methylnorepinephrine, which is then stored in the amine granules. The α-methyl group protects this compound from oxidation by MAO. Therefore, endogenous norepinephrine may be displaced from the granule, metabolized by MAO, and replaced by α-methylnorepinephrine. The α-methylnorepinephrine is released by nerve stimulation but it does not seem to be as effective at adrenergic receptors as is norepinephrine. A decrease in response to nerve stimulation occurs, which can be attributed to α-methylnorepinephrine acting as a "false transmitter." The hypotensive effect of α-methyldopa, however, is now thought to be a CNS effect.

Alpha-methyl-para-tyrosine inhibits tyrosine hydroxylase, the rate-limiting enzyme in the synthesis of norepinephrine. Norepinephrine stores are not replenished and depletion of this amine occurs after cessation of synthesis.

Monoamine oxidase inhibitors are used in human beings as "mood elevators" or antidepressants. These drugs interfere with the oxidative deamination of catecholamines; these amines accumulate in the neuron after treatment with a MAO inhibitor. Responses to peripheral nerve stimulation do not seem to be markedly augmented by MAO inhibitors. However, effects of indirect-acting sympathomimetic amines are markedly potentiated by pretreatment with MAO inhibitors. This is due to an increased concentration of amine that is available for release by the indirect-acting agent. Hypertensive crises and cerebral vascular accidents have occurred in human patients who ingested tyramine-containing foods (e.g., cheese, wine) while they were taking MAO inhibitors.

Cocaine inhibits the neuronal amine uptake pump of adrenergic nerves. This pump functions to take norepinephrine back up into the nerve. Other amines (e.g., tyramine) gain access into the neuron by this uptake mechanism. Thus cocaine potentiates the effect of norepinephrine but blocks the effect of tyramine. Imipramine and desmethylimipramine are tricyclic antidepressants; they, too, block the neuronal amine uptake mechanism.

REFERENCES

Adams, H. R. 1975. Direct myocardial depressant effects of gentamicin. Eur J Pharmacol 30:272.

Adams, H. R.; Smookler, H. H.; Clarke, D. E.; Jandhyala, B. S.; Dixit, B. N.; Ertel, R. J.; and Buckley, J. P. 1971. Clinicopathologic effects of chronic reserpine administration in mongrel dogs. J Pharm Sci 60: 1134.

Adams, H. R.; Dixit, B. N.; Smookler, H. H.; and Buckley, J. P. 1972. Clinical and biochemical effects of chronic reserpine administration in mongrel dogs. Am J Vet Res 33:699.

Ahlquist, R. P. 1948. A study of the adrenotropic receptors. Am J Physiol 153:586.

Benfey, B. G.; Kunos, G.; and Nickerson, M. 1974. Dissociation of cardiac inotropic and adenylate cyclase activating adrenoceptors. Br J Pharmacol 51:253.

Bolton, C. R. 1974. Tachyarrhythmias. In R. W. Kirk, ed. Current Veterinary Therapy V, p. 312. Philadelphia: W. B. Saunders.

Buchanan, J. W.; Dear, M. G.; Pyle, R. L.; and Berg, P. 1968. Medical and pacemaker therapy of complete heart block and congestive heart failure in a dog. J Am Vet Med Assoc 152:1099.

Chen, K. K., and Schmidt, C. F. 1930. Ephedrine and related substances. Medicine (Baltimore) 9:1.

Claborn, L. D., and Szabuniewicz, M. 1973. Prevention of chloroform and thiobarbiturate cardiac sensitization to catecholamines in dogs. Am J Vet Res 34:801.

Cornish, E. J., and Miller, R. C. 1975. Comparison of the β-adrenoceptors in the myocardium and coronary vasculature of the kitten heart. J Pharm Pharmacol 27:23.

Dale, H. H. 1906. On some physiological actions of ergot. J Physiol (Lond) 34:163.

Earl, A. E. 1956. Reserpine (Serpasil) in veterinary practice. J Am Vet Med Assoc 129:227.

Ettinger, S. 1969. Isoproterenol treatment of atrioventricular heart block in the dog. J Am Vet Med Assoc 154:398.

Fitzgerald, J. D., and Wale, J. 1971. The effects of β-blocking drugs on atrioventricular conduction and contractility. Cardiology 56:338.

Goldberg, L. I. 1972. Cardiovascular and renal actions of dopamine. Pharmacol Rev 24:1.

———. 1975. The dopamine vascular receptor. Biochem Pharmacol 24:651.

Goodman, F. R., and Weiss, G. B. 1971. Effects of lanthanum on ^{45}Ca movements and on contractions induced by norepinephrine, histamine, and potassium in vascular smooth muscle. J Pharmacol Exp Ther 177:415.

Greenway, C. V., and Lawson, A. E. 1966. The effects of adrenaline and noradrenaline on venous return and regional blood flows in the anesthetized cat with special reference to intestinal blood flow. J Physiol (Lond) 186:579.

Katz, R. L., and Katz, G. J. 1966. Surgical infiltration of pressor drugs and their interaction with volatile anesthetics. Br J Anaesth 38:712.

Lands, A. M.; Arnold, A.; McAuliff, J. P.; Luduena, F. P.; and Brown, T. G., Jr. 1967. Differentiation of receptor systems activated by sympathomimetic amines. Nature 214:597.

Langer, G. A. 1974. Calcium in mammalian myocardium—Localization, control, and the effects of digitalis. Circ Res Suppl 3, pp. 34, 35, 91.

McNay, J. L., and Goldberg, L. I. 1966. Comparison of the effects of dopamine, isoproterenol, norepinephrine and bradykinin on canine renal and femoral blood flow. J Pharmacol Exp Ther 151:23.

Moran, N. C. 1973. The classification of adrenergic receptors. In E. Usdin and S. Snyder, eds. Frontiers in Catecholamine Research, p. 291. Elmsford, N.Y.: Pergamon Press.

Moran, N. C., and Perkins, M. E. 1958. Adrenergic blockade of the mammalian heart by a dichloro analogue of isoproterenol. J Pharmacol Exp Ther 124:223.

Nickerson, M., and Nomaguchi, C. M. 1949. Mechanism of dibenamine protection against cyclopropane-epinephrine cardiac arrhythmias. J Pharmacol Exp Ther 95:1.

Powell, C. E., and Slater, I. H. 1958. Blocking of inhibitory adrenergic receptors by a dichloro analog of isoproterenol. J Pharmacol Exp Ther 122:480.

Robison, G. A.; Butcher, R. W.; and Sutherland, E. W. 1967. Adenyl cyclase as an adrenergic receptor. Ann NY Acad Sci 139:703.

———. 1971. Cyclic AMP. New York: Academic Press.

Sattler, F. P. 1968. Shock. In R. W. Kirk, ed. Current Veterinary Therapy III, p. 24. Philadelphia: W. B. Saunders.

Schaper, W. 1967. Heart. Annu Rev Physiol 29:259.

Setler, P. E.; Pendleton, R. G.; and Finlay, E. 1975. The cardiovascular actions of dopamine and the effects of central and peripheral catecholaminergic receptor blocking drugs. J Pharmacol Exp Ther 192:702.

Shore, P. A. 1972. Transport and storage of biogenic amines. Annu Rev Pharmacol 12:209.

Soma, L. R.; Burrows, C. F.; and Marshall, B. E. 1974. Shock: Etiology and management. In R. W. Kirk, ed. Current Veterinary Therapy V, p. 26. Philadelphia: W. B. Saunders.

Wagner, J.; Endoh, M.; and Reinhardt, D. 1974. Stimulation by phenylephrine of adrenergic alpha- and beta-receptors in the isolated perfused rabbit heart. Naunyn Schmiedebergs Arch Pharmacol 282:307.

Watanabe, A. M., and Besch, H. R., Jr. 1974.

Cyclic adenosine monophosphate modulation of slow calcium influx channels in guinea pig hearts. Circ Res 35:316.

Wiersig, D. O.; Davis, R. H., Jr.; and Szabuniewicz, M. 1974. Prevention of induced ventricular fibrillation in dogs anesthetized with ultrashort acting barbiturates and halothane. J Am Vet Med Assoc 165: 341.

Young, B. A., and McNeill, J. H. 1974. The effect of noradrenaline and tyramine on cardiac contractility, cyclic AMP, and phosphorylase in normal and hyperthyroid rats. Can J Physiol Pharmacol 52:375.

CHAPTER 8

PARASYMPATHOMIMETIC, PARASYMPATHOLYTIC, AND AUTONOMIC GANGLIONIC BLOCKING AGENTS

H. RICHARD ADAMS

Acetylcholine acts as the messenger between nerve endings and innervated cells of autonomic ganglia, parasympathetic neuroeffector junctions, some sympathetic neuroeffector junctions, somatic neuromuscular junctions, the adrenal medulla, and certain regions of the CNS. It has been recognized for many years that considerable therapeutic benefit could be derived from drugs that would selectively mimic the action of acetylcholine only at certain of these sites or, alternatively, that could selectively prevent only unwanted effects of this biogenic substance. Although these ideal drugs have yet to be identified, some agents have been found to be relatively more active at certain cholinergic sites than at others. In this chapter, drugs that influence postganglionic parasympathetic neuroeffector junctions and autonomic ganglia by acetylcholinelike or acetycholine blocking effects will be examined.

PARASYMPATHOMIMETIC AGENTS

"Cholinergic" is a term used to describe an acetylcholinelike effect without distinction as to anatomic site of action. "Parasympathomimetic," on the other hand, is a specific term used in reference to an acetylcholinelike effect on effector cells innervated by postganglionic neurons of the parasympathetic nervous system. Most of the cholinergic drugs discussed in this chapter are used clinically for their parasympathomimetic activities. As will be discussed below, however, the scope of pharmacologic activity of several of these compounds is not restricted to parasympathomimetic effects but include cholinergic actions throughout the body. Based on mechanism of action, drugs that cause parasympathomimetic effects can be divided into two major groups: (1) direct-acting agents, which like acetylcholine activate cholinergic receptors of the effector cells; and (2) cholinesterase inhibitors, which, by inhibition of cholinesterase, allow endogenous acetylcholine to accumulate and thereby intensify and prolong its action.

DIRECT-ACTING PARASYMPATHOMIMETIC AGENTS

These drugs consist of (1) esters of choline, and (2) naturally occurring cholinomimetic alkaloids.

CHOLINE ESTERS

Choline, a member of the B vitamin group, possesses the characteristic depressor action of a cholinergic drug when injected intravenously in large unphysiologic amounts; however, its potency is multiplied thousands of times when it is esterified with acetic acid to yield acetylcholine (Hunt and Taveau 1906).

Acetylcholine, although absolutely essential for maintenance of body homeostasis, is not used therapeutically for two important reasons. First, since it acts simultaneously at various tissue sites, no selective therapeutic response can be achieved. Second, its duration of action is quite brief due to its rapid inactivation by the cholinesterases. Several derivatives of acetylcholine, however, are more resistant to hydrolysis by cholinesterase and have a somewhat greater selectivity in their sites of action. Of several hundred choline derivatives that have been synthesized, carbachol, bethanechol, and methacholine have proved effective for certain clinical uses and will be discussed in this chapter.

MECHANISM OF ACTION

Pharmacologic effects of acetylcholine and related choline esters are mediated by activation of specific acetylcholine-responsive sites (i.e., cholinergic receptors or cholinoceptors) located on cells innervated by cholinergic nerves and, in some cases, on cells that lack cholinergic innervation. Some of the effects of choline esters, particularly those of carbachol, may be due in part to the release of endogenous acetylcholine from cholinergic nerve terminals (Takagi et al. 1968). However, most choline esters act directly on postsynaptic receptors and do not depend upon endogenous acetylcholine for their effects. Based on differential responsiveness to cholinergic agonists and antagonists, two basic types of cholinoceptors have been identified within the peripheral efferent pathways of the mammalian autonomic nervous system.

Nicotinic Receptors. Beginning with the early classical studies by Dale (1914), it has been known that nicotine in small doses mimics certain of the actions of acetylcholine, and in larger doses blocks these same cholinergic effects. As summarized in Chapter 6, nicotinic responsive sites are present in (1) autonomic ganglia, (2) adrenal medullary chromaffin cells, and also (3) the neuromuscular junctions of the somatic nervous system. Accordingly, receptors at these sites are called *nicotinic cholinergic receptors,* and effects of cholinergic drugs at these sites are referred to as *nicotinic effects.*

Muscarinic Receptors. Nicotine does not, however, mimic or block the effects of acetylcholine at postganglionic parasympathetic neuroeffector junctions, i.e., parasympathetic innervation to heart muscle, smooth muscle, and exocrine glands. The mushroom alkaloid *muscarine* was found to selectively mimic the activity of acetylcholine at these sites but not at the previously mentioned nicotinic receptors. *Muscarinic receptors,* therefore, designate the type of cholinoceptors present at postganglionic parasympathetic neuroeffector junctions.[1] Accordingly, the *parasympathomimetic,* or muscarinic, effects produced by drugs examined in this chapter are equivalent to the physiologic changes evoked by post-

1. Muscarinic receptors are also present in some smooth muscle (e.g., arterioles) that lack cholinergic innervation and at those neuroeffector junctions of the sympathetic nervous system that are cholinergic (see Chapter 6).

ganglionic parasympathetic nerve impulses, as listed in Table 6.1.

Atropine is a cholinergic blocking agent that selectively blocks muscarinic receptors without blocking nicotinic sites; whereas, hexamethonium, *d*-tubocurarine, and large doses of nicotine block nicotinic but not muscarinic receptors. Selective cholinergic blocking drugs such as these are routinely used to identify and characterize nicotinic-muscarinic properties of cholinergic drugs.

Although agonist-antagonist characteristics of cholinergic receptors have been well defined, relatively little is known about the molecular events precipitated by cholinoceptor activation. Acetylcholine evokes an excitatory response in some tissues (e.g., smooth muscle of the gastrointestinal tract) but causes inhibitory responses in other organs (e.g., myocardium). In general, excitatory effects of acetylcholine are thought to be due to depolarization of the postsynaptic membrane characterized by an increase in permeability of the membrane to both Na^+ and K^+ ions. Inhibitory effects, on the other hand, have been associated with hyperpolarization of the membrane due to a selective increase in membrane permeability to K^+ but not to Na^+ (see Chapter 6). Potential membrane configuration changes and resulting alterations in ion permeability induced by interaction of acetylcholine with a typical cholinergic receptor are covered in Chapter 9.

STRUCTURE-ACTIVITY RELATIONSHIPS

Direct-acting cholinergic agonists contain structural groupings that allow interaction of the agent with cholinergic receptors and result in similar changes in membrane configuration and, thus, ion permeability as caused by acetylcholine (Rand and Stafford 1967). The choline esters contain a quaternary nitrogen atom to which three methyl groups are attached. Except for some naturally occurring cholinomimetic alkaloids, a quaternary nitrogen moiety is usually required for a direct potent action on cholinergic receptors. Like its counterpart the ammonium ion, the quaternary nitrogen group carries a positive charge; this cationic group *electrostatically* binds with a negatively charged (*anionic*) site of the cholinergic receptor. The anionic site of the receptor is believed to be the main determinant of receptor events, and interaction of the cationic head of acetylcholine with the anionic site is the primary instigator of conformational changes that lead to alterations in membrane permeability. Even the tetramethylammonium molecule (methonium) $N^+(CH_3)_4$, which has only a cationic group, can activate anionic sites of cholinoceptors and produce a nonselective cholinomimetic effect at cholinergic receptive sites throughout the body.

Receptive macromolecules (i.e., cholinergic receptors and cholinesterases) that recognize and bind acetylcholine have, in addition to the anionic site discussed in the preceding paragraph, a region that combines with the ester component of acetylcholine (see Fig. 8.1) (Barlow 1964, 1968). In cholinesterase, this region is called the "esteratic" site and its combination with the carboxyl group results in hydrolysis of the ester (see later in this chapter). Hydrolysis of acetylcholine does not occur upon its interaction with a receptor, however, and the ester-attracting region of the receptor is called the "esterophilic" site. Acetylcholine is "ideally" arranged structurally so that it combines with the esterophilic and anionic sites of both nicotinic and muscarinic receptors (Barlow 1964, 1968). When both components of the ester moiety of acetylcholine, i.e., the carbonyl group and the ether oxygen, are replaced by methylene molecules, agonistic properties at both muscarinic and nicotinic sites are drastically reduced. If only the ether oxygen of acetylcholine is substituted by a methylene group, the muscarinic potency is markedly decreased but nicotinic properties are little affected (Ing et al. 1952; Barlow 1964). Introduction of a methyl group on the β-carbon atom of the choline segment considerably reduces nicotinic properties but does not reduce muscarinic activities. These findings indicate that the esterophilic sites are arranged somewhat differently in muscarinic than in nicotinic receptors and, therefore, influence specificity of agonistic and antagonistic properties of different drugs. The esterophilic region may contain subunits that individually attract either the ether oxygen or the carbonyl oxygen by hydrogen bonding and dipole-dipole interaction, respectively (see Fig. 8.1, part B) (Pullman and Pullman 1963; Khromov-Borisov and Michelson 1966).

The distance between the anionic and esterophilic portions of cholinergic receptors, i.e., the hydrophobic region, is also believed to be important in determining susceptibility to different agonists and antagonists. For maximum agonistic potency

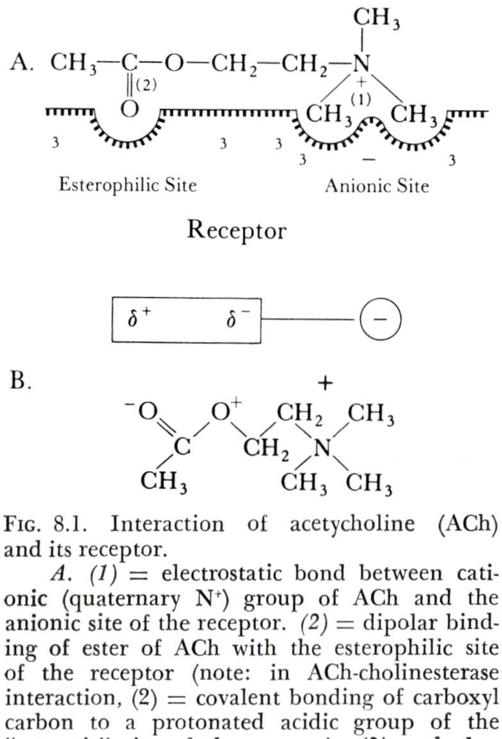

A. $CH_3—C(=O)—O—CH_2—CH_2—N^+(CH_3)_3$

(1) (2) 3 3 3 3 – 3

Esterophilic Site   Anionic Site

Receptor

B. δ^+ δ^- —— (–)

+

^-O O^+ CH_2 CH_3

C CH_2 N

CH_3 CH_3 CH_3

FIG. 8.1. Interaction of acetycholine (ACh) and its receptor.

A. (1) = electrostatic bond between cationic (quaternary N^+) group of ACh and the anionic site of the receptor. *(2)* = dipolar binding of ester of ACh with the esterophilic site of the receptor (note: in ACh-cholinesterase interaction, (2) = covalent bonding of carboxyl carbon to a protonated acidic group of the "esteratic" site of the enzyme). *(3)* = hydrophobic bonds probably exist between the various methyl groups and adjacent proteins of the receptor surface. Based on the postulated interaction of ACh and cholinesterase. (Modified from Eldefrawi 1974) *B.* Electrical charge distribution of ACh and its receptor. (Pullman and Pullman 1963; Khromov-Borisov and Michelson 1966)

at muscarinic sites, for example, at least five atoms must be in the "fourth radical" of the trimethylammonium group of acetylcholine. However, this restriction does not necessarily apply to nicotinic agonists (Ing et al. 1952; Michelson 1973). The potential importance of the distances between reactive sites on cholinergic receptors are included in Chapter 9. Rand and Stafford (1967) have examined several other aspects of the structural characteristics of parasympathomimetic agents.

Acetylcholine is the prototypical cholinergic agent; it acts at all cholinoceptor sites and, therefore, evokes both nicotinic and muscarinic effects. *Acetyl-β-methylcholine* (methacholine) is identical in structure to acetylcholine except for the substitution of a methyl group on the β-carbon atom of the choline group. This structural change yields a compound that is primarily a muscarinic receptor agonist lacking significant nicotinic effects when given in usual dosages. Further, it is more active on the cardiovascular system than on the gastrointestinal tract. The duration of action of methacholine is considerably longer than that of acetylcholine, since the former drug is hydrolyzed by acetylcholinesterase at a much slower rate than is acetylcholine, and since methacholine is almost totally resistant to breakdown by pseudocholinesterase.

Carbachol and *bethanechol* each have a carbamyl (NH_2COO^-) group substituted for the acetic moiety of acetylcholine, and bethanechol also has a β-methyl group. Both of these agents are almost completely resistant to inactivation by the cholinesterases. Their duration of action is, therefore, considerably longer than that of acetylcholine. Carbachol is active at both muscarinic and nicotinic receptor sites (therefore, it is cholinomimetic and not just parasympathomimetic), whereas bethanechol is primarily a muscarinic agonist. Dissimilar to methacholine, both of these drugs are somewhat more active on smooth muscles of the gastrointestinal (GI) tract and urinary bladder than on cardiovascular function.

TABLE 8.1. Chemical structures and scope of cholinergic receptor activating properties of some choline esters

Compound	Structure	Susceptibility to Cholinesterase		Agonistic Properties				
				Muscarinic receptors				Nicotinic receptors
		True	Pseudo	CV	GI	UB	E	
Choline	$(CH_3)_3N^+ \cdot CH_2 \cdot CH_2 \cdot OH$							
Acetylcholine	$(CH_3)_3N^+ \cdot CH_2 \cdot CH_2 \cdot O \cdot COCH_3$	+++	+++	+++	+++	++	+	+++
Methacholine	$(CH_3)_3N^+ \cdot CH_2 \cdot CH(CH_3) \cdot O \cdot COCH_3$	+	—	+++	++	++	+	±
Carbachol	$(CH_3)_3N^+ \cdot CH_2 \cdot CH_2 \cdot O \cdot CONH_2$	—	—	+	+++	+++	++	+++
Bethanechol	$(CH_3)_3N^+ \cdot CH_2 \cdot CH(CH_3) \cdot O \cdot CONH_2$	—	—	±	+++	+++	++	—

Note: CV = cardiovascular; GI = gastrointestinal; UB = urinary bladder; E = eye.

The chemical structures of these choline esters and their related pharmacologic characteristics are shown in Table 8.1.

ACETYLCHOLINE

Although acetylcholine is not used clinically, it is the prototypical cholinergic agonist and an understanding of its activity is imperative for a comprehension of the pharmacologic effects of other cholinomimetic drugs. The biosynthesis, neuronal release, cellular activities, and inactivation of endogenous acetylcholine are examined in Chapter 6 and should be reviewed in conjunction with the present chapter.

Since acetylcholine is a mixed nicotinic-muscarinic agonist, different effects can be produced by administration of this agent, depending upon the relative dominance of muscarinic (parasympathomimetic) or nicotinic actions. These effects can be differentiated by the use of small and large doses of acetylcholine and by using selective cholinergic blocking drugs. In general, parasympathomimetic effects dominate with small doses, whereas with large doses cholinergic effects at other tissue sites are also produced. Therefore, muscarinic receptors seem to be more susceptible to acetylcholine than do nicotinic receptors. The use of cholinergic blocking drugs and small and large doses of acetylcholine to differentiate muscarinic and nicotinic effects of acetylcholine is shown in Fig. 8.2. This figure is discussed in greater detail in the following sections.

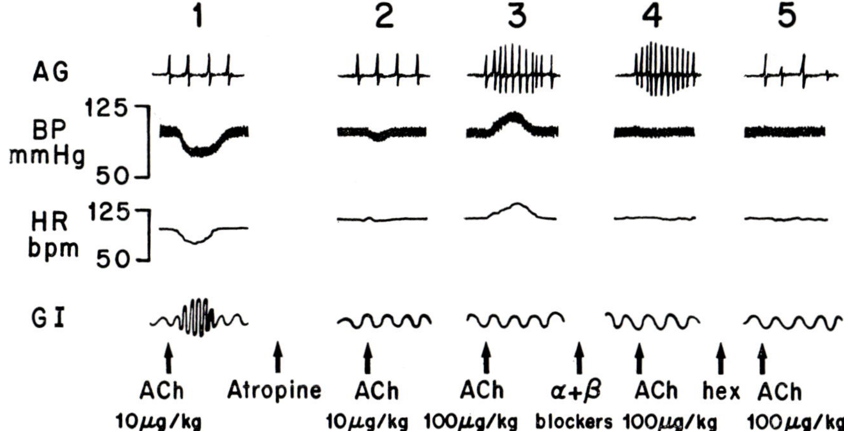

FIG. 8.2. Muscarinic and nicotinic effects of acetylcholine (ACh) on blood pressure, heart rate, intestinal motility, and autonomic ganglionic action potentials in an anesthetized dog. Schematic reproductions: *1.* A small dose of ACh (10 μg/kg) administered intravenously causes hypotension, bradycardia, and intestinal contractions due to direct stimulation of muscarinic receptors of blood vessels, heart, and intestinal smooth muscle, respectively. These effects are brief, due to rapid destruction of ACh by cholinesterase. *2.* Atropine blocks the muscarinic receptors and, thereby, prevents the effects seen in *(1)*. *3.* Large doses of ACh (100 μg/kg) stimulate, in addition to the muscarinic receptors, the nicotinic receptors of both parasympathetic and sympathetic ganglionic neurons, causing an increase in frequency and amplitude of ganglionic action potentials. Although all autonomic ganglia are activated, impulses arising from the parasympathetic ganglia do not reach their effector cells due to blockade of parasympathetic postganglionic neuroeffector junctions by atropine. Sympathomimetic responses (pressor effect and tachycardia) result. *4.* Impulses arising from sympathetic ganglia are prevented from reaching their effector cells by adrenergic blocking drugs; however, ganglionic nicotinic receptors are still activated by ACh. *5.* Hexamethonium (hex) blocks nicotinic receptors of ganglia and, thereby, inhibits the nicotinic ganglionic stimulating effect of ACh and reduces ganglionic action potentials.

AG = action potentials of an autonomic ganglionic neuron; BP = systemic blood pressure; HR = heart rate; GI = intestinal peristaltic waves.

Pharmacologic Effects. *Cardiovascular effects of small doses of acetylcholine.* Intravenous administration of small amounts of acetylcholine (5–10 μg/kg) produces a brief but rapid fall in systolic and diastolic blood pressures. This is due to a decrease in peripheral resistance resulting from direct activation of muscarinic receptors of vascular smooth muscle. These receptors subserve relaxation of vascular muscle and thus dilatation of the blood vessels.[2] Somewhat larger doses of acetylcholine (i.e., 10–30 μg/kg) produce more pronounced muscarinic effects; therefore, a greater decrease in peripheral resistance and blood pressure is produced.

In addition to the hypotension response, a slowing of the heart rate occurs after administration of acetylcholine (a transient tachycardia may initially occur but this is due to the hypotensive response affecting baroreceptor reflex activity). Atrial myocardial cells contain muscarinic receptors associated with vagal fibers that mediate negative chronotropic and inotropic effects. The chronotropic effects predominate. In addition to decreasing heart rate and force of myocardial contraction, acetylcholine can also prolong the refractory period and conduction time in cardiac conducting tissue and at the same time shorten the effective refractory period of myocardial fibers. Thus different arrhythmias and ECG abnormalities can result. These include severe bradycardia, incomplete and complete heart block, notching and decreased amplitude of the P wave, momentary ventricular asystole, and in some cases atrial tachycardia and atrial fibrillation.

Smooth muscle. GI motility and secretions are enhanced by acetylcholine in a manner identical to that seen upon stimulation of the parasympathetic innervation to the alimentary tract. These effects may be difficult to detect with small doses since the duration of action of acetylcholine is brief, due to rapid destruction by cholinesterase. Larger doses, however, markedly increase secretions and peristaltic movements of the GI tract.

Acetylcholine stimulates smooth muscle of the urinary bladder and uterus to contract. Bronchiolar smooth muscle is also contracted by acetylcholine, resulting in decreased diameter of airways. The smooth muscle effects of acetylcholine are blocked by atropine and, therefore, are due to muscarinic receptor activation.

Central nervous system. Due to its highly charged quaternary nitrogen group, acetylcholine is lipophobic and penetrates cell membranes and the blood-brain barrier poorly. Thus CNS effects are not observed when usual dosages are administered. However, intraarterial injection into cerebral arteries of large amounts of acetylcholine or its direct application into the CNS produces increased electrical activity, excitation, and possibly convulsions. Characterization of CNS cholinergic receptors as muscarinic or nicotinic is incomplete, but it seems that both types are present.

Muscarinic and nicotinic effects of large doses of acetylcholine. With high doses (i.e., 50–100 μg/kg), muscarinic effects of acetylcholine on postganglionic effector cells are accentuated. There is a profound hypotensive response, due to extensive peripheral vasodilation. The duration of this effect is prolonged. Heart rate slows dramatically and momentary asystole may even occur. The GI tract and other visceral smooth muscles are markedly activated; defecation, urination, and vomition may result.

Large doses of acetylcholine produce, in addition to the muscarinic (i.e., parasympathomimetic) effects described above, stimulation of the nicotinic receptors of autonomic ganglia (both parasympathetic and sympathetic) and the adrenal medulla. These effects are particularly evident when the muscarinic receptors of the parasympathetic neuroeffector junctions are blocked by atropine. Under these circumstances, large doses of acetylcholine stimulate nicotinic receptors of both sympathetic and

2. Blood vessels receive little or no parasympathetic innervation (see Chapter 6). Therefore, most vascular smooth muscle is different from other smooth muscle in that its muscarinic receptors are noninnervated. Some skeletal muscle vessels receive sympathetic cholinergic vasodilator fibers that terminate at typical muscarinic receptors.

parasympathetic ganglia; however, since the muscarinic receptors of the parasympathetic neuroeffector junctions are blocked by atropine, impulses originating from parasympathetic ganglia will not reach their effector cells. Only impulses originating from sympathetic ganglia will reach their effector cells and, therefore, only sympathomimetic responses will be evident. These are characterized by an increase in blood pressure, tachycardia, and other typical sympathetic-mediated effects (Fig. 8.2). These effects can be blocked by the use of appropriate adrenergic blocking drugs (Fig. 8.2) (see Chapter 7) or by the use of a ganglionic blocking agent (Fig. 8.2).

Adrenal medulla. This structure is functionally analogous to autonomic ganglia, and nicotinic receptors of adrenal medullary chromaffin cells are innervated by typical preganglionic cholinergic fibers. These receptors are stimulated by acetylcholine to cause the release of epinephrine and norepinephrine from the chromaffin cells into the circulation. This effect contributes to the overall nicotinic-mediated sympathomimetic effect evoked by large doses of acetylcholine in the presence of muscarinic blockade. In addition, acetylcholine can cause the release of endogenous norepinephrine from adrenergic nerve terminals; however, the potential for this effect is thought to be very minimal when pharmacologic characteristics of most cholinergic drugs are considered. For possible physiologic significance, see Chapter 6.

Skeletal muscle. Intraarterial injection of significant quantities of acetylcholine will produce skeletal muscle fasciculations due to penetration of some of the agent to motor end-plates and the resulting activation of the nicotinic receptors of skeletal muscle cells. Continued exposure to excessive amounts of acetylcholine causes severe fasciculations and asynchronous contractions and terminates in a depolarizing paralysis. Also, if an atropinelike drug has not been given, an increase in blood flow to the injected muscle occurs as a result of vasodilatation due to stimulation of the muscarinic receptors of blood vessels.

METHACHOLINE, CARBACHOL, AND BETHANECOL

The pharmacologic effects of these choline esters are equivalent to the previously outlined parasympathomimetic effects of acetylcholine and thus are similar to the physiologic changes evoked by stimulation of postganglionic parasympathetic nerves as listed in Table 6.1. Carbachol also has marked nicotinic agonistic characteristics; however, differences between the parasympathomimetic actions of these choline esters are primarily quantitative and vary only in relative selectivity for one organ system or another (Table 8.1).

Methacholine (acetyl-β-methylcholine) is a synthetic choline ester used occasionally in human therapeutics but infrequently employed in veterinary medicine. Methacholine causes muscarinic effects on cardiovascular function very similar to those produced by acetylcholine, but it is considerably less active on the GI system and has very few agonist properties at nicotinic receptors.

Carbachol (Lentin, Carbaminoylcholine Chloride, Doryl) is an extremely potent choline ester that is active at both muscarinic and nicotinic receptors and, therefore, causes pharmacologic effects similar to the changes evoked by acetylcholine. These are particularly prominent on the nicotinic receptors of autonomic ganglia; however, this drug is also very potent at muscarinic sites. For example, intravenous injection of doses as small as 2 μg/kg causes a transient slowing of heart rate and hypotension due to muscarinic effects.

Bethanecol (Urecholine, Carbamylmethylcholine) is somewhat similar to methacholine and carbachol in scope of pharmacologic activity. Unlike carbachol, however, it is primarily a muscarinic agonist and has little stimulant effects on nicotinic receptors.

Pharmacologic Effects

Cardiovascular effects. Methacholine is more active on the cardiovascular system than on the gastrointestinal or urinary tracts. The opposite selectivity is seen with carbachol and bethanechol. Intravenous administration of methacholine, like acetylcholine, produces a depressor response and slowing of the heart rate due to activation of muscarinic receptors of blood vessels and the heart, respectively. Cardiac rhythm is altered by methacholine, and the atrioventricular node is particularly sensitive to this agent. Conduction velocity through the atrioventricular node is decreased, which in some instances can lead to atrial fibrillation. Various degrees of heart block, including complete atrioventricular disassociation, may also occur with large doses. Intravenous administration of methacholine to normal nonanesthetized animals can produce atrial fibrillation, as can acetylcholine. These effects are completely blocked by atropine. Carbachol evokes blood pressure changes similar to those seen with methacholine except relatively less pronounced, whereas bethanechol is considerably less active on cardiovascular function.

Gastrointestinal tract. Carbachol and bethanechol are relatively more active on the GI and urinary tracts than on the cardiovascular system. Methacholine is also active on the alimentary canal but only in very large doses. Carbachol is a potent GI stimulant. It evokes profuse salivation and produces an increase in peristaltic movements of the gut, resulting in increased defecation and fluidity of feces. These responses are due to activation of muscarinic receptors of gastric and intestinal smooth muscle and related glands. GI stimulant effects of choline esters are relatively well defined in simple-stomached animals, but responsiveness of ruminants may vary. Effects of carbachol and various other autonomic drugs on the GI tract of ruminants were summarized in Table 8.2 by Stowe (1965). Ruminant pharmacology is discussed in detail in Section 9.

Other smooth muscle. Uterine musculature, in both *in-vitro* strips and the intact animal, is contracted by carbachol. This response is more evident during the latter stages of gestation. By the time a cow is 6 or 7 months pregnant, carbachol should not be used since abortion or uterine rupture might result. After parturition, however, carbachol may be useful in expelling uterine contents.

Similar to acetylcholine, carbachol also causes contraction of bronchiolar smooth muscle, resulting in a decreased airway. The urinary bladder is contracted by carbachol and bethanechol, and frequent urination results. Effects of carbachol and bethanechol on these as on other smooth muscles are muscarinic and, therefore, are blocked by atropine.

Skeletal muscle. Carbachol does not discernibly affect skeletal muscle when usual dosages are employed. If a high dose is inadvertently given, however, muscle fasciculations and even paralysis may occur. This is a nicotinic effect and is due to carbachol causing a persistent depolarization block of the postsynaptic membrane of the neuromuscular junction. Bethanechol and methacholine, due to their relative lack of agonistic effects at nicotinic sites, have little effect on voluntary muscles.

Sweating. Profuse sweating in the horse is evoked by carbachol. It is not known if this is due to a direct effect on sweat glands, a ganglionic stimulating effect, an increase in circulating catecholamines (as a result of adrenal medullary stimulation), or the local release of catecholamines from adrenergic neurons. Since sweat gland innervation in the horse seems to be adrenergic, either of the latter two mechanisms may be involved.

Other effects. Carbachol, like acetylcholine, is a mixed nicotinic-muscarinic agonist. It, therefore, has a potent stimulating effect on autonomic ganglia and the chromaffin cells of the adrenal medulla. Such an effect on the adrenal medulla would cause an increased discharge of epinephrine and norepinephrine into the bloodstream, which, in turn, could produce diffuse sympathomimetic effects. This relationship may explain why adrenergiclike effects have occasionally been encountered during the use of carbachol. Nicotinic effects of carbachol on autonomic ganglia can be demonstrated by the hypertensive response obtained with large doses after the postganglionic muscarinic receptors

TABLE 8.2. Effects of autonomic drugs on gastrointestinal tract of ruminants

Drug	*In Vitro* Muscle Strips	Reference	*In Vivo* Motility of Forestomachs and Abomasum	Reference
Epinephrine	Inhibition followed by increased motility Blocked by ergotoxine and adrenergic-blocking drugs	Dussardier and Navarro 1953 Duncan 1954	Inhibition in higher doses Inhibition No effect Inhibition Contraction in spinal ruminant No effect or inhibition in vagotomized sheep	Dougherty 1942 Duncan 1954 Quin and Van Der Wath 1938 Dussardier 1954 Dussardier 1954 Duncan 1954
Acetylcholine	Contraction Increased tonus and amplitude of abomasal strips	Duncan 1954 Dussardier and Navarro 1953	Inhibition on IV administration (epi-release?) Contraction after intraceliac artery injection Increased motility in large doses	Dougherty 1942 Duncan 1954 Dussardier 1954 Dussardier 1954 Quin and Clark 1946
Eserine			Potentiates effect of acetylcholine Increased reticular amplitude Increased frequency and amplitude	Duncan 1954 Amadon 1930 Dougherty 1942
Carbachol	Increased tone and motility	Duncan 1954	Increased tone, shallow contraction Marked depression Increased tone and frequency, sometimes tetany	Quin and Van Der Wath 1938 Dougherty 1942 Duncan 1954
Arecoline	Increased tone		Increased motility at low doses Inhibition at higher doses	Amadon 1930 Dougherty 1942
Pilocarpine	Contraction		No clearcut effect	Amadon 1930 Dougherty 1942
Methacholine	Contraction		No clearcut effect	Dougherty 1942
Histamine			Marked inhibition Marked inhibition Reversible with antihistamines	Dougherty 1942 Duncan 1954 Clark 1950
Atropine			Cessation of motility	General agreement

Source: Stowe 1965.

have been blocked with atropine (e.g., Fig. 8.2).

Clinical Uses. Methacholine and bethanechol are not used frequently in clinical veterinary medicine. In the past, methacholine has been used in human beings and animals to produce peripheral vasodilation in treating different vascular disorders such as Raynaud's disease and ergot poisoning, respectively. It has been used in human medicine to control tachycardia due to atrial or supraventricular origin. Ventricular tachycardia and nodal paroxysmal tachycardia (in which the origin is in the atrioventricular node) are not amenable to methacholine therapy. Bethanechol, 1 mg administered subcutaneously twice daily, has been used to treat urinary bladder atony in cats after incidences of urolithiasis; however, care should be taken to assure that the urethra is completely patent.

Carbachol is a very potent drug, and care should be taken to avoid overstimulation of the GI tract and uterus during its clinical use. It has been used for treatment of colic and impactions of the intestinal tract; however, its use in such cases should be closely monitored. If excessive peristaltic movements are induced in a patient suffering from severe intestinal obstruction, rupture or intussusception may occur. Before resorting to a potent cholinomimetic compound such as carbachol, consideration should first be given to more conservative approaches to GI therapy such as the use of mineral oil, saline cathartics, water, and other stool softeners. If these measures are not successful, then carbachol may be cautiously added to the therapeutic regimen. Repeated small subcutaneous doses of 1–2 mg of carbachol at 30- to 60-minute intervals have been used in treating colic in mature horses after treatment with oils and saline cathartics had been instituted. Dosages should be decreased to 0.25–0.5 mg in foals.

When administered during the middle of farrowing, carbachol (2 mg, subcutaneously) has been reported to decrease the incidence of stillbirths in litters from sows and gilts by increasing uterine contractions (Sprecher et al. 1975). However, severe GI side effects (salivation, vomiting, diarrhea) and frequent urination were objectionable. Also, a discrepancy in the experimental methodology of this study complicates accurate estimates of beneficial results.

Carbachol has been used in the treatment of rumen atony and impaction in cattle. After conservative treatment with stool softeners, repeated doses of 1–2 mg have proved effective in stimulating rumen motility. However, single doses greater than 4 mg for a 1000-lb cow may be ineffective, and in some cases may actually inhibit rumino-reticular activity. Carbachol should not be given by intravenous injection due to its potency. It can be given by the intramuscular or subcutaneous route; however, the dosage is somewhat critical. Fatalities have occurred in human patients after the intramuscular injection of carbachol (Fatal accidents from "Doryl" [carbachol] 1943).

NATURALLY OCCURRING CHOLINOMIMETIC ALKALOIDS

Pilocarpine, muscarine, and arecoline are plant alkaloids that have been found to exert parasympathomimetic effects with minimal activity at nicotinic sites. Although all three agents are frequently used in research, only pilocarpine has been used to any appreciable extent in clinical medicine.

Pilocarpine nitrate is the water-soluble salt of the alkaloid pilocarpine, obtained from leaves of the Brazilian shrubs *Pilocarpus jaborandi* and *P. microphyllus*. Arecoline is an alkaloid found in the betel nut, the seed of the betel palm, *Areca catechu*. Muscarine is found in the poisonous mushroom, *Amanita muscaria*. The chemical structures of these three compounds are given in Fig. 8.3.

Pharmacologic Mechanisms and Effects. Pilocarpine, arecoline, and muscarine are rather selective parasympathomimetic agents. That is, their cholinomimetic activity is exerted primarily at muscarinic sites with very minimal nicotinic effects.

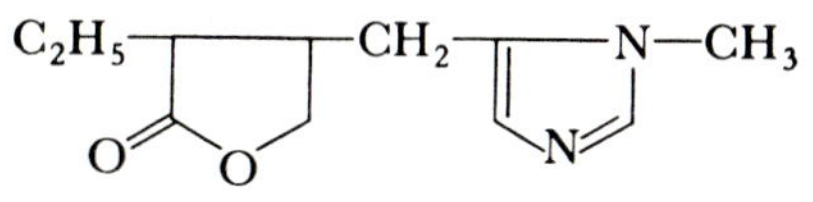

C_2H_5—CH$_2$—N—CH_3 (lactone ring with O=; imidazole ring with N)

Pilocarpine

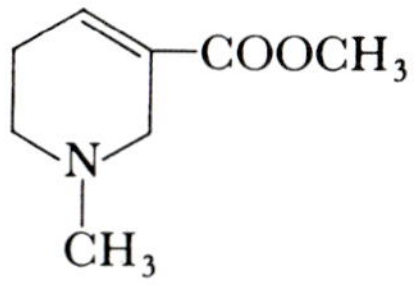

—$COOCH_3$ (tetrahydropyridine ring, N—CH_3)

Arecoline

HO—, CH_3— (tetrahydrofuran ring, O) —CH_2—$\overset{+}{N}(CH_3)_3$

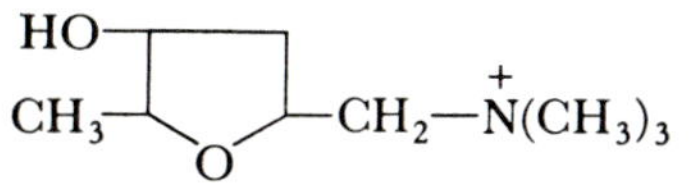

Muscarine

FIG. 8.3.

Even the slight ganglionic-stimulating effects of pilocarpine and arecoline are believed to be due to activation of the secondary muscarinic pathway involved in ganglionic transmission (see latter part of this chapter). These cholinomimetic alkaloids evoke their parasympathomimetic effects by direct stimulation of the muscarinic receptors of cells innervated by postganglionic cholinergic nerves. They do not inhibit cholinesterase. Also, since their effects are produced in chronically denervated tissue, they are not dependent upon the release of endogenous acetylcholine.

Pilocarpine is particularly effective in stimulating the flow of secretions from exocrine glands, including salivary, sweat, mucous, gastric, and digestive pancreatic secretions. Like acetylcholine, it causes contraction of gastrointestinal smooth muscle, thereby increasing smooth muscle tone and peristaltic activity. Of considerable importance, pilocarpine has a potent constrictor effect on the pupil.

Arecoline activates muscarinic receptors of cholinergically innervated effector cells of glands, smooth muscles, and myocardium and, therefore, produces the usual parasympathomimetic effects. It is similar to pilocarpine in scope of activity but is considerably more potent. Arecoline depresses heart rate and blood pressure and may produce dyspnea by constricting the bronchioles. Dyspnea generally is not marked except in cases where the dose is toxic or the animal has previously been affected with a respiratory ailment such as acute pulmonary emphysema. Arecoline stimulates secretion of the glands of the digestive tract and increases peristaltic movements of the gut. The increased flow of saliva, occurring within 5 minutes following a subcutaneous injection and lasting for an hour, is particularly noticeable. Arecoline contracts the urinary bladder.

Muscarine has been employed experimentally for many years because it has a very selective excitatory effect on the effector cells of tissues innervated by postganglionic cholinergic nerves. It does not stimulate the nicotinic receptors of autonomic ganglia or skeletal muscle as does acetylcholine.

Clinical Uses. Pupillary constriction (miosis) occurs when pilocarpine is administered systemically or applied topically to the eye. Clinically, solutions of 0.5%–2% are used for instillation into the conjunctival sac for treatment of glaucoma. Pilocarpine stimulates both the sphincter muscle of the iris and the ciliary muscle of the lens, causing pupillary constriction and spasm of accommodation. Intraocular pressure momentarily increases, followed by a persistent *decrease.* Fixation of the lens for near vision lasts only 1–2 hours; however, miosis, which develops within about 15 minutes after instillation, persists 12–24 hours. Pilocarpine is also used alternately with mydriatics to prevent synechiation, but it is contraindicated in patients with iridocyclitis.

Arecoline hydrobromide at the dosage of approximately 1.3 mg/kg has been used as a teniacide in dogs when administered orally after fasting. It has been used less successfully and with greater danger in cats. Aside from occasional use as a teniacide, arecoline has few clinical indications. At one time it was used to promote rapid evacuation of the intestines, particularly in horses; however, this nonconservative approach is now infrequently practiced.

Toxicology. Toxic doses of the cholinomimetic alkaloids evoke severe colic and diarrhea and exocrine gland secretions. The pupil is markedly constricted. Dyspnea occurs because of constriction of the bronchioles and accumulation of mucus in the airways. Hypotension and extreme cardiac slowing, complicated by excessive bronchioconstriction and bronchial secretions, lead to death. Arecoline or systemic exposure to pilocarpine is contraindicated in animals with heart failure, with depression or disease of the respiratory tract, with spasmodic colic, and during gestation. Atropine is a specific antidote to toxic doses of arecoline, pilocarpine, and muscarine. The toxic action of the poisonous mushroom in human beings results from the parasympathomimetic action of muscarine.

CHOLINESTERASE INHIBITORS

The function of acetylcholinesterase in terminating the transmitter action of endogenous acetylcholine at cholinergic synapses and neuroeffector junctions is discussed in Chapter 6. Cholinesterase inhibitors, or anticholinesterase agents, are compounds that inactivate or inhibit acetylcholinesterase and pseudocholinesterase and thereby intensify the activity of endogenous acetylcholine. In addition, the activity of those drugs that are biotransformed by cholinesterase (e.g., succinylcholine) is also prolonged by cholinesterase inhibitors. Since these drugs magnify the actions of endogenous acetylcholine at all cholinergic receptors, their scope of activity is not limited to parasympathomimetic effects but includes *cholinomimetic* actions throughout the body.

Physostigmine, neostigmine, and edrophonium are examples of the type of anticholinesterase agent that produces a "reversible" inhibition of cholinesterase, whereas organophosphate compounds like diisopropyl phosphorofluoridate (DFP) produce an "irreversible" inhibition. Although there is considerable distinction between several aspects of these two groups of anticholinesterase agents, their pharmacologic effects are quite similar, due to a common basic mechanism of action.

Pharmacologic Considerations

mechanism of action

The pharmacologic effects of cholinesterase inhibitors can be explained almost entirely by their characteristic inhibitory action on acetylcholinesterase. This results in decreased hydrolysis of neuronally released acetylcholine and intensification of its action at cholinergic receptors. This is particularly true with the irreversible organophosphate compounds and can be demonstrated by the lack of miotic effect of topically applied DFP in a chronically denervated eye, where there is no source of acetylcholine. However, neostigmine and other quaternary nitrogen anticholinesterase agents exert some direct effects (either agonistic or antagonistic) on cholinergic receptors in addition to inhibition of cholinesterase. At the somatic neuromuscular junction, for example, muscle twitch stimulant effects of neostigmine are attributed to direct receptor activation as well as to cholinesterase inhibition. However, the direct effect is not uniform throughout the body; and neostigmine, like DFP, is miotically inactive in the denervated eye. Effects of physostigmine, a tertiary amine, can be explained almost entirely by its anticholinesterase activity.

Molecular. The molecular events involved in the enzymatic interaction of acetylcholinesterase, acetylcholine, and cholinesterase inhibitors are shown schematically in Fig. 8.4 and can be summarized as follows. Acetylcholinesterase contains two active sites that recognize specific parts of the acetylcholine molecule: (1) an anionic (negatively charged) region where electrostatic binding occurs with the cationic nitrogen of the choline moiety and (2) an esteratic site where the carboxyl portion of the acetyl ester binds to it by covalent bonding. After acetylcholine-acetylcholinesterase interaction occurs, the choline portion is split off leaving the acetylated esteratic site. Acetic acid is rapidly formed as water reacts with the acetyl group, and the enzyme is thereby reactivated (Wilson 1954).

Neostigmine, physostigmine, and other carbamate derivatives are also believed to interact with both the anionic and esteratic sites of the enzyme, thereby preventing acetylcholine from affixing to the enzyme and inhibiting its destruction. Originally, it was believed that the cholinesterase inhibitors then simply disassociated from the enzyme at a slow rate, allowing its reactivation. It is likely, however, that neostigmine and physostigmine are actually hydrolyzed in a manner similar, but much slower, to that of acetylcholine (Wilson et al. 1960). That is, the alcoholic portion of the anticholinesterase compound is split off, leaving a carbamylated esteratic site. A carbamic acid is then formed upon reaction with water, and the enzyme is regenerated (Fig. 8.4). Although the rate of combination of inhibitor with acetylcholinesterase is only a few times slower than the analogous combination of acetylcholine with the enzyme, the rate of hydrolysis is probably over 10^6 times faster for acetylcholine. Therefore, neostigmine and related drugs are reversible cholinesterase inhibi-

1. ACh — Esteratic, Anionic — Acetylcholinesterase ⇌ Ch + At (10^6) H_2O ⇌ Aa +

2. NS ⇌ N + Car (1) H_2O ⇌ Cr-a +

3. Ed (10) ⇌ Ed +

4. OP (10^{-6}) → OP + ; + PAM → OP---PAM (1) ⇌ OP-PAM +

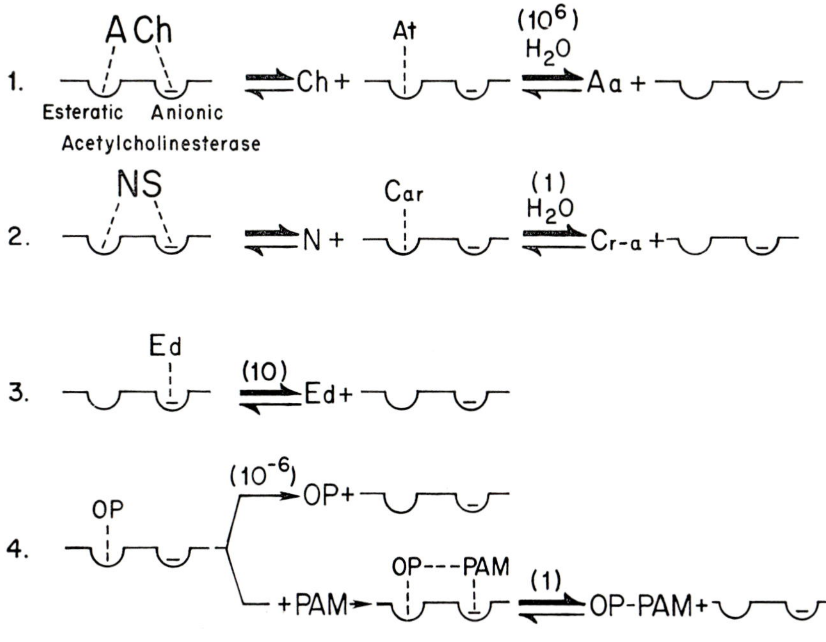

FIG. 8.4. Interactions of acetylcholinesterase (AChE), acetylcholine (ACh), and cholinesterase inhibitors. *1.* ACh and AChE form a complex of electrostatic binding of the quaternary (cationic) N^+ of the choline group with an anionic site of the enzyme and by covalent binding of the ester group of ACh with the esteratic site of the enzyme (see Fig. 8.1 for structure). Choline (Ch) is then split off, leaving the acetylated (At) enzyme, which reacts with water to yield acetic acid (Aa) and the regenerated active AChE. *2.*Neostigmine (NS) also interacts with both the esteratic and anionic sites; as the alcoholic portion of neostigmine (N) is split off, the carbamylated (Car) enzyme reacts with water to yield a carbamic acid (Cr-a) and the regenerated active enzyme. *3.* Edrophonium (Ed) reacts with the anionic site of AChE; disassociation occurs and yields Ed and the active enzyme. *4.* Organophosphate compounds (OP) irreversibly phosphorylate the esteratic site of AChE, and essentially no spontaneous disassociation of this complex occurs. However pralidoxime (PAM) and other oximes can reverse OP–AChE interaction by affecting removal of the OP from the phosphorylated-enzyme complex.

The numbers in parentheses refer to relative rates of reaction.

tors due to their acting as competitive substrates that are hydrolyzed at a much slower rate than the endogenous substrate, acetylcholine (Koelle 1970).

Edrophonium and tetraethylammonium ions are complex and simple quaternary nitrogen compounds, respectively, that interact with the anionic site of cholinesterase. Therefore, they are not hydrolyzed but act as simple competitive reversible inhibitors. Accordingly, the duration of action of edrophonium is much shorter than that of neostigmine or physostigmine.

The organophosphate compounds interact with acetylcholinesterase at the esteratic site and form an extremely stable enzyme-inhibitor complex that does not undergo significant spontaneous disassociation. Thus the esteratic site is persistently phosphorylated, and recovery of cholinesterase activity is dependent upon *de novo* synthesis of new enzyme. Some organophosphates (e.g., echothiophate) may interact with both the anionic and esteratic sites. Since cholinesterase synthesis requires days to months, organophosphates cause an irreversible inhibition. As will be discussed below, however, certain oxime compounds exhibit such high affinity for the organophosphates that they can actually cause a detachment of the inhibitor from the esteratic site, resulting in cholinesterase reactivation.

PHARMACOLOGIC EFFECTS

Effects of cholinesterase inhibitors can be reliably predicted by considering the anatomic location of cholinergic nerves and the respective physiologic processes that they modulate in their innervated cells. Thus parasympathomimetic, or muscarinic, effects of these agents are equivalent to the effects associated with postganglionic parasympathomimetic nerve impulses. Moreover, cholinesterase inhibitors also cause intensification of acetylcholine activity at nicotinic sites. Therefore, these drugs can cause the following effects: (1) stimulation of postganglionic muscarinic receptors of effector cells, resulting in typical parasympathomimetic activity; (2) stimulation of the adrenal chromaffin cells to discharge catecholamines into the circulation; (3) initial stimulation and subsequent depolarization block of nicotinic receptors of autonomic ganglia and skeletal muscle fibers; and (4) marked CNS cholinergic effects.

Although all these activities may be seen with excessive doses, therapeutic doses usually result in more selective actions. For example, neostigmine and other quaternary nitrogen compounds do not easily penetrate the blood-brain barrier and, therefore, exert little CNS activity. Also, these compounds are relatively more active at nicotinic receptors of the skeletal neuromuscular junction than at muscarinic sites of autonomic effector cells. The tertiary amines and the organophosphates are less lipophobic and can cross the blood-brain barrier and evoke CNS effects. Also, these compounds are relatively more active with low doses at autonomic receptor sites than on voluntary muscles.

REVERSIBLE INHIBITORS

PHYSOSTIGMINE AND NEOSTIGMINE

Physostigmine, or eserine, is an alkaloid extracted from the dried ripe seed of a vine, *Physostigma venenosum,* which grows in tropical West Africa. This seed, also called the Calabar or "ordeal" bean, was used by native Africans in witchcraft ordeals. A person accused of a crime was forced to eat the bean. If vomition occurred, the accused did not die and he was considered innocent. If the suspect did not vomit, however, death resulted and he was declared guilty.

Neostigmine (prostigmine) bromide is the salt of a synthetically produced substance that was discovered in a research investigation of compounds structurally related to physostigmine (Aeschlimann and Reinert 1931). Phystostigmine can also be synthesized. *Edrophonium* (Tensilon) is a synthetically derived agent that produces pharmacologic effects similar to neostigmine, except that its duration of action is considerably shorter. It is used primarily as an anticurare agent. The chemical

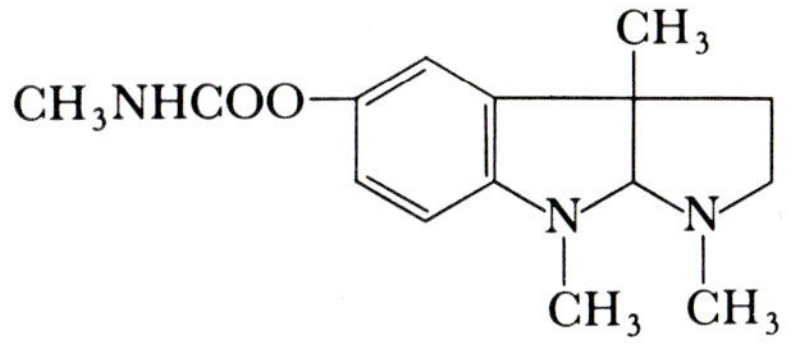

Physostigmine

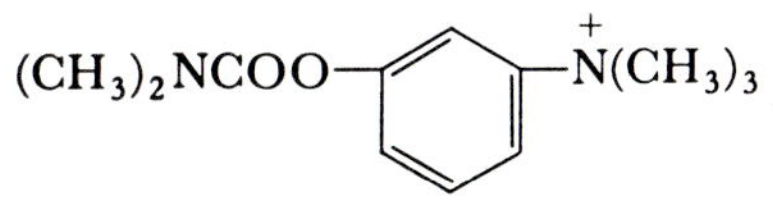

Neostigmine

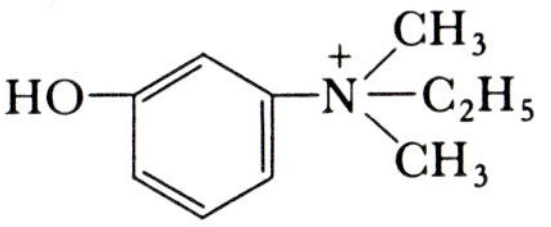

Edrophonium

FIG. 8.5.

structures of physostigmine, neostigmine, and edrophonium are shown in Fig. 8.5.

MECHANISM OF ACTION

As outlined above, these agents produce their effects by combining with cholinesterase and thereby preventing the enzyme from hydrolyzing acetylcholine. Therefore, acetylcholine released during normal cholinergic nerve impulses has a prolonged and uninterrupted action upon cholinergic receptors. The interaction of physostigmine and neostigmine with cholinesterase is reversible so that, as the inhibitor-enzyme complex breaks down, the enzyme is reactivated and it will now hydrolyze acetylcholine and terminate its activity. At certain sites, neostigmine may act directly on receptors and may evoke the release of acetylcholine from nerve endings; however these are considered to be secondary actions.

PHARMACOLOGIC EFFECTS

Digestive Tract. Physostigmine and neostigmine cause contraction of gastro-intestinal smooth muscle, thereby increasing motility and peristaltic movements of the gut. Frequency and strength of peristaltic waves are increased, and movement of intestinal contents is accelerated. Physostigmine has been used in animals for initiating peristaltic movements and for evacuating the digestive tract. Excessive peristalsis leading to intestinal spasm and colic complicates the use of this drug for this purpose. Physostigmine is given by subcutaneous or intramuscular injection; its action after oral administration is unreliable. Neostigmine is not appreciably absorbed after oral administration, due to its quaternary nitrogen structure.

Ocular Effects. Physostigmine causes pupillary constriction and spasm of accommodation when applied locally to the eye or when injected for systemic effect. Intraocular pressure decreases and physostigmine has been used in treating glaucoma to relieve elevated intraocular pressure.

Skeletal Muscle. Besides its major action of inactivating acetylcholinesterase at the somatic myoneural junction, neostigmine is believed to directly stimulate nicotinic receptors of the skeletal muscle fibers. For example, intraarterial administration of neostigmine into chronically denervated skeletal muscle still evokes muscle contraction (Riker and Wescoe 1946). Physostigmine, on the other hand, is not active in denervated muscle. The skeletal muscle effects of neostigmine are relatively more pronounced at low doses than are the smooth muscle effects of this agent. Twitching of skeletal muscles may be observed when a large dose of physostigmine or neostigmine is injected.

Physostigmine, neostigmine, and edrophonium are "anticurare" agents; they are antagonists to *d*-tubocurarine and other nondepolarizing (competitive) neuromuscular blocking agents at the somatic myoneural junction. These drugs can be used clinically to counteract an excessive dose of true curarimimetic agents but should not be used in attempts to antagonize the depolarizing neuromusclar blocking agents (e.g., succinylcholine), since synergism may actually occur (see Chapter 9).

Other Effects. A therapeutic dose of physostigmine or neostigmine does not produce pronounced effects on cardiovascular function. Effects of higher doses are complicated by concurrent ganglionic stimulation and muscarinic effects on the heart and blood vessels. Usually, hypotension and a bradycardia leading to arrhythmias are produced. The smooth muscle of the bladder is cholinergically innervated and, therefore, is contracted by cholinesterase inhibitors. Bronchiolar smooth muscle is also contracted by these agents.

CLINICAL USES

Physostigmine can be used to produce miosis of the pupil and reduce intraocular pressure in the treatment of glaucoma. A solution of 0.5%–1% physostigmine salicylate is usually applied topically three times a day. The maximum miotic effect is obtained within an hour and may persist 12–24 hours, depending upon the dosage. Physostigmine may also be used alternately with atropine to prevent or break down synechia formed between the lens and the iris, such as occurs with periodic ophthalmia in horses.

Physostigmine has been used to stimulate ruminal activity in treatment of simple impaction or nonobstructive atony in a subcutaneous dose of 30–45 mg in cattle. As mentioned, physostigmine, neostigmine, and edrophonium can be used to overcome the effects of true curarelike drugs in voluntary muscles, but the latter two agents are more commonly used for this purpose (Chapter 9). Neostigmine has been used extensively in treating myasthenia gravis in human patients. In myasthenialike syndromes in dogs, neostigmine has also proved beneficial (Hall and Walker 1962).

Impaction or other obstructions of the alimentary tract constitute a contraindication to the systemic use of cholinesterase inhibitors. The violent peristalsis that can be produced by these drugs may cause rupture or intussusception of the gut. Further, these drugs should not be used during pregnancy, particularly late in term, because of the danger of producing abortion.

TOXICOLOGY

Large doses of physostigmine first stimulate and then depress the CNS; small to moderate doses have little effect, whereas massive doses can produce convulsions. Neostigmine does not cross the blood-brain barrier to an appreciable extent. Toxic doses of these agents produce marked skeletal muscle weakness, nausea, vomiting, colic, and diarrhea. The pupil is markedly constricted and fixed. Dyspnea is characteristically seen, due to constriction of the bronchiolar musculature. Bradycardia and lowered blood pressure are also characteristic signs. Respiratory paralysis due to depolarization block of the neuromuscular junction and compounded by excess bronchiolar secretions is the usual cause of death. Atropine is the most effective pharmacologic antagonist for physostigmine or neostigmine toxicity.

ORGANOPHOSPHOROUS COMPOUNDS

Diisopropyl fluorophosphate (diisopropyl phosphorofluoridate; DFP) is the prototypical organophosphate anticholinesterase agent. Related compounds include the alkyl pyrophosphates such as hexaethyltetraphosphate (HETP), tetraethylpyrophosphate (TEPP), and octamethyl pyrophosphortetramide (OMPA). Organophosphates were originally introduced as insecticides by German scientists prior to and during World War II; however, there was considerable speculation by Allied scientists as to the potential use of these highly toxic substances as antipersonnel devices in chemical warfare. Subsequently, a wide variety of organophosphorous compounds have been synthesized and extensively investigated. Some of the more important members of this class of compounds that have been used as insecticides are parathion [Thiophos; diethyl *O*-(4-nitrophenyl)phosphorothioate]; malathion [*O,O*-dimethyl *S*-(1,2-dicarbethoxyethyl)phosphorodithioate]; ronnel [*O,O*-dimethyl *O*-(2,4,5-trichlorophenyl)phosphorothioate]; and Co-ral. Soman, tabun, and sarin are extremely potent synthetic compounds that have been referred to as "nerve gases." Dichlorvos (*O,O*-dimethyl-2,2-dichlorovinyl phosphate or 2,2-dichlorovinyl dimethyl phosphate) is commonly used as an oral anthelmentic in vet-

TABLE 8.3. Structural formulas of several organophosphate anticholinesterase agents

General Formula: $R_1R_2P(=O)X$

R_1	R_2	X	Agent
Isopropyl	Isopropyl	Fluoride	DFP
Pinacolyl	Methyl	Fluoride	Soman
Dimethylamino	Ethoxyl	Cyanide	Tabun
Isopropylamino	Isopropylamino	Fluoride	Mipafox
Ethoxyl	Ethoxyl	*S*-(2-Trimethylaminoethyl)	Echothiophate

Source: Modified from Volle 1971, p. 602.

erinary medicine; it is also impregnated in "flea collars" for use as an insecticide.

Although the chemical structures of organophosphate compounds vary considerably, the basic moiety is a phosphate with various organic groups attached to it, as described in Table 8.3. Representative structural formulas are shown in Fig. 8.6.

MECHANISM OF ACTION AND EFFECTS

Organophosphorous compounds act as irreversible inhibitors of the cholinesterases in mammals, as previously outlined. These compounds irreversibly phosphorylate the esteratic site of both acetylcholinesterase and the nonspecific or pseudocholinesterase throughout the body. Endogenous acetylcholine is not inactivated and the resulting effects are due to the excessive preservation and accumulation of endogenous acetylcholine. Therefore, organophosphate poisoning produces diffuse cholinomimetic effects: profuse salivation, vomition, defecation, hypermotility of the gastrointestinal tract, urination, bradycardia, hypotension, severe bronchioconstriction, and excess bronchial secretions. These signs reflect excess activation of muscarinic receptors of postganglionic parasympathetic neuroeffector junctions with typical parasympathomimetic actions.

In addition to the muscarinic effects, skeletal muscle fasciculations, twitching, and subsequently, muscle paralysis occur. These effects are due to persistent excessive stimulation of the nicotinic receptors of skeletal neuromuscular junctions, resulting in the depolarizing type of striated muscle paralysis. Autonomic ganglia are undoubtedly involved with consequent liberation of catecholamines, but these activities are less evident, due to cholinergic dominance. The secondary muscarinic pathway of autonomic ganglia may be activated by cholinesterase inhibitors more than the nicotinic receptors of the ganglia (Volle 1962; Takeshige et al. 1963). Convulsions are usually seen in organophosphorous poison-

Sarin: $(CH_3)_2CHO(CH_3)P(=O)F$

Tetraethyl Pyrophosphate (TEPP): $(C_2H_5O)_2P(=O)-P(=O)(OC_2H_5)_2$

Parathion: $(C_2H_5O)_2P(=S)-O-C_6H_4-NO_2$

Malathion: $(CH_3O)_2P(=S)-S-CH(C(=O)-OC_2H_5)-CH_2C(=O)-OC_2H_5$

FIG. 8.6. Representative structural formulas for organophosphate compounds.

ing, due to penetration of the agent into the CNS and subsequent intensification of the activity of acetylcholine at CNS sites.

Death from organophosphorous compounds results from the combinations of various of the above-listed effects but is usually immediately related to respiratory failure. Fatigue from CNS overstimulation, depolarizing paralysis of respiratory muscles, excess bronchiolar secretions, and bronchiolar constriction cause dyspnea and reduce the airway to the point where gaseous exchange is inadequate. Asphyxiation results.

ANTAGONISTS

Atropine. Since atropine blocks muscarinic receptors, it not only lessens the severity of the parasympathomimetic effects but also increases the quantity of organophosphate required to produce death. For example, the ratio of the LD50 of sarin in atropine-treated dogs to the LD50 in nonatropinized dogs may be 150:1 (De Candole and McPhail 1957). These ratios vary with the animal species and organophosphate, but atropine is almost invariably beneficial (Wills 1963, 1970). In addition, since atropine is a competitive antagonist to acetylcholine, large doses of atropine are effective even if administered after exposure to an organophosphate. The nondepolarizing type of nicotinic blocking agents (see Chapter 9) has also proved to be somewhat effective as partial antidotes in experimental animals; however, in clinical situations nicotinic blockers should be considered only as secondary to atropine.

Cholinesterase Reactivators. Although phosphorylation of the esteratic site of cholinesterase by the alkyl phosphates yields a normally irreversible complex, compounds have been discovered that can cause a disassociation of the enzyme bondage. Pralidoxime (pyridine-2-aldoxime-methiodide; PAM) was synthesized based on structural requirements postulated by Wilson (1958) to be necessary for a selective antidote to organophosphate-cholinesterase interaction. This compound causes an effective removal of the phosphate group from the enzyme, so that the enzyme is reactivated (see Fig. 8.4). This and related oxime compounds are undoubtedly the most valuable adjunct to atropine therapy in treating organophosphate poisoning. For example, pretreatment of animals with PAM increases by several times the LD50 of various organophosphates. If atropine is given in conjunction with PAM, the lethal dose is increased many more times (Wills 1963, 1970).

Similarly, animals previously exposed to toxic doses of organophosphates experience considerable improvement after treatment with PAM. In dogs, 10–20 mg/kg of PAM administered by slow intravenous injection is usually effective; this dose may have to be repeated. In horses and cattle, 20 mg/kg and 10–40 mg/kg, respectively, are used. Since PAM significantly reverses the combination of organophosphate with cholinesterase, the reactivated enzyme can then perform its normal function within a relatively short period of time. Although treatment with PAM alone has been used successfully in human incidences of organophosphate poisoning, atropine should always be used concurrently to block muscarinic receptor sites. Various other reactivator oximes, such as pyridine-2-aldoxime dodecaiodide (designed for CNS effects), monoisonitrosoacetone, and diacetylmonoxime, have also been investigated. The oxime reactivators are probably ineffective in antagonizing the carbamate cholinesterase inhibitors and, in some cases, apparently can act synergistically.

CLINICAL USES OF ORGANOPHOSPHATES

Organophosphorous compounds have achieved widespread use as anthelmintics and insecticides since they are highly toxic to a wide variety of internal and external parasites. Their introduction in the late 1940s and the 1950s has had considerable impact on pest control; for more detailed information, see Section 14. Concurrent with their widespread use, however, is the potential for immediate and/or delayed damage to human beings, domestic animals, and wildlife. The ecological impact of organophosphate pesticides has received considerable attention from various conservationist organizations, and there is some evidence that certain of the compounds may be carcinogenic when given in huge doses to experimental animals. On the other hand, dichlorvos-impregnated collars are routinely used on dogs and cats for control of fleas and ticks with relatively few adverse side effects. Occasional hypersensitivity skin reactions may occur on the animal's neck and, even less frequently, on pet owners.

Organophosphates such as DFP and TEPP have been used locally to constrict the pupil in human patients for treatment of glaucoma; DFP (0.1% in peanut oil) and echothiophate (phospholine iodide; 0.03%–0.25% solutions) are commonly used for this purpose in dogs. Effects of these compounds are relatively long lasting and the dosage must be carefully controlled.

Precautionary Note About Clinical Uses of Cholinesterase Inhibitors. As repeatedly emphasized in the preceding discussions, cholinesterase inhibitors are highly reactive molecules that are capable of influencing functions of cholinergic nerves throughout the body. This is particularly true with the organophosphate compounds. At no time should their clinical use be considered as an innocuous procedure. Care should always be taken by the clinician to insure that the patient is not exposed either to drugs that are metabolized by cholinesterase (e.g., succinylcholine) or to other cholinesterase inhibitors (e.g., insecticide dips or sprays) for several days before and after administering either a reversible or irreversible anticholinesterase agent. If not, serious and even fatal synergistic interactions can occur (Hines et al. 1967). Other types of drugs (e.g., phenothiazine tranquilizers) may decrease cholinesterase activity as a potential side effect; their concurrent use with anticholinesterase drugs should be avoided or very closely monitored.

Severely ill, debilitated animals should not be exposed to a cholinesterase inhibitor except in emergency situations. If hepatic disease is presented, synthesis of cholinesterase may be markedly reduced and the effects of cholinesterase inhibitors can be intensified and/or prolonged. Respiratory illness may be exacerbated, due to excessive bronchiolar constriction and secretion. Abortion may occur, particularly during the latter gestational periods. Due to the potency of the cholinesterase inhibitors, especially the organophosphate compounds, care should always be taken to closely follow the manufacturer's individual dosage recommendations and procedural directions.

PARASYMPATHOLYTIC AGENTS

Parasympatholytic drugs prevent acetylcholine from producing its characteristic effects in structures innervated by postganglionic parasympathetic nerves. They also inhibit the effects of acetylcholine on smooth muscle cells that respond to acetylcholine but lack cholinergic innervation and on those particular structures (i.e., sweat glands, some blood vessels in skeletal muscles) that are innervated by sympathetic postganglionic cholinergic fibers. In other words, these drugs inhibit the *muscarinic* actions of acetylcholine and related cholinergic agonists. In fact, "muscarinic blocking" or "antimuscarinic" is actually more completely descriptive of the effects of this group of drugs than is "parasympatholytic," since muscarinic receptors are blocked irrespective of whether or not they are innervated by a parasympathetic nerve. Clinically, however, these drugs are used almost exclusively for their parasympatholytic activities. This group of drugs includes atropine and related alkaloids and numerous synthetically derived compounds.

Atropine and Scopolamine

Atropine, the prototypical muscarinic blocking agent, is an alkaloid extracted from the belladonna plants that belong to the *Solanaceae* (potato family) and include *Atropa belladonna* (deadly nightshade), *Datura stramonium* (jimson weed), and

Hyoscyamus niger (henbane). Alkaloids obtained from *Atropa belladonna* are *atropine* (which is a racemic mixture of *d*-hyoscyamine and *l*-hyoscyamine, racemization occurring during the extraction procedure), *scopolamine* (*l*-hyoscine), and others of lesser significance. Since atropine is actually an equal mixture of dextro- and levohyoscyamine, and since the dextro form of hyoscyamine is biologically inactive, a given quantity of atropine is about one-half as potent as the same quantity of *l*-hyoscyamine. Despite the inactive dextrorotatory component, atropine is nevertheless effective in very small doses. Chemically, the atropine molecule consists of two components joined through an ester linkage: (1) tropine, an organic base, and (2) tropic acid. Other related alkaloids also contain the aromatic tropic acid moiety combined by ester linkage to either tropine or another organic base, scopine. The chemical structures of atropine and scopolamine are given in Fig. 8.7.

MECHANISM OF ACTION

Atropine, scopolamine, and other related alkaloids interact with muscarinic receptors of effector cells and by occupying these sites prevent acetylcholine from affixing to the receptor area. Physiologic responses to parasympathetic nerve impulses are thereby attenuated. Pharmacologic effects of exogenously administered acetylcholine and other muscarinic agonists are similarly blocked by atropine and scopolamine. However, blockade of muscarinic receptors of smooth muscle, cardiac muscle, and glands by atropinelike drugs involves a competitive antagonism. Therefore, large doses of acetylcholine or other cholinomimetic drugs (e.g., carbachol, cholinesterase inhibitors) can overcome or surmount the inhibitory effects of atropine at these sites,

Although atropine and related compounds act immediately distal to all postganglionic cholinergic nerve endings, this block is not equally effective throughout the body. Salivary and sweat glands are quite susceptible to small doses of atropine, whereas somewhat larger doses are required for a vagolytic effect upon the heart. Gastrointestinal and urinary tract smooth muscles are less sensitive to atropine, and even larger dosages are required to inhibit gastric secretion. Except for effects on salivation and sweating, therefore, it is quite difficult to achieve a selective action on certain structures without concurrently inducing side effects on the more susceptible sites. Also, the net pharmacologic effects of atropinic drugs in a particular organ are influenced by the relative dominance of parasympathetic or sympathetic tone in that structure. After cholinergic impulses are blocked, adrenergic nerves become dominant and sympathomimeticlike effects may contribute to the final effect. This is particularly true in the iris.

In extremely high nontherapeutic doses, atropine can also block the nicotinic receptors of autonomic ganglia and the motor end-plate of skeletal muscles; however, these sites are not affected with ordinary doses.

PHARMACOLOGIC EFFECTS

Cardiovascular System. The usual thera-

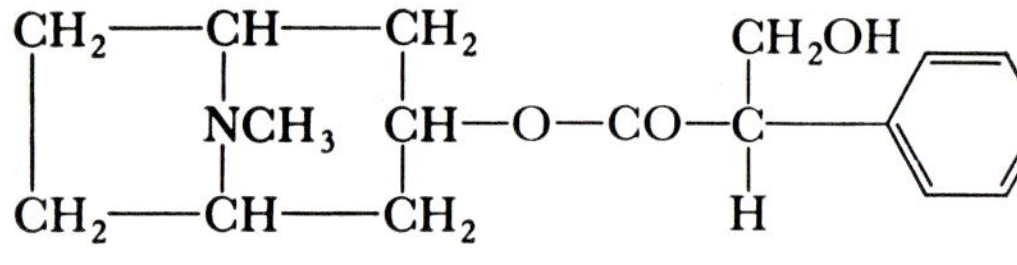

CH_2—CH—CH_2 / NCH_3 CH—O—CO—C(CH_2OH)(H)—C_6H_5 / CH_2—CH—CH_2

Atropine

O(CH—CH)—CH—CH_2 / NCH_3 CH—O—CO—C(CH_2OH)(H)—C_6H_5 / CH—CH—CH_2

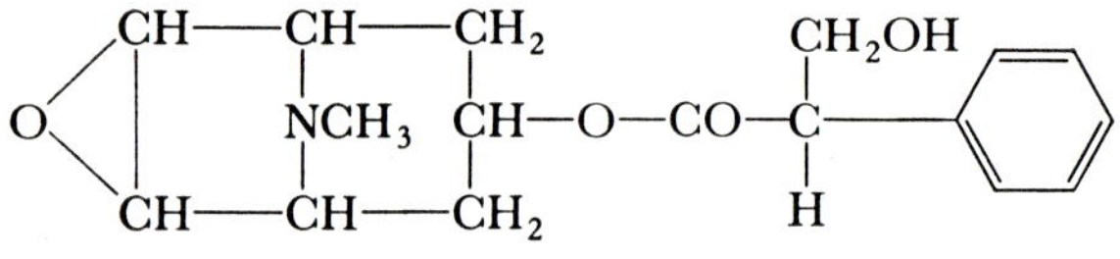

Scopolamine

Fig. 8.7.

peutic doses of atropine do not markedly affect blood pressure; however, pulse rate is altered. Tachycardia is the dominant effect and large doses of atropine invariably produce an increased heart rate. Small doses may initially produce a slight slowing of heart rate, but this effect is believed to be due to transient stimulation of vagal nuclei of the medulla oblongata and perhaps to transient stimulation of peripheral receptors prior to their block (Averill and Lamb 1959; Ashford et al. 1962). The ease with which atropine produces tachycardia is dependent, at least in part, upon the degree of "vagal tone" of the individual patient. Since atropine blocks transmission of vagal impulses to the heart, animals with a preexisting high vagal tone would show a relatively greater tachycardia than animals with a low vagal tone.

Cardiac output tends to increase with atropine, due primarily to the increase in heart rate. Arterial blood pressure either remains unchanged or increases slightly in a normal animal. In animals exposed to exogenous acetylcholine or other cholinomimetics (e.g., cholinesterase inhibitors), atropine can cause a relative increase in blood pressure since the muscarinic effects of the agonists will be blocked. Also, as mentioned previously, atropine "unmasks" the hypertensive response to high experimental doses of cholinergic agonists resulting from their nicotinic effects (see Fig. 8.2).

Since atropine blocks the cardiac vagus, it markedly reduces or abolishes the cardiac inhibitory effects of drugs acting through a vagal mechanism and will attenuate vagal-mediated reflex responses. Accordingly, the pressor effects of epinephrine and norepinephrine are accentuated in atropinized animals due to blockade of the efferent limb of vagal-baroreceptor reflexes. Large doses of atropine are directly depressant to the myocardium and also cause cutaneous dilation as a result of a direct vascular smooth muscle effect.

Gastrointestinal System. Atropine causes relaxation of GI smooth muscle by inhibiting contractile effects of endogenous acetylcholine. Smooth muscle responses to other cholineregic drugs are similarly blocked by atropine and scopolamine. Since atropine inhibits the intestinal smooth muscle contractions evoked by cholinergic nerve impulses, tone is reduced and may even be abolished. Therefore, atropine and related drugs are often effective in the treatment of intestinal spasm and hypermotility. Inhibition of smooth muscle motility extends from stomach to colon, although the degree of blockade may not be uniform. Insofar as rumen motility is concerned, adequate doses are consistently inhibitory, and atropine is one of the few agents that can be relied upon to produce cessation of rumen motility.

Secretions of the GI tract are also blocked by atropine. Salivation is reduced quite markedly. Similarly, secretions of the intestinal mucosa are inhibited; however, gastric secretions are reduced only with exceedingly high doses that also block virtually all other muscarinic sites.

Bronchioles. Cholinergic innervation to the bronchioles modulates secretion of mucus and contraction of bronchiolar smooth muscle. Atropine and other drugs of the belladonna group block the effects of cholinergic impulses and thereby decrease secretions and increase luminal diameter of the bronchioles. The dilator action of atropine is valuable in counteracting constriction of the bronchioles following overdosage of a parasympathomimetic drug.

Atropine will give temporary symptomatic relief from the dyspnea of "heaves" in horses, and it has been used by unscrupulous individuals for this purpose. A subcutaneous dose of atropine sulfate (30 mg) produces an immediate relief in the horse, which lasts 1–3 hours; however, dyspnea worsens after the effect of the drug has terminated. A crude form of the drug, such as belladonna leaves, administered orally produces its effect within 30 minutes, with a duration of about 24 hours. When atropine medication is suspected, the following signs should be detectable: a dry oral mucosa, dilated and fixed pupils, and tachycardia.

Ocular Effects. Atropine blocks the chollinergically innervated sphincter muscle of the iris and the ciliary muscle of the lens, resulting in mydriasis and cycloplegia after topical or systemic administration. Since atropine blocks cholinergic effects, adrenergic nerve impulses dominate and the pupil actively dilates. Atropine is contraindicated in the presence of increased intraocular pressure due to acute angle glaucoma because the drainage canal of Schlemm is blocked during mydriasis.

Urinary Tract. Atropine relaxes smooth muscle of the urinary tract. The spasmolytic effect on the ureters may be of some benefit in the treatment of renal colic. Atropine tends to cause urine retention, due to inhibition of smooth muscle tone. This effect may be of some use in reducing the frequency of micturition that accompanies cystitis; however, the deleterious effects of only partially emptying the bladder should be considered.

Sweat Glands. Atropine has a definite anhydrotic action in those animal species that normally sweat, and a large dose may cause a hyperpyrexic response in these species.

Central Nervous System. Therapeutic doses of atropine produce minimal effects on the CNS. Excessive doses may cause hallucinations and disorientation in human beings and mania and excitement in domestic animals. Excessive motor activity followed by depression and coma is the usual sequence of events.

Scopolamine has a slight sedative effect; when combined with morphine, it produces analgesia and amnesia (referred to as "twilight sleep") in human patients. These effects of scopolamine are not detectable in domestic animals. While small doses may be depressant in dogs and cats, larger doses produce delirium and excitement in these species and also in horses.

TOXICOLOGY

There is considerable interspecies variation in the toxicity of belladonna and atropine; the route of administration is also important. Herbivora are usually much more resistant than are Carnivora. Certain strains of rabbits are quite resistant to a diet of belladonna leaves, since an esterase (atropinase) of the liver hydrolyzes and thus inactivates atropine. However, rabbits fed on such a diet may prove toxic if eaten by dogs, cats, or human beings, because of the large amount of alkaloid present in the muscle tissues. Horses, cattle, and goats are relatively resistant to belladonna when it is administered orally; however, these species are quite susceptible to atropine when it is injected parenterally. Swine are not resistant to ingested belladonna and poisoning occurs more often in this than in other species from eating the deadly nightshade plant.

Signs of atropine poisoning are similar in all mammalian species. Dry mouth, thirst, dysphagia, constipation, mydriasis, tachycardia, hyperpnea, restlessness, delirium, ataxia, and muscle trembling may be observed; convulsions, respiratory depression, and respiratory failure lead to death. A drop of urine obtained from a patient suspected of atropine toxicosis causes mydriasis when placed in the eye of a cat. Also, the tested pupil will not constrict when exposed to light, while the untreated eye will. This simple procedure may prove helpful in the differential diagnosis of belladonna intoxication.

CLINICAL USES

Parasympatholytic drugs are frequently used to control smooth muscle spasm, i.e., they are used as antispasmodics or spasmolytics. Antispasmodics can be used to decrease or abolish gastrointestinal hypermotility and to depress hypertonicity of the uterus, urinary bladder, ureter, bile duct, and bronchioles. Parasympatholytics are not as effective as epinephrine or other adrenergic amines in dilating the bronchioles, but atropine is effective in antagonizing excessive cholinergic stimulation at these sites.

Atropine is used routinely as an adjunct to general anesthesia, particularly with inhalant anesthetics, to decrease salivary and airway secretions. Also, atropine is frequently given in conjunction with morphine to reduce salivary secretions that may be produced by the latter drug. When used prior to anesthesia, the dose of atropine sulfate in dogs is 0.088–0.11 mg/kg, administered subcutaneously. The preanesthetic use of atropine to suppress respiratory secretions is extremely important in maintaining open airways in ruminants during anesthesia at a dose of 0.044–0.088 mg/kg, administered subcutaneously. Atropine sulfate should be routinely given prior to and, if necessary, during any form of recumbent anesthesia in ruminants because of the excessive secretion and accumulation of fluids in the upper respiratory tract in these species. Also, the preoperative use of atropine probably prevents inadvertent discharge of vagal impulses that may occur during the induction and maintenance of general anesthesia.

Atropine is routinely used to facilitate ophthalmoscopic examination of internal ocular structures and functions and is also used for treatment of various ocular disorders. Homatropine hydrobromide, due to its shorter duration of action, has largely replaced atropine sulfate for ophthalmoscopic purposes in human patients. Application of a few drops of a 1%–2% solution of atropine sulfate into the conjunctival sac causes mydriasis within 15–20 minutes. Maximum pupillary dilatation occurs in about 2 hours and may be detectable for several days. The time course of the cycloplegic action of atropine is similar to that of mydriatic action. Mydriatics like atropine are helpful in preventing or breaking down adhesions between the iris and the lens when used alternately with miotics.

As discussed above, atropine is an essential antidote to anticholinesterase overdosage or poisoning.

Synthetic Muscarinic Blocking Agents

These compounds were chemically synthesized in attempts to find atropine substitutes that would act selectively at certain muscarinic sites and, therefore, would have fewer undesirable side effects than the alkaloids.

HOMATROPINE

This compound is similar in structure to atropine except that it is an ester of mandelic acid rather than of tropic acid. Homatropine closely resembles atropine in most of its pharmacologic actions, particularly the ocular effects. Mydriasis and cycloplegia are produced in the eye by topical application of a 2%–5% solution of homatropine, but these effects last for a shorter duration than those resulting from atropine. Homatropine produces fewer side effects on cardiovascular and gastrointestinal functions than atropine and is considerably less toxic than the parent drug.

METHANTHELINE, PROPANTHELINE, AND METHYLATROPINE

These compounds are quaternary amines that are used primarily as smooth muscle relaxants. Due to the charged quaternary group, these compounds do not cross the blood-brain barrier to an appreciable extent. Accordingly, they are considerably less effective than atropine as antagonists to organophosphates since the CNS effects of the latter agents would not be blocked. In addition to muscarinic blocking effects, these drugs act as autonomic ganglionic blockers, which most likely contributes to their antispasmodic effect on gastrointestinal smooth muscle.

AUTONOMIC GANGLIONIC BLOCKING DRUGS

Mechanisms

Following Langley's investigations in 1889, it has been known that small doses of nicotine stimulate autonomic ganglion cells, and larger doses block the transmitter function of acetylcholine at these same sites. Therefore, the cholinergic receptors of ganglion neurons have been classified as nicotinic. However, considerable evidence is now available indicating that impulse transmission within autonomic ganglia is much more complicated than was originally believed. Specifically, recent studies have demonstrated a secondary excitatory cholinergic pathway in autonomic ganglia that is apparently muscarinic, and an inhibitory catecholaminergic mechanism has also been recorded (Eccles and Libet 1961; Volle and Koelle 1961; Volle 1962; Libet 1970). The different putative pathways involved in synaptic transmission in sympathetic autonomic ganglia are shown schematically in Fig. 8.8 and can be summarized as follows. As the preganglionic axonal action potential arrives at the nerve terminal, it evokes the release from the neuron of acetylcholine, which then passes across the synaptic cleft and interacts with nicotinic cholinergic receptors. Depolarization of the postsynaptic membrane immediately takes place and can be measured electrically as a large action potential spike. If these nicotinic receptors are partially blocked by a ganglionic blocking agent (e.g., hexamethonium) to reduce the magnitude of the spike potential, electrical events at the postsynaptic membrane are seen to be composed of three different electrical changes.

First, there is an immediate depolarization of the postsynaptic membrane; this is termed the fast *excitatory postsynaptic potential* (epsp). It can be completely blocked by nicotinic antagonists but not by atropine and, therefore, represents activation of the "classical" nicotinic receptors of autonomic ganglia. After the fast epsp, another less pronounced and delayed depolarization of the postsynaptic membrane takes place: the *slow epsp,* which is not blocked by nicotine but is blocked by atropine; this is evidence of a muscarinic excitatory pathway.

An *inhibitory postsynaptic potential* (ipsp) is also observed; it occurs during the interval between the fast epsp and the slow epsp. The ipsp represents an inhibitory effect believed to be due to hyperpolarization of the postsynaptic membrane. Atropine reduces the ipsp and an α-adrenergic blocking drug abolishes the ipsp; however, nicotine does not block the ipsp. Thus it seems that acetylcholine released from a preganglionic fiber activates, via a muscarinic receptor, nearby catecholamine-containing chromaffin cells. These cells then release a catecholamine (epinephrine

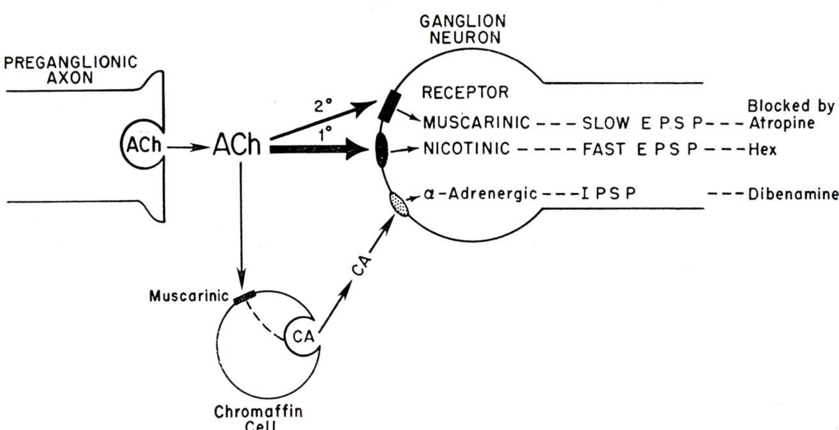

FIG. 8.8. Impulse transmission in sympathetic autonomic ganglia. Acetylcholine (ACh) is discharged from the preganglionic nerve terminal and interacts with a nicotinic receptor on the ganglionic neuron to cause a rapid depolarization measured electrically as a fast excitatory postsynaptic potential (epsp). ACh also interacts with a muscarinic receptor on the ganglionic neuron to cause a delayed depolarization measured electrically as a slow epsp. In addition, ACh activates nearby chromaffin cells through a muscarinic receptor, which results in a release of catecholamine (CA; dopamine or epinephrine). CA interacts with an α receptor on the ganglionic neuron to cause an inhibitory (hyperpolarization) response measured electrically as an inhibitory postsynaptic potential (ipsp). 1° and 2° indicate primary (nicotinic) and secondary (muscarinic) pathways of excitatory ganglionic impulses, respectively; hex = hexamethonium. (Eccles and Libet 1961; Libet 1970; Nishi 1974)

or dopamine) that acts on α-adrenergic receptors of the postganglionic neuronal cell to cause an inhibitory effect, reflected electrically as the ipsp (Fig. 8.8).

The physiologic purposes of these different ganglionic pathways are poorly understood. Evidence for the participation of different types of receptors has been gained primarily from studies of sympathetic ganglia. Parasympathetic ganglia are studied less frequently due to their poor accessibility. The nicotinic receptor and associated fast epsp represent the primary ganglionic transmission pathway present in all autonomic ganglia. The muscarinic receptors on the postganglionic neuron may facilitate impulse transmission events that are normally dominated by the nicotinic mechanisms. The adrenergic component may act as a modulator to prevent excessive impulse traffic. Various experimental drugs are being investigated in attempts to identify drugs that will selectively block or excite only the nicotinic or muscarinic ganglionic receptors. Despite these various physiologic and pharmacologic complexities, drugs that exert significant autonomic ganglionic blocking effects do so by blocking the nicotinic receptors. This generally affords an 80% or greater reduction in efficiency of impulse transmission through the ganglia. Ganglionic blocking agents act by producing either a nondepolarizing (competitive) or a depolarizing block of the postsynaptic membrane. For details of the mechanism of action of blocking agents at a nicotinic receptor, see Chapter 9.

Nicotine

Nicotine is an alkaloid obtained from leaves of the tobacco plant. Nicotine sulfate, the most commonly produced salt, is available commercially in an aqueous solution that contains 40% alkaloidal nicotine. This solution long has been designated by the proprietary name of Blackleaf 40, which has gained wide acceptance in the general literature. Nicotine was the original autonomic ganglionic blocking agent; however, it is not used clinically for this purpose. Nicotine first stimulates and then in higher doses blocks nicotinic receptors by producing a persistent depolarization of the receptor area.

Pharmacologic Effects

Central Nervous System. Alkaloidal nicotine is an extremely toxic substance that transiently stimulates and then severely depresses the CNS. Death is due to respiratory paralysis of the diaphragm and chest muscles resulting from descending paralysis and depolarization block of the nerve muscle junction of skeletal muscle. Nicotine is absorbed through the chitinous shell of insects after a direct spraying or after contacting a sprayed surface and kills by paralysis of the insect's CNS.

Cardiovascular System. Both cardioaccelerator and cardioinhibitor nerves are activated by small amounts of nicotine due to stimulation of all autonomic ganglia. Since the cardioinhibitor nerve (vagus) is predominant, the response to a small dose, or the initial response to a large dose, of nicotine is a decreased pulse rate. Due to paralysis of all autonomic ganglia, the heart rate returns toward normal after a large dose has taken full effect, and a relative tachycardia may result. Similarly, small doses of nicotine can cause a pressor response, due to stimulation of the predominating sympathetic ganglia, which furnish postganglionic vasoconstrictor fibers to the arterioles. Peripheral vasodilation, however, results after large doses, due to ganglionic block.

Gastrointestinal. Nicotine activates the smooth muscles and secretory glands of the digestive tract with the following clinical signs: excessive salivation, increased gastric secretion, vomition, increased peristalsis, and defecation.

Skeletal Muscle. Nicotine initially stimulates nicotinic receptors of the motor endplate and in large doses produces a depolarizing muscle paralysis. This effect has been used in attempts to immobilize wild animals for capture.

Acute Nicotine Poisoning. Accidental ingestion of the 40% solution of nicotine sulfate (Blackleaf 40) results in acute toxicosis characterized by excitement, hyperpnea, salivation, pulse rate irregularities, diarrhea, and emesis in those species that vomit. After this transient stimulatory phase, a depressed state occurs and is characterized by uncoordination, tachycardia, dyspnea, coma, and death from respiratory paralysis.

Synthetic Ganglionic Blocking Agents

As mentioned, nicotine is not used clinically in animals or human beings as a ganglion blocker since it activates nicotinic sites before blockage occurs and since it affects functions of various tissues throughout the body. However, several drugs have been discovered that preferentially block autonomic ganglia by a nondepolarizing (competitive) mechanism. These drugs are bis-quaternary compounds [i.e.,$(CH_3)_3\overset{+}{N}(CH_2)_n\overset{+}{N}(CH_3)_3$]; in those cases where the methonium groups are separated by 5 or 6 methylene groups (i.e., $n = 5$ or 6), a very selective site of action at autonomic ganglia is obtained. These compounds interact with the nicotinic receptors of the ganglion cells and thereby block impulse transmission across the ganglionic synapse. Dissimilar to nicotine, they do not cause initial depolarization (Paton and Perry 1953). Members of this group of ganglionic blocking agents include hexamethonium ($n = 6$; C–6), pentamethonium ($n = 5$; C–5), chlorisondamine, pentolinium, trimethidinium, and azamethonium. In addition, there are several other ganglionic blocking drugs that are not bis-quaternary compounds, such as tetraethylammonium ions, mecamylamine, and pempidine.

Pharmacologic Effects and Uses

Due to the blockade of impulse transmission at the ganglia, effects of ganglionic blocking agents are manifested on effector organs that are innervated by the postganglionic fibers of the sympathetic or parasympathetic nervous system. The overall effects of these agents on various functions are dependent upon the predominance of sympathetic or parasympathetic tone in a particular structure, as indicated in Table 8.4. For example, since the gastrointestinal system functions predominately under parasympathetic tone, ganglionic blockade will result in a relative parasympatholytic effect; decreased motility and secretions and constipation result. Similarly, since heart rate is under dominant vagal tone, a relative tachycardia may result. However, since tone of peripheral blood vessels is dominated by sympathetic impulses, vasodilation and hypotension occur after ganglionic block. Similarly, the output of catecholamines by the adrenal medulla is also reduced. Severe postural hypotension and even syncope may result. The hypotensive effect has occasionally been utilized in surgery involving highly vascular areas in order to decrease the chance of hemorrhage; however, ganglionic blocking agents have achieved no significant purpose in clinical veterinary medicine.

TABLE 8.4. Usual predominance of sympathetic or parasympathetic tone in various tissues and consequent effects of autonomic ganglionic blockade

Structures	Predominant Tone	Effects of Ganglionic Blockade
Cardiovascular		Overall depression; block reflexogenic changes
Arterioles	Sympathetic	Vasodilatation; increased peripheral blood flow; hypotension
Veins	Sympathetic	Vasodilatation; pooling of blood; decreased venous return
Heart	Parasympathetic	Tachycardia
Gastrointestinal	Parasympathetic	Decreased tone and motility; constipation
Eye		
Iris	Parasympathetic	Mydriasis
Ciliary muscle	Parasympathetic	Cycloplegia
Urinary bladder	Parasympathetic	Urinary retention
Salivary glands	Parasympathetic	Dry mouth
Sweat glands	Sympathetic	Anhidrosis

Source: Modified from Volle and Koelle 1970.

REFERENCES

Aeschlimann, J. A., and Reinert, M. 1931. Pharmacological action of some analogues of physostigmine. J Pharmacol Exp Ther 43:413.

Amadon, R. S. 1930. An experimental study of drugs stimulating the motility of the ruminant stomach. J Am Vet Med Assoc 76:65.

Ashford, A.; Penn, G. B.; and Ross, J. W. 1962. Cholinergic activity of atropine. Nature 193:1082.

Averill, K. H., and Lamb, L. E. 1959. Less commonly recognized actions of atropine on cardiac rhythm. Am J Med Sci 237:304.

Barlow, R. B. 1964. Introduction to Chemical Pharmacology, 2nd ed. London: Methuen.

———. 1968. Introduction to Chemical Pharmacology, 2nd ed. London: Methuen; New York: John Wiley & Sons.

Clark, R. 1950. A review of present knowledge of factors and drugs influencing ruminal motility. J S Afr Vet Med Assoc 21:49.

Dale, H. H. 1914. The actions of certain esters and ethers of choline and their relation to muscarine. J Pharmacol Exp Ther 6:147.

De Candole, C. A., and McPhail, M. K. 1957. Sarin and paraoxon antagonism in different species. Can J Biochem Physiol 35: 1071.

Dougherty, R. W. 1942. A study of drugs affecting the motility of the bovine rumen. Cornell Vet 32:269.

Duncan, D. L. 1954. Responses of the gastric musculature of the sheep to some humoral agents and related substances. J Physiol (Lond) 125:475.

Dussardier, M. 1954. Action *in vivo* de l'acétylcholine et de l'adrénaline sur la motricite gastrique des ruminants. J Physiol (Paris) 46:777.

Dussardier, M., and Navarro, J. 1953. Étude *in vitro* des actions motrices exercées par l'adrenaline et l'acetylcholine sur les estomacs des bovidés. J Physiol (Paris) 4:569.

Eccles, R. M., and Libet, B. 1961. Origin and blockade of the synaptic responses of curarized sympathetic ganglia. J Physiol (Lond) 157:484.

Eldefrawi, M. E. 1974. Neuromuscular transmission: The transmitter-receptor combination. In J. I. Hubbard, ed. The Peripheral Nervous System, p. 181. New York: Plenum Press.

Fatal accidents from "Doryl" (carbachol). 1943. Report: Current comment. J Amer Med Assoc 123:1051.

Hall, L. W., and Walker, R. G. 1962. Suspected myasthenia gravis in a dog. Vet Rec 74:501.

Hines, J. A.; Edds, G. I.; Kirkham, W. W.; and Neal, F. C. 1967. Potentiation of succinylcholine by organophosphate compounds in horses. J Am Vet Med Assoc 151:54.

Hunt, R., and Taveau, R. 1906. On the physiological action of certain choline derivatives and new methods for detecting choline. Br Med J 2:1788.

Ing, H. R.; Kordik, P.; and Williams, D. P. H. T. 1952. Studies on the structure-action relationships of the choline group. Br J Pharmacol 7:103.

Khromov-Borisov, N. V., and Michelson, M. J. 1966. The mutual disposition of cholinoreceptors of locomotor muscles and the changes in their disposition in the course of evolution. Pharmacol Rev 18:1051.

Koelle, G. B. 1970. Anticholinesterase agents. In L. S. Goodman and A. Gilman, eds. The Pharmacological Basis of Therapeutics, 4th ed. New York: Macmillan.

Libet, B. 1970. Generation of slow inhibitory and excitatory postsynaptic potentials. Fed Proc 29:1945.

Michelson, M. J. 1973. Structures and mutual disposition of cholinoceptors and changes in their disposition in the course of evolution. In Comparative Pharmacology, p. 357. Elmsford, N.Y.: Pergamon Press.

Nishi, S. 1974. Ganglionic transmisison. In J. I. Hubbard, ed. The Peripheral Nervous System, p. 225. New York: Plenum Press.

Pullman, B., and Pullman, A. 1963. Quantum Biochemistry. New York: Interscience.

Quin, J. I., and Clark, R. 1946. Parasympathetic control of body function and its role in veterinary practice. J S Afr Vet Med Assoc 17:140.

Quin, J. I., and Van Der Wath, J. G. 1938. Studies on the alimentary tract of the Merino sheep in South Africa. V. The motility of the rumen under various conditions. Onderstepoort J Vet Res Anim Ind 11:361.

Rand, M. J., and Stafford, A. 1967. Cardiovascular effects of choline esters. In W. S. Root and F. G. Hofman, eds. Physiological Pharmacology. Vol. 3, The Nervous System. Part C: Autonomic Nervous System Drugs, p. 1. New York: Academic Press.

Riker, W. F., Jr., and Wescoe, W. C. 1946. The direct action of prostigmine on skeletal muscle: Its relationship to the choline esters. J Pharmacol Exp Ther 88:58.

Sprecher, D. J.; Leman, A. D.; and Carlisle, S. 1975. Effects of parasympathomimetics on porcine stillbirth. Am J Vet Res 36:1331.

Stowe, C. M. 1965. Cholinergic (parasympathomimetic) drugs. In L. M. Jones, ed. Veterinary Pharmacology and Therapeutics,

3rd ed., p. 313. Ames: Iowa State Univ. Press.

Takagi, K.; Takayanagi, I.; and Maezima, Y. 1968. An analysis of the sites of action of some partial agonists. Eur J Pharmacol 3:52.

Takeshige, C.; Pappano, A. J.; DeCroat, W. C.; and Volle, R. L. 1963. Ganglionic blockade produced in sympathetic ganglia by cholinomimetic drugs. J Pharmacol Exp Ther 141:333.

Volle, R. L. 1962. The actions of several ganglion blocking agents on the postganglionic discharge induced by diisopropyl phosphorofuridate (DFP) in sympathetic ganglia. J Pharmacol Exp Ther 135:45.

———. 1971. Cholinomimetic drugs. In J. R. DiPalma, ed. Drill's Pharmacology in Medicine, 4th ed., p. 584. New York: McGraw-Hill.

Volle, R. L., and Koelle, G. B. 1961. The physiological role of acetylcholinesterase (AChE) in sympathetic ganglia. J Pharmacol Exp Ther 133:223.

———. 1970. Ganglionic stimulating and blocking agents. In L. S. Goodman and A. Gilman, eds. The Pharmacological Basis of Therapeutics, 4th ed., p. 585. New York: Macmillan.

Wills, J. H. 1963. Pharmacological antagonists of the anticholinesterase agents. In G. B. Koelle, ed. Handbuch der Experimentellen Pharmakologie. Suppl. 15, Cholinesterases and Anticholinesterase Agents, p. 883. Berlin: Springer-Verlag.

———. 1970. Toxicity of anticholinesterases and treatment of poisoning. In A. G. Karczmar, ed. Anticholinesterase Agents. Oxford, Eng.: Pergamon Press.

Wilson, I. B. 1954. The mechanism of enzyme hydrolysis studied with acetylcholinesterase. In W. D. McElroy and B. Glass, eds. Symposium on the Mechanism of Enzyme Action, p. 642. Baltimore: John Hopkins Press.

———. 1958. A specific antidote for nerve gas and insecticide (alkylphosphate) intoxication. Neurology 8:41.

Wilson, I. B.; Hatch, M. A.; and Ginsburg, S. 1960. Carbamylation of acetylcholinesterase. J Biol Chem 235:2312.

CHAPTER 9

NEUROMUSCULAR BLOCKING AGENTS

H. RICHARD ADAMS

Numerous drugs have been identified that inhibit the transmission of nerve impulses at the somatic neuromuscular junction. The neuromuscular blocking agents used clinically act primarily by interfering with the effectiveness of acetylcholine (the endogenous neurotransmitter) to activate the nicotinic cholinergic receptors of skeletal muscle cells. Based on mechanism of action, neuromuscular blocking drugs are categorized as either competitive or depolarizing agents. The *competitive* (nondepolarizing) neuromuscular blocking agents combine with the receptors and render them inaccessible to acetylcholine. *Depolarizing* neuromuscular blocking drugs interact with and depolarize the receptor areas, causing a lack of responsiveness to acetylcholine. The end results of the nondepolarizing and the depolarizing agents are skeletal muscle paralysis and profound muscular relaxation. Neuromuscular blocking agents are most often used as adjuvants to anesthesia to facilitate tracheal intubation, abdominal muscle relaxation, and orthopedic manipulations, and as part of balanced anesthesia procedures to reduce the amount of general anesthetic required.

DEVELOPMENT

The development of neuromuscular blocking drugs originated with the discovery of curare, a tarlike mixture of plant material used as a poison by South American Indians. The actual ingredients of the arrow, blowgun dart, and spear poison were known only to the local "pharmacist," who was often the tribal medicine man or witch doctor. Thus the botanical preparations obtained by explorers could not be identified as to content, so they were simply classified according to the containers in which they were packaged. Tubo-, para-, or bamboo-curare was contained in cutoff bamboo tubes; this mixture was usually obtained from southern Amazon tribes. The plant origin of tube-curare preparations was primarily Menispermaceae *(Chondodendron tomentosum).* Calabash-curare was packaged in hollow gourds or calabashes; it was the most active curare preparation. Pot-curare came in small earthenware pottery from the central part of the Amazon basin; often this concoction contained plants other than Menispermaceae. The most important constituent isolated from curare is *d*-tubocurarine. Complete discussions of the colorful and interesting history of curare were recently presented by McIntyre (1972) and by Waser (1972).

Original studies in the nineteenth century by Claude Bernard (1856) demonstrated that curare prevented the muscle contraction elicited by stimulation of the motor nerve. It did not, however, affect the CNS, prevent the response to direct stimulation of the muscle, or depress axonal conductance. It was proposed that curare acted at the nerve-muscle junction. Hundreds of reports since then have substantiated, clarified, and extended the observations concerning the neuromuscular blocking properties of the curare alkaloids. Further, early results stimulated active research into the chemical structural requirements of curarelike compounds leading to the discovery of other types of neuromuscular blocking agents.

CHEMISTRY AND STRUCTURE-ACTIVITY RELATIONSHIPS

Neuromuscular blocking agents possess chemical structural groups that allow interaction of the agent with the nicotinic cholinergic receptor. However, these drugs cause distinctly different effects from the endogenous mediator, acetylcholine. One group of neuromuscular blocking drugs is called *competitive* agents and occupies the receptor so that acetylcholine cannot act. The other group, *depolarizing* agents, acts in a more complicated manner and initially causes depolarization before blockage occurs.

Although extensive investigations into the molecular mechanisms of neuromuscular blocking agents have been carried out by many researchers, structural requirements for such activities remain somewhat equivocal. This is due in part to the dissimilar and, in some cases, similar mechanisms of the competitive and the depolarizing agents. Some neuromuscular blocking drugs were found to cause one type of block in one species and yet another type in a second species. In some cases, agents were encountered that acted dissimilarly in different muscles within the same species.

Furthermore, recent proposals question the previously accepted formula of a well-characterized and prototypical neuromuscular blocking agent, *d*-tubocurarine. Until recently, *d*-tubocurarine was believed to contain two quaternary ammonium groups, moieties considered to be important for the potency of this agent. However, Everett et al. (1970) have reported that *d*-tubocurarine actually has one quaternary nitrogen and one tertiary nitrogen group. Based on this change, the drug previously recognized as dimethyltubocurarine (and referred to as such in the following discussion) may be reclassified as trimethyltubocurarine (Pauling and Petcher 1973).

Although some problems remain to be resolved, some broad-based assumptions can be made in reference to structure-activity relationships. In general, at least one quaternary nitrogen group is required for potent blocking effects. Although some compounds that contain tertiary nitrogen groups have been shown to have blocking properties, these agents are relatively unimportant.

Based on general chemical structural characteristics, Bovet (1951) placed neuromuscular blocking agents into two large categories. One group is characterized by large, bulky, and nonflexible molecules; these agents are called *pachycurares.* Members of this group include *d*-tubocurarine, dimethyl (or trimethyl) tubocurarine, gallamine, and pancuronium. All these agents were found to produce a competitive (nondepolarizing) block. The other group, termed *leptocurares,* is characterized by long, slender, and flexible molecules. Decamethonium and succinylcholine are in this group; these agents cause a depolarizing block. The dichotomy in basic structural arrangement of the competitive and depolarizing agents has been offered as a partial explanation for the dissimilar effects evoked by interaction of these agents with the nicotinic cholinergic receptor.

The proposed arrangement of the cholinergic receptor was shown in Chapter 8. Among other requirements, adjacent receptors are believed to contain anionic (negatively charged) binding sites separated by set distances. These negative sites are essential for electrostatic bonding to the receptors of the cationic (positively charged) nitrogen moiety of acetylcholine and exogenous chemicals. Upon depolarization by acetylcholine or other depolarizing agents, it has been suggested that the distance between negative binding sites of receptors may change. This change in distance may, in fact, be a prerequisite to the depolarization. Based on this assumption, differences can be considered between the mechanism of receptor interaction of depolarizing and nondepolarizing neuromuscular blocking agents.

In relation to the depolarizing agents, Barlow and Ing (1948) and Paton and Zaimis (1949) examined a series of compounds with different length polymethylene chains and with a quaternary nitrogen group on each end, i.e., $(CH_3)_3N^+(CH_2)_nN^+(CH_3)_3$. They found maximum blocking properties when $n = 10$. This drug, decamethonium, was also more active than its monoquaternary analog, $(CH_3)_3N^+(CH_2)_9CH_3$. Due to the marked influence the length of the carbon chain had on potency, the distance between the quaternary nitrogen groups was considered critical in relation to interaction with the negative sites of the receptors.

The distance between the two quaternary nitrogen atoms in the fully extended antiplanar configuration of the decamethonium molecule is approximately 14 angstroms. Recently, however, it was suggested that when the drug is actually in solution and, presumably, in the biophase, this distance is somewhat less: 9.5–10.64 angstroms (Pauling and Petcher 1973). Depending upon preparation, the N^+-N^+ distance in succinylcholine is also reported as being approximately 10 angstroms: 7.84–11.88. In relation to the nonflexible structure of the competitive agents, the N^+-N^+ distance has also been reported to be approximately 10 angstroms (Pauling and Petcher 1973). Therefore, it seems likely that both the competitive and the depolarizing agents interact with the same anionic sites of the receptors because of similar N^+-N^+ distances and related net effects. As mentioned, it has been proposed that depolarization is preceded by or in some way brought about by some conformational change in the receptors. Pauling and Petcher (1973) proposed that with depolarization, the distance between the anionic sites of receptors decreases from the resting state value of 10.8 angstroms to 8.0–9.0 angstroms. The flexible nature of the molecular structure of the depolarizing agents would not hinder such conformational changes, and depolarization could initially occur. On the other hand, due to their molecular rigidity, the true curare agents would prevent conformational changes in the receptor and, thereby, block depolarization.

This explanation does not clarify other aspects, however. For example, a second optimal N^+-N^+ distance of about 20 angstroms was found in a series of experimental neuromuscular blocking agents. Further, many researchers believe the N^+-N^+ distance of conventional agents (e.g., decamethonium) to be about 14 angstroms. Based on the two optimal N^+-N^+ distances of 14 and 20 angstroms, Khromov-Borisov and Michelson (1966) believe that receptors are arranged in symmetrical groups of four, a tetrameric arrangement. In their model, the esterophilic portion of each receptor is located centrally, whereas each anionic binding site is located at a corner of the tetramer. The distance between the anionic sites of longitudinally adjacent receptors is 14 angstroms, and the distance between the negative sites of diagonal receptors is 20 angstroms. These distances can explain the occurrence of two optimal N^+-N^+ distances in neuromuscular blocking agents.

The negative sites of the receptors are thought to be closely associated with pores (or other transport mechanisms) of the cell membrane. Occupation of negative binding sites by acetylcholine and thus neutralization of their charge could disrupt the pores or surrounding membrane. This, in turn, would then permit influx of Na^+ and efflux of K^+ along their respective concentration gradients, resulting in depolarization of the membrane. Occupation of these sites by the molecularly rigid competitive agents can be envisioned as causing a stabilization of the receptors so that the membrane pores are not easily affected. The depolarizing agents, on the other hand, initially act similarly to acetylcholine. Due to their flexible structure, they allow changes in membrane configuration, but for some reason cause a persistent short-circuiting of the membrane so that additional changes in electrical potential are not achieved. It has also been proposed that acetylcholinesterase is actually the cholinergic receptor, but this idea has not been readily accepted (Wurzel 1967).

The fact remains that until the receptor is adequately isolated so that detailed and systematic examination can be made, proposals as to receptor configurations remain somewhat speculative. De Robertis (1971) and Miledi et al. (1971) have isolated lipoproteins from the electric eel and electric ray, respectively, that have the properties of cholinoceptors. Both substances were arranged or aggregated into tetramers, which seems to support previous chemicopharmacologic studies of Khromov-Borisov and Michelson (1966).

The chemical structures of several commonly used neuromuscular blocking agents are shown in Fig. 9.1 to demonstrate basic structural differences of the competitive and the depolarizing types.

IMPULSE TRANSMISSION AT THE SOMATIC NEUROMUSCULAR JUNCTION

Prior to discussing neuromuscular blocking agents, impulse transmission at the somatic neuromuscular junction will be reviewed in relation to sites of action of different drugs. General concepts of cholinergic transmission were mentioned in Chapter 6. Detailed examination of prac-

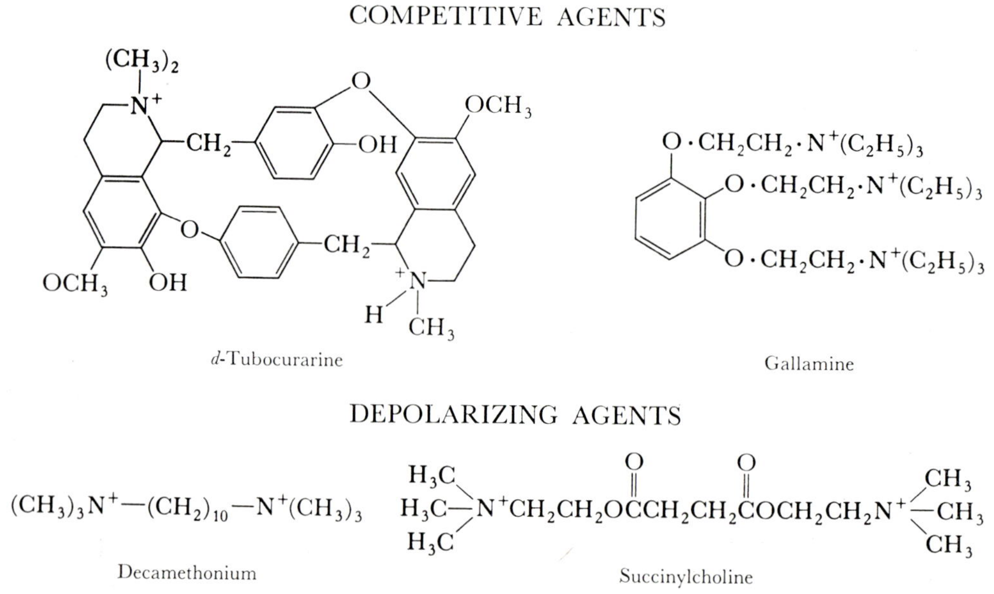

COMPETITIVE AGENTS

d-Tubocurarine

Gallamine

DEPOLARIZING AGENTS

$$(CH_3)_3N^+{-}(CH_2)_{10}{-}N^+(CH_3)_3$$

Decamethonium

$$(H_3C)_3N^+CH_2CH_2O\overset{O}{\overset{\|}{C}}CH_2CH_2\overset{O}{\overset{\|}{C}}OCH_2CH_2N^+(CH_3)_3$$

Succinylcholine

FIG. 9.1. Chemical structures of some commonly used neuromuscular blocking agents.

tical and theoretical aspects of neuromuscular anatomy, physiology, and pharmacology were recently reviewed in a two-volume text (Cheymol 1972). The interested reader is referred to this material for additional information.

Physiologic and Anatomic Considerations

The majority of investigations aimed at identifying cholinergic transmission mechanisms have utilized the somatic myoneural junction due to its accessibility in relation to other cholinergic synapses. Although the term "synapse" was originally proposed to describe a nerve-nerve junction, it is commonly used in reference to neuroeffector junctions. A representation of a somatic neuromuscular junction ("synapse") and proposed sites of drug actions are shown in Fig. 9.2.

The terminal branches of a motor axon lose their myelin sheath and embed within invaginations of the cell membrane of the skeletal muscle cell; these invaginations are termed *synaptic gutters.* A synaptic gutter, in turn, has many microinvaginations or infoldings that are called either "junctional folds" or "subneural folds." The space within the synaptic gutter between the nerve ending and the muscle cell is called the "synaptic cleft."

"Presynaptic" refers to axonal elements, whereas "postsynaptic" refers to constituents of the muscle cell. The subsynaptic membrane represents that portion of the muscle cell membrane (sarcolemma) that is imediately adjacent to the axonal

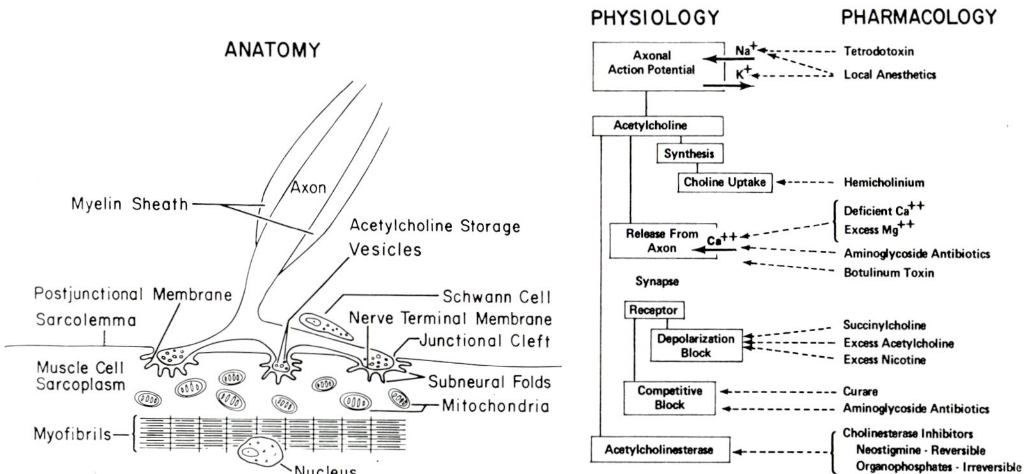

Fig. 9.2. Schematic representation of a somatic neuromuscular junction ("synapse"), related physiologic pathways, and proposed sites of action of various pharmacologic agents. An axonal action potential (AP) is characterized by an influx of Na^+ and an efflux of K^+. Tetrodotoxin and saxitoxin inactivate Na^+ pathways. Local anesthetics block Na^+ and K^+ pathways. Choline uptake into the neuron is blocked by hemicholinium; synthesis of acetylcholine (ACh) is prevented. As the AP arrives at the nerve terminal, it instigates inward movement of Ca^{++}; this triggers discharge of ACh into the junctional cleft. A lack of Ca^{++} or an excess of Mg^{++} decreases the release of ACh. Aminoglycoside antibiotics also interfere with Ca^{++}-dependent release of ACh. Botulinum toxin inhibits ACh release. Decamethonium and succinylcholine (depolarizing neuromuscular blocking agents) cause persistent depolarization block of the motor end-plate region, as do excess ACh and nicotine. Curare, gallamine, and pancuronium (competitive neuromuscular blocking agents) compete with ACh for postjunctional receptors but do not cause depolarization. Aminoglycoside antibiotics decrease the sensitivity of the postjunctional membrane to ACh. Catabolism of ACh by acetylcholinesterase is inhibited by reversible and irreversible anticholinesterase agents; ACh accumulates. (Modified from Koelle 1970 and Couteaux 1972)

terminal. The term "postsynaptic membrane" is often used synonymously; this term has also been used to designate sarcolemma adjacent to the subsynaptic membrane.

Vesicular structures localized within cholinergic nerve terminals represent storage sites for acetylcholine (see Chapter 6). As an axonal action potential arrives at the nerve terminal, it increases the release of acetylcholine from the storage vesicles into the synaptic cleft. This step (excitation-secretion coupling) is dependent upon mobilization into the neuron of extracellular Ca^{++} and/or Ca^{++} that is bound to superficial membrane areas of the nerve terminal. Released acetylcholine reacts with specialized receptor sites of the subsynaptic membrane and causes depolarization of this structure. Cholinergic receptors of somatic myoneural junctions are classified as nicotinic; they are located on the outer membrane of the muscle cell and are almost exclusively confined to the postsynaptic membrane. After denervation, sensitivity to acetylcholine spreads over the entire muscle cell.

Extraneuronal acetylcholine is rapidly metabolized by acetylcholinesterase enzyme. Acetylcholinesterase is localized in the end-plate region. Although it may be bound in part to presynaptic elements, it is concentrated at the postsynaptic membrane.

Acetylcholine-induced depolarization of the subsynaptic membrane can be measured as a change in the electrical potential of the motor end-plate region, i.e., the *end-plate potential.* If the end-plate potential is above a threshold level, it instigates a *muscle action potential,* leading to depolarization of immediately adjacent areas of the postsynaptic membrane. Subsequently, the muscle action potential is propagated along the remainder of the muscle cell membrane. Contraction of skeletal muscle is initiated by the muscle action potential causing a release of Ca^{++} into the cytoplasm from the intracellularly located sarcoplasmic reticulum. The increased free intracellular Ca^{++} binds with troponin, a protein constituent of tropomyosin that acts to inhibit sliding of the actin and myosin filaments during the resting state. Ca^{++}-bound troponin loses this function; cross-linkages are formed between actin and myosin, and sliding of these filaments occurs. The muscle contracts. *Miniature end-plate potentials* represent subthreshold depolarizations of the motor end-plate region that are due to spontaneous neuronal release of small amounts of acetylcholine; they do not instigate muscle contraction.

Pharmacologic Considerations

The neuromuscular junction is quite susceptible to alteration by selective pharmacologic agents. Various drugs, toxins, electrolytes, and other agents alter in different manners the synthesis, storage, release, receptor interactions, and catabolism of neurohumoral transmitter substances. Several important factors affecting cholinergic transmission are outlined in Fig. 9.2.

For example, hemicholinium and triethylcholine compete with choline for choline uptake into cholinergic neurons; acetylcholine synthesis is prevented due to lack of choline. Existing vesicular stores of acetylcholine are exhausted upon nerve stimulation and a gradual weakening and eventual paralysis result.

Nerve conduction is affected by only a few substances. The local anesthetics, when in high concentration and in immediate contact with the axon, act to stabilize the nerve by inactivating both Na^+ and K^+ channels so that axonal action potential propagation is halted. The pufferfish poison, tetrodotoxin, and the shellfish poison, saxitoxin, decrease the permeability of excitable membranes to Na^+ (but not K^+); thus axonal action potentials are not generated and paralysis results. These toxins do not cause an initial depolarization of nerves, they act noncompetitively, they are approximately 100,000 times more potent than cocaine or procaine, and they are frequently used in research. Clinical cases of fatal food poisoning have been attributed to ingestion of these substances.

Botulinum toxin is an extremely potent substance (lethal dose for a mouse is 4×10^7 molecules) produced by *Clostridium botulinum.* It is occasionally ingested by human beings and lower animals and is often fatal. It decreases the amount of acetylcholine released from cholinergic nerves; the molecular basis of this effect is poorly understood.

Magnesium ions (Mg^{++}) interfere with the release of acetylcholine from the nerve terminal by competing for the transport mechanisms responsible for mobilization of Ca^{++} into the nerve. Mg^{++} uncouples the excitation-secretion coupling process. An insufficient concentration of Ca^{++} produces similar effects. Mg^{++} also acts postsynaptically to decrease the effectiveness of acetylcholine to activate receptors.

Aminoglycoside antibiotics (i.e., neomycin-streptomycin group) inhibit the release of acetylcholine from motor nerves, purportedly by decreasing the availability of Ca^{++} at superficial membrane binding sites of the axonal terminal and, thereby, inhibiting the excitation-secretion coupling process (Pittinger and Adamson 1972). In addition, these antibiotics reduce the sensitivity of the postsynaptic membrane to acetylcholine.

Cholinesterase inhibitors (see Chapter 8) decrease the hydrolytic activity of acetylcholinesterase and pseudocholinesterase; acetylcholine rapidly accumulates at receptor sites. Muscle fasciculations, spasms, convulsions, and eventually apnea occur after overdosage with cholinesterase inhibitors.

POSTJUNCTIONAL MECHANISMS OF NEUROMUSCULAR BLOCKADE

The preceding examples illustrate the complexity of neuromuscular transmission and the multitude of sites susceptible to many agents and toxins. However, the pharmacologic effects of all clinically useful neuromuscular blocking drugs can best be explained by a direct alteration of the effectiveness of acetylcholine to activate postjunctional (postsynaptic) receptors. According to the mechanisms of postjunctional action, neuromuscular blocking agents are classified as either a competitive (nondepolarizing) or a depolarizing agent.

Competitive or Nondepolarizing Agents

These drugs compete with acetylcholine for available cholinergic receptors at the postsynaptic membrane and, by occupying these receptors, prevent the transmitter function of acetylcholine. A prototype of this group of drugs is *d*-tubocurarine *(Tubocurarine Chloride,* U.S.P.; Tubarine). Other similarly acting agents include dimethyl-tubocurarine *(Dimethyl Tubocurarine Iodide,* N.F.; Metubine), gallamine *(Gallamine Triethiodide,* U.S.P.; Flaxedil), and pancuronium (Pancuronium Bromide; Pavulon).

Ultrarefined experimental techniques, e.g., measurement of single-cell electrical activity and microiontophoretic application of drugs, have verified the primary site of action of the competitive blocking agents as the subsynaptic membrane (Katz 1966; Riker and Okamoto 1969; Bowen 1972; Hubbard and Quastel 1973). At this region, *d*-tubocurarine is believed to have the same or similar affinity as acetylcholine for cholinergic receptors, i.e., *d*-tubocurarine can interact with these sites as well as can acetylcholine. However, *d*-tubocurarine does not exhibit agonistic properties at these sites, whereas acetylcholine, of course, is extremely active. Although *d*-tubocurarine binds to or in some way interlocks with the cholinoceptors, it has no depolarizing activity and, therefore, does not cause an end-plate potential. Moreover, the *d*-tubocurarine-receptor interaction renders affected receptors unavailable for interaction with acetylcholine. Acetylcholine-induced end-plate potentials are reduced to subthreshold levels or abolished in curarized muscles. In the absence of acetylcholine-induced end-plate potentials and subsequent muscle action potentials, the muscle relaxes and is, in fact, paralyzed.

The lack of depolarizing action of *d*-tubocurarine and related agents has led to the use of the term "nondepolarizing" as a synonym for "competitive" in relation to neuromuscular blocking agents. The effect of curarelike agents has also been described as a "stabilization" of the postsynaptic membrane since the depolarizing activity of other drugs is inhibited.

The competitive mechanism of the nondepolarizing agents is readily demonstrable. In essence, *d*-tubocurarine blockade of receptors increases the threshold of the end-plate region to acetylcholine. Increasing the concentration of acetylcholine will overcome the blockade produced by *d*-tubocurarine and restore neuromuscular transmission. Correspondingly, reincreasing the concentration of *d*-tubocurarine will again decrease the effectiveness of acetylcholine. Other drugs that depolarize the nicotinic cholinergic receptors also antagonize in various degrees the curare effect.

Based on the competitive interaction between the nondepolarizing agents and acetylcholine, cholinesterase inhibitors were found to be effective in antagonizing the effects of these blocking agents. Cholinesterase inhibitors prevent the enzymatic catabolism of acetylcholine. More acetylcholine is available for interaction with cholinoceptors and, thereby, decreases the effectiveness of the competitive blocking agents. This relationship has been exploited clinically in successful efforts to terminate the effects of the nondepolarizing agents. However, the cholinesterase inhibitors do not antagonize the effects of the other class of neuromuscular blockers, the depolarizing drugs.

Depolarizing Neuromuscular Blocking Agents

Succinylcholine (*Succinylcholine Chloride,* U.S.P.; Diacetylcholine Chloride; Anectine; Sucostrin; Suxamethonium) and decamethonium (Syncupine; C-10) are important members of this group of agents. These drugs exert their skeletal muscle paralyzing effects by interfering with acetylcholine-mediated depolarization of the postsynaptic membrane. In contrast to the well-defined mechanism of the competitive agents, certain aspects of the mechanism(s) of depolarizing neuromuscular blockers are continually debated.

Succinylcholine and related drugs interact with the postsynaptic cholinergic receptors but cause distinctly different effects than the curarelike drugs. Initially, an end-plate potential and a corresponding muscle action potential are elicited upon exposure to succinylcholine (Burns and Paton 1951; Bovet and Bovet-Nitti 1955). These depolarization changes in membrane potential are similar to those produced by the endogenous mediator, acetylcholine. However, acetylcholine is immediately hydrolyzed by cholinesterase; the postsynaptic membrane repolarizes and is prepared for subsequent activation by additional quanta of acetylcholine. Succinylcholine, on the other hand, elicits a prolonged depolarization of the end-plate region that does not allow the subsynaptic membrane to completely repolarize and renders the motor end-plate nonresponsive to the normal action of acetylcholine.

Due to the initial depolarizing action, transient contraction of muscle cells occurs after the administration of succinylcholine and related agents. This is characterized *in vivo* as momentary asynchronous muscle twitches and fasciculations. Due to the persistent depolarization of the postsynaptic membrane, however, subsequent impulse transmissions are blocked and a flaccid type of paralysis ensues. The molecular mechanism(s) of the depolarizing neuromuscular blocking agents is not completely understood but may be biphasic.

PHASE I BLOCK

Depolarization of the motor end-plate region by acetylcholine is characterized by increased permeability of the subsynaptic membrane to Na^+ and K^+. As acetylcholine is catabolized by acetylcholinesterase, the selective permeability characteristics of the postsynaptic membrane are rapidly reestablished. Repolarization occurs. Succinylcholine, however, causes a persistent increase in the permeability of the postsynaptic membrane to Na^+ and K^+. After repeated intraarterial injection of succinylcholine for 1 hour in cats, Paton and Waud (1962) reported that depolarization of the gracilis and tibialis was approximately one-half of that recorded initially.

Although partial recovery from peak depolarization occurred, the end-plate remained depolarized in relation to normal resting membrane potential. Persistence of this state beyond a certain level tends to inactivate those Na^+ channels or transport mechanisms that are normally active in generation of an action potential. As a result, the subsynaptic membrane becomes nonresponsive to the depolarizing action of acetylcholine. The sarcolemmal membrane surrounding the motor end-plate region is similarly affected and also becomes inexcitable. Accordingly, acetylcholine cannot act as a transmitter and impulse transmission fails. It should be remembered that acetylcholine, when in excess, also causes persistent depolarization block of cholinergic synaptic junctions.

PHASE II BLOCK

Phase II block occurs in some instances after prolonged exposure to a depolarizing agent and is characterized by a change from the depolarizing block to one that in some ways resembles that caused by curare. The actual mechanisms involved are poorly understood and opinion is contradictory as to this transition. Zaimis (1959) believes, for example, that confusion has occurred because in some species some blocking agents have a "dual mechanism," i.e., they cause some effects that resemble depolarization block and cause other effects that resemble competitive blockade.

After exposure of isolated nerve-muscle preparations to succinylcholine, the initial peak level of depolarization subsides (Thesleff 1955, 1958). Subsequently, the end-plate becomes transiently sensitive to depolarizing agents. Gradually, a competitivelike blockade results that seems to be at least partially susceptible to reversal by cholinesterase inhibitors. Tachyphylaxis to depolarizing agents quickly develops and the receptors now appear to be insensitive to acetylcholine.

It must be emphasized, however, that the importance of Phase II has not been clearly defined for each depolarizing neuromuscular blocking agent. It is not known, for example, if Phase II represents a true conversion to curarization, or if it is dependent upon penetration of the blocking agent into the muscle cell, or if it represents a slow alteration of the receptors, which then become incapable of eliciting a change in ion permeability of the muscle cell membrane. In any event, development of Phase II block has been shown to be variably demonstrable, depending upon *in vitro* or *in vivo* nerve-muscle preparations, experimental conditions, species, and even different muscles in the same species.

Although dual mechanisms surely exist, the clinical applications of such complexities have not been clarified. It should be remembered that the majority of evidence indicates that as a group the depolarizing neuromuscular blocking agents act to cause depolarization of receptor areas of muscle fibers sometime during their course of action. Thus increasing the availability of acetylcholine by administration of a cholinesterase inhibitor has no effect or in some cases may actually intensify the neuromuscular block of a depolarizing agent. Just the opposite, cholinesterase inhibitors are usually quite effective in antagonizing the competitive block produced by the nondepolarizing curaremimetic agents.

PREJUNCTIONAL MECHANISMS

Recent investigations have presented evidence that neuromuscular blocking agents and some cholinesterase inhibitors have prejunctional (presynaptic) effects, i.e., under certain circumstances, these drugs alter the quantity of acetylcholine that is released from cholinergic nerves (Riker and Okamoto 1969). For example, Blaber (1973) reported that during high but not low rates of nerve stimulation, *d*-tubocurarine interfered with refilling of transmitter stores and, in this manner, decreased the quanta of acetylcholine discharged from the neuron. Just the opposite, some cholinesterase inhibitors have been shown to facilitate the discharge of acetylcholine from nerves.

In a brief report, Gergis et al. (1971)

indicated that *d*-tubocurarine, gallamine, succinylcholine, and decamethonium decreased acetylcholine output by as much as 90% from a frog nerve-muscle preparation. However, neuromuscular paralysis (i.e., decrease of muscle twitch) was not produced in their preparations by any of the agents except *d*-tubocurarine. Care should be taken in attempts to extrapolate results obtained from an atypical preparation (i.e., in relation to mammalian preparations) to those results that may be seen clinically in mammalian species.

Support for a significant presynaptic site of action of curare was obtained by Hubbard and Wilson (1973). They demonstrated that *d*-tubocurarine decreased quantal release of acetylcholine from the rat phrenic nerve–diaphragm preparation. Their studies suggest that the presynaptic and postsynaptic effects of *d*-tubocurarine develop at completely different time courses. In 1974 Galindo and Kennedy reported that succinylcholine and decamethonium caused a decreased release of acetylcholine during the initial (Phase I) neuromuscular block in *in vitro* rat phrenic nerve–diaphragm preparations. Characteristics of Phase II block were dissimilar and differed with each drug in their study. Also, they could not correlate changes in end-plate potential with the development of Phase I block.

Although presynaptic depressant effects of neuromuscular blocking agents seem likely, neither the physiologic nor pharmacologic significance has been clarified. Future studies of such aspects, however, should prove quite contributory to our understanding of basic neuromuscular mechanisms.

PHARMACOLOGIC EFFECTS OF NEUROMUSCULAR BLOCKING AGENTS

Skeletal Muscle

COMPETITIVE NEUROMUSCULAR BLOCKING AGENTS

The nondepolarizing curarelike drugs paralyze skeletal muscles due to neuromuscular blockade. As described above, these agents interact with nicotinic cholinergic receptors of skeletal muscle cells and render them inaccessible to the transmitter function of acetylcholine. Flaccid paralysis occurs. Neither axonal conductance nor the response to direct stimulation of the muscle is blocked by curare agents.

A schematic representation of an *in vivo* nerve-muscle preparation is shown in Fig. 9.3. This preparation, the sciatic nerve–gastrocnemius muscle preparation of anesthetized cats, is often used to examine actions and interactions of neuromuscular blocking agents (Adams and Mathew 1974). In this preparation, stimulation of the sciatic nerve causes contraction (kg of isometric tension) of the gastrocnemius muscle. Effects of direct stimulation of the muscle should be measured concurrently to ascertain that a new drug being tested does not directly affect the muscle fibers. The sciatic nerve can be bathed in a solution of the drug to examine for any effects on axonal conduction. Systemic blood pressure and respiratory movements can be measured concurrently.

Fig. 9.4 demonstrates the neuromuscular blocking effect of *d*-tubocurarine on indirectly stimulated muscle twitch of the sciatic nerve–gastrocnemius muscle preparation of a cat, as described in Fig. 9.3. In this example, muscle twitch quickly decreases after intravenous injection of *d*-tubocurarine, reaches peak depression within a few minutes, and then gradually returns to normal in approximately 15 minutes. Tubocurarine does not evoke an initial increase in muscle twitch; this lack of facilitation is a consistent finding with nondepolarizing agents. Gallamine, dimethyl-tubocurarine, and pancuronium produce similar characteristics of neuromuscular paralysis. Dimethyl tubocurarine is 3–10 times more active than *d*-tubocurarine, pancuronium is 5–7 times more potent than *d*-tubocurarine, whereas gallamine is somewhat less active.

Antagonism of the neuromuscular blocking effects of *d*-tubocurarine by administration of a cholinesterase inhibitor, neostigmine, is shown in Fig. 9.4. By com-

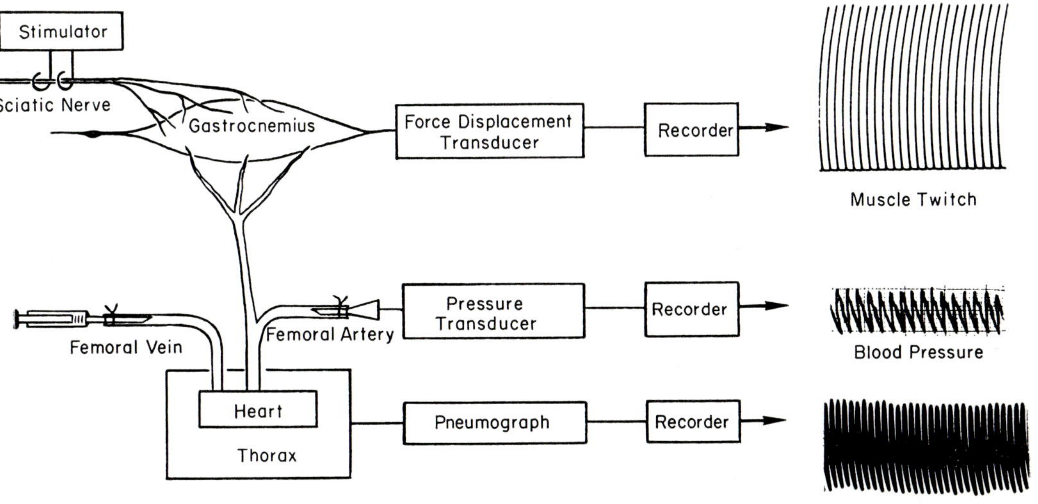

FIG. 9.3. Schematic representation of a sciatic nerve–gastrocnemius muscle preparation in an anesthetized cat. Stimulation of the isolated and decentralized sciatic nerve evokes contraction (muscle twitch) of the gastrocnemius muscle. Femoral arterial blood pressure and respiratory movements can be measured concurrently. Neuromuscular blocking drugs can be administered intravenously, and changes in muscle twitch height observed.

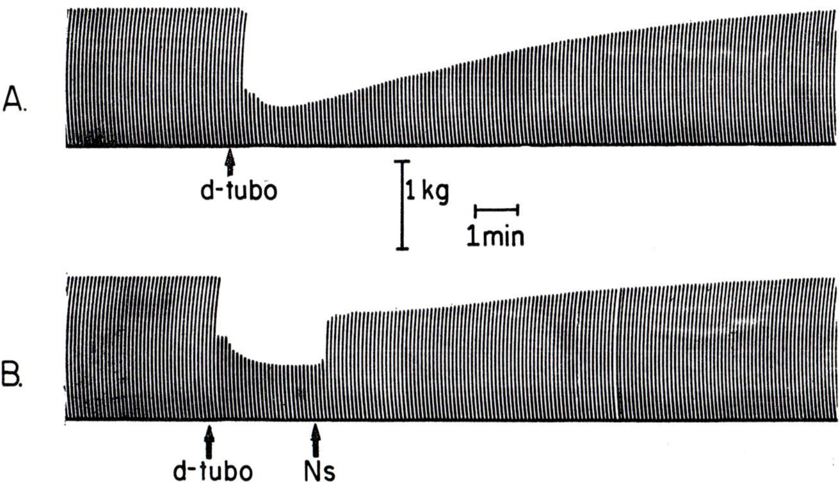

FIG. 9.4. Neuromuscular blocking effect of *d*-tubocurarine and reversal of the *d*-tubocurarine by neostigmine in a sciatic nerve–gastrocnemius muscle preparation of a cat. The cat was anesthetized with pentobarbital; muscle twitch was monitored as described in Fig. 9.3. *A*. Typical depression of muscle twitch by *d*-tubocurarine (*d*-tubo; 0.2 mg/kg) administered intravenously at designated arrow. *B*. Antagonism of *d*-tubo (0.2 mg/kg)-induced depression of muscle twitch by neostigmine (Ns; 0.1 mg/kg). Agents were administered intravenously at arrow. Notice rapid antagonism of the neuromuscular blocking effect of *d*-tubo by neostigmine. Compare this with the lack of antagonism by neostigmine of the muscle twitch depressant effect of succinylcholine in Fig. 9.5.

paring the two tracings in this figure, it is readily apparent that neostigmine markedly hastened recovery from the muscle twitch depression caused by *d*-tubocurarine. This antagonistic interaction probably depends on several factors. First, neostigmine is believed to have a direct acetylcholinelike action at the cholinergic receptors. Also, neostigmine has been reported to act presynaptically to cause an increased discharge of acetylcholine from the cholinergic fiber. However, although neostigmine may directly stimulate cholinergic receptors and also increase acetylcholine release, the interaction between this drug and *d*-tubocurarine is primarily attributed to the anticholinesterase activity of neostigmine. Inhibition of cholinesterase delays the catabolic breakdown of acetylcholine and allows its accumulation at receptor sites. Newly available acetylcholine, now in increased concentration at the postsynaptic membrane, effectively competes with *d*-tubocurarine for the cholinoceptors. Acetylcholine-mediated depolarization of the endplate, muscle action potentials, and muscle contraction are restored; muscle twitch quickly returns to normal.

DEPOLARIZING NEUROMUSCULAR BLOCKING AGENTS

Succinylcholine and decamethonium elicit transient muscle fasciculations prior to causing neuromuscular paralysis. This is due to initial depolarization of the motor end-plate and is characterized in the intact animal by asynchronous muscular contractions of the head, body trunk, and limbs. Fasciculation does not always occur in anesthetized animals.

The *in vivo* neuromuscular blocking effect of a small dose of succinylcholine in a cat nerve-muscle preparation is shown in Fig. 9.5. Initially, there is a slight and transient facilitory effect of succinylcholine on neuromuscular transmission; muscle twitch height momentarily increases by a small increment. This is due to the initial depolarizing effect of the drug. Subsequently, however, muscle twitch rapidly decreases and within 1 or 2 minutes the maximum depressant effect is obtained. Shortly thereafter, the neuromuscular effects of succinylcholine subside and muscle twitch returns to normal within an additional 5–8 minutes. The magnitude and duration of neuromuscular paralysis is de-

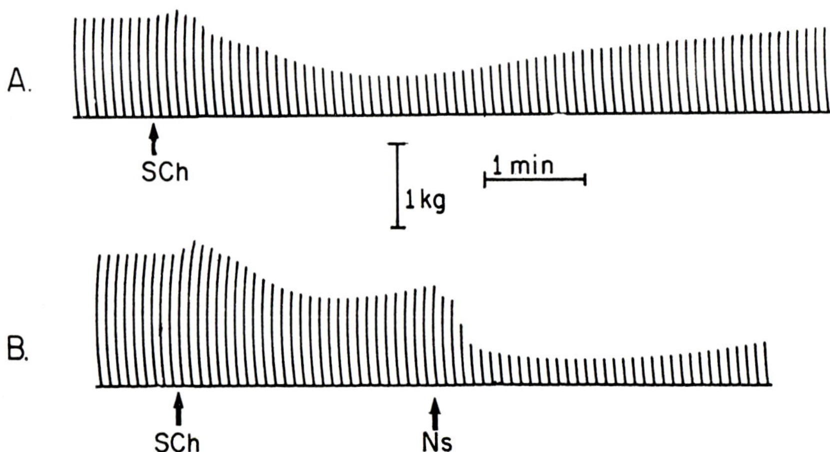

FIG. 9.5. Neuromuscular blocking effect of succinylcholine and augmentation of the effect of succinylcholine by neostigmine in a sciatic nerve–gastrocnemius muscle preparation of a cat. The cat was anesthetized with pentobarbital; muscle twitch was monitored as described in Fig. 9.3. *A*. Typical depression of muscle twitch by succinylcholine (SCh; 0.04 mg/kg) administered intravenously at designated arrow. *B*. Augmentation of the muscle twitch depressant effect of succinylcholine (0.04 mg/kg) by neostigmine (Ns; 0.1 mg/kg). Agents were administered intravenously at designated arrows. Notice augmentation of the degree and duration of effect of succinylcholine by neostigmine. Compare this with the antagonism by neostigmine of the neuromuscular blocking effect of *d*-tubocurarine in Fig. 9.4.

pendent upon the dosage of succinylcholine. The relatively short duration of succinylcholine activity is believed to be due to rapid biotransformation of this drug by plasma pseudocholinesterase. Decamethonium causes similar characteristics of neuromuscular blockade but the duration of action of this drug is considerably longer than that seen with succinylcholine. Decamethonium is not a suitable substrate for acetylcholinesterase or pseudocholinesterase.

The effects of a cholinesterase inhibitor, neostigmine, on the neuromuscular paralysis produced by succinylcholine are demonstrated in Fig. 9.5. By comparing the two tracings in this figure, it is apparent that neostigmine potentiated the muscle twitch depression evoked by succinylcholine and prolonged recovery from the effects of this agent. This synergistic interaction is primarily attributed to the anticholinesterase activity of neostigmine, resulting in decreased biotransformation of both succinylcholine and endogenous acetylcholine. Thus succinylcholine and acetylcholine are available at receptor sites for longer periods and the duration of depolarizing neuromuscular paralysis is prolonged. In addition, it seems likely that the direct depolarizing action of neostigmine at the cholinergic receptor may intensify succinylcholine-induced alterations of motor endplate potentials. Facilitation of presynaptic release of acetylcholine by neostigmine may contribute to the net effect.

The potency of the neuromuscular effects of succinylcholine varies in different species (Hansson 1958), as shown schematically in Fig. 9.6. Bovine and canine species are quite sensitive to succinylcholine, whereas horses and pigs are considerably less responsive. This difference is probably dependent upon species differences in the activity of pseudocholinesterase, the enzyme that biotransforms succinylcholine (Stowe 1955; Radeleff and Woodard 1956; Stowe et al. 1958; Palmer et al. 1965). Cattle and sheep, for example, have considerably less detectable pseudocholinesterase activity than horses and pigs. Administration of purified pseudocholinesterase preparation to dogs increases resistance to succinylcholine (Hall et al. 1953).

Autonomic Effects

Synaptic transmission at autonomic ganglia involves activation by acetylcholine of nicotinic receptors of the postganglionic nerve body (see Chapter 8). It is not surprising, therefore, that neuromuscular blocking agents (which act at somatic nicotinic sites) may also alter ganglionic transmission.

Tubocurarine is an excellent example of a drug selected for site of action at nicotinic receptors of the somatic myoneural junction that, as a side effect, also acts at ganglionic nicotinic receptors (Guyton and Reeder 1950; Alper and Flacke 1969). Tubocurarine interacts with ganglionic receptors, renders them inaccessible to acetyl-

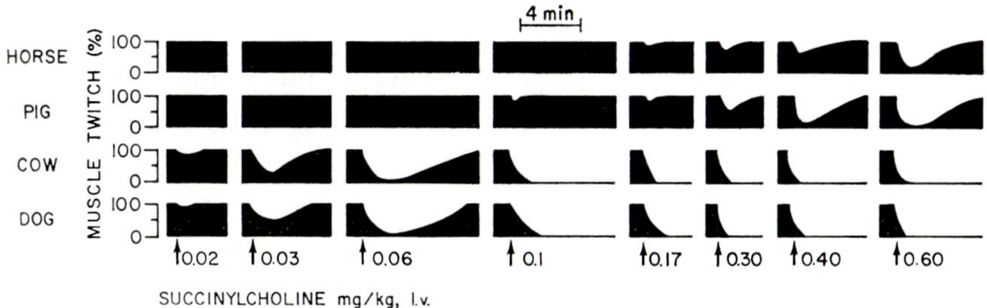

Fig. 9.6. Schematic representations of the neuromuscular blocking effect of succinylcholine iodide in nerve-muscle preparations of different species during barbiturate anesthesia. Notice interspecies differences in degree and in duration of paralysis caused by succinylcholine. (Modified from Hansson 1956; after Lumb and Jones 1973)

choline, and thereby increases the threshold of the postganglionic nerve to acetylcholine. However, as a general rule, autonomic ganglia are less sensitive than are the myoneural junctions to curare. Ganglionic impulse transmission involves, at least partially, a muscarinic pathway (see Chapter 8); *d*-tubocurarine has very little blocking effect on muscarinic receptors. Thus, in most cases, it would be anticipated that ganglionic transmission is functional during treatment with curarelike drugs. Nevertheless, hypotension that is believed to be partly dependent upon ganglionic blockade often occurs after administration of *d*-tubocurarine.

Other neuromuscular blocking drugs, both competitive and depolarizing types, have been shown experimentally to alter ganglionic transmission but in clinically insignificant amounts. Succinylcholine induces transient ganglionic stimulation prior to blockade evoked by larger doses. The former effect may partially explain hypertension that has occurred subsequent to succinylcholine administration.

Parasympathetic effects of neuromuscular blocking agents are usually minimal. Pancuronium has anticholinesterase activity. Succinylcholine and decamethonium are approximately 1000 times and 100 times less potent, respectively, than acetylcholine in eliciting contraction of guinea pig ileum. In dogs, large doses of succinylcholine induce salivation; this is antagonized by pretreatment with atropine (Hansson 1956).

Sinus tachycardia is seen after injection of gallamine. This effect seems to be dependent upon an atropinelike increase in vagal tone. A tyraminelike action (release of norepinephrine from sympathetic nerve endings) has also been proposed.

Histamine Release

Tubocurarine causes the release of histamine. The magnitude of this response varies, depending on species, dosage, and rate and route of administration. Intraarterial infusion of *d*-tubocurarine evokes histamine release in the perfused hind-limb preparation of dogs (Alam et al. 1939). Histaminelike wheals can be produced by subdermal and intraarterial administration of *d*-tubocurarine. *In vivo,* increased respiratory tract secretions and bronchospasm seen after administration of *d*-tubocurarine have been attributed to histamine release as has the hypotensive effect of *d*-tubocurarine. Pretreatment with antihistamine drugs antagonizes these side effects; they are not inhibited by atropine or neostigmine.

Dimethyl-tubocurarine, succinylcholine, decamethonium, and gallamine are very weak histamine-releasing agents.

Central Nervous System (CNS)

Although synaptic transmission in the brain is altered by direct application of neuromuscular blocking drugs into the brain, CNS effects are nondetectable when these drugs are administered by other routes. The neuromuscular blocking agents do not gain entry into the CNS to any appreciable extent due to the presence of the highly charged quaternary ammonium moieties. Therefore, neither CNS depression nor tranquilization is produced by the neuromuscular blocking agents. Nonambulation results only from peripheral myoneural paralysis. This was decisively confirmed when Smith (Smith et al. 1947) allowed himself to be paralyzed with *d*-tubocurarine. At no time during the experiment did he experience hypnosis, tranquilization, amnesia, anesthesia, or analgesia. He simply could not voluntarily breathe or move, an experience described as quite frightful.

Cardiovascular Effects

As outlined above, *d*-tubocurarine often induces hypotension, particularly if rapidly administered to dogs. Minimal tachycardia (10%–20% increase in heart rate) and an increase in cardiac output are often detected subsequent to injection of gallamine (Longnecker et al. 1973). This results primarily from a vagolytic effect that may be due to blockade of cholinergic myocardial receptors.

Several investigators have reported no significant changes in cardiovascular function with pancuronium (Brown et al. 1973). Studies in human beings indicate that this drug may cause a slight increase in blood pressure, heart rate, and cardiac output but does not affect peripheral vascular resistance during thiobarbiturate anesthesia (Coleman et al. 1972). These cardiovascular changes reportedly were absent if patients were pretreated with atropine.

Succinylcholine usually evokes minimal cardiovascular changes in dogs if administered during general anesthesia, and blood pressure remains fairly constant if artificial ventilation is provided. Subparalytic doses of succinylcholine increased the arrhythmogenicity of epinephrine during light halothane anesthesia in dogs (Tucker and Munson 1975). In dogs not treated with succinylcholine, an average dose of 4.15 μg/kg of epinephrine was required to evoke premature ventricular contractions, whereas an average dose of 1.6 μg/kg of epinephrine was the arrhythmogenic dose in dogs pretreated with 0.25 mg/kg of succinylcholine. On the other hand, *d*-tubocurarine caused a slight protection against epinephrine-induced arrhythmias. The mechanisms involved in these drug interactions were not clarified. If deemed essential, catecholamines should be used cautiously in patients treated with depolarizing neuromuscular blocking agents.

Also, succinylcholine has been reported to increase susceptibility to the myocardial irritant effects of digitalis preparations, and it has been suggested that succinylcholine may be contraindicated in digitalized patients (Dowdy et al. 1965).

Pronounced cardiovascular side effects have been reported in horses after administration of succinylcholine (Larson et al. 1959; Hofmeyer 1960; Lees and Tavernor 1969). In general, these effects seem to be more pronounced in unanesthetized and nontranquilized animals than during general anesthesia. Severe hypertension, initial bradycardia followed by tachycardia, atrioventricular conduction disturbances, and extrasystoles have been reported, and myocardial damage has been suspected. Early institution of artificial respiration has been reported to block the blood pressure effect. The hypertensive response seems to be at least partially mediated by the succinylcholine-induced dyspnea and the accompanying blood P_{O_2}-P_{CO_2} disturbances causing a reflexogenic increase in blood pressure. Direct activation of autonomic ganglia by succinylcholine may also be involved.

It should be remembered, however, that neuromuscular blocking agents do not depress the brain unless or until apnea-induced hypoxia actually causes syncope. Prior to hypoxic states, skeletal muscle paralysis affords no depression whatsoever of conscious centers of the brain of nonanesthetized animals. It seems likely, then, that the novel sensations experienced by conscious animals as they are being paralyzed evoke profound fright. This can cause activation of autonomic centers within the brain. Autonomic discharge may be markedly altered, resulting in cardiovascular side effects. Autonomic blocking agents (ganglionic block with hexamethonium; β-adrenergic block with propranolol) substantially decrease the cardiovascular side effects of succinylcholine.

Ocular Effects

Contrary to what many anesthesiology and pharmacology textbooks state, ocular muscles are not ultrasensitive to the paralyzing effects of neuromuscular blocking agents. This was demonstrated in the cat rather conclusively by Katz and Eakins (1966). The clinically important ocular effects depend upon the pronounced contracture of ocular muscles that occurs after treatment with depolarizing neuromuscular blockers. These agents are contraindicated in glaucoma since intraocular pressure may be increased.

Serum Potassium

Depolarizing neuromuscular blocking agents cause a release of K^+ from skeletal muscle. Elevation of serum K^+ may result, particularly if repeated injections are given.

Pharmacokinetics

Neuromuscular blocking agents with quaternary nitrogen groups are ionized at all levels of physiologic pH. Therefore, they are highly charged, lipophobic compounds and they cross lipoprotein membrane barriers poorly. Little if any absorption occurs after oral administration of these drugs. South American Indians were well aware of this since they ingested flesh of curare-poisoned animals without concern. Inefficient absorption after oral administration has little importance to modern medicine, however, since these agents should be given by the intravenous route so that muscle relaxation can be quickly evaluated. Whereas South American Indians were concerned only with one "end point," death, and were worried only about "underdosage," practitioners are concerned with facilitating muscle relaxation and are extremely concerned with overdosage. Administration of neuromuscular blocking agents should be closely monitored and correlated at all times with effects observed in the patient.

Intramuscular injection of neuromuscular blocking agents is occasionally used to immobilize nondomestic animals. Absorption occurs rapidly after intramuscular injection, and effective blood concentrations are obtained shortly thereafter.

Tubocurarine is distributed primarily in the extracellular space throughout body tissues, but it concentrates at myoneural junctional regions (Waser 1967). It penetrates cells poorly, due to the charged state of the molecule. The liver and kidney participate in the biologic fate of *d*-tubocurarine; however, the duration of action of this agent normally does not depend upon biotransformation. Rather, redistribution of *d*-tubocurarine away from the neuromuscular junction and into nonspecific body compartments is believed to account for the short duration of action of a single dose of this drug. Repeated treatment or excessive amounts of *d*-tubocurarine tend to saturate nonspecific sites. Under these circumstances, renal excretion becomes important as a mechanism for termination of the activity of *d*-tubocurarine. If injection has to be repeated, less drug is needed to evoke muscle relaxation. Cumulative neuromuscular blockade occurs when injections are repeated, since *d*-tubocurarine is excreted rather slowly by the kidneys.

Gallamine and dimethyl tubocurarine are probably handled similarly to *d*-tubocurarine. Gallamine is excreted virtually unchanged in the urine as are decamethonium and pancuronium. These agents are thought to bind only minimally to tissues. Renal failure markedly prolongs their duration of action.

Succinylcholine is rapidly disposed of by the body since it is a suitable substrate for plasma pseudocholinesterase. This enzyme quickly hydrolyzes succinylcholine to the considerably less active metabolite, succinylmonocholine. This metabolite is more slowly broken down by pseudocholinesterase to succinic acid and choline, natural body constituents. The interspecies potency of succinylcholine varies considerably. As mentioned, this has been attributed to species differences in the activity of pseudocholinesterase.

INTERACTIONS

Various drugs influence the pharmacologic effects of muscle relaxants. Neuromuscular blocking agents themselves alter the activity of other neuromuscular agents. As would be expected, competitive agents summate with each other. Similarly, depolarizing agents also interact synergistically with one another. However, tubocurarine decreases the muscle twitch depressant effects of succinylcholine and decamethonium. This is related to persistent occupation of a certain portion of receptors by tubocurarine, although muscle twitch may have recovered (see "Margin of safety of neuromuscular transmission" below). Depolarization of the end-plate by succinylcholine or decamethonium is partially impeded, due to the stabilizing effects of tubocurarine. Succinylcholine antagonizes the effects of curare, due to the partial agonistic characteristics of the former agent. These complex antagonistic interactions, however, have no clinical application since they depend upon complicated treatment and time and dosage schedules. During clinical situations, neuromuscular blocking agents should not be used in attempts to reverse the effects of other types of neuromuscular blocking agents since potentiation may occur despite experimental results to the contrary (Koelle 1970).

The interaction of cholinesterase inhibitors with neuromuscular blocking agents has been discussed above. Cholinesterase inhibitors decrease responsiveness to the competitive agents, while they tend to increase the intensity and duration of action of the depolarizing agents. Organophosphate insecticides and anthelmintics, carbamates, and any other cholinesterase inhibitor may cause interactions. The phenothiazine family of tranquilizers has some anticholinesterase activity. Use of succinylcholine in a patient exposed to an organophosphate may be particularly hazardous if a phenothiazine tranquilizer has also been administered.

Many general anesthetics, in addition to depressing the CNS, depress impulse transmission at somatic myoneural junctions. Ether alters neuromuscular transmission by stabilizing the postsynaptic membrane and perhaps by decreasing neuronal release of acetylcholine. Dosages of curare should be reduced by one-third to one-half during ether anesthesia. Halothane also acts synergistically with curarelike drugs but to a lesser extent than ether. Methoxyflurane and pentobarbital also have depressant effects on myoneural transmission events.

Aminoglycoside antibiotics (e.g., neomycin, streptomycin, dihydrostreptomycin, kanamycin, gentamicin,) decrease the release of acetylcholine from the nerve and also decrease the sensitivity of the endplate to acetylcholine (Pittinger and Adamson 1972). They do not cause depolarization. Their effects resemble in many ways the effects of low Ca^{++} or of excess Mg^{++}. The presynaptic effect of the antibiotics is believed to be due to interruption of Ca^{++}-dependent events at the axonal membrane (Adams 1973, 1975; Adams and Mathew 1974). Cholinesterase inhibitors, such as neostigmine, antagonize the postsynaptic depressant effect of these antibiotics. Ca^{++} antagonizes the presynaptic action and is usually more effective than neostigmine in reversing the neuromuscular paralyzing effects of the aminoglycoside antibiotics. These antibiotics interact synergistically at the myoneural junction with neuromuscular blocking agents, anesthetics, and other antibiotics. The clinical significance of neuromuscular interactions of antibiotics and other drugs has been well established in human beings and has been suggested in lower animals. These subjects were recently reviewed (Pittinger et al. 1970; Adams 1975). Other antibiotics, e.g., lincomycin and polymyxin A and B, are also neuromuscular blocking agents, but the mechanism(s) of action of these drugs is not known.

The catecholamines epinephrine and norepinephrine have some anticurare activity, probably by increasing the amount of acetylcholine discharged from the axon. This effect has little clinical importance.

Different disease states influence the pharmacologic effects of neuromuscular blocking agents. Hepatic synthesis of pseudocholinesterase is decreased in the presence of liver disease. The duration of succinylcholine activity will be prolonged if the liver is seriously affected. Administration of purified pseudocholinesterase preparation hastens recovery from the effects of succinylcholine.

Renal problems delay the excretion of *d*-tubocurarine, gallamine, pancuronium, and decamethonium. Anand et al. (1972) successfully reversed persistent gallamine-induced neuromuscular paralysis in a renally incompetent patient by use of artificial diuresis.

CLINICAL USE

Muscle paralysis proceeds at different rates in different body regions after administration of a neuromuscular blocking agent. Usually, head and neck muscles are affected first, often within 0.25–1 minute after injection. (This characteristic is employed in a biological assay, i.e., head-drop test in rabbits, for determining the potency of an unknown concentration of curare.) The tail is usually affected with the head and neck. Subsequently, muscles of the limbs are paralyzed, then the deglutition and laryngeal muscles. Abdominal muscles, intercostal muscles, and the diaphragm are then paralyzed in this order. Recovery usually proceeds in the reverse of this sequence (Hall 1971).

Attempts have been made in clinical practice to utilize the sequential development of muscle paralysis by administering doses of neuromuscular blocking agents adequate to paralyze ambulatory muscle but insufficient to affect the diaphragm. This has not always proved effective, since respiratory insufficiency may still occur, although the diaphragm is seemingly spared. Therefore, it is imperative that apparatus for administering artificial respiration be available when neuromuscular blocking agents are used clinically. In fact, to circumvent the need for immediate establishment of an adequate airway and for other emergency procedures, it would seem wise to routinely perform tracheal intubation and to institute artificial respiration whenever a neuromuscular blocking agent is used.

Muscle relaxants have been used in clinical practice for several purposes: (1) to facilitate tracheal intubation; (2) to paralyze respiratory muscle so that artificial respiration can be easily controlled; (3) to increase muscle relaxation to facilitate surgical access to difficult anatomic regions; (4) to evoke muscle relaxation to facilitate orthopedic manipulations and, particularly, fracture reduction; and (5) as part of balanced anesthesia procedures to reduce the amount of general anesthetic required.

Tracheal intubation may be performed in a nonanesthetized animal immediately after a paralyzing dose of neuromuscular blocking agent has taken effect. Prior administration of a sedative or tranquilizer is advisable both for humane reasons and to circumvent potential side effects that may be precipitated by fearful reaction to paralysis.

A wide range of dosages of neuromuscular blocking agents has been reported for the use of these drugs during anesthesia (Hansson 1956; Wright and Hall 1961; Tavernor 1971; Lumb and Jones 1973). Often this variance reflects differences in investigative procedures of the original studies, e.g., the use of different anesthetics and sedatives, different salts of the neuromuscular blocking agent, different nerve-muscle preparations, and, in some cases, the use of nonanesthetized subjects. As previously mentioned, neuromuscular blocking agents should be given to effect rather than by bolus administration of a set precalculated dose. In fact, it is advisable for these drugs to be administered by titration during anesthesia and to be continuously correlated with muscle relaxation, much in the way that barbiturates are administered for induction of general anesthesia.

In dogs, 0.4–0.5 mg/kg of *d*-tubocurarine administered intravenously will cause generalized skeletal muscle relaxation, but hypotension frequently occurs as a side effect in this species. In pigs, 0.2–0.3 mg/kg of *d*-tubocurarine will usually afford acceptable muscular relaxation; blood pressure effects are less in this species than in the dog. Tubocurarine is somewhat more potent in ruminants; doses of 0.05–0.06 mg/kg have been suggested for use in young lambs and goats.

Gallamine has been suggested as the nondepolarizing drug of choice in dogs, since adverse side effects are infrequently seen with this agent. Approximately 1 mg/kg causes complete muscle paralysis in both dogs and cats within 1 to 2 minutes after intravenous injection and lasts 15–20 minutes. A hypotensive response may be induced in cats with galamine but is infrequently observed in dogs. In young ruminants (lambs and calves), 0.4 mg/kg of gallamine is effective, whereas the dose in horses is 0.5–1.0 mg/kg.

Solutions of succinylcholine should always be refrigerated and kept on ice in the field, since this agent undergoes spontaneous hydrolysis. Hansson (1956) reported that the intravenous ED50 (dose that reduced muscle twitch by 50%) of succinylcholine in the sciatic nerve–gastrocnemius muscle preparation of anesthetized dogs was 0.045–0.060 mg/kg. This dose did not effectively paralyze the respiratory muscles, however, and 0.085 mg/kg was required to induce transient apnea, whereas 0.11 mg/kg and 0.22 mg/kg were needed to cause apnea for 18–21 minutes and for 23–27 minutes, respectively. In unanesthetized dogs, intramuscular administration of 0.12 mg/kg of succinylcholine caused ataxia in 5 minutes and caused forced abdominal respiration in 7 minutes; recovery was apparently complete in 30 minutes. In clinical situations, 0.3 mg/kg of succinylcholine administered intravenously will usually afford good muscle relaxation in dogs, whereas in the cat, 1 mg/kg may be required. In dogs Hansson (1956) reported that 0.15 mg/kg of succinylcholine was effective in paralyzing the diaphragm during thoracotomy procedures. However, Eyster and Evans (1974) suggested the use of 0.5 mg/kg of succinylcholine for muscle relaxation in dogs during thoracotomy for open-heart surgery. This dose was also reported to control muscle twitches evoked by inadvertent stimulation of nerves during use of electrocautery. Duration of paralysis varies and should be closely monitored.

In rhesus monkeys, 1–2 mg/kg of succinylcholine administered intravenously has been used for restraint for tuberculosis testing and for endotracheal intubation (Lindquist and Lau 1973). In pigs, approximately 2 mg/kg of succinylcholine is effective. Much smaller amounts, i.e., 0.01–0.02 mg/kg, are required in cattle and sheep. Hansson (1956) reported that 0.13–0.18 mg/kg of succinylcholine was required to immobilize nonanesthetized horses. Presently, however, the generally accepted dose of succinylcholine in horses, when used alone, is 4 mg/100 lb body weight (0.088 mg/kg) (Lumb and Jones 1973).

Succinylcholine has been used without anesthesia in horses for casting and restraint during brief surgical procedures such as castration. This practice should not be condoned since, as previously outlined, (1) no anesthesia is afforded for painful procedures, (2) severe fright is seemingly evoked, and (3) pronounced cardiovascular disturbances and even myocardial damage may result. Succinylcholine should not be used as a sole restraining agent during surgical procedures but should be used only in conjunction with a general or local anesthetic.

Moreover, care should always be taken during the use of neuromuscular blocking agents to insure that the patient has not recovered from the anesthetic and simply remains paralyzed. This has occurred in human patients and has led to successful lawsuits and obtainment of monetary compensation by the patient. Although lower animals cannot complain, it behooves us as veterinarians to insure that our patients are not inadvertently subjected to such excruciatingly painful incidences.

Margin of Safety of Neuromuscular Transmission

The concept of a margin of safety of neuromuscular transmission bears discussion in relation to clinical use of these drugs. It has been estimated that a relatively large percentage of the cholinergic receptors must be occupied by a curare agent before muscle twitch fails. In the cat diaphragm, for example, muscle twitch is not affected until about 80% of the receptors are blocked by *d*-tubocurarine, and twitch is not completely abolished until about 90% of the receptors are occupied (Waud and Waud 1972). A somewhat greater margin of safety was found in dogs. Accordingly, for recovery of the diaphragm from the effects of a previous injection of *d*-tubocurarine, only a small percentage (5% and 18% in dogs and cats, respectively) of the receptors need be free. Therefore, and most important, although to all outward signs recovery seems complete, over 80% of the receptors can still be blocked.

Recognition of this aspect becomes clinically important in the postoperative recovery room and should be considered in patients that have been exposed to neuromuscular blocking drugs and/or other myoneural depressants such as anesthetics. As a patient regains some control of voluntary muscles, spontaneous respiration returns and may seem completely normal. However, it must be remembered that at this time an extremely small margin of safety of neuromuscular transmission exists. That is, only a small percentage of the postsynaptic receptors are available for interaction with acetylcholine; this small fraction of receptors is now responsible for maintaining muscle contraction. Therefore, if the patient is now exposed to another drug that as a side effect depresses neuromuscular function (even though it may be minimal or even nondetectable normally), disastrous complications may result. Anesthetic mortality has occurred in human beings that can be attributed to such interactions. For example, Pridgen (1956) reported the anesthetic deaths of two children who were given neomycin intraperitoneally immediately after completion of successful appendectomies under ether anesthesia. Initially, respiration was adequate but within a short time after administration of the antibiotic, persistent apnea occurred. Death followed several hours later. It seems likely that the margin of safety of neuromuscular transmission was reduced in these infants by ether, resulting in marked augmentation of the neuromuscular blocking properties of neomycin. Pittinger et al. (1970) estimated a 9% death rate in those human patients experiencing antibiotic-induced respiratory problems in conjunction with anesthetics and neuromuscular blocking agents. Apnea and eventual death in a traumatized dog were attributed to antibiotic (dihydrostreptomycin)-induced neuromuscular paralysis (Adams and Bingham 1971); however, the clinical incidence of antibiotic-associated respiratory problems in animals is undetermined.

These examples illustrate potential problems that may be inadvertently introduced in a patient that seemingly is recovering quite well from anesthesia and surgery. The margin of safety of neuromuscular transmission should be considered any time that anesthetics, neuromuscular blocking agents, and any other drug that depresses myoneural function are used in multiple drug regimens.

Clinical Reversal of Neuromuscular Paralysis

Treatment of persistent neuromuscular paralysis and/or treatment of inadvertent overdosage of neuromuscular blocking agents should be approached conservatively. Obviously, the initial step should be immediate artificial respiration and withdrawal of administration of the involved agent. Often, prolonged artificial respiration will allow adequate time for the drug to be disposed of by the patient's system. As discussed above, exposure to other drugs that may synergistically interact with neuromuscular blocking agents should be avoided. If a competitive neuromuscular blocking agent was used, paralysis can usually be effectively antagonized by administration of a cholinesterase inhibitor, such as neostigmine or edrophonium. Neostigmine can be administered to small and large animals by slow intravenous injection at the dose of 0.1 mg/10 lb of body weight (0.022 mg/kg). It should be remembered that cholinesterase inhibitors will cause intensification of acetylcholine activity at both muscarinic and nicotinic receptors. Atropine (0.04 mg/kg) should be administered prior to or in conjunction with neostigmine to circumvent the muscarinic effects of the later drug. Care should be taken to insure that paralysis does not recur after antagonism by neostigmine; additional injection of neostigmine may be required.

Neostigmine or other cholinesterase inhibitors should not be used in attempts to reverse the effects of a depolarizing agent. At the present time, reliable chemical antidotes are not available for this group of agents. Artificial respiration may be required for a prolonged period. Injection of purified pseudocholinesterase preparation has been shown to hasten recovery from the effects of succinylcholine.

Due to the small therapeutic index of the neuromuscular blocking agents, their clinical use should always be supervised by qualified experienced personnel who are thoroughly familiar with the indications, limitations, hazards, and methods of administration of these highly active drugs.

REFERENCES

Adams, H. R. 1973. Neuromuscular blocking effect of aminoglycoside antibiotics in nonhuman primates. J Am Vet Med Assoc 163:613.

———. 1975. Acute adverse effects of antibiotics. J Am Vet Med Assoc 166:983.

Adams, H. R., and Bingham, G. A. 1971. Respiratory arrest associated with dihydrostreptomycin. J Am Vet Med Assoc 159: 179.

Adams, H. R., and Mathew, B. P. 1974. The cumulative neuromuscular blocking effect of neomycin. Arch Int Pharmacodyn 210: 288.

Alam, M.; Anrep, G. V.; Barsoum, G. S.; Talaat, M.; and Wieninger, E. 1939. Liberation of histamine from the skeletal muscle by curare. J Physiol (Lond) 95:148.

Alper, M. H., and Flacke, W. 1969. Effects of curare, atropine and halothane on ganglionic transmission in the dog. Abstr Meet Am Soc Anesthesiol (San Francisco), p. 100.

Anand, J. S.; Mehta, R. K.; Munshi, C. A.; and Mulla, D. H. 1972. Reversal of neuromuscular blockade by artificial diuresis: Case report. Can Anaesth Soc J 19:651.

Barlow, R. B., and Ing, H. R. 1948. Curare-like action of polymethylene bis-quaternary ammonium salts. Br J Pharmacol Chemother 3:298.

Bernard, C. 1856. Analyse physiologique des propriétés des systèmes musculaire et nerveux au moyer du curare. C R Hebd Seanc Acad Sci Paris 43:825.

Blaber, L. C. 1973. The prejunctional actions of some non-depolarizing blocking drugs. Br J Pharmacol 47:109.

Bovet, D. 1951. Some aspects of the relationship between chemical constitution and curare-like activity. Ann NY Acad Sci 54: 407.

Bovet, D., and Bovet-Nitti, F. 1955. Succinylcholine chloride, curarizing agent of short duration of action: Pharmacodynamic activity and clinical applications. Sci Med Ital 3:484.

Bowen, J. M. 1972. Estimation of the dissociation constant of *d*-tubocurarine and the receptor for endogenous acetylcholine. J Pharmacol Exp Ther 183:333.

Brown, E. M.; Smiler, B. G.; and Plaza, J. A. 1973. Cardiovascular effects of pancuronium. Anesthesiology 38:597.

Burns, B. D., and Paton, W. D. M. 1951. Depolarization of the motor end plate by decamethonium and acetylcholine. J Physiol (Lond) 115:41.

Cheymol, J., ed. 1972. Neuromuscular Blocking and Stimulating Agents, 2 vols. Elmsford, N.Y.: Pergamon Press.

Coleman, A. J.; Downing, J. W.; Leary, W. P.; Moyes, D. G.; and Styles, M. 1972. The immediate cardiovascular effects of pancuronium, alcuronium and tubocurarine in man. Anaesthesia 27:415.

Couteaux, R. 1972. Structure and cytochemical characteristics of the neuromuscular junction. In J. Cheymol, ed. Neuromuscular Blocking and Stimulating Agents, vol. 1, p. 7. Elmsford, N.Y.: Pergamon Press.

De Robertis, E. 1971. Molecular biology of synaptic receptors. Science 171:963.

Dowdy, E. G.; Duggar, P. N.; and Fabian, L. W. 1965. Effect of neuromuscular blocking agents on isolated digitalized mammalian hearts. Anesth Analg 44:608.

Everett, A. J.; Laue, L. A.; and Wilkinson, S. 1970. Revision of the structures of (+)-tubocurarine chloride and (+)-chondrocurine. Chem Commun 1020.

Eyster, G. E., and Evans, A. T. 1974. Open-heart surgery in the dog. In R. W. Kirk, ed. Current Veterinary Therapy V, p. 255. Philadelphia: W. B. Saunders.

Galindo, A., and Kennedy, R. 1974. Further observations on depolarizing neuromuscular block: The so-called phase II block. Br J Anaesth 46:405.

Gergis, S. D.; Dretchen, K. L.; Sokoll, M. D.; and Long, J. P. 1971. The effect of neuromuscular blocking agents on acetylcholine release. Proc Soc Exp Biol Med 138: 693.

Guyton, A. G., and Reeder, R. C. 1950. Quantitative studies of the autonomic actions of curare. J Pharmacol Exp Ther 98:188.

Hall, L. W., ed. 1971. Wright's Veterinary Anaesthesia and Analgesia, 7th ed. Baltimore: Williams & Wilkins.

Hall, L. W.; Lehman, H.; and Silk, E. 1953. Response in dogs to relaxants derived from succinic acid and choline. Br Med J 1:134.

Hansson, C. H. 1956. Succinylcholine iodide as a muscular relaxant in veterinary surgery. J Am Vet Med Assoc 128:287.

Hansson, C. H. 1958. Studies on the effect of succinylcholine in domestic animals. Nord Vet Med 10:201.

Hofmeyer, C. F. B. 1960. Some observations on the use of succinylcholine chloride (suxamethonium) in horses with particular reference to the effect on the heart. J S Afr Vet Med Assoc 31:251.

Hubbard, J. I., and Quastel, D. M. J. 1973. Micropharmacology of vertebrate neuromuscular transmission. Annu Rev Pharmacol 13:199.

Hubbard, J. I., and Wilson, D. F. 1973. Neuromuscular transmission in a mammalian preparation in the absence of blocking drugs and the effect of *d*-tubocurarine. J Physiol (Lond) 228:307.

Katz, B. 1966. Nerve, Muscle and Synapse. New York: McGraw-Hill.

Katz, R. L., and Eakins, K. E. 1966. The effects of succinylcholine, hexacarbacholine, gallamine, and dimethyl tubocurarine on the twitch and tonic neuromuscular systems of the cat. J Pharmacol Exp Ther 154:303.

Khromov-Borisov, N. V., and Michelson, M. J. 1966. The mutual disposition of cholinoceptors of locomotor muscles, and the changes in their disposition in the course of evolution. Pharmacol Rev 18:1051.

Koelle, G. B. 1970. Neuromuscular blocking agents. In L. S. Goodman and A. Gilman, eds. The Pharmacological Basis of Therapeutics, 4th ed., p. 601. New York: Macmillan.

Larson, L. H.; Loomis, L. N,; and Steel, J. D. 1959. Muscular relaxants and cardiovascular damage: With special reference to succinylcholine chloride. Aust Vet J 35: 269.

Lees, P., and Tavernor, W. D. 1969. The influence of suxamethonium on cardiovascular and respiratory function in the anaesthetized horse. Br J Pharmacol 36:116.

Lindquist, P. A., and Lau, D. T. 1973. The use of succinylcholine in the handling and restraint of rhesus monkeys *(Macaca mulatta)*. Lab Anim Sci 23:562.

Longnecker, D. E.; Stoelting, R. K.; and Morrow, A. G. 1973. Cardiac and peripheral vascular effects of gallamine in man. J Int Anesth Res Soc 52:931.

Lumb, W. V., and Jones, E. W. 1973. The muscle relaxants and other adjuvants to anesthesia. In Veterinary Anesthesia, p. 343. Philadelphia: Lea & Febiger.

McIntyre, A. R. 1972. History of curare. In J. Cheymol, ed. Neuromuscular Blocking and Stimulating Agents, vol. 1, p. 187. Elmsford, N.Y.: Pergamon Press.

Miledi, R.; Molinoff, P.; and Potter, L. T. 1971. Isolation of the cholinergic receptor protein of *Torpedo* electric tissue. Nature 229:554.

Palmer, J. S.; Jackson, J. B.; Younger, R. L.; Hunt, L. M.; Danz, J. W.; and Wunderlich, B. W. 1965. Normal cholinesterase activity of the whole blood of the horse and angora goat. Vet Med 58:885.

Paton, W. D. M., and Waud, D. R. 1962. Drug-receptor interactions at the neuromuscular junction. In A. V. S. De Reuck, ed. Curare and Curare-like Agents, p. 34. Boston: Little, Brown.

Paton, W. D. M., and Zaimis, E. J. 1949. The pharamacological actions of polymethylene bistrimethylammonium salts. Br J Pharmacol Chemother 4:381.

Pauling, P., and Petcher, T. J. 1973. Neuromuscular blocking agents: Structure and activity. Chem Biol Interact 6:351.

Pittinger, C., and Adamson, R. 1972. Antibiotic blockade of neuromuscular function. Annu Rev Pharmacol 12:169.

Pittinger, C. B.; Eryasa, Y.; and Adamson, R. 1970. Antibiotic-induced paralysis. Anesth Analg 49:487.

Pridgen, J. E. 1956. Respiratory arrest thought to be due to intraperitoneal neomycin. Surgery 40:571.

Radeleff, R. D., and Woodard, C. T. 1956. Cholinesterase activity of normal blood of cattle and sheep. Vet Med 51:512.

Riker, W. F., and Okamoto, M. 1969. Pharmacology of motor nerve terminals. Annu Rev Pharmacol 9:173.

Smith, S. M.; Brown, H. O.; Toman, J. E. P.; and Goodman, L. S. 1947. The lack of cerebral effects of *d*-tubocurarine. Anesthesiology 8:1.

Stowe, C. M. 1955. The curariform effect of succinylcholine chloride in the equine and bovine species in a preliminary report. Cornell Vet 45:193.

Stowe, C. M.; Bieter, R. N.; and Roepke, M. H. 1958. The relationship between cholinesterase activity and the effects of succinylcholine chloride in the horse and cow. Cornell Vet 48:241.

Tavernor, W. D. 1971. Muscle relaxants. In L. Soma, ed. Textbook of Veterinary Anesthesia, p. 111. Baltimore: Williams & Wilkins.

Thesleff, S. 1955. The mode of neuromuscular block caused by acetylcholine, nicotine, decamethonium and succinylcholine. Acta Physiol Scand 34:218.

———. 1958. A study of the interaction between neuromuscular blocking agents and acetylcholine at the mammalian motor end plate. Acta Anaesthesiol Scand 2:69.

Tucker, W. K., and Munson, E. S. 1975. Effects of succinylcholine and *d*-tubocurarine on epinephrine-induced arrhythmias during halothane anesthesia in dogs. Anesthesiology 42:41.

Waser, P. G. 1967. Receptor localization by autoradiography. Ann NY Acad Sci 144: 737.

———. 1972. Chemistry and pharmacology of natural curare compounds. In J. Cheymol, ed. Neuromuscular Blocking and Stimulating Agents, vol. 1, p. 205. Elmsford, N.Y.: Pergamon Press.

Waud, B. E., and Waud, D. R. 1972. The margin of safety of neuromuscular transmission in the muscle of the diaphragm. Anesthesiology 37:417.

Wright, J. G., and Hall, L. W. 1961. Veterinary Anesthesia and Analgesia, 5th ed. Baltimore: Williams & Wilkins.

Wurzel, M. 1967. The physiological role of cholinesterase at cholinergic receptor sites. Ann NY Acad Sci 144:737.

Zaimis, E. J. 1959. Mechanisms of neuromuscular blockade. In D. Bovet; F. Bovet-Nitti; and G. B. Marini-Bettòlo, eds. International Symposium on Curare and Curare-like Agents, p. 191. Amsterdam: Elsevier.

SECTION 4

Drugs Acting on the Central Nervous System

CHAPTER 10

INTRODUCTION

NICHOLAS H. BOOTH

The central nervous system (CNS) is the site of consciousness and the source of adjustment of an organism to its environment. The complex reactions of the CNS provide some of the most baffling problems of physiology and pharmacology.

PHYSIOLOGICAL CONSIDERATIONS

The CNS is more sensitive to the effects of drugs than any other system of the body. It normally has a high metabolic rate that magnifies any interference with its metabolism by a depressant drug. A variety of drugs can penetrate the blood-cerebrospinal fluid (CSF) and blood-brain barriers in animals at rates that closely parallel the lipid:water partition coefficients of the drugs. Although the blood-CSF and blood-brain barriers generally have similar permeabilities to drugs and foreign organic components, they are quite dissimilar from an anatomical standpoint. The blood-CSF barrier, for example, consists primarily of the epithelium of the choroid plexuses, whereas the blood-brain barrier appears to be either the brain capillary wall or its surrounding layer of glial cells. Despite these anatomical differences, the barriers are, from a pharmacological standpoint, not completely separate from each other. For example, a highly lipid-soluble drug can rapidly penetrate the blood-brain barrier and diffuse across the ependyma and pia mater into the CSF. This allows for greater distribution of the drug via the blood-brain barrier because of a much more extensive vascular bed compared to the choroid plexuses.

After a drug has crossed the blood-brain barrier and has gained access to the extracellular fluid, the rate of penetration into the various regions of the brain may differ. In the cat, for instance, phenobarbital is known to enter the gray matter faster than the white matter. The myelin sheath of the individual nerve fibers in white matter has a thicker lipoidal membrane than the single layer of lipoidal material in the membrane that surrounds the unmyelinated fibers of gray matter. This apparently accounts for the differences in the penetration of drugs into these two regions of the brain.

Drugs can be injected directly into the CSF and thus avoid the protective blood-brain barrier. This procedure possesses an inherent and obvious hazard in possible toxic actions upon the CNS. Some drugs such as barbiturates and volatile anesthetics act upon the cerebral cortex within a few seconds after intravenous injection or inhalation. In this short time they cannot traverse the complex route through the choroid plexus into the CSF, so they must diffuse out of the blood vessels to act directly upon the brain.

It is well established that a drug must gain entry into the extracellular fluid of the CNS to have a direct effect upon the cells of the CNS (Oldendorf 1974). To what extent an administered drug distributes into the extracellular fluid of the CNS is dependent upon a number of factors. If the drug is taken orally, its molecules must survive the chemical and enzymatic activity within the gut, penetrate the intestinal walls, pass through the liver, resist degradation by enzymes in blood plasma and other tissues, remain nonionized in solution unattached to plasma proteins, and eventually penetrate the blood-brain barrier.

Although the blood-brain barrier is nearly impermeable to macromolecules and it is quite impermeable to all known CNS transmitter substances, it is permeable to many drugs and metabolites. For example, procaine, caffeine, nicotine, opiates, L-dopamine, cyanide, barbiturates, volatile anesthetics, and many others readily penetrate the blood-brain barrier to reach the neurons. The degree of dissociation of a drug in blood plasma is a major factor in the penetration of the blood-brain barrier. If a drug is primarily nonionized at pH 7.4, its penetration into the brain is enhanced. It is generally recognized that only the nonionized component is capable of penetrating the blood-brain barrier. Inasmuch as the blood pH is quite constant and can shift in life only about ± 0.5, alterations in blood pH are not nearly so important for most drugs in altering the penetration of the blood-brain barrier as are intestinal pH changes because a very great range of pH is encountered in the gut (Oldendorf 1974). Drugs such as thiopental sodium having a pK near 7.4 may, however, undertake an extensive change in ionization with subtle shifts in blood pH characterized in conditions such as respiratory and metabolic acid-base imbalances. Such a deviation in ionization may result in atypical responses following the administration of anesthetics.

Cortical Activity

Continuous changes in electrical potential arise from the motor cortex of human and animal brains. During mental activity in human beings, electrical wave changes occur at a frequency of 50/second. During mental rest, waves occur at a frequency of 5–15/second. In very deep sleep or in coma produced by anesthetics, the wave frequency is about 4/second. Convulsive seizures produce waves of very high frequency and potential.

Sleep

The condition of sleep has long been studied not only on its own merit but because anesthesia resembles sleep in many respects. Sleep is characterized by a depression of cortical activity and is promoted by drugs that depress the activity of the higher centers. A state of apparent unconsciousness characterizes both the condition of deep sleep and of anesthesia. In both conditions there is a loss of ability to analyze changes in the environment critically. This is particularly true in poikilothermic animals where activity patterns, including the state of sleep are largely dependent upon the ambient or environmental temperature. The principal advantage of homeothermy in mammals and birds is their ability to maintain a relatively constant internal body temperature independent of environmental temperature variations so they may become awake, active, or mobile within any part of a 24-hour period. On the other hand, the homeothermic animals pay a price for this temperature independence because their food intake must be higher than that needed to maintain body heat. During food deprivation or low temperature it is well known that some warm-blooded animals are capable of converting to the poikilothermic state. For example, body temperature follows the environmental temperature within certain limits and results in states of torpor or hibernation. This permits these animals to conserve energy until the environmental conditions as well as the conditions for the acquisition of food become more favorable. A hypothesis has been advanced that sleep constitutes a period of dormancy in which energy is conserved to partially offset the increased energy demands of homeothermy (Berger 1975). This hypothesis embraces the concept that sleep is a state of reduced metabolism or form of energy conservation and may constitute a variation of dormancy, ranging from inactivity to torpor or hibernation. When depressant, neuroleptic, and anesthetic agents are used in animals in the torpid or poikilothermic state, only small amounts of these agents are required to induce severe CNS depression or deep anesthesia. Also, the recovery period can be expected to be much longer in these animals than in homeothermic animals.

Periodic sleep is a basic requirement of mammalian existence. Dogs die more quickly from loss of sleep than from loss of feed. Prolonged loss of sleep causes various phenomena, including histological changes in the contents of the CSF. This fluid will induce profound sleep in normal dogs when injected intracysternally. Alleviation of severe coughing or persistent pain so that a patient may sleep is of much therapeutic importance.

The production of sleep is favored by any treatment that depresses the cortical activity of the brain. Such treatments include bodily rest, a full stomach, external warmth, and depressants of the CNS.

Loss of Pain and Consciousness

The loss of pain and consciousness is the most important effect produced by anesthetics. Sleep produces a loss of consciousness but not a loss of pain. Depressants of the CNS, including alcohol, in one way or another have been used for centuries for pain relief. Not until the last few decades, however, has the art and science of anesthesia been developed to the point of removing pain from surgical procedures. The advent of anesthesia permitted the development of life-saving surgical techniques previously impossible because of the struggles of the patient.

The principal purpose underlying the use of anesthetics and analgesic agents is to prevent the infliction of pain when operative procedures are performed upon an animal. Theories regarding the mechanisms of how pain is perceived have changed rapidly. The theory proposed by Melzak and Wall (1965) has been useful in clinical medicine. They have proposed that cells in the substantia gelatinosa in the dorsal horn of the spinal cord act as a "gate control system" that modulates afferent patterns before they are transmitted centrally to the response system. The "gate control system" is kept open by stimuli arriving via small unmyelinated nerves that bombard the substantia gelatinosa. Nerve impulses arriving via large nerve fibers are transmitted to the central response system but also cause partial closure of the "gate," due to a negative feedback mechanism. Factors such as preconditioning, memory, and emotion may modify the system by input impulses from the cortex through afferent transmissions that may further close or open the "control gate." The perception of pain is still complex and remains difficult to define. Until more information is obtained, pain in animals should be regarded as an essentially comparable experience to pain in human patients and should be treated accordingly (Rex 1972).

Loss of consciousness is best described by what is known as the *law of descending paralysis.* This law was formulated to describe the effects of disease, but it also applies to the effects of anesthesia. It states that the more complex and more recently acquired functions of the brain are the most easily deranged by anesthesia. Thus during anesthesia there is a paralysis progressing posteriorly through the intercranial divisions to the spinal cord with the exception of the medulla. The anesthetic first depresses the anterior or cortical part of the brain at which location are the higher centers involved in conditioned reflexes and whatever powers of reasoning animals may possess. The depressant effects of the anesthetic progressively involve the more posterior parts of the brain but do not affect the medullary centers until after the spinal centers have been depressed.

The anesthetics depress *first* the cortical centers, *second* the spinal centers, and *third* the medullary centers. The existence of these various levels of nervous activity can be readily demonstrated in the laboratory by severing the brain across the central axis at the proper levels to demonstrate the progressive loss of function. This chain of behavior can be duplicated by administering an anesthetic to produce varying levels of unconsciousness in a patient. Loss of reflexes and of muscular activity is one of the more important contributions of anesthesia to veterinary medicine because the problem of restraint is of paramount importance in the treatment of animals.

Satisfactory surgical anesthesia for animals is necessary for humane treatment and for technical efficiency. Production of surgical anesthesia in animals is beset by problems arising from different species and from great variations in anatomy, physiology, and temperament as well as individual variations. The majority of human patients will cooperate with the anesthesiologist in the initial stages of anesthesia, but the veterinarian must contend with great fear and resistance from animals during the induction of anesthesia. These reactions of the animal patients necessitate preliminary restraint, which only adds to the fear and resistance of the patient. Thus, in animals receiving volatile anesthetics, a pronounced stage of voluntary excitement is often observed at the first application of the anesthetic. With the availability of highly effective and potent neuroleptic agents during the past two decades, the necessity to use forceful physical restraint procedures during the induction of anesthesia has been reduced in both small and large animals. The term "chemical restraint" was introduced when these agents were first used in veterinary medicine.

HISTORY

The earliest use of anesthetic drugs was recorded about 2250 B.C. on a Babylonian clay tablet. This ancient prescription directed the preparation of a cement for easing the pain of dental caries in man by mixing henbane seed with gum mastic. The Egyptians practiced surgery and must have used depressants such as opium and wines. The Chinese used hashish *(Cannabis sativa)* or wines containing hemp. Greek physicians recommended mandragora (belladonna alkaloids) or opium in wine.

In addition to drugs, there were many crude as well as cruel physical methods of inducing temporary insensibility. Asphyxiation was a common procedure in some countries, such as Assyria and Italy. Cerebral concussion by striking a wooden bowl placed over the head was used, but the mortality as well as the morbidity must have been very high. The somewhat more scientific procedure of compressing the carotid arteries was employed to produce cerebral anemia with consequent unconsciousness. A kind of regional anesthesia was attained by compression of the nerves and blood vessels of the region to be operated upon.

The introduction of general anesthesia for safe and painless surgery occurred between 1842 and 1847. Previous to this time surgery was a horrible, painful, and frequently fatal procedure employed only as a last resort. The surgeons attempted to shorten the agony by operating rapidly, so careful, delicate surgery was impossible.

The introduction of anesthesia had to await the development of chemistry. Joseph Priestley, a dissenting Unitarian minister, discovered oxygen (1771), nitrous oxide (1772), and carbon dioxide (date unknown). An American chemist and physician, Lantham Mitchell, administered nitrous oxide to animals with such fatal results that he concluded the gas to be poisonous. His opinions were widely accepted and no one dared use nitrous oxide until 1795 when young Humphrey Davy inhaled the gas. As a result of his experiences, Davy recommended the use of nitrous oxide for general anesthesia in surgery. Michael Faraday, a student of Davy, noted the anesthetic effects of sulfuric ether.

In 1824 Henry Hill Hickman operated without obvious pain upon animals after the administration of carbon dioxide gas. Hickman was the first to demonstrate that surgical pain could be abolished by the inhalation of a gas. He recognized that certain gases introduced into the lungs passed into the blood and circulated around the body to produce an artificial sleep suitable for surgery. While anesthetizing dogs for surgical procedures, Hickman recognized the danger of circulatory collapse.

During the period from 1825 to 1842 ether and nitrous oxide gases were variously employed by physicians in faddish treatment of respiratory disease, by showmen, and by young people at "ether-frolics" or "laughing-gas parties." At one of these "parties," Dr. Crawford W. Long of Jefferson, Georgia, noted that jubilant party participants could sustain injuries without the sensation of pain. Through this experience he recognized that ether could be used to prevent operative pain and on March 30, 1842, administered ether to permit the painless removal of a cystic tumor on the back of a man's neck. In 1846 Dr. William Morton, a dentist, used ether for the painless extraction of a tooth. He was so encouraged by his results that he requested an opportunity to anesthetize a patient undergoing major surgery at the Massachusetts General Hospital. His request was granted and on October 16, 1846, Dr. Morton publicly staged the first successful demonstration of surgical anesthesia in history. The general acceptance of ether as a surgical anesthetic by the medical world was largely due to the respected character of the surgeon-in-charge, Dr. John C. Warren, and his colleague, Dr. Henry J. Bigelow, both of whom published a report of the phenomenon in a medical journal in 1846.

Within a few months after ether was demonstrated by Morton, a demonstration was given in London. Its use also followed about 1 year later in most domestic animals and the *Veterinarian* had published a paper describing the use of the anesthetic in dogs and cats. George Dadd, an M.D., who switched from the practice of human medicine, was the first to use ether (and also chloroform) for animal surgery in the United States. He had used ether by 1852 and advocated its use in all painful operative procedures.

Dr. Horace Wells, a dentist of Hartford, Connecticut, observed the pain depressant action of nitrous oxide by a showman. Subsequently, Dr. Wells had a colleague extract a tooth while he inhaled nitrous oxide to prove to himself and others that painless dentistry was possible. Dr. Wells failed to convince medical science of the value of nitrous oxide as an anesthetic agent, but he is credited with conceiving the idea of anesthesia and publicizing its possible use in surgery.

Chloroform was discovered several years earlier than ether and had been studied by several different chemists. Early in 1847 Flourens, a French physiologist, administered chloroform to animals by inhalation and produced the same temporary type of anesthesia as that caused by ether. Soon after, Sir James Y. Simpson, a Scottish physician, began using chloroform in his obstetrical practice. His report of successful analgesia, given before the Medical Society of Edinburgh in 1847, precipitated a general controversy over the merits of analgesia in obstetrics, which was not quieted until 1853 when Queen Victoria inhaled chloroform in childbirth. Simpson was subsequently knighted by Queen Victoria.

Immediately after the first published report of Morton's successful etherization of human beings in 1846, ether was used on animal patients in the Royal Veterinary College of London. When chloroform was introduced as an anesthetic by Sir James Simpson in 1847, it was accepted widely by the veterinary profession, especially for anesthesia of horses. The use of chloroform for large animal anesthesia spread rapidly throughout the world. In small animals chloroform proved to be somewhat potent and toxic, and ether was preferred for these patients.

PHARMACOLOGICAL CONSIDERATIONS

Dr. Oliver Wendell Holmes, author and teacher of medicine, coined the term *anesthesia,* meaning "without sensation." The loss of sensation is accomplished by reversibly depressing the activity of nervous tissue either locally or generally over the body. *Local anesthesia* or *local analgesia* involves the loss of sensation of a limited area of the body. *Regional anesthesia* is the loss of sensation in a larger, although limited, area of the body. *General anesthesia* means a loss of sensation of the whole body. Anesthetizing a patient with drugs currently available results in a state of unconsciousness as well as a loss of sensation. *Surgical anesthesia* is a state of depression of the CNS characterized by a loss of all sensation and consciousness that permits painless surgery and provides the muscular relaxation necessary for various operations. *Basal anesthesia* is a lighter level of anesthesia produced generally by preanesthetic medication. The patient becomes unconscious but is not sufficiently depressed for surgery. A condition resembling normal deep sleep results from *hypnosis,* which causes moderate depression of the CNS. *Sedation* is a milder degree of central depression in which the patient is awake but calm and free of nervousness. *Analgesia* refers to the relief of pain without unconsciousness or sleep. *Nothria* refers to a torpid or stuporous state and is a term used to define mental and motor inactivity of the nervous system. *Intrathecal* or *spinal* anesthesia occurs following the introduction of a local anesthetic into the spinal fluid. *Epidural* or *extradural* anesthesia follows the administration of a local anesthetic into the epidural space. *Ataraxia* means "not disturbed," perfect peace or calmness of mind as applied to human medicine. Ataractic or neuroleptic agents are generally the same drugs as the tranquilizers. *Narcosis* is defined as analgesia accompanied by deep sleep. This is a vague and often misused term; it probably should be dropped from common medical usage. *Neuroleptanalgesia* (NLA) refers to the combined use of tranquilizers and analgesics. The drug combination is used to induce psychomotor sedation (neurolepsia) and analgesia from which the name of neuroleptanalgesia was derived. The primary objective underlying the principle of NLA is to provide a method of anesthesia for major operations to avoid the severe CNS, cardiovascular, and metabolic depressant effects of conventional anesthetics.

The major effect of the general anesthetics is to depress the CNS. In most instances the depressant effect is preceded by a period of excitement. A successful general anesthetic depresses the cortical centers first, the spinal centers next, and the medullary centers last. The vital medullary centers must be less susceptible than other areas for the general anesthetic to be clinically acceptable.

GENERAL CONSIDERATIONS IN SELECTION OF ANESTHETICS

1. The *nature of the surgery* to be performed, its *duration,* and its *location* are necessary considerations. Some operations have special anesthetic requirements as, for example, a cesarean section, in which the effect of the anesthetic upon the fetus must be considered as much as its effect upon the maternal subject. Some operations preclude the use of the most obvious anesthetic method by the nature of tissues involved. For example, a "capped" elbow in the horse cannot be effectively infiltrated by a local anesthetic because of the subdermal fibrosis. Sometimes the nearby structures produce a movement of the operative site, so general instead of local anesthesia must be used to stop the movement. An example of the latter would be an incision of a deeply situated abscess in the area of the pharynx.

2. The anatomical or physiological pe-

culiarities of the *species* or breed involved, as well as the temperament and size of the animal, influence the selection of an anesthetic.

a. Horse—Usually, the horse must be cast on the ground to insure safety of the operator and the patient in some simple operations. Some operations in the horse involving the foot or leg can be carried out in the standing position by paraneural injection. In general, the horse requires more anesthesia and restraint than most other species of animals. However, the proper use of neuroleptic, tranquilizing, and preanesthetic agents have significantly reduced the problems associated with the restraint of the large animal.

b. Ruminant—The large forestomachs, with the great amount of ingesta invariably present, render ruminants generally unsuitable for operation under general anesthesia. If general anesthetics are used, precautions should be taken to insure against regurgitation of ruminal contents and the resultant obstruction of the airway. Also, gas accumulation (bloat) must be prevented so venous return to the heart is not impeded by distension of the rumen. Local or regional anesthesia is used frequently in ruminants to avoid the complications arising from the use of general anesthetics.

c. Swine—Although local anesthesia is commonly employed in swine, it is not entirely satisfactory because of the constant squealing and struggling that is often provoked by restraint of this species. Because of the obese characteristics of the pig, the risks of administering general anesthetics are generally greater than in many of the other species. Nevertheless, thiobarbiturates given intravenously for induction of anesthesia, followed by inhalant anesthetic agents such as halothane and nitrous oxide or methoxyflurane for maintenance of anesthesia, work satisfactorily in swine. Once an airway has been established, the danger of apnea and/or hypoventilation can be avoided following the use of general anesthetics.

d. Dog and cat—General anesthetics, both parenteral and inhalant, are widely and easily used in these species. Dissociative anesthetics and neuroleptanalgesic agents have received extensive use during the last few years. Also, local anesthesia is used in the dog and cat for certain operations.

e. Avian species—Parenteral and inhalant anesthetics are used successfully in domestic fowl and in caged birds such as parakeets and canaries. Procaine is contraindicated in the parakeet because of its lethal effect.

3. *Species susceptibilities* to various depressant drugs must not be overlooked. For example, ketamine has been approved for use in only the cat and subhuman primates. The fentanyl-droperidol (Innovar-Vet) combination is usually restricted to use in the dog and various small laboratory animals. Morphine and meperidine, if not used in proper dosage, can produce severe excitement and even convulsions in the cat. In the greyhound, compared to other canine species, increased sensitivity to the thiobarbiturates is noted.

4. The *susceptibility of the patient* to toxic action of anesthetic drugs is increased by the following factors:

a. Prolonged fasting depletes the glycogen reserves in the liver, thus reducing the ability of that organ to detoxify toxic substances.

b. Many diseased conditions produce degenerative changes in vital organs of the body that render them more susceptible than usual to the toxic action of anesthetics. The liver, kidneys, lungs, and heart are especially susceptible to the toxic effects of halogenated anesthetics and certain other depressants when initially showing tissue degeneration from a disease process. In respiratory complications, irritating agents such as ether and chloroform should never be used.

Clinical laboratory tests should be made to determine the hematological status of the animal. Also, other tests should be conducted to determine the functional status of the kidneys. Urine should be examined to determine the specific gravity, presence of cell casts, albumin, and enzyme activity. Of importance in the detection of acute renal tubular damage is the conduct of enzyme tests such as glutamic oxalacetic transaminase (GOT), isocitric dehydrogenase (ICDH), and lactic dehydrogenase (LDH) in urine and serum (Szczech et al. 1974). The blood urea nitrogen (BUN) should also be determined in the assessment of renal function.

5. The clinician must be familiar with the various *drug interactions* that may jeopardize the life of the animal patient. For example, phenothiazine tranquilizers and certain neuromuscular relaxants should not be employed in animals that have been previously exposed to organophosphates. The use of barbiturate anesthetics following agents that inhibit or suppress hepatic microsomal enzyme activity must be avoided. It is well established that the sleeping time of pentobarbital sodium is prolonged following the suppression of microsomal enzyme activity by prior treatment with chloramphenicol.

6. An *elevated or low ambient temperature* may influence the toxicity of drugs (Weihe 1973). This is particularly true in the poikilothermic animals. However, homeothermic animals may also suffer adversely from drugs if extremes in temperatures exist during and following surgical anesthesia. Drug absorption following the subcutaneous and intramuscular administration of drugs may be affected by environmental temperature extremes. For example, a therapeutic dose of procaine hydrochloride may produce violent convulsive seizures in young puppies when it is used in tail docking during extremely hot weather. Recovery rooms following surgical anesthesia should not be cold. Otherwise, prolonged recovery as well as respiratory and other functional complications will occur.

7. *Legal responsibilities* exist in some countries, such as the United Kingdom where the Protection of Animals Act requires that certain operations be performed only under a general anesthetic or local analgesic. In the United States, the Animal Welfare Act as amended in 1970 requires the use of analgesic and/or anesthetic agents in all warm-blooded animal species used in experimental studies where operative procedures are involved. Only under certain conditions where the experimental results would be invalidated by the use of these agents is it permissible not to employ them. An annual report must be submitted to the U.S. Department of Agriculture by all research laboratories that use experimental animals along with information regarding the analgesic or anesthetic agents used in connection with the operative procedures undertaken.

EXAMINATION OF PATIENT

Careful examination of a patient to determine that it is a good anesthetic risk cannot be overemphasized. Many patients have died and many reputations have been damaged by administering an anesthetic to patients that were not good anesthetic risks. If an operation must be performed for the relief of disease, inquiry into the history of the case should be made. Based upon the physical condition of the animal, an anesthetic agent should be wisely selected to minimize the risks and hazards involved during and following an operative procedure.

PREPARATION OF PATIENT FOR ANESTHESIA

Some operations are performed in an emergency, when little preparation is possible. However, the majority of operations are planned, in which case the patient can be examined and put on a limited feed intake. Generally, feed is withheld 8–12 hours in small animals and 12–24 hours in large animals before the operation is to be performed under general anesthesia (Booth 1969). Also, it is recommended that liquids be withheld for 2 hours (Rawlings 1975). The presence of ingesta in the stomach or rumen may interfere with free movement of the diaphragm and predispose to respiratory difficulty. Moreover, gaseous distention occurring from fermentative processes may result in the interference of venous return to the heart in both nonruminant and ruminant animals. Animals that vomit readily must be fasted in order to decrease vomition during anesthesia with the resultant hazard of mechanical pneumonia as well as contamination of instruments and the operative field. On the other hand, excessive fasting may devitalize the tissues and expose the patient to unnecessary anesthetic risk. In some animals, particularly toxemic, dehydrated, and debilitated patients, fluid therapy to correct metabolic and acid-base balance needs should be employed during and following anesthesia. All poor-risk patients should be carefully monitored, including the assessment of central venous pressure (Jennings et al. 1967) and renal function. An indwelling catheter system for intravenous use should always be ready for any emergency eventuality.

All dogs and especially those over 4 years of age undergoing anesthesia and surgical procedures should have complete hematological evaluation, urinalysis, and BUN determination (Rosin 1974). The specific gravity of urine is valuable in identifying those surgical patients with a high risk of renal failure prior to anesthesia. A urine specific gravity of 1.008–1.012 is generally a good indicator of renal disease, especially if the specific gravity remains at this level after a water deprivation test or pitressin concentration test, or if the animal was dehydrated or uremic at the time the isosthenuric urine sample was collected (Osborne et al. 1972). Unfortunately, two-thirds of the functional kidney tissue must be diseased or nonfunctional before low specific gravity urine or isosthenuria is noted. Nevertheless, all patients with two-thirds renal dysfunction to normal function are potential subjects for renal failure following surgical anesthesia. Those patients with greater renal dysfunction are more likely to develop postsurgical uremia (Rosin 1974). To enable the maintenance of adequate renal function in the dog and to minimize post-surgical uremia, the procedure as follows is recommended (Rosin 1974):

1. Atropine sulfate (0.02–0.03 mg/lb) and acetylpromazine maleate (1 mg/20 lb) are given intramuscularly 15–20 minutes prior to induction of anesthesia.
2. An intravenous catheter is positioned into the external jugular vein and inserted to the level of the right atrium. The catheter system is then available to measure central venous pressure (Jennings et al. 1967) and to administer various fluid medications whenever needed.
3. A urinary catheter is placed in the bladder; the bladder is emptied so urine volume may be measured. The normal urine flow in the dog ranges between 0.8 and 2 ml/lb/hr.
4. The intravenous administration of lactated Ringer's solution is started at the rate of 40 ml/lb over the course of the surgical procedure.
5. Furosemide (Lasix) in a dosage of 2.5 mg/lb is administered intravenously. Diuresis should occur at an anticipated level of 2–4 ml/lb/hr. If the urine flow is inadequate, the dosage of furosemide should be repeated.
6. Induction of anesthesia is accomplished with thiamylal sodium (Surital sodium) or nitrous oxide and halothane by nose cone or mask. Endotracheal intubation is performed after induction of anesthesia and maintenance of anesthesia is continued with nitrous oxide–oxygen and halothane. Use of an intermittent positive pressure respirator (Bird Mark 6A) to assist ventilation is also recommended.

Preanesthetic Medication

Preanesthetic medication is a general term referring to the administration of some agent shortly before anesthesia is administered. The principal objective of preanesthetic medication is to permit smooth and safe induction of anesthesia as well as to permit the establishment of balanced anesthesia in the animal patient. Preanesthetics can be categorized as anticholinergic drugs, adrenergic blocking agents, tranquilizers, hypnotics, neuroleptanalgesics and narcotic analgesics. Examples of some of the preanesthetic agents are acetylpromazine, promazine, morphine, meperidine, fentanyl-droperidol mixture, xylazine, ketamine, barbiturates, chloral hydrate, atropine, and phentolamine. A summary of recommended dosages for some of the more common preanesthetic agents has been compiled for the various animal species in Table 10.1.

In the selection of the preanesthetic agents, consideration must be given to whether or not the animal species involved will respond properly to the agents selected. For example, ketamine is tolerated best in the cat and subhuman primates compared to the dog and other animal species. Conversely, the combination of fentanyl-droperidol is tolerated by dogs but has not been advocated in the cat. Also, the preanesthetics should be selected on the basis of the physical status of the patient, degree of restraint required for handling the animal, surgical procedure involved, and the complications that one is likely to encounter during the anesthetic procedure.

In addition, possible animal species interactions or idiosyncrasies to drugs and dosage levels must be considered. Morphine and meperidine, if not used in proper dosage, can produce excitement in the cat.

Inasmuch as the principal objectives in the use of anesthetic agents are directed toward the alleviation of pain during an operative procedure and to minimize the risk of the procedure to the life of the animal patient, only trained individuals who are knowledgeable with the stages and planes of anesthesia should administer anesthetics. This implies explicitly that considerable pharmacological knowledge must be obtained because anesthetics are extremely potent and toxic drugs. It also means that training must be acquired in recognizing the variations of drug reactions that occur in the different animal species. Also, training in meeting the emergencies that frequently result unexpectedly during anesthesia and postanesthesia must be included as a part of the training in veterinary anesthesiology.

With the introduction of more potent inhalant anesthetics and neuroleptanalgesic agents, it is more difficult to determine the depth of anesthesia and the condition of the animal patient. Nevertheless, the clinical signs of anesthesia still have important application in the empirical assessment of the patient's general condition. The patient must be unconscious and must not exhibit undesirable reflex activity during an operative procedure (Rex 1972). Under circumstances where the clinical signs of anesthesia are not easily assessed, major importance should be placed upon monitoring respiratory and cardiac activities. In addition, the body temperature should be closely watched to avoid hypothermic or hyperthermic responses during the course of anesthesia.

METHODS OF ADMINISTRATION OF GENERAL ANESTHETICS

General anesthetics are largely administered by inhalation or by intravenous injection. Other routes of administration are also used such as intramuscular, oral, rectal, intraperitoneal, and intrathoracic. Volatile liquids (ether, halothane, methoxyflurane, cyclopropane) anesthetize by inhalation of vapors.

Inhalation

The volatile anesthetics are primarily administered via the semiclosed system or the closed system. With excellent textbooks on anesthetic equipment available for use of volatile anesthetics, the reader is referred to these sources of information (Hall

TABLE 10.1. Recommended dosages* of commonly used preanesthetic agents in various domestic animals

Drug	Dog	Cat	Pig	Goats Sheep	Cow	Horse
Atropine sulfate	0.02 mg/lb (SC)	0.02 mg/lb (SC)	0.03–0.04 mg/lb (IM)	0.09 mg/lb (IV/15 min)	2 mg/100 lb (IM)	2 mg/100 lb (IM)
Scopolamine hydrobromide	0.005–0.01 mg/lb (SC)	0.005–0.01 mg/lb (SC)	...	...	...	...
Morphine sulfate†	0.05–1 mg/lb (SC)	0.045 mg/lb (SC)	...	...	...	...
Meperidine hydrochloride	2–5 mg/lb (IM)	2–5 mg/lb (IM)	0.5–1 mg/lb (IM)	...	300–600 mg (total dose IM)	200–400 mg (total dose IM)
Fentanyl-Droperidol (Innovar-Vet)	(1 cc/15–20 lb IM or 1 cc/25–60 lb IV)	NR	NR	NR	NR	NR
Xylazine	0.5 mg/lb (IM)	0.25–0.5 mg/lb (IM)	...	...	...	0.25–0.5 mg/lb (IV)
Acetylpromazine	1 mg/20 lb (IM or IV)	0.05 mg/lb (IM or IV)	0.01–0.04 mg/lb (IM or IV)	NR	NR	15 mg/1000 lb (IV)

* Routes of administration: SC = subcutaneous; IM = intramuscular; IV = intravenous; NR = not recommended.
† Morphine sulfate should be used in conjunction with *d*-propoxyphene (Darvon) 1 mg/lb IM or chlorpromazine 2 mg/lb IM in the cat.

1971; Soma 1971; Lumb and Jones 1973). Halothane, methoxyflurane, and nitrous oxide in combination with oxygen are the major volatile anesthetics used in the maintenance of surgical anesthesia. Preanesthetic agents and ultrashort-acting barbiturates (thiamylal, thiopental, methohexital) are usually administered to enable endotracheal intubation prior to the administration of volatile anesthetics.

INTRAVENOUS

In several animal species, depending upon the surgical procedure, only intravenous anesthetics such as the barbiturates may be employed. Barbiturate anesthesia is generally preceded by the administration of atropine sulfate; other preanesthetic agents may or may not be used. At one time pentobarbital sodium was the principal intravenous anesthetic used in veterinary medicine. However, safer procedures using the technique of balanced anesthesia have essentially replaced pentobarbital in modern veterinary practice. The ultrashort barbiturates (thiamylal, thiopental, methohexital) are used intravenously primarily to permit endotracheal intubation prior to the administration of inhalant anesthetics for maintenance anesthesia.

The intravenous route of administration may be employed in the cat when ketamine, a dissociative anesthetic, is used. In the dog, a neuroleptanalgesic agent, i.e., fentanyl-droperidol combination (Innovar-Vet), may also be administered intravenously.

INTRAMUSCULAR

Dissociative anesthetics (ketamine, phencyclidine) are administered primarily by the intramuscular route. This is advantageous in the cat and subhuman primates because the injection can usually be administered more rapidly and with minimal restraint compared to the intravenous route of administration. However, the administration of anesthetics by the intramuscular route is also a disadvantage because the depth of anesthesia is not as easily controlled compared with the intravenous or inhalational administration of anesthetic agents.

INTRAPERITONEAL

Intraperitoneal injections of general anesthetics are infrequently made. Sometimes this route of administration is preferred for barbiturates in euthanasia, as in a vicious dog or cat where giving the drug by other routes of administration may be more difficult.

INTRATHORACIC

The intrathoracic injection of barbiturates in cats is not recommended as an acceptable clinical procedure because tissue injury and necrosis of the lungs have resulted. When rapid anesthesia is essential, as in euthanasia, and an intravenous injection is difficult to make, the intrathoracic route of administration may be convenient to use.

ORAL

Oral administration of anesthetics is recommended only for sedative or hypnotic effects in several species or for anesthesia in unapproachable, vicious animals, especially wild carnivores. The drug is given in a piece of meat or other bait. Pentobarbital sodium powder has been placed in milk to capture wild domestic cats. For this purpose, it is necessary to sweeten the milk with sugar to mask the bitter taste of the barbiturate. If this is not done, most animals will refuse to drink the milk. In those that can tolerate drinking the unsweetened milk, vomition is apt to occur soon after ingestion and no drug effect is produced.

Much variation in effect is noted following oral administration apparently due to the influence of ingesta upon absorption from the gut.

PROPERTIES OF A DESIRABLE GENERAL ANESTHETIC

The ideal general anesthetic should be nonirritant and free from disagreeable odors. It must be potent; produce a pleasant, rapid, and smooth induction; and allow a rapid recovery. The margin of safety should be wide. Muscular relaxation must be adequate for surgical procedures. Capillary bleeding should not be promoted. It must be easily and inexpensively produced, and it should be nonexplosive and stable during storage. The excretion and/or metabolism of anesthetic agents should be sufficiently rapid so that residues do not persist in the edible tissues (meat, milk, eggs) of food-producing animals.

MODE OF ACTION OF GENERAL ANESTHETICS

The mode of action of anesthetics has been studied for many decades without a satisfactory explanation and there is still no clear explanation regarding the mechanism of action of anesthetic agents. In 1900 Meyer and Overton independently reported their investigations dealing with the physical and chemical properties of hundreds of compounds with varying depressive effects upon the CNS. Their data were concerned primarily with the proportional distribution of anesthetic drugs in the aqueous and lipoidal (fatty) phases of the tissues and the correlation of these ratios with the anesthetic potency of the drugs upon living organisms. Meyer and Overton contended that to be anesthetic, a drug must be soluble both in oil (lipoid) and in water. The higher the solubility in oil, the greater was its anesthetic potency. Data for the older volatile anesthetics, ether and chloroform, fit conveniently into the above hypothesis, but at present there are many objections to the Meyer-Overton theory. It was clearly a worthy contribution in 1900 because it organized unsorted data into a working hypothesis, but today the Meyer-Overton postulates are more of a statement of the distribution of anesthetics within the body than an explanation of their activity.

Of the various theories of anesthesia proposed by physiologists, biochemists, and molecular biologists, none of them has been unequivocally proved or disproved. The phenomenon of general anesthesia is distinguished from most other drug actions in that the effects produced upon the CNS are reversible. A general but descriptive definition of an anesthetic is a drug which, upon direct application to the nerve or muscle cell, reversibly blocks the action potential without appreciably affecting the resting membrane potential (within 4–5 mV) of the cell (Seeman 1972). Based upon this definition, a number of lipid-soluble compounds are anesthetics, including narcotics, sedatives, tranquilizers, anticonvulsants, antihistamines, steroids, detergents, vasodilators, and antiarrhythmic agents.

There are also irreversible anesthetics such as the haloalkylamines, which produce sustained anesthesia of the nervous tissue. The compounds alkylate the excitable membrane and remain attached to it apparently without depolarizing or damaging the nerve cell.

In 1961 molecular theories of general anesthesia were independently introduced by Pauling and Miller. In essence, Pauling's theory states that simple molecules may be linked together by hydrogen bonding as the result of instantaneous dipole moment. Clathrates, cages, or lattices are formed and their cavities or interstices may be occupied by second molecules, i.e., a gas or volatile anesthetic, to form hydrate microcrystals ("icebergs"). It is known that chloroform will form a hydrate that at 2° C decomposes to water and liquid chloroform. On the other hand, the inert gas xenon has anesthetic properties at high pressures that can stabilize a hydrate crystal with a resultant higher temperature of decomposition.

Pauling's hydrate microcrystal theory was developed from the knowledge that alkylammonium salt would interact with a clathrate structure resembling xenon hydrate. The resemblance of this salt to certain hydrophobic protein side chains suggested that brain proteins could form stable hydrates at body temperature in the presence of an anesthetic gas. Theoretical ly, the microcrystal thus formed could disrupt ionic mobility, electrical charge, and chemical and enzymatic activity of the brain so consciousness was "switched off." Interestingly, a close correlation was observed between the depressant effects of the partial pressures of anesthetics and the partial pressure required to form hydrate crystals.

It is not known whether hypothermia and the subsequent anesthesia that is maintained in the absence of an anesthetic can be ascribed to the formation of hydrate microcrystals. Apparently at a temperature of 27° C, a sufficient number of empty cages or lattices appear that are stable in the absence of an anesthetic gas. Also, it is not known if the phenomenon of hibernation in some animal species is related to the development of so-called stable or semistable lattices or clathrates when the environmental temperature declines. Other factors such as changes in metabolism and endocrine activity in addition to a lowered environmental temperature have been associated with triggering hibernation.

The hydrate microcrystal or "iceberg" theory fails to explain, at least directly, the mechanism of anesthesia induced by barbiturates and other chemical compounds. Although molecules with strong hydrogen bonds are not compatible with the theory, diethyl ether probably interacts like other nonhydrogen bonding anesthetics by its electron correlative reactivity with water molecules. There are other proposals that appear to better explain how other anesthetics, including the barbiturates, work on the CNS than Pauling's or Miller's theory. For example, it has long been speculated that biomembranes should expand in the presence of anesthetics because anesthetics can penetrate and expand films spread at the air-water interface. These observations led to the experimental finding that anesthetics do indeed expand biomembranes. In an attempt to understand the events of the anesthetic-induced biomembrane expansion, the simplest mechanism to be considered first was the observation revealing that a volume change, i.e., an increase in the volume of the membrane took place with the "burying" or peneration of the anesthetic molecules into the membrane. The amount of membrane volume expansion or membrane area expansion is of the order of 10 times the bulk volume of the anesthetic molecules that are absorbed in the membrane phase (Seeman 1972). It has been observed that surgical concentrations of halothane, chloroform, ether, and methoxyflurane expand human erythrocyte membranes about 0.4% in area, which is equivalent to about 0.6% increase in membrane volume.

The mechanisms of membrane expansion by anesthetics are not fully understood but appear to be attributable to factors as follows:

1. Membrane expansion is caused by anesthetic-induced microcrystals ("ice-formation") in the membrane as suggested previously by the theory advanced by Pauling (1961).

2. Anesthetics are known to produce conformational changes in proteins. It is possible that when the membrane expands there is an expansion or distortion of the membrane proteins.

3. Alteration in the membrane Ca^{++} may be responsible for the membrane expansion. Chlorpromazine and the amine anesthetics (procaine and tetracaine) can displace membrane-bound Ca^{++} and this leads to an unexplainable expansion of the membrane.

4. Expansion of the membrane may be induced by an anesthetic inhibition of a contractile membrane-associated ATPase. It has been shown that the phenothiazine local anesthetics have membrane-expanding actions at concentrations that only very slightly inhibit the $(Na^{+}–K^{+})$–ATPase of the membrane.

If an increase in body temperature induces membrane expansion, the question naturally arises why membrane narcosis does not occur. It may be that the anesthetic expands only the hydrophobic regions of the membrane, whereas heating the membrane results in the expansion and deformation of all membrane components (Seeman 1972).

In addition to membrane expansion, anesthetics result in a "loosening" or fluidization of the membrane components. Evidence exists that the anesthetics "melt" or fluidize the membrane-associated water. Experimental studies have revealed that neutral or charged anesthetics will increase the hydraulic flow of water molecules through the erythrocyte membrane. These findings do little to support the interesting anesthetic theory of Pauling's on the formation of ice microcrystals.

Neurosecretion is also enhanced by anesthetics and may be the result of membrane fluidization. The increased fluidity of both the cell membrane (plasmalemma) and the membranes of the secretion granules (vesicles) may lead to membrane fusion. Phenothiazine tranquilizers, reserpine, and local anesthetics release 5-hydroxytryptamine (serotonin), apparently causing membrane-membrane fusion. Anesthetic-induced neurosecretion can lead to either depressant or excitant effects, which are dependent upon the distribution of the anesthetic and upon which neurosecretory cells are most affected. Excitation or extrapyramidal disorders (i.e., Parkinsonianlike symptoms such as tremors, rigidity, salivation, and akinesia) can occur from the increased neurosecretory release of dopamine by morphine, reserpine, or chlorpromazine. Morphine administration in the cat increases the release of dopamine and may explain susceptibility of the cat to the action of this drug. Administration of phenol in the cat markedly increases nerve synaptic response. This synaptic facilitation has been observed to be both excitatory and inhibitory and supports the view that convulsant phenols act by increasing the release of neurotransmitting chemical substances. Although anesthetics stimulate neurosecretion, their major effect on synaptic or junctional transmission is to induce depression in most cases. Presumably under these circumstances the presynaptic depression of the action potential, as well as the postsynaptic inhibition of excitability, are dominant factors that have a masking effect over the enhanced neurosecretion. A summary of the membrane actions of anesthetics and tranquilizers is shown in Fig. 10.1.

An interesting aspect related to the mode of action of anesthetics is that reversal of general and local anesthesia can be produced by high atmospheric pressure. A compression pressure that reverses anesthesia has been identified to be about 0.4%, which is equal and opposite to that capable of expansion of erythrocyte membranes that have been subjected to anesthetic agents. The pressure reversal of anesthesia has led to the formulation of the critical volume hypothesis (Lever et al. 1971; Miller et al. 1973). This hypothesis refers to the induction of anethesia when the volume of a hydrophobic region is expanded beyond a certain critical volume by the absorption of an inert material. Pressure applied in opposition to this expansion will reverse anesthesia. When this hypothesis is extended to include pressures of a considerable magnitude, it includes the assumption that convulsions occur when some hydrophobic region has been compressed beyond a certain critical level (Miller 1974). In deep sea diving it is well known that nitrogen narcosis occurs despite the fact that nitrogen is a so-called inert gas. The deterrent to deep sea diving to excessive depths (i.e., 2000 feet) has been due to the adverse neurological effects of the high pressure (ca. 60 atmospheres). In human beings hyperexcitability has been observed at about 20 atmospheres of pressure, and pressures of 60 atmospheres and higher have elicited convulsive seizures in animals. Miller (1974) has shown in mice that anesthesia occurs at an expansion of 1.1% and convulsions occur at a compression of 0.85%. All the anesthetic theories that have been discussed are certainly useful and would appear to explain the variance in effect (i.e., CNS depression or CNS stimulation) of some of the newer pharmacologic agents such as the neuroleptanalgesics and dissociative anesthetics. Ketamine, for example, will produce CNS depression at a lower dosage level but will induce convulsive seizures at higher levels. In the case of some of the older drugs, high dosages of procaine, morphine, meperidine, and the phenothiazine tranquilizers will produce extrapyramidal disorders, hyper-

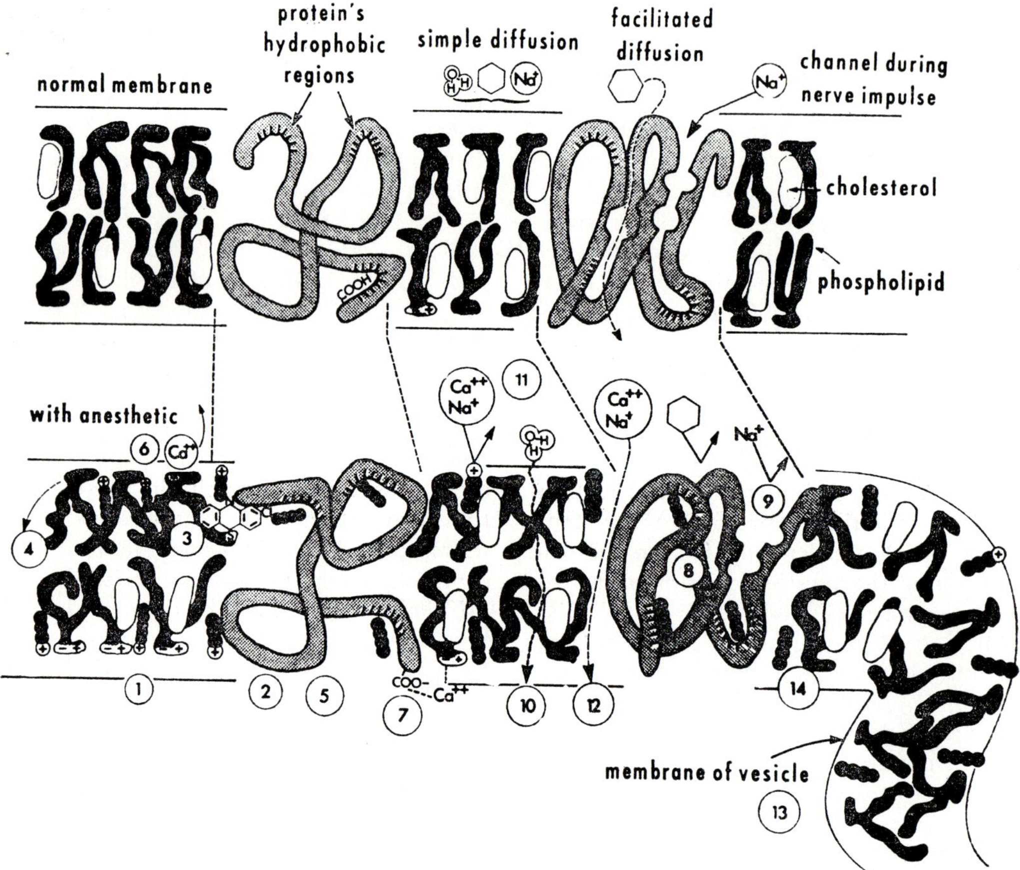

FIG. 10.1. Diagrammatic summary of the membrane actions of anesthetics and tranquilizers.

(1) Drug occupation of membrane by 0.3% in local anesthesia (0.03% in general anesthesia); *(2)* expansion of membrane by 2% in local anesthesia (0.4% in general anesthesia); membrane pressure alters; *(3)* increased rotational mobility of membrane units ("fluidization," disordering); *(4)* decreased translocation of membrane lipids; *(5)* activation or inhibition of membrane enzymes, resulting from expansion of membrane protein; *(6)* displacement of membrane Ca^{++} by anesthetic amines; *(7)* increase in membrane Ca^{++} by neutral anesthetics; *(8)* decreased facilitated diffusion of neutral solutes (glucose, choline); *(9) membrane electrostabilization* = decreased facilitated diffusion of ions during nerve impulse (Na^+, K^+); *(10)* increased passive (Fick) diffusion of neutral solutes (water, urea); *(11)* anesthetic amines decrease passive (Fick) diffusion of ions (Ca^{++} or Na^+); *(12)* neutral anesthetics increase passive (Fick) diffusion of ions Ca^{++} or Na^+); *(13)* increased membrane-membrane fusion (i.e., increased neurosecretion); *(14)* dissociation of lipid-protein complexes (at high anesthetic concentrations). (From Seeman 1972)

excitability, and convulsive seizures. From all evidence accumulated to date, the theory dealing with the deformation of biomembranes through expansion, volume change, and fluidization appears to explain best the mode of action of anesthetic agents.

REFERENCES

Berger, R. J. 1975. Bioenergetic functions of sleep and activity rhythms and their possible relevance to aging. Fed Proc 34:97.

Booth, N. H. 1969. Anesthesia in the pig. Fed Proc 28:1547.

Hall, L. W. 1971. Wright's Veterinary Anaesthesia and Analgesia, 7th ed., p. 499. Baltimore: Williams & Wilkins.

Jennings, P. B.; Anderson, R. W.; and Martin, A. M., Jr. 1967. Central venous pressure monitoring: A guide to blood volume replacement in the dog. J Am Vet Med Assoc 151:1283.

Lever, M. J.; Miller, K. W.; Paton, W. D. M; and Smith, E. B. 1971. Pressure reversal of anaesthesia. Nature (Lond) 231:368.

Lumb, W. V., and Jones, E. W. 1973. Veterinary Anesthesia, p. 680. Philadelphia: Lea & Febiger.

Melzak, R., and Wall, P. D. 1965. Pain mechanisms, a new theory. Science 150:971.

Miller, K. W. 1974. Inert gas narcosis, the high pressure neurological syndrome, and the critical volume hypothesis. Science 185:867.

Miller, K. W.; Paton, W. D. M.; Smith, R. A.; and Smith, E. B. 1973. The pressure reversal of general anesthesia and the critical volume hypothesis. Mol Pharmacol 9:131.

Miller, S. L. 1961. A theory of gaseous anesthetics. Proc Natl Acad Sci USA 47:1515.

Oldendorf, W. H. 1974. Blood-brain barrier permeability to drugs. Annu Rev Pharmacol 14:239.

Osborne, C. A.; Low, D. G.; and Finco, D. R. 1972. Canine and Feline Urology. Philadelphia: W. B. Saunders.

Pauling, L. 1961. A molecular theory of general anesthesia. Science 134:15.

Rawlings, C. A. 1975. University of Georgia. Personal communication.

Rex, M. A. E. 1972. Principles of anaesthesia. Aust Vet J 48:677.

Rosin, E. 1974. University of Georgia. Personal communication.

Seeman, P. 1972. The membrane actions of anesthetics and tranquilizers. Pharmacol Rev 24:583.

Soma, L. R. 1971. Textbook of Veterinary Anesthesia, p. 621. Baltimore: Williams & Wilkins.

Szczech, G. M.; Carlton, W. W.; and Lund, J. E. 1974. Determination of enzyme concentrations in urine for diagnosis of renal damage. J Am Anim Hosp Assoc 10:171.

Weihe, W. H. 1973. The effect of temperature on the action of drugs. Annu Rev Pharmacol 13:409.

CHAPTER 11

CLINICAL STAGES OF GENERAL ANESTHESIA

NICHOLAS H. BOOTH

The clinical response of the patient has been divided arbitrarily into various levels using the neuromuscular reflexes as criteria for classification of the depth of anesthesia. The central nervous system (CNS) may be depressed progressively through each of the clinical levels of anesthesia until death occurs. The level of depression may be reversed or approximately maintained for a period of time if administration of the depressant is readily controlled, as with a volatile anesthetic. The discussion of the clinical stages of general anesthesia in this chapter deals primarily with the progressive clinical response as observed in the administration of a volatile anesthetic. A similar response can be observed following intravenous injection of a nonvolatile anesthetic, although in clinical practice the first part of the dose is injected rapidly to minimize the early excitatory stages.

Some of the following generalizations do not fit all species of animals, i.e., nystagmus is prominent in the horse but practically absent in the dog. Even within the same species the stages and planes may vary markedly. In human beings the stages and planes of anesthesia can be delineated in approximately 90% of the subjects anesthetized.

It is generally concluded that the technique and art of employing anesthetic agents is primarily empirical and is principally gained through clinical experience. Objective methods in the assessment of the depth of anesthesia do not appear to be possible in the immediate future (Robson 1969). For example, sensory-evoked responses (i.e., auditory and visual) and electroencephalography in the determination of the depth of anesthesia do not provide ready means of assessing the depth of anesthesia within the limits of use.

General anesthesia is clinically delineated into four stages.

STAGE I: VOLUNTARY EXCITEMENT OR STAGE OF ANALGESIA

Excitement and struggling by the patient are the most characteristic features. To reduce the excitement, struggling, and undesirable reflexes of animals during induction of anesthesia, preanesthetics are employed that minimize or abolish this response; see Chapter 10 for discussion of the preanesthetic agents. Rapid-acting and potent anesthetics are generally given intravenously to avoid the excitatory response of animals so that inhalant anesthetics such as halothane or methoxyflurane may be administered to maintain surgical anesthesia.

Forced inhalation in animals of a strange, irritant gas under unusual circumstances causes great fear, with the subsequent release of epinephrine and vigorous struggling against restraint. The heart beats faster and stronger and the respiration becomes rapid and deep. Regular administration of the anesthetic is difficult, due to the struggling of the patient. The pupil dilates from the excitement. Urine and feces may be voided. This is the *stage of analgesia* without loss of consciousness.

STAGE II: INVOLUNTARY EXCITEMENT

This stage begins with depression of the cortical centers with a loss of consciousness and volitional control. The subconscious emotions, concerned primarily with survival, dictate the patient's actions. With slow induction of anesthesia that is characteristic of inhalant anesthetics, the patient reacts to any sort of external stimuli with exaggerated reflex struggling or purposeless muscular movement. The intravenous administration of rapid-acting and potent agents, such as thiamylal, thiopental, or other similar agents, avoids the undesirable characteristics of this stage of anesthesia. Occasionally, severe excitement or delirium may occur following the use of these agents when the dosage given is inadequate to carry the animal into Stage III.

If the induction of anesthesia is slow, the horse may neigh and the dog may whine or emit small barks. Vigorous "running" or "galloping" movements of the legs may occur. Occasionally some animals show little reflex activity. Respiration and pulse are influenced by the degree of excitement and exertion. Generally the pulse is rapid and strong. Commonly in the early part and sometimes throughout this stage, respiration is uneven in depth and rate, and breath holding may occur. The eyelids are wide open and the pupils are dilated because of the sympathetic stimulation. Reactivity of the eye to light (photomotor reflex) is retained. The photomotor reflex is a useful indicator in the dog during the return of consciousness when succinylcholine hydrochloride or other skeletal muscle relaxant has been administered in conjunction with a barbiturate anesthetic or ether (Croft 1961).

In the horse, orbital movement of the eyeball (nystagmus) is characteristic of the latter part of this period. Movement of the eyeball may occur in the rabbit and other species but it is never as prominent as in the horse. In the dog, reflex vomition is common unless feed has been withheld for 8 or more hours before anesthesia. Stage II may pass gradually into Stage III or the patient may suddenly relax and appear to go soundly to sleep with even, moderate breathing and strong pulse, which are characteristic of the next stage. Stage II should be passed through rapidly in most animal anesthesia to reduce the hazard of injury to the anesthetist and, in the case of a horse or other large animal, to protect the patient from injuring itself. There is, of course, a maximum limit to the rate of administering an anesthetic that must be heeded in order not to paralyze the respiratory center by excessive concentrations of anesthetic.

Stages I and II together constitute the period referred to as *induction.*

STAGE III: SURGICAL ANESTHESIA

During this stage, depressant action of the anesthetic is extended from the cortex and midbrain to the spinal cord. Consciousness, pain sensation, and spinal reflexes are abolished. Muscular relaxation occurs and coordinated movement disappears. Nearly all surgical procedures on animals are performed in this stage.

Stage III is divided into 4 different planes as shown in Table 11.1, which outlines the principal characteristics of canine anesthesia with ether. Frequently, the stage of surgical anesthesia is more simply divided into light (planes 1 and 2) and deep (planes 3 and 4) surgical anesthesia.

Light Surgical Anesthesia

In light surgical anesthesia the eyelids usually remain open and the nystagmus or oscillation of the eyeball may occur but at a slower rate than in Stage II. Nystagmus generally disappears at the termination of plane 1 or prior to entry into plane 2.

Eyeball activity following induction and maintenance of surgical anesthesia has been observed in cattle (Thurmon et al. 1968). During induction of anesthesia, a consistent pattern of ocular movement is noted when 4% halothane is used in combination with a 50:50 nitrous oxide and oxygen mixture flowing into a semiclosed respiratory system. Upon increasing the concentration of halothane to 6% or 8%, the same pattern of eye movement does not occur with a more rapid induction rate. During recovery from anesthesia, however, ocular movement appears but in reverse order.

When inhalant anesthesia is initiated in cattle, the eyeball moves dorsally or upward until the cornea is partially obscured by the upper eyelid. As the depth of anesthesia increases, the eyeball moves in the ventral direction. The cornea is then partially and sometimes completely obscured by the lower eyelid. In this ventral position, the palpebral reflex can still be elicited and these signs are interpreted with the approachment of Stage III, plane 2, anesthesia (Thurmon et al. 1968). With the advancement in the depth of anesthesia, i.e., approaching plane 3, the eyeball rotates dorsally until the cornea is centered within the palpebral opening. Major surgical procedures can be performed at this depth of anesthesia by maintenance with 1.5% to 2.5% halothane in combination with nitrous oxide and oxygen. The sequence of ocular movements is reversed in the cow upon recovery from anesthesia, i.e., the cornea first moves ventrally until it is mostly under the lower eyelid. This is followed by dorsal movement until the cornea is under the upper eyelid. With return of the eyeball to the normal position, the cattle are nearing recovery from anesthesia and are soon ambulatory.

With the continuance of plane 1 anesthesia, the corneal and palpebral reflexes are still present in the dog but slow to respond to stimulation. The pedal reflex (withdrawal of the limb on painful stimulation) disappears almost at the onset of Stage III in the dog following administration of volatile anesthetics. On the other hand, the palpebral, corneal and pedal reflexes are variable and may frequently be seen to persist throughout all planes of surgical anesthesia when the barbiturates are used.

The palpebral reflex (movement of the eyelids when the inner canthus is touched) is abolished at the end of plane 1 in all animals except the cat; initiation of this reflex in the cat is unreliable, possibly because it may be difficult to evoke (Campbell and Lawson 1958). The corneal reflex (closure of the eyelids upon lightly touching the cornea) persists longer than the palpebral reflex. In the horse the corneal reflex may be elicited under deep surgical anesthesia with most anesthetics up to the point of respiratory failure or beginning of Stage IV. Care in eliciting the corneal reflex should be exercised in order not to traumatize the eye. It is safer to rely on the palpebral reflex as a clinical sign. With a reduction in the level of anesthesia, it is important to recognize that there is often a delay in the reestablishment of the eye reflexes. The first part of plane 1 anesthesia may be reached before all the eye reflexes return in animals.

Lacrimal secretions are normal in the induction stage of anesthesia and persist in all species until the lower margin of plane 3 (Campbell and Lawson 1958). Lacrimation is increased in planes 1 and 2 in ruminants and is observed to persist longer than in other species. The corneal surface sometimes loses its normal sheen and has a glazed appearance when lower plane 3 or plane 4 is reached.

The swallowing reflex disappears in the dog at the termination of Stage II or upon entry into plane 1. The presence of this reflex in the dog is indicative of light anesthesia and/or recovery from anesthesia. In the cat, however, the swallow-

TABLE 11.1. Principal characteristics of the stages and planes of ether anesthesia in the dog

Stages of Anesthesia	Depression of Central Nervous System	Mucous Membrane Color*	Skeletal Muscle Tone	Respiration	Pulse and Blood Pressure (B.P.)	Reflexes Present†					
						Lid	Corneal	Skin	Swallowing	Cough	Pedal
I Analgesia (stage of voluntary movement)	Sensory cortex	Normal, flushed		Rapid and irregular	Rapid pulse and elevated B.P.	+	+	+	+	+	+
II Delirium (stage of involuntary movement)	Motor cortex D.R.‡	Flushed		Very irregular (erratic)	Rapid pulse and elevated B.P.	+	+	+	+	+	+
III (Surgical) Plane 1	Midbrain and spinal cord	Flushed, normal		Slow and regular	Normal pulse and normal B.P.	+	+	−	−	+	−
Plane 2	Spinal cord (increased depression)	Normal		Slow and regular	Normal pulse and normal B.P.	−	+ to − −	−	−	−	−
Plane 3§	Spinal cord (increased depression)	Normal, pale		Delayed thoracic, chiefly abdominal	Rapid pulse and fall in B.P.	−	−	−	−	−	−
Plane 4	Slight medullary depression	Pale		Abdominal (shallow)	Rapid weak pulse and fall in B.P.	−	−	−	−	−	−
IV Paralysis (death follows)	Medullary paralysis	Cyanotic	None	None	Shock level	−	−	−	−	−	−

Source: Booth and Rankin 1956.

* Cyanosis occurs in any stage of oxygen lack.

† Although significant in other species, pupillary size is too variable in the etherized dog to permit analysis. Nystagmus is not prominent in the dog as in some other species of animals.

‡ Decerebrate rigidity (extension of the limbs) is frequently observed in the dog just prior to entering Stage III; relaxation of the limbs occurs when Plane 1 is entered.

§ It has been estimated that 15 minutes in Plane 3 is as productive of shock as 2 hours in Plane 2.

ing reflex is not abolished until early plane 2 (Campbell and Lawson 1958).

Thermoregulatory function of animals is suppressed as early as the initial phases of Stage III, plane 1, with shivering only present in Stage II. The presence of shivering is quite often indicative of very light anesthesia when recovery from anesthesia is in progress.

Skeletal muscle tone, which is nearly normal at the beginning of light surgical anesthesia, decreases due to a depression of the ordinary postural reflexes. Jaw movements and licking movements ("tongue curling") are abolished in plane 1 and may be evident before return of the eye reflexes upon recovery from anesthesia (Campbell and Lawson 1958). If skeletal muscle relaxants are used in conjunction with anesthetic agents, assessment of the depth of surgical anesthesia cannot be properly determined by checking the muscular tonus, pedal, and palpebral reflexes. For this reason the photomotor reflex is a useful check to determine whether or not consciousness is returning (Croft 1961). According to Croft, both pupils react to a unilateral stimulus, and the rate of change of light intensity is the most important factor in eliciting the response. It is, therefore, important that both eyes be covered 10 seconds prior to switching a bright light suddenly onto one eye and observing the change in pupillary size. If several attempts to elicit the response are made repetitively, adaptation fatigue results and the reflex disappears. When large dosages of atropine sulfate are used for preanesthetic medication, the photomotor reflex will be impaired or abolished.

In the horse the tail becomes limp and the penis often protrudes from the sheath. Cutting of the skin or muscle does not produce reflex muscular contractions. The respiration becomes slow and regular (machinelike) and consists of both diaphragmatic and intercostal movements. The cough reflex is generally present during plane 1 of Stage III. Persistence of this reflex is of value in preventing blood and tissue debris from entering the respiratory passages when the airway is not intubated during tonsillectomies or pharyngeal or oral surgery.

Laryngospasm is probably more readily encountered in the cat during induction of anesthesia than in other species (McDonell 1972; Rex 1973). This reflex is also initiated easily in the pig, especially during endotracheal intubation. Exposure of the nasopharynx, larynx, and respiratory tract to sudden high concentrations of volatile anesthetics, especially ether or halothane, can induce laryngospasm and cause constriction or closure of the airway. In clinical anesthesia it is essential to prevent this from happening. Laryngeal spasm may also occur from mechanical stimulation of the larynx or pharynx under light anesthesia during an attempt to intubate the trachea. It also may occur from intraabdominal stimulation under deep anesthesia such as traction on mesentery and mesovarium (Campbell and Lawson 1958). Although atropine will not prevent the occurrence of laryngospasm, its use before anesthesia assists indirectly by inhibiting the formation of mucus and saliva (Rex 1973). Local anesthetic sprays (Cetacaine) are useful in minimizing the mechanical stimulation of laryngospasm during endotracheal intubation. Also, skeletal muscle relaxants are useful by producing paralysis of the laryngeal muscles. At present there are no drugs that can be used prior to surgical anesthesia to completely prevent laryngospasm (Rex 1973).

Pulse and blood pressure are essentially normal. Early in light anesthesia the pupil may be only partially dilated; however, the pupil dilates again with the approach of deep surgical anesthesia. Heavy premedication with atropine may make it difficult to assess a change in pupil size. Salivation is diminished or abolished in plane 1 in nonruminants, whereas in ruminants the formation of saliva is decreased but can persist to the terminal phase of plane 3 (Campbell and Lawson 1958).

Deep Surgical Anesthesia

In deep surgical anesthesia (planes 3 and 4), the lowly reflexes such as the palpebral, corneal, and pedal are completely depressed by the inhalant anesthetics. As pointed out above, these reflexes and especially the pedal reflex may persist throughout all planes following barbiturate anesthesia. The skeletal muscle tone rapidly disappears, leaving the patient flaccid. The pulse is rapid and weak. Feces may fall from the anus and some urine may escape from the urethra. The diaphragmatic respiration is regular but more shallow. The intercostal respiration is depressed early in plane 3 and begins to lag behind the diaphragmatic respiration progressively until it disappears in the latter part of plane 3 as the level of anesthesia becomes deeper. The disappearance of intercostal respiration indicates a dangerous depth of anesthetic depression. With the disappearance of intercostal or chest movement, the respiration is completely diaphragmatic or "rocking-the-boat" in character. This type of breathing is characteristic of deep plane 3 anesthesia. It annoys the surgeon by producing troublesome movement of abdominal viscera and may be mistaken for the jerky type of respiration characteristic of Stage II anesthesia. Such activity must not be misinterpreted for arousal or awakening from anesthesia. The proper course of action to take is to reduce, not increase, the level of anesthesia (Campbell and Lawson 1958).

The pupils are maximally dilated in plane 4 or in the latter phase of deep surgical anesthesia even in the unatropinized animal. Closure of the eyelids in the horse indicates the approximate maximum of anesthesia. Failure of diaphragmatic respiration indicates the close of deep surgical anesthesia and of Stage III.

Deep surgical anesthesia is infrequently employed in veterinary medicine. Occasionally it is produced in small animals for a few minutes but it is almost never employed in large animals. Most of the operations can be performed under light surgical anesthesia, although a few reflexes, such as those of the peritoneum, are abolished only by deep surgical anesthesia. If deep surgical anesthesia is necessary to abolish the peritoneal reflex during surgery, artificial resuscitation utilizing oxygen should be readily available in the event of respiratory depression or failure.

The hypothalamic centers are paralyzed progressively during Stage III. The direct result is to inactivate the heat-regulating mechanism so that loss of body heat fails to evoke such protective responses as shivering and vasoconstriction. The patient's temperature falls markedly unless protected against heat loss. Also, severe arterial hypotension and shock may develop.

STAGE IV: MEDULLARY PARALYSIS

Stage IV is characterized by paralysis of the vital regulatory centers of the medulla, and death soon ensues if resuscitative procedures are not readily instituted. In poor-risk patients, resuscitative efforts are often unsuccessful when this level of anesthesia is reached. Respiratory arrest and fall in arterial blood pressure to the shock level are most characteristic of Stage IV. The heart usually beats weakly for a short time after respiration ceases. As hypoxia worsens, cardiac arrest becomes increasingly imminent. There is also a complete absence of all reflexes and complete dilation of the pupil. The anal and urinary sphincters relax completely.

In summary, the veterinary anesthesiologist must be well trained and familiar with all the clinical stages and planes of surgical anesthesia so that immediate recognition of the anesthetic level as near as possible can be made in the various species. Inasmuch as the depth of anesthesia can fluctuate with considerable rapidity with most methods of administration, the need to make quick decisions to reduce or increase the depth of anesthesia or to institute immediate corrective measures in an emergency is essential.

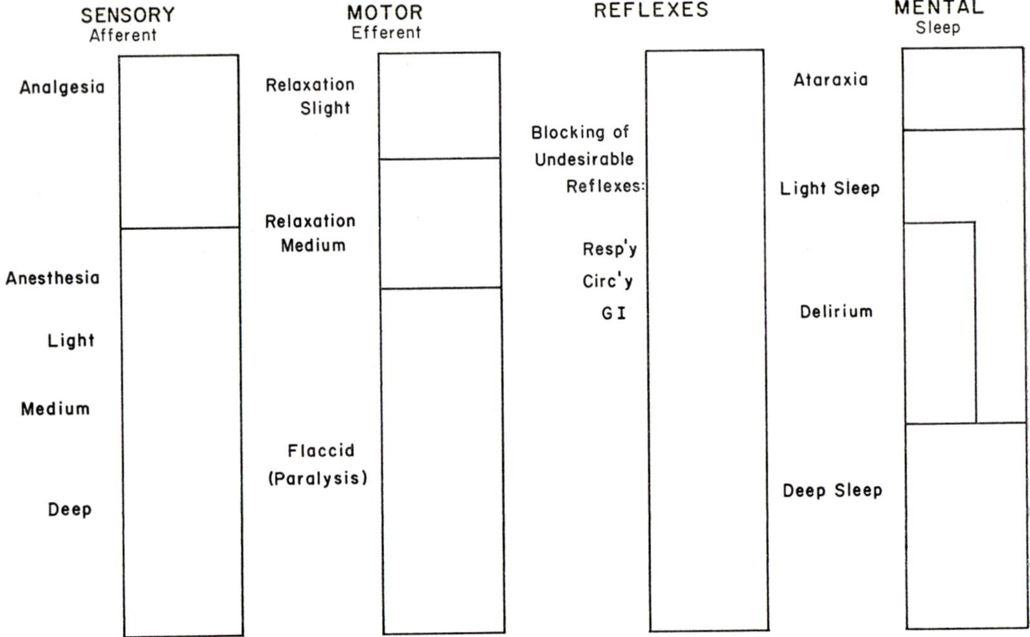

FIG. 11.1. The four components of general anesthesia or nothria. (Woodbridge 1957)

AVIAN NARCOSIS AND ANESTHESIA

The stages of narcosis and anesthesia have been classified in budgerigars (Arnall 1961); Arnall's classification for the most part appears to pertain to all birds (Graham-Jones 1965).

COMPONENTS OF BALANCED ANESTHESIA

In human anesthesiology a proposal of categorizing surgical anesthesia into four basic components has been introduced (Fig. 11.1). This categorization has real merit since pharmacologic agents such as the analgesics, hypnotics, belladonna preparations, adrenergic blocking agents, neuroleptics or tranquilizers, and skeletal muscle relaxants are customarily used in conjunction with the various anesthetics. Use of these drugs is directed toward achieving a condition referred to as *nothria* or *balanced anesthesia*. This concept is also applicable to the pharmacologic agents used in veterinary medicine (Fig. 11.2).

SENSORY

Sensory blocking is produced by the analgesic activity of xylazine, fentanyl, morphine and associated derivatives, trichloroethylene, nitrous oxide, and intravenous procaine. Analgesia also results following the administration of drug preparations having the capability of blocking all sensory perception. Pharmacologic agents such as nitrous oxide and trichloroethylene are capable of producing light anesthesia. Deep anesthesia results when intravenous barbiturates, intravenous chloral hydrate, halothane, methoxyflurane, cyclopropane, ether, chloroform, and ethyl chloride are used. Procaine and equivalent local anesthetics induce a complete blockade of sensory function.

MOTOR

A slight degree of motor blockade is produced by trichloroethylene and ethyl chloride. It is obtained to a greater degree with intravenous barbiturates, intravenous chloral hydrate, halothane, and cyclopropane. Complete relaxation occurs following ether, methoxyflurane, chloroform, curare, glyceryl guaiacolate, succinylcholine, and the use of local anesthetics for regional epidural or intrathecal anesthesia. Ether,

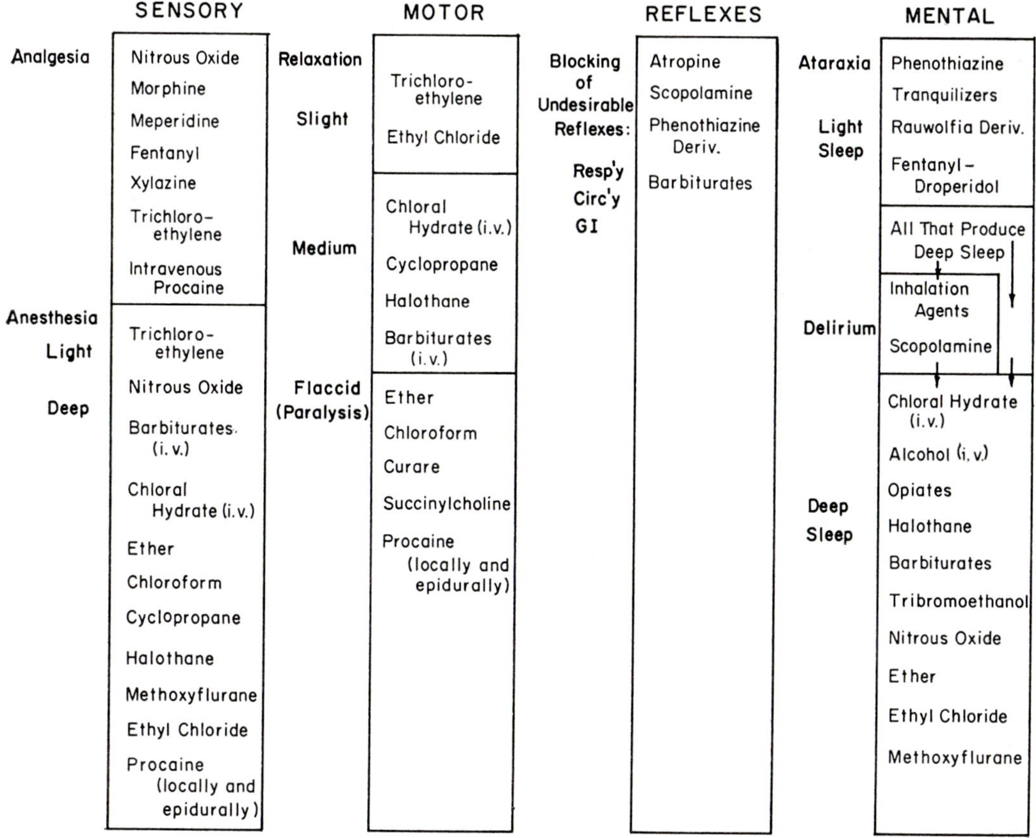

Fig. 11.2. General classification of veterinary pharmacologic agents into the four components of anesthesia or nothria. (Modified from Woodbridge 1957)

in particular, provides ideal relaxation of the skeletal musculature by virtue of its curariform activity.

Reflex

Blocking of reflex activity associated with the autonomic nervous system is an important consideration in general anesthesia. The belladonna preparations, i.e., atropine or scopolamine, are used to block the parasympathetic nervous system to lessen or prevent vomition, salivation, and the formation of mucus in the respiratory tract. In human beings, and probably in animals, these preparations are extremely important in preventing "vago-vagal" reflex activity and cardiac arrest, which is most likely to occur during surgery on the cervical and thoracic regions (Hinchey 1957). Laryngospasm readily occurs in the cat and may develop in other species during the induction of anesthesia when ether or halothane is administered in high concentrations (Rex 1973). Halothane and chloroform depress reflexes associated with salivation, mucus secretion, and vomition. Chlorpromazine and related tranquilizing agents are capable of diminishing the likelihood of vomition and cardiac arrhythmias. Acetylpromazine has α-receptor blocking effect, which is beneficial in the maintenance of renal blood flow during anesthesia. The barbiturates reduce the frequency of vomition and inhibit gastrointestinal motility.

Mental

Drugs that alter mental activity or general awareness are not only useful in anesthesia but are also important in facilitating the handling and restraint of animals. Ataractic or neuroleptic agents such as acetylpromazine and related derivatives are useful in altering animal behavior without inducing sleep. Even scopolamine, a belladonna alkaloid sometimes used in the dog, is also capable of a slight degree of tranquilization. Light sleep or hypnosis is produced by morphine, fentanyl-droperidol, and drugs that induce sleep when used in small dose levels.

REFERENCES

Arnall, L. 1961. Anaesthesia and surgery in cage and aviary birds. II. A regional outline of surgical conditions. Vet Rec 73:173.

Booth, N. H., and Rankin, A. D. 1956. Colorado State University. Personal communication.

Campbell, J. R., and Lawson, D. D. 1958. The signs and stages of anesthesia in domestic animals. Vet Rec 70:545.

Croft, P. D. 1961. The photomotor reflex as an indicator of consciousness in the immobilized dog. J Small Anim Pract 2:206.

Graham-Jones, O. (1965). Restraint and anaesthesia of small cage birds. J Small Anim Pract 6:31.

Hinchey, P. R. 1957. Cardiac arrest—The most important disaster in the operating room. Arch Surg 74:365.

McDonell, W. 1972. Anesthetic emergencies. I. Respiratory insufficiency and arrest. Mod Vet Pract 53:31.

Rex, M. A. E. 1973. Laryngeal activity during the induction of anaesthesia in the cat. Aust Vet J 49:365.

Robson, J. G. 1969. Measurement of depth of anaesthesia. Br J Anaesth 41:785.

Thurmon, J. C.; Romack, F. E.; and Garner, H. E. 1968. Excursions of the bovine eyeball during gaseous anesthesia. Vet Med Small Anim Clin 63:967.

Woodbridge, P. D. 1957. Changing concepts concerning depth of anesthesia. Anesthesiology 18:536.

CHAPTER 12

INHALANT ANESTHETICS

NICHOLAS H. BOOTH

Inhalation of a highly volatile agent was the first method of general anesthesia. Ether and chloroform were among the first general anesthetics to be used. With the introduction of the intravenous anesthetics (e.g., the barbiturates), the use of ether and chloroform declined considerably. However, with the introduction of halothane and methoxyflurane into clinical veterinary medicine, the pendulum has swung back to increased usage of the inhalant anesthetics. The barbiturates, i.e., the ultrashort-acting compounds, are used principally as induction agents, and the inhalant anesthetics such as halothane, methoxyflurane, and nitrous oxide are used in the maintenance of anesthesia. Ether is still used in small laboratory animals and chloroform is sometimes used in small animals (puppies and kittens) for euthanasia purposes.

DISTRIBUTION, METABOLISM, AND EXCRETION OF VOLATILE ANESTHETICS

A volatile anesthetic is effective by several routes of administration, provided it reaches the blood, but it is best given by inhalation. In the alveoli of the lungs, the anesthetic gas diffuses through separating membranes into the circulating blood of the lung capillaries, according to the gas laws of Dalton and Henry. Those laws state that the greater the concentration of the anesthetic gas in the alveoli, the greater is its partial pressure (Dalton's Law); and that the greater the partial pressure of the anesthetic gas, the greater will be its solubility in the blood (Henry's Law). The gaseous anesthetic dissolved in the bloodstream, according to the above gas laws, is transported over the body to lipoidal tissues into which it diffuses as a result of greater solubility in fats than in aqueous media.

Solubility is an important factor of uptake and distribution as well as the characteristic that identifies one anesthetic from another in terms of its potency, rapidity of induction, and rate of disappearance during the period of recovery. Factors affecting the solubility coefficients are the anesthetic agent itself and the solvent (e.g., solubility is greatest in lipids, less in protein, and least in aqueous medium). The most soluble anesthetic in blood is ether. Methoxyflurane, chloroform, and trichloroethylene are also quite soluble in blood but less so than ether. Cyclopropane and nitrous oxide are only slightly soluble in blood, whereas halothane has an intermediate level of solubility. This solubility characteristic of ether means that the induction of anesthesia is slower; also the level of anesthesia is not as readily changed. The lower the solubility, the more rapid the induction, as well as the level of anesthesia, can be changed.

The central nervous system (CNS) contains more lipoids than any other part of the body and therefore attracts far more anesthetic than any other system. In addition, the CNS is highly vascular so that proportionately more anesthetic is carried to that part of the body. Thus the CNS is more susceptible than other systems to the effects of an anesthetic. On the other hand, when administration ceases, the anesthetic will diffuse out of the brain more quickly than other tissues with a smaller blood supply.

During the administration of an anesthetic, the concentration gradient is higher in the arterial blood than in the tissues of the body; therefore, much of the anesthetic in the blood diffuses into the tissues. If the anesthetic were administered at a continuous rate compatible with life, an equilibrium would be reached where the anesthetic would diffuse out as fast as it diffused into tissue. Actually, true equilibrium rarely exists during clinical administration of volatile anesthetics because varying concentrations are administered to fit the needs of the situation.

At one time, it was taught that volatile anesthetics were stable within the tissues and were eliminated in the same form in which they were inhaled. New evidence during the last decade has revealed that biotransformation of the inhalant anesthetics can occur to a significant degree. Through the use of radiolabeled compounds, a number of inhalant anesthetics are partially degraded to carbon dioxide. Degradation takes place in microsomes where reduced nicotinamide adenine dinucleotide phosphate (NADPH) is essential as a cofactor in H^+ transfer. Anesthetics such as ethylene, diethyl ether, chloroform, and cyclopropane are converted to carbon dioxide. Metabolites of trichloroethylene such as trichloroacetic acid and trichloroethanol appear in urine. Evidence for the breakdown of halothane appears highly probable because bromine can be detected in urine following its use.

The excretion of a volatile anesthetic involves the same diffusion processes that were active during administration, except that they operate in the reverse direction. The rate of excretion of a volatile anesthetic is dependent upon proper ventilation of the lungs. A dangerous situation exists if an excess of anesthetic has depressed the respiratory center enough to interfere with respiration and with excretion of the anesthetic.

RECOVERY FROM ANESTHESIA

During recovery from anesthesia the patient passes through the same stages in the reverse direction as during induction. The first reflexes recovered are those that persisted the longest during induction. The patient may show a brief period of excitement just before the return of consciousness. Ordinarily, recovery is smooth and rapid without manifestation of excitement. With some nonvolatile anesthetics, the excitement period during recovery is undesirably long and the patient occasionally may throw itself about enough to necessitate rebandaging, resuturing, or other surgical repair. After consciousness has returned, the effect of the inhalant anesthetic persists to produce a hypnosis that may cause the patient to sleep for several hours.

ANESTHESIA, HYPOXIA, AND ASPHYXIA

Anesthesia as commonly and correctly practiced does not involve the condition of hypoxia or asphyxia. Anesthesia occurs when the patient is completely oxygenated. The exclusion of oxygen by strangulation, by a deficiency in a closed-system anesthesia apparatus, or by the inhalation of inert gases, such as nitrogen or helium, will produce unconsciousness. This kind of unconsciousness is characterized by hypoxemia, which is revealed clinically by a dangerous and marked cyanosis. The unconsciousness of anesthesia should be accompanied by normal oxygenation and the absence of cyanosis.

In the dog, the brain uses about 8% of the total oxygen consumption of the body at rest. These same percentages may not apply specifically to all animals, but the same principle undoubtedly applies, namely, that the metabolic level of the CNS is remarkably high compared to the rest of the body.

The high metabolic level of the brain requires a large and ready supply of oxygen. Lack of oxygen affects the brain more than any other organ of the body and constitutes one of the greatest hazards of anesthesia. Brief periods of oxygen deprivation produce CNS damage proportional to the degree of hypoxia.

MAJOR INHALANT ANESTHETICS

The three most important inhalant anesthetics used in veterinary medicine are methoxyflurane, halothane, and nitrous oxide. Other inhalant anesthetics used to a much lesser degree are ether, cyclopropane, chloroform, ethyl chloride, carbon dioxide, and tricholoroethylene.

METHOXYFLURANE

In the last decade, *Methoxyflurane,* N.F. (Metofane, Penthrane), has had extensive use in both large and small animals. Methoxyflurane has a higher anesthetic potency than halothane or nitrous oxide. The higher anesthetic potency of methoxyflurane is related to the minimal concentration of the anesthetic at the alveolar level of the respiratory system that is required in dogs to prevent gross movement to nociceptive stimuli (Eger et al. 1965). This is referred to as the minimum alveolar concentration (MAC); for methoxyflurane and halothane it is 0.23% and 0.87%, respectively. Although methoxyflurane has the highest anesthetic potency, its relatively high solubility in blood results in a slow induction as well as a slow recovery rate. Nitrous oxide has a higher MAC value than methoxyflurane or halothane. Its solubility in blood is much lower than methoxyflurane or halothane.

CHEMISTRY

Chemically, methoxyflurane is 2,2-dichloro-1,1-difluoroethyl methyl ether: $CHCl_2 - CF_2 - O - CH_3$. Prior to volatization, the liquid anesthetic is clear and colorless. However, it turns an amber color in the vaporizer. The change in color does not appear to affect its potency nor to produce adverse effects upon the animal. The boiling point of methoxyflurane is 104.8° C at 1 atmosphere of pressure, and it has a specific gravity of 1.4729. The anesthetic has a fruitlike odor and is nonexplosive and nonflammable at 20° C in all concentrations. It is not decomposed by light, air, or soda lime. Methoxyflurane contains 0.01% dibenzylamine to prevent acid formation.

EFFECT UPON THE NERVOUS SYSTEM

Methoxyflurane can induce anesthesia in large animals by inhalation within 4–11 minutes without the assistance of preanesthetic agents. However, this use is generally not advisable because the induction period is relatively slow. In determining the depth of methoxyflurane anesthesia, the conventional signs are not very reliable. Pedal and palpebral reflexes are abolished very early in the dog and cat. In the cow, abolition of the eye reflexes appears to be similar to that observed with other anesthetics (Douglas et al. 1964). The palpebral reflex does not disappear in the cow until about plane 2 or 3 and the corneal reflex may not disappear until plane 3 or 4. The swallowing reflex is ordinarily lost in the dog upon entry into Stage III, plane 1, anesthesia. Reappearance of it is usually indicative of light anesthesia (i.e., lower Stage II). The "ear flick" reflex in the cat appears before the swallowing and jaw reflexes. This reflex is stimulated by gently touching the hair on the inside of the cat's ear or by carefully blowing into the ear.

Methoxyflurane produces excellent analgesia and it appears to be quite good even at subanesthetic levels and during emergence from anesthesia. Use of postoperative analgesics is ordinarily not necessary, due to the prolonged delay in the elimination of methoxyflurane. The antianalgesic effect seen with halothane does not occur from the use of methoxyflurane.

In the cow, uninterrupted tremors (apparently of neurologic origin) have been seen throughout all stages of anesthesia. The depth of anesthesia considered to be the maximum safe level in cattle is where the corneal reflex disappears and only an abdominal type of respiratory movement is present (Douglas et al. 1964).

EEG recordings appear to have some value in monitoring the depth of anesthesia in dogs anesthetized with methoxyflurane (Prynn and Redding 1968). The progression of cerebral depression is characterized by a gradual replacement of the control patterns, i.e., high frequency and low voltage, by slow waves that initially are of high amplitudes. The slow waves persist. However, as depression progresses, there is usually reduced voltage culminating in burst suppression.

EFFECT UPON THE CARDIOPULMONARY SYSTEM

Respiratory activity is gradually dedepressed with the inhalation of an increased concentration of methoxyflurane until respiratory arrest occurs. Arrest of respiration precedes cardiac arrest. The margin between a safe anesthetic level and the dosage producing respiratory and cardiac arrest varies among the inhalant anesthetics. Chloroform has a narrow margin while methoxyflurane and halothane have an intermediate margin. Ether has a wide margin of safety between adequate anesthesia and those levels leading to respiratory and cardiac arrest.

The maximum concentration of methoxyflurane that can be given at room temperature is 3%. Induction concentrations of the anesthetic usually range between 1% and 3%. The low volatility of methoxyflurane creates some difficulty in reaching a sufficiently high initial concentration of methoxyflurane to achieve rapid stabilization of anesthesia. It is more convenient to use an ultrashort-acting barbiturate to induce anesthesia and to permit endotracheal intubation prior to the use of methoxyflurane. Maintenance of anesthesia is achieved with methoxyflurane between 0.3% and 1%.

During surgical anesthesia, the tidal volume may be reduced by about 50%. Reduction in the tidal volume to this extent makes ventilatory assistance necessary. If respiration is not assisted, respiratory acidosis occurs and the blood pH declines. In some horses, a markedly irregular respiratory rhythm has been observed throughout much of anesthesia where the depth, as judged by other signs, was considered to be plane 2 of Stage III (Douglas et al. 1964).

In general, the heart rate does not change appreciably during maintenance anesthesia in the horse. Moderate tachycardia has been observed in cattle under methoxyflurane maintenance anesthesia. Cardiac arrhythmias may occasionally occur in animals subjected to methoxyflurane anesthesia. This type of arrhythmia can usually be abolished by atropine. Also, the administration of epinephrine or norepinephrine may induce arrhythmia and ventricular fibrillation in animals during methoxyflurane anesthesia.

Cardiac output may be reduced 25%–40% during methoxyflurane anesthesia, due to direct depression of the myocardium. All halogenated anesthetics have this characteristic. Also, the arterial blood pressure is reduced considerably, especially as the depth of anesthesia increases. It is important to maintain a relatively light level of anesthesia to circumvent events leading up to circulatory shock and failure. Increase in capillary bleeding does not occur during surgery and only normal hemostatic methods are required to control hemorrhage (Heinze 1965).

EFFECT UPON THE LIVER AND KIDNEY

The results of hepatic function tests are similar to those following the use of diethyl ether. Although hepatic function may be depressed by methoxyflurane, it does not produce direct injury to liver cells like chloroform. The hepatotoxic effects of steroids and phenothiazine derivatives are increased following the use of methoxyflurane. In animals with hepatic disease, cautious use of the anesthetic is advisable. Hypoxia and hypercarbia should be avoided to reduce the possibility of liver damage.

Renal function may be altered by methoxyflurane through a reduced renal blood flow and vasoconstriction. Moreover, metabolism of methoxyflurane may result in renal damage (Mazze et al. 1971). It appears that one or both methoxyflurane metabolites (i.e., inorganic fluoride and oxalic acid), but probably inorganic fluoride, may be responsible for the renal dysfunction seen after administration of methoxyflurane.

EFFECT UPON MUSCLE

The skeletal muscle relaxation produced by methoxyflurane is quite similar to that produced by ether. Peristaltic activity of smooth muscle is decreased. Motility of the gastrointestinal (GI) tract is slowed and smooth muscle tone is diminlished. No outward effects are noted using methoxyflurane with *d*-tubocurarine or succinylcholine.

EFFECT UPON THE FETUS

Methoxyflurane can readily cross the placenta similarly to other inhalant anesthetics and enter the fetal circulation. Use of the anesthetic during cesarean section does not appear to pose any more of a problem than the use of other inhalant anesthetics. Nevertheless, minimal amounts of a barbiturate for induction and methoxyflurane for maintenance anesthesia should be used to prevent severe respiratory depression of the fetus. Surgery should be performed as rapidly as possible. The respiratory stimulatory characteristics of ether appear to be much less for methoxyflurane in newborn subjects. Barbiturates produce a tenfold higher mortality rate (i.e., 36%) of puppies delivered by cesarean section than do the inhalants (Mitchell 1966).

ADVANTAGES AND DISADVANTAGES

Methoxyflurane has the advantage that it is potent. Its potency allows it to be used in both small and large species. The MAC or the concentration of methoxyflurane at the alveolar level required to prevent a response to pain is lower than that of halothane and nitrous oxide. Moreover, the anesthetic is nonflammable at ordinary temperature conditions; methoxyflurane also produces excellent skeletal muscle relaxation and analgesia.

It has the disadvantage that the drug has a relatively high solubility in blood. This characteristic makes it more difficult to control or change the level or depth of anesthesia. Also, there is a problem in vaporizing methoxyflurane sufficiently to maintain anesthesia, particularly at temperatures below room temperature. Halothane is vaporized more rapidly and the depth of anesthesia is more easily controlled than with methoxyflurane. Halothane is generally favored over methoxyflurane by equine practitioners. Moreover, the recovery period from methoxyflurane may require several hours.

BIOTRANSFORMATION

About 1.1% of the radiolabeled methoxyflurane can be recovered from the urine of animals as nonvolatile compounds. The major substance recovered in urine is the glucuronide of $CH_2OH - CHCl_2$ occurring from $NADPH - O_2$–stimulated microsomal defluorination of the parent compound. In addition, some of the parent compound undergoes ether cleavage.

CLINICAL USE

Preanesthetic agents that have been used with methoxyflurane include atropine sulfate, acetylpromazine maleate, promazine hydrochloride, triflupromazine, droperidol-fentanyl, thiopental sodium, methohexital sodium, and thiamylal sodium. The preanesthetic agents with CNS depressant effect should be used conservatively because they can prolong recovery.

IN LARGE ANIMALS

In large animals (horse, cow) anesthesia is induced by a rapid intravenous injection of thiopental sodium, thiamylal sodium, or methohexital to permit endotracheal intubation. After intubation, methoxyflurane is administered as a maintenance anesthetic using an in-circuit oxygen vaporizer. The following procedure is commonly used in the horse (Shideler 1971): Acetylpromazine maleate (15 mg) is administered intravenously and followed 10 minutes later with an intravenous injection of thiamylal sodium (5% solution) administered in a dosage level of 2.5–3 g/1000 lb of body weight. Following intubation, methoxyflurane is administered. About 4–6 minutes are required to produce muscular relaxation and analgesia.

Although atropine is not ordinarily used prior to methoxyflurane in the horse, it is recommended in other species. Shideler (1971) believes that the use of inhalational anesthesia in the equine is one of the truly great advances of recent years and that no other drug is comparable for the production of relaxation and analgesia. Recovery of the horse from methoxyflurane anesthesia is smooth and may occur within 30–60 minutes following surgery.

IN SMALL ANIMALS

There are numerous clinical reports of the successful use of methoxyflurane in small animal practice. Methoxyflurane is used for the induction and maintenance of surgical anesthesia in the dog and cat. Methoxyflurane may also be used following xylazine in the dog and ketamine in the cat. Atropine sulfate (0.02 mg/lb of body weight) should be routinely used in both the dog and cat. Methoxyflurane may also be used following the use of phenothiazine tranquilizers in these species. Acetylpromazine maleate is recommended as a preanesthetic agent for the dog and cat at an intramuscular or intravenous dosage of 1 mg/20 lb of body weight.

IN LABORATORY ANIMALS

Methoxyflurane is also used in small laboratory animals such as the mouse, rat, guinea pig, hamster, and rabbit for both induction and maintenance anesthesia. It has been used in rabbits following ketamine hydrochloride analgesia as a maintenance anesthetic (Wass et al. 1974).

IN CAGED BIRDS

Methoxyflurane is used to produce anesthesia in parakeets and other small caged birds. The parakeet attains a surgical plane of anesthesia within 2–4 minutes (Hoge 1966). Anesthesia is induced by placing the bird inside a specially constructed cannister containing methoxyflurane. The bird is observed during the induction procedure and removed from the cannister when surgical anesthesia is reached. Anesthesia is maintained 10–15 minutes without further administration of the anesthetic. This allows time for the surgical correction for egg retention in female parakeets. Recovery of the parakeet from anesthesia requires approximately 45 minutes.

IN EXOTIC ANIMALS

Methoxyflurane has been used extensively in a number of exotic animals such as birds, skunks, and reptiles (Stunkard and Miller 1974).

HALOTHANE

Halothane, U.S.P. (Fluothane, $C_2HBrClF_3$), is a clear, volatile liquid. It is a multihalogenated ethane and is the most frequently used inhalant anesthetic. In human beings, millions of halothane anesthesias are administered every year in the United States (Cascorbi et al. 1971). Halothane is most often selected by anesthesiologists as well as preferred by surgeons because it is relatively easy to administer and it is nonexplosive. Human patients accept the anesthetic without difficulty because of its minimal unpleasant subjective effects.

CHEMISTRY

Halothane has a specific gravity of 1.86 and a boiling point of 50.2° C. The anesthetic agent has a sweetish odor and is not explosive or flammable unless used under hyperbaric conditions with 100% oxygen. It can be used with soda lime without deterioration and without the danger of the formation of toxic products. Halothane is decomposed by sunlight and should be stored in dark-colored bottles. Thymol (0.01%) is added to the anesthetic preparation to reduce decomposition.

EFFECT UPON THE NERVOUS SYSTEM

Halothane is capable of depressing all functions of the CNS at all levels or gradations until coma or death is produced without assistance from other agents. The stages and planes of anesthesia are comparable to those produced by ether. Unlike methoxyflurane, there is no postanalgesic effect produced upon recovery from halothane anesthesia. Delirium may occur in some cases in the presence of pain upon emergence from anesthesia. However, recovery from halothane anesthesia is more rapid than from methoxyflurane anesthesia. The sensorium is clear or shows little depression soon after recovery.

Postanesthetic nausea and vomiting are less frequent following the use of halothane than following the use of ether in animals that have the ability to vomit. Also, no vomition is induced during induction with halothane.

EFFECT UPON THE CARDIOPULMONARY SYSTEM

Pharmacologically, the effect of halothane upon the cardiovascular system resembles that of chloroform in many respects. As myocardial depression increases, the central venous pressure increases. Marked increases in central venous pressure have been recorded in the horse during halothane anesthesia (Sheridan et al. 1972). Halothane produces cardiopulmonary depression that is proportional to the level or depth of anesthesia.

The anesthetic is capable of eliciting a marked arterial hypotension in animals (Krantz et al. 1958). Severity of the hypotension is closely related to the depth of anesthesia. Although it has been suggested that hypotension occurs following blockade of ganglionic transmission, it has been shown that the primary circulatory action of the anesthetic is a depression of the myocardium (Severinghaus and Cullen 1958).

If it becomes necessary to combat severe hypotension, immediate return to 100% oxygen is recommended; also methamphetamine can be used safely as a vasopressor agent.

In subhuman primates, unlike the dog, the addition of nitrous oxide to halothane-oxygen anesthesia results in less depression of cardiovascular function than using halothane-oxygen alone (Steffey et al. 1974a, 1974c). This cardiovascular sparing effect of nitrous oxide is diminished in the spontaneously ventilating animal at moderate or deep levels of anesthesia.

In the horse, halothane decreases the cardiac output, stroke volume, and left ventricular work (Eberly et al. 1968). Arterial hypotension is not due to a decrease in peripheral vascular resistance and does not occur until the tension of carbon dioxide increases and arterial tension of oxygen decreases. The right ventricular diastolic pressure and central venous volume also increase slightly following halothane anesthesia.

In the horse, both chloroform and halothane decrease the arterial pressures approximately 35% during anesthesia (Wolff et al. 1968). Arterial hypotension is marked in the early phase of anesthesia and is related to high concentrations of the anesthetics. Wolff and co-workers found halothane to be 2–3 times more potent than chloroform, with recovery from halothane being smoother and shorter. Later studies revealed that the mean concentration of chloroform in the blood is approximately twice as great as that of halothane during anesthesia (Tevik et al. 1968). The concentration of chloroform 24 hours after anesthesia is 5 times greater than that of halothane and probably explains why recovery from chloroform anesthesia is slower than from halothane. Since the solubility of chloroform in blood is greater than halothane, a slower recovery from chloroform anesthesia is expected. Both halothane and chloroform can be detected in the blood in most horses as long as 1 week after anesthesia.

Cardiac arrhythmias have been observed primarily during induction. Epinephrine and norepinephrine are contraindicated during halothane anesthesia because of the risk of inducing cardiac arrhythmias or ventricular fibrillation. Bradycardia, apparently induced by cardioinhibitory activity, is another complication noted following halothane anesthesia. This effect can be eliminated or relieved in the horse by the administration of atropine sulfate (Vasko 1962).

Halothane progressively depresses the respiratory center as the level of anesthesia deepens. Respiratory arrest generally precedes cardiac arrest. However, cardiac and pulmonary activity may be arrested simultaneously. Every effort must be made not to let this happen. If it does, immediate ventilation and "washout" with 100% oxygen is necessary to lighten the depth of anesthesia as well as to correct the hypoxemia and hypercarbia.

Halothane should be administered carefully in low concentrations between 2% and 4% during induction. Rapid administration will result in respiratory depression or apnea. Even when the anesthetic is administered under normal conditions, respiratory depression may occur in the dog, cow, sheep, and horse (Fisher 1961). Respiratory depression occurs to the greatest extent in sheep, with apnea often resulting. According to Fisher, the depressed respiratory activity causes carbon dioxide retention and an elevation of the plasma carbon dioxide content. This in turn leads to a respiratory acidosis. In the horse, carbon dioxide tensions increase and pH decreases progressively during either halothane or chloroform anesthesia (Wolff et al. 1968). However, acidosis is much more severe during chloroform anesthesia.

Use of halothane in mice, dogs, and monkeys indicates that the anesthetic has a low margin of safety (Krantz et al. 1958). Difficulty is encountered in resuscitating animals subjected to respiratory paralyzing concentrations of the anesthetic. In spite of immediate resuscitative efforts, several dogs and monkeys could not be revived.

Tachypnea may also occur during halothane anesthesia. In the horse it can be abolished by the intravenous injection of 50–100 mg of meperidine hydrochloride (Wright and Hall 1961). Respiratory acidosis from increased tensions of carbon dioxide has been observed in cattle during halothane anesthesia (Gates et al. 1971). The tension of carbon dioxide increases as the level of anesthesia deepens.

Recent studies indicate that carbon dioxide differences exert much more influence on cardiovascular function than do intrapleural pressure differences (Steffey et al. 1974b). For example, there is a trend toward less cardiovascular depression with halothane anesthesia during spontaneous respiration than during controlled ventilation at equal MAC. The differences in cardiovascular responses between controlled and spontaneous ventilation were greatest when Pa_{CO_2} differences were marked and were minimal or absent when the tensions were comparable (see Fig. 12.1).

EFFECT UPON THERMOREGULATORY FUNCTION

The thermoregulatory mechanism of the hypothalamus is depressed during the course of halothane anesthesia. Depending upon the ambient temperature, the body temperature should be monitored to avoid hypothermic or hyperthermic conditions.

A condition known as malignant hyperthermia or malignant hyperpyrexia has been reported in Landrace, Poland-China, and Pietrain breeds of swine following halothane anesthesia (Allen et al. 1970; Ber-

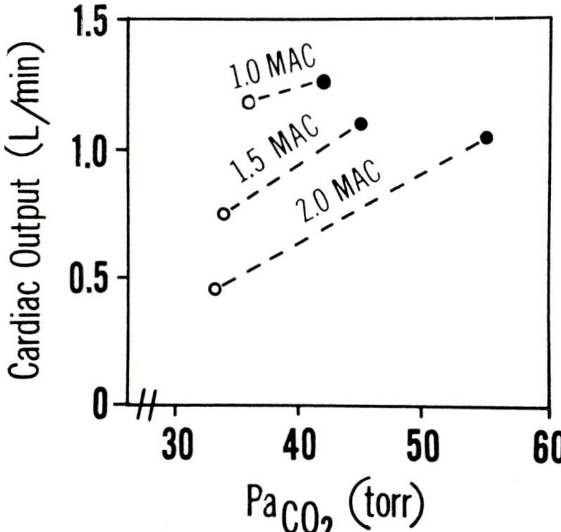

FIG. 12.1 Relationship of cardiac output to arterial CO_2 tensions (Pa_{CO_2}) during controlled (open-circle) and spontaneous (closed-circle) ventilation in the stump-tailed macaque. Halothane was administered at 1.0, 1.5, and 2.0 minimum alveolar concentrations (MAC). (From Steffey et al. 1974b)

man et al. 1970; Jones et al. 1972). An incidence as high as 25% has been noted in Landrace pigs. Body temperature may rise to 113° F (45° C). Although it is unclear why this occurs, animals studied have revealed high serum creatine phosphokinase (CPK) values. Also, animals susceptible to malignant hyperthermia were identified by increased adenosine triphosphate (ATP) depletion of biopsied skeletal muscle. Malignant hyperthermia is also triggered by succinylcholine, chloroform, and severe exercise or stress in these breeds of swine. A comparable clinical condition is seen in human beings. Genetic records of swine suggest that, as in human beings, the predilection to malignant hyperthermia is inherited as an autosomal dominant. If the hyperthermia induced by halothane is not observed in the early stages, it is difficult to reverse, and death occurs. Procaine hydrochloride has been suggested by a number of investigators for the treatment or reversal of malignant hyperthermia in human beings and the pig. However, once the clinical signs of the syndrome develop, procaine does not reverse the condition (Mitchell and Heffron 1975).

In the identification of swine that are susceptible to stress conditions, measurement of the serum level of CPK as a screening test has been suggested (Woolf et al. 1970). Tests are now conducted in young pigs (average age 15 weeks) by subjecting them to halothane (2%–4%) anesthesia up to 5 minutes (Eikelenboom and Minkema 1974). Signs of muscular rigidity are noted and the effect upon rectal temperature is determined; also, serum CPK and aldolase levels are measured.

EFFECT UPON THE LIVER

Hypercapnia appears to enhance toxicity of halothane upon liver function similar to that reported for chloroform. Adequate oxygenation and prevention of the accumulation of carbon dioxide are important throughout halothane anesthesia in minimizing hepatic injury.

In the assessment of the effects of halothane upon the liver of the horse during a period of anesthesia lasting 2 hours, serum arginase and serum isocitric dehydrogenase levels were observed to be slightly increased (Wolff et al. 1967). Also, only slight or moderate histopathological changes of the liver were noted in this study. However, after animals were subjected to chloroform anesthesia for comparable periods, these enzyme levels were markedly elevated and severe centrilobular necrosis occurred in all horses 2 days after anesthesia. The effects of halothane upon liver function of the horse have been studied, using the bromsulphalein (BSP) test (Norby and Link 1970). Following periods of anesthesia lasting 35 minutes–3.5 hours, no significant impairment of liver function could be detected 24 hours after anesthesia. However, there is some indication that halothane may damage the liver in the horse (Swerczek and Prickett 1971). Swerczek and Prickett pointed out that repeated use of halothane in horses is likely to produce liver injury similar to that reported in human beings. They warned that there may be a risk in using thiamylal in these cases because liver impairment may prevent detoxification of the barbiturate anesthetic.

In sheep, function studies indicate that the BSP clearance times have a half-life of 9 minutes after halothane anesthesia compared with 3.6 minutes on the day prior to anesthesia (Hull and Reilly 1968). This effect is not permanent because the hepatic clearance rate of BSP essentially returns to normal within 1 week.

In human beings, but not in animals, massive hepatic necrosis occasionally follows halothane anesthesia. The etiology is unknown and the effects are believed to be due to some type of "hypersensitivity reaction." Cohen et al. (1973) reported that an autoimmune response to halothane was experimentally induced in the rat. Treatment of rats twice with phenobarbital and followed by halothane resulted in multifocal hepatic necrosis. The formation of antimitochondrial antibodies resulted and is believed to be associated with the liver injury that was produced.

EFFECT UPON THE KIDNEY

Halothane is not known to have a nephrotoxic effect. Diminution of renal function is principally due to a reduction in the renal blood flow. The effect of halothane upon overall renal function appears to be no greater than that known following ether anesthesia. Blood urea may increase but returns to normal soon after recovery from anesthesia. The procedure for coping with animals that are unable to properly concentrate a high specific gravity urine was discussed under Preparation of Patient for Anesthesia in Chapter 10.

EFFECT UPON SKELETAL MUSCLE RELAXATION

Halothane ordinarily provides a satisfactory degree of skeletal muscle relaxation for surgical procedures. If additional relaxation is required, succinylcholine can be used; halothane, however, may slightly antagonize its effects. It is inadvisable to use *d*-tubocurarine chloride because it intensifies arterial hypotension. Moreover, hexamethonium, gallamine, and rauwolfia derivatives are contraindicated when halothane is used because of the risk of lowering the arterial blood pressure.

EFFECT UPON THE FETUS

Motility and tone of the uterus is progressively inhibited by halothane as anesthesia deepens. The response to oxytocic agents in inhibited by halothane. The placenta is readily penetrated by halothane. Surgical procedures should be conducted under a light level of anesthesia. Generally, respiratory activity of newborn animals is not depressed unless deep levels of halothane have been used during a cesarean section.

EFFECT UPON METABOLISM

One hour of plane 2 with halothane anesthesia in the horse significantly increases the blood glucose, lactate/pyruvate ratio, Pa_{CO_2}, and arterial oxygen tension after premedication and induction with chloral hydrate (de Moor 1968). The blood levels of both pyruvate and lactate decrease.

ADVANTAGES AND DISADVANTAGES

Halothane is a potent anesthetic and is capable of maintaining anesthesia effectively in large animals. The level and depth of anesthesia can be more rapidly changed than that noted with methoxyflurane. This characteristic can undoubtedly be ascribed to its lower solubility in blood compared to methoxyflurane. Recovery from halothane anesthesia is much more rapid than that from methoxyflurane. The principal disadvantage of halothane is the marked depression that is produced upon cardiopulmonary function. Also, the anesthetic is expensive to use and must be used in closed-anesthetic systems to prevent excessive waste.

EFFECT UPON OPERATING ROOM PERSONNEL

The potential toxic effects of inhalant anesthetics upon chronically exposed surgical personnel have been of increasing concern in recent years (Bruce et al. 1968; Linde and Bruce 1969; Whitcher et al. 1971). The incidence of death from malignancies involving the lymphoid and reticuloendothelial tissues appears to be higher among anesthesiologists than others of the general population. Also, the suicide rate appears to be more than twice that of a comparable socioeconomic group within the general population. A greater number of miscarriages have also been associated with the chronic exposure of operating room nursing personnel to trace amounts of anesthetics.

Concentrations of halothane found in surgical operating areas average about 10 ppm; anesthesiologists located near the exhaust of the anesthetic breathing circuit are probably exposed to much greater concentrations. There is concern that operating room personnel may develop deficits in cognition, perceptiveness, and motor coordination when subjected to long-term exposure to gas anesthetics. Experimentally, young animals (rats), but not adults, chronically exposed to 10 ppm of halothane during early life were noted to have deficits in learning that correlated with enduring synaptic membrane malformation in the cerebral cortex (Quimby et al. 1974).

Procedures for improvement of the exhaustion of gases from the operating theaters are now in progress to minimize exposure of the operating personnel. Veterinary anesthesiologists and personnel should also be aware of the potential hazards from long-term exposure to halogenated anesthetics.

CLINICAL USE

Halothane is the most commonly used inhalant anesthetic in veterinary medicine. It is capable of induction and maintenance of anesthesia without assistance from other CNS depressants. In most species, anesthesia is induced by ultrashort-acting barbiturates to permit endotracheal intubation. Halothane can be used in conjunction with all the preanesthetics and with other general anesthetics. Nitrous oxide is most usually combined with halothane to reduce its depressant effects upon the cardiopulmonary system.

IN LARGE AND SMALL ANIMALS

Halothane is used in both large and small animals (Fisher and Jennings 1958; Lumb 1959). Unless the drug is administered by semiclosed- or closed-circuit systems, the expense of using halothane becomes prohibitive. Because of the expense of the anesthetic, it has been used in large animals principally for maintenance anesthesia following barbiturate anesthesia and phenothiazine-derivative tranquilizers. When used in this manner, 2.2–8.7 ml/100 lb/hour of halothane are recommended (Jones et al. 1962). Halothane is an effective anesthetic in cattle. After induction of anesthesia with thiopental sodium, a 1000-lb cow can be maintained for 1 hour with 25–30 ml of halothane (Wright and Hall 1961). In calves, halothane anesthesia is successfully used during experimental cardiac surgery (Short et al. 1968). Postsurgical bloat is avoided since the calves are able to stand soon (approximately 30 minutes) after the surgical procedure.

In sheep, goats, and swine, halothane has also been used satisfactorily. For goats, atropine sulfate (0.8–2.4 mg) was given intravenously prior to the induction of anesthesia (Dhindsa et al. 1970). After rapid intravenous injection of sodium thiamylal (13–17 mg/kg of body weight), the animals were intubated and maintained on halothane using a semiclosed-circuit system. Anesthesia was maintained 18–230 minutes; the average recovery times ranged from 18 to 40 minutes. In swine, a halothane–nitrous oxide–oxygen mixture has been used satisfactorily (Vaughan 1961; Hastings et al. 1966).

Although the anesthetic is used in the dog and cat, the depth of anesthesia is sometimes difficult to control because of its high potency (Sims 1960). However, the use of a nitrous oxide–oxygen mixture in combination with halothane has minimized this difficulty. The mask induction method of anesthesia has been successfully applied with halothane and nitrous oxide in dogs and cats (Carter 1964; Goodger 1972). Initially, 70% nitrous oxide and 30% oxygen are administered without halothane (Goodger 1972). Halothane is then administered with the nitrous oxide-oxygen mixture 1 minute later at 0.5% for one-half minute. This is followed by gradually increasing the halothane by 1% increments until a concentration of 5% is reached approximately 4 minutes later. After 4 minutes, the concentration of nitrous oxide is reduced to 60%, and 40% oxygen is given for the remainder of the anesthetic procedure. All animals receive atropine intramuscularly 10 minutes prior to induction of anesthesia.

IN LABORATORY ANIMALS

Halothane is recommended for restraining monkeys and chimpanzees. An animal is placed in a transparent glass chamber and a 3.2% concentration of halothane vapor is used to induce anesthesia (Kinard and McPherson 1960). It has also been used successfully in the rabbit (Davis and Malinin 1974) and other laboratory animals (Sawyer et al. 1974).

IN CAGED BIRDS

Halothane can be used in parakeets. Surgical anesthesia is reached rapidly within 15–30 seconds. Induction is so rapid that care must be taken during the procedure because Stage IV anesthesia may be quickly reached (Grono 1961).

IN EXOTIC ANIMALS

The use of halothane in a number of exotic animals has been reported (Sawyer et al. 1974; Stunkard and Miller 1974).

Nitrous Oxide

Nitrous oxide, U.S.P. (N_2O), is a colorless, nonirritant, slightly sweet-smelling, nonflammable gas. When mixed with ether and oxygen, it will support combustion, and care must be taken to avoid violent explosions. With the introduction of halothane and methoxyflurane into veterinary medicine, the use and importance of nitrous oxide increased. It is useful when combined with the gas anesthetics, especially in the reduction of the depressant effect of halothane upon the cardiopulmonary system; when nitrous oxide is used in conjunction with halothane or methoxyflurane, the concentration of these gases can be reduced in the maintenance of anesthesia. Nitrous oxide is relatively insoluble in blood and fat compared with methoxyflurane.

From a potency aspect, nitrous oxide has weak CNS depressant properties. If nitrous oxide is used in combination with oxygen so that severe hypoxia does not occur in the induction of anesthesia, a level of anesthesia beyond plane 1 is rarely attained. With the brain being a so-called blood-rich organ, the uptake of nitrous oxide is relatively rapid during induction of anesthesia. Also, recovery from anesthesia is rapid when administration of the anesthetic is discontinued. Nitrous oxide is not metabolized and is eliminated unchanged.

Because of the low anesthetic potency of nitrous oxide, it is ordinarily preceded by intravenous barbiturates used in combination with other volatile anesthetics. Under no circumstances should nitrous oxide given for maintenance of anesthesia be more than 70% (Price and Dripps 1970). If nitrous oxide concentrations greater than this are administered at the expense of reducing the percentage of oxygen, a severe hypoxia will develop. Irreversible brain damage occurs when the concentration of oxygen is reduced to achieve higher concentrations of nitrous oxide to increase the depth of anesthesia.

Nitrous oxide is remarkably safe in the maintenance of anesthesia and has minimal side effects, providing hypoxia is excluded by the administration of no less than 30% oxygen. Thus a safe maintenance level for anesthesia is 70% nitrous oxide and 30% oxygen. Experimentally, dogs have been anesthetized continuously for 72 hours without deleterious effects. The vital functions of the body are not significantly altered provided hypoxia is not permitted to develop. Side effects such as vomition, mucus secretion, and salivation are essentially absent when nitrous oxide is used. Cardiopulmonary function is not affected and the release of catecholamines does not sensitize the myocardium to the effects of nitrous oxide. Renal and liver functions are also unaffected. The cough reflex remains active under nitrous oxide anesthesia.

Laryngospasm does not occur unless a hypoxic condition exists. Endotracheal intubation is not possible when a laryngospasm occurs without the aid of local anesthesia combined with skeletal muscle relaxants. *d*-Tubocurarine can be used with nitrous oxide. The effect of nitrous oxide upon skeletal muscle relaxation is not very great. If hypoxia is present, rigidity, spasms, and twitching of the skeletal muscles may occur.

CLINICAL USE

Nitrous oxide usually cannot be used alone in the maintenance of anesthesia. Consequently, it is ordinarily used in conjunction with other preanesthetic and anesthetic agents. Nitrous oxide has been used to maintain anesthesia in the horse, ruminant, dog, and cat.

If inhalation induction of anesthesia is preferred, nitrous oxide should be supplemented with an anesthetic that is relatively insoluble in blood, such as halothane, to attain high alveolar tensions (Carmichael 1971). According to Carmichael, induction of anesthesia with a nitrous oxide–methoxyflurane combination is satisfactory but slow in all but the smallest and debilitated animals. The relatively high blood solubility of methoxyflurane is responsible for this type of response. Preanesthetic medication should be given prior to the administration of nitrous oxide. For example, atropine sulfate, a phenothiazine tranquilizer such as acetylpromazine maleate, or a narcotic analgesic should be administered. In small animals, nitrous oxide (75%) is administered with oxygen (25%) by mask for 2–3 minutes to denitrogenate the alveoli (Carmichael 1971). Halothane is then added to the nitrous oxide–oxygen mixture in concentrations up to 3%, depending on the condition and size of the animal. The animal may then be intubated soon after surgical anesthesia is attained when jaw relaxation and other clinical signs of anesthesia are noted.

If induction of anesthesia is preferred using ultrashort-acting barbiturates, they may be used intravenously following preanesthetic medication (Carmichael 1971). Only a sufficient amount of the intravenous barbiturate to permit endotracheal intubation should be used. The semiclosed- or closed-circuit anesthetic equipment can then be connected to the endotracheal tube. Denitrogenation of the lungs is carried out similarly to the procedure referred to above, using assisted ventilation if necessary. The depth of anesthesia can be increased by adding halothane or methoxyflurane to the gas mixture.

In sick animals and in poor-risk patients, the inspired nitrous oxide may be reduced to 66% or even 50% of the inspired gas volume (Carmichael 1971). Once anesthesia is under way, there is no need to change the level or concentration of nitrous oxide unless there is an emergency that requires the discontinuance of anesthesia. When the depth of anesthesia requires changing, it is readily changed by varying the concentration of the supplemental gases (halothane or methoxyflurane) rather than changing the nitrous oxide.

Use of nitrous oxide following premedication with fentanyl-droperidol combination in the dog appears to be effective (Carmichael 1971). Also, ketamine in the cat makes excellent preanesthetic medication prior to the use of nitrous oxide and oxygen in the maintenance of anesthesia.

MINOR INHALANT ANESTHETICS

Ether

CHEMISTRY

Ether, U.S.P. (ethyl ether, diethyl ether, $C_2H_5 - O - C_2H_5$), is a colorless, highly volatile liquid with a characteristic odor and a burning, sweetish taste. It boils at 35° C. Its vapor is highly inflammable and forms an explosive mixture with air. One volume of ether will dissolve in about 12 volumes of water. It is soluble in oils and oil solvents.

Ether oxidizes slowly upon exposure to air, moisture, and light, with the formation of peroxides. Peroxides are thought to irritate the respiratory tract and to delay the onset of anesthesia. To reduce the formation of peroxides, ether should be kept in tight containers. Peroxides are known to accumulate in loosely stoppered containers or in ether vaporizer jars

(Shukys and Neeley 1958). It is considered inadvisable to leave ether in a vaporizer for more than 2 days or in an unstoppered container for over 1 week since it is known that peroxide residues remaining after volatilization may explode. Inasmuch as the peroxides formed are water soluble, rinsing vaporizer jars and wicks at 2-day intervals is recommended.

Ether should be stored in a cool place but definitely not in a refrigerator. Violent explosions and fire have occurred when only small containers of ether were stored. Ether fumes apparently are exploded and ignited by the electric relay mechanism of the refrigerator. Smoking or use of flammable devices is prohibited whenever ether is in use. Use of closed-circuit anesthetic equipment reduces the escape of ether into the surgery room and buildup of explosive concentrations of the vapors.

EFFECT UPON THE RESPIRATORY SYSTEM

Ether stimulates respiration in the early stages of anesthesia. Light etherization causes sufficient irritation of the airways to produce overventilation of the lungs reflexly with a subsequent decrease in the carbon dioxide concentration of the blood. This alkalosis or acapnia results in irregular respiration. During light surgical anesthesia (planes 1 and 2), breathing is regular and machinelike and the respiratory minute volume is increased slightly over normal. During deep surgical anesthesia (planes 3 and 4), the respiratory centers are progressively depressed until the level of anesthesia approaches Stage IV where breathing is absent.

When ether is administered by the open or drop method, it is easy to establish too high a concentration of vapor during the breath holding of induction. The inhalation of too high a concentration may produce respiratory arrest by paralysis of the respiratory centers. Artificial resuscitation will revive most such cases overcome during induction. In this respect, revival from ether is accomplished more successfully than when chloroform is used. This was demonstrated in a study where several dogs were subjected to respiratory-paralyzing concentrations of ether and chloroform (Draper and Whitehead 1942). In spite of immediate resuscitative procedures following the cessation of respiration, 0.8% and 10.3% of the animals failed to recover from ether and chloroform, respectively.

Both ether and chloroform vapors are irritating to the respiratory tract. Since the concentration of ether necessary to produce anesthesia is 4 times that of chloroform, ether produces a much greater respiratory irritation than does chloroform. Ether vapor increases the discomfort of the patient and stimulates a profuse secretion of mucus. Atropine sulfate must be used as part of the preanesthetic procedure to prevent this effect. Ether is contraindicated in animal patients suffering from pneumonia or other respiratory complications.

EFFECT UPON THE CARDIOVASCULAR SYSTEM

Anesthetic concentrations of ether have little effect upon the heart. In this respect it has a great advantage over halogenated anesthetics because there is little danger of inducing ventricular fibrillation. The heart rate and blood pressure are increased during the excitement of induction, primarily due to the release of epinephrine. There are occasional varied arrhythmias generally occurring during induction. Cardiac output during light surgical anesthesia is increased by about 20%. The increase in cardiac output probably accounts for the maintenance of blood pressure at this relatively high level.

Deep surgical anesthesia causes a progressive fall in blood pressure as a result of (1) a drop in cardiac output and (2) a progressive depression of the vasomotor centers with peripheral vasodilation. At the termination of Stage III, respiration ceases but the heart continues to beat. The circulation is inadequate because the peripheral vasodilation permits the blood to remain in the blood vessels instead of returning it to the heart in proper supply. Thus the underoxygenated myocardium ceases to beat, and death from hypoxia and asphyxiation is complete.

There are evidences of hemoconcentration during ether anesthesia, i.e., a reduction in plasma volume, and increases in cell volume, hemoglobin, and red cell counts.

EFFECT UPON THE KIDNEYS

Ether has little significant effect upon the kidneys of small animals during the relatively short time that it is usually administered in veterinary practice. The urine output is decreased probably by the antidiuretic hormone of the pituitary. Some animals may be unable to properly concentrate a high specific gravity urine either during or following anesthesia. The procedure for handling this problem was discussed in Chapter 10.

EFFECT UPON THE LIVER

Ether anesthesia of 1 hour's duration causes no depression of liver function in the dog according to the BSP tests. Prolonged etherization on successive days produces no demonstrable pathology in the livers of dogs. Liver glycogen is decreased by approximately 50% during the first hour.

EFFECT UPON THE GASTROINTESTINAL TRACT

Ether markedly depresses the tone and motility of the GI tract. During plane 3 of Stage III peristalsis and muscular tone are depressed completely. The depression continues during the postanesthetic state for a variable period, depending on the depth and duration of the etherization. Nausea followed by emesis is a common complication of light etherization that frequently occurs postanesthetically. However, this complication usually can be prevented by judicious use of preanesthetic agents.

EFFECT UPON THE SKELETAL MUSCULATURE

Ether is superior to any of the general anesthetics now in use in producing skeletal muscle relaxation. Profound muscle relaxation is achieved partly by its depressant effect upon the extrapyramidal and pyramidal pathways of the CNS. In addition, ether has a curariform blocking effect at the motor end-plate of skeletal muscle. If ether and *d*-tubocurarine chloride are used together, it is necessary to reduce the amount of *d*-tubocurarine chloride to one-third the recommended dose level to avoid paralysis of the respiratory musculature. Ordinarily the relaxation produced by ether is sufficient to obviate the use of skeletal muscle relaxants.

EFFECT UPON METABOLISM

The general level of metabolism is decreased by etherization. Hyperglycemia is characteristic. It results from decreased utilization of glucose by the tissues and also from excessive secretion of epinephrine during induction, which stimulates conversion of liver glycogen into glucose. The blood level of nonprotein nitrogen is increased.

ADVANTAGES AND DISADVANTAGES

Ether has certain disadvantages. Its vapors are inflammable. Ether boils at a low temperature and is difficult to use in hot climates. It irritates mucous membranes. Usually ether is not potent enough to avoid slow and difficult induction unless other premedication is employed.

With proper premedication ether is the safest of all general anesthetics. Ether satisfactorily depresses the CNS without undesirable effects upon other systems of the body. It permits ready control of the level of anesthesia, especially if used with oxygen, and provides good surgical anesthesia in the young pig, calf, dog, and cat.

Chloroform

In clinical practice, chloroform has been replaced by much safer inhalant and parenteral anesthetic agents. About the only justification for its continued use is as a euthanasia agent (see Section 15) or in emergency situations when other agents are unavailable. Its use in subtropical and tropical regions has been favored over the more volatile agents such as ether.

CHEMISTRY

Chloroform, N.F. ($CHCl_3$), is a clear, colorless, volatile liquid having a characteristic odor and a burning, sweet taste.

It boils at 61° C. Chloroform is relatively insoluble in water but is miscible in oils and oil solvents. Since its vapors do not burn, chloroform can be used near an open fire such as a kerosene or gasoline lamp. Chloroform to be used for anesthesia must not undergo prolonged exposure to light, air, or an open flame as it is oxidized to form traces of phosgene ($COCl_2$), a powerful irritant to the lungs. Ordinarily, 1% of ethyl alcohol is added to anesthetic chloroform to act as a reducing agent and to prevent the formation of phosgene.

Liquid chloroform is irritating to delicate tissues, especially to the conjunctiva. Chloroform vapors are as irritating to mucous membranes as ether vapors; however, since the concentration of chloroform required for anesthesia is only about one-fourth that of ether, chloroform produces less irritation to the respiratory tract during anesthesia. Even for use in euthanasia, chloroform cannot be recommended without the prior use of preanesthetic agents or tranquilizers.

Chloroform is a very powerful anesthetic. A concentration of only 2%–4% chloroform in the inspired air is necessary to induce anesthesia in an animal in a reasonable length of time (10–12 minutes). The concentration must be progressively reduced after induction to around 1.5% in inspired air to avoid depression of the respiration. The muscular relaxation under chloroform anesthesia is quite comparable to that produced by ether.

EFFECT UPON THE RESPIRATORY SYSTEM

During the induction of anesthesia, respiration is accelerated and deepened, due to struggling. From the onset of light surgical anesthesia, chloroform progressively depresses the respiration. The susceptibility of the respiratory center to stimulation by carbon dioxide is decreased and respiration becomes slow and shallow. The bronchial musculature is relaxed. Since this anesthetic is irritating to the respiratory tract, it is contraindicated in animals manifesting pneumonic and other respiratory ailments.

EFFECT UPON THE CARDIOVASCULAR SYSTEM

Chloroform is 25–30 times as poisonous as ether on direct contact with the mammalian heart. The concentration of chloroform in the blood during anesthesia is enough to injure the heart if the exposure period is long enough, whereas ether in concentrations sufficient to paralyze the respiratory center does not damage the myocardium. Chloroform is directly toxic to the heart. It sensitizes the myocardium to catecholamines such as epinephrine and norepinephrine, thus increasing the risk of serious cardiac arrhythmias and/or ventricular fibrillation. A dose level of 1–5 μg/kg of epinephrine or norepinephrine in the dog is capable of inducing ventricular fibrillation in 100% of the animals following thiobarbiturate- and chloroform-maintained anesthesia (Claborn and Szabuniewicz 1973). Preanesthetic doses of acetylpromazine maleate (1 mg/kg), chlorpromazine (2 mg/kg), and propranolol (0.5 mg/kg) prevent the fibrillatory effects of epinephrine in 100% of the animals subjected to the thiobarbiturate and chloroform anesthesia. When chloroform is used alone, epinephrine or norephinephrine induces ventricular fibrillation in 60% of the dogs. The combination of chloroform with the thiobarbiturates appears to enhance the incidence of ventricular fibrillation in animals.

Blood pressure rises somewhat during induction as a result of the excitement. Following induction with chloroform, blood pressure is markedly lowered as a result of depression of cardiac activity, depression of the vasoconstrictor center, and splanchnic vasodilation. When chloroform circulates in the blood vessels in anesthetic concentrations, the blood vessels relax. This effect, which is characteristic of the splanchnic vessels, is claimed to result from the direct depressant action of chloroform on the muscle fibers of the vessels.

Many of the adverse effects of chloroform on the cardiovascular system mentioned above doubtless can be related to the level or depth of anesthesia. Deep levels of chloroform should be avoided to prevent the injurious effect of the anesthetic upon the heart and blood vessels. Therefore caution must be exercised not to administer the anesthetic at too rapid a rate or in high concentrations during the induction phase. Rapid administration may produce cardiovascular depression or cardiac arrest through vagal inhibition. For this reason, a full therapeutic dose of atropine sulfate or a comparable anticholinergic agent should be employed in the medication prior to chloroform anesthesia. Other preanesthetic agents that should be used to reduce the potential hazard of chloroform are acetylpromazine, chlorpromazine, or propranolol.

EFFECT UPON THE KIDNEYS

Chloroform anesthesia depresses kidney function. Anuria may occur after recovery and albuminuria is often quite marked.

EFFECT UPON METABOLISM

Metabolism in general is decreased by chloroform anesthesia. Hyperglycemia results from decreased tissue metabolism of the blood sugar and also from the increased conversion of liver glycogen into blood glucose after the release of epinephrine during induction.

EFFECT UPON THE LIVER

Chloroform decreases liver efficiency as measured by dye excretion and other liver function tests. Normal dogs will excrete at least 85% of BSP injected intravenously within the first 15 minutes and the remainder is largely excreted within the next few hours. In contrast, a dog anesthetized with chloroform for 15 minutes excretes the dye for 8 days; when chloroform is administered for 2 hours, dye retention lasts 6 weeks. Three-fourths of the glycogen content of the liver is depleted during the first half hour of anesthesia. A high liver glycogen content affords some protection against the toxicity of chloroform. Protein depletion of the dog's liver renders it more vulnerable to chloroform toxicity.

Chloroform anesthesia effective for an appreciable period of time invariably causes central necrosis and fatty degeneration of the liver lobules. The susceptibility varies from animal to animal and is higher in fasted patients. Dogs fasted for 24 hours and then anesthetized for 1.5 hours show central necrosis of one-third to one-half of the liver lobules. Repair of this damage requires 7–12 days.

EFFECT UPON THE FETUS *in Utero*

In pregnant animals chloroform poisoning causes severe necrosis of the maternal liver and placenta. No damage is found in the liver or other organs of the fetus. The placenta is not a completely effective barrier against passage of chloroform into the fetal circulation. However, newborn animals delivered from females under medium depth of chloroform anesthesia move actively and breathe well, which is contrary to the effects of several nonvolatile anesthetics.

CHLOROFORM ANESTHESIA IN THE HORSE

Chloroform is sufficiently potent to anesthetize the horse. Within a few minutes of administration the animal reaches plane 1 of Stage III anesthesia. Nystagmus is prominent during Stage II and gradually diminishes in activity as anesthesia deepens. It is seen in plane 1 and disappears just as plane 2 anesthesia is entered. Frequently the eyelids close near the termination of nystagmus. To avoid the deeper planes of anesthesia and carbon dioxide accumulation, administration of the anesthetic should be discontinued when nystagmus disappears.

Chloroform should never be used in poor-risk or debilitated animals. It is contraindicated in animals suffering from cardiac or respiratory ailments. The duration of chloroform anesthesia even in a vigorous and healthy animal probably should not exceed 45 minutes (Smith 1963).

Ordinarily, recovery from chloroform anesthesia is rapid and without severe struggling or excitement. However, recovery from chloroform anesthesia is much slower than that noted when halothane is used. If excitement is imminent upon recovery, it is considered wise to maintain restraint and surveillance of the animal after completion of the surgical procedure.

DEATHS IN CHLOROFORM ANESTHESIA

Deaths from chloroform administration occur at three different times: (1) during induction, (2) during the late stages of prolonged surgical anesthesia, and (3) 24–48 hours after anesthesia, i.e., delayed chloroform poisoning.

1. *During induction.* The majority of deaths in chloroform anesthesia occur during the induction period. When this happens, the animal usually has shown considerable breath holding, excitement, and struggling. Large amounts of chloroform are inspired by irregular but deep inspirations that deliver a high concentration of anesthetic to the heart. Suddenly, without warning, the heart stops and the animal dies after a few inspiratory gasps. Death in this case is apparently the result of ventricular fibrillation.

2. *In prolonged anesthesia.* Death in the late stages of chloroform anesthesia is the result of fatal depression of the respiratory center by overdosage. The sensitivity of the center to carbon dioxide is decreased progressively and the respiratory movements become slower and more shallow and finally stop. The heartbeat stops soon after the respiration or, if previously hypoxic, the heart may stop simultaneously. Deaths in this fashion occur most often when the concentration of chloroform is not decreased sufficiently after the induction period. Premedication with another depressant agent decreases the probability of this type of death.

3. *Postanesthetically.* Delayed chloroform poisoning commonly occurs about 24–48 hours after anesthesia. Chloroform produces central lobular necrosis of the liver and marked fatty degeneration of the liver, kidneys, and heart. These vital organs may no longer be able to perform their normal metabolic and excretory functions, and thus toxins and waste products accumulate and lead to the death of the patient. Some tissue destruction always occurs in chloroform anesthesia, especially in the liver during increased P_{CO_2} concentrations. However, the regenerative powers of liver cells will replace dead liver tissue rapidly unless too much of the organ has been destroyed. The balance of these factors may not be decisive until 1–2 days and occasionally not until 7–10 days following chloroform anesthesia.

ADVANTAGES AND DISADVANTAGES

Chloroform has some advantages. It is inexpensive, easily stored, potent, nonflammable, applicable by the open-drop technique, and it provides prompt induction. These properties have led to the use of chloroform for brief periods of anesthesia in large animals and also for emergency anesthesia in many species of animals under a variety of conditions. Chloroform has been used for brief anesthesia in the castration of the mature boar and stallion, for obstetrical analgesia in the cow and mare, and for similar brief uses.

Despite some of the advantages of chloroform, it possesses serious disadvantages that weigh heavily against its use in any animal to produce surgical anesthesia. The toxic effects of chloroform upon the vital organs during surgical anesthesia and upon the life of the patient are the principal concerns. It is considered to be too potent for safe anesthesia in small animals.

CYCLOPROPANE

Cyclopropane, U.S.P. (C_3H_6), contains at least 99% by volume of C_3H_6, which is a heavy, colorless gas having a characteristic odor. The boiling point of cyclopropane is —32.9° C.

Cyclopropane was introduced in 1929 into human anesthesia. Its advantages are marked anesthetic potency, with rapid induction and recovery; relative freedom from toxicity; and lack of irritation. Disadvantages of cyclopropane are depression of respiration; less complete relaxation of abdominal muscles than provided by ether or chloroform; production of an explosive, flammable mixture on contact with air; and relatively high cost. Cyclopropane sensitizes the heart to the effects of epinephrine and certain other catecholamines and promotes cardiac irregularities. Epinephrine or norepinephrine is definitely contraindicated before or during cyclopropane anesthesia.

Cyclopropane diluted with 4 parts of oxygen is administered to small animals in a closed-circuit apparatus with total rebreathing. When administered in this fashion, the initial high cost of cyclopropane is reduced to a figure comparable with other anesthetics. Induction with cyclopropane is quiet and surgical anesthesia is produced in 1–2 minutes. Recovery is rapid even after prolonged anesthesia. Since cyclopropane causes some respiratory depression, premedication with morphine sulfate is contraindicated. However, premedication with atropine sulfate is indicated. Cyclopropane appears to have no effect upon the liver and kidneys. In animals it has little effect upon the heart.

Cyclopropane has also been used satisfactorily as a supplementary anesthetic in the horse following an intravenous thiobarbiturate. In cattle it has proved to be a most useful anesthetic for animals of all ages. It is best used when the gas is given directly to conscious, recumbent, and restrained animals. No excitement or objection results following inhalation of the cyclopropane-oxygen mixture through a face mask. Cyclopropane has also been used in swine by closed-circuit methods. It has been observed that the pig recovers rapidly from the anesthetic but some animals may vomit (Wright and Hall 1961).

The depth of cyclopropane anesthesia is best determined by the respiratory movement. In deep anesthesia, respiration is progressively depressed, but hypoxemia never exists as long as there is any respiratory movement because of the high proportion of oxygen in the anesthetic mixture. If breathing stops because of overdosage, the heart continues to beat for a reasonable period of time, during which more oxygen can be administered or the mask can be removed and artificial respiration instituted. The excess of cyclopropane is excreted with such rapidity that rarely is artificial respiration applied for more than a few seconds before the patient begins breathing.

Trichloroethylene

Trichloroethylene, U.S.P. (Trilene, Trimar), was formulated in 1864 by a German chemist. It was first used in industry as a grease solvent. Industrial grade trichloroethylene contains impurities and should not be used for anesthetic purposes. Trichloroethylene has a potent analgesic effect and has been used as an obstetrical analgesic in human medicine.

Chemistry

Trichloroethylene is a colorless, volatile liquid having an odor similar to that of chloroform. The preparation has a specific gravity of 1.47 and a boiling point of 87.6° C. It is the least volatile of the inhalant anesthetics, making open-drop administration unsatisfactory. The anesthetic grade of trichloroethylene is colored with 0.0005% waxoline blue so it can be distinguished from chloroform.

Trichloroethylene cannot be used with carbon dioxide absorbents such as soda lime. A toxic product, dichloroacetylene, forms and produces neurological injury. Cranial nerves, such as the fifth and seventh, have been most commonly damaged in human beings, but also the third, fourth, sixth, tenth, and twelfth may be affected. Knowledge of this reaction precludes the use of trichloroethylene in closed-circuit anesthesia apparatus.

Pharmacological Considerations

The primary effect of trichloroethylene upon the cardiovascular system appears to be upon cardiac rhythm. Electrocardiographic analysis reveals a bradycardia and a shift of the pacemaker favoring a nodal rhythm. This effect is ascribed to an increase in the tone of the vagus nerve. In deeper anesthesia, ventricular extrasystoles and ventricular tachycardia may occur. Epinephrine administration should be avoided during trichloroethylene anesthesia because of the danger of increasing the severity of the arrhythmia or causing ventricular fibrillation.

The vapors of trichloroethylene are only slightly irritating to the respiratory tract. Premedication with atropine sulfate or scopolamine hydrobromide is recommended to eliminate possible mucus secretions. The anesthetic typically accelerates the respiratory rate. As the tachypnea progresses, the respiratory activity becomes more rapid and shallow. Sudden bursts of tachypnea are sometimes associated directly with surgical stimulation.

Relaxation of the abdominal musculature is poor during trichloroethylene anesthesia. It is considered unsatisfactory for this type of surgery unless trichloroethylene is used in conjunction with a skeletal muscle relaxant. Trichloroethylene has very little, if any, effect upon uterine function. It readily crosses the placenta to reach the fetal circulation of sheep and goats.

DISADVANTAGES

One of the primary objections to trichloroethylene is that its anesthetic action is weak. Its low volatility appears, in part, to be responsible for this effect. Apparatus that employs bubbling oxygen assists in accelerating the volatility of the anesthetic to increase its potency. Due to its inherent weakness as an anesthetic, induction of anesthesia is slow, and surgical planes of anesthesia are not readily attained. Also, cardiac arrhythmias produced by the anesthetic are unfavorable. Trichloroethylene cannot be used in a closed circuit with soda lime because of the formation of a toxic product.

Although trichloroethylene is a potent analgesic, all the disadvantages delineated above make it virtually impossible to recommend its use in the practice of veterinary medicine.

OTHER INHALANT ANESTHETICS

Ethyl Chloride

Ethyl Chloride, N.F. (C_2H_5Cl), is a colorless, highly volatile liquid below 12° C or at a higher temperature if under increased pressure. It boils at 12°–13° C and therefore should be refrigerated when stored in glass ampules. Ethyl chloride is a potent, rapidly acting general anesthetic. It is difficult and dangerous to use for prolonged general anesthesia because of its toxic action on various organs of the body.

Since ethyl chloride is relatively nonirritating to the respiratory tract, animals such as the cat do not ordinarily object to inhaling the vapors. Ethyl chloride has a narrow margin of safety when used as an inhalation anesthetic. Caution should be observed because it is exceedingly potent. Respiratory and circulatory failures occur rapidly following overdosage.

Use of ethyl chloride for brief periods of anesthesia is primarily restricted to the cat. However, it may also be used to anesthetize birds. In anesthetizing the cat, the animal may be placed in a glass chamber with an ethyl chloride vapor concentration of 10% (Longley 1950). Light anesthesia usually occurs in approximately 2 minutes, with deep anesthesia occurring in about another 0.5–1 minute. Before respiration ceases, the animal is removed from the chamber. Anesthesia will last an additional period of 2–5 minutes before recovery.

During the induction of anesthesia in the cat, it is recommended that ethyl chloride be discontinued once a rhythmical respiratory rate is achieved (Wright and Hall 1961). Anesthesia can be continued and maintained with ether after discontinuance of the ethyl chloride.

If a glass chamber is not available for induction of ethyl chloride anesthesia, the vapors may be administered by using a face cone or mask covered with layers of cheesecloth. Ethyl chloride is sprayed on the cheesecloth until the animal loses consciousness. Some veterinarians use ethyl chloride in this manner for castration operations in the cat.

For parakeets and canaries, ethyl chloride appears to be safer than ether (Friedburg 1962). It does not irritate the respiratory mucosa of the birds. The induction period is reported to be about 5 seconds and the recovery period is about 4 minutes.

Ethyl chloride is often used as a local anesthetic. Due to its low boiling point, it evaporates very rapidly from the skin with the extraction of much tissue heat. Thus the tissues are frozen briefly and are insensitive to pain. This technique is well suited to incising the skin over an abscess or similar procedures requiring only brief surface anesthesia. Anesthetizing or freezing large areas of skin should be avoided because the marked "frostbite" pain following the anesthesia may annoy the patient. Caution must be employed in using ethyl chloride around the mouth and nose because of the danger of inhaling the volatilized anesthetic, which might produce a deep and even dangerous anesthesia.

Carbon Dioxide

Carbon Dioxide, U.S.P., is a normal gaseous constituent of air necessary for plant respiration and, in small amounts, for animal respiration, although it is a metabolic waste product in the latter. Carbon dioxide can be compressed with the loss of heat into a solid resembling snow, i.e., "dry ice."

As early as 1929, the analgesic and anesthetic properties of carbon dioxide were uncovered by experimental use in the dog (Leake and Waters 1929). Concentrations of 30%–40% carbon dioxide with oxygen produced anesthesia in the dog within 1–2 minutes, often without struggling. The analgesic and anesthetic action of carbon dioxide has been utilized in the humane and more efficient slaughter of swine, sheep, and calves for human food (Johnson 1960; Betts 1967). The swine pass through a long tube on a conveyor belt where they inhale 70% carbon dioxide and 30% air for 45–50 seconds. They are anesthetized for about 15 seconds after emerging from the tube. While unconscious, the animals are bled thoroughly, easily, and without bruising any edible tissues.

Carbon dioxide has also been used in the humane euthanasia of chickens (Cooper 1967). The chickens become anesthetized within 30–45 seconds. The birds are placed inside a chamber or bag that is filled with carbon dioxide from a gas cylinder. The author (N.H.B.) found the use of carbon dioxide to be of practical value in killing large numbers of birds in the laboratory for the collection of tissues in preparation for drug or chemical residue analysis. Compared to dislocation of the cervical vertebrae by hand or other means, the use of carbon dioxide minimizes wing flapping and the contamination of the laboratory with feathers and dust.

Solid carbon dioxide is preferred to ether or chloroform for short anesthesia periods in guinea pigs because it produces no excitement during induction and recovery (Hyde 1962). The gas has been used to perform cardiac punctures and intradermolingual inoculations. It has also been used to a limited extent in chinchillas, rabbits, and mice. The technique for inducing anesthesia consists of breaking approximately 2 lb of solid carbon dioxide into small pieces and placing them in the bottom of an open metal container (18 inches long, 12 inches wide, and 14 inches deep). The animals are placed on a removable wire platform 5 inches from the bottom of the container. Liberated carbon dioxide vapors produce general anesthesia in 10–15 seconds. Immediately following anesthesia, the animals are removed from the container. Duration of the anesthesia is 45 seconds, with recovery taking place in about 1 minute. No excitement or adverse side effects are noted other than an accelerated respiratory rate that lasts for a brief period.

Tricaine Methanesulfonate

Tricaine Methanesulfonate (Finquel, MS-222) is the most commonly used fish anesthetic and is the only one currently approved for use by the Food and Drug Administration (FDA) in food fish. The white crystals of tricaine readily dissolve in fresh or salt water. The drug enters the gills of the fish and, on this basis, is categorized with the inhalant anesthetics. An anesthetic dose of 50–100 mg/L of water is recommended. For the transport of fish, one-half the anesthetic dose is recommended. Induction of anesthesia occurs in 1–3 minutes, with recovery requiring 3–15 minutes. A toxic condition results when tricaine is used in salt water during the presence of sunlight. This effect may be avoided by keeping the container in the shade during the anesthetic period. In salmonids (lake trout and a few strains of rainbow trout), 0.01 w/w% (1 part of tricaine per 10,000 parts of water) tricaine is capable of inducing deep narcosis in less than 1 minute; recovery occurs in less than 10 minutes (McFarland and Klontz 1969). For a description of the use of tricaine in other species of fish, including the shark, the reader is referred to Healey (1964).

Tricaine has been used intramuscularly in snakes at the dosage rate of 0.18–0.27 mg/g of body weight and in American alligators at a dose level of 40–45 mg/lb of body weight (Wallach 1969).

REFERENCES

Allen, W. M.; Berrett, S.; Harding, J. D. J.; and Patterson, D. S. P. 1970. Experimentally induced acute stress syndrome in Pietrain pigs. Vet Rec 87:64.

Berman, M. C.; Harrison, G. G.; Bull, A. B.; and Kench, J. E. 1970. Changes underlying halothane-induced malignant hyperpyrexia in Landrace pigs. Nature 225:653.

Betts, A. O. 1967. The pig. In UFAW Handbook on the Care and Management of Laboratory Animals, 3rd ed., p. 666. Baltimore: Williams & Wilkins.

Bruce, D. L.; Eide, K. A.; Linde, H. W.; and Eckenhoff, J. E. 1968. Causes of death among anesthesiologists: A 20-year survey. Anesthesiology 29:565.

Carmichael, J. A. 1971. Nitrous oxide in small animal anesthesia. J Am Vet Med Assoc 159:857.

Carter, H. E. 1964. Induction of anesthesia in dogs by the inhalation of nitrous oxide, halothane and oxygen. Vet Rec 76:147.

Cascorbi, H. F.; Vessell, E. S.; Blake, D. A.; and Helrich, M. 1971. Halothane biotransformation in man. Ann NY Acad Sci 179: 244.

Claborn, L. D., and Szabuniewicz, M. 1973. Prevention of chloroform and thiobarbiturate cardiac sensitization to catecholamines in dogs. Am J Vet Res 34:801.

Cohen, A. B.; Rosenthal, W. S.; and Stenger, R. J. 1973. Autoimmune response in experimental halothane-induced liver injury. Proc Soc Exp Biol Med 142:817.

Cooper, D. M. 1967. Destruction of birds with carbon dioxide. Vet Rec 81:444.

Davis, N. L., and Malinin, T. I. 1974. Rabbit intubation and halothane anesthesia. Lab Anim Sci 24:617.

de Moor, A. 1968. Carbohydrate metabolism and hypoxia in the horse. Vet Rec 82:568.

Dhindsa, D. S.; Hoversland, A. S.; and Kluempke, R. 1970. Halothane semiclosed-circuit anesthesia in pygmy and large goats. Am J Vet Res 31:1897.

Douglas, T. A.; Jennings, S.; Longstreeth, J.; and Weaver, A. D. 1964. Methoxyflurane anaesthesia in horses and cattle. Vet Rec 76:615.

Draper, W. B., and Whitehead, R. W. 1942. Chances of resuscitation after an overdose of ether, vinyl ether and chloroform. Lancet 1:442.

Eberly, V. E.; Gillespie, J. R.; Tyler, W. S.; and Fowler, M. E. 1968. Cardiovascular values in the horse during halothane anesthesia. Am J Vet Res 29:305.

Eger, E. I., II; Brandstater, B.; Saidman, L. J.; Regan, M. J.; Severinghaus, J. W.; and Munson, E. S. 1965. Equipotent alveolar concentrations of methoxyflurane, halothane, diethyl ether, fluroxene, cyclopropane, xenon and nitrous oxide in the dog. Anesthesiology 26:771.

Eikelenboom, G., and Minkema, D. 1974. Prediction of pale, soft, exudative muscle with a non-lethal test for the halothane-induced porcine malignant hyperthermia syndrome. Neth J Vet Sci 99:421.

Fisher, E. W. 1961. Observations on the disturbance of respiration of cattle, horses, sheep and dogs caused by halothane anesthesia and changes taking place in plasma pH and plasma CO_2 content. Am J Vet Res 22:279.

Fisher, E. W., and Jennings, S. 1958. The use of halothane in horses and cattle. Vet Rec 70:567.

Friedburg, K. M. 1962. Anesthesia of parakeets and canaries. J Am Vet Med Assoc 141:1157.

Gates, J. B.; Botta, J. A., Jr.; and Teer, P. A. 1971. Blood gas and pH determinations in cattle anesthetized with halothane. J Am Vet Med Assoc 158:1678.

Goodger, W. J. 1972. Mask induction in the dog and cat using halothane and nitrous oxide anesthesia. J Am Anim Hosp Assoc 8:351.

Grono, L. R. 1961. Anaesthesia of budgerigars. Aust Vet J 37:463.

Hastings, S. G.; Booth, N. H.; and Hopwood, M. L. 1966. General anesthesia for thoracic surgical procedures in swine. In L. K. Bustad and R. K. McClellan, eds. Swine in Biomedical Research, p. 679. Seattle: Frayn Printing Co.

Healey, E. G. 1964. Anaesthesia of fishes. In O. Graham-Jones, ed. Small Animal Anaesthesia, p. 59. Elmsford, N.Y.: Pergamon Press.

Heinze, C. H. 1965. Methoxyflurane anesthesia. Proc Am Assoc Equine Pract, p. 329.

Hoge, R. S. 1966. Anesthesia and surgery for egg bound parakeets. J Am Anim Hosp Assoc 2:46.

Hull, M. W., and Reilly, M. G. 1968. Effect of repeated halothane anesthesia on sheep. Am J Vet Res 29:1161.

Hyde, D. L. 1962. The use of solid carbon dioxide for producing short periods of anesthesia in guinea pigs. Am J Vet Res 23:684.

Johnson, K. F. 1960. Humane slaughter program. J Am Vet Med Assoc 136:388.

Jones, E. W.; Vasko, K. A.; Hamm, D.; and Griffith, R. W. 1962. Equine general anesthesia-use of halothane for maintenance. J Am Vet Med Assoc 140:148.

Jones, E. W.; Nelson, T. E.; Anderson, I. L.; Kerr, D. D.; and Burnap, T. K. 1972. Malignant hyperthermia of swine. Anesthesiology 36:42.

Kinard, R., and McPherson, C. W. 1960. The use of trichloroethylene and halothane anesthesia in the restraint of laboratory primates. Am J Vet Res 21:385.

Krantz, J. C., Jr.; Park, C. S.; Truitt, E. B.; and Ling, A. S. C. 1958. Anesthesia. LVII. A further study of the anesthetic properties of 1,1-trifluoro-2,2-bromochlorethane (Fluothane). Anesthesiology 19:38.

Leake, C. D., and Waters, R. M. 1929. The anesthetic properties of carbon dioxide. Anesth Analg 8:17.

Linde, H. W., and Bruce, D. L. 1969. Occupational exposure of anesthetists to halothane, nitrous oxide and radiation. Anesthesiology 30:363.

Longley, E. O. 1950. Ethyl chloride in veterinary anaesthesia. Vet Rec 62:152.

Lumb, W. V. 1959. Closed-circuit halothane anesthesia in the dog: A report of 142 anesthetic periods. J Am Vet Med Assoc 134:218.

McFarland, W. N., and Klontz, G. W. 1969. Anesthesia in fishes. Fed Proc 28:1535.

Mazze, R. I.; Trudell, J. R.; and Cousins, M. J. 1971. Methoxyflurane metabolism and renal dysfunction: Clinical correlation in man. Anesthesiology 35:247.

Mitchell, B. 1966. Anaesthesia for caesarean section and factors influencing mortality rates of bitches and puppies. Vet Rec 79: 252.

Mitchell, G., and Heffron, J. J. A. 1975. Procaine in porcine malignant hyperthermia. Br J Anaesth 47:667.

Norby, M. A., and Link, R. P. 1970. Effect of halothane anesthesia on liver function in the horse. Vet Med Small Anim Clin 65:946.

Price, H. L., and Dripps, R. D. 1970. General anesthetics. I. Gas anesthetics: Nitrous oxide, ethylene and cyclopropane. In L. S. Goodman and A. Gilman, eds. The Pharmacological Basis of Therapeutics, 4th ed., p. 71. New York: Macmillan.

Prynn, R. B., and Redding, R. W. 1968. Electroencephalographic continuum in dogs anesthetized with methoxyflurane. Am J Vet Res 29:1913.

Quimby, K. L.; Aschkenase, L. J.; Bowman, R. E.; Katz, J.; and Chang, L. W. 1974. Enduring learning deficits and cerebral synaptic malformation from exposure to 10 parts of halothane per million. Science 185:625.

Sawyer, D. C.; Evans, A. T.; Krahwinkel, D. J., Jr.; and De Young, D. J. 1974. Anesthetic principles and techniques. Continuing Education Services, p. 1. Michigan State University, E. Lansing.

Severinghaus, J. W., and Cullen, S. C. 1958. Depression of the myocardium and body oxygen consumption with Fluothane. Anesthesiology 19:165.

Sheridan, V.; Deegen, E.; and Zeller, R. 1972. Central venous pressure (C.V.P.) measurements during halothane anaesthesia in the horse. Vet Rec 90:149.

Shideler, R. K. 1971. The practitioner's approach to equine inhalation anesthesia. Proc Am Assoc Equine Pract, p. 119.

Short, C. E.; Keats, A. S.; Liotta, D.; and Hall, C. W. 1968. Anesthesia for cardiac surgery in calves. Am J Vet Res 29:2287.

Shukys, J. G., and Neeley, A. H. 1958. Studies on the formation and decomposition of ether peroxides. Anesthesiology 19:671.

Sims, F. W. 1960. Halothane anesthesia in small animal practice. Vet Rec 72:617.

Smith, M. 1963. Maske til kloroformanaestesi af hest. Nord Vet Med 15:891.

Steffey, E. P.; Gillespie, J. R.; Berry, J. D.; and Eger, E. I., II. 1974a. Cardiovascular effects of the addition of N_2O to halothane in stump-tailed macaques during spontaneous and controlled ventilation. J Am Vet Med Assoc 165:834.

Steffey, E. P.; Gillespie, J. R.; Berry, J. D.; Eger, E. I., II; and Rhode, E. A. 1974b. Cardiovascular effects of halothane in the stump-tailed macaque during spontaneous and controlled ventilation. Am J Vet Res 35:1315.

———. 1974c. Circulatory effects of halothane-nitrous oxide anesthesia in the dog: Controlled ventilation. Am J Vet Res 35:1289.

Stunkard, J. A., and Miller, J. C. 1974. An outline guide to general anesthesia in exotic species. Vet Med Small Anim Clin 69:1181.

Swerczek, T. W., and Prickett, M. E. 1971. Post-surgical liver damage following halothane anesthesia in the horse. Proc Am Assoc Equine Pract, p. 137.

Tevik, A.; Nelson, A. W.; and Lumb, W. V. 1968. Chloroform and halothane anesthesia in horses: Effect on blood electrolytes and acid-base balance. Am J Vet Res 29: 1791.

Vasko, K. A. 1962. Preliminary report on the effects of halothane on cardiac action and blood pressure in the horse. Am J Vet Res 23:248.

Vaughan, L. C. 1961. Anaesthesia in the pig. Br Vet J 117:383.

Wallach, J. D. 1969. Medical care of reptiles. J Am Vet Med Assoc 155:1017.

Wass, J. A.; Keene, J. R.; and Kaplan, H. M. 1974. Ketamine-methoxyflurane anesthesia for rabbits. Am J Vet Res 35:317.

Whitcher, C. E.; Cohen, E. N.; and Trudell, J. R. 1971. Chronic exposure to anesthetic gases in the operating room. Anesthesiology 35:348.

Wolff, W. A.; Lumb, W. V.; and Ramsay, M. K. 1967. Effects of halothane and chloroform anesthesia on the equine liver. Am J Vet Res 28:1363.

———. 1968. Comparison of halothane and chloroform anesthesia in horses. Am J Vet Res 29:125.

Woolf, N.; Thorne, C.; Down, M.; and Walker, R. 1970. Serum creatine phosphokinase levels in pigs reacting abnormally to halogenated anaesthetics. Br Med J 3:386.

Wright, J. G., and Hall, L. W. 1961. Veterinary Anaesthesia and Analgesia, 5th ed. Baltimore: Williams & Wilkins.

CHAPTER 13

INTRAVENOUS AND OTHER PARENTERAL ANESTHETICS

NICHOLAS H. BOOTH

The Barbiturates
- **Pentobarbital Sodium**
- **Thiopental Sodium**
- **Thialbarbitone Sodium**
- **Thiamylal Sodium**
- **Methohexital Sodium**
- **Hexobarbital Sodium**

Chloral Hydrate
Chloral Hydrate and Magnesium Sulfate
Chloral Hydrate, Magnesium Sulfate, and Pentobarbital
Glyceryl Guaiacolate
Althesin
Dissociative Anesthetic Agents
- **Phencyclidine Hydrochloride**
- **Ketamine Hydrochloride**
- **Tiletamine Hydrochlorde**

Miscellaneous Agents
- **Chloralose**
- **Urethan**

In 1872 Oré of France produced a general anesthesia in human beings by an intravenous injection of chloral hydrate. Several postoperative deaths were blamed on the anesthesia and the method was discarded. The intravenous injection of chloroform and ether by Burkhardt in 1909 was unsatisfactory. Other drugs that were injected intravenously to produce general anesthesia included morphine, ethyl alcohol, avertin, urethan, and the barbiturates. Introduction of the soluble, short-acting barbiturates began a new era of general anesthesia by intravenous injection.

The stages of anesthesia are similar in a patient whether the anesthetic is injected intravenously or is administered by inhalation. However, it is possible to proceed more rapidly through induction with intravenous anesthesia than with inhalation anesthesia so that the early stages may not appear. Clinically, this rapid induction is desirable to avoid the excitement and struggling of induction.

Anesthetics administered intravenously appear to conform to the same laws of distribution within the tissues and the same theories of activity as previously discussed for other anesthetics. There is no anesthetic method or agent that produces an ideal anesthesia under all circumstances. It is desirable to know the advantages and disadvantages of different methods and drugs producing general anesthesia in order to select the kind most suited to a particular condition in a given species.

DISADVANTAGES

The depth or level of anesthesia is less readily controlled with drugs injected intravenously or parenterally, whereas it is easily controlled with volatile drugs like ether, halothane, and methoxyflurane. Unless the anesthesiologist is well trained, it is easy to inject an overdose; and, if this occurs, an overdose cannot be readily eliminated or detoxified. Volatile anesthetics are excreted rapidly after administration ceases, whereas a nonvolatile drug injected intravenously ceases to act only after it is excreted by the kidney or metabolized by the tissues. However, the introduction of the ultrashort-acting barbiturates has provided better control of intravenous anesthesia than existed earlier. The latter made possible both safe and satisfactory anesthesia for short periods and for surgery requiring only moderate muscular relaxation. The barbiturates do not provide the complete muscular relaxation required in some surgical operations in a dosage range that is entirely safe. Barbiturates given intravenously are not suitable anesthetics for cesarean section because they do not relax the abdominal muscles sufficiently and because they unduly depress the fetus *in utero,* with a high percentage of fetal deaths. Intravenous barbiturate anesthesia is contraindicated in hepatic or renal ailments since barbiturates are detoxified in the liver, excreted by the kidney, or both. When these organs are functioning improperly, the barbiturate may accumulate, causing a prolonged anesthesia with consequent toxic effects. Despite numerous advantages, the barbiturates leave much to be desired in the production of surgical anesthesia. Ether and trichloroethylene produce an effective degree of analgesia so that minor surgical procedures may be performed in Stage I; the barbiturates, by contrast, provide only a minimal analgesic effect in this stage or depth of anesthesia (Strobel and Wollman 1969).

With the inclusion of the barbiturates under the 1970 Controlled Substances Act, these preparations must be kept locked. Pentobarbital sodium is now classified as a Schedule II drug; records must be maintained indicating the species and quantities used. All other barbiturates are classified as Schedule IV compounds.

ADVANTAGES

Intravenous anesthesia has numerous advantages that justify the extensive use of this method in veterinary anesthesia. An outstanding advantage is the ease of induction, allowing the patient to pass quietly into surgical anesthesia without the usual struggling and excitement of the inductive stages. The rapidity of induction is an important feature of intravenous anesthesia, which is appreciated by the busy clinician. The rapid and easy induction by intravenous anesthesia safeguards the patient, the veterinarian, and the handlers from most of the hazards connected with restraining the animal. Compared to the administration of inhalant anesthetics, a minimum of apparatus is necessary in the administration of intravenous or parenteral anesthetic agents.

The patient receiving an intravenous injection becomes weak and drowsy and then unconscious. The ultrashort-acting barbiturates provide a brief and usually smooth recovery. Individual and species variations are noted: dogs ordinarily recover quietly but an occasional animal may show some excitement; horses often show excitement during recovery, although some regain consciousness quietly. Ordinarily vomition is absent during intravenous anesthesia in animals capable of vomiting. If vomiting occurs following the administration of a barbiturate, it is most likely to be seen in the recovery period (Chenoweth and Van Dyke 1969).

Prompt recovery with a lack of nausea and vomition will permit the majority of small animal patients to be discharged without hospitalization following minor surgery. The postanesthetic period is relatively free from complications such as may arise from irritation of the respiratory tract. Intravenous barbiturate anesthesia is indicated in the young or old, if proper precautions and care are practiced during administration.

Intravenous anesthesia has a decided advantage in operations about the head, because administration of the anesthetic intravenously does not interfere with the operative areas as would an inhalant anesthetic. Diseases of the respiratory tract, debility, and shock are usually less aggravated by intravenous anesthesia than by other forms of anesthesia. Barbiturates given intravenously are quite successful for symptomatic control of convulsive and tetanic spasms.

THE BARBITURATES

Barbital and phenobarbital were the first of the barbituric acid derivatives introduced into medicine. When used to produce anesthesia, the major limitation of the earlier barbiturates was their long period of action. In 1924 Somnifene was used intravenously to produce general anesthesia. Dial was introduced during the same year. Pernoston (Pernocton) was first used in 1927. During 1928 amobarbital sodium (Amytal sodium) was employed in animals. Pentobarbital sodium (Nembutal) was used intravenously in 1930. In 1933 Evipal sodium (Evipan-Natrium) was introduced and recognized as a marked advancement in intravenous anesthesia because of a very rapid hypnotic action of brief duration. In 1934 thiopental sodium (Pentothal sodium) was introduced and appeared to possess certain advantages over Evipal sodium. In 1946 and 1948, respectively, new ultrashort-acting barbituric acid derivatives called thialbarbitone sodium (Kemithal) and thiamylal sodium (Surital) were introduced into veterinary medicine.

There are many other barbituric acid derivatives, such as Neonal, Alurate, Ipral, Ortal, Phanodorn, Seconal, and Delvinal. These barbiturates, however, are infrequently used in veterinary medicine. Several of the barbituric acid derivatives most widely used in veterinary medicine are listed in Table 13.1, with generalizations regarding their official status, duration of action, and chemical structure.

The intermediate and long-acting barbiturates are discussed briefly in Chapter 14. These compounds should be restricted to only sedative or anticonvulsant usage. Their long action precludes using them for general anesthetic purposes.

Chemistry

The barbiturates are bitter-tasting white powders, except for the sulfur-containing thiobarbiturates, which may have a yellowish tint. Barbiturates are hygroscopic and will decompose on exposure to air, heat, and light. They should be stored in dark bottles, sealed ampules, or colored capsules. Solutions of barbiturates decom-

TABLE 13.1. Major barbiturates used in veterinary medicine

	Official Names and Synonyms	Accepted by	Approximate Duration of Action	Radicals Attached to Carbon 5	
				R_1	R_2
↑ Duration increased	Phenobarbital Sodium (soluble phenobarbital, soluble phenobarbitone, Luminal sodium)	U.S.P.	Long	Ethyl	Phenyl
	Barbital Sodium (soluble barbital, soluble barbitone, Veronal sodium)	U.S.P.	Long	Ethyl	Ethyl
	Amobarbital Sodium (Amytal sodium)	U.S.P.	Intermediate	Ethyl	Isoamyl
	Pentobarbital Sodium (Nembutal sodium)	U.S.P.	Short	Ethyl	1-Methyl butyl
	Secobarbital Sodium (Seconal sodium)	U.S.P.	Short	Allyl	1-Methyl butyl
	Thiopental Sodium* (Pentothal sodium)	U.S.P.	Ultrashort	Ethyl	1-Methyl butyl
	Thiamylal Sodium* (Surital sodium)	N.F.	Ultrashort	Allyl	1-Methyl butyl
	Thialbarbitone Sodium* (Kemithal sodium)		Ultrashort	Allyl	Cyclohexenyl
Duration decreased ↓	Methohexital Sodium† (Brevane)	N.F.	Ultrashort	Allyl	1-Methyl-2-pentynyl

* Sulfur replaces oxygen on carbon 2.
† Methyl group replaces hydrogen on nitrogen 1.

pose rapidly, unless stabilized. The boiling of aqueous solutions quickly decomposes barbiturates. Certain thiobarbiturates are relatively unstable; solutions of these may be entirely decomposed in 36 hours at room temperature but will last longer if refrigerated.

The barbiturates are derived from the nondepressant barbituric acid or malonylurea, which contains a pyrimidine nucleus.

When the hydrogens on carbon 5 are substituted with an appropriate alkyl or aryl group, depressant activity on the central nervous system (CNS) is possessed by the compound. A few barbituric acid derivatives contain a sulfur atom attached to carbon 2 in substitution for the oxygen. (See Fig. 13.1.)

Barbituric acid and its carbon 5 substituted derivatives are sparingly soluble in water. Aqueous solutions are weakly acid in reaction and will combine with sodium or other fixed alkalis to form water-soluble salts. The sodium atom joins the oxygen atom attached to carbon 2. These salts hydrolyze in water to form alkaline solutions with a pH usually between 9 and 10.

Conversion of the barbituric acid derivatives into water-soluble salts made possible the intravenous injection of barbiturates, which has been so widely and satisfactorily practiced in veterinary medicine. Furthermore, the soluble compounds are preferred for oral administration because of more regular and dependable absorption with subsequent prompt effect.

Several hundred barbituric acid derivatives have been synthesized but only a few have survived the rigors of clinical trial. From the pharmacological study of these

```
          H      O
          |     //
          N—C   H(1)
        /(1)  (6)\ /
   O=C(2)     (5)C
        \(3)  (4)/ \
          N—C   H(2)
          |     \\
          H      O
```

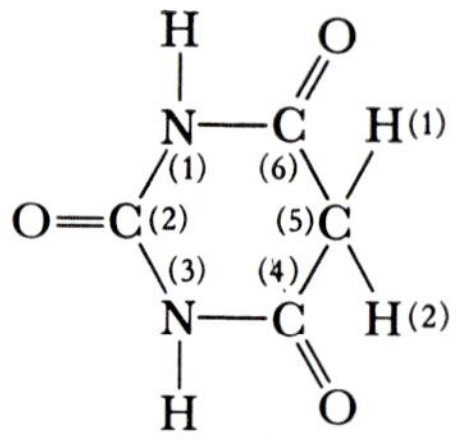

Barbituric Acid (malonylurea)

Fig. 13.1.

compounds, certain relationships of chemical structure and pharmacological response have become apparent so that certain generalities are justified.

1. To be hypnotically effective, both hydrogen atoms on carbon 5 must be replaced by an alkyl or aryl group.
2. To obtain optimal therapeutic results, the substituting radicals on carbon 5 should contain in total a minimum of 4 and a maximum of 9 carbons.
3. Unsaturated carbon chains are more readily oxidized and hence are short acting.
4. Short chains are more stable and hence are long acting.
5. Long chains are easily oxidized and are short acting.
6. Branched chains tend to be shorter in action than straight chains.
7. Only one aryl radical should be attached to carbon 5.
8. Replacement of the oxygen atom on carbon 2 by a sulfur atom increases the potency and instability and shortens the duration of action of the compound.
9. Attachment of alkyl groups to positions 1 or 3 shortens the period of action and tends to stimulate the CNS.
10. Replacement of the oxygen or carbon 2 by an HN= group destroys the hypnotic activity of the molecule.

Effect upon the Central Nervous System

The major action of the barbiturates is to depress the CNS. This effect is the reason for the extensive use of the barbiturates in medicine. Effects upon other systems become important as the toxic limitations to the use of the drug are approached.

Each of the many barbiturates depresses the CNS. Clinically they differ in respect to effective dosage, time required for initial effect, duration of action, and method of administration. The degree of depression may vary from mild sedation to surgical anesthesia.

The barbiturates depress the cortex of the brain and probably the thalamus. They depress motor areas of the brain and thus can be used to control convulsive seizures. They also depress sensory areas and induce anesthesia. Since sensory nerve fibers are less susceptible than motor nerve fibers, relatively large dosages of barbiturates are necessary to deaden the perception of pain. Barbiturates are better hypnotics than anesthetics.

The exact mechanism whereby the barbiturates depress the cellular activity of the CNS is not clear. It appears that there is a series of mechanisms, some related and some unrelated, in the depression of the CNS by barbiturates. Numerous investigations have shown a decrease in oxygen uptake by the brain following barbiturate administration. The utilization of oxygen by the cortical areas of the brain is more depressed than by other regions of the CNS. Transmission of nerve impulses at synaptic as well as at neuroeffector junctions is normally decreased by the barbiturates. The blocking effects of decamethonium and *d*-tubocurarine upon skeletal muscle are increased by the barbiturates. These effects occur because the barbiturates decrease the sensitivity of the polysynaptic junctions to the depolarizing action of acetylcholine.

It has been demonstrated in animals, particularly in cats, the barbiturates raise the threshold of spinal reflexes. Lowering of the threshold by strychnine can be overcome by barbiturates, even to the practical elimination of crossed reflexes. The barbiturates are used clinically with considerable success in the treatment of strychnine poisoning and other convulsants.

Numerous investigators have directed their work toward the effect of the barbiturates upon the reticular activating system of the CNS. This system is particularly sensitive to the barbiturates and other depressant drugs (Sharpless 1970). Animals are unable to be aroused or to maintain the wakeful state following the administration of hypnotic to anesthetic dose levels of the barbiturates.

The CNS depression produced by dose levels of the barbiturates varying in degree from mild sedation to deep anesthesia is reversible. Of interest is the effect of anesthetic agents, including the barbiturates, upon the expansion of biomembranes (Seeman 1972). This interesting aspect of the mechanism of action of anesthetics and CNS depressants was briefly discussed in Chapter 10.

Effect upon the Respiratory Center

With exception of the cat, therapeutic doses of barbiturates depress respiration slightly but no more than would be expected from the general sedation produced by the drug. In the cat, the marked susceptibility of respiratory function following barbiturate administration and especially its marked blocking effect upon the reticular formation may explain why this animal reacts adversely to barbiturates. The reticular formation of the cat apparently feeds signals or impulses into the medullary control centers governing respiration. In contrast to a single major mechanism in most other species, respiratory activity appears to be governed at two levels within the CNS. Until more is learned about the sensitivity of the cat to barbiturates, barbiturate anesthesia must be induced with particular caution.

Large doses are markedly depressant to the respiratory center in the medulla. Intravenous injection of a barbiturate produces a more severe depression of respiration than that following oral administration, due probably to the production of a higher momentary concentration of drug effective upon the center. The blood concentration inhibiting the respiratory center is considerably less than the concentration arresting the heart. Therefore, when respiratory arrest occurs during barbiturate anesthesia, attention should be devoted first to reestablishing respiration because the heart continues to function for a brief period. According to Chenoweth and Van Dyke (1969), more animals are lost from failure to maintain an adequate airway than from any other single difficulty in anesthesia. In most species, insertion of an endotracheal catheter can be accomplished so oxygen may be given when depression of respiration results from an anesthetic overdose. Pentobarbital at a dose level of approximately 4 times the level producing respiratory arrest may be administered before cardiac arrest occurs in the artificially ventilated animal (Robertson et al. 1958).

Effect upon the Cardiovascular System

One of the most important effects of pentobarbital anesthesia in the dog is upon cardiac output (Priano et al. 1969). In spite of an increase in the heart rate of 65%, these authors did not observe a change in cardiac output. Since the total peripheral resistance was not elevated, it indicated that the myocardium was severely depressed, due to a direct effect by the anesthetic. Rationale underlying this reasoning was supported by 30%–42% decreases in the contractility of the myocardium.

In the calf, cardiac output does not appear to change significantly following an intravenous injection of a relatively small dose of pentobarbital sodium (Anderson et al. 1972). However, a transient but significant effect upon the pulmonary and systemic circulations may occur following the administration of this anesthetic. A pressor response of the pulmonary circulation is observed, which may be attributable to a local vasoconstrictor effect on resistance vessels. In contrast to a pulmonary pressor effect produced by pentobarbital in the bovine, it appears to have no effect upon the resistance vessels of the pulmonary circulation in the canine. On the systemic circulation, pentobarbital sodium appears to have a varying effect (Anderson et al. 1972). These authors consistently observed tachycardia which also has been seen in other species. This effect is believed to be due to a vagolytic effect of the anesthetic agent. The vagolytic effects of barbiturates (pentobarbital and amytal in moderate doses and barbital in large doses) have been well known for some time (Linegar et al. 1936) Phenobarbital, on the other hand, does not produce this effect.

The incidence of ventricular fibrillation is increased especially when animals are subjected to both anesthesia and hypothermia (Blair 1969). Ventricular fibrillation may occur in 100% of the hypothermic animals following the administration of pentobarbital. It occurs in 50% of the animals following the administration of thiopental.

The vascular system, especially the vasomotor center, is affected more by the concentration of barbiturate acting on it than by the total dose given. Rapid intravenous injection of a relatively safe dose of a barbiturate causes a sharp but transitory fall in blood pressure because of the high concentration briefly depressing the vasomotor center. Large intravenous dosages of barbiturates depress the vasomotor center, resulting in peripheral vasodilation with a severe drop in blood pressure. Excessive intravenous concentrations of barbiturates may injure the capillary musculature directly to such an extent that sufficient capillary dilation occurs to induce vascular shock. Intraarterially, barbiturates and, in particular, thiopental produce spasm of the arterial wall to the extent that massive gangrene will occur (Kinmonth and Shepherd 1959). The accidental intraarterial injection of barbiturates has occurred on a number of occasions in the human being and has resulted in the loss of fingers or the arm due to thrombosis and gangrene (Stone and Donnelly 1961). Thiopental has been shown to cause vasoconstriction in the perfused rabbit ear; this effect was associated with the release of norepinephrine from the arterial wall (Burn 1960). Under no circumstances should the barbiturates and especially the thiobarbiturates be injected intraarterially for the induction of anesthesia. In human beings, the effects of an inadvertent, intraarterial injection can be significantly minimized or completely prevented by using a solution of thiopental no greater than 2.5% (Stone and Donnelly 1961).

A congenital porphyrin condition ("pink tooth") is sometimes observed in cattle. Also, porphyrin metabolism may be disturbed in normal animals from exposure to chemicals such as hexachlorobenzene, griseofulvin, aminopyrine, and others. In the liver, synthesis of porphyrin comes about by the condensation of succinyl coenzyme A with glycine to form aminolevulinic acid. Formation of aminolevulinic acid occurs in the mitochondria of hepatic cells through enzymic activity (i.e., aminolevulinic acid synthetase). The barbiturates stimulate the increased production of this enzyme that increases porphyrin production. Death may occur in human beings because the rise in porphyrin levels leads to neurological disturbances from demyelination of peripheral and cranial nerves.

Animals afflicted with a known or suspected metabolic disturbance should not be subjected to a barbiturate anesthetic.

Effect upon the Gastrointestinal Tract

As a group, the barbiturates appear to depress activity of the intestinal musculature. However, after an initial depression, the thiobarbiturates may increase both tonus and motility. After years of clinical use of the barbiturates, no important effects such as diarrhea or intestinal stasis have been noted.

Effect upon the Kidney

The barbiturates appear to have no direct effect upon the kidney. Indirectly, by lowering blood pressure, the barbiturates can produce oliguria or anuria. Only when prolonged, as in overmedication, does this effect become important. It may be necessary to employ the procedure discussed in Chapter 10 to maintain adequate renal function in animals that are manifesting renal impairment during and immediately following general anesthesia.

There is some evidence that phenobarbital and occasionally pentobarbital inhibit water but not saline diuresis in dogs, possibly through an influence upon the antidiuretic hormone.

Effect upon the Liver

Therapeutic doses of barbiturates have no significant effect upon liver function. In patients with liver damage, large doses of barbiturates may cause further injury. The detoxifying action of the liver will be discussed under the fate of the barbiturates.

Effect upon the Uterus and Fetus

Sedative doses of barbiturates do not influence uterine activity. Full anesthetic doses are believed, on the basis of *in vitro* studies, to depress uterine contractions during parturition (Gruber 1937). However, an equally if not more important consideration is the effect of barbiturates upon the fetus. The barbiturates readily diffuse through the placenta into the fetal circulation. Thiopental administered intravenously to a pregnant woman reaches the mixed fetal cord blood within 45 seconds and is in equilibrium with the maternal venous blood by 3 minutes (McKechnie and Converse 1955).

Pentobarbital and thiopental in concentrations that fail to produce maternal anesthesia will completely inhibit fetal respiratory movements without maternal hypoxia prevailing. Even though respiration is not completely depressed in a newborn animal following the use of a barbiturate, there is no assurance that the animal will survive. A number of studies have revealed that the liver in the newborn of a number of animals lacks the microsomal enzyme system required to biotransform or metabolize drugs such as the barbiturates. This important enzyme mechanism usually begins to develop during the first week following birth and does not attain maximal development until 8 weeks of age or older. Without this important enzyme mechanism to assist in the degradation of barbiturates, the animal must depend primarily on the renal elimination of the drugs. Even this route of elimination poses a problem because renal function in the newborn animal is less efficient than in the mature animal. Thiopental is not as depressant to the fetus as pentobarbital. Clinical experience bears out the above experimental observation. It is well known among veterinary practitioners that a cesarean section performed under general anesthesia will depress the fetus and may produce up to 100% fetal mortality.

Effect upon the Metabolic Rate

Sedative doses of barbiturates do not significantly influence the basal metabolic rate. Dosages producing surgical anesthesia depress basal metabolism, so that less body heat is produced during anesthesia concurrently with excessive heat loss as a result of vasodilation. It is important that surgical patients anesthetized with barbiturates be kept warm while depressed, especially when overmedicated. Consequently, it is always wise to monitor the effect of barbiturate anesthesia upon body temperature (Chenoweth and Van Dyke 1969). With a decline in heat production during anesthesia and an increase in heat loss due to peripheral vasodilation, the anesthetized animal drifts toward the temperature of his surrounding environment (Lutsky 1969). A definite hypothermic state is seen when the anesthetized dog is exposed to air temperatures below 27° C (Dale et al. 1968); the rectal temperature of animals in this study decreased from 1°–5° at an air temperature of 27° C to 10°–18° at an air temperature of 10° C. This not only resulted in the prolongation of recovery from pentobarbital anesthesia but deaths were also observed.

Effect upon the Skeletal Musculature

In general, the barbiturates do not completely relax the abdominal musculature. If additional relaxation is required in surgery, curariform agents may be used. Since skeletal muscle relaxants such as curare, succinylcholine, and others are not analgesics or anesthetics, caution in using them under the guise of anesthesia must be avoided for humane reasons. The photomotor reflex should be checked to determine whether or not an animal is regaining consciousness when a skeletal muscle relaxant is used in conjunction with a barbiturate anesthetic (see Chapter 10).

In the horse, postanesthetic forelimb lameness believed to be due to muscular ischemia during the recumbent phase of anesthesia has been observed in animals subjected to barbiturate and inhalant anesthetics (Trim and Mason 1973). The muscle mass and weight of large animals lying in a recumbent position for some time apparently are responsible for the initiation of the ischemia. Most clinicians in the past reported this condition to be a "postoperative radial paralysis." With an increase of serum creatine phosphokinase (CPK) occurring immediately after anesthesia, Trim and Mason (1973) felt that this response was associated with an etiology of muscular origin rather than of neurogenic origin. In addition, the blood lactate level was elevated; this condition resembled some of the characteristics seen in equine paralytic myoglobinuria. It is possible that the accumulation of lactate has a major role in the pathogenesis of both postanesthetic lameness and paralytic myoglobinuria from induction of injury to muscle cells due to a deficiency of oxygen delivery to them. The "pileup" of lactate would induce muscular spasms as well as the further reduction in blood flow and oxygen delivery to an already ischemic muscle mass. Duration of the lameness following anesthesia varies from 1 to 7 days; however, edema and swelling over the rib cage will persist for a longer period (Trim and Mason 1973).

Absorption

The barbiturates are absorbed readily from the gastrointestinal tract. The rate of absorption varies but in general is faster for the short-acting and slower for the long-acting drugs. Although the intrathoracic administration of barbiturates is not recommended, absorption following this route of administration is quite rapid.

After intravenous injection, a barbiturate remains in the blood in detectable concentrations for only a few minutes until it is taken up by the tissues.

Distribution

The barbiturates are distributed more or less generally throughout the body. Values for the specific volume of distribution (V′d) have not been determined for many barbiturates. Not only would these values differ for the different barbiturates but they would also vary among the various species. In the goat, the V′d for sodium pentobarbital (30 mg/kg) administered intravenously is 0.72 L/kg of body weight; the first-order disappearance rate kinetic constant (Kd) is 0.76 hour and the half-life ($t_{1/2}$) is 0.91 hour (Boulos et al. 1972). Thiopental and probably other barbiturates apparently pass without appreciable hindrance through the blood-brain barrier. Soon after the intravenous injection of thiopental, its concentration in the cerebrospinal fluid and plasma of the dog is found to be nearly equal (Brodie et al. 1952).

The barbiturates diffuse through the placenta into fetal tissue and may occur in the milk in small amounts. It is possible to detect minute amounts of barbiturates in body fluids such as plasma and urine as low as 500 picograms/ml using radioimmunoassay procedures (Flynn and Spector 1972).

Fate

The barbiturates are eliminated by renal excretion in the urine and/or destroyed by oxidative activity of hepatic and extrahepatic tissues. Trace amounts may be excreted in the milk of a lactating female.

Hepatic metabolism

Pentobarbital and many other barbiturates are metabolized principally by the hepatic microsomal enzyme system (Freudenthal and Carroll 1973). The thiobarbiturates are destroyed by both the liver and extrahepatic tissues. Their destruction in the extrahepatic tissues is more rapid than are any other barbiturates (see Table 13.2). Long-acting barbiturates, such as phenobarbital and barbital, are not metabolized by the liver.

The rate at which ultrashort-acting barbiturates are inactivated is not as rapid as previously thought. Originally their brief action was believed to parallel the rate of destruction by the liver and extrahepatic tissues; later, it became apparent that their systemic action was quickly terminated by localization in the body fat depots (Brodie et al. 1952).

Short-acting barbiturates are not recovered from urine following sedative doses and in only trace amounts at higher dosages. The activity of these drugs is brief because of rapid tissue oxidation. Additional evidence of the importance of the liver in destruction of many barbiturates is the clinical finding that anesthesia with a short-acting barbiturate may be prolonged many times in the presence of hepatic injury or disease. The clinician should, therefore, avoid the use of short-acting barbiturates in patients showing liver disturbances. A dose of thiopental or a comparable ultrashort-acting barbiturate producing anesthesia in a normal patient for only about 15 minutes may anesthetize a patient with impaired liver function for several hours. Studies within the last decade have shown that a number of drugs, including pentobarbital, are metabolized by hepatic microsomal enzymes (Conney 1967), which are located in the endoplasmic reticulum. The activity of the drug-metabolizing enzymes in hepatic microsomes may be affected by several factors. For instance, newborn and young animals possess only a fraction of the capability to metabolize drugs of the adult animals, and starving the animal depresses significantly the activity of hepatic microsomes to metabolize drugs. Liver microsomal activity may be

TABLE 13.2. Degradation of barbiturates by liver, brain, and muscle brei (120 micrograms of appropriate barbiturate added to all samples)

Barbiturate	Percentage Liver Destruction	Percentage Brain Destruction	Percentage Muscle Destruction
Seconal	30	0	0
Pentothal*	53	10	0
Phenobarbital	0	0	0

Source: Dorfman and Goldbaum 1947.
* Thiopental sodium.

accelerated by the administration of various drugs (e.g., phenobarbital, phenylhydantoin) to the degree that the same drug or others may be metabolized at a greater rate. For example, phenobarbital has the capability of stimulating the metabolism of other barbiturates. Consequently, animals become resistant or tolerant to these drugs because of a greater rate of metabolism of the barbiturate to inactive metabolites. This phenomenon has been noted in rats pretested with phenobarbital. The rats were anesthetized only 11 minutes by hexobarbital compared to 216 minutes for control animals (Burns et al. 1963). Chemical agents such as DDT and other chlorinated hydrocarbons can affect the duration of anesthesia produced by pentobarbital; DDT administered 2 days prior to pentobarbital reduces the duration of anesthesia in animals by 25%–50% (Conney and Burns 1972).

SPECIES VARIATION

The rate of metabolism of barbiturates varies considerably between and among the various species. For instance, the mouse metabolizes hexobarbital many times faster than human beings. In general, most of the laboratory animals metabolize drugs more rapidly than human beings. The cat, however, is an exception and requires a longer period of time to metabolize barbiturates than human beings or laboratory animals. Pentobarbital is metabolized at a rate of 4%/hour in human beings compared with 15%/hour in the dog and 50%/hour in the horse. In ruminants, particularly sheep and goats, pentobarbital is metabolized at a rapid rate (Rae 1962; Bryant 1969). In sheep, pentobarbital is cleared from the plasma at the rate of about 49%/hour and thiopental is cleared at about 17%/hour following tissue equilibrium (Rae 1962). The mean biological half-life of pentobarbital in the plasma of sheep is 66.8 $\pm$ 16 minutes (Santos and Bogan 1974).

Pretreatment of sheep with phenobarbital does not influence the *in vitro* metabolism of hexobarbital or pentobarbital (Shetty et al. 1972). According to these authors, phenobarbital in sheep is incapable of inducing a more rapid rate of metabolism in an already active microsomal enzyme system.

RENAL EXCRETION

Long-acting barbiturates, such as barbital and phenobarbital, are excreted in the urine. The substituent group on carbon 5 of these drugs is resistant to oxidation by liver or other tissues. The long-acting barbiturates are excreted slowly over a period of several days, which accounts for their prolonged periods of action. This slow excretion may lead to accumlative toxicity when an excessive dosage is administered repeatedly. In the dog about 20%–25% of the total dosage of barbital is excreted in the urine in the first 24 hours. A total of 85% is excreted in the urine in 6 days.

Renal damage interferes with the excretion of long-acting barbiturates. There is real danger of severe depression and death when these drugs are administered to a patient with impaired renal function. Dogs and cats suffering severe experimental nephrosis die in a coma after receiving an anesthetic dose of pentobarbital. Chickens will recover from pentobarbital anesthesia, but the avian kidney excretes barbital so slowly that they die in coma from respiratory failure. Since the intermediate and long-acting barbiturates are detoxified over a prolonged period, they are not recommended for anesthetic use.

Tolerance to Barbiturates

Dogs become tolerant to several barbiturates as determined by the reduction in anesthesia time of a given and frequently repeated dose. A cross-tolerance for all barbiturates occurs with a tolerance developed to one barbiturate. In a dog with tolerance to an anesthesia-inducing dose of a barbiturate, there is no change in the LD50 dose. Tolerance is soon lost by withdrawal of the drug.

Development of tolerance to barbiturates in dogs would be of interest only in cases such as eczema or chorea, where sedative doses of barbital or phenobarbital have

TABLE 13.3. Effects of certain barbiturates injected intravenously in dogs

Barbiturate	Number of Dogs	Dose	Duration of Anesthesia*	Down Time†	Return to Normal‡	Average Respiratory Rate
		(mg/kg)	*(min)*	*(min)*	*(min)*	
Pentobarbital sodium	8	25	200	252	358	11
Hexobarbital sodium	12	40	69	183	340	19
Thiopental sodium	12	26	50	69	137	15

Source: Hunt et al. 1948.
* Anesthesia = absence of pad reflex.
† Down time = from onset of anesthesia until animal stood.
‡ Return to normal = from onset of anesthesia until the dog could climb stairs without ataxia.

been given regularly for prolonged periods. It has been pointed out above that the stimulation or induction of microsomal enzyme activity in the liver markedly affects the duration of action of the barbiturates. The so-called development of tolerance that occurs after repeated use of the barbiturates is undoubtedly due to enhancement of microsomal enzyme activity.

Duration of Depressant Effect

The duration of action of two intravenous (pentobarbital and thiopental) barbiturates commonly used in veterinary medicine is illustrated in Table 13.3. The same depth of surgical anesthesia was obtained for all drugs with a dosage carefully determined by previous trials.

Duration of the depressant actions of orally administered barbiturates is illustrated in Fig. 13.2, which is based on more than 1000 trials in dogs (Swanson 1944). Other factors to be considered regarding the duration of the depressant effect of the barbiturates are nutritional status, age, and individual variations in the animal. A starved animal is much more sensitive to barbiturates because of a reduced ability to metabolize them (Chenoweth and Van Dyke 1969). Moreover, neonates and young animals are less able to metabolize barbiturates than adults and therefore will be anesthetized much longer and recover more slowly from the depressant effects. Even the influence of circadian rhythm can appreciably affect the depth of depression and duration of anesthetic action (Simmons et al. 1974). In nocturnal animals such as laboratory rodents, the hazard of drug-induced mortality is increased at night and recovery is prolonged. Individual variations exist not only because of age, sex, weight, and nutritional status but also with respect to the degree that microsomal enzyme induction is affected, which may vary qualitatively and quantitatively among individuals as well as among species (Chenoweth and Van Dyke 1969).

The duration of the depressant effect of pentobarbital sodium is prolonged by pretreatment or the concurrent administration of chloramphenicol in the mouse, rat, dog, cat, and monkey (Adams 1970; Adams and Dixit 1970; Teske and Carter 1971). Adams and Dixit (1970) found that chloramphenicol administered immediately preceding the administration of pentobarbital in the dog and cat resulted in a 120% increase in the duration of anesthesia compared to control animals. According to Teske and Carter (1971), chloramphenicol administered to the dog by the oral, intramuscular, or intravenous routes prior to or concurrently with pentobarbital-induced anesthesia resulted in the prolongation of anesthesia. This effect can be produced by relatively small quantities of chloramphenicol and can be detected as long as 24 days following the last administration of the antibiotic agent.

Sufficient evidence has been published indicating that chloramphenicol suppresses or inhibits hepatic microsomal enzyme activity. *In vitro* studies with the microsomal fraction of the liver have revealed that chloramphenicol suppresses the metabolism of hexobarbital and other drugs. The studies of Adams and Dixit (1970) strongly suggest that the prolongation of anesthesia induced by pentobarbital is attributable to

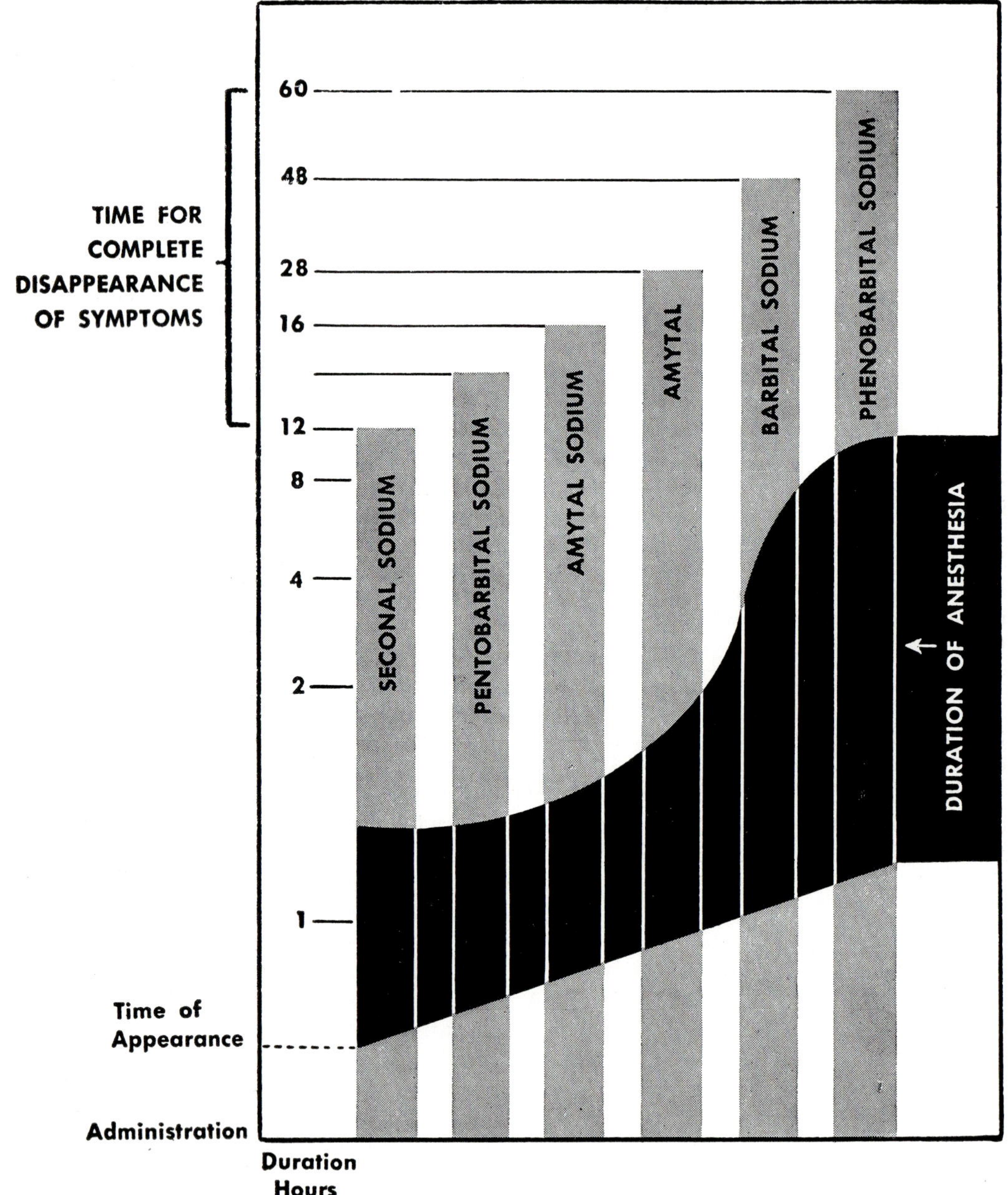

FIG. 13.2. Time of appearance, duration of anesthesia, and time needed for complete disappearance of symptoms after oral administration of equivalent single anesthetic doses in animals. (Swanson 1944. Courtesy of the Lilly Research Laboratories)

inhibition of the microsomal enzyme activity that inactivates the barbiturate by 3′–C hydroxylation.

If an animal has had a recent history of being treated with chloramphenicol, pentobarbital should not be used for the induction of anesthesia for at least 25 days after chloramphenicol. Since the duration of the anesthetic action of the thiobarbiturates does not appear to be affected by chloramphenicol (Adams and Dixit 1970), their use should be safer for induction of anesthesia followed by maintenance of anesthesia with the inhalant anesthetics.

The anesthetic action of the barbiturates, but not of other common depressants, can be potentiated by the intravenous or intraperitoneal injection of dextrose; fructose; intermediary metabolites such as lactate, pyruvate, and glutamate; and a few other substances of diverse nature. The lactate, pyruvate, and glutamate are known to increase the rate of entrance of barbital into the brain and thus increase cerebral depression. It is probable that dextrose, fructose, and the other substances act similarly. This reaction can be inhibited by administration of acetylcholine, which decreases cell permeability and the entrance of the barbital into the cortex. Clinically, about one-fourth of the dogs just recovering from pentobarbital anesthesia can be reanesthetized by an intravenous injection of 5 g of lactate (0.25 g/lb); about one-half will give a partial response, and the remaining one-fourth are refractory. The chicken, guinea pig, rabbit, rat, and mouse generally are all affected similarly (Lamson et al. 1951).

Other studies revealed that doses of glucose of 200 to greater than 600 mg/kg administered intravenously in the dog failed to influence the mode of respiration or the EEG shortly after (i.e., 6 minutes) inducing Stage III, plane 3, surgical anesthesia with pentobarbital sodium (Hamlin et al. 1965). It was concluded that the fear of embarrassing ventilation or depression of cortical activity through a "glucose effect" should not contraindicate the infusion of glucose. However, this conclusion may require modification (Hatch 1966). According to Hatch's study, the rapid intravenous administration of glucose in the dog that is regaining voluntary movement from thiopental sodium anesthesia resulted in the immobilization of 11% of the subjects. The length of this period of apparent reanesthetization represented about a 50% increase in "sleep time." Sodium lactate causes a similar reimmobilization in 39% of the dogs, with approximately a 50% increase in sleep time. Epinephrine produces reimmobilization in about 85% of the animals with an extension of about 40% in total sleep time. Hatch (1966) concluded that the possibility of producing reanesthetization with glucose, sodium lactate, and epinephrine need be of no practical concern as long as these substances are utilized properly. It was also emphasized that the improper use of these compounds, especially in the presence of longer-acting barbiturates, could lead to a dangerously prolonged period of incapacitation.

The influence of adrenergic agents upon recovery of dogs anesthetized with thiopental and methohexital was studied by Heavner and Bowen (1968). Administration of epinephrine and isoproterenol at the time the dogs were recovering from thiopental anesthesia resulted in reanesthetization. This effect was not seen in the animals recovering from methohexital anesthesia. Reanesthetization of the dogs recovering from thiopental could not be associated with α- or β- adrenergic activity. Heavner and Bowen (1968) believe there is a possibility that epinephrine produces a peripheral analgesic action that is responsible for the reanesthetization because depression of the sensory electroneurogram of the superficial radial nerve is induced.

The reinduction of thiopental anesthesia can also be brought about by the administration of high doses of aspirin and phenylbutazone in the rat (Chaplin et al. 1973). These nonsteroidal antiinflammatory agents displace the thiopental from rabbit plasma proteins *in vitro*. It is unlikely that reinduction of anesthesia by these agents would be as marked in animals that had received pentobarbital because the binding of pentobarbital to sheep plasma (36%) is less than the binding of thiopental (67%). Nevertheless, the sleep time of pentobarbital in small laboratory rodents can be significantly increased by sulfonamides (sulfanilamide, sulfamethazine, sulfaethylthiazole) salicylic acid, sodium salicylate and doxycline. All these drugs displace pentobarbital from plasma proteins, which leads to an increased blood level of unbound pentobarbital for further depressant effect upon the CNS. With the increasing number of pharmacologic agents used in therapeutic procedures, the clinician needs to be alert to these potential drug interactions.

The duration of the depressant effect of barbiturates is also generally increased (except for barbital) by hypothermia (Blair 1969). The activity of pentobarbital is greatly enhanced by hypothermia; the sleeping time in the dog at a body temperature of 27° C is 3.5 times that of the normothermic sleeping time. Consequently, about one-third of the normal dose of pentobarbital is required to maintain a specified level of anesthesia at this temperature (Blair 1969). Inadvertent hypothermia can be avoided by frequent or continuous temperature monitoring and by employing warming boards, water mattresses, or other such devices (Lutsky 1969).

Margin of Safety

All barbiturates seem to possess approximately the same margin of safety between anesthetic dose and the minimum lethal dose (MLD). Using recommended techniques of administration, 50%–70% of the MLD is needed to anesthetize an animal. Apparently no barbiturate possesses a markedly advantageous margin of safety over any other when the anesthetic dose and the MLD are compared. However, fewer postanesthetic complications follow use of the shorter-acting barbiturates because of the reduced incidence of hypostatic congestion, which often leads to pneumonia and other complications.

Toxicology

Barbiturates produce death by depression of the respiratory center, with the following symptomatology. The respiration becomes shallow and slow. The pupils dilate as hypoxia develops. The pulse becomes weak and rapid. The reflexes have disappeared and the skin is cold and cyanotic. Sometimes the respiration stops abruptly following too rapid intravenous injection of a barbiturate; following this, the heart continues to beat briefly until anoxia stops the myocardium. More often breathing continues at a progressively depressed rate and amplitude until it stops within 10–15 minutes after giving the drug. Mechanical obstruction of the airway must be avoided, especially in the brachiocephalic breeds of dogs. Artificial respiration utilizing 100% oxygen should be administered to prevent hypoxia (see Chapter 44). Although much less reliable than the use of oxygen, pentylenetetrazol or other analeptic drugs may be used to stimulate the respiratory center (see Chapter 18).

The shorter-acting barbiturates, such as pentobarbital sodium, are destroyed by the liver in large measure and therefore should not be administered to animals with hepatic disease. Patients suffering from shock and toxemia have a lesser margin of safety than normal animals. Newborn animals cannot metabolize this drug as readily as adults and consequently have a lesser margin of safety and are subject to more prolonged effect than adult animals.

When barbiturates are injected intravenously, the lethal dose varies inversely with the rate of injection. The more rapid injection results in a higher local blood concentration that is able to paralyze the vital medullary centers. The amount administered actually would not be a lethal dose if injected slowly. Fatal doses of pentobarbital cause some inflammation of the vital organs, congestion of the brain and meninges, and perivascular hemorrhage and edema. With the introduction of the antiflea collar, which is impregnated with an organophosphate compound (i.e., dichlorovos) and designed to keep dogs and cats free from fleas for 90 days, it has been alleged that animals wearing these collars fail to respond in a normal manner to anesthetics or to certain internal medication.

In uncontrolled studies, anesthetic deaths have been purportedly observed in animals that have worn flea collars following the administration of low doses of barbiturates. However, synergism between the systemic activity of dichlorovos and the intravenous administration of thiamylal sodium was found not to be significant in the dog (Ritter et al. 1970). Also, studies in the dog showed that both thiamylal sodium and pentobarbital sodium failed to produce an adverse effect when the animals had previously worn antiflea collars (Elsea et al. 1970). Even under prolonged or intense exposure conditions, the response to ultrashort-acting and short-acting barbiturates in animals wearing antiflea collars was the same as in animals not exposed to this treatment. Until more information is available, caution should be exercised in anesthetizing animals previously exposed to organophosphate compounds such as dichlorovos.

A drug interaction has been reported in mice treated with cyclophosphamide, a potent antineoplastic agent of the mustard family, and barbiturates (hexobarbital sodium, phenobarbital, pentobarbital). An increased lethality occurs when barbiturates are administered concurrently with cyclophosphamide (Rose et al. 1973). Cyclophosphamide has been investigated in sheep for removal of wool. Although the likelihood of animals having been treated with cyclophosphamide prior to the induction of barbiturate anesthesia is remote, the clinician must be alert to this possibility.

Pentobarbital Sodium

Immediately after its introduction, *Pentobarbital Sodium,* U.S.P. (Nembutal sodium), was widely accepted in veterinary medicine as a surgical anesthetic. At one time pentobarbital sodium was the most widely used anesthetic agent in small animals. With the introduction of halothane and methoxyflurane, pentobarbital declined in usage. In large animals, pentobarbital is used in combination with chloral hydrate and magnesium sulfate. Pentobarbital sodium is now rigidly controlled under the 1970 Controlled Substances Act and is classified as a Schedule II drug.

Administration and Dosage

Oral. Pentobarbital sodium can be administered orally to carnivora to produce sedation. If the stomach is empty, the drug may be given orally to produce surgical anesthesia in about one-half hour at a dosage level of 13 mg (1/5 grain)/lb of body weight. However, in average practice the routine production of anesthesia by oral administration is neither safe nor practical in the dog, cat, or other carnivora unless they are too dangerous to restrain for hypodermic injection. Vicious carnivora are best controlled by impregnating a piece of meat with capsules of pentobarbital sodium and feeding the meat to the animal. Because of the bitter taste of pentobarbital, it is easily detected and, if the capsules disintegrate, the animal may refuse to ingest the baited material. Following ingestion, the ingesta in the stomach and small intestine of most patients will cause a delayed, variable, and probably incomplete absorption of the drug.

Intraperitoneal. Intraperitoneal injection of pentobarbital sodium has been widely practiced in small animals but now is limited primarily to animals difficult to restrain for intravenous injections. The dosage generally employed is 13 mg (1/5 grain)/lb of body weight up to 35 lb, but reduced somewhat for heavier animals. Depression appears in about 15 minutes and persists in some measure 4–8 hours. The dosage must be reduced for animals showing undernourishment, toxemia, shock, and similar signs of poor condition and low resistance to anesthesia.

Intravenous. Intravenous injection of pentobarbital sodium is the most satisfactory method of administration for the production of anesthesia. The intravenous route of administration generally can be used in all species and is most often preferred in veterinary medicine where restraint of the patient is practicable. By this method the dosage is not inflexibly set by weight but can be fitted to the individual susceptibility of the patient as judged by the disappearance of normal reflexes. Routes other than intravenous (i.e., oral, intrathoracic, intramuscular, intraperitoneal, and others) have been employed in animals to induce anesthesia but they are much less reliable and there is an increased likelihood of inflicting injury to adjacent tissues.

The intravenous dose is determined by the response desired, and the drug is given until the desired effect is obtained. However, the anesthetic dose approximates 11–15 mg/lb of body weight. Once the anesthetic is injected, it cannot be removed. The duration of pentobarbital anesthesia in the dog is 1 to 2 hours (Leash 1969). Four or more hours are usually required before an animal is ambulatory after an intravenous injection. The technique for restraining and administering an intravenous anesthetic to the dog and other species has been described (Mather 1969; Soma 1971; Lumb and Jones 1973).

Injections should be made carefully to avoid accidental perivascular deposit of pentobarbital sodium since it irritates the tissues and occasionally causes a sloughing of tissues. If a perivascular injection of the barbiturate inadvertently occurs, the area should be infiltrated with 1 or 2 ml of 2% procaine hydrochloride solution (Leash 1969). If a procaine solution is unavailable, infiltration with a physiological saline solution may be of value in reducing tissue irritation and eventual sloughing.

An intravenous injection of a small dose of pentobarbital may be used to produce hypnosis or sedation to avoid the fright, excitement, and resistance to restraint that are so dangerous and objectionable in handling a patient. This sedation can be followed by local anesthesia or it may be followed by an inhalant anesthetic.

Intramuscular. Pentobarbital sodium has been suggested via the intramuscular route in the dog (Leash 1969). Dosages recommended are 20 mg/kg for basal anesthesia, 30 mg/kg for moderate anesthesia, and 40 mg/kg for general anesthesia. However, this route of administration is not recommended because of the likelihood of tissue irritation and variability in effect.

Intrathoracic. Barbiturates have been administered by the intrathoracic route to animals such as the cat. Since trauma, pleural irritation, and parenchymal necrosis of the lung tissue can occur following the intrathoracic injection of barbiturates, this route of administration is not recommended in the cat (Enold 1962; Strande 1964). This route of administration is sometimes used for euthanasia of animals when the intravenous or other routes are inaccessible.

CLINICAL USE

Although pentobarbital sodium is used in a number of species, it is approved by the Food and Drug Administration (FDA) for use only in the dog and cat.

In Dogs and Cats. Pentobarbital sodium is frequently used as an anesthetic in the dog and cat. However, it is not without toxic effects that require constant alertness by the veterinarian. For brief anesthesia, pentobarbital is surpassed by the ultrashort-acting barbiturates of more recent introduction. For intravenous anesthesia in the dog, about 11–15 mg/lb (25–35 mg/kg) of pentobarbital sodium in about 3%–6% aqueous solution should be used. In the cat, the recommended intravenous dose is 25 mg/kg of body weight with an additional 10 mg/kg of body weight if the initial dose is inadequate (Strobel and Wollman 1969).

Approximately one-half the anticipated dose should be injected at a moderately fast rate to carry the patient rapidly through the excitement stage of anesthesia into a deep hypnosis with no reflex activity. Then the anesthetist should pause for 1 minute to allow the drug to exert its full effect. Thereafter, the pentobarbital sodium must be injected slowly in repeated small amounts over a period of 2–4 minutes with continuous observation of reflexes until the desired depth of surgical anesthesia is obtained. Induction of anesthesia intravenously is generally uneventful; however, delirium or excitement may occur if the initial dose is inadequate.

Intravenous injection must be cautious and slow. Sometimes an injection must be stopped in the presence of shock or toxemia. A given level of anesthesia will persist for about half an hour, after which the depression decreases with complete recovery in 6–24 hours. Some dogs show considerable excitement during recovery, as manifested by whining, barking, and running movements. Narcotic analgesics or phenothiazine tranquilizers in combination with barbiturate anesthesia are often used to eliminate these undesirable features during recovery (Leash 1969).

Basically, the procedure for the induction of pentobarbital anesthesia in the cat is similar to that described above for the dog. However, greater skill is required in the administration of the anesthetic via the intravenous route in the cat than in the dog. The anesthetic dose of pentobarbital sodium in the cat by the intravenous route is generally not appreciably different on a body weight basis than that of the canine species. According to Clifford and Kook (1963), female cats (33 mg/kg) are more susceptible to the action of pentobarbital than males (40 mg/kg). In the newborn kitten, pentobarbital sodium is an inadequate anesthetic since the depth of anesthesia is difficult to control and the recovery time is extremely prolonged (Sis and Herron 1972). In the adult cat, recovery of the righting reflex after an intravenous dose of 30 mg/kg of pentobarbital sodium occurs in 270 $\pm$ 52 minutes; recovery of the corneal and flexor withdrawal reflexes occurs at 25 $\pm$ 8 minutes and 31 $\pm$ 11 minutes, respectively (Child et al. 1972).

Premedication. Sometimes it is difficult to inject intravenously an excitable dog or cat that has not been previously medicated with a depressant drug. Without the administration of a preanesthetic agent, the average dog requires 13 mg/lb of body weight (28.6 mg/kg) of pentobarbital sodium to become surgically anesthetized (Brodey and Thordal-Christensen 1956). Use of preanesthetic agents not only renders the animal easier to handle and treat but it also decreases the amount of barbiturate up to 50% for surgical anesthesia and reduces the likelihood of excitement during recovery. In severely toxic patients, pentobarbital sodium alone should not be used to depress a patient beyond the beginning of light surgical anesthesia. It is much safer to use preanesthetics to reduce the amount of pentobarbital needed. In many instances the safest anesthesia in toxic patients is obtained by premedication with a narcotic analgesic or a briefly acting barbiturate followed by an inhalant anesthetic. Atropine sulfate is an additional premedication preparation that should be used routinely prior to barbiturate anesthesia. The reader is referred to Chapter 10 for the various drugs and dosages recommended for premedication.

Control of Convulsions. Pentobarbital sodium is an important drug for relieving convulsive seizures, especially when caused by strychnine or other convulsants. Intravenous administration is preferable because a better balance between the convulsant and depressant influences can be obtained. In the dog, pentobarbital sodium is antidotal to as much as 35 MLD of strychnine.

Minimum Lethal Dose. The MLD of pentobarbital in the dog is 40 mg/lb (85 mg/kg) orally and 23–27 mg/lb (50–60 mg/kg) intravenously or intraperitoneally.

For Euthanasia. Several barbituric acid derivatives may be used in the euthanasia of small animals. Of the barbiturates, pentobarbital sodium is most commonly used (Am Vet Med Assoc Report 1972). The MLD for dogs, administered intravenously, is generally regarded as 23–27 mg/lb of body weight (50–60 mg/kg) or approximately double the dose used for surgical anesthesia.

In Cows and Horses. Pentobarbital sodium will produce surgical anesthesia in the horse, mule, and cow, as well as other large animals, but its use alone is not generally recommended. Some excitement may be noted, even with a rapid induction. At the completion of an intravenous injection of pentobarbital sodium alone, the horse sometimes rears and falls over backward, injuring the poll. Pentobarbital sodium produces prolonged periods of recumbency and usually excitement during recovery. Large animals make futile attempts to stand before they have recovered complete control of their locomotor activities and dangerous struggling occurs.

Pentobarbital sodium has been used with greater success in foals and small colts for sedation (e.g., while taking radiographs) and anesthesia. Minimal excitement occurs in some.

Pentobarbital sodium can be used in large animals as a sedative (0.6–1.2 g) for gynecological examination or it may be used preoperatively in combination with a local anesthetic. An intravenous dose of 1.5–2 g provides a marked sedative or hypnotic action so that with the aid of a local anesthetic several standing operations can be performed if desired.

In Swine. Pentobarbital sodium administered by slow intravenous injection provides reasonably good general anesthesia in swine weighing less than 100 lb. Above this weight pentobarbital sodium appears to have a considerably lessened margin of safety. The tendency in the United States is to administer only sedative dosages of pentobarbital sodium intravenously in heavy swine and to follow this with local anesthesia at the surgical site. Since respiratory depression is readily induced in swine following barbiturate anesthesia, hypoxia and hypoventilation can be prevented by the use of oxygen (see Chapter 44).

Intravenous dosages of pentobarbital should be fitted to each patient by observing the disappearance of reflexes. Slow injection of the solution is essential. Recovery generally requires 60–90 minutes. Pentobarbital appears to have a considerable margin of safety in pigs of 25–50 lb. It has been determined that 11 mg/lb (1/6 grain) of body weight produces anesthesia suitable for most kinds of surgery. For swine weighing over 220 lb, the intravenous dosage should be no more than 9 mg/lb (1/7 grain). For castration of a large boar where only brief light anesthesia is required, only 4.5 mg/lb (1/14 grain) is needed. Also, in castration procedures, pentobarbital is administered intratesticularly to achieve anesthesia (Henry 1968). A dose of 1 mg/15 lb of pentobarbital sodium (300 mg/ml concentration or a 30% solution) is injected into each testicle with satisfactory anesthesia being achieved within 10 minutes after administration of the anesthetic. It is recommended that the anesthetic solution be injected below the tail of the epididymis in the upper one-third of the testicle at an angle of 30 degrees from the perpendicular. To avoid fatal poisoning in dogs or other animals, the testes should be disposed of properly.

A similar clinical approach to the castration of male pigs ranging in weight from 180 to 240 lb has been reported by Dyson (1964). A "triple strength" solution of pentobarbital sodium containing 3 grains/ml is used. The total dose recommended for the larger pigs is 30 ml, and for animals weighing less than 200 lb the recommended total dose is 20–25 ml. One-half the dose required to induce anesthesia is injected into each testicle. After the injection of the anesthetic, the animals become incoordinated in a few minutes. Recumbency occurs between 5 and 15 minutes following the administration of the drug. As soon as no response is elicited upon pricking the scrotal skin with a needle, the castration procedure is conducted. Recovery from anesthesia requires 20–40 minutes.

Preanesthetic medication not only reduces the amount of anesthetic required for major surgical procedures but it facilitates handling of the pig prior to the induction of anesthesia (Booth 1969). Preanesthetic medication in the pig consists of atropine sulfate (0.07–0.09 mg/kg), meperidine hydrochloride (1–2 mg/kg), and promazine hydrochloride (2 mg/kg). All preanesthetic preparations are injected intramuscularly in separate sites 45–60 minutes prior to administration of the anesthetic. It is often necessary to administer atropine at hourly intervals during anesthesia to prevent salivation and mucus formation in the respiratory tract.

In Goats and Sheep. Surgical anesthesia in adult goats is satisfactorily produced with about 650 mg (10 grains) of pentobarbital sodium intravenously. The patients regain their feet in about 2–3 hours (Allam and Churchill 1946). According to Bryant (1969), the initial anesthetizing dose (25 mg/kg) of pentobarbital sodium in the goat should be administered slowly. The level of anesthesia will be deep for about 5 minutes and then become less until complete recovery occurs in 40–60 minutes. The duration of satisfactory anesthesia is about 20 minutes, which is sufficient time to catheterize the jugular vein for supplementary injections and to intubate the trachea. Compared to the dog, the duration of anesthesia in the goat is much shorter for an equivalent level of anesthesia. Linzell (1964) reported that the anesthetic dose of pentobarbital in the goat is about 30 mg/kg. Adult animals will stand in 20–60 minutes. However, to maintain anesthesia, 6–36 mg/kg/hour had to be administered either by intravenous infusion or doses injected every 20 minutes. Consequently, it is preferable to use pentobarbital for induction of anesthesia and then to maintain it with an inhalant anesthetic after tracheal intubation (Linzell 1964).

In adult sheep, pentobarbital is rapidly metabolized, requiring additional increments of the anesthetic to maintain anesthesia for more than 15–30 minutes. The drug is useful for induction of anesthesia; this permits intubation of the trachea, and maintenance of anesthesia is by use of an inhalant anesthetic mixture such as cyclopropane and oxygen (Harrison 1964). The average dose of pentobarbital for induction of anesthesia is about 24 mg/kg of body weight with a range of 11–54 mg/kg.

In Rabbits. The rabbit is considered to be one of the more difficult and unpredictable species of laboratory animals to anesthetize, because they vary considerably in their response to commonly used anesthetic agents and because the margin between surgical anesthesia and respiratory arrest is narrow (Morgan et al. 1966; Murdock 1969). According to Murdock, the intravenous dose of pentobarbital sodium recommended is generally 25–40 mg/kg of body weight. One-half to three-fourths of the calculated dose of a 2% pentobarbital sodium is injected slowly into the marginal ear vein until the animal becomes relaxed. The injection of more concentrated solutions is apt not only to lead to an overdose of the anesthetic but also to cause severe injury to the vessel wall to the extent that thrombosis occurs. If this occurs, vessel occlusion results, which will ultimately lead to necrosis and sloughing of the affected portion of the ear.

In comparing the anesthesia time and plasma levels between pentobarbital sodium and secobarbital sodium, there is no significant difference noted at a dose of 15 mg/kg following the intravenous administration of each of these barbiturates in the rabbit (Taylor et al. 1957). However, when a larger quantity than 25 mg/kg is administered, the animals are anesthetized for a shorter time with pentobarbital than with secobarbital.

In Mink. Intravenous injection is not practical in vicious animals such as the mink. Pentobarbital sodium, 10 mg/lb injected subcutaneously, has been reported to produce a hypnosis suitable for examining mink and for artificial insemination procedures. The hypnotic state occurs in about 10 minutes and lasts for about 40 minutes, with complete recovery in about 1.5 hours.

Pentobarbital sodium (35 or 40 mg/kg has been used intraperitoneally in ranch mink *(Mustela vision)* without mortality (Graham et al. 1967). Bemegride (40 mg/kg) administered intraperitoneally shortened the long recovery period from pentobarbital anesthesia. The use of diazepam, a neuroleptic agent, may be beneficial in mink prior to the administration of anesthetics. Diazepam has been of value in calming aggressive and vicious animals prior to mating (see Chapter 17).

In Birds. According to a number of literature sources, pentobarbital sodium administered alone and intravenously has not been satisfactory as an anesthetic for the chicken because of the narrow margin of safety. However, Hollingsworth and Howes (1965) felt that pentobarbital proved to be the best general anesthetic when compared with thiopental sodium, ether, methoxyflurane, and Equithesin in spite of its individual variability in dosage required for surgical anesthesia. These authors found that the critical dose of pentobarbital varied greatly in chickens of the same strain, age, sex, and weight. Also, they observed that dose levels fatal for some birds produced only light anesthesia in others.

Pentobarbital readily depresses the respiration or may paralyze respiratory activity of the chicken. However, it has been the experience of the author and another investigator (Herin 1959) that pentobarbital sodium (7 mg/lb) administered through the external thoracic vein provides safe anesthesia when oxygen is continuously administered to prevent hypoxia. Pentobarbital sodium has been used in mature chicken hens for induction of light narcosis prior to the inhalation of ether for maintenance anesthesia (Fussell 1969). The barbiturate was administered intraperitoneally at an average dose level of 25 mg/kg of body weight; doses greater than this frequently produced respiratory and cardiac failure. Pentobarbital has a hypotensive action in fowl; soon after its administration there is a decline of 30–50 mm Hg in the arterial blood pressure but this is followed by a partial recovery in a few minutes (Sykes 1964).

Pentobarbital sodium has also been satisfactorily used in the turkey by injecting 12 mg/lb of body weight via the radial or saphenous veins (Durant 1953). It is recommended that the birds be fasted 12–18 hours prior to general anesthesia. Use of pentobarbital sodium in the Aylesbury domestic duck by intravenous injection (30–60 mg/kg) produces unsatisfactory anesthesia (Desforges and Scott 1971). Equithesin produces a safer level of anesthesia in the duck; dose levels of 3–3.5 ml/kg of body weight administered intravenously were found to be satisfactory.

An anticholinergic agent such as atropine sulfate (0.02 mg/lb intramuscularly) should be administered prior to the use of barbiturates in birds to prevent bronchial secretion. Pentobarbital sodium (1%) has been administered intramuscularly at a dose level of 0.01 cc (0.1 mg)/2 g of body weight to canaries, sparrows, parakeets, and chickens (Donovan 1958). Induction of anesthesia occurred in about 2 minutes; 5–9 minutes following the injection there was no skeletal muscle resistance to extension of the extremities. Surgical anesthesia lasted for approximately 30 minutes; the birds were standing within 90 minutes after the injection.

Chickens, grackles, pigeons, and parakeets are also anesthetized with a commercial preparation (Equithesin) containing 21.3 g of chloral hydrate, 4.8 g of pentobarbital, and 10.6 g of magnesium sulfate/500 ml. The drugs are mixed in an aqueous solution of propylene glycol with 9.5% alcohol. The anesthetic preparation is injected into the pectoral muscles of the bird in dosimetric levels of 0.22–0.25 ml/100 g of body weight (Gandal 1956; Gandal and Saunders 1959). Compared to other anesthetics, Equithesin is not surpassed for overall safety and efficiency (Gandal 1969).

Equithesin has been used in a number of surgical procedures in the chicken, including the devocalizing of the rooster (Madsen 1967). Pet roosters are sometimes brought to the veterinarian to be silenced to prevent annoyance of the neighbors who like to sleep after 4 o'clock each morning. The dose of Equithesin recommended for cross-bred meat birds and bantams is 1 cc/lb of body weight; this dose can be administered intravenously or intramuscularly.

In falconiform birds, Equithesin has not been satisfactorily used for anesthetizing prairie falcons, red-tailed hawks,

Swainson's hawks, marsh hawks, and golden eagles (Seidenstricker and Reynolds 1969). However, deaths produced in some birds suggest that the anesthetic has a narrow margin of safety.

In Subhuman Primates. With the introduction of ultrashort-acting barbiturates (thiopental, thiamylal) the use of pentobarbital in primates has declined; however, pentobarbital is essentially safe and effective in monkeys (Bywater and Rutty 1964). In the rhesus monkey, most anesthetic failures in healthy animals following pentobarbital sodium administration are attributable to an excessively rapid rate of injection or to the use of a highly concentrated solution (Domino et al. 1969). The commercially available pentobarbital sodium solution containing 60 mg/ml is too concentrated and should be diluted 1:2 or 1:4 just prior to use. Moreover, the solution must be injected by slow, steady infusion at a rate not to exceed 2 ml/minute until the corneal reflexes are abolished and respiration becomes slow, deep, and regular. Monkeys so treated can be expected to remain in surgical anesthesia for a minimum of 2 hours; recovery ordinarily does not occur in less than 6 hours (Domino et al. 1969).

Pentobarbital sodium has been used following phencyclidine (Sernylan) in the baboon and other primates for the induction of surgical anesthesia (Vice et al. 1965). In addition, this barbiturate has been very useful as a restraint and anesthetic agent in the chimpanzee (Day 1965); a dose of 30 mg/kg of body weight is administered intravenously to effect. The dose of pentobarbital recommended for mature and young chimpanzees is 11–13 mg and 13–18 mg/lb of body weight, respectively. A 5% pentobarbital sodium solution is used in both age groups. Anesthesia occurs in most instances in 6–15 minutes. Complete recovery usually results within 6–8 hours, with the younger animals recovering in less time.

In Guinea Pigs and Gerbils. Although the usual intravascular routes, i.e., intravenous and intracardiac, for administering anesthetics are available in the guinea pig, they are infrequently utilized (Hoar 1969); the intraperitoneal route is most commonly used because of its easy and ready accessibility. A number of literature sources indicate that the anesthetic level for pentobarbital sodium is 15–30 mg/kg of body weight, administered by the intraperitoneal route. In the gerbil, pentobarbital sodium in a dose of 5 mg/100 g of body weight is recommended intraperitoneally (Stunkard and Miller 1974).

In Rats and Mice. Pentobarbital sodium diluted in sterile physiological saline solution is usually given intraperitoneally at a dose level of 30–40 mg/kg of body weight to the adult albino male rat (Ben et al. 1969). Female rats are usually less capable of metabolizing pentobarbital and may require less of the barbiturate than the male. Pentobarbital may be administered by the intravenous route in the rat; however, the dose level and rate of administration must be carefully observed (Ben et al. 1969). In mice, pentobarbital is the most commonly used parenteral anesthetic agent and is generally given intravenously or intraperitoneally in doses of 40–70 mg/kg of body weight (Taber and Irwin 1969). Intraperitoneally, this dose range induces anesthesia of 20–30 minutes duration following a latency interval of 5–10 minutes with less than 10% mortality. A number of literature sources indicates that male mice are more sensitive to the effect of barbiturates than females. In the neonatal subject (1–4 days old), an intraperitoneal dose of 5 mg/kg of pentobarbital produces anesthesia of approximately 1 hour's duration (Taber and Irwin 1969).

In Amphibians and Reptiles. Frogs *(Rana pipiens)* can be satisfactorily anesthetized with pentobarbital administered through the dorsal lymph sac at a dose of 60 mg/kg of body weight (Kaplan 1969). Surgical anesthesia is attained in about one-half hour and will last for as long as 9 hours. Turtles *(Pseudemys)* can also be anesthetized with pentobarbital by an intravenous or intracardiac injection at a dose level of 15.5–17.5 mg/kg of body weight. The induction time of anesthesia is approximately 30–53 minutes by these routes of administration; the animals may remain in deep anesthesia as long as 3 hours. Also, *Pseudemys* turtles may be anesthetized by the intraperitoneal route of administration with pentobarbital at a dose of 16 mg/kg of body weight (Kaplan 1969). Pentobarbital sodium has also been used in crocodiles weighing 200–400 lb (Pleuger 1950).

In Bears and Large Cats. Pentobarbital sodium has been used intravenously (17–27 mg/lb) in bears following intramuscular administration of morphine sulfate (4 mg/lb) and promazine hydrochloride (2 mg/lb) (Clifford et al. 1962). For safe handling and minor surgery, a mean intravenous dose of 13.5 mg/kg of pentobarbital sodium is recommended in bears; supplemental increments of the anesthetic agent will maintain the animals up to 6 hours in anesthesia (Clarke et al. 1963). The principal disadvantage in using pentobarbital as an anesthetic in bears is the necessity for immobilizing the animals so a venipuncture can be made; once venipuncture is achieved following a quota of good fortune, the pentobarbital sodium (12–15 mg/kg) is administered as rapidly as possible (Day 1965). This dose is about 50%–75% of the anesthetizing dose. The portion of the dose remaining is then given until an adequate level of anesthesia is reached.

Phencyclidine (Sernylan) at a dose of 0.7–1.5 mg/kg may be administered intramuscularly to assist in immobilizing animals (Day 1965). After 15–20 minutes, the animals enter a cataleptoid state that permits pentobarbital sodium (10–12 mg/kg) to be administered intravenously. The oral administration of pentobarbital in soft drinks or ice cream will induce vomiting in black and grizzly bears (Martyn 1955).

Pentobarbital sodium is contraindicated in any of the large cats in the zoo because of their apparent inability to metabolize the drug (Fisher 1965). The large

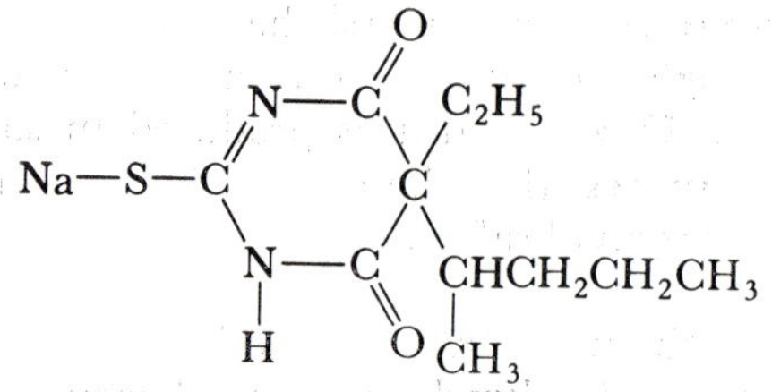

O, N—C, C_2H_5, Na—S—C, C, N—C, $CHCH_2CH_2CH_3$, H, O, CH_3

Thiopental Sodium

O, N—C, C_2H_5, Na—O—C, C, N—C, $CHCH_2CH_2CH_3$, H, O, CH_3

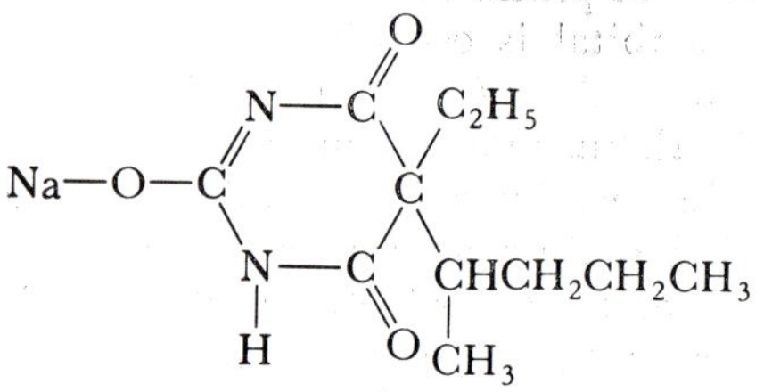

Pentobarbital Sodium

Fig. 13.3.

cats may be anesthetized for 6 or 7 days following the use of pentobarbital. When ultrashort barbiturates (thiamylal or thiopental) are administered, these animals sleep 6–24 hours.

Thiopental Sodium

As the name indicates, *Thiopental Sodium,* U.S.P. (Pentothal sodium), is a sulfur-containing barbiturate or a thiobarbiturate. Instead of having the R-O-Na, which is characteristic of most other sodium salts of the barbituric acid derivatives, thiopental possesses a sulfur atom, R-S-Na, in substitution for the oxygen atom. Except for the sulfur atom, thiopental sodium is similar chemically to pentobarbital sodium (see Fig. 13.3).

Storage and Stability

Thiopental sodium is available only as a powder buffered with sodium carbonate in sealed ampules. The powder in evacuated or nitrogen-filled ampules should be stored away from light and in a cool place. It is unstable in aqueous solution or when exposed to moisture of the atmosphere. Steady deterioration occurs in proportion to the temperature of the solution. For maximum effect and safety, aqueous solutions of thiopental should be prepared just prior to use. When large amounts are used, as in a hospital, a bulk solution of thiopental sodium may be prepared if careful attention is given to its expiration date. A 5% bulk solution of thiopental sodium can be stored in a refrigerator at 5°–6° C (41°–42° F) until turbidity appears, but for no longer than 7 days. At room temperature of 18°–22° C (64°–71° F) a solution should be kept no longer than 3 days. Solutions kept beyond the above limits contain clinically active thiopental sodium, but the progressive loss of action at any given period cannot be easily determined. When aged solutions are used, the same characteristic action of the drug is obtained by injecting larger volumes of solution. However, from the standpoint of maintaining a reliable anesthetic and surgical routine, it is desirable to use fully potent, fresh solutions of thiopental sodium.

PHARMACOLOGICAL CONSIDERATIONS

In the horse, thiopental sodium elevates the blood glucose level and induces a leukopenia (Tyagi et al. 1964). The cardiac rate increases while the cardiac output decreases. No significant change in the arterial pressure or in the packed cell volume occurs in the horse following the administration of thiopental sodium. The respiratory rate is slowed and frequently becomes irregular in character for brief periods. This leads to an elevated arterial P_{CO_2} and concomitant decrease in blood pH (Tyagi et al. 1964). Plasma levels of thiopental sodium do not correlate well with the clinical signs or the EEG in the horse or in other species.

In the dog, thiopental has an arrhythmogenic effect with an incidence of about 40%. This is lower than the incidence (i.e., 85%) of arrhythmia produced in the dog by thiamylal sodium (Pedersoli and Brown 1973). Anesthetics such as the ultrashort-acting barbiturates (thiopental, thiamylal, methohexital) and others (halothane, methoxyflurane) that trigger cardiac arrhythmia set the stage for the heart to go into ventricular fibrillation, especially if endogenous or exogenous catecholamines appear on the scene at the right time. Although the fibrillatory effect of epinephrine and norepinephrine is potentiated in dogs anesthetized with a combination of ultrashort-acting barbiturates and halothane, both catecholamines may be used safely if the dog is treated with acetylpromazine or chlorpromazine prior to induction of anesthesia (Wiersig et al. 1974).

METABOLISM

Thiopental is metabolized primarily by the hepatic microsomal enzyme system. Studies in the monkey with thiopental containing labeled sulfur, S^{35}, indicate that at least twelve metabolic products are excreted in the urine. Within 4 days after an intravenous injection of 16 mg/lb, the monkey excretes about 86% of the dose in the urine. Additional small amounts are found in the feces and the tissues (Taylor et al. 1952).

In human beings only about 0.3% of the administered thiopental is excreted unchanged, indicating that the drug is almost totally transformed (Brodie et al. 1950). Oxidation of one of the alkyl side chains to yield thiopental carboxylic acid, a metabolite of thiopental, is almost completely metabolized, with only traces of this metabolite appearing in the urine. The metabolite has little if any anesthetic activity.

In clinical anesthesia, a small dose of thiopental sodium has a brief duration of action not because of its rapid metabolic destruction but because of the rapid distribution of the drug from plasma into the various tissues. Actually, the metabolic conversion of thiopental is slow (10%–15%/hour). Since fat is capable of localizing thiopental, the plasma level of the anesthetic is below that required to maintain anesthesia, and the animal recovers soon after the injection. Following large doses or repeated small doses of thiopental, the plasma level remains near that of the fat and tissues and anesthesia persists for a longer period because of the slow metabolism of the anesthetic (Brodie et al. 1952).

In sheep thiopental sodium is cleared

from the plasma at the rate of 17%/hour after tissue equilibrium is reached. Pentobarbital sodium, on the other hand, is cleared at a rate of approximately 49%/hour. Also, binding of the two barbiturates to sheep plasma proteins occurs to the extent of 67% for thiopental sodium and 36% for pentobarbital sodium (Rae 1962).

The phenomenon of microsomal enzyme induction has been demonstrated in calves pretreated with phenobarbital (Sharma et al. 1970). Plasma levels of thiopental sodium disappear at a more rapid rate as a result of enzyme induction. The development of enzyme induction should be thought of while treating domestic animals because animals are frequently exposed to potent inducers of microsomal enzymes such as the halogenated hydrocarbons and other compounds. Such induction may be responsible for wide variation in the metabolism of certain drugs and may greatly affect an animal's response (Sharma et al. 1970).

TOXICITY

The major toxic effect of thiopental sodium is a marked depression of the respiratory centers. The rate is slowed and the amplitude decreased. Ordinarily the respiratory rate is a good indication of the condition of the animal and of the dosage of drug. When given properly, thiopental has little toxic action upon the cardiovascular system. About 16 times as much thiopental sodium is needed to stop the myocardium as is needed to paralyze respiration. As long as the cardiovascular system functions well, there is every opportunity for recovery of a patient if proper oxygenation is maintained by artificial respiration.

In general, thiopental sodium possesses a wide margin of safety. The twice daily intravenous injection of 9 mg/lb of thiopental sodium into dogs for 2–3 weeks results in only slight depression of liver function.

GENERAL USE

The brief duration of effect of thiobarbiturate can be employed advantageously for numerous conditions, including setting of fractures; gynecological, radiographical, and other kinds of examinations; short surgical procedures; and premedication to an inhalant anesthetic. The rapid, complete recovery permits quick return of the patient to the owner if hospitalization is undesirable. The minimal hypnotic dose of thiopental injected intravenously produces anesthesia for only about one-fourth as long as pentobarbital under the same conditions. Although an outstanding advantage of thiopental is its brief duration of effect, it may be used for prolonged anesthesia by repeatedly injecting small amounts as needed. During World War II, thiopental came into wide use as a routine general anesthetic in human beings in front-line hospitals where equipment was limited.

ADMINISTRATION AND DOSAGE

Thiopental sodium is administered only by intravenous injection. Subcutaneous or intramuscular injections are irritating and may result in a slough of tissue. The anesthetic is too irritant to inject into a cavity of the body. An equal volume of 1% procaine hydrochloride infiltrated into the perivascular tissue where the thiopental may have been injected by accident is claimed to obviate the usual tissue reaction (Elder and Harrison 1944). Thiopental sodium is usually prepared as a 2.5% solution for intravenous injection in the smaller animals. In the larger animals the concentration should be increased to 5%, although 10% solutions have been used. It should be borne in mind that the injection of the more concentrated solution (5% or 10%) will produce serious complications if the barbiturate anesthetic is accidentally administered intraarterially (Burn 1960; Stone and Donnelly 1961). Also, the "quick-shot" administration of thiopental sodium in the horse via the external jugular vein may result in the inadvertent injection of the anesthetic extravascularly. This often results in a severe tissue reaction, including abscessation and necrosis of the involved tissue (Neal 1963; Jones 1968). In the event thiopental sodium is accidentally injected perivascularly, normal saline should be injected to dilute the drug; in addition, hyaluronidase should be added to the normal saline to promote dispersion of the thiopental and absorption (Jones 1968). This hazard has been discussed above.

The amount of thiopental needed varies with the disposition of the patient and the nature of the operation. Of the several factors seeming to influence the depth and duration of anesthesia, the most important is the rate of injection. When small animals are injected rapidly, as within one-half minute, the onset of anesthesia is abrupt and sometimes alarming. Rapid injection usually induces anesthesia in less than a minute and lowers the dosage needed to produce anesthesia, but the anesthesia is of brief duration. The duration of anesthesia is directly proportional to the time taken for injection of the anesthetic dose. The duration of anesthesia can be varied from 2–3 minutes to 25–30 minutes by the rate and amount of drug injected. At either extreme, the same depth of depression can be produced. When prolonged anesthesia is found necessary, repeated injections of thiopental sodium at progressively longer periods, depending upon the need of the patient, give good results in small animals. It is possible and practicable in some circumstances to keep patients under thiopental anesthesia for hours at a time. It must not be forgotten that too rapid intravenous injection depresses the vasomotor center and results in a vascular dilation with sudden drop in blood pressure.

In the dog the anesthetic dose of thiopental sodium approximates 15–17 mg/kg intravenously; for the cat it is 9–11 mg/kg of body weight (Mark et al. 1968). However, each dose should be adjusted to the patient to compensate for individual differences. Regardless of the dose, the initial injection of a solution of thiopental sodium in small animals should consist of about 6 mg/lb (1/10 grain) followed by a pause of 30–60 seconds. The remainder of the desired dose can be injected during the next 1–2 minutes to produce the desired depth of anesthesia.

For brief anesthesia of 7–10 minutes, suitable for radiography, minor surgery, and examinations, a dose of 6–8 mg/lb (1/10–1/8 grain) is suggested. For anesthesia of 10–15 minutes, as might be needed for reducing a fracture, a dose of 8–10 mg/lb (1/8–1/6 grain) is desirable. For anesthesia of 15–25 minutes to permit major surgery, a dose of 10–13 mg/lb (1/6–1/5 grain) is needed in most small animals. For longer periods this initial dose may be increased or, better, it may be repeated as needed. However, thiopental is not strongly recommended for extended periods of anesthesia. Thiopental may be used to induce anesthesia, followed then by safer agents such as inhalant anesthetics for prolonged effect. A small dose of thiopental injected rapidly produces anesthesia briefly.

If desired, morphine can be administered preanesthetically to thiopental as it is to pentobarbital. However, morphine does not cause a significant extension of thiopental-induced anesthesia in the dog (Dobkin 1961). Prolongation of thiopental-induced anesthesia by a therapeutic dose of the narcotic analgesics appears to be less significant than that observed with most of the phenothiazine tranquilizers. Atropine sulfate should be routinely used preceding thiopental anesthesia to prevent parasympathetic side effects. Atropine sulfate, but not atropine methylnitrate, nonspecifically reduces the anesthetic dosage of thiopental sodium as well as the thiopental plasma level at awakening (Hatch 1972).

RECOVERY

The recovery period varies with the dosage from 15 minutes to 6 to 8 hours before full leg coordination appears and may not be complete in less than 24 hours in the dog following an intravenous dose (15–25 mg/kg) of thiopental sodium (Chenoweth and Van Dyke 1969). With repeated administration of the drug, recovery time is prolonged to the extent that there is little advantage over the use of pentobarbital. According to Hatch (1966), the rapid intravenous administration of glucose in the dog that is regaining voluntary movement from thiopental anesthesia resulted in the reanesthetization of 11% of the animals. Sodium lactate and epinephrine also produced an increase in the "sleep time." However, it was concluded that the possibility of producing reanesthetization with these substances is of little practical concern as long as these compounds are administered properly.

Old animals may exhibit hind-leg weakness for 1 to 2 days after thiopental anesthesia. Incoordination of the legs, especially the rear legs, causes the patient to stagger about for an hour or so when disturbed during recovery. If the patient is not disturbed, recovery ordinarily is uneventful. Complete recovery requires approximately 2 hours and is usually free from excitement. Vomition or other signs of postanesthetic toxicity have seldom been noted.

RESUSCITATION

As is the case with the other barbiturates, excessive amounts of thiopental produce severe respiratory depression. Continuous administration of oxygen is more beneficial than any other therapeutic measure for combating the respiratory depression from barbiturate overdosage.

CLINICAL USE

Thiopental sodium is approved by the FDA for use only in the dog and cat.

In Small Animals. The anesthesia produced by thiopental in small animals is very similar to that by pentobarbital. Although muscular relaxation is fair, it is inferior to that produced by ether and other inhalant anesthetics. The respirations are regular but slow and shallow. The heart beat is fast but strong. Excitement is generally absent during the induction and recovery periods if the patient is kept quiet. The anesthetic dose of thiopental sodium for the dog is 15–17 mg/kg of body weight administered by the intravenous route; for the cat it is 9–11 mg/kg of body weight (Mark et al. 1968). These dose levels are generally considered to be on the conservative side. For example, some authors recommend an intravenous dose level of 25–30 mg/kg of thiopental sodium for both the dog and cat (Mitchell 1966; Strobel and Wollman 1969). Strobel and Wollman reported that 30 mg/kg of the drug will produce 10–20 minutes of anesthesia and 2 hours of somnolence. In the greyhound, compared to other breeds of dogs, the recovery rate from thiopental sodium anesthesia is more prolonged (Fabry 1963). The greyhound can metabolize methohexital sodium, an ultrashort-acting oxybarbiturate, much more rapidly than the thiobarbiturate anesthetics.

Doses of 12 and 24 mg/kg of thiopental sodium administered intravenously in the cat require 27 $\pm$ 8 minutes and 63 $\pm$ 6 minutes after the barbiturate is injected before recovery of the righting reflex (Child et al. 1972). Because of considerable variability in the anesthetic dose level for the dog and cat, thiopental should be administered cautiously and "to effect." In the cat, the administration of increasing amounts of thiopental does not allow EEG patterns to be related to the clinical depth of anesthesia or to plasma thiopental concentration (Hatch et al. 1970).

In Swine. Thiopental sodium, in 5% solution intravenously, has been used satisfactorily in swine varying in weight from 10 to 600 lb (Muhrer 1950). Although the dose levels of thiopental generally used in clinical practice can differ considerably from those recommended by Muhrer (1950), the information provided by him is nevertheless useful for determining the initial quantity of drug needed for induction. Swine weighing 5–50 kg usually require doses of 10–11 mg/kg of body weight (Booth 1969). In pregnant sows weighing 165–323 kg, induction of anesthesia without premedication is accomplished by the intravenous injection of thiopental sodium (2.5–6.25 g) "to effect"; no reliable dosage-weight relationship is observed (Cummings et al. 1972). After endotracheal intubation, a gas mixture of oxygen and nitrous oxide in a ratio of 1:1 or 1:2 can be delivered to the animals. The flow rate is 6–8 L/minute, the tidal volume varies from 900 to 1800 ml, and the inspiratory pressure is maintained between 15 and 20 cm

TABLE 13.4. Suggested intravenous dosage of thiopental sodium in swine*

Weight	Dosage	Dosage in 5% Solution
(lb)	*(mg/lb)*	*(mg/lb)*
10–50	5.0	0.1
50–100	4.5	0.09
100–200	4.0	0.08
200–300	3.5	0.07
300–400	3.0	0.06
400–600	2.5	0.05

Source: Muhrer 1950.

* Unthrifty animals require less drug for a comparable effect.

of H_2O. *d*-Tubocurarine (30 mg) is administered intravenously soon after the administration of the nitrous oxide–oxygen mixture. This results in muscular paralysis, including interference with respiration; positive pressure mechanical respiration is used throughout the entire surgical procedure.

Thiopental is more expensive but superior to ether, chloroform, and barbital sodium as a depressant for castration, removal of tusks, and the application of nose rings. The suggested dosage decreases with the weight of the animal, as indicated in Table 13.4.

One-half the dosage should be injected rapidly to carry the animal quickly through the period of excitement. The remainder of the intravenous injection should be given slowly until the desired effect is produced. The dosage injected can be adapted to the individual susceptibility of the patient.

The dosage suggested in the table produces little depression of respiration, but if it is exceeded, marked respiratory depression occurs.

About 1 hour is required before swine can move about satisfactorily after thiopental administration. This period is ordinarily longer than in human beings, dogs, rabbits, and some other animals where approximately 15 minutes are usually required for recovery. In general, swine show a slower recovery rate from the effects of any CNS depressant than other species. The obese condition of swine is apparently contributory to a slower recovery period because thiopental is known for its ability to localize in fat.

Satisfactory anesthesia has been obtained by the author using thiopental for thoracic and abdominal surgery in swine lasting as long as 3 hours. The anesthesia is preceded by parenteral medication using atropine sulfate (0.03–0.04 mg/lb), chlorpromazine hydrochloride (0.5 mg/lb), and meperidine hydrochloride (0.5 mg/lb).

Thiopental sodium is best given intravenously via the anterior vena cava by an indwelling catheter. Since respiratory depression readily occurs in swine, endotracheal intubation is necessary for oxygen administration and/or artificial respiration. In addition, intubation of the pig provides an excellent means for supplementing thiopental with inhalant anesthetics.

In Cattle. Thiopental sodium has been used, with satisfactory results, to produce surgical anesthesia for laparotomy in calves under 2 weeks of age. A 6.5% solution (1 grain/ml) should be injected slowly during 4–5 minutes until complete muscular relaxation occurs. The total dose varies from 7 to 10 mg/lb (1/9 to 1/6 grain). The stage of light surgical anesthesia usually exists 10–12 minutes. Partial recovery follows rapidly, with complete recovery of limb coordination in 2 hours.

A transient stage of deep hypnosis or light surgical anesthesia results from rapid injection of a small dose of thiopental sodium. Three g/lb (1/15–1/13 grain) in 10% solution injected intravenously within 10 seconds produce deep hypnosis in 600- to 800-lb steers (Henderson 1944). The full effect is apparent within 1–2 minutes and persists 5–10 minutes. The steers fall to the ground at the close of fairly rapid injection. The animals assume a normal recumbent position in about one-half hour and stand within 2–3 hours. The phlegmatic disposition of the bovine ordinarily results in a quiet recovery and only slight incoordination of movement when the animals stand. This anesthetic technique has been used in cattle for such minor operations as dehorning, which in the United Kingdom must be performed under general anesthesia because of the regulations of the Animal Anesthetics Act.

In Horses. The rapid intravenous injection of thiopental sodium without the benefit of preanesthetic agents or tranquilizers has been tried in horses. While anesthesia may occur briefly, the recovery period in the horse is so marked by excitement and incoordination that the use of thiopental sodium alone is contraindicated (Henderson and Brooksby 1950; Ford 1951). The adverse effects may arise partly from the action of the drug, but much of the difficulty undoubtedly results from the nervous and excitable disposition of the horse in comparison to the phlegmatic disposition of the bovine.

A dose of 9–17 mg/kg of thiopental sodium has been used to anesthetize 8 horses (Tyagi et al. 1964). A single dose within the dosage range produces anesthesia lasting 21–33 minutes. Considerable variation was observed in the clinical signs of anesthesia. Nystagmus was not seen in 3 of the 8 animals; when it was present, it was a good indicator of the depth of anesthesia. Muscular relaxation of the limbs, abdomen, and jaw is the most dependable sign of the level and depth of surgical anesthesia. More recent clinical experience with thiopental in the horse indicates that the rapid intravenous injection of a dose (10 mg/kg) that will induce anesthesia is accompanied by a moderate tachycardia, a slight reduction in arterial pressure, and a brief period of apnea lasting one-half minute to more than 1 minute (Tavernor and Lees 1970). In addition, a transient reversal in the T wave of the ECG is seen in some animals. Thiopental sodium is considered to be a relatively safe drug for general anesthesia in the horse, providing the rate and character of respiration are carefully observed (Tyagi et al. 1964). Thiopental sodium is often used intravenously for rapid ("crash" or "quick-shot") induction of anesthesia in the horse at the rate of 3 g/1000 lb of body weight in a tranquilized animal (Short 1974). Without tranquilization, the dosage of thiopental required to induce anesthesia may increase as much as 25%. Induction of anesthesia usually requires one-half–1 minute after injection of the drug and corresponds to the speed or rate of injection of the anesthetic agent. A more gradual approach to induction of anesthesia may be preferred by the use of thiopental sodium in combination with glyceryl guaiacolate. This involves the intravenous administration of 1000 ml of 5% glyceryl guaiacolate plus 2 g of thiopental sodium for a horse weighing 1000 lb. The anesthetic can be used in the horse satisfactorily if promazine hydrochloride is injected intravenously in a dose of 0.25 mg/lb of body weight prior to the use of the barbiturate. The prior use of the tranquilizer is doubtless responsible for smoother recovery from the anesthetic.

Thiopental sodium has been used intravenously in a dose of 2.7 g/1000 lb of body weight as maintenance anesthesia in the horse following promazine and chloral hydrate administration (Gable 1962).

In Goats. Thiopental sodium (5%) has been satisfactorily used in the goat for adrenalectomy procedures lasting about 2 hours. Since the animal detoxifies the anesthetic at a rapid rate, the dose level required for anesthesia varies greatly. An initial intravenous dose of 9–10 mg/lb of body weight is usually effective in anesthetizing the goat. Maintenance anesthesia is achieved by repeated administration of the anesthetic via an indwelling catheter placed in the external jugular vein.

Atropine sulfate is capable of controlling salivation in the goat following barbiturate anesthesia. However, larger doses (15 mg/50 lb) of atropine, injected intramuscularly, are required than are customarily used in other species. To maintain control of salivation, it is necessary to repeat the atropine sulfate, administered by the intravenous route, at 15-minute intervals at a dose level of 3–6 mg in animals weighing 65–85 lb.

An endotracheal catheter is routinely used to protect the airway from possible regurgitated ruminal contents. The tracheal intubation is valuable for administration of oxygen in the event of respiratory depression or arrest from an overdose of anesthesia.

In Birds. Thiopental sodium has been administered intravenously via the wing vein to geese, ducks, chickens, and pigeons for induction of anesthesia (Lee 1953). Anesthetic dosages used on a per lb body weight basis were 6–10 mg for native Chinese geese, 8–12 mg for ducks, and 6–8 mg for chickens and pigeons. It was observed that sudden death often occurred in pigeons during administration of the anesthetic agent. In the chicken, the injection of 6 mg/lb of body weight of thiopental is without satisfactory results and death occurs if the dose exceeds 8 mg/lb. It appears that the relative lack of safety and short duration of anesthesia make this agent unsatisfactory for poultry surgery.

In Subhuman Primates. When short-term surgical procedures are indicated and rapid recovery is preferred, thiopental sodium is a useful anesthetic agent in subhuman primates (Day 1965; Sawyer 1965a; Domino et al. 1969). In the chimpanzee, thiopental sodium is the choice of agents for long-term (i.e., 3–4 hours), light-stage anesthetic procedures and short-term surgical procedures, i.e., 30–45 minutes (Day 1965). According to Day, the initial dose of thiopental is 33 mg/kg of body weight; this dose produces light Stage III anesthesia.

In the rhesus monkey, thiopental sodium is administered intravenously at a dose level of 25–30 mg/kg of body weight (Sawyer 1965a; Domino et al. 1969). According to Sawyer, the excitatory phase during induction of anesthesia is not as turbulent as it is in the canine species and the slow rate of administration of the barbiturate can be readily performed. This type of response during induction of anesthesia reduces the possibility of administering an overdose to the animal. Sawyer (1965a) advocates the intramuscular administration of atropine sulfate (0.04 mg/kg) prior to or at the time of anesthesia induction.

Unless reinforced, the duration of thiopental anesthesia from a single administration is not more than 10 minutes in the rhesus monkey and recovery generally is complete within 45–60 minutes (Domino et al. 1969).

In Rabbits. Thiopental sodium (2.5%) is used as the intravenous anesthetic of choice in the rabbit (Sawyer 1965b). Sawyer recommends the slow administration of the anesthetic agent via the ear vein while the respiratory rate and oral and palpebral reflexes are observed. He also emphasizes that the pedal reflex should not be used to determine the depth of anesthesia; when this reflex is severely depressed or absent, the animals may be in the terminal stage of anesthesia. The intravenous dose level of thiopental sodium recommended for the rabbit is 50 mg/kg of body weight; this will produce anesthesia for 5–10 minutes and full recovery usually occurs in 15 minutes (Murdock 1969).

In Snakes. Experimentally, skin grafting procedures have been conducted in bull snakes *(Pituophis catenifer)* and Texas rat snakes *(Elaphe quadrivittata)* using thiopental sodium and thiamylal sodium 2–6 mg/kg intraperitoneally for induction of surgical anesthesia (Kraner et al. 1965). It is necessary to administer both in dosages near the lethal level to be effective. Moreover, recovery is observed to be extremely slow, taking 48–72 hours even when analeptic agents are used (Kraner et al. 1965). A large number of snakes fail to survive barbiturate-induced anesthesia. For this reason, Kraner et al. (1965) found the use of inhalant anesthetics more satisfactory than thiopental or thiamylal.

THIALBARBITONE SODIUM

Thialbarbitone Sodium (Kemithal sodium) is a sulfur-containing barbiturate (Fig. 13.4). Its duration of action is intermediate between the short-acting and the ultrashort-acting barbiturates. Thialbarbitone has a potency of approximately one-half that of thiopental and has similar pharmacological characteristics.

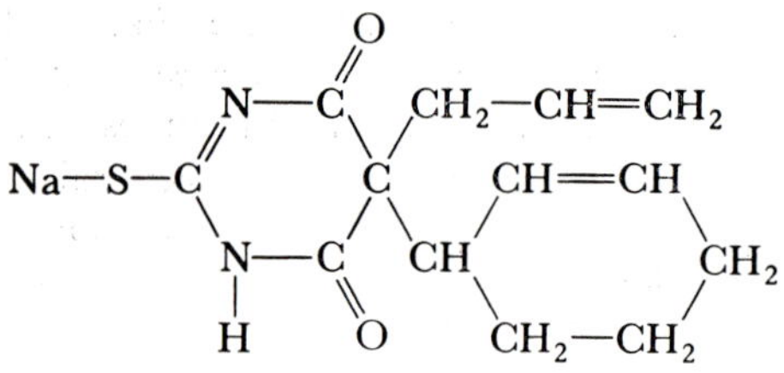

Thialbarbitone Sodium

FIG. 13.4.

Chemically this compound is a sodium salt of 5-(2-cyclohexen-1-yl)-5-allyl-2-thiobarbituric acid. Thialbarbitone sodium is used in about a 10% buffered aqueous solution. Unbuffered solutions have a pH of 10.6. Thialbarbitone sodium is almost entirely detoxified by the body tissues.

CLINICAL USE

Thialbarbitone sodium is approved by the FDA for use in the dog, cat, horse, cow, sheep, and pig.

In Dogs and Cats. Thialbarbitone sodium is considered a satisfactory agent in the dog and cat for anesthesia lasting about 15 minutes. The drug is administered intravenously in a 10% solution to give the desired effect. Doses of 33–40 mg/lb of body weight are indicated for surgery lasting 1 hour or more, while a dose of 20 mg/lb of body weight is satisfactory for minor surgery in the dog (Aranēz and Forteza 1955).

The intravenous dosage levels in the dog have been categorized into the various body weight ranges as follows (*Code of Federal Regulations,* 135b. 79, April 1, 1974):

Weight (lb)	*Dose (mg/lb)*
Over 50	14.1
30–50	18.8
10–30	23.5
Under 10	28.2

The intravenous dose of thialbarbitone specified for the cat in the *Code of Federal Regulations* is 31.3–37.6 mg/lb of body weight. Although only slight salivation occurs during thialbarbitone anesthesia, atropine sulfate (0.02 mg/lb) should be routinely employed prior to surgical anesthesia.

TABLE 13.5. Average dosages of thiobarbiturates administered to sheep (44–66 lb)

	Thiopental Sodium	Thialbarbitone Sodium
	(5%)	(10%)
Induction dose	0.56 g	1.3 g
Time from induction dose to first maintenance dose	20 min	13 min
Maintenance dose	0.2 g	0.37 g
Interval between maintenance doses	26 min	14 min

Source: Titchen et al. 1949.

In Calves, Cattle, and Swine. The intravenous dosage levels are as follows (*Code of Federal Regulations,* 135b. 79, April 1, 1974):

Species	*Dose (mg/lb)*
Calves	9.4–11.8
Cattle	6.7– 9.4
Swine	6.7–9.4

In Sheep. Thialbarbitone sodium produces rapid and smooth surgical anesthesia of short duration in sheep following the intravenous injection of about 25 mg/lb (Titchen et al. 1949). Table 13.5 gives the average dosages necessary to induce anesthesia in lambs with thialbarbitone sodium and thiopental sodium. Induction, which was accomplished without excitement, was produced by an initial rapid and then a slower injection of the drugs over a period of 30–60 seconds until apnea resulted. The apnea lasted only about 15 seconds and was terminated by a "sighing respiration," which was then followed by rapid, shallow breathing of 30–40 respirations/minute.

The sheep invariably defecated during anesthesia, and many regurgitated ruminal contents. Regurgitation was more frequent after thiopental anesthesia than after the thialbarbitone sodium anesthesia. These investigators concluded that both anesthetics in sheep provided a rapid, smooth induction without excitement, a satisfactory and controlled anesthesia, and quiet and rapid postanesthetic recovery. Recovery from thialbarbitone was more rapid and constituted a significant advantage in sheep because prolonged recumbency induces regurgitation with the hazard of inhalation of foreign matter leading to aspiration pneumonia.

The intravenous dose for sheep recommended by the *Code of Federal Regulations* (135b. 79, April 1, 1974) is 9.4–11.8 mg/lb of body weight.

In Horses. Thialbarbitone sodium is an unsatisfactory anesthetic in the horse if it is not preceded 30 minutes by a preanesthetic agent such as acetylpromazine. A dose of thialbarbitone sodium (6.3–7.8 mg/lb) is injected rapidly following this time (*Code of Federal Regulations,* 135b. 79, April 1, 1974). Thialbarbitone must not be used without a preanesthetic because recovery is most unsatisfactory and dangerous. Recovery may last up to an hour, even with small dosages, and is characterized by great ataxia and struggling on the part of the patient with considerable self-injury when a preanesthetic has not been used.

THIAMYLAL SODIUM

Thiamylal Sodium, N.F. (Surital sodium), is an ultrashort-acting thiobarbiturate (see Fig. 13.5). It is prepared for use in a mixture with sodium carbonate, a buffering agent. It consists of pale yellow, hygroscopic masses of crystals.

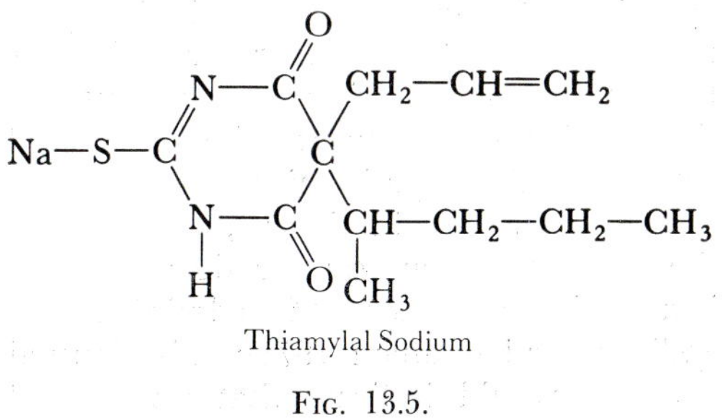

```
              O
             //
        N—C    CH₂—CH=CH₂
       //     \ /
Na—S—C        C
       \      / \
        N—C    CH—CH₂—CH₂—CH₃
        |   \\  |
        H    O  CH₃
```

Thiamylal Sodium

Fig. 13.5.

CHEMISTRY

Thiamylal is the thiobarbiturate analogue of secobarbital. Thiamylal sodium is freely soluble in water with a pH of about 10.5. The solution of thiamylal sodium is clear, bright, and yellow, with a pungent odor. The pH of the solution decreases slowly when carbon dioxide is absorbed from the atmosphere. Air should not be bubbled through the solution during preparation. The solution should be discarded if a precipitate forms in it.

STABILITY

Thiamylal sodium is relatively stable as a dry powder mixed with sodium carbonate and stored in air-tight vials.

Aseptic procedures must be used in the preparation of thiamylal solutions; sterile water or diluent must be used in dissolving the sterile, dry thiamylal powder. Solutions of thiamylal sodium cannot be subjected to heat or sterilization because of deterioration. Refrigeration or storage in a cool, dark place is necessary once the preparation is in the form of a solution. The thiamylal solution should be used within 24 hours.

PHARMACOLOGIC CONSIDERATIONS

Cardiac arrhythmias and an increase in the arterial blood pressure have been reported to develop in 85% of the dogs injected with thiamylal sodium (Pedersoli and Brown 1973). The arrhythmogenic effect produced by this thiobarbiturate is thought to be elicited through the release of epinephrine from the adrenal medulla during the course of anesthesia. Administration of atropine, procainamide, lidocaine, or oxygen failed either to prevent or to completely arrest the arrhythmias. However, autonomic ganglionic blocking agents such as phenoxybenzamine or hexamethonium prevented the development of the arrhythmias. Inasmuch as autonomic blocking agents can produce severe arterial hypotension, their use clinically to prevent cardiac arrhythmia is not advisable.

As previously discussed for thiopental, the ability of anesthetics to induce cardiac arrhythmia increases the hazard for the initiation of ventricular fibrillation, especially when critical levels of catecholamines are released or administered in clinical procedures. Recent studies in the dog indicate that epinephrine or norepinephrine may be used safely if the animal is premedicated with acetylpromazine or chlorpromazine before induction of anesthesia (Wiersig et al. 1974).

Thiamylal sodium (20 mg/kg) administered intravenously in the dog increases the systemic arterial pressure and decreases coronary blood flow (Goldberg et al. 1968). All these effects appear to be produced by vasoconstriction. Goldberg et al. also noted a vasoconstrictor effect of thiamylal upon the pulmonary bed of the dog; pentobarbital did not produce a significant effect upon pulmonary circulation. However, pentobarbital produced a late effect and an increase in systemic arterial pressure. The results obtained by these investigators indicate that pentobarbital and, particularly, thiamylal would be unacceptable for sedation or anesthetic purposes to determine the functional status of the pulmonary or systemic circulation through cardiac catheterization.

Excessive salivation is noted in some animals following the administration of thiamylal sodium. It can be controlled readily by the use of atropine sulfate given in premedication. Emesis with thiamylal sodium occurs infrequently.

ADMINISTRATION

Thiamylal sodium is administered in veterinary medicine in aqueous solution approximating 4% concentration. In human medicine a 2.5% solution is used. The administration is by intermittent intravenous injection. An inadvertent extravascular injection may produce pain, swelling, and necrosis of tissues. Also, the intraarterial injection of thiamylal should be avoided as discussed under Thiopental Sodium. Intravenous administration of thiamylal sodium in solution is comparable to the technique employed with other barbiturates, particularly pentobarbital sodium and thiopental sodium. The drug solution is injected intravenously in prescribed fashion until the desired depressant effect is obtained.

Thiamylal sodium may be administered alone or in combination with other anesthetic agents. It may follow premedication with acetylpromazine maleate and atropine as commonly employed with other depressants. It may be used to induce anesthesia, which is then maintained under some other agent, and it may be used for extension of anesthesia. Thiamylal sodium may also be employed with several curare-type compounds.

DURATION OF ACTION AND RECOVERY

Thiamylal sodium is an ultrashort-acting barbiturate particularly indicated for intravenous anesthesia of short duration. Thiamylal produces a smooth, rapid induction of anesthesia with little excitement. The recovery period is at least equal to and perhaps shorter than that for thiopental sodium. The potency of thiamylal sodium approximates 1.5 times that of thiopental in the dog. Thus a smaller amount of thiamylal sodium is required to produce anesthesia of equal depth and duration. Anesthesia generally occurs in 20–60 seconds, and recovery may be expected within 10–30 minutes following the last injection, depending on the amount of drug administered.

METABOLISM

Thiamylal sodium is metabolized primarily by the liver. It should not be employed in the presence of hepatic disease. This barbiturate accumulates more slowly in dogs than thiopental sodium, so it would appear to be detoxified by the liver more rapidly. Induction of microsomal enzymes in the liver markedly affects the duration of barbiturate anesthesia. The phenomenon of resistance or tolerance that develops following repeated use of the barbiturates is due to the accelerated activity of the hepatic microsomal enzyme system. However, in the cat, tolerance to the barbiturates appears to decrease with increased frequency of administration (Wilson and Graham 1971); this unusual response would indicate that microsomal enzyme activity may possibly be suppressed by barbiturates in this species.

TOXICITY

Thiamylal sodium possesses less cardiotoxicity than thiopental sodium when both compounds are administered intravenously to dogs (Woods et al. 1949). Studies in human beings on the effect of thiamylal sodium on respiration and blood pressure confirm the findings in dogs, namely, that no significant decrease of respiratory rate or volume was noted during anesthesia and no stimulative or depressive effect upon blood pressure was observed (Dornette and Tuohy 1951).

Thiamylal sodium should be employed cautiously in the presence of hepatic diseases, respiratory disease or obstruction, obesity, anemia or severe cardiovascular disturbances, and traumatic shock. Any condition interfering with the intake and distribution of oxygen contraindicates the use of this and other barbiturates.

CLINICAL USE

Thiamylal sodium is approved by the FDA for use in the dog, cat, pig, cow, and horse.

In Small Animals. Thiamylal sodium was originally employed by Reutner and Gruhzit (1948) to produce surgical anesthesia in dogs. Although originally recommended for dogs alone, thiamylal sodium is also employed satisfactorily in cats for routine operations. Thiamylal has been used for a wide variety of operations and examinations in the dog and cat, such as are encountered in routine practice. It appears to have the same general indications and uses as pentobarbital sodium and thiopental sodium.

The dosage of thiamylal sodium in dogs intravenously is determined by the effect produced. An average dose of 8 mg/lb of body weight will produce surgical anesthesia for about 15 minutes (Roberts et al. 1951). This dosage may have to be increased slightly for puppies and decreased slightly for aged dogs. If longer anesthesia is required, one-fourth the original dose can be administered to prolong the operative period up to 45 minutes of satisfactory anesthesia. Other authors have reported that an intravenous dose of 10–20 mg/kg of body weight of thiamylal sodium in the dog and cat will produce 10–15 minutes of anesthesia and up to 2 hours of sleep (Strobel and Wollman 1969). In the Siamese cat, thiamylal sodium has been reported to have a greater CNS depressant effect than other breeds of cats (Wilson and Graham 1971). Induction of anesthesia in the dog has been accomplished by Short (1970) by the intravenous administration of thiamylal sodium (22 mg/kg) following preanesthetic medication with atropine sulfate and morphine sulfate or meperidine hydrochloride. This permitted endotracheal intubation soon afterward so anesthesia could be maintained with either halothane or methoxyflurane.

In the rabbit, a dilute (1%) solution of thiamylal sodium is considered to be a safer concentration to administer. An intravenous dose of thiamylal sodium of 30 mg/kg of body weight will induce anesthesia for 5 minutes; complete recovery usually requires 15 minutes (Murdock 1969).

In the rhesus monkey, the initial intravenous dose for induction of anesthesia is recommended at 25 mg/kg of body weight (Domino et al. 1969). One-fourth of this dose is rapidly administered, followed by a slow injection of as much of the maximal dose as is necessary to depress or inhibit corneal reflex activity. According to Domino et al. (1969), useful anesthesia with thiamylal without reinforcement is not more than 10 minutes.

In Large Animals. Thiamylal is used to induce rapid anesthesia in the horse prior to the use of inhalant anesthetics. A dose of 1 mg/lb of body weight is injected rapidly by the intravenous route. Immediately after the animal becomes recumbent, it is restrained securely and prepared for endotracheal intubation.

Thiamylal sodium is also used intravenously in the horse at a dose level of 2.7 g/1000 lb of body weight following promazine hydrochloride and chloral hydrate (Gabel 1962). A combination of 0.2% thiamylal sodium and 5% glyceryl guaiacolate has been used in the horse (Jackson and Lundvall 1972). This is recommended in the horse as an intravenous induction agent for general anesthesia with inhalant anesthetics. Following an intravenous injection of promazine hydrochloride (0.25 mg/lb), the 5% glyceryl guaiacolate and 0.2% thiamylal sodium mixture is given at a dose level of 1 ml/lb (2.2 mg/kg) of body weight; this produces a recumbent, cooperative patient for about 18–25 minutes (Heath and Gabel 1970). The animals are then intubated for the administration of halothane anesthesia. Although this procedure permits effective restraint and anesthesia, the primary disadvantage is the relatively large volume of glyceryl guaiacolate–thiamylal solution needed for restraint and anesthesia.

Thiamylal sodium is also used for "crash" or "quick-shot" induction of anesthesia in the horse (Short 1974). The dosage for this purpose is also similar to that of thiopental sodium previously mentioned for the horse.

Thiamylal sodium is also used intravenously for induction of anesthesia in calves and adult cattle. The thiobarbiturate is given "to effect"; a dose of 7 mg/kg of body weight is recommended for induction of anesthesia. Prior to the administration of thiamylal, atropine sulfate (0.05 mg/kg) is recommended for control of bradycardia and salivation; for control of excitation, propiopromazine hydrochloride (0.4 mg/kg) is used on occasion.

In swine thiamylal sodium has been used for brief periods of anesthesia. The barbiturate is administered by the cranial vena cava and intraperitoneal route or by the ear vein. The intravenous dosage for swine weighing 11.25–31.5 kg is 1 ml of a 4% solution of thiamylal sodium for each 2.25 kg of body weight; a similar schedule is used for the intraperitoneal route of administration (Dunne and Benbrook 1954).

Miller and Gudmundson (1964) used a 10% solution of thiamylal via the ear vein in boars weighing 112.5–405 kg. The weight of each animal is estimated to the nearest 100 lb (45 kg), and 2 ml of the anesthetic is administered for each 45 kg up to 180 kg. Over this weight, an additional 0.5 ml is administered for each 45 kg above 180 kg, to a maximum of 10 ml. The intravenous injection is made rapidly (3 seconds); induction of anesthesia requires 15–45 seconds but is usually produced within 20–30 seconds after completion of the injection. Induction occurs without excitement; a short period of apnea is observed occasionally, but never exceeds 15 seconds. Most pigs regain their feet in 10–15 minutes. Some animals, if not disturbed, sleep for an hour or more but can be aroused easily and can stand.

Thiamylal anesthetic lasts approximately 10–12 minutes (Dunne and Benbrook 1954). The animals recover quickly and within 30–40 minutes after the onset of anesthesia are again standing. Overdosage is probably the result of inaccurate estimation of the weight of the animal; cessation of respiration occurs but vigorous cardiac action continues. When prompt artificial respiration is applied, no deaths occur.

Methohexital Sodium

Several hundred barbiturates have been synthesized in an effort to find an ultrashort-acting barbiturate with greater potency and a shorter duration of action than the thiobarbiturates, viz., thiopental and thiamylal. As the result of this effort, an oxybarbiturate (methohexital sodium) was also synthesized by pharmaceutical chemists. *Methohexital Sodium,* N.F. (Brevane, Brevital), has been approved by the FDA for use only in the dog and cat.

CHEMISTRY

Chemically, methohexital sodium is α-*dl*-1-methyl-5-allyl-5-(1-methyl-2 pentynyl) barbituric acid sodium (see Fig. 13.6). This anesthetic agent resembles secobarbital and pentobarbital, the oxygen analogues of thiamylal and thiopental, respectively.

STABILITY

Methohexital sodium is stable in an aqueous solution at room temperature for

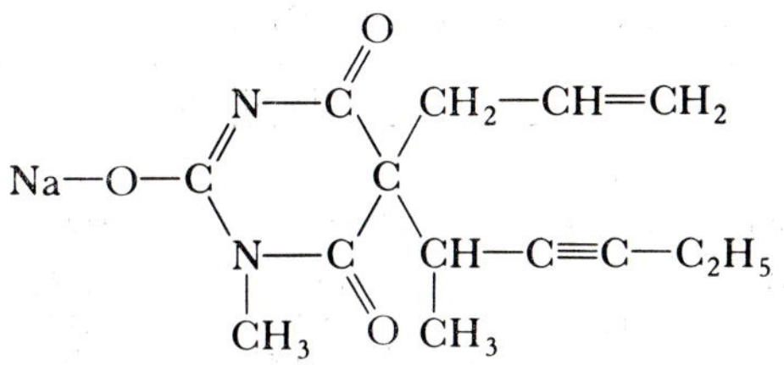

```
                 O
                 //
          N—C   CH2—CH=CH2
         //    \  /
Na—O—C          C
        \       / \
          N—C   CH—C≡C—C2H5
          |    \\   |
         CH3    O  CH3
```

Methohexital Sodium

FIG. 13.6.

at least 6 weeks at a pH of 11. It is readily dissolved in saline or distilled water.

ADMINISTRATION

Methohexital sodium is administered as a 1% solution in the dog and cat by the intravenous route (Fowler and Stevenson 1961). According to these authors, perivascular injection does not produce tissue irritation. The rate of administration of methohexital plays an important role in the depth and duration of anesthesia. It is recommended that the drug be injected as rapidly as possible, consistent with safety, to reach a suitable plane of anesthesia. Fowler and Stevenson injected 1% methohexital sodium at approximately 1 ml/second. If a slow injection rate is used, muscular tremors frequently occur. Similar findings have been reported in human beings.

When methohexital is injected rapidly, induction of anesthesia is smooth and rapid. Animals are able to lift their heads or can sit up within 5–10 minutes. Complete recovery occurs within 30 minutes. When promazine hydrochloride (1.5 mg/lb) is administered intramuscularly and preceding methohexital by 1 hour, the duration of methohexital anesthesia is slightly prolonged but recovery is smoother (Fowler and Stevenson 1961).

In the greyhound, recovery from thiopental sodium anesthesia is prolonged compared to other breeds of dogs and requires twice as long as the longest comparable period with methohexital sodium (Fabry 1963). The effective intravenous dose of methohexital sodium for induction of anesthesia in the greyhound is 9–11 mg/kg (4–5 mg/lb). The recommended rate of injection for the greyhound is about 25 mg/second (1 ml/second of a 2.5% solution). The inadvertent extravascular injection of this concentration of the anesthetic solution does not result in any untoward effects when left untreated as compared to a 5% solution of thiopental sodium, which causes swelling, lameness, and even sloughing of tissues (Fabry 1963).

In human beings the anesthetic is considered to be an ideal preparation for rapid induction of hypnosis when inhalation anesthesia such as cyclopropane, ether, or halothane is used. Since the drug is rapidly metabolized, it does not interfere with the use of these inhalant anesthetics.

TOXICITY

It has been observed in human beings that respiratory depression is more severe following the use of methohexital than with thiamylal or thiopental at a comparable level of narcosis (Taylor and Stoelting 1960). Inasmuch as respiratory depression is prevalent throughout the course of anesthesia in the human subject, it is necessary to assist respiration by artificial means. Also, in human beings pain at the injection site occurs in 60% of the patients.

In the normal, healthy dog and cat at least twice the calculated dose of methohexital can be given with safety (Fowler and Stevenson 1961).

DOSAGE

A dosimetry schedule for the dog and cat is recommended as follows (Fowler and Stevenson 1961):

(1) Body weight up to 30 lb:

$$\frac{\text{Body weight}}{3} = \text{ml of 1\% solution required}$$

(2) Body weight over 30 lb:

$$\frac{\text{Body weight}}{4} = \text{ml of 1\% solution required}$$

In a more recent clinical report (Clifford and Soma 1969), a dose of 2.6 mg/lb of body weight (5.8 mg/kg) is recommended for the cat. This dose is slightly less than the dose (i.e., 3.3 mg/lb) previously recommended.

TABLE 13.6. Median anesthetic dose and average duration of anesthesia in animals

	Methohexital Sodium			Thiopental Sodium		
Animal	Number of animals	AD50 ± S.E.*	Duration of anesthesia	Number of animals	AD50 ± S.E.*	Duration of anesthesia
		(mg/kg)	*(min)*		*(mg/kg)*	*(min)*
Dogs	15	9.74 ± 0.93	29	15	16.0 ± 0.97	142
Cats	20	5.78 ± 0.54	39	15	10.4 ± 0.92	58
Monkeys	15	4.43 ± 0.21	15	15	9.95 ± 1.39	44

Source: Taylor and Stoelting 1960.
* Standard error.

CLINICAL USE

Comparison of the potency of methohexital and thiopental for several species has indicated that it is twice as potent as thiopental. Table 13.6 gives the median anesthetic doses and average durations of anesthesia in the dog, cat, and monkey.

Methohexital sodium is used in the horse as a 2.5% solution at a dose level of 2.27 mg/lb of body weight (Tavernor 1962). The anesthetic preparation is injected intravenously at a rapid rate. The horse falls to the ground within 15–20 seconds, with the period of anesthesia not exceeding 5 minutes. This permits enough time to insert an endotracheal catheter so inhalant anesthetics can be administered.

Methohexital sodium should not be used alone because excitation during recovery limits its use in the horse (Grono 1966). Premedication with neuroleptic agents (acetylpromazine, promazine) in conjunction with narcotic analgesics (meperidine, morphine) reduces the severity of excitation upon recovery.

Methohexital is used on occasion in swine for detusking boars, hoof trimming, foot inspection, and other minor procedures not requiring more than a few minutes. A dose of 5 mg/kg of body weight is recommended for these purposes (Emberton 1966).

This ultrashort-acting oxybarbiturate has also been used for performing a ventriculocordectomy in swine held in biomedical research facilities (Mackey et al. 1970). The recommended intravenous dose of methohexital sodium is 8 mg/kg of body weight; surgical anesthesia of approximately 10–15 minutes is produced by this dosage. If additional anesthesia is necessary to complete the surgery, inhalant anesthetic (ether) has been used. With this combination of anesthetic agents the animals are usually standing within 10 minutes following surgery.

The pig characteristically shakes its head vigorously during recovery from most barbiturates, including methohexital. The animals should recover in a well-padded area and not on concrete floors or other hard surfaces.

In the domestic duck, methohexital sodium administered intravenously has no apparent effect when given in doses of 5–10 mg/kg initially or when followed with additional dosages every 3–4 minutes. It is unclear whether the large fat depots are responsible for this unresponsive effect or if a hyperactive hepatic microsomal enzyme system exists in ducks.

SECOBARBITAL SODIUM

Secobarbital Sodium, U.S.P. (Seconal Sodium) (sodium 5-allyl-5-[1-methylbutyl] barbiturate), is a short-acting oxybarbiturate and is the chemical analogue of thiamylal sodium (see Fig. 13.7).

Secobarbital has been used in dogs as

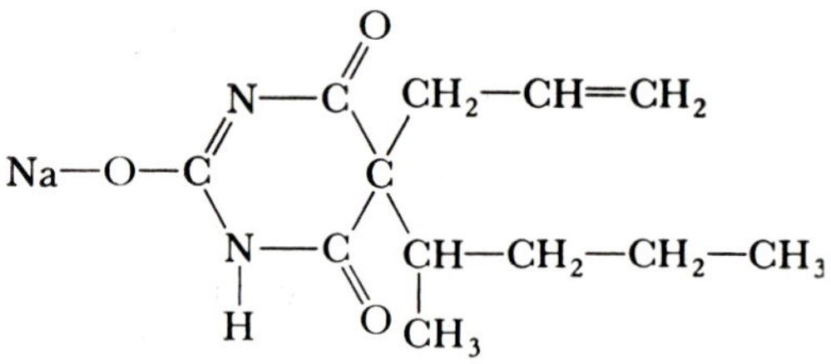

Secobarbital Sodium

FIG. 13.7.

an intravenous anesthetic in combination with mephenesin, a skeletal muscle relaxant. However, this barbiturate appears to be better suited to preanesthetic, basal anesthetic, and sedative uses. Since abdominal relaxation is not satisfactory following mephenesin, its use in combination with barbiturate anesthetics has been virtually discarded. Secobarbital has been used as a sedative prior to EEG recordings because it is purported to have less neurophysiologic effect than many other barbiturates (Strobel and Wollman 1969).

HEXOBARBITAL SODIUM

Hexobarbital Sodium, N.F. (Evipal Sodium), is an ultrashort-acting oxybarbiturate that is infrequently used for clinical purposes. A distinct disadvantage of hexobarbital is the uncontrollable excitement and ataxia exhibited during recovery in the dog. In the small laboratory animal, hexobarbital is occasionally used for short surgical procedures. For use in the rabbit, an intravenous dose of 40 mg/kg of body weight will produce anesthesia for 5–10 minutes, with complete recovery occurring in 15 minutes (Murdock 1969). In the adult albino rat, hexobarbital is usually administered intraperitoneally at a dose of 100 mg/kg of body weight for induction of anesthesia (Ben et al. 1969).

CHLORAL HYDRATE

Chloral Hydrate, U.S.P. ($CCl_3CH[OH]_2$), was introduced into medicine as a hypnotic in 1869 by Liebrich because it released chloroform *in vitro* and was thought to do the same *in vivo*. Subsequent investigation revealed the error of this assumption. It was among the first of the depressants of the CNS to be used in veterinary surgery. It still is one of the best hypnotics available for large animals when evaluated from the viewpoint of general practice. It is rarely used in small animals.

Chloral hydrate was first injected intravenously into experimental animals in 1872 by Oré. Three years later Humbert injected 30–70 g intravenously into horses. Chloral hydrate has since been injected intravenously to produce surgical anesthesia in large animals, especially horses.

The drug is classified as a Schedule IV compound under the 1970 Controlled Substances Act.

Chemistry

When acetic aldehyde is chlorinated, trichloroacetaldehyde (CCl_3CHO) is formed. The end product is chloral, a heavy, acrid oil. Chloral combines with one molecule of water to form chloral hydrate. It occurs as colorless, translucent crystals containing not less than 99.5% of $CCl_3CH(OH)_2$. Chloral hydrate volatilizes on exposure to air with an aromatic, penetrating odor. It has a slightly bitter, caustic taste. One g is soluble in 0.25 ml of water and in 1–2 ml of the common fat solvents.

Administration

Chloral hydrate in solution can be injected intravenously or intraperitoneally and is administered orally in solution or by capsule. Simple-stomached animals generally have little fluid in their stomachs, so the drug is better administered in dilute solution to these species to decrease the local irritation to the gastric mucosa. Vomition is often produced in the carnivorous animals from irritation of the gastric mucosa. The presence of food in the stomach reduces the irritant effects of the drug upon the mucosa and decreases the likelihood of vomition.

Chloral hydrate is not a satisfactory anesthetic because it has low pain-relieving power. In addition, so-called anesthetic dosages severely depress the respiratory and vasomotor centers. The anesthetic dosage approaches the MLD and therefore is hazardous.

Chloral hydrate is best employed for its hypnotic action. The intravenous injection for hypnotic effect provides the advantage of almost immediate action as compared to a delay of 15–30 minutes following oral administration. The intraperitoneal injection gives a slower response and is employed in swine where an intra-

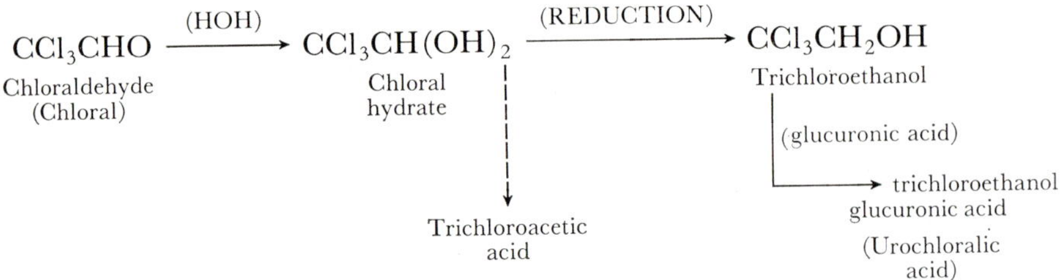

FIG. 13.8. Formation and fate of chloral hydrate.

venous injection would be more difficult. A desirable effect is obtained from the combined use of chloral hydrate and a local anesthetic. Preanesthetic medication with chloral hydrate for hypnotic effect renders the patient less fearful and more cooperative. Since the advent of the tranquilizers, the preanesthetic use of promazine hydrochloride reduces the amount of chloral hydrate needed to induce anesthesia in the horse.

Various concentrations have been injected intravenously, but it seems advisable to inject no greater than a 7% solution. Despite good intention, the perivascular injection of chloral hydrate solution does occur sometimes. Chloral hydrate is quite irritating to the tissues, especially in the horse. Severe pain, swelling, and necrosis of tissues result, including sloughing and destruction of the external jugular vein. Furthermore, there appears to be a latent period in the action of chloral hydrate given intravenously. When higher concentrations are injected at the usual rate until the desired effect is observed clinically, the animal will exhibit further depression within 10–15 minutes after the injection is stopped. Avoiding solution in excess of about 7% concentration diminishes the hazard involved in the latent action of chloral hydrate.

Absorption, Fate, and Excretion

Chloral hydrate is absorbed well and readily from the gastrointestinal tract. It causes some irritation of the gastric mucosa, especially if not well diluted by water. Vomition is readily induced in the dog after oral administration of the drug.

When chloral hydrate is injected intravenously in the dog, a small amount (3%–4%) is oxidized to trichloroacetic acid, and the major portion remaining is reduced to trichloroethanol (Fig. 13.8). The plasma concentration of trichloroethanol is sufficient to account for most of the hypnotic effect following the administration of chloral hydrate (Butler 1948; Marshall and Owens 1954). It is reported by these investigators that trichloroethanol is rapidly and completely absorbed when given orally to the dog. A peak concentration in the plasma is attained in 15–30 minutes, and as much metabolized drug is excreted in the urine in 2 hours from oral administration as from intravenous administration.

Trichloroethanol is conjugated, principally in the liver, with glucuronic acid to form urochloralic (trichloroethanol-glucuronic) acid, which is not hypnotic. A small part of the chloral hydrate is excreted unchanged in the urine. However, the major excretory form is urochloralic acid (Fig. 13.8). In the presence of liver damage, more chloral hydrate and less urochloralic acid are excreted. Urochloralic acid found in the urine gives a false positive test for sugar, which has led occasionally to the incorrect conclusion that chloral hydrate causes glucosuria.

Local Action

Chloral hydrate is irritating to the stomach, especially when empty. In simple-stomached animals it should be well diluted when administered. The local irritating property has led to its incorporation in rubefacient liniments.

Effect upon the CNS

Chloral hydrate and trichloroethanol produce depression of the cerebrum. Reflex excitability is reduced by chloral hydrate but not completely abolished in the horse (Booth and Rankin 1953). Even when curare is used as an adjunct to chloral hydrate anesthesia, spinal reflex activity persists. Persistence of reflex activity may be due to the eserinelike effect of chloral hydrate (Brown 1962). Brown reports that the neuromuscular blocking action of tubocurarine on isolated rat diaphragm preparation is completely and rapidly reversed by chloral hydrate.

Motor and sensory nerves are not affected except by large doses, which may produce anesthesia. Chloral hydrate is a good hypnotic but a poor anesthetic because of a narrow margin of safety. It produces a deep anesthesia that lasts for several hours. The depressant action of a hypnotic dose is limited to the cerebrum. The vital medullary centers are not affected.

Chloral hydrate has only very weak analgesic action, so its power to relieve pain is minimal. However, in combination with a local anesthetic, chloral hydrate is quite valuable in veterinary surgery for overcoming nervousness and excitability in large animals so that they are more cooperative.

Massive doses of chloral hydrate will induce anesthesia. Unfortunately, the margin of safety is too narrow to recommend widespread use of chloral hydrate as a surgical anesthetic. Fatal doses of chloral hydrate cause death by a progressive depression of the respiratory center.

Effect upon the Cardiovascular System

Following hypnotic dosages of chloral hydrate, the blood pressure and pulse are only a little more depressed than by ordinary sleep. Following anesthetic dosages, the central vasomotor center is severely depressed, resulting in a fall in blood pressure. The mean arterial pressure of the horse can drop from a normal 170 mm Hg to about 80 mm Hg following an anesthetic dose (5 g/100 lb) of chloral hydrate (Booth and Rankin 1953).

Limited cardiac depression may occur with any of the halogenated hydrocarbons, including chloral hydrate, but this has become serious only in those animals with previous heart defects. Hypnotic dosages of chloral hydrate clearly do not injure the myocardium. However, sudden death occurs occasionally in horses under chloral hydrate depression and is claimed to result from stimulation of the vagus nerve, which causes a cardiac block. Since chloral hydrate has an eserinelike action mentioned above, marked vagal stimulation can be attributed to this pharmacologic effect. In the light of this information, routine use of atropine sulfate as a preanesthetic agent is recommended.

Effect upon Respiration

A hypnotic dose of chloral hydrate depresses respiration somewhat more than does normal sleep. A large anesthetic dose markedly depresses the respiratory centers of the medulla so that too narrow a margin of safety exists for satisfactory clinical use.

Effect upon the Liver

Earlier, degeneration of the liver was presumed to result from large doses of chloral hydrate because the drug was thought to release chloroform, which is injurious to the liver. Repeated attempts to verify this claim have been unsuccessful, so it now appears that chloral hydrate has little or no detrimental effect upon the liver in the absence of hypercapnia and hypoxia.

Clinical Use

Chloral hydrate is best employed as a hypnotic in large animals. When administered in premedication, it overcomes the patient's fear of restraint and reduces risk of accidental injury to the patient and the operator. Chloral hydrate greatly facilitates the surgical technique under local or regional anesthesia.

It probably is used more for hypnosis preceding local or regional anesthesia in large animals than for any other purpose. It is an excellent hypnotic and possesses a wide margin of safety when used in this way. When a patient is premedicated with chloral hydrate, the induction of general anesthesia is more regular and there is less voluntary and involuntary activity. A uniform depth of anesthesia is easier to maintain following premedication with chloral hydrate, and less general anesthetic is required.

Chloral hydrate has not been used as successfully in ruminants as in horses and swine. In fact, *chloral hydrate has been used with continued satisfaction only in the horse and only for hypnosis.* Chloral hydrate has been used in cattle to depress the nervous excitement or even mania that may accompany acetonemia.

DOSAGE

About 5 g/100 lb of body weight in the horse, administered orally in solution, provides good hypnosis within 10–20 minutes. This dose should be increased slightly in nervous, light horses and perhaps decreased in phlegmatic draft horses and debilitated animals. Individual variation is very prominent following the oral administration of chloral hydrate. There is also a breed variation: the high-strung thoroughbred horse may require 60 g/1000 lb, whereas the standardbred may need only 50 g to produce comparable levels of hypnosis.

Less variation is noted following intravenous injection because the drug is given to produce the desired effect with less attention to dosage. The intravenous dose level for nonfasted horses weighing 900–1300 lb is 5.9 g/100 lb of body weight (Wright and Hall 1961). A slightly reduced dose will produce a similar anesthetic effect in the heavier animal; in lighter horses it is necessary to increase the dose. A yearling animal requires up to 6.35 g/100 lb of body weight.

Promazine hydrochloride is a useful adjunct to chloral hydrate anesthesia in the horse (Wright and Hall 1961). According to these authors, a dose level of 30–40 mg/100 lb of body weight given intravenously 15 minutes preceding the chloral hydrate reduces the struggling of the animal upon casting.

The oral dosage employed in maniacal acetonemia in cattle sometimes approaches twice the hypnotic dose listed above for the horse.

In the calf, chloral hydrate anesthesia can be used for abdominal surgery (Wilde 1962). Fasting of the animals for 18 hours prior to surgical anesthesia is recommended. Also, preanesthetic medication with atropine sulfate is strongly advised. Chloral hydrate in intravenous dose levels of 58–125 mg/lb of body weight induces anesthesia lasting 16–52 minutes. In young calves, chloral hydrate has been considered superior to other anesthetics for routine splenectomy (Berger 1966).

In cattle and swine, Bemis et al. (1924) used chloral hydrate orally preceding inhalant anesthesia. For mature cattle Bemis and co-workers gave 1–2 ounces of chloral hydrate dissolved in 1 quart of warm water by stomach tube or drench. In swine, Bemis et al. recommended chloral hydrate in practically all surgical procedures where general anesthesia was indicated. They administered chloral hydrate (12 g/50 lb) by stomach tube; satisfactory anesthesia was obtained in 80% of the animals approximately 20–30 minutes after administration of the drug. In 20% of the pigs, anesthesia was not attained after 30 minutes and then an inhalant anesthetic was administered to induce as well as to maintain anesthesia.

A method of combined chloral hydrate, halothane, and nitrous oxide anesthesia has been used in Colorado mule deer (Wolff et al. 1965). The animals were fasted 24 hours prior to surgery and 7% chloral hydrate was administered slowly by the intravenous route until most voluntary movement was abolished. Wolff and coworkers found the average dose of chloral hydrate to be 210 ml/200 lb of body weight or 73.5 mg/lb of body weight. Also, atropine sulfate was administered at a dose of 0.5–0.75 grain/animal to eliminate the excessive salivation; although the route of administration was not described, the drug was probably given subcutaneously or intramuscularly.

In the dog a 30% solution of chloral hydrate given intravenously in a dose of 300 mg/kg produces anesthesia for 60–85 minutes; salivation, vomition, urination, and defecation may occur following the injection (Lumb 1965). Respiration is depressed and arterial blood pressure falls; in addition, the heart may be sensitized to sudden vagal arrest or arrhythmias (Strobel and Wollman 1969). Atropine sulfate should be routinely employed prior to the induction of deep hypnosis or surgical anesthesia in all animal patients.

Chloral hydrate has been used also in domestic fowl (geese, ducks, chickens, pigeons) for induction of anesthesia (Lee 1953). The hypnotic drug was administered orally after the birds had been fasted; anesthesia was produced within 30 minutes after administration. Anesthesia was maintained 0.5, 2.5, and 4.5 hours in geese, ducks, and chickens, respectively. The anesthetic dose is 100–150 mg/lb of body weight for geese, 125–150 mg/lb for ducks, and 80–150 mg/lb for chickens. The body temperature of the birds dropped 1°–2.4° C during the course of anesthesia. In the pigeon, Lee (1953) reported that the oral administration of chloral hydrate failed to produce general anesthesia. They exhibited only depression and ataxia when chloral hydrate was administered in a dose below 225 mg/lb of body weight; dosage levels greater than this resulted in repeated vomiting within 0.5 hour after administration.

CHLORAL HYDRATE AND MAGNESIUM SULFATE

A mixture of 12% chloral hydrate and 6% magnesium sulfate in solution for intravenous injection has been advocated for anesthesia in large animals (Danks 1943). This mixture of chloral hydrate and magnesium sulfate is stable indefinitely. The solution is administered intravenously in horses at a rate not exceeding 30 ml/minute to avoid excessive depression of the CNS. Administration is discontinued when the stage of surgical anesthesia appears, as indicated by the slowing or absence of nystagmus and other significant reflexes. Anesthesia usually lasts over 30 minutes.

The addition of magnesium sulfate was originally thought to enhance the depressant action of the drug mixture through its own depressant effect upon the CNS. It is now known that the magnesium ion exerts little, if any, direct depressant effect on the CNS (Bowen et al. 1970). The primary effect of magnesium is its neuromuscular blocking action similar to the curariform agents. From this standpoint, magnesium is beneficial in producing skeletal muscle relaxation. Chloral hydrate produces poor skeletal muscle relaxation. Inasmuch as magnesium sulfate alone produces only neuromuscular blockade and death due to asphyxia, it is considered inhumane to use the drug in the euthanasia of animals (Bowen et al. 1970).

Chloral hydrate and magnesium sulfate in the concentrations given above are injected intravenously from a gravity flow apparatus until the desired stage of depression is produced. Amounts used in the horse vary from 200 to 400 ml of the above solution, depending on the size and condition of the animal.

For swine the solution of chloral hydrate and magnesium sulfate has been used by intraperitoneal injection to produce surgical anesthesia. The dosage employed of the above solution has been about 1 ml/lb of body weight.

According to Bhargava and Vyas (1967), there is still a need for relatively simple and inexpensive methods of administering anesthetics in many parts of the world. For example, the camel is economically important in several of the less developed countries and a less expensive but effective method of anesthesia is needed that requires only simple equipment for field conditions. The combination of chloral hydrate (12%) and magnesium sulfate (12%) has proved useful in anesthetizing the camel *(Camelus dromedarius)*. An intravenous dose of 12 g/220 lb of body weight of the mixture (i.e., 6 g each of chloral hydrate and magnesium sulfate are administered for each 220 lb of body weight).

Some veterinary clinics have modified Dank's formulation by using a mixture containing 8% each of chloral hydrate and magnesium sulfate.

CHLORAL HYDRATE, MAGNESIUM SULFATE, AND PENTOBARBITAL

The combination of *chloral hydrate, magnesium sulfate,* and *pentobarbital sodium* (Chloropent, Equithesin) provides some of the desirable depressant actions of each compound without the pronounced toxicities of each drug. The original combination proposed by Millenbruck and Wallinga (1946) for anesthesia in horses and cattle consists of chloral hydrate, 30 g; magnesium sulfate, 15 g; and pentobarbital sodium, 6.6 g; dissolved in 1000 ml of water.

Stability

The pentobarbital sodium cannot be added to the solution of chloral hydrate and magnesium sulfate unless it is to be used within about 1 hour. After 2 hours a precipitate forms from the exposure of chloral hydrate to the alkalinity of pentobarbital sodium. Commercially, stable solutions have been prepared by substituting the relatively insoluble pentobarbituric acid for the soluble sodium salt. The solubility of the acid compound has been increased by the use of propylene glycol and alcohol in the solvent. Present specifications for two commercial preparations are based on a United States *Federal Register* publication (CFR 135b. 57) of January 3, 1974. The contents of these anesthetic mixtures are described in each ml as follows: (1) *Anesthetic Mixture A*—chloral hydrate, 42.51 mg; pentobarbital, 9.72 mg; and magnesium sulfate, 21.25 mg. The drugs are dissolved in sterile aqueous solution containing 44.34% propylene glycol and 11.5% ethyl alcohol. (2) *Anesthetic Mixture B*—chloral hydrate, 42.5 mg; pentobarbital, 8.86; and magnesium sulfate, 21.2 mg. The drugs are dissolved in sterile aqueous solution containing 33.8% propylene glycol and 14.25% ethyl alcohol.

Mixture A contains slightly more pentobarbial than Mixture B. The chloral hydrate and magnesium sulfate content of both mixtures are nearly the same. Although the pentobarbital content in Mixture B is slightly less than Mixture A, its alcohol content is greater than that of Mixture A. Apparently, there is no difference in the level of CNS depression produced by either mixture because the recommended dosages of both preparations are identical. These two preparations have been approved by the FDA for intravenous use only for general anesthesia and a sedative-relaxant effect in cattle and horses.

Administration and Dosage

The mixture is injected intravenously by gravity to the desired level of clinical depression. The dose necessary to produce general anesthesia is 20–50 ml/100 lb of body weight. The drug preparation is administered until the desired effect is obtained as indicated by the degree of CNS depression produced as well as the effect produced upon respiration, eye activity, and other signs characterizing surgical anesthesia. Compared to the horse, cattle usually require a reduced dosage of the drug preparation due to weight contributed by the rumen contents. In both the horse and cow, use of the preparation for sedative and relaxant effects requires the administration of one-fourth to one-half of the anesthetic dosage level or less. The anesthetic preparation is not used in lactating cows because of the danger of the animal falling and bruising the udder.

The period of surgical anesthesia lasts about 30 minutes in an average horse. There is a fair margin of safety. Additional amounts prolong the anesthesia. Relaxation of the patient is good.

Recovery

Usually recovery from this anesthetic is satisfactory. The patient regains consciousness at about the same rate as it regains muscular coordination so that in most cases the legs will support the patient when it tries to stand. This is an advantage over chloral hydrate or pentobarbital sodium alone because the patient may struggle during the recovery period.

CLINICAL USE

In addition to the use of this drug mixture for anesthesia in cattle, horses, and birds, it is used for sedation purposes to assist in the restraint and handling of the horse for a number of clinical and diagnostic procedures (Swanson 1973). In physical examinations, Swanson uses 20 ml of chloropent and 30 mg of acetylpromazine maleate for each 1000 lb of body weight intravenously. Also, this drug mixture is used to restrain animals in the treatment of wounds; 15 ml of chloropent, 30 mg of acetylpromazine maleate, and 8 ml of pentazocine are administered intravenously for each 1000 lb of body weight. In addition, these three drugs are used for standing castrations. Some clients do not want their animals cast or placed in a recumbent position by anesthesia. Fifteen minutes after the administration of chloropent, acetylpromazine, and pentazocine, a local anesthetic, mepivacaine, is injected into each testicular cord and along the median raphe. The nose twitch may be required during the injection of the local anesthetic.

Chloropent (40 ml/1000 lb or "to effect") administered intravenously is useful 15 minutes following acetylpromazine maleate (30 mg/1000 lb) to assist in positioning the horse next to the operating table; this is then followed with an intravenous dose (2 g/1000 lb) of thiamylal sodium (Swanson 1973). After the animal is anesthetized and secure on the operating table, the trachea is intubated for inhalation anesthesia.

GLYCERYL GUAIACOLATE

Glyceryl Guaiacolate, N.F. (Gecolate), has been used as a therapeutic agent for over seven decades. An excellent review of the historical development of the medical uses of glyceryl guaiacolate has been written by Funk (1970). The drug was first used for its analgesic, antipyretic, and expectorant properties. Glyceryl guaiacolate is chemically similar to mephenesin and meprobamate; it is designated as 3-phenoxy-1,2-propanediol (Fig. 13.9).

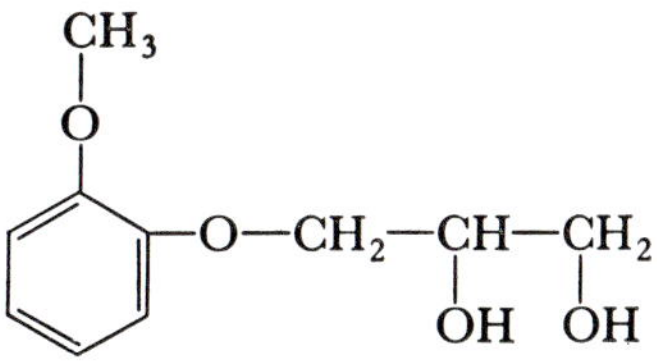

CH_3–O– (on benzene ring) –O–CH_2–CH(OH)–CH_2(OH)

Glyceryl Guaiacolate

FIG. 13.9.

Glyceryl guaiacolate has been used as an adjunct to anesthesia in the horse since 1949; in the United States it was first used in 1965. The compound increases the potency of preanesthetic agents and barbiturates. In addition, glyceryl guaiacolate is a central-acting skeletal muscle relaxant that selectively depresses or blocks nerve impulse transmission at the internuncial neuron level of the spinal cord, brainstem, and subcortical areas of the brain.

Glyceryl guaiacolate is approved as a muscle relaxant by the FDA for use in the horse. It must not be used in horses intended for human consumption. A 5% concentration of the compound is prepared by dissolving the powder (50 g/L) in sterile water.

STABILITY

Glyceryl guaiacolate is a white powder with a bitter taste. It is not readily soluble and partially precipitates out of solution at 72° F or lower (Funk 1973). Heating and agitation usually eliminate the precipitate. Only freshly prepared solutions should be used.

ADMINISTRATION AND DURATION OF ACTION

Although glyceryl guaiacolate has been administered by all parenteral routes, it is best administered intravenously. Orally, the drug must be administered in high dosages to produce a perceptible effect. The accidental perivascular injection of 5% glyceryl guaiacolate does not result in a severe tissue reaction. However, thrombophlebitis of the jugular vein was noted several days after anesthesia; this effect may be associated with the use of glyceryl guaiacolate (Schatzman 1974).

The primary disadvantage in the use of glyceryl guaiacolate is the large volume of solution required parenterally to produce relaxation. The effect of the drug is brief (Tavernor and Jones 1970). The duration of action of a single muscle relaxant dose is 15–30 minutes (Pedersoli 1972).

Pharmacological Considerations

Polysynaptic reflexes are more effectively blocked by glyceryl guaiacolate than the monosynaptic reflexes. A number of literature sources indicate that by itself glyceryl guaiacolate has sedative, hypnotic, and analgesic effects. There is evidence that the sedative and hypnotic effects of the drug are due to the depressant effect upon the reticular formation of the brainstem.

The side effects produced by the drug include a transient decline in the systemic arterial pressure when used (200 mg/kg) intravenously in the dog with thiopental and halothane anesthesia (Tavernor and Jones 1970). When used alone in the dog, the effect upon systemic arterial pressure is slight. A tachycardia occurs after the drug is administered but the heart rate returns to normal within 5 minutes after the injection.

In the horse the intravenous administration of glyceryl guaiacolate (160 mg/kg) produces recumbency; minor effects in the cardiac and respiratory rates, along with a slight drop in mean systemic arterial pressure and in arterial P_{O_2}, occur (Tavernor 1970). When glyceryl guaiacolate (80 mg/kg) is administered intravenously in the horse with thiopental sodium (3.5 mg/kg), recumbency and a slight decline in the mean systemic arterial pressure occur. The heart and respiratory rates increase in conjunction with a moderate fall in arterial P_{O_2}.

Glyceryl guaiacolate in therapeutic amounts does not lead to the hazard of paralysis of the muscles (intercostal and diaphragm) of respiration like the peripheral-acting skeletal muscle relaxants. Respiratory activity usually remains normal after a therapeutic dose. In the dog, an intravenous dose (200 mg/kg) has only a slight effect on arterial P_{O_2}, indicating that aveolar ventilation is unaltered (Tavernor and Jones 1970). Only when doses greater than those recommended are used in therapeutics will respiratory paralysis become a problem. Approximately 3–4 times the quantity required to produce recumbency of the horse can be administered before death occurs (Funk 1973).

Hemolysis is induced when concentrations of glyceryl guaiacolate in excess of 5% are used. This effect is related to the concentration of the glyceryl guaiacolate rather than to the total dosage used.

The kinetics of disappearance of glyceryl guaiacolate from blood plasma in the pony have been studied by Davis and Wolff (1970). Of particular interest is the sex difference in the rate of disappearance of glyceryl guaiacolate. The rate of disappearance ($t_{1/2} = 59.6 \pm 4.8$ minutes) in the female is more rapid than in the male ($t_{1/2} = 84.4 \pm 7.9$ minutes). This indicates that the drug would need to be administered more frequently to maintain effect in the female, and recovery would be more rapid.

Clinical Use

Glyceryl guaiacolate has been used in human beings, domestic animals, and in various species of laboratory animals. However, it is approved by the FDA as a muscle relaxant for use only in the horse. Its use is not permitted in horses intended for human consumption The intravenous dose approved for the use of 5% glyceryl guaiacolate in the horse is at a fixed level of 1 ml/lb (50 mg/lb) of body weight. Most clinical uses of glyceryl guaiacolate in the horse are in line with this dose level (Gertsen and Tillotson 1968; Heath and Gabel 1970; Coffman and Pedersoli 1971; Jackson and Lundvall 1972; Pedersoli 1972).

Preanesthetic preparations used intra-

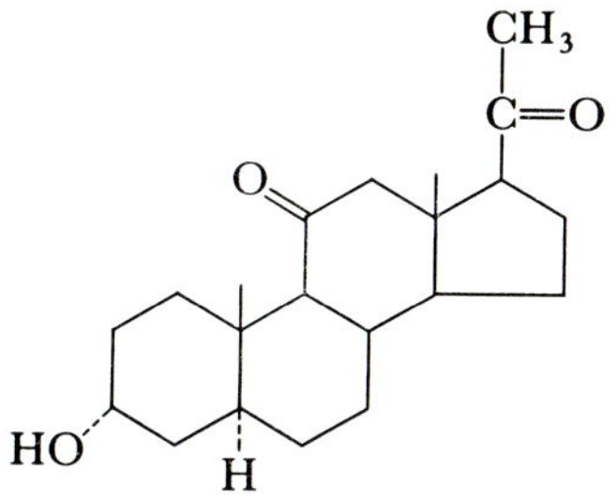

Steroid I
(3α-hydroxy-5α-pregnane-11,20, dione)

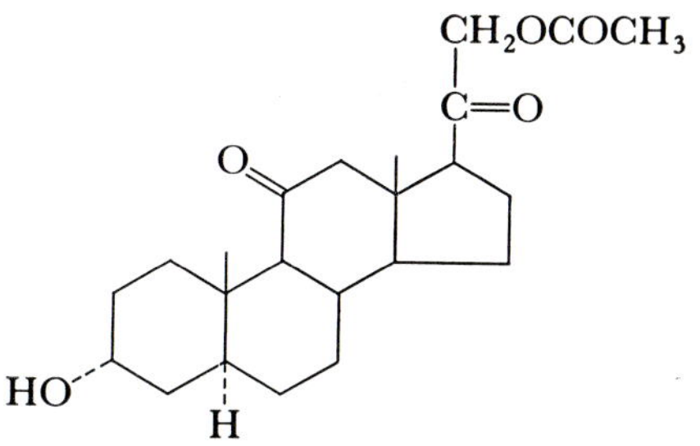

Steroid II
(21-acetoxy-3α-hydroxy-5α-pregnane-11,20, dione)

FIG. 13.10.

venously and recommended prior to the administration of glyceryl guaiacolate offer a number of options as follows (Pedersoli 1972):

1. Chloral hydrate (4 g/50 kg)
2. Promazine hydrochloride (300 mg/1000 lb)
3. Acetylpromazine maleate (4 mg/100 lb)

Usually, glyceryl guaiacolate (5%) plus an ultrashort-acting barbiturate such as thiamylal sodium (0.2%) is administered rapidly by the intravenous route 10–15 minutes following a preanesthetic level of promazine or acetylpromazine. Glyceryl guaiacolate (60 g) has also been used with pentobarbital sodium (3 g) and 50% dextrose (125 ml) in water up to 1 L (Keeran 1972). A total of 1 L of this preparation is used by rapid intravenous injection for ovariectomy in mares weighing 800–1000 lb.

Glyceryl guaiacolate as the sole induction agent followed by halothane anesthesia has been used successfully in the horse (Schatzman 1974). When it is used alone (i.e., not with an ultrashort-acting barbiturate for induction), a higher average respiration rate and a lower, more balanced pulse rate is noted. However, it requires a higher average concentration of halothane to induce and maintain anesthesia. Schatzman (1974) recommends the sole use of glyceryl guaiacolate for routine as well as for high-risk cases.

ALTHESIN

Althesin (Saffan, CT 1341) is a new steroidal preparation containing two pregnanediones for the induction of anesthesia (Child et al. 1972). The anesthetic is in current use within the United Kingdom; it has not been approved by the FDA for use in the United States. Based on the studies by Child and co-workers, the preparation produces immediate induction of anesthesia of short duration when it is administered intravenously into experimental animals; also, they have observed that recovery is rapid and without complications.

CHEMISTRY

Althesin contains two pregnanediones referred to as steroid I and steroid II (Fig. 13.10) (Child et al. 1972). The anesthetic preparation contains 0.9% w/v of steroid I and 0.3% w/v of steroid II. Each ml of althesin contains 12 mg of both steroids, i.e., 9 mg of steroid I and 3 mg of steroid II. Dosage is expressed as ml/kg of body weight; this expression of dosage is preferable because the solution may sometimes be diluted with physiological saline prior to administration (Child et al. 1972).

PHARMACOLOGICAL ACTIVITY

In the cat, 1.2 mg/kg of body weight of althesin administered intravenously produces a transient drop in systemic arterial blood pressure and tachycardia within a few seconds after the injection (Child et al. 1972). This is then succeeded by a slight rise in blood pressure during recovery from anesthesia. Within 6–9 minutes following the injection, Child and co-workers reported that the animals were able to stand and, after a period of ataxia, a rapid return to normal was observed. It was also reported that an intravenous dose of 7.2 mg/kg of althesin administered 5–10 minutes prior to the use of inhalant anesthetics proved to be a compatible procedure. The cats were satisfactorily maintained for 50 minutes by halothane, methoxyflurane, chloroform, trichloroethylene, diethyl ether, or cyclopropane (Child et al. 1972). Also, neuromuscular agents such as succinylcholine, *d*-tubocurarine, or gallamine with althesin proved to be compatible. Preanesthetic agents administered intramuscularly such as atropine sulfate (1 mg/kg) and meperidine (7.5 mg/kg) 1 hour before induction with althesin (7.2 mg/kg) proved to be satisfactory (Child et al. 1972).

Irrespective of the dosage of althesin, Child et al. (1972) observed no injury to the veins and no vomiting in the cat. The intramuscular route of administration of althesin (15–18 mg/kg) was useful in kittens where venepuncture was difficult to perform (Hall 1972).

Clinical Use

For induction of anesthesia in the cat, a single intravenous dose of althesin (9 mg/kg) has been used clinically for castration and dental operative procedures (Evan et al. 1972). Duration of anesthesia is 10–12 minutes; surgical procedures requiring more than 5–10 minutes may be extended by the injection of additional small amounts of the anesthetic preparation.

Althesin may also be administered intramuscularly (9 mg/kg) for clinical procedures such as radiography, dematting, and examination of the mouth (Evan et al. 1972). This dose level of the anesthetic will produce sedation of the animal in approximately 7 minutes after injection, and sedation will last for about 5 minutes. According to Evan and co-workers (1972), 12 mg/kg of althesin administered intramuscularly will result in deep sedation or light anesthesia that is sufficient to permit a number of minor surgical procedures such as drainage of an abscess or suturing small superficial wounds. The maximum response produced by this dose level occurs in 7–8 minutes and has a duration of action of about 15 minutes. Light sedation produced by an intravenous dose of 4 mg/kg has been suggested in premedication prior to the induction of full anesthesia with althesin or other anesthetic agents (Evan et al. 1972).

Althesin can be used to maintain surgical anesthesia for a prolonged period in the cat by repeated supplementary injections of one-half the intravenous induction dose without significant cumulative anesthetic or respiratory depressant effects (Dodds and Twissell 1973). However, isolated clinical reports have indicated that cessation of respiration occasionally occurs and efforts to revive these animals are unsuccessful.

In the Chicken

Cooper and Frank (1973) concluded that althesin is of value in the chicken when it is administered by the intravenous route. Analgesia, muscle relaxation, and speed of recovery were considered to be excellent at an intravenous dose level up to 14 mg/kg. However, Cooper and Frank (1973) suggested an intravenous dose for birds of 10 mg/kg. Althesin appears to be a safe drug even in recently captured birds of prey unaccustomed to restraint. Given by the intramuscular and intraperitoneal routes, the drug is of limited value because large volumes are required to induce analgesia (Cooper and Frank 1973).

Contraindications and Drug Interactions

Use of althesin in the dog is contraindicated because the nonionic surface active agent (i.e., Cremophor EL or polyoxyethylated castor oil) in the preparation causes the release of histamine (Stock 1973). This results in cardiovascular collapse in this species. Apart from the barbiturates, any preoperative and postoperative medicant and inhalational agent can be used in conjunction with althesin (Stock 1973). Anesthetic adjuvants, including pressor agents, adrenergic blocking agents, and analeptics have been used without adverse effects (Stock 1973). Skeletal muscle–paralyzing drugs have also been used in the cat during althesin analgesia and anesthesia. Only a slight reduction in the activity of succinylcholine chloride is noted during a prolonged infusion of althesin. No effect on the activity of other neuromuscular blocking agents has been observed.

DISSOCIATIVE ANESTHETICS

There are three drugs in this category that have current interest in veterinary medicine. They are phencyclidine hydrochloride (CI-395) and its congeners, ketamine hydrochloride (CI-581) and tiletamine (CI-634). A cataleptic-type state referred to as "dissociative anesthesia" is typical of phencyclidine and its derivatives and is accompanied by marked analgesia in most species (Thurmon et al. 1972). The term *dissociative anesthetic* originated from the use of ketamine in human medicine. Use of ketamine in human beings causes what has been described as dissociative anesthesia because, during induction, the patient feels dissociated from or unaware of his environment (Price 1975). The mechanism of action of these anesthetics has not been elucidated.

Thurmon et al. reported that in some animals analgesia is not profound, and supplemental anesthesia may be necessary if surgical procedures are conducted. Phencyclidine hydrochloride is approved for use by the FDA in laboratory animals, and ketamine hydrochloride is approved for use in the cat and subhuman primates. Tiletamine remains unapproved by the FDA for use in animals.

Phencyclidine Hydrochloride

Chemically, *Phencyclidine Hydrochloride* (Sernylan, Sernyl, GP-121, CI-395) is 1-(1-phenylcyclohexyl) piperidine hydrochloride (Fig. 13.11). It is a white, glistening solid with a high degree of solubility in water. Phencyclidine is a Schedule III drug subject to the Controlled Substances Act of 1970.

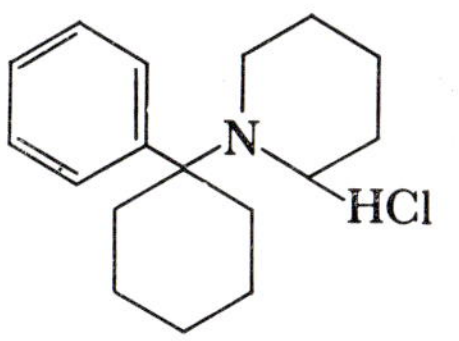

N
HCl

Phencyclidine Hydrochloride

Fig. 13.11.

Pharmacological Considerations

Phencyclidine differs greatly from general anesthetics in that the absence of responses to nociceptive stimuli is not accompanied with the loss of corneal, pupillary, and other reflexes. In most, if not all species, phencyclidine in high dosages produces a generalized increase in skeletal muscular tone and catalepsy. The neurophysiologic responses of animals to phencyclidine and related derivatives have not been completely elucidated or, for that matter, very well understood. The experimental procedures for the evaluation of the effects of drugs upon the CNS are far from a precise science.

The primary pharmacologic effect of phencyclidine is depression or stimulation of the CNS or a combination of these effects (Chen et al. 1959; Stoliker 1965). According to Stoliker, the quality of the effect produced by phencyclidine is highly species specific. In the domestic chicken *(Gallus domesticus)* phencyclidine hydrochloride does not induce sedation or anesthesia when administered in high dosages by the intravenous or intramuscular route (Wright and Jordan 1963). In mice the principal initial effect is excitation and not depression (Chen et al. 1959). However, in the dog and other species depression is produced by phencyclidine at low dosages; excitation leading to convulsive seizures may occur following large doses (Stoliker 1965).

In carefully controlled studies, the intramuscular administration of 2 mg/kg of phencyclidine hydrochloride was evaluated upon the heart rate, arterial pressure, and other physiological parameters in the rhesus monkey (Popovic et al. 1972). A significant decrease in the heart rate occurred about 3 minutes after the intramuscular injection and lasted 2 hours. Also, a corresponding decrease in the systolic and diastolic arterial pressures, along with a drop in central venous pressure, was measured. These changes were only significant for the initial 90 minutes of the study. ECG irregularities, along with prominent changes in the QRS amplitude, were also recorded.

Popovic et al. (1972) noted a decrease in pH during the initial 3 hours and an increase in Pa_{CO_2} without a significant change in the respiratory rate following the administration of phencyclidine. In addition, significant decreases in Pa_{CO_2} were noted during the first 45 minutes, whereas a decrease in hemoglobin concentration and oxygen content of the blood prevailed for the duration of the experiment; significant changes in oxyhemoglobin saturation were not seen.

The EEG of the phencyclidine-treated monkeys was affected within 3 minutes following the injection. Decreases in the amplitude of alpha rhythm and, occasionally, delta waves appeared to be reestablished (Popovic et al. 1972).

Three hours later, upon repeated administration of phencyclidine up to one-half the dose (i.e., 1 mg/kg) by the intravenous route, the drug produced an immediate but temporary decline in arterial pressure, change in the ECG, and catalepsy (Popovic et al. 1972).

In contrast to this effect and after the drug was repeated intramuscularly at one-half the recommended dose 2–3 hours after the original injection (i.e., 2 mg/kg), a marked long-lasting elevation in arterial pressure without a noticeable change in the central venous pressure was recorded. Additional intramuscular injections appeared to produce similar effects. No explanation was offered by Popovic and coworkers regarding these different, but interesting, effects of phencyclidine upon the cardiovascular system of the rhesus monkey.

A number of authors in the current literature have referred to the effect of phencyclidine and other central-acting drugs upon the behavioral qualities of the offspring following the use of these agents in pregnant animals. It is suggested by Tonge (1973) that the developing brain of neonates may be particularly susceptible to phencyclidine.

CLINICAL USE

In Subhuman Primates. The greatest benefit of phencyclidine has been its use in the primates. Bywater and Rutty (1964) believe that phencyclidine has a definite place in simian medicine, but rather for its tranquilizing properties than for its usefulness as an anesthetic. Also, Soma (1971) stated that the use of phencyclidine as a total anesthetic should be questioned because of the tremors and inferior relaxation of the skeletal musculature.

Stoliker (1965) has described the use of phencyclidine in a number of different subhuman primates as well as in many other exotic species. In the monkey, phencyclidine can be administered intramuscularly into either the forelimbs or rear limbs while the animal is in the cage; this permits easy removal of the animal from the cage in 5–10 minutes without danger to the handler (Spalding and Heymann 1962). By using an intramuscular dose of 3 mg/kg, Spalding and Heymann reported a satisfactory level of anesthesia for about 1 hour and almost full recovery within 4–5 hours. Also, 3 mg/kg of phencyclidine administered intramuscularly for smaller species and 0.25 mg/kg for larger species are recommended in the immobilization or restraint of infrahuman primates (Domino et al. 1969). For induction of analgesia to surgical anesthesia, dosages of 0.5–1.5 mg/kg have been recommended intramuscularly in the *Macaca mulatta* (Melby and Baker 1965).

Clifford (1971) reported that calming and sedation occur in the monkey following 0.3–0.5 mg/kg and a "cataleptoidlike" state and immobilization occur with higher doses of phencyclidine. An intramuscular dose level of phencyclidine hydrochloride as low as 0.25 mg/kg has been recommended for producing calmness in the *Macaca mulatta;* the average time for recovery is 30 minutes (Melby and Baker 1965). According to Joffe (1964), an intravenous dose of 0.5 mg/kg will restrain a chimpanzee without obscuring the physiological effects of an experimental drug upon the cardiopulmonary systems. Phencyclidine has been used in juvenile and adolescent rhesus monkeys in a dose of 1.5 mg/kg intramuscularly; 4–10 minutes after the administration of phencyclidine, pentobarbital sodium (5 mg/kg) was administered intravenously (Kuroda and McNamara 1972). In the baboon an average dose level of 1.2 mg/lb was administered intramuscularly for immobilization of the animals (Vondruska 1965). Also, phencyclidine hydrochloride (1 mg/kg) was given intramuscularly as a preanesthetic with atropine (0.05 mg/kg and produced recumbency in the baboon within 10 minutes (Rawlings and Dean 1971). Anesthesia was then maintained with nitrous oxide, halothane, and oxygen. For the collection of liver and spleen biopsy samples in marmoset monkeys (*Saguinus oedipus* and *Callithrix jacchus*), Voss (1970) used 1 mg/kg of phencyclidine via the intramuscular route. In the owl monkey *(Aotus trivirgatus),* phencyclidine is not recommended because of the prolonged time that is required before recovery (Bone 1970).

In Other Exotic Species. Phencyclidine was used to capture and transport animals in East Africa in the late 1950s. Dr. A. M. Harthoorn was one of the first veterinarians to use phencyclidine and other agents for this purpose. Phencyclidine has also been used in combination with diazepam, chlorpromazine, and thiopental sodium in the African lion for restraint and anesthetic purposes (Harthoorn et al. 1971).

A drug mixture containing phencyclidine (23 mg), thiambutene (330 mg), and hyoscine (11 mg) in each cc has been used for the capture and immobilization of hippopotami and topi (Buck et al. 1963). The use of phencyclidine has been advocated in wild *Felidae* (leopard and tiger) at a dose level of 1–1.8 mg/kg of body weight by the intramuscular route of administration (Bennett and Tillotson 1969). According to Soma (1971), the simultaneous administration of a neuroleptic agent is desirable to reduce the muscular tremors and oculogyric movements. In addition, atropine sulfate should always be administered to prevent salivation. In fact, a neuroleptic agent (i.e., 10 mg of acetylpromazine maleate), atropine sulfate (1/50 grain), and phencyclidine hydrochloride (50 mg) have been successfully used intramuscularly for performing a laparotomy in a black panther weighing 90 lb (Miller and Peddie 1970).

In the domestic cat, phencyclidine produces surgical anesthesia; however, the recovery period may last more than a day in some animals (Chen and Ensor 1968). Phencyclidine has also been used intramuscularly in the American alligator for immobilization at a dose level of 5–10 mg/lb of body weight. Duration of its effects is 6–7 hours (Walach 1969).

Ketamine Hydrochloride

Ketamine Hydrochloride (Ketalar, Ketaset, Vetalar, CI-581) is a congener of phencyclidine and is chemically designated as 2-(o-chlorophenyl)-2-(methylamino) cyclohexanone hydrochloride (Fig. 13.12).

The adverse effects produced by phencyclidine such as oculogyric activity, tremors, tonic spasticity, and convulsive seizures are ordinarily less pronounced with ketamine. Although ketamine has been approved for use only in the cat and

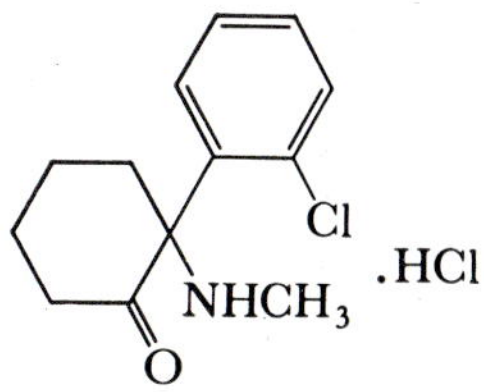

Cl
$NHCH_3$ .HCl
O

Ketamine Hydrochloride

Fig. 13.12.

subhuman primates, it has been used in sheep, swine, and laboratory animals. Ketamine and other phencyclidine derivatives have not been approved for use in animals intended for human consumption.

PHARMACOLOGICAL CONSIDERATIONS

In human beings, ketamine has been used primarily in children for the rapid induction of analgesia. According to Virtue et al. (1967), there is presently no more rapid method for induction of analgesia than the intravenous administration of ketamine hydrochloride. Compared to most anesthetic agents in use, ketamine produces an increase in cardiac output and arterial blood pressure with little alteration in the peripheral resistance (Virtue et al. 1967). The increase in cardiac output is due almost entirely to an accelerated cardiac rate because the stroke volume remains unchanged.

Because of the hallucinogenic effect that ketamine produces in the adult, its use is considered more satisfactory in children. If the drug is used in human adults, droperidol is administered to prevent hallucinations and postanesthetic disturbances (Szappanyos et al. 1971); also, in adults, ketamine is contraindicated in visceral surgery unless it is used in combination with conventional anesthetics. However, one clinical report referred to the use of ketamine alone administered intravenously for cesarean section procedures; the authors (Meer et al. 1973) indicated that the drug apeared to be well tolerated by the mother and infant.

Clinical case reports in human beings have suggested that an interaction occurs between the thyroid hormones and ketamine. Two cases of human patients on thyroid replacement therapy were reported to have developed a severe hypertension and tachycardia following ketamine administration (Kaplan and Cooperman 1971). If such an adverse action occurs, Kaplan and Cooperman suggest that β-adrenergic blocking agents may be of value. Other interactions reported in human beings following ketamine administration have involved the potentiation of respiratory depression and/or paralysis following the use of succinylcholine and propanidid (Bovill et al. 1971).

Similar interactions between *d*-tubocurarine have been observed using the cat sciatic nerve–gastrocnemius muscle preparation (Cronnelly 1972; Cronnelly et al. 1973). Also, the potentiation of skeletal muscle twitch of the cat by edrophonium chloride (Tensilon chloride) was antagonized by ketamine in doses of 1 and 2 mg/kg of body weight administered by the intravenous route (Cronnelly 1972). However, the administration of ketamine alone produced no significant effect upon the muscle twitch (Cronnelly et al. 1973). The authors pointed out that this is to be expected since ketamine produces only a 30% reduction of end-plate sensitivity.

In the dog experimental studies have been conducted with intravenous dose levels of ketamine (5 mg/kg) for the induction of anesthesia, with recovery occurring after 2 hours (Traber et al. 1970a). In this study the vasopressor response to ketamine was completely blocked by hexamethonium and there was no longer either a positive chronotropic response or an increase in the cardiac output. This confirms previous work by Traber and his associates showing that ketamine is devoid of direct sympathomimetic effects and that the drug does not have an action on the sympathetic nerve endings and the adrenal medulla to initiate release of the adrenergic neurotransmitting humors. In addition, Traber and co-workers (1970b) have shown that atropine completely blocks the positive chronotropic effects of ketamine and decreases by about 50% the elevated cardiac output and blood pressure produced by ketamine. It was suggested that ketamine must produce at least a portion of its cardiovascular effect by vagal blockade or by stimulation of the so-called muscarinic sites of the stellate ganglia. The fact that the positive chronotropic effects of ketamine cannot account for all its cardiostimulatory effects means that the drug must have other unexplained effects because ketamine still produces some increase in cardiac output and arterial pressure in the dog after vagal blockade (Traber et al. 1970b). It was suggested that the stimulatory effect could be brought about by augmentation of activity in sympathetic fibers to capacitance vessels (e.g., the cranial and caudal venae cavae), which would produce an increased venous return and cardiac output, or by enhancement of the discharge of sympathetic activity to the heart. Later studies by Traber et al. (1971) in the dog revealed that the pressor response to ketamine is produced by augmentation of neural α-adrenergic activity and blockade of the vagus nerve. Moreover, the elevation in arterial pressure induced by ketamine is secondary to the acceleration in cardiac rate and cardiac output.

Ketamine hydrochloride, 2 mg/kg administered intravenously, increases the cerebral blood flow in the dog 80% and the cerebral oxygen consumption 16%; also, EEG changes accompany those of increased cerebral oxygen consumption in that the wave frequency increases after the injection of the drug (Dawson et al. 1971). Dawson and associates concluded that ketamine is a cerebral metabolic stimulant and a cerebral vasodilator. They were able to block these pharmacologic effects by the prior administration of thiopental.

In the cat body temperature declined by an average of 2.9° F following clinical dose levels of ketamine (Beck et al. 1971). Also, ketamine did not abolish the pedal and pinnal reflexes; in addition, the photic and corneal reflexes persisted in the cat as well as the laryngeal and pharyngeal reflexes.

Ketamine is currently recommended for use in the domestic cat but not in the canine species because of its excessive stimulatory effect upon the CNS. The current knowledge of the pharmacologic activity of ketamine raises uncertainty as to what surgical procedures may be carried out in an animal in which this drug is the only agent employed (Rex 1972). It has also been pointed out by Rex (1972) that in human anesthesiology the consensus is that it is unreasonable to use ketamine as the only anesthetic for surgical procedures even of a minor nature. Although ketamine has been used as a sole anesthetic agent for major surgery in the cat, it is not considered to be a prudent or recommended practice (Evans et al. 1972). Until more information is acquired, other intravenous or inhalation anesthetics should be used in conjunction with ketamine. According to Kayama and Iwama (1972), EEG recordings in the cat indicated that ketamine has a concurrent stimulatory effect upon the neocortex, hippocampus, and other subcortical nuclei with the eventual development of seizure activity. This activity seems to challenge the concept of ketamine as a dissociative anesthetic.

When ketamine, 3–5 mg/kg, is used intravenously and as the only agent in cats, their eyes remain completely open, with a fixed stare, and the pupils are dilated (Kayama and Iwama 1972). Other clinical signs produced are licking of their lips and profuse salivation. Also, slow movements of the head are observed; rigidity or extension of the forelimbs is also seen and opisthotonus occurs after an intravenous dose of 8–10 mg/kg of body weight. Convulsive seizures have been reported in 5.3% (Beck et al. 1971) and in 20% of the cats that received clinical dose levels of ketamine (Stock 1973). According to Beck et al., dose levels of ketamine less than 10 mg/lb of body weight administered intramuscularly produce basic chemical restraint without total analgesia but are satisfactory for physical examination and minor procedures. Dosages of 10–20 mg/lb (22–44 mg/kg) administered intramuscularly produce cataleptoid anesthesia, a comatose state that is similar to decerebrate rigidity (Beck et al. 1971). It is reported that this effect is adequate for performing short, simple diagnostic procedures and short surgical procedures and that the duration of surgical cataleptoid anesthesia ranges from 20 to 40 minutes. Although recovery from ketamine is frequently prolonged and may be accompanied by excitement, the cat is ordinarily able to attain the sitting position after 2 hours (Massey 1973).

The mechanism of ketamine-induced

catalepsy has not been extensively investigated and, consequently, is not clearly understood. With the plethora of literature on catalepsy and other mobility disorders, there is indication that most of these may be due to a deficiency of dopamine function or to an imbalance in cholinergic-dopaminergic function. Moreover, other neurotransmitting chemicals cannot be ignored from consideration in catalepsy. For example, serotonin is also associated with the extrapyramidal system and can induce catalepsy when it is administered intracerebroventricularly in the cat.

When an antiserotonin neuroleptic agent (i.e., methiothepin maleate) is administered in the cat prior to ketamine, it is interesting that the ketamine-induced catalepsy is not observed (Hatch 1973a). Instead of muscle tonus and the presence of limb rigidity, which typifies the action of ketamine in the cat, muscle flaccidity is observed. Another agent that is an antidopamine neuroleptic (i.e., pimozide) was also employed by Hatch (1973a). The only effect of pimozide on ketamine was that it prevented the sporadic stimulus-induced paw twitch often seen in the cat. The blocking effect of methiothepin upon serotonin suggests that serotonergic mechanisms are involved in ketamine-induced catalepsy whereas the blocking effect of pimozide suggests that dopamine is involved in the ketamine-induced sporadic movements of muscles and limbs.

The pharmacologic effects of ketamine can be antagonized or shortened almost immediately by the administration of a mixture of l-amphetamine and yohimbine (Hatch and Ruch 1974). Yohimbine is believed to enhance the release of serotonin or to directly stimulate central serotonin receptors. The ability of yohimbine to shorten the effects of ketamine is consistent with the finding that serotonin may mediate acute tolerance to the effect of ketamine in the cat (Hatch 1973a).

CONTRAINDICATIONS AND PRECAUTIONS

Ketamine must not be used in animals intended for human consumption. The use of this drug as the sole agent for abdominal and orthopedic surgery cannot be recommended; use of ketamine in major surgical procedures must be supplemented with general anesthesia. Ketamine is contraindicated in animals afflicted with hepatic or renal dysfunction. Precautions should be taken to control hemorrhage after surgery because arterial hypertension from the use of ketamine occurs; this precaution is especially important following the declawing of mature cats, particularly if the paws are not bandaged (Evans et al. 1972).

CLINICAL USE

In the Cat. Prior to the administration of ketamine, atropine sulfate should be administered subcutaneously or intramuscularly at a dose level of 0.02 mg/lb of body weight to prevent salivation and other autonomic nervous system effects. Also, it is recommended that a bland ophthalmic ointment be used soon after the peak effect of ketamine to prevent drying and irritation of the cornea.

It is felt that ketamine is most valuable as an immobilizing agent for examinations, radiographic procedures, and prior to the induction of general anesthesia with conventional agents (Glen 1973). The recommended intramuscular dosage range is from 5 to 15 mg/lb of body weight; however, some clinicians use an intramuscular dose as high as 20 mg/lb of body weight; 3–5 minutes are required for the animal to become anesthetized (DeYoung et al. 1972). Pain is elicited during the intramuscular injection of ketamine hydrochloride at the dose level of 5–20 mg/lb (Evans et al. 1972).

After the routine administration of atropine sulfate (0.02 mg/lb), intramuscular dosages of ketamine hydrochloride are used as follows (DeYoung et al. 1972):

Dose Level (mg/lb)	*Indicated Clinical Procedures*
15	Major surgery such as ovariohysterectomy, cesarean section, abdominal laparotomy, and orthopedic repair in healthy cats; all

these procedures must be supplemented with inhalant anesthesia.

10 Minor surgery such as castrations and onychectomy and restraint of wild cats.

5 Minor restraint; used in sick cats to aid in the induction of anesthesia that will be maintained under inhalant anesthesia.

The duration of the effects of ketamine following an intramuscular injection of 5–20 mg/lb of body weight may last 20–45 minutes (DeYoung et al. 1972) and can vary from 15 to 60 minutes (Evans et al. 1972). Recovery may not be complete for 10 hours after the administration of ketamine; however, most animals are able to stand within 2 hours (Evans et al. 1972).

The use of ketamine as the sole agent for abdominal surgery in the cat cannot be recommended (Evans et al. 1972). Endotracheal intubation can be achieved during the effects of ketamine followed by inhalant anesthetics such as halothane and methoxyflurane in conjunction with nitrous oxide and oxygen. Also, the ultrashort-acting barbiturates (thiamylal or thiopental) can be used in small dosages (2–4 mg/lb) intravenously to supplement the effect of ketamine.

When ketamine is used without the intervention of other pharmacologic agents, undesirable side effects occur in a large number of animals (Reid and Frank 1972). By using a combination of oxymorphone (Numorphan) at a dose level of 0.075 mg/lb and triflupromazine (0.5 mg/lb) prior to the administration of ketamine, the side effects of ketamine can be effectively blocked. The dosage of ketamine is reduced by 2.5% to 10% of the recommended intramuscular dose and is not given until after the peak effect of oxymorphone and triflupromazine has been reached. Both oxymorphone and triflupromazine may be administered subcutaneously, intramuscularly, or intravenously. Once the peak effect of these agents is attained, ketamine hydrochloride is administered intravenously at a dosage of 0.5–1 mg/lb of body weight (Reid and Frank 1972).

Xylazine (Rompun) has been used prior to ketamine in the cat to prevent muscular hypertonicity (Amend et al. 1972). A dose level of 0.25–0.5 mg/lb of xylazine administered intramuscularly effectively sedates the cat and renders it relatively insensitive to the subsequent injection of ketamine. Twenty minutes after the administration of xylazine, 5–10 mg/lb of ketamine hydrochloride are given intramuscularly. Premedication with xylazine prolongs the duration of analgesia, reduces the dosage of ketamine required, and shortens the recovery time. In addition, disturbances of recovery often noted when ketamine was used alone are eliminated with the combined use of xylazine (Amend et al. 1972).

Another clinical approach in the reduction of ketamine side effects involves the intramuscular injection of acetylpromazine maleate (1 mg/20 lb) and atropine sulfate (0.02–0.03 mg/lb) about 15–20 minutes prior to the intramuscular administration of 10 mg/lb of ketamine hydrochloride (Rosin 1974). This procedure reduces the dosage of ketamine about 50%.

When ketamine is used in conjunction with meperidine or morphine in the cat, the effects of ketamine are neither improved nor complicated by these agents (Hatch 1973b). Both meperidine and morphine do not appear to have any value as sedative or anticataleptic agents given prior to the administration of ketamine.

In Subhuman Primates. Ketamine hydrochloride is recommended for restraint and minor surgical procedures in a number of subhuman primates (Beck and Dresner 1972). The usual therapeutic dose level of ketamine recommended for primates is 3–15 mg/kg administered intramuscularly. However, an intramuscular dose level as high as 20 mg/kg has been used in patas monkeys (Britton et al. 1974). This dosage produced safe and adequate sedation for 30 minutes with minimal respiratory depression. The successful use of ketamine in the infant pigtail monkey *(Macaca* *nemestrina)* has been reported (Bowden et al. 1974). It was used at a dose level of 18 mg/kg intramuscularly prior to the administration of an intravenous injection of thiamylal sodium (15 mg/kg). According to Bowden et al. (1974), the intramuscular administration of ketamine prior to thiamylal had three advantages: it simplified the venepuncture procedure for the administration of thiamylal; it reduced the amount of thiamylal required for induction of anesthesia; and it shortened the recovery time. For example, the recovery time until the infant monkeys were alert enough to ingest fluids decreased from a mean of 9.4 hours when thiamylal alone was administered to 4.8 hours when the combination with ketamine was used.

In the Dog. Ketamine has not been approved by the FDA for use in the dog. However, there are some practitioners who feel that ketamine can be used as safely and as effectively in dogs as in cats.

In the previous discussion of the pharmacologic action of ketamine in the cat it was pointed out that serotonin may function in the mediation of catalepsy and that dopamine may mediate ketamine-induced muscle jerking (Hatch 1973a). Studies in the dog indicate that brain mechanisms involved with the various effects of ketamine could be quite different and more complex than those suggested in the cat (Hatch 1974). It appears that dopaminergic and nicotinic chlolinoceptive receptors could be involved in mediation of ketamine "anesthesia" in the dog. This is particularly suggested because ketamine was antagonized by a subsequent dose of the antidopaminergic neuroleptic pimozide and was partly antagonized by the nicotinic cholinoceptor blocking agent mecamylamine (Hatch 1974). Also, ketamine-induced muscle jerking and emergent delirium are both enhanced by a subsedative dose of pimozide, by atropine, and by small dosages of chlorpromazine. It is known that chlorpromazine possesses both antidopaminergic and anticholinergic actions. All these drug effects suggest that dopaminergic and muscarinic cholinoceptive receptors could both have a role in modulating the myoclonic and deliriant effects of ketamine in the dog (Hatch 1974).

In Sheep and Swine. Although ketamine has not been approved for food-producing animals, it can be used in animals such as sheep and swine that are maintained for experimental purposes.

In the use of ketamine in sheep, doses of 22–44 mg/kg of body weight administered intravenously or intramuscularly were adequate for short surgical and diagnostic procedures (Thurmon et al. 1973). Preanesthetic treatment with atropine sulfate (0.2 mg/kg) via the intramuscular route of administration was carried out 20–25 minutes before the administration of ketamine. Also, acetylpromazine maleate (0.55 mg/kg) was given intravenously 15 minutes following the administration of atropine and then ketamine was administered 10 minutes later.

According to Thurmon et al. (1973), the administration of atropine reduced the volume of saliva secreted in sheep. Acetylpromazine reduced the dosage of ketamine required for a given period of analgesia, increased skeletal muscle relaxation, and prevented reflex movement of the limbs. Conversely, the recovery period in sheep was longer with the use of acetylpromazine than with the use of ketamine alone.

In swine, ketamine hydrochloride has been used intramuscularly at a dose of 9.2 $\pm$ 0.42 mg/lb of body weight for surgical procedures lasting 10–20 minutes (Thurmon et al. 1972). In surgical procedures lasting longer than this, ketamine was supplemented with local infiltration of the surgical site with 2% lidocaine, or thiopental sodium was administered intravenously at a dosage level of 3–5 mg/lb of body weight.

In Avian and Exotic Species. In pigeons, ketamine alone did not produce a state of anesthesia even when used in dose levels of 400 mg/kg (Bree and Gross 1969). Anesthesia was, however, achieved by using pentobarbital sodium (20 mg/kg), followed 10 minutes later with 16, 32, and

64 mg/kg of ketamine hydrochloride. Both drugs were administered into the pectoral muscles. Induction of anesthesia occurred smoothly and varied from 5 to 30 minutes after the administration of ketamine. The mean duration of anesthesia following pentobarbital and ketamine (i.e., after 16, 32, and 64 mg/kg) was 20, 40, and 109 minutes, respectively. Anesthesia was maintained for as long as 15 hours in some birds by the successive administration of ketamine in dosages of 32 mg/kg at 1- to 3-hour intervals. Recovery from anesthesia was uneventful (Bree and Gross 1969).

In the parakeet, ketamine hydrochloride is considered to be a safe anesthetic (Mandelker 1973). A dosage rate of 0.05 mg/g–0.1 mg/g of body weight administered intramuscularly appears adequate. The lethal dosage of ketamine for the parakeet is approximately 0.5 mg/g of body weight (Mandelker 1973).

Ketamine has also been used in wildfowl for immobilization purposes (Kittle 1971; Borzio 1973). The recommended initial intramuscular dose of ketamine hydrochloride for most wildfowl is 15–20 mg/kg of body weight supplemented with increments of 10 mg/kg (Borzio 1973). Immobilization is produced in 1–5 minutes to 6 hours, depending upon the total dose administered.

For dosages of ketamine hydrochloride recommended in the exotic species, see Table 13.7.

TABLE 13.7. Intramuscular dosages of ketamine hydrochloride recommended for some of the exotic species

Species	Dose	Reference
	(mg/kg)	
Lion cub	4*	Cannon and Higgins 1972
Kangaroo	15–19	Denny 1973
Tiger	11–13†	Johnston 1974
Pinnipeds	4.5–11	Geraci 1973
Snakes	55–88‡	Glenn et al. 1972

* Administered in conjunction with acetylpromazine maleate (0.25 mg/kg).

† Used in combination with acetylpromazine maleate (0.22 mg/kg) and atropine sulfate in the same projectile syringe.

‡ Effects last 1–3 days.

Tiletamine Hydrochloride

Fig. 13.13.

Tiletamine Hydrochloride

Tiletamine Hydrochloride (CI-634) is also a congener of phencyclidine. The adverse effects that are characteristic of phencyclidine are considered to be less pronounced following the administration of tiletamine. In most respects the pharmacologic effect elicited by tiletamine is quite similar to that produced by ketamine.

Chemically, tiletamine hydrochloride is designated as 2-(ethylamino)-2-(2-thienyl) cyclohexanone hydrochloride (Fig. 13.13).

Currently, tiletamine is unapproved for use in animals by the FDA.

PHARMACOLOGIC ACTIVITY

Pharmacologic studies have been conducted with tiletamine in the mouse, rat, pigeon, guinea pig, rabbit, dog, cat, and monkey by Chen et al. (1967). A species variation was observed by these authors in the CNS effects of tiletamine; in mice and rats, excitation was observed but was not so marked in other species. Moreover, with large doses of the drug, analgesia and general anesthesia were produced in mice, rats, pigeons, cats, and monkeys. In the guinea pig and rabbit, only depression was produced by tiletamine; anesthesia was not induced in these two species (Chen et al. 1967). Upon approach of the lethal level of tiletamine, brief and mild clonic seizures were seen in some cats and monkeys. It was concluded by Chen and associates that tiletamine, like phencyclidine, was more effective in the induction of general anesthesia in primates and in the cat than in other species.

In the unanesthetized dog, an intravenous injection of 2 mg/kg of tiletamine resulted in an increase of the arterial pressure and heart rate that lasted about

30 minutes (Chen et al. 1967). A similar dose level of tiletamine in dogs anesthetized with pentobarbital also produced arterial hypertension; at higher dose levels (4–8 mg/kg) hypotension occurred. Further studies by Chen and co-workers revealed that premedication with tiletamine did not potentiate the hypertensive response to norepinephrine. Also, no anticholinergic effects were noted when tiletamine was compared with the arterial hypotensive effects produced by acetylcholine and histamine, respectively.

In the cat, after a surgical plane of anesthesia is attained, the eyelids remain open and the pupils are slightly dilated (Bennett 1969). Since the eyelids remain open as they do following the administration of ketamine, it is advisable to use a bland ophthalmic ointment to prevent undue drying and irritation of the cornea. Bennett (1969) also observed involuntary rotation of the eyeball following tiletamine anesthesia; other effects observed were retention of the pinnal, corneal, and palpebral reflexes. In addition, 10% of the anesthetized cats salivated. Atropine sulfate (0.02 mg/lb) is also recommended as a premedicant to tiletamine administration for the prevention of salivation and possibly other undesirable autonomic effects as described above for ketamine administration.

Although it has been reported (Bennett 1969) that tiletamine has moderate to no perceptible effect upon the respiratory activity in the cat, Calderwood et al. (1971) are not in agreement with these findings. According to these authors, an irregular respiratory rate frequently tending toward an inspiratory breath-holding pattern (i.e., apneustic-type pattern) is seen, and conversion to a normal respiratory pattern may be attained by the intravenous administration of a neuroleptic (a phenothiazine type, such as promazine, or a benzodiazepine type such as diazepam).

Tiletamine has an anesthetic induction time similar to ketamine, ranging between 2 and 3 minutes following intramuscular injection (Soma 1971). The duration of the peak effect of tiletamine is about 60 minutes or about 3 times longer than ketamine.

The effect of tiletamine upon the cardiovascular system of the cat has been described by Soma (1971). A decrease in the heart rate and systemic arterial pressure occurs following an intramuscular injection that declines to a maximum level within 20–30 minutes, with a gradual return toward normal thereafter. Following an intravenous injection, an elevated arterial pressure and heart rate are observed; also, arrhythmias are frequent following the intravenous route of administration of tiletamine. According to Soma (1971), the arrhythmias include coupled premature ventricular beats that appear as a bigeminal and trigeminal rhythm. Also, there are fused ventricular beats with an increase in the amplitude of the P wave.

When dose levels of 10 mg/kg of body weight and up were administered intramuscularly in the cat, evidence of increased CNS activity was reported (Garmer 1969). This included clonic muscle spasms, particularly in the face and limbs. The duration of these effects varied, dependent on the dose level used, between 0.5 and 1 hour. Garmer (1969) observed in a cat given 30 mg/kg of tiletamine that the muscle spasms progressed into a convulsive state requiring the use of thiopental sodium for control of the seizure. Despite these neurological disturbances, no adverse effects were seen upon recovery of the cats. Tiletamine elicits a severe metabolic acidosis in cats manifesting clonic muscular spasms (Garmer 1969). A marked drop in the body temperature from 38.5° to 36° C was observed in an animal following the intramuscular administration of 30 mg/kg of body weight.

Garmer (1969) stated that it is unlikely that tiletamine will be a satisfactory anesthetic agent in the cat, but in small dose levels the drug may be of value as an induction and sedative agent prior to general anesthesia. Bennett (1969) also reported that tiletamine could be used to induce anesthesia in the cat. Inasmuch as skeletal muscle relaxation may not be sufficient for abdominal and orthopedic surgical procedures, Bennett pointed out that methoxyflurane can be used to obtain adequate muscle relaxation.

A safe anesthetic dose range for tiletamine in the cat appears to be 15–100 mg/kg of body weight; general anesthesia occurs within 3 minutes after intramuscular injection (Chen and Ensor 1968; Bennett 1969). Bennett (1969) reported that surgical anesthesia lasted between 55 and 140 minutes and that recovery (i.e., the ability to stand) required between 160 and 210 minutes following the injection of tiletamine. Some ataxia is observed even following the recovery period.

According to Chen and Ensor (1968), the minimal anesthetic dose of tiletamine that produces anesthesia lasting 1–1.5 hours occurs from an intramuscular injection of 10–15 mg/kg of body weight; in some animals 20 mg/kg are necessary to induce anesthesia for 1.5–2.75 hours. Ensor and Chen also reported that there are no marked differences in the duration of anesthesia in cats given 20–40 mg/kg. When they administered 100 mg/kg of body weight, more than 7 hours of anesthesia were produced.

Chen and Ensor (1968) reported that the onset of tiletamine anesthesia after an intramuscular injection is 1–3 minutes. They first observed the appearance of akinesia, which was followed by motor paralysis of the rear limbs and then of the forelimbs. Upon recovery these effects disappeared in a reverse order and the time of recovery varied from 1 to 5 hours in cats given dose levels of 10–40 mg/kg of tiletamine. Chen and Ensor also reported that tiletamine anesthesia produced no emetic effect in the cat.

Tiletamine has also been used in other species. In the rabbit the drug has been used in conjunction with chloral hydrate anesthesia (Chen 1968). Chen used 20 mg/kg of tiletamine intramuscularly, followed by 250 mg/kg of chloral hydrate injected via the intravenous route. This dose of chloral hydrate was found to be the minimum necessary to produce surgical anesthesia regardless of the dose of tiletamine. According to Chen, tiletamine enhances the depth and the duration of chloral hydrate anesthesia. However, anesthesia induced by tiletamine (20 mg/kg) given intramuscularly and thiamylal sodium (12.5–30 mg/kg) given intravenously was reported to be similar to that induced by thiamylal alone. Bree (1972) has evaluated the use of tiletamine in six subhuman primate species. After an intramuscular injection of tiletamine (3–6 mg/kg), induction of anesthesia occurred smoothly and without excitement in 1–3 minutes. According to Bree, the mean anesthesia time is 83 minutes at the higher dose level for one species (i.e., *Macaca nemestrina*).

Tiletamine hydrochloride in combination with zolasepam (diazepinone tranquilizer) is presently in the investigative phase. The two drugs are combined in a 1:1 ratio and are designated by the symbol CI-774. The drug preparation has been evaluated following parenteral administration in a number of laboratory species (Ward et al. 1974). Except for the pigeon, the drug appears to have a wide safety margin. Dosages of 13 mg/kg in sheep, 6–13 mg/kg in cats and dogs, and 20–30 mg/kg in rats produce satisfactory anesthesia for surgical procedures lasting 30–60 minutes. In the guinea pig and rabbit, the lack of muscle relaxation and their response to external stimuli make CI-744 alone unsatisfactory (Ward et al. 1974).

CI-744 has also been used in the chinchilla (Schulz and Fowler 1974). Surgical anesthesia is produced by intramuscular dose levels of 22–110 mg/kg of body weight. However, some deaths occurred at dosages of 66 mg/kg and above.

MISCELLANEOUS AGENTS

Chloralose (Alpha Chloralose, Monochloral *d*-Glucose)

The family of compounds called chloraloses are prepared by condensing anhydrous glucose with chloraldehyde (chloral) in the presence of sulfuric acid. A mixture, 3 dichloralglucoses and 2 monoglucochloraloses (i.e., α-chloralose and β-chloralose), is formed. α-Chloralose has been used in the experimental laboratory more frequently than any of the other chloralose preparations. It is usually administered intravenously in a concentration of 1%. However, concentrations of 10% have been prepared by using an inert dispersing agent such as polyethylene glycol (Bass and Buckley 1966).

Chloralose is difficult to dissolve in an aqueous medium without simultaneous heating. Because of deterioration, chloralose solutions should not be boiled. After solution is accomplished, the preparation is allowed to cool to the approximate body temperature of the animal before it is injected intravenously.

Chloralose is metabolized to chloraldehyde or chloral. Chloraldehyde is mainly transformed into trichloroethanol. The hypnosis and anesthesia produced by chloral hydrate and chloralose are quite similar because of the formation of trichloroethanol.

Chloralose has a pharmacologic action more like morphine than like chloraldehyde. It possesses hypnotic characteristics by depressing the mental component of CNS activity while increasing reflex activity. Spinal reflex activity may increase to the degree that convulsions similar to those of strychnine develop in the dog and cat (Lees 1972). As an anesthetic agent, chloralose is restricted in use to laboratory animals in which recovery from anesthesia is not necessary. It is used primarily in physiological experimentation because it does not interfere with respiratory and cardioreflexes, e.g., baroceptor and chemoceptor activities.

In the dog and cat, the intravenous dose level of chloralose is between 40 and 100 mg/kg; anesthesia lasts 6–10 hours (Lees 1972). It is usually administered with ether to reduce the spinal reflex activity and "convulsivelike" actions associated with the use of chloralose. The cardiovascular responses following the intravenous administration of α-chloralose (100 mg/kg) have been studied extensively in the dog (Cox 1972). With the exception of brief effects immediately after the injection, which last about 15 minutes, there are no changes in systemic hemodynamics.

Chloralose has been used in sheep at a dose level of 22–25 mg/lb of body weight (Phillipson and Barnett 1939). The onset of action is delayed following chloralose administration and does not attain its full effect for at least 20 minutes. In swine, following premedication with small dose levels of morphine sulfate, the intravenous dose of chloralose required to induce a hypnotic effect is 25–39 mg/lb of body weight (Booth et al. 1960). Paddling movements of the limbs are observed in the pig similar to those reported in sheep by Phillipson and Barnett.

In the United Kingdom, α-chloralose is employed for killing rats and is available to the general public (Lees 1972). Cases of suspected chloralose poisoning have been reported in the dog and cat (Copestake 1967). The drug apparently is also being illegally used in baits against crows, gulls, and foxes (Conder 1973). However, other birds (golden eagle, buzzard, hen harrier), whether intended or not, also receive the bait and have died from its use.

Urethan

Urethan, N.F. (NH_2 $COOC_2H_5$), is known also as ethyl carbamate. It is chemically related to urea and is readily soluble in water and alcohol. Urethan is only occasionally used as an anesthetic in laboratory animals. The drug can be administered intravenously (1 g/kg) or intraperitoneally (1–2 g/kg). In small laboratory animals such as the rat, urethan (1.25 g/kg) is administered intraperitoneally. Urethan produces anesthesia that lasts many hours. It is metabolized slowly into carbamic acid and ethyl alcohol.

Urethan apparently produces a variable or little effect in the domestic duck (Desforges and Scott 1971). It is not used clinically because there are safer anesthetics available for use. Liver injury is produced by urethan. In addition, urethan has a carcinogenic effect in several species.

REFERENCES

Adams, H. R. 1970. Prolongation of barbiturate anesthesia by chloramphenicol in laboratory animals. J Am Vet Med Assoc 157:1908.

Adams, H. R., and Dixit, B. N. 1970. Prolongation of pentobarbital anesthesia by chloramphenicol in dogs and cats. J Am Vet Med Assoc 156:902.

Allam, M. W., and Churchill, E. A. 1946. Pentobarbital sodium anesthesia in swine and goats. J Am Vet Med Assoc 109:355.

Amend, J. F.; Klavano, P. A.; and Stone, E. C. 1972. Premedication with xylazine to eliminate muscular hypertonicity in cats during ketamine anesthesia. Vet Med Small Anim Clin 67:1305.

American Veterinary Medical Association Council. 1972. Report of the AVMA panel on euthanasia. J Am Vet Med Assoc 160: 761.

Anderson, F. L.; Kralios, A. C.; Tsagaris, T. J.; and Kuida, H. 1972. Hemodynamic effects of sodium pentobarbital in the bovine. J Surg Res 13:182.

Arañez, J. B.; and Forteza, T. F. 1955. Kemithal sodium as a general anesthetic for dogs. J Am Vet Med Assoc 127:122.

Bass, B. G., and Buckley, N. M. 1966. Chloralose anesthesia in the dog: A study of actions and analytical methodology. Am J Physiol 210:854.

Beck, C. C., and Dresner, A. J. 1972. Vetalar (ketamine HCl): A cataleptoid anesthetic agent for primate species. Vet Med Small Anim Clin 67:1082.

Beck, C. C.; Coppock, R. W.; and Ott, B. S. 1971. Evaluation of Vetalar (Ketamine HCI): A unique feline anesthetic. Vet Med 66:993.

Bemis, H. E.; Guard, W. F.; and Covault, C. H. 1924. Anesthesia, general and local. J Am Vet Med Assoc 64:413.

Ben, M.; Dixon, R. L.; and Adamson, R. H. 1969. Anesthesia in the rat. Fed Proc 28:1522.

Bennett, R. R. 1969. The clinical use of 2-(ethylamino)-2-(2-thienyl) cyclohexanone HCl (CI-634) as an anesthetic for the cat. Am J Vet Res 30:1469.

Bennett, R. R., and Tillotson, P. J. 1969. Cyclohexanone as an anesthetic for the leopard and the bengal tiger. J Am Vet Med Assoc 155:1098.

Berger, J. 1966. A comparison of some anaesthetic techniques in young calves. Br Vet J 122:65.

Bhargava, A. K., and Vyas, U. K. 1967. "Chloral-Mag" anaesthesia in the camel. Vet Rec 80:322.

Blair, E. 1969. Generalized hypothermia. Fed Proc 28: 1456.

Bone, J. F. 1970. Letters to the editor. Lab Anim Sci 20:289.

Booth, N. H. 1969. Anesthesia in the pig. Fed Proc 28:1547.

Booth, N. H., and Rankin, A. D. 1953. Studies on the pharmacodynamics of curare in the horse. II. Curare as an adjunct to chloral hydrate anesthesia. Am J Vet Res 14:56.

Booth, N. H.; Bredeck, H. E.; and Herin, R. A. 1960. Baroceptor reflex mechanisms in swine. Am J Physiol 199:1189.

Borzio, F. 1973. Ketamine hydrochloride as an anesthetic for wild fowl. Vet Med Small Anim Clin 68:1364.

Boulos, B. M.; Jenkins, W. L.; and Davis, L. E. 1972. Pharmacokinetics of certain drugs in the domesticated goat. Am J Vet Res 33:943.

Bovill, J. G.; Coppel, D. L.; Dundee, J. W.; and Moore, J. 1971. Current status of ketamine anaesthesia. Lancet 1:1285.

Bowden, D. M.; Holm, R.; and Morgan, M. K. 1974. General anesthesia for surgery in the infant pigtail monkey, *Macaca nemestrina.* Lab Anim Sci 24:675.

Bowen, J. M.; Blackmon, D. M.; and Heavner, J. E. 1970. Effect of magnesium ions on neuromuscular transmission in the horse, steer, and dog. J Am Vet Med Assoc 157: 164.

Bree, M. M. 1972. Clinical evaluation of tiletamine as an anesthetic in six nonhuman primate species. J Am Vet Med Assoc 161:693.

Bree, M. M., and Gross, N. B. 1969. Anesthesia of pigeons with CI-581 (ketamine) and pentobarbital. Lab Anim Sci 19:500.

Britton, B. J.; Wood, W. G.; and Irving, M. H. 1974. Sedation of sheep and patas monkeys with ketamine. Lab Anim Sci 8:41.

Brodey, R. S., and Thordal-Christensen, A. 1956. Chlorpromazine hydrochloride as a preanesthetic agent for pentobarbital sodium anesthesia in the dog. J Am Vet Med Assoc 129:410.

Brodie, B. B.; Bernstein, E.; and Mark, L. C. 1952. The role of body fat in limiting the duration of action of thiopental. J Pharmacol Exp Ther 105:421.

Brodie, B. B.; Mark, L. C.; Papper, E. M.; Lief, P. A.; Bernstein, E.; and Rovenstine, E. A. 1950. The fate of thiopental in man and a method for its estimation in biological material. J Pharmacol Exp Ther 98:85.

Brown, D. A. 1962. An eserine-like action of chloral hydrate. Br J Pharmacol 19:111.

Bryant, S. H. 1969. General anesthesia in the goat. Fed Proc 28:1553.

Buck, N.; Fry, P.; Green, C.; Gwynn, R.; Keen, P.; Pout, D.; Pressland, D.; and Suddes, H. 1963. The use of a thiambutene-phencyclidine-hyoscine mixture for the immobilization of the topi *(Damaliscus korrigum)* and the hippopotamus *(Hippopotamus amphibius).* Vet Rec 75:630.

Burn, J. H. 1960. Why thiopentone injected into artery may cause gangrene. Br Med J 2:414.

Burns, J. J.; Conney, A. H.; and Koster, R. 1963. Stimulatory effect of chronic drug administration on drug-metabolizing enzymes in liver microsomes. Ann NY Acad Sci 104:881.

Butler, T. C. 1948. The metabolic fate of chloral hydrate. J Pharmacol Exp Ther 92:49.

Bywater, J. E. C., and Rutty, D. A. 1964. Simple techniques for simian anesthesia. In O. Graham-Jones, ed. Small Animal Anaesthesia, p. 9. Elmsford, N.Y.: Pergamon Press.

Calderwood, H. W.; Klide, A. M.; Cohn, B. B.; and Soma, L. R. 1971. Cardiorespiratory effects of tiletamine in cats. Am J Vet Res 32:1511.

Cannon, J. E., and Higgins, W. Y. 1972. Pyothorax in a lion cub. Mod Vet Pract 53:40.

Chaplin, M. D.; Roszkowski, A. P.; and Richards, R. K. 1973. Displacement of thiopental from plasma proteins by nonsteroidal anti-inflammatory agents. Proc Soc Exp Biol Med 143:667.

Chen, G. 1968. Surgical anesthesia in the rabbit with 2-(ethylamino)-2-(2-thienyl) cyclohexanone HCl (CI-634) and chloral hydrate. Am J Vet Res 29:869.

Chen, G., and Ensor, C. R. 1968. 2-(ethylamino)-2-2(2-thienyl) cyclohexanone HCl (CI-634): A taming, incapacitating and anesthetic agent for the cat. Am J Vet Res 29:863.

Chen, G.; Ensor, C. R.; Russell, D.; and Bohner, B. 1959. The pharmacology of 1-(1-phenylcyclohexyl) piperidine HCl. J Pharmacol Exp Ther 127:241.

Chen, G.; Ensor, C. R.; and Bohner, B. 1967. The pharmacology of 2-(ethylamino)-2-(2-thienyl) cyclohexanone HCl (CI-634). J Pharmacol Exp Ther 168:171.

Chenoweth, M. B., and Van Dyke, R. A. 1969. Choice of anesthetic agents for the dog. Fed Proc 28:1432.

Child, K. J.; Davis, B.; Dodds, M. G.; and Twissell, D. J. 1972. Anaesthesia, cardiovascular and respiratory effects of a new steroidal agent CT 1341: A comparison with other intravenous anaesthetic drugs in the unrestrained cat. Br J Pharmacol 46:189.

Clarke, N. P.; Hukeey, M. J.; and Martin, W. M. 1963. Pentobarbital anesthesia in bears. J Am Vet Med Assoc 143:47.

Clifford, D. 1971. Restraint and anesthesia of subhuman primates. In L. R. Soma, ed. Textbook of Veterinary Anesthesia, p. 385. Baltimore: Williams & Wilkins.

Clifford, D. H., and Kook, C. C. 1963. Pentobarbital anesthesia in the dog following preanesthetic administration of promazine and meperidine in clinical practice. Cornell Vet 53:199.

Clifford, D. H., and Soma, L. R. 1969. Feline anesthesia. Fed Proc 28:1479.

Clifford, D. H.; Good, A. L.: and Stowe, C. M. 1962. Observations on the use of ataractic and narcotic preanesthesia and pentobarbital in bears. J Am Vet Med Assoc 140: 464.

Code of Federal Regulations. 1974. Title 21, Food and Drugs. Parts 130–40. Washington, D.C.: U.S. Government Printing Office.

Coffman, M. T., and Pedersoli, W. M. 1971. Glyceryl guaiacolate as an adjunct to equine anesthesia. J Am Vet Med Assoc 158:1548.

Conder, P. 1973. Illegal use of alphachloralose. Vet Rec 92:325.

Conney, A. H. 1967. Pharmacological implications of microsomal enzyme induction. Pharmacol Rev 19:317.

Conney, A. H., and Burns, J. J. 1972. Metabolic interactions among environmental chemicals and drugs. Science 178:576.

Cooper, J. E., and Frank, L. 1973. Use of the steroid anaesthetic CT 1341 in birds. Vet Rec 92:474.

Copestake, P. 1967. Suspected chloralose poisoning. Vet Rec 80:81.

Cox, R. H. 1972. Influence of chloralose anesthesia on cardiovascular function in trained dogs. Am J Physiol 223:660.

Cronnelly, R. 1972. Interaction of ketamine HCl with neuromuscular agents. Survey Anesthesiol 16:372.

Cronnelly, R.; Dretchen, K. L.; Sokoll, M. D.; and Long, J. P. 1973. Ketamine: Myoneural activity and interaction with neuromuscular blocking agents. Eur J Pharmacol 22:17.

Cummings, J. N.; Harris, W. H.; and Agar, J. L. 1972. Anaesthetic regime for prolonged operations in swine. Can Anaesth Soc J 19:557.

Dale, H. E.: Elefson, E. E.; and Niemeyer, K. H. 1968. Influence of environmental temperature on recovery of dogs from pentobarbital anesthesia. Am J Vet Res 29:1339.

Danks, A. G. 1943. Anesthesia in horses and swine. Cornell Vet 33:344.

Davis, L. E. and Wolff, W. A. 1970. Pharmacokinetics and metabolism of glyceryl guaiacolate in ponies. Am J Vet Res 31: 469.

Dawson, B.; Michenfelder, J. D.; and Theye, R. A. 1971. Effects of ketamine on canine cerebral blood flow and metabolism: Modification by prior administration of thiopental. Anesth Analg 50:443.

Day, P. W. 1965. Anesthetic technics for the chimpanzee. In D. C. Sawyer, ed. Experimental Animal Anesthesiology, p. 289. Brooks Air Force Base, Texas: USAF School of Aerospace Medicine.

Denny, M. J. S. 1973. The use of ketamine hydrochloride as a safe, short duration anaesthetic in kangaroos. Br Vet J 129:362.

Desforges, M. F., and Scott, H. H. 1971. Use of anaesthetics in the Aylesbury domestic duck. Res Vet Sci 12:596.

DeYoung, D. W.; Paddleford, R. R.; and Short, C. E. 1972. Dissociative anesthetics in the cat and dog. J Am Vet Med Assoc 161:1442.

Dobkin, A. B. 1961. Prolongation of thiopental-induced sleep in dogs by narcotic analgesics. Anesthesiology 22:291.

Dodds, M. G., and Twissell, D. J. 1973. CT 1341 and thiopentone compared in feline anaesthesia by an intermittent injection technique. J Small Anim Pract 14:487.

Domino, E. F.; McCarthy, D. A.; and Deneau, G. A. 1969. General anesthesia in infrahuman primates. Fed Proc 28:1500.

Donovan, C. A. 1958. Restraint and anesthesia of caged birds. Vet Med 53:541.

Dorfman, A., and Goldbaum, L. R. 1947. Detoxification of barbiturates. J Pharmacol Exp Ther 90:330.

Dornette, W. H., and Tuohy, E. B. 1951. Clinical trial of Surital sodium in 1200 cases of general anesthesia. Anesth Analg 30:159.

Dunne, H. W., and Benbrook, S. C. 1954. A note on the use of Surital sodium anesthesia in swine. J Am Vet Med Assoc 124:19.

Durant, A. J. 1953. Removing the vocal cords of fowls. J Am Vet Med Assoc 122:14.

Dyson, J. A. 1964. Castration of the mature boar with reference to general anaesthesia induced by intratesticular injection of pentobarbitone sodium. Vet Rec 76:28.

Elder, C. K., and Harrison, E. M. 1944. Pentothal sodium slough. Prevention by procaine hydrochloride. J Am Med Assoc 125:116.

Elsea, J. R.; Cloyd, G. D.; Gilbert, D. L.; Perkinson, E.; and Ward, J. W. 1970. Barbiturate anesthesia in dogs wearing collars containing dichlorovos. J Am Vet Med Assoc 157:2068.

Emberton, G. A. 1966. Methohexitone sodium anaesthesia in pigs. Vet Rec 78:541.

Enold, G. L. 1962. Pathologic effects of intrathoracic barbiturate anesthesia in cats. J Am Vet Med Assoc 140:795.

Evan, J. M.; Aspinall, K. W.; and Hendy, P. G. 1972. Clinical evaluation in cats of a new anaesthetic, CT 1341. J Small Anim Pract 13:479.

Evans, A. T.; Krahwinkel, D. J.; and Sawyer, D. C. 1972. Dissociative anesthesia in the cat. J Am Anim Hosp Assoc 8:371.

Fabry, A. 1963. Methohexital sodium anaesthesia in greyhounds. Vet Rec 75:1049.

Fisher, L. E. 1965. General and chemical restraint technics used in a zoologic garden. In D. C. Sawyer, ed. Experimental Animal Anesthesiology, p. 379. Brooks Air Force Base, Texas: USAF School of Aerospace Medicine.

Flynn, E. J., and Spector, S. 1972. Determination of barbiturate derivatives by radioimmunoassay. J Pharmacol Exp Ther 181:547.

Ford, E. J. H. 1951. Some observations on the use of thiopentone in large animals. Vet Rec 63:636.

Fowler, N. G., and Stevenson, G. E. 1961. The use of methohexital sodium in small animal anaesthesia. Vet Rec 73:917.

Freudenthal, R. I., and Carroll, F. I. 1973. Metabolism of certain commonly used barbiturates. Drug Rev 2:265.

Funk, K. A. 1970. Glyceryl guaiacolate: A centrally acting muscle relaxant. Equine Vet J 2:173.

———. 1973. Glyceryl guaiacolate: Some effects and indications in horses. Equine Vet J 5:15.

Fussell, M. H. 1969. A method for the separation and collection of urine and faeces in the fowl *Gallus domesticus*. Res Vet Sci 10:332.

Gabel, A. A. 1962. Promazine, chloral hydrate and ultrashort-acting barbiturate anesthesia in horses. J Am Vet Med Assoc 140:564.

Gandal, C. P. 1956. Satisfactory general anesthesia in birds. J Am Vet Med Assoc 128:332.

———. 1969. Avian anesthesia. Fed Proc 28:1533.

Gandal, C. P., and Saunders, L. Z. 1959. The surgery of subcutaneous tumors in parakeets *(Melopsittacus undulatus)*. J Am Vet Med Assoc 134:212.

Garmer, N. L. 1969. Effects of 2-(ethylamino)-2-(2-thienyl) cyclohexanone HCl (CI-634) in cats. Res Vet Sci 10:382.

Geraci, J. R. 1973. An appraisal of ketamine as an immobilizing agent in wild and captive pinnipeds. J Am Vet Med Assoc 163:574.

Gertsen, K. E., and Tillotson, P. J. 1968. Clinical use of glyceryl guaiacolate in the horse. Vet Med Small Anim Clin 63:1062.

Glen, J. B. 1973. The use of ketamine (CI-581) in feline practice. Vet Rec 92:65.

Glenn, J. L.; Straight, L. R.; and Snyder, C. C. 1972. Clinical use of ketamine hydrochloride as an anesthetic agent for snakes. Am J Vet Res 33:1901.

Goldberg, S. H.; Linde, L. M.; Goal, P. G.; Momma, K.; Takahashi, M.; and Sarna, G. 1968. Effects of barbiturates on pulmonary and systemic hemodynamics. Cardiovasc Res 2:136.

Graham, D. L.; Dunlop, R. H.; and Travis, H. F. 1967. Barbiturate anesthesia in ranch mink *(Mustela vison)*. Am J Vet Res 28:293.

Grono, L. R. 1966. Methohexial sodium anaesthesia in the horse. Aust Vet J 42:398.

Gruber, C. M. 1937. On certain pharmacologic actions of newer barbituric acid compounds. Am J Obst Gynecol 33:729.

Hall, L. W. 1972. The anaesthesia and euthanasia of neonatal and juvenile dogs and cats Vet Rec 90:303.

Hamlin, R. L.; Redding, R. W.; Rieger, J. E.; Smith, R. C.; and Prynn, R. B. 1965. Insignificance of the "glucose effect" in dogs anesthetized with pentobarbital. J Am Vet Med Assoc 146:238.

Harrison, F. A. 1964. The anaesthesia of sheep using pentobarbitone sodium and cyclopropane. In O. Graham-Jones, ed. Small Animal Anaesthesia, p. 149. Elmsford, N.Y.: Pergamon Press.

Harthoorn, A. M.; Harthoorn, S.; and Sayer, P. D. 1971. Two field operations on the African lion *(Felis leo)*. Vet Rec 89:159.

Hatch, R. C. 1966. The effect of glucose, sodium lactate and epinephrine on thiopental anesthesia in dogs. J Am Vet Med Assoc 148:135.

———. 1972. Effect of autonomic blocking agents on development of acute tolerance to thiopental in dogs. Am J Vet Res 33: 365.

———. 1973a. Prevention of ketamine catalepsy and enhancement of ketamine anesthesia in cats pretreated with methiothepin. Pharmacol Res Commun 5:311.

———. 1973b. Effects of ketamine when used in conjunction with meperidine or morphine in cats. J Am Vet Med Assoc 162: 964.

———. 1974. Ketamine catalepsy and anesthesia in dogs pretreated with antiserotonergic or antidopinergic neuroleptics or with anticholinergic agents. Pharmacol Res Commun 6:289.

Hatch, R. C., and Ruch, T. 1974. Experiments on antagonism of ketamine anesthesia in cats given adrenergic, serotonergic and cholinergic stimulants alone and in combination. Am J Vet Res 35:35.

Hatch, R. C.; Currie, R. B.; and Grieve, G. A. 1970. Feline electroencephalograms and plasma thiopental concentrations associated with clinical stages of anesthesia. Am J Vet Res 31:291.

Heath, R. B., and Gabel, A. A. 1970. Evaluation of thiamylal sodium, succinylcholine and glyceryl guaiacolate prior to inhalation anesthesia in horses. J Am Vet Med Assoc 157:1486.

Heavner, J. E., and Bowen, J. M. 1968. Influence of adrenergic agents on recovery of dogs from anesthesia. Am J Vet Res 29: 2133.

Henderson, W. M. 1944. Pentothal sodium as a narcotic in cattle. J Comp Pathol 54: 245.

Henderson, W. M., and Brooksby, J. B. 1950. Thiopentone as an anaesthetic in the horse. Vet Rec 62:38.

Henry, D. P. 1968. Anaesthesia of boars by intratesticular injection. Aust Vet J 44: 418.

Herin, R. A. 1959. Thermoregulatory effects of the abdominal air sacs on spermatogenesis in domestic fowl. M.S. thesis. Colorado State University.

Hoar, R. M. 1969. Anesthesia in the guinea pig. Fed Proc 28:1517.

Hollingsworth, H., and Howes, J. R. 1965. A comparison of some new anesthetics for avian surgery. Poult Sci 44:1380.

Hunt, W. H.; Fosbinder, R. J.; and Barlow, O. W. 1948. Anesthetic effects of some new barbituric acid derivatives administered to dogs. J Am Pharm Assoc 37:1.

Jackson, L. L., and Lundvall, R. L. 1972. Effect of glyceryl guaiacolate-thiamylal sodium solution on respiratory function and various hematologic factors of the horse. J Am Vet Med Assoc 161:164.

Joffe, M. H. 1964. An anesthetic for the chimpanzee: 1-(1-phenyl-cyclohexyl) piperidine HCl. Anesth Analg 43:221.

Johnston, N. L. 1974. Techniques for anesthetizing and vaccinating exotic felidae. Vet Med Small Anim Clin 69:1243.

Jones, R. S. 1968. The effects of extravascular injection of thiopentone in the horse. Br Vet J 124:72.

Kaplan, H. M. 1969. Anesthesia in amphibians and reptiles. Fed Proc 28:1541.

Kaplan, J. A., and Cooperman, L. H. 1971. Alarming reactions to ketamine in patients taking thyroid medication-treatment with propranolol. Anesthesiology 35:229.

Kayama, J., and Iwama, K. 1972. The EEG, evoked potentials and single-unit activity during ketamine anesthesia in cats. Anesthesiology 36:316.

Keeran, R. J. 1972. Equine ovariectomy: Anesthesia and positioning. Proc Am Assoc Equine Pract, p. 41.

Kinmonth, J. B., and Shepherd, R. C. 1959.

Accidental injection of thiopentone into arteries. Br Med J 2: 914.

Kittle, E. L. 1971. Ketamine HCl as an anesthetic for birds. Mod Vet Pract 52:40.

Kraner, K. L.; Silverstein, A. M.; and Parshall, C. J., Jr. 1965. Surgical anesthesia in snakes. In D. C. Sawyer, ed. Experimental Animal Anesthesiology, p. 374. Brooks Air Force Base, Texas: USAF School of Aerospace Medicine.

Kuroda, T., and McNamara, J. A., Jr. 1972. The effect of ketamine and phencyclidine on muscle activity in nonhuman primates. Anesth Analg 51:710.

Lamson, P. D.; Grieg, M. E.; and Hobdy, C. J. 1951. Modification of bariturate anesthesia by glucose, intermediary metabolites and certain other substances. J Pharmacol Exp Ther 103:460.

Leash, A. M. 1969. Intravascular and other routes for anesthesia in the dog. Fed Proc 28:1436.

Lee, C. C. 1953. Experimental studies on the action of several anesthetics in domestic fowls. Poult Sci 32:624.

Lees, P. 1972. Pharmacology and toxicology of alpha chloralose: A review. Vet Rec 91:330.

Linegar, C. R.; Dille, J. M.; and Koppanyi, T. 1936. Studies on barbiturates. XVIII. Analysis of a peripheral action of barbiturates. J Pharmacol Exp Ther 58:128.

Linzell, J. L. 1964. Some observations on general and regional anaesthesia in goats. In O. Graham-Jones, ed. Small Animal Anaesthesia, p. 163. Elmsford, N.Y.: Pergamon Press.

Lumb, W. V. 1965. The intravenous anesthetic agents. In D. C. Sawyer, ed. Experimental Animal Anesthesiology, p. 99. Brooks Air Force Base, Texas: USAF School of Aerospace Medicine.

Lumb, W. V., and Jones, E. W. 1973. Veterinary Anesthesia, p. 680. Philadelphia: Lea & Febiger.

Lutsky, I. 1969. Immediate postanesthetic care of the dog. Fed Proc 28:1477.

McKechnie, F. B., and Converse, J. G. 1955. Placental transmission of thiopental. Am J Obst Gynecol 70:639.

Mackey, W. J.; Anderson, W. D.; and Kubicek, W. G. 1970. Ventriculocordectomy technic for use on research swine. Lab Anim Sci 20:992.

Madsen, D. E. 1967. A surgical procedure for devocalizing the rooster. Vet Med Small Anim Clin 62:114.

Mandelker, L. 1973. A toxicity study of ketamine HCl in parakeets. Vet Med Small Anim Clin 68:487.

Mark, L. C.,; Perel, J. M.; Brand, L.; and Dayton, P. G. 1968. Studies with thiohexital, an anesthetic barbiturate metabolized with unusual rapidity in man. Anesthesiology 29:1159.

Marshall, E. K., Jr., and Owens, A. H., Jr. 1954. Absorption, excretion and metabolic fate of chloral hydrate and trichloroethanol. Bull Johns Hopkins Hosp 95:1.

Martyn, E. 1955. Pentobarital sodium as an anesthetic for bears. J Am Vet Med Assoc 127:415.

Massey, G. M. 1973. Anaesthesia in the dog and cat. Aust Vet J 49:207.

Mather, G. W. 1969. Restraint of the laboratory dog. Fed Proc 28:1423.

Meer, F. M.; Downing, J. W.; and Coleman, A. J. 1973. An intravenous method anaesthesia for caesarean section. II. Ketamine. Br J Anaesth 45:191.

Melby, E. C., Jr., and Baker, H. J. 1965. Phencyclidine for analgesia and anesthesia in simian primates. J Am Vet Med Assoc 147:1068.

Millenbruck, E. W., and Wallinga, M. H. 1946. A newly developed anesthesia for large animals. J Am Vet Med Assoc 108: 148.

Miller, A. E., and Gudmundson, J. 1964. Use of thiamylal sodium in mature swine. Can Vet J 5:217.

Miller, R. M., and Peddie, J. 1970. Phencyclidine hydrochloride as a general anesthetic. Vet Med Small Anim Clin 65:131.

Mitchell, B. 1966. Anaesthesia in small animal practice. Vet Rec 79. Clin Suppl 3, v.

Morgan, W. W.; Morlan, S. L.; Krupp, J. H.; and Rosenkrantz, J. G. 1966. Pentobarbital anesthesia in the rabbit. Am J Vet Res 27:1133.

Muhrer, M. E. 1950. Restraint of swine with Pentothal sodium. J Am Vet Med Assoc 117:293.

Murdock, H. R., Jr. 1969. Anesthesia in the rabbit. Fed Proc 28:1510.

Neal, P. A. 1963. Aneurysmal-varix in the horse: A sequel to the perivascular injection of thiopentone sodium. Vet Rec 75: 289.

Pedersoli, W. M. 1972. Glyceryl guaiacolate as an adjunct to equine anesthesia. Auburn Vet 29:6.

Pedersoli, W. M., and Brown, M. K. 1973. A new approach to the etiology of arrhythmogenic effects of thiamylal sodium in dogs. Vet Med Small Anim Clin 68:1286.

Phillipson, A. T., and Barnett, S. F. 1939. Anaesthesia in sheep. Vet Rec 51:869.

Pleuger, C. A. 1950. Gastrotomy in a crocodile —A case report. J Am Vet Med Assoc 117: 297.

Popovic, N. A.; Mullane, J. F.; Vick, J. A.; and Kobrine, A. 1972. Effect of phencyclidine hydrochloride on certain cardiorespiratory values of rhesus monkey *(Macaca mulatta)*. Am J Vet Res 33:1649.

Priano, L. L.; Traber, D. L.; and Wilson, R. D. 1969. Barbiturate anesthesia: An abnormal physiologic situation. J Pharmacol Exp Ther 165:126.

Price, H. L. 1975. Intravenous anesthetics. In L. S. Goodman and A. Gilman, eds. The Pharmacological Basis of Therapeutics, p. 97. New York: Macmillan.

Rae, J. H. 1962. The fate of pentobarbitone and thiopentone in the sheep. Res Vet Sci 3:399.

Rawlings, C. A., and Dean, D. F. 1971. An anesthetic technic for primates during emplacement of a flow sensor about the middle cerebral artery. Lab Anim Sci 21:520.

Reid, J. S., and Frank, R. J. 1972. Prevention of undesirable side reactions of ketamine anesthesia in cats. J Am Anim Hosp Assoc 8:115.

Reutner, T. F., and Gruhzit, O. M. 1948. Surital sodium, a new anesthetic and hypnotic. J Am Vet Med Assoc 113:357.

Rex, M. A. E. 1972. Principles of anaesthesia. Aust Vet J 48:677.

Ritter, C.; Hughes, R.; Snyder, G.; and Weaver, L. 1970. Dichlorvos-containing dog collars and thiamylal anesthesia. Am J Vet Res 31:2025.

Roberts, H. B.; Wendt, W. E.; Wagner, C. C.; and Reutner, T. F. 1951. Surital sodium anesthesia in canine surgery. J Am Vet Med Assoc 118:151.

Robertson, A. C.; Foulks, J. G.; and Daniel, E. E. 1958. The effects of pentobarbital-induced myocardial depression on cardiac electrolytes distribution. J Pharmacol Exp Ther 122:281.

Rose, W. C.; Munson, A. E.; and Bradley, S. G. 1973. Acute lethality for mice following administration of cyclophosphamide with barbiturates. Proc Soc Exp Biol Med 143:1.

Rosin, E. 1974. University of Georgia. Personal communication.

Santos, M. D., and Bogan, J. A. 1974. The metabolism of pentobarbitone in sheep. Res Vet Sci 17:226.

Sawyer, D. C. 1965a. Anesthetic technics of the *Macaca mulatta*. In D.C. Sawyer, ed. Experimental Animal Anesthesiology, p. 321. Brooks Air Force Base, Texas: USAF School of Aerospace Medicine.

———. 1965b. Anesthetic technics of rabbits and mice. In D. C. Sawyer, ed. Experimental Animal Anesthesiology, p. 344. Brooks Air Force Base, Texas: USAF School of Aerospace Medicine.

Schatzman, U. 1974. The induction of general anaesthesia in the horse with glyceryl guaiacolate. Comparison when used alone and with sodium thiamylal (Surital). Equine Vet J 6:164.

Schulz, T. A., and Fowler, M. E. 1974. The clinical effects of CI-744 in chinchillas, *Chinchilla villidera* (Laniger). Lab Anim Sci 24:810.

Seeman, P. 1972. The membrane actions of anesthetics and tranquilizers. Pharmacol Rev 24:583.

Seidenstricker, J. C., and Reynolds, H. V. 1969. Preliminary studies on the use of a general anesthetic in falconiform birds. J Am Vet Med Assoc 155:1044.

Sharma, R. P.; Stowe, C. M.; and Good, A. L. 1970. Alteration of thiopental metabolism in phenobarbital treated calves. Toxicol Appl Pharmacol 17:400.

Sharpless, S. K. 1970. Hypnotics and sedatives. I. The barbiturates. In L. S. Goodman and A. Gilman, eds. The Pharmacological Basis of Therapeutics, 4th ed., p. 98. New York: Macmillan.

Shetty, S. N.; Himes, J. A.; and Edds, G. T. 1972. Enzyme induction in sheep: Effects of phenobarbital on *in vivo* and *in vitro* drug metabolism. Am J Vet Res 33:935.

Short, C. E. 1970. Advances in small animal anesthesiology. J Am Vet Med Assoc 157: 1719.

———. 1974. Technic and equipment for equine inhalation anesthesia. Mod Vet Pract 55:393.

Simmons, D. J.; Lesker, P. A.; and Sherman, N. E. 1974. Induction of sodium pentobarbital anesthesia. A circadian rhythm. J Interdiscipl Cycle Res 5:71.

Sis, R. F., and Herron, M. A. 1972. Anesthesia of the newborn kitten. Lab Anim Sci 22:746.

Soma, L. R. 1971. Textbook of Veterinary Anesthesia, p. 621. Baltimore: Williams & Wilkins.

Spalding, V. T., and Heymann, C. S. 1962. The value of phencyclidine in the anaesthesia of monkeys. Vet Rec 74:158.

Stock, J. E. 1973. Advances in small animal anaesthesia. Vet Rec 92:351.

Stoliker, H. E. 1965. The physiologic and pharmacologic effects of Sernylan: A review. In D. C. Sawyer, ed. Experimental Animal Anesthesiology, p. 148. Brooks Air Force Base, Texas: USAF School of Aerospace Medicine.

Stone, H. H., and Donnelly, C. C. 1961. The accidental intra-arterial injection of thiopental. Anesthesiology 22:995.

Strande, A. 1964. Intrapulmonary anaesthesia with pentobarbitone sodium in cats. J Small Anim Pract 5:153.

Strobel, G. E., and Wollman, H. 1969. Pharmacology of anesthetic agents. Fed Proc 28: 1386.

Stunkard, J. A., and Miller, J. C. 1974. An outline guide to general anesthesia in exotic species. Vet Med Small Anim Clin 69: 1181.

Swanson, E. E. 1944. Therapy with Barbiturates. Indianapolis: Eli Lilly.

Swanson, T. D. 1973. Restraint in treatment. Proc Am Assoc Equine Pract, p. 147.

Sykes, A. H. 1964. Some aspects of anaesthesia in the adult fowl. In O. Graham-Jones, ed. Small Animal Anaesthesia, p. 117. Elmsford, N.Y.: Pergamon Press.

Szappanyos, G.; Gemperle, M.; and Rifat, K. 1971. Selective indications for ketamine anaesthesia. Proc R Soc Med 64:1156.

Taber, R., and Irwin, S. 1969. Anesthesia in the mouse. Fed Proc 28:1528

Tavernor, A. D. 1962. Recent trends in equine anaesthesia. Vet Rec 74:595.

Tavernor, W. D. 1970. The influence of guaiacol ether on cardiovascular and respiratory function in the horse. Res Vet Sci 11: 91.

Tavernor, W. D., and Jones, E. W. 1970. Observations on the cardiovascular and respiratory effects of guaiacol glycerol ether in conscious and anaesthetized dogs. J Small Anim Pract 11:177.

Tavernor, W. D., and Lees, P. 1970. The influence of thiopentone and suxamethonium on cardiovascular and respiratory function in the horse. Res Vet Sci 11:45.

Taylor, C., and Stoelting, V. K. 1960. Methohexital sodium—A new ultrashort-acting barbiturate. Anesthesiology 21:29.

Taylor, J. D.; Richards, R. K.; and Tabern, D. L. 1952. Metabolism of S^{35} thiopental (Pentothal). J Pharmacol Exp Ther 104: 93.

Taylor, J. D.; Swenson, E. M.; Davin, J. C.; and Richards, R. K. 1957. Relationship between sleep, biotransformation rates, and plasma levels of pentobarbital and secobarbital in animals. Proc Soc Exp Biol 95:462.

Teske, R. H., and Carter, G. G. 1971. Effect of chloramphenicol on pentobarbital-induced anesthesia in dogs. J Am Vet Med Assoc 159:777.

Thurmon, J. C.; Nelson, D. R.; and Christie, G. J. 1972. Ketamine anesthesia in swine. J Am Vet Med Assoc 160:1325.

Thurmon, J. C.; Kumar, A.; and Link, R. P. 1973. Evaluation of ketamine hydrochloride as an anesthetic in sheep. J Am Vet Med Assoc 162:293.

Titchen, D. A.; Steel, J. D.; and Hamilton, F. J. 1949. Clinical observations on thiobarbiturate anaesthesia in sheep. Aust Vet J 25: 257.

Tonge, S. R. 1973. Catecholamine concentrations in discrete areas of the rat brain after the pre- and neonatal administration of phencyclidine and imipramine. J Pharm Pharmacol 25:164.

Traber, D. L.; Wilson, R. D.; and Priano, L. L. 1970a. Blockade of the hypertensive response to ketamine. Anesth Analg 49: 420.

———. 1970b. A detailed study of the cardiopulmonary response to ketamine and its blockade by atropine. South Med J 63: 1077.

———. 1971. The effect of alpha-adrenergic blockade on the cardiopulmonary response to ketamine. Anesth Analg 50:737.

Trim, C. M., and Mason, J. 1973. Post-anesthetic forelimb lameness in horses. Equine Vet J 5:71.

Tyagi, R. P. S.; Arnold, J. P.; Usenik, E. A.; and Fletcher, T. F. 1964. Effects of thiopental sodium (Pentothal sodium) anesthesia on the horse. Cornell Vet 54:583.

Vice, T. E.; Claborn, L. D.; and Ratner, R. A. 1965. Anesthetic technics in the baboon with some observations on other primates. In D. C. Sawyer, ed. Experimental Animal Anesthesiology, p. 301. Brooks Air Force Base, Texas: USAF School of Aerospace Medicine.

Virtue, R. W.; Alanis, J. M.; Mori, M.; Lafargue, R. T.; Vogel, J. H. K.; and Metcalf, D. R. 1967. An anesthetic agent: 2-(orthochlorophenyl)-2-(methylamino) cyclohexanone HCl (CI-581). Anesthesiology 28:823.

Vondruska, J. F. 1965. Phencyclidine anesthesia in baboons. J Am Vet Med Assoc 147: 1073.

Voss, W. R. 1970. Primate liver and spleen biopsy procedures. Lab Anim Sci 20:995.

Wallach, J. D. 1969. Medical care of reptiles. J Am Vet Med Assoc 115:1017.

Ward, G. S.; Johnsen, D. O.; and Roberts, C. R. 1974. The use of CI-744 as an anesthetic for laboratory animals. Lab Anim Sci 24:737.

Wiersig, D. O.; Davis, R. H., Jr.; and Szabuniewicz, M. 1974. Prevention of induced ventricular fibrillation in dogs anesthetized with ultrashort-acting barbiturates and halothane. J Am Vet Med Assoc 165:341.

Wilde, J. K. H. 1962. Chloral hydrate anaesthesia in calves. Br Vet J 118:206.

Wilson, J. W., and Graham, T. C. 1971. Acquired hyperreaction to barbiturate anesthesia in cats. Vet Med Small Anim Clin 66:30.

Wolff, W. A.; Davis, R. W.; and Lumb, W. V. 1965. Chloral hydrate-halothane-nitrous oxide anesthesia in deer. J Am Vet Med Assoc 147:1099.

Woods, L. A.; Wyngaarden, J. B.; Rennick, B.; and Seevers, M. H. 1949. Cardiovascular toxicity of thiobarbiturates: Comparison of thiopental and 5-allyl-5-(1-methylbutyl)-2-thiobarbiturate (Surital) in dogs. J Pharmacol Exp Ther 95:328.

Wright, A., and Jordan, F. T. W. 1963. 1-(1-phenylcyclohexyl) piperidine HCl in avian anaesthesia. Vet Rec 75:471.

Wright, J. G., and Hall, L. W. 1961. Veterinary Anaesthesia and Analgesia, 5th ed. Baltimore: Williams & Wilkins.

CHAPTER 14

HYPNOTICS, SEDATIVES, AND ANTICONVULSANTS

NICHOLAS H. BOOTH

Hypnotics and Sedatives
- **Barbital Sodium**
- **Phenobarbital Sodium**
- **Amobarbital Sodium**
- **Secobarbital Sodium**
- **Pentobarbital Sodium**
- **Chloral Hydrate**
- **Sodium Bromide**
- **Paraldehyde**
- **Tribromoethanol**

Motor Depressant Anticonvulsants
- **Phenobarbital**
- **Mephobarbital**
- **Diphenylhydantoin Sodium**
- **Primidone**

Hypnotics are drugs used to moderately depress the central nervous system (CNS) of animals so that they are less responsive to stimuli. The stimulus may be pain, itching, dyspnea, or it may be a form of restraint applied by the veterinarian. Hypnotic drugs in small doses generally exert a a sedative action. A sedative may be used to quiet an animal that is excited by a change in its surroundings or by some unfamiliar procedure such as a rectal or vaginal examination. Hypnotics do not relieve pain but they dull the conscious perception of pain.

Hypnotic and sedative drugs have been used in all species of animals. In the dog, hypnotic and sedative drugs are usually given subcutaneously or orally. In large animals, chloral hydrate is administered orally in capsule or solution as a hypnotic or sedative. When barbiturates are employed in herbivores, they are usually administered intravenously because the large amount of ingesta in the digestive tract would interfere with absorption. Under some circumstances the barbiturates might be injected intraperitoneally.

Any drug that depresses the CNS may be used for its anticonvulsant activity. However, specific drugs are selected and used in the control of epileptiform convulsions.

HYPNOTICS AND SEDATIVES

Barbital Sodium

In 1903 Fischer and von Mering introduced the first of the barbiturates, barbital, under the trade name Veronal. *Barbital Sodium,* N.F. (soluble barbitone, Medinal, Veronal sodium), is still one of the better hypnotics available and is particularly valuable for its prolonged depressive action. Barbital was the first of the barbiturates of clinical value that was synthesized. The sodium salt was soon produced to make the compound water soluble. Numerous other derivatives of barbituric acid have been synthesized and tested on animals. Several have been found suitable for clinical use.

Barbital sodium is used primarily as a a sedative and hypnotic. It has a slightly shorter duration of action than does phenobarbital. Since the anesthetic dose of barbital sodium in the dog (0.09 mg/lb) approached the minimum lethal dose (MLD) (0.11 mg/lb), the use of this drug for anesthesia cannot be recommended (Sharaf 1947). When injected intravenously, barbital sodium tends to paralyze the vital medullary centers too easily to justify its administration by this route. The oral sedative dose of barbital sodium in the dog is 150–1000 mg (2.5–15 grains) daily, depending on the indication and size of the animal. The total oral sedative dose of barbital in the cat is 100–300 mg, and the average lethal dose is 300 mg/kg of body weight (Milks 1949). Barbital and phenobarbital have exceptionally long periods of action in the cat (Clifford and Soma 1969). In the rat, the plasma level of barbital has a biological half-life of 19.3 hours after an intraperitoneal injection of 200 mg/kg of body weight; in contrast, the plasma level of pentobarbital has a biological half-life of only 1.7 hours following an intraperitoneal injection of 30 mg/kg of body weight (Flynn and Spector 1972). In both instances these dosages are essentially equivalent in their CNS depressant effects.

Phenobarbital, which was synthesized several years after barbital, has largely replaced barbital in therapeutic usage.

Phenobarbital Sodium

Phenobarbital Sodium, U.S.P. (soluble phenobarbitone, Luminal sodium), was the second barbituric acid derivative of clinical importance to be developed. It was synthesized in 1912 in Germany and patented under the trade name of Luminal. Phenobarbital was only slightly soluble in water, so a readily soluble sodium salt was soon prepared.

ENZYME INDUCTION

As discussed in Chapter 13, hepatic microsomal enzyme activity is accelerated by phenobarbital. For some unknown reason, the long-acting barbiturates are better inducers of microsomal enzyme activity than the short-acting compounds. If rats are treated with phenobarbital, the weight of their livers is increased (Dollery 1972). An increase occurs in the amount of microsomal protein per g of liver as well as in the content of cytochrome P-450. The result of the increased level of enzyme is a more rapid rate of drug metabolism in treated animals. Treatment with phenobarbital stimulates hepatic drug-metabolizing enzymes in several animals, including swine, sheep, and cattle (Conney and Burns 1972). The administration of low doses of phenobarbital to lactating cows given DDT for several days results in a significant decline in the content of DDT metabolites in the milk (Alary et al. 1971). A 7- to 9-fold increase occurs in the toxicity of carbon tetrachloride after treatment of sheep with phenobarbital and DDT (Seawright et al. 1972). This is an undesirable drug interaction that the veterinarian should avoid if carbon tetrachloride is used for anthelmintic purposes.

Treatment of animals with phenobarbital also increases the activity of microsomal enzymes that hydroxylate estrogens, androgens, progestational steroids, and adrenocortical steroids. The accelerated hydroxylation of the steroidal hormones by microsomal enzymes is influenced *in vivo* by an increased metabolism and altered physiologic action of the steroids. Other compounds such as diphenylhydantoin (Dilantin), chlorcyclizine, phenylbutazone, and several halogenated hydrocarbon pesticides also stimulate steroid hydroxylase activity (Conney and Burns 1972).

Zoxazolamine, a skeletal muscle relaxant, is metabolized by liver microsomal enzymes to an inactive compound. A large dose level of this drug paralyzes the rat for over 11 hours (Conney and Burns 1972). However, if the animals have been pretreated with phenobarbital, they are paralyzed for only a fraction of this time (i.e., about 1.7 hours).

ADMINISTRATION

Phenobarbital sodium is administered extensively by the oral route, but comparatively little by the intravenous route. The oral use of phenobarbital sodium for sedation and hypnosis was well established before the intravenous route was investigated. This tradition plus the availability of short-acting barbiturates has limited phenobarbital sodium to oral administration.

Impens (1912) studied the effects of intravenous injections of phenobarbital sodium in cats, and Gruber and Baskett (1925) conducted a parallel study on dogs. Adams (1944) concluded that intravenous injection of phenobarbital sodium as an anesthetic is of little or no value, whether alone or in combination with another agent. The prolonged recovery from its anesthetic effects is much too long and its use as an anesthetic is hazardous as well as contraindicated. Administered orally, phenobarbital sodium is valuable as a sedative, a hypnotic, and an anticonvulsant. These effects are obtained from safe dosages having no deleterious effect on the body.

DOSAGE

The recommended oral dose depends upon the usage and varies from 30 to 300 mg in the dog and from 15 to 60 mg in the cat. A common dose in a 15- to 25-lb dog is 15 mg (1/4 grain) orally every 6 hours. Some clinicians prefer to use initially a so-called loading dose of 30 mg/20 lb in the dog. This is then followed and maintained with 15 mg/20 lb of body weight every 6–24 hours to attain the effect needed.

CLINICAL USE

Phenobarbital is frequently used for a general sedative effect in nervous, irritable dogs that have to be hospitalized or restrained. It is indicated in dogs suffering from pruritis to depress the itching sensation that results in scratching or even biting, with considerable mechanical damage to the skin. Phenobarbital will serve also as a gastric sedative in small animals. In slightly larger doses, phenobarbital serves as a hypnotic. Its duration of effect exceeds all other common barbiturates. The depressant effect of phenobarbital lasts for about 24 hours, depending upon the dose.

Phenobarbital has a more specific depressant effect upon convulsive seizures than does any other barbiturate. It has long been used in the symptomatic or prophylactic control of the convulsive seizures of chorea or epilepsy. Phenobarbital specifically antagonizes the production of canine hysteria from wheat gluten treated with nitrogen trichloride (Agene) (Radomski and Woodard 1949). Phenobarbital has been used to control convulsive seizures of varied origin, such as from chorea and eclampsia.

Amobarbital Sodium

Amobarbital Sodium, U.S.P. (Amytal sodium) (5-ethyl-5-isoamylbarbituric acid), is metabolized by oxidation to form a 3′-hydroxy metabolite. About 40% of a hypnotic dose of amobarbital is excreted in the urine within 2 days as the hydroxylated metabolite. Very little of the parent compound is excreted unchanged in the urine. Consequently, most of the drug is subjected to biotransformation.

As applied in veterinary practice, amobarbital sodium is used primarily for its hypnotic or sedative action. Since it is an intermediate-acting barbiturate, it is not suitable as a general anesthetic agent in mammals. Because of its longer action, amobarbital has been replaced by pentobarbital and the ultrashort-acting barbiturates.

The dosimetry of amobarbital for sedative or basal anesthetic effect in all species is 2–5 mg/lb of body weight. Except in carnivores and occasional omnivores, the intravenous route of administration is preferred in all animals.

Amobarbital sodium has been used in some species of freshwater and saltwater fish for anesthesia (Keys and Wells 1930). The optimum dosage for fish is 40–54 mg/kg of body weight administered intraperitoneally as a 1% or 2% solution. The duration of anesthesia is 4–18 hours. Anesthesia is complete within 20 minutes after the injection in saltwater fish; the effects in freshwater fish are not very great until after 30 or 90 minutes.

Secobarbital Sodium

The action of *Secobarbital Sodium,* U.S.P. (Seconal sodium) (sodium 5-allyl-5-[1-methylbutyl] barbiturate), resembles that of barbital except that it is more potent and shorter acting. Secobarbital is used primarily as a short-acting hypnotic and sedative in veterinary medicine. It can be used orally in anesthetic dosage but it is better suited to preanesthetic and basal anesthesia.

The oral dosage in dogs and cats varies from about 30 to 200 mg, depending on the purpose and the size of the animal.

Pentobarbital Sodium

The oral and intravenous sedative dose level of *Pentobarbital Sodium,* U.S.P. (Nembutal), for most species is approximately 2 mg/lb of body weight. When pentobarbital sodium is administered intravenously, it requires less than the oral dose and it is given only to the desired effect.

Chloral Hydrate

Chloral Hydrate, U.S.P., is one of the oldest sedatives. Yet it is one of the most dependable drugs used for induction of sedation in large animals. The drug is also used for its hypnotic and anesthetic effect (see Chapter 13).

Chloral hydrate for sedative use may be administered intravenously or orally. Inasmuch as chloral hydrate has a pungent odor and bitter taste, placement of the drug in drinking water is an unsatisfactory way to administer it because most animals will refuse to drink the water. The sedative effects of chloral hydrate have been useful in quieting the horse for shoeing or other procedures lasting 30–60 minutes (Fraser 1967). Administered by the intravenous route, the dose of chloral hydrate is 22.5–30 g/1000 lb of body weight; with the effect being quite rapid, the administration of the drug can be discontinued when the desired effect is attained. By the oral route of administration, 60 g/1000 lb of body weight administered by stomach tube (mix the chloral hydrate in 1 L of warm water) usually produces sedation in 10–15 minutes. If the animal has been fasted the previous night, sedation occurs more rapidly. Tavernor (1961) believes that chloral hydrate can best be used as a sedative in the horse by the oral administration of small dosages (2.5–3.5 g/50 kg). Converted to body weight in lb, this dose range is equivalent to 22.7–31.8 g/1000 lb of body weight. The difference between the dose level recommended by Fraser (1967) and Tavernor (1961) is primarily related to the temperament of the horse; this will vary considerably with the age, breed, sex, and general condition of the animal.

The sedative effects produced by chloral hydrate in the horse are as follows (Fraser 1967): the head droops, the eyes may close, and incoordination of the rear limbs occurs particularly when turning the animal. Recovery from chloral hydrate progressively occurs over a period of 30–60 minutes. Animals that receive large sedative doses may become recumbent. Although it may be an inconvenience, this poses no hazard to the animal. The horse characteristically goes down on its rear limbs first and usually rolls into the lateral recumbent position. The animal should not be forced to stand but should recover and stand of its own volition. Forcing a horse to stand prematurely can lead to considerable floundering and injury to the animal and attending personnel. According to Fraser (1967), chloral hydrate can be used satisfactorily with acetylpromazine. When acetylpromazine is administered following chloral hydrate, the dose level is reduced by one-half.

If *cattle* require sedation prior to local anesthesia for surgery in the standing position, a 7% chloral hydrate solution is given to effect (Gabel 1964). Depending upon the physical condition and temperament of the animal, 150–250 ml of a 7% chloral hydrate solution (10.5–17.5 g) is required intravenously for a cow weighing 1000 lb. In debilitated and sick cattle, a reduced dose should be administered. The dosage administered should not make the animal incoordinated or cause the animal to become recumbent. To determine whether or not the cow has received a sufficient sedative dose of chloral hydrate, the animal is pushed to the side at the tuber coxae; if the animal is easily moved or stumbles, a sufficient dose has been administered without the animal becoming recumbent (Gabel 1964).

Sodium Bromide

The bromide ion depresses both the motor and the sensory areas of the cerebral cortex. It is sedative in action and does not relieve pain significantly. The depressant action of the bromide ion is characteristic only of those inorganic salts releasing the ion, i.e., sodium, potassium, ammonium, and calcium. Various salts, often as mixtures, have been used for many decades for their sedative action upon the cerebral cortex. In recent years the bromides have been largely replaced for this effect by the barbiturates, especially phenobarbital. The sedative action results from the bromide ion and none of the above bromide salts is known to be better than another.

Sodium bromide unfortunately has a slow onset of action, requiring several hours after its administration before an effect occurs. It has been used to calm horses for traveling long distances by surface transportation or to reduce excitation when working around vehicular traffic or crowds of people (Fraser 1967). The drug can be administered in the feed; flavoring with molasses or other appetizer may be necessary to prevent the animal from refusing to eat the mixture. Fraser (1967) recommended a dose of 45 g (1.5 oz)/1000 lb of body weight. The effect is not noted for several hours and its duration of action is about 12 hours. Sodium bromide is administered twice daily to maintain the sedative effect. Use of the sedative in the horse does not appear to affect its normal locomotor activity and no adverse effects occur.

Paraldehyde

Paraldehyde, N.F. ($[CHCH_3]_3O_3$), is a polymer of acetaldehyde formed by three molecules of the latter joining in cyclic structure. Paraldehyde has a wide margin of safety when used in hypnotic doses because it depresses only the cerebrum and not the vital medullary centers. It is not as potent as chloral hydrate but is less toxic. It has little analgesic or anesthetic value. Paraldehyde by rectum has been used widely in human obstetrics.

Tribromoethanol

Tribromoethanol, N.F. (CBr_3CH_2OH), is a white crystalline powder having a slight aromatic odor. The drug is chemically similar to chloral and ethanol. It is a basal anesthetic preparation that decomposes in the presence of light or air. A dose of 135 mg/lb of body weight in a 3% aqueous solution, given rectally, induces deep basal anesthesia in the healthy cat (Wright and Hall 1961). Since the advent of halothane, methoxyflurane, and the ultrashort-acting barbiturates, tribromoethanol is infrequently used in the cat.

MOTOR DEPRESSANT ANTICONVULSANTS

Chorea and various epileptiform disturbances of the CNS in small animals have been treated symptomatically with several drugs, including the bromides.

Phenobarbital

Phenobarbital, U.S.P., specifically depresses the motor centers of the cerebral cortex. Electroshock experiments in cats and in other species establish phenobarbital as one of the most potent anticonvulsants available. Phenobarbital is the only barbiturate that in anesthetic dosage can completely abolish the electrical excitability of the motor cortex in monkeys. It is the least toxic of all antiepileptic drugs. Its action begins within 1–2 hours after administration. Antiepileptic dosage causes more drowsiness and central depression than does diphenylhydantoin. The dose of phenobarbital used for anticonvulsant effect is about 1 mg/lb of body weight administered 2–3 times daily (Redding 1969).

Mephobarbital

Mephobarbital, N.F. (Mebaral, *N*-methylphenobarbital, slowly releases two molecules of phenobarbital by demethylation that depress the motor areas of the cortex and effectively control epileptiform convulsions. Phenobarbital is detectable in plasma for several days after the mephobarbital has disappeared. It is questionable both therapeutically and economically whether mephobarbital should be used instead of phenobarbital, because (1) mephobarbital is expensive, (2) it is poorly absorbed and therefore must be given in large dosage, and (3) conversion to phenobarbital is much more rapid than the rate of elimination of phenobarbital.

Of all the above drugs with an anticonvulsant action, phenobarbital sodium is probably used more extensively than any other in veterinary medicine.

Diphenylhydantoin Sodium

Diphenylhydantoin Sodium, U.S.P. (Dilantin sodium), depresses the motor areas of the cortex (antiepileptic action) without depressing the sensory areas. It is not a general anticonvulsant, as is phenobarbital, and is not used for emergency treatment of poisoning by convulsant drugs or tetanic seizures. It is administered orally only and is easily absorbed. Anticonvulsant activity occurs only after accumulation of the drug from a series of doses. It has a wide margin of safety and is successful in preventive treatment of severe epileptic seizure in the dog.

The chemical structure of diphenylhydantoin (Fig. 14.1) is quite similar to diazepam, a psychotropic agent. Diazepam is also used in the treatment of status epilepticus in the dog (see Chapter 17). Diphenylhydantoin has been approved for use in the dog by the Food and Drug Administration (FDA).

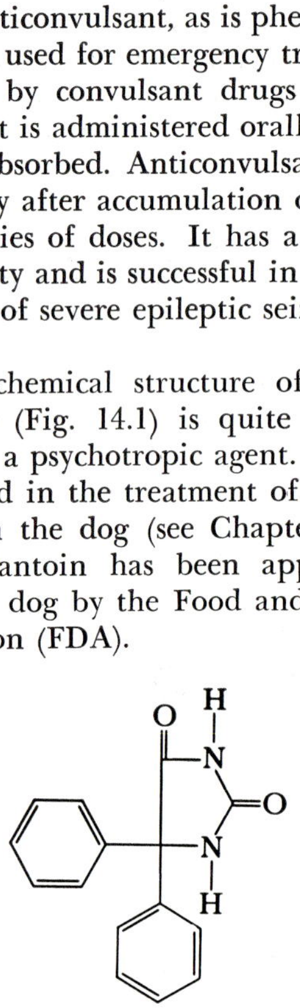

Diphenylhydantoin

Fig. 14.1.

Pharmacologic Activity

Diphyenylhydantoin produces a stabilizing effect upon synaptic junctions that ordinarily allow nerve impulses to be readily transmitted at lower thresholds. Consequently, the level of synaptic excitability that permits impulses to be transmitted easily is reduced and/or stabilized. This stabilizing effect appears to be associated with the active extrusion of the Na^+ from neurons and a decrease of posttetanic potentiation or spread of nerve impulses to adjacent neurons. A reduction in spread of the "burst" activity associated with epilepsy prevents the genesis of the cortical seizure. The activity of diphenylhydantoin in stabilizing hyperexcitable neurons so epileptic seizure does not develop occurs without causing general depression of the CNS (Toman 1970).

Diphenylhydantoin becomes bound to the plasma proteins of a number of species (Baggot and Davis 1973). The percentage of diphenylhydantoin bound to plasma proteins decreases in the rabbit and in the ruminant, dog, cat, pig, and horse. Only a 10% difference exists in the binding of diphenylhydantoin between human beings and the pony (Baggot and Davis 1973).

It has been known for almost three decades that diphenylhydantoin has a long duration of action in the cat. This prolonged anticonvulsant effect in the cat is due to the long plasma half-life (ca. 41.5 hours) of the drug in this species (Tobin et al. 1973). A plasma half-life of 108 hours, following the oral administration of diphenylhydantoin (10 mg/kg) in the cat, has been reported (Roye et al. 1973). In the dog, despite relatively large single daily doses of diphenylhydantoin (50 mg/kg) administered orally, the plasma concentration of the drug was low. Paralleling this observation, the plasma half-life of a single 50-mg/kg dose of diphenylhydantoin in the dog is only 6–7.8 hours (Dayton et al. 1967). Roye et al. (1973) found the plasma half-life was 4–6 hours after an intramuscular injection of diphenylhydantoin (50 mg/kg). The apparent discrepancy between the results of these two studies may be due to pretreatment of the dogs for 9 days with diphenylhydantoin by Roye et al. (1973). Induction of hepatic microsomal enzyme activity may have accounted for this shorter plasma half-life of diphenylhydantoin. The long plasma half-life of diphenylhydantoin probably explains the prolonged antiepileptic effect of the drug and prolonged effect upon the brain. In addition to long exposure of the brain to levels of the drug, high concentrations (3 times the level in blood) accumulate in the liver. Also, high concentrations of diphenylhydantoin appear in cardiac, renal, pulmonic, and adipose tissues.

Another logical reason for the long duration of action of diphenylhydantoin in animals is the very slow clearance of the drug by the kidney. The marked affinity of the drug for plasma proteins undoubtedly is largely responsible for this effect. In addition, the prolonged effect observed in the cat over some of the other species may also be related to the inability of the cat to conjugate compounds with glucuronic acid. Diphenylhydantoin is excreted after the formation of a hydroxylated derivative and conjugation with glucuronic acid or sulfate. The inability of the cat to conjugate aspirin and salicylate compounds with glucuronic acid also results in a slow detoxification rate and prolonged effect from these compounds (see Chapter 16).

In the chicken, rickets, hypocalcemia, decreased duodenal calcium transport, and the reduction of calcium binding protein have been produced in birds treated with diphenylhydantoin (Villareale et al. 1974). These findings suggest that close attention should be given to the calciferol intake in patients requiring epileptic seizure treatment. Calciferol metabolism apparently is altered by diphenylhydantoin, which in turn leads to a functional vitamin D deficiency.

The pleasure-type behavioral response of the cat to nepetalactones in catnip *(Nepeta cataria)* is blocked by pretreatment with diphenylhydantoin (Hatch 1972). The response is blocked for more than 4 weeks after the drug is administered and then it gradually returns. Why this effect involves olfactory acuity and possibly other neurophysiological mechanisms associated with the action of diphenylhydantoin remains unclear.

In laboratory mice, a single dose of diphenylhydantoin administered to pregnant animals on the 9th–14th day of gestation produces various fetal anomalies (Harbison and Becker 1969). Also, fetal growth and embryolethal effects were reported. However, the intraperitoneal dose required to produce this teratogenic effect in mice was exceedingly large (150 mg/kg). The teratogenic effect in the dog from the use of diphenylhydantoin has not been identified or reported in veterinary literature. Diphenylhydantoin also has cardiac antiarrhythmic properties and is useful in correcting or preventing clinical arrhythmias (see Chapter 24).

DRUG INTERACTIONS

Diphenylhydantoin and phenobarbital are used in combination for the treatment of epilepsy in both human beings and dogs. At present the combined use of diphenylhydantoin and phenobarbital is considered optimal therapy for epilepsy in human beings. The therapeutic rationale of this combination has not been clearly established (Morselli et al. 1971). Use of both drugs is particularly questioned because phenobarbital induces hepatic microsomal enzyme activity that accelerates the metabolism (i.e., hydroxylation) of diphenylhydantoin. In addition, diphenylhydantoin is an enzyme inducer that speeds up the metabolism or hydroxylation of phenobarbital. This "see-saw" effect in the metabolism of both drugs is apparently involved during the course of treatment. Yet, despite the interaction between the two compounds, they appear to work satisfactorily in the prevention of epileptic seizures.

The inhibition of diphenylhydantoin metabolism by other drugs has been observed in human beings. Prolongation of the effect of diphenylhydantion has been reported following the simultaneous administration of dicoumarol, chloramphenicol, phenylbutazone, and the phenothiazines. Also, *in vitro* inhibition of diphenylhydantoin metabolism has been noted in the presence of diazepam and propoxyphene. The significance of this *in vivo* has not been determined.

The metabolism of a number of chemicals or drugs is enhanced by diphenylhydantoin. These include digitoxin, dexamethasone, DDT, dieldrin, and cortisol (Conney and Burns 1972).

BLOOD LEVELS AND ASSOCIATED TOXICITY

In human beings, clinical therapeutic effects and intoxication are related to the blood level of diphenylhydantoin (Kutt 1971). According to Kutt, a reduction in the number of seizures occurs when diphenylhydantoin blood levels exceed 10 μg/ml. This level (i.e., 10 μg/ml) is an average achieved following the oral administration of the commonly used adult daily dose of 300 mg. Assuming that the drug kinetics for the attainment of a blood level in a 7-kg dog are comparable to those of a 70-kg person, the human dose of diphenylhydantoin would be equivalent to 30 mg/7 kg or 1.2 mg/lb of body weight/day in the dog. Actually, an initial oral dose of 1–2 mg/lb of body weight, 4 times daily, is suggested for the dosages of diphenylhydantoin in the dog. The blood level of diphenylhydantoin required to reduce or prevent seizures in the dog is unknown. However, it probably is similar to the level required in human beings.

In human beings, mild signs of intoxication, such as nystagmus, develop with blood levels of 20 μg/ml; patients with levels over 40 μg/ml have marked nystagmus and are incoordinated and lethargic (Kutt 1971). Blood levels in the dog would probably have to increase a comparable 100%–400% as in human beings before serious signs of intoxication develop.

CLINICAL USE IN THE TREATMENT OF GRAND MAL, PSYCHOMOTOR, AND FOCAL SEIZURES

Diphenylhydantoin is approved for use by the FDA in the dog for the control of epileptiform convulsions. An initial oral dose of 4–8 mg/lb of body weight in divided doses is suggested with the dose then gradually increased or decreased to the daily minimum required to maintain control or prevention of the convulsive seizure. The above dose range for diphenylhydantoin is generally divided into 3 or 4 doses per day.

Several days are required to achieve a sufficient anticonvulsant level of diphenylhydantoin at the suggested or recommended clinical dosages. A typical initial dose in the dog is 2 mg/lb orally, 4 times daily, progressively increased if necessary until seizures are controlled or toxicity supervenes. Transition from other anticonvulsant drugs, e.g., from phenobarbital to diphenylhydantoin, should be gradual. A sudden discontinuance of therapy, including withdrawal of phenobarbital, should be avoided to properly control the likelihood of the development of seizures.

According to Oliver and Hoerlein (1965), three basic drugs form the "backbone" of medical therapy in epilepsy. They are phenobarbital, diphenylhydantoin, and primidone. It is preferable to initiate the therapy with phenobarbital, then increase the dosage until the sedative effect is attained. Oliver and Hoerlein (1965) emphasized that the anticonvulsive effects produced by phenobarbital occur at a level far below that necessary for sedation. In the event phenobarbital therapy fails to control the seizures, diphenylhydantoin is added to the regimen in gradually increasing dosages until control is successfully attained. Should the seizures continue, primidone is then included in the treatment (see the last part of this chapter for the suggested dosage schedule). With the addition of primidone, reduced dosages of phenobarbital and diphenylhydantoin may be necessary to elevate the level of primidone for effective control of the seizure. The principal side effects noted from this therapeutic procedure are oversedation and ataxia.

Since diphenylhydantoin requires several days for the blood levels to reach therapeutic proportions, Oliver and Hoerlein (1965) also caution against changing the medication too rapidly. *Reserpine* and the *phenothiazine* tranquilizers are considered to be *contraindicated* in the treatment of epileptic conditions because they can induce seizures.

CLINICAL USE IN THE TREATMENT OF STATUS EPILEPTICUS

Treatment of status epilepticus in the dog is regarded as an emergency (Oliver and Hoerlein 1965). It is known that death or permanent neurologic deficit can occur if the seizures persist too long. Immediate intravenous administration of pentobarbital sodium is considered to be the most efficacious procedure for abolishing the seizure (Redding 1969). However, the animal's tolerance for barbiturates from microsomal enzyme activity may have developed from previous treatments of seizure. After the seizures have been abolished, maintenance therapy consists of the intramuscular injection of barbiturates or intravenous medication with diphenylhydantoin. The dose level of diphenylhydantoin for treatment of status epilepticus is essentially similar to that discussed above in the treatment of other forms of epileptic seizures. Six to 8 hours are necessary for the complete effect to occur following the administration of diphenylhydantoin. Consequently, barbiturates will need to be continued during this time (Oliver and Hoerlein 1965). As the medication is reduced to enable the dog to regain consciousness, oral medication is continued.

PRIMIDONE

Primidone, U.S.P. (Mylepsin, Mysoline) (5-phenyl-5-ethylhexahydropyrimidine-4, 6-dione) (Fig. 14.2), is a close congener of phenobarbital (Goodman et al. 1953). The drug is a white, crystalline, tasteless substance.

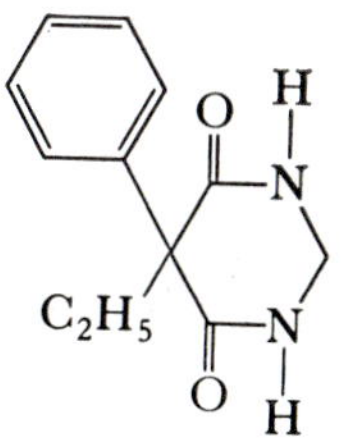

C_2H_5 O H N N O H

Primidone

FIG. 14.2.

Primidone is approved by the FDA for use in the dog for the control of convulsions associated with true epilepsy, epileptiform seizures, virus encephalitis, distemper, and "hardpad" disease.

PHARMACOLOGIC ACTIVITY

Primidone is much less neurotoxic in mice and rats than phenobarbital (Goodman et al. 1953). A dose of the magnitude of 20 times that of phenobarbital is necessary to produce a comparable degree of neurotoxicity (Bogue and Carrington 1953). Although primidone is less potent than phenobarbital as a general CNS depressant, primidone is more potent than phenobarbital in the protection of animals against maximal seizures induced by electroshock and pentylenetetrazol. Primidone is more toxic in cats or rabbits than in rats or mice (Goodman et al. 1953).

CLINICAL USE

Primidone was used in veterinary medicine for the control of convulsive seizures in the dog soon after it was introduced into human medicine for clinical use (Archibald 1953; Lambert 1953). The use of primidone in conjunction with diphenylhydantoin was previously discussed. According to Oliver and Hoerlein (1965), primidone has been the most effective agent in the dog for the control of seizures, particularly those associated with postdistemper convulsions. Inasmuch as the effectiveness of anticonvulsant therapy declines from prolonged medication possibly due to the development of tolerance (probably related to microsomal enzyme induction), primidone is recommended for use as a last resort. This procedure is followed because clinical experience has revealed that once the seizure of a dog cannot be controlled with primidone, none of the other anticonvulsants is likely to be any better (Oliver and Hoerlein 1965).

Primidone is administered orally at a daily dose level of 25 mg/lb of body weight. The daily dose should be divided and administered at intervals that best control the convulsive seizures according to good clinical judgment. The primidone tablets may be administered directly to the dog; the tablet can be placed inside a small meat ball, or the tablet can be pulverized for placement in or upon food. If convulsions develop only every few days, or less frequently, the daily dosimetry should be administered at one time. It is recommended that the reduction in dosage be made gradually and therapy should never be discontinued abruptly.

REFERENCES

Adams, R. C. 1944. Intravenous Anesthesia. London: Paul B. Hoeber.

Alary, J.-G.; Guay, P.; and Brodeur, J. 1971. Effect of phenobarital pretreatment on the metabolism of DDT in the rat and the bovine. Toxicol Appl Pharmacol 18:457.

Archibald, J. 1953. Clinical trials of Mysoline, a new anticonvulsant drug. North Am Vet 34:870.

Baggot, J. D., and Davis, L. E. 1973. Comparative study of plasma protein binding of diphenylhydantoin. Comp Gen Pharmacol 4:399.

Bogue, J. Y., and Carrington, H. C. 1953. The evaluation of "Mysoline"—A new anticonvulsant drug. Br J Pharmacol 8:230.

Clifford, D. H., and Soma, L. R. 1969. Feline anesthesia. Fed Proc 28:1479.

Conney, A. H., and Burns, J. J. 1972. Metabolic interactions among environmental chemicals and drugs. Science 178:576.

Dayton, P. G.; Cucinell, S. A.; Weiss, M.; and Perel, J. M. 1967. Dose dependence of drug plasma level decline in dogs. J Pharmacol Exp Ther 158:305.

Dollery, C. T. 1972. Enzyme induction. Br J Anaesth 44:961.

Flynn, E. J., and Spector, S. 1972. Determination of bariturate derivatives by radioimmunoassay. J Pharmacol Exp Ther 181: 547.

Fraser, A. C. 1967. Restraint in the horse. Vet Rec 80:56.

Gabel, A. A. 1964. Practical technics for bovine anesthesia. Mod Vet Pract 45:39.

Goodman, L. S.; Swineyard, E. A.; Brown, W. C.; Schiffman, D. O.; Grewal, M. S.; and Bliss, E. L. 1953. Anticonvulsant properties of 5-phenyl-5-ethylhexahydropyrimidine-4, 6-dione (Mysoline), a new antiepileptic. J Pharmacol Exp Ther 108:428.

Gruber, C. M., and Baskett, R. F. 1925. I. The effect of phenobarital (Luminal) and sodium phenobarbital (Luminal sodium) upon blood pressure and respiration. J Pharmacol Exp Ther 25:219.

Harbison, R. D., and Becker, B. A. 1969. Relation of dosage and time of administration of diphenylhydantoin to its teratogenic effect in mice. Teratology 2:305.

Hatch, R. C. 1972. Effects of drugs on catnip *(Nepeta cataria)*-induced pleasure behavior in cats. Am J Vet Res 33:143.

Impens, E. 1912. Pharmakologisches über Luminal oder Phenyläthylbarbitursäure. Dtsch Med Wochenschr 1:945. (Quoted in Adams, R. C. 1944. Intravenous Anesthesia. London: Paul B. Hoeber.)

Keys, A. B., and Wells, N. A. 1930. Amytal anesthesia in fishes. J Pharmacol Exp Ther 40:115.

Kutt, H. 1971. Biochemical and genetic factors regulating Dilantin metabolism in man. Ann NY Acad Sci 179:704.

Lambert, N. H. 1953. Some experiences with "Mysoline" in dogs. Vet Rec 65:123.

Milks, H. J. 1949. Practical Veterinary Pharmacology, Materia Medica and Therapeutics, 4th ed., p. 188. Chicago: Alex Eger.

Morselli, P. L.; Rizzo, M.; and Garattini, S. 1971. Interaction between phenobarbital and diphenylhydantoin in animals and in epileptic patients. Ann NY Acad Sci 179: 88.

Oliver, J. E., Jr., and Hoerlein, B. F. 1965. Convulsive disorders of dogs. J Am Vet Med Assoc 146:1126.

Radomski, J. L., and Woodard, G. 1949. Pharmacological studies on the causative agent of canine hysteria. J Pharmacol Exp Ther 95:429.

Redding, R. W. 1969. The diagnosis and therapy of seizures. J Am Anim Hosp Assoc 5:79.

Roye, D. B.; Serrano, E. E.; Hammer, R. H.; and Wilder, B. J. 1973. Plasma kinetics of diphenylhydantoin in dogs and cats. Am J Vet Res 34:947.

Seawright, A. A.; Steele, D. P.; Mudie, A. W.; and Bishop, R. 1972. The effect of diet and drugs on hepatic microsomal aminopyrine N-demethylase activity *in vitro* and susceptibility to carbon tetrachloride in sheep. Res Vet Sci 13:245.

Sharaf, A. E. A. 1947. Medical (soluble Veronal) hypnosis anaesthesia and toxicity in dogs. Vet J 103: 358.

Tavernor, W. D. 1961. Equine anaesthesia. Br Vet J 117:392.

Tobin, T.; Dirdjosudjono, S.; and Baskin, S. I. 1973. Pharmacokinetics and distribution of diphenylhydantoin in kittens. Am J Vet Res 34:951.

Toman, J. E. P. 1970. Drugs effective in convulsive disorders. In L. S. Goodman and A. Gilman, eds. The Pharamacological

Basis of Therapeutics, 4th ed., p. 204. New York: Macmillan.

Villareale, M.; Gould, L. V.; Wasserman, R. H.; Barr, A.; Chiroff, R. T.; and Bergstrom, W. H. 1974. Diphenylhydantoin: Effects on calcium metabolism in the chick. Science 183:671.

Wright, J. G., and Hall, L. W. 1961. Veterinary Anaesthesia and Analgesia, 5th ed. Baltimore: Williams & Wilkins.

CHAPTER 15

NEUROLEPTANALGESICS, NARCOTIC ANALGESICS, AND ANALGESIC ANTAGONISTS

NICHOLAS H. BOOTH

The analgesic drugs play an important role in the practice of veterinary medicine and have increasing importance in laboratory animal medicine. Guidelines were issued January 1975 by the U.S. Department of Agriculture (USDA), which has the responsibility for enforcing the U.S. Animal Welfare Act, to assure the appropriate use of pain-relieving drugs by biomedical research laboratories. The regulations of the act place a considerable amount of responsibility upon the attending doctor of veterinary medicine in assuring the appropriate use of analgesic agents in experimental animals.

Within the last decade, new analgesic agents such as fentanyl, oxymorphone, etorphine, and others have been introduced for use in animals. These agents are important in the alleviation of pain and they are valuable in facilitating restraint and handling of animals. The increasing practice of combining an analgesic agent with neuroleptic drugs (droperidol and the phenothiazine tranquilizers) has expanded the number of preparations that the veterinarian can use for neuroleptanalgesic purposes. The older analgesics such as morphine, codeine, meperidine, and others still have an important use in clinical practice; they will be discussed in the latter part of the chapter along with the narcotic antagonists.

NEUROLEPTANALGESICS

The term neuroleptanalgesia is derived from two words, i.e., neurolepsia and analgesia. When the combination of droperidol (a neuroleptic or tranquilizing agent) and fentanyl (analgesic agent) as well as comparable agents were first administered in human beings to induce psychomotor sedation (neurolepsia) and analgesia, the genesis of this term evolved.

DROPERIDOL-FENTANYL CITRATE (INNOVAR-VET)

Droperidol is classified as a neuroleptic, tranquilizer, or psychotropic agent. A discussion of this agent has been presented in Chapter 17 under the heading of butyrophenone derivatives. The chemical structure of droperidol is also included in

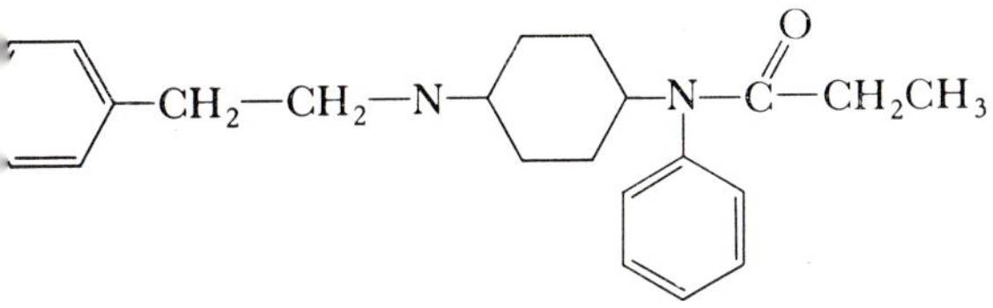

$-CH_2-CH_2-N-$ ... $-N-C(=O)-CH_2CH_3$

Fentanyl

FIG. 15.1.

Chapter 17; the chemical structure of *fentanyl* is shown in Fig. 15.1.

Droperidol is not available for use as a single agent but is available only in combination with fentanyl citrate. The combination of droperidol:fentanyl is in a 50:1 ratio. Each cc of the mixture contains 20 mg of droperidol and 0.4 mg of fentanyl citrate. The pH is adjusted to 3.1 ± 0.4 with lactic acid. By virtue of the fentanyl citrate component in this preparation, it is a Schedule II drug subject to the Controlled Substances Act of 1970.

Fentanyl is an analgesic with a potency of about 100 times that of an equivalent quantity of morphine. Droperidol does not produce analgesia but is a potent neuroleptic agent. Yelnosky and Gardocki (1964) suggest that each compound in the droperidol-fentanyl mixture exerts its own pharmacologic actions without any well-defined antagonistic or potentiating interactions. However, there is one exception; droperidol does enhance the analgesic potency of fentanyl through a potentiative rather than an additive effect. The mechanism of this potentiating effect is unknown.

In human beings, the combination of droperidol and fentanyl (Innovar) is administered to induce psychomotor sedation (neurolepsia) and analgesia. The primary objective underlying the principle of neuroleptanalgesia is to provide a method of anesthesia for major operations and to avoid the severe central nervous system (CNS), cardiovascular, and metabolic depressant effects of conventional anesthetics (Tornetta and Wilson 1969). In veterinary medicine, the combination of droperidol and fentanyl (Innovar-Vet) has been approved by the Food and Drug Administration (FDA) for use only in the dog for various clinical procedures requiring analgesia and tranquilization.

SIDE EFFECTS

Adverse effects of droperidol and fentanyl are dose related and are encountered most frequently at maximum therapeutic or high dosages (Krahwinkel et al. 1972). Bradycardia and respiratory depression, with occasional tachypnea, salivation, and defecation frequently observed within 10 minutes after intramuscular injection, are induced by the fentanyl component of the combination (Gardocki and Yelnosky 1964). Atropine sulfate administered subcutaneously (0.02 mg/lb) 15 minutes prior to droperidol and fentanyl minimizes or prevents the bradycardia and controls other autonomic effects related to the parasympathetic system.

If droperidol and fentanyl are used alone in the dog, the animal can be aroused at any point during a minor surgical procedure; loud noises often elicit an involuntary "startled" movement when the dog has not received adjunctive general anesthesia (Franklin and Reid 1965). Occasionally, an animal may exhibit convulsive seizures but this is not the usual response at lower dosage levels (Krahwinkel et al. 1972).

It has been reported that the Australian terrier may not properly respond to the droperidol-fentanyl mixture. However, Dorn (1972) reported that there was no appreciable difference in the response of this breed from that of other breeds. A side effect that he observed, which had not been previously reported in this breed, was muscular tremor and twitching; this effect did not appear to influence the duration of neuroleptanalgesia. Other side effects seen in the Australian terrier were excessive salivation, diarrhea, and bradycardia. Dorn (1972) reported that fentanyl-droperidol should never be administered without atropine as a preanesthetic agent.

Other side effects noted in the dog include nystagmuslike activity of the eyes. Also, some discomfort is manifested following an intramuscular injection of the drug combination, and whining may occur after an intravenous injection. The discomfort produced may be due to the effect of the low pH (i.e., 3.1 ± 0.4) of the droperidol-fentanyl mixture (Leash et al. 1973). In the guinea pig, Leash and associates reported that swelling, lameness, and self-mutilation of the injected leg developed several days to 1 week later in 33% of the animals. The intramuscular dose that produced this effect was 0.88 ml/kg; despite the excellent anesthesia, it was concluded that the intramuscular injection of the drug into guinea pigs at this dose level cannot be recommended.

CONTRAINDICATIONS

Droperidol and fentanyl must not be used in food-producing animals. Although its use has been approved by the FDA only in the dog, the drug combination is used in a number of species (see Table 15.1). Because of its undesirable central nervous stimulant effects in cats, horses, and ruminants, droperidol-fentanyl is not recommended. In cesarean section, it is recommended that droperidol-fentanyl not be used with barbiturates because this may be hazardous to the neonate; use with inhalant anesthetics is considered to be a much safer procedure.

TABLE 15.1. Summarization of the intramuscular dosage levels of droperidol-fentanyl for induction of neuroleptanalgesia in laboratory animals

Species	Dose*	Reference
	(ml/kg)	
Mouse	0.002–0.005†	Lewis and Jennings 1972
Rat	0.016–0.02‡	Jones and Simmons 1968; Thayer et al. 1972
Guinea pig§	0.66–0.88	Rubright and Thayer 1970
Rabbit	0.22	Strack and Kaplan 1968
Hamster	0.01–0.016‡	Moller 1968
Primates	0.0275–0.22	Field et al. 1966
Opossum	0.5	Feldman and Self 1971

Source: Leash et al. 1973.

* Each ml of the combination contains 0.4 mg of fentanyl and 20 mg of droperidol.

† The fentanyl-droperidol mixture was diluted to 10% in physiological saline and administered in ml/g of body weight.

‡ Administered as ml/100 g of body weight.

§ A dose level of 0.88 ml/kg produces swelling and lameness and cannot be recommended.

CLINICAL USE

Atropine sulfate should be administered subcutaneously (0.02 mg/lb) 15 minutes prior to droperidol and fentanyl to prevent bradycardia and salivation.

In the Dog. In a clinical study by Franklin and Reid (1965), which included most of the major breeds of dogs varying in age from 6 weeks to 16 years and in weight from 3 to 150 lb, intramuscular dose levels of fentanyl-droperidol of 1 ml/20 lb (0.11 ml/kg) and, in a few instances, 1 ml/15 lb (0.146 ml/kg) or 1 ml/40 lb (0.055 ml/kg) were used in 567 animals. The drug combination was used either alone or in conjunction with local or general anesthesia. When the neuroleptanalgesic preparation is used with either thiamylal or methoxyflurane, induction is smooth, muscular relaxation is marked, and recovery time is shortened and free of an excitatory phase (Franklin and Reid 1965). The amount of thiamylal necessary to induce and maintain general anesthesia is decreased 80%–90%.

The use of droperidol-fentanyl in cesarean sections does not produce neonatal depression in puppies when used alone or when it is used with 1% procaine (Franklin and Reid 1965). If supplemental analgesia is necessary during a cesarean section beyond 30–40 minutes, an additional dose of droperidol and fentanyl from one-half to the full dose can be administered to maintain analgesia.

The dose levels[1] recommended in the dog for analgesia and tranquilization are as follows:

Route of Administration	*Weight of Animal (lb)*	*Dose Level*
Intramuscular	15–20	1 cc
Intravenous	25–60	1 cc

1. Each cc contains 20 mg of droperidol and 0.4 mg of fentanyl citrate.

Dosages recommended in the dog for general anesthesia are as follows:

Route of Administration	*Dose Level*	*Follow-up Procedure*
Intramuscular	1 cc/ 40 lb	After 10 min give pentobarbital sodium (3 mg/lb) i.v.
Intravenous	1 cc/ 25–60 lb	Within 15 sec give pentobarbital sodium (3 mg/lb) i.v.

Some clinicians prefer to deviate from the procedure described above in the use of droperidol and fentanyl. In addition to the use of atropine sulfate recommended for premedication, pentobarbital sodium (Nembutal) is considered a useful preanesthetic preparation (Krahwinkel et al. 1972). A dose level of 2–3 mg/lb is administered intramuscularly 15 minutes prior to droperidol and fentanyl. Pentobarbital produces a mild sedation and tends to reduce the undesirable effects of droperidol and fentanyl such as muscle tremors, convulsions, and responses to noise.

In the recent literature, nitrous oxide (50%–70%) with oxygen is considered to be an excellent anesthetic for concurrent administration with droperidol and fentanyl (Krahwinkel et al. 1972). This procedure produces muscle relaxation and anesthesia that cannot be provided by the sole use of droperidol and fentanyl; also, the stabilization of cardiovascular function makes this approach well suited for the poor-risk or shock-prone patient.

Inhalant anesthetics such as halothane or methoxyflurane may be used in conjunction with droperidol and fentanyl (Krahwinkel et al. 1972). It is advisable to use these agents cautiously and at reduced levels to prolong or increase the depth of anesthesia. Moreover, small dosages of the thiobarbiturates may be used to supplement or maintain general anesthesia to produce the desired effect.

In Laboratory Animals. For the summarization of dosages of droperidol and fentanyl recommended in laboratory animals see Table 15.1.

DURATION OF EFFECT AND RECOVERY

At the dose level (0.11 cc/kg) recommended for the dog by the intramuscular route, analgesia lasts 30–40 minutes (Soma and Shields 1964); this produces sufficient neuroleptanalgesia for minor surgical procedures lasting no longer than this period. The majority of dogs regain their righting and mobility functions within 2 hours following the administration of droperidol-fentanyl. However, most animals will appear tranquilized and will remain quiet for several hours unless they are agitated or disturbed. Following the recommended dosage for intravenous administration, the majority of dogs recover from the principal effects of the drug preparation in about 1.5 hours.

TREATMENT OF OVERDOSAGE

Overdosage due to the excessive administration of droperidol and fentanyl that leads to tremors, rigidity of the neck, and tonoclonic convulsions may be antagonized by an intravenous dose of pentobarbital sodium (3 mg/lb). Also, nalorphine (Nalline) has been used to reverse the action of fentanyl citrate in the dog. A dose of 1 mg/kg administered intravenously was capable of antagonizing the lethal effect of 2–7 mg/kg of fentanyl citrate (Gardocki et al. 1964). In addition, *n*-allylnoroxymorphone (Naloxone) has been used intravenously at a dose of 0.4 mg for each 0.4 mg of fentanyl citrate (Franklin and Reid 1965). Nalorphine and *n*-allylnoroxymorphone do not have an effect in reversing the action of droperidol.

Etorphine and Neuroleptic Combinations

In 1973 etorphine hydrochloride and its antagonist, diprenorphine hydrochloride, were approved by the FDA for immobilization of wild and exotic animals. These agents must not be used in animals, domestic or wild, intended for human consumption or in animals that might be used

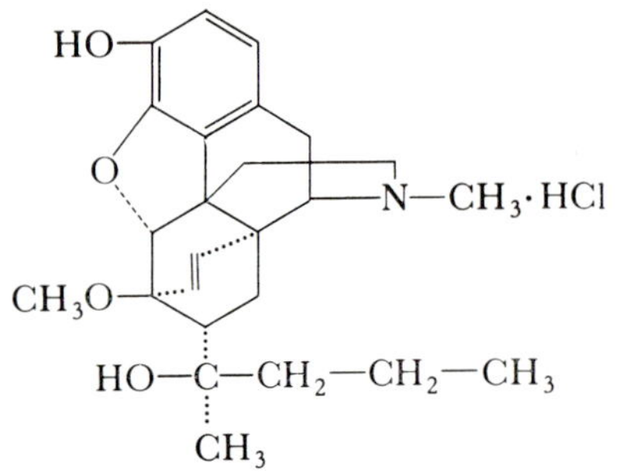

Etorphine

FIG. 15.2.

for food during the hunting season. Both etorphine and diprenorphine are subject to the Controlled Substances Act of 1970 and are classified as Schedule II drugs.

Etorphine, alone or in combination with a neuroleptic agent (primarily acetylpromazine), has been used primarily for immobilization of various domestic and exotic species in Europe, Africa, and other countries.

ETORPHINE HYDROCHLORIDE

Etorphine Hydrochloride (M-99, oripavine) is a semisynthetic opiate derivative having up to 10,000 times the analgesic potency of morphine (Harthoorn 1965a). It has been referred to as M-99 Reckitt and/or oripavine and chemically is 6, 14-endoetheno-7α-(2-hydroxy-2-pentyl)-tetrahydrooripavine hydrochloride (Fig. 15.2).

USE IN EXOTIC SPECIES

In the early 1960s, Dr. A. M. Harthoorn began using etorphine for field investigations in the immobilization and capture of exotic species (Harthoorn 1965b), and for over a decade etorphine has been used extensively in the field of animal conservation (Harthoorn 1972). According to Harthoorn, the principal uses are:

1. Ecological work involving identification, weighing, examination, and sampling of wild animals.
2. Translocation of rare and valuable species to areas of minimum conflict with human beings.
3. Humane capture of animals for zoological gardens and parks.
4. Physiological and biochemical studies.
5. Diagnostic work such as blood sampling and examination for lesions of disease such as foot-and-mouth disease.
6. Direct therapeutic and surgical interference to injured and incapacitated animals.

The potency of etorphine is extremely impressive. One mg is capable of immobilizing a rhinoceros weighing approximately 2000 kg; this is equivalent to 0.5 μg/kg of body weight. A dose level of 4 mg is capable of immobilizing an African elephant weighing about 5000 kg; this amounts to less than 1 μg/kg (Harthoorn and Bligh 1965).

Immediately following the injection of animals with projectile equipment containing etorphine, acetylpromazine, and hyoscine, nervous animals (sable antelope) will run with the herd for variable distances; other animals such as the zebra may trot or walk for only a few yards (Harthoorn and Bligh 1965). The first effects noted following the adminstration of etorphine, acetylpromazine, and hyoscine usually occur within 3–4 minutes. Slight ataxia and the predilection of the affected animal to move from the herd are characteristic. After these effects are apparent, the opportunity to track the animal without losing it is favorable; progress of the animal becomes erratic and consists in circling about.

As the effects of the etorphine mixture progressively increase, the posture and gait of the animal appear to be similar to the effect of morphine (Harthoorn and Bligh 1965). The forelimbs are lifted high at every step, and steps become shorter. The head of some animals, such as the giraffe, is carried far back so that visual capability is impaired. Often the animal may stop when it comes in contact with a bush or tree. Visual accommodation is lost from the effect of etorphine and hyoscine. At this stage, the animal may be captured by seizing an ear or horn because it will approach a stationary person. Any overt movement by a person is readily detected and may cause the animal to run for several yards before returning to a walk. Also, auditory perceptivity remains acute; alarming noises will initiate an immediate flight response (Harthoorn and Bligh 1965).

With the increased absorption of the drug mixture, or when large doses are given, most animals stand with their heads down. Often they will find an object to lean on. Sometimes, animals such as the antelope lie down in sternal recumbency and, if aroused, are usually able to stand voluntarily. It is rare for an animal to assume the lateral recumbent position and this occurs only after the administration of excessive dosages. The normal behavior of wild animals involves curiosity, which is counterbalanced by apprehension and fear. However, under the effects of the etorphine mixture, the elements of apprehension and fear are abolished, leaving the element of curiosity unaffected. According to Harthoorn and Bligh (1965), affected animals will circle and approach a vehicle close enough to be captured by a passenger's hand extended through the window. With capture of the animal, resistance is rarely attempted and the majority of animals will stand quietly when held by an ear or horn. Animals such as the zebra and rhino will permit one to sit on their backs while unrestrained but under the effects of etorphine.

Most animals injected with the etorphine mixture do not lie down unless excessive dosages are administered. This has the advantage that the standing animal can be more easily seen in "short" grass 3–4 feet high). If the animal goes down, it usually assumes sternal recumbency. This is important in ruminants because they will regurgitate ruminal contents and aspirate the contents into the trachea during lateral recumbency but not in the sternal recumbent position. Moreover, the sternal recumbent position permits the eructation of gas from the rumen so bloating does not occur despite abolition of ruminal contractability by etorphine (Harthoorn and Bligh 1965).

The action of etorphine can be antagonized or reversed by nalorphine or diprenorphine (cyprenorphine, nororipavine, M-285, M50-50). Used by itself in exotic species, the intramuscular dose levels of etorphine hydrochloride that usually result in rapid immobilization, sedation, and analgesia are as follows (Alford et al. 1974):

Species Classification	*Dose (mg/100 lb)*
Equidae (Mongolian horse, zebra)	0.44
Ursidae (black, grizzly, polar bear)	0.5
Cervidae (fallow deer, moose)	0.98
Bovidae (antelope, bighorn sheep)	0.09

According to Harthoorn (1966), the dose of etorphine for most exotic animals is about 1–2 mg (total dose); for example, the zebra requires about 1.5 mg and the rhinoceros 1–1.5 mg (total dose). The intramuscular dose level of etorphine alone for chimpanzees is 0.3–0.8 μg/lb of body weight; for small primates it is 0.2–0.6 μg/lb of body weight (Wallach 1969).

The combination of etorphine with either acetylpromazine or phencyclidine and hyoscine (scopolamine) has been recommended for effective immobilization of wild and exotic species (Harthoorn and Bligh 1965; Wallach 1966; Wallach et al. 1967; Williamson and Wallach 1968). Two combinations (A and B) successfully used by Harthoorn and Bligh (1965) are as follows:

Combination A
- Etorphine 1–1.5 mg/animal
- Acetylpromazine 20 mg/250 kg of body weight
- Hyoscine 2.5 mg/250 kg of body weight

Combination B
- Etorphine 1–1.5 mg/animal
- Phencyclidine 100 mg/250 kg of body weight
- Hyoscine 2.5 mg/250 kg of body weight

Harthoorn and Bligh (1965) used combination A for the more placid species that were not greatly excited upon injection, such as the zebra, wildebeest, waterbuck, and impala. For larger animals such as the hippo, white rhino, and elephant, which may require acetylpromazine to reduce excitation, the effective dosage of this tranquilizer is too bulky in volume to administer; only small amounts of acetylpromazine can be administered due to volume limitations of the projectile syringe.

Combination B was used by Harthoorn and Bligh (1965) on nervous animals such as the black rhino, kudu, and eland because their behavior indicated the need for a more potent neuroleptic agent (i.e., phencyclidine). Favorable results are obtained with phencyclidine, provided the dose level administered is not excessive and will permit the animal to stand soon after the antagonist (diprenorphine or nalorphine) is administered. There is some overlap in the choice of A or B combination and either is satisfactory for the immobilization and capture of 250–300-kg antelope, immature zebras, and rhinos. In extremely nervous antelope such as kudu and nyla, the substitution of acetylpromazine for the more potent chlorpromazine (3–4 mg/kg) is indicated (Harthoorn and Bligh 1965).

Observations made by Wallach and Anderson (1968) in the African elephant indicated that the combination of hyoscine (scopolamine) with etorphine prolongs the recovery period unnecessarily. Their results indicated that etorphine alone will immobilize the adult African elephant satisfactorily; safe and effective results were obtained with a dose of 6 mg of etorphine in animals ranging in weight from 4000 to 15,000 lb. Use of etorphine alone in the Asiatic working elephant at dosages of 5–8 mg have also proved satisfactory for immobilization; the drug was administered by a projectile syringe (Jainudeen et al. 1971).

In Defassa waterbuck, unfavorable reactions have occurred from the combined use of etorphine, acetylpromazine, and hyoscine (Short and Spinage 1967). It is believed that the toxic reaction produced in this species of waterbuck may be attributable to the acetylpromazine component of the mixture. Etorphine and hyoscine produced satisfactory effects when acetylpromazine was excluded from the mixture (Keep and Keep 1967).

Etorphine has been used to immobilize the American alligator, red-ear turtle, and Galapagos tortoise (Wallach and Hoessle 1970). Immobilization of these poikilothermic animals was satisfactory. However, the total dose required to attain a desired effect was much greater on a body weight basis than those required in homeothermic species.

USE IN DOMESTIC SPECIES

Etorphine has been approved by the FDA in the United States for use only in wild or exotic species. Information is incomplete on the tissue residue patterns as well as excretion of etorphine and its metabolites in the food-producing animals. In the United Kingdom, etorphine in combination with acetylpromazine has been extensively investigated as a neuroleptanalgesic agent for use in the pig, cow, horse, and other animals. The proprietary name for this combination is "Immobilon." Immobilon contains 2.25 mg of etorphine hydrochloride and 10 mg of acetylpromazine maleate in each ml.

PHARMACOLOGIC CONSIDERATIONS

Etorphine produces a bradycardia and arterial hypotension in a number of species such as the rat, cat, dog, and monkey. However, in some large species a tachycardia has been observed and an explanation for this difference is unclear. In the horse, tachycardia is more severe initially following the administration of etorphine but is not maintained (Daniel and Ling 1972). In addition, the heart rate declines to 50%–75% of its maximum by 30 minutes after injection of etorphine.

Premedication with propranolol reduces the tachycardia but does not abolish it completely (Daniel and Ling 1972). The action of the β-adrenergic blocking agent (propranolol) indicated to Daniel and Ling that the tachycardia induced by the etorphine-acetylpromazine combination resulted from the release of catecholamines. The turnover rate of dopamine, a neurotransmitter catecholamine, is increased by the phenothiazines of which acetylpromazine is a member. Acetylpromazine is 5–10 times more potent than chlorpromazine as an α-adrenolytic agent. Consequently, it is not too surprising that arterial hypotension is noted following a drug such as acetylpromazine. With a drop in arterial pressure, a reflex tachycardia is expected because pressoreceptor activity in the carotid sinus and aortic arch would be activated.

Use in the Horse. The combination of etorphine and acetylpromazine is administered intramuscularly or intravenously at a dose rate of 0.5 ml/100 lb of body weight, which corresponds to 22.5 μg/kg of etorphine and 100 μg/kg of acetylpromazine (Jenkin, 1972). Tachycardia and respiratory depression are side effects associated with the use of this combination and, in 80% of the cases studied, muscular tremors in varying intensity were observed. Immobilization and analgesia were reversed rapidly by an intravenous injection of the antagonist, diprenorphine (30 μg/kg); within 30 seconds of its administration, Jenkin (1972) observed an increase in the respiratory rate, and muscular tremors were no longer present. Following this, the animals would usually roll into sternal recumbency and immediately stand. Jenkin (1972) found that the intravenous route for administering the mixture of etorphine and acetylpromazine immobilized the animal in less than 1 minute and as rapidly as 20 seconds after the injection. The circling movements that are seen in the induction stage following an intramuscular injection were not seen when the intravenous route of administration was used. According to Jenkin, use of this drug combination has radically changed the approach to the surgical treatment of horses. Schlarmann et al. (1973) do not favor the use of etorphine-acetylpromazine because of its numerous and potentially dangerous side effects. Until more information is available, the safety and efficacy of this mixture in the horse are uncertain.

Use in Cattle. The potential value of an etorphine-acetylpromazine mixture for analgesia and restraint was assessed in cattle by Dobbs (1973). The concentration of the mixture, as well as dose level used, is identical to that used in the horse by Jenkin (1972). Following an intramuscular injection of the etorphine-acetylpromazine mixture (0.5 ml/100 lb), the cattle become recumbent in about 6 minutes after a period of excitement (Dobbs 1973). Dobbs reported that the excitation is absent when the mixture is administered intravenously and the time to recumbency is reduced to less than 1 minute. Fifteen minutes after administration of the mixture by the intramuscular or intravenous route, the animals do not respond to audible, visual, and certain painful stimuli. Dobbs (1973) also reported that the body temperature remained constant but that the respiratory and cardiac rates increased. He found 6 hours to be the minimum time that should elapse between a normal immobilization-remobilization cycle before an animal could again be immobilized with a full dose of the mixture. Reappearance of excitement was occasionally seen 8 hours after an immobilization-remobilization cycle and was attributed to enterohepatic cycling of etorphine. Although the information on the safety of this mixture has not been well documented, 1 animal was given 10 times the normal recommended dose and survived (Jenkin 1972). Another 2 animals were immobilized and remobilized every day for 30 successive days without fatalities. No immediate or delayed overt signs of tissue reaction at the injection site were observed. With the need for more complete data, both from experimental and clinical standpoints, judgment regarding the safety and efficacy of this preparation in cattle should be withheld. Also, the problem of whether or not tissue residues exist in animals that are slaughtered for food purposes will need to be resolved before a mixture such as this can obtain FDA approval.

Use in the Pig. Etorphine-acetylpromazine combination has been used on an experimental basis in the pig (Cox et al. 1973). A combination of 2.25 mg/ml of etorphine hydrochloride and 10 mg/ml of acetylpromazine maleate was used in 116 pigs ranging in age from 8 to 17 weeks and in 10 adult pigs. The dose level of the mixture used in the young pigs was less than 0.375 ml/50 kg to over 0.625 ml/50 kg of body weight. The average dose rate was 0.515 ml/50 kg of body weight or near the manufacturer's recommended dose of 0.5 ml/100 lb.

The characteristic effect produced by the drug preparation after an intramuscular injection is an unsteady gait after about 1 minute, with a twitching movement of the legs (Cox et al. 1973). Soon afterward, the pig loses control of the rear limbs and sits down. About 2 minutes after the injection, the animal assumes sternal recumbency. Slight involuntary movements of the head, neck, and limbs are also seen in most pigs. Five minutes after the administration of the drug, the animals can be placed in lateral recumbency without resistance; this is the earliest they can be disturbed without evoking a response from them. The fully immobilized pigs are usually unaffected by external stimuli; however, some respond to noise and others move their ears and heads slightly in response to stimuli applied to the ear region (Cox et al. 1973). There were 15 deaths in this study, which included all deaths associated with the use of the etorphine-acetylpromazine mixture. Considerably more information, both experimental and clinical, will be needed to determine the safety and efficacy of this preparation in the pig before it can be recommended. In addition, the matter of determining the residue patterns of these drugs in edible tissues will also need to be evaluated before it can be approved for use in food-producing animals.

Use in Other Domestic Animals. Etorphine has also been used in combination with methotrimeprazine as a neuroleptanalgesic preparation in the dog (Crooks et al. 1970). Claims made by the originators of this drug combination are that consistent effects are produced, a wide margin of safety exists, and side effects such as convulsions are absent.

Etorphine in combination with triflupromazine was evaluated in the goat by Thurmon et al. (1974). Dosages of etorphine of 0.07 ± 0.018 mg/kg and triflupromazine (1.98 ± 0.396 mg/kg) were administered intramuscularly and supplemented with local anesthesia (2% lidocaine). Several surgical procedures were conducted such as laparotomy, rumenotomy, splenectomy, nephrectomy, enucleation of the eye, dehorning, and amputation of the claw. Upon completion of surgery, diprenorphine (0.140 ± 0.025 mg/kg) was administered intravenously to reverse the action of etorphine.

According to Thurmon et al. (1974), the onset of immobilization occurred in 1–8.5 (mean of 3) minutes and the duration of immobilization was 60–120 (mean of 87) minutes. Reversal of immobilization of the etorphine by the antagonist was complete within 2–25 (mean of 13.5) minutes.

There will undoubtedly be more combinations of neuroleptic and analgesic agents developed in the future. Many referred to in this chapter will in all probability fall by the wayside as more effective combinations are developed.

THE OPIUM ALKALOIDS

Opium has been used in medicine since the dawn of history. It was recommended for relief of pain in the *Papyros Ebers,* written about 1500 B.C. The Greek, Arabian, and Roman physicians were well versed in the uses of opium. Arabian traders introduced opium into the Orient. Opium has been widely used by physicians throughout the world from the times of earliest record down through the Dark Ages in Europe to the Renaissance and to the present day. During the eighteenth century, Portuguese merchant shippers promoted the use of opium in China solely for economic exploitation. Armed conflict resulting from this and other exploitations led to international regulation of opium commerce by the former League of Nations and now by the United Nations.

Within the United States the Drug Enforcement Agency of the Justice Department maintains a large work force to regulate and control the importation, processing, sale, and dispensing of all opium and its alkaloids, since opium is capable of producing addiction in human beings. On May 1, 1971, the Controlled Substances Act was implemented; it superseded the Harrison Narcotic Act of 1914. With the exception of heroin and some other opiate derivatives, morphine and all derivatives are classified as Schedule II drugs. Heroin is classified as a Schedule I drug because it has no accepted medical use in the United States.

The addictive property of morphine is of little direct importance in animal medicine because ordinarily animals are not given the opportunity to develop a drug dependence. However, the development of addiction in human beings has led to restrictions that have caused many veterinarians to forego the use of morphine in their practice. This is unfortunate because morphine and morphine substitutes have valuable applications in veterinary medicine.

Source and Composition

Opium is the air-dried milky exudate obtained from the incised unripe seed capsules of the poppy plant, *Papaver somniferum,* which is indigenous to Asia Minor. The plant is cultivated in other countries such as China, India, Persia, and Egypt. After the flower petals fall from the poppy, the green seed capsule is incised. The milky juice dries on the capsule to form a brownish, gummy mass, which is collected, dried further, and powdered to make *Opium,* U.S.P.

Pharmacologically, the active constituents of opium are alkaloids. Opium contains about 24 alkaloids but only 2, morphine and codeine, have much clinical usage. The principal alkaloid of opium is morphine.

Morphine Sulfate

Morphine was the first of the plant alkaloids to be isolated. Morphine was crystallized from crude opium by F. W. A. Sertürner in 1805. *Morphine Sulfate,*

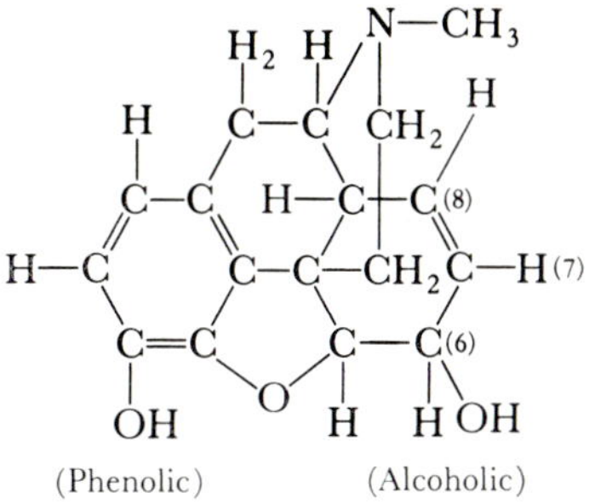

(Phenolic) (Alcoholic)

Morphine

Fig. 15.3.

U.S.P., is the principal salt of morphine. The pharmacopeias generally based the standard for opium upon its morphine content. The *United States Pharmacopeia* states that the official powdered opium shall contain not less than 10% nor more than 10.5% of anhydrous morphine. In addition to the alkaloids, opium contains pharmacologically inert substances such as organic acids, resins, gums, and sugars, which comprise about 75% of the weight of dried powdered opium.

Chemistry

The morphine molecule consists of a partially hydrogenated phenanthrene nucleus, an oxide link, and a nitrogen-containing structure (ethenamine,—CH_2CH_2—NCH_3). In addition, two hydroxy groups (alcoholic and phenolic, Fig. 15.3) are important in maintaining the pharmacological integrity of the morphine molecule.

The synthesis of morphine has been accomplished with considerable difficulty. Semisynthetic derivatives of morphine are relatively easy to manufacture by substitution of chemical radicals in place of the hydrogen atoms at one or both hydroxy positions of the morphine molecule. The chemical relationships of the natural and semisynthetic opiates are given in Table 15.2.

When substitutions are made in place of one or both hydrogen atoms at the phenolic and alcoholic hydroxy position, the pharmacodynamic activity of the morphine molecule is altered in an interesting manner. Alteration of the phenolic hydroxy group reduces the analgesic potency,

TABLE 15.2. Natural and semisynthetic opiates

Drug	Phenolic Position	Alcoholic Position
Morphine	H	H
Methylmorphine (codeine)	CH_3	H
Hydromorphone* (Dilaudid)	H	O
Diacetylmorphine (heroin)	$COCH_3$	$COCH_3$
Oxymorphone† (Numorphan)	H	O

* Hydrogenation of carbons 7 and 8 occurs with the double bond being removed; an oxygen atom replaces the H and OH groups in position 6.

† With exception of an OH group replacing the H atom in carbon 14 position (opposite or to the left of carbon 8), the chemical structure is identical to hydromorphone.

respiratory depression, and likelihood of constipation. A stimulant activity upon the CNS is noted when substitution is made in this position. The lessened analgesic potency and increased stimulant effect typifies the pharmacodynamic activity of codeine. If substitution is made at the alcoholic hydroxy position, narcotic and respiratory depression are enhanced. Consequently, dilaudid is more potent as an analgesic agent than morphine. Substitution in either of the hydroxy positions lessens the emetic activity of the parent molecule. As a result, both codeine and dilaudid are less potent than morphine in producing emesis.

Other semisynthetic derivatives of morphine are apomorphine hydrochloride, a potent emetic agent, and nalorphine hydrochloride, a morphine antagonist. Apomorphine hydrochloride is formed by treating morphine with concentrated hydrochloric acid. Nalorphine differs from morphine by replacement of the methyl radical in the ethenamine chain by an allyl branch ($-CH_2-CH=CH_2$).

PHARMACOLOGICAL ACTIONS OF MORPHINE

Effect upon the Brain. The action of morphine upon the brain and entire CNS is curiously irregular. In small doses, morphine produces CNS depression and, in large doses, CNS stimulation and even convulsive seizures. The greatest irregularity of effect is found among the different species, although individual variation within a species is rather frequent. Considerable controversy has existed over the years regarding whether or not morphine should be used in the cat because of its inability to consistently produce sedation. Relatively recent work indicates that morphine sulfate is effective in obtunding intense pain (Davis and Donnelly 1968). According to Davis and Donnelly, the excitatory response frequently observed in the cat may be the effect of overdosage with morphine. When dose levels of morphine hydrochloride of 5, 10, and 20 mg/kg of body weight are injected intraperitoneally in conscious cats, a manic response characterized by hyperexcitement and aggressive behavior is observed (Dhasmana et al. 1972). This manic response can be prevented by pretreatment of the animals with either CNS catecholamine depletors (i.e., reserpine, tetrabenazine) or central dopaminergic receptor blocking agents such as those produced by chlorpromazine and halperidol. It was concluded by Dhasmana et al. (1972) that morphine releases dopamine in the CNS, which in turn excites the central dopaminergic receptors to induce the manic response. Other investigators (Mullin et al. 1973) have reported that morphine enhances the release of acetylcholine from the lateral ventricles and the cerebral cortex and the excitant action of morphine in the cat parallels the release of acetylcholine.

Swine, goats, sheep, cattle, asses, and horses are generally stimulated by morphine, although the effects of morphine in the horse and the ox are somewhat irregular. In these species it may be that the dose levels used are higher than required to produce analgesia similar to that observed in the cat. Moreover, the release of dopamine following morphine administration may also be involved in the production of restlessness and CNS excitation in these species similar to that in the cat. If this is true, dopaminergic blocking agents such as the phenothiazines or droperidol should effectively prevent the excitation as it does in cats. CNS depression does not necessarily need to occur prior to, or concomitantly with, the development of the state of analgesia. In fact, morphine is capable of producing a high degree of analgesia without accompanying narcosis or respiratory depression in animals such as the hamster (Chen et al. 1945).

The dog shows a brief preliminary period of central excitement marked by restlessness, panting, salivation, nausea, vomition, urination, and defecation. These symptoms gradually disappear and are followed by a stupor indicating depression of the cerebral cortex. Inasmuch as morphine induces CNS depression and accompanying analgesia in the dog, clinicians have used it almost entirely in this species. Morphine is preferred by clinicians primarily for preanesthetic medication in the dog over its use in other animals because the drug facilitates handling for the induction of general anesthesia.

Although morphine is used principally for its analgesic effect in human beings and other animals, very little is known about sites in the CNS that mediate the analgesic action of the drug (Jacquet and Lajtha 1973). Efforts to study the distribution characteristics of morphine in the CNS in relation to its analgesic actions in the normal, intact animal following systemic administration have all led to negative results. To circumvent interference of the blood-brain barrier following a systemic-administered dose of morphine, studies have been conducted by injecting morphine into the subcortical sites of the brain using fine-gauge implanted cannulae. By circumventing the blood-brain barrier in this manner, precise amounts of morphine can be delivered to selected anatomical sites in the brain. When a few μg of morphine are injected into the posterior hypothalamus, a significant degree of analgesia is induced; yet, the same dose injected into the medial septum, the caudate, and periaqueductal gray matter induces hyperalgesia (Jacquet and Lajtha 1973). Consequently, intracerebral injections of morphine produce different effects from those administered systemically (i.e., analgesia or hyperalgesia is produced, depending on the CNS site).

Not only have the anatomical sites within the CNS been difficult to pinpoint and relate to the analgesic effect produced but it has not been clear just how morphine produces analgesia. One procedure used in studying the mechanism of analgesia has been to study the electrical activity of the cat's cortex and brainstem during and after either electrical stimulation of the skin or chemical stimulation by the intraarterial injection of bradykinin. The bradykinins are among the most potent agents in the induction of pain known; a dose level of 2 μg or less administered intraarterially produces a markedly evoked response that can be detected in the caudate nucleus to the mesencephalic and medullary reticular formation but not in the cortical area of the brain. These evoked central responses from bradykinin can be blocked in the dog by morphine (1 mg/kg) administered intravenously; the central blocking action of morphine involves synaptic transmission of the excitatory pathway linking with the reticular formation (Lim 1970). Any factor that interferes with the proper function of the brainstem reticular formation will also affect the ability of an animal to perceive pain (Breazile and Kitchell 1969). Analgesic agents such as morphine decrease the activity of the reticular formation and simultaneously decrease the ability of an animal to respond to or perceive pain.

Administration of morphine or ethanol to rats produces a drop in the brain calcium (Ross et al. 1974). The alteration in the brain calcium level by morphine may be related to general CNS depression. Not all CNS depressants are capable of lowering the calcium level of the brain. For example, pentobarbital sodium does not reduce the calcium level.

Other mechanisms implicated in the induction of analgesia have been associated with the increased activity of central cholinergic mechanisms. For example, the administration of pilocarpine on a mg/kg basis was reported to be comparable in potency to morphine; physostigmine was 35 times as potent (Dayton and Garrett 1973). The central analgesic effect of these cholinergic agents can be blocked by atropine or scopolamine. Release of acetylcholine by morphine in the unanesthetized cat has been associated with CNS excitation; the analgesic effect of acetylcholine release was not discussed (Mullin et al. 1973). According to these investigators, a dose of morphine (0.5 mg/kg) administered parenterally resulted in the animals becoming more "alert."

Until the synthesis of methadone, morphine was the most effective analgesic known for dogs and human beings. However, with the ban on the use of methadone except in the treatment of human drug addicts, it is no longer available for veterinary use. Information on the effectiveness of morphine in relieving pain comes primarily from use of the drug in human patients because of the ease of noting the subjective response. Morphine will relieve pain without blocking motor activity or consciousness. The pain threshold is increased so that moderate pain disappears and sharp pain is dulled. Morphine is most useful in human beings in relieving pain arising from the viscera and from trauma. Anxiety and alarm disappear. Sleep may be produced during the period of morphine analgesia. In human patients, morphine is used almost exclusively for the relief of pain. These observations give some indication as to the probable effectiveness of morphine in relieving pain in the dog. The analgesic effects of morphine are decreased slightly in intensity and in duration by therapeutic doses of atropine or scopolamine (Christensen and Gross 1948).

Effect upon the Spinal Cord. Morphine has a biphasic effect upon the cerebrospinal axis, i.e., a depressant and a stimulant effect upon the CNS. In dogs and human patients, morphine seems to depress the anterior end of the cerebrospinal axis and to stimulate the posterior end, i.e., the spinal cord. A laboratory animal with only the spinal cord intact will show strychninelike tetany following administration of morphine. This cord-stimulating activity is the reason that morphine is strictly contraindicated in the treatment of strychnine poisoning, despite the depressant effect of morphine upon the cerebrum. Apparently the cerebral depressant activity of morphine neutralizes to some degree the stimulant effects upon the spinal cord because in the intact animal an excessive dose of morphine is required to produce a spinal convulsion. The author has induced spinal convulsions in the dog and rabbit with large doses of morphine sulfate (500 mg/kg).

Effect upon the Emetic Center. Considerable species variation occurs with respect to effect of morphine upon vomition in animals. For example, swine and chickens do not respond to central-acting emetics (i.e., morphine, apomorphine) but do respond to local emetic agents (i.e., copper sulfate, zinc sulfate). Both dogs and cats will respond to central- and local-acting emetics. However, the cat requires considerably higher doses of morphine or apomorphine to induce vomiting than the dog. For example, morphine and apomorphine dosages 740–2800 times greater are required in the cat over the level that stimulates vomition in the dog (Brand and Perry 1966). The horse and ruminant do not vomit following the administration of central- or local-acting emetics. The emetic center in the dog is readily stimulated by small to moderate dosages of morphine. Within 5–10 minutes after subcutaneous injection of morphine sulfate, the majority of dogs will vomit profusely unless the stomach was previously emptied, in which case only saliva and bile may be lost. The act of vomition is preceded by salivation and nausea and is accompanied usually by defecation. The emetic center appears to be stimulated directly.

A trace of morphine applied directly to the floor of the fourth ventricle will produce simulated vomition in dogs from which the entire gastrointestinal tract has been removed. This effect would seem to exclude gastric irritation as a causative factor as was previously believed. Following stimulation of the emetic center in the dog, depression soon develops secondarily even to the extent of overcoming the emetic action of apomorphine.

Effect upon the Cough Center. The cough center appears to be more susceptible to morphine than do the other medullary centers. Morphine is an excellent cough sedative, and were it not for its addictive properties to dogs as well as to human beings, the drug probably would be the most widely used and effective control available for dry, nonproductive coughs. Generally, morphine is used only in those patients in which codeine previously was ineffective.

Effect upon Thermoregulation. A variation in the effect upon body temperature is seen in different species following the administration of morphine. Generally, the heat regulatory function of the hypothalamus is altered by morphine to the degree that most animals develop a decrease in body temperature. Panting is noted initially in the dog after administration of morphine but finally stops with a decline in the body temperature. The response to morphine in the cat is comparable to the dog; however, at high dosages a marked hyperthermic response occurs that does not subside until the effects of morphine disappear. The hyperthermic response may be related to the increase in the catecholamine level in the midbrain. In the midbrain of the rat and mouse, the concentration of the catecholamines increases rapidly following the administration of morphine (Heinrich et al. 1971). Sweating and a hyperglycemic response in the horse following the administration of morphine is believed to be associated with an increased circulating level of epinephrine (Alexander 1960).

Another species variation with respect to the effect of opiate derivatives upon the thermoregulatory mechanism pertains to the interesting response of the rabbit to apomorphine (Quock and Horita 1974). Apomorphine has been well established as a dopaminergic agonist. Dopamine is one of a number of catecholamines found in the brainstem that have a thermoregulatory role in the rabbit. Experimental evidence exists indicating that central dopaminergic mechanisms are activated prior to a temperature response in animals following the administration of *d*-amphetamine or apomorphine; both of these drugs induce hyperthermia, and the hyperthermic response can be blocked by a dopaminergic receptor blocking agent such as pimozide.

The studies of Quock and Horita (1974) also indicate that 5-hydroxytryptamine (serotonin,) another catecholamine derivative related to dopamine and other monoamines, has an important role in the mediation of the hyperthermic response of rabbits to apomorphine. Their conclusion was based upon the observation that after depletion of the cerebral serotonin pool by *p*-chlorophenylalanine, apomorphine does not have the ability to evoke the hyperthermic response. With reestablishment of the serotonin pool to normal levels, apomorphine is again able to produce hyperthermia. Inasmuch as morphine has effects similar to those of apomorphine upon neurotransmitter substances in the brain, its mechanism of action upon thermoregulatory control mechanisms should be comparable to those of apomorphine.

Effect upon the Iris. Morhpine produces a variable effect upon the size of the pupil in animals. The pupillary size of the cat and most other domestic animals increases after morphine. This is probably related to an increase in the circulating catecholamine levels following the administration of morphine. The iris of the bird is not affected because it contains nonresponsive skeletal muscles. The pupil of human beings decreases following the administration of morphine, producing what is called the "pinpoint pupil." The effects on the involuntary muscle fibers of the iris arise centrally from the oculomotor center.

Effect upon the Respiratory System. The respiratory center of the dog is initially stimulated; panting is seen and is attributable to the initial rise in body temperature. As the body temperature declines and CNS depression increases, respiratory activity is depressed by morphine, resulting in a decreased minute volume of respired air. The threshold of response to carbon dioxide stimulation is increased and the alveolar concentration of carbon dioxide is higher. Respirations become slower and shallower. In deep sedation, Cheyne-Stokes type of breathing may occur. In normal, healthy dogs, small doses of morphine may not decrease the respiratory minute volume and the oxygen consumption by more than about 10%. Following large doses of morphine that lead to convulsive seizures, the respiration rate is markedly increased. Eventually depression and paralysis of the respiratory center develop ostensibly from overstimulation. Moreover, moderate to large doses are known to produce bronchiolar constriction in the dog. A significant bronchoconstriction occurs following an intravenous dose of 1 mg/kg and a more marked effect is produced following a dose of 2.5 mg/kg; a decrease in lung capacity at the latter dose averaged 24% (Shemano and Wendel 1965).

Morphine can be used therapeutically in certain forms of cardiac dyspnea because of its ability to depress the central sensation of respiratory need, i.e., by raising the threshold of response to carbon dioxide stimulation. In cardiac dyspnea resulting from a pulmonary complication and treated with morphine, the normal sensory perception of respiratory need is depressed, with the result that both the heart and respiration function more slowly and easily. The patient experiences suboptimal but adequate oxygenation for an inactive existence. Thus a slight depression of respiratory activity may be used therapeutically to relieve the symptom of cardiac dyspnea.

Effect upon the Cardiovascular System. Experimental studies conducted in the dog indicate that morphine improves ventricular performance; this effect on the heart is an indirect one and is the result of sympathoadrenal discharge (Vasko et al. 1966). In the last few years, the use of large intravenous doses (up to a total of 600 mg) of morphine in human beings is being advocated as the sole anesthetic agent for open-heart surgery in high-risk patients (Lowenstein et al. 1969; Hasbrouck 1970). Clinical observations in human beings indicate, as in the intact animal, that morphine produces a rise in systemic arterial pressure and pulse rate. These effects appear to be mediated through an increase in sympathetic activity because the blood levels of norepinephrine and epinephrine rise. It is, therefore, assumed that this rise in the circulating catecholamines increases the inotropic state of the heart (Hasbrouck 1970).

An arterial hypotensive effect is associated with the use of morphine following a rapid intravenous injection (15–20 mg/minute) in human beings; diluted infusions of morphine administered slowly obviate this problem. Presumably the hypotension in human beings occurs due to the release of histamine (Hasbrouck 1970). In high-risk patients, the development of a severe systemic arterial hypotension can be potentially hazardous in a patient with a reduced or marginal coronary blood flow. If this occurs, the systemic arterial hypotension can be rapidly corrected by vasoconstrictor drugs and by being ready to expand the blood volume. Although morphine possesses this disadvantage, it still outweighs the use of inhalant anesthetics for open-heart surgery. Unlike morphine, inhalant anesthetics produce severe cardiovascular depression, which makes recovery of the cardiac patient from a surgical procedure more difficult.

The author has administered morphine sulfate (0.5 mg/lb or more) by a rapid intravenous injection into the dog; a transient excitatory period occurs that can be quite violent. However, if the dose is administered slowly over a 2- to 3-minute period, no excitement is observed. The animal is immediately depressed and rarely vomits.

Effect upon the Urinary Tract. The initial effects of morphine along with salivation, nausea, vomiting, and defecation may also include urination. As the effect progresses, morphine can decrease urine secretion in the dog to 10% or less of normal by liberating an excess of the antidiuretic hormone from the posterior lobe of the pituitary gland. This hormone, in excess, stimulates intensive reabsorption of the glomerular filtrate by the cells of the renal tubules. To produce the above effect, the dose of morphine must approach 1.1 mg/lb intravenously or 2.3 mg/lb subcutaneously (De Bodo 1944).

Morphine increases the muscular tone of the bladder, which, among other effects, results in spasm of the sphincter. This effect may make urination difficult. Conversely, animals seem to be less affected and have less difficulty in this respect than human beings.

Effect upon the Gastrointestinal Tract. Emptying of the gastrointestinal tract is the dog's first response to morphine. Morphine is known to promote vomition by directly stimulating the emetic center. Defecation usually accompanies or follows vomition, probably as a reflex response of the intestines to gastric hypermotility.

Following initial emptying of the digestive tract, morphine causes constipation of the dog and other animals.

Morphine has a spasmogenic effect upon intestinal smooth muscle by a direct action, partly by a cholinergic and partly by a histaminergic mechanism (Türker and Kaymakcalan 1971). Atropine partially inhibits the spasmogenic effect of morphine. Mepyramine partially blocks or antagonizes the spasmogenic activity of morphine; apparently this is related to the histamine-releasing action of morphine. Release of serotonin occurs in the isolated intestine of the dog when it is perfused with morphine. Intestinal smooth muscle has two types of serotonin receptors, i.e., "M" and "D." M receptors ostensibly located on nerve terminals are blocked by morphine, whereas D receptors presumably located on smooth muscle membranes are blocked by dihydroergotamine and lysergic acid diethylamide.

By virtue of the spasmogenic action, the primary effect of morphine is to increase the tonus of the smooth muscles of the entire gastrointestinal tract. The sphincters exhibit a spastic tonus. The propulsive motility of the tract is markedly depressed, apparently as a result of the excessive tonus that interferes with normal peristaltic waves. The tonus may become great enough to close or constrict the intestinal lumen in the conscious dog (Vaughn-Williams and Streeten 1951). Thus the passage of food through the tract is delayed. The delay results in increased absorption of water from the ingesta, which contributes to constipation. The tonus of the anal sphincter is increased by morphine. In addition, morphine depresses mental perception of the ordinary sensory stimuli for the defecation reflex.

The effect of morphine upon the enzyme secretions of the digestive tract of the dog is variable but slight. Biliary secretion appears to be reduced to one-third of normal. Morphine causes an initial delay in gastric secretion of HCl, which is later compensated by excessive secretion (Table 15.3).

TABLE 15.3. Estimated constipative action of morphine (2.7 mg/lb) on the gastrointestinal tract of the dog (administered before feeding)

A. Delay in stomach		13 hr
1. Initial failure of HCl secretion	1 hr	
2. Initial decrease in stomach motility and constriction of sphincter *antri pylorici*	4 hr	
3. Closure of pylorus—initially maintained, later interrupted but more prominent than normal	9 hr	
4. Delayed increase in HCl secretion	—1 hr	
B. Delay in small intestine		7 hr
1. Decreased digestion due to decrease in bile and pancreatic secretion	2.5 hr	
2. Decreased propulsive motility	2 hr	
3. Increased viscosity brought about by increased absorption of water due to increased pressure applied to intestinal contents	1.5 hr	
4. Closure of ileocolic sphincter	1 hr	
C. Delay in colon		4 hr
1. Motility effects increasing dryness of contents	2 hr	
2. Presence of excessively dried material which cannot be passed through closed sphincter	2 hr	
3. Loss of defecation reflex	? hr	
Total delay		24 hr

Source: Krueger 1937.

ABSORPTION, FATE, AND EXCRETION

Although morphine is considered to be one of our oldest and most efficacious drugs, pharmacokinetic information regarding its fate has not been clearly determined in animals or human beings. One of the primary reasons for this has been the lack of a sensitive analytical method for the detection of morphine and its various metabolites (Spector and Vesell 1971). In recent years, the development of radioimmunoassay methodology has improved the sensitivity for the detection of compounds such as morphine over 1000-fold.

Morphine is readily absorbed from the small intestine and some may be absorbed from the stomach. It is absorbed promptly following subcutaneous injection. Morphine is not absorbed through the intact skin, but a scarified epithelium permits slow entrance to the circulation.

The biotransformation of morphine to morphine 3-*O*-glucuronide is the primary metabolic pathway for the inactivation and eventual elimination of the drug (Sanchez and Tephly 1974). The principal catalyst in the formation of morphine glucuronide is a hepatic microsomal uridine diphosphate (UDP)-glucuronyl transferase, which transfers a glucuronic acid moiety from UDP-glucuronic acid (UDPGA) to morphine. With exception of the cat, approximately 50% of the morphine administered to most mammals appears in the urine as the glucuronide form. In the cat, a deficiency in UDPGA and its associated glucuronyl transferase enzyme does not favor glucuronidation of morphine. The increased toxicity of aspirin and salicylate drugs is linked to the failure of the cat to conjugate the compounds with glucuronic acid. The biological half-life of morphine would be expected to be longer in the cat, due to its inability to form glucuronides. Surprisingly, the biological half-life in plasma is only 3.05 hours in the cat following subcutaneous injection of morphine (1 mg/kg) (Davis and Donnelly 1968). The biological half-life of morphine in other species is probably shorter than in the cat; these values were not located in the literature.

In human beings, morphine was studied after a single intravenous dose (10 mg/70 kg); a rapid initial decline of morphine in the blood occurred during the first 6 hours after its administration (Spector and Vesell 1971). After the rapid initial decline of the drug, levels of morphine could be detected in the blood for several hours, which may be attributable to enterohepatic recirculation, the persistence of metabolites, or a combination of these and other factors. During the first 6 hours, the half-life of morphine ranged from 1.9 to 3.1 hours. Following this, the disappearance of the drug was slow, with a half-life of 10–44 hours (Spector and Vesell 1971).

MORPHINE TOXICITY

The toxic dose of morphine for the dog appears to be variable. Subcutaneously or intravenously, the fatal dose of morphine sulfate is 50–100 mg/lb of body weight. Spinal convulsive seizures quite similar to strychnine occur in most species following the administration of higher dosages of morphine. Thebaine (dimethylmorphine), a component of opium, is also well known for its strychninelike seizures.

The author has induced convulsive seizures in a fox terrier with a total of 29 grains of morphine (500 mg/kg). The animal survived this dose level following treatment with pentobarbital sodium and the use of oxygen to support ventilation. In the small rodent (mouse), acute toxicity and death from morphine are produced by the intravenous administration of 221–311 mg/kg of body weight; subcutaneously, a dose level of morphine between 420 and 526 mg/kg of body weight produces death (Gardocki and Yelnosky 1964).

The condition and age of the animal seem to make considerable difference. Toxicity data for other species have been compiled by Krueger et al. (1941). Swine apparently are quite susceptible to the stimulant action of morphine. The author injected a pig (ca. 40 lb) with a total dose of 2 grains of morphine sulfate by the intramuscular route to observe the pharmacodynamic effects of the opiate. The animal manifested a marked period of excitation and eventually succumbed approximately 3 hours after the injection.

Poisoning in cattle from eating stems and capsules of *Papaver somniferum* has been noted. Symptoms consisted of CNS stimulation and gastrointestinal disturbances, without fatality (Lagneau and Gallard 1946).

Several narcotic antagonists such as nalorphine, naloxone, and others are valuable in the reversal of the CNS depressant effects of morphine.

ADDICTION

The marked addicting properties of morphine and related derivatives are well known in human beings. This problem is rarely encountered in the animal because the narcotic drugs are not ordinarily administered for prolonged periods. There is a clinical report of addiction due to the prolonged (6–8 months) use of paregoric (camphorated tincture of opium) in the dog by an overzealous owner (Segall 1964).

The veterinarian has the responsibility of properly recording the use of all narcotic analgesics in accordance with the Controlled Substances Act of 1970. Also, adequate security measures are required under this act to avoid theft of these compounds for misuse. Prior to, and following, the implementation of the Controlled Substances Act, the record of the veterinary medical profession in maintaining proper control and use of these drugs was exceptionally good. Rarely is a veterinarian indicted for the improper handling or use of narcotic drugs. All veterinary medical students should familiarize themselves with the serious consequences associated with addiction in human beings. A good source of information on addiction is available in most human pharmacology textbooks.

TOLERANCE

In human beings, tolerance and physical dependence as well as psychological dependence with chronic or repeated use of the opiates and other narcotic analgesics are well-known patterns of these compounds (Jaffe 1970). Two major factors that appear to explain the development of tolerance are the adaptation of the cells of the CNS and increased metabolism of the drug (Berkowitz and Spector 1972). CNS adaptation is related to the tolerance that develops following the continued use of narcotic analgesics. In addition, an immunelike mechanism may be associated with the development of tolerance. For example, some forms of tolerance last for many months; serum and tissues of adapted or tolerant animals possess a substance that can be passively transferred to another animal, which will affect narcotic activity; and the development of tolerance can be suppressed by chemicals that inhibit synthesis of protein. Berkowitz and Spector (1972) have evidence that the serum of mice can be actively immunized with a morphine immunogen that can bind dihydromorphine. The effects of morphine are decreased in these "immunized" animals and the level of morphine in their plasma is altered.

CLINICAL USES OF MORPHINE

Morphine has been used for a wide variety of clinical conditions since the beginning of recorded history. Several of these uses are still valid indications. When an opiate is used to relieve pain or to control diarrhea or coughs, only symptomatic therapy is administered. The underlying etiology and pathology are still present. Furthermore, the unwise use of alkaloids may obscure the symptomatic progress of the disease.

In the Dog. Morphine is important in canine surgery to relieve pain, to facilitate handling the patient for local or general anesthesia, and to decrease the amount of CNS depressants necessary to produce surgical anesthesia. The peak effect of morphine is usually reached between 30 and 45 minutes following subcutaneous injection. Duration of the analgesic effect has not been accurately determined but appears to last 1–2 hours. The subcutaneous dose levels of morphine sulfate recommended for preanesthetic medication vary from 0.05 to 1 mg/lb of body weight. The preanesthetic dose is usually reduced to one-half that used for other purposes. The onset of action after an intramuscular or subcutaneous injection is within a few minutes. Atropine sulfate (0.05 mg/kg) is routinely administered subcutaneously or intramuscularly at the same time as morphine to prevent salivation and bronchial secretions. Very young, aged, and debilitated dogs are more susceptible to morphine than normal, middle-aged, vigorous dogs. A dog depressed by morphine should be handled gently because roughness may awaken it and provoke hypnotic excitement. The emetic action of morphine may cause great inconvenience if it is not anticipated. On the other hand, it is a definite advantage to have the stomach emptied preoperatively by morphine.

Premedication with sufficient morphine will decrease the total amount of general anesthetic required for surgical anesthesia to one-half or perhaps even to one-third the anesthetic dose required when morphine is not used. This supports the concept of balanced anesthesia and increases the safety of the anesthetic procedure.

Morphine is of value postoperatively for overcoming the recurring excitement stage observed in dogs recovering from anesthesia with pentobarbital sodium. Without a depressant such as morphine, a dog may, by its struggles, induce hemorrhage, injury, or fracture or open a surgical inincision.

Traditionally, morphine has been used cautiously in cesarean section of the dog because of fetal respiratory depression. It now appears that fetal respiratory movements are not abolished by dosages of morphine that depress maternal respiration and produce maternal analgesia. However, fetal respiratory movements may be depressed by large doses of morphine. A large dose of morphine also interferes with uterine contraction and parturition (Snyder and Lim 1941).

Morphine may be used in the dog for symptomatic relief of "cardiac dyspnea." Dyspnea is associated with a ventricular deficiency and arises from inability of the heart to supply the amount of oxygen desired by the respiratory centers. Morphine sulfate may be used in the dog in a dosage of about 0.5 mg/lb of body weight.

Contraindications. Morphine should be used with care in acutely uremic and toxemic dogs. By stimulating secretion of the antidiuretic hormone, morphine increases reabsorption of the renal filtrate. A large dose of morphine may decrease urine flow in the dog by 90%.

Morphine cannot be used to control convulsive disorders such as strychnine poisoning, tetanus, and running fits. Doses of morphine sufficient to depress the motor excitability of the cortex are large enough to stimulate the spinal reflexes, which would make the condition worse.

Morphine should not be administered to dogs suffering from traumatic shock because it further lowers blood pressure, cardiac output, and oxygen consumption (Powers et al. 1947). This is important if provisions are not available to expand the blood volume and if vasoconstrictors are not included to restore systemic arterial pressure.

In the Cat. An effective analgesic dose of morphine subcutaneously in the cat is 0.1–1 mg/kg (0.045 mg–0.45 mg/lb) of body weight (Davis and Donnelly 1968). Other investigators have found that the subcutaneous administration of morphine sulfate (0.1 mg/kg) produces effective analgesia in the cat (Watts et al. 1973). Inasmuch as the evidence is convincing that the phenothiazine tranquilizers (e.g., chlorpromazine, promazine) block the central dopaminergic receptors, this probably explains the satisfactory effect of these drugs in combination with morphine as observed in the cat by Davis and Donnelly (1968) and Jacobsen (1970). Davis and Donnelly (1968) reported that morphine in combination with *d*-propoxyphene (Darvon) administered intramuscularly in a dose level of 2.2 mg/kg is an effective analgesic combination in the cat. Chlorpromazine (4.4 mg/kg) with morphine (0.1 mg/kg) is administered intramuscularly. For postoperative use, Heavner (1970) recommends morphine in the cat up to 0.1 mg/kg intravenously for management of pain. He noted that recovery from anesthesia was smoother, and upon awakening the animals lay quietly.

In the Guinea Pig and Rat. Morphine may be used subcutaneously or intramuscularly as a preanesthetic agent in the guinea pig and rat (Strobel and Wollman 1969) prior to parenteral or inhalational anesthetics; the recommended dose level of morphine in these species is 2–5 mg/kg of body weight. According to Strobel and Wollman (1969), the usual analgesic and sedative doses of morphine exert an effect within 15 minutes of subcutaneous administration and last several hours.

In the Rabbit. Morphine has a profound depressant effect in the rabbit. Gardner (1964) recommends the intramuscular use of morphine (8 mg/kg) in the rabbit 30 minutes prior to intravenous thiamylal sodium (20 mg/kg anesthesia. Atropine sulfate (0.2 mg/kg) is also administered intramuscularly at the same time as the morphine injection.

In the Pig. As in the cat and other species (goats, sheep, cattle, horses), morphine has more CNS stimulant than depressant effects in the pig. However, morphine sulfate is used successfully for analgesic effect in the pig prior to chloralose and barbiturate anesthesia (Booth et al. 1960; Booth 1969); the recommended intramuscular dose is 0.2–0.9 mg/kg of body weight. The mechanism of the excitatory effect produced by morphine in the pig is similar to that described in the cat by Dhasmana et al. (1972). Thus phenothiazine tranquilizers in the cat are useful when combined with morphine in the prevention of the excitation (Davis and Donnelly 1968; Jacobsen 1970).

In Subhuman Primates. Comparatively large doses (1–3 mg/kg) of morphine are necessary for "chemical restraint" and sedation of the chimpanzee (Clifford 1971). The dose range for the dog is recommended for adequate sedation and safe management of the subhuman primate (Soma 1971). In the baboon, Newsome and Robinson (1957) reported that the only effects produced by morphine were a very severe skin irritation, especially of the palms and soles, and the loss of appetite. They administered morphine hydrochloride up to 1 grain orally and by injection (route not specified) in animals of all ages weighing up to 26 kg; no noticeable sedation was observed.

In the Horse. Morphine and other opiates have been used in the horse for various ailments, but particularly to relieve the acute pain of spasmodic colic. Although some patients were relieved, many horses showed central stimulation and excitement that were undesirable and dangerous. Some clinicians contend that overdosing is the reason morphine has fallen into disrepute in the treatment of spasmodic colic in the horse. It is recommended that no more than 120 mg (2 grains) be given to a heavy draft horse. Experimental observation indicated that all natural or synthetic alkaloids of opium used to date were unsatisfactory as sedatives for the horse (Amadon and Craige 1937). Phaneuf and co-workers (1972) reported the intravenous use of morphine chlorhydrate (1 mg/kg) in two ponies with classical forms of colic. The analgesic effect produced by the drug resulted in a hyperactive but uniform contraction of the jejunum. The jejunal spasms disappeared, motility of the colon became prominent, and the stomach remained quiescent. According to Phaneuf and associates, the intravenous administration of morphine chlorhydrate to a normal horse will result in the induction of intense and sustained activity of the colon. On the other regions of the intestinal tract, the action of morphine has a moderate and transitory effect in the normal animal.

With the new information that in the cat morphine induces the release of dopamine in the CNS, which in turn excites the central dopaminergic receptors (Dhasmana et al. 1972), the use of phenothiazine or butyrophenone tranquilizers in combination with morphine should be evaluated in the horse. Both chlorpromazine and halperidol are capable of blocking the central dopaminergic receptors in the cat so the excitant effects of dopamine are prevented.

MORPHINE DERIVATIVES

Codeine Phosphate. *Codeine Phosphate,* U.S.P. (methylmorphine), occurs in opium to the extent of around 0.5%. Most of it is produced semisynthetically from morphine. The phosphate salt is more widely used than codeine sulfate despite respective solubilities in water of 2.3 and 30 parts.

Codeine is metabolized rapidly by the tissues of human beings, dogs, and rats. Metabolic alteration followed by rapid urinary excretion begins a few minutes after intramuscular injection and after a slight delay following oral administration. About one-half an ordinary dose is eliminated within 6 hours and all within 24 hours. In the dog about 50% of the dose is excreted in a conjugated (glucuronide) form in the urine. Limited conversion of codeine to morphine does not occur in the dog as in human beings (Woods and Muehlenbeck 1954). The excretion products in human beings include norcodeine, conjugated codiene, morphine, and traces of codeine in the feces.

Codeine is widely used to depress the cough center. On this center codeine is about one-third as depressant as morphine, but on the other cortical centers codeine is one-twentieth as depressant. Relatively, codeine has a more specific depressant effect upon the cough center than does morphine. The dose of codeine should be increased proportionately over that of morphine to produce the desired depression of the cough reflex with less undesirable side action. Unfortunately, codeine possesses some of the constipating action of morphine; therefore, a large dose or prolonged administration may result in constipation. Since the analgesic action of codeine is less than morphine, codeine is not used for analgesia. Addiction to codeine is uncommon.

Codeine phosphate is used in an expectorant and cough syrup mixture at 0.5–1 mg/lb to allay irritating coughs in dogs; this level is administered orally 3–4 times daily.

Hydromorphone Hydrochloride. *Hydromorphone Hydrochloride,* U.S.P. (Dilaudid), is about 5 times more potent as an analgesic than morphine. In the dog it produces less nausea, emesis, and gastrointestinal disturbance than morphine. It is soluble in 3 parts of water. The subcutaneous dose for the dog is 0.5–1 mg/lb of body weight.

Oxymorphone Hydrochloride. *Oxymorphone Hydrochloride* (Numorphan) is approximately 2.5 times as potent as Dilaudid and about 10 times more potent than morphine on a mg/mg basis. This narcotic analgesic is potent when used alone or in combination with neuroleptic agents or barbiturates in the dog and cat (Palminteri 1963; Nytch 1964). Oxymorphone is approved by the FDA for use in the dog and cat.

In the cat, a combination of oxymorphone (0.075 mg/lb) and triflupromazine (0.5 mg/lb) has proved satisfactory (Reid and Frank 1972). This neuroleptanalgesic mixture was followed with intravenous ketamine (0.5–1 mg/lb). According to Reid and Frank (1972), the combination of oxymorphone and triflupromazine can be administered subcutaneously, intramuscularly, or intravenously. They recommend that ketamine not be administered until after oxymorphone and triflupromazine have taken effect because the simultaneous administration of all three drugs induces prolonged apnea resembling the "locked chest" syndrome described in human beings.

When used alone, the preanesthetic effectiveness of oxymorphone is limited in the dog and cat because its CNS depressant effects are slight (Palminteri 1963). Also, it produces a mild ataxia and hyperesthesia in the cat when used by itself. In combining the narcotic analgesic with a neuroleptic drug such as triflupromazine, a greater degree of neurolepsia or transquilization is achieved. Oxymorphone (1.5 mg/cc) is used

TABLE 15.4. Parenteral doses of a mixture of equal volumes of oxymorphone* and triflupromazine† required to produce analgesia in small animals

Animal	Body Weight	Volume of Narcotic-Tranquilizer Mixture
	(lb)	*(cc)*
Dogs	2–5	1.0
	5–15	1.0–2.0
	15–30	2.0–4.0
	30–60	4.0–6.0
	60+	6.0–8.0
Cats	Small	0.5–1.0
	Large	1.0–2.0

Source: Palminteri 1963.
* 1.5 mg/cc
† 20.0 mg/cc

in combination with triflupromazine (20 mg/cc) by mixing equal volumes of both drugs in the same syringe for intravenous, intramuscular, or subcutaneous administration. For the dosage schedule recommended in the dog and cat, see Table 15.4.

In the dog, premedication with oxymorphone reduced the amount of thiamylal sodium required to produce surgical anesthesia by one-third to two-thirds (Nytch 1964). Use of the analgesic agent prior to thiamylal sodium required intramuscular or subcutaneous doses of oxymorphone varying from 0.03 to 0.2 mg/lb of body weight. The lower doses were administered to the large breeds. For all dogs, the average dose was 0.09 mg/lb of body weight. Thiamylal sodium (2.5%) was administered intravenously to effect 45–90 minutes after the administration of oxymorphone.

Etorphine Hydrochloride. *Etorphine Hydrochloride* (M-99, oripavine) is a semisynthetic opiate derivative that possesses up to 10,000 times the analgesic potency of morphine. It is used extensively in the capture and restraint of exotic species. In addition, etorphine has been combined with acetylpromazine for use in large domestic species; this neuroleptanalgesic preparation has been discussed in this chapter.

MORPHINE SUBSTITUTES

A number of morphine substitutes have been synthesized in an effort to find an analgesic agent without the addictive properties of morphine. Essentially all the potent analgesics advocated for replacement of morphine have resulted in addiction either equivalent to or greater than that produced by morphine. For example, methadone was introduced because it not only was a potent analgesic agent but appeared initially to be without the addictive effects of morphine. However, the nonaddicting effects of methadone proved later to be untrue. Methadone is not available for human or veterinary use. The decision to remove methadone from general medical use was reached jointly by the Drug Enforcement Agency and the FDA in 1973. The only approved use is treatment of abstinence or withdrawal symptoms of addicts who have been dependent upon "hard drugs," including methadone.

Of the many analgesic substitutes for morphine that have been synthesized, meperidine hydrochloride is the only nonmorphine derivative used extensively in the United States for veterinary purposes. In the United Kingdom and other countries, thiambutene is also used for its analgesic effect. Thiambutene has not been approved by the FDA for use in the United States.

Meperidine Hydrochloride. *Meperidine Hydrochloride,* U.S.P. (Demerol, pethidine, dolantin) (Fig. 15.4), was synthesized in Germany during a search for an atropine-like drug with spasmolytic activity (Eisleb and Schaumann 1939). Meperidine is not only spasmolytic but also analgesic and sedative. The hydrochloride salt is used in medicine. It is a colorless crystalline powder with a neutral reaction, a slightly bit-

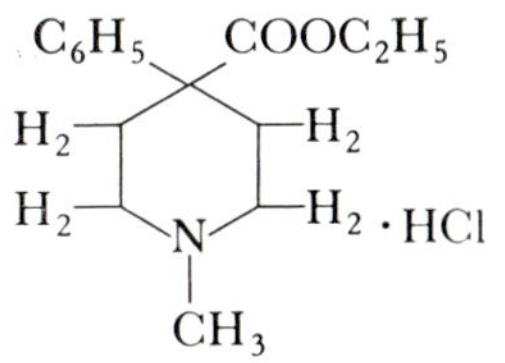

C_6H_5 $COOC_2H_5$
H_2 H_2
H_2 N $H_2 \cdot HCl$
CH_3

Meperidine Hydrochloride

FIG. 15.4.

ter taste, and ready solubility in water. The aqueous solution is not decomposed by a short period of boiling.

Administration. Meperidine is best administered intramuscularly in animals. The subcutaneous route is not preferred because local irritation and pain may be produced. Oral administration is not advised in large animals because of the cost. If the drug contacts the buccal mucosa, particularly in the cat, considerable irritation and salivation result. Intravenous injection must be made slowly to avoid drug shock and prostration. Following intramuscular or subcutaneous administration in the cat, emesis does not occur but defecation occurs in some animals.

Metabolism and fate. Meperidine is absorbed rapidly following subcutaneous, intramuscular, or oral administration. The drug is largely inactivated in the liver (Way et al. 1947). According to studies with C^{14}-labeled meperidine, a small amount is excreted unchanged in the urine. The major part of a given dose is demethylated (normeperidine) and hydrolyzed before being excreted in the urine. Neither the demethylated nor hydrolyzed form possesses analgesic activity (Plotnikoff et al. 1952).

In human beings, only about 5% of meperidine administered is excreted unchanged; the remaining portion undergoes *N*-demethylation to normeperidine acid or conjugation with glucuronic acid. About 60% of the administered meperidine in human beings can be recovered (Greene 1968); 5% of the drug is unchanged, 5% is in the form of normeperidine, 20% is meperidine acid, 7% normeperidine acid, and 12% each is recovered as bound meperidine and normeperidine. The disposition of the remaining 40% of the parent compound is unknown. The biotransformation of meperidine in human beings occurs at the rate of 10%–20%/hour; *N*-demethylation occurs through hepatic microsomal enzyme activity together with NADPH and oxygen. Only the unchanged meperidine molecule can be metabolized by the liver; all other metabolic changes or degradation occur to some degree in extrahepatic tissues.

When meperidine hydrochloride (22 mg/kg) is administered intravenously, Davis and Donnelly (1968) found the plasma half-life to be 0.7 hour in the cat. Despite the short half-life in plasma, the analgesic effect of 11 mg/kg of the drug given intramuscularly is apparent at 2 hours but not at one-half hour or 4 hours after administration. Because the duration of effective plasma levels of meperidine are short, and the biotransformation is rapid, Davis and Donnelly (1968) stated that meperidine probably will serve better as a preanesthetic drug than in the management of severe pain in cats.

Thermoregulatory effect. In the cat, following the subcutaneous injection of large doses (13.5–22.5 mg/lb) of meperidine, a marked rise to 105°–107° F occurs in the rectal temperature. This response may be indicative of an accelerated metabolic rate (Booth and Rankin 1954). Since a hyperthermic response can occur following administration of morphine and apomorphine through activation of central dopaminergic mechanisms, it is possible that meperidine produces a similar effect.

Cardiopulmonary effect. Following an intramuscular dose of 10 mg/kg of meperidine, a reduction in the heart rate and a drop in the systemic arterial pressure occur in dogs (Robbins 1945). Generally, the fall in blood pressure is moderate and occurs 10–20 minutes after the intramuscular injection, with return to the control level in 30 minutes. The decline in systemic arterial pressure is probably the result of peripheral vasodilation.

A significant degree of bronchoconstriction occurs in the dog following an intravenous dose of 0.5 mg/kg (Shemano and Wendel 1965). Also, meperidine administered at 2.5 mg/kg intravenously produces a 22% decrease in lung capacity. Shemano and Wendel (1965) suggested that the bronchoconstrictor effect of meperidine and morphine may be due to a combination of central vagal stimulation and histamine release.

Analgesic action. The analgesic effect of meperidine is intermediate between codeine and morphine. In dogs, meperidine depresses the cough reflex satisfactorily and is useful in cardiac "asthma." Success follows the intramuscular injection of 2 mg/lb every 3–6 hours, as indicated (Schnelle 1949). In the horse, meperidine produces analgesia within a few minutes following intravenous administration and 15–25 minutes after an intramuscular injection (Archer 1947).

Spasmolytic action. The spasmolytic activity of meperidine is significant but considerably less than morphine and methadone. Meperidine will relax the intestine, the bronchi, the ureter, and, to some degree, the uterus. Meperidine, morphine, and methadone depress intestinal peristalsis in the dog. The ratio of doses producing the same degree of intestinal inhibition is morphine 1 and meperidine 750. Because the ratio of doses producing a given analgesic effect is 1:10, meperidine has an advantage of 75 to 1 over morphine when an analgesic drug is needed that does not depress intestinal motility (Vaughn-Williams and Streeten 1950a). It is apparent that meperidine possesses a marked advantage over morphine for relief of postoperative pain because it can be given in many times (up to 750) the dose of morphine before it depresses intestinal propulsion as much as morphine (Vaughn-Williams and Streeten 1950b).

Meperidine is distributed widely throughout the body, including the placental and fetal tissues. It is used to allay parturition pains in women because it does not depress fetal respiration.

Toxicity. Subcutaneous dosages in excess of 10–15 mg/lb of body weight can produce excitement and clonic convulsions in cats (see Table 15.5). These convulsions can be controlled by the injection of pentobarbital sodium (Mayer 1945; Booth and Rankin 1954). The barbiturates can be used successfully to antagonize the lethal convulsive effects of meperidine. However, meperidine potentiates the depressant effect of the barbiturates upon respiration and will only increase the certainty of death if administered in barbiturate intoxication (Way 1946). Nalorphine is an antagonist of the respiratory depressant and toxic effects of meperidine.

Meperidine is rapidly destroyed and eliminated so cumulative toxicity is not observed. Prolonged administration of meperidine to dogs in amounts up to 6 times the recommended therapeutic dose produced no toxic effects other than a slight anorexia and loss of weight (Gruber et al. 1941). Although no addiction to meperidine has been demonstrated in animals, addiction manifested by withdrawal symptoms has been noted in human beings.

Clinical use. In veterinary medicine the main use of meperidine is control of pain. Although meperidine is an effective analgesic, it is not a potent CNS depressant or sedative. However, it will significantly augment the activity of other depressants. In dogs, meperidine given preanesthetically eliminates the period of excitement and reduces the amount of anesthetic needed (Rovenstine and Batterman 1943).

TABLE 15.5. Effect of varying dose levels of meperidine hydrochloride in the cat

Dose	Number of Cats Tested	Number Showing Excitation	Number Showing Muscular Spasms	Number Showing Convulsions	Deaths
(mg/kg)					
5	10	0	0	0	0
10	25	5 (slight)	0	0	0
20	15	8	0	0	0
30	15	15	9	6*	0
40	15	15	13	11†	0
50	10	10	10	9‡	0

Source: Booth and Rankin 1954.

Pentobarbital sodium (15–20 mg/kg) was used as an anticonvulsant in 3 cats,* 1 cat,† and 7 cats‡ of these respective groups.

TABLE 15.6. Dosages and indications of meperidine hydrochloride for use in laboratory animals

Species	Dose	Route of Administration	Major Indications	Reference
	(mg/kg)			
Mouse	40	I.P.	Analgesia	. . .
Rat	50	I.P.	Analgesia	. . .
Hamster	2	I.M.	Preanesthetic	. . .
Guinea pig	2	I.M.	Preanesthetic	Maykut 1958
Rabbit	25	I.M.	Preanesthetic	Gardner 1964
Subhuman primates	11	Unspecified (probably i.m.)	Combination with promazine (4.4 mg/kg)	Clifford 1971

There is individual variation in the depressant effects of meperidine.

Meperidine has been used successfully in prolonging pentobarbital sodium anesthesia. Anesthetic mortality data indicate that meperidine is much preferred over ether because of a lower death rate (Albrecht and Blakely 1951). Either is preferred over pentobarbital sodium because of the tendency for the barbiturates to paralyze the respiratory centers in excessive dosages.

In the dog and cat. In the dog, meperidine hydrochloride is used intramuscularly for preanesthetic medication varying from 2.5 to 6.5 mg/kg of body weight (Soma 1971). The postanalgesic dose recommended in the dog is 5–10 mg/kg intramuscularly. In the cat, the intramuscular dose of meperidine is 2–5 mg/lb of body weight for preanesthetic medication. For general use of meperidine in the relief of pain for both the dog and cat, an intramuscular dose of 5 mg/lb is recommended, repeated safely every 8–12 hours. A small repeated dose of 2 mg/lb can be given every 3–6 hours to depress a cough and "cardiac dyspnea." Effective analgesia is produced in about 30–40 minutes after meperidine is administered.

In the pig. Meperidine hydrochloride (10 mg/kg) administered subcutaneously in large sows and boars contributes little toward restraint (Vaughn 1961). However, as an analgesic the drug is beneficial in obtunding pain following major surgery. For preanesthetic medication in the pig, meperidine hydrochloride (1–2 mg/kg), promazine hydrochloride (2 mg/kg), and atropine sulfate (0.07–0.09 mg/kg) work satisfactorily prior to barbiturate and inhalant anesthesia (Booth 1969). All these preanesthetic preparations are administered intramuscularly in separate sites 45–60 minutes prior to the induction of anesthesia.

In the horse and cow. The total intravenous and intramuscular doses recommended for the adult horse are 500 and 1000 mg, respectively (Archer 1947). Archer also uses meperidine in cattle at a dose level of 500 mg. Although it was unreported by Archer, the intramuscular route of administration is probably used in cattle. Meperidine is used to treat equine colic, especially acute spasmodic conditions. In cattle, the drug is used for calving to calm the "nervous" heifer and to provide analgesia during parturition. Meperidine does not inhibit uterine contractions in cattle.

In laboratory animals. Meperidine is useful as an analgesic in laboratory species. Dose levels have been compiled in Table 15.6.

Thiambutene Hydrochloride. *Thiambutene Hydrochloride* (Themalon) (3-diethylamino-1, 1-dithienylbut-1-ene hydrochloride) is available in the United Kingdom where it is recommended for use only in the dog because it has analgesic and pharmacologic properties similar to morphine. Thiambutene produces untoward effects such as tetanic muscle spasms, tremors, and excitation.

The incidence of violent tetanic spasms in the dog after an intramuscular injection of thiambutene hydrochloride (5 mg/lb) is 3.6%–4.6% without and with acetylpromazine (Cansfield 1968). The tetanic spasms occur 15–20 minutes after administration of the drug. Thiopental sodium has been used to control the spasms.

The usual procedure employed in the use of thiambutene to avoid the tetanic spasms following an intravenous dose (2 mg/lb) is to follow up immediately with either pentobarbital sodium or thiopental sodium at the same dosage rate intravenously (Kneen 1968). In the experience of Hayes (1968), the tetanic effect can arise following administration by either route, but it is noted more commonly after intravenous administration, particularly if the drug is administered rapidly. Also, the tetanic spasms appear to involve dogs under 6 months of age; thiambutene should not be used in animals below this age (Hayes 1968).

Thiambutene has been successfully used with local anesthesia for cesarean section in the bitch (Spira 1960). The drug is usually administered intravenously; the dose recommended varies from 1 to 2 mg/lb of body weight depending on the obstetrical status of the animal. Although healthy or nontoxic animals may need up to 2 mg/lb of thiambutene, a dose of 0.5 mg/lb produces satisfactory analgesia and narcosis in the toxic animal (Spira 1960). The puppies are active at delivery; consequently, placental transfer of thiambutene does not appear to be significant. If the bitches have littered previously, they accept their pups readily after recovery from thiambutene. Spira (1960) believes the long recovery period causes some dulling of the maternal instinct.

In the dog following the intravenous administration of 2 mg/lb of body weight, thiambutene narcosis develops rapidly and is usually complete within 1–2 minutes. The depth of the depression varies (medium to deep) and lasts up to 2.5 hours. Following intramuscular administration of 5 mg/lb of body weight, complete thiambutene narcosis usually occurs after 10–15 minutes and reaches a peak effect after approximately 30 minutes. The analgesic and narcotic actions of thiambutene are rapidly terminated in the dog by an intravenous injection of 0.45 mg/lb of body weight of nalorphine (Owen 1955).

In pigs thiambutene produces excitement and convulsions (Owen 1955). Intramuscular dosages of 10–30 mg/kg were observed to produce little or no quieting effect in them; they responded violently to restraint (Vaughan 1961). Untoward effects such as muscle spasms, tremors, and excitation also occur in the cat, horse, and cow following thiambutene. According to Watts et al. (1973), morphine produced superior analgesic effect in the cat. Watts and coworkers concluded that thiambutene is not suitable for clinical use in the cat because of toxic effects at doses slightly higher than those required to produce the desired analgesic effect.

Prior to the use of etorphine in the capture and restraint of large wild animals, thiambutene hydrochloride was administered per 1000 lb of body weight as follows (Harthoorn 1969): thiambutene (1.5 g); hyoscine (25–50 mg); and acetylpromazine (10 mg). Due to the necessity of having to estimate body weight of wild game in the field, the variation in dosage between the minimum effective dose and the maximum dose used was several hundred percent. According to Harthoorn (1969), thiambutene use was not discontinued in large wild animals for reasons of safety. It was superseded by etorphine since the onset of action was faster, due to a more rapid absorption rate.

ANALGESIC ANTAGONISTS

The narcotic antagonists of current importance in veterinary medicine are nalorphine hydrochloride, naloxone hydrochloride, and diprenorphine hydrochloride. *Levallorphan Tartate,* U.S.P. (Lorfan), is only occasionally used in clinical practice. Other narcotic antagonists that have been under study for possible use are nalbuphine hydrochloride and nalmexone hydrochloride.

Nalorphine Hydrochloride

Nalorphine Hydrochloride, U.S.P. (*N*-allylnormorphine, Nalline), is a morphine

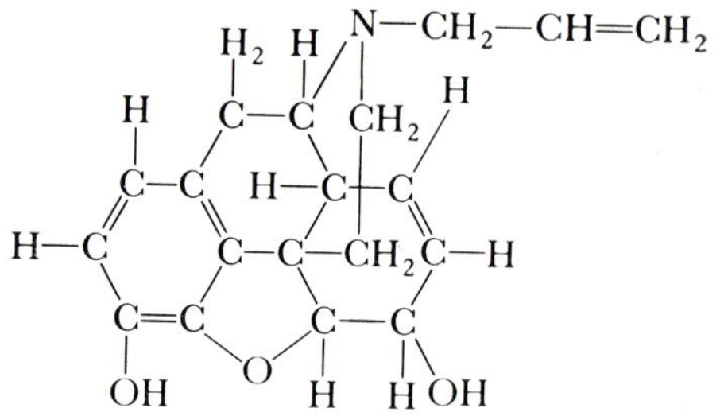

Nalorphine (N-allylnormorphine)

FIG. 15.5.

derivative in which an *N*-methyl group has been replaced with an *N*-allyl group (Fig. 15.5). Surprisingly, this compound antagonizes many of the reactions of morphine and its congeners.

ADMINISTRATION

Nalorphine hydrochloride is available as a liquid (5 mg/ml) and is subject to the Controlled Substances Act of 1970 as a Schedule III drug. It is injected subcutaneously, intramuscularly, or intravenously. Nalorphine cannot be mixed with meperidine because a precipitate will form.

ABSORPTION AND FATE

Nalorphine is relatively ineffective after oral administration but is promptly absorbed after subcutaneous or intramuscular injection. The biotransformation of nalorphine probably is quite similar to that of morphine because it is conjugated by liver tissue as is morphine. The duration of action of nalorphine appears to be briefer than morphine.

ACTION

During the action or effect of narcotics, nalorphine acts as a narcotic antagonist. However, in its absence, it acts like a narcotic and may produce CNS depression and analgesia. Also, nalorphine does not antagonize mild respiratory depression and may actually aggravate it. Very large doses will paralyze respiration in the dog, but lower dosages have little effect. Nalorphine is not constipative in the dog as is morphine. It has little effect upon the cardiovascular system.

The most prominent and valuable pharmacological action of nalorphine is in preventing or relieving the typical respiratory-depressant activity of morphine and all its derivatives plus meperidine and fentanyl. The analgesic and narcotic actions of thiambutene are rapidly terminated by an intravenous injection of nalorphine. It is ineffective against the respiratory depression of barbiturates, cyclopropane, and ether (Eckenhoff et al. 1952). In fact, nalorphine may increase the respiratory depressant effects on nonnarcotic CNS depressants. Also, nalorphine does not antagonize the effects of xylazine, a nonnarcotic analgesic.

The ability of nalorphine to antagonize the respiratory-depressant action of morphine is demonstrated in Fig. 15.6. A subsequent injection of morphine is ineffective in depressing respiration. A subsequent injection of nalorphine has little effect in increasing respiratory rate.

The fetal respiratory depression of morphine in pregnant rabbits is antagonized by nalorphine with no effect upon uterine motility, labor, or incidence of stillbirths. Apnea in the newborn, induced by morphine sedation of the mother, is corrected by administering nalorphine to the newborn. Nalorphine will produce typical withdrawal symptoms in a morphine-addicted persons.

DOSAGE

One mg of nalorphine is recommended for every 10 mg of morphine or 20 mg of meperidine for reversal of narcotic effects (Aronson and Gans 1959b). For reversal of the effects of etorphine, a ratio of 10–20 mg of nalorphine to 1 mg of etorphine is required (Alford et al. 1974). The intravenous route is recommended for administration of nalorphine.

TOXICITY

Nalorphine appears to possess about the same toxicity as morphine but provides less relief from pain. The subcutaneous injection of 5–10 mg/lb of nalorphine in the dog produces little analgesia and no depression of the brain or respiration. This

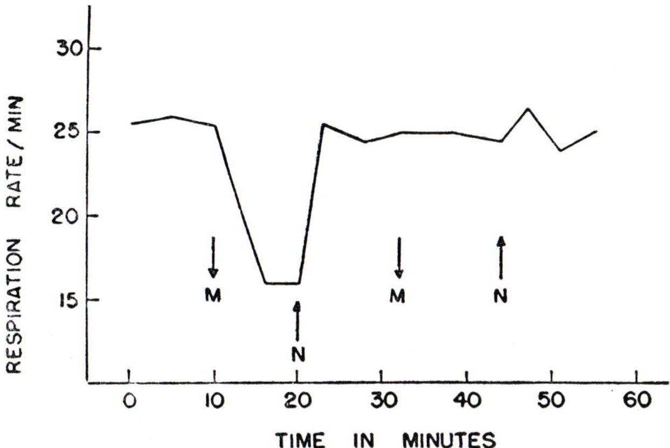

FIG. 15.6. The antagonistic action of nalorphine (N) to the respiratory depressant effect of morphine (M). (Unna 1943)

dose prevents any response to morphine (2.5–5 mg/lb) administered within 1 hour. It also arouses dogs intoxicated with morphine (2.5 mg/lb) so that they are almost normal within 15 minutes. Although nalorphine effectively antagonizes the sedative and respiratory depressant effects of morphine and meperidine in the dog, it will not reliably prevent arterial hypotension (Aronson and Gans 1959a).

Cats exhibit no significant response to subcutaneous injections of 5–10 mg/lb of nalorphine. Subcutaneous injections of morphine (2.5 mg/lb), which usually cause restlessness, extreme mydriasis, marked irritability, and incoordination, cause no apparent reaction in cats when given 30 minutes following nalorphine (Unna 1943).

Caution should be observed to ensure proper dose levels of nalorphine. Should the first dose fail to produce an effect on the depression, additional dosages are contraindicated. In the event of an overdosage of nalorphine, respiratory supportive measures must be instituted, including the establishment of a patent airway and oxygen administration.

NALOXONE HYDROCHLORIDE

Naxloxone Hydrochloride (*N*-allylnoroxymorphone hydrochloride, Narcan) is approved by the FDA for use in the dog. Chemically, naloxone hydrochloride is 17-allyl-4,5α-epoxy-3,14-dihydroxymorphinan-6-one hydrochloride (Fig. 15.7).

Naloxone has a potency 10–30 times that of nalorphine. Unlike nalorphine, it lacks the agonistic effect that is highly desirable if the drug is to be depended on as an antagonist of narcotic analgesics. Consequently, naloxone does not produce respiratory depression, which commonly occurs with other narcotic antagonists.

ACTION

In the dog and cat, one part of naloxene will antagonize respiratory depression produced by 15–20 parts of oxymorphone hydrochloride (Palminteri 1966). The reversal of all actions of oxymorphone, including its analgesic effect, occurs when a ratio of 0.4 mg of naloxone to 1.5 mg of oxymorphone is administered. The effects of morphine and meperidine are reversed by naloxone to a lesser degree than those of oxymorphone. According to Palminteri (1966), naloxone does not antagonize the effect of inhalant anesthetics, barbiturates, procaine, or tranquilizers. Moreover, he observed no adverse reactions in 300 dogs

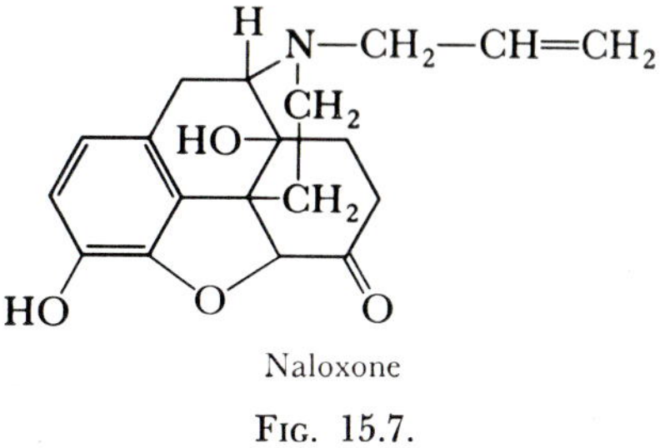

Naloxone

FIG. 15.7.

and cats when naloxone was used with ether, methoxyflurane, pentobarbital, thiamylal, procaine, oxymorphone, morphine, meperidine, or with many commercially available phenothiazine tranquilizers.

In the dog, naloxone hydrochloride will also adequately reverse the fentanyl component of Innovar-Vet (Paddleford and Short 1973).

ADMINISTRATION AND DOSAGE

Naloxone can be administered by all of the parenteral routes. However, the intravenous route of administration is preferred to attain immediate effect from the drug. The respiratory depressant effects of overdosages of oxymorphone in dogs and cats can be reversed with a ratio of 0.1 mg of naloxone to 1.5 mg of oxymorphone (Palminteri 1966). If the narcotic antagonist is administered intramuscularly or subcutaneously, the onset of action occurs in 1–5 minutes; intravenously the onset is immediate and lasts 1–2 hours.

In the reversal of the narcotic effects of morphine and fentanyl in the dog, 0.016–0.1 mg/0.45 kg of naloxone hydrochloride was used intravenously (Paddleford and Short 1973). This quantity of naloxone antagonized the effects of 0.02–0.03 mg/0.45 kg of fentanyl administered intramuscularly and 0.01 mg/0.45 kg of fentanyl administered intravenously. Also, this same quantity of naloxone antagonizes the effect of 0.5 mg/0.45 kg of morphine sulfate intravenously.

The parenteral dosage of naloxone approved by the FDA for the dog is 0.04 mg/kg of body weight. When the drug is administered intravenously, this dose level may be repeated at 2- to 3-minute intervals to produce the desired effect.

Diprenorphine Hydrochloride

Chemically, *Diprenorphine Hydrochloride* (nororipavine, cyprenorphine, M-285, M50-50) is *N*-(cyclopropylmethyl)-6,7,8,14-tetrahydro-7-α-(1-hydroxy-1-methylethyl)-6,14-endo-ethano-nororipavine hydrochloride (Fig. 15.8).

Diprenorphine

Fig. 15.8.

Like nalorphine, diprenorphine has an agonistic effect and in the presence of a mild respiratory depression it may be further aggravated. Diprenorphine at double the dose level of etorphine is capable of immobilizing wild animals (Alford et al. 1974). The same general precautions mentioned above for nalorphine apply to diprenorphine.

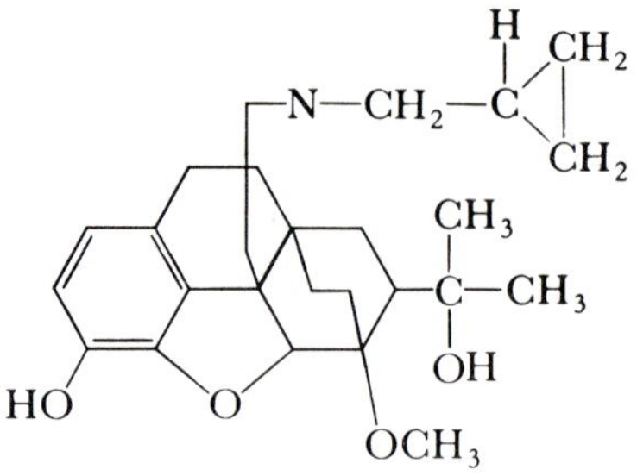

Diprenorphine hydrochloride (2 mg/ml) was approved by the FDA in 1973 for use in wild and exotic animals to specifically reverse the effects of etorphine hydrochloride. It is administered intravenously or intramuscularly. Diprenorphine must not be used in animals intended for human consumption or in animals that might be used for food during the hunting season. The drug is subject to the Controlled Substances Act of 1970 like other narcotic antagonists.

ADMINISTRATION AND DOSAGE

Most consistent results are obtained when an etorphine to diprenorphine ratio of 1:2 is used, i.e., 1 mg of etorphine is antagonized by 2 mg of diprenorphine. Reversal of the narcotic effects of etorphine is obtained by intravenous administration with either diprenorphine or nalorphine (Alford et al. 1974). The residual narcosis after the administration of diprenorphine is less than that from the use of nalorphine. If diprenorphine is administered intramuscularly to reverse the effect of etorphine, 5–20 minutes are required before the CNS depressant effects are reversed.

Diprenorphine (30 μg/kg) is also recommended intravenously for reversal of the effects of etorphine (22 μg/kg) when employed in combination with acetylpromazine for immobilization of the horse (Jenkin 1972). Thurmon et al. (1974) used diprenorphine (0.140 ± 0.025 mg/kg) intravenously in the goat to reverse the action of etorphine (0.07 ± 0.018 mg/kg) when used in combination with triflupromazine.

REFERENCES

Albrecht, D. T., and Blakely, C. L. 1951. Anesthetic mortality: A five-year survey of the records of the Angell Memorial Animal Hospital. J Am Vet Med Assoc 199:429.

Alexander, F. 1960. The effect of centrally acting drugs on the concentration of glucose and eosinophils in horse blood. Res Vet Sci 1:355.

Alford, B. T.; Burkhart, R. L.; and Johnson, W. P. 1974. Etorphine and diprenorphine as immobilizing and reversing agents in captive and free-ranging mammals. J Am Vet Med Assoc 164:702.

Amadon, R. C., and Craige, A. H. 1937. The actions of morphine on the horse. Preliminary studies: Diacetylmorphine (heroin), dihydrodesoxymorphine-D (desomorphine) and dihydrohetercodeine. J Am Vet Med Assoc 91:674.

Archer, R. K. 1947. Pethidine in veterinary practice. Vet Rec 59:401.

Aronson, A. L., and Gans, J. H. 1959a. The narcotic analgesics and their antagonists as adjuncts to barbiturate anesthesia. I. Physiological and pharmacological considerations. Am J Vet Res 20:909.

———. 1959b. The narcotic analgesics and their antagonists as adjuncts to barbiturate anesthesia. II. Clinical applications. J Am Vet Med Assoc 134:459.

Berkowitz, B., and Spector, S. 1972. Evidence for active immunity to morphine in mice. Science 178:1290.

Booth, N. H. 1969. Anesthesia in the pig. Fed Proc 28:1547.

Booth, N. H., and Rankin, A. D. 1954. Evaluation of meperidine hydrochloride in the cat. Vet Med 49:249.

Booth, N. H.; Bredeck, H. E.; and Herin, R. A. 1960. Baroceptor reflex mechanisms in swine. Am J Physiol 199:1189.

Brand, J. J., and Perry, W. L. M. 1966. Drugs used in motion sickness. Pharmacol Rev 18:895.

Breazile, J. E., and Kitchell, R. L. 1969. Pain perception in animals. Fed Proc 28:1379.

Cansfield, C. J. 1968. The use of thiambutene hydrochloride. Vet Rec 83:475.

Chen, K. K.; Powell, C. E.; and Maze, N. 1945. The response of the hamster to drugs. J Pharmacol Exp Ther 85:348.

Christian, E. M., and Gross, E. G. 1948. Analgesic effects in human subjects of morphine, meperidine and methadon. J Am Med Assoc 137:594.

Clifford, D. 1971. Restraint and anesthesia of subhuman primates. In L. R. Soma, ed. Textbok of Veterinary Anesthesia, p. 385. Baltimore: Williams & Wilkins.

Cox, J. E. 1973. Immobilization and anaesthesia of the pig. Vet Rec 92:143.

Cox, J. E.; Meese, G. B.; and Ewbank, R. 1973. The use of large animal Immobilon in pigs. Vet Rec 93:354.

Crooks, J. L.; Whiteley, H.; Jenkins, J. T.; and Blane, G. F. 1970. The use of a new analgesic-tranquilizer mixture in dogs. Vet Rec 87:498.

Daniel, M., and Ling, C. M. 1972. The effect of an etorphine-acepromazine mixture on the heart rate and blood pressure of the horse. Vet Rec 90:336.

Davis, L. E., and Donnelly, E. J. 1968. Analgesic drugs in the cat. J Am Med Assoc 153: 1161.

Dayton, H. E., and Garrett, R. L. 1973. Production of analgesia by cholinergic drug. Proc Soc Exp Biol Med 142:1011.

De Bodo, R. C. 1944. The antidiuretic action of morphine and its mechanism. J Pharmacol Exp Ther 82:74.

Dhasmana, K. M.; Dixit, K. S.; Jaju, B. P.; and Gupta, M. L. 1972. Role of central dopaminergic receptors in manic response of cats to morphine. Psychopharmacologia 24:380.

Dobbs, H. E. 1973. Reversible immobolization and analgesia in the bullock. Vet Rec 93: 11.

Dorn, A. S. 1972. Fentanyl citrate and droperidol in the Australian terrier. Aust Vet J 48:54.

Eckenhoff, J. E.; Hoffman, G. L.; and Dripps, R. D. 1952. *N*-allyl normorphine: An antagonist to the opiates. Anesthesiology 13:242.

Eisleb, O., and Schaumann, O. 1939. Dolantin, ein neurartiges spasmolytikum und analgetickum. Dtsch Med Wochenschr 65:967.

Feldman, D. B., and Self, J. L. 1971. Sedation and anesthesia of the Virginia opossum *Didelphis virginiana*. Lab Anim Sci 21: 717.

Field, W. E.; Yelnosky, J.; Mundy, J.; and Mitchell, J. 1966. Use of droperidol and fentanyl for analgesia and sedation in primates. J Am Vet Med Assoc 149:896.

Franklin, I. I., and Reid, J. S. 1965. Clinical use of a combination of fentanyl and droperidol in dogs. Vet Med 60:927.

Gardner, A. F. 1964. The development of general anesthesia in the albino rabbit for surgical procedures. Lab Anim Sci 14:214.

Gardocki, J. F., and Yelnosky, J. 1964. A study

of some of the pharmacologic actions of fentanyl citrate. Toxicol Appl Pharmacol 6:48.

Gardocki, J. F.; Yelnosky, J.; Kuehn, W. F.; and Gunster, J. C. 1964. A study of the interaction of nalorphine with fentanyl and Innovar. Toxical Appl Pharmacol 6:593.

Greene, N. M. 1968. The metabolism of drugs employed in anesthesia. Anesthesiology 29: 327.

Gruber, C. M.; Hart, E. R.; and Gruber, C. M., Jr. 1941. The pharmacology and toxicology of the ethyl ester of 1-methyl-4-phenylpiperidine-4-carboxylic acid (Demerol). J Pharmacol Exp Ther 73:319.

Gupta, B. N.; Moore, J. A.; and Conner, G. H. 1970. The use of promazine hydrochloride in cesarean section in the dog. Lab Anim Sci 20:474.

Harthoorn, A. M. 1965a. Wildlife monographs. Application of pharmacological and physiological principles in restraint of wild animals, p. 40. Washington D.C.: Wildlife Society.

———. 1965b. The use of a new oripavine derivative for restraint of domestic hoofed animals. J S Afr Vet Assoc 36:45.

———. 1966. Restraint of undomesticated animals. J Am Med Assoc 149:875.

———. 1969. The use of thiambutene hydrochloride. Vet Rec 84:151.

———. 1972. Restraint and neuroleptanalgesia in ungulates. Vet Rec 91:63.

Harthoorn, A. M., and Bligh, J. 1965. The use of a new oripavine derivative with potent morphine-like activity for the restraint of hoofed wild animals. Res Vet Sci 6:290.

Hasbrouck, J. D. 1970. Morphine anesthesia for open-heart surgery. Ann Thorac Surg 10:364.

Hayes, M. J. 1968. The use of thiambutene hydrochloride. Vet Rec 83:528.

Heavner, J. E. 1970. Morphine for postsurgical use in cats. J Am Vet Med Assoc 156:1018.

Heinrich, U.; Lichtensteiger, W.; and Langemann, H. 1971. Effect of morphine on the catecholamine content of midbrain nerve cell groups in rat and mouse. J Pharmacol Exp Ther 179:259.

Hillidge, C. J.; Lees, P.; and Serrano, L. 1973. Investigations of azaperone/metomidate anaesthesia in the horse. Vet Rec 93:307.

Jacobsen, C. E. 1970. Morphine-promazine: A better preanesthetic. Mod Vet Pract 51:29.

Jacquet, Y. F., and Lajtha, A. 1973. Morphine action at central nervous system sites in rat: Analgesia for hyperalgesia depending on site and dose. Science 182:490.

Jaffe, J. H. 1970. Narcotic analgesics. In L. S. Goodman and A. Gilman, eds. The Pharmacological Basis of Therapeutics, 4th ed., p. 237. New York: Macmillan.

Jainudeen, M. R.; Bongso, T. A.; and Perera, B. M. O. A. 1971. Immobilization of aggressive working elephants *(Elephas maximus).* Vet Rec 89:686.

Jenkin, J. T. 1972. The use of etorphine-acepromazine (analgesic-tranquilizer) mixtures in horses. Vet Rec 90:207.

Jones, J. B., and Simmons, M. L. 1968. Innovar-Vet as an intramuscular anesthetic for rats. Lab Anim Sci 18:642.

Keep, M. E., and Keep, P. J. 1967. Immobilization of waterbuck. Vet Rec 81:552.

Kneen, J. E. 1968. The use of thiambutene hydrochloride. Vet Rec 83:502.

Krahwinkel, D. J.; Sawyer, D. C.; and Evans, A. T. 1972. Neuroleptanalgesia and neuroleptanesthesia. J Am Anim Hosp Assoc 8:368.

Krueger, H. 1937. The action of morphine on the digestive tract. Physiol Rev 17:618.

Krueger, H.; Eddy, N. B.; and Sumwalt, M. 1941. The pharmacology of the opium alkaloids. US Public Health Rep, Supl 165, Parts 1, 2.

Lagneau, F., and Gallard, P. 1946. Intoxication des bovins par l'oeillette. Rec Med Vet 122:310.

Leash, A. M.; Beyer, R. D.; and Wilber, R. G. 1973. Self-mutilation following Innovar-Vet injection in the guinea pig. Lab Anim Sci 23:720.

Lewis, G. E., Jr., and Jennings, P. B., Jr. 1972. Effective sedation of laboratory animals using Innovar-Vet. Lab Anim Sci 22:430.

Lim, R. K. S. 1970. Pain. Ann Rev Physiol 32:269.

Lowenstein, E.; Hallowell, P.; Levine, F. H.; Daggett, W. M.; Austen, W. G.; and Laver, M. B. 1969. Cardiovascular response to large doses of intravenous morphine in man. N Eng J Med 281:1389.

Mayer, K. 1945. Demerol hydrochloride as a sedative for cats. N Am Vet 26:477.

Maykut, M. O. 1958. The combined action of pentobarbital and meperidine and of procaine and meperidine in guinea pigs. Can Anaesth Soc J 5:161.

Moller, A. W. 1968. Diseases and management of the golden hamster *(Mesocricetus auratus).* In R. W. Kirk, ed. Current Veterinary Therapy. Vol. 3, Small Animal Practice, p. 421. Philadelphia: W. B. Saunders.

Mullin, W. J.; Phillis, J. W.; and Pinsky, C. 1973. Morphine enhancement of acetylcholine release from the brain in unanesthetized cats. Eur J Pharmacol 22:117.

Newsome, J., and Robinson, D. L. H. 1957. Sedatives and anaesthetics for baboons. Br Vet J 113:163.

Nytch, T. F. 1964. Clinical observations on the preanesthetic use of oxymorphone and its antagonist, *N*-allylnoroxymorphone, in dogs. J Am Vet Med Assoc 145:127.

Owen, L. N. 1955. The narcotic effects in the dog and its antagonism by nalorphine. Vet Rec 67:561.

Paddleford, R. R., and Short, C. E. 1973. An evaluation of naloxone as a narcotic antagonist in the dog. J Am Vet Med Assoc 163:144.

Palminteri, A. 1963. Oxymorphone, an effective analgesic in dogs and cats. J Am Vet Med Assoc 143:160–61.

———. 1966. Clinical appraisal of the narcotic antagonist *N*-allylnoroxymorphone. J Am Vet Med Assoc 148:1396.

Phaneuf, L. P.; Grivel, M. L.; and Ruckebusch, Y. 1972. Electromyoenterography during normal gastro-intestinal activity, painful or non-painful colic and morphine analgesia, in the horse. Comp Med 36:138.

Plotnikoff, N. P.; Elliott, H. W.; and Way, E. L. 1952. The metabolism of N-$C^{14}H_3$ labelled meperidine. J Pharmacol Exp Ther 104:377.

Powers, S.; Reed, C.; and Gregersen, M. I. 1947. The effects of morphine on dogs in hemorrhagic and traumatic shock. Am J Physiol 148:269.

Quock, R. M., and Horita, A. 1974. Apomorphine: Modification of its hyperthermic effect in rabbits by *p*-chlorophenylalanine. Science 183:539.

Reid, J. S., and Frank, R. J. 1972 Prevention of undesirable side reactions of ketamine anesthesia in cats. J Am Anim Hosp Assoc 8:115.

Robbins, B. H. 1945. Studies on cyclopropane. IX. The effect of premedication with Demerol upon the heart rate, rhythm and blood pressure in dogs under cyclopropane anesthesia. J Pharmacol Exp Ther 85:198.

Ross, D. H.; Medina, M. A.; and Cardenas, H. L. 1974. Morphine and ethanol: Selective depletion of regional brain calcium. Science 186:63.

Rovenstine, E. A., and Batterman, R. C. 1943. The utility of Demerol as a substitute for the opiates in preanesthetic medication. Anesthesiology 4:126.

Rubright, W. C., and Thayer, C. B. 1970. The use of Innovar-Vet as a surgical anesthetic for the guinea pig. Lab Anim Sci 20:989.

Sanchez, E., and Tephly, T. R. 1974. Morphine metabolism. I. Evidence for separate enzymes in the glucuronidation of morphine and *p*-nitrophenol by rat hepatic microsomes. Drug Metab Dispos 2:248.

Schlarmann, B.; Görlitz, B.-D.; Wintzer, H.-J.; and Frey, H.-H. 1973. Clinical pharmacology of an etorphine-acepromazine preparation. Experiments in dogs and horses. Am J Vet Res 34:411.

Schnelle, G. B. 1949. Bronchial or cardiac asthma. N Am Vet 30:190.

Segall, S. 1964. Opium addiction in the dog. J Am Vet Med Assoc 144:603.

Shemano, I., and Wendel, H. 1965. Effects of meperidine hydrochloride and morphine sulfate on the lung capacity of intact dogs. J Pharmacol Exp Ther 149:379.

Short, R. V., and Spinage, C. A. 1967. Drug immobilization of the Defassa waterbuck. Vet Rec 81:336.

Soma, L. R. 1971. Textbook of Veterinary Anesthesia, p. 621. Baltimore: Williams & Wilkins.

Soma, L. R., and Shields, D. R. 1964. Neuroleptanalgesia produced by fentanyl and droperidol. J Am Vet Med Assoc 145:897.

Spector, S., and Vesell, E. S. 1971. Disposition of morphine in man. Science 174: 421.

Seal, U. S., and Erickson, A. W. 1969. Immobilization of carnivora and other mammals with phencyclidine and promazine. Fed Proc 28:1410.

Spira, H. R. 1960. Thiambutene for caesarean section in bitches and its antagonism by nalorphine. Aust Vet J 36:232.

Strack, L. E., and Kaplan, H. M. 1968. Fentanyl and droperidol for surgical anesthesia of rabbits. J Am Vet Med Assoc 153:822.

Strobel, G. E., and Wollman, H. 1969. Pharmacology of anesthetic agents. Fed Proc 28:1386.

Synder, F. F., and Lim, K. T. 1941. Effect of morphine on labor. Proc Soc Exp Biol Med 48:199.

Thayer, C. B.; Lowe, S.; and Rubright, W. C. 1972. Clinical evaluation of a combination of droperidol and fentanyl as an anesthetic for the rat and hamster. J Am Vet Med Assoc 161:665.

Thurmon, J. C.; Nelson, D. R.; and Kumar, A. 1974. Etorphine and triflupromazine as immobilizing agents in the goat. J Am Vet Med Assoc 165:168.

Tornetta, F. J., and Wilson, F. S. 1969. Innovar-nitrous oxide-oxygen: A four-year clinical appraisal of neuroleptanalgesia. Anesth Analg 48:850.

Türker, R. K., and Kaymakcalan, S. 1971. Effect of morphine and nalorphine on the intestinal motility of the cat. Arch Int Pharmacodyn Ther 193:397.

Unna, K. 1943. Antagonistic Effect of *N*-allylnormorphine upon morphine. J Pharmacol Exp Ther 79:27.

Vasko, J. S.; Henney, R. P.; Brawley, R. K.; Oldham, H. N.; and Morrow, A. G. 1966. Effects of morphine on ventricular function and myocardial contractile force. Am J Physiol 210:329.

Vaughan, L. C. 1961. Anaesthesia in the pig. Br Vet J 117:383:

Vaughn-Williams, E. M., and Streeten, D. H. P. 1950a. The action of morphine, pethidine and amidone upon the intestinal motility of conscious dogs. Br J Pharmacol 5:584.

———. 1950b. Relief of postoperative pain and intestinal motility. Lancet 259:213.

———. 1951. The mode of action of morphine upon the intestine. Br J Pharmacol 6:263.

Wallach, J. D. 1966. Immobilization and translocation of the white (square-lipped) rhinoceros. J Am Vet Med Assoc 149:871.

———. 1969. Etorphine (M 99), a new analgesic-immobilizing agent, and its antagonists. Vet Med Small Anim Clin 64:53.

Wallach, J. D., and Anderson, J. L. 1968. Oripavine (M 99) combination and solvents for immobilization of the African elephant. J Am Vet Med Assoc 153:793.

Wallach, J. D., and Hoessle, C. 1970. M 99 as an immobilizing agent in poikilotherms. Vet Med Small Anim Clin 65:163.

Wallach, J. D.; Frueh, R.; and Lentz, M. 1967. The use of M 99 as an immobilizing and analgesic agent in captive wild animals. J Am Vet Med Assoc 151:870.

Watts, S. J.; Slocombe, R. F.; Harbison, W. D.; and Stewart, G. A. 1973. Assessment of analgesia and other effects of morphine and thiambutene in the mouse and cat. Aust Vet J 49:525.

Way, E. L. 1946. Barbiturate antagonism of isonipecaine convulsions and isonipecaine potentiation of barbiturate depressions. J Pharmacol Exp Ther 87:265.

Way, E. L.; Swanson, R.; and Gimble, A. I. 1947. Studies *in vitro* on the influence of the liver on isonipecaine (Demerol) activity. J Pharmacol Exp Ther 91:178.

Williamson. W. M., and Wallach, J. D. 1968. M 99-induced recumbency and analgesia in a giraffe. J Am Vet Med Assoc 153: 816.

Wise, C. D.; Berger, B. D.; and Stein, L. 1972. Benzodiazepines: Anxiety-reducing activity by reduction of serotonin turnover in the brain. Science 177:180.

Woods, L. A., and Muehlenbeck, H. 1954. Urinary excretion of codeine and its metabolites in the dog. J Pharmacol Exp Ther 110:54.

Yelnosky, J., and Gardocki, J. F. 1964. A study of some of the pharmacologic actions of fentanyl citrate and droperidol. Toxicol Appl Pharmacol 6:63.

CHAPTER 16

NONNARCOTIC ANALGESICS

NICHOLAS H. BOOTH

- Salicylate Analgesics
  - Acetylsalicylic Acid
  - Sodium Salicylate
  - Salicylic Acid
- Para-Aminophenol–Derivative Analgesics
  - Acetanilid and Acetophenetidin (Phenacetin)
  - Acetaminophen
- Pyrazolon-Derivative Analgesics
  - Phenylbutazone
  - Dipyrone
  - Aminopyrine
- Other Nonnarcotic Analgesics
  - Xylazine Hydrochloride
  - Pentazocine Lactate
  - Propoxyphene Hydrochloride

SALICYLATE ANALGESICS

Salicylates, such as aspirin and sodium salicylate, relieve pain without causing unconsciousness as do the general anesthetics. They are of value in relief of mild to moderate pain only. The salicylates are effective in relieving pain such as cephalagia, myalgia, arthralgia, and other pains arising from integumental structures rather than from viscera (Woodbury 1970). They do not relieve deep-seated visceral pain or sharp, intense pain as will morphine. Morphine relieves severe pain by raising the pain threshold of the cerebral cortex. Salicylate analgesics are believed to act on the brain at a subcortical level because analgesic doses do not affect mental function in human beings nor do they produce hypnosis or alter sensory perception other than pain (Woodbury 1970). The salicylates do not appear to interfere with reticular function involved in arousal or in alerting an animal's attention to the presence of pain. The most common salicylate analgesic drugs are aspirin and sodium salicylate. The chronic use of these agents does not result in tolerance or addiction and the toxicity is lower than that of more potent narcotic analgesics.

The salicylate analgesics also have an antipyretic action; i.e., they lower elevated temperatures to normal. They do not lower the normal temperature. Antipyretic drugs have little or no influence on heat production but do increase heat elimination in feverish patients so that the body temperature is reduced. Quinine derived from the bark of the cinchona tree was the first antipyretic discovered.

Antipyretic drugs appear to raise the threshold of stimuli relayed from the heat-regulating center located in the hypothalamus to the cortex. The heat center controls body temperature by sympathetic nervous impulses to the cutaneous blood vessels, the pilomotor muscles, and the sweat glands. Consequently, the hypothalamus regulates peripheral mechanisms (i.e., vasoconstriction, vasodilation, shivering, sweating) concerned with the production and loss of body heat. The hypothalamus is the "thermostat" of the body (Woodbury 1970). In the febrile state, the balance between heat production and heat loss still persists except that the thermostat is set at a higher level. The salicylates act to reset the thermostat for the normal temperature range.

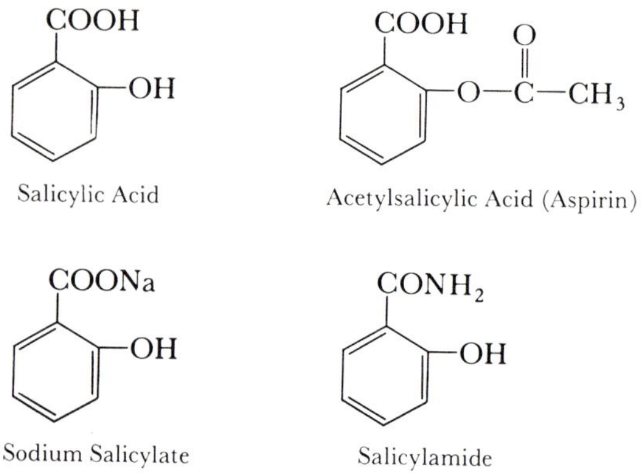

FIG. 16.1.

Heat loss is augmented by increased peripheral blood flow and sweating.

ACETYLSALICYLIC ACID

Acetylsalicylic Acid, U.S.P. (aspirin) is a member of the salicylate group of compounds such as salicylic acid, salicylamide, and sodium salicylate (Fig. 16.1).

PHARMACOLOGICAL CONSIDERATIONS

In addition to analgesic and antipyretic activity, aspirin has other interesting pharmacologic effects. The finding in 1971 that the biosynthesis of prostaglandins (PGs) is inhibited by large doses of aspirin has been of particular interest. Now that this effect is known, it is not difficult to understand why aspirin has some beneficial effect in the alleviation of asthma. It is known that $PGF_2\alpha$ is a potent bronchoconstrictor and that an anaphylactoid type reaction develops, including an asthmalike condition, following the administration of minute dosages (Said 1973). Aspirin and aspirinlike drugs are all potent inhibitors of PG synthetase (Flower 1974); inhibition of this enzyme prevents the biosynthesis of the PGs. Inhibition of the formation of PGs is a unique action mainly of aspirinlike drugs. A number of drugs studied have been ineffective in the inhibition of PG formation such as morphine, droperidol, fentanyl, chlorpromazine, phenergan, mepyramine, atropine, methysergide, phenoxybenzamine, propranolol, disodium cromoylycate, and others. In addition, the corticosteroids are inactive against PG formation in the dog spleen; however, in rat skin these compounds at high concentrations will inhibit PG synthetase by 50%. The antiinflammatory effects associated with the aspirinlike drugs and the corticosteroids are undoubtedly linked to the inhibition of PG.

Another effect of aspirin-type drugs is their inhibitory effect upon the release of PGE_2 and $F_2\alpha$ from thrombin-stimulated platelets; as a result, platelet aggregation is inhibited. For years it has been known by clinicians that the bleeding time is prolonged following the long-term administration of aspirin, acetaminophen, and sodium salicylate. However, this mechanism was not understood until recent years. According to Willis (1974), aspirin-type drugs may inhibit clumping or aggregation of blood platelets by blocking the enzymatic conversion of arachidonic acid to a hitherto undiscovered factor, i.e., labile aggregation-stimulation substance, which triggers aggregation of platelets. Also, serotonin release from blood platelets can be inhibited by aspirin (Willis and Kuhn 1974). It is believed that irreversible aggregation of platelets may be a terminal pathway in the pathogenesis of arterial thromboembolism and that aspirinlike drugs could be clinically useful in prophylactic treatment of arterial thrombosis in human beings.

ASPIRIN TOXICOSIS

Aspirin is a derivative of phenol; phenol is known to be especially toxic to cats. Daily doses of 2 grains and 5 grains of aspirin (33–63 mg/kg and 81–130 mg/kg, respectively) produced clinical signs of drug intoxication and pathologic changes in the organs and tissues when given to two groups of cats (on an experimental basis) for an average of 35 and 12 days, respectively (Larson 1963). The low dose of aspirin induced toxic hepatitis in 50% of the animals. Both levels of aspirin induced clinical signs of depression, poor appetite, vomiting, weight loss, and, at high doses, death. The high dose, according to Larson (1963), caused anemia, gastric lesions, toxic hepatitis, and suppression of erythropoiesis in the bone marrow in some but not all the animals. Severe anemia before death has been reported following up to 7 daily doses of aspirin (110 mg/kg) as well as bone marrow hypoplasia and the formation of Heinz bodies on the day of death in cats (Penny et al. 1967). A clinical case of aspirin poisoning in the cat given 2.5 grains 4 times daily was reported by Herrgesell (1967). The outstanding clinical signs of toxicity were hyperpnea (due to acid-base balance disturbance), hyperpyrexia (an elevated body temperature as high as 107.2° F), depression, and death.

Aspirin produces severe gastric hemorrhage when in suspension form at pH 3 in the dog (Davison et al. 1966). However, the same drug in solution, as well as salicylic acid, salicylamide, methylsalicylate, and acetaminophen, produced no significant effect. In addition, aspirin administered intravenously in high doses produces no gastric effect in the dog.

Of considerable interest is the finding that buffered aspirin produces more severe gastrointestinal lesions than does pure aspirin in the dog (Taylor and Crawford 1968). However, the lesions were fewer and less extensive than in animals given an equivalent level of pure aspirin and it was concluded that the long-term use of buffered aspirin was less irritating. Moreover, Taylor and Crawford (1968) felt that aspirin can do more injury than the benefit derived. Preexisting gastritis, enteritis, or gastroenteritis may contraindicate the use of aspirin.

Hematemesis and gastric ulcer perforation have been reported in dogs receiving 100–300 mg/kg/day of aspirin orally for 1–4 weeks (Lev et al. 1972). The common histopathological findings were degenerative changes or necrosis of the surface epithelium and mucosal hemorrhages. Also, intracellular mucin was reduced in both damaged and regenerating epithelium.

DOSAGE

In the Cat. It is known that the hepatic microsomal system of the cat does not rapidly metabolize certain drugs, particularly those that primarily require conjugation with glucuronic acid for detoxification and excretion. Aspirin is conjugated by the transfer of glucuronic acid from uridine diphosphate glucuronic acid (UDPGA) via enzyme action (i.e., glucuronyl transferase) in the hepatic microsomes. Glucuronyl transferase is present in the liver of most adult mammals except the cat (Greig 1957). Also, the fetal liver and livers of all newborn animals are often unable to synthesize glucuronides (Boyland and Booth 1962).

As it was aptly pointed out by Yeary and Swanson (1973), it is not surprising that drug dosages extrapolated from other species to the cat frequently lead to the induction of toxicosis. Considering the cat's inability to conjugate drugs with glucuronic acid, the potential of toxicosis development from the use of extrapolated dosages should not be surprising. This additional burden explains the susceptibility of the cat over other species to the effects of a drug like aspirin. As has been recommended in a number of published reports, the cat would become a "therapeutic orphan" if the logic was applied "across the board" not to use drugs such as aspirin in this species (Yeary and Swanson 1973). Consequently, aspirin toxicosis appears more likely to be associated with nonrecognition of the size of the cat in relation to dosage size, as well as to the cat's inability to rapidly metabolize the drug, rather than to be due to an increased sensitivity of the animal's tissues to the effects of aspirin.

Yeary and Swanson (1973) used levels of aspirin to attain the therapeutic range in human beings (i.e., 10–30 mg/100 mg of

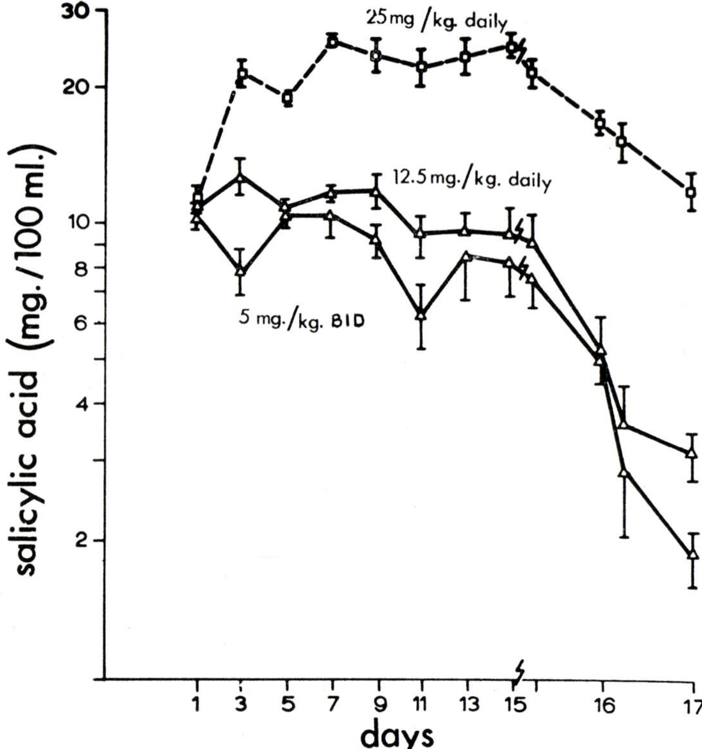

FIG. 16.2. Serum concentrations of salicyclic acid in cats given acetylsalicylic acid. (From Yeary and Swanson 1973)

serum). A dose of 25 mg/kg was given as a priming dose to three groups of cats. They were then maintained with 25 mg/kg, 12.5 mg/kg, and 5 mg/kg of aspirin daily for 15 days (see Fig. 16.2).

The 25-mg/kg daily dose maintained a serum concentration between 10 and 25 mg/100 ml (10 and 25 mg%) during a 24-hour period. The other two levels of aspirin resulted in serum concentrations between 5 and 12 mg%. The calculated half-lives were found to be dose dependent (5 mg/kg twice daily = 21.8 hr; 12.5 mg/kg daily = 26.8 hr; 25 mg/kg daily = 44.6 hr). It is apparent from this study that in the cat the biological half-life of aspirin is exceedingly long as well as dose dependent. To attain a therapeutic level of aspirin in the serum comparable to human beings (between 10 and 30 mg%), an oral daily dose level of 25 mg/kg of aspirin is required in the cat (Yeary and Swanson 1973). None of the aspirin dosages used in this study produced evidence of clinical toxicosis.

In the Dog. When an oral dose level of 50 mg/kg of aspirin was administered every 12 hours, emesis within approximately 2 hours occurred in most dogs (Yeary and Brant 1975). To avoid emesis, a maintenance dosage of 25 mg/kg was administered every 12 hours. However, this dosage and frequency of administration did not maintain the serum salicylate level within the desired therapeutic range (Yeary and Brant 1975). The biological half-life calculated for this level and frequency of drug administration is 7.5 hours. This is in sharp contrast to the biological half-life (i.e., 44.6 hours) calculated in the cat at a dose level of 25 mg/kg/24 hours; refer to the discussion above regarding the dose level of aspirin in the cat.

Inasmuch as the administration of aspirin (25 mg/kg/12 hours) did not maintain the desired therapeutic concentration in the serum of the dog, the dosage interval was decreased by Yeary and Brant to every 8 hours (the dose level of aspirin was still maintained at 25 mg/kg of body weight).

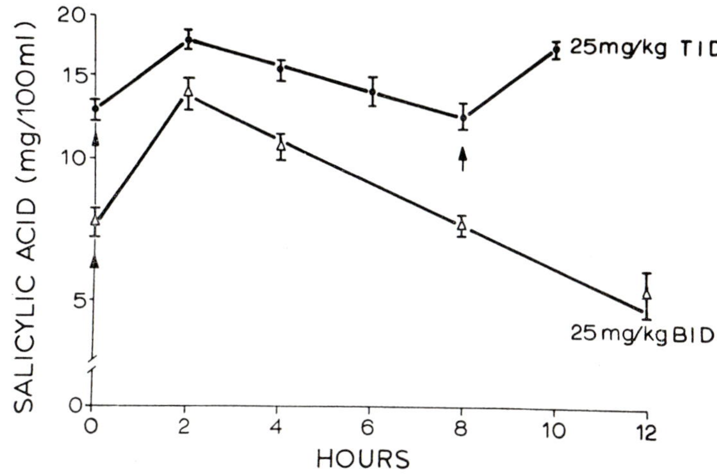

FIG. 16.3. Serum salicylate concentrations after oral administration of aspirin at the rate of 25 mg/kg of body weight every 8 hours (t.i.d.) or every 12 hours (b.i.d.). The dots and triangles represent the mean values for 6 dogs and the bars indicate ± 1 standard error of the mean. The arrows indicate time of drug administration. (From Yeary and Brant 1975)

Serum concentrations of aspirin were approximately 17–19 mg% at the peak level when 25 mg/kg were administered every 8 hours (see Fig. 16.3); the biological half-life was calculated to be 12.2 hours (Yeary and Brant 1975). Like the cat, the biological half-life of aspirin in the dog was dose dependent. From the results obtained in this study and those published in other studies, Yeary and Brant (1975) stated, "It would appear that the upper limit for aspirin dosage in the dog would be 50 mg/kg every 8 to 12 hours."

SODIUM SALICYLATE

Sodium Salicylate, U.S.P., is readily absorbed from the digestive tract, and its tendency to irritate the mucous membranes can be decreased by simultaneous administration of an equal amount of sodium bicarbonate. Salicylates are absorbed from the skin when applied as ointments.

After absorption, sodium salicylate is distributed widely and uniformly in the body. The salicylates do not affect the heart, but they will relax the smooth muscles of the blood vessels. Renal excretion of urates is increased by the salicylates.

The salicylates are excreted primarily by the kidney. About 40% of a dose is excreted unchanged and another 40% is excreted in the urine conjugated with glucuronic and sulfuric acids. Massive doses of salicylates may have a nephrotoxic action in dogs.

The mechanism of action of sodium salicylate is comparable to that of other salicylates, including aspirin. The primary actions of sodium salicylate are those of analgesia and antipyresis. Sodium salicylate has antirheumatic action, which is important in animals and human beings. The mechanism of action of sodium salicylate and other salicylates as an antirheumatic agent is not well understood. Ostensibly, the main mechanism of the salicylates is the nonspecific effect they have upon capillary permeability. The permeability of the capillaries resulting from inflammatory processes is reduced by salicylates. Inasmuch as the primary characteristic of acute inflammation is fluid exudate secondary to increased capillary permeability, considerable effort in experimental studies has been directed toward the possibility that injuries of all kinds might cause the local tissue release or activation of substances or factors ("mediators") that increase capillary permeability. Many mediators have been proposed such as serotonin, histamine, prostaglandins, and bradykinin. Experimentally, it has been found that salicylates do not inhibit or suppress bradykinin formation or prevent the inflammatory processes that it induces and they do not antagonize serotonin or histamine. Evidence indicates that the salicylates have a stabilizing effect upon cell lysosomes. This effect may be responsible for part of the anti-inflammatory effect that is produced by the salicylates since the release of hydrolases and proteases by lysosomes is prevented.

The salicylates also suppress a variety of antigen-antibody reactions, including anaphylactic reactions produced by foreign protein. An understanding of the immunosuppressive effect induced by the salicylates is complex. Its clarification will be difficult and will entail a considerable amount of additional investigation.

In a number of infectious diseases, the sedimentation rate of the blood cells is increased. Salicylate therapy frequently will reverse this characteristic by markedly reducing the sedimentation rate or by returning it to normal. This trend occurs regardless of the disease process involved. Salicylates may reduce the fibrinogen levels of whole blood by 50%, which concomitantly increases the blood-clotting time. The aggregation or clumping of blood platelets is also inhibited similarly to that for aspirin.

The metabolic rate is increased after the administration of salicylates; an increased oxygen consumption and carbon dioxide production occur. A drop in the protein-bound iodine (PBI) also follows salicylate treatment as well as a concomitant increase in free serum thyroxin (Korsgaard Christensen 1959). In addition, there is a depression of thyroid function along with a low uptake of iodine.

Pharmacokinetic studies in the pony, pig, goat, dog, and cat following an intravenous injection of sodium salicylate (44 mg/kg) revealed plasma half-lives of 1, 5.9, 0.78, 8.6, and 37.6 hours, respectively (Davis and Westfall 1972). The biologic half-lives of the dog and cat for sodium salicylate at this dose level are remarkably similar to those of aspirin (25 mg/kg). Refer to the previous discussion on the biologic half-lives of aspirin.

The pharmacokinetic studies on sodium salicylate by Davis and Westfall (1972) indicated that the elimination rate of sodium salicylate was most rapid in herbivores, slowest in carnivores, and intermediate in the omnivores. On the basis of the type of urinary salicyl metabolites as well as the rate of disappearance of sodium salicylate from the plasma of swine, a marked similarity exists in the way human beings and swine metabolize and excrete the salicylates. Davis and Westfall (1972) suggested that further studies of other drugs in swine may reveal that domesticated swine have greater predictive value in the preclinical testing of drugs intended for use in human beings than do the laboratory species in present use.

In newborn animals, the plasma half-lives of sodium salicylate (44 mg/kg) following intravenous administration decrease as a function of age (Davis et al. 1973). By 30 days of age, except in puppies, the plasma half-lives are similar to those in the adult of the same species (Davis and Westfall 1972). Puppies seem to excrete free salicylate with difficulty and they lack the capability to synthesize salicylurate. The primary conjugates of salicylate, salicyl glucuronide, and salicylurate are present in the urine of newborn animals, but compounds are synthesized at a low rate.

As previously pointed out, the adult cat has difficulty in metabolizing drugs such as aspirin, due to its inability to conjugate compounds with glucuronic acid. This defect is due to a deficiency in glucuronyl transferase, which is necessary in the transfer of glucuronic acid from UDPGA to salicylate for conjugation purposes. Also, neonates of any species are deficient in this enzyme found in the liver and kidney. The adult cat may be a useful model for studying drug metabolism typical of the newborn animal (Davis et al. 1973).

As previously mentioned for aspirin, sodium salicylate gives no relief to visceral or to sharp, excruciating pain. The suggested daily oral dosages are as follows:

Horse and cow	8–50 g
Sheep and swine	1–3 g
Dog	0.15–1 g
Cat	0.1–0.3 g

The above dosages for the dog and cat may be higher than desirable for safe use. Every precaution should be taken to avoid the problem of toxicosis described for aspirin. Salicylates administered to animals prior to 30 days of age could constitute a toxicologic hazard if certain precautions are not followed (Davis et al. 1973). However, once the animals have attained an age of 30 days or more, the same dose levels recommended for adult animals of the same species should be safe to use.

Sodium salicylate is not used to any great extent in the horse and other large species. The need to administer the drug orally is an inconvenience and sufficient reason to discourage its use. In addition, there appears to be a pharmacological basis for not using the salicylates in the horse because of their rapid disappearance from the plasma and excretion in the urine. Literature sources indicate that the salicylate compounds are excreted almost 4 times faster than in human beings. This rapid rate of excretion in the urine may be related to the alkaline pH of the equine urine (Alexander and Nicholson 1970). From a physiological standpoint, it has been observed in several species that pH has an important function in the excretion rate of drugs. For example, ionized molecules of a drug are not reabsorbed by the renal tubules inasmuch as they are less lipid soluble than non ionized molecules. Consequently, the ionized molecules are excreted in the urine. The majority of drug or chemical compounds are bases and, therefore, ionize in an acid medium. However, salicylates are weak acids, with the resultant formation of salts that ionize in an alkaline medium. Inactive, lightly exercised or stabled horses ordinarily have an alkaline urine, whereas the thoroughbred undergoing vigorous training or exercise has an acid urine. The pharmacologic action of salicylates would be expected to have a longer duration of action in animals excreting an acid urine. Studies in horses have, in fact, shown that an acid or low pH urine extends the excretion time of phenylbutazone over 100%.

Salicylic Acid

Salicylic Acid, U.S.P., is restricted almost entirely to external application because it is extremely irritating to the gastric mucosa. Its principal use internally is in cattle as an antifermentative agent. For this purpose, an oral dose of 16–24 g of salicylic acid has been used in cattle to decrease the amount of gas produced by bacterial fermentation. The efficacy of salicylic acid as an antifermentative agent in cattle does not appear to have been firmly established. More modern trends to prevent excess gas production (bloat) in cattle are the use of agents that affect the surface tension of the ruminal fluid contents. For example, poloxalene is approved for use in cattle for the prevention and treatment of bloat due to alfalfa and other legumes such as clover (*Code of Federal Regulations,* 135 c. 23 and 135 e. 60, April 1, 1973).

Salicylic acid (3%) and benzoic acid (6%) in combination are used externally in ointments and alcoholic solutions for their marked antifungal action. Whitfield's ointment, which has been employed for a number of years for its antifungal activity, still remains in use for the treatment of dermatomycotic infections. The ointment contains 3 g of salicylic acid, 6 g of benzoic acid, 5 g of lanolin (wool fat), and white petrolatum (white vaseline) to make a total weight of 100 g. Salicylic acid is a relatively weak antifungal agent and is important primarily for its keratolytic action. Benzoic acid is a much better antifungal agent. The combination of salicylic and benzoic acids is comparable to the antifungal activity of undecylenic acid.

PARA-AMINOPHENOL–DERIVATIVE ANALGESICS

The para-aminophenol–derivative analgesics consist of acetanilid, acetophenetidin, and acetaminophen (Tylenol).

Acetanilid and Acetophenetidin (Phenacetin)

Acetanilid and acetophenetidin (phenacetin) are also classified as analgesics and antipyretics. In clinical usage, the salicylates will hold a more prominent position because they are less toxic than acetanilid and phenacetin. Chemically, this group of drugs is related to aniline; aniline is a dye that had widespread use

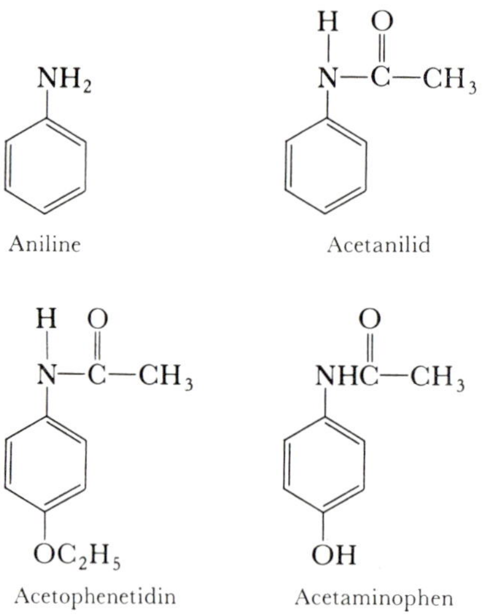

NH_2 Aniline

H O | $\|$ N—C—CH_3 Acetanilid

H O | $\|$ N—C—CH_3 OC_2H_5 Acetophenetidin

O $\|$ NHC—CH_3 OH Acetaminophen

FIG. 16.4.

at one time (e.g., it was an important ingredient in liquid shoe polish). Until it was discontinued, a number of infants developed severe methemoglobinemia, some cases being fatal, as a result of licking polish from shoes or drinking the polish. Structural formulas are shown in Fig. 16.4.

MECHANISM OF ACTION AND DOSAGE

The analgesic and antipyretic actions resemble those of the salicylates. The toxic effects of acetanilid and phenacetin are greater than those of the salicylates. Prolonged use of these drugs can lead to the induction of methemoglobinemia. The dye, aniline, is highly toxic and readily converts hemoglobin into methemoglobin following absorption through the skin or after accidental ingestion. The excess toxicity of acetanilid has resulted in its removal from the list of official drugs in the *National Formulary*.

Phenacetin is not as potent as acetanilid in the production of analgesia. Its analgesic potency is roughly equivalent to aspirin. Phenacetin is incorporated in the well-known APC (aspirin, phenacetin, caffeine) tablets. Clinically, phenacetin has been used in the dog at a suggested dosage of 0.13–2 g; the drug is administered orally in divided dosage 2–3 times daily. Until further information on safety and efficacy can be provided, use of phenacetin and other para-aminophenol derivatives is not recommended at any dose level in the cat (Finco et al. 1975).

ACETAMINOPHEN

The use of *Acetaminophen,* N.F. (Tylenol), in the cat is not recommended at any dose (Finco et al. 1975). In a case report published by Finco and associates, acetaminophen produced severe illness in 1 adult Burmese cat and death in a 2nd animal of the same breed. Three 325-mg (5-gr) tablets were administered orally by the owner to each of the animals.

In an experimental study, acetaminophen was administered to 4 adult cats (Finco et al. 1975). A marked degree of cyanosis was noted in these animals within 4 hours after the administration of a single tablet containing 325 mg of acetaminophen. The cyanotic condition induced by acetaminophen was believed to have been due to hypoxia associated with conversion of hemoglobin to methemoglobin. In addition, anemia, hemoglobinuria, and icterus were eventually seen in the cats. Hemolysis of the red blood cells was responsible for the development of the anemia and hemoglobinuria. Icterus was attributed to both lysis of erythrocytes and hepatic necrosis. Facial edema was also observed in 3 of the 4 experimental cats. Inasmuch as phenacetin is metabolized to acetaminophen, comparble clinical signs of toxicosis are likely to develop in the cat. Like acetaminophen, phenacetin is not recommended for use in the cat (Finco et al. 1975).

PYRAZOLON-DERIVATIVE ANALGESICS

The pyrazolon derivatives have analgesic and antipyretic activity; they share similar pharmacological characteristics with the salicylates and para-aminophenol derivatives. However, the pyrazolon derivatives differ in the type of toxic effects produced. This occurs in human beings perhaps to a higher degree than in animals.

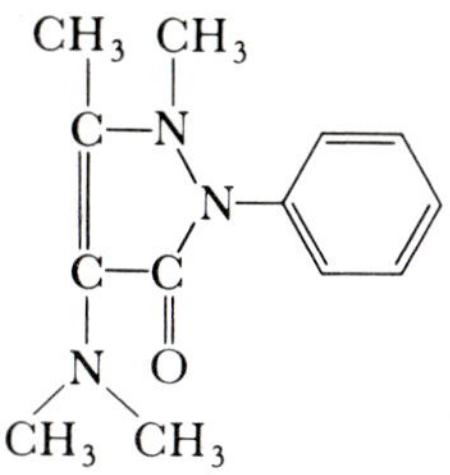

Aminopyrine

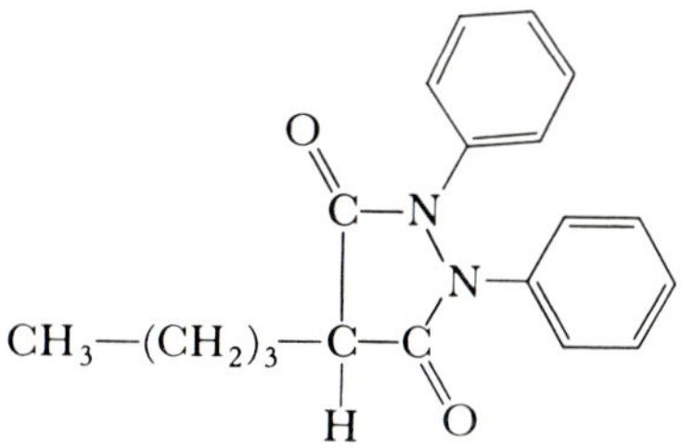

Phenylbutazone

FIG. 16.5.

In human beings, fatal agranulocytosis can occur following the use of these derivatives (i.e., phenylbutazone, dipyrone, aminopyrine). Clinically, agranulocytosis in animals has not been a serious concern.

Structural formulas of the pyrazolon derivatives are shown in Fig. 16.5.

PHENYLBUTAZONE

Phenylbutazone, U.S.P. (Butazolidin) (3,5-dioxo-1,2-diphenyl-4-*n*-butylpyrazolidine) (Fig. 16.6), is insoluble in water. This drug was synthesized as the result of a search for a compound having therapeutic attributes of aminopyrine but without its toxicity.

Phenylbutazone is an antiinflammatory agent resembling cortisone in activity. The antiinflammatory mechanism of action produced by phenylbutazone is unknown. It may act similarly to the salicylates in the reduction of capillary permeability by having a stabilization effect upon lysosomes.

Clinically, phenylbutazone is used for its analgesic and antipyretic activity in the treatment of painful arthritis and skeletal muscular disorders. It is approved by the Food and Drug Administration (FDA) for use in the dog and horse (*Code of Federal Regulations,* 135 b. 47, 135 c. 57, and 135 c. 75, April 1, 1973). Hemacytological disturbances reported in human beings have not been observed in animals to the same degree or extent. Horses that have received phenylbutazone continuously for 2–3 years have no major changes in hemacytological function (Dunn 1972). Prolonged daily administration of 2 g of phenylbutazone for 32 days in the horse is associated with necrotizing phlebitis of the portal veins (Gabriel and Martin 1962). Since sodium chloride retention can occur following phenylbutazone therapy, the drug is contraindicated in animals suffering from congestive heart failure.

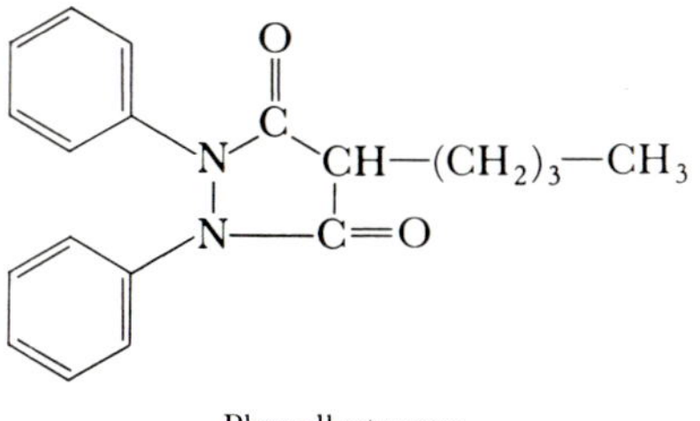

Induction or stimulation of hepatic microsomal enzyme activity is produced so that continuous administration of phenylbutazone results in progressively lower plasma levels (Piperno et al. 1968). According to Piperno and associates, the prolonged effect of phenylbutazone may possibly be due to an active metabolite, oxyphenbutazone. In human beings this metabolite has significant analgesic and antiinflammatory effects. The presence of this metabolite (i.e., oxyphenbutazone) has also been reported in the urine of the horse (Finocchio et al. 1970).

At the recommended clinical dose of 2 g/1000 lb of body weight (4.4 mg/kg) intravenously, the half-life of phenylbutazone is 3.5 hours in the horse (Piperno et al. 1968). Dose levels at double and quadruple the recommended clinical doses resulted in half-life values from 3.5 to 6 hours. The biological half-life reported by Piperno et al. at the higher dose levels was

Phenylbutazone

FIG. 16.6.

similar to that reported by Gandal et al. (1969). For other species the half-life for phenylbutazone is as follows (Dayton et al. 1973):

Species	*Half-life (hr)*
Human beings	72
Baboon	5
Dog	6
Rat	6
Rabbit	3

Using a sensitive GLC method of detection, the average plasma half-life in the horse following a single oral dose of phenylbutazone (8.9 mg/kg) was 4 hours (Bruce et al. 1974). In the dog, the average plasma half-life following a single oral dose of 150 mg was 2.5 hours; the dogs varied in weight from 8 to 15.2 kg. Oxyphenbutazone persists in the urine for at least 48 hours following a single oral dose of 8.9 mg/kg; in 72-hour urine samples, none could be detected. The unchanged drug (i.e., phenylbutazone) could not be detected in the 36-hour urine samples.

Inasmuch as phenylbutazone is a weak acid, it has been generally suspected that the drug would be preferentially excreted at a more rapid rate in an alkaline urine, whereas in an acid urine a slower, more prolonged excretion rate would occur. As mentioned earlier, thoroughbreds during training, and definitely at the termination of a race, excrete a low pH or acid urine, whereas during rest or light exercise a higher pH or more alkaline urine is produced (Moss 1972). In determining whether or not the differences in the pH would influence the length of time of phenylbutazone elimination in the urine, studies were conducted by Moss and Haywood (1973) using unlabeled and C^{14}-labeled phenylbutazone. Unlabeled phenylbutazone (5 mg/kg) administered orally to a pony revealed the presence of phenylbutazone up to 11 hours after dosing and oxyphenbutazone up to 48 hours. In the same animal treated with ammonium chloride to acidify the urine, phenylbutazone was detected up to 48 hours (4 times longer than in alkaline urine) and oxyphenbutazone was present up to 57 hours. C^{14}-phenylbutazone (5 mg/kg) administered to the horse by stomach tube also indicated that the drug persisted longer (nearly 150 hours) in acid urine as compared to over 60 hours for alkaline urine (see Fig. 16.7).

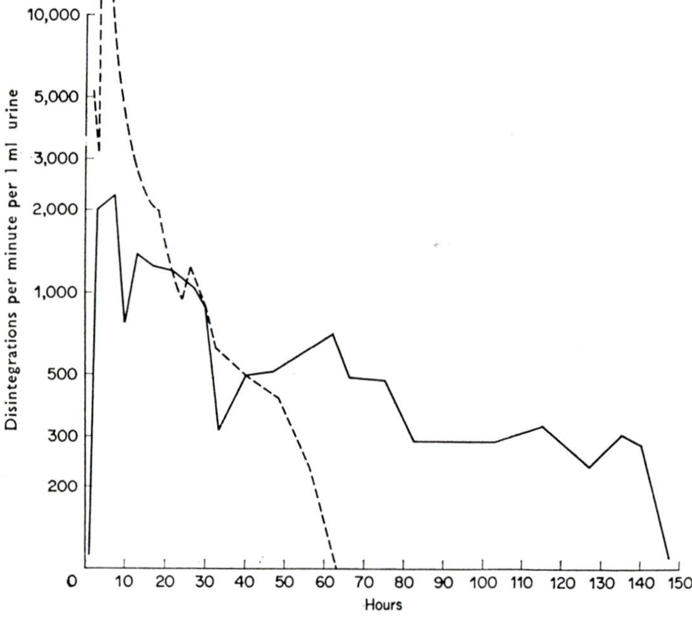

FIG. 16.7. Concentrations of radioactivity in urine following administration of ^{14}C-phenylbutazone to a horse while producing acidic urine (continuous line, pH range 4.6–5.5) and while producing alkaline urine (discontinuous line, pH range 7.5–8.9). (From Moss and Haywood 1973)

A therapeutic dose of phenylbutazone can become 99% bound to plasma proteins. It can displace other drugs that bind to plasma proteins such as warfarin to the extent that severe hemorrhage may occur. Pharmacologic agents are therapeutically inert in the bound state, whereas their displacement enables the drug to diffuse to its active receptor site(s), and this also exposes the unbound drug to metabolism and excretion.

Unlike aspirin and aspirinlike drugs, the metabolism of phenylbutazone is accelerated by pretreatment of the dog with phenobarbital, pentobarbital, and diphenhydramine through induction of microsomal enzyme activity. Like aspirin and aspirinlike compounds, phenylbutazone inhibits the formation of prostaglandins such as PGE_2 and $PGF_{2}\alpha$. However, its effect or potency is about one-tenth that of aspirin in the inhibition of PG biosynthesis.

TOXICITY

Idiosyncrasy has been reported in a Dachshund following treatment with phenylbutazone (Tandy and Thorpe 1967). A fatal condition characterized by severe hemorrhages, biliary stasis, and renal tubular degeneration was observed in this clinical case. In the cat, the administration of phenylbutazone (44 mg/kg) twice daily resulted in the death of 4 of 5 animals following 13–20 doses (Carlisle et al. 1968). Death of the animals was preceded by gradual loss of appetite, loss of body weight, dehydration, and severe depression. Renal pathology was a constant finding on postmortem examination. A downward trend was noted in the percentage of erythroblasts in some animals; also, erythroid hyperplasia was observed.

CLINICAL USE

Approximately 62% of the racehorses running on the track in California are receiving phenylbutazone (Cannon 1974). California permits the controlled use of phenylbutazone within 24 hours of the race, if the veterinarian declares the dosage rate and is prepared to certify the horse as "raceably fit." Such animals are expected to be positive for phenylbutazone in the urine; however, levels of the drug above 50 μg/ml (50 ppm) are interpreted as evidence of administration of phenylbutazone within 24 hours. Some states within the United States will not permit the use of phenylbutazone in the racehorse; the presence of any level of the drug in the urine is illegal. A serious problem the veterinarian faces with the use of phenylbutazone in the racehorse is to know where therapy ends and doping begins (Bierhaus 1970; Hopes 1972).

In 1971 the Stewards of the Turf Authorities of Great Britain, France, and Ireland issued a statement affirming that the presence of phenylbutazone in the body fluids of racehorses was illegal. The Turf Authorities pointed out that the elimination time of phenylbutazone depended on many variable factors and, therefore, they could not provide a stated time that the drug would need to be discontinued in the treatment of a racehorse prior to the race event. They did state, "If a veterinarian recommends the discontinuance of any drug *not less than eight days before racing* (although such a period may be longer than is necessary in many instances), he should be able to feel sure that he has catered for all but the most exceptional case." The suggestion of 8 days for the discontinuance or withdrawal of treatment with phenylbutazone is probably not an overconservative one because phenylbutazone can be detected in acid urine for over 6 days (Moss and Haywood 1973). Similar problems confront the veterinarian in the use of phenylbutazone in racing dogs.

Use of phenylbutazone but avoiding its misuse is a most perplexing problem for the equine practitioner (Dunn 1972). For example, the use of phenylbutazone by unscrupulous individuals to mask a lame horse for examination for soundness or for sale creates serious problems for the examining veterinarian. According to Dunn (1972), it is possible for a complete examination for soundness to fail in the detection of the lame or "footy" horse that is under phenylbutazone therapy. Three to

4 days after the examination and after the horse has been with its new owner, signs of lameness may appear following phenylbutazone therapy. Although legislation banning the use of phenylbutazone in horses to be sold needs to be considered, a rapid detection method is needed to determine the illegal use of the drug (Dunn 1972).

Commercially, phenylbutazone is provided in three forms: (1) an injectable preparation, (2) tablets and boluses, and (3) a granular form. Injectable preparations, tablets, and boluses are provided for the dog and horse. The granular form of phenylbutazone is provided only for the horse.

Phenylbutazone has not been approved by the FDA for use in other species. The drug cannot be used in animals intended for human food. Administration of phenylbutazone by the subcutaneous or intramuscular route is contraindicated.

INJECTABLE PHENYLBUTAZONE

Phenylbutazone is used for the relief of inflammatory conditions associated with the musculoskeletal system in dogs and horses. The drug is administered intravenously *(slowly)* to dogs at a dosage level of 10 mg/lb of body weight but not to exceed 800 mg/animal/day regardless of weight. Intravenous injections in the dog should be limited to 2 successive days but may be followed by oral medication. Phenylbutazone is administered intravenously to horses at a dosage level of 1–2 g/1000 lb of body weight for a maximum of 5 days.

PHENYLBUTAZONE TABLETS AND BOLUSES

Tablets of phenylbutazone are provided in two sizes, i.e., 100 mg and 1000 mg (1 g) in each tablet. Each bolus contains 4 g of phenylbutazone. Phenylbutazone tablets or boluses are used for the relief of inflammatory conditions associated with the musculoskeletal systems in dogs and horses. Phenylbutazone is administered orally to dogs at a dosage level of 20 mg/lb of body weight in 3 divided doses daily, with a maximum dosage level of 800 mg/day regardless of body weight. The drug is used at a relatively high dosage level for the first 48 hours and then reduced gradually to a maintenance level, at the lowest dosage capable of producing a desired clinical response.

In the horse phenylbutazone is used at a dosage level of 1–2 g/500 lb of body weight (2–4 g/1000 lb) but not to exceed 4 g/animal/day with a relatively high dose level given for the first 48 hours, which is reduced gradually to a maintenance level that is maintained at the lowest dose level capable of producing the desired clinical response. Because of the relatively short half-life of the drug, administration every 8 hours appears to be satisfactory. If there is no significant clinical effect in 5 days, a reevaluation of the diagnosis and treatment should be made.

GRANULAR FORM OF PHENYLBUTAZONE

Each 27-g package contains 8 g of phenylbutazone. The drug is administered orally to horses at the rate of 1–2 g/500 lb of body weight; dosage should not exceed 4 g daily. A relatively high dose is used for the first 48 hours. The dose is then reduced gradually to a maintenance level and is maintained at the lowest level capable of producing the desired clinical response.

CONTRAINDICATIONS

Phenylbutazone must not be administered to animals afflicted with serious cardiac, renal, or hepatic injury or those with evidence of a hemacytological disorder. Care should be taken to avoid the perivascular administration of phenylbutazone during an intravenous injection; severe swelling or necrosis at the site of injection may occur.

DIPYRONE

Dipyrone (Novin, Methampyrone) is used as an analgesic and antipyretic agent. It has also been widely used by equine practitioners to treat equine colic and other conditions of gastrointestinal spasm or hypermotility in both small and large animals (Gray and Yano 1975).

Commercially, dipyrone (Novin) is

supplied in 100 cc bottles in a concentration of 500 mg/cc.

CLINICAL USE

In the Horse. Dipyrone is injected intravenously *(slowly)*, subcutaneously, or intramuscularly at a dose level of 10–20 cc (5–10 g). Doses may be repeated 1 or 2 times daily at 8-hour intervals. The efficacy of dipyrone in the treatment of spasmodic conditions in small and large animals has been challenged (Lowe 1969; Gray and Yano 1975). According to Lowe (1969), dipyrone is valueless as an analgesic in the treatment of equine colic.

In the Dog and Cat. The same routes of administration as specified in the horse are used; the dose administered is 0.25 cc (125 mg)/10 lb of body weight. Doses may be repeated similarly to the procedure described above for the horse. When dipyrone is given *in vivo* or *in vitro,* it has no effect upon spontaneous intestinal motility or upon intestinal spasms produced by nerve stimulation, cholinergic drugs, ganglionic stimulant drugs, histamine, or morphine (Gray and Yano 1975). Conversely, the drug does antagonize bradykinin-induced intestinal spasms as do other members of the pyrazolon class of compounds.

PRECAUTIONS AND CONTRAINDICATIONS

The hemacytological condition of the animal should be monitored when prolonged periods of use are necessary; agranulocytosis and leukopenia may result under conditions of prolonged use. Overdosage can result in convulsive seizures. Dipyrone is contraindicated for use in conjunction with barbiturates or phenylbutazone because of drug interaction involving the microsomal enzyme system. The drug is contraindicated in food-producing animals, including lactating dairy animals. Dipyrone apparently can interfere with, or mask the presence of, prohibited drugs in race animals for 5 days after its use (Bierhaus 1970). This would indicate that the drug should not be used in racing animals for at least 5 days prior to a race event.

More recent information indicates that the use of dipyrone with chlorpromazine can result in serious hypothermia (Woodbury and Fingl 1975). This simultaneous use of these drugs is contraindicated. Also, dipyrone has a tendency to increase bleeding, due to the suppression of the formation of prothrombin.

AMINOPYRINE

Aminopyrine, N.F. (Pyramidon), possesses more antipyretic and analgesic activity than acetanilid and acetophenetidin. It is absorbed rapidly following oral administration and produces a prompt analgesia. Aminopyrine is excreted in the urine unchanged or conjugated with glucuronic and sulfuric acids. Numerous cases of agranulocytosis have been reported in human patients following continued use of the drug. However, experiments designed to produce this condition in dogs and other laboratory animals following both oral and parenteral use have been unsuccessful. The oral daily dosage in the dog is 0.13–0.4 g given in divided dosage.

OTHER NONNARCOTIC ANALGESICS

XYLAZINE HYDROCHLORIDE

Xylazine Hydrochloride (Rompun, Bay Va 1470) was first synthesized in 1962 and was given the code name of Bay Va 1470. Chemically, xylazine hydrochloride is 2(2,6-dimethylphenylamino)-4H-5,6-dihydro-1,3-thiazine hydrochloride (Fig. 16.8). Pharmacologically, xylazine is classified as an analgesic as well as a sedative. It is not a neuroleptic or tranquilizer or an an-

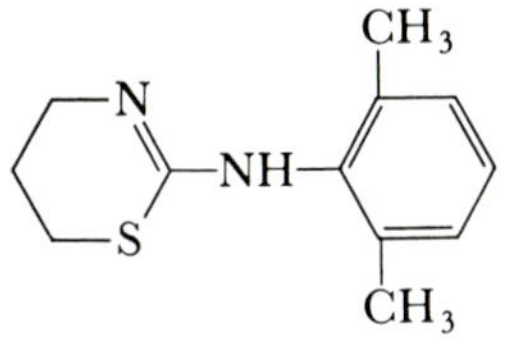

CH_3 N NH S CH_3

Xylazine

FIG. 16.8.

esthetic agent. Xylazine is approved by the FDA for use in the dog, cat, and horse.

PHARMACOLOGICAL CONSIDERATIONS

Xylazine has a number of pharmacological characteristics in common with morphine but it will not substitute for morphine in dependent rats and its effect is not antagonized by nalorphine or levallorphan. Xylazine does not produce central nervous system (CNS) excitation usually induced by narcotic analgesics in mice, rats, and cats. Instead, it produces depression and sedation in these species. In addition to analgesia and sedation, the drug has an inhibitory effect upon adrenergic and cholinergic neurons.

Xylazine also produces muscle relaxation by inhibition of the intraneuronal transmission of impulses at the central level of the CNS. Apparently due to direct stimulatory effect upon the emetic center, emesis is commonly induced by xylazine in the cat and occasionally in the dog. Cardiac output is decreased 5–10 minutes following the intravenous injection of xylazine (0.3 mg/lb) in the pony and then returns to normal in 15 minutes (Garner et al. 1971a). No significant alteration in the systemic arterial pressure and cardiac rate was noted 2 minutes after the administration of xylazine in the pony. The sinoatrial node of the 2nd degree type was blocked consistently in the pony within 0.5–1.5 minutes. A transient 2nd degree block is also induced by xylazine in the horse with intravenous doses of 0.55, 1.1, and 2.2 mg/kg of body weight (Kerr et al. 1972b). Atropine sulfate (0.011 mg or more/kg) administered immediately before the administration of xylazine prevents the heart block. In a clinical evaluation of xylazine in the horse, no cardiac alterations other than bradycardia were reported (Hoffman 1974). It is well known that horses have "functional" heart block or 2nd degree heart block, especially in young animals. Its incidence may be as high as 16% and it is not considered a pathological entity because it disappears following excitement and the administration of atropine sulfate.

In the pony, no statistically significant alterations occurred in the arterial pH, P_{CO_2}, or P_{O_2} following an intravenous injection of xylazine (0.3–0.5 mg/lb); also no significant change was noted in tidal and minute volumes at this dose level (Garner et al. 1971b).

There was little alteration in the serum electrolytes following the intravenous administration of xylazine (0.5 mg/lb) in the horse (Short et al. 1972). Electrolyte values were affected only by a decline in the potassium level. Serum protein levels remained unchanged.

Ruminants are considered to be the most sensitive of the domestic animals to the action of xylazine. In cattle, dose levels of the drug that produces deep sedation and analgesia are one-tenth those required to produce this effect in horses, dogs, and cats (Hopkins 1972). Also, the pig is less affected than any of these species, and dose levels are reported to be 20–30 times greater than those required in cattle. Toxicity trials in cattle have shown that the minimum lethal dose (MLD) of xylazine in adult cattle was 3 times the highest recommended intramuscular dose of 0.3 mg/kg. According to Hopkins (1972), this is 6 times the dose rate indicated for the majority of clinical cases. The type of sedation produced by xylazine in cattle closely resembles that produced by chloral hydrate (Clarke and Hall 1969). Moreover, analgesia is not present except in the deeply sedated animals; supplementation with a general or local anesthetic is necessary to prevent movement in response to a nociceptive stimulus. It appears that more information is needed to establish the efficacy and safety of xylazine in cattle.

ONSET OF ACTION, DURATION OF EFFECT, AND RECOVERY

In the horse, doses of about 2 mg/kg of xylazine have been given by intramuscular injection 15–20 minutes prior to thiopental sodium or methohexital sodium anesthesia (Clarke and Hall 1969). Two to 3 mg/kg are reported to produce a rapid, deep sedation lasting about 30 minutes, followed by rapid recovery. Other clinical reports in the horse pertaining to the duration of effect are essentially in agreement with the observations of Clarke and Hall (1969). After an intravenous injection of xylazine (0.5 mg/lb), the onset of effect is noted in 1–1.5 minutes after the injection; in 3 minutes the head droops; in 6–6.5 minutes the drug exerts its maximum effect and will continue 10–15 minutes (McCashin and Gabel 1971).

Maximum sedation occurs 3 minutes after an intravenous injection of xylazine (1.1 mg/kg) in the horse (Hoffman 1974). The duration of this effect is 30–40 minutes.

Onset of action after an intramuscular or subcutaneous injection is within 10–15 minutes and after intravenous administration it occurs within 3–5 minutes in dogs and cats (Newkirk and Miles 1974). A sedative or sleeplike effect occurs and appears to be dose dependent; this effect usually lasts 1–2 hours. The analgesic effect lasts only 15–30 minutes. Complete recovery from xylazine varies with the dose administered. Recovery is usually complete within 2–4 hours in the dog and cat and 2–3 hours in the horse after recommended dosages of xylazine are administered intramuscularly or intravenously.

PRECAUTIONS AND CONTRAINDICATIONS

Animals should be handled carefully after the drug is administered. A false sense of security may result in injury to personnel because animals can respond by kicking or by reacting in other defensive ways. Intraarterial injection of xylazine should be avoided. The problems associated with intraarterial injection of anesthetic or tranquilizer agents have been previously discussed (see Chapters 13 and 17).

Xylazine cannot be used in conjunction with neuroleptics or tranquilizers. Additive depressant effects occur from the use of xylazine and the barbiturates; the use of barbiturates to induce anesthesia must be at a reduced dose level and slowly administered when injected by the intravenous route. Debilitated animals with depressed respiration, cardiac disease, renal and liver impairment, shock, or any other stress conditions should be carefully monitored whenever xylazine is administered. The drug is contraindicated in animals within the last month of pregnancy except at parturition since it precipitates an early parturition or abortion (Jones 1972).

CLINICAL USE

In the Dog and Cat. A commercial preparation containing 20 mg/ml of xylazine hydrochloride is available for intravenous (0.5 mg/lb), intramuscular, or subcutaneous (1 mg/lb) administration in the dog and cat. In dogs weighing over 50 lb, a dose level of 0.5 mg/lb of body weight administered intramuscularly is usually recommended for sedation and analgesia. The analgesic effect produced is pronounced over the head, neck, and body but is minimal in the extremities. With intravenous barbiturates and inhalant anesthetics, a smooth, rapid induction of anesthesia is achieved along with an uneventful recovery. The amount of intravenous barbiturate anesthetic needed to induce anesthesia is decreased by about one-half or more in the dog and cat. Inhalant anesthetics are also reduced but administered to effect.

For restraint of the dog in cystometry, xylazine (2.2 mg/kg) administered subcutaneously was the only drug that proved adequate without interfering with the micturition reflex (Oliver and Young 1973). Xylazine significantly decreases (26%–71%) the amount of pentobarbital sodium required to induce general anesthesia in the dog (Lacuata and Subang 1973). The depth of analgesia produced by xylazine alone is insufficient to permit endotracheal intubation before the administration of an inhalant anesthetic; after the administration of xylazine, the inhalant anesthetic can be delivered easily with a face mask and then can be followed by intubation (Moye et al. 1973).

Emesis occurs in the majority of the cats 3–5 minutes following the administration of xylazine at any dose level (Moye et al. 1973). A dose of 0.5 mg/lb administered intramuscularly is considered an optimum level for the inducement of emesis in the cat; however, analgesic effects are not observed at this dosage (Amend and Klavano 1973).

In the dog emesis may also occur following xylazine administered in large dosages. The emetic effect of xylazine is clinically beneficial in emptying the stomach; this prevents the likelihood of vomitus from being aspirated into the trachea prior to and during surgery. Xylazine can be used to perform a cesarean section under local anesthesia without a depressant effect developing in the puppies (Yates 1973).

Xylazine premedication is recommended to eliminate muscular hypertonic effects in cats during ketamine anesthesia (Amend et al. 1972; Amend 1973). A combination in which xylazine (0.25–0.5 mg/lb) is given intramuscularly as a preanesthetic, followed 20 minutes later with an intramuscular injection of ketamine (7–10 mg/lb), provides analgesia and relaxation on an average of 30 minutes. Xylazine renders the cat relatively insensitive to the pain often associated with the injection of ketamine.

In the Horse. A commercial preparation containing 100 mg/ml of xylazine hydrochloride is available for intravenous (0.5 ml/100 lb) or intramuscular (1 ml/100 lb) use in the horse. Xylazine must not be used in horses or other animals intended for human food consumption.

According to McCashin and Gabel (1971), xylazine is more dependable and has resulted in a higher percentage of quieter recoveries in the horse from surgical anesthesia than when promazine or acetylpromazine is used for preanesthetic medication. They concluded that the most satisfactory dosage of xylazine is 0.5 mg/lb intravenously or 1 mg/lb intramuscularly. However, weak or debilitated animals should be given a slightly lower dose, particularly if the drug is administered intravenously. Considerably higher doses of xylazine than those recommended rarely produce recumbency in a horse; however, the animals may become incoordinated so that it is difficult to work on them (McCashin and Gabel 1971).

Within a very short time after an intravenous injection in the horse, the head characteristically drops or droops. The only disadvantage to this effect is the difficulty in examination of the mouth or passage of the endoscope (McCashin and Gabel 1971). In order that the examination of the mouth can be conducted, assisting personnel can hold up the head for the examination. Hypostatic congestion of the nasal mucosa sometimes occurs in the head-down position. The muscle tone of the animal is decreased after the administration of xylazine; difficulty in walking is noted soon after the drug is administered intravenously. In colts and geldings prolapse of the penis sometimes occurs but paraphimosis does not; the effect upon the retractor muscle of the penis is less than that seen with promazine (McCashin and Gabel 1971).

The intravenous (1.1 mg/kg) or intramuscular (2.2 mg/kg) administration of xylazine prior to the induction of anesthesia either with thiamylal sodium or with thiamylal sodium and halothane is a satisfactory preanesthetic agent in the horse; less respiratory depression and greater cardiovascular stability followed the use of xylazine than followed the intravenous administration of 0.66 mg/kg of acetylpromazine maleate (Kerr et al. 1972a). Of the drugs evaluated in the horse, xylazine in the presence of epinephrine release is less likely to produce tachycardia than acetylpromazine (Aitken and Sanford 1972).

For preanesthetic purposes in the horse, xylazine is administered intravenously at a dose level of 0.25–0.5 mg/lb of body weight (Short 1974). In addition, atropine sulfate (0.02 mg/lb) is administered subcutaneously or intramuscularly.

Hoffman (1974) found the sedative and analgesic effects to be good to excellent in 88% and 81% of the horses, respectively, following the intravenous administration of xylazine; optimal dosage is 1.1 mg/kg of body weight. The quantity of general anesthetic needed was the same as when promazine hydrochloride was used as a preanesthetic medication. Although recovery was rapid and smooth after general anesthesia of short duration, it was too rapid and often violent when anesthesia was prolonged for 45 minutes or more (Hoffman 1974).

In Cattle. Although xylazine is not approved by the FDA for use in cattle, it shows promise experimentally of being useful in bovine diagnostic and surgical procedures when combined with local anesthesia (Rickard et al. 1974). Rickard and co-workers administered xylazine (0.22 mg/kg) and atropine (0.044 mg/kg) intramuscularly in bulls of mixed breeding; the ages of the animals were 15–24 months and the body weights were 500–600 kg. Ten to 15 minutes after administration of the xylazine, the animals became recumbent in the sternal position. The animals were then placed in lateral recumbency and restrained with a halter and leg ropes in preparation for electroejaculation and semen collection. In a fourth series of semen collections, xylazine in a dosage of 0.22 mg/kg of body weight was observed to be less effective. Inasmuch as the animals attempted to stand during the electrostimulation, an additional 20–40 mg of the drug were administered to maintain restraint. With the semen collection period extending through a 3-week period that required repeated administration of xylazine, this additional dosage of the drug could possibly indicate that the induction of microsomal enzyme activity had occurred. If so, a more rapid degradation and metabolism of the drug would result.

A dose level of xylazine (0.09–0.35 mg/kg) administered intramuscularly produces light to deep sedation in cattle (Hopkins 1972). Intravenously, xylazine (0.05–0.1 mg/kg) produces basal narcosis in cattle for 1–2 hours (Clarke and Hall 1969). Also, sedation and slight muscle relaxation with the animal in the standing position were reported following an intramuscular dose of 0.05 mg/kg of body weight (Jones 1972). Xylazine (0.1 mg/kg) at increased intramuscular dose levels produces good sedation, marked muscle relaxation, and some analgesia; this dose level ordinarily allows the animal to remain in the standing position but may result in recumbency. At still higher intramuscular dose levels of xylazine (0.2 mg/kg), deep sedation and a useful level of analgesia are induced with the animal usually lying down. Following the administration of this dose level, the first effects are noted within 5 minutes and the maximal effect is induced 10 minutes later (Jones 1972).

In Avian and Exotic Species. Xylazine has been used in 9 avian species (Levinger et al. 1973). Following intramuscular injection, xylazine produced a marked sedative effect in birds. Intramuscular doses of 1–2 mg/kg of xylazine produced no changes in behavior. At dosages above 5 mg/kg, all birds exhibited signs of CNS depression. Light sedation was induced with xylazine in the chicken and turkey at 10 mg/kg of body weight administered intramuscularly (Levinger et al. 1973).

Xylazine has been used in a large number of exotic species (Bauditz 1972). Sedation and immobilization dosages of xylazine administered by projectile syringe or intramuscularly are listed for some of the species on page 368.

Pentazocine Lactate or Hydrochloride (Talwin)

With the knowledge that one of the narcotic antagonists, nalorphine, possesses potent analgesic effects, other compounds are needed with antagonistic effects and little abuse potential. Nalorphine cannot be used in human beings for analgesic purposes because of undesirable side effects. In the search for antagonists with a benzomorphan structure, pentazocine emerged as an analgesic with few side effects. Consequently, pentazocine has received a considerable amount of attention in human beings because of its potential as a nonaddicting and effective analgesic. Chemically, pentazocine is 2′-hydroxy-5,9-dimethyl-2-(3,3-dimethylallyl)-6,7-benzomorphan (Fig. 16.9).

Pharmacological Considerations

The pharmacological characteristics of pentazocine are quite similar to those of

Species (common name)	*Genus and Species*	*Xylazine Dosage*	
		Sedation	*Immobilization*
		(mg/kg)	
Fallow deer	*Dama dama*	1–2	5–8
Red deer	*Cervus nippon*	2	3–4
Roe deer	*Capreolus capreolus*	0.5–1	1.5–3
White-tailed deer	*Odocoileus virginianus*	0.5–1	3–4
Elk	*Alces alces*	0.5	1.5
Reindeer	*Rangifer tarandus*	0.5	2
Greater kudu	*Tragelaphus strepsiceros*	1	3
Bushbuck	*Tr. spekei*	1.5	3
Eland	*Taurotragus oryx*	1	3
Sable antelope	*Hippotragus niger*	1.5	3
Gazelle	*Gazella* sp.	1	2–4
Water buffalo	*Bubalis arnee*	0.5–1	1–2(?)
Yak	*Bos mutus*	0.3	0.6–1
American bison	*Bison bison*	0.1–0.3	0.6–1
Musk ox	*Ovibos moschatus*	<0.5	0.5–1.5
Dromedary	*Camelus dromedarius*	0.1	0.5
Llama	*Lama guanicoë glama*	0.2–0.5	1–2
Bear	Most species	2–6	8–10
Striped hyena	*Hyaena striata*	3–5	7–8
Wolf	*Canis lupus*	3–5	7–8
Puma	*Puma concolor*	. . .	8
Jaguar	*Panthera onca*	. . .	8
Lion	*Panthera leo*	. . .	8–10
Leopard (spotted)	*Panthera pardus*	. . .	8–10
Cheetah	*Acinonyx jubatus*	. . .	2(?)
Zebra	*Equus quagga*	3–5	. . .
Subhuman primates	Many species	0.5–1	2–5

$N—CH_2—CH=C(CH_3)_2$; CH_3; CH_3; OH

Pentazocine

FIG. 16.9.

the opiate compounds. Consequently, the principal effects of the analgesic agent are upon the CNS and smooth muscle. The analgesic potency of pentazocine is approximately one-half that of morphine and about 5 times more potent than that of meperidine. The hourly utilization rates of meperidine and pentazocine are essentially equivalent in maintaining an analgesic effect in human beings; this may be due to a more rapid metabolization rate of pentazocine compared to meperidine (Ahlgren and Stephen 1966). Based upon this clinical observation, the analgesic potency of pentazocine is considered to be equivalent to meperidine mg for mg.

Paired animal studies have been conducted in the dog to compare the respiration and cardiovascular actions of pentazocine, meperidine, and morphine (Ahlgren and Stephen 1966). These drugs in equianalgesic doses (i.e., 5 mg/kg of pentazocine, 5 mg/kg of meperidine hydrochloride, or 0.5 mg/kg of morphine, all administered intravenously) depressed the respiratory rate. Although respiration was depressed, a challenge with 5% carbon dioxide indicated an increased response in respiratory activity. In the case of pentazocine, an elevation in the tidal volume occurred over the preanalgesic or control level.

The most significant response of pentazocine in the dog was its effect upon systemic arterial pressure (Ahlgren and Stephen 1966). Following pentazocine and morphine administration, an 18% and a 25% decrease in the systolic pressure occurred, respectively. The drop in arterial pressure produced by meperidine was 75%. The blood pressure drop following morphine and pentazocine was only transient and returned to the original level in less than 1 minute. The decrease in arterial pressure by meperidine eventually returned to control levels about 5 minutes after the drug was administered; this prolonged hypotensive effect was believed to be related to the initial release of histamine.

FATE AND METABOLISM OF PENTAZOCINE

The kinetics of the disappearance of pentazocine from plasma following an intramuscular injection of 3 mg/kg of body weight were determined in ponies, goats, swine, dogs, and cats (Davis and Sturm 1970). This dose level of pentazocine (3 mg/kg) was higher than that employed in human patients (i.e., 0.6 mg/kg). However, according to Davis and Sturm (1970), the dose of pentazocine used in their studies was considerably below the amount reported to induce toxic effects in animals. With the exception of the dog, disappearance of pentazocine from plasma follows first-order kinetics. The peak plasma concentrations of pentazocine after its administration occur at 15 minutes in dogs, goats, and swine; at 30 minutes in ponies; and at 1 hour in cats (Davis and Sturm 1970). The plasma half-life values ranged from 22 minutes in dogs to 97 minutes in ponies (see Table 16.1). In human beings the plasma half-life of pentazocine is about 2 hours after intravenous (20–25 mg/70 kg) or intramuscular (45 mg/70 kg) administration (Berkowitz 1971). Also, in human patients the peak analgesic effect occurs between 30 and 60 minutes after an intramuscular dose of pentazocine and lasts 2–3 hours. It is obvious that the plasma half-life of pentazocine and duration of action in human beings are longer than in domestic animals.

TABLE 16.1. Kinetic constants for the disappearance of pentazocine from the blood plasma of domesticated animals

Species	C_0	$T_{1/2}$	K′d	V′d
	(mg/L)	*(min)*	*(hr^{-1})*	*(L/kg)*
Ponies	0.59	97.1	0.0071	5.09
Goats	0.52	51.0	0.0136	5.77
Swine	0.63	48.6	0.0143	4.76
Dogs	0.85	22.1	0.0313	3.66
Cats	1.08	83.6	0.0083	2.78

Source: Davis and Sturm 1970.

Note: C_0 = plasma concentration of drug at zero time; $T_{1/2}$ = plasma half-life; K′d = apparent first-order disappearance rate constant; V′d = apparent specific volume of distribution of the drug.

Pentazocine is metabolized in human beings to a large degree with little of the unchanged (<5%) or parent compound appearing in the urine. The fate of pentazocine is probably quite similar to morphine and its derivatives. Its conjugation with glucuronic acid and excretion as a glucuronide have been established. Trace amounts of pentazocine and its metabolites can be detected in the urine for several days after a single administration of the drug.

CLINICAL USE

The clinical pharmacological experience with pentazocine in veterinary medicine has not been extensive. Pentazocine has been essentially restricted to preanesthetic medication use because of its lack of profound sedation in animals (Soma 1971). According to Soma, use of pentazocine for postanalgesic effect in both small-animal and equine anesthesia was inconclusive. A dose of pentazocine in the dog of 1.5–3 mg/kg was suggested and was presumably administered intramuscularly. In the horse Soma (1971) indicated that the total intravenous dose of pentazocine was 200–400 mg. Dose levels of 6–10 mg/kg in the dog (presumably via the intramuscular route) produced tremors and convulsions reminiscent of the morphine-like compounds (Soma 1971). Side effects were also observed in the pony when 1–2 mg/lb of body weight of pentazocine were administered intravenously or intramuscularly (Lowe 1969). The side effects consisted of incoordination, muscular tremors, hypertonicity of muscles, and hypersensitivity to noise. In one trial, a dose of 3 mg/kg administered intramuscularly caused the animal to fall backard to the floor; it paddled its feet in the lateral recumbent position and in a few seconds returned to the standing position. However, the pony was very ataxic for another 10 minutes.

The analgesic action of pentazocine in the pony provided a more prolonged and consistent effect than meperidine; the duration of analgesia for pentazocine was 48 minutes and for meperidine it was 21 minutes (Lowe 1969). An intravenous dose of pentazocine (0.25–0.5 mg/lb) produced analgesia lasting 10–20 minutes; an intramuscular or intravenous dose of 0.75–1 mg/lb produced an analgesic effect varying from 15 to 60 minutes (Lowe 1969).

In the clinical evaluation of pentazocine and meperidine in the relief of postoperative pain, a blind study was conducted in the dog by Short et al. (1971). It was concluded that meperidine was more effective than pentazocine for surgery of the extremities and thorax, whereas pentazocine was more effective for ocular surgery. In the case of both pentazocine and meperidine, the relief of pain varied most in obtunding moderate pain but both drugs were comparable in the relief of severe pain (Short et al. 1971).

Propoxyphene Hydrochloride

The analgesic potency of *Propoxyphene Hydrochloride,* U.S.P. (Darvon), is less than that of codeine. It has not been used to any great extent in clinical veterinary medicine. A dose level of 2.2 mg/kg of propoxyphene hydrochloride administered intramuscularly and in combination with morphine is an effective analgesic combination in the cat (Davis and Donnelly 1968). The therapeutic efficacy of propoxyphene has not been determined in most species.

REFERENCES

Ahlgren, E. W., and Stephen, C. R. 1966. Laboratory and clinical experience with a new analgesic—Pentazocine. Anesth Analg 45:673.

Aitken, M. M., and Sanford, J. 1972. Effects of tranquillizers on tachycardia induced by adrenaline in the horse. Br Vet J 128:vii.

Alexander, F., and Nicholson, J. D. 1970. Drugs and doses in equine practice. Equine Vet J 2:183.

Amend, J. F. 1973. Rompun (Bay Va 1470), an effective pre-medication for ketamine anesthesia in the cat. Vet Med Rev No. 2:142.

Amend, J. F., and Klavano, P. A. 1973. Xylazine: A new sedative-analgesic with predictable emetic properties in the cat. Vet Med Small Anim Clin 68:741.

Amend, J. F.; Klavano, P. A.; and Stone, E. C. 1972. Premedication with xylazine to eliminate muscular hypertonicity in cats during ketamine anesthesia. Vet Med Small Anim Clin 67:1305.

Bauditz, R. 1972. Sedation, immobilization and anaesthesia with Rompun in captive and free-living wild animals. Vet Med Rev No. 3/4:204.

Berkowitz, B. 1971. Influence of plasma levels and metabolism of pharmacological activity: Pentazocine. Ann NY Acad Sci 179: 269.

Bierhaus, G. M. 1970. Modern medicine and testing. Proc Am Assoc Equine Pract, p. 199.

Boyland, E., and Booth, J. 1962. The metabolic fate and excretion of drugs. Ann Rev Pharmacol 2:129.

Bruce, R. B.; Maynard, W. R., Jr.; and Dunning, L. K. 1974. Oxyphenbutazone and phenylbutazone determination in plasma and urine by GLC. J Pharm Sci 63:446.

Cannon, J. H. 1974. Excerpts from AAEP meeting reports. Phenylbutazone. J Am Vet Med Assoc 164:367.

Carlisle, C. H.; Penny, R. H. C.; Prescott, C. W.; and Davidson, H. A. 1968. Toxic effects of phenylbutazone on the cat. Br Vet J 124:560.

Clarke, K. W., and Hall, L. W. 1969. "Xylazine"—A new sedative for horses and cattle. Vet Rec 85:512.

Davis, L. E., and Donnelly, E. J. 1968. Analgesic drugs in the cat. J Am Vet Med Assoc 153:1161.

Davis, L. E., and Sturm, B. L. 1970. Drug effects and plasma concentrations of pentazocine in domesticated animals. Am J Vet Res 31:1631.

Davis, L. E., and Westfall, B. A. 1972. Species differences in biotransformation and excretion of salicylate. Am J Vet Res 33: 1253.

Davis, L. E.; Westfall, B. A.; and Short, C. R. 1973. Biotransformation and pharmacokinetics of salicylate in newborn animals. Am J Vet Res 34:1105.

Davison, C.; Hertig, D. H.; and DeVine, R. 1966. Gastric hemorrhage induced by nonnarcotic analgetic agents in dogs. Clin Pharmacol Ther 7:239.

Dayton, P. G.; Israili, Z. H.; and Perel, J. M. 1973. Influence of binding on drug metabolism and distribution. Ann NY Acad Sci 226:172.

Dunn, S. 1972. A clinician's views on the use and misuse of phenylbutazone. Equine Vet J 4:63.

Finco, D. R.; Duncan, J. R.; Schall, W. D.; and Prasse, K. W. 1975. Acetaminophen toxicosis in the cat. J Am Vet Med Assoc 166:469.

Finocchio, E. J.; Ozog, F. J.; Oehme, F. W.; Johnson, J. H.; and Osbaldiston, G. W. 1970. Detection of phenylbutazone and oxyphenbutazone in the urine of thoroughbreds. J Am Vet Med Assoc 156: 454.

Flower, R. J. 1974. Drugs which inhibit prostaglandin biosynthesis. Pharmacol Rev 26: 33.

Gabriel, K. L., and Martin, J. E. 1962. Phenylbutazone: Short-term versus long-term administration to thoroughbred and standardbred horses. J Am Vet Med Assoc 140: 337.

Gandal, C. P.; Dayton, P. G.; Weiner, M.; and Perel, J. M. 1969. Studies with phenylbutazone, oxyphenbutazone and para-paradichloro phenylbutazone in horses. Cornell Vet 59:577.

Garner, H. E.; Amend, J. F.; and Rosborough, J. P. 1971a. Effects of Bay VA 1470 on cardiovascular parameters in ponies. Vet Med Small Anim Clin 66:1016.

———. 1971b. Effects of Bay VA 1470 on respiratory parameters in ponies. Vet Med Small Anim Clin 66:921.

Gray, G. W., and Yano, B. L. 1975. A study of the actions of methampyrone and a commercial intestinal extract perparation on intestinal motility. Am J Vet Res 36: 201.

Greig, C. G. 1957. Observations on the distribution of glucuronide synthesis in tissues. Biochem J 66:52.

Herrgesell, J. D. 1967. Aspirin poisoning in the cat. J Am Vet Med Assoc 151:452.

Hoffman, P. E. 1974. Clinical evaluation of xylazine as a chemical restraining agent sedative and analgesic in horses. J Am Vet Med Assoc 164:42.

Hopes, R. 1972. Uses and misuses of antiinflammatory drugs in racehorses. Equine Vet J 4:66.

Hopkins, T. J. 1972. The clinical pharmacology of xylazine in cattle. Aust Vet J 48:109.

Jones, R. S. 1972. A review of tranquillization and sedation in large animals. Vet Res 90:613.

Kerr, D. D.; Jones, E. W.; Holbert, D.; and Huggins, K. 1972a. Comparison of the effects of zylazine and acetylpromazine maleate in the horse. Am J Vet Res 33: 777.

Kerr, D. D.; Jones, E. W.; Huggins, K.; and Edwards, W. C. 1972b. Sedative and other effects of xylazine given intravenously to horses. Am J Vet Res 33:525.

Korsgaard Christensen, L. K. 1959. The metabolic effect of salicylate and other hydroxybenzoates. Acta Pharmacol Toxicol 16:129.

Lacuata, A. Q., and Subang, P. M. 1973. A preliminary study on the preanesthetic value of Rompun given intravenously in dogs prior to pentobarbital sodium anesthesia. Philipp J Vet Med 12:143.

Larson, E. J. 1963. Toxicity of low doses of aspirin in the cat. J Am Vet Med Assoc 143:837.

Lev, R.; Siegel, H. I.; and Glass, G. B. J. 1972. Effects of salicylates on the canine stomach: A morphological and histochemical study. Gastroenterology 62:970.

Levinger, I. M.; Kedem, J.; and Abram, M. 1973. A new anaesthetic-sedative agent for birds. Br Vet J 129:296.

Lowe, J. E. 1969. Pentazocine (Talwin-V) for the relief of abdominal pain in ponies—A comparative evaluation with description of a colic model for analgesia evaluation. Proc Am Assoc Equine Pract, p. 31.

McCashin, F. B., and Gabel, A. A. 1971. Rompun—A new sedative with analgesic properties. Proc Am Assoc Equine Pract, p. 111.

Moss, M. S. 1972. Uses and misuse of antiinflammatory drugs in racehorses. Equine Vet J 4:69.

Moss, M. S., and Haywood, P. E. 1973. Persistence of phenylbutazone in horses producing acid urines. Vet Rec 93:124.

Moye, R. J.; Pailet, A.; and Smith, M. W., Jr. 1973. Clinical use of xylazine in dogs and cats. Vet Med Small Anim Clin 68:236.

Newkirk, H. L., and Miles, D. G. 1974. Xylazine as a sedative-analgesic for dogs and cats. Mod Vet Pract 55:677.

Oliver, J. E., Jr., and Young, W. O. 1973. Evaluation of pharmacologic agents for restraint in cystometry in the dog and cat. Am J Vet Res 34:665.

Penny, R. H. C.; Carlisle, C. H.; Prescott, C. W.; and Davidson, H. A. 1967. Effects of aspirin (acetylsalicylic acid) on the haemopoietic system of the cat. Br Vet J 123:154.

Piperno, E.; Ellis, D. J.; Getty, S. M.; and Brody, T. M. 1968. Plasma and urine levels of phenylbutazone in the horse. J Am Vet Med Assoc 153:195.

Rickard, L. J.; Thurmon, J. C.; and Lingard, D. R. 1974. Preliminary report on xylazine HCl as a sedative agent in bulls for electroejaculation and semen collection. Vet Med Small Anim Clin 69:1029.

Said, S. I. 1973. The lung in relation to vasoactive hormone. Fed Proc 32:1972.

Short, C. E. 1974. Technic and equipment for equine inhalation anesthesia. Mod Vet Pract 55:393.

Short, C. E.; Hoppingardner, J.; Bendick, F.; and Greenwald, W. 1971. Comparative responses of pentazocine and meperidine for control of postoperative pain in dogs. Vet Med Small Anim Clin 66:586.

Short, C. E.; Tumbleson, M. E.; and Merriam, J. G. 1972. Comparative effects of Bay VA 1470 (xylazine), promazine and halothane on serum electrolytes in the horse. Vet Med Small Anim Clin 67:747.

Soma, L. R., ed. 1971. Preanesthetic medication. In Textbook of Veterinary Anesthesia, p. 121. Baltimore: Williams & Wilkins.

Tandy, J., and Thorpe, E. 1967. A fatal syndrome in a dog following administration of phenylbutazone. Vet Rec 81:398.

Taylor, L. A., and Crawford, L. M. 1968. Aspirin-induced gastrointestinal lesions in dogs. J Am Vet Med Assoc 152:617.

Willis, A. L. 1974. An enzymatic mechanism for the antithrombotic and antihemostatic actions of aspirin. Science 183:325.

Willis, A. L., and Kuhn, D. C. 1974. Acetylenic analog of arachidonate that acts like aspirin on platelets. Science 183:327.

Woodbury, D. M. 1970. Analgesic-antipyretics, anti-inflammatory agents, and inhibitors of uric acid synthesis. In L. S. Goodman and A. Gilman, eds. The Pharmacological Basis of Therapeutics, 4th ed., p. 314. New York: Macmillan.

Woodbury, D. M., and Fingl, E. 1975. Analgesic-antipyretics, anti-inflammatory agents and drugs employed in the therapy of gout. In L. S. Goodman and A. Gilman, eds. The Pharmacological Basis of Therapeutics, 5th ed., p. 348. New York: Macmillan.

Yates, W. D. 1973. Clinical use of xylazine, a new drug for old problems. Vet Med Small Anim Clin 68:483.

Yeary, R. A., and Brant, R. J. 1975. Aspirin dosages for the dog. J Am Vet Med Assoc 167:63.

Yeary, R. A., and Swanson, W. 1973. Aspirin dosages for the cat. J Am Vet Med Assoc 163:1177.

CHAPTER 17

PSYCHOTROPIC AGENTS

NICHOLAS H. BOOTH

In the 1950s reserpine and the phenothiazine derivatives (chlorpromazine, promazine, and others) were introduced into clinical veterinary medicine and were referred to as ataractics or tranquilizers; the latter term is still commonly used. French pharmacologists and chemists, who discovered the phenothiazines, have used the term "neuroleptics" to denote that their most prominent pharmacologic effects are upon certain functions of the central nervous system (CNS). This pharmacological effect differentiated the phenothiazine derivatives and related drugs from other psychotropic compounds.

In veterinary medicine the phenothiazines have been valuable in the "chemical restraint" of animals for various diagnostic and clinical procedures. Their value in quieting and calming unfriendly and apprehensive animals has been beneficial in the preparation of animals for neurolept-analgesia and general anesthesia.

The psychotropic drugs of major importance in veterinary medicine are the phenothiazine derivatives, thioxanthene derivative, butyrophenone derivatives, and rauwolfia preparations. This chapter will discuss these classes of drugs and others of lesser importance such as meprobamate and the benzodiazepine derivatives.

PHENOTHIAZINE DERIVATIVES

Phenothiazine is the parent compound for all the derivatives in this group (Fig. 17.1). Substitution is made primarily in the phenothiazine nucleus at the 2 and 10 positions.

MECHANISM OF ACTION OF THE PHENOTHIAZINES

The majority of pharmacologic actions discussed for the phenothiazines pertain to chlorpromazine. However, the mechanisms of action for other phenothiazines are also similar to chlorpromazine except for variations primarily referable to

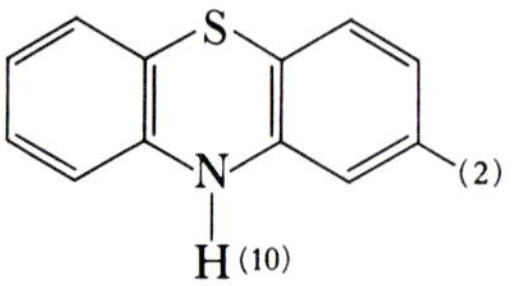

Phenothiazine

FIG. 17.1.

potency and duration of action. In clinical practice greater potency of a drug does not necessarily imply greater effectiveness. This is true of the phenothiazines because controlled investigations have been unable to show any significant difference in the effectiveness of these agents when administered in equipotent dosage levels.

The phenothiazines have a broad spectrum of activity ranging from suppression of protozoan motility to the alteration of the pecking order and behavior of birds. Except for variations in potency and duration of action, all the phenothiazines exert a sedative action by depresssing the brainstem and the connections to the cerebral cortex. The sedative effect differs from the barbiturates since it does not affect appreciably the coordinated motor responses of the animal. Moreover, arousal is easily accomplished. Reduced or no sedative action is observed when a piperazine structure (e.g., in the case of prochlorperazine) is linked to position 10 of the molecule.

It is believed that the principal central activity of the neuroleptics is the blockade of dopamine, a neurotransmitter catecholamine, principally found in the basal ganglia complex (Iversen 1975). A deficiency of dopamine within the basal ganglia has been shown to be associated with a definite dysfunction of this neuroanatomical system, namely, the Parkinsonian syndrome in human beings and catalepsy in experimental animals (Hornykiewicz 1973).

All the phenothiazines decrease spontaneous motor activity in animals. At high dosages, cataleptic effects may be produced so that the animals will remain immobile in a fixed position for long periods. Most phenothiazine derivatives increase the rate of dopamine turnover, i.e., synthesis and destruction, in the brain (Hornykiewicz 1973; Matthysse 1973). Extrapyramidal symptoms (rigidity, tremor, akinesia) or cataleptic symptoms are observed as prominent side effects of the phenothiazines in animals, particularly at high dose levels.

Chlorpromazine increases the concentration of the dopamine metabolite, homovanillic acid, in the caudate nucleus of the cat and rabbit. This effect appears to be related to the potency of of these compounds in eliciting extrapyramidal symptoms (catalepsy) in animals. The prototype phenothiazine derivative, promethazine, has antihistaminic activity and does not increase the concentration of homovanillic acid like chlorpromazine; the increased synthesis and disappearance of dopamine is also unaffected by promethazine, whereas chlorpromazine, perphenazine, and chlorprothixene all increase its synthesis and destruction (Matthysse 1973). Trimeprazine, a nonpsychotropic phenothiazine, produces a slight increase in the dopamine metabolite level within the corpus striatum of the rabbit. The effect of administering chlorpromazine, promethazine, trimeprazine, and other compounds upon the level of homovanillic acid in the brain of a single monkey is shown in Fig. 17.2; all drugs were injected intramuscularly at a dose of 10 mg/kg of body weight in procaine solution to prevent pain.

In addition to blockade of the central effect of catecholamines (viz., dopamine), the phenothiazines are known to block the peripheral actions of catecholamines. Chlorpromazine and other related compounds can prevent and reverse a number of actions of epinephrine ("epinephrine reversal"). The administration of epinephrine hydrochloride is contraindicated whenever the phenothiazine derivatives are used. However, norepinephrine (levarterenol) can be used without risk of aggravating the arterial hypotensive effects of the phenothiazines. Chlorpromazine and, to a lesser degree, acetylpromazine prevent epinephrine-induced ventricular fibrillation during the use of

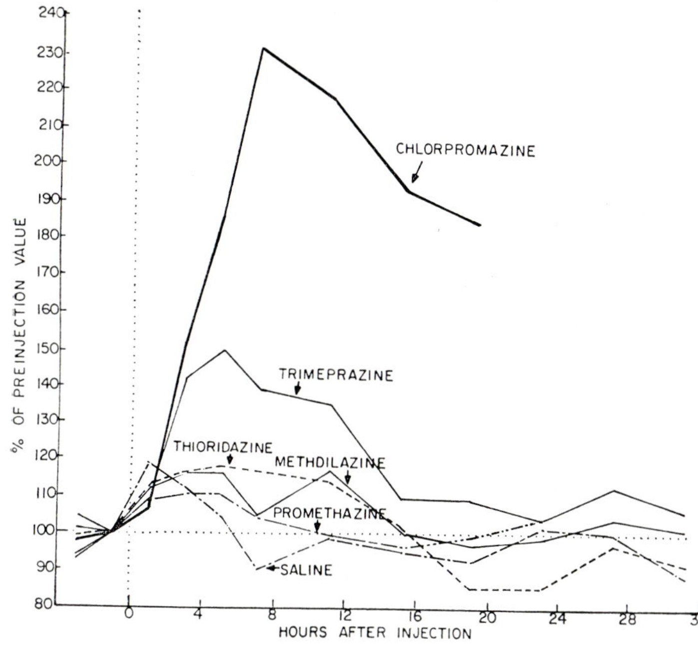

FIG. 17.2. Comparison of phenothiazine effects on lateral ventricular homovanillic acid. (From Matthysse 1973)

halogenated anesthetics (halothane, methoxyflurane, and others) similar to the α-adrenergic blocking agents.

Amphetamine and many sympathomimetic compounds structurally similar to catecholamines are blocked centrally by phenothiazine derivatives. In amphetamine overdosage, chlorpromazine is recommended as one of the antidotes for treatment of CNS excitation and convulsions. Serotonin is also blocked by chlorpromazine. In addition, it blocks the locomotor hyperactivity and stereotyped motor behavior evoked by apomorphine in animals (Hornykiewicz 1973). Morphine-induced hyperexcitement and manic behavior in the cat can be prevented by pretreatment with chlorpromazine (Dhasmana et al. 1972). It is believed that morphine enhances the release of dopamine in the CNS, which in turn stimulates central dopaminergic receptors to induce the manic response.

Hypothermic effects appear to be induced by the phenothiazines, due to depletion of catecholamine substances within the hypothalamus where thermoregulation is controlled centrally. The effects of chlorpromazine upon metabolism and autonomic nervous activity under conditions of environmental temperature changes and other types of "stress" have been the target of many studies. In the transportation of animals to abattoirs for slaughter, this so-called antistress effect of the neuroleptics was investigated to reduce weight losses ("shrinkage") and bruising in transport (Ginsberg et al. 1963). This use is not approved by the Food and Drug Administration (FDA) because of the possibility that tissue residues will persist above the accepted tolerance levels permitted in food for human consumption.

Chlorpromazine affects pituitary activity only in quantities that exceed those required to induce depressant effects (de Wied 1967). At high dosages chlorpromazine appears to block the release of the follicle-stimulating hormone (FSH) and the luteinzing hormone (LH). Also, ovulation is blocked and the estrus cycle is suppressed. Recent work has shown that chlorpromazine, acetylpromazine, and perphenazine increase the plasma level of prolactin in a number of species, i.e., rat, sheep, goat, and human being (Blackwell et al.

1973). Other endocrine effects include inhibition of the release of the melanocyte-stimulating hormone (MSH) and the antidiuretic hormone (ADH), and it may inhibit the release of oxytocin.

Hyperglycemia has been observed following the administration of chlorpromazine and other phenothiazines in several species, including human beings. The principal mechanism of the phenothiazine-evoked hyperglycemia is believed to be due to the release of epinephrine via the adrenal medulla; this in turn mobilizes liver glycogen. Inasmuch as the relative effectiveness of the phenothiazines in elevating the blood glucose does not correlate well with their capability to stimulate secretion of adrenal catecholamine, questions arose about the actual mechanism(s) involved. The phenothiazines do indeed elevate blood glucose through the release of epinephrine from the adrenal medulla because extirpation of the adrenal medullae abolishes or reduces the glycemic responses. However, extraadrenal mechanisms are also involved and appear to be more important in the overall effect upon blood glucose; for example, inhibition or blockade of the effect of insulin is a major factor in determining the degree of the hyperglycemic effect produced by certain phenothiazines (Proakis and Borowitz 1974).

Other important effects of chlorpromazine apart from its central influences are its adrenergic blocking action in conjunction with weak anticholinergic, antihistaminic, and antispasmodic effects. Chlorpromazine also potentiates the effect of analgesics, hypnotics, and local and general anesthetics. Although the blocking effect of local anesthetics is enhanced by chlorpromazine, the phenothiazines are contraindicated in epidural anesthetic procedures because they potentiate the arterial hypotensive effects of local anesthetics. In addition, chlorpromazine produces local analgesic, autonomic ganglion blocking, and arterial hypertensive effects along with reduction in capillary permeability, inhibition of blood clotting, and potentiation of the effect of neuromuscular blocking agents. Chlorpromazine and other phenothiazines have a paralyzing action upon skeletal muscle similar to that produced by *d*-tubocurarine. Its action can be antagonized to some extent by eserine or neostigmine. Antipyretic, hypothermic, hypometabolic, and anticonvulsive actions are produced by chlorpromazine and related derivatives.

Although the phenothiazine tranquilizers will antagonize the CNS-stimulating effects of sympathomimetic amines (e.g., amphetamine and related drugs), it does not prevent the convulsive action of strychnine, pentylenetetrazol (metrazol), and picrotoxin. The phenothiazines in therapeutic dosages suppress conditioned avoidance behavior, inhibit spontaneous motor activity, and reduce aggressive behavior and hostility. At higher dosages, interference with locomotor function is observed. Moderate dosages produce sedation and drowsiness and, in larger concentrations, the phenothiazines induce ataxia and somnolence.

Clinical levels of the phenothiazines ordinarily have little effect upon respiratory activity. If arterial hypotension occurs, respiratory activity may be reflexly accelerated through the decreased activity of the carotid and aortic pressoreceptors. Large dosages, however, will depress respiratory activity. Vasomotor activity controlled via the hypothalamus or at the medullary level is depressed by low levels of chlorpromazine.

Activity upon the brainstem by the phenothiazines appears to be more complex than that produced by barbiturates. For example, chlorpromazine produces only a slight increase in the threshold for arousal. Barbiturates, on the other hand, produce deeper levels of depression and impair arousal activity.

Chlorpromazine and other phenothiazines markedly reduce the hematocrit of animals, the mechanism apparently being related to a hemodilution effect or an increased plasma volume. Blood samples drawn from chlorpromazine-treated animals for diagnostic purposes will be interpreted incorrectly as anemic unless one is familiar with this effect of chlorpromazine (Collette and Meriwether 1965).

Chlorpromazine Hydrochloride

Chemically, *Chlorpromazine,* U.S.P. (Thorazine, Largactil), is 2-chloro-10-(3-dimethylaminopropyl)-phenothiazine (Fig. 17.3). In the hydrochloride salt form, it is a grayish white crystalline powder that is very soluble in water. Although it decomposes in light, it can be boiled without decomposition. The chemical synthesis of chlorpromazine soon followed the observation that an antihistaminic agent (i.e., promethazine), also a phenothiazine compound, produced CNS depression. Chlorpromazine has slight antihistaminic activity being 1/100 as potent as promethazine.

ADMINISTRATION

In most species, chlorpromazine is administered primarily by the intramuscular and intravenous routes. Intramuscular injections are slower, somewhat irritating, and less reliable in action. In the rabbit, the intramuscular injection of chlorpromazine produces severe myositis, lameness, swelling, muscular atrophy, and paralysis. Intramuscular use of this drug is contraindicated in the rabbit for preanesthetic medication (Bree et al. 1971).

METABOLISM

Chlorpromazine is metabolized slowly in the dog. The biologic half-life is about 6 hours. In human beings, and probably in the dog, hydroxylation in the 3 and 7 positions and conjugation with glucuronic acid represent the major metabolic pathways in the degradation of chlorpromazine. Sulfoxide is the next important product of metabolic biotransformation of chlorpromazine. The sulfoxide form of chlorpromazine possesses about one-eighth the sedative action of the parent drug in the dog.

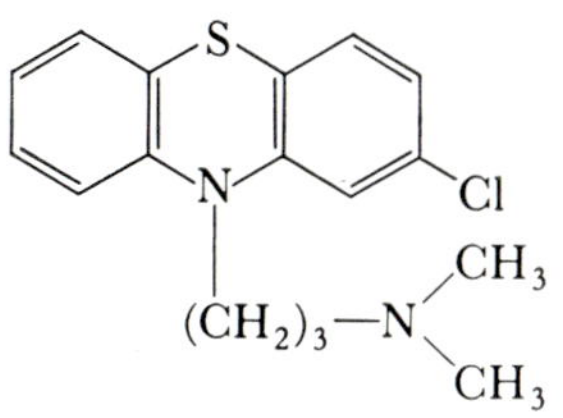

S
N
Cl
$(CH_2)_3—N$
CH_3
CH_3

Chlorpromazine

Fig. 17.3.

In mental patients, chlorpromazine and various metabolites may be detected in urine 6–18 months after termination of treatment (Jarvik 1970). In food-producing animals, drug residues may possibly persist in edible tissues for long periods; information on this subject is lacking.

EXCRETION

Little or no chlorpromazine is eliminated in the urine of the dog. The primary excretory product is chlorpromazine sulfoxide, but only 10%–15% of the dose is eliminated as such. In other species, there is little information about the excretion patterns of chlorpromazine and its metabolites.

Limited studies of the excretion patterns have been conducted in the horse following the intramuscular and oral administration of chlorpromazine (Weir and Sanford 1972). After intramuscular injection, metabolites were detected in the urine up to 96 hours. Following oral administration, metabolites were no longer detected after 80–96 hours. The percentage of the dose recovered in equine urine was low, with the average being 10% after intramuscular and 27% after oral administration. Unconjugated metabolites excreted in the horse represented only 1%–1.5% of the dosage after either route of administration; these were excreted entirely as sulfoxide derivatives. Glucuronide-conjugated metabolites were predominately excreted by the horse in a ratio to unconjugated metabolites of approximately 7:1 after intramuscular injection and 18:1 after oral administration. The sulfate-conjugated metabolites made up about 5% of the total after oral administration but were detected only in trace amounts after intramuscular injection. With the use of spectroscopic analytical methodology, phenothiazine derivatives in the feces of horses were not detected (Weir and Sanford 1972).

ANTEMETIC EFFECT

In the dog, but not in the cat, chlorpromazine is effective in antagonizing apomorphine-induced emesis (Brand et al. 1954). It also protects against vomiting induced by morphine, but it is ineffective against intravenous copper sulfate, digitalis glycosides and veratrum and oral copper sulfate. The antemetic effect of chlorpromazine in dogs indicates that the mechanism of action is a selective depression of the emetic chemoreceptor trigger zone located in the brainstem.

SIDE EFFECTS

Cardiac arrhythmias are induced in the unanesthetized and anesthetized dog by either chlorpromazine or promazine in parenteral dosages ranging from 2.5 to 5 mg/kg of body weight (Santos-Martinez et al. 1972). Atropinization reverts the arrhythmia to the characteristic anticholinergic effects such as sinus and atrial tachycardia. High doses of chlorpromazine in the cat produce tremors of one or more extremities or the head (Kaelber and Joynt 1956). Also, variable degrees of shivering, lethargy, relaxation of the anal sphincter, diarrhea, and diminution or loss of righting reflexes occur. Rigidity of the extremities and trunk without evident alteration in postural and righting reflexes may also occur in the cat. Upon discontinuance of medication, the rigidity and other side effects disappear within 10 days and the cat appears to be fully recovered and normal.

In the horse, chlorpromazine produces undesirable effects in many animals and is no longer advocated in equine practice. After a few minutes of initial sedation following the administration of the drug, the animal becomes unsteady, sinks backward on its hocks, and then lunges forward in an uncoordinated manner. The horse may stumble and fall, then stand and continue lunging and rearing. This violent reaction alternates with periods of sedation.

TOXICITY

In the dog, a subcutaneous dose of 1.5 mg/kg of chlorpromazine produces no gross signs of toxicity (Brand et al. 1954). However, when the dosage is administered intravenously, moderate depression and ataxia occur, which last 6–12 hours. When a dose of 3 mg/kg is injected intravenously, marked CNS depression and ataxia are noted for 24–48 hours.

In the Beagle and American foxhound, chlorpromazine hydrochloride given orally at 30 mg/kg/day produces ocular lesions within 73 days in both breeds whether exposed to natural daylight or maintained under ultraviolet-free artificial light (Barron et al. 1972). Granular corneal deposits are produced by chlorpromazine and persist for many weeks even after withdrawal or discontinuance of treatment. Clinically, the phenothiazines are used intermittently and usually do not entail a protracted period of therapeutic use in veterinary medicine. The likelihood that ocular lesions would develop under short-term therapeutic use is improbable.

CONTRAINDICATIONS AND PRECAUTIONS

The administration of epinephrine hydrochloride is contraindicated whenever the phenothiazines are used. Phenothiazine derivatives are contraindicated in epidural anesthetic procedures because they potentiate the arterial hypotensive activity of local anesthetics. Their use in the control of strychnine, pentylenetetrazol, and picrotoxin convulsive seizures is contraindicated because of their ineffectiveness.

Package inserts of drug firms caution against the use of phenothiazines when animals have been exposed to organophosphates because they may potentiate the toxicity of the organophosphates. Repeated administration of chlorpromazine and promazine increases the toxicity of parathion in the rat. The anthelmintic phenothiazine does not seem to potentiate the toxic effects of organophosphates such as malathion, coumaphos, ronnel, crufomate, dichlorvos, and others (Schlinke and Palmer 1973). In addition, caution against the use of phenothiazines in conjunction with procaine hydrochloride is listed on package inserts; the activity of procaine may also be potentiated.

The use of chlorpromazine hydrochloride alone in the horse is contraindicated because of the violent incoordination and excitement that often occurs following its administration. In the air transport of horses, the administration of phenothiazines appears to be contraindicated due to the variable effects that may be produced such as incoordination, anxiety, and excitement.

Precautions in the use of phenothiazine derivatives include their careful use in debilitated and cardiac disease patients. In addition, caution must be taken in animals suffering from hypovolemic shock as well as those that have sympathetic blockade following epidural anesthesia.

CLINICAL USE

In the Dog and Cat. Chlorpromazine hydrochloride is approved as a prescription item by the FDA for use in only the dog and cat. At one time, chlorpromazine was the most extensively used neuroleptic agent in these species. However, promazine hydrochloride (Sparine) and acetylpromazine maleate (acepromazine) are now preferred for use in the dog and cat.

Clinically, chlorpromazine has been used in the dog and cat at 0.25 to 2 mg/lb of body weight by intravenous injection for immediate effect. The sedative effect is especially helpful in nervous or aggressive animals. By the intramuscular route of administration, the dose recommended for the dog and cat is 0.5–3 mg/lb of body weight. The oral dosage recommended consists of 1 tablet containing 10 mg/7 lb of body weight or 1 tablet containing 25 mg/17 lb of body weight. For all routes of administration (intravenous, intramuscular, oral), chlorpromazine is administered 1–4 times daily, depending on the size of the dosage used within the ranges given and the needs of the patients.

For preanesthetic purposes in the dog and cat, chlorpromazine should be injected intramuscularly 1–1.5 hours prior to anesthesia for surgery at a dose not to exceed 0.5 mg/lb of body weight. The clinical effects are prominent for 4–5 hours but total action may persist for 24 hours. Premedication with chlorpromazine decreases the amount of barbiturate anesthetic (thiopental sodium) required to produce anesthesia by approximately 50% but does not alter the duration of anesthesia (Hatch 1967). However, the combination of atropine sulfate and chlorpromazine has been shown to reduce the amount of thiopental needed by about 50% but increases the "sleep time" by 33%.

The most consistent clinical effects of chlorpromazine premedication include drowsiness and disinclination to move. When aroused, the animal takes a normal interest in its surroundings. Body temperature may fall several hours later. The pulse rate does not change appreciably nor is respiration markedly depressed.

Chlorpromazine is safe to use in obstetrical procedures because it does not depress the respiratory center of the puppy nor inhibit labor in the bitch. Phenothiazines, including chlorpromazine, readily cross the placenta. In newborn pups, tissue levels of the phenothiazines are found in the liver, lung, kidney, and brain.

In the cat, chlorpromazine hydrochloride administered intramuscularly at 4.4 mg/kg with morphine sulfate (0.1–1 mg/kg) is an effective neuroleptanalgesic combination (Davis and Donnelly 1968). Chlorpromazine blocks central dopaminergic receptors and reduces the excitatory response often observed in the cat following morphine administration. Little, if any, analgesic effect is contributed by chlorpromazine or other phenothiazines.

The manufacturer makes the claim that chlorpromazine has antemetic action in the cat and dog. The claim is questionable in the cat because chlorpromazine fails to inhibit apomorphine-induced emesis; in the dog, chlorpromazine does prevent emesis induced by apomorphine (Brand et al. 1954). However, emesis is not prevented by chlorpromazine in animals that are subjected to vestibular stimulation.

In Food-Producing Species. Use of the phenothiazines in most food-producing animals has not been approved by the FDA because of the possibility that residues may persist in the edible tissues such as meat, milk, and eggs. A tissue tolerance level for chlorpromazine has not been published; the only one that has been published is for promazine hydrochloride.

In Breeding Animals. Chlorpromazine is sometimes used in animals not scheduled for food use or slaughter, such as breeding animals. The pig is easily restrained for intravenous injections 45–60 minutes following an intramuscular injection (0.5 mg/lb) of chlorpromazine. It is recommended in excitable sows following farrowing, especially in those reluctant to accept their newborn. Intravenous doses of 75–100 mg have been used in sows weighing 275–300 lb. If the drug is used immediately prior to parturition, the sow will farrow naturally. To prevent venous thrombosis, chlorpromazine should be given in dilute solution when it is used intravenously (Jones 1972).

Chlorpromazine has been useful as an adjunct to treatment of agalactia, which is a frequent clinical problem following parturition in swine (Lewis and Oakly 1971). Chlorpromazine has also been used experimentally in swine to protect them from heat stress. It is suggested that the neuroleptic diminishes the stressful response of the pituitary-adrenal axis due to the hyperthermia.

In Exotic Species. Chlorpromazine has been used in the capture of African lions (Campbell and Harthoorn 1963). Also, it has been used as an adjunct to restraint and anesthesia in lions (Harthoorn et al. 1971). For induction of neuroleptanalgesia in bears, the drug is administered via a projectile syringe dart in combination with analgesic preparations (Kuntze 1967). According to Bolz (1962), neuroleptics are effective agents in zoo practice; intramuscular doses of chlorpromazine recommended for several species are listed as follows:

	mg/kg
Tiger	4.0
Jackal	2.0
Bear	2.5
Rhesus monkey	2.0
Dromedary	1.5–2.5
Water buffalo	2.5
Bison	2.5

Chlorpromazine has been used in reptiles intramuscularly (10 mg/kg) prior to barbiturate anesthesia (Calderwood 1971).

Promazine Hydrochloride

Chemically, *Promazine,* N.F. (Sparine), is 10-(3-diethylaminopropyl) phenothiazine (Fig. 17.4). It is used in the hydrochloride form, and 1 g is soluble in about 3 ml of water. The drug is incompatible with alkalies, heavy metals, and oxidizing agents.

Although promazine has been used in nearly all domestic animals, monkeys, and small laboratory rodents, it is approved by the FDA for use only in the dog, cat, and horse Promazine cannot be used in animals intended for food; a zero tolerance has been established in tissues of food-producing animals.

excretion and metabolism

Excretion patterns of promazine hydrochloride have been studied in the horse (Weir and Sanford 1972). When 10 mg/kg of body weight were given orally, the excretion rate reached maximums of about 55 mg/hr within 8 hours of dosing and about 25 mg/hr between 16 and 24 hours. Metabolites could not be detected in urine after 72 hours (Weir and Sanford 1972). The percentage of promazine recovered in urine averaged 10%. Glucuronide-conju-

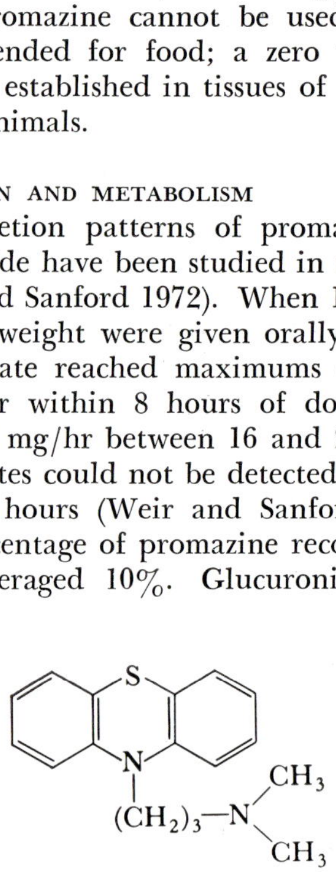

S
N
$(CH_2)_3$—N
CH_3
CH_3

Promazine

Fig. 17.4.

gated metabolites were predominant; conjugated metabolites were excreted almost entirely in the form of sulfoxide.

CONTRAINDICATIONS AND PRECAUTIONS

In general, the contraindications described for chlorpromazine apply to promazine. However, unlike chlorpromazine, promazine can be administered to horses with less likelihood of producing excitation. Some animals may be unusually reactive to noise and may respond violently to disturbances.

Caution must be taken to avoid the intracarotid injection of promazine, otherwise the horse may become violent and exhibit muscular tremors, stertorous respiration, and pupillary dilatation; eventually recumbency and convulsions appear (Christian et al. 1974). Large-caliber needles, especially 14 or 16 gauge, favor the pulsatile flow of arterial blood whereas smaller-bore needles do not with the result that the walls of the external jugular vein are easily passed through and the external carotid artery is inadvertently penetrated (Gabel and Koestner 1963).

Neuroleptics are contraindicated for quieting and calming animals for show rings and fairs. They are sometimes used unscrupulously in show horses to assist them in winning their classes. Also, in the sale of horses, tranquilizers must not be administered. Riding horses or ponies that have been tranquilized to overcome a vicious habit such as biting, kicking, rearing, and bucking have been sold. Purchase of such animals is hazardous and could result in serious injury or death to the rider. The veterinarian must be cautious in the examination of animals for sale purposes and recognize those that show signs of tranquilization.

CLINICAL USE

In the Dog. The major use of neuroleptics, including that of promazine is as a preanesthetic agent to facilitate handling through its sedative action. This permits smoother induction of anesthesia and reduces the amount of anesthetic required by 30%–50%. In the dog, the dose recommended by the parenteral routes (intramuscular or intravenous) is 1–3 mg/lb. For antemetic use, the above parenteral dose should be reduced by one-third to one-half (Leash 1969). Promazine may be repeated as necessary at 4- to 6-hour intervals.

Promazine is indicated in animals manifesting nervous behavior and excitability. It has value in the alleviation of self-inflicted mutilation associated with otitis, pruritis, and eczemic conditions. The drug assists in the handling of animals for radiographic diagnosis or therapy and in other procedures where restraint is required.

Promazine hydrochloride (3 mg/lb intravenously) has been used for cesarean section in 1- to 6-year-old Beagle bitches in conjunction with infiltration of 6 ml of 2% lidocaine hydrochloride or mepivacaine hydrochloride into the abdominal wall (Gupta et al. 1970). In the event this dosage of promazine does not produce complete relaxation, additional promazine is given subcutaneously at the rate of 1–2 mg/lb of body weight for the latent effect during surgery. Of the puppies delivered by this procedure, Gupta et al. reported that 98% lived and nursed with no signs of tranquilization.

In the Cat. The clinical indications and recommended parenteral dosage for the cat are similar to those for the dog. Compared to chlorpromazine, twice as much promazine is generally required to produce a comparable effect in the cat. Arterial hypotension and other cardiovascular effects produced by promazine in the cat are considerably less than those of chlorpromazine (Clifford and Soma 1969).

One of the therapeutic claims made by the manufacturer of promazine is that its administration before a vermifuge will prevent emesis in the cat. This claim is debatable because studies have shown that chlorpromazine fails to antagonize emesis induced by apomorphine in cats (Brand et al. 1954).

In the Horse. The recommended dosage of promazine hydrochloride is 0.2–0.5 mg/lb of body weight via the intravenous or intramuscular route. When 0.4 mg/lb of promazine hydrochloride is administered intramuscularly to a horse weighing 1000 lb (total dose of 400 mg), the effect of the drug is apparent in 10–15 minutes and lasts about one-half hour (Fraser 1967). According to Fraser, promazine takes effect less rapidly than acetylpromazine in the horse.

Promazine is also useful in the treatment of tetanus and in facilitating dental operations such as "floating the teeth" of horses. In loading and surface transportation of colts, promazine is valuable.

Promazine is used in conjunction with chloral hydrate and ultrashort-acting barbiturates in the horse (Gabel 1962). The procedure used by Gabel consists of administering promazine hydrochloride intravenously in a dose level of 333–500 mg/1000 lb of body weight. Ten minutes following intravenous injection, 7% chloral hydrate is administered intravenously at a dose level of 333 ml/1000 lb. After casting the animal, a catheter is placed in the external jugular vein so thiopental or thiamylal sodium can be injected to maintain surgical anesthesia. Barbiturates should not be used intravenously in the horse without preanesthetic sedation. An intravenous dose of 250 mg of promazine hydrochloride per 1000 lb of body weight is recommended (Jones 1961).

Promazine is also provided in granular form for use in the feed of horses. The oral dose is 0.75–1.25 mg/lb of body weight. The granular as well as the injectable preparation of promazine must not be used in horses intended for human food consumption.

In Cattle. The granular form of promazine hydrochloride can be used in feed of nonlactating cattle, 0.75–1.25 mg/lb of body weight. Unless the drug has been withdrawn from the feed for at least 72 hours prior to slaughter, the animals cannot be sold for human consumption. The established tolerance level for promazine in food is zero.

In Swine. Promazine hydrochloride (2 mg/kg) along with atropine sulfate (0.07–0.09 mg/kg) and meperidine hydrochloride (1–2 mg/kg) is useful as a preanesthetic in swine used for experimental purposes (Booth 1969). Promazine provides a mild tranquilizing effect and assists in restraint of the pig prior to general anesthesia.

In Exotic Species. Promazine has been used in tranquilizing bears (Clifford et al. 1962). An intramuscular injection of 2 mg/lb of body weight of promazine is effective in potentiating morphine sulfate. Promazine has been useful in combination with phencyclidine for immobilization of bears, with the exception of the polar bear, and for big cats, except tigers, as well as other exotic species (Seal and Erickson 1969).

The preparturient and postparturient use of promazine hydrochloride was successful in a hippopotamus weighing about 5000 lb (Graham-Jones 1962); 2 mg/lb or a total of 10 g were used in the feed and administered daily for 1 week prior to parturition. Parturition occurred normally, with the survival of the calf.

Acetylpromazine Maleate

Acetylpromazine Maleate (Acepromazine, Atrovet, Notensil) is approved by the FDA for use in the dog, cat, and horse. This phenothiazine derivative is the one most extensively used in veterinary medicine. Acetylpromazine is 2-acetyl-10-(3-dimethylaminopropyl) phenothiazine (Fig. 17.5). The drug is a yellow, odorless, crystalline powder with a bitter taste; the powder melts at 135°–138° C.

PHARMACOLOGICAL CONSIDERATIONS

Most of the pharmacologic effects of

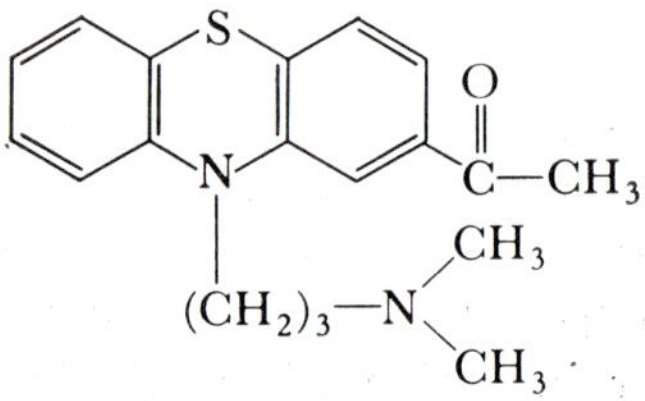

S

N

O

$C—CH_3$

CH_3

$(CH_2)_3—N$

CH_3

Acetylpromazine

FIG. 17.5.

acetylpromazine are similar to those of the other phenothiazine derivatives. Acetylpromazine is more potent than chlorpromazine or promazine and is effective parenterally in small dosages. The contraindications are the same as those for promazine and chlorpromazine.

Experimentally, acetylpromazine maleate decreases the arterial blood pressure in the dog 3 minutes after 1 mg/kg of the drug is administered by the intramuscular route (Popovic et al. 1972); this effect lasts 2 hours. A significant increase in central venous pressure occurs 90 minutes after administration of the drug and generally persists for the duration of its effect. Intermittent bradycardia was reported by Popovic and co-workers (1972). Sinoatrial arrest occurred at 3.5 minutes following the injection of acetylpromazine and lasted about 8 seconds; recovery was spontaneous with no apparent permanent cardiac injury. Atropine sulfate (0.02 mg/lb) should always be used in conjunction with acetylpromazine prior to the administration of a general anesthetic to minimize or prevent the vagal effects that may induce bradycardia or sinoatrial arrest.

Acetylpromazine markedly decreases the respiratory rate in the dog. Despite this, however, no significant alterations were noted in the Pa_{CO_2}, pH, Pa_{O_2} and oxyhemoglobin saturation (Popovic et al. 1972). Significant drops in the level of hemoglobin concentration were first observed 45 minutes after drug administration; this persisted for the duration (2 hours) of the experimental study.

ADVERSE REACTIONS

Clinically, a few case reports have revealed adverse reactions following administration of acetylpromazine in dogs (Garland and White 1968; White 1968). Within 5–10 minutes after the intramuscular injection of 0.25 mg/lb of acetylpromazine, sudden collapse was observed. Initially, the animals manifested apnea, then a slow pulse and unconsciousness.

Caution in the administration of acetylpromazine to weak, debilitated, aged, and cardiac disease patients must be observed to minimize adverse effects. Also, a drug interaction with the organophosphates must be avoided because the toxicity of the phenothiazines is enhanced.

CLINICAL USE

The primary use of acetylpromazine has been as a preanesthetic agent in the dog, cat, and horse. It markedly potentiates barbiturates where handling and restraint of animals may be facilitated.

In the Dog. Acetylpromazine may be administered intravenously, intramuscularly, subcutaneously, or orally in the dog. The recommended dose for the parenteral routes ranges from 0.25 to 0.5 mg/lb; for oral administration in tablet form, the recommended dose is 0.25–1 mg/lb of body weight. All dosages may be repeated, depending on the degree and duration of tranquilization required. Usually it is necessary to repeat the dose every 6–8 hours to maintain tranquilization.

According to Pugh (1964), the oral administration of 1–3 mg/kg of acetylpromazine in a single dose produces deep sedation in the dog. This is also accompanied by lethargy and reduced motor activity as evidenced by some posterior ataxia. Onset of the effect is noted by changes in facial expression. The skin overlying the frontal portion of the skull appears more pliable and wrinkled; the upper eyelid droops (ptosis); and the nictitating membrane is relaxed and protruded. The first indication of posterior ataxia is usually evident at this time. Recumbency soon follows and the animal frequently goes into a somnolent state.

The clinical signs of acetylpromazine usually begin to regress after 3–4 hours but may be present after 7 hours (Pugh 1964). As in other species, a drop in rectal temperature occurs. This effect is shown in Fig. 17.6.

For preanesthetic use, the dosage of acetylpromazine maleate is 1 mg/20 lb of body weight intramuscularly (Rosin 1974). Also, atropine sulfate (0.02–0.03 mg/lb) is administered intramuscularly or subcutaneously. After the peak effect (usually

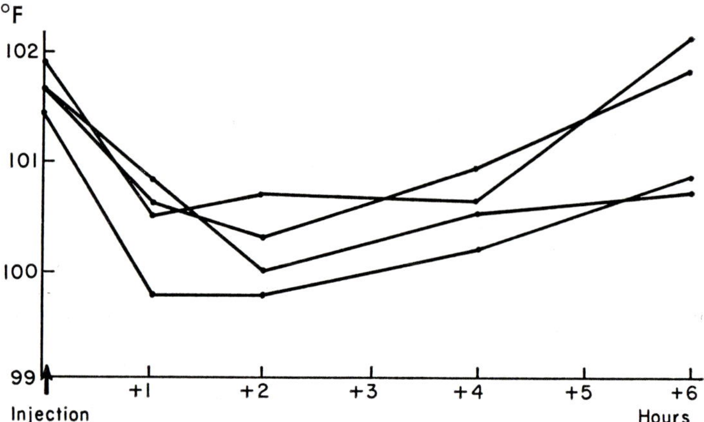

FIG. 17.6. Changes in rectal temperature of four dogs following intramuscular injection of acepromazine at a dose rate of 0.25 mg/kg. (From Pugh 1964)

15–20 minutes) of acetylpromazine has been attained, thiamylal sodium is then administered "to effect" to produce general anesthesia; this permits endotracheal intubation so inhalant anesthetics may be administered. The dosage of thiamylal sodium necessary to produce general anesthesia is reduced by about 50%. Like other phenothiazines (chlorpromazine, promazine), acetylpromazine produces a moderate degree of blockade of the α-adrenergic receptors. This effect is needed to prevent renal ischemia, to maintain an adequate kidney function during general anesthesia, and to minimize postsurgical uremia (Rosin 1974).

In the Cat. Acetylpromazine maleate may be administered intravenously, intramuscularly, subcutaneously, and orally in the cat. The recommended dosage for the parenteral and oral routes ranges from 0.5 to 1 mg/lb of body weight. It is usually necessary to repeat the dosage every 8–12 hours to maintain tranquilization. Many of the drug effects produced in the dog are also seen in the cat (refer to the discussion above).

Clinically, acetylpromazine is important as a preanesthetic agent in the cat. The dose successfully used in clinical practice is 1 mg/20 lb of body weight administered intramuscularly (Rosin 1974). Atropine sulfate (0.02–0.03 mg/lb) is also injected intramuscularly or subcutaneously. General anesthesia with an ultrashort-acting barbiturate or inhalant anesthetic may be administered 15–20 minutes after the peak effect of acetylpromazine has been reached. As in the dog, the amount of general anesthetic is reduced significantly.

Acetylpromazine maleate is used as a preanesthetic agent (1 mg/20 lb) prior to ketamine hydrochloride (10 mg/lb) anesthesia. Both acetylpromazine and ketamine are administered intramuscularly. Acetylpromazine in the dosage mentioned above will reduce the dose of ketamine by by about 50% (Rosin 1974).

In the Horse. Acetylpromazine must not used in horses intended for human consumption. Acetylpromazine maleate may be administered intravenously or intramuscularly. The recommended dose ranges from 2 to 4 mg/100 lb of body weight.

According to Fraser (1967), acetylpromazine administered intramuscularly at a dose level of 30 mg/1000 lb is effective in 2–3 minutes; its action persists for about 30 minutes. Clinical signs noted are drooping of the upper eyelid, slight protrusion of the nictitating membrane, and dropping of the head below its normal level. An overdose of the drug produces ataxia and may interfere with the clinical procedure.

Acetylpromazine reduces excitability so the animal can be easily handled. For example, rectal examinations and exploration of the genitalia are facilitated. However, tranquilization of dangerous animals may lead to a false sense of security; painful procedures should be avoided because the phenothiazines provide little, if any, analgesic effect.

Horses medicated with acetylpromazine retain auditory and visual acuity; loud sounds or rapid movements should be avoided.

Acetylpromazine maleate, even in high therapeutic doses, infrequently produces recumbency in the horse. Although horses may appear to be somnolent, they will usually remain standing. In the event the animal lies down, it can ordinarily be persuaded to stand. The risk of the animal stepping or falling on the attending veterinarian is minimal.

An important use of acetylpromazine is as a preanesthetic agent. Acetylpromazine maleate (a total dose of 15 mg) is administered intravenously and followed 10 minutes later with an intravenous injection of thiamylal sodium administered in a dose of 2.5–3 g/1000 lb of body weight (Shideler 1971). This permits endotracheal intubation so methoxyflurane can be administered for maintenance of surgical anesthesia.

Acetylpromazine maleate has been useful in the treatment of equine colic. A dose of 30 mg/1000 lb of body weight intravenously brings about prompt relief (Frank 1970). This effect is due to the antispasmodic activity of acetylpromazine. According to Frank, less severe cases of colic respond to an intramuscular dose of 1 mg/10 kg of body weight.

Acetylpromazine maleate in combination with meperidine hydrochloride, an analgesic and antispasmodic drug, is an effective neuroleptanalgesic agent in the horse (Jones 1972). Approximately a two-thirds dosage of each drug is recommended in the combination. Many equine colic cases should respond favorably to this mixture.

A combination of acetylpromazine and another analgesic agent (etorphine) has been advocated in the horse and other domestic animals in the United Kingdom. Acetylpromazine maleate in a concentration of 10 mg/ml is combined with 2.25 mg/ml of etorphine; this neuroleptanalgesic preparation, referred to as Immobilon, is sometimes used for minor surgery in the horse (Jenkin 1972).

Prochlorperazine Edisylate

Prochlorperazine Edisylate, U.S.P. (Darbazine, Compazine) is a piperazine derivative of phenothiazine (Fig. 17.7). Extrapyramidal symptoms, especially at high dose levels, are characteristic of the piperazines more than the nonpiperazine derivatives (e.g., chlorpromazine, promazine, acetylpromazine). The antemetic properties of the piperazine phenothiazine derivatives are greater than the nonpiperazine derivatives.

Pharmacologically, the sedative effect of prochlorperazine is moderate compared to the greater sedative effects of chlorpromazine and triflupromazine. Consequently, only a slight effect upon consciousness is elicited by prochlorperazine. The hypotensive and respiratory effects are low compared to promazine.

Prochlorperazine edisylate has been approved as an injectable preparation by the FDA for use in combination with isopropamide iodide. Isopropamide is a potent, long-acting anticholinergic drug that suppresses both gastrointestinal motility and secretions for about 12 hours after a single oral dose. This injectable combination has been approved for use in the dog and cat.

CLINICAL USE

In the dog (but not the cat) a sustained release capsule for oral use has been approved by the FDA. The capsule contains the combination of prochlorperazine dimaleate and isopropamide iodide to provide control of gastrointesti-

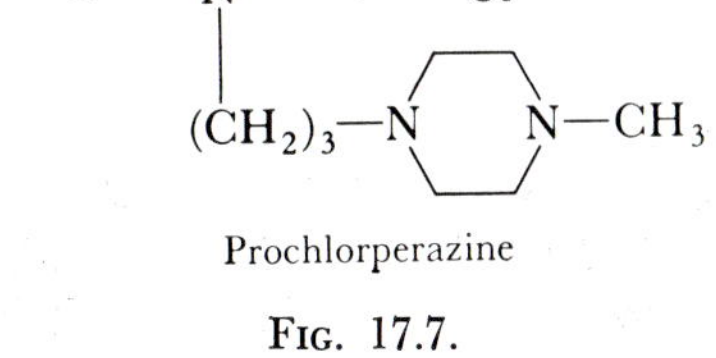

S
N
Cl
$(CH_2)_3$—N N—CH_3

Prochlorperazine

FIG. 17.7.

nal disturbances associated with emotional stress.

The injectable preparation contains 6 mg/ml of prochlorperazine edisylate or the equivalent of 4 mg of prochlorperazine and 0.38 mg/ml of isopropamide iodide or the equivalent of 0.28 mg of isopropamide. The drug combination in the dog and cat is based on subcutaneous injection twice daily at a dosage rate as follows (*Code of Federal Regulations,* 135b. 55, April 1, 1974):

Animal Weight (lb)	*Dosage (ml)*
Up to 4	0.25
5–14	0.5–1
15–30	2–3
30–45	3–4
45–60	4–5
Over 60	6

In the event medication needs to be continued in the dog, a change to the oral form or sustained release capsules can be made following the last injection. Two capsule sizes are available for dogs, the small size for animals weighing up to 30 lb and the large size capsule for dogs weighing 30 lb and over. The small capsules contain 3.33 mg of prochlorperazine dimaleate and 1.67 mg of isopropamide iodide; the dose is administered by the oral route twice daily as follows:

Animal Weight (lb)	*Number of Capsules (small size)*
Less than 4	Less than 1 or fraction thereof
4–15	1
15–30	1–2

The large capsules contain 10 mg of prochlorperazine dimaleate and 5 mg of isopropamide iodide; the dose is administered by the oral route twice daily as follows:

Animal Weight (lb)	*Number of Capsules (large size)*
30 lb and over	1

Perphenazine

Perphenazine, N.F. (Trilafon), solution (colorless) is sensitive to light and turns brown upon deterioration; it is soluble in water. Chemically it is 1-(2-hydroxyethyl)-4-[3-(2-chloro-10-phenothiazinyl) propyl] piperazine (Fig. 17.8).

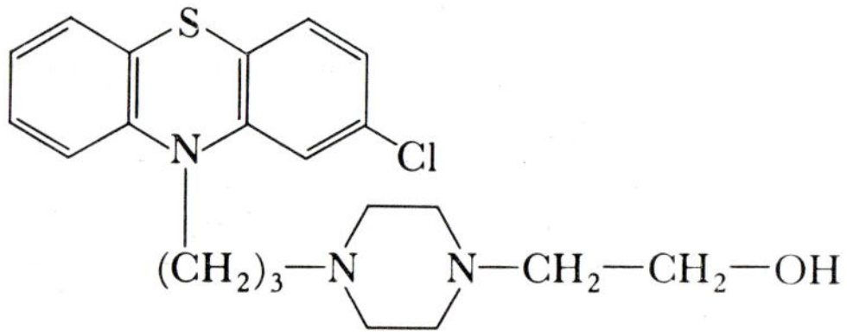

Perphenazine

Fig. 17.8.

Pharmacologically, perphenazine produces marked extrapyramidal and antemetic effects; its effect as a sedative is low compared to chlorpromazine and triflupromazine. Also, the degree of arterial hypotension produced by perphenazine is less than promazine. The majority of the effects are characteristic of all the piperazine phenothiazine derivatives.

Most phenothiazines, including perphenazine, increase plasma prolactin in the rat (Blackwell et al. 1973). The effect of perphenazine appears to be depletion of hypothalamic catecholamine stores and decreased synthesis of the prolactin-inhibiting factor. Perphenazine is capable of inhibiting the rat estrous cycle.

Clinical Use

Use of this tranquilizer in the horse is contraindicated because it produces excitatory reactions and it must not be used in animals intended for human consumption. Perphenazine has limited use in the dog and cat.

Perphenazine can be administered orally twice daily to the dog and cat in a dose of 0.4 mg/lb of body weight. Intravenously or intramuscularly, the dose for the dog and cat is 0.25 mg/lb. The peak effect occurs in about 5–15 minutes for the intravenous route and 15–30 minutes for the intramuscular route. Therapeutic levels of perphenazine have a duration of 6 hours or longer.

An overdose of perphenazine may produce prolonged depression or tonoclonic convulsions leading to death from respiratory paralysis. Autonomic side effects such as constipation and xerostomia may also occur. The drug is contraindicated via the subcutaneous route of administration. Other contraindications that have been described for the phenothiazines also generally apply to perphenazine.

Ethylisobutrazine Hydrochloride

Chemically, *Ethylisobutrazine* (Diquel) is 2-ethyl-10-(3-dimethylamino-2-methylpropyl) phenothiazine (Fig. 17.9).

Ethylisobutrazine hydrochloride has been approved for use in the dog by the FDA. The oral and intramuscular dose is 2–5 mg/lb; 1–2 mg/lb is the recommended intravenous dose. The neuroleptic agent is administered once daily by the oral route for maintenance of tranquilization.

In general, the contraindications for other phenothiazines also apply to ethylisobutrazine. Untoward effects have been observed frequently in the horse and other species. The drug must not be used in animals intended for human food.

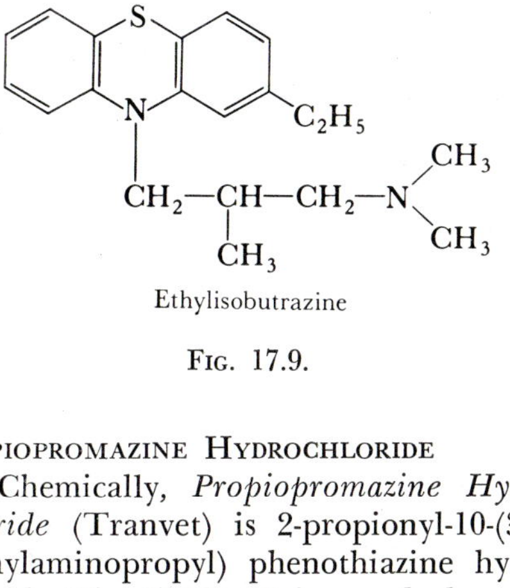

S, N, C_2H_5, CH_3, CH_2—CH—CH_2—N, CH_3, CH_3

Ethylisobutrazine

Fig. 17.9.

Propiopromazine Hydrochloride

Chemically, *Propiopromazine Hydrochloride* (Tranvet) is 2-propionyl-10-(3-dimethylaminopropyl) phenothiazine hydrochloride (Fig. 17.10). It is an odorless, yellow powder that is readily soluble in water.

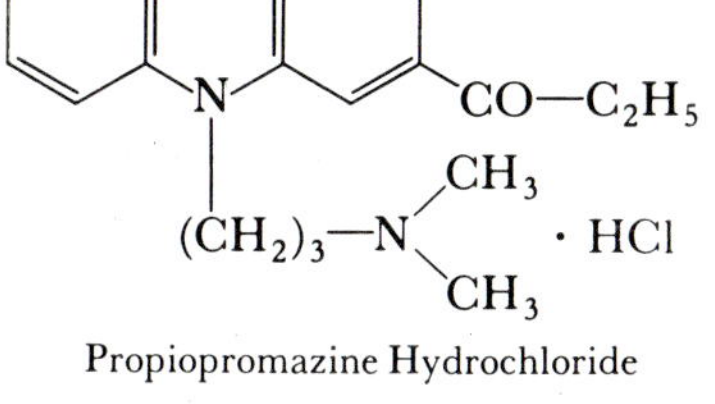

S, N, CO—C_2H_5, CH_3, $(CH_2)_3$—N, · HCl, CH_3

Propiopromazine Hydrochloride

Fig. 17.10.

When propiopromazine was first introduced for clinical use, it was used as a tranquilizer and restraint agent in the horse (Gillespie and Tyler 1963). However, in the stallion an irreversible paralysis of the penis occurs (Wheat 1966). Penile paralysis has been observed up to 18 months after the administration of propiopromazine and following castration the penis had failed to retract completely 2 years later.

Propiopromazine has been used also in other species. It is approved by the FDA for use only in nonfood-producing animals such as the dog and cat.

Clinical Use

In the Dog and Cat. Propiopromazine hydrochloride is available for use in the dog and cat parenterally and orally. For preanesthetic use, it is used intravenously in both at a dosage rate of 0.25 mg/lb. In tranquilization of the dog and cat, a dose level of 0.05–0.5 mg/lb is recommended either intravenously or intramuscularly.

For oral use, the drug is available in the form of chewable tablets containing 10 and 20 mg of propiopromazine hydrochloride. The oral dose is 0.5–2 mg/lb. The level of tranquilization required to produce the desired effects is dependent on the dosage level and frequency of its administration.

Propiopromazine has been recommended as an aid in handling and restraint of animals in need of "attitude adjustment." It is of value in controlling nervous animals prior to routine examinations, diagnostic procedures, and general anesthesia.

Triflupromazine Hydrochloride

Triflupromazine, N.F. (Vetame, Vesprin) (2-trifluoromethyl-10-[3-dimethylamino]propyl) phenothiazine, in the hydrochloride salt form is available for parenteral use in the dog, cat, and horse; tablets are available for oral use in the dog and cat.

The neuroleptic has been approved by the FDA for use only in the dog, cat,

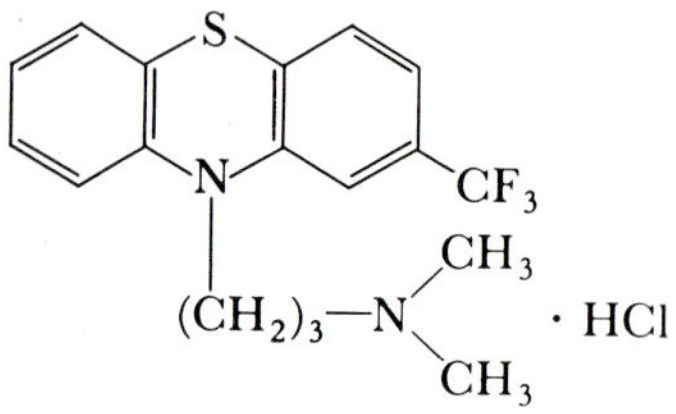

$$\text{(phenothiazine ring, 2-}CF_3\text{)}-N-(CH_2)_3-N(CH_3)_2 \cdot HCl$$

Triflupromazine Hydrochloride

FIG. 17.11.

and horse. Contraindications are similar to other phenothiazines.

CLINICAL USE

In the Dog, Cat, and Horse. Triflupromazine is recommended for the control of psychomotor overactivity, preanesthetic medication, and other clinical or diagnostic procedures requiring restraint of the dog, cat, and horse. The dose schedule and parenteral routes of administration are summarized as follows (the maximum daily dose in the horse should not exceed 100 mg/animal):

Animal	*Route of Administration*	*Daily Dose (mg/lb)*
Dog	Intravenous	0.5–1
	Intramuscular	1–2
Cat	Intramuscular	2–4
Horse	Intravenous or Intramuscular	0.1–0.15

The initial oral dose suggested for the dog and cat is 2 mg/lb followed by daily levels of 1 mg/lb. Generally, treatment is discontinued after 4–5 days; the drug effects are noted for several hours after withdrawal.

For radiographic examination of the gastrointestinal tract, the effect of triflupromazine hydrochloride upon the transit time of barium sulfate through the stomach and duodenum has been evaluated in the dog (Zontine 1973). Triflupromazine gave the most satisfactory clinical response when compared to pentobarbital sodium, halothane, methoxyflurane, fentanyl-droperidol, meperidine hydrochloride, promazine hydrochloride, and acetylpromazine maleate. Most of these were unsatisfactory because of prolonged depression of intestinal motility.

The triflupromazine hydrochloride intravenous dose is 0.5 mg/lb (Zontine 1973). The drug produces adequate restraint, is effective over 3 hours, and decreases peristalsis sufficiently for proper radiographic examination.

TRIMEPRAZINE TARTRATE

Trimeprazine, N.F. (Temaril) (dl-10-[3-dimethylamino-2-methylpropyl]-phenothiazine) (Fig. 17.12), in addition to having a tranquilizing effect, is antipruritic, antitussive, and antihistaminic.

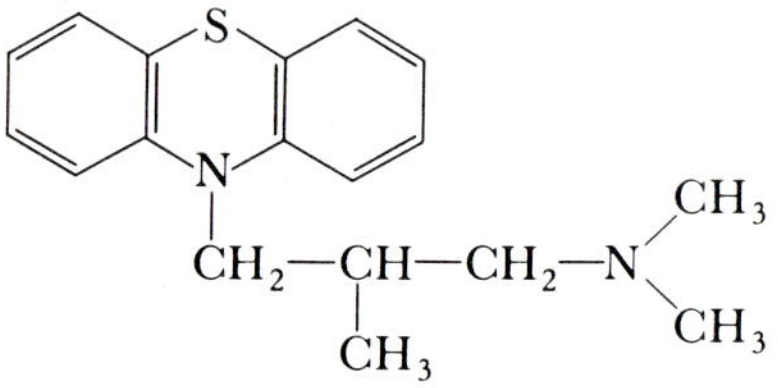

$$\text{(phenothiazine ring)}-N-CH_2-CH(CH_3)-CH_2-N(CH_3)_2$$

Trimeprazine

FIG. 17.12.

Trimeprazine tartrate (5 mg) is combined with prednisolone (2 mg) in tablet form for oral administration in the dog. The dog is the only species in which this combination product (Temaril-P) has been approved by the FDA. Twice-daily oral dosages for the dog are:

Weight of Animal (lb)	*Number of Tablets Administered Twice Daily*
Up to 10	0.5
11–20	1.0
21–40	2.0
Over 40	3.0

Following 4 days of treatment, the dose is decreased to about one-half the initial dose, which is sufficient to prevent the return of symptoms. Because of individual variation, dosages will need to be regulated in accordance with the clinical response desired.

Temaril-P is indicated for the alleviation of pruritis, irrespective of the etiology, and for reduction of inflammatory reactions associated with skin disorders such as eczema, otitis, and allergic dermatitis. The drug combination has been advocated as an adjunctive treatment in cough conditions such as "kennel cough" and various forms of bronchitis.

With incorporation of prednisolone into the tablet, the drug preparation must not be used in viral infections or ulceration of the cornea. Healing of the cornea will be delayed or inhibited. Moreover, prednisolone should not be used in the last trimester of pregnancy because it may induce premature parturition with accompaniment of dystocia, fetal death, retained placenta, and metritis. *(Note: Drug withdrawn from market July 19, 1976.)*

TRIFLUOMEPRAZINE MALEATE

Trifluomeprazine Maleate (Nortran) (10-[3-dimethylamino-2-methylpropyl]-2 trifluoromethyl phenothiazine) (Fig. 17.13) is approved by the FDA for oral use in the dog (Johnston and Cairy 1961). Trifluomeprazine is more than twice as potent as chlorpromazine.

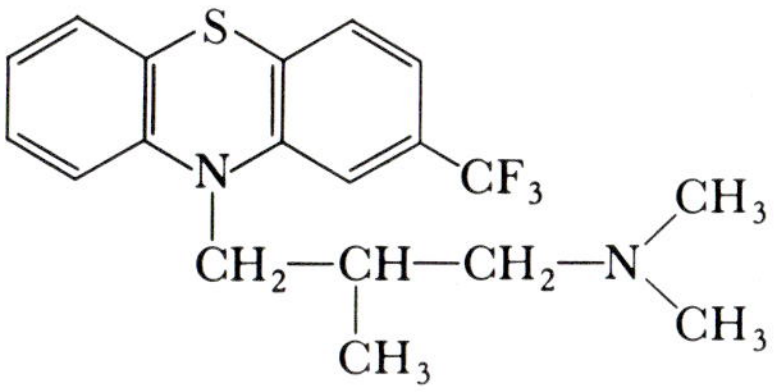

Trifluomeprazine

FIG. 17.13.

SIDE EFFECTS

Oral dosages of 9 mg/lb of body weight and higher produce untoward effects such as ataxia (Johnston and Cairy 1961). Also, vomiting, miosis, relaxation of the nictitating membrane, and lacrimation may be observed following oral administration of therapeutic levels of the drug. Posterior paresis is produced, lasting about 45 minutes following large parenteral doses. The animals appear alert and frightened and become more irritable. Ataxia is prominent prior to and following the temporary paresis. All dogs affected in this manner recover uneventfully.

CLINICAL USE

Trifluomeprazine maleate is available in 10-mg tablets for oral administration in the dog. For tranquilization and "chemical restraint" purposes, a dose level of 0.25–1 mg/lb is recommended once or twice daily. Contraindications for use of the drug are similar to chlorpromazine and other phenothiazines.

MEPAZINE HYDROCHLORIDE

Chemically, *Mepazine,* N.N.D. (Paxital), is 10-[(1-methyl-3-piperidyl)methyl] phenothiazine (Fig. 17.14). Mepazine hydrochloride is photosensitive and should be protected from light to prevent deterioration of the compound. The drug is slightly soluble in water and has a bitter taste.

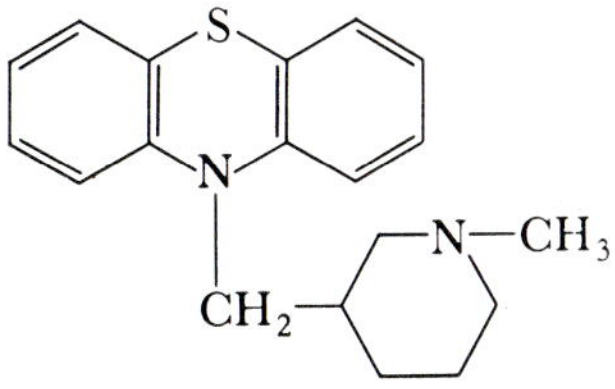

Mepazine

FIG. 17.14.

The tranquilizer is approved by the FDA for oral use in the dog. It is approximately one-half as potent as chlorpromazine. Mepazine produces an increase in the arterial pressure of animals, whereas the other phenothiazine derivatives produce some degree of hypotension.

The duration of action is approximately 8–12 hours. Orally the dose for the dog is 1.5–2.5 mg/lb 2–3 times daily. The recommended intramuscular or intravenous dose for preanesthetic sedation is 1 mg/lb.

PIPERACETAZINE HYDROCHLORIDE

Chemically, *Piperacetazine* (Psymod, Quide) is 2-acetyl-10-(3[4-(beta-hydroxyethyl)-piperidino] propyl) phenothiazine (Fig. 17.15). Piperacetazine possesses pharmacologic properties similar to chlorpromazine. The antihistaminic activity of piperacetazine is moderately effective in the guinea pig (Weaver et al. 1963). However, it fails to alter the convulsant properties of pentylenetetrazol (metrazol) in mice.

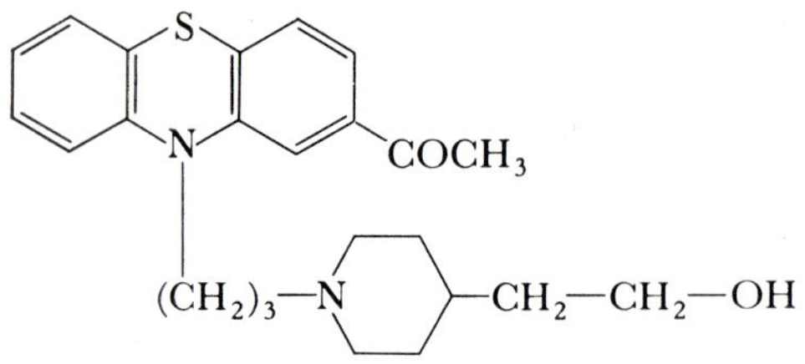

Piperacetazine

FIG. 17.15.

TOXICITY

Chronic toxicity studies were conducted in the dog at dose levels of piperacetazine of 0.25, 1, and 5 mg/kg/day for about 1 year (Weaver et al. 1963). All animals gained weight; the effect upon weight appeared to be unrelated to the dose level of the drug. Animals that received 0.25 mg/kg/day were quiet and appeared to be depressed longer during the early phase. In dogs that had received 1 mg/kg/day, scleral congestion, slight ataxia, and drowsiness were observed. At the 5 mg/kg/day, all animals showed varying degrees of depressed activity and lacrimation. Also, ataxia and considerable drowsiness occurred. Some of the animals were mated and all pups appeared to be normal. At all dosages, histopathologic and clinical laboratory evaluations did not reveal any abnormal effects (Weaver et al. 1963).

CLINICAL USE

Piperacetazine is approved by the FDA for use in the dog and cat as a tranquilizer, sedative, and antemetic agent. In addition, it is approved for the symptomatic relief of pruritis. Parenteral and oral forms of the drug are available.

The parenteral administration of piperacetazine in the dog and cat is recommended with a dose range from 0.5 to 2 mg/10 lb (0.05 to 0.2 mg/lb) of body weight. The dose level used is dependent on the response desired. After a response is observed from the initial administration of the drug, subsequent dosages may be decreased or increased as required. Parenteral therapy may be followed and maintained by oral administration for tranquilization and/or sedation as follows:

Indicated Use Orally	*Dosage (mg/lb)*	*Frequency of Administration*
Tranquilization	0.05	Repeat in 6–12 hr
Sedation	0.1–0.2	Repeat in 8–12 hr

Frequency of administration of piperacetazine to maintain tranquilization or sedation may be adjusted to obtain the optimum clinical effect.

THIOXANTHENE DERIVATIVE

CHLORPROTHIXENE

Chlorprothixene, N.F. (Taractan), is not approved by the FDA for use in animals in the United States; it is used in the United Kingdom. Chlorprothixene is related chemically to the phenothiazine tranquilizers. Chemically, chlorprothixene is α-2-chloro-9-ω-dimethylamino-propulidene)-thioxanthene (Fig. 17.16). It is a yellow crystalline substance possessing a slightly fishy odor. The salts of chlorprothixene are freely soluble in water.

Chlorprothixene has a greater depressant and anticholinergic activity than chlorpromazine. It also possesses antemetic and antihistaminic activity.

CLINICAL USE

In the Dog. Clinically, chlorprothixene has been used in the dog (Sumner-Smith 1962). The intravenous or intramuscular dose for the dog is 1–2 mg/lb; intractable animals are rendered manageable. The tranquilizing agent can be used prior to barbiturate anesthesia, facilitating preoperative preparation and induction of anesthesia.

In Small Ruminants. Chlorprothixene is recommended in sheep and goats for seda-

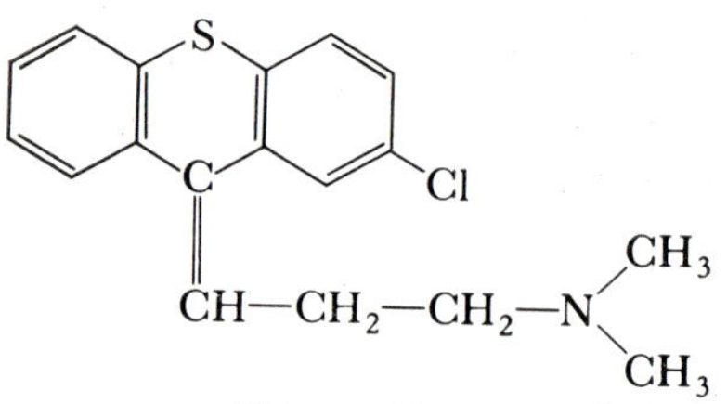

Chlorprothixene

FIG. 17.16.

tive use (Jones 1972). A dose of 0.5 mg/kg by the intravenous route permits surgical procedures in conjunction with local or regional anesthesia.

In Swine. A dose level of 0.3–1 mg/kg is recommended intravenously in swine ranging in weight from 10 to 325 kg for cesarean section, amputation of digits, foot examination, surgery of the prolapsed rectum, and incision of abscesses. Chlorprothixene decreases the body temperature of the pig 1°–2° F (Jones 1972).

Jones reported the following effects of chlorprothixene: within 5 minutes the pig was lying down and appeared somnolent; or, less commonly observed, the pig showed excitement within a few minutes after the injection. The excitement was of short duration; then the animal lay down quietly in lateral recumbency.

Chlorprothixene is considered an ideal drug for cesarean section as the sedation allows the operation in conjunction with local infiltration anesthesia (Jones 1972). The action of the drug in sows that do not accept their offspring has been spectacular. Within 10 minutes following an injection, the piglets can be reintroduced and are able to play and crawl near the mouth of the sow without hazard; the optimum dose for the adult pig is 0.4–0.5 mg/kg (Jones 1972).

BUTYROPHENONE DERIVATIVES

The butyrophenone derivatives of major importance in clinical veterinary medical usage are droperidol (Inapsine, dehydrobenzperidol) and azaperone (Stresnil, Suicalm). Another butyrophenone derivative, haloperidol, has only limited use in veterinary medicine.

Mechanism of Action

The butyrophenones and piperazine-substituted phenothiazines (perphenazine, prochlorperazine) have a number of related neuroleptic properties in animals: motor activity is reduced; cataleptic effects may be produced; mortality from stress or trauma is decreased; apomorphine emesis is blocked; and the fatal effects of catecholamines are prevented.

The central actions of dopamine and norepinephrine as well as other catecholamines are blocked by the butyrophenones. Penetration of catecholamine neurotransmitters through the membranes of neuronal cells is blocked so that activation of cell receptors cannot take place. In the extrapyramidal system, the butyrophenones may act by mimicking the action of gamma-aminobutyric acid or by preventing the effect of glutamic acid on synaptic junctions (Selye and Szabo 1972).

Droperidol

The chemical structure of *droperidol* (Inapsine, dehydrobenzperidol) (Fig. 17.17) has been described by Yelonsky and Field (1964).

Pharmacological Considerations

Droperidol is 400 times more active in dogs than chlorpromazine or chlorprothixene and 10 times more active than haloperidol (Marsboom and Mortelmans 1964). Droperidol has the shortest action of the butyrophenones. It is the most potent antemetic known, being up to 1000 times more active than chlorpromazine and chlorprothixene.

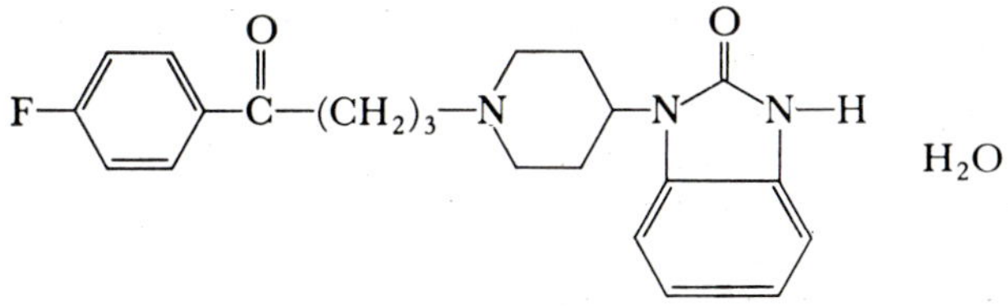

F—C—$(CH_2)_3$—N—N N—H H_2O

Droperidol

Fig. 17.17.

As cataleptic immobility-producing drugs and inhibitors of spontaneous and conditioned learning behavior in rats, the butyrophenones are several times more effective than chlorpromazine and chlorprothixene (Marsboom and Mortelmans 1964). Also, they are several times more effective as protagonists of amphetamine and apomorphine actions in the rat than chlorpromazine or chlorprothixene. Quite unlike the butyrophenones, the phenothiazines are potent hypotensive and hypothermic agents as well as antagonists of epinephrine. Also, the phenothiazines induce ataxia at much lower dosages and are quantitatively more toxic in action than the butyrophenones. The wide safety margin of droperidol is related to its brief duration of action. Droperidol as well as chlorprothixene may be classified among the most potent antitraumatic shock agents known (Marsboom and Mortelmans 1964). There seems to be an interrelationship between the antitraumatic shock activity and the ability of these agents to inhibit arterial vasoconstriction.

In the dog, droperidol has a wide safety margin; tremors, muscle spasticity, and hyperirritability occur only after intravenous administration and at high dosages, i.e., 11–22 mg/kg of body weight (Soma and Shields 1964). At an intravenous dose rate of 0.5 mg/kg, droperidol has little or no effect on cardiac output but decreases arterial pressure, total peripheral resistance, and heart rate (Yelonsky et al. 1964). Yelonsky et al. observed that adrenergic blockade was one of the principal pharmacologic actions of droperidol (0.125 mg/kg, intravenously) in the dog. The slight hypotensive effect at this dosage was believed to have been the result of peripheral vasodilation at least due in part to adrenergic blockade. Droperidol (4 mg/kg, intravenously) caused slowing of the respiration and heart rate, hypotension, and a drop in cardiac output, as well as a decrease in the force of myocardial contraction (Yelonsky et al. 1964). In the United States droperidol is unavailable for veterinary use as a single agent. It is available only in combination with fentanyl citrate (see Chapter 15).

Azaperone

Azaperone (Stresnil, Suicalm) is a neuroleptic agent belonging to the butyrophenone derivatives. It has not been approved for use in the United States but is being used increasingly in Belgium and the United Kingdom. Azaperone is chemically 4′-fluor-4-[4-(2-pyridyl)-1-piperazinyl]-butyrophenone (Fig. 17.18).

Pharmacologic considerations

Azaperone is a relatively nontoxic, short-acting drug that is rapidly detoxified and eliminated. The drug is active 2–3 hours and is nearly eliminated from body tissues within 16 hours (Callear and Van Gestel 1973). Its effect appears to be specific for use in ungulates.

Studies have been conducted upon the hemodynamic and pulmonary effects of azaperone following intramuscular and intravenous administration in swine (Clarke 1969). Intramuscular doses of 0.54–3.5 mg/kg reduced the arterial pressure to between 70% and 84% of control values and reflexly stimulated respiration. The severity of the drop in blood pressure appears to be related to the dosage level and usually occurs within 5–10 minutes after administration. The skin of the pig becomes pink, ostensibly due to cutaneous vasodilation (Clarke 1969).

Administration of 0.03 mg/kg of azaperone by the intravenous route results in a greater drop in the arterial pressure (42% of the control value). In addition, initial violent excitement occurs with good sedation following later. The respiration rate becomes elevated during the period of sedation, and a fall in the Pa_{CO_2} is observed (Clarke 1969). Other cardiovascular effects of azaperone include reduction in heart rate and cardiac output.

Inasmuch as azaperone has a number

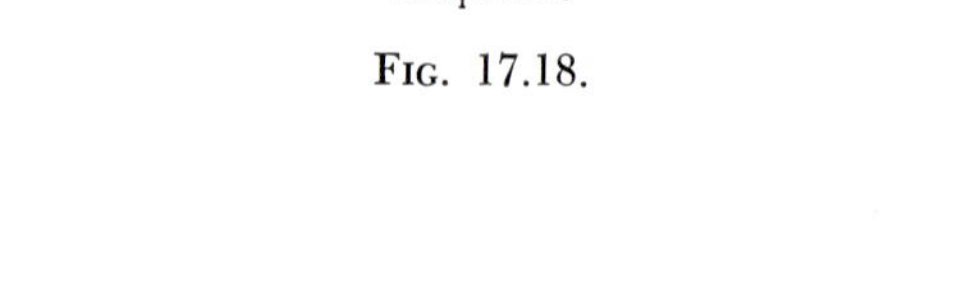

F—C₆H₄—C(=O)—$(CH_2)_3$—N(piperazine)N—(2-pyridyl)

Azaperone

Fig. 17.18.

of other pharmacologic properties similar to droperidol, the reader is referred to the mechanism of action and pharmacologic effects of this butyrophenone derivative.

CLINICAL USE

In the Pig. Azaperone is used in swine to prevent "population stress" and the aggressiveness and fighting that occur upon mixing litters (Symoens and Van Den Brande 1969). It is indicated in the reduction of excitement during parturition and in prevention of sows from overt mistreatment and abuse of their young. In Pietrain pigs azaperone is used for the prevention of excitement and for the reduction of mortality from the "overloading of the heart" syndrome common to this breed. Also, it is used prior to minor and major surgical procedures conducted under local, regional, and general anesthesia (Jones 1972).

The efficacy of azaperone against aggressiveness in the pig was evaluated in animals brought together in small unfamiliar groups (Symoens and Van Den Brande 1969). After an intramuscular dose of less than 1.5 mg/kg, the piglets and adult pigs would lie down in 3 and 10 minutes, respectively, for 30–60 minutes. Despite the influence of the azaperone, violent fighting followed whenever they were startled by the closing of a door or a disturbance in an adjacent pen. A few animals treated at dosages lower than 1.5 mg/kg died following episodes of fighting (Symoens and Van Den Brande 1969). When dosages of 1.5–3 mg/kg were administered intramuscularly, sedation was observed within 5–15 minutes. This effect lasted about 2 hours after which the pigs moved about without difficulty and without manifesting aggressiveness. Although occasional fighting occurred to establish a "pecking order," it usually was of short duration and intensity. None of the animals treated at these dosages died (Symoens and Van Den Brande 1969). The untreated or control animals fought more than twice as frequently and four times as long.

The remarkable action of azaperone in inhibiting aggressiveness in the pig not only occurs during sedation but appears to be somewhat permanent. Perhaps by the time the sedative effects have waned or disappeared, the animals have adapted to each other by the exchange of sensory information (smell) and acceptance of one another occurs (Symoens and Van Den Brande 1969).

In a field study involving a large number of pigs, azaperone was classified into three types of effect following intramuscular administration (Callear and Van Gestel 1973):

(1) *Low Dosages* (0.4–1.2 mg/kg) for "stress" conditions such as anxiety and nervousness. This dose range permitted the animals to remain ambulatory and calm.

(2) *Median dosages* primarily for the "socializing" effect at a level of 2 mg/kg. The animals eventually lay down and appeared somnolent but moved around if disturbed.

(3) *High dosages* of 4 mg/kg in adult pigs and 8 mg/kg in piglets for their "knock-down" effect for minor surgical procedures. The animals were recumbent and unable to stand.

To avoid untoward effects, it is recommended that 2 mg/kg not be exceeded in large boars (Callear and Van Gestel 1973).

Recommendations of the manufacturers for azaperone in the pig intramuscularly are 1 mg/kg for the production of sedation, 2.5 mg/kg for reduction of aggressiveness, and 5–10 mg/kg for a "knock-down" or immobilization effect (Cox 1973). Azaperone must be administered by the intramuscular route or it will be ineffective. A disadvantage in the use of azaperone for immobilization of adult swine is the large volume that must be administered.

Azaperone and a hypnotic drug, metomidate (Hypnodil), are used in combination to produce a condition resembling neuroleptanalgesia in the pig. Azaperone is given intramuscularly at a dose level of 2 mg/kg and is immediately followed by metomidate intraperitoneally at 10 mg/kg of body weight (Cox 1973). As an alternative method, azaperone (2.5 mg/kg) is given intramuscularly, and 20–30 minutes later the metomidate (2.5 mg/kg) is administered intravenously (Jones 1972). This dosage combination produces deep sedation for over 1 hour and is satisfactory for surgical procedures such as amputation of a digit or cesarean section in conjunction with regional or local anesthesia. If it is necessary to extend or increase the period of sedation, another dose of metomidate (1 mg/kg) may be administered intravenously. When general anesthesia is required, and to enable endotracheal intubation, 5 mg/kg of metomidate are recommended following the administration of azaperone (Jones 1972).

In the Horse. Limited studies with azaperone-metomidate have been conducted in the horse (Hillidge et al. 1973). Hemolysis was observed in samples of venous plasma collected between 5 minutes and 6 hours following the administration of metomidate. Until more information is gained about the hemolytic effect, this drug combination should not be used in the horse (Archer 1973).

RAUWOLFIA DERIVATIVES

The rauwolfia derivatives of primary importance in veterinary medicine are reserpine and metoserpate hydrochloride. Reserpine is approved by the FDA for use in the dog and in turkey poults; metoserpate is approved for use in chickens. A tolerance of zero has been established by the FDA for residues of reserpine in edible tissues and eggs of turkeys. The negligible residue tolerance level for metoserpate hydrochloride in tissues of chickens has been established by the FDA at 0.02 ppm.

Reserpine

Reserpine is the primary alkaloid of the derivatives having therapeutic importance (Fig. 17.19). The alkaloid is obtained from shrubs, *Rauwolfia serpentina* and *R. vomitoria,* that grow in India and Africa, respectively. For centuries the medicine men of India used the ground root or tea of rauwolfia for conditions such as snake bite, insanity, and cholera. In human beings rauwolfia is used primarily as an antihypertensive agent.

Administration

The onset of action of reserpine is delayed regardless of the route of administration. Even following an intravenous injection, tranquilizing effects are not attained for approximately 30 minutes. Its peak effect is reached in about 2 hours and is sustained for nearly 6 hours, followed by an eventual return to normal over 24 hours or longer. Following an intramuscular injection, the onset of action and duration of effect are similar to an intravenous injection. Oral administration results in a much slower onset of action.

Effect upon Animal Behavior

After the parenteral administration of reserpine in the dog, the first effects noted are hyperpnea and slight tremors, occasionally accompanied by some excitement with eventual tranquilization (Earl 1956). At higher levels, the animal appears torpid or stuporous, yet it can be aroused. Monkeys can be placed unrestrained in unusual positions and will remain in position unless disturbed.

Depletion of brain catecholamines by

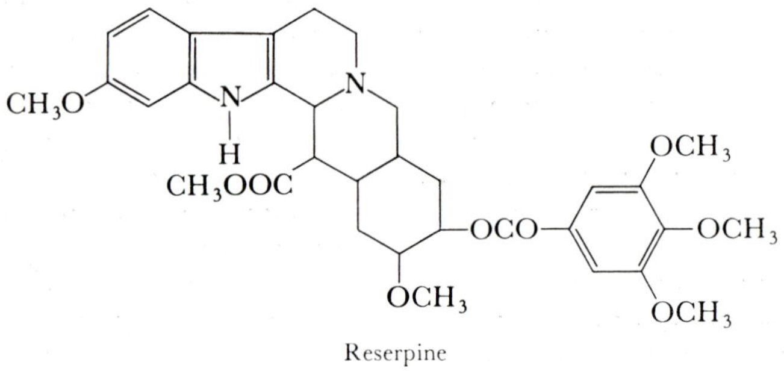

Reserpine

Fig. 17.19.

reserpine plays an important role in the behavioral changes manifested in animals. Depending on the dosage of reserpine, animals may be sedated or they may manifest hyperactive behavior concomitant with increased tyrosine hydroxylase activity in the midbrain and in the caudate (Segal et al. 1971).

The manic behavior manifested by the cat following morphine overdosage can be prevented by pretreatment of the animals with reserpine (Dhasmana et al. 1972). An intraperitoneal injection of morphine hydrochloride at a dose level of 20 mg/kg will produce a manic response in 100% of the cats. Treatment with reserpine (2.5 mg/kg) intraperitoneally 24 hours prior to morphine effectively prevents this response.

EFFECT UPON THE NERVOUS SYSTEM

Reserpine induces a state of rigidity and akinesia; these actions contribute to what is referred to as reserpine-induced catalepsy (Hornykiewicz 1966). Tremor is a common effect. Under the influence of reserpine, animals manifest reduced activity and response to environmental stress. This is noted in highly nervous animals. With an average daily dose of reserpine (18–39 μg/kg) for up to 1 year in the dog, CNS depression, muscle tremors, and a pronounced Parkinsonianlike syndrome occur; these central effects, in contrast to alterations in peripheral autonomic activity, appear to increase in intensity as the duration of reserpine treatment increases (Adams et al. 1971). The frequency response to sympathetic nerve stimulation decreases following chronic low-dosage reserpine treatment in the dog; this neuronal depression, however, can be reversed by the administration of norepinephrine (Clarke et al. 1970).

Reserpine depletes or releases serotonin (5-hydroxytryptamine), dopamine, and norepinephrine from depots in the brain and other parts of the body. The reserpine-induced deficiency of dopamine in the brain occurs in the striatum, substantia nigra, and pallidum (Hornykiewicz 1966). Restoration of serotonin to normal levels is prolonged. After a single dose to a rabbit, the brain serotonin is depressed to 10% of normal within 4 hours and remains at this level for 36 hours, after which it increases gradually over a period of 7 days before premedication values are regained (Pletscher et al. 1956).

EFFECT UPON THE BODY TEMPERATURE

Reserpine produces a hypothermic effect that can be prevented by elevating the environmental temperature. Apparently, this thermoregulatory effect is related to a serotonin depletion of the hypothalamic region. The hypothalamus contains one of the highest concentrations of serotonin found in the nervous system (Himwich 1958).

EFFECT UPON THE EYE

Reserpine produces a marked miosis in the cat and dog and, to a lesser extent, in the monkey. Relaxation of the nictitating membrane is seen in the dog and cat.

EFFECT UPON THE CARDIOVASCULAR AND RESPIRATORY SYSTEMS

Reserpine produces bradycardia in the dog. A hypotensive effect may be produced as a result of vasodilation. Reserpine decreases the respiratory rate of the cat, dog, rabbit, and monkey.

Clinical trials in human beings have suggested that antihypertensive therapeutic levels of reserpine can adversely affect myocardial function and evoke signs of right-congestive heart failure. A number of studies in animals also have indicated that reserpine adversely affects cardiac function. In the dog fatalities following reserpine (0.1 mg/kg) were believed due to cardiac failure because cardiac hypertrophy, ascites, and pulmonary edema were present upon postmortem examination. Circulatory failure has also been observed in the cat within 24 hours following 1 mg/kg of reserpine. Too, the short-term treatment of dogs with 25 μg/kg of reserpine intramuscularly for only 4 days can alter the ultrastructure of the myocardium (Wilcken et al. 1967). Mitochondrial abnormalities occurred at the 5th and 14th days, but all changes were reversible.

Adams et al. (1971) found a possible adverse myocardial effect in dogs subjected to an oral dose of reserpine between 18 and 39 μg/kg for periods up to 1 year. Right ventricular dilation was observed in 55% of the dogs. In addition, the hematocrit, hemoglobin content, and total leukocyte count decreased.

Anesthesiologists recommend that treatment with reserpine and other rauwolfia derivatives be discontinued at least 2 weeks before elective surgery. Human patients who have been on long-term therapy with the reserpine preparations often develop severe bradycardia and arterial hypotension when general anesthetics are administered. Animals similarly pretreated with reserpine are more sensitive to the hypotensive effects of thiopental sodium. Other anesthetics induce this effect in animals that have been treated with reserpine. Discontinuance of reserpine 2 weeks before elective surgery should be observed in animals.

Reserpine is used as an antihypertensive agent in turkeys over 4 weeks of age to lessen the risk of aortic rupture. Arterial blood pressure increases at a rapid rate with age and growth in the turkey and aortic aneurysm and rupture of the aorta can occur during rapid growth. Arterial pressures are highest in male birds with systolic and diastolic values as high as 270 and 167 mm Hg, respectively (Ferguson et al. 1969).

When reserpine is incorporated in the feed of turkeys at levels between 0.1 and 0.3 ppm, the arterial pressure is reduced (Speckman and Ringer 1961). At levels above 0.3 ppm (i.e., 1 and 4 ppm), the arterial pressure is reduced but signs of toxicity are noted as evidenced by a reduction in weight gain. Feeding reserpine at 0.25 ppm prevents aortic rupture in the rapidly growing turkey.

EFFECT UPON THE GASTROINTESTINAL TRACT

In the dog and cat, superpurgation, dehydration, and death may occur in 2–5 days following large doses (in excess of 0.227 mg/lb of body weight) of reserpine. Atropine sulfate decreases the activity of reserpine upon the gastrointestinal tract.

Gastric ulcers have been experimentally induced in the dog, cat, and pig following reserpine. In the dog and cat, gastric ulcers and erosions occur in about 6.5 and 5 days, respectively, following daily administration. Apparently, reserpine is just as potent as histamine in the production of experimental peptic ulceration (Nicoloff et al. 1961).

Reserpine at a level of 55 μg/kg/day is the lowest intramuscular dose that consistently produces ulcers in the pig after 5–15 days of treatment (Muggenberg et al. 1966). The incidence of ulcers produced experimentally was over 81%. The pig is quite sensitive to reserpine; most swine die within 15 days after intramuscular doses of 0.22 mg/kg/day.

EFFECT UPON ENDOCRINE AND REPRODUCTIVE ACTIVITY

In the rat, reserpine inhibits estrus and fertility but not lactation; large doses on the 9th or 10th day of gestation are teratogenic (Goldman and Yakovac 1965). Disturbance in catecholamine metabolism by reserpine may be an important factor in teratogenicity.

Reserpine given to 1-month-old male chickens for 3 months produces hypoplasia of the seminiferous tubules and atrophy of the testes (Hagen and Wallace 1961). In adult roosters 2 large doses of reserpine given 1 month apart also caused atrophy of the testes. No adverse effects were apparent on semen volume, fertility, hatchability of fertile eggs, body weight, and feed consumption in adult roosters fed 1 and 7 ppm of reserpine (Arscott and Parker 1967). However, in turkeys, adverse effects have been reported on egg production, fertility, and hatchability when 2 ppm of reserpine were fed continuously. In the duck, egg production is partially suppressed with 0.5 ppm of reserpine and completely suppressed at dosages of 2.5 and 10 ppm (Greene et al. 1961).

CLINICAL USE

Reserpine is not used extensively in the practice of veterinary medicine. *The phenothiazine derivatives are preferred because their onset of action is more rapid and recovery is quicker.*

In Dogs and Cats. With a daily oral dose of 4.5–9 μg/lb, satisfactory effects are usually not obtainable until 48 hours. Some animals may require total daily doses of 13.5–16 μg/lb of body weight. Initially, 2–3 divided doses are recommended; however, maintenance levels may consist of a single daily dose. Oral doses up to 16 μg/lb have been well tolerated. Dogs may be maintained chronically on a daily oral dose up to 45 μg/lb of body weight. However, it is generally not recommended to exceed a total maintenance dose level of 0.25 mg/day in the average-size dog (i.e., 25–30 lb). Cats tolerate slightly higher doses than dogs with less gastrointestinal disturbance (Earl 1956).

In Turkeys. Reserpine (3,4,5-trimethoxybenzoyl methyl reserpate) at 0.00002% (0.2 ppm) to 0.0001% (1 ppm) levels in the feed is approved for use in turkeys over 4 weeks of age to aid in the prevention of aortic rupture. For the 0.2 ppm level, 182 mg/ton of feed are required to reach a concentration of 0.00002%. This level is fed through 8 or more weeks of age to prevent rupture of the aorta. At the 1 ppm level in feed, 908 mg/ton of feed are required to attain a concentration of 0.0001%. This level must not be fed beyond 5 days for the purpose of reducing the incidence of aortic rupture in the flock.

In conjunction with the above approved uses of reserpine, it is approved for use in the feed at 0.2 ppm combined with penicillin (4–50 g/ton), penicillin plus bacitracin (6–50 g/ton), and bacitracin (4–50 g/ton) for growth promotion and feed efficiency.

In Exotic Species. It is reported that chinchillas are highly sensitive to reserpine and that daily doses as low as 1–2 μg produce tranquilization, ptosis, and general lethargy (Earl 1956). Tranquilization of the monkey has been maintained with daily dose levels of 3 mg/kg orally for long periods of time (Strobel and Wollman 1969). Reserpine has been used to facilitate the transportation of wild turkeys from hatcheries to their releasing grounds. An intramuscular injection of 2 μg/10 g of body weight permitted delivery of the birds where the mortality rate previously was 30%–40% (Earl 1956).

Side Effects and Toxicity. The horse is sensitive to reserpine. Total parenteral doses of 5 mg have produced violent colic in some animals. However, a total daily oral dose of 4 mg produces a tranquilizing action in the Thoroughbred horse without evidence of colic but with increased frequency in defecation (Earl 1956).

Reserpine has a potent effect in cattle. A total intravenous dose of 50 mg was considered to be responsible for the death of a 3-year-old purebred Holstein-Friesian bull weighing approximately 2000 lb (Gassner cited by Earl 1956). An intravenous dose of 7–7.5 mg/1000 lb will produce a satisfactory response in cattle.

Metoserpate Hydrochloride

Metoserpate Hydrochloride (methyl-*o*-methyl-18-epireserpate hydrochloride) is approved by the FDA for use only in the chicken. It is used as a tranquilizer for flock treatment of birds prior to handling at a dose level of 568.5 mg/gal of drinking water or at a concentration of 0.015% (150 ppm). The drug is used as a one-time treatment for replacement chickens in the flock up to 16 weeks of age. Water should be withheld for a sufficient time prior to treatment to assure that an adequate level of medicated drinking water is consumed. Metoserpate must not be used in egg-laying chickens. There is a 72-hour withdrawal time for human consumption.

Metoserpate hydrochloride is approved by the FDA for use in the treatment of chickens up to 16 weeks of age as an aid in the control of hysteria. Water should be withheld for a sufficient time before treatment to assure that an adequate level of medicated drinking water is consumed. The drug should be administered at a dose level of 4 mg/kg on the first day (equivalent to about 27 cc of 0.015%

metoserpate hydrochloride for each kg of body weight). This is followed by two treatments at 4-day intervals at one-half the above dosage (i.e., 2 mg/kg). The same restricted uses apply in laying chickens or slaughter chickens.

PSYCHOTROPIC AGENTS OF LESSER IMPORTANCE IN VETERINARY MEDICINE

The propanediol derivatives and benzodiazepine derivatives are occasionally used in clinical veterinary practice. These have been used to calm nervous and hysterical dogs and cats frightened by thunderstorms and to alleviate anxiety in female mink that refuse to mate. None has been approved by the FDA for use in animals. Moreover, these drugs must not be used in animals intended for human consumption.

Meprobamate, a propanediol derivative, is classified as a Schedule IV drug by the Controlled Substances Act of 1970. Diazepam (Valium) and chlordiazepoxide (Librium), both benzodiazepine derivatives, have been undergoing review to determine if they are to be controlled substances. If they are ruled controlled substances, they will be placed in Schedule IV.

PROPANEDIOL DERIVATIVES

Of the propanediol derivatives, meprobamate has been used most frequently in human medical practice. In veterinary medicine, meprobamate has not been used as extensively because its use in animals has not been entirely satisfactory (Wright and Hall 1961).

Meprobamate

Chemically, *Meprobamate* (Equanil) is 2-methyl-2-propyl-1,3-propanediol dicarbamate. It is a white crystalline powder and has a bitter taste. Meprobamate is soluble in water to the extent of only 0.79% at 37° C. The drug is stable in dilute alkali and acid solutions and does not decompose in gastric or intestinal juices.

Administration, Duration of Action, and Absorption

Meprobamate can be administered only by the oral route; meprobamate is absorbed from the gastrointestinal tract and does not provoke nausea or emesis (Berger 1954). Parenteral preparations are unavailable because of solubility difficulties in aqueous solutions. The duration of action is 5–6 hours, about 8 times longer than mephenesin.

Effects on Skeletal Muscle and the Nervous System

Pharmacologically, meprobate is similar in action to that of mephenesin. It produces a reversible paralysis of voluntary musculature without significantly altering autonomic functions. Like mephenesin, meprobamate decreases or may completely prevent transmission of nerve impulses at internuncial junctions of the spinal cord. It counteracts the action of strychnine. Meprobamate also resembles mephenesin in having little direct action on skeletal muscle, in not altering transmission at the motor end-plate, and in not interfering with conduction in the peripheral nervous system (Berger 1954).

Effect in the Monkey

Within 30 minutes after an oral dose of meprobamate (90 mg/lb), the monkey becomes more tractable. It does not object to being handled and shows no sign of fear. When offered food, the monkey readily eats. Approximately an hour after this dose level has been given, the animal suffers some loss of coordination and gradually becomes paralyzed. It rests calmly on its side and is unable to ambulate. There is an absence of excitation or restlessness. This effect lasts 5–6 hours. Recovery occurs completely and uneventfully. When doses of 182–272 mg/lb of body weight are used, complete flaccid paralysis lasts 7 or more hours. The respiratory and cardiac rates remain normal even with these large doses. Complete recovery occurs without any immediate or delayed ill effect (Berger 1954).

EFFECT IN THE DOG

Meprobamate has been administered orally to a limited number of dogs at a dose level of 1 g daily for 60–75 days with no gross evidence of toxicity. Hematological values, urine analysis, and phenosulfonphthalein excretion tests, as well as blood urea nitrogen and urea clearances, were all within normal limits (Berger 1954).

An acceptable therapeutic level of meprobamate used in veterinary practice is 100–400 mg administered orally 2–4 times daily.

EFFECT IN THE PIG

The author has used this ataractic agent on two occasions in one pig. A single dose of 1600 mg was administered by stomach tube to a gilt weighing 81 kg. It was difficult to determine if any degree of tranquilization was achieved. If anything, the animal appeared less tractable and became somewhat irritable following use of the drug.

BENZODIAZEPINE DERIVATIVES

Two benzodiazepine derivatives are used in the practice of veterinary medicine. They are diazepam (Valium) and chlordiazepoxide (Librium).

Diazepam

Of the benzodiazepine derivatives (i.e., diazepam and chlordiazepoxide), *diazepam* is about 20 times more potent than chlordiazepoxide in blocking decerebrate rigidity in animals. The principal site of CNS depression produced by diazepam is in the brainstem reticular formation. There is evidence indicating that the benzodiazepines and barbiturates decrease the turnover of serotonin and norepinephrine and other biogenic amines in the brain.

Diazepam and other related derivatives have anticonvulsant activity in animals. Unlike the phenothiazines and reserpine, these derivatives are capable of antagonizing convulsive seizures induced by pentylenetetrazol and strychnine. Extrapyramidal side effects are absent.

In decerebrate cats, polysynaptic reflexes elicited by sciatic nerve stimulation can be depressed to 50% or less by the intravenous administration of diazepam (0.05–0.2 mg/kg), chlordiazepoxide (10–30 mg/kg), meprobamate (20–40 mg/kg), mephenesin (10–50 mg/kg), and pentobarbital (24 mg/kg); blockade of the polysynaptic reflexes by these drugs is immediate and lasts up to 4 hours (Ngai et al. 1966). Diazepam, chlordiazepoxide, meprobamate, and mephenesin do not alter significantly the monosynaptic reflexes. Pentobarbital, cyclopropane, and nitrous oxide reduce the monosynaptic reflexes. According to Ngai et al. (1966), these findings suggest that central depressants, such as diazepam, chlordiazepoxide, meprobamate, mephenesin, and some anesthetics act upon supraspinal structures, most likely the reticular facilitatory system, in blockade of the spinal polysynaptic reflexes.

In the rat, it has been suggested that the benzodiazepines may elicit their anxiety-reducing effects by a reduction of serotonin activity in a behaviorally suppressive punishment system; furthermore, they may evoke their depressant effects by a reduction of norepinephrine activity in a behaviorally facilitatory reward system (Wise et al. 1972). In support of this, it is known that the anxiety-reducing effects of the benzodiazepines in the rat conflict test are mimicked by serotonin antagonists and by *p*-chlorophenylalanine, an inhibitor of serotonin synthesis. Also, it is known that the depressant effects of the benzodiazepines are mimicked by norepinephrine antagonists.

CLINICAL USE

In the Dog and Cat. Diazepam sodium has been used as an antianxiolytic agent in the dog and cat and for sedative purposes. It has been used in the treatment of status epilepticus in dogs (Averill 1970). Dosages are 5 and 10 mg intravenously. This dosage produces a mild generalized weakness and tranquilization lasting about 3 hours in the healthy adult dog.

The procedure for the treatment of clinical cases of status epilepticus has been described by Averill (1970). A dose of 5 mg of diazepam sodium is administered slowly by the intravenous route. In the event this dose level does not abolish the seizure in 1–2 minutes, the dose is repeated. If a response has not occurred following the second dose of the drug, pentobarbital sodium (7.5 mg/lb) is slowly administered intravenously. Those patients that respond to the first and/or second dosages of diazepam are carefully monitored, and, if status epilepticus returns in 2–4 hours after the initial treatment, the regimen is repeated. Oral anticonvulsant treatment with 100 mg of diphenylhydantoin (Dilantin) sodium every 8 hours is started as soon as the seizures are abolished. Out of 14 dogs treated for status epilepticus by the above method, 12 animals responded promptly and satisfactorily to a single dose of diazepam. One dog (13th animal) required repeated treatment for lasting effect and the 14th animal needed barbiturate anesthesia but died within minutes due to respiratory failure.

Diazepam sodium has been used to abolish ketamine-induced convulsive seizures in the cat (Reid and Frank 1972). A dose of 0.2 mg/lb intravenously has been used for this purpose. Diazepam has also been used in the control of "epileptic" disorders or "fits" in the cat regardless of the etiology (Kay 1975).

Generally, an intravenous dose (5–10 mg) of the drug is given to effect. A dose as high as 20 mg may be necessary; if high dosages are used, they must be injected slowly. The procedure commonly followed is to administer 2–10 mg intravenously, and then wait 10 minutes. In the event seizures persist, Kay (1975) recommends the intravenous administration of phenobarbital sodium (5–60 mg). Caution must be taken not to oversedate or depress the animal when these drugs are administered close together. Should the animal manifest refractoriness to diazepam and phenobarbital as in status epilepticus, pentobarbital sodium anesthesia is then carefully administered to effect.

Once the seizures have been brought under control, oral anticonvulsant therapy should be initiated. Regulation of oral anticonvulsant therapy in the cat can be difficult (Kay 1975). Phenobarbital (8–32 mg) is given orally 2–3 times daily; diazepam may be used in place of phenobarbital in animals that react unfavorably to barbiturate therapy. Diazepam is given orally in dosages of 2–5 mg 2 or 3 times daily. Phenobarbital dosages may be adjusted by increasing or decreasing in 4-mg to 8-mg increments and diazepam may be increased or decreased in increments of 2 mg (Kay 1975).

In Other Species. Diazepam has been used in mink to prevent conditions of anxiety and aggressiveness (Sandelien 1966). In white mink of the Hedlund strain, the animals are totally deaf and are extremely restless and excitable when handled. Pure breeding of this valuable strain is extremely difficult. The females frequently refuse to mate during normal estrus and may initiate vicious and even fatal fights. In the reduction of this aberrant behavior, various drugs such as sedatives, hypnotics, bromines, morphine, alcohol, barbiturates, and phenothiazines, including chlorpromazine, have been used with variable success (Sandelien 1966). Trials with diazepam administered in the feed indicate that it is possible to improve mating in mink and during whelping to prevent the females from killing their kits. For improvement of mating, the oral dosage of diazepam consisted of 1 mg/animal/day for 2 successive days followed by a maintenance level of 0.66 mg/animal/day. In the use of diazepam in standard dark mink during whelping, 0.66 mg/animal/day was fed for 1 month or more.

Chlordiazepoxide

The pharmacologic activity of *chlordiazepoxide* (Librium) is comparable to that of diazepam. Chlordiazepoxide has less overall potency than does diazepam. In the treatment of anxiety and related conditions in human beings, its long-term use is ordinarily free from most complications. Several publications report liver damage, including icterus, from the long-term ad-

TABLE 17.1. Dosages of chlordiazepoxide used in zoological species

Species	Dosage	Route of Administration	Effects Produced
	(mg/kg)		
European lynx	6	Oral	Calm in 2–3 hr; drowsiness and ataxia noted for several hr
Dingo	3	Oral	Onset of action in about 2 hr; no ataxia noted; allowed petting
	7	Oral	Ataxia produced
Guinea baboon	13	Oral	Docile in 2.5 hr to allow i.v. pentobarbital
Sea lion	7	Oral	Lethargy and calmness noted 4 hr later
Burmese macaque	5	I.M.	Calmed for anesthesia
Red kangaroo	11	Oral	Calm in 1.5 hr for radiographs
Mule deer	2.2	I.V.	Calm within a few min
Gnu	4	I.M.	Calm in 45 min
Gerenuk	5	I.M.	Calm in 45 min

ministration of chlordiazepoxide. In the rat, studies on the isolated perfused liver revealed that the drug decreases bile flow and the biliary excretion of sulfobromophthalein (Abernathy et al. 1975). Most of the veterinary medical uses of chlordiazepoxide in animals do not extend over long periods. The probability of the development of liver impairment in animals following short-term treatment is unlikely.

CLINICAL USE

Although chlordiazepoxide produces a satisfactory effect in a number of exotic animals, it failed to produce a desired effect in the Sumatran tiger, Hensel's cat, the tapir, and klipspringer (Heuschele 1961). However, the lynx and dingo were converted from hostile, aggressive animals to docile animals. Dosages of chlordiazepoxide reported by Heuschele (1961) that have produced favorable responses in zoological species are summarized in Table 17.1.

REFERENCES

Abernathy, C. O.; Smith, S.; and Zimmerman, H. J. 1975. The effect of chlordiazepoxide hydrochloride on the isolated perfused rat liver. Proc Soc Exp Biol Med 149:271.

Adams, H. R.; Smookler, H. H.; Clarke, D. E.; Jandhyala, B. S.; Dixit, B. N.; Ertel, R. J.; and Burkley, J. P. 1971. Clinicopathologic effects of chronic reserpine administration in mongrel dogs. J Pharm Sci 60:1134.

Archer, R. K. 1973. Investigations of azaperone-metomidate anaesthesia in the horse. Vet Rec 93:379.

Arscott, G. H., and Parker, J. E. 1967. Effect of reserpine in the diet of adult male chickens. Poult Sci 46:1019.

Averill, D. R. 1970. Treatment of status epilepticus in dogs with diazepam sodium. J Am Vet Med Assoc 156:432.

Berger, F. M. 1954. The pharmacological properties of 2-methyl-2-*n*-propyl-1,3-propanediol dicarbamate (Miltown), a new interneuronal blocking agent. J Pharmacol Exp Ther 112:413.

Barron, C. N.; Rubin, L. F.; and Steelman, R. L. 1972. Chlorpromazine and the eye of the dog. III. Natural daylight versus artificial light. Exp Mol Pathol 16:158.

Blackwell, R.; Vale, W.; Rivier, C.; and Guillemin, R. 1973. Effect of perphenazine on the secretion of prolactin *in vivo* and *in vitro*. Proc Soc Exp Biol Med 142:68.

Bolz, W. 1962. Neuroleptica und potenzierte narkose speziell bei zootieren. Nord Vet Med 14: [Suppl 1] 17.

Booth, N. H. 1969. Anesthesia in the pig. Fed Proc 28:1547.

Brand, E. D.; Harris, T. D.; Borison, H. L.; and Goodman, L. S. 1954. The antiemetic activity of 10-γ-dimethylaminopropyl)-2-chlorophenothiazine (chlorpromazine) in the dog and cat. J Pharmacol Exp Ther 110:86.

Bree, M. M.; Cohen, B. J.; and Abrams, G. D. 1971. Injection lesions following intramuscular administration of chlorpromazine in rabbits. J Am Vet Med Assoc 159:1598.

Calderwood, H. W. 1971. Anesthesia for reptiles. J Am Vet Med Assoc 159:1618.

Callear, J. F. F., and Van Gestel, J. F. E. 1973. An analysis of the results of field experiments in pigs in the U.K. and Eire with the combination anaesthetic azaperone and metomidate. Vet Rec 92:284.

Campbell, H., and Harthoorn, A. M. 1963. The capture and anaesthesia of the African lion in his natural environment. Vet Rec 75: 275.

Chatterton, R. T., Jr.; Chien, J.; and Ward, D. A. 1974. Effect of perphenazine treatment of rats on serum ovarian and adrenal steroids. Proc Soc Exp Biol Med 145:874.

Christian, R. G.; Mills, J. H. L.; and Kramer, L. L. 1974. Accidental intracarotid artery injection of promazine in the horse. Can Vet J 15:29.

Clarke, D. E.; Adams, H. R.; and Buckley, J. P. 1970. Chronic reserpine treatment on adrenergic neuronal and receptor function in the isolated perfused mesenteric blood vessels of the dog. Eur J Pharmacol 12:378.

Clarke, K. W. 1969. Effect of azaperone on the blood pressure and pulmonary ventilation in pigs. Vet Rec 85:649.

Clifford, D. H., and Soma, L. R. 1969. Feline anesthesia. Fed Proc 28:1479.

Clifford, D. H.; Good, A. L.; and Stowe, C. M. 1962. Observation on the use of ataractic and narcotic preanesthesia and pentobarbital in bears. J Am Vet Med Assoc 140: 464.

Code of Federal Regulations. 1974. 21 CFR 131.11 U.S. Government Printing Office, Washington, D.C.

Collette, W. L., and Meriwether, W. F. 1965. Some changes in the peripheral blood of dogs after administration of certain tranquilizers and narcotics. Vet Med Small Anim Clin 60:1223.

Cox, J. E. 1973. Immobilization and anaesthesia of the pig. Vet Rec 92:143.

Davis, L. E., and Donnelly, E. J. 1968. Analgesic drugs in the cat. J Am Vet Med Assoc 153:1161.

Dawson, H. A.; Lickfeldt, W. E.; and Brengle, L. A. 1959. Promazine in equine practice. J Am Vet Med Assoc 135:69.

de Wied, D. 1967. Chlorpromazine and endocrine function. Pharmacol Rev 19:251.

Dhasmana, K. M.; Dixit, K. S.; Jaju, B. P.; and Gupta, M. L. 1972. Role of central dopaminergic receptors in manic response of cats of morphine. Psychopharmacologia 24:380.

Earl, A. E. 1956. Reserpine (Serpasil) in veterinary practice. J Am Vet Med Assoc 129: 227.

Ferguson, T. M.; Muller, D. H.; Bradley, J. W.; and Atkinson, R. L. 1969. Blood pressure and heart rate of turkeys 17–21 months of age. Poult Sci 48:1478.

Frank, C. J. 1970. Equine colic—A routine modern approach. Vet Rec 87:497.

Fraser, A. C. 1967. Restraint in the horse. Vet Rec 80:56.

Gabel, A. A. 1962. Promazine, chloral hydrate and ultrashort-acting barbiturate anesthesia in horses. J Am Vet Med Assoc 140:564.

Gabel, A. A., and Koestner, A. 1963. The effects of intracarotid artery injection of drugs in domestic animals. J Am Vet Med Assoc 142:1397.

Garland, J. E., and White, K. B. 1968. Unusual reactions to acetylpromazine. Vet Rec 83:641.

Gillespie, J. R., and Tyler, W. S. 1963. Surgical restraint hobbles for the horse. J Am Vet Med Assoc 143:511.

Ginsberg, A.; French, P.; and McManus, D. 1963. The use of tranquillisers in the transport of slaughter stock. Vet Rec 75: 996.

Goldman, A. S., and Yakovac, W. C. 1965. Teratogenic action in rats of reserpine alone and in combination with salicylate and immobilization. Proc Soc Exp Biol Med 118:857.

Graham-Jones, O. 1962. Tranquillisation of a pregnant hippopotamus. Vet Rec. 74:1021.

Greene, D. E.; Eaton, R. C.; Wilcke, H. L.; and Bethke, R. M. 1961. Species differences in the effect of reserpine on reproductive performance. Poult Sci 40:1410.

Gupta, B. N.; Moore, J. A.; and Conner, G. H. 1970. The use of promazine hydrochloride in cesarean section in the dog. Lab Anim Sci 20:474.

Hagen, P., and Wallace, A. C. 1961. Effect of reserpine on growth and sexual development of chickens. Br J Pharmacol 17:267.

Harthoorn, A. M.; Harthoorn, S.; and Sayer, P. D. 1971. Two field operations on the African lion (*Felis leo*). Vet Rec 89:159.

Hatch, R. C. 1967. Restraint, preanesthetic medication and postanesthetic medication of dogs with chlorpromazine and atropine. J Am Vet Med Assoc 150:27.

Heuschele, W. P. 1961. Chlordiazepoxide for calming zoo animals. J Am Vet Med Assoc 139:996.

Hillidge, C. J.; Lees, P.; and Serrano, L. 1973. Investigations of azaperone/metomidate anesthesia in the horse. Vet Rec 93:307.

Himwich, H. E. 1958. Psychopharmacologic drugs. Science 127:59.

Hornykiewicz, O. 1966. Dopamine (3-hydroxytyramine) and brain function. Pharmacol Rev 18:925.

———. 1973. Dopamine in the basal ganglia. Br Med Bull 29:172.

Iverson, L. L. 1975. Dopamine receptors in the brain. Science 188:1084.

Jarvik, M. E. 1970. Drugs used in the treatment of psychiatric disorders. In L. S. Goodman and A. Gilman, eds. The Pharmacological Basis of Therapeutics, 4th ed., p. 163. New York: Macmillan.

Jenkin, J. T. 1972. The use of etorphine-acepromazine (analgesic-tranquilizer) mixtures in horses. Vet Rec 90:207.

Johnston, R. F., and Cairy, C. F. 1961. Effects of trifluomeprazine on dogs and cats. Vet Med 56:430.

Jones, E. W. 1961. Equine anesthesia-maintenance by inhalation techniques. J Am Vet Med Assoc 139:785.

Jones, R. S. 1963 . Methylamphetamine as an antagonist of some tranquillising drugs in the horse. Vet Rec 75:1157.

———. 1972. A review of tranquillisation and sedation in large animals. Vet Rec 90:611.

Kaebler, W. W., and Joynt, R. J. 1956. Tremor production in cats given chlorpromazine. Proc Soc Exp Biol Med 92:399.

Kay, W. J. 1975. Epilepsy in cats. J Am Anim Hosp Assoc 11:77.

Kuntz, A. 1967. Neuroleptanalgesia in bears. Vet Rec 80:278.

Leash, A. M. 1969. Intravascular and other routes for anesthesia in the dog. Fed Proc 28:1436.

Lewis, C. J., and Oakley, G. A. 1971. The use of chlorpromazine in swine agalactia. Vet Rec 88:380.

Marsboom, K., and Mortelmans, J. 1964. Some pharmacologic aspects of analgesics and neuroleptics and their use for neuroleptanalgesia in primates and lower monkeys. In O. Graham-Jones, ed. Small Animal Anaesthesia, p. 131. Elmsford, N.Y.: Pergamon Press.

Matthysse, S. 1973. Antipsychotic drug actions: A clue to the neuropathology of schizophrenia? Fed Proc 32:200.

Muggenberg, A.; Kowalczyk, T.; Hoekstra, W. G.; and Grummer, R. H. 1966. Experimental production of gastric ulcers in swine by reserpine. Am J Vet Res 27:1663.

Ngai, S. H.; Tseng, D. T. C.; and Wang, S. C. 1966. Effect of diazepam and other central nervous system depressants on spinal reflexes in cats: A study of site of action. J Pharmacol Exp Ther 153:344.

Nicoloff, D. M.; Stone, N. H.; Leonard, A. S.; Doberneck, R.; and Wangensteen, O. H. 1961. Effect of reserpine on peptic ulceration and gastric blood flow in dogs. Proc Soc Exp Biol Med 106:877.

Pletscher, A.; Shore, P. A.; and Brodie, B. B. 1956. Serotonin as a mediator of reserpine actions in brain. J Pharmacol Exp Ther 116:84.

Popovic, N. A.; Mullane, J. F.; and Yhap, E. O. 1972. Effects of acetylpromazine maleate on certain cardiorespiratory responses in dogs. Am J Vet Res 33:1819.

Proakis, A. G., and Borowitz, J. L. 1974. Blockade of insulin release by certain phenothiazines. Biochem Pharmacol 23:1693.

Pugh, D. M. 1964. Acepromazine in veterinary use. Vet Rec 76:439.

Raker, C. W., and Sayers, A. C. 1959. Promazine as a preanesthetic agent in horses. J Am Vet Med Assoc 124:23.

Reid, J. S., and Frank, R. J. 1972. Prevention of undesirable side reactions of ketamine anesthesia in cats. J Am Anim Hosp Assoc 8:115.

Rosin, E. 1974. University of Georgia. Personal communication.

Sandelien, H. 1966. Oral administration of "Valium" to restless and aggressive mink. Nord Vet Med 18:271.

Santos-Martinez, J.; Aviles, T. A.; and Laboy-Torres, J. A. 1972. Arrhythmic effects of phenothiazine derivatives. Survey Anesth 16:373.

Schlinke, J. C., and Palmer, J. S. 1973. Combined effects of phenothiazine and organophosphate insecticides in cattle. J Am Vet Med Assoc 163:756.

Seal, U. S., and Erickson, A. W. 1969. Immobilization of carnivora and other mammals with phencyclidine and promazine. Fed Proc 28:1410.

Segal, D. S.; Sullivan, J. L., III; Kuczenski, R. T.; and Mandell, A. J. 1971. Effects of long-term reserpine treatment on brain tyrosine hydroxylase and behavioral activity. Science 173:847.

Selye, H., and Szabo, S. 1972. Protection against halperidol by catatoxic steroids. Psychopharmacologia 24:430.

Shideler, R. K. 1971. The practitioner's approach to equine inhalation anesthesia. Proc Am Assoc Equine Pract, p. 119.

Slinger, S. J.; Pepper, W. F.; and Sibbald, I. R. 1962. Interrelationships between methionine, choline, sodium chloride and reserpine in growing turkeys. Poult Sci 41:974.

Soma, L. R., and Shields, D. R. 1964. Neuroleptanalgesia produced by fentanyl and droperidol. J Am Vet Med Assoc 145:897.

Speckman, E. W., and Ringer, R. K. 1961. Hemodynamic responses following reserpine feeding to turkeys. Poult Sci 40:1292.

Strobel, G. E., and Wollman, H. 1969. Pharmacology of anesthetic agents. Fed Proc 28:1386.

Sumner-Smith, G. A. 1962. A preliminary report on the clinical use of chlorprothixene as a sedative, narcotic and premedicant in the dog. J Small Anim Pract 3:13.

Symoens, J., and Van Den Brande, M. 1969. Prevention and cure of aggressiveness in pigs using the sedative azaperone. Vet Rec 85:64.

Weaver, L. C.; Mitchell, F. E.; and Kerley, T. L. 1963. Toxicopathologic and pharmacologic properties of piperacetazine, a potent tranquilizing agent. Toxicol Appl Pharmacol 5:49.

Weir, J. J. R., and Sandford, J. 1972. Urinary

excretion of phenothiazine tranquillisers by the horse. Equine Vet J 4:88.

Wheat, J. D. 1966. Penile paralysis in stallions given propiopromazine. J Am Vet Med Assoc 148:405.

White, K. 1968. Unusual reactions to acetylpromazine. Vet Rec 83:688.

Wilcken, D. E. L.; Brender, D.; Shorey, C. D.; and McDonald, G. J. 1967. Reserpine: Effect on structure of heart muscle. Science 157:1332.

Wise, C. D.; Berger, B. D.; and Stein, L. 1972. Benzodiazepines: Anxiety-reducing activity by reduction of serotonin turnover in the brain. Science 177:180.

Wright, J. G., and Hall, L. W. 1961. Veterinary Anaesthesia and Analgesia, 5th ed. Baltimore: Williams & Wilkins.

Yelnosky, J., and Field, W. E. 1964. A preliminary report on the use of a combination of droperidol and fentanyl citrate in veterinary medicine. Am J Vet Res 25:1751.

Yelnosky, J.; Katz, R.; and Dietrich, E. V. 1964. A study of some of the pharmacologic actions of droperidol. Toxicol Appl Pharmacol 6:37.

Zontine, W. J. 1973. Effect of chemical restraint drugs on the passage of barium sulfate through the stomach and duodenum of dogs. J Am Vet Med Assoc 162:878.

CHAPTER 18

STIMULANTS

NICHOLAS H. BOOTH

A large number of drugs possess the ability to stimulate the central nervous system (CNS). Stimulant drugs vary markedly in their total pharmacological action. Some can be used for therapeutic stimulation within narrow limits of dosage; others are only poisons. Some, such as ephedrine, influence the function of the CNS only secondarily while primarily affecting another system of the body. Toxic drugs, such as phenol, stimulate the CNS as a manifestation of poisoning. Many of these are considered as poisons and accordingly are discussed under other headings.

Some drugs affecting the CNS have a specific type of action that limits their clinical application. Apomorphine, for example, stimulates the emetic center in the medulla more than other parts of the brain, so it is used clinically to induce emesis. Stimulants of the CNS, such as caffeine, are used by human beings to stimulate the sensory areas of the brain to combat mental fatigue.

Other drugs that stimulate the CNS are those that act directly or reflexly upon the respiratory center to counteract respiratory collapse. These drugs are employed in the treatment of barbiturate poisoning, drowning, neonatal asphyxia, heat or lightning shock, and threatened respiratory collapse during anesthesia. Examples of this latter category of CNS stimulants are doxapram, pentylenetetrazol (metrazol), picrotoxin, nikethamide (Coramine), and bemegride.

The term *respiratory analeptic* refers to drugs that stimulate a depressed respiratory center to produce increased respiratory exchange. Drugs used for this purpose, with the exception of carbon dioxide, exert an "arousal" effect characterized by a partial return of consciousness of the patient. Oftentimes animals do not return to a state of normal cerebration or locomotion but bump and bruise themselves in a severe fashion. The period of stimulation is brief. Most respiratory analeptics are of doubtful value in animals following the development of severe respiratory paralysis by the barbiturates. The best therapy consists in applying artificial ventilation using oxygen until the excess barbiturate is detoxified. The extensive use of the ultrashort-acting barbiturates and inhalants in recent years has decreased the value of, and interest in, the respiratory analeptic drugs. These analeptic agents may have some value as adjuncts in shortening respiratory depression. In many instances, the use of analeptics may be more of a liability than an asset because severe complications such as tremor, convulsive seizures, arterial hypotension, and poststimulatory depression, including paralysis of respiration, can occur.

Some CNS stimulants such as amphetamine and methamphetamine are subject to the Controlled Substances Act of 1970. In 1974 the approval of the animal drug application for amphetamine sulfate was withdrawn by the Food and Drug Administration (FDA) at the request of the manufacturer. This occurred after the FDA had advised the manufacturer that data were needed to establish the absence of unsafe residues in the edible tissues of treated cattle. Also, amphetamine has a record high abuse incidence in human beings and more recent regulatory action has resulted in the removal of the drug for medical use.

In animals, misuse and abuse of the CNS stimulants have been complex problems involving the racing dog or horse. Many of the stimulants have been illegally used by individuals to improve the performance of racing animals. The sensitivity of the analytical methodology used for the identification of stimulants has improved considerably within the last decade so that it is now more difficult for unscrupulous individuals to use these drugs without detection. The use of drugs such as phenylbutazone for doping and local anesthetics to reduce pain from limb injuries and lamenesses has been previously covered. Other motives for doping animals relate to the illegal use of CNS depressants in a competitor's animal to slow it down.

The stimulant value obtained by doping horses to win a race is subject to considerable debate. It is not possible to stimulate the animal to the extent that it is certain to win; even if it were possible, other factors, such as injury, stumbling, or overexcitation, present hazards (Bogan and Smith 1968).

DOXAPRAM HYDROCHLORIDE

Doxapram Hydrochloride, N.F. (Dopram), is approved by the FDA for use in the dog, cat, and horse. It has not been approved for use in food-producing animals intended for human consumption. Chemically, doxapram hydrochloride is 1-ethyl-4-(2-morpholinoethyl)-3,3-diphenyl-2-pyrrolidinone hydrochloride (Fig. 18.1).

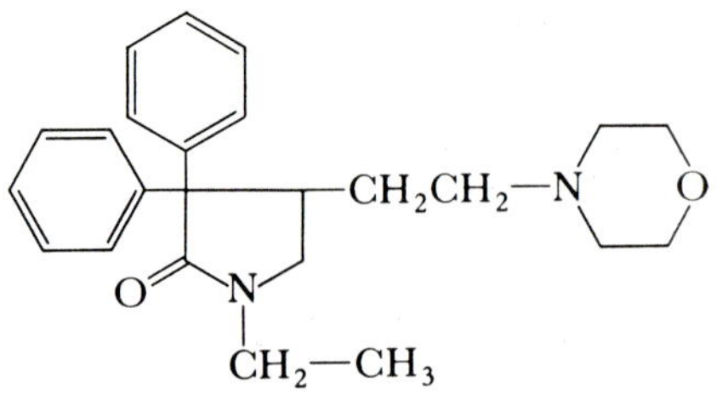

FIG. 18.1.

PHARMACOLOGICAL CONSIDERATIONS

Doxapram is primarily used to stimulate respiratory activity in the postanethetic or recovery period. The stimulation effect is believed to be related to a direct action upon the chemoreceptors of the carotid and aortic regions as well as stimulation of the medullary respiratory center. The principal effect upon ventilation is upon the tidal volume; an increase in the tidal volume occurs after the administration of doxapram. Stimulation of other portions of the CNS occurs only when high dose levels are used. Convulsions or alterations in the EEG patterns are not seen with therapeutic levels (Soma and Kenny 1967). The convulsant dose of doxapram is 70–75 times the dose that stimulates respiratory center activity.

In the evaluation of doxapram with various combinations of analeptic agents, doxapram was superior to all the combinations evaluated; the respiratory minute volume was increased 200% within 1 minute after the administration of doxapram in the dog (Klemm 1966). Other studies of a clinical pharmacological nature have been conducted to determine the ventilatory effects of doxapram in the dog (Soma and Kenny 1967). When doxapram (2 mg/kg) is administered intravenously, the change in the expired minute volume is marked and rapid. The ventilatory and cardiovascular stimulatory effects occur within one circulation time of the drug. According to Soma and Kenny (1967), the initial marked increase in the expired minute volume is due to an increase in tidal volume and respiration rate. However, the increase in tidal volume is not maintained and diminishes in 5–6 minutes. The overall improvement in ventilation is reflected by changes in the acid-base status of the blood as well as in the oxygen tension of arterial blood.

The pressor response of doxapram occurs rapidly and concurrently with the respiratory effects (Soma and Kenny 1967). This response is said to be mediated through activation of the sympathetic nervous system. An arterial hypotensive effect of brief duration occurs after the intravenous administration of a large dose (4 mg/kg); this effect does not occur when a dose of 2 mg/kg or less is administered. The pressor and respiratory responses occur when the dose level of doxapram is not higher than 2 mg/kg (Soma and Kenny 1967).

Studies in the cat anesthetized with pentobarbital sodium have been conducted to determine the effects of bilateral or unilateral pneumotaxic center ablation upon doxapram-induced respiratory changes (St. John et al. 1973). Following the unilateral or bilateral ablation of the pneumotaxic center in the cat, the tidal volume is "reset" at a higher level while the frequency is "reset" at a lower level. In these ablated animal preparations, doxapram stimulation of respiration causes only minor changes in the tidal volume but the frequency of respiratory activity is increased (St. John et al. 1973). The intravenous dosages of doxapram (1–2.5 mg/kg) used by St. John and associates were adequate to stimulate effects through both peripheral chemoreceptor and medullary respiratory area activation. Doxapram-induced stimulatory influences arising from one or both of these areas (i.e., chemoreceptor and/or medullary respiratory center) are integrated by the pontile pneumotaxic center. The study did not distinguish between the components of respiratory activity produced by peripheral chemoreceptor and medullary respiratory area stimulation and it did not provide direct information as to the mechanism of action in the induction of the respiratory stimulant effects. The study did reveal that the respiratory stimulatory effect of doxapram is integrated by the same neuroanatomical structure that regulates the respiratory responses evoked by neurochemical stimulation of carbon dioxide (St. John et al. 1973).

Doxapram has also been experimentally used in the pig, rabbit, sheep, and chicken; sheep and rabbits appear to be far less sensitive than other species to the effects of analeptic agents (Beretta et al. 1973). Although there are variations in the degree of responses produced by different analeptics in various species, doxapram, when used alone or in combination with other analeptics, always elicits a marked improvement in respiratory activity.

Clinical Use

Use of doxapram in clinical practice is specified for the reversal of central respiratory depression due to barbiturates and inhalant anesthetics. Doxapram hydrochloride is used intravenously and is recommended as follows:

	Species	*Dosage (mg/lb)*	*Clinical Use*
(1)	Dog and cat	2.5–5	Barbiturate depression
(2)	Dog and cat	0.5	Depression due to inhalant anesthetics
(3)	Horse	0.25	Depression from chloral hydrate and pentobarbital sodium
(4)	Horse	0.20	Depression produced by inhalant anesthetics

Dosages of doxapram can be repeated within 15–20 minutes to achieve the desired effect. Although second injections are effective in both the dog or cat, it is not as effective as the first injection (Jensen and Klemm 1967).

In the horse, a clinical evaluation of doxapram (0.25 mg/lb) as a respiratory stimulant was conducted during and after general anesthesia with intravenous injections of chloral hydrate alone and chloral hydrate in combination with pentobarbital and magnesium sulfate (Short et al. 1970). The arousal time was reduced; respiratory volume and rate increased immediately following administration of the drug. No toxic or adverse effects were noted. A similar clinical evaluation of doxapram (0.21 mg/lb) in the horse during and after general anesthesia with halothane and methoxyflurane revealed comparable effects (Short and Cloyd 1970).

BEMEGRIDE

Chemically, *Bemegride,* U.S.P. (metharimide, Megimide, Mikedimide), is 3-ethyl-3-methylglutarimide and is soluble in water only to the extent of approximately 1:200 (Fig. 18.2).

Effect upon the Nervous System

Bemegride is a stimulant of the CNS and is a specific antagonist to the barbiturate group of drugs. Large doses produce muscular twitching, tremors, and convulsions. Convulsive seizures occur more readily in the cat than in the dog; doses of bemegride (15–30 mg/kg) produced convulsions in cats that had been pretreated with an anesthetizing dose of pentobarbital sodium (Aizstrauts et al. 1962).

In therapeutic amounts, barbiturate depression is reversed and awakening of the animal occurs. The intravenous administration of 11 mg/lb of body weight of the analeptic in sheep that are deeply anesthetized with pentobarbital restores them immediately to consciousness (Turner and Hodgetts 1956). In the cat, barbiturate depression is decreased and respiration and circulation are improved, but consciousness is not restored even with convulsive dose levels.

Respiratory and Circulatory Responses

In dogs deeply anesthetized with pentobarbital sodium, bemegride is superior to several analeptic agents in stimulating ventilatory activity (Cairy et al. 1961). Also, in animals suffering from barbiturate depression and hemorrhagic shock, the drug has a greater effect in reversing arterial hypotension and respiratory depression (Cairy and Ramaswamy 1962).

Dosage

The suggested intravenous dose of bemegride sodium for the cat and dog is 7–9 mg/lb of body weight (MacFarlane and Bentley 1957).

PENTYLENETETRAZOL

Pentylenetetrazol, N.F. (metrazol, leptazol), is a synthetic organic compound occurring as white crystals that are freely soluble in water (Fig. 18.3).

Effect upon the Nervous System

Pentylenetetrazol acts promptly and primarily upon the CNS. The medulla and midbrain are the most responsive parts of the brain. Larger doses of this drug stimulate the cerebral cortex and also the spinal cord. Pentylenetetrazol appears to stimulate directly and not reflexly. Clinically, it has been used for stimulation of the respiratory centers, although there is also an effect upon the vasomotor and vagal centers.

Respiratory Response

Respiration appears to be controlled by a series of respiratory centers located in

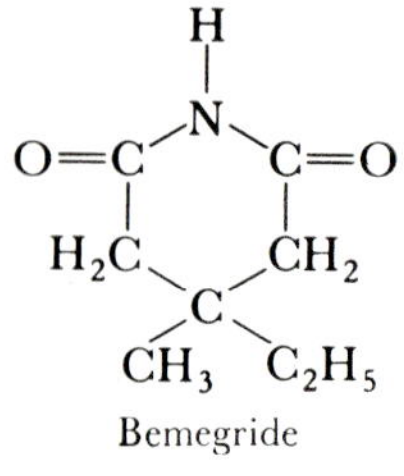

H
N
O=C C=O
H_2C CH_2
C
CH_3 C_2H_5

Bemegride

Fig. 18.2.

H_2C—CH_2—CH_2
N—N
H_2C—CH_2—C
N—N

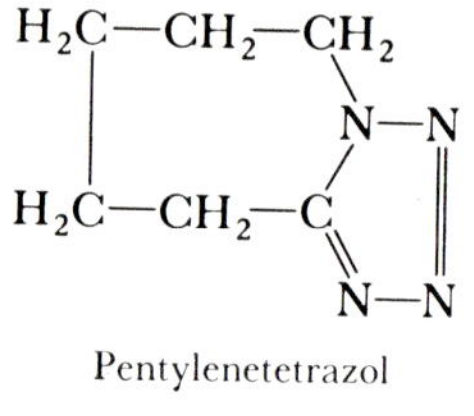

Pentylenetetrazol

Fig. 18.3.

the medulla, the upper pons, and the frontal lobes of the cortex. Pentylenetetrazol stimulates these respiratory centers directly, particularly those of the medulla. It increases the depth and to some degree the rate of respiration.

Circulatory Response

There is no convincing evidence to prove that pentylenetetrazol produces any direct effect upon the circulatory system. However, during respiratory depression the circulatory system is apt to show a parallel depression. In this case, an improvement in respiration would result reflexly in improvement of circulation.

Convulsant doses of pentylenetetrazol clearly increase arterial blood pressure in dogs. In this case, vasoconstriction appears to be a negligible factor because the increased blood pressure is principally the result of contractions of skeletal muscles during the convulsive seizures. The convulsive muscular contractions increase the extravascular pressure over most of the body areas, and this compresses blood vessels and increases the arterial pressure.

Absorption, Fate, and Excretion

Pentylenetetrazol is rapidly absorbed following oral or parenteral administration. In dogs and cats most of the drug is detoxified by the liver. The kidney has little or no effect on detoxification. Only traces of pentylenetetrazol are excreted unchanged in the urine of dogs after large doses. No conjugated form of the drug has been found in the urine or feces. Pentylenetetrazol is distributed equally at all times in the tissues, in the blood, liver, muscle, and brain. No particular tissue affinity is noted. The rate of detoxification is proportional to the concentration of the drug in the tissues.

Clinical Use

Pentylenetetrazol is used principally as a respiratory stimulant in emergencies to counteract depression from barbiturates, morphine, chloral hydrate, and certain other CNS depressants. It may also be of benefit in some other types of conditions involving depression of the CNS.

Pentylenetetrazol may be administered orally in liquid or tablet form as well as subcutaneously, intramuscularly, or intravenously. It is absorbed almost as rapidly following oral administration as by any other route. An outstanding advantage of pentylenetetrazol is a relatively wide margin of safety and shorter duration of action compared to some other CNS stimulants.

Pentylenetetrazol administered with nikethamide shows neither synergistic nor additive effect. In fact, the total action is less than additive, perhaps because different parts of the CNS are stimulated.

Dosage

The dosage of pentylenetetrazol for dogs is about 3–5 mg/lb of body weight, subcutaneously or intramuscularly. This dose may be repeated in 15–30 minutes, as indicated. Pentylenetetrazol is relatively nontoxic, although excessive dosage will stimulate the CNS and produce convulsions followed by respiratory paralysis.

NIKETHAMIDE

Nikethamide, N.F. (Coramine), is a synthetic pyridine derivative (Fig. 18.4). It is a clear to pale yellow liquid with a characteristic odor and ready solubility in water.

Effect upon the Nervous System

Nikethamide stimulates chemoreceptor activity in the carotid and aortic bodies. These receptor organs reflexly stimulate the respiratory centers primarily and the vasoconstrictor and vagal centers secondarily. The carotid and aortic bodies are

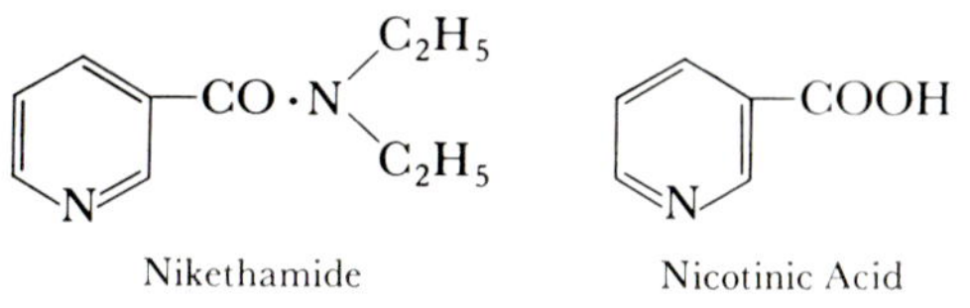

C_2H_5
—CO · N
C_2H_5
N
—COOH
N

Nikethamide   Nicotinic Acid

Fig. 18.4.

composed of undifferentiated tissues of embryonic origin and are sensitive to stimuli that will not provoke a response from the more highly specialized cells of the medulla during such unfavorable conditions as hypoxia. Thus it is possible to stimulate the respiratory centers indirectly through the carotid bodies at a time when direct medullary stimulation of the centers would not be effective.

An excessive dose of nikethamide stimulates the cerebral cortex and the spinal cord, resulting in convulsions. However, a CNS depressant effect follows the stimulant action of nikethamide. This shortcoming of the drug reduces its value as an effective analeptic agent.

Circulatory Effects

Nikethamide produces an increase in blood pressure, preceded by a brief decrease. This response appears to be secondary to improvement of the respiratory mechanism.

Absorption and Fate

Nikethamide is readily absorbed following any route of administration. It is ordinarily injected intramuscularly but is most potent when injected intravenously. Nikethamide is converted to nicotinamide and excreted as nicotinamide methochloride.

Clinical Use

The primary therapeutic use of nikethamide is to stimulate respiration in the presence of excessive depression of the CNS. However, Nikethamide is viewed as being less efficacious than other available analeptic agents. When compared with caffeine and sodium benzoate, pentylenetetrazol, and bemegride, nikethamide is least effective in stimulating ventilatory activity in the deeply anesthetized dog (Cairy et al. 1961).

It is interesting to note that nikethamide possesses antipellagrous activity, which would indicate that the drug is probably of therapeutic value in the treatment of blacktongue in dogs.

Dosage

The suggested dose of nikethamide for the dog is 10–20 mg/lb administered orally, intravenously, intramuscularly, or subcutaneously. This dose may be repeated as indicated.

PICROTOXIN

Picrotoxin, N.F. (Fig. 18.5), is the active principle found in the seeds of *Anamirta cocculus,* a climbing shrub indigenous to the East Indies. The seeds of this plant contain 1.5%–5% of picrotoxin. The natives call the fruit of the plant "fish berries" because they toss the bruised berries onto the water where the fish eat them; the fish are immediately paralyzed and float to the surface where they are caught and eaten without harm to the natives. Under proper conditions in water, picrotoxin hydrolyzes into picrotin and the slightly more potent picrotoxinin. Even the aqueous pharmaceutic preparation deteriorates slowly.

Effects upon the Nervous System

Picrotoxin stimulates the CNS strongly, especially the medulla oblongata. With the exception of picrotoxin and strychnine, the mechanism of action of most convulsants is unknown. Picrotoxin blocks the gamma-aminobutyric acid receptor within the CNS (Smythies 1974). Gamma-aminobutyric acid normally functions to inhibit neurotransmission in synaptic or interneuronal junctions. Picrotoxin allows nerve impulse transmission to proceed unimpeded following blockade of the inhibitory transmitter, i.e., gamma-aminobutyric acid.

Picrotoxin has been employed to stimulate the respiratory centers and the en-

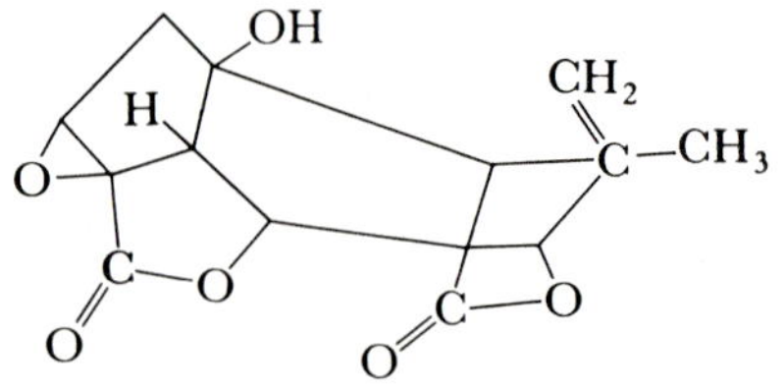

Picrotoxin

Fig. 18.5.

tire CNS in patients depressed by anesthetic drugs. It is particularly beneficial in antagonizing barbiturate depression and clinically has been limited almost entirely to this use.

Fate

Picrotoxin is rapidly destroyed in the body. A therapeutic dose of picrotoxin appears to be metabolized within 15–20 minutes. Since only 10% of a given dose is excreted in the urine, picrotoxin is believed to be metabolized by the tissues.

Dosage

The dose of picrotoxin for the adult dog is 1–3 mg intravenously. The drug may be readministered at one-half the previous dose in 15 minutes.

Therapeutic Use

Picrotoxin has been used almost entirely to counteract barbiturate poisoning. It is extremely potent and is a hazardous drug to use, especially when the dosage is repeated. It should not be used to speed recovery from normal anesthesia.

Disadvantages

Picrotoxin is too potent to be the drug of choice in treatment of barbiturate poisoning. Since picrotoxin is apt to produce a convulsant seizure, there is a tendency to employ safer drugs. Another major disadvantage of picrotoxin is the latent period. In dogs, as much as 5–8 minutes may pass from the time of intravenous injection before the stimulant action is observed. This is too long in critical cases to permit recovery. Failure to allow for this latent period may lead to overdosage and picrotoxin convulsions.

METHYLXANTHINE DERIVATIVES

Three compounds containing the xanthine nucleus are used medicinally: caffeine, theophylline, and theobromine (Fig. 18.6). These compounds are used to some extent in small animal medicine but rarely in large animals. Caffeine is found in coffee beans to the extent of about 1%.

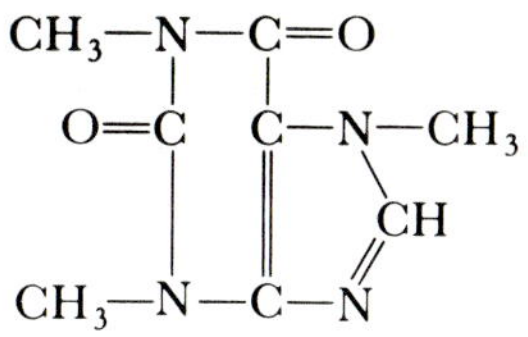

```
CH3—N—C=O
    |  |
  O=C  C—N—CH3
    |  ||  \
    |  ||   CH
    |  ||  //
CH3—N—C—N
```

Caffeine

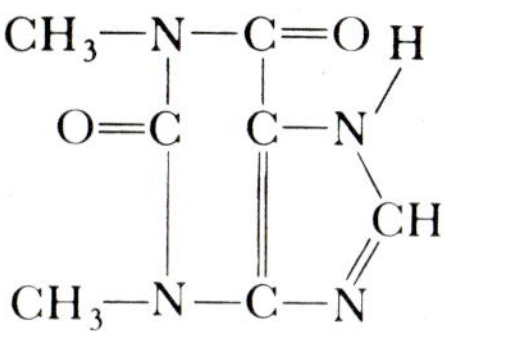

```
CH3—N—C=O H
    |  |  /
  O=C  C—N
    |  ||  \
    |  ||   CH
    |  ||  //
CH3—N—C—N
```

Theophylline

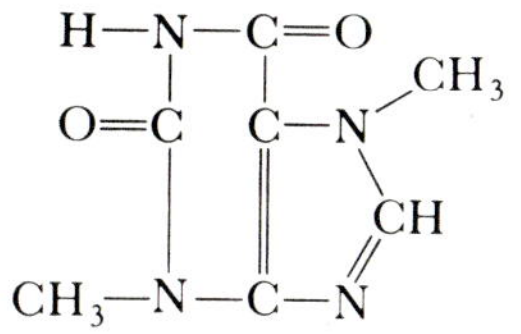

```
   H—N—C=O
    |  |   CH3
  O=C  C—N/
    |  ||  \
    |  ||   CH
    |  ||  //
CH3—N—C—N
```

Theobromine

Fig. 18.6.

Theophylline and caffeine are present in tea leaves to around 3%. Theobromine is found in small amounts in cacao beans.

The above methylxanthine compounds affect the same organs but to a varying degree. They all stimulate the CNS, dilate the coronary blood vessels, and promote diuresis. However, caffeine is primarily a CNS stimulant. Theophylline is better for dilation of the coronary vessels, and theobromine is preferred for inducing diuresis because its action is more prolonged than that of theophylline.

Caffeine and Sodium Benzoate

Caffeine and Sodium Benzoate, U.S.P., make up the preparation of choice for parenteral administration, primarily because this preparation is more soluble in water than caffeine citrate.

ACTION

Caffeine increases the irritability of the sensory cortex, which results in increased mental alertness. Caffeine is a potent cerebral stimulant that may superimpose exceptional muscular activity over fatigue and temporarily increase the performer's capacity for muscular work. Large doses cause an increased motor activity that may lead to exaggerated responses to normal stimuli.

Caffeine will stimulate the respiratory centers directly when they are depressed by such drugs as chloral hydrate, ethanol, or morphine. It has been suggested that caffeine may act by rendering the respiratory centers more sensitive to carbon dioxide.

METABOLISM

Caffeine is readily absorbed from the digestive tract or from the site of injection in small animals. It is partially demethylated and excreted in the urine. About 80% is metabolized to urea.

DOSAGE

The dosage of caffeine and sodium benzoate administered hypodermically in the dog varies from 0.1 to 1 g, depending on the weight.

TOXICITY

Caffeine has a remarkably wide margin of safety. An excessive dosage can produce convulsions, but the amount is of such magnitude as to render the clinical occurrence unlikely. At first the convulsions are epileptiform, but later they become tonic as the effect of caffeine descends to the spinal cord. The convulsive effect may be counteracted by administration of a barbiturate. A lethal dose of caffeine administered parenterally in the dog and cat is 110–175 mg/kg and 80–150 mg/kg, respectively.

AMINOPHYLLINE

Aminophylline, U.S.P. (theophylline ethylenediamine), is one of the more soluble forms of theophylline. It has a brief but potent action in stimulating diuresis. In laboratory animals theophylline has been shown to dilate the coronary blood vessels. This effect is highly beneficial because the increased blood flow that it brings to the myocardium increases the mechanical efficiency of the heart.

In recent years, it has been learned that theophylline is a potent inhibitor of phosphodiesterase, an enzyme that destroys cyclic AMP (cyclic adenosine, 3′,5′-monophosphate, or 3′, 5′ AMP). This leads to the accumulation of cyclic AMP and the stimulation of lipolysis. Consequently, the lipolytic effect of the methylxanthines, including theophylline, is related to their inhibitory activity of phosphodiesterase. In addition, it appears that the excessive accumulation of cyclic AMP in bone tissue as induced by theophylline also inhibits bone resorption of calcium, which in turn leads to the development of hypocalcemia (Luthman et al. 1972). An intravenous infusion of theophylline (1–2 mg/kg/minute for 40 minutes) induces a marked hypocalcemia in intact sheep. Moreover, the lipolytic but not the hypocalcemic effect of the theophylline in sheep could be completely inhibited by nicotinic acid (Luthman et al. 1972).

Another interesting effect of theophylline is its effect as a phase "resetter" (zeitgeber) of the body temperature of the rat (Ehret et al. 1975). When pharmacologic agents are used immediately before or during the early active phases of the circadian cycle, the rhythm may be set back; this is referred to as a phase delay. If the drugs are applied later in the cycle beyond the highest peak of the body temperature, theophylline shifts the rhythm ahead; this is referred to as a phase advance. Pentobarbital, on the other hand, by virtue of its depressant rather than stimulant effect will not shift the rhythm ahead. However, if pentobarbital is administered before or during the early active phase of the circadian cycle, the rhythm is set back or a phase delay occurs (Ehret et al. 1975). Inasmuch as theophylline and pentobarbital can alter the biological time relationship by rephasing the circadian rhythm, they are now identified as chronobiotics.

TOXICITY

Large dosages of methylxanthines are required to produce toxic effects in animals. A clinical case of aminophylline toxicity occurred in swine from the inadvertent packaging of this product by a manufacturer (Haxby 1962). The owner believed he was administering piperazine adipate to his pigs for anthelmintic purposes. After administering the recommended dosage, 5 out of a total of 8 pigs died. Some of the clinical signs of the survivors consisted of intense excitement and incoordination. In addition, the animals walked in a staggering manner and then lay down to thrash or paddle their feet (Haxby 1962).

CLINICAL USE

Although theophylline or aminophylline is not commonly used in veterinary medicine, it is sometimes recommended for "broken wind" in horses and, with cardiac glycosides, in the treatment of congestive heart failure in the dog (Haxby 1962). Aminophylline has been advocated to prevent or relieve bronchial spasm during anesthetic emergencies (Hall 1964). Limited clinical experience with the use of aminophylline in the cat indicates that it may be valuable as an adjunct to steroid therapy in the treatment of bronchial asthma. The dosage recommended is 50 mg orally every 6 hours (Carpenter 1971). In human beings aminophylline is considered one of the most effective bronchodilating agents (Ritchie 1970).

Therapeutic dosages of theophylline are unavailable in the literature. Aminophylline is administered orally in human beings in tablets of 0.25 g 3–4 times daily. The aqueous form is administered intravenously or intramuscularly in about the same dosage.

Theobromine Sodium Acetate

Theobromine Sodium Acetate is readily soluble in water, whereas theobromine is insoluble. Theobromine possesses mild central action and has little effect upon the blood vessels but exerts considerable diuretic action. Theobromine does not produce the acute diuresis observed following the use of theophylline but theobromine is used clinically as a diuretic because its action is prolonged.

The diuretic action of theobromine is less pronounced and less dependable than the mercurial diuretics but it is less toxic than the mercurials. At one time theobromine was used in edema accompanied by renal insufficiency, where the toxic action of a mercurial diuretic on the impaired kidneys had to be avoided. However, furosemide and other potent diuretic agents have lessened the need for theobromine as a diuretic agent.

Tolerance to the drug may be developed by a patient, but this can be broken by a short withdrawal period. In the human being, theobromine sodium acetate is given to produce the desired effect, although a daily dose of 3–4 g is sometimes necessary for full diuretic action.

In the dog, theobromine sodium salicylate is listed in the *British Veterinary Codex* (1965) at an oral dosage of 0.3–1 g as a diuretic in the treatment of edema of cardiac and renal origin.

CARBON DIOXIDE

Carbon Dioxide, U.S.P. (CO_2), is considered physiologically and pharmacologically to be one of the most potent stimulants of respiration. Specifically, it influences the carotid and aortic bodies, which reflexly affect the respiratory centers. In addition, CO_2 has a direct effect upon the respiratory center.

Carbon dioxide in high concentrations has been discussed as an anesthetic agent in the chapter on inhalant anesthetics and as an agent for induction of euthanasia in Section 15. Its role as a therapeutic gas has been covered in Chapter 44.

MISCELLANEOUS STIMULANTS OF TOXICOLOGICAL IMPORTANCE

Camphor

Camphor has been used for centuries in oriental medicine. It is of interest only from a toxicity standpoint. Because of its odor, camphor has been used extensively as a medicinal agent. Despite its long background of medicinal usage, camphor is of limited value as a stimulant. Traditionally, camphor in oil (20% solution) was injected intramuscularly to obtain a prolonged reflex stimulant effect upon the CNS. Experimentally, this cannot be demonstrated. Despite its long usage, it is doubtful that camphor in oil possesses any valuable stimulant action on the CNS.

Camphor can produce fatal poisoning. Deaths in children and in puppies occur from the ingestion of camphorated mothballs. Death results from respiratory paralysis.

Locally, camphor is weakly antiseptic and has a rubefacient action when applied to the skin. It is a common ingredient of many liniments.

STRYCHNINE

Although *strychnine* was once used extensively in animal and human therapeutics, it no longer has a rational place in the therapeutic armamentarium of the veterinarian or physician. Its only interest is from a veterinary toxicology standpoint because animals are sometimes poisoned inadvertently or intentionally with strychnine. For a discussion on the toxicology and the treatment of strychnine poisoning, the reader is referred to Section 15.

REFERENCES

Aizstrauts, A.; Dixon, R. T.; and Larsen, L. H. 1962. A clinical evaluation of "megimide" (bemegride) and N.P. 274 in the dog and cat. Aust Vet J 38:424.

Beretta, C.; Faustini, R.; and Gallina, G. 1973. Analeptic medication in domestic animals: Species differences observed with doxapram and combinations of it with other stimulants. Vet Rec 92:217.

Bogan, J., and Smith, H. 1968. Drugs and racing greyhounds. Vet Rec 82:658.

British Veterinary Codex. 1965. London: Pharmaceutical Press, p. 406.

Cairy, C. F., and Ramaswamy, V. M. 1962. Comparison of treatments of hemorrhagic shock under deep pentobarbital anesthesia. J Am Vet Med Assoc 140:576.

Cairy, C. F.; Leash, A.; and Sisodia, C. S. 1961. Comparison of several drugs in treating acute barbiturate depression in the dog. I. Single drugs. J Am Vet Med Assoc 138:129.

Carpenter, J. L. 1971. Bronchial asthma in cats. In R. W. Kirk, ed. Current Veterinary Therapy, 4th ed., p. 123. Philadelphia: W. B. Saunders.

Ehret, C. F.; Potter, V. R.; and Dobra, K. W. 1975. Chronotypic action of theophylline and of pentobarbital as circadian zeitgebers in the rat. Science 188:1212.

Hall, L. W. 1964. Anaesthetic accidents and emergencies. Vet Rec 76:713.

Haxby, D. L. 1962. Aminophylline poisoning in pigs. Vet Rec 74:832.

Jensen, E. C., and Klemm, W. R. 1967. Clinical evaluation of the analeptic, doxapram, in dogs and cats. J Am Vet Med Assoc 150:516.

Klemm, W. R. 1966. Evaluation of effectiveness of doxapram and various analeptic combinations in dogs. J Am Vet Med Assoc 148:894.

Luthman, J.; Jonson, G.; and Persson, J. 1972. Theophylline-induced hypocalcemia in sheep. Acta Vet Scand 13:484.

MacFarlane, A. W., and Bentley, G. A. 1957. The application of bemegride in pentobarbitone anaesthesia in the dog and cat. Vet Rec 69:304.

Ritchie, J. M. 1970. Central nervous system stimulants. II. The xanthines. In L. S. Goodman and A. Gilman, eds. The Pharmacological Basis of Therapeutics, 4th ed., p. 358. New York: Macmillan.

St. John, W. M.; Cunningham, M. H.; Johnson, J. W.; and Glasser, R. L. 1973. Pontile pneumotaxic center regulation of doxapram-induced respiratory alterations. Proc Soc Exp Biol Med 142:1215.

Short, C. E., and Cloyd, G. D. 1970. II. The use of doxapram hydrochloride with inhalation anesthetics in horses. Vet Med Small Anim Clin 65:260.

Short, C. E.; Cloyd, G. D.; and Ward, J. W. 1970. I. The use of doxapram hydrochloride with intravenous anesthetics in horses. Vet Med Small Anim Clin 65:157.

Smythies, J. R. 1974. Relationships between the chemical structure and biological activity of convulsants. Ann Rev Pharmacol 14:9.

Soma, L. R., and Kenny, R. 1967. Respiratory, cardiovascular, metabolic, and electroencephalographic effects of doxapram hydrochloride in the dog. Am J Vet Res 28:191.

Turner, A. W., and Hodgetts, V. E. 1956. Barbiturate antagonism: The use of "megimide" and of "daptazole" in curtailing "nembutal" anaesthesia, and in treating apnoeic "nembutal" intoxication in sheep. Aust Vet J 32:49.

SECTION 5

Drugs Anesthetizing the Peripheral Nerves

CHAPTER 19

LOCAL ANESTHETICS

NICHOLAS H. BOOTH

Local Anesthetic Agents
- **Procaine Hydrochloride**
- **Hexylcaine Hydrochloride**
- **Lidocaine Hydrochloride**
- **Tetracaine Hydrochloride**
- **Piperocaine Hydrochloride**
- **Phenacaine Hydrochloride**
- **Proparacaine Hydrochloride**
- **Prilocaine Hydrochloride**
- **Mepivacaine Hydrochloride**
- **Cetacaine**
- **Dyclonine Hydrochloride**

Other Local Anesthetic Agents
- **Cocaine Hydrochloride**
- **Butethamine Hydrochloride**
- **Cyclomethycaine**
- **Dibucaine Hydrochloride**
- **Naepaine Hydrochloride**

Slightly Soluble Local Anesthetics
- **Ethyl Aminobenzoate**
- **Butyl Aminobenzoate**
- **Butesin Picrate**

Local anesthetic drugs, when applied locally to nerve tissue in effective concentrations, provide relief from pain by blocking the conduction of a sensory nerve impulse from the receptor to the cortex of the brain. Contrary to the action of general anesthetics, the local anesthetics have no effect upon consciousness. Any portion of the nervous system and every type of nerve fiber can be affected by these drugs.

A local anesthetic contacting a mixed nerve trunk in sufficient concentration will paralyze the smallest fibers first because of a greater surface area exposure per unit of volume. Nerve fibers are paralyzed in the following general order when present in an exposed nerve trunk: autonomic, sensory, and motor. The sensations disappear in the following order: pain, cold, warmth, touch, joint, and deep pressure. Recovery of sensation is in the reverse order. The outstanding advantage of local anesthetics lies in a reversibility of effect; i.e., paralysis of the nerve is followed by complete recovery of function with no apparent damage to the nerve tissue.

Many drugs will paralyze nerve fibers and endings, but only a limited number can paralyze without injuring the surrounding tissues. Phenol will anesthetize tissues to which it is applied, but unfortunately it kills all forms of protoplasm. Quinine is also a general protoplasmic poison. Drugs employed clinically as local anesthetics produce a temporary and reversible paralysis of sensory nerve fibers or endings in concentrations much less than those required to affect other tissues of the body.

The first clinically significant local anesthetic to be used was cocaine. It is an alkaloid and was first obtained from the leaves of *Erythroxylon coca,* a tree indigenous to Chile, Peru, and Bolivia. The native runners of this area chewed coca leaves to allay hunger and fatigue and to produce psychic stimulation while they carried messages through the forests. Native Peruvians still use the leaf. The tree is cultivated now in several tropical countries. It was imported to Europe as a botanical curiosity. In 1860 Niemann isolated alkaloidal cocaine from the leaves of the tree. The local anesthetic effect of the alkaloid was noted but not utilized until Karl Koller used cocaine to anesthetize the eye in 1884. Thereafter, cocaine was accepted as a local anesthetic. It was used in dental and surgical procedures by the methods of infiltration and nerve blocking. In 1885 Corning injected cocaine intrathecally (intraspinally) in a dog and paralyzed the posterior spinal nerves to produce spinal anesthesia. It was nearly 15 years later before the technique was successfully employed on human beings. Also in 1885 cocaine was first successfully used for nerve blocks of the limbs in the horse by McLean, a veterinarian of Meadville, Pennsylvania.

The chemical structure and final synthesis of cocaine were completed in 1902 by Willstätter. It became apparent that cocaine possessed at least two undesirable properties, namely, a marked toxicity and drug addiction. Chemists began searching for substitutes for cocaine that possessed the local anesthetic properties of this compound. Three years later, Einhorn synthesized procaine hydrochloride. Many other preparations have been synthesized for use as local anesthetics. No local anesthetic is entirely free from undesirable properties. Many differ little in therapeutic efficacy. Procaine hydrochloride has been accepted and used more widely than any other local anesthetic.

TYPES OF LOCAL ANESTHESIA

Local anesthesia is produced in several ways. *Surface* or *topical anesthesia* results when the drug is applied to the skin or mucous membrane to cause loss of sensation by paralyzing the sensory nerve endings. Local anesthetics are widely used on mucous membranes of the eye, nose, and mouth. They are ineffectively used on the unbroken skin because the cornified epidermis limits penetration.

Infiltration anesthesia is perhaps the most common method of producing local anesthesia. This method consists of making numerous subcutaneous injections of small volumes of a local anesthetic solution into the tissues. The anesthetic diffuses into surrounding tissue from the site of injection and anesthetizes the nerve fibers and endings. Large amounts of relatively dilute solutions are often infiltrated into operative sites.

Conduction or *nerve-block anesthesia* is produced by injecting a local anesthetic solution into the immediate vicinity of a nerve. The anesthetic diffuses to the nerve trunk and anesthetizes the area innervated by preventing any further conduction of nerve impulses along the nerve. A small amount of local anesthetic solution of relatively high concentration is used for nerve-block anesthesia.

Epidural or *extradural anesthesia* is produced by injecting a local anesthetic solution into the epidural space of the spinal canal posterior to the end of the spinal cord. The needle is usually inserted into the first intercoccygeal space. The local anesthetic acts upon the posterior spinal nerves before they leave the vertebral column and are distributed to the posterior body.

Paravertebral anesthesia is a special form of conduction anesthesia wherein the local anesthetic is applied to the spinal nerves as they emerge from the intervertebral foramina.

Intrathecal or *spinal anesthesia* is seldom used to induce local anesthesia in animals. Intrathecal anesthesia has been accomplished in sheep by injecting the local anesthetic into the spinal fluid. Frequently, intrathecal or spinal anesthesia is confused with epidural or extradural anesthesia or vice versa.

Regional anesthesia is a term used rather loosely to refer to anesthesia of a large area or region. It may be produced by several methods, including epidural, intrathecal, paravertebral, or conduction anesthesia.

Local anesthesia may occur in ways other than by the administration of drugs to paralyze sensory nerve fibers or endings. Local anesthesia was practiced centuries ago by application of pressure to nerve trunks. Pressure upon blood vessels also was used to produce a tissue ischemia that resulted in local anesthesia. In both cases the affected area was peripheral to the point where pressure was applied.

The application of cold *(refrigeration anesthesia)* has been employed during recent years for regional anesthesia of an appendage or local anesthesia of a tissue. Local anesthesia of small and superficial areas of the body results from spraying some highly volatile liquid such as ethyl chloride onto the skin. It evaporates very rapidly and, in doing so, absorbs heat from the skin. The superficial layers of tissue are frozen and insensitive. The duration of insensibility is brief but adequate for minor incision. This "freezing" of the skin is followed by the typical sensation experienced from a frostbite.

REQUIREMENTS OF AN IDEAL LOCAL ANESTHETIC

The ideal local anesthetic would possess many desirable properties. It should produce a reversible paralysis of the sensory nerves but not of other tissues. The agent should have nonaddictive properties. It should be readily soluble and stable in water. The local anesthetic should possess a pH near neutrality and be nonirritating to the tissues. It should possess a minimum of systemic local toxicity, as evidenced by absence of tissue damage at the injection site. The local anesthetic should be absorbed slowly to minimize danger of systemic toxicity and to prolong the effect at the site of injection. After systemic absorption, the compound should be readily and rapidly detoxified. It should be compatible with epinephrine so that its anesthetic action might be prolonged by this or some other vasoconstrictor. There should be no hyperesthesia following the recovery of sensation by the tissues. The local anesthetic should withstand heat sterilization and be relatively inexpensive.

MODE OF ACTION

Local anesthetics are generally water-soluble acid salts. When these salts are injected into the slightly alkaline body tissues, they appear to hydrolyze slowly, releasing the alkaloidal base, which then acts upon the nerve tissue. *In vitro,* a small amount of alkali added to a solution of a local anesthetic increases its anesthetic potency. After alkalinization, the solution becomes turbid and the free base precipitates out.

Alkalinization of anesthetic solutions to increase their potency is not a practical procedure. Nevertheless, this reaction is believed to occur in the tissue fluids. Clinical confirmation is found in the inability of local anesthetics to anesthetize when injected into tissues having an acid reaction from the accumulation of pus. The accumulation of pus with a slightly acid pH prevents hydrolysis of the acid salt and the freeing of the potent alkaloidal base. This is confirmed circumstantially by the observation that an abscessed area is difficult or impossible to anesthetize thoroughly.

The manner in which the alkaloidal base of a local anesthetic interferes with the ability of nerves to conduct an impulse is better understood now than a decade ago. Local anesthetics decrease cell membrane permeability. The amino groups of the classic local anesthetic drugs, such as procaine and others, interact with the polar groups of the cell membrane to decrease membrane permeability of the nerve cell and to stabilize the membrane forces. As a result, the diffusion of postassium and sodium ions cannot occur, and the changes that give rise to the nerve impulse are blocked. With the cell membrane of nerve cells stabilized in the resting state, the generation and transmission of the nerve impulse cannot occur.

Another mechanism of importance, along with the stabilization of the cell membrane and the lack of sodium and potassium ion diffusion, involves the influence of local anesthetics upon membrane calcium. Many authoritative sources indicate that both calcium and local anesthetics have a stabilization effect upon excitable membranes. For example, the threshold of electrical stimulation of the membrane is elevated by calcium and local anesthetics.

Consequently, there is a blockade in the transmission or conduction of nerve impulses with no change in the resting membrane potential. It has been suspected that calcium has a crucial role in the generation of the nerve impulse (Ritchie and Greengard 1966). Speculation suggests that it is the displacement or removal of calcium ions from the nerve membrane sites by depolarization that results in a transient increase in the permeability of the cell membrane to sodium ions during the action potential. Calcium ions and local anesthetics act upon the same mechanism that is necessary for the conveyance of sodium ions through the nerve cell membrane. As previously discussed under the Mode of Action of General Anesthetics in Chapter 10, all anesthetic agents, including local anesthetics, produce deformation or expansion of the cell membrane that results in anesthesia (Seeman 1972). The alteration in the membrane Ca^{++} may be responsible for this.

FATE

The liver is the most important organ involved in the destruction of local anesthetics after absorption. The rate of destruction varies greatly and is the major factor in determining the safety of any anesthetic. From a practical standpoint, the toxicity of a local anesthetic is determined by the ratio between the rate of absorption and the rate of destruction. Differences between various local anesthetics in rate of absorption can be reduced by the use of a vasoconstrictor such as epinephrine in the anesthetic solution.

Local anesthetics can be divided into two general groups: those detoxified rapidly (e.g., procaine); and those detoxified slowly (e.g., cocaine). One LD50 of the former may be detoxified in the body in about 20 minutes, whereas 1 LD50 of the latter may require about 60 minutes. Variation in the rate of detoxification by the liver and other tissues of the body is one of the main reasons for varying toxicities among local anesthetics.

TOXICITY

Lethal doses of local anesthetics vary widely, but the signs of toxicity are the same. The symptoms arise primarily from stimulation of the central nervous system (CNS) and consist chiefly of restlessness and muscular tremors that progress into clonic convulsions. Depression follows the stimulation. Death usually results from respiratory failure. Susceptibility to convulsions is related to the degree of development of the CNS; primates are more susceptible than other species (Strobel and Wollman 1969).

Resuscitory measures include (1) a short-acting barbiturate for intravenous injection to control the CNS stimulation and (2) a source of oxygen for promoting respiration exchange. When barbiturates are administered prophylactically, the LD50 of a local anesthetic is increased 3–4 times.

When infiltrating a local anesthetic into vascular areas, there is a constant hazard of making an intravenous injection. Immediately after an intravenous injection, premonitory signs of death from respiratory paralysis may appear. After the tissues have been penetrated by the hypodermic needle, the plunger of the syringe should be aspirated slightly to determine that the needle is not within a blood vessel.

An elevated ambient temperature may influence the toxicity of drugs, including the local anesthetics (Weihe 1973). Drug absorption following the infiltration of a local anesthetic into the tissues may be affected by environmental temperature extremes. For example, an analgesic blocking dose of procaine hydrochloride may produce violent convulsive seizures in young puppies when it is used in tail docking during hot weather.

In domestic animals, deaths caused by local anesthetics are uncommon. Stimulation of the CNS, pronounced muscular tremors, and muscular weakness are observed in animals following the injection of local anesthetics (Jones 1951a). For example, death is produced in a cat if procaine hydrochloride (45 mg/kg) is injected rapidly by the intravenous route, whereas the same animal can tolerate a dose 10 times this amount when the drug is administered slowly (Ott 1969).

POTENTIATION BY VASOCONSTRICTORS

Constriction of blood capillaries near the site of injection of a local anesthetic decreases the rate of absorption and thereby prolongs the period of action of the local anesthetic. Addition of epinephrine hydrochloride or other vasoconstrictors to a solution of the drug will prolong the action of a local anesthetic. Cocaine is an exception in that it constricts blood vessels itself and therefore delays its own absorption. A vasoconstrictor is never administered with cocaine. The sterile 1:1000 solution of epinephrine hydrochloride is added to a local anesthetic solution following sterilization and shortly before use. A concentration of 1 part of epinephrine in 50,000 parts of local anesthetic solution should not be exceeded, and 1 in 100,000 is preferred. For intracutaneous injection, a concentration of 1 part of epinephrine in 200,000 parts of local anesthetic solution gives longer duration of anesthesia.

In addition to prolonging the anesthetic action, a vasoconstrictor decreases the toxicity of a local anesthetic by delaying absorption and preventing high blood concentrations. Slower absorption provides more time for destruction of a local anesthetic by the tissues of the body. Thus a toxic concentration in the bloodstream is less probable.

POTENTIATION BY HYALURONIDASE

Hyaluronic acid is a viscous polysaccharide found in the interstitial spaces of the tissues, where it normally obstructs the diffusion of foreign materials. Hyaluronidase, a mucolytic enzyme, hydrolyzes hyaluronic acid and increases the diffusion of injected substances. Normally, the injection of a solution into the tissue provides sufficient interstitial pressure to promote diffusion of the injected material. Within limits, the rate at which an injected substance diffuses through tissues is proportional to the amount of hyaluronidase. The area through which it diffuses is proportional to the volume of solution injected. The natural tissue barrier of hyaluronic acid is partly restored in 24 hours and completely restored in 48 hours.

Hyaluronidase solution should not be injected into inflamed tissue because it will promote spreading of microorganisms.

INFILTRATION ANESTHESIA

Hyaluronidase may be added to local anesthetic solutions injected subcutaneously to promote tissue diffusion and thereby to increase the area of skin anesthetized (Table 19.1). This enzyme decreases the duration of anesthesia, apparently as the result of more extensive absorption of the local anesthetic (Table 19.2). The increased absorption can be counteracted by the addition of epinephine to the solution. Presumably, the vasoconstrictor decreases the absorption of hyaluronidase, thus permitting it to exert its maximal spreading

TABLE 19.1. Spreading effect of hyaluronidase on procaine injected subcutaneously

Number of Subjects	Solution Injected	Average Area of Skin Anesthesia
		(sq cm)
28	Procaine 1% (3 ml)	8.8
25	Procaine 1% + hyaluronidase (1.6 mg %)	15.7
13	Procaine 1% + hyaluronidase + epinephrine (1–100,000)	17.5

Source: Kirby et al. 1950.

TABLE 19.2. Effect of hyaluronidase and epinephrine on duration of anesthesia

Number of Subjects	Solution Injected	Average Duration of Anesthesia to Pinprick
		(min)
28	Procaine (1%)	32
25	Procaine + hyaluronidase (3.2 mg %)	23
13	Procaine + epinephrine (1–100,000)	188
13	Procaine + hyaluronidase + epinephrine	180

Source: Kirby et al. 1950.

action. The overall effect of adding hyaluronidase and epinephrine (1:100,000) to a solution of procaine hydrochloride for subcutaneous infiltration is roughly to double the skin area anesthetized and to increase the duration of anesthesia by about 5 times (Kirby et al. 1950).

A concentration of 150 units (turbidity reducing units) per 100 ml of local anesthetic solution seems to be as effective as twice that amount.

Conduction Anesthesia

Eckenhoff and Kirby (1951) investigated the effectiveness of hyaluronidase in promoting diffusion of a local anesthetic into nerve trunks. These investigators found that hyaluronidase did not increase the incidence of successful nerve blocks. The addition of hyaluronidase to a solution of local anesthetic is not a substitute for anatomical knowledge in conduction anesthesia. Moore (1950) reached much the same conclusion after the use of hyaluronidase in a large series of nerve-block anesthesias. However, adequate nerve blocks could be produced with smaller volumes of local anesthetic when hyaluronidase was incorporated into the anesthetic solution.

Clinical Disadvantages

The rapid spreading effect produced by hyaluronidase may enhance the absorption and toxicity of local anesthetics. This effect plus the relatively high cost of using the enzyme preparation has limited the use of hyaluronidase in veterinary medicine.

LOCAL ANESTHETIC AGENTS

Procaine Hydrochloride

CHEMISTRY

Procaine Hydrochloride, U.S.P. (Novocain), is a white crystalline powder dissolving in an equal weight of water (Fig. 19.1). It is relatively stable while exposed to the air and also in aqueous solution. Solutions of procaine hydrochloride can be sterilized repeatedly by boiling without loss of anesthetic potency. However, alkalis and their carbonates, tannic acid, and various metals are incompatible with procaine hydrochloride. Solutions should not be boiled in metal vessels or in glass that contains alkali. Nonalkaline, heat-resistant glasswares should be used. If the water for dissolving procaine contains carbon dioxide, deterioration occurs. A minor degree of deterioration in a solution of procaine hydrochloride is indicated by a yellowish tint. A distinct yellowing or a darkening of the solution indicates that it should be discarded.

The preceding remarks on stability and coloration do not apply to a solution of procaine hydrochloride containing epinephrine. Epinephrine hydrochloride is

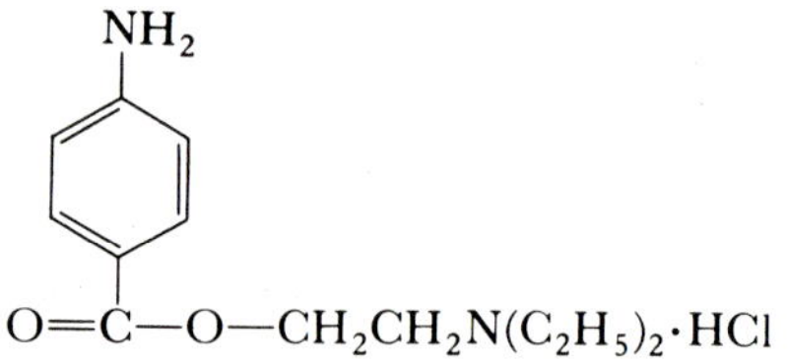

NH_2

$O{=}C{-}O{-}CH_2CH_2N(C_2H_5)_2 \cdot HCl$

Procaine Hydrochloride

Fig. 19.1.

very sensitive to the influence of heat, air, and sunlight, so that decomposition occurs rapidly from boiling and also from exposure to air and sunlight. A pinkish discoloration, i.e., the formation of adrenochrome, is the first sign of decomposition of epinephrine. Epinephrine hydrochloride in sterile solution is added to a procaine solution after the procaine has been sterilized.

A solution of procaine hydrochloride in water has a pH of approximately 6.0. After standing, the solution becomes more acid. Procaine hydrochloride may be dissolved in either water or physiological saline for subcutaneous injection. The amount of tissue irritation following injection is determined by the tissue osmotic pressure changes, by the pH of the solution, and by preservatives that may be added to the preparation.

ACTION

Procaine was synthesized after cocaine was discovered to be habit forming and relatively toxic. Procaine hydrochloride is the most widely used and the most satisfactory of all the local anesthetics. A large number of local anesthetic compounds have been studied and, in general, there appears to be an increased toxicity associated with increased anesthetic efficiency. Procaine is not as active as cocaine. However, it is considerably less toxic than cocaine and most other commonly used local anesthetics.

The solution of procaine hydrochloride is nonirritant and promptly effective when injected subcutaneously. Anesthesia is relatively brief because the drug is absorbed rapidly and destroyed quickly by the liver. Anesthesia with procaine is commonly prolonged by the addition of a vasoconstrictor to the solution to delay absorption of the local anesthetic from the site of injection.

METABOLISM

Procaine is hydrolyzed primarily in the liver and, to some extent, in other tissues of the body. In the cat the liver is responsible for up to 40% of the procaine

NH_2 (benzene ring) $CO \cdot OCH_2CH_2N(C_2H_5)_2$ $\xrightarrow{(HOH)}$ NH_2 (benzene ring) $COOH$

Procaine PABA

$+ \ HOCH_2CH_2—N(C_2H_5)_2$

Diethylaminoethanol

FIG. 19.2.

metabolization. An enzyme hydrolyzes procaine to *p*-aminobenzoic acid (PABA) and diethylaminoethanol. The enzyme, procaine esterase, is the same as plasma cholinesterase (Kalow 1952). The kidneys play no significant part in the reduction of procaine blood levels, but they excrete PABA rapidly and to a considerable extent.

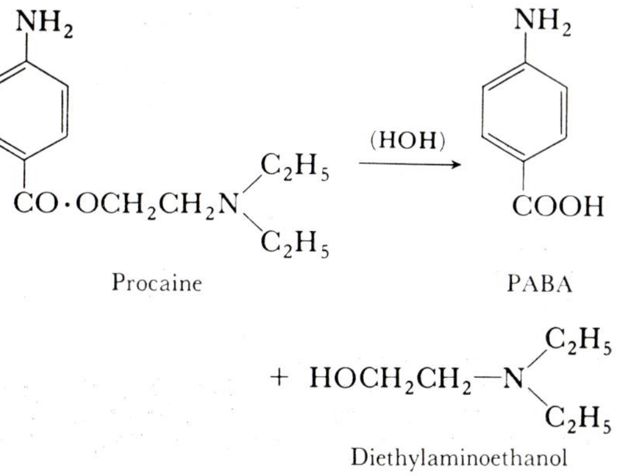

PABA exhibits no local anesthetic action. Diethylaminoethanol possesses only a part of the full anesthetic activity of procaine. (See Fig. 19.2.)

COMPARATIVE ANESTHETIC POTENCY

Information on the clinical effectiveness of four common local anesthetics is given in Table 19.3 for intracutaneous, subcutaneous, corneal, and conduction anesthesia. The comparative potency of the local anesthetics is listed for cattle (Table 19.4).

TOXICITY

A rapid intravenous injection of procaine (45 mg/kg) in the *cat* or *rabbit* produces a lethal effect; if the drug is administered slowly or by the subcutaneous route, the dose required to produce death is about 10 times greater.

The greatest difference between the toxicities of procaine hydrochloride and a potent local anesthetic such as cocaine hydrochloride is the rate of metabolism. Cocaine is slowly metabolized, whereas procaine hydrochloride is rapidly detoxified by the liver. An LD50 of procaine hydro-

TABLE 19.3. Comparative anesthetic potency of four common local anesthetics

Drug	Threshold Anesthetic Concentrations			Duration of Anesthesia			Toxicity in Rabbits	
	(1)	(2)	(3)	(4)	(5)	(6)	(7)	(8)
		(%)			*(min)*		*(mg/kg)*	
Procaine	0.250	4.0	0.04	0–2	16	171	460	55
Butacaine	0.125	0.31	0.02	30	45	200	50	12
Dibucaine	0.004	0.003	0.0025	51*	100	221	10	2.5
Cocaine	0.125	0.32	0.02	22	12	...	126	15

Source: Goodman and Gilman 1955.
Note: (1) Sensory nerve block (frog sciatic); (2) rabbit cornea; (3) intracutaneous wheal (human); (4) rabbit cornea—1% solution; (5) intracutaneous (human) 0.5%; (6) intracutaneous (human) 0.5% + epinephrine 1:50,000; (7) subcutaneous LD50; (8) intravenous LD50.

chloride is detoxified in the cat within 20 minutes, whereas an LD50 of cocaine is metabolized in 60 minutes.

The use of procaine when the ambient temperature is high may lead to increased absorption from subcutaneous infiltration sites to the extent that CNS stimulation or convulsions occur. Vasoconstrictor agents should be employed with the local anesthetic to reduce or prevent this problem. If convulsions occur, the use of ultrashort-acting barbiturates intravenously to effect are indicated. Should shock and respiratory complications develop, the administration of oxygen and the application of supportive therapy to correct these complications will be required.

When injected alone in high concentration, procaine produces a fall in blood pressure. However, a small dose of procaine given in conjunction with epinephrine causes a rise in blood pressure higher than that produced by epinephrine alone.

Table 19.5 gives average minimum lethal dose (MLD) data for procaine hydrochloride in four species of animals.

TABLE 19.4. Comparative potency of some local anesthetics* in cattle

Mode of Administration	Anesthetic	Number of Animals	Average Duration
			(hr)
Epidural	Hexylcaine	8	4.9
	Lidocaine	11	4.2
	Pyribenzamine	10	4.3
	Procaine	8	1.7
Paravertebral	Hexylcaine	9	5.2
	Lidocaine	8	4.3
	Pyribenzamine	8	4.7
	Procaine	9	2.0
Infiltration	Hexylcaine	9	3.3
	Lidocaine	8	2.7
	Pyribenzamine	...	2.9
	Procaine	...	1.6

Source: Link and Smith 1956.
* Although not stated in the publication, it is assumed that all local anesthetics used were hydrochloride salts.
The concentration of each local anesthetic was 2 percent in 1:100,000 epinephrine hydrochloride. Dose levels were approximately 1.25 ml/100 lb of body weight when injected epidurally and 7 ml in the vicinity of each nerve when injected paravertebrally. Although the quantity was not given, the volume of each local anesthetic infiltrated into the tissues was the same in all experiments.

CONTRAINDICATIONS

Large quantities of anesthetic solution injected into the lumbosacral space of the dog or cat will generally produce a marked drop in systemic arterial pressure, especially if the preparations do not contain vasoconstrictor drugs. Because of this potential hazard, epidural anesthesia in the dog or cat is contraindicated where shock may be a major factor during or following surgery (Ott 1969).

TABLE 19.5. Average minimum lethal dose of procaine hydrochloride (g/kg)

Species	Route of Administration	
	Subcutaneous	Intravenous
Guinea pig	0.43	0.05
Rabbit	0.46	0.055
Cat	0.45	0.045
Dog	0.25	...

Source: Graubard and Peterson 1950.

Procaine is contraindicated in the parakeet because of its lethal effect.

CLINICAL USE

Local anesthesia by tissue infiltration with a procaine hydrochloride solution is a routine clinical technique employed for the relief of pain. The majority of these clinical applications are to relieve pain of the skin. Anesthesia is produced by anesthetizing a major nerve supply of specific areas, such as perineural injection of the mandibular nerve for a dental operation in the dog (Ott 1969), of the cornual nerve for dehorning in the goat (Mitchell 1966) or cow (Gabel 1964), and of the last thoracic and first two lumbar nerves on the left side for rumenotomy or cesarean section in the cow (Farquharson 1940). Procaine is also used to induce analgesia or anesthesia for tail docking in the lamb (Bradley 1966) or dog, for nerve blocks in the bovine foot (Raker 1956; Gabel 1964), and for enucleation of the eye in cattle referred to as the Peterson eye block (Gabel 1964). In recent years, procaine has been used intravenously to produce retrograde regional anesthesia of the forelimbs of ruminants (Manohar et al. 1971; Tyagi et al. 1973). Actually the technique of intravenous regional anesthesia into a limb whose circulation has been disrupted by a tourniquet is not new because it was used in human beings almost seven decades ago.

In cattle, procaine is used epidurally to produce anesthesia for obstetrical procedures and perineal operations. Its use in small animals has not been as frequent because of the problem with restraint of the animal during surgery. In animal surgery, credit for using epidural anesthesia belongs to Retzgen, Pape, Pitzschk, and Silbersiepe of the Berlin Clinic; they published reports on the technique in 1925. During the next year, Benesch of Austria, while pursuing graduate studies at Cornell University, demonstrated epidural anesthesia in cattle at the national AVMA meeting in Lexington, Kentucky. In 1927–1929, Frank of Kansas State University developed the epidural technique in the horse. For additional information pertaining to epidural anesthesia, the reader is referred to Chapter 20.

Procaine hydrochloride is used in veterinary medicine for infiltration, conduction, and epidural anesthesia. For infiltration in small animals, a concentration of 1% is generally employed, whereas in larger animals 2% is preferable. About 2–5 ml of a 2% solution are used for nerve-block or conduction anesthesia in small animals. In large animals, 5–10 ml of a 4% solution are most commonly employed for this purpose. Epinephrine hydrochloride solution may be added to give a concentration of 1:100,000, i.e., 1 ml of epinephrine hydrochloride solution (1:1000), to each 99 ml of anesthetic solution.

Procaine hydrochloride is rarely used for surface anesthesia because it is less effective than other local anesthetics. However, high concentrations of 10%–20% of procaine will produce brief surface anesthesia of the eye, the ureter, and similar tissue surfaces.

INTRAVENOUS INJECTION

In the dog and human beings, intravenous injection of procaine hydrochloride depresses cardiac irritability induced by general anesthetics and thereby decreases the incidence of cardiac arrhythmia and ventricular fibrillation. This effect of procaine led to the development of *Procainamide Hydrochloride,* U.S.P., which is used prophylactically and therapeutically for treatment of cardiac arrhythmias occurring in heart disease or from general anesthesia. Inasmuch as procainamide is classified as an antiarrhythmic agent, additional information is provided in Chapter 24.

Intravenous procaine hydrochloride has been used as a treatment of spasmodic colic in horses (MacKellar 1967) and is suited to this type (i.e., "spasmodic") of colic. This terminology means that the animal has intermittent acute pain, elevated pulse and respiratory rates, usually violent borborygmal sounds, an empty rectum, and no signs of impaction of the lower intestinal tract. The etiologic factors can frequently be related to a sudden change of feed or water supply, overfeeding, or overwatering, particularly after prolonged exercise. Upon making a diagnosis of spasmodic colic, MacKellar (1967) administers procaine hydrochloride by a slow intravenous injection in the form of a 5% solution at the rate of 0.6–0.8 ml/100 lb. No adverse effects have been noted at this dose level except a slight increase in heart rate. Without any other treatment, relief of pain is apparent in 5–10 minutes; return of the appetite appears in 10–15 minutes (MacKellar 1967). MacKellar has concluded that this form of treatment is simple and enables the common type of colic to be dealt with rapidly in one call.

Procaine hydrochloride was used intravenously quite frequently at one time in the treatment of intractable pain in human beings. It was employed particularly in treatment of inflammatory conditions such as arthritis, neuritis, and bursitis.

In veterinary medicine, it was used intravenously in control of pruritus of various types in dogs (Pickett 1951). Clinical analgesia occurs irregularly in dogs and only following excessive dosages (Jones 1951a). The analgesia produced in a dog by procaine given intravenously does not seem to parallel that observed in human patients. On the contrary, reactions to painful stimuli may be exaggerated in the dog (Allen and Safford 1948).

Use of procaine intravenously in human patients appears to have declined recently. The side effects of tachycardia, dyspnea, anxiety, and disorientation contraindicate its use (Ritchie et al. 1970).

STIMULANT ACTION

The horse seems to be more sensitive to the CNS stimulation of procaine hydrochloride than other species of domestic animals. Reactions of a horse stimulated with procaine resemble those of a horse doped with an opiate. Considerably larger doses are necessary to produce central stimulation in the cow, whereas the pig falls intermediately between the horse and the cow (Jones 1951b).

Due to its CNS stimulant and analgesic actions, procaine has been used illegally in race animals to improve their performance and/or to mask lamenesses in track and racing events. For years procaine was the most common agent detected following a race. As pointed out in Chapter 18, the likelihood of an animal winning a race under the effects of stimulant drugs is improbable. The unscrupulous use of procaine or other blocking agents to mask lameness in horses is an occasional problem in horses offered for sale. The veterinarian must be alert to this possibility when examining a horse for soundness.

HEXYLCAINE HYDROCHLORIDE

Hexylcaine Hydrochloride, N.F. (Cyclaine), is approved by the Food and Drug Administration (FDA) for use as a long-lasting anesthetic for epidural anesthesia of mature cattle, horses, and dogs. It is approved for infiltration anesthesia ("field blocking") in cattle, horses, and dogs and for nerve-block anesthesia in cattle and horses.

CHEMISTRY

Hexylcaine hydrochloride (Fig. 19.3) is soluble in water to a concentration of 12%. The 1% solution is stable to boiling and autoclaving for sterilization. This solution is clear and colorless. It can be stored for 3 months at room temperature in indirect sunlight with no apparent change in appearance or effectivness. The pH of the 1% solution is 3.9.

DURATION

Hexylcaine is reported to be 4–8 times as active as procaine in producing conduction or nerve-block anesthesia. In-

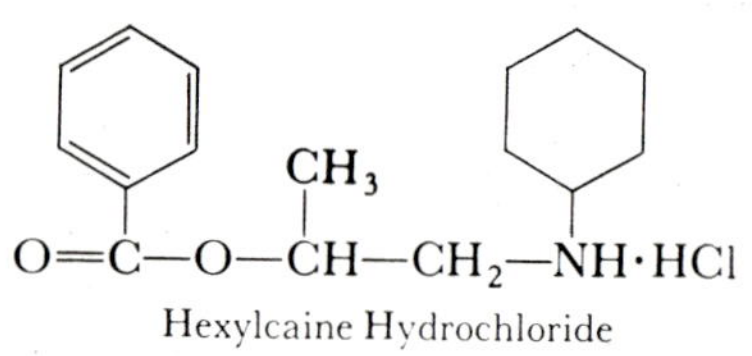

$$O{=}C{-}O{-}CH(CH_3){-}CH_2{-}NH{\cdot}HCl$$

Hexylcaine Hydrochloride

FIG. 19.3.

vestigations by Orkin and Rovenstine (1952) indicated that hexylcaine is hydrolyzed slower than procaine. This may explain its prolonged action.

TOXICITY

Intravenously, hexylcaine compares with piperocaine and cocaine in lethal toxicity. Subcutaneously, hexylcaine is slightly more toxic than piperocaine. Subconvulsive dosages cause ataxia, salivation, and vomition. Convulsions produced by larger doses may be controlled by a barbiturate given intravenously.

CLINICAL USE

Hexylcaine is used for production of nerve-block anesthesia and topical anesthesia. It ranks with cocaine in effectiveness as a topical anesthetic. Solutions are available in concentrations of 5% and 1% for topical and infiltration use, respectively.

Hexylcaine has been used in posterior epidural anesthesia in the cow. An injection of 100 mg (5 ml of 2% or 10 ml of 1% solution) produces satisfactory anesthesia. Also, in cattle, dose levels of 1.25 ml/100 lb of body weight of a 2% solution in 1:100,000 epinephrine hydrochloride produces epidural anesthesia lasting an average of 4.9 hours (Link and Smith 1956).

Hexylcaine has been used for paravertebral nerve blocks in the cow with an injection of 5–7 ml of a 1%–2% solution around each nerve (Table 19.4). Rumenotomy and cesarean section are performed satisfactorily under this anesthesia (Wheat 1952).

In the dog (depending upon its size), epidural anesthesia is accomplished with 0.5–2 ml of a 5% solution and lasts 6–12 hours (Bone and Peck 1956).

DOSAGE

In accordance with the *Code of Federal Regulations,* 135b. 90, April 1, 1974, the dose level for epidural anesthesia in mature cattle is 0.2–0.6 mg/lb, in horses is 0.2–0.4 mg/lb, and in dogs is 0.5–1 mg/lb. For infiltration anesthesia, a 1% or 2% solution is recommended in appropriate dosages to produce the desired effect.

LIDOCAINE

Lidocaine, U.S.P. (Xylocaine, lignocaine) (α-diethylaminoaceto-2,6-xylidide), is a white or slightly yellow powder with a characteristic odor. It is relatively stable but nearly insoluble in water. Lidocaine hydrochloride is available as a sterile aqueous solution from 0.5% to 5% with or without epinephrine and in a gel preparation from 2.5% to 5%.

METABOLISM AND FATE

Lidocaine is metabolized primarily in the liver at a rate nearly as rapid as that for procaine. The unchanged form is excreted in the urine of the dog (McMahon and Woods 1951) in a concentration of 10%–20%.

There is no evidence *in vivo* that hydrolysis of the amide linkage or oxidation of the ortho-methyl groups occurs. A large amount of lidocaine is conjugated with sulfate and excreted in this form.

Following the intravenous administration of lidocaine (10 mg/kg) in pregnant guinea pigs, it rapidly crosses the placenta (Finster et al. 1972). High concentrations are found in the fetal liver, heart, and brain. The liver of the fetal guinea pig is the only organ in which lidocaine was found in higher concentration than in the maternal subject. High myocardial levels of the drug in the fetus may possibly account for the marked depressant effects that local anesthetics produce.

The kinetics and oral absorption rate of lidocaine have been determined in the dog (Boyes et al. 1970); 78% of the administered dose of lidocaine reaches the general circulation. Emesis occurs regularly at 2.5 hours after the administration of lidocaine.

ACTION

Lidocaine hydrochloride is a water-soluble, local anesthetic that produces more prompt, potent, and extensive anesthesia than an equal concentration of procaine hydrochloride; in fact, the anesthetic potency and area of anesthesia are about twice those of procaine hydrochloride.

Lidocaine hydrochloride is used for infiltration, nerve conduction, epidural, and topical anesthesia. Depending on the concentration of solution and the procedure, the onset of mucosal anesthesia appears in about 5 minutes and the effect persists for 30 minutes or more.

Lidocaine hydrochloride is effective at about one-half the concentration of procaine. For infiltration anesthesia, 0.5% is normally used in small animals and 1% in large animals with a 1:100,000 solution of epinephrine hydrochloride. For conduction anesthesia, a concentration of 1%–2% in small animals and 2%–3% in large animals is used, usually with a vasoconstrictor. In the horse 50 and 30 ml of a 2% solution are effective in blocking the thoracic and pelvic limbs, respectively (Getty et al. 1956). A concentration of 1%–2% lidocaine hydrochloride is suggested for epidural injections, although 50 ml of 3% have been used in the cow without toxicity and with good clinical effect.

CLINICAL USE

In Dogs and Cats. The epidural use of lidocaine hydrochloride (1 ml of a 2% solution per 10 lb or 20 mg/10 lb) will block cranially to lumbar vertebra 1 (L_1) and 1 ml of a 2% solution per 7.5 lb (20 mg/7.5 lb) will block to thoracic vertebra 5 (T_5) in the "average" dog or cat (Klide and Soma 1968). According to Klide and Soma, the onset of epidural analgesia with lidocaine is relatively rapid (3–12 minutes) and the duration of action is 45–90 minutes. In the treatment of cardiac arrhythmia, lidocaine is used intravenously at the rate of 2 mg/kg every 20–30 minutes (McDonell 1972). Also, after defibrillation of the canine, lidocaine (0.5 mg/lb) is administered intravenously to control arrhythmias (Paddleford and Short 1973). Lidocaine has been recommended for use as a topical anesthetic for endotracheal intubation in the cat (Lawson 1965). Following general anesthesia, the vocal cords as well as the immediate parts of the larynx are sprayed with lidocaine hydrochloride (total of 20 mg) using an aerosol device; within 30 seconds the vocal cords are anesthetized and the intubation is easily accomplished.

In Pigs, Goats, and Sheep. In the pig, the dose of lidocaine required to produce epidural anesthesia to T_{10} to permit a laparotomy has been determined (Strande 1968). Dosage was determined by the length (in cm) of the animal measured from the external occipital protuberance to the first coccygeal vertebra. The recommended dose of 2% lidocaine up to 40 cm in length is 1 ml; after this an additional 1.5 ml are administered for every 10 cm increase in the vertebral column of the pig. This dose-length relationship also applies to the dog (Strande 1968).

Lidocaine hydrochloride (1% or 2%) has been used in cornual nerve blocks of the goat; 2 ml of the local anesthetic are injected at each site to block the lacrimal and infratrochlear branches of the cornual nerve (Mitchell 1966). In adult sheep, lidocaine (2%) has been used for epidural anesthesia (Hopcroft 1967). About 10 minutes prior to the epidural injection, a phenothiazine tranquilizer such as chlorpromazine hydrochloride (25–50 mg) is administered intramuscularly. The dose of lidocaine varies from 8 to 12 ml; onset of anesthesia occurs 2–10 minutes after the injection. The analgesia produced by lidocaine in sheep is preceded by a short period of muscular twitching, which is followed by profound relaxation. Hopcroft (1967) performed operations up to 80 minutes in duration with excellent analgesia; after the surgery, recovery required 1.5 hours.

For use as a spinal (intrathecal) anesthetic, a 2% lidocaine solution (5 ml) is injected into the lumbosacral space of sheep (Grono 1966). Anesthesia lasts an average of more than an hour.

In Cattle. In cattle, lidocaine is preferred for a number of surgical procedures in conjunction with tranquilizers (Gabel 1964; Heinze 1970). For low epidural analgesia, 4 ml of a 2% solution has been used without and with 1:80,000 epinephrine (Rülcker 1965). The duration of analgesia without and with epinephrine was 96 ± 10 and 116 ± 14 minutes, respectively; there was no significant difference statistically ($P < 0.05$). In cattle where high epidural analgesia was produced, 60 ml of a 2% lidocaine hydrochloride solution were used (Rülcker 1965); this dose produced recumbency in all animals. Analgesia lasted 220–360 minutes. For anesthesia with lidocaine involving the lower portion of the limbs of cattle, a tourniquet is placed around the limb just below or above the hock (Weaver 1972). Then 10–20 ml of 2% lidocaine hydrochloride are injected into any superficial vein below the tourniquet. According to Weaver, rapid anesthesia develops and normal sensation and limb movements return about 5 minutes after release of the tourniquet.

In Horses. Lidocaine is probably the most commonly used local anesthetic for nerve blocks in the equine (Owen 1973). Ten to 20 ml of 2% xylocaine block the mandibular nerve and desensitize the mandible, lower molars, incisors, and lower lips. Blockade of other major nerves usually does not require as great a volume of anesthetic.

TOXICITY

When injected without epinephrine, sufficient lidocaine is absorbed from the site of a nerve block or regional anesthesia to depress the CNS, producing a general drowsiness. Local irritation is rare. Overdosage will cause muscular twitching, hypotension, nausea, and vomition.

The toxicity of 0.5% lidocaine approximates that of 0.5% procaine. However, lidocaine is progressively more toxic than procaine as the concentration increases, i.e., at 2% concentration lidocaine is 50% more toxic than procaine.

Tetracaine Hydrochloride

Tetracaine Hydrochloride, U.S.P. (Pontocaine Hydrochloride) (Fig. 19.4), is a white crystalline powder readily soluble in water.

Tetracaine is more potent than procaine or cocaine in concentrations of 0.5%–2%. It does not possess the vasoconstrictor action of cocaine. Epinephrine hydrochloride may be added to a solution of tetracaine when indicated.

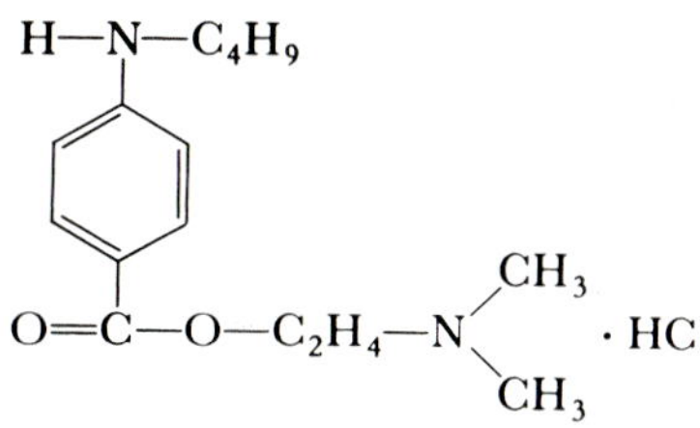

$H{-}N{-}C_4H_9$ (para-substituted benzene ring) $O{=}C{-}O{-}C_2H_4{-}N(CH_3)_2 \cdot HCl$

Tetracaine Hydrochloride

Fig. 19.4.

CLINICAL USE

Tetracaine may be used for surface, conduction, infiltration, and spinal anesthesia. It can be used topically in the eye at a concentration of 0.5% in small animals and 1% in large animals. A concentration of 2% is recommended for application to mucous membranes to produce surface anesthesia. Tetracaine can be employed for infiltration anesthesia, but there is still a tendency to use procaine.

A few drops of 0.5%–1.0% tetracaine on the eye of the rabbit will produce excellent anesthesia for minor procedures such as the cannulation of the tear duct (Murdock 1969). Veterinary ophthalmologists seldom use tetracaine on the eye of the dog in surgical procedures because it appears to delay postsurgical wound healing. Also, the various ophthalmic ointments containing tetracaine are seldom used for the same reason.

Tetracaine has been used in human medicine for abolishing the laryngeal and esophageal reflexes preparatory to introduction of a bronchoscope or esophagoscope. In anesthesia of human beings there has been strict adherence to the rule of not spraying more than 2 ml of a 1% solution or 1 ml of a 2% solution into the trachea or esophagus previous to instrumentation. This admonition is important in order to avoid serious toxic manifestations because of the complete and rapid absorption of tetracaine from the tracheal mucosa.

Piperocaine Hydrochloride

Piperocaine Hydrochloride, U.S.P. (Metycaine Hydrochloride) (Fig. 19.5), is a white crystalline powder freely soluble in water. Piperocaine in solution can be auto-

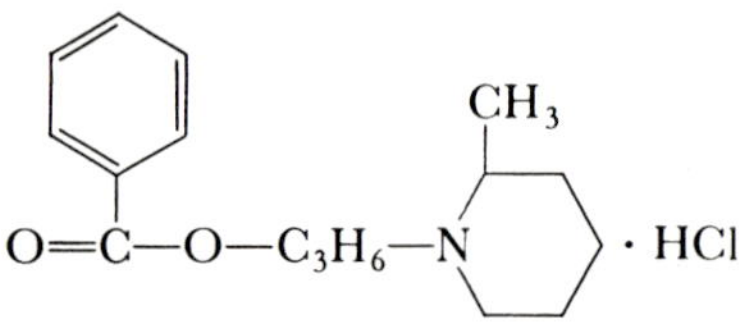

$O{=}C{-}O{-}C_3H_6{-}N$ (2-methylpiperidine) $\cdot HCl$

Piperocaine Hydrochloride

FIG. 19.5.

claved repeatedly without loss of potency.

CLINICAL USE

Piperocaine is adapted to surface infiltration and conduction anesthesia. For infiltration anesthesia and nerve-block procedures in small animals, concentrations of 0.5%–1% are used. Concentrations of 1% and 2% are preferable in large animals. For anesthetization of mucous membranes, concentrations of 2%–10% are used. An ophthalmic ointment containing 2%–4% piperocaine is used for anesthesia of the eye.

It is roughly 3 times as toxic as procaine when injected intravenously. Subcutaneously, piperocaine compares with procaine in toxicity.

Phenacaine Hydrochloride

Phenacaine Hydrochloride, N.F. (Holocaine Hydrochloride) (Fig. 19.6), is a white crystalline powder. It was one of the earliest of the local anesthetics to be introduced. Phenacaine is a derivative of phenetidin and varies greatly from the majority of the local anesthetics.

TOXICITY

Phenacaine is not used by injection because it is too toxic. Intravenously, phenacaine is as toxic as cocaine. Subcutaneously, phenacaine is twice as toxic as cocaine.

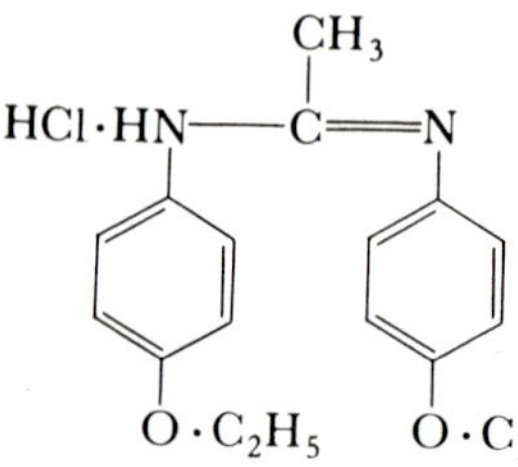

$HCl \cdot HN{-}C(CH_3){=}N$, each N bearing a phenyl ring with $O \cdot C_2H_5$

Phenacaine Hydrochloride

FIG. 19.6.

CLINICAL USE

Its use is limited to surface anesthesia. The chief advantage of phenacaine over cocaine is its prompt action when applied topically. A 1% solution of phenacaine applied to the eye is irritating, but it results in prompt and prolonged local anesthesia.

Proparacaine Hydrochloride

Proparacaine Hydrochloride, N.F. (Ophthaine, Ophthetic) (Fig. 19.7), is comparable to tetracaine. Unlike some topical anesthetics, it produces little or no tissue irritation (Ritchie et al. 1970). Proparacaine has been approved by the FDA for use as a topical anesthetic in animals. The drug is available in an aqueous solution containing 0.5% proparacaine hydrochloride, 2.45% glycerin as a stabilizer, and 0.2% chlorobutanol and 1:10,000 benzalkonium chloride as preservatives.

CLINICAL USE

Proparacaine is used as an anesthetic during cauterization of corneal ulcers and removal of foreign bodies and sutures from the cornea (*Code of Federal Regulations,* 135a. 10, April 1, 1974). In addition, it is used in the measurement of intraocular pressure (tonometry) when glaucoma is suspected. The topical application of proparacaine may be used as an adjunct in the removal of foreign bodies from the ear canal and nose as well as an aid in the treatment of painful otitis, in minor surgery, and prior to catheterization. Uses and indications of proparacaine are summarized as follows:

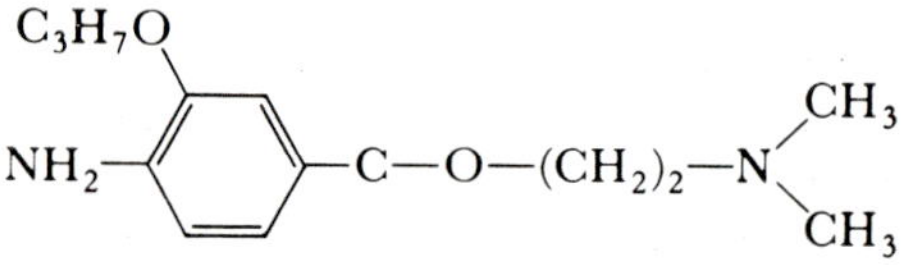

C_3H_7O, NH_2 on phenyl ring $-C{-}O{-}(CH_2)_2{-}N(CH_3)_2$

Proparacaine

FIG. 19.7.

Clinical Use or Indication	*Recommended Number of Drops*
(1) Suture removal	(1) Instill 1–2 drops 2 or 3 minutes prior to removal of the sutures.
(2) Foreign body removal from eye, ear, and nose	(2) Eye: Instill 3–5 drops. Ear: Instill 5–10 drops. Nose: Instill 5–10 drops in each nostril every 3 minutes for 3 doses.
(3) Tonometry	(3) Instill 1–2 drops immediately before measurement of the pressure.
(4) Adjunct treatment of otitis	(4) Instill 1–2 drops into the affected ear every 5 minutes for 3 doses.
(5) Minor surgery	(5) Instill 1 or more drops as needed.
(6) Catheterization	(6) Instill 2–3 drops with a blunt needle (20 ga.) or similar device prior to insertion of the catheter.

PRILOCAINE HYDROCHLORIDE

Prilocaine Hydrochloride, N.F. (Citanest) (Fig. 19.8), is available in aqueous solution varying in concentration (1%, 2%, and 3%) for injection. It resembles lidocaine chemically and pharmacologically. However, the onset and duration of action are longer than lidocaine (Ritchie et al. 1970). Similar to the action of lidocaine, prilocaine may produce drowsiness. A side effect of prilocaine that is unusual is the formation of methemoglobin; the extent or degree of the methemoglobinemia apparently is of little consequence provided therapeutic levels are not exceeded.

In sheep prilocaine has been compared with lidocaine to determine the duration of anesthesia produced by the two anesthetics following intrathecal and epidural administration (Grono 1966). A 2% concentration and an equal volume (5 ml) of each drug were used in the comparative study. The duration of anesthesia with prilocaine varied from 39 to 69 minutes following its epidural use, while the variation with lidocaine was 35–60 minutes. Also, the anesthetic period following the intrathecal use of prilocaine was longer than that produced by lidocaine.

Prilocaine is primarily used in human medicine for all types of infiltration and regional nerve-block anesthesia as well as for spinal anesthesia (Ritchie et al. 1970).

MEPIVACAINE HYDROCHLORIDE

Mepivacaine Hydrochloride, N.F. (Carbocaine) (Fig. 19.9), is about 2–2.5 times as potent in producing analgesia as procaine. It has the equivalent potency of lidocaine. The toxicity of mepivacaine is about 1.5–2 times that of procaine but slightly less toxic than lidocaine. The onset of anesthesia following mepivacaine (ca 11–12 minutes) is slower than lidocaine (ca 5 minutes) or prilocaine (ca 8 minutes). The duration of anesthesia is about 2–3 times that of procaine.

In human beings mepivacaine has been used for all types of infiltration and regional nerve-block anesthesia as well as for spinal anesthesia (Ritchie et al. 1970). The dose of mepivacaine in human beings is up to 8 mg/kg of body weight. Concen-

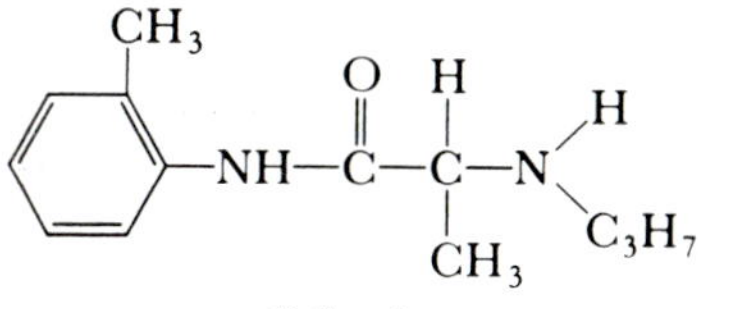

CH_3; O H; —NH—C—C—N; H; CH_3; C_3H_7

Prilocaine

FIG. 19.8.

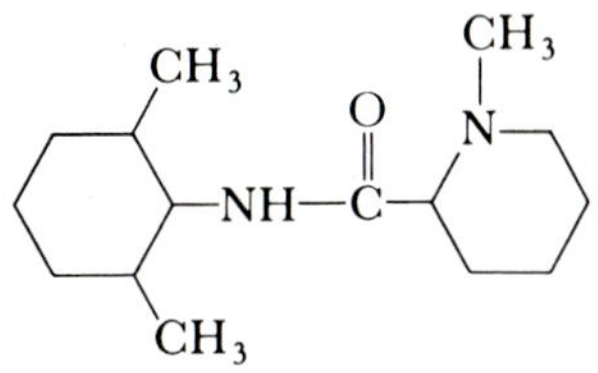

CH_3; CH_3; O; N; —NH—C—; CH_3

Mepivacaine

FIG. 19.9.

trations of 1% and 2% with 1:200,000 epinephrine hydrochloride are available.

Mepivacaine hydrochloride with epinephrine hydrochloride is commonly used for epidural anesthesia in the dog (Persson 1970); a 1% solution of mepivacaine with 1:200,000 epinephrine is preferred over other concentrations. Persson (1970) administered the local anesthetic in the lumbosacral space with the dog in the standing position. The anesthetic solution was given at the rate of 0.5 ml every 30 seconds and was continued until the toe reflexes disappeared, indicating that surgical analgesia up to T_5 had been attained.

Cetacaine

Cetacaine contains a combination of tetracaine 2%, benzocaine 14%, and butylaminobenzoate (Butesin), as well as stabilizers and preservatives such as benzalkonium chloride 0.5% and cetyldimethyl ammonium bromide 0.005%. Cetacaine is restricted to topical use and must not be injected or infiltrated into tissues. Moreover, it must not be used in the eyes.

Cetacaine is used as a topical anesthetic spray for the mucous membranes and is used on the gums in dentistry. Onset of anesthesia is about 30 seconds. Only small quantities of the spray should be used. In a 70-kg person, tetracaine in excess of 20 mg is contraindicated.

Dyclonine Hydrochloride

Dyclonine Hydrochloride, U.S.P. (Dyclone), is used for topical anesthesia, local infiltration anesthesia, field-block, nerve-block, or epidural anesthesia (Ott 1969). It may be used in 0.5% concentration as a topical anesthetic for the eye or on mucous membranes. For field-block, nerve-block, local infiltration, or epidural anesthesia, a 0.5%–1% solution may be used; a dose of about 1 ml/5–7 lb of body weight as an epidural agent will produce anesthesia up to 2 hours (Ott 1969).

OTHER LOCAL ANESTHETIC AGENTS

Cocaine is subject to the Controlled Substances Act of 1970 and is a Schedule II drug. It is highly addictive in human beings. With many other local anesthetics now available with equivalent potency and effect upon the mucous membranes for topical anesthesia, there is little justification for its use in therapeutics.

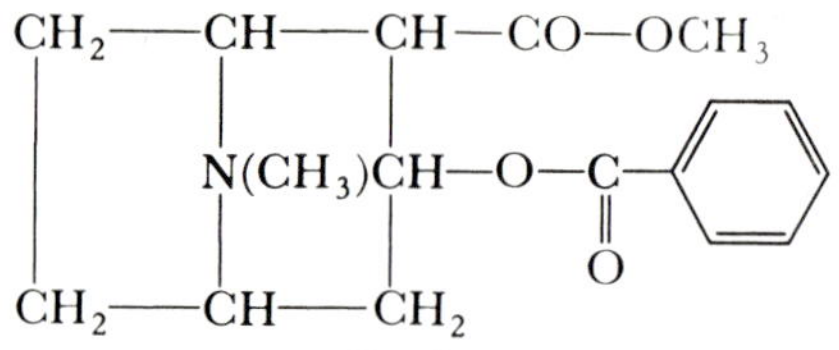

CH_2—CH—CH—CO—OCH_3
N(CH_3)CH—O—C(=O)—C_6H_5
CH_2—CH—CH_2

Cocaine

Fig. 19.10.

Cocaine Hydrochloride

chemistry

Cocaine Hydrochloride, U.S.P. (Fig. 19.10), is a white crystalline substance readily soluble in water. The alkaloidal form of cocaine is sparingly soluble in water but freely soluble in organic solvents. Alkaloidal cocaine is not used orally or parenterally.

Local anesthetics chemically related to cocaine are esters of PABA, with the alkyl amine introduced into the alkyl group (Fig. 19.11). In Fig. 19.11 R represents various alkyl groups according to the derivative. The relation of this formula to that of cocaine is apparent.

administration

Cocaine hydrochloride anesthetizes when infiltrated into the tissues, but it is no longer employed in this manner because of its high tissue toxicity. Cocaine is not sufficiently effective when applied to the intact skin because it penetrates the horny epidermis slowly. It will anesthetize if there is an abrasion, desquamation, or hyperemia of the skin. Surface anesthesia

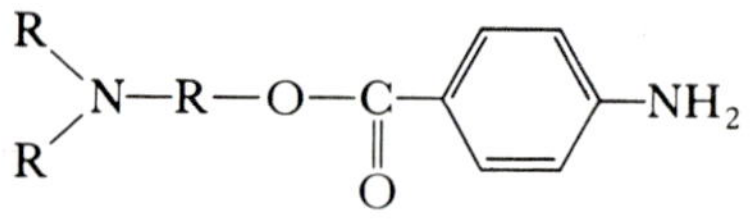

R(R)N—R—O—C(=O)—C_6H_4—NH_2

Fig. 19.11.

with cocaine is generally confined to the mucous membranes of the body. Cocaine is not administered orally because gastric secretions destroy its activity.

ACTION

Sensory nerve endings are completely and reversibly paralyzed upon local contact with cocaine. For a number of years this drug was looked upon as the most effective of the local anesthetics for the production of surface anesthesia. However, local anesthetics with comparable potency and no addicting potential have equaled or surpassed cocaine. Several of these agents are safer to use than cocaine.

Local vasoconstriction characteristically occurs following the application of cocaine to tissue. Cocaine is the only common local anesthetic possessing this action. In addition, it sensitizes the sympathetic effector mechanism so that the effector cells give an exaggerated response to epinephrine. Cocaine inactivates amine oxidase and phenol oxidase, enzymes that oxidize and destroy epinephrine. Through its ability to inactivate these enzymes, cocaine permits more intensified action by the neurohomone released at the postganglionic adrenergic nerve endings.

DURATION

The duration of local anesthesia from cocaine depends on the concentration and the site of application of the solution. Concentrations as low as 0.02% applied locally to susceptible tissues will produce fleeting anesthesia. Higher concentrations may produce local anesthesia lasting as long as half an hour.

THERAPEUTIC USE

Cocaine should be used only for topical anesthesia and it must not be injected into tissues. Cocaine hydrochloride in a 5% solution has been used for many years for instillation into the eye of the horse preparatory to surgery or examination. Concentrations of 3%–5% have been employed in the dog for this purpose. Good local anesthesia of the conjunctiva and many parts of the eyeball results. The conjunctival blood vessels are constricted, giving the mucosa a blanched or pale appearance. The pupil dilates and the power of accommodation may be diminished. The light reflex and the response of the iris to drugs acting on the parasympathetic innervation remain.

Cocaine hydrochloride solutions in concentrations of 5%–10% are used to anesthetize the mucous membranes of the nose, larynx, and buccal cavity in large animals. In smaller species, concentrations of 5% are adequate. The use of cocaine hydrochloride for local anesthesia has decreased following the introduction of a number of safer but just as effective topical anesthetics.

TOXICITY

Acute toxicity from cocaine can occur clinically from overdosage, too rapid absorption, or improper administration. Adverse or toxic effects from the subcutaneous use of cocaine in the horse can occur at a dosage as low as 10 grains (600 mg). However, excitant toxic effects have been reported when only 3 grains (180 mg) of cocaine were injected hypodermically. Severe toxic effects without fatality occur in the horse following the intravenous administration of cocaine at a dose of 0.93–1.13 mg/kg. The maximum dose of cocaine that can be injected into the horse with safety and without causing muscular spasms is 600 mg. A dose as low as 2–3 grains (120–180 mg) of cocaine (presumably injected by the intravenous route) can be lethal in the horse. On a body weight basis (i.e., mg/kg), the horse is more sensitive to cocaine than human beings. The computed range of safety that should not be exceeded when cocoaine is used on mucous membranes of the horse is 5–7 grains (300–420 mg). Cocaine is cumulative upon repeated injection; no tolerance develops from its continued use.

The following quantities of cocaine may be considered LD100 doses following subcutaneous (s.c.) and intravenous (i.v.) injection (Westhues and Fritsch 1964):

Species	*Route of Adminis-tration*	*Dose (g/kg)*
Rabbit	s.c.	0.1
Rabbit	i.v.	0.02–0.025
Cat	s.c.	0.03–0.033
Cat	i.v.	0.015
Dog	s.c.	0.02–0.035
Dog	i.v.	0.012
Goat	s.c.	0.015
Horse and cattle	s.c.	0.018

The first toxic effect of cocaine is stimulation of the CNS followed by violent convulsive seizures. If sufficient cocaine is given, the stimulation is followed by a period of depression that may terminate in unconsciousness and death from respiratory paralysis.

Chronic poisoning or addiction to cocaine may occur in animals under unusual conditions, but generally addiction is limited to human beings.

Butethamine Hydrochloride

Butethamine Hydrochloride, N.F. (Monocaine Hydrochloride), is a fine, white crystalline powder soluble in water to the extent of 3%. Its solutions are bitter, but they possess considerable surface anesthetic properties when applied to mucous membranes. Monocaine possesses local anesthetic properties similar to those of cocaine upon injection. At one time it was popular for nerve-block anesthesia in human dentistry, where it was employed in concentrations not to exceed 1%.

Cyclomethycaine

Cyclomethycaine (Surfacaine) is a white crystalline powder that dissolves poorly in water. It has been used mostly in the form of creams or ointments for application to burns, pruritic areas, and skin lesions of various sorts.

Dibucaine Hydrochloride

Dibucaine Hydrochloride, U.S.P. (Nupercaine Hydrochloride), is one of the most toxic and most potent of the local anesthetics. Its high potency provides only a fair margin of safety. Dibucaine has been used for all types of local anesthetic purposes. It provides anesthesia of longer duration than most other local anesthetics. In ointment form, dibucaine can be applied to the surface of the body to produce anesthesia in immediately underlying tissues. However, there is considerable hazard in the use of dibucaine ointment because of extensive absorption. In view of its high toxicity, dibucaine should be used only by individuals familiar with the action of the drug.

Naepaine Hydrochioride

Naepaine Hydrochloride, N.N.D. (Amylsine Hydrochloride), is recommended for use in the eye in 2%–4% solution. It produces anesthesia without mydriasis.

SLIGHTLY SOLUBLE LOCAL ANESTHETICS

A few compounds possess a limited local anesthetizing property and are relatively insoluble in water. These agents are applied to mucous surfaces, wounds, and pruritic or eczematous areas of the skin to produce a slight to moderate local anesthesia of considerable duration. These agents may be applied as dusting powders, oily liquids, and ointments.

Ethyl Aminobenzoate, Butyl Aminobenzoate, and Butesin Picrate

Ethyl Aminobenzoate, N.F. (Anesthesin, Benzocaine), *Butyl Aminobenzoate,* N.F. (Butesin), and *Butesin Picrate* are the outstanding examples of this group of compounds. The first two agents are employed to some extent in dentistry for anesthesia of the gums as well as of the entire buccal mucosa. Butesin picrate combines the moderate antiseptic action of picric acid with the local anesthetic action of butesin. It has been employed almost entirely in the treatment of minor skin burns in the form of a 1% ointment. The yellow picric acid stain cannot be removed from animal fibers and will permanently discolor the hair of a light-skinned animal.

REFERENCES

Allen, F. M., and Safford, F. K. 1948. Animal experiments with procaine and related drugs. Anesth Analg 27:121.

Bone, J. K., and Peck, J. G. 1956. Epidural anesthesia in dogs. J Am Vet Med Assoc 128:236.

Boyes, R. N.; Adams, H. J.; and Duce, B. R. 1970. Oral absorption and disposition kinetics of lidocaine hydrochloride in dogs. J Pharmacol Exp Ther 174:1.

Bradley, W. A. 1966. Epidural analgesia for tail docking in lambs. Vet Rec 79:787.

Eckenhoff, J. E., and Kirby, C. K. 1951. The use of hyaluronidase in regional nerve blocks. Anesthesiology 12:27.

Farquharson, J. 1940. Paravertebral lumbar anesthesia in the bovine species. J Am Vet Med Assoc 97:54.

Finster, M.; Morishima, H. O.; Boyes, R. N.; and Covino, B. G. 1972. The placental transfer of lidocaine and its uptake by fetal tissues. Anesthesiology 36:159.

Gabel, A. A. 1964. Practical technics for bovine anesthesia. Mod Vet Pract 45:40.

Getty, R.; Sowa, J. A.; and Lundvall, R. L. 1956. Local anesthesia and applied anatomy as related to nerve blocks in horses. J Am Vet Med Assoc 128:583.

Goodman, L. S., and Gilman, A., eds. 1955. The Pharmacological Basis of Therapeutics, 2nd ed. New York: Macmillan.

Graubard, D. J., and Peterson, M. C. 1950. Clinical Uses of Intravenous Procaine. Springfield, Ill.: Charles C Thomas.

Grono, L. R. 1966. Spinal anaesthesia in the sheep. Aust Vet J 42:58.

Heinze, C. D. 1970. Surgical procedures. In W. J. Gibbons, E. J. Catcott, and J. F. Smithcors, eds. Bovine Medicine and Surgery and Herd Health Management, p. 795. Wheaton, Ill.: American Veterinary Publications.

Hopcroft, S. C. 1967. Technique of epidural anesthesia in experimental sheep. Aust Vet J 43:213.

Jones, L. M. 1951a. The toxic and analgesic effect of procaine hydrochloride administered intravenously in the dog. Vet Med 46:93.

———. 1951b. Miscellaneous observations on the clinical effects of injecting solutions and suspensions of procaine hydrochloride into domestic animals. Vet Med 46:435.

Kalow, W. 1952. Hydrolysis of local anesthetics by human serum cholinesterase. J Pharmacol Exp Ther 104:122.

Kirby, C. K.; Eckenhoff, J. E.; and Looby, J. P. 1950. The use of hyaluronidase with local anesthetic agents in surgery and dentistry. Ann NY Acad Sci 52:1166.

Klide, A. M., and Soma, L. R. 1968. Epidural analgesia in the dog and cat. J Am Vet Med Assoc 153:165.

Lawson, J. 1965. Intubation of cats. Vet Rec 77:912.

Link, R. P., and Smith, J. C. 1956. Comparison of some local anesthetics in cattle. J Am Vet Med Assoc 129:306.

McDonell, W. 1972. Anesthetic emergencies. II. Cardiovascular insufficiency and arrest. Mod Vet Pract 53:37.

MacKellar, J. C. 1967. Procaine hydrochloride in the treatment of spasmodic colic in horses. Vet Rec 80:444.

McMahon, F. G., and Woods, L. A. 1951. Further studies on the metabolism of lidocaine (xylocaine) in the dog. J Pharmacol Exp Ther 103:354.

Manohar, M.; Kumar, R.; and Tyagi, R. P. S. 1971. Studies on intravenous retrograde regional anesthesia of the forelimb in buffalo calves. Br Vet J 127:401.

Mitchell, B. 1966. Local analgesia of the horn and horn base in the goat. Vet Rec 79:135.

Moore, D. C. 1950. An evaluation of hyaluronidase in local and nerve block analgesia: A review of 519 cases. Anesthesiology 11: 470.

Murdock, H. R., Jr. 1969. Anesthesia in the rabbit. Fed Proc 28:1510.

Orkin, L. R., and Rovenstine, E. A. 1952. Hexylcaine (Cyclaine): Usefulness in regional and topical anesthesia—Preliminary report. Anesthesiology 13:465.

Ott, R. L. 1969. Local anesthesia in the dog. Fed Proc 28:1450.

Owen, D. 1973. Local nerve block. Proc Am Assoc Equine Pract, p. 153.

Paddleford, R. R., and Short, C. E. 1973. Cardiopulmonary resuscitation following arrest from vagovagal stimulation. Vet Med Small Anim Clin 68:973.

Persson, F. 1970. Epidural analgesia in dogs with special reference to the intraarterial blood pressure. Acta Vet Scand 11:186.

Pickett, D. 1951. Intravenous procaine hydrochloride for treatment of pruritus in dogs. Vet Med 46:271.

Raker, C. W. 1956. Regional anesthesia of the bovine foot. J Am Vet Med Assoc 128:238.

Ritchie, J. M., and Greengard, P. 1966. On the mode of action of local anesthetics. Ann Rev Pharmacol 6:405.

Ritchie, J. M.; Cohen, P. J.; and Dripps, R. D. 1970. Cocaine, procaine and other synthetic local anesthetics. In L. S. Goodman and

A. Gilman, eds. The Pharmacological Basis of Therapeutics, 4th ed., p. 371. New York: Macmillan.

Rülcker, C. 1965. Lignocaine hydrochloride with and without adrenaline for epidural analgesia in cattle. Vet Rec 77:1180.

Seeman, P. 1972. The membrane actions of anesthetics and tranquilizers. Pharmacol Rev 24:583.

Strande, A. 1968. Epidural anaesthesia in young pigs, dosage in relation to the length of the vertebral column. Acta Vet Scand 9:41.

Strobel, G. E., and Wollman, H. 1969. Pharmacology of anesthetic agents. Fed Proc 28:1386.

Tyagi, R. P. S.; Kumar, R.; and Manohar, M. 1973. Studies on intravenous retrograde regional anesthesia for the forelimbs of ruminants. Aust Vet J 49:321.

Weaver, A. D. 1972. Intravenous local anesthesia of the lower limb in cattle. J Am Vet Med Assoc 160:55.

Weihe, W. H. 1973. The effect of temperature on the action of drugs. Ann Rev Pharmacol 13:409.

Westhues, M., and Fritsch, R. 1964. Principles of local anaesthesia. In Local Anaesthesia, vol. 1, p. 25. Philadelphia: J. B. Lippincott.

Wheat, J. D. 1952. The clinical use of Cyclaine (hexylcaine HCl) as a local anesthetic. A preliminary report. J Am Vet Med Assoc 120:71.

CHAPTER 20

INTRATHECAL AND EPIDURAL ANESTHESIA

NICHOLAS H. BOOTH

INTRATHECAL ANESTHESIA

Intrathecal, or spinal, anesthesia is accomplished by the introduction of a local anesthetic solution into the spinal fluid. The drug temporarily paralyzes the spinal nerve roots in the subarachnoid space it contacts and anesthetizes the tissues innervated by the affected nerves. Spinal anesthesia was first performed in a dog by Corning in 1885 with cocaine.

Many years ago French veterinarians also attempted the intrathecal injection of local anesthetics in several species of domestic animals. This technique has never become popular because of the difficulties and dangers associated with it. Intrathecal injection has been made in dogs, cats, and sheep, but it has not been accepted in general clinical use. Intrathecal injection can be performed more readily in the dog and cat than in other species because the curvature of the spinal column can be modified to permit ready introduction of the needle. The vertebrae in animals are fitted closely together so that the spinal column does not bend as readily as in human beings. Animals are far from cooperative and will not bend their spinal columns to facilitate penetration of the spinal needle. In large animals, improper restraint makes it difficult to employ intraspinal injections effectively. The response of the animal patient may be so vigorous at times as to break the needle, and the broken end is not always found for extraction.

EPIDURAL ANESTHESIA

Epidural, or extradural, anesthesia is attained by injecting the local anesthetic solution into the epidural space. In this case, the meninges are not penetrated by the needle and the solution remains outside or upon (epi-) the dura mater. This method of inducing local anesthesia is much safer than using the intrathecal technique. When the epidural technique is employed, there is less risk of traumatic injury to the nervous system and of the anesthetic reaching the medullary centers. Actually, contact of the anesthetic with the vital centers in the medulla is obviated by the epidural space terminating at the foramen magnum.

Application of epidural anesthesia in veterinary medicine is most important in large animal practice. Although it can be applied in small animals, the method is not used as frequently because of the preference to use general anesthetics. On the other hand, in small animals that are considered poor risks with the use of general anesthetics, epidural anesthesia is distinctly advantageous.

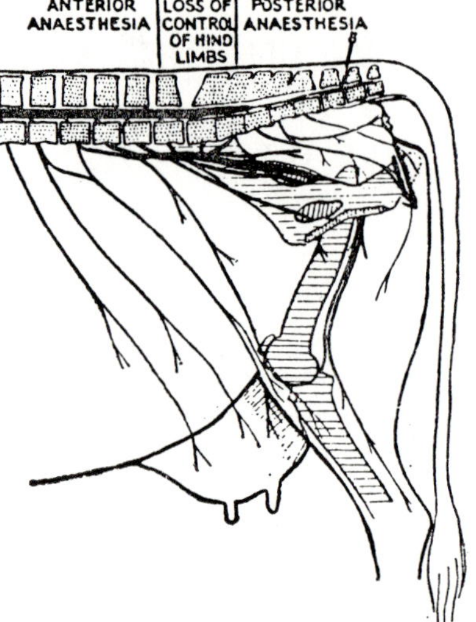

Fig. 20.1. A schematic diagram showing general distribution of nerves and approximate levels of epidural anesthesia in the cow. (By permission from Wright, Veterinary Anaesthesia, Ballière, Tindall and Cox, Ltd., 1947)

Nature of Epidural Anesthesia

Epidural injection was accepted slowly when cocaine was the only drug available, and it proved to be rather toxic. With the introduction of less toxic local anesthetics, epidural anesthesia became widely employed in some species.

By using this technique in cattle, sensory anesthesia can be produced as far forward as the flank and abdominal wall without affecting the respiration or circulation (see Fig. 20.1). More frequently, however, this technique is limited to regional anesthesia of the posterior part of the animal for operations involving the udder and the perineal and penile areas.

The epidural space is the cavity between the dura mater covering the spinal cord and the periosteum lining the spinal canal. From the foramen magnum, the epidural space extends posteriorly to about the fourth coccygeal vertebra. Located in the epidural space are the internal venous plexus and loose connective tissue containing variable amounts of fat.

The amount of anesthetic solution injected is generally small compared with the volume of the epidural space. A solution injected at the junction of the first and second coccygeal vertebrae flows forward. The distance the solution will traverse depends largely on the volume of the solution and on the posture of the animal following injection. If the rear end is lower than the fore end of the animal, the solution will stay in the posterior epidural space. If the reverse plane is assumed, the solution will gravitate forward.

There is no natural tissue barrier preventing the flow of anesthetic solution forward in the epidural space except excessive fat deposits. However, the normal position of recumbent herbivora is with the rear end of the animal lower than the fore end. If 10 ml of anesthetic solution are injected in a prone cow, only the nerves of the coccygeal and perineal area are anesthetized. If 40 ml are injected, the anesthetic solution flows forward to block all nerves as far as about the fourth lumbar nerve (McLeod and Frank 1927–28).

Volumes of 150 ml and occasionally of 200 ml are injected epidurally for anesthetizing areas as far forward as the umbilicus. These larger amounts are rarely used in the United States. It is possible to fill the epidural space with anesthetic solution and to anesthetize every spinal nerve from the tail to the foramen magnum. Such extensive conduction anesthesia could conceivably result in death from paralysis of the spinal nerves innervating the respiratory muscles of the thorax and from vascular collapse caused by paralysis of vasoconstrictor nerves to the visceral blood vessels. However, the author has obtained anesthesia up to the foramen magnum of the dog with the head down in the sternal position by injecting large volumes of 2.5% procaine hydrochloride containing 1:10,000 ephedrine sulfate. In no instance did the animals manifest any evidence of toxic symptoms. This technique cannot be recommended for clinical application until definitive studies determine its actual safety.

An improvement in the technique of epidural injection has been introduced through the adaptation of epidural anesthesia to the human being in so-called caudal anesthesia. Small-bore plastic tubing is introduced through a large-bore needle into the epidural space. The needle can then be withdrawn from the tissue, leaving the plastic tubing intact and communicating with the epidural space. A hypodermic needle or a needle base can be inserted into the end of the plastic tubing and connected to a syringe for injection of anesthetic solution. The tubing stays in place so that small amounts of solution can be injected intermittently into the epidural space during the surgical procedure as needed. Such technique gives the anesthetist better control over the condition of the patient and tends to avoid the initial injection of excessive amounts of local anesthetic.

This method of intermittent injection would disregard the fixed dosage schedule suggested in Table 20.1 in favor of a dose-to-effect technique. This technique adapts the dosage of anesthetic to the needs of the patient much better and tends to avoid undesirable reactions.

TABLE 20.1. Duration of posterior epidural anesthesia in the bovine

Drug	Dosage	Duration of Good to Fair Anesthesia
	(mg/lb)	*(hr)*
1% Procaine hydrochloride	0.16–0.18	1.9
1% Procaine hydrochloride with epinephrine hydrochloride, 1:50,000–1:100,000	0.16–0.17	2.4
2% Procaine hydrochloride	0.20–0.25	1.9
2% Procaine hydrochloride with epinephrine hydrochloride, 1:25,000–1:50,000	0.16–0.20	3.5
1% Tetracaine hydrochloride (Pontocaine)	0.06–0.10	4.6
5% Hexylcaine (Cyclaine)	0.33–0.45	8.8

Source: Roberts 1950.

MECHANISM OF ACTION IN THE EPIDURAL SPACE

Procaine hydrochloride, and probably other local anesthetics, diffuse from the epidural space through the dura mater into the subarachnoidal space. It appears that a local anesthetic injected epidurally may exert a depressant action upon (1) a spinal nerve by diffusing through the covering of dura as it crosses the epidural space, (2) a spinal nerve rootlet emerging from the spinal cord by diffusing into the subarachnoid space, and (3) the spinal cord by similar diffusion if present in sufficient concentration or time interval to penetrate deeply.

Injection of 10 ml of 2% or 3% procaine hydrochloride epidurally in the dog resulted in concentrations of procaine in the subarachnoid space varying between 0.3 and 0.8 mg/ml of cerebrospinal fluid; this was the result of direct penetration and not the result of secondary diffusion via the bloodstream. Spinal cord function in the dog is depressed by subarachnoidal procaine concentrations varying from 0.1 to 1 mg/ml.

Although individual variation occurs, experimental data indicate that routine epidural injection of procaine hydrochloride in the dog results in subarachnoidal concentrations of procaine that act directly upon the spinal cord as well as upon the spinal rootlets to depress the function of both (Rudin et al. 1951). Procaine hydrochloride has been found in the cerebrospinal fluid of calves following epidural injection of a 1.5% solution.

The sensory nerves in the spinal nerve trunks are paralyzed more readily than are the motor nerves. The sensory nerves are smaller in cross section and have a greater surface exposure in proportion to the volume of contained nerve fibers than do the motor nerves. The large motor nerves, with a smaller surface exposed to the action of a local anesthetic and a greater volume, are anesthetized only by higher concentrations of local anesthetic.

ONSET AND DURATION OF EPIDURAL ANESTHESIA

A delay of at least 5 minutes and sometimes 20 minutes is observed before epidural anesthesia reaches the maximum. However, the rapidity of onset varies with age as well as species. Brook (1935) noted that the appearance of epidural anesthesia is most rapid in the sheep and the calf, followed by the ox, the pig, and the foal. It is less rapid in the dog and cat and is slowest in the horse. The onset of anesthesia can be speeded somewhat by adding hyaluronidase to the anesthetic solution; this undoubtedly promotes diffusion of the anesthetic through the dura mater.

Epidural anesthesia is characterized by paralysis of the sensory nerve fibers. A sensory block generally will persist 1–2 hours. Partial to complete paralysis of motor nerve fibers may occur.

When epinephrine is added to a procaine solution in a concentration of 1:50,000, the duration of intrathecal anesthesia in dogs is prolonged 60% (Prickett et al. 1945). The duration of posterior epidural anesthesia in the bovine is prolonged, roughly, an equivalent length of time by the addition of epinephrine hydrochloride (Table 20.1).

METABOLISM

The procaine hydrochloride injected epidurally probably is absorbed by the blood and lymph vessels of the epidural space and then metabolized. At least, intrathecal injections of procaine are known to be absorbed as such rather than to undergo chemical decomposition in the spinal fluid (Helrich et al. 1950).

Drugs for Epidural Anesthesia

For successful epidural anesthesia a drug should rate highly with respect to the following requirements: (1) low absolute and relative toxicity, (2) a high degree of potency, (3) a short latent period, (4) a prolonged duration, and (5) a high degree of diffusability.

Procaine hydrochloride has been more or less universally employed for epidural anesthesia. Hexylcaine and lidocaine are finding increasing use. Tutocaine and tetracaine have been used to a lesser degree.

The relative values of lidocaine and hexylcaine for epidural anesthesia are similar, although one representative report lists the following agents in order of preference: hexylcaine hydrochloride (2%), lidocaine hydrochloride (2%), and procaine hydrochloride (Blundell et al. 1955). The concentration of procaine hydrochloride solutions has varied between 1% and 2% depending on the volume employed (see Table 20.1). Concentrations of procaine up to 5% can be used, but the volume of solution injected must be decreased so that approximately the same weight of drug is injected. However, the volume of solution and therefore the concentration of the solution are influenced by the forward extent of anesthesia desired and the size of the animal. The volume of anesthetic solution is increased as the size of the animal and forward extent of anesthesia increase.

Epidural Anesthesia in the Cow

Epidural anesthesia has been divided arbitrarily into the anterior level and the posterior level of regional anesthesia.

POSTERIOR EPIDURAL ANESTHESIA

This plane provides sensory anesthesia for the skin areas of (1) the tail and croup as far as the mid-sacral region; (2) the anus, vulva, and perineum; and (3) the posterior aspects of the thighs. Motor control of the hind legs is not affected, although there may be paralysis of the motor fibers to the anal sphincter. From 10 to 15 ml of 2% procaine hydrochloride solution can be injected epidurally in the cow with reasonable assurance that motor control of the hind legs will be unaffected (Table 20.2). If motor paralysis of the adductor muscles of the hind legs does appear, the cow simply lies down and shows no excitement or tendency to throw itself about as does the

TABLE 20.2. Epidural anesthesia in the bovine by procaine hydrochloride

Indications	Concentration	Dose	
Posterior epidural anesthesia			
			(ml)
Tail operation	2%	small animal medium animal large animal	5–10
To overcome straining for obstetrical manipulation and simple embryotomy; operation of parturient injuries; reduction of prolapsed rectum, vagina or uterus	1%	small animal medium animal large animal	10 12 15
Repair of anus, vulva, perineum; manipulation of genital organs in fractious patients	2%	small animal medium animal large animal	10 12 15
Anterior epidural anesthesia			
Examination and surgery of the penis	1–1.5%	small animal medium animal large animal	25 50 70
Difficult obstetrical manipulation; extensive embryotomy; uterine amputation, castration; surgery of prepuce and inguinal area	1–1.5%	small animal medium animal large animal	40 75 100
Amputation of a rear digit or udder; cesarean section*	1–1.5%	small animal medium animal large animal	90 120 150

Source: Wright 1947.
* Frank and Roberts (1940) reported that 40–50 ml of 2% procaine hydrochloride anesthetizes for ventral incision.

horse. Defecation is inhibited. The posterior rectum tends to balloon. Stretching of the vulva arouses no response, and the vagina dilates. The parturient cow stops the "straining" movement, but contractions of the uterus are not affected.

Duration. Posterior epidural anesthesia reaches its peak in about 15–20 minutes following injection and persists for about an hour after injection. Progressive recovery occurs during the second hour following injection, with the animal approaching normality at the end of the second hour. No response to a pin prick in the skin of the tail occurs within 2–3 minutes following injection; this provides reliable evidence that the injection was properly made.

A comparison of the posterior epidural anesthesia produced by solutions of local anesthetics in the bovine has been reported by Roberts (1950). Satisfactory anesthesia consisted of suitable anesthetic effect without causing the animal to stagger, to become paralyzed in the hind quarters, or to fall to the ground. A "good" anesthesia was indicated by paralysis of the tail, suspended defecation, and no sensory reaction to pinching of the vulva. A "fair" anesthesia was indicated by paralysis of the tail, limited defecation, and slight to partial sensory response to pinching of the vulva. The duration of "good" to "fair" posterior epidural anesthesia in the bovine is indicated in Table 20.1.

ANTERIOR EPIDURAL ANESTHESIA

This level of anesthesia involves a loss of skin sensation in the areas (1) spreading progressively forward over the croup; (2) between the hind limbs to the inguinal areas, prepuce, scrotum, and mammary glands; (3) over the hind legs; and finally, (4) the flanks and abdominal areas forward to the region of the umbilicus. The motor paralysis of the hind limbs varies from partial to complete. In the case of partial paralysis, some moderate restraint may be necessary. If motor paralysis of the hind legs is complete, the patient should be kept on its sternum 10–15 minutes during the onset of anesthesia to provide a bilateral instead of unilateral anesthesia. If only unilateral anesthesia is necessary, the animal should be restrained with the side downward that is to be anesthetized. After the spinal nerves on one side are anesthetized, the patient may be turned to expose the operative area. See Table 20.1 for suggested dosages of procaine hydrochloride.

Duration. The duration of anterior epidural anesthesia is longer because of the larger amount of local anesthetic solution injected. The patient ordinarily cannot stand for at least 2 hours. Incoordination may persist 3–4 hours or longer.

Toxicity. Toxic reactions can be produced by the epidural injection of excessive amounts of any local anesthetic. Roberts (1950) mentions the effects of giving 6 ml of a 4% solution of tetracaine epidurally to each of two cows and 10 ml of a 2% solution to another. Each cow became unsteady and fell to the ground about 1 hour after injection. One cow got up in 7 hours and another in 12 hours. The third cow was down 60 hours, when she was assisted to her feet by slings. Persistent motor paralysis was noted in all three cows 10 days after the injection by the absence of voluntary tail movement. The cow that was aided by slings finally had to be slaughtered because of persisting partial paralysis. The sensory responses suffered less damage than the motor reactions, because sensory stimulation elicited a response even though the cow was unsteady on her feet from partial motor paralysis.

LUMBAR EPIDURAL ANESTHESIA

Lumbar epidural anesthesia is a technique proposed for accomplishing anesthesia of the last thoracic and first two lumbar nerves for rumenotomies. This technique supposedly has an advantage over earlier methods in that only one injection site is necessary to accomplish anesthesia of the left flank (St. Clair and Hardenbrook 1956). However, Aanes (1963) has encountered considerable difficulty in using this method in dairy and beef cattle.

DISADVANTAGES OF EPIDURAL ANESTHESIA

Not all cattle respond satisfactorily to epidural anesthesia. Occasionally, a patient is not anesthetized by an epidural injection of a local anesthetic. Two inherent faults of the method may have a bearing on this problem. Careful study by Brook (1935) indicated that some of the intervertebral foramina of the spinal column occasionally are not closed. When the local anesthetic solution is injected epidurally in these animals, the solution escapes through the foramina into the peritoneal space and does not exert its action on the spinal nerves as desired. Animals with such a defect cannot be identified from the exterior; therefore, this handicap constitutes one of the disadvantages of epidural anesthesia that apparently must be expected.

Another disadvantage is the tendency for fat to be deposited in the epidural space in fattened cattle. The heavy deposit of fat can block the flow of the anesthetic solution from the point of injection forward through the epidural space to paralyze the spinal nerves.

An additional disadvantage occurring with anterior epidural anesthesia is the pooling of blood in the viscera, which results from the blocking of the vasoconstrictor fibers contained in the spinal nerves.

Epidural Anesthesia in the Horse

Epidural anesthesia in the horse has not been as successful as in the cow. In the first place, the spinal column of the horse is somewhat more depressed than in the cow, making the site for epidural injection more difficult to identify. Many horses are temperamentally unsuited to needle punctures, especially in the area of the rear quarters. Of more importance, however, is the tendency for the horse to become excited and to throw itself with the first signs of impending motor paralysis of the adductor muscles of the hind legs. This disturbance is dangerous to the horse as well as to the veterinarian and attendants. The only way to avoid this hazard is to cast the horse before making the epidural injection. Unless the cast animal is carefully arranged on its back with side supports, the anesthetic solution will gravitate to one side of the epidural space and produce unilateral instead of bilateral nerve block.

Epidural anesthesia has been employed for numerous operations in horses, including tail setting, perineal operations, and numerous other kinds of surgery on the rear part of the animal. However, there appears to be an increasing tendency on the part of the more active practitioners of the United States to avoid epidural anesthesia in the horse. For more information on epidural anesthesia in horses the reader is referred to Brook (1935) and to *Veterinary Anaesthesia and Analgesia* by Wright and Hall (1961).

Epidural Anesthesia in the Dog

Epidural anesthesia in the dog has been effectively used by some veterinarians. Since the introduction of the barbiturates, the use of epidural anesthesia has decreased in the United States until now it is infrequently used in the dog. Epidural anesthesia in the dog offers certain advantages that should be used more widely. One of the most useful applications of epidural anesthesia is in the old dog. When combined with effective sedation, epidural anesthesia is definitely safer than general anesthesia in old patients. Epidural anesthesia can be routinely considered in all ages of dogs in select cases of cesarean section; hysterectomy; painful manipulation of the rear leg; and rectal, vaginal, or perineal surgery.

TECHNIQUE

The epidural space is entered at the lumbosacral junction with a 20-gauge, 2.5- to 3-inch hypodermic needle, as described by Frank (1927) and Riddell (1952). The needle is introduced into this area with or without a procaine wheal at the site of injection. The needle is pressed downward until it reaches the floor of the spinal canal and then is withdrawn about one-quarter of an inch. After aspiration with a syringe to be sure the needle is not within a venous sinus, the anesthetic solution can be injected with no resistance.

The injection period should take 1–2 minutes. It is advisable to inject about one-half the calculated amount of anesthetic solution and then to pause 30–60 seconds to watch for relaxation of the anal sphincter and to note the respiratory activity.

Anatomic study of many breeds of dogs indicates that the lumbosacral space used for epidural injection is absent or undeveloped in one-eighth of all dogs (Grafe and Schulze 1949).

DRUG AND DOSAGE

Several local anesthetics can be used, but the most satisfactory drug is procaine hydrochloride in 2% solution. The dose is about 4 mg/lb (1 ml of 2% solution per 5 lb) for dogs up to 20 lb of body weight. Above this weight the dose should be decreased slightly (Riddell 1952). A vasoconstrictor, such as ephedrine sulfate, is beneficial in prolonging and increasing the safety of anesthesia.

SYMPTOMS AND DURATION

Regional anesthesia should begin during or at the close of the injection. Absence of immediate anesthesia suggests faulty location of the needle. The usual signs of anesthesia in order of appearance are relaxation of the tail, of the anal sphincter, and of the skeletal muscles, with loss of all sensory and motor function in the rear quarters. Surgical anesthesia ordinarily lasts about 30 minutes. The dog usually is walking with only slight difficulty within 1 hour from the time of injection.

INDICATIONS

Epidural anesthesia has many applications for postumbilical anesthesia in the dog. It is especially indicated in cesarean section. In this condition it is a desirable substitute for ether anesthesia, especially when the veterinarian does not have a capable assistant to administer the anesthetic. The client can assist by comforting the dog, which is restrained during the operation with a minimum of tapes. Meperidine hydrochloride is also useful in assisting in the restraint of the animal as well as providing satisfactory general analgesia. After the operation, the client can take the dog and the puppies home if there are no complications. The dog can be returned as an outpatient for further treatment, including removal of sutures.

Epidural anesthesia has also been used successfully for ovariohysterectomy, hernia, rectal prolapse, cystic and urethral calculi, and tail amputation. Epidural anesthesia allows easy reduction of fracture and hip luxation, but the muscular relaxation is so complete that the lack of muscle tone frequently permits the reduction to slip out of position again (Riddell 1952).

Epidural Anesthesia in Other Species

Epidural anesthesia can be employed in sheep and swine, but it is less satisfactory than in the cow, dog, and even the horse.

Epidural anesthesia can be used in the cat (Frank 1927), but it is not entirely adaptable to cats because of the temperament of this species (Riddell 1952).

Cesarean section can be successfully performed in the chinchilla under epidural anesthesia. The lumbosacral space is comparatively large in this species and easily found by the same landmarks (Riddell 1952).

Autonomic Nervous System and Epidural Anesthesia

Epidural anesthesia involves reversible and temporary paralysis of spinal nerves, which carry not only sensory and motor fibers but also efferent autonomic fibers in many instances. The autonomic nervous system is divided into the sympathetic and parasympathetic divisions, which are largely antagonistic in their innervation of viscera. The parasympathetic division is divided into the cranial and sacral parts. The cranial part, comprised primarily of the tenth or vagus cranial nerve, arises from the medulla and leaves the spinal canal immediately. The vagus, therefore, is not affected by epidural injections. The sacral part of the parasympathetic nerves arises from the second and third sacral nerves and is distributed chiefly by the internal pudic nerve. Paralysis of the sacral parasympathetic nerves occurs with all but the lightest of epidural anesthesia with resultant inhibition and dilation of the colon and rectum and relaxation of the urinary bladder and retractor penis muscle.

Paralysis of Vasoconstrictor Fibers

Efferent fibers of the sympathetic division of the autonomic nervous system leave the spinal cord in the ventral horn of the spinal nerves in the thoracolumbar area. These white (medullated), preganglionic fibers carry vasoconstrictor impulses to the blood vessels. The effect of an epidural injection of a local anesthetic solution, large in volume and concentration, may extend forward to paralyze the sympathetic vasoconstrictor fibers contained in the spinal nerves. Vasodilation results in a pooling of blood, which is more marked in the splanchnic area than elsewhere, because the vascular bed of the splanchnic vessels is subject to the greatest variation. The vasoconstrictor fibers controlling the spanchnic blood vessels arise primarily from the last thoracic and first lumbar spinal nerves. Posterior epidural anesthesia ordinarily does not affect this forward area and has no depressant effect upon the vascular system. The larger volume of local anesthetic solution necessary for anterior epidural anesthesia usually reaches and affects the spinal nerves of the thoracolumbar junction.

Protective Effect of Ephedrine Sulfate

Occasionally, vascular shock occurs and is manifested by a very rapid heart rate, weak pulse, and rapid, shallow respirations. Swangarde (quoted by Wright 1947) observed this condition in bulls following the epidural injection of 150–200 ml of 2% solution of procaine hydrochloride. European investigators have adequately demonstrated that the depression of blood pressure in cattle subject to anterior epidural anesthesia is much less marked with a 1% solution of procaine hydrochloride than a 2% concentration. This reaction is guarded against in human beings by the preanesthetic oral administration of 25 mg of ephedrine sulfate, which antagonizes the vasodilation. In dogs the premedicative or simultaneous intraspinal administration of 1–2 mg of ephedrine sulfate per lb of body weight with an intraspinal anesthetic prevents the hypotensive action of the anesthetic. Similar administration of ephedrine to dogs under the influence of a spinal anesthetic usually causes a rise in blood pressure, increased cardiac output, and decreased susceptibility to hemorrhage (Burch and Harrison 1931).

Commercially there are preparations of procaine hydrochloride for veterinary medical use that contain ephedrine sulfate usually in 1:10,000 concentration. Premedication with ephedrine sulfate probably should be a routine procedure prior to epidural anesthesia. This is especially true any time an epidural injection is made that is apt to produce paralysis of the sympathetic nerve outflow tracts or vasoconstrictor fibers.

REFERENCES

Aanes, W. A. 1963. Personal communication.

Blundell, A. E.; Bodell, B.; Andorko, J. E.; Sweeney, J. C., Jr.; and Ansbro, F. P. 1955. Clinical evaluation of drugs used in obtaining lumbar epidural anesthesia. Anesthesiology 16:386.

Brook, G. B. 1935. Spinal (epidural) anaesthesia in the domestic animals: A review of our knowledge at the present time. Vet Rec 15:549, 576, 597, 631, 659.

Burch, J. C., and Harrison, T. R. 1931. The effect of ephedrine on the circulation of dogs during spinal anaesthesia. Surg Gynecol Obstet 52:953.

Frank, E. R. 1927. Regional anesthesia in the dog and cat. J Am Vet Med Assoc 72:336.

Frank, E. R., and Roberts, S. J. 1940. Cesarean section in the bovine. N Am Vet 21:516.

Grafe, W., and Schulze, W. 1949. Zur Technik der lumbosacren Extraduralanaesthesie beim Hund. Berl Munch Tierarztl Wochenschr 10:140.

Helrich, M.; Papper, E. M.; Brodie, B. B.; Fink, M.; and Rovenstine, E. A. 1950. The fate of intrathecal procaine and the spinal fluid required for surgical anesthesia. J Pharmacol Exp Ther 100:78.

McLeod, W. M., and Frank, E. R. 1927–28. A preliminary report regarding epidural anesthesia in equines and bovines. J Am Vet Med Assoc 72:327.

Prickett, M. D.; Gross, E. G.; and Cullen, S. C. 1945. Spinal analgesia with solutions of procaine and epinephrine: A preliminary report of 108 cases. Anesthesiology 6:469.

Riddell, W. K. 1952. Caudal anesthesia in canine surgery. J Small Anim Med 1:159.

Roberts, S. J. 1950. A comparison of anesthetics used in the bovine animal. J Am Vet Med Assoc. 116:282.

Rudin, D. O.; Fremont-Smith, K.; and Beecher, H. K. 1951. Permeability of dura mater to epidural procaine in dogs. J Appl Physiol 3:388.

St. Clair, L. E., and Hardenbrook, H. J. 1956. Lumbar epidural anesthesia in cattle. J Am Vet Med Assoc 129:405.

Wright, J. G. 1947. Veterinary Anaesthesia, 2nd ed. London: Baillière, Tindall & Cox.

Wright, J. G., and Hall, L. W. 1961. Veterinary Anaesthesia and Analgesia, 5th ed. Baltimore: Williams & Wilkins.

SECTION 6

Drugs Acting on the Cardiovascular System

CHAPTER 21

HISTAMINE, SEROTONIN, KININS, PROSTAGLANDINS, AND ALLERGY-ANAPHYLAXIS PHENOMENA

MICHAEL SZABUNIEWICZ and
J. D. McCRADY

HISTAMINE

Histamine and other agents described in this chapter are extractable from the body tissues. For this reason they have been called local hormones, autacoids, or autopharmacologic agents.

Formation and Tissue Distribution

Histamine, 2-(4-imidazolyl) ethylamine, may be considered to be the decarboxylation product of histidine and has the structure shown in Fig. 21.1.

Histamine in the body is present primarily in at least 3 pools: mast cells and circulating basophils, mucosal layer of the gastrointestinal (GI) tract, and the central nervous system (CNS). In these pools it reacts differently with depleting and antagonizing agents. There is a species variation in the concentration of histamine in particular tissues. In human beings van Arsdel (1960) found high concentrations in the lungs (33 μg/g), face skin (30.4 μg/g), basophils (1080 μg/10^9 cells), stomach and duodenum (14 μg/g), spleen (3.4 μg/g), CNS (0.2 μg/g), and whole blood (16–89 μg/L). Blood of the goat and rabbit is relatively high in histamine, whereas blood of the horse, dog, cat, and rat is relatively low. Histamine is nearly always present in damaged tissue, decomposing tissue extract, and putrefying ingesta rich in protein.

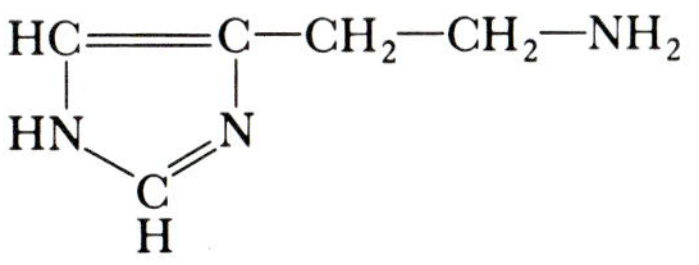

```
HC=====C—CH2—CH2—NH2
 |     |
HN     N
  \\  //
    C
    H
```

Histamine

Fig. 21.1.

Release

Histamine is readily released by degranulating agents from the mast cells in a two-step process: (1) extrusion of the granules and (2) release of histamine from these granules as an ionic exchange between granule histamine and the cations (probably sodium ions) in the extracellular fluid. It also has been postulated that part of the histamine is released without a concomitant expulsion of granules (Slorach 1971), e.g., without direct communication to the extracellular medium. A large number of "stressors" can liberate histamine from its tissue stores. These include (1) mechanical trauma, (2) cold and heat, (3) ultraviolet radiation, (4) many chemicals, and (5) antibody-antigen or allergen reaction. The mechanisms of mast cell damage during antigen-antibody reactions are not yet known. Some drugs are known to cause the release of histamine: alkaloids (curare, morphine, atropine), sympathomimetic amines, procaine, tetracycline, penicillins, polymyxin, dextran, and the experimental compound 48/80. Additionally, histamine is released by certain toxins, venoms, and proteolytic enzymes.

Pharmacologic Effects

Histamine administered orally has little effect, if any, because it is rapidly destroyed in the GI tract and in the liver. However, when injected intravenously, it causes marked pharmacologic effects, which are quite variable between species. Responses in human beings and dogs are similar and may be summarized as (1) stimulation of exocrine glands, (2) contraction of nonvascular smooth muscle, (3) cardiovascular effects, and (4) action on other systems. Large doses of histamine (in mg/kg), administered intravenously to animals experimentally, may produce histamine shock, frequently with fatal termination.

The following exocrine glands are listed in a descending order of response to histamine: gastric, salivary, pancreatic, bronchial, and lacrimal. Only the gastric secretion of hydrochloric acid, and to a lesser degree pepsinogen, is of physiological and medicinal importance.

Histamine causes contraction of the intestine, uterus, and bronchial smooth muscles. However, there is a great variation in susceptibilities of species to this action, as shown in Table 21.1.

Cardiovascular effects are manifested by (1) vasodilation, (2) reduction in arterial pressure, and (3) increased capillary permeability. In the human patient small doses (10 μg) of histamine administered by intradermal injection cause a "triple response" (Lewis and Grant 1924): (1) a localized bluish red area around the injection site within a few seconds, (2) an edema (or wheal) around the injection site, and (3) a slowly developing area (diffuse) of reddening, which is termed "flare." The first two responses correspond to action on vessels. The third phenomenon, which is accompanied by itching, is due to stimulation of sensory nerve fibers and can be eliminated by sensory denervation. The triple response of human skin may be similar to manifestations of urticaria in animals. The fall of blood pressure is a sequence of arteriole, vein, and capillary dilation and consequent reduction of effective blood volume. However, in some species (rabbit), systemic or pulmonary arterial pressure may increase (Table 21.1). Arterial pressure may be efficiently supported by sympathetic amines; whereas the antihistamines have only minor cardiovascular effects during acute histamine reactions. The cardiac effects of histamine include tachycardia, probably as a reflex phenomenon, from the histamine-induced hypotension. Some changes in the ECG may be observed, such as premature systoles, changes in T-wave polarity and amplitude, and P-Q interval (↑ or ↓). In the rat and rabbit constriction of the pulmonary arterioles may be so pronounced

TABLE 21.1. Summary of histamine actions on vascular bed and smooth muscle in different species

Species	Effect on: Pulmonary arterioles	Bronchial smooth muscles	Uterine smooth muscles	Systemic blood pressure
Human being	+−	++	+	−
Dog	+	++	+	−
Cat	+	+	+	+−
Rat	+−	+	−	+−
Rabbit	++	+	+	+
Guinea pig	+−	+++	+	+

Note: Information for larger domestic animals is lacking. (+) Denotes smooth muscle constriction or increase in blood pressure; (−) denotes relaxation, dilatation, or decrease in blood pressure; (+−) denotes no significant effect.

that it may cause dilation of the right side of the heart. In the guinea pig histamine administered hypodermically (0.4 g/kg) or as a spray rapidly induces acute bronchoconstriction and collapse of the animal. This effect, however, can be prevented by the prior administration of an antihistaminic drug and can be alleviated by the administration of epinephrine or isoproterenol. Histamine also causes atony of the rumen and inhibits eructation.

The clinical signs of histamine are expressed by salivation, lacrimation, vomition, constriction of the pupil, abdominal pain, and diarrhea; other signs are dilation of the skin vessels, rapid pulse, polypnea, dyspnea or apnea, lower body temperature, and decreased blood volume (hemoconcentration) due to the loss of fluid into the tissue.

Metabolism and Excretion

Histamine administered orally is poorly absorbed; however, via parenteral routes absorption is complete. It is readily metabolized. Probably it is incorporated to a minor degree into body pools of the endogenous histamine.

The biotransformation of histamine involves, as shown in Fig. 21.2, (1) methylation, (2) oxidation, and (3) acetylation. Histamine is N′-methylated to 1-methylhistamine; most of this is oxidized to methylimidazole acetic acid by action of monoamine oxidase (MAO) enzyme (> 50%). The second pathway is oxidative deamination (amino group) by diamine oxidase (histaminase) to form imidazoleacetic acid, which is conjugated with ribose (as riboside, > 25%). Only a small percentage of the primary amine can be acetylated in the GI tract, absorbed, and secreted in the urine (1%). Some free histamine is also excreted in the urine (2%–3%).

Role in Health and Disease

The physiological role of histamine is not fully understood. Its action as a powerful stimulant of gastric secretion and its role in the release of catecholamines in patients with pheochromocytoma are well documented. The roles of histamine in synaptic transmission and as a neurohumoral mediator of pain are still debatable.

Histamine has been incriminated as a causative agent in certain vascular headaches of human beings and in various types of shock. In domestic animals it has been suggested that histamine released from damaged tissue may play a role in the following: allergic reactions to some drugs (e.g., sulfonamides, penicillin), ruminant bloating, overeating and other intestinal disorders of ruminants, laminitis, azoturia, endotoxic shock, gangrenous mastitis, metritis, retained placenta especially associated with toxemia, pneumonia, gut edema of the pig, and various types of

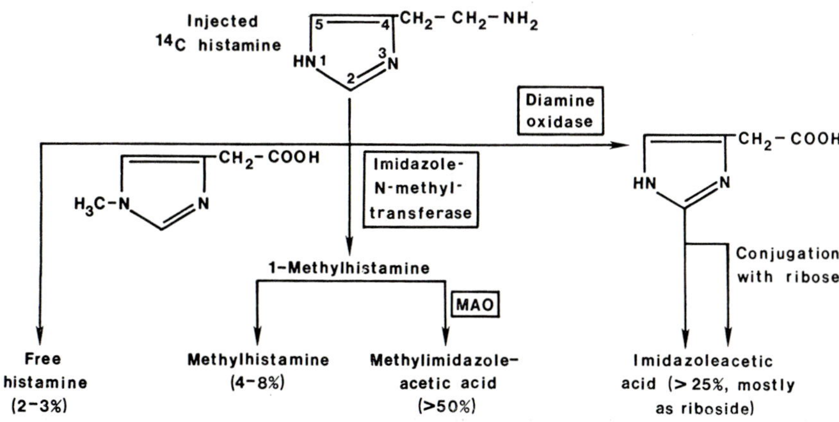

Fig. 21.2. Synthesis, metabolism, and urinary metabolites of histamine, recovered in 12 hours following intradermal injection of ^{14}C-histamine in a human male (% values from Schayer and Cooper 1956).

shock. However, the role of histamine in all these conditions is more empirically based than experimentally founded.

Medical Use

Clinical applications in human beings are limited to (1) its use as a test agent for gastric achlorhydria, (2) the diagnosis of pheochromocytoma, and (3) the production of the triple reaction to evaluate the integrity of sensory innervations. Clinical uses in animals are not documented. Histamine phosphate and histamine dihydrochloride preparations are available. Dosage is expressed in terms of the equivalent amount of free base.

ANTIHISTAMINES

The pharmacodynamic actions of histamine may be antagonized by (1) physiological antagonists, (2) metabolic antagonists, and (3) competitive antagonists. One group of physiological antagonists, sympathomimetic amines (epinephrine, isoproterenol, ephedrine, and others), produce physiologic effects opposite those of histamine, thus restoring function. These are usually the first to be considered in anaphylactic shock. Another physiological antagonist, aminophilline (xanthine), is often effective in the treatment of pulmonary edema and some types of bronchial asthma. The metabolic antagonist of histamine is the enzyme histaminase, which destroys endogenously produced histamine. However, its action is too slow to be of therapeutic value. The competitive antagonists, antihistamines or antihistaminics, have been developed and their role in therapeutics is described below.

Development of Antihistamines

Historically Bovet and Staub (1937) of the Pasteur Institute in Paris first dem-

TABLE 21.2. Preparations and dosages of some antihistamines in veterinary use

Generic Name	Trade Name	Single Dose and Route (in mg/kg unless indicated otherwise)	Preparation Available	Special Properties
Diphenhydramine HCl., U.S.P.	Benadryl, Caladryl (lotion)	L.A.: 0.5–1 S.A.: 1–2 p.o., i.v./12 hr	Inj. 10, 25, 50 mg/ml Elix. 10 mg/4 ml	Marked sedation; antimotion sickness
Pyrilamine maleate, N.F.	Histosol,* Neoantergan	L.A., S.A.: 1–2 i.m., i.v., s.c.	Inj. 20–25 mg/ml Tab. 25–50 mg	Prominent sedation
Tripelennamine HCl, U.S.P.	Pyribenzamine	L.A.: 1–2 p.o., i.v. S.A.: 1–1.5 p.o., t.i.d.	Inj. 20 mg/ml Tab. 25–50 mg Bolus 500 mg	Sedation; if overdose, ataxia; convulsions
Chlorpheniramine maleate, N.F.	Telodron,† Teldrin	S.A.: 1 span. for dogs $>$ 8–40 lb/12 hr 2 span. for dogs $>$ 40 lb/12 hr	Spansule 8 mg., sustained release form	Moderate sedation
Dimenhydrinate, U.S.P.	Dramamine	L.A., S.A.: 1–1.5 p.o., i.m., s.c.	Inj. 50 mg/ml Tab. 50 mg Liquid 12.5 mg/4 ml	Prominent antimotion sickness
Promethazine HCl, U.S.P.	Phenergan	L.A., S.A.: 0.2–1 i.m., i.v., p.o., t.i.d.	Inj. 25–50 mg/ml Tab. 25, and 50 mg Also available as cream for topical use	Long acting, marked sedation; antimotion sickness

Note: Trade names are capitalized.

Abbreviations: L.A., large animal; S.A., small animal; p.o., orally; s.c., subcutaneously; i.m., intramuscular; i.v., intravenous.

* Also available: Pyrazine with ephedrine (injectable and oral); Antiphrine with ephedrine (injectable and granules to administer in feed); Novahistine with phenylephrine HCl.

† Metrevet and Predmaton with prednisone for oral use in dogs and cats.

onstrated that two phenolic esters, designated by their discoverer, Fourneau, as compounds 929F and 157F, possessed antihistaminic activity. One of these compounds, 929F (thymoxyethyldiethylamine), protected guinea pigs against several lethal doses of histamine. These agents, however, were too toxic for therapeutic use but led the way to the development of many modern antagonists of histamine. The most frequently used experimental and therapeutic antihistaminic drugs are listed in Table 21.2.

Chemistry

The chemical structure of nearly all the antihistaminic drugs can be depicted by the structural formula shown in Fig. 21.3. In this formula it is apparent that the nucleus is an ethylamine ($—CH_2CH_2N=$), which is also present in histamine. Therefore, it may be postulated that this part of the molecule competes with histamine for specific cell receptors.

Three types of antihistaminics are known in which the element *X* (as depicted in Fig. 21.3) may be nitrogen, oxygen, or carbon. The *X* represents a nitrogen for the ethylenediamine (pyrilamine, Neoantergan) class, oxygen for the ethanolamine (diphenhydramine, Benadryl) class, and carbon for the alkylamine (chlorpheniramine, Teldrin) class. The fourth class of antihistaminics contains a piperazine in place of the conventional ethylenediamine linkage (cyclizine, Marezine). The representative of the fifth class (promethazine, Phenergan) is not related to the previous drugs as it is a phenothiazine derivative. These chemical differences may influence the potency of action as well as produce a variety of side effects, e.g., Antergen protects the guinea pig against 60, Neoantergan against 80, and Phenergan against 1000 lethal doses of histamine.

$$\begin{matrix} R_1 \\ \quad \end{matrix}\!\!>\!X-\overset{|}{\underset{|}{C}}-\overset{|}{\underset{|}{C}}-N\!<\!\begin{matrix} R \\ R \end{matrix} \quad (R_2 \text{ on } X)$$

Fig. 21.3. General formula of most of the antihistaminic agents.

Pharmacologic Effects

Antihistaminics are satisfactorily absorbed following oral administration in monogastric animals but not in ruminants. Effects are usually expected within 20–45 minutes, and the duration of action of a therapeutic dose ranges from 3 to 12 hours, as shown in Table 21.2. The intravenous administration elicits immediate effects but this route is not frequently recommended because of resulting CNS stimulation and other side effects. However, the intramuscular route rarely gives rise to side effects and this route is commonly used. Topical application may be suitable in certain skin conditions.

Antihistamines act as competitive antagonists for specific receptors in the tissue cells and their binding to the cell receptors evokes no pharmacologic action. This mechanism of action is based on quantitative considerations; therefore, histamine in excess may displace antihistaminics. Generally, antihistaminics are more effective against exogenously released histamine than against endogenously released histamine. They are also more effective in preventing the actions of histamine than in reversing them.

The antihistaminics are most efficient in countering the action of histamine on bronchial, intestinal, and uterine smooth muscle, and to a lesser degree on the vascular bed. The antihistaminics antagonize both the vasoconstrictor effects (on systemic vessels in the rabbit and pulmonary vessels in the cat), and vasodilator effects of histamine. However, the vascular effects are less marked than effects on other smooth musculature. Yet, even this reduced effect on smooth muscle of vessels has great clinical importance for both augmentation of the tonus of arterioles and capillary vessels, as well as for reduction of capillary permeability and reduction of formation of edema in response to histamine. This antihistaminic effect counteracts urticaria, whealing, and other types of edema formation in response to injury, antigens, allergens, or histamine-liberating drugs in many species. Antihistaminics also suppress itching and "flare" in human beings and greatly reduce the itching of allergic reactions.

The antihistiminics only partially antagonize histamine-induced arterial hypotension. They do not block the stimulant effect of histamine on gastric secretion, but some stimulant effects on salivary and other exocrine glands may be antagonized. Antihistamine does not prevent histamine-liberating drugs from releasing histamine and, in fact, some antihistaminics possess histamine-liberating properties. This latter action may be of clinical significance in therapeutic uses of these drugs. The antihistaminics do not prevent the release of histamine during the antigen-antibody reaction. Their therapeutic action, however, may be useful, due to competitive antagonistic effects at receptor sites.

Side Effects and Interactions

Each antihistaminic produces certain side effects. Those of clinical importance are (1) sedation or excitement, (2) GI disturbances, (3) parasympatholytic action, (4) local anesthetic properties, (5) allergenic properties, and (6) teratogenic effects.

Antihistaminics elicit a sedative effect in therapeutic doses, which is expressed by drowsiness or ataxia. In higher doses they may produce irritability, convulsions, hyperpyrexia, and even death. GI disorders may be seen as anorexia, nausea, vomiting, constipation, or diarrhea when antihistamines are administered orally for a prolonged period of time. The antichloliner-gic effects are expressed by a dry mouth, pupillary dilation, blurred vision, and tachycardia. Local anesthetic properties are of value when these agents are used as antipruritic drugs in topical application. Paradoxically, antihistaminics may be also allergenic when applied to the skin. The teratogenic effects of some, demonstrated in animals, suggest caution in the use of these drugs during pregnancy. These agents possess antiserotonin properties and also cocainelike effects on catecholamine uptake.

Interaction of antihistamines with other agents may result in an additive or potentiative effect with other CNS depressants such as tranquilizers, narcotic anesthetics, and in human beings with alcohol, reserpine, and monoamine oxidase inhibitors. Atropinism may occur with combined parasympatholytic and phenothiazine derivative agents. Antihistamines decrease the effects of steroids, androgens, progesterone, and hydrocortisone. They may also interfere with allergic diagnostic tests, particularly with the tuberculin test.

Toxicity

In recommended doses antihistamines are nontoxic; however, overdosage or combinations with the above potentiating agents may elicit toxic effects. These effects are expressed by hyperexcitability and even convulsions. The treatment of acute toxicity is symptomatic; sedative or ultrashort barbiturates may be of value, but caution is indicated because additive effects are possible.

Therapeutic Uses

Clinically, these agents are used in certain allergic reactions and, in combination with physiologic antagonists, in anaphylactic shock. These considerations will be discussed at the end of this chapter under Allergy and Immunity.

Nonallergic but suspected histamine-related phenomena, which via empirical experience prove to respond to antihistaminic therapy in animals, include many pathologic conditions. Those in which antihistaminics are reported to be of therapeutic value are pruritus, urticaria, various types of dermatitis, moist eczema, acute eczematous otitis, insect stings, nutritional type of laminitis, pregnancy laminitis, paroxysmal myoglobinuria or azoturia, periodic ophthalmia, and pulmonary emphysema in horses. Also, they are considered to be of value in the treatment of bovine asthma (pulmonary emphysema), some types of bloat and acetonemia in ruminants, acute septic and gangrenous mastitis, septic metritis and retained placenta, pregnancy toxemia, and gut edema of pigs. In addition, these agents are helpful in some types of asthma and motion and/or seasickness.

The action of antihistaminics is symptomatic in character. Therefore, they are not a panacea for all maladies, and the removal of etiological factors must be the goal of therapy. The most frequently used antihistaminics in animals and their posology are shown in Table 21.2.

SEROTONIN

The unidentified vasoconstrictor agent appearing in serum was known for about a century and was called *vasotonin*. Rapport et al. (1948) isolated this vasoconstrictor from the serum in a crystalline form and gave it the name *serotonin*. These investigators discovered that, chemically, serotonin was 5-hydroxytryptamine (5-HT). Independently, another group of researchers studying histochemical properties of the intestinal mucosa discovered an active agent in enterochromaffin (argentaffin) cells and gave it the name *enteramine* (Erspamer 1946; Erspamer and Asero 1952). After the discovery of 5-HT in the blood, it was soon confirmed that enteramine had the same chemical structure as serotonin (5-HT). When Hamlin and Fischer (1951) made this agent synthetically, considerable research on the action of 5-HT followed.

Chemistry

Serotonin is synthesized from dietary tryptophan in a two-stage chemical reaction. First, tryptophan is hydroxylated by the enzyme tryptophan 5-hydroxylase to give 5-hydroxytryptophan (5-HTP). The substrate for 5-HTP decarboxylase yielding serotonin is shown in Fig. 21.4. Like histamine, 5-HT is widely distributed in animals and plants. It occurs in high concentration in some fruits such as bananas, pineapples, and plums and is also present in stings (common stinging nettle) and venoms.

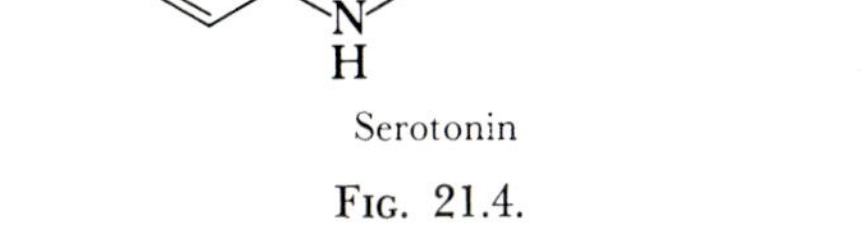

HO— (indole ring) —CH_2—CH_2—NH_2; N—H

Serotonin

Fig. 21.4.

In mammals endogenous 5-HT is synthesized from about 1% of the dietary tryptophan and found in 3 essential pools, where it is also formed (1) in argentaffin cells of the intestine (about 90%), (2) in a small number of neurons in the CNS, and (3) in the mast cells of rodents (rats, mice, and hamsters) along with histamine and heparin. Although serotonin (thrombocytin) is concentrated in the blood platelets, which contain about 8% serotonin, it is not synthetized there because of the lack of decarboxylase. Serotonin appears to be bound within cytoplasmic granules. It is also continually produced and destroyed in the pool of the intestine and brain. In platelets it appears to be released only upon their destruction.

Most serotonin is metabolized by oxidative deamination to form 5-hydroxyindoleacetic acid (5-HIAA); the enzyme catalyzing this reaction is a MAO. The end product, 5-HIAA, of metabolism is excreted in the urine. However, in the pineal gland, *N*-acetylation and 5-methylation form the hormone *melatonin*.

Pharmacologic Effects

Serotonin may have multiple mechanisms of action and great variation in different species. However, its essential actions are on smooth muscle, CNS, and peripheral nerves, including afferent nerve endings. Given orally, it is quickly degraded and produces no effect.

Fast intravenous injection of serotonin-creatine sulfate produces a triphasic response: (1) initial fall of systemic arterial pressure accompanied by paradoxical bradycardia, due mainly to reflex chemoreceptor stimulation (Bezold-Jarish effect); (2) a short period of pressor effect (similar to epinephrine effect); and (3) a prolonged fall in systemic blood pressure attributed to the vasodilator effect in the vascular bed of skeletal muscle. It also causes a fall in pulmonary arterial pressure (pulmonary depressor reflex). A continuous infusion of 5-HT (drip method, experimentally), which most closely resembles the release of this agent endogenously, causes a prolonged fall in arterial pressure due to vascular bed dilation. Only in rodents, serotonin increases small vessel permeability similar to that of histamine.

The nonvascular smooth muscle of the bronchi and intestines is stimulated. Intestinal effects are direct and are mediated via excitation of ganglion cells in the myenteric plexus. This action has an important role in regulating intestinal motility. In some species serotonin causes contraction of the ureter and uterus (rodent). On repeated doses of serotonin, tachyphylaxis is a common phenomenon.

When serotonin is injected, it has no effect on the CNS because it is strongly polar and cannot cross the blood-brain barrier. However, 5-HTP can penetrate into the brain and be decarboxylated to serotonin; this may produce behavioral changes. Serotonin also can stimulate afferent nerve endings, ganglion cells, and adrenal medullary cells.

Role in Physiologic and Pathologic Processes

The finding that serotonin is present in the CNS (hypothalamic and other areas) and that reserpine may release serotonin from these areas led to the hypothesis of the role of serotonin as a central neurotransmitter. Serotonin influences sleep, intestinal motility, and temperature regulaation, and it affects the mood and behavior of human beings. While the functions of serotonin in the brain are not yet well defined, it seems that an excess of this agent brings about stimulation of CNS activity and that a deficiency produces a depressant effect. The role of serotonin in platelets may be related to the mechanism of hemostasis (via vasoconstriction). However, a recent study using a depletor agent (reserpine) places this hypothesis (Harper 1971) in doubt.

There is evidence that serotonin exerts an inhibitory effect on a variety of behaviors (Green and Harvey 1974). The role of serotonin in the mental disorders of human beings has been speculative; its role has not been well established. The only disease where serotonin probably plays an important role is in the carcinoid syndrome (argentaffinoma). The disease is characterized by the widespread development of a serotonin-producing tumor in the argentaffin cells of the GI tract. Symptoms are related to the action on smooth muscle of the blood vessels and the digestive and respiratory tracts. The serotonin in the blood of a carcinoid subject is 0.5–2.7 μg/ml (while normal is 0.1–0.3 μg/ml). The urinary metabolite has significant diagnostic value; excretion of 5-HIAA has been reported as 76–850 mg in 24 hours (normal is 2–8 mg). This results in 60% of the dietary intake of tryptophan being converted to serotonin. Consequently, a deficiency may develop producing symptoms of pellagra and negative nitrogen balance. The effectiveness of several serotonin antagonists in the prevention of migraine in human beings emphasizes its role in this condition (vascular headaches). Serotonin's role in allergy anaphylaxis is discussed at the end of this chapter.

Antagonists

The actions of serotonin are countered by two groups of antagonists. Neural effects on smooth muscle of the digestive tract are antagonized by morphine, atropine, and cocaine; the direct effects on smooth muscle are antagonized by phenoxybenzamine and two derivatives of ergot alkaloids, LSD and methysergide. An antihistamine, cyproheptadine, is also a powerful antiserotonin agent. Chlorpromazine and phenoxybenzamine are weak blocking agents. Reserpine and the experimental agent known as 48/80 are examples of drugs that deplete serotonin in the CNS. Another antagonist frequently used experimentally is *p*-chlorophenylamine. This agent acts via inhibition of serotonin synthesis. For clinical use, especially in human beings, methysergide (oral dose 2–4 mg t.i.a.) and cyproheptadine (oral dose 4 mg t.i.a.) are the only available effective antagonists.

KININS

Kinins, are the most potent vasodilators released into the plasma by action of various proteolytic enzymes. The first was named by Kraut et al. (1930) "kallikrein" from the Greek word *kallikreas* (pancreas) when this agent was isolated from the pancreas. These authors found that kallikreins were present in saliva and plasma. In 1948 Werle and Berek named the active agent "kallidin" and its precursor "kallidinogen"; kallikrein, an enzymelike substance, activates a precursor present in blood. Rocha e Silva et al. (1949) discovered a new polypeptide agent acting on plasma globulin by trypsin. This substance was named "bradykinin" from the Greek words *bradys* (slow) and *kinein* (to move) to express the characteristic action of slowly developing contractions in the smooth muscle of the isolated guinea pig ileum. Their potent effects on smooth muscle were the first properties studied. This effect is not inhibited by atropine, cholinesterase inhibitors, or ganglionic blocking agents.

Chemistry

Bradykinin and kallidin are formed from the same substrate, an α-2-globulin of plasma, via the action of several proteolytic enzymes. This created some confusion about identity of these agents. However, Elliot (1963) suggested that bradykinin or killidin-9 be retained for the nanopeptide and that kallidin-10 be retained for the decapeptide. The addition of methionine to the *N*-terminal lysine of kallidin-10 results in the formation of the third biologically active plasma kinin called methionyl-kallidin or methionyl-lysyl-bradykinin. The release of these kinins is normally controlled in the body by many factors because the principal kininogen-activating enzyme is in an inactive form, kallikreinogen. The enzyme may be activated by a change in pH (lowered) or by the Hageman factor (same as in clotting mechanism).

The kinins, initially isolated from tissue, have been synthesized. Kinins are soluble in water and resistant to boiling temperature, but dilute solutions deteriorate as they are adsorbed to glass surfaces. In the body, kinins are short lived (a halflife of only seconds to minutes) because blood contains the enzyme aminopeptidase, which converts kallidin to bradykinin, and another enzyme, carboxypeptidase-*N*, which degrades both kinins to inactive products. Some kinins are excreted in the urine unchanged. Formation of kinins and their destruction are illustrated in Fig. 21.5*A*.

Pharmacologic Effects

The principal effects of kinins are depicted in Fig. 21.5*B*. These are (1) arteriolar, capillary, and venular dilation and, ultimately, venous constriction (due to reflex catecholamine liberation), (2) increase in capillary permeability (more potent than histamine), (3) production of pain (on intradermal injection), (4) constriction of nonvascular smooth muscle (bronchi, intestine, uterus), and (5) migration of leukocytes (granulocytes). However, the effects of kinins on vascular and other smooth muscle depend on both the anatomic location and species and, probably, on the interaction with other vasoactive substances such as catecholamines and angiotensin. Kinins also can cause release of catecholamines (from the adrenal medulla) and histamine and stimulate the autonomic ganglia.

Tachyphylaxis is a common phenomenon following repeated administration of kinin (pain in human patients and bronchoconstriction in guinea pigs). The future role of kinins in different physiopathological states awaits results from more intensive biochemical and molecular studies.

Role in Physiologic and Pathologic Conditions

The role of kinins, even where they exist in large quantities (parotid gland, pancreas, and plasma), has not yet been determined. Melman et al. (1968) suggested that kinins may play a role by constricting umbilical vessels and the ductus

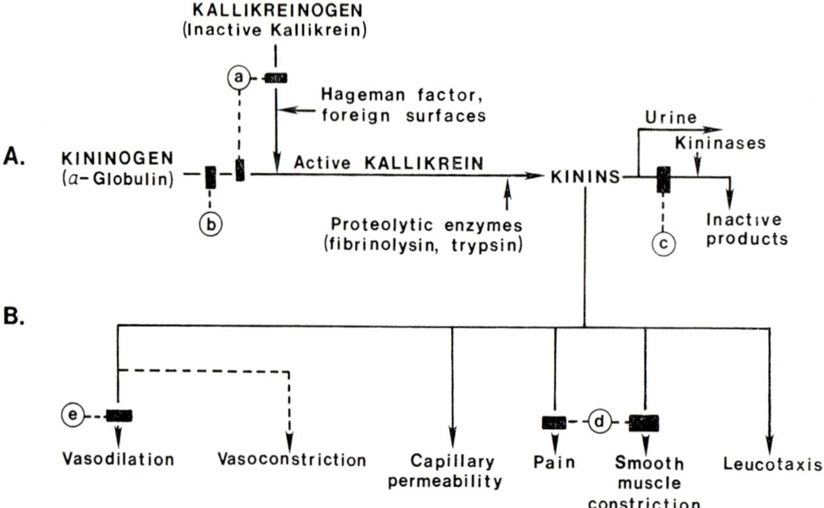

C.

a - Corticosteroids (?)
b - Aprotinin (protein from parotid gl. of ox.)
Pancreatic trypsin inhibitor
c - BAL (Dimercaprol), EDTA, acid pH
d - Aspirin, Phenylbutazone
e - Chlorpromazine

FIG. 21.5. Schematic presentation of the mechanism of kinin: *(A)* formation and destruction; *(B)* pharmacologic actions; and *(C)* antagonistic agents.

arteriosis in neonates. Their role as neurotransmitter substances in the CNS still awaits elucidation.

Pathological conditions in which kinins may be active are acute inflammation associated with burns, rheumatoid arthritis, hereditary angioneurotic edema (in human beings) and carcinoid syndrome, pancreatitis, migraine headache (in human beings), reactions after transfusion of plasma products, allergic diseases, endotoxin shock, and anaphylactic shock. In several other conditions, the role of kinins is less certain.

In the carcinoid syndrome, the tumor secretes not only serotonin but also kinins and histamine. However, the exact molecular interaction between kinins and the target organ in all these conditions is unknown.

Inhibitors of Kinins

At present, there is no known antagonist of kinins. However, several chemicals or drugs may inhibit particular actions or the formation of kinins. These agents are enumerated in Fig. 21.5*C*, and their sites of action are depicted in *A* and *B* in the same figure. Trasylol (aprotinin) has been used in the treatment of pancreatitis in human beings with variable results. The corticosteroids, inhibitors of activated kallikrein and its substrate, may be useful in these conditions where overproduction of kinins is likely to occur (as in endotoxin shock). Aspirin and other analgesics, as well as chlorpromazine, may alleviate pain and bronchoconstriction due to the inhibition of action of kinins but they do not alter vascular effects. Other agents such as British antilewisite (BAL) and ethylenediaminetetraacetic acid (EDTA) acting as kininase inhibitors may augment kinins in target organs and/or in plasma. The role of kinin deficiency in pathological conditions is unknown.

Other Peptides

Several other peptides, of which the actions and role in pathological states are less known, are substance P, eledoisin, physalaemin, and coerulein.

Substance P was first extracted from horse intestine and brain, and the structure is not yet known (von Euler and Gaddum 1931). It has, however, bradykininlike action (i.e., powerful vasodilator), it contracts smooth muscle, and it has an inhibitory effect on the CNS. Eledoisin (from the octopus), physalaemin (from amphibian skin), and coerulein are also examples of active peptides. These are derived from lower animals and have bradykininlike actions in mammals.

Angiotensin is still another polypeptide chemically related to the kinins. It can be released by the enzyme renin from the ischemic juxtaglomerular cells in the kidney. Renin forms angiotensin I (decapeptide) from a plasma α-globulin precursor, angiotensinogen. Angiotensin I is converted to angiotensin II (octapeptide) by another enzyme.

Angiotensin is a powerful vasoconstrictor, in contrast to all previously described peptides that were essentially vasodilators. Angiotensin also contracts smooth muscle of other organs. Its function is related to (1) the maintenance of renal circulation and (2) the control of aldosterone secretion. It is postulated that the renin-angiotensin-aldosterone mechanism may play a role in the etiology of some forms of hypertension in human beings. No effective antagonists for angiotensin are known. Angiotensin amide (N.F.), synthetic octapeptide, is recommended in treatment of shock; the human dose is 2.5 mg in 250 ml of isotonic saline solution administered intravenously.

Other vasoactive polypeptides, including oxytocin and vasopressin, will be discussed in Section 8.

PROSTAGLANDINS

In 1930 Kurzrok and Lieb reported that the human uterus contracted or relaxed upon instillation of fresh human semen. This report generated new studies in the search for an active agent. Almost simultaneously, Goldblatt in England (1933) and von Euler in Sweden (1934) published observations on the strong smooth muscle–stimulating activity of human seminal fluid. von Euler (1935) found similar effects were related to seminal fluid from the monkey, sheep, and goat and named the then unknown active agent "prostaglandin." About 30 years later, Bergström et al. (1962) established the structure of the first two prostaglandins, PGE_1 and $PGF_{1\alpha}$. A few years later, synthesis was accomplished. This discovery initiated numerous studies and publications on the physiologic and pharmacologic effects of prostaglandins as well as speculations on their future therapeutic role.

Chemistry

Prostaglandins are found in virtually all tissues. High concentrations occur in human and sheep seminal plasma with values reported up to 200 μg/ml. The concentration in other tissues is much lower, i.e., about 1 μg/g.

Prostaglandins are derived enzymatically from arachidonic acid (and some other related 20-carbon essential fatty acids) by cyclization and oxidation. Prostanoic acid, an intermediate product, is inactive. The carbon chains in prostanoic acid are bonded at positions 8 and 12 by a 5-membered ring. The variations in this ring give rise to 4 major groups of prostaglandins: E, F, A, and B (Fig. 21.6). Six variations of E and F are known and are referred to as primary prostaglandins. These in turn may be converted in the body to 8 secondary prostaglandins. Of 14 naturally occurring prostaglandins, there are 3 PGE, 3 PGFα, 4 PGA, and 4 PGB. Also about 500 synthetic analogs have been developed.

Labeled prostaglandins, when administered intravenously to human beings, disappear from the blood within 10 minutes. About 60% of the administered dose is excreted in the urine, 20% in the feces, and the remainder unknown.

Pharmacologic Effects

Prostaglandins are the first chemical derivatives of fatty acid known to be pharmacologically active. The synthetic compounds are 40–400 times more potent than the natural compounds because they are

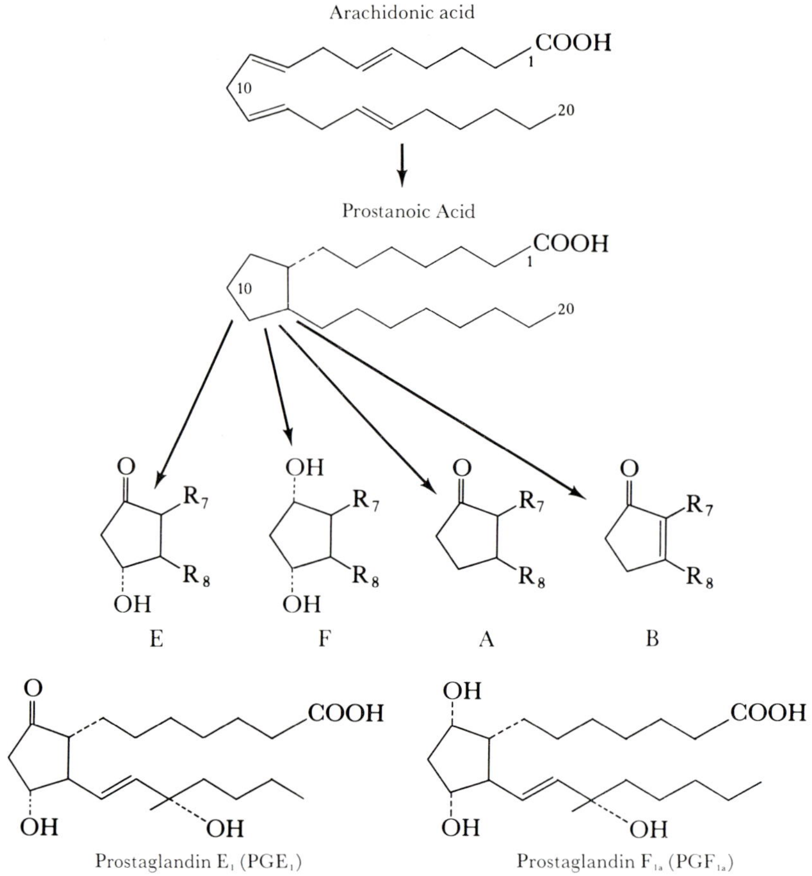

Arachidonic acid

Prostanoic Acid

E F A B

Prostaglandin E_1 (PGE_1)

Prostaglandin $F_{1\alpha}$ ($PGF_{1\alpha}$)

FIG. 21.6. Schematic presentation of the structure and nomenclature of the four groups of naturally occurring prostaglandins.

not metabolized. They are active *in vitro* at 0.01 μg/ml and *in vivo* at 10 μg/kg concentration, respectively; all are readily absorbed from the vaginal mucosa.

Natural and synthetic prostaglandins exhibit hormonelike actions and are among the most potent agents known. However, the actions of prostaglandins vary among themselves, both qualitatively and quantitatively. Their actions also vary in the different species. They possess a myriad of biological activities; the most characteristic are exerted on the smooth muscle of the following organs: uterus (nongravid: PGE—relaxes, PGF—contracts; gravid: PGE and PGF—contract); cardiovascular (vasodilation, in a few exceptions PGE and PGF produce vasoconstriction); GI tract (stimulation); and bronchi (PGE relaxes and PGF contracts). In the CNS (stimulation and/or inhibition) they may release transmitter impulses. They also play some role in metabolism of lipids and carbohydrates, inhibition of platelet aggregation and inflammatory and immune mechanisms (Ramwell and Shaw 1971), and inhibition of gastric secretion. The mechanism of prostaglandin formation and release is brought about by nerve activity, both central and peripheral.

Prostaglandins interact with many drugs and with other endogenously produced substances. They potentiate actions of vasopressin, catecholamines, acetylcholine, and serotonin, but they antagonize morphine. Aspirin blocks the synthesis of PGs in human platelets, guinea pig lung, and some other tissues. Therefore, it has been postulated that the antiinflammatory action of aspirin may be related to the inhibition of prostaglandins. Recently it was shown that indomethacin reduces pituitary and hypothalamic levels of PGF (Orczyk and Behrman 1972).

The role of prostaglandins in reproductive physiology is a complex interrelationship between ovarian function and the hypothalamic-pituitary axis that regulates the reproductive process. At this time the best established action of PGF_{2a} is its role as the "uterine luteolysin" responsible for causing regression of corpora lutea in many nonprimate mammalian species (Inskeep 1973). See Chapter 32.

Therapeutic Use

Prostaglandins are still under investigation. Their possible therapeutic uses have been explored as inducers of labor at term, as abortifacients, and as postconceptional fertility control agents. In cattle, F_{2a} and analogs are being used to induce luteolysis for estrus synchronization and, in mares, to induce estrus and ovulation in animals during diestrus. Also, PGE_1 has been used in conjunction with follicle-stimulating hormone (FSH) to induce multiple ovulation in rhesus monkeys. For clinical use they are approved in the United Kingdom for mares and cattle and for mares in United States.

Their usefulness in asthma, hypertension, peptic ulcers, and control of inflammation is still under investigation. It is also postulated that inhibitors of PG synthesis, when elucidated, may play a role in male fertility and in control of sickle cell anemia in human beings.

Other Fatty Acid Derivatives

Feldberg and Kellaway (1938) discovered a substance in perfused lungs exposed to cobra venom that caused slowly developing vasodilation. Human bronchioles are very sensitive to it and react by sustained contraction. The active principle has not been identified. However, it appears to be a group of unsaturated fatty acids. It has been postulated that this substance may play a role in anaphylaxis. Due to its character of action and participation in anaphylaxis, this agent was named "slow reacting substance of anaphylaxis" (SRS-A).

Preparations

Preparations available in the United Kingdom are *Equimate* and *Estrumate* (ICI), analogs of PGF_{2a}, and in the United States *Veterinary Prostin* F_{2a} (Upjohn).

ALLERGY AND IMMUNITY

The antigen-antibody reaction is a basic phenomenon of allergy and immunity. The immunologic mechanism is expressed by the body's recognition of, response to, and disposition of foreign material within living cells and tissue to chemicals, drugs and antigenic substances. The recognition and response are expressed by the production of antibodies or cells with specific affinity to antigen. The immunoglobulins are mediators of antigen-antibody reactions, while the mechanism of cellular immunity is associated with circulating macrophages and/or lymphocytes. Some foreign substances may be classified as strong antigens that produce the classical immune (therapeutic immunity) or hypersensitive effect in the host. Weak antigens induce only a weak response. However, a second contact with the same antigen (strong or weak) may cause an antigen-antibody reaction that elicits an allergic response in susceptible subjects. Once hypersensitivity to an allergen is established, it can persist for years. The most severe reaction of the sensitized subject to renewed contact with an antigen (especially of protein origin) is termed anaphylaxis (systemic as opposed to cutaneous) or anaphylactic shock. An additional mechanism related to the disposition of antigenic substances is inflammation. This develops by the toxic or irritant effect of many substances, which induce vascular permeability, and in consequence, edema. However, in immunized subjects small quantities of antigens, via release of mediators, may also induce increased vascular permeability with rapid accumulation of monocytes.

Antigens or allergens may include not only foreign proteins but practically any foreign substance. Nonprotein substances are called haptens, as in the case of many drugs, which may combine with the host's body proteins and subsequently produce the allergens; e.g., penicillin or its metabolite such as penicillenic acid that readily conjugates *in vivo* with protein, forming an antigen-hapten. The penetration of allergens into the body may be accomplished by various means such as inhalation (dust, plant pollens), ingestion (food, drugs), skin contact (antibiotic ointment, poisons), or deliberate introduction of the antigen by injection. Infections or parasitic diseases may also provide the source of protein or other substances that may evoke allergy.

Chemical Mediators

The chemical mediators that are released from their storage sites in the tissue of sensitized animals as the result of an antigen-antibody reaction are histamine, serotonin, bradykinin, and SRS-A. The pharmacologic effects, storage, and release of these substances were previously discussed. The role of heparin, acetylcholine, prostaglandins, and other substances in the antigen-antibody reaction remains uncertain.

The species variation in manifestations of anaphylaxis is partly due to varying amounts of histamine, serotonin, and SRS-A in different stores, as in mast cells, basophils, and platelets; also, there are differences in response of the so-called shock tissues, such as skin, smooth muscle, blood vessels and bronchioles, mucus-secreting cells, and mast cells.

Allergic Reactions

von Pirquet (1906) used the term allergy (from Greek "altered action") to describe any altered response to a foreign material (antigen) induced by previous exposure to the same antigen. Therefore, increased resistance, called immunity, and increased susceptibility, called hypersusceptibility, were considered as two opposite forms of allergy. From this original definition, the terms allergy and hypersensitivity have become synonymous. From a clinical aspect, allergic reactions are classified as immediate (acute) and delayed (protracted).

The immediate-type reactions develop in minutes. They are mediated by antibodies that react with antigenic substances or allergens and cause the rapid release of histamine as well as other pharmacologically active substances. The most important allergic responses of this type are systemic anaphylaxis, cutaneous anaphylaxis, Arthus reaction, and serum sickness syndrome. The delayed-type reactions develop in hours or days. They are mediated by sensitized lymphocytes or macrophages (cellular immunity). This type of allergy is due to microbial antigen, purified proteins, and chemicals and drugs. The best example of delayed-type allergic reaction is the positive tuberculin test, contact dermatitis, some serum sickness syndromes, and rejection of homografts.

Another type of hypersensitivity is autoallergy (autoimmunity), which is expressed by an immune response against components of the body's own tissue, e.g., autoimmune hemolytic anemia, lupus erythematosus in dogs, and milk allergy in cattle. In milk allergy casein may be absorbed from the udder, which produces an allergic response exhibited as urticaria and respiratory distress. Anaphylactoid reaction is produced in normal subjects by injection of any material capable of releasing mediators without activation of the antigen-antibody response (clinical aspect may be indistinguishable from true anaphylaxis). Atopic allergy is the group of naturally occurring allergies to atopic reagins as pollens, foods, and insect stings, i.e., hay fever, urticaria, and atopic eczema.

Clinical Allergies

Allergic reactions most frequently recognized clinically are not due to microbial antigens but to environmental allergens (dust, pollens, chemicals) as well as autoantigens (such as red cells or erythroglobulins) in autoimmune diseases. In addition, allergic responses may arise from medicinal interventions such as blood transfusions or organ transplants (homografts). Allergies to drugs and biologic agents (vaccines, toxoids) probably occur in animals more often than they are recognized. In Canada, 80 veterinary surgeons diagnosed varying degrees of reactions in 1200 cattle injected with the following antibiotics: penicillin-streptomycin combination, neomycin, and oxytetracycline (Brisbane 1963). Recently it has been shown that some allergic reactions in cows and horses observed after administration of some penicillins were due to the presence of carboxymethylcellulose in these preparations (Szabuniewicz 1973). Of all antibiotics in use, penicillin has the highest incidence of severe (720 cases) and fatal (8 cases) anaphylactoid reactions. All animals reacted within a few minutes to one-half hour after injection. Anaphylactic reaction was characterized by dyspnea, salivation, staggering, and collapse. Milder forms were described as urticaria, with swelling of the eyelids and rectum and a papillary edema; a local reaction produced discomfort or pain at the site of injection, which disappeared in one-half hour. Also, a significant number of clinicians believe that allergic reactions may occur after the animal's first exposure to particular allergens.

Occurrence of allergy and anaphylaxis in domestic animals is accepted but not well documented. A number of pathological conditions is believed to be related to an allergic reaction. In dogs the most frequently reported forms of allergic dermatitis are contact, atopic, flea bite, and medicamentosa. Other disorders associated with allergy are eczema, urticaria, food-induced allergy, hemolytic anemia, specific allergic enteropathies, allergic rhinitis, asthmatic coughs, edema (angioneurotic), conjunctivitis, otitis (externa), and acute gastritis.

Allergy in cattle may be manifested by acute respiratory signs such as dyspnea, pulmonary emphysema, asthma, and hay fever. Causes of allergic reactions have been attributed to inhalant agents, certain feeds (in allergic laminitis), end products of protein disintegration (in retained placenta and metritis, acute gangrenous mastitis), enterotoxins (in atony and bloat of the rumen), and distension of the udder with milk (autoallergic reaction). All these conditions may produce only a mild syndrome of urticaria (also called hives or "bunches") or severe anaphylactic reactions, as in the case of penicillin injections or vaccination.

In horses a variety of endogenous and exogenous allergens may produce urticaria (so-called wheals, nettlerash) and contact dermatitis; physical urticaria due to hot or cold stimuli is a rare condition. Other entities in which an allergic etiology is suspected are acne, purpura hemorrhagica, rhinitis, heaves or pulmonary edema, laminitis, parturient laminitis, insect stings, and streptococcal infections.

In swine the most frequently reported reaction was urticaria that resulted from serum injection, a change of diet, or GI disorders. However, this condition must be differentiated from the clinical picture of swine erysipelas, purpura hemorrhagica, and other dermal manifestations.

Treatment of Allergy

The symptoms of allergy vary with the different species. The most frequently observed signs are restlessness, anorexia, yawning, salivation, lacrimation, nasal discharge, coughing, edema, urticaria, eczema, necrosis, hemorrhage, inflammation of the mucous membranes and eyes, contraction of smooth muscle (bronchoconstriction), cardiovascular disturbances, and hematocytogical alterations. In case of acute or delayed anaphylaxis, the clinical signs occur quickly and, if not treated, are followed by collapse and death in minutes. For the treatment of shock see Chapter 29.

Diagnosis is dependent on the anamnesis, specific symptoms, feed tests, eosinophil count, and skin tests; in large animals, skin tests are of questionable value. Eosinophilia is evident in several allergic conditions; some authorities believe that eosinophilia in parasitic diseases also may be allergy related.

Treatment consists of further avoidance of allergens, emergency measures, administration of antihistaminics, and desensitization. It is often difficult to prevent allergy because the allergen has not been identified. Occasionally, however, an owner can pinpoint the allergen by the process of elimination. Intradermal allergy test kits are available from a commercial source; the reliability of such tests have not been fully assessed. A routine skin test prior to pencillin administration could safeguard against immediate hypersensitivity reactions. It is anticipated that reagents for this test will be available commercially within the near future for human use.

Anaphylactic syndrome requires emergency treatment because it may progress rapidly to irreversible cardiovascular collapse. The drug of choice is epinephrine. The dose for large animals is 1–5 ml of a 1:1000 solution subcutaneously or intramuscularly; for small animals, 1–5 ml of a 1:10,000 solution subcutaneously or 0.2–1 ml intravenously. Epinephrine does not act as an antagonist of mediators but reverses the effects of the mediator. Thus epinephrine acts as a physiologic antagonist. Other sympathomimetic drugs, ephedrine and isoproterenol, are used in a variety of acute and chronic allergic reactions. Aminophylline may be beneficial, especially in small animals, as a smooth muscle relaxant in bronchoconstriction and in edema of the bronchial mucosa. The oral dose for the dog is 11 mg/kg/6 hours. Other emergency treatment may require oxygen or even tracheotomy in the presence of laryngeal edema.

Corticosteroids are used as suppressants of allergic inflammation, especially in pruritus in dogs (see Section 8). Although corticosteroids have little indication in emergency treatment, their use may prevent the late development of skin reactions. Drugs frequently used include hydrocortisone sodium succinate (Solu-Cortef), dexamethasone sodium phosphate (Azium), or others.

Desensitization, also called hyposensitization, is a method of treatment of allergy with small repeated doses of appropriate allergens or antigens subcutaneously; this method of therapy is under experimental study in animals.

Immunosuppressive Drugs

Immune injury in human beings and animals has considerable experimental and clinical interest in tissue or organ transplantation. Several types of immune injury mechanisms are recognized such as anaphylaxis, cytolysis, immune-complex reactions, and delayed hypersensitivity. For suppression of these complicated immune reactions to transplanted tissues or organs, several groups of drugs have been used clinically: corticosteroids, cytotoxic drugs (antimetabolites, alkylating agents, and folic acid antagonists), and antilymphocytic serum. Radiation also has a practical application as a potent immunosuppressant procedure.

REFERENCES

Bergström, S.; Ryhge, R.; Samuelsson, B.; and Sjövall, J. 1962. The structure of prostaglandin E, F, and F_2 Acta Chem Scand 16:501.

Bovet, D., and Staub, A. M. 1937. Action protectrice des ethers phénoliques au cours de l'intoxication histaminique. C R Soc Biol 124:547.

Brisbane, W. P. 1963. Antibiotic reactions in cattle. Can Vet J 4:234.

Elliot, D. F. 1963. Introductory remarks. Ann NY Acad Sci 104:4.

Elliot, D. F.; Lewis, G. P.; and Horton, E. W. 1960. The structure of bradykinin—A plasma kinin from ox blood. Biochem Biophys Res Commun 3:87.

Erspamer, V. 1946. Ricerche farmacologie sull'enteramina. Arch Sci Biol 31:86.

Erspamer, V., and Asero, B. 1952. Identification of enteramine, the specific hormone of the enterochromaffin cell system, as 5-hydroxytryptamine. Nature 169:800.

Feldberg, W., and Kellaway, C. H. 1938. Liberation of histamine and formation of lysocithin-like substance by cobra venom. J Physiol 94:187.

Goldbatt, M. W. 1933. A depressor substance in seminal fluid. J Soc Chem Ind (Lond) 52:1056.

Green, T. K., and Harvey, J. A. 1974. Enhancement of amphetamine action after interaction of ascending serotogenic pathways. J Pharmacol Exp Ther 190:109.

Hamlin, K. E., and Fischer, F. E. 1951. The

synthesis of 5-hydroxytryptamine. J Am Chem Soc 73:5007.

Harper, H. A. 1971. Physiological Chemistry. San Francisco: Lange Medical Publications.

Inskeep, E. K. 1973. Potential uses of prostaglandins in control of reproductive cycles of domestic animals. J Anim Sci 36:1149.

Kraut, H.; Frey, E. K.; and Werle, E. 1930. Der Nachweis eines Kreislaufhormons in der Pankreasdrüsse. Hoppe Seylers Z Physiol Chem 189:87.

Kurzrok, R., and Lieb, C. C. 1930. Biochemical studies of human semen. II. The action of semen on the human uterus. Proc Soc Exp Biol Med 28:268–72.

Lewis, T., and Grant, R. T. 1924. Vascular reactions of the skin to injury. Heart 11: 209.

Melmon, K. L.; Cline, M. J.; Hughes, T.; and Nies, A. S. 1968. Kinins: Possible mediators of neonatal circulatory changes in man. J Clin Invest 47:1295.

Orczyk, G. P., and Behrman, H. R. 1972. Ovulation blockade by aspirin or indomethacin: *In vivo* evidence for a role of prostaglandin in gonadotrophin secretion. Prostaglandins 1:3.

Ramwell, P. W., and Shaw, J. E. 1971. Prostaglandins. Ann NY Acad Sci 180:10.

Rapport, M. M.; Green, A. A.; and Page, I. H. 1948. Serum vasoconstrictor (serotonin). IV. Isolation and characterization. J Biol Chem 176:1243.

Rocha e Silva, M.,; Beraldo, W. R.; and Rosenfeld, G. 1949. Bradykinin, a hypotensive and smooth muscle stimulating factor released from plasma globulin by snake venoms and by trypsin. Am J Physiol 156: 261.

Schayer, R. W., and Cooper, J. A. D. 1956. Metabolism of C^{14} histamine in man. J Appl Physiol 4:481.

Slorach, S. A. 1971. Histamine and heparin release from isolated rat mast cells exposed to compound 48/80. Acta Physiol Scand 82:91.

Szabuniewicz, M.; Bailey, E. M.; and Wiersig, D. O. 1973. Drug actions and interactions. Vet Med Small Anim Clin 9:1048.

van Arsdel, P. P., Jr., and Beall, G. N. 1960. The metabolism and functions of histamine. Am Med Assoc Intern Med 106:714.

von Euler, U. S. 1934. Sur Kenntnis der pharmakologishen Wirkung von Nativsecretin und Extracten mannlicher accesorischer Geschlechtsdrüssen. Arch Exp Pathol Pharmakol 175:78.

———. 1935. Über die spezifische blut-drucksenkende Substanz des menschlichenkende prostataund Samen-blasensekretes. Klin Wochenschr 14:1182.

von Euler, U. S., and Gaddum, J. H. 1931. An unidentified depressor substance in certain tissue extracts. J Physiol (Lond) 72:74.

von Pirquet, C. 1906. Allergie. Munch Med Wochenschr 53:1457.

Waksman, B. H. 1970. Atlas of Experimental Immunology and Immunopathology. New Haven and London: Yale University Press.

Werle, E., and Berek, V. 1948. Zur Kenntnis des Kallikreins. Angew Chem 60A:53.

CHAPTER 22

HEMOSTASIS, HEMOSTATIC, ANTICOAGULANT, AND FIBRINOLYTIC AGENTS

MICHAEL SZABUNIEWICZ and
J. D. McCRADY

HEMOSTASIS

Blood and Its Fractions

Whole blood from healthy animals is frequently used for transfusions to supply the physiological components and immune bodies needed by sick animals. Plasma may also be used for transfusion. Plasma and serum in the natural or dehydrated states (lyophilized) are widely used in human medicine but not in veterinary medicine.

Several other blood products are used as therapeutic agents: fibrin, thrombin, and thromboplastin. Their roles in the blood coagulation phenomenon and in therapeutics are discussed below.

Hemorrhage and Hemostasis

Hemorrhage is characterized by arterial, venous, or capillary discharge of blood. Hemorrhage occurs from wounds, incisions, and lacerations. Many factors may interfere with the normal clotting mechanism and result in various degrees of hemorrhage, such as liver disease, chemical poisoning (heparin, dicumarol), estrogen therapy, exposure to various venoms, coagulation disorders (hemophilia, thrombocytopenia), and anaphylaxis. Spontaneous hemorrhage may also occur in vascular disorders (allergic purpura, scurvy, symptomatic purpura).

Control of hemorrhage is essential. Uncontrolled hemorrhage may cause serious hypotension and hypoxia. The physiologic mechanisms controlling hemorrhage are referred to as hemostatic phenomena (Fig. 22.1). These involve the response of blood vessels, blood platelets, and multiple factors of blood plasma in the coagulation phase. In the vascular phase, bleeding is reduced by local vasoconstriction (reflex response initially, followed by epinephrine and serotonin release) and by mechanical pressure on the injured vessels by extravasated blood in the surrounding tissue. The initial role of platelets in hemostasis is manifest by adhesion to the surface of the blood vessels (collagen affinity) and to one another (aggregation). They also produce temporary hemostasis with a small plug or a platelet thrombus (white thrombus) at the site of injury. This interaction in the vessel walls results in the release of platelet constituents (e.g., adenosine diphosphate [ADP], serotonin, histamine, and platelet factor 3, the phospholipids) that play an essential role in the coagulation phase. The blood vessel response and

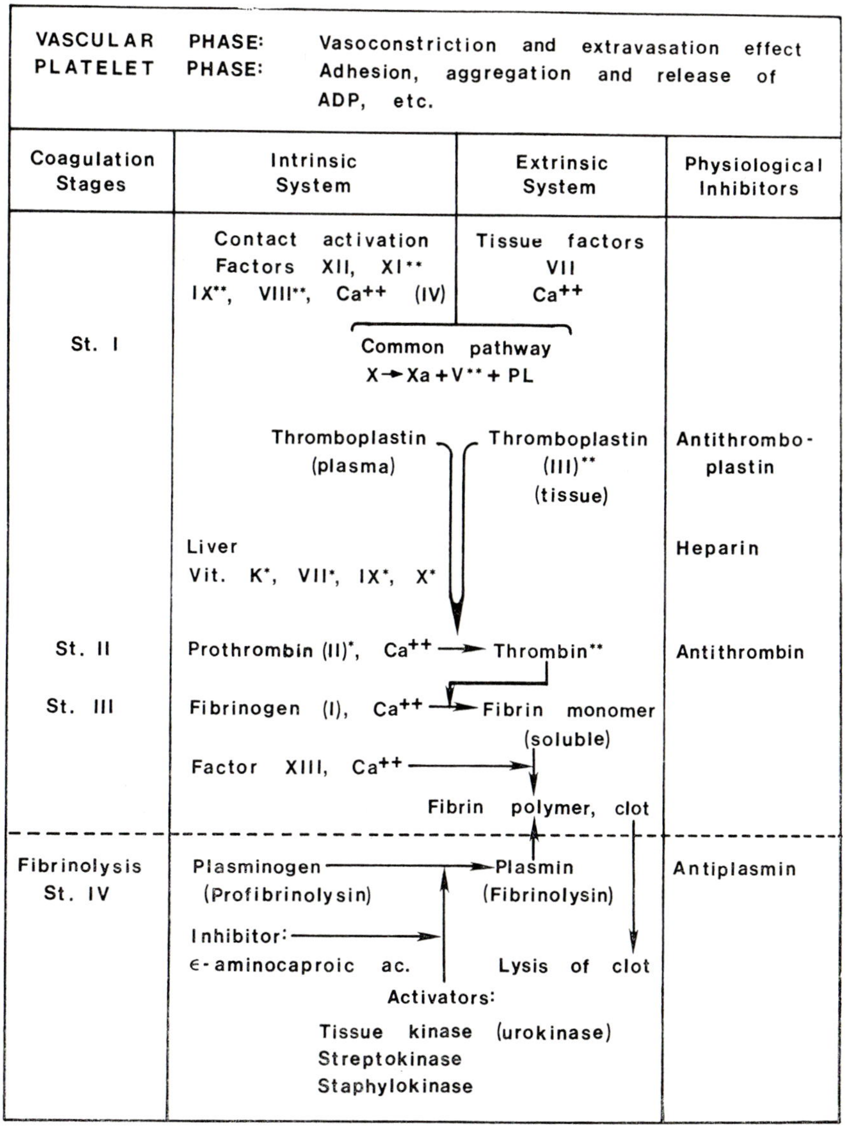

VASCULAR PHASE:	Vasoconstriction and extravasation effect		
PLATELET PHASE:	Adhesion, aggregation and release of ADP, etc.		
Coagulation Stages	**Intrinsic System**	**Extrinsic System**	**Physiological Inhibitors**
	Contact activation Factors XII, XI** IX**, VIII**, Ca^{++} (IV)	Tissue factors VII Ca^{++}	
St. I	Common pathway X → Xa + V** + PL		
	Thromboplastin (plasma)	Thromboplastin (III)** (tissue)	Antithrombo-plastin
	Liver Vit. K*, VII*, IX*, X*		Heparin
St. II	Prothrombin (II)*, Ca^{++} → Thrombin**		Antithrombin
St. III	Fibrinogen (I), Ca^{++} → Fibrin monomer (soluble)		
	Factor XIII, Ca^{++} → Fibrin polymer, clot		
Fibrinolysis St. IV	Plasminogen (Profibrinolysin) → Plasmin (Fibrinolysin) → Lysis of clot		Antiplasmin
	Inhibitor: ε-aminocaproic ac.		
	Activators: Tissue kinase (urokinase) Streptokinase Staphylokinase		

FIG. 22.1. Simplified scheme of hemostasis and fibrinolysis. PL = phospholipids from platelets. The sites of action of coumarin derivative antagonists (*) and those of heparin (**).

platelet adhesion, aggregation, and release of chemical factors are initiated within seconds following vascular injury. These phases of hemostasis may be influenced by several agents, inducers, or inhibitors of the platelet and vascular functions. Known inducers are ADP, epinephrine, norepinephrine, serotonin, vasopressin, thrombin, collagen, estrogens, and prostaglandin E_2; known inhibitors are prostaglandin E_1 and aspirin. Aspirin may be transferred to the platelet membrane (20 minutes from ingestion) and may irreversibly inhibit any release of factors from platelets for their life span. It appears that there are specific receptors on the surface membrane of platelets for each inducer or inhibitor. The activity of the initial phase of hemostasis is tested by the bleeding time test, which may be indicative of pathological changes in vasculature or of the number and activity of circulating platelets. However, this test has no value in estimation of activity of blood-clotting factors.

Terminal hemostasis occurs when the platelet plug becomes organized and bound together by strands of fibrin during the development of the coagulation phase.

Coagulation of Blood

Hemostasis is sometimes confused with coagulation. Control of bleeding is an integrated mechanism. The initial step resides in the vessels and platelets, whereas coagulation is a late stage, constituting a third phase of defense against hemorrhage (Quick 1970). The role of platelets is intimately associated with the vascular phase via vasodilator/constrictor action (histamine and serotonin). Platelets also bridge the vascular phase with the coagulation phase, the last step in the hemostasis phenomenon.

Coagulation, or blood clotting, whether intravascular or extravascular, involves the interactions of several plasma proteins known as coagulation factors (Table 22.1). Calcium is required and has a status as factor IV. The sequence of events in coagulation is described as the cascade or waterfall theory since each step in sequence activates the next. The clotting mechanism (Fig. 22.1) involves intrinsic and extrinsic pathways. In the intrinsic pathway, upon injury to tissue, the contact activation between shed blood and vascular surface converts inactive factor XII to its activated form XIIa. This in turn converts XI to XIa, etc. In the extrinsic pathway, tissue factors released interact with factor VII and the product of this step converts X to Xa. Both the intrinsic and the extrinsic pathways lead to activation of the common pathway, in which factors Xa and V plus phospholipids interact to form thromboplastin. All these steps, complicated and even controversial, are referred to as stage I coagulation, which supplies activated thromboplastin (enzyme). In stage II thromboplastin in the presence of Ca^{++} converts prothrombin (produced in the liver) to thrombin (proteolytic enzyme). With entry into stage III, thrombin activates a soluble protein, fibrinogen (also produced in the liver), into a monomer of fibrin (soluble); then by action of factor XIII (activated by thrombin and Ca^{++}) this is converted into a fibrin polymer (referred to as fibrin threads). The threads of fibrin, bound together with the platelet thrombus, form the strong, insoluble fibrin clot, which terminates the events of the hemostasis phenomenon. Subsequent clot retraction is due to a contractile protein from the platelets. The function of this event is not well understood; however, it may act as a "physiologic suture." Coagulation is a complicated process that is not yet fully understood.

Blood is maintained in the fluid condition, even when a clot is formed locally, by physiological inhibitors of intermediate products of coagulation: antithromboplastin, antithrombin, and heparin. These inhibitors maintain the hemostatic balance and prevent the occurrence of fatal thromboses and embolisms in vital organs.

TABLE 22.1. Numerical system and synonyms for nomenclature of blood-clotting factors*

Factor Number	Names
I	Fibrinogen
II	Prothrombin
III	Thromboplastin, tissue extract
IV	Calcium ions
V	Proaccelerin, labile factor, accelerator (Ac^-) globulin
VI	Existence questionable
VII	Proconvertin, stable factor, serum prothrombin conversion accelerator (SPCA), cothromboplastin, autoprothrombin I
VIII	Antihemophilic Factor (AHF), antihemophilic globulin AHG, platelet cofactor I
IX	Christmas Factor, plasma thromboplastin component (PTC), platelet cofactor II, autothrombin II
X	Stuart-Prower Factor, Koller's factor
XI	Plasma Thromboplastin Antecedent (PTA)
XII	Hageman Factor, glass activation factor (not present in birds)
XIII	Fibrin Stabilizing Factor, Laki-Lorand factor (LLF)

* Recommended numerical system by the International Committee for the Standardization of Nomenclature of Blood-clotting Factors (1972). The most commonly used synonym is capitalized.

TABLE 22.2. Hemostasis, fibrinolysis defects, and common causes of hemorrhagic disorders in animals

Vascular defects
1. Equine purpura hemorrhagica, frequent in *Streptococcus equi* infection
2. Symptomatic purpura, drug and systemic disorders
3. Allergic purpura, autoerythrocyte sensitization
4. Scurvy (deficiency of vitamin C), rare in animals
5. Vascular wall anoxia, cardiocirculatory disorders or anemia

Platelet defects
1. Thrombocytopenic purpura (TP) in the dog and cow
   a. Idiopathic TP due to autoimmune sensitization to own tissue
   b. Secondary TP due to chemicals, drugs, leukemia and aplastic anemia, disorders involving spleen (acromegaly), and other diseases
2. Thrombasthenia (Glanzmann's disease), platelet disfunction in otterhounds
3. Thrombocytopathy, defective release of platelet phospholipids, hereditary and acquired
4. Thrombocythemia, unknown pathogenesis

Coagulation defects
1. Hereditary
   a. Hemophilia in human beings: deficiency of factors I–XIII; in animals: deficiency of factor VIII (hemophilia A), identified in numerous breeds in dogs and in horses; deficiency of factor VII (not related to vitamin K deficiency), in beagle hounds; deficiency of factor IX (hemophilia B), in cairn terriers and black and tan coonhounds
   b. van Willebrand's disease (similar to hemophilia): deficiency of factor VIII, in pigs and in a family of German shepherds
2. Acquired (secondary)
   a. Deficiency of vitamin K–dependent coagulation factors II, VII, IX, and X
   b. Defibrination syndrome (hypofibrinogenemia) in septicemia, shock, etc.
   c. Abnormal ratio of inhibitors of coagulation
   d. Miscellaneous causes in trauma, shock, sepsis, hemolytic conditions, neoplastic diseases, hepatic and renal diseases, snake venoms, etc.

Fibrinolysis defects
1. Hyperactivity, due to variety of vasoactive drugs
2. Hypoactivity, due to overactivity of inhibitors of plasmin

Clinically, there are many conditions characterized by an abnormal tendency to bleed. The classification of hemorrhagic disorders is summarized in Table 22.2.

Fibrinolysis

Fibrinolysis is the physiological converse of the coagulation phenomenon and its function is a defense against overactivity of the coagulation mechanism. Therefore, it is reasonable to consider fibrinolysis as a fourth stage (stage IV) of the coagulation process as shown in Fig. 22.1. It is apparent that patency of the vascular bed depends on the balanced equilibrium between coagulation and fibrinolysis.

The fibrinolytic mechanism, which is the same in all mammals, is depicted in Fig. 22.1. Plasminogen, a β-globulin, is a normal component of plasma but also an inactive precursor of plasmin. Several endogenous and exogenous agents, known as activators, may convert plasminogen to plasmin (enzyme), which exerts proteolytic activity on fibrin, fibrinogen, and factors V, VIII, and X. The breakdown products of fibrinolysis to soluble polypeptides prevent further fibrin polymerization. Activators of plasminogen (kinases) are present in blood, the body fluids (also in urine), the walls of blood vessels, and most tissues of the body.

HEMOSTATICS

Agents that primarily hasten blood clotting are coagulants, whereas hemostatics include coagulants as well as other agents that arrest bleeding via action on blood vessels. Surgical methods in the control of hemorrhage from large vessels include the application of pressure, ligation, or suturing. Oozing of blood from the capillaries and veins can obscure the surgical field and delay wound healing. Suturing individual blood vessels in such an area is not practical. Use of electrical cautery is helpful but not adequate when many tiny vessels are involved. However, several locally applied chemicals and substances may be of value in capillary bleeding if blood clotting is normal. In the case of hemostasis and fibrinolysis defects (see Table 22.2), local agents may be of little or no value and replacement therapy will be indicated (see Chapter 27). Lyophilized concentrates of factor VIII (Hemophil) and factors II, VII, IX, and X (Konyne) are available for experimental use. Few systemic hemostatic agents are available. Some antifibrinolytic agents also may reduce bleeding. Prototypes of hemostatic agents are subdivided into topical and systemic agents.

Topical Hemostatics

THROMBIN

Thrombin, U.S.P., a physiological coagulant, is a white, sterile powder prepared by interaction of thromboplastin and calcium on prothrombin of bovine or human origin. It is applied topically as a powder or isotonic saline solution to control capillary bleeding during surgery. Thrombin may be used also as an adhesive in plastic surgery and, orally, after neutralization of stomach acid to arrest bleeding in the upper gastrointestinal (GI) tract. Due to its high potency, thrombin should not be given by injection because subcutaneous administration may produce local ischemia and intravenous injection may promote intravascular clotting. Thrombin is an antigenic substance and may evoke allergic reactions when injected experimentally. It transforms fibrinogen to fibrin by direct action. Failure of blood to clot occurs when fibrinogen is low or absent. Thrombin is an effective hemostatic agent and may be used in conjunction with fibrin foam or gelatin sponge.

Vials containing 5000 or 10,000 N.I.H. (National Institutes of Health) units are diluted in sterile saline to 1000 units or less per ml just before using. For gastric bleeding, the oral use of 10,000 units dissolved in 25 ml of phosphate buffer solution has been recommended following neutralization of stomach acid.

THROMBOPLASTIN

Thromboplastin, U.S.P., is produced naturally by platelets and damaged tissue. Commercially, it is extracted from cattle brains. It accelerates blood clotting and stops bleeding. Topical administration is by spray or direct application in a sponge.

FIBRINOGEN

Fibrinogen, U.S.P., is prepared by purification and fractionation from human plasma and is available as a white powder. It is readily soluble in normal saline. It is used principally in skin grafts (as a 2% solution) and on mucous membranes. For its action, an adequate amount of thrombin is essential. It may be used also via injection to restore blood fibrinogen levels after extensive surgery or in hemorrhagic complications with hypofibrinogenemia.

FIBRIN FOAM

Fibrin Foam is a spongelike material, prepared by the action of thrombin on fibrinogen from human blood. It is an insoluble substance marketed as strips of fine white sponge. It may be applied directly, with pressure, to the hemorrhagic area or applied after presoaking the foam in thrombin solution. This preparation acts as a preformed network to trap oozing blood from the surface area.

ABSORBABLE GELATIN SPONGE

Absorbable Gelatin Sponge, U.S.P. (Gelfoam), is a sterile, water-insoluble, gelatin-base sponge that may be cut to the desired size. It is nonantigenic and will absorb several times its weight of whole blood. This denaturized gelatin is usually soaked in bovine thrombin and may be left in place following closure of the operative wound. It is completely absorbed in 4–6 weeks, without inducing a reaction or excessive scar tissue formation. When applied to the surface of the body or to the mucosal surfaces, it liquefies within 3–5 days. It is used primarily for capillary or venous bleeding.

OXIDIZED CELLULOSE

Oxidized Cellulose, U.S.P., is a specially treated form of surgical gauze or cotton that adheres to tissue and has a hemostatic effect on oozing of blood. The hemostatic action depends on its acidic (cellulosic acid) affinity to hemoglobin and tissue fluids to form a gummy matrix for clot formation. When buried in tissue it may take up to 6 weeks to be absorbed. Clinically, it is used only as a temporary implant. Cellulosic acid inhibits epithelization and for this reason oxidized cellulose should not be used for surface dressings, except for immediate control of bleeding. Its acidity may inactivate thrombin; therefore, unless it is neutralized (using sodium bicarbonate), the addition of thrombin is not advised. When *sodium alginate* (derived from seaweed) is added, it hastens the clotting process by contact with blood and serum and the formation of calcium alginate, which "clots" to form a tenacious layer.

Oxidized cellulose, gelatin sponge, or fibrin foam may be inserted into alveolar sockets with firm pressure for control of hemorrhage after dental extractions.

MICROCRYSTALLINE COLLAGEN

Microcrystalline Collagen is a new surface hemostatic agent and is presently limited by federal law for investigational use. Collagen crystals adhere to each other. A suitable amount of this preparation may be picked up by ordinary tissue forceps and applied to a bleeding surface. A valuable property of this substance is its affinity for wet surfaces, to which it quickly adheres. Microcrystalline collagen is absorbed in about 6 weeks with minimal tissue reaction. It is slightly antigenic and effective in the presence of clotting factor deficiencies but less effective in low platelet counts. It has also been shown to be effective in systemically heparinized patients (Abbott 1974). Surface hemostasis obtained with this agent appears to be most effective and reliable in such cases as venoarterial anastomoses or in surgery of the spleen and liver.

EPINEPHRINE OR NOREPINEPHRINE

Topically, *Epinephrine,* U.S.P., and *Norepinephrine,* U.S.P., produce an immediate but transitory vasoconstriction, which may be of value in control of bleeding. However, they are rapidly absorbed via the intact mucosa, despite vasoconstriction, and they may interact with halogenated anesthetics. For example, they may induce arrhythmia (Wiersig et al. 1974) or other undesirable cardiovascular effects.

MISCELLANEOUS LOCAL HEMOSTATICS

Local Hemostatics, also known as styptics, are the oldest blood-clotting drugs. The styptics include such agents as ferric chloride, ferric sulfate, ferric subsulfate, alum, tannic acid, chromium trioxide, silver nitrate, zinc chloride, cotarnine chloride, and a variety of other astringent substances. Some of these drugs are used locally in full strength as powders dusted onto a bleeding area; in solution they are used in concentrations from 1% to 20%. The action of these drugs depends upon precipitation of the protein of blood and soft tissue, and they supposedly seal off the ruptured vessel. However, many of these agents, especially if used in high concentration, may damage the tissue, resulting in sloughing and even recurrence of bleeding. Therefore, they should be used with care and only on superficial areas.

SYSTEMIC HEMOSTATICS

NORMAL BLOOD

Fresh Serum is indicated for emergency treatment in cases of acute hemorrhagic syndromes due to deficiency of clotting factors and in thrombocytopenia. For example, sweet-clover poisoning produces a severe clotting deficiency due to the development of hypoprothrombinemia.

VITAMIN K

Vitamin K found in alfalfa (K_1) differs from the vitamin formed by gram-positive bacteria in the GI tract (K_2). Both chemical compounds are related to 2-methyl-1,4-naphthoquinone, which possesses activity of vitamin K. Several synthetic compounds containing the same radical, such as menadione (vitamin K_3, in Fig. 22.2), exhibit vitamin K activity.

Vitamin K is essential for the formation of prothrombin and factors VII, IX, and X by the liver. Deficiency of vitamin K may result in a decrease of these coagulation factors and is characterized by hemorrhage into tissue following minor injuries. Vitamin K deficiency results from dietary deficiency (rare), limited absorption or utilization of vitamin K (sprue,

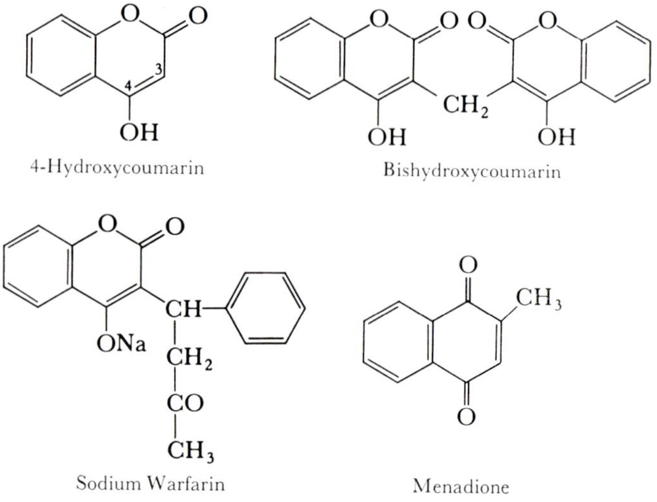

FIG. 22.2. The structure of 4-hydroxycoumarin, the two most commonly used coumarin type anticoagulants (bishydroxycoumarin and warfarin), and synthetic vitamin K (Menadione).

ulcerative colitis, intestinal resection, regional enteritis, hepatic disease), ingestion of anti–vitamin K compounds (bishydroxycoumarin and warfarin). Vitamin K deficiency also may be secondary to drug therapy (e.g., salicylates, antibacterials).

Clinical uses of vitamin K are indicated most frequently in the dog, cow, swine, and birds. In the dog and swine hypoprothrombinemia may be caused by warfarin, a commercial rodenticide. In cattle this condition is seen only as the result of the consumption of bishydroxycoumarin formed on spoiled and moldy sweet clover. In birds vitamin K deficiency is more likely to occur because of the relatively poor absorption of vitamin K by the large intestine or when a sulfonamide is administered for a prolonged period of time for the control of coccidiosis. Vitamin K may be helpful in preventing excessive hemorrhage in patients with known disease of the liver. In human patients an important therapeutic use of vitamin K is as an antidote to the anticoagulant drugs (coumarin derivatives). Prothrombin time, which is augmented by coumarins, will usually return to normal in 12–36 hours after treatment with vitamin K.

The intramuscular dose of vitamin K (natural or synthetic) for an adult dog is 0.25–2.5 mg/kg and for large animals it is 0.5–2.5 mg/kg. However, synthetic vitamin K administered orally, subcutaneously, or intramuscularly usually is absorbed too slowly to save the life of patients in an acute condition. A stable emulsion of 5% vitamin K_1 in 5% dextrose injected intravenously will reverse hypoprothrombinemia in dogs within 30–60 minutes; the reversal is complete within 2–6 hours (see Fig. 22.3). An intravenous dose of 50–60 mg produces no toxic effect in dogs and exerts a moderate prothrombin-stimulating action for as long as 10 days after injection (Shoshkes et al. 1950). The parenteral form that contains natural vitamin K_1 is effective for the treatment of hemorrhagic disease due to anticoagulant-induced prothrombin deficiency.

Preparations. Vitamin K preparations for clinical use may be obtained from synthetic and natural sources. The synthetic preparations are (1) *Menadione,* N.F. (2-methyl-1, 4-naphthoquinone), a yellow crystalline powder that is relatively insoluble in water, for oral and intramuscular use; and (2) *Menadione Sodium Bisulfite,* U.S.P., and *Menadione Sodium Diphosphate,* U.S.P. (Synkayvite), for oral and parenteral use in ampuls of 5 mg/ml, 10 mg/ml, and 75 mg/2 ml as well as 5-mg tablets.

A natural source is *Phytonadione,* U.S.P. (Aquamephyton), a fat-soluble natural vitamin K_1 that can be given orally as well as parenterally. It is more prompt, potent, and prolonged in action than the

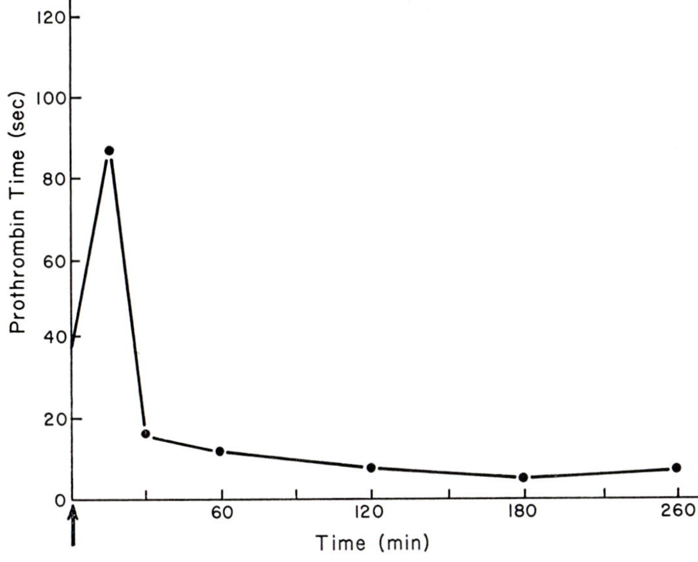

FIG. 22.3. The reversal of bishydroxycoumarin - induced hypoprothrombinemia in the dog by an emulsion of vitamin K administered intravenously. (Shoshkes et al. 1950)

vitamin K analogs. It is available in a concentration of 10 mg/cc and in 5-mg tablets.

ERGONOVINE MALEATE

Ergonovine Maleate (Ergonil) is obtained from ergot and has been shown to possess all the oxytocic activity of ergot itself. Intramuscular injection produces contraction of the uterus in 10–15 minutes. Relaxation gradually occurs over a period of about 1.5 hours but vigorous rhythmic contractions continue for 3–4 hours.

Dosage. Each ml of solution contains 0.2 mg of ergonovine maleate. The intramuscular dose for large animals is 1–3 mg; in the bitch and cat it is 0.2–0.5 and 0.07–0.2 mg, respectively. In severe bleeding the dosage may be repeated after 2–4 hours. The drug is contraindicated in pregnant animals.

CARBAZOCHROME SALICYLATE

Carbazochrome Salicylate (Adrenosem Salicylate, Hemostop) is a water-soluble salt of adrenochrome that is an oxidation product of epinephrine. It is used orally or intramuscularly to control hemorrhage preoperatively or postoperatively. The dose of carbazochrome for the dog is 0.33 mg/kg every 3–4 hours as needed.

In 1970 the National Academy of Sciences–National Research Council and the Food and Drug Administration (FDA) classified the drug as "less-than-effective" for the indications stated.

PROTAMINE SULFATE

Protamine Sulfate, U.S.P., is a low-molecular-weight protein found in the sperm of certain fish. It is strongly basic and combines with acidic heparin to form a stable salt that prevents any further anticoagulant activity of heparin. Protamine sulfate is used as an antagonist only to heparin-evoked hemorrhages. It also arrests the action of heparin *in vitro.* Protamine itself has anticoagulant properties probably due to interference with the reaction of thrombin and fibrinogen. This would imply that the clinician must take care not to "overneutralize" the heparin.

Protamine sulfate is available as a 1%–2% solution. It is administered slowly by the intravenous route at a rate no greater than 50 mg over a 10-minute period. The average dose is 1–1.5 mg to antagonize each 1 mg of heparin. The dose is related to the lapse of time from administration, e.g., 30 minutes after heparin injection only 0.5 mg of protamine may be required to antagonize each 1 mg of heparin.

ANTICOAGULANTS

The principal uses of anticoagulant agents are (1) *in vitro* to prevent clotting of blood for transfusion or laboratory use and (2) *in vivo* to prevent enlargement of thrombi. The most frequent forms of thromboembolism in human patients are pulmonary embolism, myocardial infarction, and cerebrovascular and disseminated intravascular coagulation. The use of anticoagulants is also important for prophylaxis against thromboembolism during surgery or following other trauma. An additional category of drugs is made up of fibrinolytic agents, which also may be used in control of thromboembolism.

In Vitro Anticoagulants

A variety of chemicals have been used to prevent coagulation of shed blood. Essentially two categories of chemicals are used: (1) those employed as anticoagulants in samples of blood intended for physical or chemical examination and (2) those employed to preserve blood for transfusion. In the first category of chemicals, some will prevent clotting *in vitro* but may cause clotting *in vivo* (citrates), others may prevent clotting both *in vitro* and *in vivo* (heparin), and still others may be good for use *in vitro* but are not practical *in vivo* because of their toxicity (oxalates).

1. Anticoagulant agents used in laboratory examination of blood:
   - (a) *Sodium Oxalate* in a concentration of 20% is used at the level of 0.01 ml/ml (2 mg/ml) of blood.
   - (b) *Sodium Citrate* in a concentration of 25% is used at the rate of 0.01 ml/ml (2.5 mg/ml) of blood.
   - (c) *Sodium Edetate* (NaEDTA, Endrate, ethylenediaminetetraacetic acid) is used to prevent coagulation, i.e., 1 mg/5 ml of blood. Moreover, it is used for the emergency treatment of hypercalcemia and for the control of ventricular arrhythmias associated with digitalis and oleander toxicity. Sodium calcium edetate is in use as a systemic antidote in lead poisoning (see Chapter 58). The anticoagulant property is related to its ability to chelate calcium.
   - (d) *Heparin Sodium* prevents coagulation by the addition of 75 units to each 10 ml of whole blood.

   All the above anticoagulants may be added to sample tubes in the desired amounts and evaporated to dryness. Sterile vacuum tubes that contain appropriate anticoagulants and double needles for ease in blood collection are now available.

2. Anticoagulant agents used for blood and blood plasma transfusion:
   - (a) *Sodium Citrate* solution formulated with sodium citrate 2.5 g, sodium chloride 0.9 g, and distilled water to make a total volume of 100 ml is used at the rate of 10 ml/90 ml of blood for the direct transfusion of blood.
   - (b) *Acid Citrate Dextrose* (A.C.D. solution), U.S.P., consists of sodium citrate 25 g, citric acid 8 g, dextrose 24.5 g, and distilled water to make a total volume of 1000 ml; it is used at the level of 15 ml/100 ml of blood. Several commercial firms prepare vacuum bottles containing these or comparable ingredients. The toxicity of citrated blood injected intravenously varies with the rate of injection and total dose. The lethal dose of sodium citrate for the dog is estimated to be 60 mg/lb after extensive hemorrhage; in the normal intact dog the lethal dose is 130 mg/lb.
   - (c) *Heparin Sodium,* U.S.P., prevents coagulation by the addition of 400–600 U.S.P. units/100 ml of whole blood. Hepa-

rinized blood should not be used for isoagglutination, complement, or erythrocyte fragility tests.

Other means also may prevent or retard coagulation. These are cold, at 2°–5° C (35.6°–41° F), and collection of blood into a receptacle having smooth and unwettable walls, as paraffin or silicone coated. Silicone coating is the most effective method used for many types of gadgets for implantation, transfusion, and dialysis.

SYSTEMIC ANTICOAGULANTS

At present, two types of anticoagulants are used therapeutically for prevention of enlargement of thrombi. Heparin used parenterally has a direct and almost instantaneous action on the coagulation process whereas the coumarin derivatives (for oral administration) have an indirect effect (vitamin K antagonists) on the coagulation system. Therefore, action of the coumarin derivatives is delayed for several hours. For emergency treatment heparin is used first and then may be followed by the coumarin derivatives.

There are other anticoagulants. These include sodium edetate, sodium oxalate, and sodium citrate, which hinder coagulation by combining with calcium. However, these agents are not effective *in vivo* because lowering ionized calcium to the anticoagulant level is incompatible with life. Dextran sulfate has anticoagulant properties but its activity is variable; its use is limited to a plasma expander. Malayan pit viper venom, which removes fibrinogen and inhibits clot formation, is under clinical investigation.

Both categories of the systemic anticoagulants act by inhibition of the action or formation of one or more clotting factors (see Fig. 22.1). This implies that these drugs exert their action by evoking a clotting defect similar to that of clinical diseases. Consequently, there is a relatively narrow therapeutic ratio because hemorrhage may occur, due to individual susceptibility or an interaction with other drugs used simultaneously.

HEPARIN

Heparin, U.S.P., is the only anticoagulant drug used parenterally. It is present in mast cells together with histamine and serotonin and is produced for therapeutic use from porcine intestinal mucosa.

Chemistry. Heparin is a mucopolysaccharide consisting of a high-molecular-weight polymer of 30 monosaccharides in which the repeating units contain sulfuric acid. Its high content of sulfuric acid radicals makes it strongly acidic; therefore, the sodium salt of heparin is used therapeutically. Sodium heparin is a white amorphous powder, readily soluble in water and nearly neutral in aqueous solution. Its chemical structure has not been definitely established. Several synthetic analogs are under investigation at this time.

Action. Heparin, per se, is not an anticoagulant. The acidic property of heparin dissociated from the sodium ion allows it to react with basic groups of enzyme proteins active in the blood-clotting system. Thus heparin first combines with a cofactor, probably α-globulin; in the next step it inhibits the action of thrombin and also blocks the activation of factor IX by activated factor XI in the early stages of the blood coagulation mechanism. Its antithrombin effect may also partially inhibit the activation of factors VIII and V. In high concentration it may inhibit platelet aggregation. *In toto,* heparin acts as an antithrombin, antiprothrombin, and antithromboplastin. It acts as an anticoagulant immediately both *in vivo* and *in vitro.* Heparin also causes a clearing effect on alimentary hyperlipemia. Its use in lowering the cholesterol level in plasma is still in the investigational phase.

An increase in clotting time is directly proportional to the concentration of heparin. The clotting time test is a satisfactory method of monitoring the effect of heparin. A second laboratory monitoring method is the activated partial thromboplastin time (PTT) also called the Lee-White clotting time. Because heparin does not cross the placenta, it is a treatment of choice for thromboembolic episodes during pregnancy (in human beings). At this time, the physiological role of heparin in mast cells is not fully understood.

Heparin is inactivated by the enzyme heparinase in the liver, and about 20% is secreted in the urine. It does not appear in milk. The plasma half-life is approximately 1.5 hours. Clinically, use of heparin intermittently via the intravenous route of administration is the preferred method of treatment.

Clinical Use. Clinical evidence of heparin efficiency in human patients has been rated as *effective* in the following conditions: for prophylaxis and treatment of venous thrombosis and pulmonary embolism; for atrial fibrillation with embolization; for diagnosis and treatment of chronic consumptive coagulopathies; as an anticoagulant in blood transfusion; for prevention of clotting in arterial and heart surgery; and for prevention of cerebral thrombosis in evolving stroke. It has been rated *probably effective* for prophylaxis and treatment of peripheral arterial embolism; for prevention of recurrent arterial embolism as an adjunct in the treatment of coronary occlusion with myocardial infarction; and for treatment of arterial occlusion due to embolism. Heparin has been rated *ineffective* for the treatment of cerebral thrombosis. For frostbite heparin is recommended at double the normal dose while bishydroxycoumarin therapy is being initiated.

The principal adverse effect of heparin is its tendency to induce hemorrhage. For this reason it is contraindicated in patients with internal bleeding or cerebral hemorrhage. However, in case of overactivity of heparin, protamine sulfate, along with whole fresh blood transfusion, is used successfully to reverse or antagonize the anticoagulant effect. Two other antagonists, toluidine blue and hexadimethrine, are obsolete heparin antagonists. Other rare side effects include allergic reactions, thrombocytopenia, osteoporosis, and alopecia.

Several drugs may interact with heparin and may cause augmented or lowered activity. Such drugs are acetylsalicylic acid, digitalis, antihistamines, and tetracyclines. Heparin is incompatible with polymyxin B.

Administration. Heparin administered orally loses its electronegativity by action of sulfatases. This results in its loss of anticoagulant activity. It is active only parenterally; the intravenous route of administration is preferred. Also, heparin may be used intramuscularly in a repository form. The repository form is prepared in a gelatin-dextrose medium and has a duration of action up to 24 hours. Its use in this form is recommended reluctantly because absorption is irregular and hematomas frequently form at the site of injection. The dosage of heparin is not established for the various species. However, the human dose applied on a weight basis may be used as a guide.

In human beings continuous infusion or intermittent injection of heparin via an indwelling needle or infusion tube is recommended. With the infusion technique, a solution of 20,000–40,000 units of heparin in 1 L of 5% dextrose is administered at a rate of about 1 ml/minute. The infusion rate is controlled by determining the clotting time at periodic intervals. With the intermittent method, 3000–6000 units are injected every 4 hours or 5000–10,000 units every 6 hours; the dose is adjusted in accordance with the results of the clotting time prior to administration of the next dose.

Heparin Sodium, U.S.P. (Lipo-Hepin, Liquaemin), for injection contains 10 mg (or 1000 units) or more in each ml. For intravenous administration, dilution is made with normal saline or 5% glucose (10 mg/1000 ml) and is dripped slowly as needed. One thousand units, or 10 mg of heparin, are sufficient to prevent clotting of 5000 ml of plasma for 4 hours *in vitro.* In experimental pharmacology, heparin (5 mg/kg) produces no significant side effects.

VITAMIN K ANTAGONISTS

Vitamin K antagonists (coumarins) are administered orally. There are two groups of antagonists: (1) coumarin derivatives and (2) indandione (or indanedione) derivatives. These derivatives no longer have clinical significance because their use is too hazardous.

Coumarin, normally present in some species of sweet clover, has no anticoagulant action. However, bishydroxycoumarin, a derivative of moldy or spoiled sweet clover, which was synthesized by Link (1943–1944), is responsible for hemorrhagic disease in cattle. Other drugs have been synthesized with the 4-hydroxycoumarin structure.

Bishydroxycoumarin. Of the several coumarin derivatives, bishydroxycoumarin (dicoumarin) was the first oral anticoagulant and 3-(α-acetonyl-benzyl)-4-hydroxycoumarin *(warfarin)* was the second compound used. These two coumarin preparations are examples of the first group of vitamin K antagonists.

Chemistry. Dicoumarin is a colorless, crystalline solid; it is relatively insoluble in water but forms soluble salts with strong alkalies. The chemical structures of coumarin, bishydroxycoumarin, warfarin, and menadione (vitamin K_3) are shown in Fig. 22.2. The structure of vitamin K suggests the competitive relation between vitamin K and these inhibitors. Bioavailability of warfarin is much greater than dicoumarin because it is approximately 75,000 times more soluble than dicoumarol in aqueous media. Warfarin is also extensively used as a rodenticide because it produces fatal internal bleeding in rodents. Domestic animals also may be poisoned accidentally (see Section 15).

Action. All coumarins have essentially the same action except for some quantitative differences, e.g., the speed of onset and duration of action may vary. Consequently, only the action of bishydroxycoumarin will be discussed below.

Bishydroxycoumarin does not act as an anticoagulant *in vitro* and its effect *in vivo* is delayed 24–48 hours. Its maximum effect is produced in 3–5 days; after cessation of therapy, it lasts 4–14 days. The drug acts as a competitive antagonist of vitamin K. It inhibits the synthesis of the four vitamin K–dependent clotting factors in the liver: factor II (prothrombin), VII, IX, and I (see Fig. 22.1). There is no action upon circulating prothrombin. The drug's principal effect is upon inhibition of synthesis and not upon the release or destruction of prothrombin. The mechanism of action of the bishydroxycoumarin is unclear. Experimental evidence indicates that vitamin K and bishydroxycoumarin are mutually antagonistic (O'Reilly 1972). Administration of vitamin K can reverse hypoprothrombinemia. This action is clinically important where there is an unusual response to bishydroxycoumarin as in overdose. The antidotal effect of vitamin K and its clinical use were discussed above. The characteristics of coumarin derivatives and those of heparin are shown in Table 22.3.

Absorption and metabolism. Bishydroxycoumarin, as other coumarin derivatives, is absorbed from the GI tract; over

TABLE 22.3. Characteristics of heparin and coumarin derivative anticoagulants

	Heparin	Coumarin Derivatives
Onset of action	Immediate	Mean half-life of 44 hours*
Duration of action	4 Hours	2–5 Days
Route of administration	Parenteral	Oral
Laboratory control method	Clotting time, PTT (partial thromboplastin time)	Prothrombin time
Antidotal treatment	Protamine sulfate, fresh blood	Fresh blood, plasma, vitamin K
Active *in vitro*	Yes	No
Cost	Expensive	Inexpensive

* Half-life for warfarin in an individual subject is independent of size of the dose; half-life for dicoumarol is proportional to the dose administered.

90% is bound to plasma protein and some of it is stored in the liver. This binding is reversible and is in part responsible for the long plasma half-life of these drugs. Despite this property, the drug displays great variability in action. This may be due to variable metabolic transformation, GI absorption, a possible influence of diet (amount of vitamin K), and interaction with other drugs. Bishydroxycoumarin is hydroxylated by hepatic enzymes to inactive compounds, which are excreted in the urine. Their metabolites have no anticoagulant effect. Variations in rate of metabolism are due in part to genetic factors. A small quantity, if any, appears unchanged in the urine. However, coumarins cross the placenta and are probably secreted in the milk.

Laboratory control. Due to variability in the individual and species response to dicoumarin, laboratory monitoring of prothrombin activity is essential in its clinical use. Tests used in regulating the dosage of the drug are (1) Quick one-stage prothrombin time, often referred to as prothrombin time, and (2) Thrombotest. Both tests are sensitive enough to detect depressed levels of prothrombin as well as factors VII and X. During therapy it is essential to maintain prothrombin concentration at 20%–25% of normal.

Clinical use. Clinical use of bishydroxycoumarin and evidence of efficiency in human patients have been rated as *effective* for prophylaxis and treatment of venous thrombosis. All coumarin derivatives may cause one principal side reaction, hemorrhage. However, bleeding rarely occurs if the dose is regulated in relation to prothrombin test results. Contraindications include bleeding from any cause, purpura of any type, or a severe state of malnutrition.

Drug interactions. The simultaneous administration of other drugs with dicoumarin may lead to interaction with vitamin K. Drug interactions may be associated with the process of absorption, distribution, binding, metabolism, and excretion. An astonishing number of interactions may potentiate or inhibit the action of this group of anticoagulant drugs. The most important prescribed drugs that may increase the response are phenylbutazone, heparin, salicylates, quinine, clofibrate, broad-spectrum antibiotics, and anabolic steroids. Among those that may decrease the response are barbiturates (via induction of liver microsomal enzymes), alcohol, chloral hydrate, and griseofulvin. Experimentally, it has been shown that the hypoprothrombinemic activity of orally administered bishydroxycoumarin is nullified in sheep injected with phenobarbital (Shetty et al. 1972). Also, coumarins may inhibit the metabolism of tolbutamide and diphenylhydantoin. Some physiologic factors may increase the action of coumarins. These are hepatic dysfunction, hypermetabolism, and vitamin K deficiency due to poor GI absorption. Other physiologic factors may also decrease the response to anticoagulants, e.g., pregnancy and diuresis.

Administration. The dosage of oral anticoagulants in dogs is based on the schedule used in human beings. Bishydroxycoumarin is given on the first day at 5 mg/kg of body weight; the average daily maintenance is ⅓–⅔ of the first day's dose and is dependent on daily prothrombin time determinations. When prothrombin activity is reduced to less than 25%, the drug must be discontinued.

Bishydroxycoumarin, U.S.P. (dicumarol), is available in 25-, 50-, and 100-mg capsules and tablets. *Warfarin Sodium,* U.S.P. (Panwarfin, Coumadin), is available in tablet form (2–25 mg) and for parenteral use (25 mg/ml).

FIBRINOLYTIC AGENTS

The process of fibrinolysis is presented in Fig. 22.1. Fibrinolysis has an inherent capacity to dissolve clots deposited in small vessels. In rabbits clotted blood has been injected repeatedly without harmful effects. This indicates that clotted blood may be dissolved via the fibrinolysis process. The presence of plasmin in peripheral blood indicates a pathological fibrinolytic state. Such a condition may be the result of overactivation of plasminogen, which may overcome the neutralizing capacity of antiplasmin.

Fibrinolytic activity can be activated or inhibited by several additional endogenous and exogenous agents. Common activators are hormones (androgens, corticosteroids, growth hormone, TSH), enzymes (streptokinase, staphylokinase), epinephrine (exercise, stress), and agents from the body fluids (urokinase, thrombin). Inhibition may result by (1) preventing the activation of plasminogen (ϵ-aminocaproic acid, calcium, and antibodies to streptokinase, staphylokinase) or (2) preventing the action of plasmin (antiplasmins α_1, α_2-globulin).

Clinical Aspect

Overactivity or underactivity of the fibrinolytic mechanism may result in hemorrhage or vascular occlusion. Overactive fibrinolysis has been recognized in a variety of pathological conditions in human patients, such as shock, blood disorders, hepatic cirrhosis, snakebite, and following lung surgery. In these conditions, excessive fibrinolytic activity may be present, due to the rapid digestion of prothrombin by plasmin or inhibition of other factors (V, VII, and VIII). Two drugs are now available for treatment of hyperfibrinolytic conditions; they are ε-aminocarproic acid (Amicar) and a biologic inhibitor, Trasylol (a kallikrein inhibitor).

In human beings underactive fibrinolysis is postulated to play a role in occlusive vascular disease, as in myocardial infarction, pulmonarythromboembolic disease, massive postsurgical adhesions, and in such unrelated processes as inflammation and malignancy. It appears possible to enhance fibrinolytic activity with drugs. Those undergoing clinical trials for human use are sulphonylurea in nondiabetic subjects (tolbutamide, chlorpropamide), anabolic steroids (ethylestrol, methenolone), clofibrate (Atromid-S), and biguanidine (phenformin, metformin).

Experimentally, postoperative adhesions have been successfully prevented in the dog with urokinase (Gervin et al. 1973). Anticoagulants (heparin or coumarins) are only effective in the prevention of thrombi and have little or no effect on fibrin already formed. The effectiveness of fibrinolytic therapy is still in an investigative phase. It should be regarded as an adjunct to and not a replacement for anticoagulant therapy.

Streptokinase-streptodornase (Varizyme) is available for clinical use. It is a stable, vacuum-dried powder containing streptococcal enzymes combined with plasminogen of human placental origin. Streptokinase activates human plasminogen to the humoral proteolytic enzyme, plasmin. Plasmin liquefies fibrin or clotted blood. The conversion of animal plasminogens to plasmins by streptokinase is variable. Human plasminogen is added to assure the activation of plasminogen to plasmin in all domestic species. Streptodornase liquefies purulent, caseous, and other viscous exudates by its action on deoxyribonucleoprotein.

Local use is indicated whenever removal of fibrin or a viscous exudate is desired and drainage can be achieved. Clinical trials have demonstrated its usefulness in the treatment of wounds not responding to antibacterial therapy, burns, ulcers, chronic eczema, ear hematoma, otitis externa, sinusitis, cysts, fractures with fistulous tracts, and osteomyelitis. Locally, it can be administered as a powder or wet pack by infusion or by irrigation. Therapy can be repeated as often as necessary since normal cells are not affected. The liquefaction of blood clots and fibrinous exudates may occur in 30 minutes to 12 hours.

Parenteral use in all species is indicated in the treatment of ulcers, eczema, dermatitis, edema, cellulitis, hematoma, trauma, and pneumonia. For parenteral use, the solution may be administered intramuscularly or intravenously. The daily dose for large animals is 5000–10,000 units/100 lb of body weight. The recommended total daily dose for small animals is 5000–10,000 units. Therapy may be given 1 or 2 times daily for up to 5 days.

Streptokinase-streptodornase is available in vials containing 100,000 streptokinase units, 25,000 streptodornase units, and 500 plasminogen units.

It is recommended that antibacterial agents be administered simultaneously with the enzyme preparation. Anaphylactic reactions may occur following parenteral use. The product is contraindicated in the presence of a blood dyscrasia.

Fibrinolysin (Thrombolysin, Actase) is an enzyme preparation derived from a fraction of human plasma. It is prepared by the action of streptokinase on human profibrinolysin and is potentially useful in the treatment of thrombosis and embolism. The drug has several unpleasant side effects. In human patients a dose of 50,000 to 100,000 units/hour by intravenous drip for 1–6 hours/day is recommended; this dose may be given 3–4 days. An effective antagonist of fibrinolysin is ε-aminocaproic acid.

Urokinase (Win-Kinase), excreted in human urine, is an activator of plasminogen. It is believed that this preparation may have some advantages over streptokinase. The drug is available only for experimental use. It purportedly prevents serosal postoperative adhesions in 80% of the dogs when administered as a lavage in a dose of 5000 to 10,000 units/kg into the peritoneal cavity.

Bisorbin Lactate (EN 1661) is a synthetic fibrinolytic drug in the investigational phase; it resembles urokinase in action.

REFERENCES

Abbott, W. M. 1974. Microcrystalline collagen aids vessels anastomosis. J Am Med Assoc 229:1270.

Gervin, A. S.; Puckett, C. L.; and Silver, D. 1973. Serosal hypofibrinolysis. Am J Surg 125:80.

Hall, D. E. 1972. Blood Coagulation and Its Disorders in the Dog. Baltimore: Williams & Wilkins.

Link, K. P. 1943–44. The anticoagulant from spoiled sweet clover hay. Harvey Lect 39: 162.

Macfarlane, R. G. 1970. The Homeostatic Mechanism in Man and Other Animals. London: Academic Press.

O'Reilly, R. A. 1972. Vitamin K and oral anticoagulant drugs as competitive antagonists in man. Pharmacology 7:149.

Poler, L. 1969. Recent Advances in Blood Coagulation. Boston: Little, Brown.

Quick, A. J. 1970. Bleeding Problems in Clinical Medicine. Philadelphia: W. B. Saunders.

Shetty, S. N.; Himes, J. A.; and Edds, G. T. 1972. Effect of phenobarbital on bishydroxycoumarin plasma concentration and hypoprothrombinemic responses. Am J Vet Res 33:825.

Shoshkes, M.; Geyer, R. P.; Yee, G. S.; and Stare, F. J. 1950. The treatment of dicoumarol-induced hypoprothrombinemia in dogs with emulsified vitamin K, administered intravenously. J Lab Clin Med 36: 531.

Wiersig, D. O.; Davis, R. H.; and Szabuniewicz, M. 1974. Prevention of induced ventricular fibrillation in dogs anesthetized with ultrashort-acting barbiturates and halothane. J Am Vet Med Assoc 165:341.

CHAPTER 23

ANEMIA AND HEMATINIC DRUGS

MICHAEL SZABUNIEWICZ and
J. D. McCRADY

Erythropoiesis is responsible for the maintenance of a normal level of circulating red blood cells (RBCs) and hemoglobin for optimal oxygen transport. A decrease in blood oxygen concentration normally results in increased RBC production via (1) stimulation of erythroid tissue by erythropoietin, (2) augmentation of the iron supply, and (3) acceleration of erythroid-generating tissue.

Anemia may be defined as a reduction in circulating RBCs or hemoglobin or both below the normal physiological range. It may occur as a primary condition or, more frequently, secondary to some other disorder. Clinically, the degree of anemia may be determined by measurements of hemoglobin concentration, packed red cell volume (PCV), or total red cell count.

The pathophysiologic effects of anemia are related to tissue hypoxia and to compensatory mechanisms activated to reduce this hypoxia. In acute cases, regardless of cause, signs include weakness; apathy, staggering; lowered surface temperature; pallor of the visible mucous membranes; weak, rapid pulse; labored respiration; muscular weakness or tremors; and finally debilitation or collapse. In the chronic state, some degree of weakness, loss of appetite, decreased milk production, decreased physical performance, or general malaise may be the only symptom. The major effect of anemia on the circulatory system is an increased cardiac output. This is due to (1) a fall of the blood viscosity and (2) a dilation of blood vessels as a result of hypoxia that further increases venous return. Increased cardiac output may alleviate hypoxia of the tissue when there is a decrease in activity but not during intensive physical activity.

CLASSIFICATION OF ANEMIAS

Morphologic and etiologic classifications of the anemias are presented in Table 23.1. Anemias are classified morphologically by calculation of the red cell indices: mean corpuscular volume (MCV), mean corpuscular hemoglobin (MCH), and mean corpuscular hemoglobin concentration (MCHC).

Etiologically, anemias are caused by one of two mechanisms: (1) failure of erythropoiesis to restore losses or destruction of RBCs or (2) failure of erythropoiesis to compensate for normal daily losses of erythrocytes. Of the uncomplicated anemias, those most commonly seen are (1) anemia from blood loss, (2) hemolytic anemia, (3) anemias due to nutritional deficiencies, and (4) hypoplastic or aplastic anemia.

TABLE 23.1. Comparison of the morphologic and etiologic classifications of the anemias

Morphologic Classification		
Size of erythrocyte	Hemoglobin content	Etiologic Classification
Macrocytic anemias		
Type I macrocytic	Normochromic	1. Cobalt deficiency (vitamin B12 deficiency) 2. Congenital porphyrinuria
Type II macrocytic	Hypochromic	1. Transitory condition occurring during the active phase of erythrocytic regeneration following acute blood loss or erythrocyte destruction a. Spontaneous hemorrhages from hypoprothrombinemia caused by spoiled sweet clover b. Bacillary hemoglobinuria c. Leptospirosis d. Parturient hemoglobinuria e. Anaplasmosis f. Piroplasmosis g. *Haemobartonella* infection
Normocytic or normochromic anemias		
Normocytic	Normochromic	1. Subacute and chronic inflammatory diseases 2. Acute blood loss unaccompanied by intense bone marrow response 3. Nephritis with terminal uremia
Normocytic	Hypochromic	4. Stomach worm infection (excluding *Haemonchus,* which causes blood loss)
or		5. Leukemia or other marrow displacements 6. Hypoplastic anemias
Microcytic	Normochromic	a. Bracken fern poisoning b. Poisoning from soybean meal extracted with trichloroethylene c. Radiation injury
Microcytic	Hypochromic	1. Deficiency of iron a. Chronic blood loss from injury to vascular bed which does not heal b. Heavy infection with blood sucking parasites (*Haemonchus,* lice, ticks, etc.) c. Dietary iron deficiency 2. Defect in utilization of iron stores of body a. Copper deficiency b. Molybdenum poisoning

Source: Coles 1974.

Blood Loss Anemia

Blood loss anemia from acute or chronic hemorrhage is seen frequently in animals. Acute hemorrhage may be due to a variety of injuries, surgical procedures, or interference with clotting mechanisms, i.e., sweet clover, warfarin, or bracken fern poisoning. Chronic hemorrhage may develop from bloodsucking internal and external parasite infestations. Chronic hemorrhage may also result from gastrointestinal (GI) lesions and coagulation defects. Following acute blood loss, the anemia is normocytic and normochromic, while chronic blood loss anemias are usually microcytic hypochromic; this latter occurs from the lack of iron for production of hemoglobin. Blood loss anemias are commonly characterized by a low PCV, marked reticulocytosis, and thrombocytopenia. Prothrombin levels may be low in sweet clover or warfarin poisoning, in some hepatic disorders, or in vitamin K deficiency.

Hemolytic Anemia

Hemolytic anemia results from the destruction of erythrocytes (hemolysis) by a variety of diseases. Blood parasites (*Anaplasma, Babesia, Haemobartonella,* and *Eperythrozoon*) are the most frequent pathogens, followed by bacterial infections (*Leptospira* and *Clostridium haemolyticum*) and some viral infections (equine infectious anemia). Anemia can occur following exposure to chemical agents (arsenic, lead, copper, phenothiazine, saponins, some snake venoms, and certain drugs), a variety of poisonous plants, metabolic diseases (postparturient hemoglobinuria), physical agents (skin burns), excessive ingestion of cold water (calves), and isoimmunization phenomena in several species.

In hemolytic anemia the RBCs present in the peripheral blood may contain normal amounts of iron and hemoglobin. The bone marrow may be hyperplastic, especially in an anemia due to erythrocyte parasitism, and the peripheral blood may show marked reticulocytosis. Hemolytic anemias associated with hemoglobinuria (usually parasitic) result in the loss of both iron and protein and recovery will therefore be prolonged.

In some poisonings Heinz bodies are present in great numbers. In the cat hemolytic anemia characterized by Heinz bodies has been associated with use of urinary antiseptics containing methylene blue (Schechter et al. 1973). Similar anemias have been described following overdosage of phenothiazine in horses and ingestion of onion (wild or cultivated) in sheep, cattle, and horses (Pierce et al. 1972). All these intoxications were characterized by hemolytic anemia, icterus, hemoglobinemia, and hemoglobinuria. The morphologic alterations in erythrocytes were expressed by the presence of Heinz bodies in damaged erythrocytes. Heinz body hemolytic anemia has also been observed in severe postparturient hemoglobinuria of cows (Martinovich and Woodhouse 1971).

In the racehorse hemolytic anemia may be associated with the stress of excessive exercise. This has been attributed to splenic contraction resulting in an increase in RBCs and PCV. This was accompanied by an increase in erythrocyte fragility and rate of disintegration (Clarkson 1968).

Hemolytic anemia may also develop in cattle, swine, and cats as a result of genetically defective hemoglobin metabolism (porphyrinuria, pink tooth). This condition is characterized by an excessive amount of porphyrins (porphyria) in the nuclei of forming normoblasts and marked basophilic stippling. The human types of hemolytic hereditary anemias, such as sickle cell, thalassemia (Mediterranean), and glucose-6-phosphate dehydrogenase deficiency, are not well documented in animals.

Nutritional Anemia

Nutritional anemia may be produced by mineral, vitamin, or protein deficiencies. This type of anemia is rare as a primary entity but is likely to be secondary to anorexia, metabolic disorders, and debilitation, all of which influence digestion and absorption of essential elements.

MINERALS

Minerals, both organic and inorganic forms, are involved in (1) skeletal development, (2) physicochemical actions (i.e., maintenance of acid balance, osmotic pressure), and (3) biochemical activity (in hemoglobin, enzymes, hormones). Iron, copper, and cobalt deserve particular attention because of their frequent relationship to anemia.

Iron deficiency is a rare entity in adult animals but does occur in baby pigs and calves on a low-iron milk diet. Inadequate iron absorption and utilization, increased requirements (or, in rare circumstances, increased excretion), or a combination of these factors will result in iron nutritional anemia. Molybdenum poisoning may interfere with iron utilization via an interference with copper metabolism. The end result of iron deficiency is a reduction of hemoglobin synthesis and a deficit of RBCs. Generally, iron deficiencies are characterized by a microcytic, hypochromic anemia.

Copper, as a trace element, has a role in the formation of the porphyrin nucleus of hemoglobin and in the normal growth of bone and epithelial structures. It is also present in the structure of cytochrome oxidase. Even though iron is absorbed, it is not efficiently utilized for the formation of hemoglobin in the absence of copper. In the body, copper is found in the serum and red cells. In pigs, copper (up to 250 ppm) may be included in rations as a growth stimulant. Copper is combined in serum with an α_2-globulin, forming ceruloplasmin. A small amount may be linked to siderophilin.

Copper deficiency may be primary or secondary to an excess of molybdenum (which is usually phytogenous in origin) or due to excess of copper sulfate in the ration. Both of these agents lower copper solubility and reduce its absorption. Thus the complex interaction among copper, molybdenum, and sulfates may enhance or mask the clinical signs of various conditions.

Primary copper deficiency has been reported in ruminants where the soil (marshy or sandy) is deficient in this element (Florida and several foreign countries). Copper-deficient animals may display growth disorders, bone malformations, lack of hair pigmentation, diarrhea, disorders of myelinization, and myocardial lesions. Lameness and abnormal bone development of distal growth plates of the metacarpus and metatarsus have been reported with secondary copper deficiency in young cattle. Treatment with copper glycinate subcutaneously at a dose of 0.5 mg/kg eliminates lameness and improves the condition; however, bone enlargements remain (Smith et al. 1975). Copper deficiency anemia is characterized by microcytic and hypochromic erythrocytes.

Cobalt is an indispensable element in animals. It is a structural component of vitamin B_{12} and may be important in other ways as a trace mineral. Body requirements normally are well within the amount obtained in green leafy plants, cereals, and milk. The cobalt requirement for ruminants is 0.07–0.10 ppm of ration.

Deficiencies have been reported in cattle and sheep in Wisconsin, Michigan, New Hampshire, New York, and Florida, as well as in many countries of the world. A deficiency of this element in ruminants is accompanied by a deficiency of vitamin B_{12}. Cobalt stimulates erythropoietin production, but an overdose may depress erythrocyte production. Morphologically, the RBCs are macrocytic and normochromic from a cobalt deficiency.

VITAMINS

Cyanocobalamin (vitamin B_{12}) and folic acid are well known as hematopoietic vitamins. Their deficiency in human beings is expressed by ineffective erythropoiesis, resulting in an anemia characterized by the production of enlarged, somewhat oval macrocytes (megaloblastic hemopoiesis). These macrocytes have a short life span and may even be destroyed before they can circulate. Although the exact mechanism of action of vitamin B_{12} is not known, its deficiency seems to be responsible for diminished DNA synthesis. This affects the cells of the bone marrow, GI tract, and the antibody-forming lymphoid cells. Due to some other mechanism, vitamin B_{12} deficiency also produces neurologic abnormalities, particularly demyelination.

Vitamin B_{12} is synthesized by microorganisms. Its existence in higher plants is still questionable. It is stored principally in the liver; however, it is also present in the kidneys, heart, spleen, and brain. The biological half-life of vitamin B_{12} in the liver of some species is about 1 year (Albanese 1967).

Absorption of vitamin B_{12} from the ileum requires the presence of the *intrinsic factor,* a glycoprotein found in normal gastric juice. A deficiency of this glycoprotein results in true *pernicious anemia* in human beings but has not been documented in animals. In the absence of intrinsic factor, vitamin B_{12} can be partially absorbed but only if massive amounts are given. The mechanism for absorption in the absence of intrinsic factor is not understood. Porcine stomach, in particular the mucosal layer of the pyloric section, is the richest source of this glycoprotein and is used for its commercial production.

In human beings vitamin B_{12} deficiency may be either nutritional in origin or due to the lack of intrinsic factor secretion. Animals have not been known to be deficient like human beings in the secretion of intrinsic factor. In nutritional anemia, oral administration of B_{12} is efficient, while in pernicious anemia oral absorption of B_{12} is negligible. In human beings large oral doses (3000 mg) of vitamin B_{12} in the absence of intrinsic factor have been effective in the treatment of pernicious anemia. However, saturation of body stores of vitamin B_{12} may be accomplished more rapidly with parenteral treatment. The significance of vitamin B_{12} deficiency as expressed by a macrocytic normochromic anemia is unclear.

Normal adult ruminants and other species are not dependent on a supply of vitamin B_{12} in their diet since the rumen or enteric bacteria synthesize all the B-complex vitamins needed. However, a sufficient supply of cobalt is essential. Experimentally, cobalt given in excess may produce a polycythemia.

Folic acid (pteroylglutamic acid) occurs extensively in green leafy plants. It is also synthesized by bacteria in the large intestine. The presence of cyanocobalamin is required for the release of free or hydrolyzed folic acid; ascorbic acid is necessary to reduce folic acid to the intermediate coenzyme involved in one-carbon transfer in the synthesis of pyrimidines, purines, and amino acids.

The major site of folate storage is the liver. The kidney contains about one-third of the amount found in the liver; erythrocytes and leukocytes contain one-tenth as much as the liver (Albanese 1967). Folates are excreted in the urine; it has been recently suggested that an enterohepatic circulation may contribute to the development of folate deficiency.

Folate deficiency may be related to dietary deficiency, malabsorption (due to a variety of conditions affecting the small and large intestines), inadequate utilization (liver disease, B_{12} deficiency), increased requirement (pregnancy, tumors), or increased excretion (B_{12} deficiency). Folic acid deficiency may be present as a complication of chronic hemolytic anemia. This implies that increased hematopoiesis results in an increased folate requirement. In recent years, emphasis has been placed on the interrelationship among folate, B_{12}, and ascorbate deficiency in the magaloblastic type anemia in human beings and animals. There is evidence that a deficiency of folic acid has induced anemia in horses fed rations that did not contain fresh grass (Seckington et al. 1967). The presence of macrocytic erythrocytes characterizes the anemia induced by folic acid deficiency. Also, the MCV is greater than normal. An associated leukopenia, thrombocytopenia, and impaired synthesis of immune globulin also may be present. Folic acid will correct many of the hematological defects due to deficiency of B_{12} but has no effect on neurological changes.

Niacin (nicotinic acid) deficiency is known to occur in the dog (blacktongue syndrome) and in pigs fed a low tryptophan diet. In both species anemia may be present. A macrocytic anemia accompanied by leukopenia is seen in the dog; in the pig normocytic anemia occurs without associated leukopenia (Coles 1974).

Riboflavine and *pyridoxine* (B_6) deficiencies are rare in occurrence, and a clinical picture of anemia in animals is recognized only experimentally. In human beings "pyridoxine deficiency" refers to an anemia responsive to pyridoxine treatment. Pyridoxine deficiency in swine (experimental) results in a microcytic, hypochromic anemia.

Ascorbic acid (vitamin C) deficiency may be associated with anemia. Vitamin C is necessary to prevent the conversion of ingested ferrous iron into ferric iron, which is not absorbed in some species. The dog and many other species seem to absorb ferrous and ferric iron equally well. The role of vitamin C does not appear to have as important a role in most animals because they can synthesize their own ascorbate.

Vitamin E is required for the synthesis of heme. Anemia has been occasionally reported in porcine selenium–vitamin E deficiency. Experimental rations low in selenium and vitamin E produced anemia and death in swine (Piper et al. 1975). Much evidence has been accumulated indicating that incorporation of selenium–vitamin E may reduce death loss in pigs fed practical corn-soy diets. Because of this the Food and Drug Administration (FDA) approved (Feb. 7, 1974) the use of sodium selenite or sodium selenate as an additive in the feed of swine but at a level not to exceed 0.1 ppm of selenium.

Recent studies in the United Kingdom and the Scandinavian countries have shown that vitamin E–selenium–deficient pigs have a lower tolerance for iron. However, experimental iron toxicity could not be demonstrated in pigs with a low vitamin E–selenium reserve when they were fed a diet of corn and soybeans (Miller et al. 1973).

PROTEIN

Protein in adequate amounts is essential for a normal rate of hemoglobin and RBC production. A primary deficiency of protein in the ration, a secondary deficiency from serum loss, or severe digestive disorders may contribute to the development of anemia. However, protein deficiency alone in animals has not been demonstrated to produce anemia. Treatment with protein alone has failed to correct anemia in animals. In human beings a disease called kwashiorkor is mainly due to a protein deficiency. This condition is also frequently associated with a deficiency of iron and of various B vitamins. In the treatment of many types of anemia, protein may be supplemented orally or parenterally with balanced concentrates of pure crystalline amino acids (Bal-Con, Proteplex with B complex).

HYPOPLASTIC ANEMIA

Anemia associated with bone marrow dysfunction may reveal a variety of clinical signs. For example, if all three essential cell types are affected, *pancytopenia* may be present. If there is a deficiency of RBC production, the term *hypoplastic* or *aplastic* anemia is applied. With a deficiency of white cell production, *agranulocytosis* results; and with a deficiency of platelets, *thrombocytopenia* may be present. An overlap of all these entities may occur.

Hypoplastic or aplastic anemia may occur as an idiopathic disorder. However, the causes are most frequently due to physical factors (irradiation), chemical (including drugs), and toxic substances (bracken fern, arsenicals). Anemia also may follow infectious diseases (equine infectious anemia, panleukopenia in *Felidea*). It is also seen in chronic infections, both of bacterial and parasitic origin (especially of the kidneys and liver), endocrine disorders, and neoplastic malignancies. Bone marrow is affected by many drugs and industrial chemicals. In human beings and some animals, development of blood dyscrasias, including pancytopenia, leukopenia, and thrombocytopenia, may occur following the use of chloramphenicol, tetracycline plus penicillin, sulfonamides, phenothiazines, insecticides (chlordane, lindane, DDT), acetophenetidin, and acetylsalicylic acid.

Morphologically, the bone marrow may appear hypercellular, normocellular, or hypocellular. However, even hypercellular marrow may be hypofunctional because of a failure to produce or release formed elements. In most cases the marrow is hypocellular and has an excessive amount of fat. Typically the RBCs are normocytic and normochromic; however, slight macrocytosis is also found, but not reticulocytosis (Robbins 1968). Bone marrow biopsy may be helpful in diagnosis and prognosis.

POLYCYTHEMIA

Polycythemia, physiologically the converse of anemia, refers to a relative or absolute increase in the number of circulating red cells per unit volume of blood. This increase in RBC numbers is usually associated with a corresponding increase in hemoglobin.

Relative polycythemia, erythrocytosis, results from loss of the fluid component of the blood. Frequently, it is only a transient state, accompanied by dehydration, as a result of continual vomiting, persistent diarrhea, polyuria, thermal burns, excessive sweating, shock, or insufficient fluid intake. This type of hemoconcentration may be superimposed upon an existing anemia and may mask the true disease. Because of hemoconcentration, an anemic animal may have a "normal" PCV, hemoglobin, and RBC count. A so-called normal blood picture can lead to misinterpretation and an erroneous diagnosis.

Absolute polycythemia is characterized by an increase in the total RBC mass and is usually associated with hyperplasia of bone marrow elements. It may be idiopathic, as a primary disorder, called *polycythemia vera.* However, it may also be secondary to diseases associated with chronic hypoxia as in right to left circulatory shunts, chronic pulmonary disease, or residence at high altitude. Transient polycythemia in the racehorse occurs with exercise or excitement and is believed to be due to a release of stored RBCs (Archer and Clabby 1965).

The etiology of polycythemia vera (also known as erythremia) is unknown in human beings and animals. Although rare in animals, it has been reported in the dog (Donovan and Loeb 1959) and in cattle (Fowler et al. 1964). Laboratory findings in polycythemia include an increase of RBCs, PCV, and hemoglobin. The white cell count is also elevated, and the alkaline phosphatase level is above normal. The hypervolemia and hyperviscosity may produce arterial hypertension and a tendency to thrombosis. Paradoxically, the thrombotic tendency is associated with an abnormal bleeding tendency (Robbins 1968).

IRON

Iron is utilized chiefly in the synthesis of hemoglobin and is commonly involved in the development and treatment of anemia. It is no less vital as a component of myoglobin and in the process of cellular respiration. The iron-bearing portion of hemoglobin includes iron molecules in the ferrous state, incorporated in a porphyrin ring, as an iron protoporphyrin, or *heme.* Heme is then combined with a protein known as *globin* to form hemoglobin. Heme is also found in enzymes, such as the cytochromes; catalase; and peroxidase.

Dietary iron requirements are increased during growth or pregnancy or as a result of several types of anemias. Normally there is adequate iron in the diet of the adult animal and human being. However, only a small part (ca 10%) of the iron present in the ingesta is absorbed from the digestive tract.

Absorption and Metabolism

Use of radioactive isotopes has advanced the knowledge of iron metabolism. Many phenomena, including erythropoietic rate, iron stores, anemia, and chelating and complexing agents are known to have marked influence on iron absorption and metabolism.

Absorption of iron, which occurs primarily in the duodenum and upper jejunum, may be modified by many intraluminal and extraluminal factors. Important intraluminal factors are the amount of iron in the diet, form of iron, and the presence of other dietary components. Generally, with higher levels of iron in the diet, the proportion of the iron absorbed decreases, but the absolute amount of iron absorbed may increase. In human patients iron administered as ferrous salts appears to be utilized more efficiently than ferric salts. However, experiments with rats and chicks have shown no consistent difference between these two salts. Many dietary components may affect iron absorption. Those improving absorption, by increasing solubility, are sugars (fructose and sorbitol), several amino acids, and a number of other organic acids including ascorbic, succinic, lactic, pyruvic, and citric. Those components depressing absorption are phosphates, phytates, oxalate, pancreatic secretions, and bicarbonate. Gastric hypoacidity or other diseases of the intestine may also depress iron absorption.

Other factors that may play a role in iron absorption (extraluminal) are erythropoiesis, body iron stores, and anemia. It is known that the rate of erythropoiesis may be increased by hemorrhage, ascent to higher altitudes, and following a decrease in the ambient oxygen tension. All these factors tend to increase iron absorption. Conversely, a return to normal oxygen tension, an oversupply of RBCs (as in multiple transfusions), or large doses of radiation may cause a decrease in erythropoiesis and in iron absorption. Body iron stores may also contribute to the rate of absorption. It has been found that absorption is greater, even with normal hemoglobin content, when iron stores are low, whereas a high level in the body stores has a tendency to decrease absorption. Anemia may also influence iron uptake. For example, dogs suffering from iron deficiency will absorb up to 66% of radioactive iron following oral administration (Stewart 1953).

The role of intraluminal and extraluminal factors is well documented. However, all these factors may be considered only as stimuli to some "primary control system." Inasmuch as the mechanism for transfer of information to the control system remains unknown, the "mucosal block" theory (Granick 1946) is still valid. This theory is based on the observation that when the body does not require iron, only a small amount of this element entering the mucosal cell is moved into the plasma. Therefore, the major barrier to absorption of excess iron apparently is the mucosal cell. However, the means by which information regarding the plasma level of iron is transmitted to the mucosal cells is unknown. Information may be transmitted by humoral factors or other mechanisms (Van Campen 1974).

The fate of iron in the mucosal cell (its distribution and excretion) is presented schematically in Fig. 23.1. Ingested iron salts are reduced to the ferrous state by microbial fermentation. Ferrous iron is readily absorbed in the duodenum and passes into the blood. After oxidation to the ferric state by a copper-containing protein, it combines with β_1-globulin and becomes *transferrin,* also called siderophilin. Transferrin is responsible for conveying iron among various sites of absorption, storage, and utilization.

An excess of iron within the villous epithelial cells is oxidized to the ferric state. This form of iron combines with a protein, called *apoferritin,* to yield *ferritin,* which forms small granules when stored in the cytoplasm of the epithelial cells. The participation of ferritin in iron absorption and its role in the mucosal block theory have recently been questioned. However, ferritin releases iron into the circulating blood, where it combines with transferrin. In this form it may be transported to the tissues to be stored again as ferritin. As the iron content of a cell, represented by ferritin, grows larger, amorphous aggregates of ferric ions combine with hydroxide ions, various polysaccharides, and proteins to form the compound *hemosiderin.* Hemosiderin may also be a product of the degradation of ferritin and is a convenient storage form of iron.

Recently, a new cytoplasmic iron transport agent, with the proposed name of siderochelin, was discovered within the RBC itself. This proteinlike agent appears to pick up the iron from the cell membrane receptors and in turn makes it available to the hemoglobin synthesis process within the blood cell (Workman and Bates 1974). However, the exact mechanism of iron absorption or its transfer through the membranes of RBCs by siderochelin is not fully understood.

Distribution

Iron in the body is in a dynamic state. It is distributed in several pools: (1) the circulating pool, i.e., hemoglobin (60%–70%) and plasma transferrin (0.1%); (2) stored, i.e., ferritin and hemosiderin (25%); (3) stored in myoglobin (3%–7%); and (4) as a constituent of respiratory enzymes (0.1%).

Dietary, or exogenous, iron is stored as ferritin and hemosiderin in the reticuloendothelial cells, chiefly in the liver, spleen, and bone marrow. Also, added to this pool is the salvage iron (endogenous) from the breakup of old RBCs; the life span of erythrocytes is 100–120 days. Iron from recently degraded heme is preferentially used for erythropoiesis. The normal concentration of iron in plasma is about 100 μg/100 ml, which is approximately one-third the binding capacity of the transferrin pool. In hemochromatosis and transfusion hemosiderosis, β_1-globulin (transferrin) becomes 100% saturated. Even though

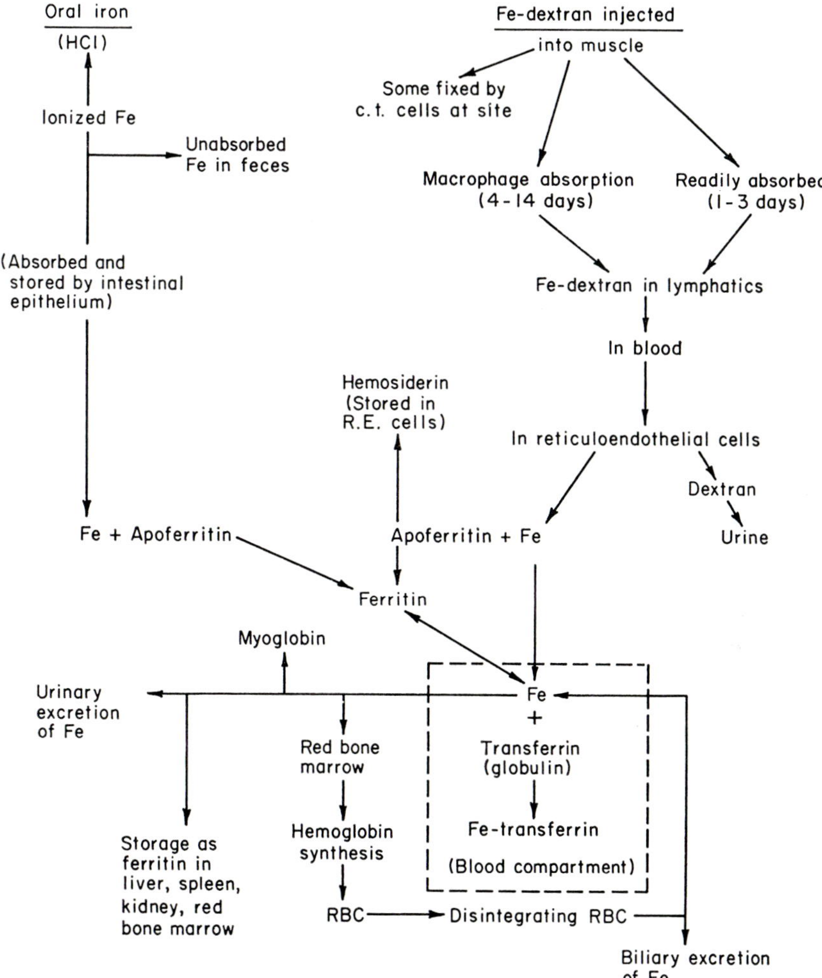

Fig. 23.1. Iron metabolism.

transferrin-bound iron is only 0.1% of the total pool, 50% may be utilized metabolically every hour. Transferrin molecules are active between erythropoietic precursors and reticuloendothelial cells. In a hypoplastic condition, where iron utilization is depressed, plasma iron clearance is decreased from 1 to 3 hours. In iron deficiency the clearance is more rapid, and plasma iron level diminishes to about 10%.

Excretion

The body excretes only minimal amounts of iron. In human beings the daily loss of iron is about 1–2 mg; the same amount of iron is also absorbed from the diet. There is no specialized mechanism for iron excretion. Small amounts are lost via epithelial desquamation, bile, urine, feces, and sweat. Approximately 1%–2% of an intravenously administered dose of iron may be detected in the urine. Due to this limited excretory ability, iron homeostasis is maintained primarily by adjusting the amount of iron absorbed ("mucosal block").

The metabolism of iron in the dog has been studied extensively. In other species there is a lack of information.

Iron Overload

The mucosal block effect may be exceeded by the administration of large doses of iron, which may lead to iron overload. Also, an accumulation of iron may occur with excessive destruction of RBCs, decreased formation of RBCs, and prolonged administration of iron.

The accumulation of iron in the body may be expressed by two known conditions: (1) hemosiderosis or (2) hemochromatosis. Hemosiderosis is referred to as a localized process of abnormal pigmentation due to increased amounts of hemosiderin in the tissues. It usually follows hemorrhage into tissues or body cavities. Hemochromatosis, a systemic disease of uncertain etiology, is characterized by a systemic hemosiderosis, accompanied by cirrhosis of the liver; in human patients bronzing of the skin and diabetes also occur. Classically, it is found in the excessive breakdown of RBCs as seen in hemolytic anemia, in multiple transfusions, in transfusion reactions, and after prolonged ingestion of large doses of iron. This indicates that some secondary transport system of iron may be operative or the mucosal block is not functioning efficiently.

In rats it has been shown that the placenta protects the fetus from iron overload. When large doses of iron were administered to female rats, the maternal blood iron concentration was significantly elevated whereas the fetal iron content was not appreciably affected (Fish et al. 1975).

Iron Toxicity

Iron salts are incompatible with many chemicals and drugs. It is advisable not to use other drugs with iron salt preparations. An example of such a combination is ferrous sulfate and tetracycline; a chelating interaction occurs with a reduction in absorption of both agents.

All iron preparations are probably equally toxic per unit of soluble iron. Orally administered iron is known to be relatively safe for human beings and animals, provided excessive amounts or unphysiologic doses are not administered. The clinical signs of iron toxicosis in baby pigs may be expressed by a pale skin, corrosion of the mucosa, dark feces, bloody diarrhea, tachycardia, arterial hypotension, shock, dyspnea, and lethargy.

An interesting case of iron toxicity has been reported in the bovine (Reagor 1975); Simmental heifers were treated with a large dose of the commercial iron preparation produced for use in racehorses. Twenty of 36 heifers died within 72 hours following treatment with the iron preparation. Postmortem examination revealed multiple organ petechial hemorrhages, severe centrolobular necrosis of the livers, and over 500 μg of elemental iron per 100 ml of blood. In the use of parenteral iron preparations, caution must be exercised to avoid an iron overload because the body does not have an efficient mechanism for iron excretion or degradation.

Treatment of Iron Poisoning

Local treatment is aimed at preventing absorption by the mucosal cells and may require use of an emetic or a local-acting antidote. Sodium bicarbonate (6% solution) may be used as a lavage, followed by oral administration of deferoxamine, a specific chelating drug. For systemic treatment, the most effective means of removing iron is by chelation. For this action, deferoxamine is administered intramuscularly (20 mg/kg/4 hours). If shock is present, the preparation is injected intravenously (40 mg/kg drip over a 4-hour period); it is then followed by 20 mg/kg/12 hours.

Deferoxamine (Desferal) may also be effective in treatment of hemochromatosis. In human beings it promotes renal excretion of chelated iron (1–3 mg/day up to 50 mg/day). Deferoxamine is an experimental drug. Its safety and efficacy remain to be established in different species.

TREATMENT OF ANEMIA

Blood Loss

Treatment of anemia from acute blood loss is directed toward arresting hemorrhage and restoration of blood volume (via transfusion of whole blood or plasma). Subsequent treatment may require a high protein ration as well as vitamin and iron supplementation for up to 30 or more days. Depending upon the causative agent, chronic blood loss requires specific treatment. Blood transfusions may be indicated if the chronic anemia becomes severe. Hematinic drugs also may be indicated. Chronic blood loss is seen more commonly than any other type of clinical anemia in animals.

The therapeutic use of iron is indicated only in the treatment of iron deficiency. Use of iron for other conditions is strictly empirical and has no proven clinical value. Administration of iron to healthy animals may result in iron-storage disease or iron toxicity.

Hemolytic Anemia

In hemolytic anemia, blood transfusion, as a lifesaving procedure, may be the first choice of treatment. Specific treatment should be aimed at elimination of the causative agent. Specific treatments for particular diseases are considered elsewhere. In the treatment of hemolytic anemia of unknown etiology, corticosteroids may be useful. The maintenance of renal function and fluid balance, cardiovascular system support, and general supportive therapy also has great importance in handling these cases.

Nutritional Anemia

Nutritional anemia due to iron deficiency may be treated either by oral or parenteral administration of any of several organic or inorganic iron preparations. However, deficiencies of copper, cobalt, various vitamins, and protein may also play an important role in the development of anemia. In the treatment of anemia, not only iron but the trace elements (copper and cobalt), vitamins (especially those essential for hematopoiesis), and protein are also administered. Some commonly available preparations of these agents and their posology are presented in Table 23.2.

Anemia in Suckling Pigs

Anemia in suckling pigs is a frequently encountered clinical entity. It is ordi-

TABLE 23.2. Hematinic drugs for veterinary use

Generic Name	Trade Name and Ingredients
Oral preparations	
Ferrous sulfate, U.S.P.*	Dose: horse 2–8 g; cattle 8–15 g; sheep, swine 0.5–2 g; dog 0.06–0.3 g; cat 0.03–0.2 g; daily for 2 weeks or more
	Livibron: vitamin B-complex, Manganese
	Vi-Natura: vitamin B-complex (for horses)
	Ferratin: arsenic, strychnine, copper, cobalt
	E-Kwine: vitamin B-complex, cobalt (for horses)
	Ironate: vitamin B-complex, vitamin C, copper
	Ferro-Folic-500: folic acid, controlled release
Ferrous lactate	*Ferro Drops:* 25 mg/ml for small animals
Ferrous gluconate, N.F.	*Triple A & N Tab:* strychnine, arsenic, nucleic acid
	V-L-I-B: desiccated liver, vitamin B-complex (for small animals)
Ferrous fumarate, U.S.P.	*V-Sorbits:* vitamin B-complex, folic acid, vitamins A, D, E
	Livitamin: vitamin B-complex, vitamin C, desiccated liver
Dextran-iron	*Tongy-Tab:* vitamin B-complex, vitamins A, D, E, copper, magnesium, manganese
Ferric pyrophosphate	*Vi-Sorbin:* vitamin B-complex, folic acid, sorbitol
Ferric ammonium citrate	*Ferrisol:* vitamin B-complex, copper, cobalt
	Allane: vitamin B-complex
Ferric chloride	*Caco-Copper:* arsenic, copper
Ferric citrochloride	*Ferrogen:* strychnine, cobalt, copper
Parenteral preparations	
Iron-dextran, U.S.P.	*Ferrextran, Nonemic, Dexiron*
Ferric hydroxide, polymaltose complex	*Iro-Jex* (for treatment of anemia in pigs)
Colloidal ferric oxide	*Felac:* iron dextrin complex

* Dosage is given only for ferrous sulfate as the standard drug. Ferrous sulfate and other iron salts are commercially available under a variety of trade names; all of these contain iron and other hematinic or tonic drugs.

narily due to iron deficiency and, at times, a coexisting lack of copper. Pigs are born with a limited store of iron and copper; sow's milk supplies only one-seventh of the daily requirement of iron. If newborn pigs do not have access to extra sources of these elements, anemia develops in 2–3 weeks.

The suckling pig can obtain only about 1 mg of iron per day from the milk of its mother during the first 3 weeks of life, or a total of 21 mg. To grow at a normal rate during this period and at the same time maintain its normal hemoglobin concentration, the pig must absorb and retain a total of about 300 mg of iron. Pigs ingest some iron (no more than 100 mg) from their surroundings during the first 3 weeks even when kept on clean concrete floors. Pigs raised on concrete are apt to be lacking nearly 200 mg of iron at the end of the first 3 weeks and will probably show clinical symptoms of anemia. The baby pig must take in 7 mg of iron daily to maintain the concentration present in its tissue at birth (Venn et al. 1947). A daily intake of 7 mg must continue for the first 5 weeks of life until baby pigs consume sufficient creep feed to supply the needed iron.

Incidence and susceptibility of suckling pigs to iron-deficiency anemia have increased in parallel with an increase in the average weaning weight because rapidly growing pigs are the most susceptible. A deficiency of iron and copper in baby pigs may augment the susceptibility to infections such as navel-ill and diarrhea diseases (Pullar 1959).

Anemia of suckling pigs is of the hypochromic, microcytic type and the clinical signs are quite characteristic. The pigs may be well developed and apparently well nourished, but they show poor growth, listlessness, rough haircoat, wrinkled skin, and drooping ears and tail. They may also exhibit labored respiration, dyspnea, fatigue, pale skin, and pale mucous membranes. The mortality rate may be high. Some pigs may appear healthy but die suddenly. Surviving pigs are permanently unthrifty. The anemia occurs more frequently when the litters are housed on concrete floors than when the pigs are reared on pasture, since vegetation and soil normally provide sufficient amounts of iron and copper.

Anemia of baby pigs can be prevented by a variety of methods. Because of the labor involved in multiple oral administrations of iron, a single intramuscular injection of an iron compound on the 2nd or 3rd day of life is the preferred method of prevention. In 3 days after iron administration, hemoglobin values increase markedly (Fig. 23.2); recipients ingest more milk and grow more rapidly than nontreated pigs. The iron requirement of the baby pig up to 60 days of age is approximately 60 ppm of dry matter intake.

Pigs raised with free access to soil have more iron in their tissues than pigs treated with iron; soil contains about 1.5% iron. Also, bluegrass sod will prevent anemia because it contains iron and copper. Application of iron-copper preparations to the sow's udder will also prevent anemia.

A high rate of stillbirths have been observed in swine herds that had a significant reduction of hemoglobin. These herds were located in an area with soil that produced iron chlorosis in plants. The stillbirth rate was reduced markedly by the addition of 100 ppm of ferrous sulfate to the ration (Archibald and Hancock 1939; Moore et al. 1965).

Iron dextrans are the most frequently used iron supplements in newborn pigs; these are absorbed into the lymphatic system within 3 days following intramuscular injection. Most of the absorption and transfer of iron dextran from the injection site into the lymphatic system is achieved by macrophage cells. A variable portion of the iron-dextran remains fixed in the connective tissue at the injection site as a less available depot of iron. Iron dextran passes rapidly from the lymphatics into the bloodstream; then it readily enters the reticuloendothelial cells throughout the body. Here the first separation of free iron from the polysaccharide occurs. The dextran is largely excreted in the urine; some of it may be metabolized to glucose. The free iron may pass into the

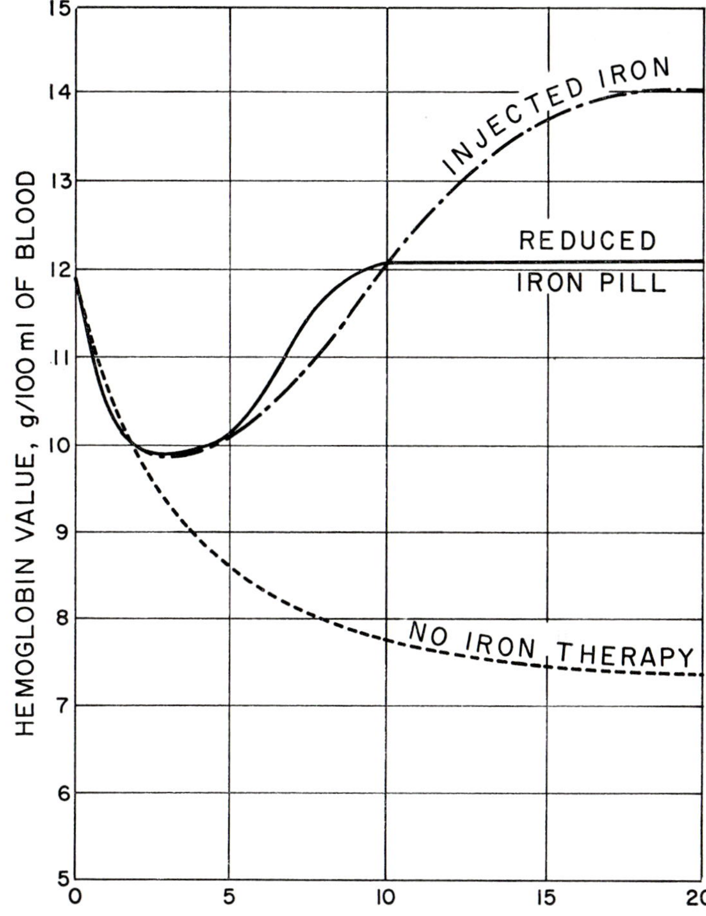

FIG. 23.2. The influence of iron therapy upon the hemoglobin value of newborn pigs. (Hubbard et al. 1952)

bloodstream to combine with β-globulin (transferrin) for transport throughout the body (Fig. 23.2).

The utilization efficiency of three iron preparations (iron dextran, iron hydrogenated dextran, and iron dextrin complex) has been compared in swine. These preparations were administered as a single intramuscular injection of 100 mg of iron to each nursing pig at 3 days of age; prior to treatment their hemoglobin averaged 8 g/100 ml of blood. Iron from the two dextrans was utilized at an efficiency of 90%–100%, while the iron from the dextrin preparation was utilized at an efficiency of 74% (Miller 1973).

There is no established indication for iron therapy in swine weighing 50 lb or more. Should anemia occur in older swine, it is more likely to be associated with an infective agent than with a simple deficiency of iron. Unfortunately, there has been some unjustifiable use of injectable iron preparations to prevent tail biting and other "social vices" induced by confinement. Administration of iron preparations in older swine has caused condemnation or discoloration of hams at slaughter.

Most species of newborn animals are not kept in such rigid confinement as suckling pigs. Usually the young have access to other sources of iron besides their mother's milk. Furthermore, the newborn of other species seem to be better fortified than pigs by the fetal storage of iron in their livers.

Hypoplastic Anemia

This type of anemia can be diagnosed

by bone marrow aspiration biopsy and examination of the peripheral blood. Treatment of this type of anemia should include the elimination of the underlying cause. When this is not feasible or the immediate cause cannot be determined, the administration of corticosteroids and antibiotics may be beneficial.

HEMATINIC DRUGS

Hematinic drugs are properly used when the exact nature of the blood disorder is known. Treatment rests upon a clear understanding of the pharmacological properties of the hematinic. Along with the hematinic drugs, supplemental protein or amino acids and control of parasites are also essential. Many commercial preparations frequently include excessive amounts of cobalt, copper, B-complex vitamins, vitamins C and E, and even some "tonic" drugs. The efficacy of these "shotgun" remedies remains to be determined.

The *United States Pharmacopeia* lists a large number of iron preparations. These may be classified as (1) reduced iron: the finely divided metal (this form is rather obsolete); (2) soluble ferrous salts: ferrous sulfate, ferrous gluconate, ferrous fumarate, and iron chelate compounds; (3) soluble ferric salts of organic acids: ferric ammonium citrate, ferric phosphate with sodium citrate; (4) parenteral iron preparations; saccharated iron oxide, colloidal solution of ferric hydroxide in complex with partially hydrolyzed dextrin, iron-dextran complex, and iron-sorbitol-citric acid complex.

In the treatment of iron-deficiency anemia, an increase of 1% daily in hemoglobin is a satisfactory response. This response is optimal and diminishes as the hemoglobin level improves. Medication should not be discontinued with an improvement in the level of hemoglobin because an iron deficiency in the tissues may still exist.

The hematinic drugs available for veterinary use are listed in Table 23.2. Posology is given only for a standard drug, i.e., ferrous sulfate. Many other ferrous and ferric salts are effective in the treatment of iron-deficiency anemia. For the treatment of other types of anemia, a number of proprietary products are available that contain iron and other hematinic or "tonic" substances or combinations. The posology of these drugs is always given in the package insert as required by the FDA.

REFERENCES

Albanese, A. A. 1967. Newer Methods of Nutritional Biochemistry, vol. 3. New York: Academic Press.

Archer, R. K., and Clabby, J. 1965. The effect of excitation and exertion on the circulating blood of horses. Vet Rec 77:689.

Archibald, R. M., and Hancock, E. E. 1939. Iron deficiency as the probable cause of stillbirths in swine. Can J Comp Med 3: 134.

Clarkson, G. T. 1968. Hematology and serum iron in the race horse. Thesis, Univ. of Melbourne, Australia.

Coles, E. H. 1974. Veterinary Clinical Pathology, 2nd ed. Philadelphia: W. B. Saunders.

Donovan, E. F., and Loeb, W. F. 1959. Polycythemia rubra vera in the dog. J Am Vet Med Assoc 134:36.

Fish, R. O.; Deinard, A. S.; Dish, L. J.; and Krivit, W. 1975. Potential toxicity of iron overload in successive generations of rates. Am J Clin Nutr 28:136.

Fowler, M. E.; Cornelius, C. E.; and Baker, N. F. 1964. Clinical and erythrokinetic studies on a case of bovine polycythemia vera. Cornell Vet 54:154.

Granick, S. 1946. Ferritin: Increase of the protein apoferritin in the gastrointestinal mucosa as a direct response to iron feeding. J Biol Chem 164:737.

Hubbard, E. D.; Bauriedel, W. R.; Picken, J. C.; and Hoerlein, A. B., III. 1952. Nutritional Anemia of Suckling Pigs. A report of progress in veterinary medical research. Iowa State Univ., Ames.

Martinovich, D., and Woodhouse, D. A. 1971. Post-parturient haemoglobinuria in cattle: A Heinz body haemolytic anemia. NZ Vet J 19:259.

Miller, E. R. 1973. Injectable iron comparison. Mich Agr Exp Sta Rep 232, AH-SW-7309.

Miller, E. R.; Hitchcock, J. P.; Kuan, K. K.; Ku. P. K.; Ullrey, D. E.; and Keahey, K. K. 1973. Iron tolerance and E-Se status of young swine. J Anim Sci. 37:287 (Abstr).

Moore, R. W.; Redmond, H. E.; and Livingston, C. W. 1965. Iron deficiency anemia as a cause of stillbirths in swine. J Am Vet Med Assoc 147:746.

by an old woman in Shropshire, England. He recognized the purple foxglove *(Digitalis purpurea)* as the active ingredient and employed it experimentally, at first on his charity patients. After 10 years, Withering published the results of his clinical observations on the use of the drug in the now classical *An Account of the Foxglove.* Although he was aware that digitalis could slow the pulse rate, Withering considered it a diuretic that acted primarily on the kidneys and did not distinguish congestive heart failure from other conditions producing edema.

It is not clear when foxglove was introduced into veterinary medicine. In 1841 Delabere Blaine wrote of its use in ascites of the dog, attributing its value to a diuretic action and declaring its effect in a very few cases to be both "salutary and durable."

PHARMACOGNOSY

Digitalis is defined in the *United States Pharmacopeia* as the "dried leaf of *Digitalis purpurea* Linné." One-tenth g of the dried leaf is equivalent to 1 U.S.P. Digitalis Unit. *Digitalis purpurea* contains three well-known glycosides: (1) digitoxin, (2) gitoxin, and (3) gitalin. *Digitalis lanata* Ehrh. is recognized by the *United States Pharmacopeia* as an official source of digoxin. There are many glycosides from sources other than digitalis plants with a similar cardiac action: (4) ouabain and (5) strophanthidin are derived from species of *Strophanthus.* Other sources of cardioactive glycosides of no therapeutic value include *Urginea maritima* (squill), *Thevetia neriifolia* (yellow oleander), *Convallaria majalis* (lily of the valley), and *Helleborus niger* (Christmas rose). In the animal kingdom, cardiac glycosides are found in the venoms of certain toads (Chen et al. 1951).

CHEMISTRY

The active principles of these plants are nitrogen-free compounds (and therefore cannot be termed alkaloids) containing sugar components (mono-, di-, tri-, or tetrasaccharides); thus they are designated glycosides. Cardioactive alkaloids are

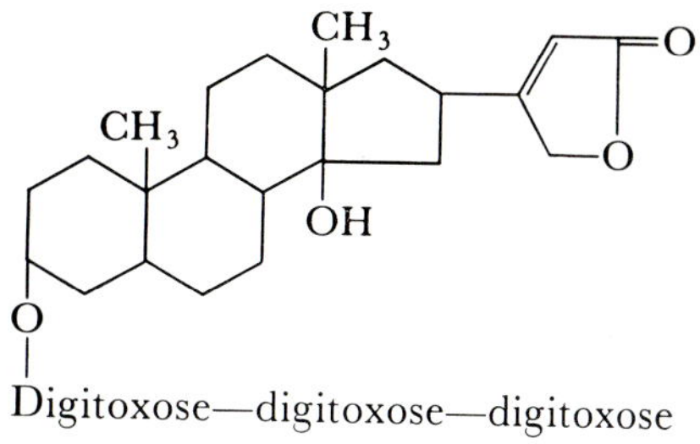

CH_3 CH_3 OH O O O

Digitoxose—digitoxose—digitoxose

Digitoxin

FIG. 24.1.

known from certain African plants and a nitrogen-containing progesterone derivative (progesterone bis-guanyl-hydrazone) possesses cardiotoxic activity (Gero 1971) despite the absence of a lactone ring.

Digitalis glycosides consist of the cyclopentanoperhydrophenanthrene (steroid type) nucleus to which are attached an unsaturated lactone ring at carbon atom 17 and 3 glucose molecules at carbon atom 3. The structure of digitoxin is shown in Fig. 24.1.

The sugar residues at C 3 render the compound soluble and influence potency and duration of activity. The sugar-free compounds, aglycones or genins, have prompter but weaker and briefer actions than the glycosides. The unsaturated butyrolactone group in the genin was considered essential for cardiotonic activity. However, it has been demonstrated that when the double bond is removed by reduction with hydrogen, some digitalis glycoside action remains (Vick et al. 1957). Thus the digitalis aglycones share the basic nucleus found in various steroids, such as the adrenal cortical and sex hormones and cholesterol, but differ in having a lactone ring, which is ordinarily unsaturated, attached at C 17. Simple lactone compounds do not have digitalislike effects on the mammalian heart (Walton et al. 1950a). Certain lactones, however, can inhibit digitoxin action, presumably by competing with the glycoside for some myocardial cell receptor site (Cosmides et al. 1956). The effect of lactones on the frog heart resembling cardiac glycoside action results from peroxide formation (Krayer et al. 1943; Mendez 1944). Thus the common features of digitalis genins related to their positive inotropic effects include the steroid nucleus, an unsaturated lactone ring (of 5 or 6 members) attached to C 17 in beta orientation, hydroxyl group at C 14, and a cis junction of rings C and D of the steroid nucleus. Reduction or destruction of cardiac action occurs with opening the lactone ring, saturating its double bond, or removing the OH at C 14. Stereochemistry of the digitalis genins clearly determines effective attachment to target organ receptors; e.g., reversal of the direction of the lactone ring relative to the 5-membered ring of the steroid nucleus can destroy cardiac action (Gero 1971). Acetylation of the genin may confer faster and shorter action (e.g., acetyl strophanthidin acts more rapidly and briefly than strophanthidin).

Standardization

Animal bioassay is required for standardizing digitalis preparations since there is no chemical measurement equivalent to the biologic activity of different glycosides, mixtures of glycosides, and crude plant extracts. For the purified glycosides of known biologic activity, chemical analysis is sufficient to assure uniformity. The so-called cat unit of digitalis biologic activity is the lethal dose (LD) per kg of body weight in etherized cats. The Digitalis Unit is the activity equal to 0.1 g of the International Digitalis Standard powder and is determined by comparing LDs of standard and unknown in lightly etherized pigeons. One U.S.P. Digitalis Unit equals about 1.2 "cat units."

Pharmacodynamic Actions

Digitalis glycosides *affect* the heart chiefly by (1) increasing effective vagal tone, (2) sympatholytic action at the sinoatrial (SA) node and atrioventricular (AV) junction, and (3) exerting a direct positive inotropic effect on myocardial cells. The most important *results* of these digitalis actions in the failing heart are (1) slowing of the heart rate (SA node), (2) decreasing AV conduction (which slows ventricular rate in atrial fibrillation), and (3) increasing the strength of ventricular contraction. In the failing heart these actions result in improved systolic emptying of the ventricles, marked decrease in ventricular rate when atrial fibrillation is present, reduction in cardiac size, and an increase in cardiac output toward the optimal for bodily needs.

Direct Cardiac Actions

Cardioactive glycosides (1) increase the strength of contraction of atrial and ventricular muscle (positive inotropic action), (2) decrease excitability of the atria, (3) first increase and then decrease ventricular excitability, (4) increase automaticity (i.e., activation of ectopic pacemakers), (5) decrease conduction velocity in both atria and ventricles, (6) prolong the refractory period of atrial muscle, (7) increase the total refractory period of ventricular muscle, (8) increase mobilization of intracytoplasmic Ca^{++} for excitation-contraction coupling, and (9) inhibit Na^+-K^+–activated membrane ATPase (toxic levels decrease intracellular K^+ and increase intracellular Na^+) (Mendez and Mendez 1957; Lee and Klaus 1971).

The most important action of digitalis in the failing heart is the strengthening of contractile force, i.e., the positive inotropic effect. This action is most pronounced in the failing or hypodynamic heart. It may be demonstrated on isolated strips of cardiac tissue (Cattell and Gold 1938) and in intact, normal animals (Walton et al. 1950b).

Metabolic Actions

Earlier studies (Modell 1966) indicated the positive inotropic effect of digitalis is unique in that, in contrast with catecholamines, it can increase contractile strength without a measurable concomitant increase in oxygen consumption, thus increasing myocardial efficiency, i.e., improving the efficiency of conversion of chemical to mechanical energy. However, in more recent studies with normal tissues (Skelton and Sonnenblick 1972), oxygen consumption and high energy phosphate utilization (ATP and creatine phosphate [CP]) increased commensurately with elevated mechanical activity. Thus in the normal myocardium, efficiency is not increased. Cardiac glycosides increase myocardial oxygen consumption and contractile force simultaneously at the positive inotropic stage of activity; the increase in oxygen consumption is the direct result of the increase in cardiac work induced by the positive inotropic effect (Lee and Klaus 1971). When the contractility of the myocardium is depressed and the ventricles are concomitantly dilated, digitalis may effect a substantial reduction in ventricular volume, owing to its positive inotropic action. In accordance with the LaPlace relation (tension $\approx$ pressure $\times$ radius), ventricular wall tension for a given intraventricular pressure would decrease with decreasing intraventricular volume. In the failing and dilated heart, digitalis through increasing the contractile state can reduce ventricular radii and thus decrease wall tension for a given pressure. When digitalis has this effect, myocardial oxygen consumption may decrease for a given work load owing to the geometrical reduction in intraventricular radii. Thus in the dilated and failing heart, digitalis can and does increase mechanical efficiency.

The consensus is that congestive heart failure represents a disturbance in energy utilization and that cardiac glycosides in some way tend to correct this defect, i.e., increase the ability of the contractile protein to convert chemical energy into mechanical work. This does not necessarily mean that the biochemical disturbance responsible for heart failure is specifically corrected by digitalis glycosides. Thus the cause of failure and the mechanism of improvement by glycosides may be different (Hajdu and Leonard 1959).

There are types of heart failure attributable to primary interference with energy production (myocardial hypoxia, thiamine deficiency, thyrotoxicosis). Although some clinical improvement may occur, these types of congestive heart failure are generally resistant to the action of digitalis glycosides.

Ouabain increases the ATP-induced shortening of skeletal muscle actomyosin threads (Robb and Mallov 1953), and digoxin, in the presence of Ca^{++}, brings the depressed contractility of actomyosin bands from hearts in failure to within the normal range (Hajdu and Leonard 1959). Since the contractility of actomyosin bands and fibrils from failing hearts is reduced, the hypothesis is supported that the deficiency in heart failure is in the contractile mechanism (Olson 1962).

Effects on Membrane Ion Exchanges

Because digitalis glycosides are known to alter ionic exchanges across the myocardial cell membrane, investigators have studied closely these effects in relation to digitalis action on contractility and excitability.

TRANSMEMBRANE POTENTIALS

Some current views regarding ionic exchanges during the action potential can be considered first for the Purkinje fiber (Fig. 24.2). Myocardial cell membrane permeability and conductance to Na^{+}, K^{+}, Ca^{++}, and Cl^{-} largely account for transmembrane potentials. The approximate concentration ratios for intracellular:extracel-

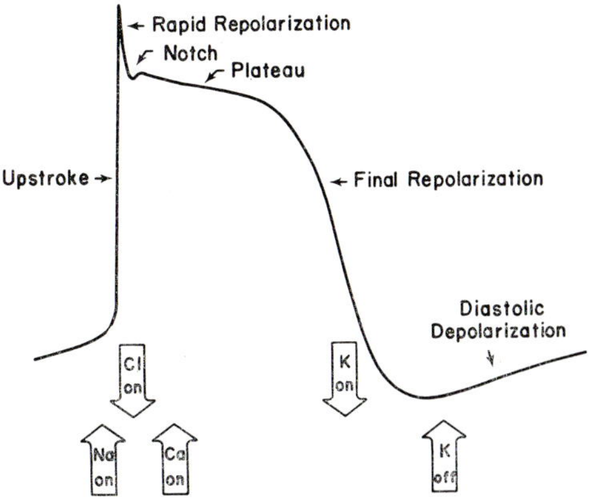

Fig. 24.2. Action potential of a Purkinje fiber illustrating the sequence of ionic influences governing changes in membrane potential. The arrows point in the direction of the effect on membrane potential—upward for depolarization and downward for repolarization. Upstroke (spike depolarization or phase 0); rapid repolarization (phase 1); notch; plateau (phase 2); final repolarization (phase 3); diastolic depolarization (phase 4). (Fozzard and Gibbons 1973)

lular for sodium, potassium, and chloride ions in heart muscle cells are Na^+, 1:10; K^+, 40:1; and Cl^-, 1:30. The distribution of Na^+ and K^+ across the cell membrane is maintained by a metabolically active Na/K membrane pump *(vide infra)*. When the cell is at rest, the membrane is more permeable to K^+ than to the other ions, and K^+ has been identified as the major ion species chiefly responsible for maintaining resting potentials. With excitation, the action potential at a given membrane site results from sequential changes in membrane ion permeability. For descriptive purposes the action potential is divided into various phases, which are identified in Fig. 24.3 and in the legend under Fig. 24.2. At the onset of excitation, the mem-

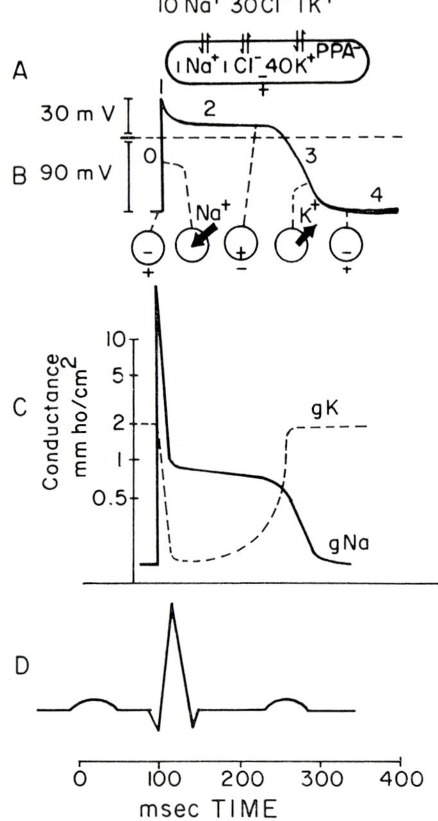

FIG. 24.3. Schematic representation of ionic distribution and exchanges during the action potential in a single myocardial cell (*A* and *B*) related to the transmembrane potential changes (*B*), sodium and potassium conductance curves (*C*) and the electrocardiogram *(D)*. *A*. Ionic distribution between the cell interior and extracellular fluid. The numbers represent the relative concentrations of each ion inside and outside the cell. PPA represents the negative charges of protein, phosphate, and amino acids. The signs + and − indicate the net charge across the resting cell membrane. *B*. A schematic tracing of a typical TMP from a ventricular muscle fiber. The initial rapid upstroke (spike) is labeled phase 0; phase 1 is the early period of rapid repolarization; phase 2 is the prolonged phase of slow repolarization or plateau; phase 3 is the final period of rapid repolarization; and phase 4 is the period of diastole. Immediately below the action potential tracing, the exchanges of Na^+ and K^+ during excitation and recovery are represented. Charges across the cell membrane are indicatd by + and − signs. *C*. Na^+ and K^+ conductance curves (gNa and gK) expressed in millimhos/cm^2. *D*. Electrocardiogram tracing to show the relationship between the overall electrical activity of the heart and these cellular events. (Tracings adapted from Trautwein 1963)

brane conductance (expressed as mhos) to Na^+ increases and that to K^+ decreases (Fig. 24.3). This rapid upstroke (phase 0) lasts only a few milliseconds and is followed by a period of rapid repolarization (phase 1), which slows to a plateau potential (phase 2). In Purkinje fibers a notch often appears on transition to the plateau. A final period of rapid repolarization (phase 3) follows and the transmembrane potential (TMP) returns to its resting value. In working ventricular muscle fibers, the resting potential remains constant during diastole (phase 4, Fig. 24.3), while in pacemaker tissue such as Purkinje fibers a gradual depolarization occurs (diastolic depolarization, Fig. 24.2). The period of rapid repolarization (phase 2) is the result of a rise in inward Cl^- current as well as the inactivation of the Na^+ current. A notch often appears in Purkinje fiber TMP at this point and has been attributed to an inward moving Ca^{++} current. This Ca^{++} current may contribute to the maintenance of the plateau (phase 2); and its inactivation, if this occurs, would contribute to termination of the plateau as the rapid repolarization of phase 3 begins (Fozzard and Gibbons 1973). This inward calcium flow also may serve to supply intracellular calcium stores from which Ca^{++} are released for excitation-contraction coupling (Lee and Klaus 1971; Entman et al. 1972).

The inward movement of Na^+ and outward movement of K^+ are passive movements requiring no energy, the ions flowing down their respective electrochemical gradients. At each activation, minute amounts of Na^+ and K^+ are transferred across the cell membrane. The metabolically active Na^+-K^+ pump mechanism is located in the cell membrane. It consumes energy from ATP, which is split by a Mg^{++}-dependent Na^+-K^+–activated ATPase. The mechanism is appropriately polarized since the ATPase is activated by an increase of Na^+ inside the membrane and by an increase in K^+ outside the membrane. This pump is known to be inhibited by, among other agents, cardioactive glycosides (e.g., ouabain, digoxin) that show asymmetry of action too, inhibiting K^+ transport from the outside to the inside of the fiber, thus decreasing intracellular K^+ concentration.

PACEMAKER POTENTIAL

Pacemaker cells depolarize progressively during phase 4 (Fig. 24.2). The chief cause of this diastolic depolarization is a time-dependent and voltage-dependent fall in potassium conductance (gK, Fig. 24.3), i.e., potassium conductance decreases with elapsed time and with decrease in TMP. Outward movement of Cl^- contributes to diastolic depolarization. When the threshold potential is reached, gNa increases suddenly and markedly, producing the spike potential (phase 0).

The sequence of changes in the TMP of isolated dog Purkinje fibers exposed to cardioactive glycosides is as follows: (1) an increased duration of action potential owing to the prolongation of phase 3; (2) a progessive decrease in action potential duration owing to the shortening of phase 2; (3) further shortening of phase 2, development of phase 4 depolarization characteristic of pacemaker cells, decrease in amplitude of maximum diastolic potential, and decrease in the rate of rise of phase 0; (4) onset of spontaneous activity owing to phase 4 depolarization and further decrease in maximum diastolic potential; and (5) progressive decrease in maximum diastolic potential, leading to the arrest of action potential formation and inexcitability of cells (Hoffman 1969). The effects on ventricular fibers are similar to those on Purkinje fibers. Low concentrations of cardiac glycosides cause a positive inotropic effect before any TMP change is seen (Hoffman 1972). The effects on action potentials of atrial muscle fibers are like those for Purkinje and ventricular fibers.

In SA nodal cells of rabbits, ouabain caused no decrease in the spontaneous rate of pacemaker (phase 4) depolarization. In the rabbit AV node, lower concentrations in the "therapeutic" range did not decrease diastolic potential or action potential amplitude; higher (toxic) concentrations did decrease diastolic potential and action potential amplitude (Hoffman 1972).

Potassium. There is a net loss of potassium from myocardial cells in the presence of digitalis glycosides. This appears to be due to the decrease of the reentry rate of potassium into the cell during the recovery phase of the contraction cycle. This change is a function of drug concentration, occurring at high (toxic) levels but not at low (therapeutic) levels. There is no disagreement that toxic doses of digitalis reduce potassium concentration in the myocardial cells and in myocardium as a whole. The cause of the potassium loss is attributed to the specific Na^+-K^+–ATPase inhibition by cardiac glycosides, mentioned above. The positive inotropic action of digitalis could be influenced by this loss of intracellular potassium, since a net decrease in intracellular monovalent cation content (sodium plus potassium) increases contractility. There is some evidence that the inotropic effect occurs without a decrease in intracellular potassium (Hajdu and Leonard 1959; Leonard and Hajdu 1962). However, there is more general agreement that changes in myocardial automaticity are related to intracellular potassium loss (Hajdu and Leonard 1959; Trautwein 1963). This increase in automaticity results in the appearance of various cardiac arrhythmias, owing to the development of ectopic pacemakers. When the extracellular potassium concentration is increased or the intracellular K^+ concentration decreased, the resting membrane potential is reduced toward threshold, i.e., reduced toward the critical level at which the action potential is triggered. While potassium fluxes are in some way related to the induction of digitalis-induced arrhythmias and their abolition to the administration of potassium salts, the nature of the underlying changes is not understood fully.

Calcium. Calcium ions are thought to play an integral role in the coupling of excitation and contraction in muscle and are known to be essential for inotropic cardiac glycoside action. Depolarization in itself does not directly initiate muscle contraction since electrical but not mechanical activity is maintained in hearts perfused with calcium-free solutions. Apparently, excitation frees Ca^{++} from a bound form in or on the muscle fiber, and the Ca^{++} in turn establish the link between excitation and contraction. The mechanism of cardiac glycoside action may involve this process in some way (Nayler 1963). Both calcium and digitalis have similar inotropic effects on hypodynamic hearts. Cardioactive glycosides may enable the heart to utilize intracellular stores of calcium since the glycosides restore depressed contractility in frog hearts perfused with calcium-free Ringer solution, provided the perfusion has not been continued long enough to deplete the store of calcium in the heart. Presumably, digitalis glycosides can make available Ca^{++} for excitation-contraction coupling by mobilizing previously bound calcium and also can increase calcium uptake from the extracellular fluid (Broadbent 1962; Klaus and Kuschinsky 1962).

Significance of Ion Effects and Digitalis Actions

Currently, the consensus is that the positive inotropic action of cardiac glycosides is related to an increase in the availability of intracellular Ca^{++} for excitation-contraction coupling; i.e., on the distribution *and* state of binding and release of intracellular Ca^{++}. They do not appear to accomplish their inotropic effect by influencing energy metabolism. The specific inhibitory effects on Na^+-K^+ ATPase produce action potential changes that favor toxic arrhythmias. There is substantial correlation between inotropic potency and Na^+-K^+–ATPase inhibitory potency, suggesting that the two may be interrelated. Thus it has been suggested that inhibition of Na^+-K^+–coupled transport could serve to increase Na^+-Ca^{++}–coupled transport and thus account for both inotropic and electrophysiological effects of these drugs (Langer 1972).

Vagal Action and the Vagal Component of Digitalis Action

Vagal fibers innervate the atria and AV junctional tissues primarily. The general effect of vagal stimulation is to slow or temporarily stop the SA node pacemaker and increase the refractory period of the AV conduction system. The SA pacemaker cells have an unstable resting potential and spontaneously depolarize during diastole until the TMP reaches threshold, when an action potential occurs. Vagal stimulation decreases the rate of this diastolic depolarization, thus slowing the frequency of discharge of the pacemaker cell. If strong enough, vagal stimulation may hyperpolarize the cell and stop its pacemaker activities. The effect of vagal stimulation on the atrial cells is to accelerate repolarization and thus decrease the duration of the action potential, increase slightly conduction velocity, produce a small increase in resting potential, and shorten the refractory period (Hoffman and Cranefield 1960). In addition, it decreases the strength of atrial contraction. Although vagal nerve stimulation can exert a weak negative inotropic effect on the ventricle, this effect is negligible in the dog (Kissling et al. 1969) and probably effective only in certain diving species.

Cardiac glycosides increase vagal tone. This vagal component of their action can be abolished by atropine. Three mechanisms have been advanced to explain the elevation of vagal action: (1) sensitization of the heart to the effect of vagal stimulation, (2) direct stimulation of the vagal centers in the medulla, and (3) sensitization of the carotid sinus to the effect of pulse pressure (Gaffney et al. 1958).

Sympatholytic Actions of Digitalis

In experiments on dogs, acetyldigitoxin has been shown to inhibit the influence of sympathetic innervation and epinephrine on AV conduction (Mendez et al. 1961a). Thus in intact animals the prolonging effect on AV conduction is presumed to result from (1) elevated vagal tone, (2) decreased sympathetic tone and antiepinephrine effect, and (3) direct glycoside action on the conduction tissue. This latter direct effect is probably of minor importance (Schaal et al. 1968, see below).

There is evidence also that digitoxin diminishes the reactivity of the SA and AV nodes to the chronotropic action of epinephrine and sympathetic stimulation (Mendez et al. 1961b). Thus the sympatholytic action of cardiac glycosides participates both in cardiac slowing by action on the SA node and in increasing the refractory period of the AV node. The positive inotropic action of cardiac glycosides occurs in reserpinized dogs and in the presence of β-adrenergic blockade; thus it is independent of catecholamine release or potentiation (Fawaz 1967). Adrenergic blockade inhibits digitalis-induced ventricular ectopic beats and fibrillation.

Direct Effect of Digitalis Glycosides on Conduction and Refractory Period

In addition to their positive inotropic effects, digitalis glycosides affect other functional properties of the cardiac musculature and AV conduction tissues. These can be distinguished from the vagal effects by study of the denervated heart. In the denervated heart, active glycosides decrease excitability of the atria and, after an initial increase, decrease ventricular excitability. It is necessary to distinguish between excitability as measured by the strength of electrical stimulus required to excite the heart and the tendency to develop ectopic beats (automaticity). With increasing doses of digitalis, electrical excitability is diminished below normal levels at the time when ventricular ectopic systoles increase in frequency and ventricular fibrillation is likely to develop (Moe and Mendez 1951).

Conduction velocity is slowed and the total refractory period prolonged in both atria and ventricles. The delay in intraventricular conduction is due primarily to slowing of conduction velocity in the Purkinje system rather than in the ventricular myocardial cells (Moe and Mendez 1951; Swain and Weidner 1957).

Combined Vagal, Sympatholytic, and Direct Components of Digitalis Action

When digitalis is administered to intact animals or human beings, the effects caused by the elevation in vagal tone can be abolished by atropinization. With an intact cardiac innervation, digitalis favors the appearance of atrial fibrillation, presumably owing to the influence of vagal action in shortening the refractory period of atrial fibers. Denervation of the heart converts digitalis glycosides from drugs that favor the occurrence of atrial fibrillation to agents that oppose its development (Mendez and Mendez 1957).

In patients with atrial fibrillation, digitalis slows the ventricular rate by increasing the refractory period of the AV conduction tissues. This action is the result of the vagal, sympatholytic, and direct components of digitalis action. The relative importance of the vagal component in this action can be determined by eliminating vagal effects with atropine (Gold et al. 1939). Data from trials in human beings are presented schematically in Fig. 24.4.

It will be noted that most of the effect on AV conduction of smaller doses of digitalis results from vagal action. With increasing doses, this action becomes relatively less and less important until finally the nonvagal effect accounts for almost all the ventricular rate slowing. Apparently, this so-called nonvagal effect of cardiac glycosides in intact animals is largely the sympatholytic action described in the foregoing.

The effect of digitalization on ventricular rate in atrial fibrillation in the horse, ox, and dog can be seen in Fig. 24.5. Table 24.1 summarizes various actions of digitalis and vagal stimulation on the heart.

Digitalis Effects on the Electrocardiogram

Digitalis glycosides can slow the heart rate, increase the PR interval, decrease the QT interval, cause deviation of the ST segment, alter the direction of the T waves, flatten the P wave, and produce various types of ectopic arrhythmias. In fact, most types of conduction disturbances and arrhythmias that have been described in diseased animals (Detweiler 1961; Patterson et al. 1961) can be produced in normal animals by the action of digitalis. These include SA block, various grades of AV block, and atrial and ventricular ectopic rhythms (atrial premature beats, atrial tachycardia, paroxysmal atrial tachycardia with block, atrial fibrillation, AV nodal rhythm, coupled premature ventricular beats, paroxysmal ventricular tachycardia, ventricular fibrillation, parasystole, and AV dissociation).

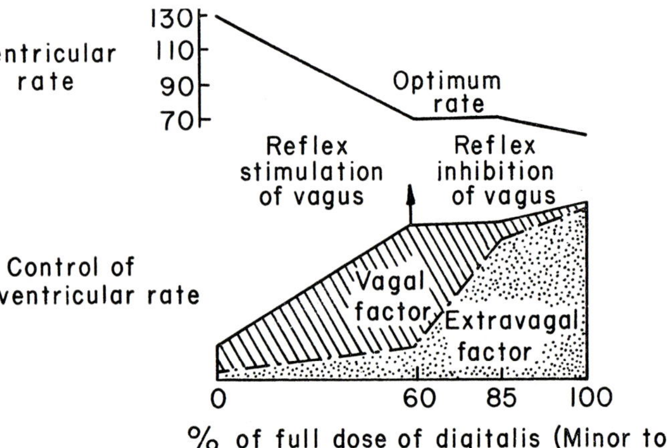

Fig. 24.4. Schematic representation of the mechanism by which digitalis slows the ventricular rate in patients with atrial fibrillation and congestive heart failure, and the relative importance of the vagal and extravagal effects. (Gold et al. 1939)

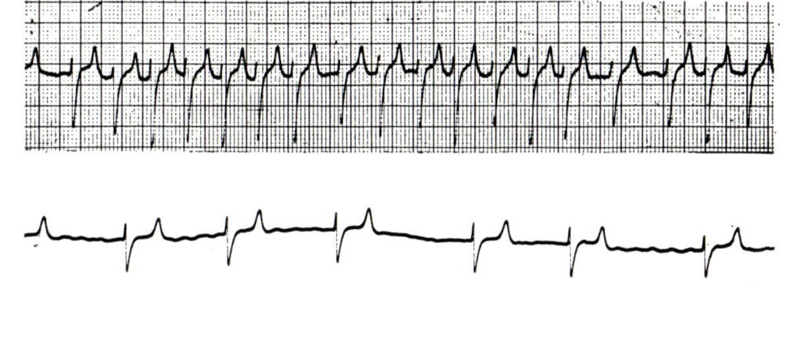

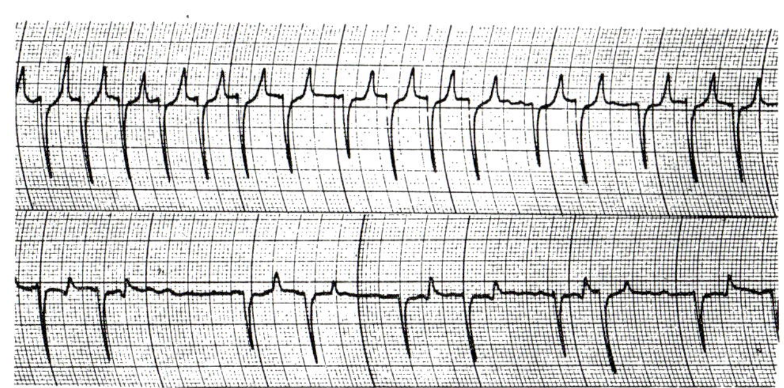

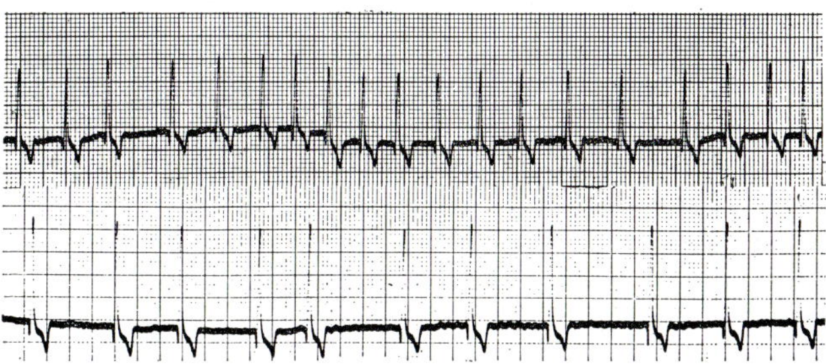

FIG. 24.5. Digitalis glycoside action in atrial fibrillation. The effect of digitalization on the ventricular rate in three species. *A:* Horse. Lead CV_6LL electrocardiogram. Above: before intravenous digitalization with ouabain, ventricular rate approximately 160/minute. Below: following digitalization, rate approximately 53/minute. *B:* Cow. Lead base-apex electrocardiogram. Above: before intravenous digitalization with ouabain, ventricular rate approximately 140/minute. Below: following digitalization, ventricular rate approximately 78/minute. *C:* Dog. Lead AVF electrocardiogram. Above: before digitalization, ventricular rate approximately 160/minute. Below: following oral digitalization, ventricular rate approximately 90/minute.

The ECG effects of various digitalis glycosides during chronic administration in normal cats indicate the types of changes to be expected in mammals. In cats the P wave is flattened. PR interval prolongation occurs but is not dependent on dosage and is not a good criterion for the evaluation of glycosidal activity. The duration of QRS is not changed in the absence of ectopic rhythms, although its amplitude may be decreased. The earliest occurring and most constant ECG change is relative shortening of the QT interval. An early sign of toxic action is deviation of the ST segment, which appears in association with other signs of toxicosis such as vomiting and weight loss. The T wave may show various form changes, including reversal of direction. The ST segment, T-wave changes, and QT shortening represent the characteristic effects on ventricular repolarization; additionally, a slight elevation of the U-wave amplitude may occur (Surawicz and Lasseter 1970). These ST, T, and QT effects are due to phase 2 shortening, decreased slope of phase 3, and shortening of the TMP duration. Various arrhythmias develop, especially in the more advanced stages of poisoning. Digitoxin produces a higher incidence of arrhythmias

TABLE 24.1. Digitalis effects in intact animals

Structure	Dose	Automaticity	Excitability	Conductivity	Refractoriness	Contractile Strength	Components	Results
SAN	Rx	—					V,S	No direct (D) effect
	T	——						Bradycardia
SA junction	Rx			—			V,S(D?)	SA block
	T			——				
AVN	Rx	±		—				AV junctional rhythm
AV junction	T	++		——	++		V,S(D?)	AV block (↑ PR) slows ventricular rate in atrial fibrillation
Purkinje fibers	Rx	±	±	—	±		S,D	Ventricular ectopic rhythms
	T	+++	++	——	++			
Atria	Rx	—	—	—	+	+	D	
	T	++	+	+	—	—	V	Favors atrial fibrillation
Ventricles	Rx	—	+→—			++	D	
	T	++	+	——			D	Ventricular ectopic rhythms

Definitions:
Automaticity, ability to initiate impulse spontaneously.
Excitability, ability to respond to a simulus.
Conductivity, speed of conduction.
Refractoriness, duration of total (not necessarily absolute) refractory period; for AVN rate of conduction and duration of refractory period.

Abbreviations:
SAN, sinoatrial node; SA, sinoatrial.
AVN, atrioventricular node; AV, atrioventricular.
Rx, therapeutic dose (level).
T, toxic dose (level).
+, increased.
—, decreased.
V, S, D, vagal, sympatholytic, and direct components of digitalis action.
PR, interval of electrocardiogram.

in cats than the other glycosides studied; when these occur, the stage of intoxication is usually irreversible and lethal. With acetyldigitoxin, lanatoside A, lanatoside C, and K-strophanthoside, the intoxication stage at which arrhythmias develop is ordinarily reversible (Rothlin and Bircher 1961).

In anesthetized experimental dogs, the duration of AV conduction (PR interval) is progressively prolonged by various digitalis glycosides until complete AV block occurs at about 65%–75% of the LD (Moe and Mendez 1951). In dogs with congestive heart failure, minimal therapeutic dose levels often fail to produce PR interval prolongation. Although prolongation of the PR interval is not consistently observed, it occurs in the ECGs of many digitalized dogs sometimes beyond normal limits (Wallace and Hamilton 1962).

Occurrence of ectopic cardiac arrhythmias is reliable evidence of digitalis toxicosis in the normal dog; in toxicosis from digoxin, a major percentage of the dogs that develop ectopic rhythm do not survive more than a few days (Fillmore and Detweiler 1973). In a survival study of subacute digoxin toxicosis in normal Beagles, the following ECG signs were accepted as reliable evidence of digoxin action (Fillmore and Detweiler 1973):

1. Signs unlikely to occur spontaneously in normal resting dogs: *sinus tachycardia exceeding 200 beats/minute,* and *sinus bradycardia less than 50 beats/minute.*

2. Signs occasionally observed in normal dogs but also characteristic of digoxin action in dogs in which they do not occur spontaneously: *first degree AV block; AV block with dropped beats.*

3. Signs never occurring in normal dogs: *AV dissociation; paroxysmal atrial tachycardia; paroxysmal atrial tachycardia with block;* occasional *ectopic atrial beats; fusion beats; intraventricular block; ventricular ectopic beats.*

Actions on Certain Other Organs

Digitalis glycosides produce arteriolar and venous constriction by direct action (Brender et al. 1969). In anesthetized dogs this results in elevated arterial pressure and generalized systemic venous constriction. The latter appears to be more intense in the hepatic veins, causing portal venous pooling with decreased venous return. This overall hemodynamic response increases resistance to left ventricular output and decreases venous return, and cardiac output usually decreases (Mason et al. 1972). The blood pressure rise can also be seen in dogs with congestive heart failure (Fig. 24.6). In unanesthetized dogs, there is no significant change in arterial blood pressure, and cardiac output is increased (Kumar et al. 1972).

The coronary vessels do not appear to be importantly affected by digitalization in the unanesthetized dog. In both anesthetized and unanesthetized dogs, cardiac glycosides increase pulmonary vascular resistance, and pulmonary arterial pressure increases to a variable extent (Linde et al. 1968). Plasma and extracellular fluid volumes are not altered (Cotten and Williams 1961).

The diuretic effect of digitalis in congestive heart failure is largely the result of compensation of the failing heart. In dogs with congestive heart failure, hemodynamic improvement is associated with a reduction in aldosterone secretion by the adrenal cortex within 90 minutes after intravenous digitalization (Fig. 24.6). This effect is not observed in dogs in the absence of congestive heart failure. The importance of aldosterone in the sodium retention of congestive heart failure is discussed later (see Chronic Congestive Heart Failure). Digitalis glycosides also have direct actions on the kidney. In experimental dogs, both with and without induced congestive heart failure, digitoxin given through a catheter in one renal artery (dose inadequate for a systemic effect) produces sodium and water diuresis in only this one kidney (Tanabe et al. 1961). On the basis of this and other studies, as well as *in vitro* studies, it has been suggested that Na^{+}-K^{+} ATPase plays an important role in urine concentration mechanisms (Martinez-Maldonado et al. 1969; Robin-

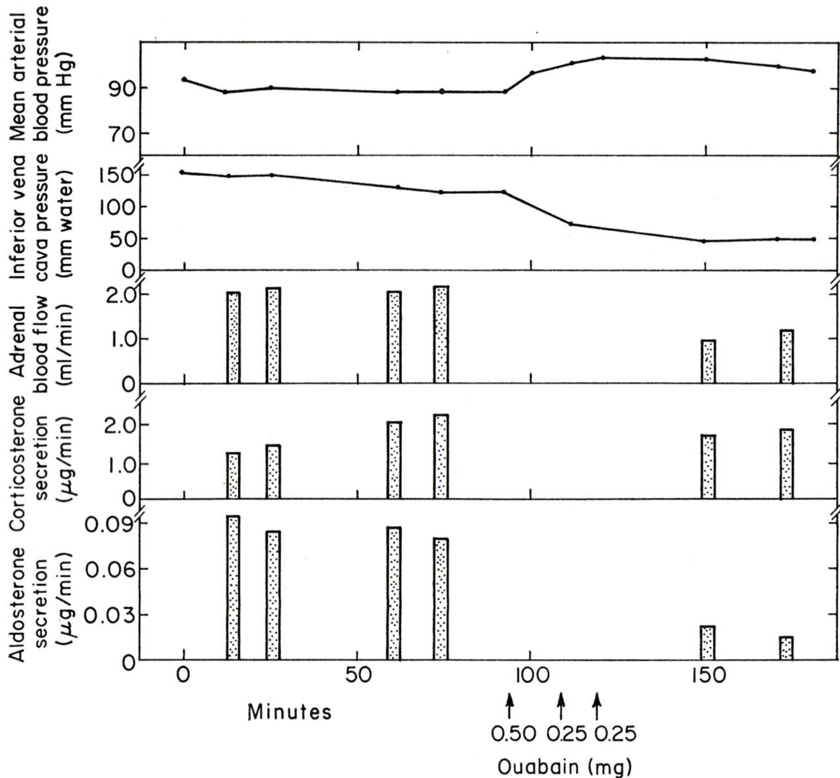

FIG. 24.6. The effects of intravenous ouabain injection (total dose 0.05 mg/kg) in an 8-year-old, 20-kg male pointer with naturally occurring congestive heart failure. Following injection, the mean arterial blood pressure increased from 88 mm Hg to a maximum of 110 mm Hg, and inferior vena cava pressure fell from a control value of 150–140 mm water to a minimum of 38 mm water; these changes started within 5 minutes after beginning the ouabain injection and reached a maximum 40–50 minutes postinjection. Following drug administration, there was also a marked fall in adrenal corticosterone and aldosterone secretion. (Carpenter et al. 1962)

son 1972). In persons with congestive heart failure, a saluretic effect following digitalis injection precedes any hemodynamic action (Werkö et al. 1958). The two suggested explanations for this action are that digitalis glycosides have an antialdosterone effect at renal tubular receptor sites or that they block a renal tubular enzyme system (e.g., Na^+-K^+ ATPase) and thus decrease sodium and water reabsorption. The latter appears to be the better explanation (Cahill 1962).

Emesis following digitalis is largely due to a central action and appears even following parenteral injection in the eviscerated animal preparation (Hatcher and Eggleston 1912–13). Vomiting produced within 30 minutes of an intravenous injection in the dog or cat is due to stimulation of the chemoreceptor trigger zone (CTZ), which in turn excites the medullary emetic center (Borison and Wang 1951). Destruction of the CTZ area on the dorsal surface of the ala cinerea abolishes this early emetic effect, but delayed emesis, occurring 90 minutes or more after intravenous injection, still occurs (Rothlin and Bircher 1961). This delayed action presumably is a direct effect on the emetic center. Local gastric irritation can also play a role in producing emesis following oral administration.

In addition to the foregoing extracardiac actions of digitalis glycosides, pharmacologists have demonstrated a variety of other effects in experiments on laboratory animals or isolated tissues. These are of little clinical or therapeutic importance and often require doses or concentrations in excess of those that could be employed in patients (Lendle and Mercker 1961). Included among these actions are stimulation followed by depression of the central nervous system (CNS); increase in contractile strength of striated and smooth muscle at certain concentrations and paralysis with higher concentrations or doses; depression of thyroid gland activity; actions similar to and competitive with those of certain adrenal cortical steroids; decrease in blood coagulation time; acceleration of wound healing with local application; and antagonism of the mitosis inhibitory action of colchicine.

Absorption, Distribution, Fate, and Excretion

The principal site of digitalis absorption following oral administration is the small intestine. The rate of intestinal absorption varies with different glycosides. In cats it is estimated that 100% of digitoxin is absorbed in 80–100 minutes following duodenal administration, while only 60% of ouabain is absorbed after 5 hours. Passage through the stomach reduces the amount of ouabain absorbed in 5 hours to 10% of the administered dose (Reinert 1952). In experimental cats, the dose required to produce cardiac standstill by intraduodenal infusion exceeded the dose required by intravenous infusion by the following multiples for various glycosides: digitoxin 1.33, acetyldigitoxin 1.51, digoxin 2.30, and ouabain 11.0 (Rothlin and Bircher 1961). For dogs, the emetic dose for intrajejunal administration exceeded the dose required by intravenous infusion by the following multiples: digitoxin 1.36, acetylstrophanthidin 1.38, lanatoside E 2.12, and ouabain 20.5 (Herrmann et al. 1962). These differences in intestinal absorbability are dependent on the relative polarity of the compound. The more nonpolar or nonionized compounds are more lipid soluble and more readily penetrate the lipoid membrane of the intestinal mucosa, whereas the more polar and highly ionized compounds are more water soluble and less well absorbed. Thus digitoxin, one of the most nonpolar glycosides, is well absorbed (about 80% for the dog and cat); digoxin, a more polar glycoside, is less well absorbed (about 43% in the cat); and ouabain, one of the most polar glycosides, is absorbed poorly (about 5%–10% in the dog and cat).

Experiments have shown that chlortetracycline-sensitive microorganisms in rumen fluid can inactivate 37%–73% of digitalis *in vitro* within 48 hours (Westermarck 1959). In sheep, an oral dose 7–10 times the intravenous dose is required to produce the same ECG effects (Westermarck 1956). Owing to this variable and marked inactivation in the rumen, oral digitalization can be expected to be unreliable in ruminants.

Digitalis glycosides are transported by the blood, in part bound to plasma proteins, particularly albumin, and in part free. Dog serum binds certain glycosides less firmly than human serum (Rothlin and Bircher 1954). The glycosides leave the vascular system rapidly. There is an initial fall in serum concentration owing to mixing in the vascular compartment and tissue uptake, followed by a slower exponential decline. In the dog, following 0.1 mg/kg of digoxin intravenously, serum digitalis concentrations peaked at between 70 and 90 ng/ml, fell rapidly to below 1/3 these levels during the first hour, and continued to fall rapidly over the next 2 hours. After 5 hours blood levels declined slowly and exponentially; the mean serum half-life for this latter phase was 26.9 hours (Barr et al. 1972).

Tissue distribution is not primarily to the heart, i.e., there is no selective concentration of cardiac glycoside in its chief target organ. In general, the highest concentrations are found in the excretory organs (liver, bile, intestinal tract, kidney); moderate concentrations in the heart, lung, and spleen; and lower concentrations in the blood, skeletal muscle, and brain

(Beck 1969a; Okita 1969). Insignificant amounts of digitoxin are found in extravascular fluids of human patients and in ascitic fluid of dogs in congestive heart failure (Beck 1969b). Thus the idea that toxic digitalis effects following diuresis are caused by mobilization of digitalis in edema fluids is improbable. Electrolyte concentration alterations associated with the diuresis probably account for the toxic effects observed.

Digitalis glycosides are metabolized chiefly in the liver, and both parent glycosides and biotransformation products are excreted in the bile. There is considerable species difference in metabolism of cardiac glycosides, so that results from one species cannot be generalized. Dogs metabolize at least some glycosides, e.g., digoxin (Marcus et al. 1967), similar to human beings. In human beings, there is a relationship between the percentage of glycoside excreted as metabolic products and relative polarity: 80% of the nonpolar digitoxin is excreted as metabolites; 10% of the more polar digoxin excreted is excreted as metabolites; and the polar glycoside ouabain is excreted unchanged (Okita 1969).

Cardioactive glycosides and their metabolites follow an *enterohepatic cycle* in which absorbed compounds reach the liver, parent compound and metabolites are excreted in the bile, and some parent glycoside and metabolites are subsequently reabsorbed (Okita 1969). This enterohepatic cycle accounts in part for differences in duration of action for a given glycoside in various species and aids in maintaining glycoside concentration within a species (e.g., biliary fistula dogs lose digitoxin at about double the rate of control dogs) (Okita 1969).

The primary route of digitoxin and digoxin excretion in the human being and the dog is reported to be via the kidney (Okita 1969). However, fecal excretion of orally administered digitoxin or digoxin may be substantial in the dog, even exceeding urinary excretion (Beck 1969b).

The absorption, metabolic fate, and excretion of digitoxin in experimental rats, rabbits, cats, and dogs appear to be as follows (Fig. 24.7): absorption occurs chiefly in the small intestine and there is rapid removal of the drug from the bloodstream with the greatest deposition occurring in

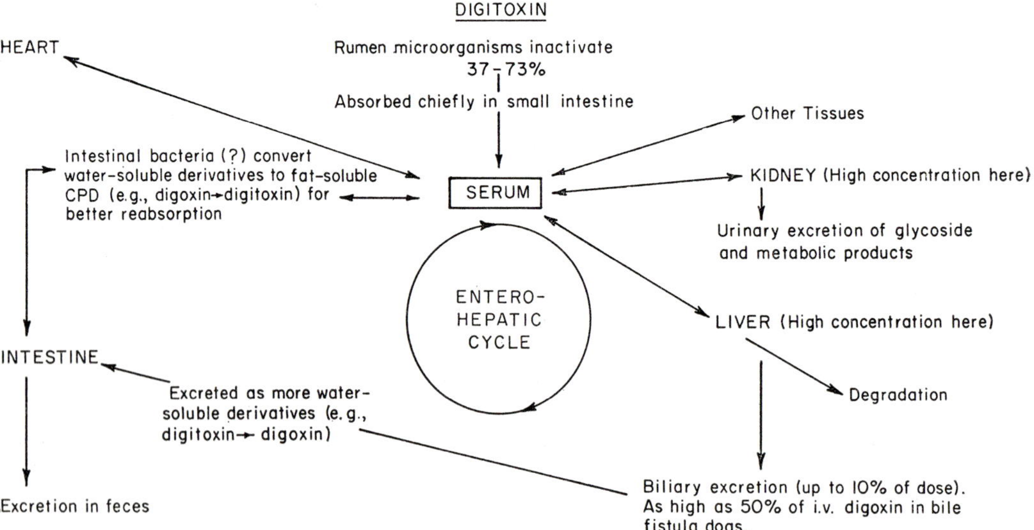

FIG. 24.7. Summary of absorption, distribution, fate, and excretion of digitoxin.

the liver and the kidney, lesser amounts in the heart and lungs, and still less in the skeletal muscles. Absorbed glycosides and metabolites from the intestine are excreted in the bile and reabsorbed to some extent *(enterohepatic cycle)*. The enterohepatic system has the highest concentration of glycosides and the organs of lower concentration follow the half-life of the gastrointestinal (GI) tract. Biotransformation to more water-soluble (polar) glycosides occurs for biliary excretion (e.g., digitoxin to digoxin). Intestinal bacteria can convert water-soluble (polar) to fat-soluble (nonpolar) compounds (e.g., digoxin to digitoxin) for better reabsorption. The chief organ of biotransformation is the liver. Excretion occurs via the bowel and urine, with the distribution between these routes variable in different species. In the rat and guinea pig, the chief portal of excretion is the bowel; in the dog and human being, the kidney (Okita 1969). However, the dog can excrete a greater percentage of digitoxin and digoxin in the bowel than in the urine (Beck 1969a).

Beck (1969b) found the biological half-life for tritiated digitoxin in the dog to be about 21.3 hours, with roughly 54% of the amount in the body excreted in 24 hours, as contrasted to a biological half-life of 9 days in the human being (Okita 1969). For digoxin in dogs, a daily elimination of about 30% of the amount in the body can be estimated from published data (Marcus et al. 1967). Thus both digitoxin and digoxin are rapidly eliminated in dogs, especially digitoxin, while in human beings digoxin is eliminated far more rapidly than digitoxin (Okita 1969).

Serum Digitalis Assay Techniques

A major advance in recent years has been the development of accurate radioimmune assay methods for determining serum concentrations of digitalis glycosides (Smith 1972). These techniques permit monitoring serum levels of digitalis glycosides in treated patients and their correlation with therapeutic and toxic effects. In human beings therapeutic serum levels for digitoxin ranged from 17 to 44 ng/ml and for digoxin from 0.76 to 2.4 ng/ml, while toxicity was observed with levels from 34 to 67 ng/ml for digitoxin and 1.7 to 5.7 ng/ml for digoxin (Smith and Haber 1973). Note that there is some overlapping of the toxic and therapeutic blood levels. In healthy Beagle dogs, digoxin serum levels of up to 2.5 ng/ml produced no or only mild signs of toxicosis. Levels exceeding this limit were associated with moderate-to-severe toxic signs. On postmortem examination, cardiac lesions found included coronary arteritis, myocardial necrosis, and degeneration or necrosis of renal proximal tubules and collecting ducts. These were associated with elevation of blood urea nitrogen, serum creatinine, and serum electrolyte changes (Fillmore and Detweiler 1973; Teske et al. 1976). From these data it would appear that therapeutic serum levels of digoxin should not exceed 2.5 ng/ml in dogs. As yet, data on digitalis glycoside levels in dogs treated for congestive heart failure have not been reported.

Toxic Action

The characteristic manifestations of digitalis toxicosis in animals consist of such GI disturbances as inappetence, diarrhea, and emesis; weakness and depression; and cardiac arrhythmias and conduction disturbances. In the experimental cat and dog, a feature of chronic toxicosis is continued weight loss (Rothlin and Bircher 1961; Fillmore and Detweiler 1973; Teske et al. 1976).

Inappetence and mild-to-moderate diarrhea are frequent side actions that are no cause for alarm and ordinarily do not require reducing the dose. Following the intravenous injection of digitalization doses of ouabain in dogs, emesis may occur within 10 or 20 minutes. This reaction is not uncommon, does not appear to be related to dosage, and may not necessarily occur with subsequent injections in the same animal. The onset of emesis in dogs receiving oral digitalis is often a sign of more severe toxic action. Incomplete AV block with dropped beats, ST-segment shifts, and the occurrence of coupled ventricular ectopic beats are ECG changes indicating toxic action on the heart. The coupled unifocal ventricular premature systoles are an early evidence of toxicosis; multifocal ventricular ectopic beats, paroxysmal ventricular tachycardia, parasystole, and paroxysmal atrial tachycardia with block are signs of more severe toxic action. When these ECG changes develop, administration should be stopped until they disappear before continuing at lower dose levels.

Toxic doses of digitalis can produce myocardial necrosis. This result has been reported in dogs (Kyser et al. 1946; Teske et al. 1975), cats (Buchner 1934; Dearing et al. 1943), rabbits (Friedman 1957), and rats (Selye 1961). This type of necrosis has certain similarities to that produced in rats by excess of various sodium salts and simple potassium deficiency. Desoxycorticosterone (which causes hypokalemia) aggravates the necrosis produced by potassium deficiency and decreases the threshold of digitalis toxicity in human beings (Selye 1958). Both digitalis and desoxycorticosterone deplete the myocardium of potassium. Thus it appears that the myocardial necrosis caused by digitalis could be related to its decrease of myocardial potassium.

In dogs the acute toxic intravenous dose of digoxin has been determined to be 0.177 mg/kg $\pm$ SE $=$ 0.008 (Beck 1969b). In healthy Beagle dogs, subacute digoxin toxicosis can be induced and maintained with an intravenous loading dose of 0.125–0.150 mg/kg given in divided doses at 0, 1, 4, and 24 hours, followed by a daily intravenous maintenance dose of 0.015–0.025 mg/kg (or for more severe toxicity up to 0.035 mg/kg daily) (Fillmore and Detweiler 1973; Teske et al. 1976). An ECG scoring system to monitor digoxin toxicosis was found reliable in these two investigations and superior to serum enzyme changes (e.g., creatinine phosphokinase [CPK], alkaline phosphatase, serum glutamic-oxalacetic transaminase, and lactic dehydrogenase [LDH]) in detecting mild to moderate toxicosis. It was found that with serum digoxin concentrations less than 2.5 ng/ml toxic signs were mild or absent, concentrations of 2.5 to 6 ng/ml caused moderate toxicoses, and concentrations above 6 ng/ml produced severe toxicosis and some deaths. The latter high serum digoxin levels caused reductions in body temperature (1°–3° F); elevations in blood urea nitrogen (BUN), serum creatinine, serum potassium, serum CPK, and LDH levels; and reductions in serum sodium and chloride levels (Teske et al. 1976). An unexpected finding in this study was evidence that toxic doses of digoxin compromised renal function (elevated serum creatinine and BUN levels; serum electrolyte alterations). These changes were associated with degeneration and necrosis of proximal tubular and collecting duct epithelium, the severity of which was directly related to the elevation of BUN and serum creatinine levels. The latter, in turn, were directly related to the height and persistence of the serum digoxin levels. Thus it appears that digoxin, in toxic doses, can inhibit its own renal excretion, thus creating a vicious cycle if dosage is continued.

In addition to monitoring the ECG, serum enzymes, and plasma electrolytes to detect digitalis toxicosis, measurement of salivary calcium and potassium concentrations has proved useful in human beings (Swanson et al. 1973). Cardiac glycosides increase Ca^{++} and K^{+} concentration in the saliva by an unknown mechanism. It was found that the product of salivary Ca^{++} concentration $\times$ K^{+} concentration exceeded 300 mEq/L in patients with other signs of digitalis toxicity.

Various neurotoxic effects occur in human beings following large therapeutic and toxic doses. The reactions observed include stupor, ataxia, psychotic episodes, confusion, headache, neuralgia, restlessness, visual hallucinations, delirium, and coma (Lyon and DeGraff 1963). The cardiac glycosides are less neurotoxic than the corresponding genin. For example, digitoxigenin produces convulsions in cats at lower doses than digitoxin, while the latter produces lethal cardiac toxicity in the same species at a lower dose than the former. The rat is relatively insensitive to the cardiotoxic action of digitalis but develops neurotoxicity. In dogs, typical neurotoxic effects with therapeutic doses have not been reported or at least not distinguished from the weakness and depression accompanying cardiac toxicosis. These untoward CNS effects have been attributed to intracellular potassium depletion (Lyon and DeGraff 1963); see the discussion below.

There are marked species differences in sensitivity to acute toxic effects of digitalis glycosides (Detweiler 1967). For example, the relative LD50 in various species, taking the cat as unity, are cat, 1; rabbit, 2; various frog species, 2–8; various toads, > 400; and rat, 671. The sensitivity or resistance appears to reside in the heart and depend on the relative sensitivity of Na^+-K^+ membrane ATPase to glycoside (ouabain) inhibition (Akera et al. 1969; Allen and Schwartz 1969).

Cations and Digitalis Cardiac Toxicosis

The sensitivity of the heart to the toxic effects of digitalis glycosides can be modified by the influence of K^+, Ca^{++}, and Mg^{++}. The digitalis-antagonizing effect of K^+ and Mg^{++} has led to the use of their salts in digitalis poisoning, and the production of hypocalcemia with chelating agents protects the heart against the toxic actions of digitalis.

POTASSIUM

Potassium controls arrhythmias and conduction disturbances caused by digitalis but does not abolish its therapeutic action. In dogs the toxic dose of digitalis is increased to approximately 240% of the control toxic dose when the serum potassium level is raised to between 7 and 8 mEq/L, and it is decreased to 40% of the control toxic dose when the serum potassium level is decreased to 2 mEq/L. However, it appears to be the cellular rather than the extracellular level of potassium that governs the sensitivity to digitalis toxicity. Two groups of dogs were segregated on the basis of their significantly differing digitalis tolerance. One group required twice as much acetylstrophanthidin as the other group for the production of ventricular tachycardia, but both groups had nearly identical mean serum potassium levels (Lown 1961). Digitoxin in doses of 0.2–0.4 mg daily (intravenously or subcutaneously) reduces intracellular myocardial potassium in dogs by inhibiting potassium flux into the cell (Conn 1956), although digitalis intoxication is not associated with a reduction in serum potassium concentration (Lown et al. 1960). It may be that the intracellular-extracellular potassium gradient is the critical factor in determining the threshold to digitalis toxic action. Thus depletion of intracellular potassium may enhance the toxic effect of digitalis without a decrease in extracellular potassium level.

CALCIUM

The actions of Ca^{++} on the contractility and excitability of the myocardium are similar to those of digitalis. As with digitalis, the initial effects on heart rate and AV conduction are the result of increased vagal tone and can be abolished by atropine. Presumably the two drugs could have an additive effect on the heart and there is experimental evidence to indicate this (Nalbandian et al. 1957). However, in experiments in dogs, no increased sensitivity to calcium injections was found when the degree of digitalization with ouabain varied from 0% to 90% of toxicity. Digitalislike arrhythmias were induced by calcium only when the animals had received more than 95% of the toxic dose of ouabain (Lown et al. 1960). Likewise, the lethal dose of digitalis was decreased only in dogs given calcium in doses large enough to produce ECG changes. Thus in the normal dog a synergistic or additive effect of calcium and digitalis could not be demonstrated. Whether or not this is true in unanesthetized dogs with congestive heart failure has not been established. The use of calcium injections in the dog as a tolerance test for digitalis to assess the level of digitalization is not justified on the basis of this work (Beume et al. 1961).

Lowering the serum calcium with sodium salts of the chelating agent ethylenediaminetetraacetic acid (EDTA) controls the ECG changes caused by toxic doses of digitalis. At the pH of blood, EDTA has a selective affinity for calcium. This antiarrhythmic action of EDTA is not specific and will abolish arrhythmias caused by factors other than calcium or digitalis (Lown et al. 1960). Lowering ionized serum calcium with sodium citrate will also abolish digitalis-induced cardiac arrhythmias in dogs (Cordey and Skelton 1964).

MAGNESIUM

This cation is taken up selectively by the myocardium and at high serum concentrations depresses cardiac contractility and excitability. It has a transient and inconstant protective action against digitalis-induced arrhythmias, and magnesium depletion sensitizes the heart to digitalis (Lown et al. 1960).

Estrogens exert a protective effect against the toxic effects of digitalis on the myocardium. Entire female dogs and spayed female dogs treated with estrogen are more resistant to digitalis toxicity than are spayed female and male dogs. A nonestrogenic steroid with this protective action has been described (Grinnell and Smith 1957; Grinnell and Johnson 1961). A protective effect of estrogens and a similar effect of elevated serum cholesterol have been demonstrated in rabbits (Rodensky and Wasserman 1964). Although a segregation of resistant and susceptible dogs to acetylstrophanthidin toxic arrhythmias has been reported, neither this nor a sex difference in susceptibility was found in dogs with digoxin (Beck 1969b).

Treatment of Digitalis-Induced Arrhythmias

Although there has been much experimental work on antidotes for digitalis toxicosis in normal dogs, there is little information to go on regarding dogs with clinical congestive heart failure. Ordinarily, cardiac arrhythmias and other toxic manifestations of digitalis overdosage disappear with cage rest or the use of diphenylhydantoin (Mosey et al. 1952). If there is no kidney impairment, potassium chloride may be administered in dogs: 0.6–1 g orally as the initial dose, followed by 0.3–0.5 g every 1–2 hours for 2 doses and continued at 4-hour intervals, as necessary, to control the arrhythmia. Other agents such as magnesium, procaine amide, quinidine, EDTA, and saturated lactones have had little use in clinical digitalis poisoning in animals, and general recommendations for their administration will not be made (Somlyo 1960). Of the antiarrhythmic agents, diphenylhydantoin and lidocaine appear to be the most effective against digitalis-induced arrhythmias (Hoffman and Bigger 1971).

Separability of Toxic (Arrhythmic) and Inotropic Effects

In the intact experimental dog, it has been shown that with ouabain, when toxic arrhythmias developed, the contractile strength increased about 65%. When these arrhythmias were abolished with K^+, and additional K^+ and digitalis were given together, a further 20% increase in contractile strength was induced (Williams et al. 1966). Thus potassium permitted additional inotropic effect without further toxicity. This same effect has been demonstrated with diphenylhydantoin (Helfant et al. 1967a) and sodium or potassium canrenoate (Yeh and Lazzara 1973). Since potassium is a myocardial depressant and digitalis toxicity is associated with a decreased inotropic response following further increments in dosage, the clinical application of this finding could be hazardous (Greenspan and Edmands 1969). Further, arrhythmias are only part of the dangerous effects of digitalis toxicity. We now know (Teske et al. 1976) that digoxin at least produces renal damage at serum levels associated with only mild signs of toxicity. Thus abolishing cardiac arrhythmias so as to permit use of higher doses of digitalis glycosides for their additional inotropic effect might very well result in serious renal damage.

CHRONIC CONGESTIVE HEART FAILURE

Chronic congestive heart failure is a clinical syndrome that develops when the cardiac output is reduced below that required to provide blood circulation adequate for bodily needs, and there is a resultant retention and accumulation of extracellular fluid.

THE HEART

1. *Mechanical factors.* Ventricular hypertrophy usually precedes chronic congestive heart failure. It has been shown that myocardial contractile strength is reduced per unit of myocardial tissue although compensation is maintained by the increase in total muscle mass. Ventricular dilation (magnitude of ventricular radii r_1, r_2) results in increased wall tension (T) per unit of intraventricular pressure (P), in accordance with the LaPlace relation $P = T/r_1 + r_2$. While the Starling mechanism (increase in cardiac output with increase in end-diastolic volume) serves, within limits, to support the dilated heart, maximal tension developed declines in both hypertrophy and the failure state. The cardiac mechanical deficits in congestive heart failure include decreased velocity and extent of cardiac muscle shortening, reduced maximal tension, and increased wall tension per unit pressure maintained. The development of these deficits is a continuum from hypertrophy to failure, beginning with reduction in unit contractile strength during hypertrophy and the progression of the unfavorable pressure to wall tension (LaPlace) relationship as dilation proceeds. These changes are accompanied by a progressive reduction in developed active tension.

In the intact, diseased heart, in addition to the effect of ventricular dilation, other geometrical factors (such as valvular stenosis or regurgitation) and cardiac arrhythmias decrease effective cardiac work.

2. *Biochemical factors.* Congestive heart failure has been variously attributed to defects in energy production, energy storage, or energy utilization (see Metabolic Actions earlier in this chapter). Deficits in energy production or energy storage have not been identified. Although the efficiency of energy utilization appears unimpaired, the rate of conversion of chemical to mechanical energy is slowed because of reduced myofibrillar ATPase activity in the failing myocardium. A fundamental defect in excitation-contraction coupling related to inadequate release of Ca^{++} for optimal contraction is a possible defect having neither been proved nor refuted (Harris and Opie 1971).

3. *Supporting factors.* In the failing myocardium, norepinephrine stores and biosynthesis are reduced and response to sympathetic nerve stimulation is curtailed. β-Adrenergic receptor blockade intensifies cardiac failure. Possibly the failing myocardium is dependent on circulating catecholamines to maintain function.

SUMMARY

The myocardial deficits in congestive heart failure include (1) depression of contractility, (2) reduction in rate of energy utilization, (3) reduction in effective cardiac work owing to geometrical factors, and (4) possibly an excitation-contraction–coupling defect.

CONSEQUENCES OF CARDIAC FAILURE

MECHANISMS

Edema formation in congestive heart failure results because of renal retention of sodium and water (volume imbalance). There is an associated elevation of venous pressure causing an increase in capillary hydrostatic pressure (pressure imbalance) favoring the extravascular accumulation of the fluid retained by the kidneys. There are at least two processes that account for renal reabsorption of sodium and water in congestive heart failure: the direct effect of underperfusion on renal function and a humoral sequence triggered by this hemodynamic insufficiency. Some of the mechanisms involved are represented in Fig. 24.8. Certain unresolved and conflicting views are not represented and will not be discussed.

Fig. 24.8. Cardiac failure.

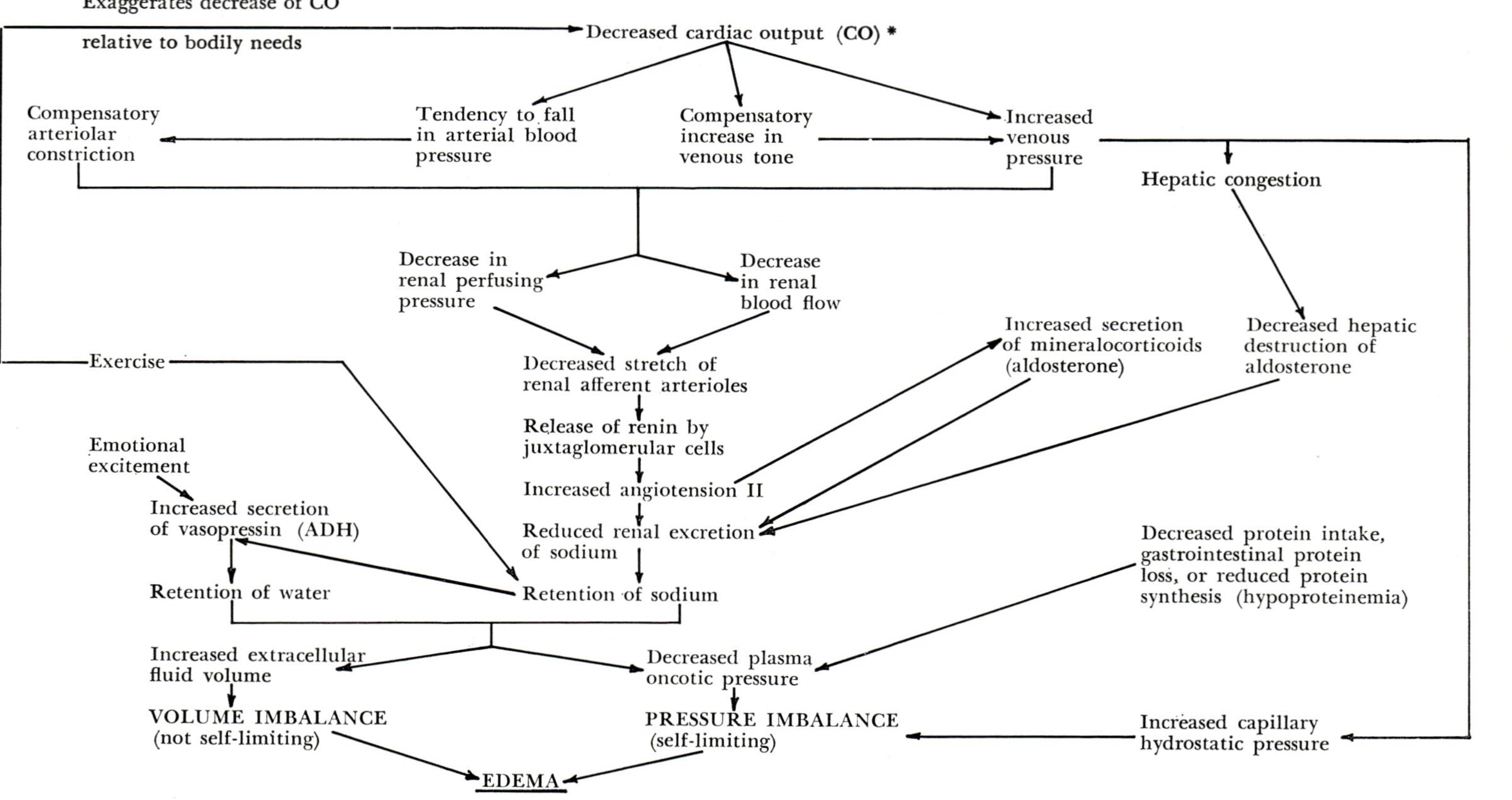

* In high output failure (hyperthyroidism, anemia) the CO is elevated but still relatively insufficient to meet bodily needs.

The principal factors thought to operate in bringing about altered renal function and expansion of the extracellular fluid volume in congestive heart failure are as follows: the initial causative event is an absolute or relative fall in cardiac output below that required to maintain adequate circulation of blood. This may occur only at intervals when increased demands are placed on the heart, as during muscular exercise, or may be present even at rest. There is a tendency for the arterial blood pressure to fall, but this is prevented largely by compensatory arterial and arteriolar constriction involving, among others, the preglomerular vessels. In dogs with experimental congestive heart failure, there is an increase in sympathetic tone reducing renal blood flow (Davis et al. 1955; Barger et al. 1961). This may be part of a baroreceptor reflex associated with the tendency for a decrease in arterial pressure. Presumably, decreased stretch of the renal afferent arterioles occurs. Located in the media of these vessels are the juxtaglomerular (JG) cells that produce renin (Tobian 1960; Davis 1962). The decrease in stretch causes the JG cells to release renin, which acts on renin substrate (a protein in the α2-globulin fraction of blood plasma) to produce angiotensin I (a decapeptide), which is converted to angiotensin II (an octapeptide) by a converting enzyme. The chief site of this conversion is the lung, although a varying degree of conversion can take place in the kidney, hind legs, and intestine. Angiotensin II (hypertensin or angiotonin) acts on the zona glomerulosa cells of the adrenal cortex causing increase in aldosterone secretion. When hepatic congestion is severe enough, the decreased rate of metabolic destruction of aldosterone in the liver contributes to the elevation of its blood level (Ayers et al. 1962). Aldosterone increases reabsorption of sodium, acting primarily on the distal renal tubule. It is generally thought that the initial event in sodium-water retention is sodium retention. This increases the electrolyte concentration of extracellular fluid that could be expected to stimulate osmoreceptors in the hypothalamus. This stimulation would bring about the release of antidiuretic hormone (vasopressin) by the posterior pituitary gland. Vasopressin causes increased reabsorption of water in the renal tubule, acting primarily at the distal tubule and collecting ducts. There is evidence that the role of antidiuretic hormone is nonessential in edema formation, although its release may occur and would promote the accumulation of fluid (Laragh 1962).

The retention of sodium and water produces a volume imbalance with an increase in extracellular fluid volume. The increased venous pressure, which may occur only after the retention of sodium and water has been initiated, is a major factor accounting for the extravascular accumulation of fluid retained by the kidneys owing to its effect of increasing capillary hydrostatic pressure (pressure imbalance). The rise in venous pressure may augment renal retention of sodium and water, while the retention of sodium and water can promote a rise in venous pressure. The renal mechanism (i.e., sodium retention) has been shown to precede the hydrostatic effect of increased venous pressure in experimental congestive heart failure (Barger et al. 1959). Exercise increases the work of the heart and causes renal retention of sodium in human beings (Barger 1956), although this has not been observed in normal dogs (Kruhoffer 1960). In forced exercise in dogs, antidiuresis occurs, but this effect disappears with training. Thus it appears to be emotional stress rather than exercise itself that is responsible for the antidiuretic effect (Harris 1962).

The plasma protein concentration is reduced in congestive heart failure (Wallace and Hamilton 1962). One reason for this is the dilution of the extracellular fluid by the retained sodium and water. A similar effect can be produced in dogs simply by injecting physiological saline solution (O'Connor 1962). Also there is loss of plasma protein from the vascular system since the ascitic fluid is found to contain substantial amounts. The total amount of plasma protein in ascitic fluid alone may exceed that in the circulating blood. A further cause of reduced plasma protein level may be attributed to reduced food intake (inappetence), poor GI absorption, GI loss of protein, or interference with hepatic protein synthesis owing to liver damage. The relative importance of these factors has not been determined in dogs, but in human beings, at least in certain cases, plasma protein deficiency primarily owing to intraenteric loss has been recognized (Davidson et al. 1961). Despite the decrease in plasma protein level in the blood in congestive heart failure, the total amount of plasma protein, including that in blood and extracellular fluids, may exceed the total blood protein in normal dogs (Wallace and Hamilton 1962). The low plasma protein level reduces the plasma oncotic pressure. This further alters the balance of forces in the capillaries in the direction of fluid loss from the plasma into the interstitial fluid compartment.

The result of these various effects is the production of a volume imbalance, because of the retention of sodium and water, and a pressure imbalance because of increased hydrostatic pressure and decreased plasma oncotic pressure in the capillaries. The pressure imbalance component cannot account for the relatively enormous accumulation of edema fluid that may occur in congestive heart failure. These processes tending to cause edema (increased hydrostatic pressure, decreased oncotic pressure) would limit themselves as blood concentration increased, capillary hydrostatic pressure decreased, and tissue hydrostatic pressure increased with the transudation of plasma fluid into the interstitial compartment. Increased capillary permeability due to capillary injury resulting from the venous congestion is another hypothetical factor that can be involved. If these pressure imbalance factors were the only ones acting, a volume of edema fluid exceeding that of the plasma compartment could not occur. It is the volume imbalance brought about by retention of water and salt that causes the relatively unlimited accumulation of edema fluid found in congestive heart failure.

From the foregoing, a body of evidence emphasizes the central role of the kidney and adrenal cortex in congestive heart failure (Urquhart and Davis 1963). The chronic renal retention of sodium is largely the result of increased tubular resorption caused by increased aldosterone secretion. Decreased destruction of the hormone by the liver may be a secondary factor accounting for increased plasma levels. The increased aldosterone secretion appears to be regulated by the kidney itself, acting through the renin-angiotensin system. Presumably the renal afferent arterioles and the macula densa act as receptors in a negative feedback control mechanism that responds to a decrease in wall tension by causing an increased renin release from the JG cells. The resultant retention of sodium and fluid would serve to increase blood volume, resulting in decreased renal arterial blood pressure and flow. Thus the stimulus to enhanced renin release would be removed and aldosterone secretion returned to normal. This mechanism is outlined in Fig. 24.9. In normal animals aldosterone release increases retention of salt and water. Any retained fluid increases the extracellular fluid volume, including plasma volume, and thus tends to elevate blood pressure, circulating blood volume, and renal blood flow. These changes presumably can decrease renin release by the negative feedback loop depicted in Fig. 24.9.

One aspect of this response has not been explained. In normal animals the sodium-retaining effects of aldosterone are transient, lasting only 1 or 2 days in dogs despite continued administration of the hormone (Urquhart and Davis 1963). In congestive heart failure, some factor maintains the kidneys in a state of continued responsiveness to the sodium-retaining effects of aldosterone and the fluid retention continues indefinitely. The nature of this factor appearing to sensitize the renal tubule to aldosterone action is unknown (Davis et al. 1964).

Possibly in congestive heart failure the retained fluid fails to restore renal arteriolar hemodynamics to normal, despite the increase in blood volume, thus accounting for the continued hypersecretion of renin

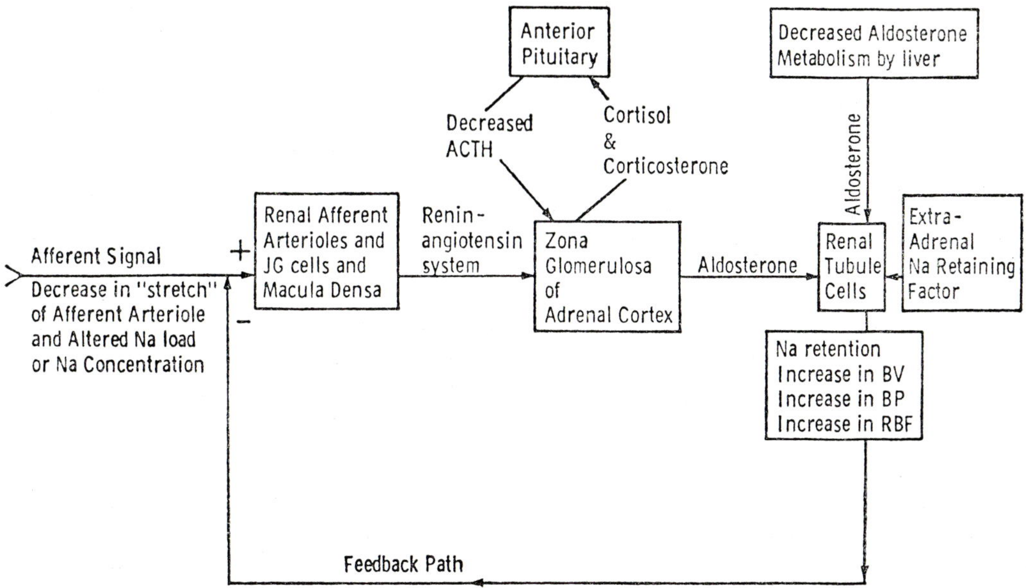

Fig. 24.9. Negative feedback diagram to explain the renin-angiotensin-aldosterone system. Two intrarenal receptors are postulated: (1) a stretch in the renal afferent arterioles and (2) the macula densa, which are sensitive to signals leading to renin release by juxtaglomerular apparatus cells. The vascular stretch receptor responds to changes in wall tension and the macula densa to changes in sodium load or transport. (JG, juxtaglomerular; BP, blood pressure; BV, blood volume; RBF, renal blood flow.) (Davis 1974)

and aldosterone (Davis 1971). Therefore, the failing heart might be considered the "unknown factor" that permits the renin-angiotensin-aldosterone mechanism to maintain its effectiveness on the tubule and sustain the abnormally increased extracellular fluid volume. In any case, in congestive heart failure, renal hemodynamics are not improved by the retention of fluid, and elevated secretion of aldosterone continues.

Effect of Digitalis Glycosides in Congestive Heart Failure

cellular level

Digitalis glycosides do not appear to act by modifying energy production or storage nor is there clear evidence that they improve energy utilization by direct effects on enzyme systems. Although still speculative, the consensus is that digitalis action in congestive heart failure is at the level of excitation-contraction coupling. This is associated with an increased availability of Ca^{++} for excitation-contraction coupling during activation, which may be linked in some manner with effects on Na^{+}-K^{+} membrane transport (Na^{+}-K^{+}–ATPase inhibition).

myocardial level

Digitalis increases contractile force in both the normal and failing myocardium. An important component of digitalis action in the failing myocardium is reduction in size of the dilated ventricle. Another important action is slowing of the ventricular rate in atrial fibrillation. Depression of myocardial contractile strength by drugs (halothane, barbiturates, potassium) is combated by digitalis. Cardiac glycosides have also been shown to protect rats against the development of experimental ventricular hypertrophy induced by constriction of the aorta but not that produced by swimming exercise (Williams and Braunwald 1965; Aldinger 1970). In mice digitoxin afforded some protection against hypoxia-induced ventricular hypertrophy (Heinz et al. 1968). Thus digitalis glycosides appear to protect against the pathological hypertrophy of aortic constriction and chronic hypoxia but not against the physiologic hypertrophy produced by chronic exercise.

Digitalization

The decompensated or failing heart is ordinarily dilated beyond optimal limits. When it decreases in size, there is often an improvement in ventricular emptying with a consequent increase in stroke volume and cardiac output. According to the law of LaPlace, the improvement in ventricular emptying is attributed to the positive inotropic action of digitalis and to the mechanical advantage of the reduction in cardiac diameter.

The effect of digitalis on heart rate in the decompensated heart has been overemphasized because of generalizations made from the influence of the drug on ventricular rate in atrial fibrillation. In atrial fibrillation, marked decrease in ventricular rate is one of the primary effects of digitalis that accounts for its therapeutic action. On the other hand, in the presence of normal sinus rhythm, therapeutic effects of digitalis may develop without any important change in heart rate as determined under clinical conditions. When sinus tachycardia is associated with decompensation, however, hemodynamic improvement may be accompanied by a substantial reduction in heart rate. The increase in myocardial contractile strength can be demonstrated in both normal (Walton et al. 1950b) and decompensated hearts, although the effect is most consistently demonstrable in the failing myocardium.

The belief that digitalis is harmful to the nonfailing heart has not been supported (Rodman and Pastor 1963). Evidence has accumulated indicating that digitalization may be of value prophylactically in normal hearts about to undergo unusual strain as in cardiac surgery or manual resuscitation of the heart in ventricular fibrillation or standstill. It has also been shown to protect the heart against depressant effects of anesthetic agents. Further, both in the failing heart and in dogs not showing evidence of failure, abnormal cardiac arrhythmias may be abolished by digitalization. Thus in recent years belief in the concept that there was only one indication for digitalis therapy, i.e., overt congestive heart failure, has waned. There is an increasing tendency to digitalize patients in the absence of reliable signs of congestive heart failure and to use the drug when severe cardiac strain is anticipated. Thus preoperative digitalization in older dogs has been advocated, especially when the heart is enlarged or the clinical history suggests a lowered cardiac reserve. Experimental results indicate that prophylactic digitalization protects dogs from myocardial weakening in hemorrhagic shock and thus prolongs survival time in normal animals (Braunwald and Kahler 1964). Whether or not prophylactic digitalization of animals without cardiac disease is justified in infectious diseases remains controversial, since there is no evidence as to whether it would be helpful or detrimental.

The clinical use of digitalis was discovered because of its diuretic effect in congestive heart failure and this is an outstanding feature of its therapeutic action. A decrease in aldosterone secretion is responsible, at least in part, for this effect in dogs with cardiac decompensation (Carpenter et al. 1962) (see Actions on Certain Other Organs earlier in this chapter). In normal animals and those with noncardiac edema, the diuretic effect is negligible.

Dosage and Choice of Preparation

Species and individual differences in response to digitalis glycosides are remarkably great. Individual variation is marked in dogs and probably in other species as well. In experiments with normal dogs, it was possible to select two groups, one of which required twice as much acetylstrophanthidin as the other to produce ventricular tachycardia (Lown 1961). In dogs with congestive heart failure, the dose required for digitalization also varies widely. It is for this reason that strict limits regarding digitalization and maintenance dosages cannot be made and each animal must be given the drug to effect.

In the choice of digitalis preparations it is best to become familiar with a limited number rather than attempt to use a wide variety. Qualitatively, the cardiac actions of various preparations are the same, but there are differences in absorption, potency, rapidity of onset of action, and duration of effect. These factors determine the clinical action. Since most aims of digitalis therapy can be accomplished by the official preparations of digitalis, digitoxin, digoxin, and ouabain, only these will be discussed.

Of the three glycosides, ouabain is the most potent and acts most rapidly and its effect disappears most quickly. Thus it is well suited for emergency therapy. It is absorbed too irregularly and poorly to be given orally.

Digoxin is suitable for both oral and parenteral digitalization and for maintenance therapy. In the dog, its clinical effects are more rapid than digitoxin. Therapeutic action is observed more quickly and toxic effects are more common than with digitoxin. Because its effects disappear relatively rapidly, toxic reactions ordinarily are controlled simply by ceasing treatment for a few days and then resuming therapy at a lower dose level.

Digitoxin may be employed either parenterally or orally. Its slow disappearance makes it especially well suited for prolonged maintenance therapy in human beings. In dogs it is excreted more rapidly than digoxin and far more rapidly than in human beings. Digitalis leaf combines the effects of several glycosides, most notably digitoxin. It causes more nausea and vomiting in human beings than the more purified glycosides.

Generalizations regarding the most suitable preparation for different species under various circumstances cannot be made because well-controlled clinical studies are lacking. In the dog digoxin is preferred over digitoxin and digitalis when a more rapid effect with oral administration is desired. Ouabain is recommended for rapid parenteral digitalization. In horses and cattle there has been more experience with ouabain and digoxin by the parenteral route, and information on oral medication is inadequate.

The principle followed in digitalis therapy is the administration of an initial amount over a relatively short period of time, sufficient to produce the desired therapeutic effect, and then to continue with smaller doses daily to maintain this effect. The amount of drug required to produce the initial effect is called the digitalization dose. The daily dose required to continue this level of therapeutic action is called the maintenance dose. Owing to the marked individual variation in response to the digitalis glycosides, the digitalization dose cannot be calculated with precision. Therefore, determining the proper amount for each subject is a trial and error attempt to administer a therapeutically effective dose without producing serious toxic effects. To accomplish this, a trial digitalization dose is arbitrarily estimated from a knowledge of the dose ranges for different drugs and this is administered over a short period of time in divided doses. The rate of administration is continued until either a therapeutic response is attained or signs of toxic action supervene, even though the amount originally estimated as appropriate might be exceeded. When the desired therapeutic effect is reached, the drug is continued at a lower dose rate, sufficient to maintain the therapeutic action. Since most preparations are cumulative, therapy must be guided by the response of the subject and adjustments in dosage made as necessary. In estimating the digitalization dose required, body weight resulting from edema fluid should be discounted. The elimination rate of digitalis glycosides depends on the total quantity accumulated in the body, since the amount lost tends to be a fixed percentage of the quantity in the body, e.g., normal dogs excrete daily roughly 30% of the total digoxin in the body (Marcus et al. 1967). Over the long term

TABLE 24.2. Average dose ranges of digitalis preparation for dogs

Preparation	Total Digitalization Dose	Daily Maintenance Dose
Oral		
Digitalis, U.S.P. (powder, tablets)	0.015–0.05 g/lb	1/8–1/3 the total digitalization dose
Digitalis Tincture, U.S.P.	0.15–0.45 ml/lb	
Digitoxin, U.S.P. (tablets)	0.05–0.15 mg/lb	
Digoxin, U.S.P. (tablets)	0.03–0.10 mg/lb	
Parenteral		
Ouabain, U.S.P.	0.01–0.015 mg/lb	The same dose daily for 3–4 days.
Digoxin, U.S.P.	0.02–0.03 mg/lb	This usually must be reduced thereafter

the size of the initial digitalization or "loading" dose is less important than the maintenance dose, which is decisive. Further, larger "loading" doses result in high serum levels and may be toxic, while an adequate maintenance dose without an initial loading dose will accumulate and eventually digitalize, although this may require many days. Because of the importance of renal excretion, animals with renal disease may develop toxicosis unexpectedly following "loading" doses.

DOG

Dose ranges for dogs are given in Table 24.2. These doses can be employed only as guides. For example, in the author's experience, two dogs with similar heart conditions and atrial fibrillation were being treated after digitalization with digoxin. One was a 35-lb cocker spaniel and the other a 160-lb Irish wolfhound. Each required 0.25 mg of digoxin daily to maintain an optimal ventricular rate, despite the great disparity in weight.

THE TIME COURSE OF DIGITALIZATION

Rigid schedules for digitalization should not be recommended. Rather, it is important to emphasize that the time course of digitalization is an individual matter that must be adjusted to the subject's needs. However, the patterns of therapy can be classified into three general types.

Intensive digitalization. One-half of the calculated amount is given at once; 6 hours later, one-fourth of the total dose is given; then one-eighth of the total dose is continued at 4- to 6-hour intervals until a therapeutic or toxic effect becomes evident.

Rapid digitalization. In general, this method is preferred to avoid dangerous toxic effects. The estimated amount is divided into 3 equal doses given at 6-hour intervals.

Slow digitalization. This method is suitable for dogs with mild failure that are to be treated at home and under other circumstances in which conservative therapy is satisfactory. One-third of the calculated digitalization dose is given daily until the desired response is attained. The patient should be examined on the 2nd and 4th days of treatment and then at intervals governed by the response.

For digoxin in dogs, Beck (1969b) calculated on the basis of the excretion data of Marcus et al. (1966, 1967) the probable amounts retained during different oral dosage schedules (Fig. 24.10). Note that a loading dose of 0.03 mg/lb daily for 2 days (total 0.06 mg/lb) would produce high body levels initially, whereas a loading dose of 0.03 mg/lb for 1 day would not. The calculated amount retained with loading doses, followed by a maintenance of 0.01 mg/lb or with maintenance doses alone would be about the same after 10–14 days. While these calculations are purely speculative, a regime now often successful in the dog consists of giving digoxin 0.03 mg/lb in 3 divided doses on day 1 of therapy and continuing with a daily maintenance dose of 0.01 mg/lb.

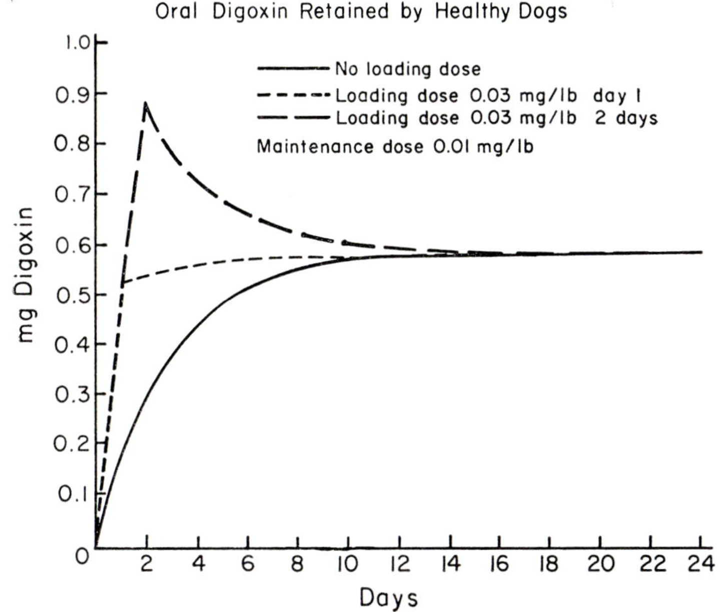

FIG. 24.10. Calculated retention of digoxin with different dosage schedules. (Beck 1969b)

It is probable that the oral dose recommended for digitoxin in Table 24.2 is too low. Ettinger (1966) employed digitoxin loading doses of 0.2 mg/lb given in divided doses over 48 hours and daily maintenance doses of 0.05 mg/lb. From Beck's (1969a) calculations based on excretion data for digitoxin in dogs, this maintenance dose would be expected to be adequate, but the digitalization dose seemed excessive. Unfortunately, the question of adequate oral digitoxin dosage in dogs remains unsolved, although the consensus is that this glycoside is less reliable than digoxin in clinical practice (Ettinger and Suter 1970).

SIGNS OF EFFECTIVE DIGITALIZATION IN DOGS

The earliest evidence may be an amelioration of coughing, dyspnea, and fatigability. In dogs with atrial fibrillation, the ventricular rate is a useful guide to therapy. The ventricular rate in untreated animals usually exceeds 190/minute and a reduction to 150/minute is a satisfactory early effect. The final aim is to reduce the heart rate to between 80 and 120/minute. In the absence of atrial fibrillation, the cardiac rate may change little or, if tachycardia is marked, there may be slowing. Diuresis should develop and, if urine volume cannot be measured, body weight loss may serve as a guide to treatment (Figs. 24.11, 24.12). Ascites and peripheral edema should be reduced or disappear. See also ECG changes.

PARENTERAL DIGITALIZATION IN DOGS

This is indicated when an emergency exists or animals do not retain oral medication. With ouabain, the onset of action is rapid (i.e., within minutes). Fig. 24.6 shows the effect of ouabain in a dog with congestive heart failure (Carpenter et al. 1962). Within 5 minutes following the first injection, there was an increase in arterial pressure and a decrease in right atrial pressure. These changes reached a maximum 40–50 minutes after the beginning of administration. Note also the marked fall in aldosterone secretion rate following digitalization. Parenteral digitalization is more dangerous than the oral route and this must be considered in electing its use. To reduce the danger of intravenous administration, the calculated amount may be injected intramuscularly in 2 divided doses. A disadvantage of intramuscular injections is that ouabain is irritating and marked swelling may occur even

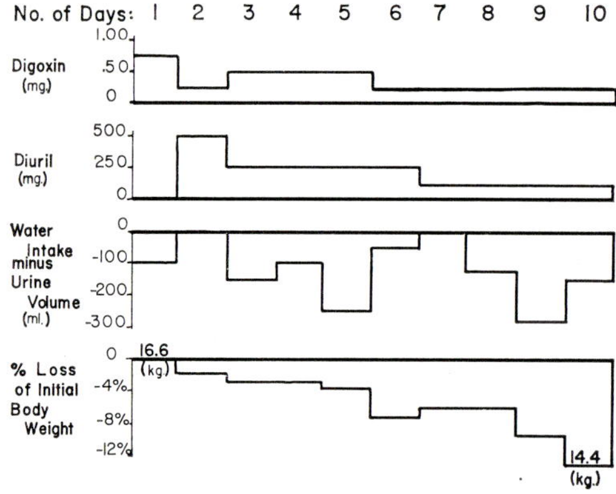

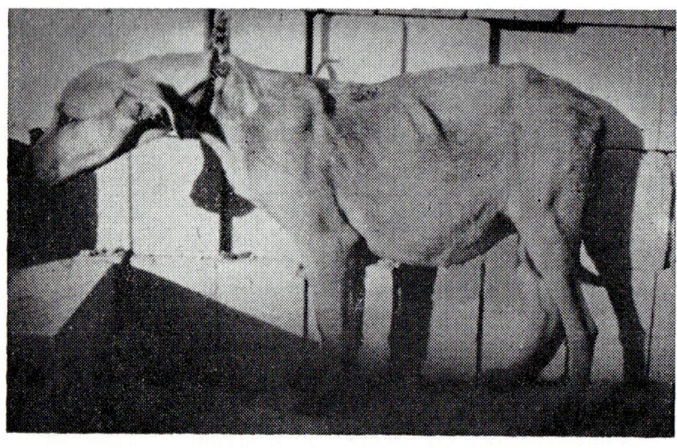

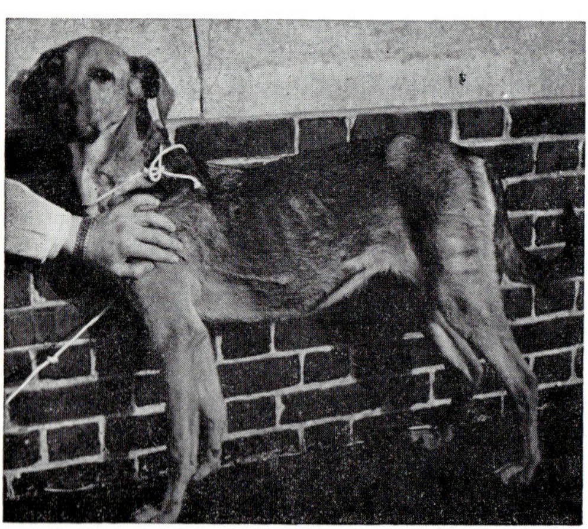

FIG. 24.11. The effect of digitalis and chlorothiazide (Diuril) therapy on a 2-year-old female mongrel with pulmonic stenosis and right heart failure. Top: chart showing the course of therapy, water loss, and weight loss. Middle: patient before treatment. Bottom: patient after treatment.

with dilute solutions. Digoxin may also be given parenterally, if desirable, in the digitalization doses indicated in Table 24.2.

After parenteral digitalization has been continued with ouabain given at 24- to 36-hour intervals for 3–5 days, oral maintenance therapy may be started. Digoxin may be used for this purpose, and not infrequently the oral maintenance dose of digoxin is found to approximately equal the total daily intravenous digitalization dose of ouabain, e.g., 0.01 mg/lb of body weight.

MAINTENANCE THERAPY IN DOGS

After the initial digitalization has been accomplished as judged by clinical signs, a daily maintenance dose is prescribed. This may range from one-eighth to one-third of the digitalization dose. The required maintenance dose cannot be predicted with any greater precision than the digitalization dose. In general, the larger the amount employed for digitalization, the larger is the maintenance dose required. When the maintenance dose is inadequate, signs of congestive heart failure return, and if it is too high, toxic effects develop. If signs of returning failure occur (increased weight, pitting edema, cough, fatigability) the maintenance dose may be doubled for several days and then a new dose level established. In dogs with atrial fibrillation, the resting heart rate may be used as a guide to adequate maintenance. When toxic signs appear (inappetence, vomiting, ECG changes), the daily dose should be omitted for several days and then treatment continued at perhaps one-half the former level.

HORSE

Dosage recommendations for digitalization of horses are based on meager clinical and experimental work and should be considered provisional (Detweiler and Patterson 1963). Dose ranges that have been employed in horses are given in Table 24.3.

The total oral digitalization amounts may be given in 6 divided doses over a

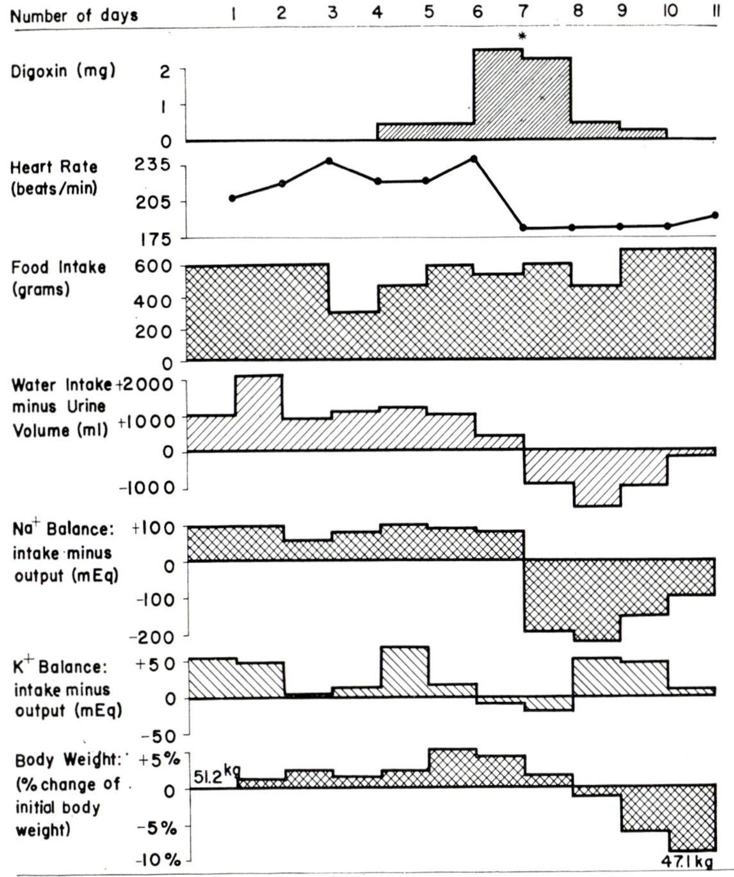

FIG. 24.12. The effect of digitalization on a 6-year-old Weimaraner with mitral insufficiency and chronic myocardial disease and atrial fibrillation. Note the reduction of heart rate and the markedly negative sodium and water balances associated with weight loss following digitalization.

period of 48 hours. On the third day, if no effect has been observed, continue with digitalization, giving one-third the total calculated dose. This daily dose may be continued until a therapeutic effect is produced or signs of digitalis toxicosis occur. Diarrhea may develop and, unless severe, is not a contraindication to continued treatment. The daily maintenance dose selected following digitalization should be from one-eighth to one-fifth the originally calculated digitalization dose and may be increased or decreased as needed.

When ouabain is employed for intravenous digitalization, the dose required for a 1000-lb animal may be determined by injecting 3 mg intravenously at 2-hour intervals until cardiac slowing or other signs of effective digitalization appear or a total of 10 mg has been given. If this total dose appears inadequate, additional 1-mg amounts may be injected at 2-hour intervals until a therapeutic or toxic effect is produced. The dose required can then be given daily for several days to maintain digitalization, provided the animal is carefully observed for evidence of toxic action.

TABLE 24.3. Digitalization doses for horses

Preparation	Total Digitalization Dose
Oral	
Digitalis, U.S.P. (powder)	1.5–3.0 g/100 lb
Digitalis Tincture, U.S.P.	15–30 ml/100 lb
Digitoxin, U.S.P.	1.5–3.0 mg/100 lb
Digoxin, U.S.P.	3.0 mg/100 lb
Parenteral	
Ouabain, U.S.P.	0.6–1.0 mg/100 lb
Digoxin, U.S.P.	1.0–1.5 mg/100 lb

OX

Doses of digitalis preparations that have been employed clinically in cattle vary widely (Mayer 1938; Davis and Garb 1953; Hostettler 1959; Will 1963). Only provisional recommendations for digitalization doses can be made as follows:

Intramuscularly	
Digitoxin, U.S.P.	1.4 mg/100 lb
Intravenously	
Digoxin, U.S.P.	0.4 mg/100 lb
Ouabain, U.S.P.	0.6–1 mg/100 lb

Maintenance doses would probably average one-eighth–one-fifth of the total digitalization doses of digoxin and digitoxin. Ouabain is rapidly dissipated in the ox as in other species and would have to be repeated at 24- to 36-hour intervals.

DIURETICS

Effective diuretics act on the renal tubule to oppose the relative increase in electrolyte and water reabsorption characteristic of congestive heart failure. The pharmacology, dosage, and administration of these agents are discussed in Chapter 27.

Diuretics may deplete the body of potassium. Since potassium depletion can precipitate or aggravate digitalis toxicity, it is desirable to prescribe potassium chloride when diuretic therapy is given over a long period. Daily oral doses of 0.25–0.5 g potassium chloride may be given for this purpose in the dog.

LOW SODIUM DIET

Sodium intake should be restricted. In dogs this may be accomplished for a short period by feeding boiled rice flavored with unsalted meat gravy or a mixture of equal parts soybean oil meal and meat cooked together. An experimental diet containing 28 mg of sodium and 136 mg of potassium/100 g has proved effective in dogs with congestive heart failure. Low-salt canned dog foods are now available commercially for canine cardiac patients.

RESTRICTION OF EXERCISE

It is desirable to diminish bodily exercise as much as possible by confinement and, if necessary, the administration of sedatives.

FLUIDS

In general, it is unnecessary to restrict drinking water unless excessive. When, because of fluid losses (excessive vomiting and diarrhea, posttraumatic syndromes), parenteral fluid therapy is considered, special problems arise requiring serum electrolyte determinations and fluid balance studies. Ordinarily, physiological saline solution should not be administered unless there is evidence that hyponatremia has developed. When intravenous infusions are necessary, they must be given slowly and with special care to avoid overloading the work capacity of the heart and precipitating acute cardiac failure.

MORPHINE SULFATE

In dogs with dyspnea in the absence of cyanosis, labored breathing can sometimes be relieved with small doses (8–15 mg) of morphine sulfate. Morphine is useful in acute pulmonary edema.

OXYGEN

Animals suffering from severe cardiovascular failure and hypoxia should be placed in an oxygen chamber (see Chapter 44).

MISCELLANEOUS THERAPY

Paroxysmal coughing may occur in dogs with mitral insufficiency and marked pulmonary congestion (so-called left heart failure). Along with digitalis, codeine may be given to ameliorate coughing; see Chapter 43 regarding the recommended dosage of codeine.

EMERGENCY TREATMENT

When death appears imminent in congestive heart failure, the following measures should be taken: oxygen therapy, intravenous digitalization with ouabain (in animals not already digitalized), paracentesis (remove all the fluid in the thorax and only sufficient ascitic fluid to relieve discomfort and interference with breathing), morphine sulfate in dogs (to reduce dyspnea and anxiety), and phlebotomy (use extreme caution). Phlebotomy can lead to circulatory collapse and is ordinarily a last resort. In a 30-lb dog, from 40 to 100 ml of blood may be removed—small quantities being taken over 30–60 minutes.

PREPARATIONS

Digitalis, U.S.P. The dried leaf of *Digitalis purpurea* Linné (Fam. Scrophulariaceae). The potency of digitalis is such that 100 mg are equivalent to not less than 1 U.S.P. Digitalis Unit.

Powdered Digitalis, U.S.P.

Digitalis Tablets, U.S.P. Tablets available: 60 and 100 mg.

Digitoxin, U.S.P. A cardiotonic glycoside obtained from *Digitalis purpurea* Linné, *Digitalis lanata* Ehrh., and other suitable species of *Digitalis.*

Digitoxin Injection, U.S.P. A sterile solution of digitoxin in 5%–50% alcohol. Injections available: 0.2 mg digitoxin in 1 ml.

Digitoxin Tablets, U.S.P. Tablets available: 0.1 and 0.2 mg.

Digoxin, U.S.P. A cardiotonic glycoside obtained from the leaves of *Digitalis lanata* Ehrh. (Fam. Scrophulariaceae).

Digoxin Injection, U.S.P. A sterile solution of digoxin in 10% alcohol. In jections available: 0.5 mg in 2 ml.

Digoxin Tablets, U.S.P. Tablets available: 0.25 and 0.5 mg.

Ouabain, U.S.P. (G-strophanthin).

Ouabain Injection, U.S.P. Injections available: 0.25 mg in 1 ml; 0.5 mg in 2 ml.

ANTIARRHYTHMIC DRUGS

Cardiac arrhythmias may be caused by changes in automaticity (pacemaker activity) of cardiac cells (which produce ectopic rhythms), alterations in conductivity, or a combination of automaticity and conduction disturbances. A large number of drugs suppress cardiac arrhythmias through acting on one or both of these properties. The classes of compounds found to possess antiarrhythmic activity include certain antimalarial, local anesthetic, antispasmodic, antihistaminic, and sympatholytic agents as well as various cations (magnesium, calcium, potassium, barium). For a number of compounds electrophysiologic studies have identified depression of automaticity coupled with either a decrease, no change, or an increase in conduction velocity as actions that can account for antiarrhythmic effects (Hoffman and Bigger 1971; Bassett and Hoffman 1971; Rosen and Hoffman 1973). These agents include: quinidine, procainamide, lidocaine, propranolol, and diphenylhydantoin. Many actions of these antiarrhythmic compounds are currently explained by their effect on certain features of the cardiac action potential, viz., (1) phase 4 (diastolic) depolarization, i.e., pacemaker function or automaticity; (2) slope of phase 0, i.e., rate of depolarization which governs conduction rate; and (3) membrane responsiveness, i.e., the relationship between the slope of phase 0 and the membrane potential at which the action potential is elicited (Hoffman and Bigger 1971). This latter concept, originated by Weidmann (1955), is pertinent to the understanding of antiarrhythmic drug effects on action potential of myocardial cells. Conduction velocity is determined, for a given fiber, by the maximum rate of rise (maximum dv/dt) of phase 0 spike action potential (V_{max}.). This, in turn, is dependent in part on the level of the negative intracellular potential at the moment of excitation (see Fig. 24.13). The maximum rate of rise of phase 0 increases as the intracellular potential becomes more negative. When this relation is plotted for the period from the end of the absolute refractory period to completion of repolarization, an S-shaped curve (Fig. 24.14) is obtained. This electrophysiological property of cardiac cells relates conduction velocity to TMP at the time of excitation. When resting potential (greater negative charge intracellularly) is increased, the rate of rise of the

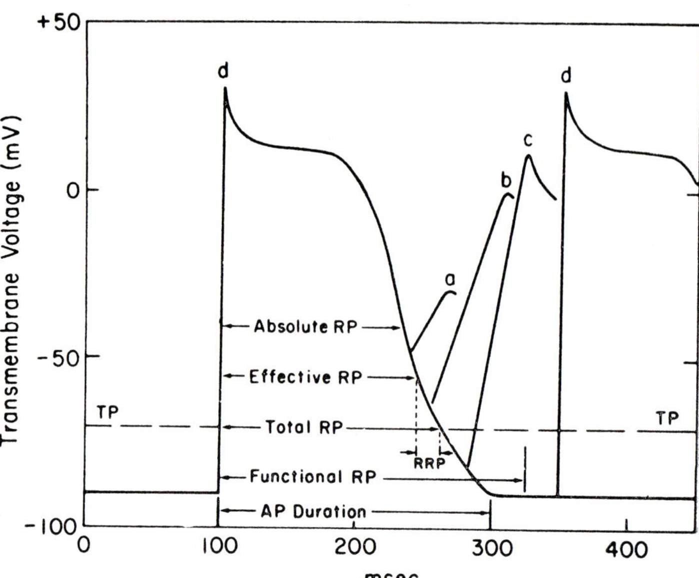

FIG. 24.13 Diagram of TMP of a working ventricular muscle cell. The maximum rate of rise of the action potentials labeled *a, b, c,* and *d* depends on the level of the action potential at the time of excitation. Thus electrical V_{max} is least *(a)* at low levels of membrane potential, becomes progressively greater as TMP increases (*b, c*), and finally reaches a maximum at the resting potential *(d)*. (RP, refractory period; RRP, relatively refractory period; AP, action potential; TP, threshold potential.) (Mason et al. 1973)

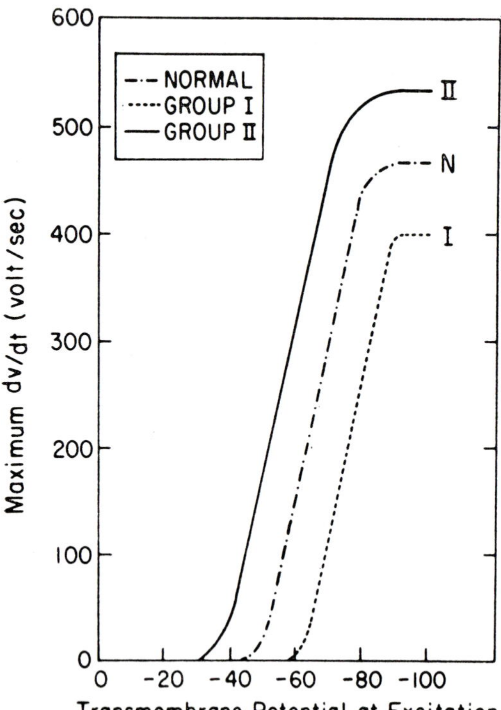

FIG. 24.14. Diagram showing the relationship between maximum rate of rise (dv/dt) of the action potential (ordinate) and the transmembrane potential (abscissa) at the moment of activation. Curve *N* represents the normal relationship. The curve is shifted to the right by Group I drugs (quinidine, procainamide, propranolol) and to the left by Group II agents (lidocaine, diphenylhydantoin). (Mason et al. 1973)

spike potential (phase 0) is enhanced and conduction velocity increased, while excitability is decreased. Thus automaticity, excitability, responsiveness, and conduction velocity are interrelated properties depending on the level of resting potential and excitation threshold.

The characteristics of antiarrhythmic drugs may be described from quantitative electrophysiological studies in terms of their qualitative effects on these interdependent variables: membrane responsiveness, conduction velocity, automaticity, action potential duration, and duration of refractoriness to electrical stimulation.

Automatic or pacemaker cells are those in which diastolic depolarization occurs spontaneously; they are found in the SA node, the His-Purkinje system, some parts of the specialized atrial internodal tracts, and portions of the AV node (AN cells located between the atrial cells and central AV nodal cells and NH cells located below the central nodal region at the origin of the His bundle) but not in the mid-portion of the AV node. The term *automaticity* describes the spontaneous generation of action potentials by these various cells. Following each action potential, they repolarize to a point of maximum diastolic depolarization and immediately begin to depolarize progressively. If this phase 4 depolarization reduces the TMP to a

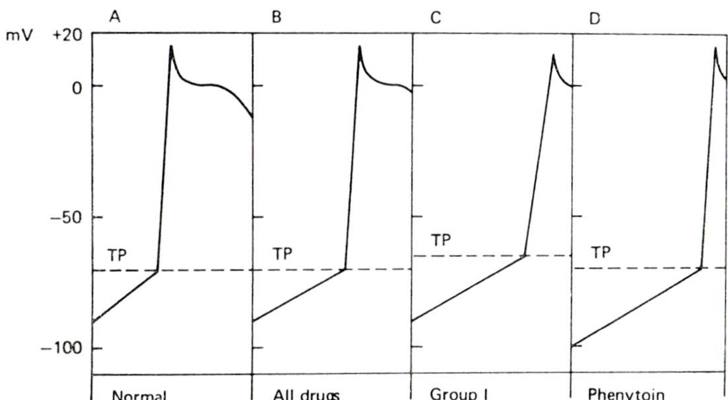

FIG. 24.15. Diagram *A* depicts phase 4 (see Fig. 24.2) diastolic depolarization of a normal pacemaker cell, threshold potential (TP), spike potential (phase 0), rapid repolarization (phase 1), plateau (phase 2), and the beginning of terminal repolarization (phase 3). The remaining diagrams (*B, C, D*) illustrate the mechanisms of action of antiarrhythmic drugs. All antiarrhythmic drugs decrease rate of diastolic depolarization (*B*). Group I agents (see text) extend cycle length by raising excitation threshold (lowering threshold potential, TP) (*C*). Diphenylhydantoin prolongs the diastolic period in part by increasing maximal diastolic intracellular negativity (*D*). (Mason et al. 1973)

threshold potential (TP), a conducted impulse is initiated. The rate at which an automatic cell reaches threshold depends on the slope of phase 4 depolarization, the level of the maximum diastolic potential, and the level of the TP.

Drugs that decrease automaticity act to prolong the diastolic period required for pacemaker cells to reach the TP at which a conducted impulse is initiated. The variables involved are illustrated in Fig. 24.15. The frequency at which a pacemaker cell may reach threshold is dependent on three factors: (1) the slope of diastolic depolarization (phase 4, Fig. 24.15 *A*); (2) the level of the TP (Fig. 24.15 *C*); and (3) the level of maximal diastolic potential (Fig. 24.15 *D*). All antiarrhythmic drugs decrease the rate of diastolic depolarization (Fig. 24.15 *B*). Quinidine, procainamide, and propranolol (Group I agents) also raise TP (Fig. 24.15 *C*). Diphenylhydantoin increases maximal diastolic intracellular negativity. All antiarrhythmic drugs decrease the slope of diastolic depolarization (phase 4), in part by depressing Na^+ influx during this phase (Mason et al. 1973).

Normally, SA nodal cells reach threshold first and thus determine heart rate, the resultant propagated excitation reaching all other potential pacemaker cells before they attain threshold values. In ectopic arrhythmias other pacemaker cells reach threshold and "fire," initiating the heartbeat from an abnormal locus. Such ectopic pacemaker function is ordinarily limited to these normally automatic cardiac cells and is not found in working muscle fibers of the atria or ventricles. However, various drugs, certain cations (e.g., calcium, potassium), injury, ischemia, etc., can result in the generation of abnormal action potentials affecting any type of myocardial cell (Bassett and Hoffman 1971).

The term *excitability* describes the sensitivity of the myocardium to external stimuli and is usually measured as a quantity of pulsed electric current required to stimulate at specific phases of the resting and action potential. *Automaticity* and *excitability* do not represent equivalent properties of cardiac muscle, and certain drugs (e.g., digitalis q.v.) may affect them in opposite directions. Some antiarrhythmic compounds (e.g., quinidine, procainamide) can be shown to depress excitability as well as automaticity in certain concentrations, but the suppression of diastolic depolarization (automaticity) can occur independently of significant alterations in refractoriness, excitability, or conductivity (Bassett and Hoffman 1971). The level of diastolic depolarization at which a cell is excited governs the rate of rise of phase 0 and thus determines conduction velocity (Fig. 24.13). Depressant drugs such as quinidine, during one phase of their action, may suppress diastolic depolarization, thus increasing the TMP at the time of excitation. When this action occurs at a concentration that does not reduce membrane responsiveness, the rate of rise of phase 0 is increased and the magnitude and conduction rates of the action potential are increased. Thus enhanced action potential propagation may play a role in antiarrhythmic action of primarily depressant drugs such as quinidine and procainamide. The primary effect of certain antiarrhythmic agents (e.g., diphenylhydantoin, lidocaine) is to increase membrane responsiveness. In contrast to quinidine, procainamide, and propranolol, which depress electrical excitability, diphenylhydantoin and lidocaine have little effect on excitability.

During much of the action potential (Fig. 24.13), myocardial cells will not respond to stimulation. This initial phase is called the *absolute refractory period.* Ordinarily, excited myocardial cells do not respond to stimulation until the membrane potential reaches —55 mV during the repolarization of phase 3. As the magnitude of the TMP increases with phase 3 repolarization, the evoked response (action potential) to stimulation increases progressively in amplitude and rate of rise (phase 0). The term *relative refractory period* is applied to the phase during which submaximal responses result only from stimuli exceeding the resting threshold. The *effective refractory period* (ERP) is the minimum interval of time between two propagated impulses (Hoffman 1969) and is a useful measure of refractoriness for comparison of drug effects. Factors determining ERP include the duration of the action potential and the relationship between membrane potential and responsiveness (i.e., the TMP level to which repolarization must proceed before a propagated response can be induced). Quinidine and procainamide increase ERP by increasing action potential duration (slowing repolarization phase 3) and by shifting the relationship between membrane potential and responsiveness so that repolarization must progress further before a propagated response can be evoked. Thus ERP is increased relatively more than action potential duration. Propranolol, on the other hand, decreases action potential duration but has the same effect as quinidine on the membrane potential and responsiveness relationship, so that the duration of ERP is increased relative to the action potential. Diphenylhydantoin and lidocaine decrease the duration of both ERP and action potential, but ERP is not reduced in proportion to reduction in action potential duration. The various differing characteristics of several antiarrhythmic drugs were employed by Hoffman and Bigger (1971) to classify these agents into two groups based on their effects on conduction rate, action potential duration, and membrane responsiveness. Group I drugs (quinidine, procainamide, propranolol) depress conduction and responsiveness; Group II drugs (diphenylhydantoin, lidocaine) do not depress and may enhance conduction and responsiveness (Table 24.4).

Quinidine and procainamide decrease excitability, prolong refractoriness, decrease conduction velocity, and suppress ectopic automaticity. Propranolol, like quinidine and procainamide, decreases excitability and conduction velocity, suppresses automaticity, but shortens both action potential duration and ERP. However, the relative ERP is increased. In addition it blocks β-adrenergic activity in the heart. Lidocaine and diphenylhydantoin suppress automaticity but decrease refractoriness, have little or no effect on excitability and either have no effect on or increase conduction velocity. In addition, the latter two drugs can shorten AV conduction time.

Since antiarrhythmic drugs in Groups I and II have opposite effects on membrane responsiveness and conductivity *(vide supra),* a consideration of the mechanism of reentry in producing tachyarrhythmias has been used to explain their effects (Fig. 24.16). The Purkinje network has multiple branchings at its junctions with the ventricular myocardium. Thus retrograde or circular activation is theoretically possi-

TABLE 24.4. Characteristic electrophysiologic and antiarrhythmic actions

	Group I		Group II
	Procainamide Quinidine	Propranolol	DPH Lidocaine
Electrophysiologic properties			
Purkinje fibers:			
Automaticity	↓	↓	↓
Responsiveness	↓	↓	→ or ↑
Conduction velocity	↓	↓	→ or ↑
ERP	↑	↓	↓
APD	↑	↓	↓
Δ ERP relative to APD	↑	↑	↑
Excitability	↓	↓	→
Atrioventricular conduction time	→ or ↑	→ or ↑	→ or ↓
Experimental arrhythmias			
Digitalis induced	+	++	+++
Coronary ligation	++	+	++?

Source: Hoffman and Bigger 1971.

Abbreviations: DPH, diphenylhydantoin; ERP, effective refractory period; APD, action potential duration; +, moderately effective; ++, effective; +++, highly effective; ↑, increased; ↓, decreased; →, no change. (Arrows indicate the direction and not the magnitude of change.)

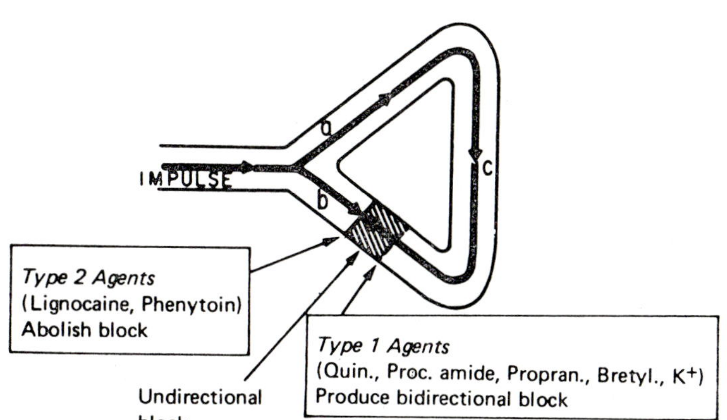

Fig. 24.16. Diagram of the mechanism postulated for reentrant or reciprocating rhythms producing tachyarrhythmias. The impulse entering terminal Purkinje system branches ordinarily would pass down branches *a* and *b* and meet in branch *c* where conduction would be extinguished owing to refractoriness of the cells just excited. In a reentrant conduction disorder, unidirectional block at the shaded area stops the impulse coursing over branch *b*, but allows the impulse arriving later from branch *c* to be conducted retrogradely. Thus a circus movement is set up, which could continuously excite the rest of the heart at rapid rates. Group I drugs could break up this circus movement by establishing complete bidirectional block at the shaded area. Group II agents could have the same effect by abolishing the antegrade block. (Quin., quinidine; Proc. amide, procainamide; Propran., propranolol; Bretyl., bretylium tosylate; Lignocaine, lidocaine; Phenytoin, diphenylhydantoin.) (Mason et al. 1973)

ble if a unidirectional block could prevent a portion of the network from being activated in an antegrade direction. As illustrated in Fig. 24.16, an impulse that ordinarily travels down branches *a* and *b* may encounter an area of unidirectional block (shaded section) in pathway *b*. If this area subsequently recovers sufficiently to conduct by the time an impulse coursing over *c* reaches it, the conditions exist for a circular conduction pathway that would conduct continuously (reentry or reciprocal excitation). Group I drugs that depress conduction velocity and membrane responsiveness could abolish such a reentrant tachycardia by producing complete bidirectional block at the shaded area; Group II drugs that increase conduction velocity and membrane responsiveness could act by abolishing the antegrade block.

Clinically, in human patients, quinidine and procainamide have been found most effective against atrial fibrillation and moderately effective in other supraventricular arrhythmias; procainamide, diphenylhydantoin, and lidocaine are considered superior to the other agents in ventricular arrhythmias; and diphenylhydantoin and lidocaine are the most effective of these five agents in digitalis-induced arrhythmias (Hoffman and Bigger 1971). Diphenylhydantoin specifically antagonizes the toxic electrophysiologic effects of digitalis; thus it can reverse automaticity and may reverse AV block induced by digitalis. Consequently, it can effectively widen the toxic to therapeutic dosage ratio of digitalis. Lidocaine is similarly effective against digitalis-induced arrhythmias.

Of the antiarrhythmic drugs mentioned, there is substantial clinical experience only with quinidine in the treatment of atrial fibrillation in horses and, to a lesser extent, in dogs.

Quinidine Sulfate

Quinidine Sulfate, U.S.P., is the *d* isomer of quinine and occurs naturally in cinchona bark. Quinine was introduced for the treatment of atrial fibrillation by Wenckebach in 1914 after one of his patients observed that when he took quinine for malaria his coincidental atrial fibrillation was abolished. Quinidine proved to be more effective than quinine and became the drug of choice in atrial fibrillation.

Quinidine is rapidly absorbed from the GI tract and also following intramuscular injection. Serum levels correlate well with toxic effects but not with therapeutic action. Much of the drug is destroyed in the liver and 10%–40% is excreted in the urine. Toxic doses injected intravenously in dogs anesthetized with pentobarbital sodium produce a sinus bradycardia, reduction in cardiac output (with little change in stroke volume), a striking fall in blood pressure, pronounced peripheral vasodilation, a decrease in ventricular contractility, and a relative increase in the PR, QRS, and QT intervals of the ECG (Luchi et al. 1963).

Quinidine acts on the heart to prolong the effective refractory period of cardiac muscle, apparently by altering the relationship between membrane potential and the ability of the cell to increase its permeability to sodium ions. It depresses the diastolic depolarization of spontaneously active Purkinje fibers but, in the same concentrations, not that of SA node pacemaker cells (Hoffman and Cranefield 1960). Thus quinidine does not greatly alter the frequency of normal cardiac pacemaker cells. Further, while it prolongs the refractory period of atrial and ventricular muscle, moderate doses have little effect on the refractory period of normal pacemaker tissue. Presumably, the ability of quinidine to increase the refractory period of atrial fibers can account for its effectiveness in abolishing atrial fibrillation (Moe and Mendez 1962). If the supposition is true that the site of ectopic impulse formation in the heart is spontaneously active Purkinje fibers, then the depression of diastolic depolarization of these fibers by quinidine in concentrations that do not have this effect on normal pacemaker cells explains its action in suppressing ectopic arrhythmias.

Quinidine has a vagal blocking action and antagonizes acetylcholine. Further, it is particularly effective in treating atrial arrhythmias because, unlike other agents, it prolongs the atrial refractory period directly and by its anticholinergic actions, indirectly (Moss and Patton 1973). One result of these effects is tachycardia in normal dogs if sufficient drug is given. In studies on unanesthetized dogs before and after cardiac denervation, it was learned that conduction across the AV node itself was little affected by either vagolytic or direct actions of quinidine (Wallace et al. 1966). Conduction was slowed in the Purkinje system below the AV node, thus prolonging ventricular activating time, and there was a decrease in excitability. Clinically, in supraventricular arrhythmias such as atrial flutter and atrial fibrillation, an untoward effect of quinidine is a sometimes dangerous acceleration of ventricular rate before the arrhythmia is abolished. This results from improved AV conduction of the rapidly occurring atrial impulses and has been attributed to the vagolytic action of quinidine. The observations of Wallace et al. (1966) fail to support the interpretation that conduction through the AV node is improved by vagolytic effects during normal sinus- or atrial-paced rhythms. Another explanation of this effect is based on the concept of "concealed conduction." It is assumed that the irregular ventricular responses in atrial fibrillation result from penetration of the AV junctional tissue by atrial impulses that, after passing some distance, are blocked. These "concealed" impulses influence conduction of subsequent beats by increasing refractoriness of the cells they have depolarized. Any increase in atrial rate would cause more concealed responses and greater refractoriness of the AV junctional tissue. Slowing of the atrial rate, as occurs with quinidine in both flutter and fibrillation, would result in fewer concealed impulses and better AV conduction, the effect of which would be an absolute increase in the number of impulses per minute reaching the ventricles. Large doses of quinidine can produce SA and AV block.

THERAPEUTIC USE

The chief use of quinidine sulfate in veterinary medicine is the treatment of atrial fibrillation (Fig. 24.17) in horses (Detweiler 1957; Detweiler and Patterson 1963, 1972). The following dose schedule for oral administration by capsule or stomach tube is recommended:

Day 1 5 g (test dose)
Day 2 10 g 3 times daily at 3-hour intervals
Day 3 10 g 4 times daily at 2-hour intervals
Day 4 10 g 4 times daily at 2-hour intervals

If conversion does not occur by day 4 of this regimen, continuously increase the dose. Up to 90 g daily have been administered (9 consecutive 10-g doses at hourly intervals) but such high doses are clearly within the toxic range and therefore dangerous.

The toxic effects of quinidine sulfate in horses are urticarial wheals, GI disturbances (inappetence, colic, diarrhea), erythema and edema of the nasal mucosa (with respiratory embarrassment), vascular collapse, laminitis, congestive heart failure, and sudden death. The development of mild urticaria and GI disturbances do not require cessation of therapy. The other toxic effects are dangerous and necessitate stopping drug administration. If severe edema of the nasal mucosa develops, respiration may be seriously impeded. This reaction is dose related and usually subsides if administration is halted for 12 hours and the dose reduced to the level tolerated on previous days. Serious laminitis may be prevented by prompt administration of antiinflammatory steroids at the earliest sign of discomfort. Vascular collapse may be heralded by the onset of restlessness, sweating, muscular fasciculations, and incoordination. Congestive heart failure requires intravenous digitalization with ouabain.

Oral administration of quinidine sulfate for a prolonged period is tedious and in some subjects difficult. Intravenous administration, although possibly more dangerous than oral therapy, avoids these dif-

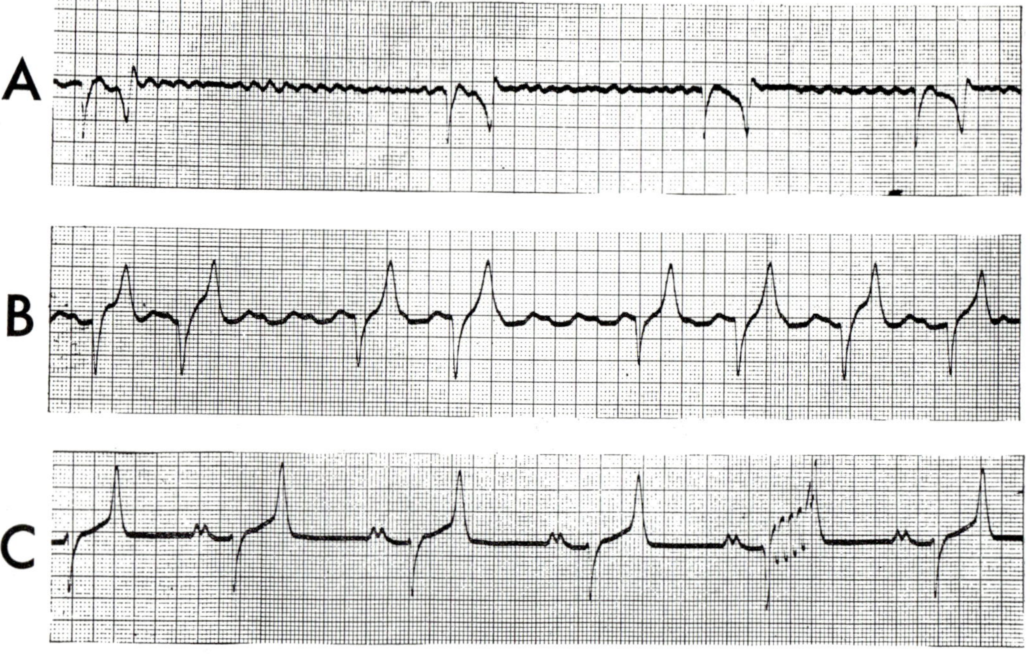

FIG. 24.17. Quinidine sulfate in atrial fibrillation. The effect of quinidine sulfate on atrial fibrillation in a 4-year-old thoroughbred. All ECGs are base-apex lead. *A*. On the previous day, a 5-g test dose of quinidine sulfate had been given. This record was taken 24 hours later when the quinidine blood level was 0.8 mg/L. *B*. Record taken on the 4th day of treatment. The quinidine level in the morning was 8.0 mg/L. Forty grams of quinidine were given in 2 divided doses 3 hours apart, and this record was taken 6 hours after the last dose. The quinidine blood level was 13.8 mg/L. Note the rapidly occurring P waves (atrial tachycardia) with variable ventricular response. An additional 20-g dose of quinidine sulfate was given at the time of the tracing in *B*, and 4 hours later the blood level reached 16 mg/L. This had fallen to 8.4 mg/L 12 hours later on the morning of the 5th day. Forty-five grams of quinidine sulfate in 2 divided doses 3 hours apart were given on this day, and the blood level reached 15.8 mg/L. *C*. During the evening of the 5th day, the rhythm returned to normal, and this record was taken on the 6th day after the initiation of treatment, when the blood level had dropped to 7.3 mg/L.

ficulties. For intravenous therapy, dihydroquinidine gluconate (available in 0.3-g ampules, Honde, Paris) has been employed (Gerber 1971). It is administered by slow intravenous infusion (10 g/L of physiological saline solution at the rate of 50 ml/minute). With this therapy, conversion to normal rhythm has occurred with doses of 5.5–18 g. Severe ventricular tachycardia may occur during infusion, an obviously dangerous side effect.

In dogs with atrial fibrillation, quinidine proved unsatisfactory in the smaller breeds (Detweiler 1957). More recently it has been ascertained that in giant breeds (e.g., Great Dane, St. Bernard, Newfoundland, Irish Wolfhound) with atrial fibrillation, abolition of the arrhythmia is possible (Pyle 1967; Bohn 1970; Bohn et al. 1971). This appears to be related to the observation that atrial fibrillation occurs in giant breeds with less severe degrees of underlying heart disease than in smaller breeds and that susceptibility to atrial fibrillation increases with increasing atrial mass.

As a test dose, 50–100 mg orally may be given. Several hours later or on the following day, the course of quinidine may be started. A dose of 3–6 mg/lb of body weight is given every 2 hours for 4–5 doses daily. This dosage level is continued for 3 days. Thus the daily amount can be elevated at 3-day intervals until the arrhythmia is abolished or toxic signs appear.

Other than with quinidine sulfate, there is not substantial clinical experience with the other antiarrhythmic agents mentioned in the foregoing. The information available is for the most part based on clinical use in human beings and experimental studies on normal anesthetized dogs and on isolated tissues. Accordingly, dosage and use recommendations can be considered only provisional. Since these agents can initiate myocardial depression and arterial hypotension, their use is accompanied by hazards requiring ECG and blood pressure monitoring (Freundlich et al. 1972). Thus their clinical application in diseased animals is still in the experimental stage. While their use can be justified in the control of dangerous arrhythmias, their possible favorable effects must be carefully weighed against their potential dangers.

Procainamide Hydrochloride

Procainamide Hydrochloride, U.S.P., differs from procaine in that an imido group replaces the oxygen linkage in the procaine molecule. Its actions resemble those of procaine topically and its cardiac effects are like those of quinidine (Hoffman and Cranefield 1960). Untoward effects, as with quinidine sulfate, include myocardial depression, hypotension, and ventricular arrhythmias or asystole. For dogs weighing 25–35 lb, doses of 250 mg every 4–6 hours and intramuscular doses of 250 mg as frequently as every 2 hours have been employed (Ettinger and Suter 1970). For treating dangerous ventricular tachycardias, Huisman and Teunissen (1963) recommended intravenous infusion at the rate of 100 mg/minute. ECG and blood pressure monitoring should be practiced with cessation of administration upon the appearance of changes indicating toxic effects (widening of QRS complex, additional arrhythmias, bradycardia, tachycardia, or hypotension).

In human patients, procainamide has been found more effective in treating ventricular arrhythmias than those originating in the atria.

Diphenylhydantoin Sodium

Originally employed as an antiepileptic agent, *Diphenylhydantoin Sodium,* U.S.P. (Dilantin), was found effective in abolishing ectopic ventricular activity in dogs with experimental infarction (Harris and Kokernot 1950) and following toxic doses of ouabain (Mosey et al. 1952). These actions have been amply confirmed in later experimental studies in animals and clinical observations in human beings. It is considered particularly effective in digitalis-induced arrhythmias of all types and in ventricular arrhythmias from other causes. Most atrial arrhythmias other than those caused by digitalis do not respond well (Hayes 1972). It specifically antagonizes certain toxic electrophysiological actions of digitalis. Thus it can reverse digitalis-induced automaticity and AV block in doses that do not abolish the positive inotropic effect of digitalis (Scherlag et al. 1968). In normal experimental dogs, prior administration of diphenylhydantoin sodium intravenously increased the amount of acetylstrophanthidin required to produce toxicity by 72%–224% without altering the positive inotropic effect of the cardiac glycoside (Helfant et al. 1967b). Given intravenously in experimental dogs, diphenylhydantoin can be injected in doses of 5–10 mg/kg at a rate of 25–50 mg/minute with little depressant effect on myocardial function. This dose range is effective in abolishing digitalis-induced arrhythmias (Helfant et al. 1967b; Damato 1969). Oral doses employed in human beings for antiarrhythmic action amount to approximately 14 mg/kg on day 1, 7 mg/kg on days 2 and 3, and 6 mg/kg daily thereafter.

Lidocaine Hydrochloride

The therapeutic advantages of *Lidocaine Hydrochloride,* U.S.P. (Xylocaine), in cardiac arrhythmias are its rapid onset and brief duration of action. In large doses in dogs, it has hypotensive and marked negative chronotropic, dromotropic, and inotropic actions. In doses below 2 mg/

kg intravenously, these depressant effects are not profound (Lieberman et al. 1968) but, nevertheless, substantial hypotensive and myocardial depressant actions remain (Austen and Moran 1965). It is not recommended for the treatment of supraventricular arrhythmias and has been employed in human beings primarily to control ventricular arrhythmias during cardiac surgery and following myocardial infarction. Experimentally, it shares an efficacy similar to diphenylhydantoin against digitalis-induced arrhythmias. Owing to its brief duration of action it is not effective orally nor for maintenance therapy. The preparations of lidocaine containing epinephrine should not be used in antiarrhythmic therapy.

PROPRANOLOL

Propranolol is a β-adrenergic blocking agent, is effective against catecholamine-induced arrhythmias, and possesses, unlike some other β-adrenergic antagonists, quinidinelike actions on myocardial cells. In human beings, it has been found most useful in arrhythmias precipitated by emotion, exercise, or digitalis toxicosis (Gibson and Sowton 1969). In atrial flutter and atrial fibrillation, propranolol frequently fails to restore normal rhythm, but its depression of AV conductivity slows ventricular rate. This effect has been beneficial when digitalis failed to control ventricular tachycardia in human beings with atrial fibrillation (Theilen and Wilson 1968). Toxic effects include myocardial depression, arterial hypotension, and marked bradycardia; these actions can precipitate congestive heart failure when cardiac reserve is limited by disease.

In experimental dogs, 0.3 mg/kg of propranolol intravenously is effective in preventing cyclopropane-epinephrine–induced ventricular tachycardia (Gutgesell et al. 1969). In conscious dogs intravenous doses of 1 and 3 mg/kg of propranolol ameliorated or prevented epinephrine-induced arrhythmias before and on the 2nd, 3rd, and 4th days after ligation of the anterior descending branch of the left coronary artery; intravenous doses of 1.0 mg/kg failed to suppress spontaneous ventricular arrhythmias 24 hours after coronary occlusion as did larger doses (3 mg/kg and 5 mg/kg), which were fatal (Shanks and Dunlop 1967). These intravenous doses are large compared to those (0.1 mg/kg) employed clinically in human beings (Kerber and Harrison 1971). In human patients approximately 0.5–1 mg/kg/day orally in divided doses every 6–8 hours is recommended, although up to 4 times this amount daily has been employed (Kerber and Harrison 1971). In experimental dogs, suppression of catecholamine-induced arrhythmias requires smaller doses (0.1–1 mg/kg intravenously) than reversal of ouabain-induced arrhythmias (3–5 mg/kg intravenously). The β-blocking dose of propranolol is 1 mg/kg, and β blockade accounts for its effectiveness against catecholamine-induced arrhythmias at low doses. Larger doses are required for the treatment of digitalis-induced arrhythmias presumably because this action depends also on its quinidinelike membrane effects. It would appear that the latter necessitate higher concentrations. That some of propranolol's antiarrhythmic actions are related to its membrane effects is supported by the finding that *d*-propranolol, which has insignificant β-blocking properties, is also an effective antiarrhythmic agent. However, in ouabain-induced arrhythmias, *l*-propranolol is superior to *d*-propranolol, indicating that both β blockade and quinidinelike activity are involved in this action (Florez et al. 1969). In any case, the higher doses required for abolition of digitalis arrhythmias produce cardiovascular depression, which can be profound at doses exceeding 10 mg/kg intravenously (Baum et al. 1971). Propranolol is contraindicated in bronchial asthma, sinus bradycardia, AV block, and congestive heart failure.

PREPARATIONS

Quinidine Sulfate, U.S.P. Obtained from Cinchona and their hybrids and from *Remijia pedunculata* Flückiger (Fam. Rubiaceae) or prepared from quinine.

Quinine Sulfate Tablets, U.S.P. Tablets available: 200 mg.

Procainamide Hydrochloride, U.S.P.

Procainamide Hydrochloride Capsules, U.S.P. Capsules available: 250 mg.

Procainamide Hydrochloride Injection, U.S.P. Injections available: 1 g in 10 ml.

Propranolol Hydrochloride (Inderal). Tablets available: 10 mg and 40 mg. Injections available: 1 mg in 1-ml ampules.

Sodium Diphenylhydantoin, U.S.P. (Dilantin). Capsules available: 100 mg, 50 mg, and 30 mg. Suspensions available: 125 mg and 30 mg in each 5 ml.

Sterile Sodium Diphenylhydantoin, U.S.P. Vials available: 100 mg and 250 mg with special solvent to be added.

Lidocaine Hydrochloride, U.S.P. (Xylocaine). Use only epinephrine-free solutions. *Xylocaine Hydrochloride* 2% for intravenous use in cardiac arrhythmias: 5-ml ampules; 50-ml single dose container, ampules, or vials for preparing intravenous infusion.

REFERENCES

Akera, T.; Larsen, F. S.; and Brody, T. M. 1969. The effect of ouabain on sodium and potassium-activated adenosine triphosphatase from the hearts of several mammalian species. J Pharmacol Exp Ther 170:17.

Aldinger, E. E. 1970. Effects of digitoxin on the development of cardiac hypertrophy in the rat subjected to chronic exercise. Am J Cardiol 25:339.

Allen, J. C., and Schwartz, A. 1969. A possible biochemical explanation for the insensitivity of the rat to cardiac glycosides. J Pharmacol Exp Ther 168:42.

Austen, W. G., and Moran, J. M. 1965. Cardiac and peripheral vascular effects of lidocaine and procainamide. Am J Cardiol 16:701.

Ayers, C. R.; Davis, J. O.; Lieberman, F., Carpenter, C. C. J.; and Berman, M. 1962. The effects of chronic hepatic venous congestion on the metabolism of *d, l*-aldosterone and *d*-aldosterone. J Clin Invest 41: 884.

Barger, A. C. 1956. The pathogenesis of sodium retention in congestive heart failure. Metabolism 5:380.

Barger, A. C.; Muldowney, F. P.; and Lubowitz, M. R. 1959. Role of the kidney in the pathogenesis of congestive heart failure. Circulation 20:273.

Barger, A. C.; Yates, T. E.; and Rudolph, A. M. 1961. Renal hemodynamics and sodium excretion in dogs with graded valvular damage. Am J Physiol 200:601.

Barr, I.; Smith, T. W.; Klein, M. D.; Hagemeijer, F.; and Lown, B. 1972. Correlation of the electrophysiologic action of digoxin with serum digoxin concentration. J Pharmacol Exp Ther 180:710.

Bassett, A. L., and Hoffman, B. F. 1971. Antiarrhythmic drugs: Electrophysiological action. Ann Rev Pharmacol 11:143.

Baum, T.; Eckfield, D. K.; Shropshire, A. T.; Rowles, G.; and Varner, L. L. 1971. Observations on models used for the evaluation of antiarrhythmic drugs. Arch Int Pharmacodyn Ther 193:149.

Beck, A. M. 1969a. Selective studies on digoxin and digitoxin in dogs. M.S. thesis, Univ. of Pennsylvania.

———. 1969b. Digoxin therapy and toxicity in dogs. Proc Am Anim Hosp Assoc 36:23.

Beume, R. B.; Menashe, V. D.; and Griswald, H. E. 1961. Animal experience with the calcium-digitalis tolerance test. Am J Med Sci 242:177.

Blaine, D. 1841. Canine Pathology. A Description of Diseases of the Dog, 4th ed. London: Longman, Orme.

Bohn, K. 1970. Unpublished observations.

Bohn, K.; Patterson, D. F.; and Pyle, R. L. 1971. Atrial fibrillation in dogs. Br Vet J 127:485.

Borison, H. L., and Wang, S. C. 1951. Locus of the central emetic action of cardiac glycosides. Proc Soc Exp Biol Med 76:335.

Braunwald, E., and Kahler, R. L. 1964. The mechanism of action of cardiac drugs. Physiol Physicians 2:1.

Brender, D.; Vanhoutte, P. M.; and Sheperd, J. T. 1969. Potentiation of adrenergic venomotor responses in dogs by cardiac glycosides. Circ Res 25:597.

Broadbent, J. L. 1962. Importance of calcium in the actions of some drugs that stimulate the isolated, hypodynamic frog heart. Br J Pharmacol Chemother 19:183.

Buchner, F. 1934. Herzmuskelnekrosen durch hohe Dosen von Digitalis-glykosiden. Arch Exp Pathol Pharmacol 176:59.

Cahill, K. M. 1962. Digitalis as a diuretic. Lancet 2:445.

Carpenter, C. S. J.; Davis, J. O.; Wallace, C. R.; and Hamilton, W. F. 1962. Acute effects of cardiac glycosides on aldosterone secretion in dogs with hyperaldosteronism secondary to chronic right heart failure. Circ Res 10:178.

Cattell, M., and Gold, H. 1938. Influence of digitalis glycosides on force of contraction of mammalian cardiac muscle. J Pharmacol Exp Ther 62:116.

Chen, K K.; Anderson, R. C.; and Henderson, F. G. 1951. Comparison of cardiac action of bufalin, cinobufotalin and telocinobufagin. Proc Soc Exp Biol Med 76:372.

Conn, H. L., Jr. 1956. Effects of digitalis and hypoxia on potassium transfer and distribution in the dog heart. Am J Physiol 184:548.

Cordey, E., and Skelton, R. B. T. 1964. The use of citrate salts for testing digitalis-induced cardiac arrhythmias in the experimental animal. Am Heart J 67:237.

Cosmides, G. J.; Miya, T. S.; and Carr, C. J. 1956. A study of the effects of certain lactones on digitoxin toxicity. J Pharmacol Exp Ther 118:286.

Cotten, M. deV., and Williams, B. J. 1961. Effect of cardiac glycosides on blood volume in the dog. Am J Physiol 201:112.

Damato, A. N. 1969. Diphenylhydantoin: Pharmacological and clinical use. Prog Cardiovasc Dis 12:1.

Davidson, J. D.; Waldman, T. A.; Goodman, D. S.; and Gordon, R. S., Jr. 1961. Protein-losing gastroenteropathy in congestive heart failure. Lancet 1:899.

Davis, J. O. 1962. Adrenocortical and renal hormonal function in experimental cardiac failure. Circulation 25:1002.

———. 1971. The renin-angiotensin system in the control of aldosterone secretion. In J. W. Fisher, ed. Kidney Hormones, p. 173. New York: Academic Press.

———. 1974. The renin-angiotensin system in the control of aldosterone secretion. In I. H. Page and F. M. Bumpus, eds. Handbuch der experimentellen Pharmakologie. Vol. 37, Angiotensin, p. 322. Berlin: Springer-Verlag.

Davis, J. O.; Hyatt, R. E.; and Howell, D. S. 1955. Right-sided congestive heart failure in dogs produced by controlled progressive constriction of the pulmonary artery. Circ Res 3:252.

Davis, J. O.; Holman, J. E.; Carpenter, C. C. J.; Urquhart, J.; and Higgins, J. T. 1964. An extra-adrenal factor essential for chronic renal sodium retention in presence of increased sodium-retaining hormone. Circ Res 14:17.

Davis, L. E., and Garb, S. 1953. Treatment of a cow with congestive heart failure. J Am Vet Med Assoc 142:255.

Dearing, W. H.; Barnes, A. R.; and Essex, H. E. 1943. Experiments with calculated therapeutic and toxic doses of digitalis. I. Effects on myocardial cellular structure. Am Heart J 25:648.

Detweiler, D. K. 1957. Electrocardiographic and clinical features of spontaneous auricular fibrillation and flutter (tachycardia) in dogs. Zentralbl Veterinaermed 4:509.

———. 1961. Cardiovascular disease in animals: Clinical consideration. In A. A. Luisada. Cardiology, vol. 5, p. 10. New York: McGraw-Hill.

———. 1967. Comparative pharmacology of cardiac glycosides. Fed Proc 26:1119.

Detweiler, D. K., and Patterson, D. F. 1963. Diseases of the cardiovascular system. In J. F. Bone, ed. Equine Medicine and Surgery. Wheaton, Ill.: American Veterinary Publications.

———. 1972. The cardiovascular system. In E. J. Catcott and J. F. Smithcors, eds. Equine Medicine and Surgery, 2nd ed., p. 277. Wheaton, Ill.; American Veterinary Publications.

Entman, M.; Bressler, R.; and Schwartz. A. 1972. Proposed mechanisms for the positive inotropic effect of digitalis. In B. N. Marks and A. M. Weissler, eds. Basic and Clinical Pharmacology of Digitalis, p. 144. Springfield, Ill.: Charles C Thomas.

Ettinger, S. 1966. Therapeutic digitalization of the dog in congestive heart failure. J Am Vet Med Assoc 148:525.

Ettinger, S., and Suter, P. F. 1970. Canine Cardiology. Philadelphia: W. B. Saunders.

Fawaz, G. 1967. The effect of reserpine and pronethalol on the therapeutic and toxic actions of digitalis in the dog heart–lung preparation. Br J Pharmacol 29:302.

Fillmore, G. E., and Detweiler, D. K. 1973. Maintenance of subacute digoxin toxicosis in normal Beagles. Toxicol Appl Pharmacol 25:418.

Florez, J.; Pomar, J. L.; and Malpartida, F. 1969. Beta-adrenergic blockage and acute arrhythmic activity of (−) and (+) propranolol. R Esp Fisiol 25:287.

Fozzard, H. A., and Gibbons, W. R. 1973. Action potential and contraction of heart muscle. Am J Cardiol 31:182.

Freundlich, J. J.; Detweiler, D. K.; and Hance, H. E. 1972. Indirect blood pressure determination by the ultrasonic Doppler technique in dogs. Curr Ther Res 14:73.

Friedman, M. 1957. The fate and deposition of digitoxin in animal and man. In E. G. Dimond, ed. Digitalis. Springfield, Ill.: Charles C Thomas.

Gaffney, T. E.; Kahn, J. B., Jr.; Van Maanen, E. F.; and Acheson, G. H. 1958. The mechanism of the vagal effect of cardiac glycosides. J Pharmacol Exp Ther 122:423.

Gerber, H. 1971. Unpublished observations.

Gero, A. 1971. Cardiac glycosides 1: Chemistry. In J. R. Di Palma, ed. Drill's Pharmacology in Medicine, 3rd ed., p. 773. New York: McGraw-Hill.

Gibson, D., and Sowton, E. 1969. The use of beta-adrenergic blocking drugs in dysrhythmias. Prog Cardiovasc Dis 12:16.

Gold, H.; Kwit, N. T.; Otto, H.; and Fox, T. 1939. Physiological adaptations in cardiac slowing by digitalis and their bearing on problems of digitalization in patients with auricular fibrillation. J Pharmacol Exp Ther 67:224.

Greenspan, K., and Edmands, R. E. 1969. The inotropic effects of digitalis. In C. Fisch and B. Surawicz, eds. Digitalis, p. 65. New York: Grune & Stratton.

Grinnell, E. H., and Johnson, J. R. 1961. Oestrogen protection against acute digitalis toxicity in dogs. Nature 190:1117.

Grinnell, E. H., and Smith, P. W. 1957. Effect of estrogens on myocardial sensitivity to toxic effects of digitalis. Proc Soc Exp Biol Med 94:524.

Gutgesell, H. P.; Temte, J. V.; and Murphy, Q. R. 1969. The effect of propranolol on epinephrine induced changes in cardiac rhythm and arterial potassium in dogs anesthetized with cyclopropane. J Pharmacol Exp Ther 170:281.

Hajdu, S., and Leonard, E. 1959. The cellular basis of cardiac glycoside action. Pharmacol Rev 11:173.

Harris, A. S., and Kokernot, R. H. 1950. Effects of diphenylhydantoin sodium and phenobarbital sodium upon ectopic ventricular tachycardia in acute myocardial infarction. Am J Physiol 163:505.

Harris, G. W. 1962. Central control of pituitary secretion. Handbook of Physiology. Washington, D.C.: American Physiological Society.

Harris, P., and Opie, L. H. 1971. Calcium and the Heart. New York: Academic Press.

Hatcher, R. S., and Eggleston, C. 1912–13. The emetic action of the digitalis bodies. J Pharmacol Exp Ther 4:113.

Hayes, A. H., Jr. 1972. The actions and clinical use of the newer antiarrhythmic drugs. Ration Drug Ther 6:1.

Heinz, N.; Haan, D.; and Tilsner, V. 1968. Beeinflussung der experimentellen durch Hypoxie induzierten Herzhypertrophy der Maus durch Digitoxin. Z Kreislaufforsch 57:675.

Helfant, R. H.; Scherlag, B. J.; and Damato, A. N. 1967a. Protection from digitalis toxicity with the prophylactic use of diphenylhydantoin sodium. Circulation 36:119.

———. 1967b. Use of diphenylhydantoin sodium to dissociate the effects of procainamide on automaticity and conduction in the normal arrhythmic heart. Am J Cardiol 20:820.

Herrmann, R. G.; Parker, R. J.; Henderson, F. G.; and Chen, K. K. 1962. Intestinal absorption of cardiac steroids. Proc Soc Biol Med 109:646.

Hoffman, B. F. 1969. Effects of digitalis on electrical activity of cardiac fibers. In C. Fisch and Surawicz, eds. Digitalis, p. 93. New York: Grune & Stratton.

———. 1972. Effects of digitalis on electrical activity of cardiac membranes. In B. H. Marks and A. M. Weissler, eds. Basic and Clinical Pharmacology and Digitalis, p. 118. Springfield, Ill.: Charles C Thomas.

Hoffman, B. F., and Bigger, J. T. 1971. Antiarrhythmic drugs. In J. Di Palma, ed. Drill's Pharmacology in Medicine, 3rd ed., p. 284. New York: McGraw-Hill.

Hoffman, B. F., and Cranefield, P. E. 1960. Electrophysiology of the Heart. New York: McGraw-Hill.

Hostettler, D. 1959. Personal communication.

Huisman, G. H., and Teunissen, G. H. B. 1963. Paroxysmal ventricular tachycardia in the dog. Zentralbl Veterinaermed 10:273.

Kerber, R. E., and Harrison, D. C. 1971. Beta-adrenergic blocking drugs in the treatment and prophylaxis of cardiac arrhythmias. In Circulatory Effects and Clinical Uses of Beta-adrenergic Blocking Drugs, p. 49. Amsterdam: Exerpta Medica.

Kissling, G.; Jacob, R.; Peiper, U.; and Bauereisen, E. 1969. Inotrope Wirkungen der Nervus Vagus am Hundeventrikel *in situ*. Pfluegers Arch 310:64.

Klaus, W., and Kuschinsky, G. 1962. Ueber die Wirkung von Digitoxigenin auf den cellulären Calcium-Umsatz in Herzmuskelgewebe. Naunyn Schmiedebergs Arch Pharmakol 244:237.

Krayer, O.; Linstead, R. P.; and Todd, D. 1943. Pharmacology and chemistry of substances with cardiac activity. II. Effect of L-ascorbic acid and some related compounds of hydrogen peroxide on the isolated heart of the frog. J Pharmacol Exp Ther 77:113.

Kruhoffer, P. 1960. Handling of alkali metal ions by the kidney. In O. Eichler and A. Farah, eds. Handbuch der experimentellen Pharmacologie. Vol. 13, The Alkali Metal Ions, p. 233. Berlin: Springer-Verlag.

Kumar, R.; Hood, W. B., Jr.; Gilmore, D. P.; and Abelman, W. H. 1972. Effect of acetylstrophanthidin on cardiovascular function in intact, conscious dogs. J Pharmacol Exp Ther 180:24.

Kyser, F. A.; Ginsberg, H.; and Gilbert, N. C. 1946. The effect of certain drugs upon the cardiotoxic lesions of digitalis in the dog. Am Heart J 31:451.

Langer, G. A. 1972. Effects of digitalis on myocardial ionic exchange. Circulation 46:180.

Laragh, J. H. 1962. Hormones and the pathogenesis of congestive heart failure: Vasopressin, aldosterone, and angiotensin. Circulation 25:1015.

Lee, K. S., and Klaus, W. 1971. The subcellular basis for the mechanism of inotropic action of cardiac glycosides. Pharmacol Rev 23:193.

Lendle, L., and Mercker, H. 1961. Extrakardiale Digitaliswirkungen. Ergeb Physiol 51:199.

Leonard, E., and Hajdu, S. 1962. Action of electrolytes and drugs on the contractile mechanism of cardiac muscle cell. Handbook of Physiology. Vol. 1, Circulation, p. 151. Washington, D.C.: American Physiological Society.

Lieberman, N. A.; Harris, R. S.; Katz, R. L.; Lipschutz, H. N.; Dolgin, M.; and Fisher, V. J. 1968. The effects of lidocaine on the electrical and mechanical activity of the heart. Am J Cardiol 22:375.

Linde, L. M.; Goldberg, S. J.; Gaal, P.; Momma, K.; Takahashi, M.; and Sarna, G. 1968. Pulmonary and systemic hemodynamic effects of cardiac glycosides. Am Heart J 76: 356.

Lown, B. 1961. The clinical use of digitalis drugs. In A. A. Luisada, ed. Cardiology, vol. 5, p. 154. New York: McGraw-Hill.

Lown, B.; Black, H.; and Moore, D.F. 1960. Digitalis, electrolytes and the surgical patient. Am J Cardiol 6:309.

Luchi, R. J.; Helwig, J., Jr.; and Conn, H. L., Jr. 1963. Quinidine toxicity and its treatment. Am Heart J 65:340.

Lyon, A. F., and DeGraff, A. C. 1963. The neurotoxic effects of digitalis. Am Heart J 65: 340.

Marcus, F. I.; Burkhalter, L. A.; Cuccia, C. M.; Palovich, J.; and Kapadia, G. G. The administration of tritiated digoxin with and without a loading dose. A metabolic study. Circulation 34:865.

Marcus, F. I.; Pavlovich, J.; Burkhalter, S. L.; and Cuccia, C. M. 1967. The metabolic fate of tritiated digoxin in the dog: A comparison of digitalis administration with and without a "loading dose." J Pharmacol Exp Ther 156:548.

Martinez-Maldonado, M.; Allen, J. C.; Eknoyan, G.; Suki, W.; and Schwartz, A. 1969. Renal concentrating mechanism: Possible role for sodium-potassium activated adenosine triphosphatase. Science 165:807.

Mason, D. T.; Lelis, R.; and Amsterdam, E. A. 1972. Unified concept of the mechanism of action of digitalis: Influence of ventricular function and cardiac disease on hemodynamic response to fundamental contractile effect. In B. H. Marks and A. M. Weissler, eds. Basic and Clinical Pharmacology of Digitalis, p. 206. Springfield, Ill: Charles C Thomas.

Mason, D. T.; DeMaria, A. N.; Amsterdam, E. A.; Zelis, R.; and Massumi, R. A. 1973. Antiarrhythmic agents. I. Mechanisms of action and clinical pharmacology. Drugs 5:261.

Mayer, E. 1938. Der Einfluss von Digitalis und Strophanthin am Elecktrokardiogramm des Rindes mit Untersuchungen zur Klärung der Natur der darin auftretenden Strecke h. Dissertation, Munich.

Mendez, C., and Mendez, R. 1957. The action of cardiac glycosides on the excitability and conduction velocity of the mammalian atrium. J Pharmacol Exp Ther 121:402.

Mendez, C.; Aceves, I.; and Mendez, R. 1961a. The anti-adrenergic action of digitalis on the refractory period of the A-V transmission system. J Pharmacol Exp Ther 131: 199.

———. 1961b. Inhibition of adrenergic cardiac acceleration by cardiac glycosides. J Pharmacol Exp Ther 131:191.

Mendez, R. 1944. Pharmacology and chemistry of substances with cardiac activity. III. The effect of simple unsaturated lactones and *t*-butyl hydrogen peroxide on the isolated frog heart. J Pharmacol Exp Ther 81:151.

Modell, W. 1966. The pharmacologic basis of the use of digitalis in congestive heart failure. Physiol Pharmacol Physicians 1:1.

Moe, G. K., and Mendez, C. 1962. Basis of pharmacotherapy of cardiac arrhythmias. Mod Concepts Cardiovasc Dis 31:739.

Moe, G. K., and Mendez, R. 1951. The action of several cardiac glycosides on conduction velocity and ventricular excitability in the dog heart. Circulation 4:729.

Mosey, S.; Tyler, M. D.; and Bauer, R. O. 1952. Effect of diphenylhydantoin sodium (Dilantin) on digitalis arrhythmias. Fed Proc 11:377.

Moss, A. J., and Patton, R. D. 1973. Antiarrhythmic Agents. Springfield, Ill.; Charles C Thomas.

Nalbandian, R. M.; Gordon, D.; and Campbell, R. 1957. A new, quantitative digitalis tolerance test based upon the synergism of calcium and digitalis. Am J Med Sci 233: 503.

Naylor, W. G. 1963. The significance of calcium ions in cardiac excitation and contraction. Am Heart J 56:404.

O'Connor, W. J. 1962. Renal Function. Baltimore: Williams & Wilkins.

Okita, G. T. 1969. Distribution, disposition, and excretion of digitalis glycosides. In C. Fisch and B. Surawicz, eds. Digitalis. New York: Grune & Stratton.

Olson, R. E. 1962. Physiology of cardiac muscle. Handbook of Physiology. Vol. 1, Circulation, p. 199. Washington, D.C.: American Physiological Society.

Patterson, D. F.; Detweiler, D. K.; Hubben, K.; and Botts, R. P. 1961. Spontaneous abnormal cardiac arrhythmias and conduction disturbances in the dog. Am J Vet Res 22:355.

Pyle, R. L. 1967. Conversion of atrial fibrillation with quinidine sulfate in a dog. J Am Vet Med Assoc 151:582.

Reinert, H. 1952. Die enterale Resorption des g-Strophanthins, k-Strophantols- α and Digitoxins bei der Katze. Arch Exp Pathol Pharmakol 215:1.

Robb, J. S., and Mallov, S. 1953. Effect of ouabain on actomyosin threads. J Pharmacol Exp Ther 108:251.

Robinson, J. W. L. 1972. The inhibition of glycine and beta-methylglucoside transport in dog kidney cortex slices by ouabain and ethacrynic acid: Contribution to the understanding of sodium pumping mechanisms. Comp Gen Pharmacol 3:145.

Rodensky, P. L., and Wasserman, F. 1964. The possible role of sex in digitalis tolerance. Am Heart J 68:325.

Rodman, T., and Pastor, B. H. 1963. The hemodynamic effects of digitalis in the normal and diseased heart. Am Heart J 65:564.

Rosen, M. R. and Hoffman, B. F. 1973. Mechanisms of action of antiarrhythmic drugs. Circ Res 32:1.

Rothlin, E., and Bircher, R. P. 1954. Pharmakodynamische Grundlagen der Therapie mit herzwirksamen Glykosiden. Ergeb Inn Med Kinderheilkd 5:457.

———. 1961. Pharmacology of cardiac glycosides. In A. A. Luisada, ed. Cardiology, p. 133. New York: McGraw-Hill.

Schaal, S. F.; Sugimoto, T.; Wallace, A. G.; and Sealy, W. C. 1968. Effects of digitalis on the functional refractory period of the AV node: Studies in awake dogs with and without cardiac denervation. Cardiovasc Res 4:356.

Scherlag, B. J.; Helfant, R. H.; Ricciutti, M. A.; and Damato, A. N. 1968. Dissociation of the effects of digitalis on myocardial potassium flux and contractility. Am J Physiol 215:1288.

Selye, H. 1958. The Chemical Prevention of Cardiac Necroses. New York: Ronald Press.

———. 1961. The Pleuricausal Cardiopathies. Springfield, Ill.: Charles C Thomas.

Shanks, R. G., and Dunlop, D. 1967. Effect of propranolol on arrhythmias following coronary artery occlusion in dogs. Cardiovasc Res 1:34.

Skelton, C. L., and Sonnenblick, E. H. 1972. The response of the heart to digitalis. In B. A. Marks and A. M. Weissler, eds. Basic and Clinical Pharmacology of Digitalis, p. 193. Springfield, Ill.: Charles C Thomas.

Smith, T. W. 1972. Contribution of quantitative assay technics to the understanding of clinical pharmacology of digitalis. Circulation 46:188.

Smith, T. W., and Haber E. 1973. Digitalis. N Engl J Med 289:945.

Somlyo, A. P. 1960. The toxicology of digitalis. Am J Cardiol 5:523.

Surawicz, B., and Lasseter, K. C. 1970. Effect of drugs on the electrocardiogram. Prog Cardiovasc Dis 13:26.

Swain, H. H., and Weidner, C. L. 1957. A study of substances which alter intraventricular conduction in the isolated dog heart. J Pharmacol Exp Ther 120:137.

Swanson, M.; Cacace, L.; Chun, G.; and Itano, M. 1973. Saliva calcium and potassium concentrations in the detection of digitalis toxicity. Circulation 47:736.

Tanabe, T.; Tsunemi, I.; Abiko, Y.; and Dazai, H. 1961. On the diuresis from the unilateral kidney produced by ouabain injected directly into the renal artery. Arch Int Pharmacodyn Ther 133:452.

Teske, R. H.; Bishop, S. P.; Righter, H. F.; and Detweiler, D. K. 1976. Subacute digoxin toxicosis in the Beagle dog. Toxicol Appl Pharmacol 35:283.

Theilen, E. O., and Wilson, W. P. 1968. Beta-adrenergic receptor blocking drugs in the treatment of cardiac arrhythmias. Med Clin North Am 52:1017.

Tobian, L. 1960. Interrelationship of electrolytes, juxtaglomerular cells and hypertension. Physiol Rev 40:280.

Trautwein, W. 1963. Generation and conduction of impulses in the heart as affected by drugs. Pharmacol Rev 15:277.

Urquhart, J., and Davis, J. O. 1963. Role of the kidney and the adrenal cortex in congestive heart failure. Mod Concepts Cardiovasc Dis 32:787.

Vick, R. L.; Kahn, J. B., Jr.; and Acheson, G. H. 1957. Effects of dihydro-ouabain, dihydrodigoxin and dihydrodigitoxin on the heart-lung preparation of the dog. J Pharmacol Exp Ther 121:330.

Wallace, A. G.; Cline R. E.; Sealy, W. C.; Young, W. G., Jr.; and Troyer, W. G. 1966. Electrophysiologic effects of quinidine. Circ Res 19:969.

Wallace, C. R., and Hamilton, W. F. 1962. Study of spontaneous congestive heart failure in the dog. Circ Res 11:301.

Walton, R. P.; Cotten, M. deV.; and McCord, W. M. 1950a. Absence of digitalis-like cardiac effects in the action pattern of several lactones. Proc Soc Exp Biol Med 74: 548.

Walton, R. P.; Leary, J. S.; and Jones, H. P. 1950b. Comparative increase in ventricular contractile force produced by several cardiac glycosides. J Pharmacol Exp Ther 98:346.

Weidmann, S. 1955. The effect of the cardiac membrane potential on the rapid availability of the sodium-carrying system. J Physiol 127:213.

Werkö, L.; Bucht, H.; Ek, J.; and Varnaukas, E. 1958. Studies on the renal function in mitral valvular disease. IV. Effect of a single intravenous dose of lanatoside C. Cardiologia 29:305.

Westermarck, H. 1956. Electrocardiographic changes in sheep following intravenous and oral administration of digitalis. Zentralbl Veterinaermed 3:727.

———. 1959. Digitalis inactivation *in vitro* due to rumen microbes in sheep. Acta Vet Scand 1:67.

Will, D. H. 1963. Personal communication.

Williams, J. F. Jr., and Braunwald, E. 1965. Studies on digitalis. XI. Effects of digoxin on the development of cardiac hypertrophy in the rat subjected to aortic constriction. Am J Cardiol 16:534.

Williams, J. F., Jr.; Klocke, F. J.; and Braunwald, E. 1966. Studies on digitalis. XIII. A comparison of the effects of potassium on the inotropic and arrhythmia-producing actions of ouabain. J Clin Invest 45:346.

Withering, W. 1785. An account of the foxglove and some of its medical uses with practical remarks on dropsy and other diseases. Reprinted in Willius, F. A., and Keys, T. E. 1961. Classics of Cardiology, vol. 1, p. 231. New York: Dover.

Yeh, B. K., and Lazzara, R. 1973. Reversal of ouabain induced electrophysiological effects by potassium canrenoate in canine Purkinje fibers. Circ Res 32:501.

SECTION 7

Drugs Acting on Fluid and Electrolyte Balance

CHAPTER 25

PHYSIOLOGICAL BASIS

DAVID R. GROSS and J. D. McCRADY

BODY WATER

Body water and certain selected electrolytes are in a state of continuous flux among various compartments within the animal body. Water turnover is the term used to describe the input and output of water in the body over any period, usually 24 hours. In general, water input must balance water output, i.e., the body water volume is held constant. The control of water turnover is regulated centrally by the thirst and drinking control centers. These centers are located in the ventromedial and anterior areas of the hypothalamus and the osmoreceptors are located in the lateral hypothalamus of vertebrates (Andersson 1952, 1956, 1960). As the the osmolarity of the blood changes, the central sensors detect this change. The thirst and drinking control centers are stimulated or depressed, depending on whether the osmolarity is increased or decreased (negative feedback). The osmoreceptors are stimulated or depressed in the same manner and control the release of antidiuretic hormone (ADH); ADH exerts its effect on the distal tubules of the kidney, and water is retained or excreted. Other secondary water conservation mechanisms also may be involved, i.e., peripheral vasoconstriction, anhidrosis, and urine concentration.

Values for water turnover per 24 hours in various domestic animals resting in metabolism cages or stalls range from about 25 to 60 ml /lb/day. The range is influenced by species, age, and physiological state (Adolph 1939; Leitch 1944; Smith 1970). Water demands may change markedly during extremes of temperature, psychological state, disease, and other variables. For most purposes one can assume that the water turnover in mature animals is 30 ml/lb/day (65 ml/kg/day), while immature and lactating animals may turn over approximately twice that amount.

For practical reasons, which will become more apparent later in this discussion, it is desirable to know the amount of water present in an animal's body. These values are usually expressed as a percentage of the total body weight of the animal. The method most commonly employed uses dilution techniques and the Fick principle. With this method, a known quantity of a marker that will distribute evenly throughout the water volume is injected. A wide variety of dyes or radioisotopes attached to diffusable substances can be used as markers. Perhaps the best marker is tri-

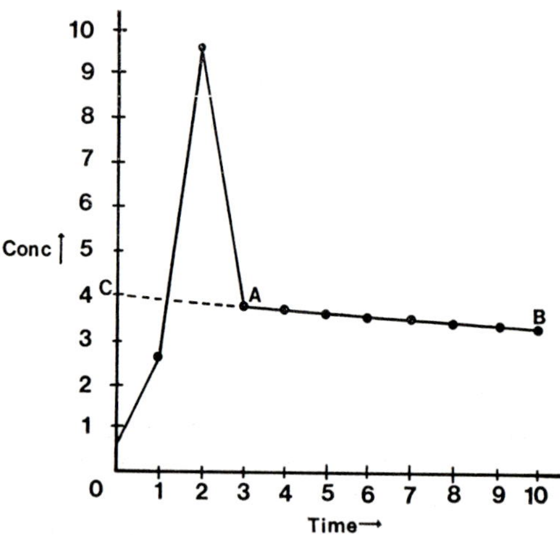

FIG. 25.1. Sample plot of concentration of a water marker decay curve used for the calculation of total body water.

tiated water (^3H_2O radioactive water or deuterium oxide), which distributes completely. The technique involves sampling of the marker following its injection. The concentration at various sampling periods is plotted against time (Fig. 25.1). The slope of the decay curve (line *A–B*) is determined and the concentration at time 0 (*A–C*) is then graphically extrapolated. The volume of distribution is calculated from the relationship:

$$C_{t0} = \frac{I}{V_D}$$

where

C_{t0} = concentration at time 0
I = amount of marker injected
V_D = volume of distribution

Other methods of calculating total body water also exist and involve calculations of "apparent volumes of distribution," using other techniques wherein the marker is administered either orally or parenterally and samples are taken until equilibrium is reached. This usually requires about 2 hours.

Using these techniques, it has been found that the water content of mature animals varies from approximately 55% to 60% of their body weight. Similar measurements made in immature animals indicate they are about 70%–75% water and obese animals about 50% water (Lassiter and Gottschalk 1974).

Similarly, it is possible to measure other body compartments of water. This is done by using markers that distribute only within those various volumes or by measuring a specific compartment and calculating another compartment from the various relationships that exist. For example,

TBW − ECF = ICF
ECF − PV = ISF

TBW = total body water; can be measured with ^3H_2O or by other substances.
ECF = extracellular fluid; can be measured as inulin space or with markers that only enter the ECF.
ICF = intracellular fluid.
PV = plasma volume; can be measured with radioactive albumin or Evans blue dye markers.
ISF = interstitial fluid.

Table 25.1 gives experimentally derived blood volumes for various species (Smith 1970).

Fig. 25.2 represents the various fluid compartments as a percentage of body weight. Semipermeable membranes separate the majority of these compartments.

TABLE 25.1. Approximate values for blood volumes of various animals expressed as a percentage of total body weight

Animal	Total Volume Blood	Plasma Volume	RBC Volume
Dog	8.5	4.5	4.0
Cat	6.7	4.7	2.0
Chicken	6.5	4.5	2.0
Cattle	5.7	3.8	1.9
Goat	7.0	5.4	1.6
Horse			
Draft	7.0	4.0	3.0
Thoroughbred	10.0	6.0	4.0
Saddle	7.7	5.2	2.5
Pig	7.5	4.8	2.7
Sheep	6.5	4.5	2.0

Source: Smith 1970. (Values represent averages from approximately 30 references.)

Normally, the rate of passage of water through these membranes in both directions is equal and equilibrium is maintained. As can be seen in Fig. 25.2, the ICF is the largest water compartment and represents about 40% of the total body weight. The ECF is made up of 3 separate subcompartments: (1) plasma water (PW), approximately 5% of the body weight, which represents the water within the cardiovascular system; (2) ISF, which constitutes about 14% of the body weight, and (3) the transcellular fluid, which can vary between 1% and 6% of the body weight. The transcellular fluid is found in separated locations, i.e., cerebrospinal fluid, pleural cavity, gastrointestinal (GI) tract, bladder, synovia, aqueous humor, and peritoneal cavity. This fluid is separated from the plasma by a capillary membrane and an additional synovial, serous or mucous membrane. In diseases, these membranes can separate in one direction and the compartment can undergo a dramatic change, i.e., ascites, hydropericardium, urinary blockage, hydrothorax, synovitis, and hydrochephalus. The transcellular compartment cannot be considered a part of the functional reserve. The ECF, therefore, comprises about 20% of the total body weight.

Since the water content of some tissues is large, loss of, or injury to, these tissues can cause a serious loss of body water. Blood

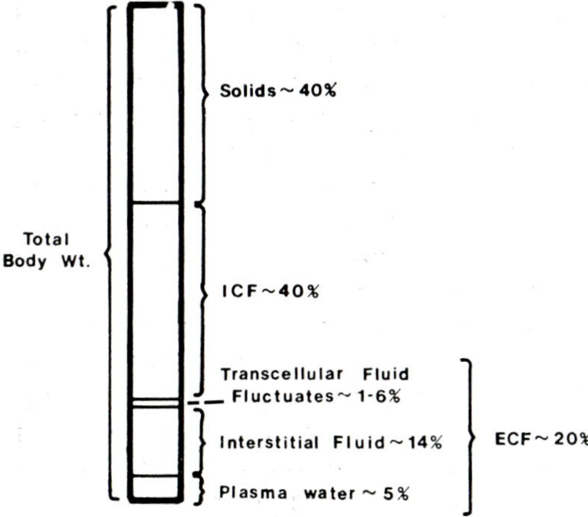

FIG. 25.2. Fluid compartments expressed as a percentage of body weight.

is approximately 76% water; liver 70%; muscle 76%; skin 69% in dogs, 72% in human beings, and 70% in horses and cows. Fat, on the other hand, is only 10%–13% water, bone and cartilage 20%–30% water (Lassiter and Gottschalk 1974).

Skin, aside from its obvious role in protection, serves some important functions in regulation of body water. The skin is approximately 16% of the body weight and is about 70% water so it is a rather vast water reservoir, as well as a reservoir for Na^+ and Cl^-. Clinically, one can measure the degree of dehydration by observing the loss of turgor, elasticity, and dryness of the skin. Overhydration is often demonstrated by subcutaneous edema.

The body surface area is important in the functioning of water reserve. It is true that the metabolic rate of any animal is directly proportional to the body surface area. That is, the more area, the more energy expended and the more water lost. As body size increases, body mass increases at a more rapid rate than does the body surface area. A puppy represented by a cube 10 cm on each side would have a surface area of $10 \times 10 \times 6 = 600$ cm². The same puppy's volume would be $10 \times 10 \times 10 = 1000$ cm³ The surface area/volume (SA/V) ratio would be 6:10. A mature dog might measure 100 cm on a side, if represented by a cube. His surface area would be $100 \times 100 \times 6 = 60{,}000$ cm², his volume would be $100 \times 100 \times 100 = 1{,}000{,}000$ cm³, and his SA/V ratio would then be 6:100. The puppy has 10 times the SA/V ratio as the adult dog, therefore it has a much larger basal metabolic rate, the evaporative water loss from the skin is much greater per unit volume, and the daily water turnover per unit of body weight may be twice that of an adult animal. This is very important clinically and helps to explain why dehydration is so much more serious in a young animal than in a mature animal. Calf scours, puppy diarrhea, and feline panleukopenia are some examples of diseases of immature animals in which dehydration assumes critical importance.

CONCEPT OF MILLIEQUIVALENTS (ELECTROCHEMICAL EQUIVALENCE)

Electrolytes combine in proportion to their ionic valence rather than in proportion to their weights. One equivalent of a substance is the atomic weight divided by the ionic valence and provides a quantitative index of the combining proportions of all ionic species. The electrolyte concentrations found in the body fluids are rather dilute and are therefore more easily expressed as milliequivalents (1 mEq = 1/1000 Eq). Example:

1 mM Na = 23 mg
1 mM Cl = 35.5 mg

$$\underset{1\ \text{mM}}{23\ \text{mg}\ Na^+} + \underset{1\ \text{mM}}{35.5\ \text{mg}\ Cl^-}\ \underset{1\ \text{L}}{\text{in}\ H_2O} \rightarrow \underset{1\ \text{mM}}{58.5\ \text{mg NaCl}}$$

If 35.5 mg Na^+ are added to 35.5 mg Cl^-, we have 58.5 mg NaCl + 12.5 mgNa^+, i.e., electrolytes do not combine mg for mg, they combine mEq for mEq. In the case of univalent ions, 1 Eq = 1 M and 1 mEq = 1 mM.

Multivalent ions have a greater chemical combining power than univalent ions. One divalent ion will react with 2 univalent ions. Therefore, 1 mM divalent ion supplies 2 mEq and 1 mM of a trivalent substance will contain 3 mEq.

Dividing the number of milligrams of a univalent electrolyte by its atomic (molecular) weight yields the number of mEq. With multivalent substances, the weight of the substance must be mutiplied by its valence and then divided by the atomic weight. Since laboratory results are often expressed as mg% (mg/100 ml), the conversion to mEq/L can be made from the following formula:

$$\frac{\text{mg}/100\ \text{ml}}{\text{atomic wt}} \times \text{valence} \times 10 = \text{mEq/L}$$

The utility of expressing most of the electrolyte concentrations in mEq/L is apparent from Table 25.2. The values given are average normals for dogs. Other species may vary slightly from these values. It is evident that the total concentration of cations is equal to that of the anions and electroneutrality exists. If these ions were expressed as mg%, nothing useful could be learned about their chemical interrelationships. The largest component, by weight, in the anion column is protein, which in terms of acid-base balance is seldom of importance.

However, mEq/L is not ideally applicable to all the electrolytes in all circumstances. In problems of calcium and phosphorus metabolism, these ions are properly measured as millimoles/L. The ionized (diffusible) calcium fraction depends on the proportion of calcium not bound to plasma proteins. Since the usual laboratory determinations include all the serum calcium, including those ions protein bound, it would not be proper to express these ions as mEq/L. Serum "phosphorus" consists of variable proportions of phosphate and monohydrogen and dihydrogen phosphate so that no valence can be assigned to this substance. Plasma proteins are usually expressed as g% or g/100 ml plasma. Although they are included in the anion column in Table 25.2, their electrochemical equivalence is affected by pH and other factors and at times they may even act as weak cations.

TABLE 25.2. Electrolyte composition of body fluids

Electrolytes	ICF mEq/L	ECF mEq/L
Cations		
Na^+	143	10
K^+	5	150
Ca^{++}	5	
Mg^{++}	2	40
Total	155	200
Anions		
Cl^-	106	
HCO_3^-	20	10
HPO_4^-	2	140
$SO_4^=$	2	10
Organic acids	10	
Protein	15	40
Total	155	200

Note: Values cited are approximate and represent general levels for all species.

OSMOLARITY AND OSMOSIS

An understanding of osmolarity and osmosis is essential to an understanding of homeostasis, disturbances in body water balance, and fluid therapy. All the fluid compartments are separated by semipermeable membranes. These membranes allow free passage of water in either direction but restrict particles, ions, crystalloids, and colloids in the water. The number of individual particles in solution is all important. This is independent of electrical charge, valence, or chemical formula. This explains why 5% dextrose, 0.89% NaCl, and 1.3% Na bicarbonate are all isotonic.

For substances that do not dissociate into smaller parts (i.e., glucose), 1 M = 180 g (1 osmole) and 1mM = 1 mOsm (1 milliosmole). The same is true of ions (1 mM Na, i.e., 23 mg, = 1 mOsm). Divalent and trivalent ions exert no more osmotic pressure than univalent ions. Therefore, 1 mM Mg^{++} (24.5 mg) = 1 mOsm = 2 mEq and 1 mM PO_4^{-3} (95 mg) = 1 mOsm = 3 mEq. One gram molecular weight of NaCl (58.5 mg) dissociates into Na^+ and Cl^- in solution and contributes twice as many osmotically active particles as a nonionized substance, so that 1 mM = 2 mEq = 2 mOsm.

Osmolarity is usually expressed as the number of milliosmoles (or osmoles) per L of body fluid. All isotonic solutions equal approximately 300 mOsm. Hypertonic solutions are $>$ 300 mOsm and hypotonic solutions $<$ 300 mOsm.

ROLE OF THE KIDNEY IN WATER AND SALT REGULATION

Approximately 20%–90% of the water filtered through the kidney is reabsorbed passively from the proximal convoluted tubules. Sodium ions and other substances follow the water back into the circulation. Some active reabsorption (energy utilizing) of sodium and other ions occurs in the proximal tubule, and water follows these processes. In the thick portion of the loop of Henle, intense active reabsorption of Na^+ occurs. In the distal nephron, the concentration of urine (i.e., the reabsorption of water from provisional urine) is a function of the countercurrent mechanism and ADH.

A major mechanism for conservation of water in the animal is urine concentration. The canine kidney can concentrate urine as much as 2400 mOsm. Human beings, by comparison, can concentrate to 1400 mOsm. Some species of desert mice are able to concentrate to greater than 10,000 mOsm. Urine volume in a healthy animal is a rather accurate index of water intake.

Water excretion by the kidney is essentially controlled by ADH in the circulating blood. As the ADH concentration in the renal blood increases, the distal nephron becomes more permeable to water. If the ADH concentration decreases, the distal nephron becomes less permeable and more water is passed out of the body as urine. Injury or disease of the posterior pituitary causes decreased levels of ADH, less water is reabsorbed from the distal nephron, and the urine is dilute and copious (diabetes insipidus). Under normal circumstances, the levels of ADH released from the posterior pituitary are controlled by the osmoreceptors in the hypothalamus. These sensors are sensitive to changes in the osmolarity of the fluids surrounding them. As the osmolarity of these fluids increases, more ADH is released and more water is reabsorbed, thereby causing the fluids to become more dilute and the osmolarity to decrease. With an increase in the volume of ECF, release of ADH decreases and more water is allowed to pass until equilibrium is reestablished (negative feedback). The interactions of the ADH mechanisms are illustrated in Fig. 25.3.

The ECF volume is more under the control of the Na^+ concentration in this compartment. Each 150 mEq of Na^+ in the ECF will normally be accompanied by 1 L of water. The kidney will excrete or retain Na^+ depending on the volume of ECF; therefore, control of the ECF volume is dependent on the control of Na^+. The rate of excretion or retention of Na^+ by the kidney is determined by the concentration of aldosterone (ALD) in the renal blood. Fig.

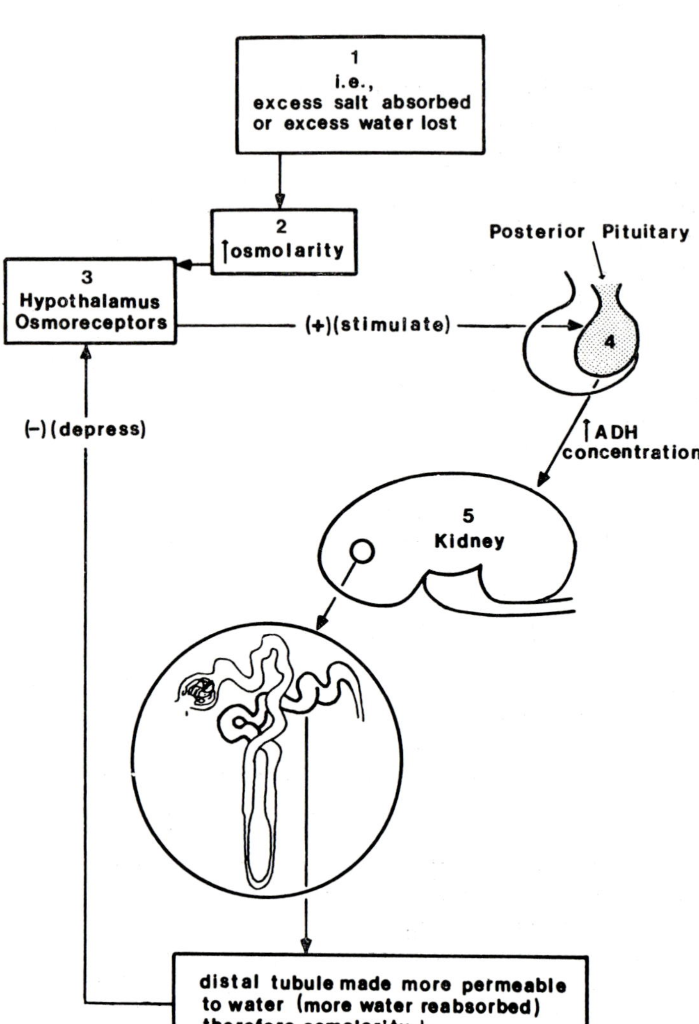

Fig. 25.3. The role of ADH in the regulation of osmolarity of extracellular fluids.

25.4 depicts the role of ALD. Volume receptors in the cardiovascular system, located in the aortic arch, the atria, and possibly other places, sense changes in circulating blood volumes, i.e., ECF volumes. Decreases in ECF volume cause increases in the rate of ALD secretion and vice versa. An increase or decrease of ALD concentration causes a similar increase or decrease in the reabsorption of Na^+ from the filtrate and thereby contributes to Na^+ and water regulation.

Renal corrections for disturbances in volume are dependent upon retention or excretion of sodium, whereas corrections for concentration (osmolarity) are dependent upon excretion or retention of water. In reality the ADH-ALD mechanisms are two components of the same control system and the corrections for volume and osmolarity require the same renal response, i.e., solute concentration and body fluid volume are interdependent. However, in certain abnormal states, such as water deprivation, the corrections for hyperosmolarity and hypovolemia are directly opposed. In this instance the body responses to correct this situation are, of necessity, much slower.

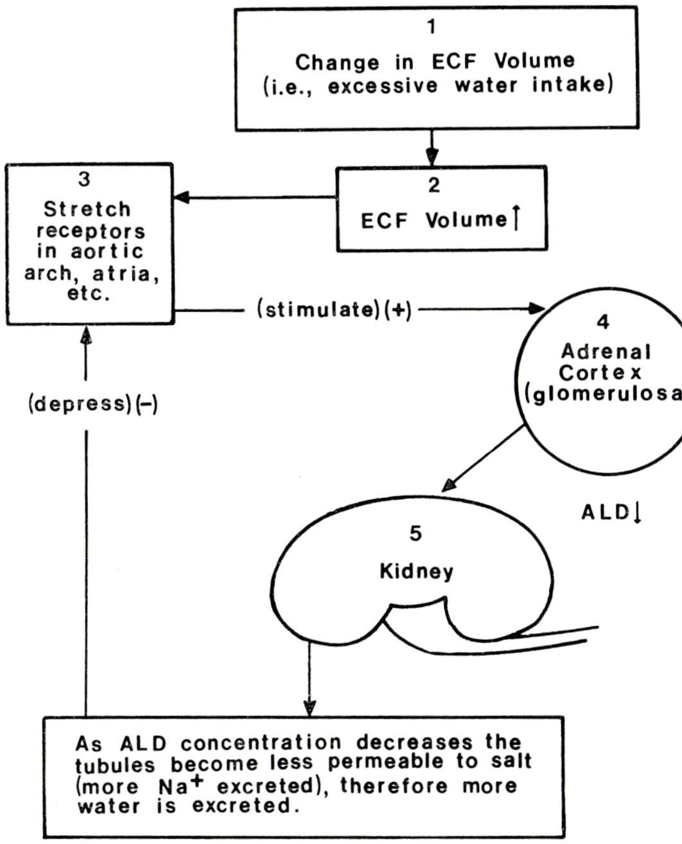

FIG. 25.4. The role of aldosterone in the regulation of extracellular fluid volume.

The kidney also plays a major role in the regulation of H^+ concentration, but this will be dealt with in more detail later in the discussion of body buffer systems. Normally, more than one-half the total acid excretion is in the form of ammonia via renal mechanisms. When circumstances dictate that acid excretion is maximal, this may approach three-fourths the total acid excretion (Pitts 1968).

The kidney can adjust volume, osmolarity, ion content, and pH of body fluids. The administration of fluids that are far from corrective in one or all of these respects can be compensated for by normally functioning kidneys. If the kidneys are not capable of normal function, problems increase exponentially.

ACID-BASE REGULATION

Pulmonary and renal function are necessary for precise regulation of the pH of the body fluids. It is important not to be concerned with only the pH of the blood. It is equally important to know what is happening in the extravascular tissues of the body.

There is a logarithmic relationship between pH and H^+ activity:

$$pH = -\log a_{H^+}$$

or

$$H^+ = \frac{1}{\text{antilog pH}}$$

Therefore, H^+ activity can be calculated from the pH (usually measured with a glass membrane electrode only porous to H^+). The H^+ concentration cannot be measured directly but is assumed equal to the hydrogen activity as measured by the electrode.

An acid is defined as a substance that

can supply H^+ (protons) and a base as a substance that can accept H^+. In aqueous solutions, H^+ is hydrated; therefore, H_3O^+ is considered an acid and is implied by the symbol H^+. Bases include water, hydroxyl ions, ammonia (NH_3), and the anions of the salts of weak acids, all of which can find free H^+.

BUFFER SYSTEMS

In general, acid-base regulation can be divided into a five-part system:

1. Intrinsic buffering (chemical) involves ECF buffer interactions:

$$pH = pK_1 + \log \frac{NaHCO_3}{H_2CO_3}$$

$$= pK_2 + \log \frac{NaHPO_4}{NaH_2PO_4}$$

$$= pK_3 + \log \frac{B^+Pr}{H^-Pr}$$

$$= pK_4 + \log \frac{B^+ \text{ organic}}{H^- \text{ organic}}$$

The carbonic acid and base bicarbonate portion of the intrinsic buffer system, although not the most efficient, is the most important by reason of its large distribution and availability. This system is normally expressed chemically by the following equation:

$$H_2O + CO_2 \overset{CA}{\rightleftarrows} H_2CO_3 \rightleftarrows H^+ + HCO_3^-$$

One part H_2CO_3 to 20 parts HCO_3^- is normal. When this ratio is disturbed, the result is either acidosis or alkalosis. The carbonic anhydrase (CA) enzyme catalyzes this reaction. This enzyme is found in moderate-to-high concentrations in tissues associated with electrolyte exchange or transport (i.e., lungs, kidneys). This is a more or less instantaneous reaction.

2. The early cellular component takes place during the first stages of the development of the abnormal state. With acidosis, K^+ are extruded from the cells and H^+ enter the cells. During early alkalosis, the reverse process occurs, i.e., K^+ move in and H^+ move out. There also occurs, on the cellular level, a Cl^- shift between cells and the ECF to adjust for marked changes in Cl^- concentration or HCO_3^- concentration. This reaction normally takes 2–4 hours.

3. The respiratory component involves changes in respiratory rate and volume. An increase in respiratory rate and volume accelerates the removal of CO_2 causing a shift in the

$$H_2O + CO_2 \overset{CA}{\rightleftarrows} H_2CO_3$$

equilibrium. By the removal of CO_2, it is obvious that less H_2CO_3 will be present. Conversely, H^+ may be retained by decreasing respiratory rate and volume. Initiation of these processes requires only minutes.

4. The renal component involves selective reabsorption. During periods of acidosis, H^+ is excreted and Na^+ and HCO_3^- are retained. During alkalosis, K^+ is excreted and Na^+ and HCO_3^- are retained; however, H^+ secretion is depressed, i.e., less H^+ is extruded than normally. This process is slower and requires hours to days to produce an effect.

5. The late cellular component exerts its effect after prolonged alkalosis. Because of the loss of K^+ from the renal component in prolonged alkalosis, the ECF-K^+ concentration decreases. Potassium ions then move out of the cells into the ECF. It has been theorized that for every K^+ that leaves the cells 2 Na^+ and 1 H^+ enter the cell. The end result is to make the ECF even more alkalotic and the ICF more acidotic.

True chemical buffering, biological buffering (cellular exchange), and physiological buffering (respiratory and/or renal adaptation) are occurring simultaneously when the body fluids are confronted with an acid or alkaline load. Therefore, in health the mechanisms available for regulation of acid-base balance are capable of maintaining the proper H^+ concentration.

ACID-BASE PARAMETERS AND TERMINOLOGY

Disorders of acid-base equilibrium can result from a primary disturbance in the pulmonary regulation of the concentration of carbonic acid (H_2CO_3) in body fluids, by metabolic changes in the concentration of bicarbonate, or from a combination of these mechanisms. The partial pressure of carbon dioxide is generally accepted as the best measure of respiratory disturbances. The uptake of CO_2 in the tissues and its loss in the lungs are dependent on the rapidity of the hydration and dehydration reactions of CO_2, i.e.,

$$H_2O + CO_2 \overset{CA}{\rightleftarrows} H_2CO_3$$

The concentration of H_2CO_3 for any given P_{CO_2} is defined by the solubility constant of CO_2. For plasma at body temperature, the constant relating the concentration of dissolved CO_2 in millimoles per L and P_{CO_2} in mm of Hg (torr) is 0.03, i.e.,

$$H_2CO_3 = 0.03\ P_{CO_2}$$

The Henderson-Hasselbalch equation further defines the relationship among pH, P_{CO_2}, and HCO_3^-, as defined by the pK_1 of H_2CO_3. A simplification of the Henderson-Hasselbalch equation shows this relationship as:

$$pH = pK_1 + \log \frac{[HCO_3^-]}{[0.03\ pCO_2]} \quad \text{or}$$

$$pH = pK + \log \frac{[HCO_3^-]}{[H_2CO_3]}$$

Since the pK_1 of H_2CO_3 is 6.1, which is far below the physiologic pH compatible with life (6.8–7.7), H_2CO_3 almost completely dissociates to $HCO_3^- + H^+$. At pH = 7.4, the ratio $HCO_3^-/H_2CO_3 = 20{:}1$.

Whole-Blood Buffer Base

This concept was introduced by Singer and Hastings (1948) as a parameter for measurement of metabolic disturbances that would be uninfluenced acutely by the P_{CO_2}. The term was defined as the sum of the concentrations of buffer anions contained in whole blood, i.e., those components of the intrinsic buffering system. To calculate the whole-blood buffer base, one needs to determine only 2 of the 3 parameters of the Henderson-Hasselbalch equation (pH, P_{CO_2}, or HCO_3^-) and either the hemoglobin concentration or the hematocrit. With the use of a nomogram the whole-blood buffer base can then be calculated.

Standard Bicarbonate and Base Excess

This concept was proposed by Astrup and co-workers (1960). Standard bicarbonate is defined as the concentration of bicarbonate after fully oxygenated whole blood has been equilibrated with CO_2 at a P_{CO2} of 40 mm Hg at 38° C. The measurement of HCO_3^- at a normal fixed P_{CO2} of 40 mm Hg "eliminates" the influence of respiration on the plasma [HCO_3^-]. Any deviation from the normal range established for the species being measured, therefore, represents only metabolic changes in the acid-base balance. Given a value for standard bicarbonate, one can estimate the "base excess" (the amount of strong base or acid added per L of blood) by multiplying the deviation of standard bicarbonate by an empirical factor of 1.2; this factor supposedly accounts for the greater buffer content of red cells as opposed to plasma. Base excess is equivalent to the deviation of whole-blood buffer base from normal values (Maxwell and Kleeman 1972).

Acidosis and Alkalosis

Deviation of the arterial pH from 6.8 to 7.35 is referred to as acidosis; from 7.45 to 7.8 it is referred to as alkalosis. Any arterial pH < 6.8 or >7.8 is usually incompatible with life.

Hydrogen Ion Balance

Most of the fat and carbohydrate metabolized in the metabolic pool is burned

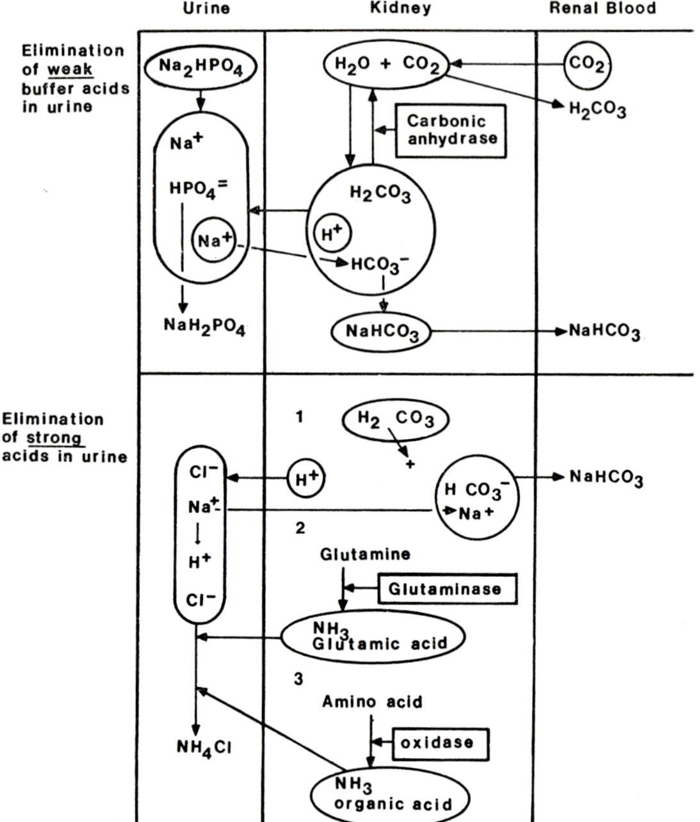

Fig. 25.5 Mechanisms of acid urine production.

completely to CO_2 and H_2O. As long as the CO_2 generated is excreted via the lungs, no excess H^+ is produced from this source. Carbonic acid is a volatile acid end product of metabolism; its concentration can be regulated by ventilatory adjustments of the P_{CO_2}. There appear to be three other sources of acid end products of metabolism. These metabolically generated H^+ originate from (1) a small amount of fat and carbohydrate that is incompletely oxidized to organic acids, (2) oxidation of the sulfur-containing amino acids to sulfonic acids, and (3) the oxidation and hydrolysis of isoelectric phosphoprotein residues to phosphoric acids. These fixed-acid end products of metabolism must be excreted by the kidneys to maintain normal pH levels.

ROLE OF THE KIDNEY IN H^+ EXCRETION

The kidney regulates acid-base balance by maintaining the appropriate HCO_3^- in the plasma. The kidney accomplishes this by reclaiming virtually all filtered HCO_3^- and excreting an amount of acid that equals the amount of ingested or of endogenously generated nonvolatile acid. The sequential mechanisms for the elimination of weak and strong acids in the urine are shown in Fig. 25.5. In the formation of acid urine, NH_3 production may increase tenfold over normal.

REFERENCES

Adolph, E. F. 1939. Measurements of water drinking in dogs. Am J Physiol 125:75.

Andersson, B. 1952. Polydipsia caused by intrahypothalamic injections of hypertonic NaCl solutions. Experimentia 8:157.

Andersson, B., and McCarrn, S. M. 1956. The effect of hypothalamic lesions on the water intake of the dog. Acta Physiol Scand 35: 312.

Andersson, B.; Larsson, S.; and Persson, N. 1960. Some characteristics of the hypothalamic "drinking centre" in the goat as shown by the use of permanent electrodes. Acta Physiol Scand 50:140.

Astrup, P.; Jorgensen, K.; Anderson, O. S.; and Engel, K. 1960. Acid-base metabolism: New approach. Lancet 1:1035.

Cooke, R. E.; Segar, W. E.; Cheek, D. B.; Conille, F. E.; and Darrow, D. C. 1952. The extrarenal correction of alkalosis associated with potassium deficiency. J Clin Invest 31:798.

Lassiter, W. E., and Gottschalk, C. W. 1974. Volume and Composition of the Body Fluids in Medical Physiology, 13th ed. St. Louis: C. V. Mosby.

Leitch, I., and Thomson, J. S. 1944. Nutr Abstr Rev 14:197.

Maxwell, M. H., and Kleeman, C. R. 1972. Clinical Disorders of Fluid and Electrolyte Metabolism, 2nd ed., p. 303. New York: McGraw-Hill.

Pitts, R. F. 1968. Physiology of the Kidney and Body Fluids, 2nd ed. Chicago: Year Book Medical Publishers.

Singer, R. B., and Hastings, A. B. 1948. Improved clinical method for estimation of disturbances of acid-base balance of human blood. Medicine 27:223.

Smith, C. R. 1970. Unpublished data. Ohio State University.

CHAPTER 26

GENERAL CONCEPTS OF FLUID THERAPY

DAVID R. GROSS and J. D. McCRADY

Six questions are to be considered when fluid therapy is under consideration: (1) When should fluid therapy be instituted? (2) What kind(s) of solution(s) should be used? (3) How much fluid should be administered? (4) How fast should the solution be given? (5) What route of administration should be used? and (6) How is the success of the therapy evaluated?

Answers to these questions are individual in character and dependent on a knowledge and understanding of normal homeostatic mechanisms; also, they are dependent on the history of the patient, on a basic understanding of how a particular disease affects water and electrolyte balance, and on the diagnosis. In making a diagnosis, one must include a good initial and continuous clinical reevaluation and supplementary clinical laboratory tests with repeated determinations.

INSTITUTION OF THERAPY

The purpose of fluid and electrolyte therapy is to correct dehydration or overhydration and/or electrolyte imbalance. These states may occur as a result of intestinal, renal, cardiac, or hepatic disease; trauma; or a host of other diseases. Fluid therapy may be indicated to correct a condition of acidosis or alkalosis, to treat shock, to give parenteral nourishment, or even to stimulate organ function, i.e., the kidneys. Causes of fluid, electrolyte, and/or protein loss include situations wherein substances are not available from a lack of supply or because of the condition of the animal. For example, an animal with a fractured mandible may be unable to take in food or liquid, or an animal with a central nervous system (CNS) disturbance may be unable to eat or drink due to the primary disease state. Other causes of fluid, electrolyte, and/or protein imbalances may involve excessive elimination.

Fig. 26.1 depicts the electrolyte imbalances associated with vomiting and diarrhea and the compensatory reactions that occur as a result of this excessive loss. Obviously, the fluid loss associated with these disease states may be considerable. Excessive salivation may cause imbalances as may kidney disease, either of which may be responsible for marked fluid and electrolyte changes. Specific disease conditions such as diabetes insipidus and mellitis may also cause excessive fluid loss. Excessive panting, hyperventilation or pulmonary disease and inhalation anesthesia may all cause dramatic changes in acid-base balance and, via compensatory mechanisms, other electrolyte shifts. Great imbalances may result from abnormalities of the skin and cutaneous glands and losses from body exudates and wounds.

To determine when fluid and/or electrolyte therapy is needed, it is necessary to

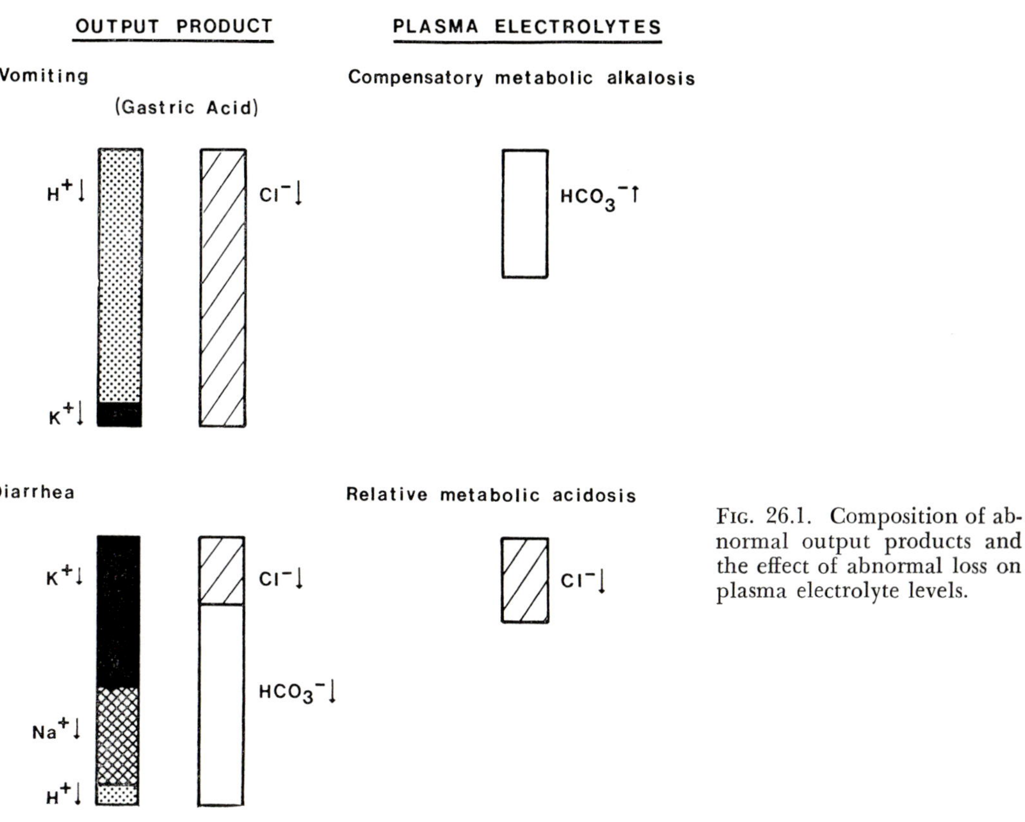

FIG. 26.1. Composition of abnormal output products and the effect of abnormal loss on plasma electrolyte levels.

recognize the various clinical signs that herald these needs. A lack of water will cause the osmolarity and Na^+ concentration of the blood to increase and the urine will be highly concentrated, providing the kidneys are functional. The animal will be thirsty, there may be oliguria, fever, circulatory collapse, dry mucous membranes, a lack of skin pliability, constipation, weight loss, and sunken eyes. Also, muscular twitching may appear toward the terminal phase and the animal may eventually lapse into coma and finally die. Too much water will cause the reverse; osmolarity and Na^+ decrease, urine is dilute, and there is polyuria. If fluids are administered, despite these early signs, intracranial hypertension may develop, causing mental confusion. Pulmonary edema may develop as well as nausea, vomiting, and generalized weakness. The animal may eventually begin convulsing, then lapse into coma, and fifinally die.

Lack of adequate Na^+ is associated with a decrease in extracellular fluid (ECF), hemoconcentration, loss of tissue elasticity, muscular weakness, depression, a lack of thirst, a loss of appetite, and eventually uremia and circulatory collapse. Conversely, too much Na^+ causes the ECF to increase, edema to form, congestive heart failure to develop, and K^+ deficiency to occur.

Hypopotassemia (hypokalemia) will result in inactivity, muscular weakness, possible changes in the electrocardiogram (ECG) (the development of U waves as described in human beings has not been documented in animals), ileus or diarrhea, metabolic alkalosis, and abdominal distention. Potassium depletion also tends to impair carbohydrate tolerance curves, which appear to be diabetic (Eliel et al. 1952). Hyperpotassemia (hyperkalemia) is characterized by classical changes in the ECG (wide QRS intervals and a peaking of the T waves), muscular weakness, and eventually cardiac arrest. Hyperphosphatemia is associated with hypocalcemia and tetany, whereas hypophosphatemia is characterized only by low blood levels of phosphorus. Hypocalcemia will result in tetany, circulatory failure, and abnormalities of muscle contraction. Hypercalcemia will result in calcium deposits within the body and, when overdosed parenterally, can result in cardiac fibrillation or arrest during systole.

Too little carbohydrate causes an increase in catabolism of protein, greater water and electrolyte loss, and ketosis. Overintake of carbohydrate results in hyperglycemia, glucosuria, obesity, and eventually hepatic failure.

A lack of adequate protein results in weakness, loss of appetite, tissue edema, arterial hypotension, sluggishness, hydroperitoneum (ascites), hydrothorax, and delayed wound healing; an overdose of protein can result in nephrosis.

History taking and clinical examination must include the following information: the duration of signs, duration and frequency of vomiting and/or diarrhea, consistency of stools, frequency of urination, color of urine, thirst, fluid and dietary intake, dryness or elasticity (turgor) of the skin, the nature and color of the mucous membranes and sclera, the odor of the breath (acetone, ammonia odor), and weight loss or gain.

Various laboratory tests that are essential to the proper handling of the case as well as any others that might provide useful information should be considered. A urinalysis should be run, including tests for specific gravity, glucose, acetone, pH, albumin, and a microscopic sediment examination. During a state of dehydration, if the kidneys are functioning normally, the specific gravity will increase and the urine volume will decrease. If the specific gravity of the urine is unchanged or lowered and the animal shows other clinical signs of dehydration, the kidneys are probably not functioning properly and other renal function tests should be employed. The specific gravity of the urine should be monitored during the treatment period; if this parameter begins to decrease, it would indicate that hydration is taking place. If the animal has not yet received treatment with a solution containing glucose and glucose is found in the urine, it is possible that diabetic acidosis is the cause of the dehydration. The urine glucose should also be monitored during treatment. If the animal is receiving glucose and the urine glucose reaches +3 or +4, the dosage must be lowered. Acetone in the urine is a frequent finding during dehydration and/or carbohydrate starvation. If the pH of the urine, in species with normally acid urine, tests alkaline, a diagnosis of alkalosis may be indicated, provided no kidney nor urinary tract disease is present. Presence of urinary albumin and sediment may be an indication of renal disease. If the kidneys are functioning properly, they can adjust markedly to insult. However, in the presence of renal impairment, therapy must be specific or it may be fatal.

Laboratory examination of the blood should include a hematocrit, plasma CO_2 combining power (bicarbonate), serum CL^-, serum Na^+, blood urea nitrogen (BUN), and creatinine determinations. The hematocrit is an indicator for the state of hydration and an estimate of blood volume. This test is important initially but is even more essential as a monitor of the effectiveness of therapy. When the degree of hydration is increasing, the hematocrit should decrease. If hydration increases and the hematocrit decreases below normal, blood therapy must be considered. If the animal is in critical condition, monitoring the arterial pH, P_{O_2}, and P_{CO_2} must be considered essential to proper handling of the case. If readily available, serum levels of K^+, Ca^{++}, Mg^{++}, HPO_4^-, $SO_4^=$ organic acid, and plasma protein may be very useful in the management of the animal.

FLUIDS TO BE USED

By using the history, clinical signs, and laboratory examinations just described, the need for fluid and/or electrolyte therapy may be determined. The type of solution used is dictated by these same considerations. Table 26.1 gives examples of commonly used fluids. Good management is aimed at treating the specific condition as it exists and adjusting the treatment as necessary. Various disease states dictate different types of treatment. Some commonly encountered situations and the appropriate treatment for each are discussed next.

TABLE 26.1. Composition of and formula for solutions commonly used in fluid therapy

	Na	K	Cl	HCO_3 (or lactate)
1. Normal plasma	140	4.0	100	24
2. 5% Dextrose	0	0	0	0
3. Ringer's solution:				
6.0 g NaCl	103		103	
0.3 g KCl		4	4	
0.22 g $CaCl_2$			6	
distilled water, q.s. 1 L				
	103	4	113	0
Alkalinizing solutions:				
4. Lactated Ringer's solution:				
6.0 g NaCl	103		103	
0.3 g KCl		4	4	
0.22 g $CaCl_2$			6	
5.0 ml 60% sodium lactate (Merck #5082)	27			27
distilled water, q.s. 1 L				
	130	4	113	27
5. 1.3% $NaHCO_3$:				
13.0 g $NaHCO_3$	155			155
distilled water, q.s. 1 L				
6. High Na^+, high K^+ solution:				
1 L lactated Ringer's	130	4	113	27
1 g KCl		14	14	
5 g $NaHCO_3$	60			60
	190	18	127	87
7. High Na^+ solution:				
1 L lactated Ringer's	130	4	113	27
5 g $NaHCO_3$	60			60
	190	4	113	87
Acidifying solutions:				
8. Isotonic saline:				
8.9 g NaCl	154		154	
distilled water, q.s. 1 L				
9. 1.9% NH_4Cl (hypotonic):				
19 g NH_4Cl			71	
distilled water, q.s. 1 L				
10. High K^+ solution:				
1 L isotonic saline	154		154	
2.5 g KCl		34	34	
	154	34	188	0
Spiking products:				
11. (each 1 g adds)				
$NaHCO_3$	12			12
KCl		14	14	
NH_4Cl			19	
$CaCl_2$			18	

Note: Electrolytes are expressed as mEq/L, approximates.

Fig. 26.2 depicts the changes that occur in plasma electrolytes with a theoretically "pure" state of metabolic acidosis (an excess of H^+ and characterized by a deficit of HCO_3^- in the ECF). This condition may be associated with (1) extreme diarrhea, causing a loss of $NaHCO_3$ via the digestive juices; (2) ketosis, associated with diabetes mellitis or starvation; (3) renal insufficiency; (4) chemical and drug poisonings such as an excess of NaCl solution, NH_4Cl excess, and thallium poisoning; (5) severe infectious disease; (6) shock; and (7) congestive heart failure.

The clinical signs most commonly associated with metabolic acidosis are hyperpnea and CNS depression. Laboratory analysis of blood and urine reveals a lowered urine pH, lowered blood pH, decreased serum HCO_3^- (<20 mEq/L), and a variable serum Cl^-.

The pathogenesis of this condition is that ketones and excess Cl^- replace HCO_3^-, thus lowering the pH. Various disease states that cause renal failure result in additional acid buildup since the kidney is unable to excrete and a positive feedback cycle is initiated. The compensatory mechanisms for metabolic acidosis include hyperactive respiration to remove H_2CO_3 and the kidneys' ability to save HCO_3^- and excrete H^+.

Therapy for metabolic acidosis should include $NaHCO_3$ (1 mEq/lb/15 minutes of treatment); Na lactate (1/6 molar), which is metabolized in the liver to form HCO_3^-; lactated Ringer's solution; Na gluconate; or some other supply of HCO_3^-.

Metabolic alkalosis (Fig. 26.2) is characterized by an excess of HCO_3^- due to a deficit in the ECF of H^+. This state may be caused by (1) excessive vomiting, especially when due to gastrointestinal (GI) obstruction; (2) excessive alkaline therapy or use of diuretics that can create iatrogenic metabolic alkalosis; or (3) excessive loss of potassium due to hyperadrenal corticoidism or the administration of large quantities of K^+-free solutions. Clinical signs of metabolic alkalosis are depressed breathing

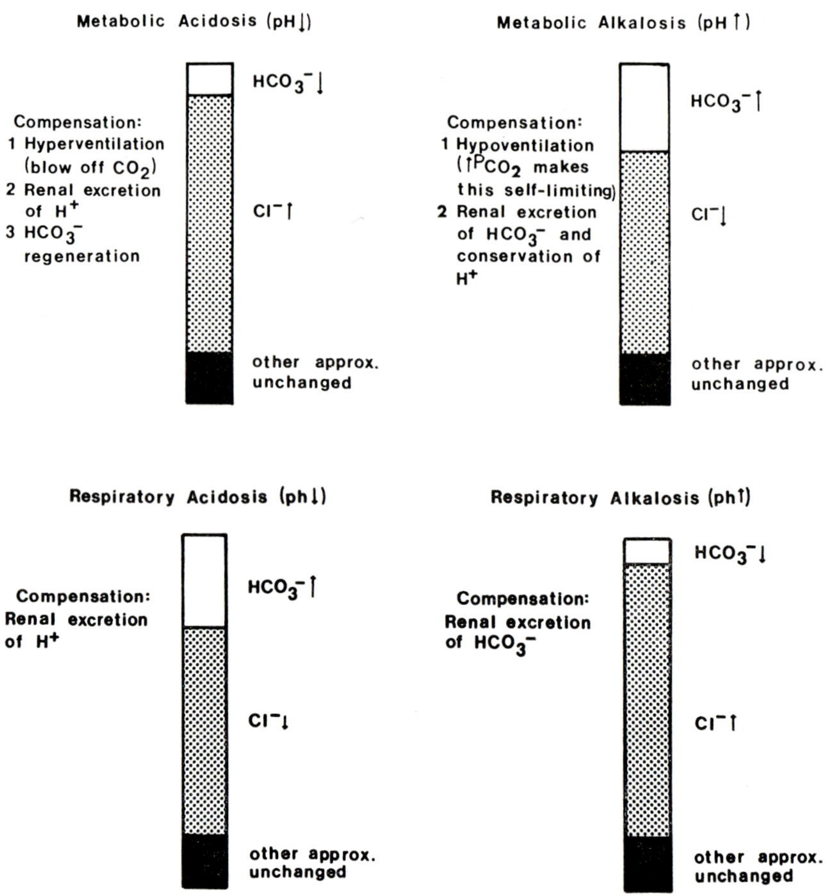

FIG. 26.2. Plasma electrolytes in acidosis and alkalosis as they occur in "theoretically pure" conditions.

(slow and shallow), nervous excitement including tetany, and even convulsions and muscular hypertonicity. The respiratory compensation is relatively ineffective.

Values for serum electrolytes usually reveal an elevated HCO_3^-, lowered Cl^-, and a variable Na^+. There is usually a low serum K^+ in this condition and a peculiar relationship exists between K^+ loss and metabolic alkalosis. Each can result in the other (positive feedback). In ruminants the situation is much more complex and metabolic alkalosis is much more common. The compensatory mechanism requires the kidneys to excrete HCO_3^- and retain H^+.

Therapy for metabolic alkalosis involves the use of acidifying solutions: NaCl (0.9%); NH_4Cl (1.9%) (NH_4^+ is conjugated to urea in the liver which frees the Cl^-); Ringer's solution (without lactate), which supplies Na^+, K^+, Ca^{++}, and Cl^- (the Cl^- is in demand).

Respiratory acidosis (Fig. 26.2) involves the retention of CO_2 as a consequence of alveolar hypoventilation. The fall in pH is predictable from the Henderson-Hasselbalch equation. Impaired respiration can be caused by pneumonia, pulmonary edema, emphysema, pneumothorax, respiratory muscle paralysis, morphine or barbiturate poisoning, or airway occlusion.

Clinical signs include respiratory distress; CNS depression with progressive disorientation, weakness, and finally coma

(CO_2 narcosis); and cyanosis in the advanced stages. Laboratory analysis of blood and urine will show a decreased urine pH, decreased blood pH, increased serum HCO_3^- (due to tissue buffers and renal reabsorption of HCO_3^-), and a decrease in serum Cl^- because of renal excretion. The pathogenesis is the hypoventilation resulting in CO_2 retention and excess of H_2CO_3 and thereby excess H^+, while the compensatory mechanism is for the kidneys to conserve HCO_3^- and excrete H^+.

Treatment for this condition involves, most importantly, proper ventilation of the animal. The use of alkalyzing solutions (to increase the pH) may aid in cases of lung disease when ventilation alone will not correct the condition. Whenever possible, therapy should be directed at the removal of the causative factor. Also, Na lactate, $NaHCO_3$, Na gluconate, or other HCO_3^- donators may be used.

Respiratory alkalosis, a deficiency of H_2CO_3 and thereby H^+, is depicted in Fig. 26.2. The causes of this disease are fever, stimulation of respiratory centers by encephalitis, salicylate intoxication, a deficiency of O_2 (hypoxia), heat prostration, hysteria, or a host of conditions causing chronic hyperventilation (excessive "blowing off" of CO_2).

Clinical signs include hyperpnea (with or without panting), hyperactive tendon reflexes, and CNS stimulation with or without convulsions. Laboratory analysis reveals increased urine pH, increased blood pH, decreased serum HCO_3^-, and serum Cl^- normal to slightly increased. The pathogenesis is the excessive "blowing off" of CO_2. The compensatory mechanism depends on the kidneys for excretion of HCO_3^- and retention of H^+.

Treatment for this condition should involve the same acidifying solutions as used for metabolic alkalosis: NaCl, NH_4Cl, or Ringer's solution. The underlying etiological factors also must be eliminated.

The preceding discussion of acidosis and alkalosis has purposely dealt with single etiologic processes in the genesis of acid-base abnormalities in the "pure" sense. Such states rarely exist in "real life." Mixed disturbances occur much more frequently and treatment will often convert one type of acid-base disturbance into another type. With careful appraisal of repeated laboratory determinations and close observation of the clinical situation, these mixed disturbances can be identified, evaluated, and managed successfully.

The most conservative fluid therapy consists of using a "balanced" electrolyte solution. This fluid should be incapable of inducing abnormalities in the patient and should be isotonic. Since bicarbonate cannot be autoclaved, most commercial solutions do not contain this substance. Lactate or acetate ions are metabolized by the liver to bicarbonate and these substances are usually incorporated commercially. Obviously, if substantial liver disease exists, these compounds are not easily converted and their beneficial effects are not realized. The conservative approach is indicated when there are no particular electrolyte disturbances or when there is no way to determine which, if any, electrolyte imbalance exists. Use of such a balanced solution is not an effective means of correcting severe acidosis, alkalosis, hyponatremia, or hypokalemia.

When metabolic acidosis is present, an unphysiologically high concentration of bicarbonate must be given. When additional sodium is also required a very useful solution is obtained by adding 3–5 g of sodium bicarbonate to each L of lactated Ringer's solution. Nearly pure sodium bicarbonate can be purchased in bulk from a laboratory supply house. The powder can then be measured into 3- and 5-g individual packets. These packets can be gas sterilized. Most human hospitals now have access to gas sterilization. The packets can then be stored until needed. If the sodium value is not abnormally low, the fluid given should be high in bicarbonate but not abnormally high in Na^+. In this case, a slightly hypertonic solution of sodium bicarbonate (1.3%, approximately 300 mOsm) can be made by adding sterile distilled water (q.s. to 1 L) to 13 g of sterile sodium bicarbonate powder. If it is impossible to monitor the patient, a crude estimate of the amount of bicarbonate needed can be made. An animal in severe acidosis will usually have bicarbonate levels of 10–15 mEq/L. Normal bicarbonate levels for most species vary between 20 and 30 mEq/L. Therefore, animals in acidosis will have deficits of about 10–15 mEq/L of ECF. Since the ECF is about 20% of the body weight, it is possible to calculate the volume of ECF for each case. The number of mEq of bicarbonate needed is calculated by multiplying the bicarbonate deficit by the ECF volume.

Example A: a 450-kg horse with estimated bicarbonate deficit of 10 mEq/L ECF; 450 kg × 20% × 10 mEq/L = 900 mEq needed.

Example B: a 20-kg dog with estimated bicarbonate deficit of 10 mEq/L ECF; 20 kg × 20% × 10 mEq/L = 40 mEq needed.

In cases of severe acidosis associated with anesthesia, surgery, and/or shock, it may be desirable to administer a bolus of sodium bicarbonate. Commercial solutions containing 1 mEq/ml are available or a solution of this concentration can be made by mixing 84 g of gas-sterilized sodium bicarbonate q.s. to 1000 ml with sterile water. This solution should be given at the rate of 1 mEq/lb every 15 minutes as needed. The solution should be injected intravenously at the rate of approximately 10 ml/minute.

Horses present some special problems in acid-base management. In cases of severe diarrhea, shock, and intestinal obstruction, the horse seems predisposed to rather severe metabolic acidosis. Respiratory acidosis is a very common sequela to closed-circuit inhalation anesthesia in the horse. An abnormally low sodium concentration is also a common problem in dehydrated horses. Severe hypokalemia, with blood potassium values less than 2.5–3 mEq/L, may require treatment with high potassium solutions. Dangerous hyperkalemia, with blood levels greater than 6–7 mEq/L may be associated with acidosis in foals. Prompt correction of the acidosis will usually correct the hyperkalemia.

Ruminants also present special fluid and electrolyte management problems. When a diagnosis of abomasal disease is coupled with an obvious fluid balance disorder, usually hypochloremia, hypokalemia, and alkalosis are present. These should be confirmed by appropriate laboratory tests. Grain overloading will result in severe dehydration and metabolic acidosis. Calf diarrhea also results in severe dehydration and metabolic acidosis with dangerous hyperkalemia in some cases. If hyperkalemia exists, one should guard against the administration of even more potassium.

When dealing with herbivores, it is important to remember that normal feed contains high levels of potassium. When these animals are anorexic, they frequently become potassium depleted. The best way to replace potassium deficits is by consumption of hay or grass, but potassium must be added parenterally when the situation dictates.

Special problems in fluid and electrolyte management for all species are presented by heat exhaustion, heat prostration, and burns. Heat exhaustion is due to an excessive loss of Na^+. The compensatory reaction of the body is to pass K^+ from the intracellular fluid (ICF) to the ECF to replace the lost Na^+. Renal excretion of Na^+ ceases but water excretion continues. Heat prostration, on the other hand, involves the loss of both Na^+ and Cl^-. There is usually an associated respiratory alkalosis due to hyperventilation. In these conditions, the clinician must continuously monitor the patient, using the indicated laboratory tests, and correct the disturbances as they exist. With burns, relatively more electrolyte than water is lost. The end result is a hypotonic dehydration of the ECF. With the loss of ECF electrolytes, fluid moves into cells, causing swelling and edema. The latest forms of therapy involve the use of hypertonic electrolytes that replace Na^+ (usually NaCl). The goal of this therapy is a gradual restoration of ECF volume by replacing the electrolytes and draining water out of the cells (Monajo et al. 1973).

HOW MUCH FLUID TO USE

The calculation of how much fluid to use must be based on a total of the normal turnover of water plus replacement of the abnormal losses. The average resting animal at standard conditions of humidity and temperature has a rather constant rate of water turnover. Obviously, these requirements must be adjusted according to prevailing conditions. We can use, for practical purposes, 65 ml/kg/24 hours average water turnover for mature animals and 130 ml/kg/24 hours for immature animals of all species. From these assumptions, an average mature dog weighing 44 lb (approximately 20 kg) requires about 1300 ml for a daily maintenance supply of water. A horse weighing 1000 lb (approximately 445 kg) would require about 29 L/day.

The replacement of abnormal losses must be in addition to the maintenance requirements. To calculate this quantity, one must estimate the degree of dehydration present. This is accomplished by application of the following guidelines.

An animal with 4% dehydration (mild or no evidence of clinical dehydration) will have a history of fluid loss (vomiting, diarrhea), the skin will be slightly leathery, the mucous membranes will still be moist, and there will be evidence of a history of thirst. These signs dictate the replacement of water to 4% of body weight, i.e., a 20-kg dog = 0.8 L (800 ml).

With a 6% dehydration (moderate) level, the animal's skin will be leathery. When the skin is picked up, or lifted, it will peak but will return to normal slowly; the hair coat will be dull and the mucous membranes dry but the tongue will still be moist. In this case, fluid replacement to 6% of the body weight for a 20-kg dog = 1.2 L (1200 ml).

Animals with severe dehydration, i.e., 8% dehydration, will show a lack of skin pliability and elasticity. When picked up, the skin will peak and stay, both the mucous membranes and tongue will be dry, and the eyeballs will be soft and sunken. These animals require replacement of water to 8% of body weight, i.e., a 20-kg dog = 1.6 L (1600 ml).

Circulatory insufficiency is the severe extension of the dehydration syndrome. All the classical signs of a circulatory collapse are evidenced. Water is replaced up to 12% of body weight, i.e., a 20-kg dog = 2.4 L (2400 ml). In classical signs of acute shock, water is replaced up to 15% of the body weight, i.e., a 20-kg dog = 3 L (3000 ml).

If the animal being treated continues to lose water during the treatment period, this additional amount must be estimated and added to the replacement and maintenance figures.

Example A: a 2-month-old, 20-kg St. Bernard, 6% dehydrated clinically, is losing approximately 120 ml of water a day while undergoing treatment for a rather severe diarrhea. This animal needs:

1. Maintenance
   130 ml/kg × 20 kg — 2600 ml
2. Replacement
   0.06 × 20 kg = 1.2 L or 1200 ml
3. Continuing loss = 120 ml

Total fluid required over the first 24 hours = 3920 ml

Example B: a mature 450-kg horse with severe obstructive colic and 8% dehydration clinically is presented. This animal needs:

1. Maintenance
   65 ml/kg × 450 kg = 29,250 ml
2. Replacement
   0.08 × 450 kg = 36 L or 36,000 ml

Total during the first 24 hours = 62,250 ml

Additional circumstances that must be considered are:

1. Dehydration affects young animals much faster than adults.
2. Old patients with chronic diseases (especially impaired renal function) require more water than other animals.
3. Animals need more fluids if they are very active or if the weather is hot and/or humid.
4. Drugs, such as corticosteroids and diuretics, will alter fluid and electrolyte requirements.

5. Animals that have been under various forms of anesthesia may require additional water for a few days.

RATE OF ADMINISTRATION

The rate of fluid and/or electrolyte replacement should parallel the severity of dehydration. Fluids should be administered rapidly at first and then at decreasing rates until the condition is corrected. A general guideline for the intravenous route is to administer fluids at the rate of 13–14 ml/kg/hour (6 ml/lb/hour) until urine flow is restored or for the first 40–60 minutes. After urine flow is established, the rate is reduced to about 10 ml/kg/hour. If urine is not voided by 60 minutes, it is appropriate to reduce the rate by approximately one-third, i.e., to 9 ml/kg/hour (approximately 4 ml/lb/hour). Table 26.2 gives examples of rates of intravenous fluid administration. A 20–kg dog, from the previous criteria, should receive approximately 275 ml for the first hour, approximately 180 ml for the next hour, and then the amount is gradually decreased. A 450-kg horse would require about 6 L in the first hour and about 4 L/hour after that. It would require almost 14 hours of continuous therapy to administer all the fluid to the horse in Example B above. Also, note that a kitten weighing 1 kg should not be given more than 13–14 ml/hour intravenously at this rate (Table 26.2).

In the administration of fluids, common sense and clinical judgment must be exercised. If an animal is severely dehydrated and in shock, it is almost impossible to administer the fluids too fast. If, however, an animal is almost normally hydrated and the aim is only to maintain hydration, the rate should be slowed considerably. The importance of renal function has been repeatedly emphasized. A commonly used method of determining if

TABLE 26.2. Approximate rates of intravenous fluid administration, based upon body weight

Animal Weight	First Hour	Second and Subsequent Hours with Good Urine Flow	Second Hour without Urine Flow	Third Hour without Urine Flow	Fourth and Subsequent Hours without Urine Flow*
(kg)	*(ml/hr)*	*(ml/hr)*	*(ml/hr)*	*(ml/hr)*	*(ml/hr)*
1	14	12–10	9	5	2
5	70	60–50	45	25	10
10	140	120–100	90	50	20
15	210	180–150	135	75	30
20	280	240–200	180	100	40
25	350	300–250	225	125	50
30	420	360–300	270	150	60
35	490	420–350	315	175	70
40	560	480–400	360	200	80
45	630	540–450	405	225	90
50	700	600–500	450	250	100
60	840	720–600	540	300	120
70	980	840–700	630	350	140
80	1120	960–800	720	400	160
90	1260	1080–900	810	450	180
100	1400	1200–1000	900	500	200
125	1750	1500–1250	1125	625	250
150	2100	1800–1500	1350	750	300
175	2450	2100–1750	1575	875	350
200	2800	2400–2000	1800	1000	400
250	3500	3000–2500	2250	1250	500
300	4200	3600–3000	2700	1500	600
350	4900	4200–3500	3150	1750	700
400	5600	4800–4000	3600	2000	800
450	6300	5400–4500	4050	2250	900
500	7000	6000–5000	4500	2500	1000

* Every attempt must be made to establish renal function if no urine flow is detected.

the kidneys are capable of functioning is to inject a small bolus (1–25 ml, depending on the size of the animal) of 50% glucose. The urine is then checked every 5 minutes for the presence of glucose. The presence of glucose indicates glomerular filtration is occurring.

ROUTE OF ADMINISTRATION

The route of fluid administration depends on (1) the type of illness being dealt with and the severity of the condition, (2) degree of dehydration, (3) the condition of the patient, (4) the type of electrolyte imbalance, (5) the organic functions of the patient, and (6) the time and equipment available.

Probably the easiest, most physiologic, and the most overlooked route of administration of fluid and electrolytes is the oral or nasogastric route. The oral route is the least dangerous since the solution can be administered without strict attention to tonicity, volume, and asepsis.

A relatively unused route of administration that might be considered, especially in very young animals, is per rectum. Warm water, K^+, Na^+, and Cl^- are well absorbed via this route. It may be difficult, however, to get the animal to retain material given in this manner, especially with GI disease.

The most commonly used and perhaps most practical routes of fluid and electrolyte administration are the parenteral routes: intravenous, subcutaneous, or intraperitoneal.

The intravenous route is the most versatile. Severe disturbances of fluid and electrolyte balance demand this route. Nearly all the toxicity of solutions administered in this manner is more related to the rate of administration than the volume administered or its composition. To date no indications for hypotonic solutions have been found, but many indications for isotonic and hypertonic solutions exist. Some of the problems associated with intravenous administration include those associated with maintenance and asepsis of indwelling catheters, clotting, and hematomas, as well as the location of a vein on very small or very ill animals. Obviously, both the fluids administered and the equipment used must be sterile. Large volumes of fluid administered rapidly may overload the circulatory system, causing pulmonary edema and even death. However, the intravenous route is preferred for blood, blood plasma, and plasma volume expanders.

The subcutaneous route is often overlooked. The technique is known as hypodermoclysis. In human beings the technique is not commonly used because it causes subcutaneous hematomas and is very painful; the solutions are, for the most part, poorly absorbed; and the risk of infection is great. In large animals the technique is not used because of the huge volumes of fluids that must be administered. For small animals none of these drawbacks exist. The technique is rapid and easy to use. Fluids are absorbed more slowly than by the intravenous route. If the animal is not in critical condition, this is of no real consequence. Only *isotonic* solutions should be used in this manner. Dextrose of any tonicity or any solutions lacking electrolytes in isotonic levels are contraindicated; they may produce a rapid diffusion of major extracellular electrolytes to the area initially causing additional problems, including death, if the animal is in severe shock.

Hypodermoclysis is extremely valuable in very young or very small animals. If the animal is difficult to restrain long enough for a prolonged intravenous infusion, this is a useful technique. Although hyaluronidase is sometimes recommended to aid absorption with hypodermoclysis, its use is unnecessary in animals. When edema is present, absorption will not occur and this route of administration is contraindicated. If the animal is chilled by a cold environment or by injection of a cold fluid, absorption by this route will be delayed.

Intraperitoneal infusion of fluids has the same restrictions as those in effect for hypodermoclysis. This technique may predispose to peritonitis; aseptic procedures must be used. It is faster than subcutaneous administration and is potentially more hazardous (puncture of abdominal organs). Nevertheless, this is a good route for electrolyte and water absorption. Plasma and a large percentage of red blood cells can be absorbed in this manner; in large animals it can be a very practical method of treatment since a large quantity of fluid can be administered rapidly with few adverse effects. Perhaps the greatest application of this technique is in peritoneal lavage.

EVALUATION OF TREATMENT

The only effective method for evaluation of the success of fluid therapy is the application of clinical judgment and experience. One must observe a return to normalcy of the clinical signs presented by the patient and a return to normal of the various physiological parameters being monitored.

REFERENCES

Eliel, L. P.; Pearson, D. H.; and White, F. C. 1952. Postoperative potassium deficit and metabolic alkalosis: The pathogenic significance of operative trauma and of potassium and phosphorus deprivation. J Clin Domest 31:419.

Monajo, W. W.; Chuntrasakul, C.; and Aynazian, V. H. Dec. 1973. Hypertonic sodium solutions in the treatment of burn shock. Am J Surg 126:778.

CHAPTER 27

TRANSFUSIONS AND OTHER SPECIAL CONSIDERATIONS

DAVID R. GROSS and J. D. McCRADY

WHOLE BLOOD AND PLASMA

Use of whole blood, blood plasma, and blood serum occupies an important place in veterinary therapy. Four major indications for whole blood therapy include (1) hemorrhage or shock, (2) anemia, (3) coagulation abnormalities, and (4) the provision of specific and nonspecific antibodies. Whole blood is also known to supply substances of metabolic benefit.

Donor Selection

Although five isoantibodies have been demonstrated in blood serums of transfused dogs (Young et al. 1952), the only known blood factor causing transfusion reactions of clinical significance is the A factor. Approximately 63% of all dogs seem to be positive for factor A and 37% negative. Unless the practitioner is able to type each donor and recipient before transfusion, it is desirable to keep A-negative donor dogs (universal donors) that have never received a transfusion. Blood from these animals can be given safely to any other dog, whereas A-positive blood can be given only to A-positive recipients (Thornton 1974).

Although A-negative donors are the most desirable, finding them may be difficult. Interpretation of blood types requires a technician with training and experience. The inexperienced clinician is not likely to be able to make the readings that are necessary. In addition, serum for typing dogs for the A factor is almost impossible to obtain. The best sources for this serum are large research facilities or large institutional hospitals with well-managed laboratory animal facilities. Serum for typing human blood is not adequate for dogs.

Cross matching is of limited value in dogs since an incompatible recipient will not be detected unless it or the donor has previously had a transfusion with incompatible blood. Confusing results are often obtained with cross matching since blood factors other than A cause production of antibodies easily detected with this technique. These other factors are apparently not important in transfusion incompatibilities. From a practical standpoint, however, cross matching will prevent the use of incompatible types and is essential when repeated transfusions from unknown donors are used.

The dangers in using A-positive blood for an A-negative recipient are (1) delayed destruction of the transfused cells, 7–10 days following the first transfusion, (2) sensitization of the animal to subsequent transfusions of A-positive blood, (3) immediate transfusion reaction if the recipient has been previously sensitized, and (4) hemolytic disease in A-positive pups from an A-positive sire and A-negative bitch transfused with A-positive blood. This can be avoided if the pups are not allowed to suckle during the first 24 hours of life.

There is little information on blood typing in cats. It appears that most cats have the same blood type but complications after single or repeated transfusions have been experienced by many clinicians. For practical purposes, blood usually will be used in emergency situations only and rarely more than once. The likelihood of experiencing a transfusion reaction under these circumstances is greatly reduced. Cross matching in cats has been difficult at best but should be used if repeated transfusions are indicated.

First blood transfusions of incompatible blood will seldom cause severe illness or death in horses. Hemolysis occurs, due to the incompatibility, and the spleen, liver, and reticuloendothelial system may be stressed in removing the lysed blood cells and hemoglobin. With extensive hemolysis, lower nephron nephrosis may occur. The second and subsequent transfusions of incompatible blood are more likely to cause serious reactions. If the transfusion history of either the donor or recipient is unknown, cross matching should be done. Cross matching should always be done before giving a transfusion to foals with hemolytic icterus. It should also be done before giving blood, especially repeated transfusions, to a mare that may be used for future breeding. Introduction of reactive cells into a mare will cause her to produce antibodies and may increase her chances of producing a foal with hemolytic icterus. A mare who has produced a foal with hemolytic icterus probably already has antibodies and therefore has a much greater chance for a transfusion reaction. Antibodies can also develop following the administration of equine tissue origin vaccines. If cross matching is impossible, it may be safer to use donors from different breeds or bloodlines to minimize the risk of reaction.

Hemolytic reactions have been reported in cattle (Ferguson 1947), swine (Bruner et al. 1949), and most other species. This would indicate that blood groupings probably exist in all animals.

Cross-Matching Technique

Blood samples are collected from both the recipient and donor and allowed to clot. The serum is removed from each tube and labeled. A suspension of erythrocytes from each animal is made by resuspending cells from the clot in several ml of saline. The cell suspension should be the consistency of thin tomato juice. One drop of donor cell suspension is mixed with 2 drops of recipient serum (major test). One drop of recipient cell suspension is mixed with 2 drops of donor serum (minor test). The tubes are incubated 5–8 minutes at 37° F in a water bath or for 30 minutes at room temperature. The tubes are then centrifuged at 1000 rpm for 1 minute. The cells are then resuspended by jarring the tubes sharply against the hand or flipping with a finger. A strong agglutination can be detected macroscopically. A drop of the contents is placed on a microscope slide without a coverslip and examined at a magnification of 100. Results are reported as strong, weak, or negative agglutination. If there is doubt that agglutination has occurred, the slide is rotated from side to side for a few minutes. If agglutination is occurring, it will become stronger; if not, any clumps that have formed will break up.

Blood Collection

Direct transfusions are usually unsatisfactory in veterinary medicine for two reasons: lack of patient cooperation and clotting in the collection and/or administration apparatus. The general technique of collection is the same whether the blood is to be stored or used directly. Commercially available collection equipment with disposable evacuated bottles containing ACD solution is available and is practical for small animal use. In cats, blood may be drawn directly into a syringe with heparin and injected into the recipient after cross matching. Blood with heparin cannot be stored for more than a few hours. Collection bottles should be stored in the refrigerator before collection to reduce initial hemolysis and they must be rotated gently during the entire collection period. For all species, blood should be collected under sterile conditions. For large animals, 1-gal containers can be autoclaved and partially filled with 400 ml of a 4% solution of sodium citrate (40 g sodium citrate q.s. to 1 L sterile water). Blood can be collected by gravity flow from the jugular vein through a 10-gauge needle in larger species or the collection can be speeded with the use of a suction device.

Collected blood should be stored in the refrigerator at a temperature of 42°–44° F. Dog blood can be stored safely for 21 days; however, it is best to remove the plasma for future use after 16 days. Cat blood is usually collected only as needed, as are horse and cattle blood.

Plasma can be aspirated from the top of a stored container of blood after at least 12 hours in the refrigerator to allow for good separation. The plasma can then be stored in the refrigerator for several months or frozen and kept for as long as 2 years. All containers should be adequately identified.

ADMINISTRATION AND DOSAGE

Inexpensive, sterile, disposable equipment is commercially available for transfusion purposes. Filter-type transfusion apparatus is available in a variety of designs; use of this type of equipment is encouraged. The speed of administration is best controlled by the gauge of the needle or catheter through which the blood or plasma is administered and the height of the supply bottle above the site of injection. Devices that force the blood in more rapidly, by positive pressure, are potentially dangerous. It is felt that a venous cutdown and insertion of a larger bore cannula is a much preferred method if a more rapid injection rate is indicated.

The rate of administration is determined by the severity of the signs and the calculated dose. A large animal may be able to handle rates of 40–60 ml/minute or more in a case of severe shock, whereas a 10-kg dog or a 5-kg cat could probably not tolerate a rate much above 5–10 ml/minute. Again, there is no substitute for good clinical judgment. The usual recommended dose of blood or plasma is 10–20 ml/kg of body weight, depending on the severity of the condition. At this dose, a 450-kg mature horse will require a minimum of 4.5 L of blood.

Interspecies Transfusions

It is known that 50% of the transfused canine red blood cells (RBCs) are destroyed in the cat within 6 hours after injection (Thornton 1974). There is no reason to believe that this phenomenon does not occur in other species as well. The hemolyzed cells are not beneficial to the animal and cause additional problems in excretion of the breakdown products by already stressed liver and kidneys. More than one transfusion of blood from one species into another may cause severe anaphylactic reaction and death.

PLASMA VOLUME EXPANDERS

It has been assumed that plasma itself is an ideal expander of blood volume in shock therapy because it is well retained in the vascular space. Studies in dogs and human beings indicate that this is not the case where heterologous plasma transfusions are used. In the dog only 50% of heterologous plasma is retained in the vascular space, whereas homologous plasma is completely retained. Incomplete retention is frequently accompanied by urticaria, which may be prevented by the use of antihistamines or corticosteroids (Bliss et al. 1959).

Artificial plasma volume expanders are generally considered to be somewhat inferior to plasma itself. The two most commonly used agents in veterinary medicine are dextran and gelatin.

Dextran is a polysaccharide obtained by bacterial fermentation of sucrose. It is administered intravenously as a 6% solution in physiological saline. Approximately 50% is excreted by the kidney within the first 24 hours; the remainder traverses the capillary wall very slowly and is oxidized within a few weeks. Dextran appears to have no significant deleterious effects on renal, hepatic, or other vital functions but does have some antigenic action that may result in mild pruritus, urticaria, joint pain, and other minor side effects.

Sterile gelatin solutions are also available for use as infusion colloids. These agents are excreted rapidly by the kidneys, which may produce extra stress for that organ. The use of these agents is not recommended for animals with renal disease. Gelatin is antigenic and minor allergic type reactions occur following its use in some animals.

A wide variety of other artificial plasma volume expanders have been used experimentally and clinically but none of these is currently recommended for veterinary use.

PARENTERAL ALIMENTATION

The first continuous intravenous delivery technique for long-term administration of nutrients was employed in dogs (Rhode et al. 1949a,b); however, this technique was used clinically in human medicine before it was used in veterinary medicine. Indications for this type of therapy include a wide variety of gastrointestinal (GI) diseases that preclude the administration of nutrients orally. This technique is especially useful in inflammatory lesions of the bowel requiring healing time that can be gained only by placing the gut completely at rest. Hypermetabolic states associated with extensive burns, severe infections, or multiple injuries all respond to this therapy.

Meticulous care of an indwelling central venous catheter is essential to safe long-term parenteral feeding. The catheter tip must extend into the anterior vena cava or even the right atrium, a region of high velocity and high flow. The size of the catheter will depend on the size and dose requirements of the animal to be maintained. In very small animals a jugular vein cutdown will be necessary and the catheter should be exteriorized through a subcutaneous tunnel to a point on the dorsal aspect of the neck or between the scapulae. Catheter placement must be done under aseptic conditions. Withdrawal or administration of blood through the catheter should be avoided since blood in the lumen is more likely to increase the possibilities of contamination, sludging, or clotting.

The ideal solution for parenteral alimentation should contain the same nutrients as a well-balanced oral diet. It seems to make little difference whether the required calories are given as fat, alcohol, or carbohydrates, but at least 150 calories must be supplied for each g of nitrogen infused. At the present time, fat emulsions and alcohols are being used on a trial basis in the United States but hypertonic glucose in the presence of adequate insulin seems to offer the most inexpensive and practical caloric source at present. Nitrogen is usually supplied as protein hydrolysates from enzymatic hydrolysis of casein or acid hydrolysis of fibrin. These solutions provide about two-thirds of the available nitrogen as amino acids and one-third as dipeptides and tripeptides. When combined with sufficient calories, minerals, and vitamins, these hydrolysates are capable of supplying the necessary substrates for protein synthesis (Dudrick et al. 1970).

Alimentation solutions cannot be autoclaved because of caramelization at elevated temperatures. However, most large hospital pharmacies are equipped to prepare these solutions using a laminar-flow filtered-air hood for mixing and a small micropore membrane filter for sterilization. For adult animals the following formula has been practical: 250 ml of 5% glucose, 500 ml of 5% fibrin hydrolysate, plus 350 ml of 50% glucose. The resulting 1100 ml of solution contains 5.25 g of nitrogen, 212 g of glucose, 7 mEq of sodium, 13 mEq of potassium, and approximately 1000 calories. To this basic solution are added 50 mEq of NaCl (2.93 g) and 40 mEq of KCl

(2.98 g). Multivitamins containing both fat-soluble and water-soluble vitamins are added according to the calculated dose for each individual animal. Vitamin B_{12}, folic acid, and vitamin K are also added to the solution. Calcium gluconate and potassium acid phosphate are added to supply extra calcium and phosphorus if blood chemistry studies indicate they are needed. Iron is usually supplied as iron dextran intramuscularly. Immature animals may require higher concentrations of glucose, vitamins, and minerals for maintenance.

For maximum metabolic benefit and safety, the alimentation solution must be infused into a large-diameter, high-flow vein at a constant rate for 24 hours every day or until clinical improvement occurs. To accomplish this, a peristaltic or roller type constant infusion pump is used. A constant infusion rate can be maintained despite fluctuations in central venous pressure. If the alimentation solution is infused not faster than 1.2 g/kg/hour for immature animals and 0.5 g/kg/hour for mature animals, hyperglycemia, glycosuria, diuresis, and dehydration can be prevented. Since each ml of basic solution contains approximately 0.2 g of glucose, a 20-kg adult dog would require a rate of 10 ml/hour. Water requirements must be supplied in addition to the above metabolic requirements.

Relative glucose intolerance often occurs during periods of increased stress and at the onset of this form of therapy. Glucose overload during these periods may cause osmotic diuresis. The urine glucose is therefore monitored closely during parenteral alimentation and the rate of infusion is adjusted to maintain a 3+, or less, urine glucose. As the normal pancreas responds by increasing its output of insulin, the rate of infusion can be gradually increased as needed. If the pancreas is unable to respond, supplementation with exogenous insulin may be indicated.

An abrupt hypoglycemia may occur if parenteral alimentation is stopped suddenly. It is generally recommended that patients be gradually weaned to oral feeding over a 12- to 24-hour period (Sherman et al. 1971). In all species, particularly herbivores, potassium levels must be carefully monitored and supplements given as indicated.

It is strongly recommended that at least every 4–5 days the patient's blood be examined for white blood cell count (WBC), differential blood count, hemoglobin, hematocrit, serum protein, blood urea nitrogen (BUN), blood sugar, and electrolytes. Appropriate adjustments should be made as indicated. In some animals a persistent, and as yet unexplained, anemia will develop. This phenomenon has been observed in experimental animals with indwelling catheters not receiving parenteral alimentation, so it may be a reaction to the catheter.

MISUSE OF ADRENAL HORMONES

At present a bewildering array of corticosteroid compounds is marketed for a wide variety of clinical indications in veterinary medicine. The overzealous use of these agents can easily result in severe water and electrolyte imbalances. In general, corticosteroids, to a greater or lesser degree, depending upon the specific compound, cause a retention of sodium and loss of potassium. Water is retained in conjunction with the sodium. Typically, these animals consume huge quantities of water and suffer abnormal weight gains as a result of water retention. A possibly overlooked aftermath of long-term steroid therapy is that the adrenal cortex is depressed and hypocorticism may develop. This may result in extraordinary loss of sodium and water and a state of hyperkalemia.

PERITONEAL DIALYSIS

As the diagnostic techniques and skills of the veterinary clinician become more sophisticated, there is an increasing awareness of the beneficial effects of special therapeutic techniques such as peritoneal dialysis. During the intraperitoneal administration of fluids for this purpose, the equilibration of a large percentage of solutes between the plasma and dialysate occurs within about 1 hour. By repeating this technique 5–7 times in uremic dogs, Parker et al. (1972) were able to reduce the BUN from 250 to 100 mg%, the plasma creatinine from 15 to 6 mg%, the plasma potassium from 7.9 to 4.8 mEq/L, and to improve significantly existing metabolic acidosis.

The surgical technique for placement of the indwelling catheter deemed necessary for the effective use of this form of therapy has been adequately described (Parker et al. 1972). The prewarmed dialysate fluid can be infused at about 200 ml/minute. After about 1 hour the fluid is withdrawn at the rate of about 60–70 ml/minute.

Commercial solutions for human use can be used in dogs but require the addition of 1 g of NaCl for each L of solution to more nearly equal the increased osmolality of the uremic animal. Each 20 ml of sterile 50% glucose added to a L of stock dialysate solution will increase the osmolality about 50 mOsm. If the osmolality of the dialysate is not greater than that of the animal, plasma water will diffuse rapidly into the system. In an already overhydrated animal, this may cause a water overload and perhaps pulmonary edema. Hypoosmotic dialysates may be used to aid in hydration of the patient. In the latter instance, the recovery of dialysate will be lowered because water will be taken up by the animal. This may be beneficial in initiating a water diuresis. If it is not possible to measure plasma osmolality, adjustments in the dialysate must be made empirically, based on the patient's degree of hydration and the BUN. An increase of 200 mg% in the BUN has been correlated with an approximate 50 mOsm increase in plasma osmolality. Dehydration by itself has not been shown to increase the plasma osmolality significantly, but in the presence of renal disease this may cause significant change. From this discussion it should be obvious that the degree of hydration of the animal must be constantly evaluated while the patient is undergoing repeated dialysis. Initially, the choice of dialysate might be hypoosmotic to aid water diuresis and hydration. After urine flow has been established and the animal well hydrated, an osmotic or perhaps a hyperosmotic solution should be used.

REFERENCES

Bliss, J. Q.; Johns, D. G.; and Burgen, A.S.U. 1959. Transfusion reactions due to plasma incompatibility in dogs. Circ Res 7:79.

Bruner, D. W.; Brown, R. G.; Hull, F. E.; and Kinkaid, A. S. 1949. Blood factors and baby pig anemia. J Am Vet Med Assoc 115:94.

Dudrick, S. J.; Long, J. M.; Steiger, E.; and Rhoads, J. E. 1970. Intravenous hyperalimentation. Med Clin North Am 54:577.

Ferguson, L. C. 1947. The blood groups of cattle. J Am Vet Med Assoc 111:466.

Parker, H. R.; Gourley, I. M.; and Bell, R. L. Sept. 17, 1972. Current developments in peritoneal and hemodialysis. Gaines 22nd Veterinary Symposium, Stillwater, Oklahoma, p. 3.

Rhode, C. M.; Parkins, W.; Tourtellotte, D.; and Vars, H. M. 1949a. Method for continuous intravenous administration of nutritive solutions suitable for prolonged metabolic studies in dogs. Am J Physiol 159:409.

Rhode, C. M.; Parkins, W. M.; and Vars, H. M. 1949b. Nitrogen balances of dogs continuously infused with 50 per cent glucose and protein preparations. Am J Physiol 159:415.

Sherman, J. O.; Egan, T.; and Macalad, F. V. 1971. Parenteral hyperalimentation, a useful surgical adjunct. Surg Clin North Am 51:37.

Thornton, G. W. 1974. Blood transfusions. In Robert W. Kirk, ed. Current Veterinary Therapy, 5th ed., p. 47. Philadephia: W. B. Saunders.

Young, L. E.; O'Brien, W. A.; Swister, S. N.; Miller, G.; and Yuile, C. L. 1952. Blood groups in dogs—Their significance to the veterinarian. Am J Vet Res 13:207.

CHAPTER 28

DRUGS AFFECTING FLUID AND ELECTROLYTE BALANCE

DAVID R. GROSS and J. D. McCRADY

POSTERIOR PITUITARY HORMONES

The neurohypophysis stores and releases neurohumors that have vasoactive, antidiuretic, and oxytocic properties. The material first isolated was separated into two fractions (Kamm et al. 1928). One of the fractions was found to contain most of the vasoactive and antidiuretic portion and was called vasopressin or antidiuretic hormone (ADH). The other fraction was found to act primarily on the myometrium and myoepithelial cells of the mammary gland and was named oxytocin.

The chemical structures of both ADH and oxytocin are known (du Vigneaud et al. 1953 a,b). Both neurohumors contain eight amino acids; however, the structures may vary in different species (see Section 8).

Antidiuretic Hormone

The only clearly established physiological function of *antidiuretic hormone* (vasopressin) is its antidiuretic effect. It requires doses many times larger than the antidiuretic dose to exert any pressor (vasoconstrictor) effects. The use of this agent for its pressor effects is discouraged because of the intense vasoconstriction of the coronary vessels and the profound effects on the renal system caused by the massive doses required.

The antidiuretic action of ADH is exerted on the mechanism of water reabsorption by the distal convoluted tubules and collecting ducts of the kidneys. In physiologic doses, the hormone apparently does not influence electrolyte reabsorption. In larger doses, increased reabsorption of sodium and chloride has been shown, but this is probably an indirect effect.

ADH originates from the paired supraoptic and paraventricular nuclei in the hypothalamus; it is transported down the axoplasm to the posterior lobe of the pituitary gland where it is stored awaiting release. Release is governed by the osmolarity of the extracellular fluid and may be influenced directly by many drugs. Pain and psychic stimuli have been shown to affect the release of ADH. Osmoreceptors located within the hypothalamus are the sensing devices that respond to changes in osmolarity of the extracellular fluid. By these mechanisms, dilution of the extracellular fluid inhibits ADH secretion, whereas hypertonicity promotes ADH release.

Diabetes insipidus is characterized by a lack of ADH and occurs in animals as a result of disease or injury to the hypothalamic and/or posterior pituitary structure. Animals thus afflicted drink copiously and urinate large quantities of dilute urine.

Experiments have shown that injections of acetylcholine or diisopropylfluorophosphate into the supraoptic nuclei cause release of ADH (Pickford 1952). Release of ADH occurs during general anesthesia and following the injection of histamine, morphine, and barbiturates, other than thiopental (Aprahamian et al. 1959). Many other drugs known to alter neural activity or to act as stressful stimuli may influence ADH release. Certain metastic neoplasms and injuries to the head may also be associated with abnormal ADH response.

ADH is marketed in several forms. *Posterior pituitary injectable,* which also contains oxytocin activity, is available. *Vasopressin injectable* (Pitressin), which contains 10 pressor units/ml, and *vasopressin tannate injectable* (Pitressin tannate), a suspension in peanut oil of the insoluble tannate of the hormone (5 pressor units/ml), are also available.

Oxytocin

Oxytocin differs chemically from ADH as previously described. In therapeutic doses, it has no effect on water diuresis but is a potent stimulator of uterine contractions, especially at term and during the immediate postpartum period. It is responsible for milk let-down, due to its effects on the myoepithelial cells of the mammary gland. Its activity is further discussed with the other drugs acting on the uterus (Chapter 32).

ADRENAL STEROIDS

Although the adrenal steroids are discussed in detail elsewhere (Section 8), some of these compounds have significant mineralocorticoid activity and influence fluid and electrolyte balance. Over thirty steroid compounds have been isolated from the adrenal cortex but probably only three of these are significant physiologically: corticosterone, cortisol, and aldosterone.

Aldosterone is the primary mineralocorticoid of the adrenal cortex. Its primary effect is to cause a *retention of sodium* and *excretion of potassium* by the kidney. Aldosterone also influences chloride and hydrogen ion balance. Via this regulation of ion concentration, water is retained or excreted and the circulating volume of the extracellular fluid is regulated.

Adrenalectomized animals will usually die unless given special treatment. Death results from circulatory collapse or severe hyperkalemia. The most widely utilized mineralocorticoid for replacement is desoxycorticosterone acetate (DOCA or DOC), which has less mineralocorticoid activity than aldosterone and is available commercially. DOCA also has some glucocorticoid activity, but additional glucocorticoid must be given to adrenalectomized animals to maintain optimal vigor and resistance to stress.

Many variants of the basic steroid structure are now marketed, primarily for their metabolic and antiinflammatory action. It is important to remember, however, that many of these agents also possess mineralocorticoid, i.e., sodium retention and potassium depletion activity. A comparison of the sodium-retaining activity of some steroids is made in Table 28.1. It can be seen that the 9 α-halogenated steroids have the greatest action in this regard.

DIURETIC AGENTS

General Considerations

The physiological basis of fluid and electrolyte balance is discussed in detail in Chapter 25. The reader is referred to that discussion.

The kidney, acting under both endocrine and neurologic control, has a primary

TABLE 28.1. Comparison of sodium-retaining activity

Steroid	Approximate Retention Activity*
Cortisol	1
Cortisone	0.8
Prednisone	0.8
Prednisolone	0.8
Methylprednisolone	0
Triamcinolone	0
Dexamethasone	0
Paramethasone	0
Betamethasone	0
Desoxycorticosterone acetate	20
9α-Fluoro-11β-hydroxyprogesterone	34
9α-Fluoro-11β,17d-dihydroxy-progesterone	16
9α-Fluorocorticosterone acetate	360–720
9α-Fluoro F acetate	180
9α-Chloro F acetate	46–90
9α-Fluoroprednisolone	400–800
Aldosterone	400–800

Source: Swingle et al. 1955; Goth 1972.

* Sodium retention units are arbitrary. A comparison is made with cortisol assigned a value of 1 unit and the activities of all other agents are compared to this.

role in the coordination of electrolyte, primarily sodium, and water balance between the external and internal environment. That part of the fluid portion of the blood consisting of molecules of molecular weights less than approximately 68,000 is filtered through the capillary loops of the glomerulus. The afferent and efferent renal arterioles act as variable resistors to maintain a relatively constant filtration pressure. If there is a decrease in aortic pressure, the afferent arterioles constrict to help restore the aortic pressure. This causes a decrease in renal blood flow. If a drug induces diuresis more rapidly than the blood can be rehydrated from the transcellular fluid spaces (see Fig. 25.2), arterial hypotension will occur and the afferent arterioles will constrict. Prerenal azotemia will result from constriction of the afferent renal arterioles. Prerenal azotemia can be induced by any mechanism that effectively reduces cardiac output for a prolonged period of time (congestive heart failure).

Decreases in circulating blood volume induced by diuretics may assume added importance in the presence of liver disease. In patients with hepatic disease, a small decrease in circulating blood volume may have catastrophic effects on perfusion of the liver. Chronic liver disease is usually associated with a decrease in the colloidal osmotic pressure of the plasma, due to a low serum albumin, and with a slow rate of rehydration of the blood from other fluid spaces. Small decreases in arterial perfusion, which would go unnoticed under most circumstances, may precipitate hepatic coma and the hepatorenal syndrome in patients with extensive liver disease.

All diuretics, except water and osmotic diuretics, exert their action by preventing the establishment of a normal ion gradient by the tubular cells. This interference with normal transport mechanisms, which principally move sodium back into the system from the provisional urine, results in natriuresis. Since normal gradients are not established in the tissues surrounding the loops of Henle, distal tubules, and collecting ducts, water does not move out of the provisional urine in normal quantities and diuresis results. Inasmuch as many edematous conditions are associated with a positive sodium balance, diuretics that interfere with sodium transport mechanisms are most effective in the treatment of this class of edema.

Water and Osmotic Diuretics

Criteria for agents that have diuretic effects as a result of osmotic activity are: (1) the substances pass through the glomerular filter freely, (2) they undergo limited tubular reabsorption, and (3) they are pharmacologically inert.

The administration of water in excess of the homeostatic needs of the body will result in the excretion of a larger quantity of dilute urine. In this respect, *water is a true physiological diuretic* and is commonly used in clinical veterinary medicine. The obvious example is in compensated chronic interstitial nephritis of dogs where a ready supply of water is essential for maintenance of the compensated state.

A significant increase in the amount of any osmotically active solute in the provisional urine is usually accompanied by an increase in the volume of urine voided. When the renal circulation is acutely compromised as a result of hypovolemic shock, dehydration, or trauma, the solutes of the glomerular filtrate undergo more complete reabsorption, and water is thereby conserved. Diuretics that normally act by inhibiting tubular transport of ions may be ineffective in this situation. Under these circumstances osmotic diuretics will maintain their activity. This characteristic accounts for the clinical indications for the use of osmotic diuretics: (1) prophylaxis of acute renal failure, (2) differential diagnosis of acute oliguria, (3) regulation of cerebrospinal and intraocular fluid pressures, (4) mobilization of edema fluid, and (5) induction of polyuria to aid in the elimination of certain toxic substances. This explains the rationale, for example, for the use of mannitol to reduce intracranial pressure in the treatment of traumatic cerebral edema when the animal is, in all probability, also suffering from hypovolemic shock.

Mannitol, U.S.P., undergoes very little tubular reabsorption and is likewise poorly absorbed from the gastrointestinal (GI) tract. It must, therefore, be administered parenterally. Mannitol is available in 50-ml ampules for intravenous injection as a 25% solution. Under normal circumstances this amount is diluted with other parenteral fluids just prior to administration. The dose varies with the disease and renal response. For most purposes, 1–2 ml/kg of a 5%–10% solution are administered to effect at a rate of 4 ml/minute.

Other sugars and sugar alcohols, i.e., glucose, sucrose, sorbitol, and isosorbitol, may be used in hypertonic concentrations for their osmotic diuretic effect. In general, the sugars must be given intravenously in hypertonic solutions at high doses to produce diuresis. Isosorbitol is absorbed from the GI tract but its clinical use is not well documented.

Salts

In veterinary clinical practice, *sodium chloride* occupies a unique role as a diuretic. It is used in the control of urolithiasis, especially in sheep, range calves, and cats with cystitis-urolithiasis. The inclusion of salt in the ration assures, along with readily available drinking water, adequate water intake and thereby adequate flushing of the urethra.

Sodium bicarbonate, when given in excess, will exert a diuretic effect. However, this is due to the excess of the salt administered and edema fluid is not mobilized. Systemic alkalosis may result from the misuse of bicarbonate.

Sodium sulfate acts as a cathartic when given orally, since the sulfate is not absorbed from the GI tract. When it is given as a parenteral solution, urine volume is augmented because the renal tubules have only limited capacity for the reabsorption of sulfate. Complex reactions with divalent cations occur with the parenteral use of sulfates and this type of diuresis results in a marked rise in the excretion of calcium and other divalent cations. This effect has been used in the treatment of hypercalcemia and radiostrontium toxicity (Walser et al. 1961).

Potassium salts have been used in the past as diuretics but they are potentially dangerous and their use is discouraged. *Acid-forming salts,* such as ammonium chloride, ammonium nitrate, and calcium chloride, tend to produce acidosis and have a transient diuretic effect. The ammonium salts form acid via the conversion of ammonia to urea in the liver. This conversion results in a net accumulation of hydrogen ion, which reacts with body buffers. Until full compensation by the homeostatic mechanisms for acid-base balance is achieved and the kidney is excreting the same quantity of acid-forming salt relative to that administered, the composition of extracellular fluid is altered by changes in the chloride and bicarbonate concentrations. This results in an acute chloride load for the renal tubules. Some of the chloride will escape reabsorption and pass out in the urine with an equivalent amount of cation, usually sodium, and an isoosmotic amount of water. After compensation is achieved, the diuretic effects are no longer experienced. However, the development of subclinical acidosis and resulting production of acid urine are utilized in the treatment of certain types of cystitis, especially those characterized by basic-reacting urine from species that normally produce acid urine.

MERCURIAL DIURETICS

These agents, with the possible exception of *Chlormerodrin,* N.F. (Neohydrin), are more important historically than clinically. They are pH dependent and appear to act by liberation of a small amount of mercuric ion. This combines with cysteine found in enzymes associated with transport systems located in the proximal and beginning distal tubules. The sodium reabsorption and potassium excretion produced by aldosterone are not blocked by the administration of mercurials. Misuse of mercurial diuretics can cause acute renal insufficiency of a temporary or permanent nature. Commonly available mercurial diuretics are listed in Table 28.2.

CARBONIC ANHYDRASE INHIBITORS

Transport mechanisms that exchange sodium and potassium ions in the provisional urine for excess hydrogen ion in the extracellular fluid exist in many locations along the renal tubular system. Hydrogen ions become available for this exchange by the conversion of carbon dioxide and water to carbonic acid in the presence of carbonic anhydrase. Carbonic anhydrase is present in large concentrations, especially in the tubular epithelial cells. Drugs that inhibit carbonic anhydrase will inhibit ion exchange mechanisms. This causes a retention of sodium and potassium ions in the provisional urine. An isoosmotic quantity of water is excreted with the ions. The diuretic effect of these agents is lost after a few days, since in that time enough hydrogen ion accumulates to allow the exchange process to proceed. Because formation of aqueous humor is highly carbonic-anhydrase dependent, the greatest clinical use of these agents is in the treatment of chronic glaucoma. These diuretic agents have been used for the treatment of udder edema (Gauge et al. 1959). Commonly available carbonic-anhydrase inhibitor diuretics are listed in Table 28.3.

TABLE 28.2. Mercurial diuretics

Nonproprietary and Trade Names	Dosage and Route of Administration
Mercurous chloride (Calomel)	Historical only, displaced by organic mercurials because of cathartic effects and uncertain intestinal absorption
Merbaphen (Novasurol)	Historical only, first introduced as an antisyphilitic agent
Meralluride, U.S.P. (Mercuhydrin)	0.25 mg Hg/kg body wt, i.m.
Mercurophylline (Mercupurin)	0.25 mg Hg/kg body wt, i.m.
Mersalyl (Salyrgan)	0.25 mg Hg/kg body wt, i.m.
Mersalyl with theophylline (Salyrgan theophylline)	0.25–2 mg Hg/kg body wt, i.m.
Merethoxylline (Dicurin)	0.25 mg Hg/kg body wt, i.m.
Mercumatilin (Cumertilin)	0.25 mg Hg/kg body wt, i.m.
Mercaptomerin (Thiomerin)	0.25 mg Hg/kg body wt, i.m. or s.c.
Chlormerodrin, N.F. (Neohydrin)	0.1–0.4 mg Hg/kg body wt, orally

BENZOTHIADIAZIDES (THIAZIDES)

Many compounds in this class of diuretics are orthochlorosulfonamides; in some compounds, a trifluoromethyl group is substituted for the chloride group. Most agents are derivatives of either chlorthiazide or hydrochlorthiazide and differ in their duration of action and potency. They exert their effect primarily on the proximal tubule to prevent the reabsorption of sodium. There is also evidence that some of the thiazides directly influence water reabsorption, perhaps through carbonic anhydrase inhibition (Dies et al. 1963).

TABLE 28.3. Carbonic-anhydrase inhibitor diuretics

Nonproprietary and Trade Names	Dosage and Route of Administration
Acetazolamide (Diamox)	1–3 mg/kg/24 hr, orally 1 mg/kg/24 hr, i.m.
Dichlorphenamide, U.S.P. (Daramide)	2–4 mg/kg/24 hr, orally
Methazolamide, U.S.P. (Neptazane)	2–4 mg/kg/24 hr, orally
Ethorzolamide, U.S.P. (Cardrase, Ethamide)	2–15 mg/kg/24 hr, orally, in divided doses

These agents appear to work proximally to the site of the aldosterone-stimulated sodium-potassium exchange. A possible side effect of their use is profound potassium loss in the presence of high aldosterone activity as seen in congestive heart failure. The thiazide diuretics have some diabetogenic effect, especially in subclinical cases of diabetes mellitus. Hyperuricemia and acute pancreatis also have been reported following their use in human beings (Gantt 1972).

Although fluid accumulation associated with chronic hepatic or renal disease responds favorably to the thiazides, these drugs have been useful also in the management of edema associated with congestive heart failure. Paradoxically, the thiazides may also be used in the treatment of diabetes insipidus. They appear to be effective in diabetes insipidus of nephrogenic as well as pituitary origin. They induce a change from a copious polyuria to a smaller volume of nearly isotonic urine. The mechanism of this action is not well understood but most investigators agree that the natriuretic nature of these drugs plays the dominant role. The continuous administration of thiazides to a nonedematous patient results in an initial loss of sodium, chloride, and water, which eventually results in a moderate state of electrolyte and water depletion. Under these circumstances, a more complete absorption of glomerular filtrate occurs in the proximal tubules. This results in a reduced amount of sodium, chloride, and water in the provisional urine arriving at the distal tubular network. The commonly available benzothiadiazide diuretics are shown in Table 28.4.

TABLE 28.4. Benzothiadiazide diuretics

Nonproprietary and Trade Names	Dosage and Route of Administration
Chlorothiazide, U.S.P. (Diuril)	12–15 mg/kg, orally, b.i.d. 10 mg/kg, i.v.
Hydrochlorothiazide, U.S.P. (Hydrodiuril, Esidrix, Oretic)	1 mg/kg, orally, b.i.d. 1 mg/kg, i.v.
Flumethiazide, N.N.D. (Ademol)	12–15 mg/kg, orally, b.i.d.
Hydroflumethiazide, N.F. (Saluron, Hydro Ademol)	1 mg/kg, orally, b.i.d.
Trichloroflumethiazide (Naqua)	0.15 mg/kg, orally, b.i.d.
Bendroflumethiazide, N.N.D. (Naturetin)	0.15 mg/kg, orally, b.i.d.
Benzthiazide	0.10–0.15 mg/kg, orally, b.i.d.
Hydrobenzthiazide	0.10–0.15 mg/kg, orally, b.i.d.
Trichlormethiazide	0.10–0.15 mg/kg, orally, b.i.d.
Methylclothiazide	0.10–0.15 mg/kg, orally, b.i.d.
Polythiazide	0.10–0.15 mg/kg, orally, b.i.d.
Cyclothiazide	0.10–0.15 mg/kg, orally, b.i.d.

Xanthines and Aminouracils

The diuretic activity of the xanthines has been known for some time. Of the various xanthines, *theophylline* has the greatest renal activity. More recently a large number of heterocyclic nitrogenous compounds tenuously related to the xanthines have been synthesized and their diuretic actions have been studied. *Amisometradine* (Rolicton) and *chlorazanil* (Daquin) are examples of the newer aminouracils. Along with theophylline, more familiar members of this group of compounds include *caffeine, theobromine,* and *aminophylline.*

The drugs in this group stimulate cardiac function and it is possible that a portion of their diuretic activity may stem from the resultant increase in renal blood flow and thereby an increase in glomerular filtration rate. However, these agents all appear to exert a direct action on the renal tubule. The renal response is manifested by an increase in the levels of sodium and chloride in the urine. No significant change in the urine pH occurs and potassium excretion appears to be relatively unaffected. There is some evidence that these agents have the action of weak steroidal antagonists (Shulan and Shideman 1965).

In modern veterinary clinical practice, these agents have received little attention. In general, they are not as effective as other agents available. Their continued use often leads to loss of effectiveness, and gastric irritation may become a problem. Cardiovascular manifestations also may not be desirable.

Aldosterone Antagonists

Two drugs that manifest this action are currently available; however, their modes of action and side effects differ. Spironolactone is an oral preparation often marketed in combination with a thiazide diuretic. This combination is rational, since the potassium excretion encountered with the thiazide diuretics is mainly the result of the exchange of sodium for potassium in the distal tubule, an exchange that is almost entirely under the control of aldosterone. Therefore, this combination of agents enhances the diuretic action and controls the untoward side effects of the thiazide agents.

Spironolactone (Aldactone) is a true competitive antagonist of aldosterone. Aldosterone enhances the direct reabsorption of sodium in the more proximal areas of the distal tubule of the nephrons. In the more distal areas of the distal tubular network, aldosterone promotes sodium reabsorption by enhancement of exchange mechanisms with either potassium or hydrogen ions. Spironolactone blocks both of these actions of aldosterone. The drug has a very slow onset of action, which is not dose dependent and which cannot be overcome by increasing the dosage. This agent does not prevent the excretion of uric acid.

Spironolactone may exert some estrogenlike activity but is not diabetogenic.

The usual oral dose of spironolactone is 0.5–1.5 mg/kg alone or in combination with a thiazide or other diuretic. No parenteral form is available. Since potassium excretion is impeded by spironolactone, it is important that additional potassium is not administered to the patient. Increased serum potassium levels stimulate the release of aldosterone, and the higher aldosterone levels then stimulate potassium excretion. Apparently this is the mechanism by which hyperkalemia is avoided with prolonged spironolactone treatment. In patients with diminished renal function, i.e., blood urea nitrogen (BUN) above 40 or 50 mg%, this agent must be used with care. If hyperkalemia does develop, it must be remembered that the effects of the drug may persist up to 3 days following discontinuation of therapy. During the withdrawal period, it may be necessary to continue the use of a thiazide or other diuretic 48–72 hours to promote potassium excretion.

Heparin prevents the release of aldosterone by the adrenal gland. When indicated for therapy of other conditions, one may take advantage of this diuretic action as well.

Potassium-retaining Agents

Triamterene (Dyrenium) is presumed to act directly on tubular transport of sodium. This effect appears to be independent of the plasma level of aldosterone. It is not an inhibitor of carbonic anhydrase. Because the action of this drug is independent of plasma aldosterone levels, the incidence of hyperkalemia with prolonged administration is greater. Triamterene is not diabetogenic but may be associated with an increase in serum uric acid levels. The reduced rate of potassium excretion associated with the use of this compound has been attributed to an inhibition of potassium secretion in the distal tubular network.

The usual oral dose is 0.5–3 mg/kg. Onset of action is usually within 2–3 hours and may last 6–8 hours. With 3 times a day administration, the action of the drug seems to become more pronounced on the 2nd to 3rd day of treatment. No parenteral form is available.

Amiloride slightly increases the renal excretion of sodium and chloride without causing a significant change in the glomerular filtration rate. This natriuresis is associated with only a slight increase and in some cases an absolute decrease in the rate of potassium excretion. Many diuretics, including the thiazides, furosemide, and ethacrynic acid, normally cause marked increases in potassium output, but this response is depressed with the simultaneous use of amiloride as well as with triamterene. Clinical dosages in animals have not been established for amiloride.

Loop of Henle Diuretics

At present there are two compounds

available that act by affecting the reabsorption of sodium primarily in the ascending limb of the loop of Henle. Since the mechanisms by which sodium reabsorption occurs in this portion of the nephron are poorly understood, the exact mode of action of these agents is likewise unknown. The agents also exert pharmacological action on the proximal and distal tubules. Use of one of these drugs, *furosemide* (Lasix), has become widespread in veterinary medicine in recent years. The other drug in this group, *ethacrynic acid* (Edecrin), is apparently equally potent. These two drugs are the only diuretic agents currently available that have a significant effect on patients with impaired renal function. In human beings they have been reported as useful in patients with serum creatinine levels of 3–8 mg% (Gantt 1972). The diuretic response to these agents is not significantly altered by changes in the acid-base balance of the patient. The ability of the kidney to regulate bicarbonate reabsorption is apparently not altered.

Both of the compounds are readily absorbed from the GI tract. They do not accumulate in organs other than in the liver where biliary excretion occurs. Following intravenous injection, approximately one-third of the dose is excreted by the liver and two-thirds by the kidneys. The net rate of urinary secretion is dependent on urinary pH, which may account for variations in duration of action and dosage recommendations between herbivores and carnivores. Elimination of these compounds is rapid enough so that cumulation of the drug does not occur with normal dosages. These compounds do not inhibit carbonic anhydrase or affect aldosterone activity. Renal potassium output is augmented as the result of increased distal potassium secretion.

Metabolic alkalosis may result from the misuse of these agents. This side effect is attributable to (1) the urinary excretion of chloride (most significantly), (2) the urinary excretion of potassium, and (3) an increase in the rate of hydrogen ion excretion. The action of these drugs on the renal excretion of uric acid is variable. In low doses urates tend to be retained while at higher doses urates are excreted.

Both furosemide and ethacrynic acid are potent diuretic-saluretics. If used excessively, they may result in dehydration and electrolyte imbalance. Excessive loss of potassium in patients also receiving digitalis glycosides may precipitate digitalis toxicity (see Chapter 24).

Indications for the use of these agents include, but are not limited to, the treatment of edema, pulmonary congestion, ascites, hydrothorax, pulmonary edema, or any pathological accumulation of noninflammatory fluid. Dosage for both drugs must be adjusted to the individual animal's response. In severe edematous or refractory cases, the dose may be doubled or increased at the rate of 2 mg/kg of body weight per dose. The established effective dose should be administered 1 or 2 times daily as indicated. Mobilization of edema in chronic cases, i.e., congestive heart failure, may require an intermittent dosage schedule. A regimen might be every other day or on consecutive days with varying periods without treatment interceding. Chronic cases, which necessitate a continued use of these agents, require frequent reexamination for signs of dehydration and electrolyte disturbance. These reexaminations should include periodic evaluations of BUN, plasma or serum creatinine, potassium sodium, or other electrolytes. Other tests may be indicated by the clinical signs.

Both drugs are contraindicated in anuria. Therapy should be discontinued in cases of progressive renal disease with increasing azotemia and oliguria. As previously pointed out, hepatic coma may result from sudden changes in fluid and electrolyte balance in animals with liver disease. Because of this, the use of these agents in the presence of liver disease requires close monitoring. If potassium-depleting steroids have been used, diuretics must be utilized with extreme care and potassium supplementation may be necessary.

Furosemide

Furosemide (Lasix) is also an ortho-

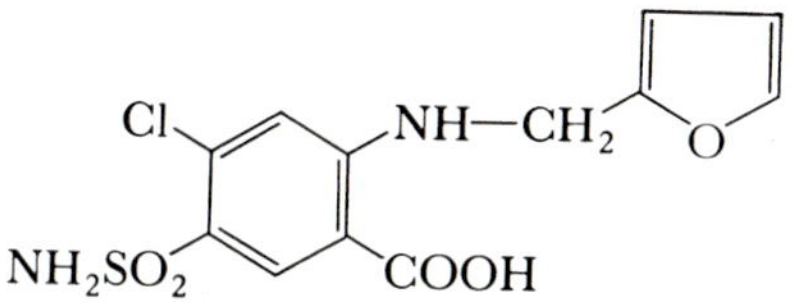

Cl, $NH-CH_2$, O, NH_2SO_2, COOH

Furosemide

FIG. 28.1.

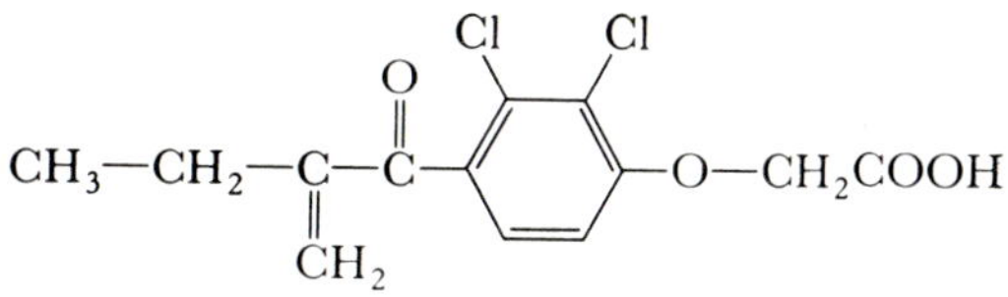

Cl, Cl, O, CH_3-CH_2-C-C, $-O-CH_2COOH$, CH_2

Ethacrynic Acid

FIG. 28.2.

chlorosulfonamide compound but has an additional carboxyl group that differentiates it from the thiazides. It has the structural formula shown in Fig. 28.1. It is possible that the action on sodium transport is in some way dependent on the strong acidic property of this compound as well as that of ethacrynic acid because both compounds contain the carboxyl group. Furosemide is available in 12.5-mg and 50-mg tablets for oral administration. A 5% (50 mg/ml) injectable form is available for parenteral use.

Dosage of furosemide for dogs and cats is approximately 5 mg/kg of body weight. This dose may be increased as indicated up to 10 mg/kg. Following oral administration, a diuretic response is often seen within 30 minutes. It may be repeated each 6–8 hours as needed. The parenteral use of furosemide results in a dramatic and almost immediate diuretic response.

The effective dosage of furosemide for horses is 1.5–3 mg/kg, and this too may be doubled as needed. At present, furosemide is not approved by the Food and Drug Administration in animals used for food. Nevertheless, it is being used for udder edema in dairy cattle and to rid show animals of excessive tissue water in order to more clearly delineate musculature. It is also used on race tracks in horses as prophylactic therapy for epistaxis. The rationale for its use in epistaxis is not well documented.

ETHACRYNIC ACID

Although the site of action of *ethacrynic acid* (Edecrin) is apparently very similar to that of furosemide, its chemical structure is quite different, except for the carboxyl group common to both agents. The structural formula for ethacrynic acid is given in Fig. 28.2.

Mechanisms of elimination and side effects for this compound and furosemide are essentially the same. Its misuse may produce profound hypokalemia. It is apparently not diabetogenic and it blocks the excretion of uric acid.

Ethacrynic acid is available for both oral and parenteral administration. For dogs and cats, the dosage is the same as for furosemide, 5 mg/kg. It is marketed in tablets of 25 and 50 mg for oral use and the sodium salt is available only for intravenous use. The dosage for large animals has not been established.

REFERENCES

Aprahamian, H. A.; Vanderneen, J. L.; Bunker, J. P.; and Crawford, J. D. 1959. The influence of general anesthetics on water solute excretion in man. Ann Surg 150:122.

Dies, F.; Suarez, A.; and Rivera, A. 1963. Treatment of diabetes insipidus with orally administered compounds. Clin Pharmacol Ther 4:602.

du Vigneaud, V.; Lamler, H.; Popenoe, C.; and Popenoe, E. A. 1953a. Enzymatic cleavage of glycinamide from vasopressin and a proposed structure for this pressor-antidiuretic hormone of the posterior pituitary. J Am Chem Soc 75:4880.

du Vigneaud, V.; Ressler, C.; Swan, J. M.; Roberts, C. S.; Katsoyannis, P. G.; and Gordon, S. 1953b. The synthesis of an octapeptide amide with the hormonal activity of oxytocin. J Am Chem Soc 75:4879.

Gantt, C. L. 1972. Rational Drug Therapy, vol. 6. Philadelphia: W. B. Saunders.

Gauge, H. E.; Shor, A. L.; and Johnson, W. P. 1959. Control of udder edema in dairy cows. Vet Med 54:342.

Goth, A. 1972. Medical Pharmacology, p. 458. St. Louis: C. V. Mosby.

Kamm, O. H.; Aldrich, T. B.; Grottee, I. W.; Rowe, L. W.; and Bugbee, E. P. 1928. The active principles of the posterior lobe of the pituitary gland. J Am Chem Soc 50: 573.

Pickford, M. 1952. Antidiuretic substances. Pharmacol Rev 4:254.

Shulan, T. W., and Shideman, F. E. 1965. Natriuretic and antiglycogenic activities of a series of symmetrical triazine and pteridine derivatives. J Pharmacol Exp Ther 148:356.

Swingle, W. W.; Baker, C.; Eisler, M.; LeBrie, S. J.; and Brannich, L. J. 1955. Efficacy of 9 alpha-halo adrenal steroids for maintenance of adrenalectomized dogs. Proc Soc Exp Biol Med 88:193.

Walser, M.; Payne, J. W.; and Browder, A. A. 1961. Ion association. IV. Effect of sodium sulfate infusion on renal clearance and body retention of injected radio-strontium in dogs. J Clin Invest 40:234.

CHAPTER 29

TREATMENT OF CIRCULATORY SHOCK

DONALD R. CLARK and J. D. McCRADY

MAJOR CHARACTERISTICS OF SHOCK

Circulatory shock may be defined as an acute circulatory insufficiency in which cardiac output is not adequate to provide for the normal perfusion of tissues. The syndrome involves complex derangements in physiologic and metabolic mechanisms. Metabolic and cellular changes are sequential, and their severity varies with time as well as with the degree of the initial disturbance. Once shock is evoked, the progression of events is largely independent of the initiating mechanism.

Common to all forms of shock is circulatory inadequacy. Diminished blood flow results in insufficient tissue oxygenation. Cellular functions decline, including basic cellular metabolism. Maintenance or loss of oxidative mechanisms determines the reversibility or irreversibility of a state of shock. Therefore, in a broad sense, the treatment of shock centers on prevention and correction of cellular hypoxia.

Circulatory shock is related initially to generalized excessive changes in peripheral resistance, to a diminished effective blood volume, or to an acute loss of cardiac function. The end result in each instance is similar, namely, inadequate flow of blood to provide sufficient organ or tissue perfusion. The clinical signs observed generally reflect the direct effect of the initiating disturbance, the physiologic response to that disturbance, and the consequences of prolonged tissue hypoxia. Commonly observed signs include:

1. Tachycardia
2. Weak, "thready," or nonpalpable arterial pulse
3. Collapse of peripheral veins
4. Cold, pale mucous membranes
5. Prolonged capillary refilling time
6. Dry, shriveled tongue

7. Mental depression or unconsciousness
8. Increased respiration
9. Subnormal temperature and lack of surface warmth
10. Oliguria or anuria

Except in cardiogenic shock, there is collapse of peripheral veins. Digital pressure applied to gingival membranes is followed by an extended capillary refilling time. Arterial hypotension, although a relatively constant finding, is not synonymous with shock but is rather only one feature of shock. The implications of hypotension are less direct and less vital than is the lack of peripheral perfusion and tissue oxygen delivery. Accordingly, therapy designed to increase arterial pressure must not do so at the cost of reducing tissue blood flow.

ETIOLOGY AND TYPES OF SHOCK

Circulatory shock may be classed as three major types according to primary etiology. This basic classification includes (1) hypovolemic shock, (2) vasculogenic shock, and (3) cardiogenic shock. The scheme of classification is as follows:

A. Shock due to Reduction in Blood Volume (Hypovolemic Shock)
   1. Loss of whole blood
      a. External hemorrhage
      b. Internal hemorrhage
   2. Loss of plasma
      a. Surface exudation—thermal or chemical burns
      b. Exudation into body cavities—inflammatory processes
   3. Loss of water and electrolytes
      a. Acute water deprivation
      b. Excessive sweating, vomition, diarrhea, and fluid loss in acute intestinal obstruction

B. Shock Due to Primary Changes in Venous Capacitance or Peripheral Resistance (Vasculogenic Shock)
   1. Endotoxin
   2. Anaphylaxis or acute hypersensitivity
   3. Vasomotor paralysis due to central nervous system (CNS) trauma or depression

C. Shock Due to Acute Changes in Cardiac Pumping Effectiveness (Cardiogenic Shock)
   1. Interference with effective cardiac filling
      a. Cardiac tamponade
      b. Positive pressure ventilation
   2. Improper ventricular emptying
      a. Acute cor pulmonale
      b. Abrupt increase in systemic vascular resistance
      c. Rupture of chordae tendinae
      d. Severe toxic myocardial depression
      e. Significant cardiac dysrhythmias

Shock Due to Reduction in Blood Volume (Hypovolemic Shock)

Hypovolemic shock follows severe volume loss from the circulation. In a healthy animal, the rapid loss of 30% or more of the normal blood volume induces signs of circulatory shock. Frequently, such a fall in circulating volume is the consequence of major tissue trauma; for example, fractures of the pelvis or femur, rupture of the liver or spleen, or severance of a principal artery. Plasma loss of similar magnitude occurs when increased capillary permeability develops over a large area, such as with superficial burns or in acute intestinal obstruction where transudation of plasma into the intestinal lumen and peritoneal cavity takes place. Significant depletion of plasma volume also occurs in rapid dehydration due to excessive sweating, prolonged diuresis, or persistent vomition and diarrhea. These rapid reductions in circulatory volume may induce shock similar to that associated with major physical trauma.

Shock Due to Changes in Venous Capacitance or Peripheral Resistance (Vasculogenic Shock)

Bacterial toxins may be a direct cause of shock due principally to their effect in producing widespread vascular alterations. Severe bacterial infections, particularly but not exclusively those caused by gram-negative organisms, are a significant cause of shock. Endotoxins, which are lipopolysaccharides derived from cell walls of certain bacterial inhabitants of the gastrointestinal (GI) tract, are especially capable of inducing shock. Thus in septicemia, endotoxins from organisms such as *Escherichia coli, Proteus* spp., and *Klebsiella* spp. may be introduced into the general circulation. The endotoxins result in an increase in portal vein pressure because of hepatic vein constriction and an increase in pulmonary arterial pressure because of pulmonary venoconstriction. Cardiac output falls progressively and large quantities of blood are sequestered in the hepatoportal system. The sequestering of large volumes of blood in the splanchnic area removes this fluid as a part of the effective circulatory volume. To this extent, endotoxic shock is similar to hypovolemic shock.

Vasomotor paralysis ensues from depression or trauma to special areas of the CNS, particularly the medulla and thoracolumbar region of the spinal cord. These areas are involved with maintenance of normal vascular tone. Various pharmacologic agents, including those that interfere with sympathetically mediated vasoconstriction, also may be involved in the genesis of circulatory shock. Anaphylaxis as a cause of circulatory shock is discussed below.

Shock Due to Acute Changes in Cardiac Pumping Effectiveness (Cardiogenic Shock)

Circulatory shock resulting from spontaneous, acute disturbance in cardiac pumping capacity is less common in domestic animals than in human beings. However, in animals it may result from the heart failing to fill properly, as in cardiac tamponade or excessive intrathoracic pressure during positive pressure ventilation, or from the heart failing to empty properly. Incomplete emptying may be due to rupture of the chordae tendinae, severe depression of myocardial contractility, or the onset of certain cardiac dysrhythmias. Cardiogenic shock is characterized by low cardiac output, arterial hypotension, increased systemic resistance, and elevated central venous pressure. Pronounced jugular distension, often with pulsation, and evidence of cardiac failure on auscultation or ECG examination are likely to be present. Decrease in effective circulating blood volume may occur in cardiogenic shock. Myocardial depression is now recognized as a contributing factor to advanced shock from other causes as well (Lefer 1970).

PATHOPHYSIOLOGY OF SHOCK

A decrease in effective circulating blood volume is the primary disorder in shock resulting from hemorrhage or trauma. This is also an important feature of septic shock, because of extensive vascular pooling and sequestering of blood. There is a marked reduction in venous return. Central venous pressure, an indicator of right ventricular filling pressure, is low. Cardiac output and arterial pressure decrease, resulting in inadequate tissue perfusion and stagnant hypoxia.

In response to the hypoxia and arterial hypotension, reflex neuroendocrine stimulation results. Pain accentuates the response. Intense sympathetic activity occurs. Catecholamine release at neuroeffector endings and from the adrenal medulla is enhanced, as is the pituitary release of antidiuretic hormone (ADH). The renin-angiotensin-aldosterone mechanism is also activated. Sympathetic cardiac stimulation results in greatly increased heart rate and contractility. Hepatic glycogenolysis results in hyperglycemia and some degree of hyperkalemia.

Sympathetic vasoconstrictor tone increases, particularly in the skin, mucous membranes, skeletal muscles, kidneys, and splanchnic areas. Muscular weakness is evident. Mucous membranes are pale and dry, and the body surface, particularly in the extremities, lacks warmth. Blood is redistributed so that those organs with the least sympathetic vasoconstrictor response, the heart and brain, are preferentially, although not adequately, perfused. Reduced renal blood flow results in decreased glomerular filtration and in consequent oliguria or anuria. Prolonged renal ischemia may lead to tubular necrosis, a process accentuated by the hemoglobinemia or myoglobinemia, which may occur with trauma. Renal shutdown is marked by azotemia, hyperkalemia, and metabolic acidosis.

With the lack of adequate tissue perfusion, decreased aerobic oxidation occurs, and along with this an increase in anaerobic glycolysis by the Embden-Meyerhof pathway. Increases in circulating pyruvate and particularly lactate occur. Blood pH falls as metabolic acidosis develops. A decrease in P_{CO_2} indicates ventilatory compensation in response to the metabolic acidosis. The progression of metabolic acidosis, through local autoregulatory mechanisms, reduces somewhat the degree of arteriolar constriction while the postcapillary venules maintain their constriction; this results in the extravasation of fluids from capillaries into tissue spaces.

Cerebral depression may be attributed to the acidotic state and to limited cerebral blood flow. Cerebral blood flow diminishes because of arterial hypotension and because of cerebral vasoconstriction in response to hypocapnia. The hypocapnia, in turn, occurs as alveolar ventilation is increased in response to metabolic acidosis. The compensatory hypocapnia effects a partial correction of the bicarbonate buffer imbalance.

Other changes having profound effects on the patient in circulatory shock include progressive myocardial depression (Hackel et al. 1974); microcirculatory sludging of blood and development of disseminated intravascular coagulation (Hardaway 1967); generalized disruption of cells and of cellular organelles, including release of lytic enzymes from lysosomes (Schumer and Sperling 1968); GI ischemia with loss of effective enteric epithelium; loss of blood and fluids into the intestinal lumen (Jacobson 1968); and increased absorption of bacterial endotoxins (Fine 1967). The increased absorption of enteric toxins occurs in the presence of a greatly decreased ability of the reticuloendothelial cells to inactivate circulating toxins.

THERAPY OF SHOCK

Blood, Fluids, and Volume Replacement

Early correction of volume deficits in shock is mandatory. The need for fluid or blood administration to the hypovolemic patient is urgent. Although volume expansion in hypovolemic shock is standard therapy, its usefulness in patients with septic shock and even cardiogenic shock is now more clearly recognized. The early and more desperate need is not for red cells but for fluid. In fact, the packed cell volume (PCV) may be high because of the loss of plasma and interstitial fluid. In general, the red cell mass is usually adequate to support life if the effective circulating volume can be restored. Yet restoration of the plasma volume to an optimal degree often requires significantly greater quantities than can be accounted for by known or calculated losses.

The requirements for large quantities of replacement fluids center around the following considerations: (1) certain losses may be hidden or inapparent, especially in traumatic shock with fractures of the femur or pelvis; (2) loss of vascular tone, particularly of veins, necessitates a greater than normal filling volume; (3) loss of capillary wall integrity results in continuous loss of fluid into tissues; and (4) moderate overfilling of the vascular system (hypervolemia) results in the enhancement of cardiac output if the heart is adequately competent.

Fluids may be administered according to some predetermined dosage based on estimated need or can be given until the physical signs and the results of patient monitoring indicate that a satisfactory quantity has been given. The choice of fluids depends on the prevailing state of shock.

BLOOD

Administration of whole blood may be-indicated if there has been significant hemorrhage or hemolysis. The PCV may or may not be low, depending on the length of time since the loss of blood and on the degree of fluid shift from extravascular compartments. In general, blood should be administered intravenously at a rate of approximately 20–40 ml/kg, except where blood loss is continuing. In virtually all circumstances where a shock state exists, administration of whole blood should be accompanied by balanced electrolyte solutions in a ratio of 1 part of blood to between 2 and 6 parts of fluid. This is especially true in traumatic shock and in advanced, severe shock from any cause. In these circumstances, the additional fluid volume is vital for replacement of fluid lost into extravascular spaces because of traumatized capillary beds and loss of capillary endothelial integrity. Should the animal have a history of previous blood transfusion, cross matching is required to prevent the possibility of a transfusion reaction.

PLASMA

Plasma, serum, and fractionated protein solutions should be considered where there is need to expand blood volume without additional cells. Two to 5 ml/kg of plasma may be given intravenously somewhat rapidly, then more slowly to a total quantity of 5–20 ml/kg. Principal limitations on use of plasma are cost and availability. Canine plasma albumin solutions (Canalb) are commercially available and have been described as effective in treatment of shock in dogs (Fish and Cooksey 1970).

PLASMA EXPANDERS

Several types of plasma expanders are available. Those of most importance in the treatment of shock are clinical dextran solution (Dextran 70 Injection) and low molecular weight dextran solution (Dextran 40 Injection). It has been shown that the higher molecular weight dextrans may result in accentuated sludging of blood in microcirculatory vessels, an effect reversed by low molecular weight dextran (Gronwall and Ingelman 1945).

The usefulness of low molecular weight dextran in shock patients has not been conclusively established. Its principal benefit may be due to its prevention of capillary sludging and disseminated intravascular coagulation. The action of low molecular weight dextran (average molecular weight = 40,000) in preventing or reversing cell aggregation can be attributed in part to its induction of rapid hemodilution by osmotic attraction of extravascular water and by a direct coating of the erythrocyte membranes to prevent cell aggregation. The initial intravenous dosage rate of Dextran 40 is 10–15 ml/kg. The total dose should not exceed 20 ml/kg over a 24-hour period. It is particularly important to administer electrolyte solutions when plasma or dextrans are employed in the treatment of shock. Otherwise, fluid shifts from tissues may be excessive and compensatory mechanisms become exhausted.

ELECTROLYTE SOLUTIONS

The concept of hypervolemic therapy has evolved in the management of patients in shock. The early administration of sufficient quantities of electrolyte solutions is perhaps the most vital measure in shock therapy. Treatment should be based on achieving volume expansion sufficient to effect satisfactory arterial pressure, adequate urine output, and good peripheral perfusion without excessive elevation of central venous pressure. In experimental hemorrhagic shock, optimal survival of bled dogs occurred when treatment consisted of reinfusion of one-half the shed blood along with a volume of Ringer's lactate equal to 4 times the volume of blood lost (Dillon et al. 1966).

The administration of various types of electrolyte solutions has been advocated, particularly isotonic saline and Ringer's lactate. One advantage to the use of Ringer's lactate instead of isotonic saline is the prevention of a further lowering of pH because of buffer dilution when large amounts of saline are given. One potential disadvantage to the use of Ringer's lactate, the accentuation of an existing lactacidemia, does not materialize as a real problem. It has been shown that as cardiac ouput and tissue perfusion are normalized the excess lactate is quickly metabolized (Baue et al. 1967).

Because Ringer's lactate may have a pH of 7 or less, it may be buffered by addition of 0.75 g of bicarbonate to each L. Additional steps in correction of metabolic acidosis are important. Sodium bicarbonate solution (7.5%) available in 50-ml ampules containing 44.6 mEq of sodium bicarbonate is particularly useful in correcting bicarbonate deficit. Methods of determining and correcting acid-base imbalances have been discussed in Chapter 26.

The dosage of fluids should be in accordance with the intensity of shock and the circulatory response to the fluids received. In hypovolemic shock, a quantity of 2%–4% of body weight, or approximately 20–40 ml/kg, is often required. Electrolyte solutions should be administered as rapidly as the patient can tolerate them. This will commonly require the use of large-gauge needles and, particularly in large animals, may require the simultaneous use of several intravenous sets or delivery by pressure of a roller-pump device.

The principal danger from the use of fluids is pulmonary edema and the secondary danger is acute congestive heart failure. The central venous pressure (CVP) provides a reliable indication of the capability of the heart to accept the additional volume load. Fluid administration should cease, at least temporarily, if (1) auscultation and clinical signs indicate developing pulmonary edema, (2) administration of 2 ml/kg in 10 minutes causes a rise in CVP of 5 cm H_2O or more, or (3) CVP exceeds 15 cm H_2O.

Oxygen and Ventilatory Assistance

The failure of respiratory gas exchange has been described as a significant contributor to the shock state (Weil and Shubin 1969; Brasmer 1972) and may be a direct cause of death in shock. Although it would seem advantageous to empirically provide oxygen for breathing, it is not always of appreciable value. The additional oxygen will not necessarily improve either arterial oxygen saturation or oxygen delivery to tissues. However, in patients that suffer from a lack of adequate alveolar ventilation or in which there is interference with diffusion of gases across the respiratory epithelium, oxygen administered by the inhalation of a 40% or 100% atmosphere by mask, tent, or endotracheal tube is highly beneficial. In the majority of patients suffering from shock, the limitations in tissue oxygenation result primarily from reduced cardiac output and from arteriovenous shunting in poorly ventilated pulmonary capillaries. The latter condition is corrected most successfully by steps to improve alveolar ventilation, steps that should include the provision of a patent airway and ventilatory assistance.

Cardiostimulatory and Vasoactive Drugs

sympathetic agonists

Vasoactive drugs such as norepinephrine, epinephrine, and isoproterenol, which are also cardiostimulants, have been used to treat shock, particularly when other measures such as administration of blood and fluids have failed to satisfactorily raise arterial pressure. Such agents are nearly always successful in elevating arterial pressure, at least transiently, even though the animal may not ultimately survive. However, apart from their use in anaphylaxis, adrenergic agents are of value only in limited circumstances in the treatment of shock and may even be contraindicated in certain situations.

The catecholamines may be of benefit in cardiogenic shock because of their positive inotropic and chronotropic effects. The administration of norepinephrine might be beneficial if used early in hypovolemic shock when endogenous sympathetic activity is not at its maximum. In addition, pressor agents may act to correct hypotension caused by anesthetic agents such as halothane or by high spinal anesthesia.

Levarterenol or *l*-norepinephrine (Levophed) is most valuable as a pressor agent.

When diluted to a concentration of 8 μg/ml in 5% dextrose, it may be given as a continuous intravenous drip at a rate of 0.5–1 ml/minute to dogs of average size or at a rate sufficient to achieve appropriate arterial pressure. For cardiac stimulation and vasomotor effects, 0.1–0.5 ml of 1:1000 epinephrine (Adrenalin) may be given intravenously to dogs of average size. Isoproterenol (Isuprel) is also effective in improving cardiac output and in lowering CVP through cardiac stimulation. This agent, because of its β-adrenergic actions, has a marked inotropic effect, greatly accelerates heart rate, and causes vasodilation, particularly in skeletal muscle. It should be diluted to a concentration of 10 μg/ml in 5% dextrose and given by continuous intravenous drip at a rate of 5–10 μg/minute to dogs of average size. Alternately, it may be administered at a rate that produces a pulse rate of 125–175. Dopamine, a precursor of norepinephrine and epinephrine, possesses β-adrenergic and only minor α-adrenergic effects. Like isoproterenol, its principal usefulness is in the treatment of cardiogenic shock.

Evidence has accumlated in recent years to support the concept that sympathetic stimulation and intense, prolonged vasoconstriction are harmful in hemorrhagic and other forms of hypovolemic shock. In fact, the catecholamines, epinephrine and norepinephrine, have been shown to potentiate circulatory failure (Greisman and Michaelis 1963), to fail to protect against lethal shock following hemorrhage (Closs et al. 1957), and even to induce fatal shock (Yard and Nickerson 1956). The potentially harmful effects of catecholamines include (1) intensification of tissue ischemia through excessive vasoconstriction, (2) reduction in plasma volume because of increased capillary filtration, (3) increase in oxygen requirements resulting from their direct calorigenic effect, and (4) induction of tachyarrhythmias and ventricular fibrillation. The routine use of vasopressor drugs in hypovolemic shock should be abandoned unless their α-adrenergic effects are blocked and they are used primarily as inotropic agents.

SYMPATHETIC ANTAGONISTS

The reduction of excessive vasoconstriction by agents blocking α-adrenergic receptors may be helpful in otherwise unresponsive patients in which the circulating fluid volume has been restored. Both phenoxybenzamine (Dibenzyline) and phentolamine (Regitine) have been described as beneficial in sustained, deep shock characterized by excessive vasoconstriction. Chlorpromazine (Thorazine) has also been used as a mild vasodilator. With chlorpromazine, as with other α blocking agents, the therapeutic goal is to effect a lessening of vasoconstriction to improve peripheral capillary flow, minimize capillary sludging, and increase venous return.

Uncertainty exists as to the choice of patients that should receive these drugs and to what degree these agents provide improvement in recovery from shock. However, their use should be restricted to patients in which full circulatory volume replacement has been achieved.

STEROIDS

To an increasingly greater degree, the administration of massive doses of corticosteroids has become a principal step in shock therapy. Although some controversy still exists regarding the benefits of steroid administration, there remains a growing emphasis on the incorporation of steroids into the routine regimen for shock. Evidence, both clinical and experimental, points to the efficacy of glucocorticoids in the treatment of septic and cardiogenic shock, which are both characterized by very high mortality rates (Sambhi et al. 1965; Motsay et al. 1970; Mills 1971). Benefit from corticoid therapy has also been described in cases of hemorrhagic shock (Weil and Whigham 1965).

Steroids in very large doses affect the microcirculation, producing sustained vasodilation and significantly improved tissue perfusion. Improvement of cardiac output also occurs. If only standard doses of steroids are used, these effects are not evident. Because of their substantial effects on microcirculatory vessels and lack of side effects in most patients, steroids may be considered in the treatment of shock as the most nearly ideal vasodilators available to the practitioner.

Other effects of steroids that are beneficial in the therapy of shock include protection of capillary endothelial integrity during hypoxia, stabilization of lysosomal membranes, and reduction in sensitivity to endotoxin. Improved cardiac performance results from a decrease in vascular resistance rather than from a direct inotropic effect. Corticoids induce the entrance of amino acids into the metabolic oxidative cycle and provide an increase in cellular energy mechanisms (Wajchenburg et al. 1964). Enhanced conversion of lactic acid to glucose and glycogen occurs, moderating the lactacidemia and increasing available carbohydrate.

Dosages of corticosteroids that produce a maximal effect in shock treatment are large compared to those generally used in therapeutics. An optimal dose for use in shock is 4–6 mg/kg of dexamethasone (Azium) or equivalent doses of methylprednisolone (25–30 mg/kg), prednisolone (35–40 mg/kg), or other glucocorticoid. Following adequate fluid volume replacement, the steroids should be given as a single intravenous injection (bolus) over a 1- to 3-minute period. The more soluble succinate and phosphate salts of steroids are purported to have a more rapid onset of action. Improvement in circulation may be noted in some patients within 5–10 minutes and may persist for as long as 4 hours. If arterial pressure is not reestablished following volume replacement and vasodilator therapy, positive inotropic agents such as levarterenol, epinephrine, or isoproterenol may be used more effectively and at lower dosage than when not preceded by steroid-induced vasodilation. See the discussion in Chapter 33 concerning steroids.

Other Therapeutic Measures

ANTIBIOTICS

The use of broad-spectrum antibiotics is specifically indicated whenever shock is the result of sepsis or trauma. Antibiotics are important for the prophylactic management of shock from other causes as well. It is advisable to consider the possible adverse effects, including moderate circulatory depression, that are attributed to certain antibiotics, especially the aminoglycoside antibiotics (Adams 1975).

HEPARIN

Administration of heparin should be restricted to those patients in which disseminated intravascular coagulation (DIC) has been demonstrated. DIC is the syndrome of widespread thromboses in microcirculatory vessels due to the combined effects of capillary stagnation and stimulation of the coagulation process. The latter may occur due to acidosis, hemolysis, bacterial toxins, or the presence of tissue damage and necrosis. DIC may be ameliorated by correction of the acidosis, volume expansion, vasodilator therapy, or administration of heparin. Heparin is administered intravenously at a dosage of 250 units/kg and may be repeated every 4 hours.

HYPOTHERMIA

Hypothermia as an adjunct in treatment of shock is of uncertain benefit. While it has been a long-accepted procedure to maintain or restore normal body temperature, recent evidence suggests that a moderate hypothermia (33° C) may be effective in increasing the survival rate in both hemorrhagic and endotoxic shock (Halmagyi et al. 1973). In any event, one should not attempt rapid restoration of body temperature in a shock patient by devices or procedures supplying large quantities of heat to the body surface. Rapid surface warming results in diversion of blood flow to the skin from more critical areas.

OTHER CARDIOTONICS

Cardiotonic agents, other than the sympathomimetics described above, may be of use in strengthening cardiac contractility. Calcium salts are capable of increasing circulatory performance through their positive inotropic effects, particularly when hyperkalemia exists. Calcium gluconate is safer than the more highly ionized calcium salts. Intravenously, the dosage of calcium gluconate is 10–20 mg/kg administered slowly.

Glucagon is a polypeptide hormone with significant cardiostimulatory activity that produces a moderately sustained inotropy and chronotropy. It has been reported to be of value in the treatment of experimental cardiogenic shock in dogs (Matloff et al. 1970). Because of a marked action in stimulating cardiac output and the absence of arrhythmogenic effects, glucagon is potentially a useful drug in management of circulatory shock (Clark et al. 1974). Glucagon may be administered at a dosage of 50 μg/kg intravenously and may be repeated at 30-minute intervals.

Rapid-acting digitalis glycosides such as deslanoside (Cedilanid) or digoxin (Lanoxin) may be employed. If cardiac glycosides are elected for use, rapid digitalization should be achieved by intravenous administration (Chapter 24).

MANNITOL

Urine output tends to be clearly reduced at arterial pressures of less than 80 mm Hg and generally ceases at arterial pressures below 50 mm Hg. In shock, following restoration of effective circulatory volume and the normalization of arterial pressure, renal function may not necessarily recover promptly or adequately. Mannitol effects a return of urine flow by further increasing intravascular volume, promoting increased renal blood flow, retaining glomerular filtrate within renal tubules, and reducing cellular edema in the renal tubular epithelium. Dosages of 1–3 g/kg enhance urine flow in oliguric or anuric animals that have received adequate fluid replacement. An inotropic effect of mannitol is due to a slight increase in plasma extracellular osmolarity (Atkins et al. 1973).

SPECIAL CONSIDERATIONS IN SHOCK THERAPY

Acute Adrenocortical Insufficiency

An acute shocklike state occurs in animals that develop sudden loss of adrenocortical function. The disease complex is marked by weakness, prostration, hypovolemia, and electrolyte imbalances. There is hyperkalemia and, usually, hyponatremia, along with an absolute sodium deficit. ECG changes include P-wave suppression, widening of the QRS interval, and increased amplitude of T waves. Because acute adrenal crisis represents a medical emergency, intravenous fluids and corticosteroids must be administered immediately. Fluids containing potassium should be avoided. Use of 5% dextrose in normal saline may be used for volume expansion and correction of sodium deficit.

Cortisol hemisuccinate preparations administered intravenously are ideal for rapid supplementation of glucocorticoids. In addition, mineralocorticoids such as desoxycorticosterone acetate are required. Extended therapy includes mineralocorticoids and increased dietary salt intake.

Anaphylactic Shock

Anaphylaxis is an acute systemic reaction that occurs upon administration of an antigen to any suitably sensitized subject and is mediated by pharmacologically active substances. Anaphylactic reactions are the result of the interaction of antigen and antibody (IgE) and the subsequent release of mediators from mast cells and basophils. These pharmacologically active substances are principally histamine, serotonin, and slow-reacting substance of anaphylaxis (SRS-A), in addition to plasma kinins. These agents, through their own effects and by initiating certain physiologic reflexes, result in the clinical syndrome known as anaphylaxis. This subject is discussed more fully in Chapter 21.

The most important step in treatment of anaphylaxis is the prompt administration of epinephrine. Epinephrine, with its α- and β-adrenergic effects, is clearly the treatment of choice. Intramuscular administration of 0.1 ml of 1:1000 epinephrine is used in dogs of average size. Hypotension, bronchospasm, pruritus, and urticaria are commonly relieved if epinephrine is employed early. If the clinical signs persist, epinephrine may be repeated at 15- to 20-minute intervals.

Diphenhydramine (Benadryl) administered intravenously at a dosage of 2 mg/kg is suggested when the sympotoms of anaphylaxis are severe or when the response to epinephrine is not satisfactory. In mild reactions, antihistamines may be given orally. Specific antagonists of mediators other than histamine are recognized and may become useful in treatment of anaphylaxis in which histamine is not the primary mediating substance (Eyre 1972). Aminophilline, 10 mg/kg intravenously, is indicated when bronchospasm persists. Corticosteroids should not be considered as primary therapy in anaphylaxis but employed as adjunctive therapy where shock persists.

If anaphylaxis proceeds to a state of circulatory collapse and shock, the measures described above for the management of shock are indicated. These measures include volume expansion, massive quantities of corticoids, and the vasoactive and inotropic agents.

Acute Colitis Syndrome in Horses

A particularly malignant form of circulatory shock is observed in horses afflicted with the acute colitis (colitis X) syndrome. The disease onset is extremely rapid. Its specific etiology is uncertain but its development may relate to exhaustion and other forms of physical and physiological stresses. There is early elevation of body temperature, which later falls to normal or below. A profuse diarrhea develops, but at times death occurs so quickly that the diarrhea is not observed. There are dark, congested mucous membranes; focal areas of sweating; shallow, rapid respiration; and, commonly, outward signs of colic. Hemoconcentration is marked by a rise in PCV. In more advanced stages, the animals exhibit signs of extreme distress, central nervous depression, and mania (Vaughn 1973). The survival rate is low and clinical management must begin early and be pursued vigorously.

The principal consideration in treating acute colitis is in maintaining an adequate circulatory fluid volume. Balanced electrolyte solutions in quantities as great as 12 L/hour (1 L/5 minutes) may be required for expansion and maintenance of adequate circulatory volume. Metabolic acidosis is best corrected by first measuring the negative base excess (base deficit) and administering sodium bicarbonate in appropriate amounts. Alternatively, in presumed severe acidosis, the base deficit may be estimated to be 10–12 mEq/L of bicarbonate in the extracellular fluids.

As in other forms of shock, a comprehensive regimen also requires use of steroids, antibiotics, vasoactive drugs where indicated, and other forms of supportive therapy as discussed above.

REFERENCES

Adams, H. R. 1975. Acute adverse effects of antibiotics. J Am Vet Med Assoc 166:983.

Atkins, J. M.; Wildenthal, K.; and Horwitz, L. D. 1973. Cardiovascular responses to hypertonic mannitol in anesthetized and conscious dogs. Am J Physiol 225:132.

Baue, A. E.; Tragus, E. T.; Wolfson, S. K., Jr.; Cary, A. L.; and Parkins, W. M. 1967. Hemodynamic and metabolic effects of Ringer's Lactate Solution in hemorrhagic shock. Ann Surg 166:29.

Brasmer, T. H. 1972. Shock—Basic pathophysiology and treatment. Vet Clin North Am 2:219.

Clark, D. R.; Webb, T. J.; and McCrady, J. D. 1974. Physiologic actions and clinical usefulness of glucagon in veterinary medicine. Southwest Vet 27:255.

Closs, A. S.; Wagner, J. A.; Kloehn, R. A., Jr.; and Kory, R. C. 1957. The effect of norepinephrine on survival in experimental acute hemorrhagic hypotension. Surg Forum 8:22.

Dillon, J.; Lynch, L. J., Jr.; Myers, R.; and Butcher, H. R., Jr. 1966. The treatment of hemorrhagic shock. Surg Gynecol Obstet 122:967.

Eyre, P. 1972. Acute bovine pulmonary emphysema. Vet Rec 91:38.

Fine, J. 1967. Intestinal circulation in shock. Gastroenterology 52:1967.

Fish, J. G., and Cooksey, J. L. 1970. Use of canine plasma protein solution in small animal practice. Vet Med Small Anim Clin 65:133.

Greisman, S. E., and Michaelis, M. 1963. Effect of catechol amines during traumatic shock in the rat. J Surg Res 3:268.

Gronwall, A., and Ingelman, B. 1945. II. Untersuchungen über Dextran und sein Verhalten bei parenteraler Zufer. Acta Physiol Scand 9:1.

Hackel, C. B.; Ratliff, N. B.; and Mikat, E. 1974. The heart in shock. Circ Res 35:805.

Halmagyi, D. F. J.; Frazer, T. A.; and Varga, D. 1973. Treatment of volume resistant experimental shock by hypovolemia and hypothermia. Surgery 74:370.

Hardaway, R. M. 1967. Disseminated intravascular coagulation in experimental and clinical shock. Am J Cardiol 20:161.

Jacobson, E. D. 1968. A physiologic approach to shock. N Engl J Med 278:834.

Lefer, A. M. 1970. Role of a myocardial depressant factor in the pathogenesis of circulatory shock. Fed Proc 29:1189.

Matloff, J. M.; Parmley, W. W.; Manchester, J. M.; Berkovits, B.; Sonnenblick, E. H.; and Harken, D. E. 1970. Effects of glucagon in canine myocardial infarction and shock. Am J Cardiol 25:675.

Mills, L. C. 1971. Corticosteroids in endotoxic shock. Proc Soc Exp Biol Med 138:507.

Motsay, G. J.; Alho, A.; Jaeger, T.; Dietzman, R. H.; and Lillehei, R. C. 1970. Effects of corticosteroids on the circulation in shock: Experimental and clinical results. Fed Proc 29:1861.

Sambhi, M. P.; Weil, M. H.; and Vasant, N. U. 1965. Acute pharmacodynamic effects of glucocorticoids. Circulation 31:523.

Schumer, W., and Sperling, R. 1968. Shock and its effect on the cell. J Am Med Assoc 205:75.

Vaughn, J. T. 1973. The acute colitis syndrome. Colitis X. Vet Clin North Am 3:301.

Wajchenburg, B. L.; Pereira, V. G.; and Pupa, A. A. 1964. On the mechanism of insulin hypersensitivity in adrenocortical insufficiency. Diabetes 13:169.

Weil, M. H., and Shubin, H. 1969. The "VIP" approach to the bedside management of shock. J Am Med Assoc 207:337.

Weil, M. H., and Whigham, H. 1965. Corticosteroids in reversal of hemorrhagic shock in rats. Am J Physiol 209:815.

Yard, A. C., and Nickerson, M. 1965. Shock produced in dogs by infusions of norepinephrine. Fed Proc 15:502.

SECTION 8

Endocrine Pharmacology

CHAPTER 30

INTRODUCTION

LESLIE E. McDONALD

Endocrinology has been one of the latest of the medical sciences to develop. It is truly a twentieth-century science; most of the advances have been made since the 1930s. It has been an outgrowth from physiology, much as was biochemistry some years previously.

The endocrine system is one of the two great control or integrating forces in the body. The nervous system was the first to gain attention and it still remains an important coordinating system, but the endocrine system, which depends on a humoral mediator, has now taken its place alongside the nervous system. In fact, it is now evident that these two great control systems work together within the body. For example, the nervous system may serve as an afferent branch, bringing the impulse to the hypothalamus, wherein the endocrine system (hypophysis) then releases humoral substances that act peripherally to complete the reflex.

In the nervous system, the signal that travels throughout the body is similar regardless of the eventual effect, but it is the choice of pathways that determines the end result. In the case of the endocrine system, the pathway the mediator travels is always the same, namely, the circulatory system, but the humoral mediator varies to bring about the intended effects. This humoral substance travels rather slowly because it is dependent on the circulatory system for transportation. It has been named *hormone*.

Hormone is a Greek word meaning "I stir up or stimulate" and was first used by Bayliss and Starling in 1902. *A hormone is a chemical substance produced in one part of the body (restricted area) that diffuses or is transported to another area, where it influences activity and tends to integrate component parts of the organism.* It should be pointed out that *hormones regulate* (decrease or increase) the rates of specific processes but do not contribute energy to the process or initiate metabolic reactions. Instead, hormones influence an existing reaction, usually one involving enzymes. Consequently, an excess of hormone may be as detrimental as a deficiency since an existing reaction could be stimulated to excess. Starling's original definition of a hormone must now be broadened to include other "local hormones" or parahormones. These chemical messengers or regulators that are not hormones in the strictest sense include (1) prostaglandins, present in many tissues, but having important local effects on reproduction other systems, (2) erythropoietin, released by the anoxic kidney, stimulating bone marrow production of red blood cells (RBCs), and (3) histamine produced by injured tissues but acting locally on the surrounding tissue.

The restricted area where the hormone acts has been properly termed the *target organ* because it alone is responsive to the hormone. It is now known in some cases what constitutes or determines which shall be the target organ of a specific hormone. For example, the uterus is the target organ for estrogen because it contains an estrogen-dependent enzyme, pyridine nucleotide transhydrogenase. This estrogen-dependent transhydrogenase, when activated by estrogen, causes an increased production of biologically useful energy. This biologically useful energy can be used for myometrial growth, contraction, or even uterine gland secretion. It is of interest to note that the placenta, mammary gland, and anterior pituitary also contain this enzyme, whereas the liver does not. Target organs function at a minimal rate in the absence of the regulatory hormones.

MECHANISM OF HORMONE ACTION

A specific receptor site in a target organ selectively "binds," "takes up," or "traps" a particular hormone to the membrane or other part of the cell as the first step in hormone action (see Fig. 30.1).

The second step in this hormone action is the subsequent stimulation of the enzyme, adenyl cyclase, in the cell membrane to convert adenosine triphosphate (ATP) to the nucleotide adenosine monophosphate, cyclic 3′, 5′-AMP or cAMP. The cAMP (second messenger) provides energy for protein synthesis. Parathyroid hormone (PTH), adrenocorticotropic hormone (ACTH), luteinizing hormone (LH), thyroid-stimulating hormone (TSH), glucagon, epinephrine, and vasopressin produce some of their effects by this cAMP route. Some steroid production is regulated by cAMP. In fact, injection of cAMP will often mimic the effects of LH or ACTH to some degree. The cAMP then affects protein synthesis, and the inducer protein causes the mitochondrion to produce a hormone (third messenger).

Since different cells contain receptors

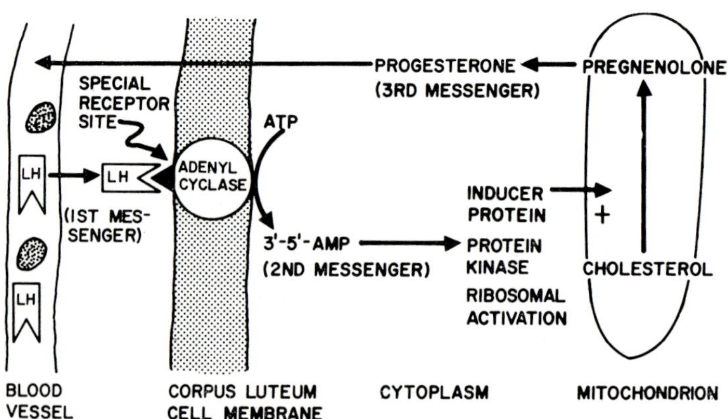

FIG. 30.1. Model to show how a specific receptor site binds a particular hormone (LH in this case). The target organ (corpus luteum cell membrane) contains a *hormone-specific receptor protein* as part of its adenyl cyclase system. Binding of LH results in activation of adenyl cyclase with a resulting increase in the production of cAMP (second messenger). The cAMP then activates the protein kinase in that particular cell, which leads to progesterone (third messenger) production by the mitochondrion.

for different hormones, one might postulate that cAMP could be the common denominator of all hormone action. Each cell would have different enzymes to be affected by cAMP.

Although the above scheme explains the mechanism of action of many hormones, there are still some additional possibilities such as (1) a hormone may affect the permeability of, or transport across, the cell membrane or subcellular structures, thereby making substrate more available, such as insulin increasing the uptake of glucose by muscle cells or the way somatotropin facilitates the entrance of amino acids through the cell membrane; (2) hormones may act by activating or suppressing certain genes. The ecdysone (a steroid) work in insects showed the hormone caused puffing of the salivary chromosomes. This puffing was on the transverse bands (deoxyribonucleic acid [DNA] bundles) and was actually the site where ribonucleic acid (RNA) and protein were being synthesized. The RNA was then transferred to the cytoplasm where it served as a template for the synthesis of particular proteins such as enzymes (Fig. 30.2).

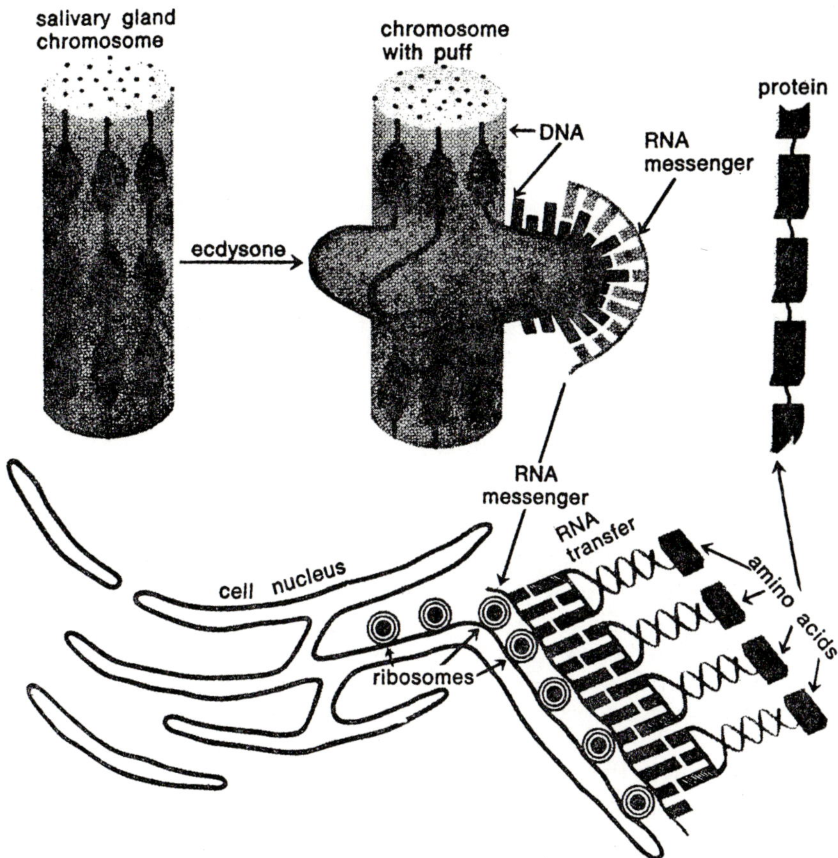

Fig. 30.2. Mechanism of action of ecdysone upon the giant salivary gland chromosomes of certain insects. The hormone is believed to act first on the DNA to produce a puff, which is the site of RNA synthesis. The messenger RNA carries the information necessary for the alignment of amino acids in the synthesis of specific proteins (e.g., certain enzymes). These enzymes presumably evoke within the target cells the biochemical changes involved in the molting process. (From Karlson, P., New concepts on the mode of action of hormones. Rassegna 42:7, 1965)

CHEMICAL CLASSES OF HORMONES

Hormones may be classified in two groups from the chemical point of view: (1) glycoproteins and (2) steroids.

Glycoproteins

The first group includes the peptide, protein, or glycoprotein hormones that are varied in structure and represent those hormones produced by the neurohypophysis and adenohypophysis, the thyroid and parathyroid glands, and islets of Langerhans. Building blocks for these hormones obviously are amino acids, and production of the hormone is dependent on the proper substrate, presence of an energy supply, and necessary biological stimulation. These hormones must be administered parenterally since oral administration would lead to their destruction by the digestive enzymes. Thyroxin is an exception since it is slightly active following oral administration.

Steroids

Steroid hormones constitute the second group and include all the gonadal and adrenal cortical hormones. The steroid structure is quite complex; the building blocks are acetate leading to cholesterol, with delicate alterations determining which steroid is finally released. The accompanying figures, 30.3 and 30.4, show the routes of steroidogenesis according to our present knowledge. Biogenesis of steroids by the endocrine organs probably involves each steroidogenic organ producing varying amounts of many related steroids. The tropic hormones from the pituitary, such as ACTH, favor a certain pathway, thereby causing that target organ (i.e. adrenal cortex) to produce primarily the end steroid intended and desired, cortisol (hydrocortisone). The substrate used may be any of the immediate substances circulating to the target organ such as acetate, cholesterol, or even another hormone such as progesterone, produced elsewhere by the corpus luteum. Furthermore, it can be seen how derangement of steroidogenesis may cause abnormal production of a hormone, such as the adrenal cortex producing excessive androgens in adrenal virilism.

Attention should be drawn to the structural similarity of several steroid hormones that have widely different physiological-pharmacological effects within the body. For example, the chemical differences between a potent androgen (testosterone) and a life-giving mineralocorticoid (aldosterone) are very minor.

Recognizing that the state of our knowledge at this time is imperfect and that other intermediates and pathways most probably will be found upon further investigation, we now will consider the conversion of immediate precursors into biologically active hormones. (1) *Adrenal corticoids.* (a) *Mineralocorticoids.* The three major mineralocorticoids are deoxycorticosterone (DOC), 11-deoxycortisol, and aldosterone. Fig. 30.4 shows that DOC and aldosterone both probably arise from progesterone, while 11-deoxycortisol probably comes from 17α-hydroxyprogesterone. (b) *Glucocorticoids.* The 11-oxygenated corticosteroids are the most potent in affecting carbohydrate and protein metabolism and include cortisol, corticosterone, 11-dehydrocorticosterone, and cortisone. It can be seen in Fig. 30.4 that cortisone can be derived from cortisol, which in turn is obtained from 17αOH progesterone via 11-deoxycortisol. Dehydrocorticosterone can be obtained from progesterone via two intermediates, deoxycorticosterone and corticosterone. (2) *Androgens.* The major androgens listed in order of increasing biological potency are dehydroepiandrosterone, androstenedione, and testosterone. Dehydroepiandrosterone is derived from pregnenolone via the intermediate 17α-hydroxypregnenolone. Dehydroepiandrosterone could then be secreted or further metabolized. If not secreted and if oxidation at C-3 took place, the product would be androstenedione. Another pathway for androstenedione biosynthesis would be by splitting of the side chain and oxidation at C-17 of 17α-hydroxyprogesterone. Testosterone is formed via the enzyme 17β-steroid dehydrogenase that reduces the ketone

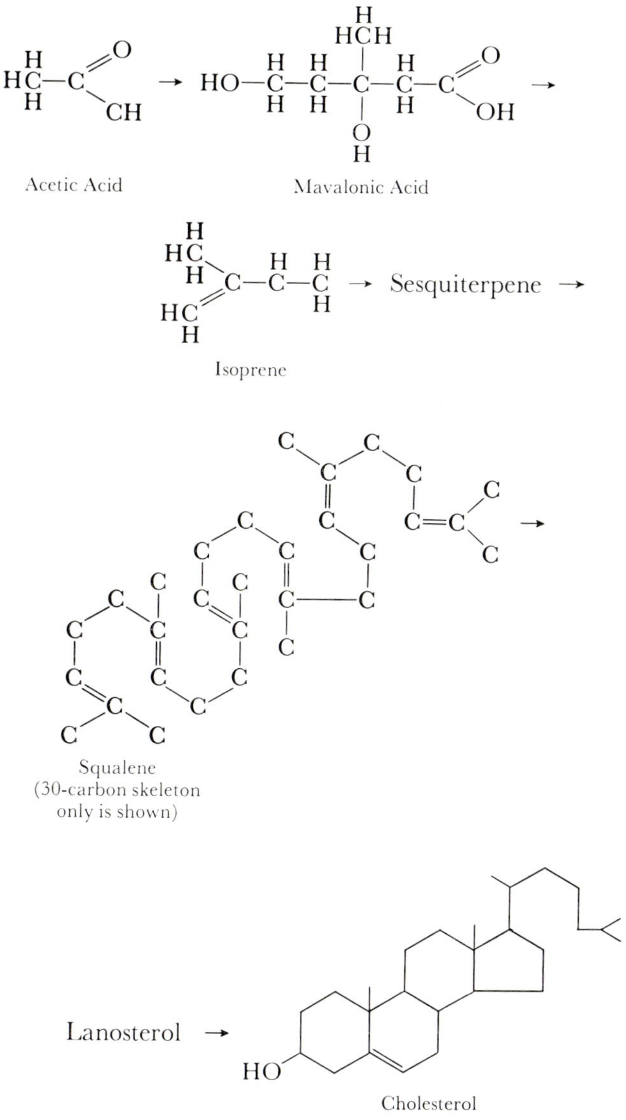

Acetic Acid

Mavalonic Acid

Isoprene

Sesquiterpene

Squalene (30-carbon skeleton only is shown)

Lanosterol

Cholesterol

FIG. 30.3. Steps in the synthesis of cholesterol from acetate via the linking of small units to form the unsaturated aliphatic hydrocarbon squalene and the closure of rings to form the cyclic sterols. (From A. Gorbman and H. A. Bern 1962)

to hydroxyl at C-17. (3) *Estrogens.* The primary ovarian estrogens are estradiol-17β and estrone. It is interesting that estrogens probably arise from androgens. Estrone and estradiol-17β are interconvertable and probably exist in equilibrium with one another. Estradiol-17β can arise from testosterone by hydroxylation at C-19 and aromatization (complete unsaturation) of ring A. Estrone on the other hand most likely arises from androstenedione via hydroxylation at C-19 and aromatization of ring A.

In summary, it appears that the differences between several steroid-secreting glands are largely quantitative rather than qualitative. This concept could be used to explain various natural phenomena that to this date are not clearly understood. For example, this could explain the change from secretion of estrogens by the ovarian follicle to progesterone secretion by the

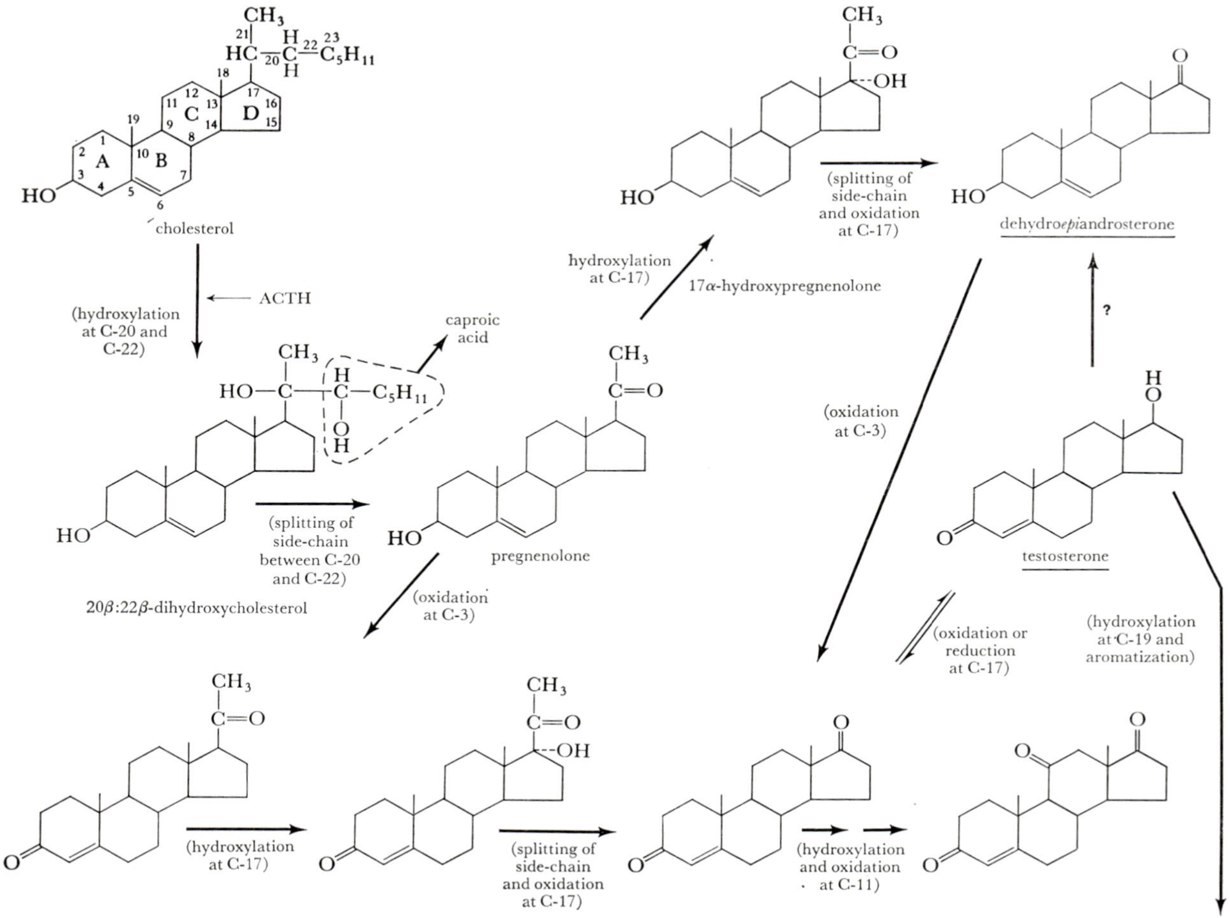

Fig. 30.4. Major metabolic pathways involved in biogenesis of steroid hormones. The principal secretory products of the steroidogenic organs are underlined. Specific enzymes have been characterized, and mitochondrial or microsomal participation has been determined for many of the steps shown. The 17- and 21-hydroxylations appear to require mitochondria; the 11-hydroxylation, microsomes. Also, various cofactors have been specified for many of the steps. For example, reduced nicotinamide adenine dinucleotide phosphate (NADPH) and molecular O_2 are required for the various hydroxylations and for the side-chain splitting (desmolase enzyme activity). In addition, certain ions are known to be required for the conversion of corticosterone to aldosterone by the zona glomerulosa cells of the adrenal cortex. Most of the products of catabolism of the major steroid hormones are not shown. (From A. Gorbman and H. A. Bern 1962)

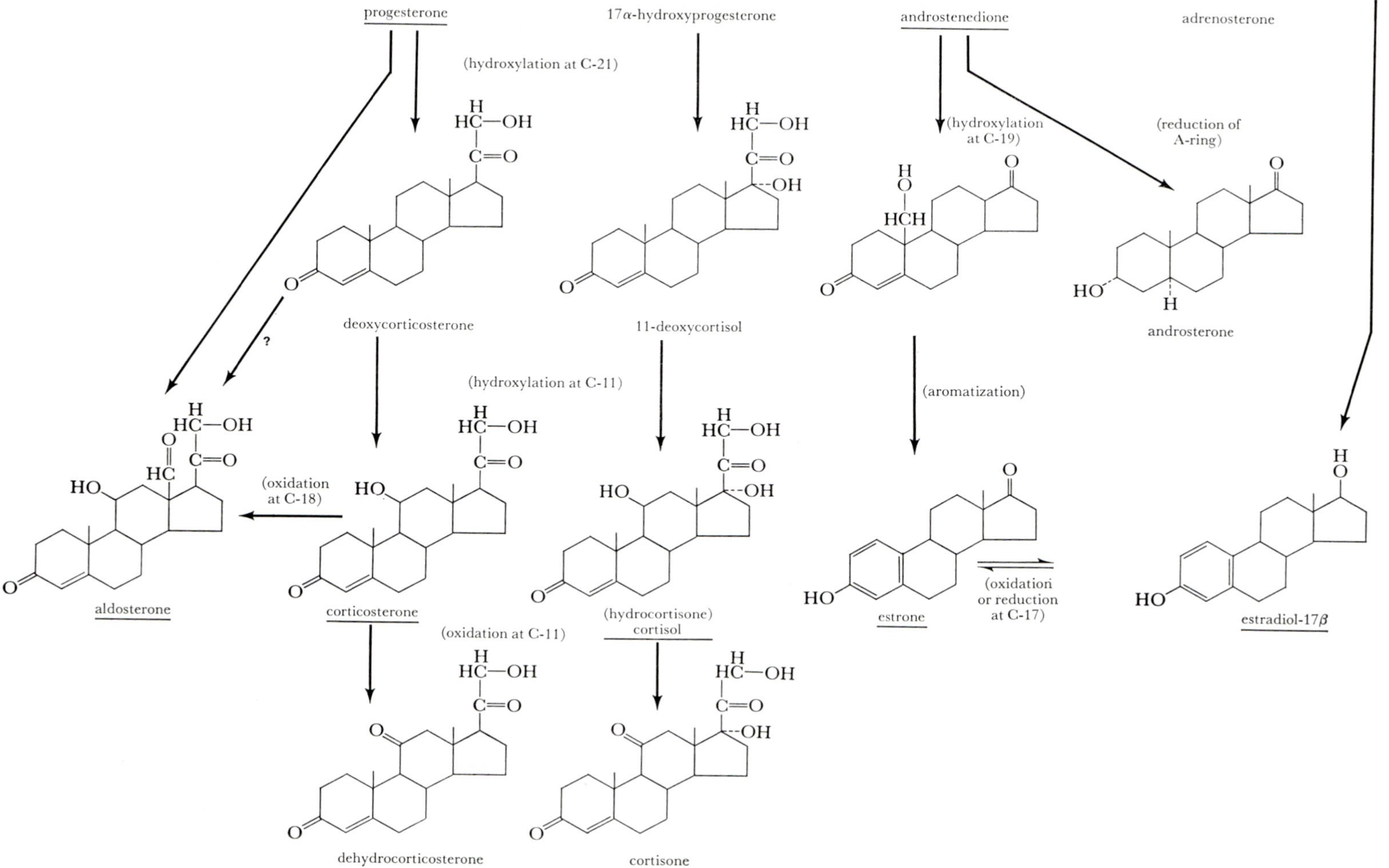
progesterone
17α-hydroxyprogesterone
androstenedione
adrenosterone
(hydroxylation at C-21)
(hydroxylation at C-19)
(reduction of A-ring)
deoxycorticosterone
11-deoxycortisol
androsterone
?
(hydroxylation at C-11)
(aromatization)
(oxidation at C-18)
aldosterone
corticosterone
(hydrocortisone) cortisol
estrone
(oxidation or reduction at C-17)
estradiol-17β
(oxidation at C-11)
dehydrocorticosterone
cortisone

TABLE 30.1. Common nomenclature conventions of the steroids

Suffix or Prefix	Meaning	Example
-ane	Saturated chain or ring system	Androst*ane*
-ene	Unsaturation, one or more double bonds	Pregn*en*olone
-ol	Hydroxy group	Cholester*ol*
-one	Keto group	Aldoster*one*
hydroxy-	α-OH (below plane of ring, indicated by dashed line as — — —)	α-Estradi*ol*
α-, β-	β-OH (above plane of ring, indicated by solid line as ———)	β-Estradi*ol*
keto-	Ketone group	17-*keto*steroid
Δ^3-	Double bond between C-3 and C-4	Δ^3-Isopentenyl pyrophosphate
nor-	One less carbon in side chain	19-*Nor*testosterone
allo-	Another form, rings A and B are trans	*Allo*pregnane
cis-	Two groups on same side of plane	. . . . . .
trans-	Two groups on opposite sides of plane	. . . . . .
oxy- (oxo)-	Additional oxygen	19-*Oxo*testosterone
deoxy-	Less one oxygen	11-*Deoxy*corticosterone
hydro- (dihydro)-	Two additional hydrogens	*Hydro*cortisone (cortisol)
dehydro-	Two less hydrogens	7-*Dehydro*cholesterol
epi-	Isomeric to named compound (usually at C-3)	*Epi*androsterone

corpus luteum. If such a difference is due solely to levels of key enzymes, this radical change in steroid secretion pattern could be understood as a relative loss of activity of an enzyme in the pathway between progesterone and estrogens. If the enzyme for 17-hydroxylation of progesterone became inactive as the follicle cells are replaced by luteal cells, progesterone rather than estrogen would subsequently be produced.

The steroid hormones, either natural or synthetic, are active when administered orally since intestinal destruction is minimal. Obviously, the dosage must be increased when this route is used because the net absorption is reduced.

DETERMINANTS OF SUCCESS WITH HORMONE THERAPY

One of the main purposes of this chapter is to acquaint the practitioner with some of the possible reasons why endocrine therapy is not always satisfactory. Our knowledge is deficient in many areas insofar as the endocrine system is concerned. We must consider the possible ways that endocrine pharmacology may differ from more classical pharmacology. We shall consider several possible causes of these differences.

OVERLAPPING OF EFFECTS BY HORMONES

The chemical structures of many of the hormones are so similar that there is an overlapping of effects when the hormone reaches the target organ. For example, hydrocortisone, which is primarily a glucocorticoid and is not essential for the immediate life of the animal, has only minor biochemical differences in its massive steroid structure from aldosterone, a life-preserving electrolyte-influencing adrenal corticoid. Differences in saturation, methylation, or oxygenation of the steroid structure alter biological activity sufficiently to determine life or death of an adrenal-deficient animal. On the other hand, the chemical similarity may be such that a target organ cannot distinguish the difference completely, hence a glucocorticoid may have some sodium-retaining and potassium-eliminating effects on the renal tubule similar to a mineralocorticoid.

Steroid chemistry has advanced sufficiently that many structural alterations are possible in the laboratory, thereby bringing a virtual flood of steroids on the market, each with specific effects, some of which are unnatural to the recipient animal.

ADMINISTRATION OF HORMONES

In the administration of hormones it should be established early whether or not the course of action constitutes *replacement therapy* of a failing organ with a naturally occurring hormone administered at a *physiological* level to bring about the usual physiological effects. For example, insulin is administered only to bring about physiological effects that would be occurring if functional islet cells were present. Other hormones administered at physiological levels for replacement therapy include vasopressin, thyroxin, gonadotropins, and ACTH.

In contrast to the above, we must consider that occasionally *additive therapy* will be instituted, using either naturally occurring hormones or the newer synthetic hormones, either of which is administered at higher or *pharmacological levels to bring about effects not usually related to natural metabolic functions.* In this case, unnatural effects are desired, consequently one may encounter side effects or untoward reactions. This should be kept in mind during the course of therapy. For example, it is a common practice to administer a progestin, usually a synthetic one that is biochemically slightly different from the natural substance. If administered in high dosage, there is an interference with pituitary gonadotropin release and inhibition of follicular growth, and anestrus and infertility ensue. This contraceptive effect is desired sometimes in the case of the bitch or the mare. Another example involves the administration of potent synthetic androgens to bring about anabolism and nitrogen retention to fight wasting disease of aged or debilitated animals. This is brought about to an extent that is unnatural or unphysiologic in the domestic animal, yet is desirable. Perhaps the many glucocorticoids are the hormones most commonly used pharmacologically, because of their antiinflammatory effects.

Critical Dosage

Many hormones are unique in that different effects may be brought about depending on whether a small or a large dose is administered. This is rather unique when we consider the use of drugs. For example, a small amount of progesterone, such as 10 mg in a dairy cow, favors the release of the ovulatory hormone from the pituitary gland, whereas high levels of progesterone administered to the same animal would inhibit the release of the ovulatory hormone. Furthermore, low levels of estrogen, such as the dairy cow experiences between periods of estrus, favor lactation by stimulating lactiferous tissue, whereas high estrogen levels, such as the cow experiences during estrus or after an injection of estrogen, tend to suppress milk secretion. A low level of estrogen has a favorable effect upon the anestrous ovary, bringing about stimulation of ovagenesis, whereas a high level of estrogen tends to block pituitary gonadotropins, thereby causing ovagenesis to decrease. This points out that there is an extremely critical dosage range in the use of many hormones and that the response one gets may be not only dependent upon the hormone selected but the amount given.

Duration of Action

The duration of hormone action within the animal body after entering the circulation varies considerably with the natural hormone. For example, progesterone has a biological half-life of 4 minutes and ACTH 6 minutes, whereas thyroxin has a half-life of 10 days. This means that a given molecule of the circulating hormone may be eliminated quickly in the case of progesterone but circulate for a considerable length of time, bringing about more prolonged effects in the case of thyroxin.

The onset of action is somewhat dependent on the routes of administration. For example, intravenous administration of a hormone, if feasible, brings about the quickest response, followed by the intraperitoneal, intramuscular, subcutaneous, and, finally, oral routes. The parenteral absorption rate is directly related to the adequacy of the blood supply to the injection site. Not all hormones can be injected intravenously; for example, the oily preparations cannot be administered this way, whereas protein hormones cannot be administered orally because of digestive breakdown.

Attempts have been made to prolong the short half-life of many hormones. The metabolic destruction rate has been decreased by altering the structure, such as acetylation of steroid hormones. The acetylated steroid is unnatural within the body and is more slowly metabolized because the destructive enzyme system is not adapted to the altered steroid. This means that the steroid will circulate longer, have a more prolonged effect, and consequently be a more potent hormone. Oily preparations of the fat-soluble hormones delay absorption following intramuscular injection. Of considerable importance in veterinary medicine is the implanting of hormones, which consists of depositing the hormone along with a slowly disintegrating filler in a poorly vascularized area such as subcutaneously, thereby slowing absorption and more closely simulating natural release of the hormone.

AUGMENTATION

Protein hormones may be combined with certain substances such as copper, zinc, or the iron of heme to bring about a more prolonged effect. This augmentation by a foreign substance is probably brought about because the destructive enzyme system associated with hormone metabolism is not able to cope with the altered substance as quickly as it would otherwise. Pharmacologists have taken advantage of this phenomenon as in the addition of zinc to insulin, thereby prolonging its activity.

Synergism is another phenomenon that may occur when two or more hormones are administered simultaneously. Synergism means that the total response when the hormones are administered simultaneously is greater than the sum of the effects of the same hormones when given separately. Follicle-stimulating hormone (FSH) and LH (or interstitial cell–stimulating hormone [ICSH]) are good examples of hormones causing this phenomenon.

ANTIHORMONES

Most of the protein hormones, such as the pituitary gonadotropins and the thyroid-stimulating hormone (TSH), are able to induce refractoriness to the injected hormone from a heterologous species. This means that continued administration of a protein hormone from another species may bring about antibody production to the extent that neutralization of the injected hormone may occur. This may or may not be a typical antibody. Maddock (1949) found that the administration of sheep pituitary FSH to infertile men elicited sufficient antibody within a few months to neutralize the daily injections and eventually to neutralize the endogenous pituitary gonadotropin being produced.

Antihormone production has been demonstrated when TSH is administered to the normal rabbit, guinea pig, dog, and horse. In the rabbit, Mahaux (1939) found that basal metabolic rate (100) rose rapidly (to 129) for approximately 1 week following daily injections of TSH, then the basal metabolic rate (BMR) fell for approximately 1 week until the normal BMR (100) was again reached. Thereafter, continued administration of exogenous TSH caused sufficient antibody production to neutralize the animal's own endogenous TSH, bringing about profound hypothyroidism (BMR of 76). This is illustrated in Fig. 30.5.

In addition to the hormone neutralization occurring when heterologous hormones are administered, there may be additional side effects such as dermal reactions, respiratory distress, or severe anaphylactic shock. This is especially true when pregnant mare serum is administered as a source of a FSH-like substance. The foreign plasma proteins can elicit a severe anaphylactic shock if the animal is injected again within the sensitive period.

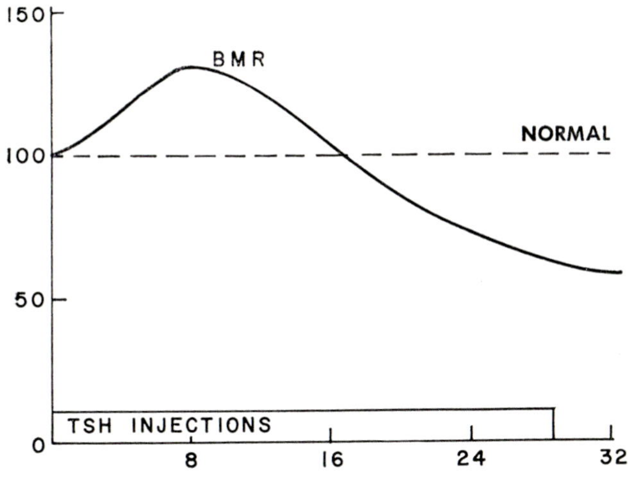

FIG. 30.5. The effect of daily injections of TSH on BMR in the rabbit. (After Mahaux 1939)

ANTAGONISTS OR ANALOGS

Endocrine pharmacology has been primarily concerned with the treatment of hormonal deficiencies, leaving hormonal excesses to treatment by surgical removal or radiation destruction of the hyperactive gland. Some progress is being made in developing selective inhibitors of the hormone or the synthesis of the hormone within the body, although progress is limited.

An adrenocorticolytic agent, *o,p'*DDD (Schechter et al. 1973), reduces adrenal corticosteroid output (Calif Biochem).

Thyroxin synthesis by the thyroid can be interfered with by certain substances such as the thioureas. Some of the tranquilizers can block ovulation in laboratory animals (Barraclough and Sawyer 1957). Progress in this field will be slow, but the practitioner can look forward to eventual help in this area.

HORMONE TRANSPORT

After production by a particular gland, the protein hormones are usually stored within that gland until needed. Upon call, they are then secreted into the efferent capillaries. Steroid hormones are not stored, instead they are released as produced.

Few, if any, of the steroid hormones circulate in the blood as the pure hormone after having been released from the endocrine organ that formed it. Plasma contains specific carrier proteins for the steroid hormones and thyroxin. These are thyroxin-binding globulin (TBG), corticosteroid-binding globulin (CBG) (also called transcortin), and sex-hormone–binding globulin (SHBG). This binding to plasma proteins restricts diffusion through the tissues but at the same time prolongs their action since the binding is a storage and buffer scheme to some extent. The bound form of a hormone is inactive at the intracellular level and must be in the free form before it can act. Pregnancy causes an increase in the protein-bound thyroid hormone or iodine (PBI) but the BMR remains essentially the same because the hormone is held in the blood and only the usual amount gets to the tissues in the free state to stimulate metabolism.

The sex steroids are firmly bound to SHBG, thus increasing the solubility of the steroid in the aqueous medium of the blood. The bound steroid is biologically inactive but it is in equilibrium with the free form, which is the form taken up by the target cells.

Thyroxin has a much shorter period of action in the chicken than in mammals. This may be due to the fact that the bird has a low ability to bind thyroxin to its plasma proteins, consequently thyroxin is lost from the avian body by metabolism more quickly than from mammals, which have a greater ability to bind thyroxin to the plasma proteins.

TARGET CELL SPECIFICITY—RECEPTOR SITES

The effector tissues have a particular ability to "trap" or "bind" the hormone concerned with their function and hold it firmly at the receptor site. This is especially true in the case of insulin since we know that those tissues that use insulin, namely, muscle and adipose and mammary tissues, take up insulin with such an affinity that it is difficult to wash away. This is not true of brain tissue or RBCs since these tissues do not use insulin and consequently do not hold it. Likewise, the gonads appear to "trap" the gonadotropins and hold them in close association so that the effector tissue has an opportunity to be acted upon by the hormone. This "trapping" mechanism means that the hormone is attached to the receptor site.

Although most hormones have a target organ that responds to a greater extent than any other tissue, most hormones affect other tissues to varying degrees. For example, the female sex hormone from the ovarian follicle, estradiol, has as its target organ the accessory sex organs such as the uterus and vagina. Estradiol exerts a most profound influence on their growth, development, and function. But other tissues such as skin, hair, and bone also have receptor sites and respond to estrogen. Thus it is important to keep in mind that a hormone may have several effects in the body even though its main effect may be on the primary target organ.

Target organs can function at a minimal level even in the absence of the hormone. Thus nature has provided a base level of function that may be sufficient to maintain life in the absence of the hormone. *In vitro* slices of the thyroid, adrenals, or even gonads produce some of their respective hormones; likewise all tissues are able to use carbohydrates at a minimal level even in the absence of insulin. It is of interest to note that nerve tissue and RBCs do not respond to insulin, consequently not all cells of the body are dependent on insulin for their normal functions.

Some physiological processes need more than one hormone for full function. Development of full lactation potential by the mammary gland requires a sequential effect by estrogen, progesterone, and possibly some adenohypophyseal hormones. In addition, thyroxin and adrenal corticoids are essential. Thus lactation is a response to several hormones.

REGULATION OF HORMONE SECRETION

The endocrine glands are important regulators of many processes in the body, therefore it is obvious that careful regulation of endocrine output is critical. Regulation of hormone secretion depends on several mechanisms. A particular hormone output may depend on more than one control mechanism. Some are fairly well understood while others are still being studied. With current information we can categorize these (Table 30.2).

Humoral control is the mechanism we usually think of first and the category of *metabolite concentration* is one of the simplest control schemes we have. For example, a rising level of blood glucose signals for a blood sugar–lowering hormone, insulin, to be released. Insulin facilitates glucose movement through the cell membrane and it is either metabolized or stored for later use, usually in the form of glycogen. Either route lowers blood glucose. Should the blood glucose level drop below normal, a blood glucose–raising hormone, glucagon, which acts to stimulate

TABLE 30.2. Types of control of endocrine secretion

Humoral
Concentration of a metabolite
Concentration of another hormone
Nervous
Peripheral nerve connection
Hypothalamic connection (pituitary)
Genetic

Source: Gorbman and Bern 1962.

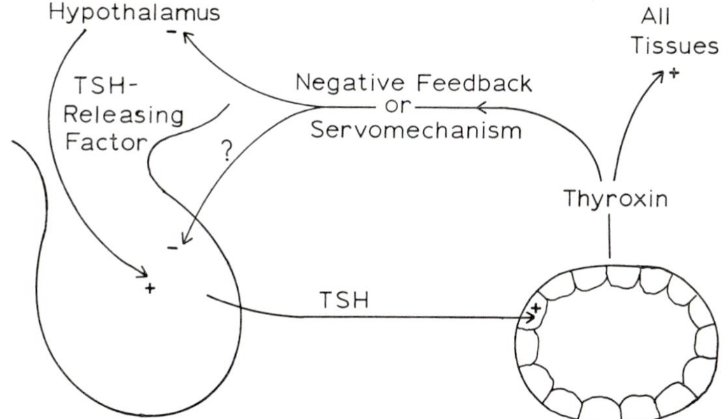

FIG. 30.6. A typical "negative feedback" or "servomechanism" type of regulation of hormone output. There is a continuing effort by the hypothalamus to produce TSH-releasing factor. This causes TSH to be released, which in turn causes thyroxin output. Thyroxin "feeds" back to inhibit the hypothalamus from producing TSH-releasing factor. If thyroxin levels fall, then the brake is released and TSH production rises.

the release of sugar from the glycogen stores of the liver thereby raising the glucose level back to normal, is released from the alpha cells of the pancreatic islets.

Regulation of hormone output by *concentration of another hormone* is best depicted via the adenohypophysis, which secretes some 5 hormones that regulate other glands. This is a *feedback mechanism* or *servomechanism.* The anterior pituitary is in turn inhibited directly or indirectly (via the hypothalamic releasing factors) by those hormones produced by the target endocrine organs. Therefore, a balance is finally achieved between the continual stimulating effects of the adenohypophyseal hormone and the resultant inhibitory effects on adenohypophyseal hormone output by the target organ hormone (Fig. 30.6). A *servomechanism* as used in endocrinology is an automatic means of correcting the hormone output of a gland to a desired level by a level-sensing feedback of another hormone.

Peripheral nervous control of hormone output is difficult to separate entirely except in the case of the adrenal medulla where a peripheral nerve connection (pregangionic sympathetic fiber) can cause increased output of epinephrine. This impulse could have arisen in the cerebral cortex after the animal recorded a frightful image on the visual cortex.

Another method involves the *hypothalamic connection* as a means of mediating *nervous control.* A good example of this is the way light affects the reproductive cycle of certain animals. In some species, increasing day length signals the hypothalamus, which in turn increases the output or changes the ratio of adenohypophyseal gonadotropins (FSH and LH). This awakens the gonad, causing germ cell and sex hormone production to resume.

Finally, we must consider, especially in domestic animals, the influence of the *genetic makeup* of the animal on endocrine secretion. The possible effects of genetic coding on hormone output and the effect of hormones on protein synthesis were considered earlier. The practical aspect of this in terms of pituitary somatotropin content is the increased output present in fast-growing animals.

Thus one can see that the endocrine system serves as an important control mechanism but it in turn is controlled by and is obedient to other forces. There does not appear to be any central control and the old reference to the anterior pituitary as being "the master gland" is no longer tenable. There are so many external influences on the function of the adenohypophysis that we cannot look upon it as a control headquarters but instead we must consider it as an important link in a circuitous control scheme.

REFERENCES

Banting, F., and Best, C. H. 1922. The internal secretion of the pancreas. J Lab Clin Med 7:251.

Barraclough, C., and Sawyer, C. H. 1957. Blockade of the release of pituitary ovulating hormone in the rat by chlorpromazine and reserpine. Endocrinology 61:341.

Bayliss, W. M., and Starling, E. H. 1902. The mechanism of pancreatic secretion. J Physiol 28:325.

Gorbman, A., and Bern, H. A. 1962. A Textbook of Comparative Endocrinology, p. 239. New York: John Wiley & Sons.

Hector, O., and Halkerson, I. D. K. 1965. Effects of steroid hormones on gene regulation and cell metabolism. Annu Rev Physiol 27:133.

Jacob, F., and Monod, J. 1961. Genetic regulatory mechanisms in the synthesis of proteins. J Mol Biol 3:318.

Kleinsmith, L. J. 1972. Molecular mechanisms for the regulation of cell function. Bioscience 22:343.

Maddock, W. O. 1949. Antihormone formation complicating pituitary gonadotropin therapy in infertile men. I. Properties of the antihormones. J Clin Endocrinol 9:213, 355.

Mahaux, Jacques. 1939. Action de l'"hormone thyréotrope" sur le métabolisme basal de lapins normaux et de lapins ayant présente précédement une période d'inversion d' action de l'"hormone thyréotrope." C R Soc Biol 132(23–25):97–99.

Schechter, R. D.; Stabenfeldt, G. H.; Gribble, D. H.; and Ling, G. V. 1973. Treatment of Cushing's syndrome in the dog with an adrenocorticolytic agent (*o,p'*DDD). J Am Vet Med Assoc 162:629.

Starling, E. H. 1905. The chemical correlation of the functions of the body. Lancet 2:339.

Sutherland, E. W. 1972. Studies on the mechanism of hormone action. Science 177:401.

CHAPTER 31

HORMONES OF THE PITUITARY GLAND

LESLIE E. McDONALD

The pituitary gland is divided into two major components according to the embryologic derivation: the adenohypophysis, which came from the oral ectoderm; and the neurohypophysis, which came from the neural ectoderm. The adenohypophysis is further divided into the pars distalis or anterior lobe; the pars tuberalis; and a minor part, the pars intermedia, which is of no currently known significance in domestic animals. The neurohypophysis is of physiologic importance in domestic animals and will be considered later in the chapter.

TABLE 31.1. Tentative cell source of adenohypophysis hormones

Cells	Secretion
Chromophobes	None (resting or precursor cell)
Chromophils	
Acidophils	
somatotrophs	STH
lactotrophs	Prolactin
Basophils	
FSH gonadotrophs	FSH
LH gonadotrophs	LH
thyrotrophs	TSH
corticotrophs	ACTH

ADENOHYPOPHYSIS

The hormones of the anterior lobe of the pituitary can be divided into two main groups according to their method of action. In the first group are those hormones acting directly on the soma, whereas in the second group are those hormones acting indirectly by first stimulating another endocrine organ to release a hormone, thereby bringing about an effect (Fig. 31.1). In the first group, acting directly on the soma, are the somatotropic, or growth hormone, and prolactin, or lactogenic hormone, which acts on the mammary tissue affecting milk secretion. In the second group are the thyrotropic, adrenal corticotropic, and gonadotropic hormones that act on the various endocrine organs concerned. A summary of the various hormones from the pituitary, their source, site of action, and activity within the body are shown in Table 31.2.

The effects of removal of the anterior lobe of the pituitary or of total hypophysectomy are varied and not specific since

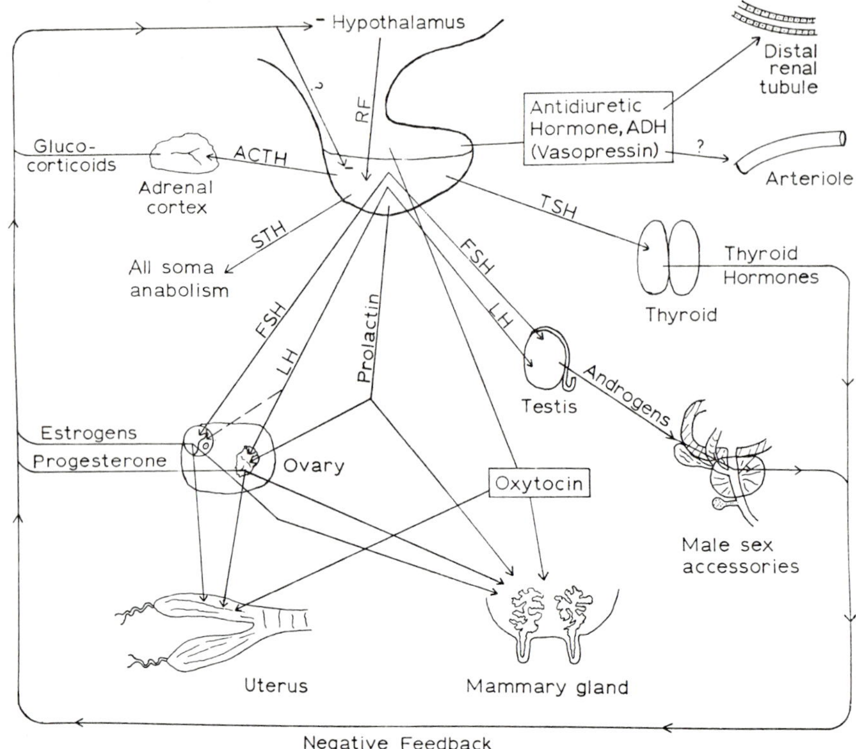

FIG. 31.1. Diagram of hormones of pituitary gland, their target organs, and interrelationships.

the anterior pituitary regulates the function of so many other organs.

Age has considerable effect on the manifestations of hypophysectomy since the prepubertal animal would show primarily a deficiency in the rate of growth with accompanying decrease in the activity of the thyroid and adrenal glands. Since the gonads have not reached a peak of function, gonadal insufficiency would be less recognizable.

If hypophysectomy occurs after puberty, growth would not be affected since the animal would have reached adult proportions, but deficiencies in thyroid and adrenal functions would appear, as well as reproductive abeyance and lactation cessation. In general, the clinical picture would be one of subsistence or maintenance level of bodily activities that had been influenced by the adenohypophysis. (See Fig. 31.1.)

It is of importance to note that the pituitary gland is not essential for life, that the essential organs such as the adrenal cortex are capable of continued function to the extent that the basic life processes are preserved. It is those functions above the maintenance level of the body that are most drastically affected, such as growth, reproduction, and lactation.

Releasing Factors (Hormones)

The last two decades can be referred to in the endocrinology story as the period of releasing factors. This truly has been an exciting chapter in endocrinology because it explained the functional role of the anatomical oddity, the hypophyseal portal system. At the same time the anatomical and functional relationships of the adenohypophysis to the hypothalamus and the central nervous system (CNS) were brought into a clear perspective. This miss-

TABLE 31.2. Hormones of the pituitary gland

Lobe	Part	Hormone		Site of Action (target organ)	Biologic Activity
Adenohypophysis	Pars distalis (anterior lobe)	Somatotropin (STH, growth hormone)		General soma	Body growth (bone, muscle, organs), protein synthesis, carbohydrate metabolism, regulation of renal functions (GFR) and water metabolism, increase cell permeability to amino acids
		Adrenocorticotropic hormone (ACTH, corticotropin)		Adrenal cortex	Maintenance of structural integrity of adrenal cortex, regulation of glucocorticoid secretion by zona fasciculata
		Thyrotropic hormone (TSH, thyrotropin)		Thyroid	Maintenance of the normal structure and function of the thyroid gland, production of thyroxin and analogs
		Prolactin (lactogenic hormone)		Mammary gland	Possibly favoring lactation
		Gonadotropins	Follicle-stimulating hormone (FSH)	Ovary	Growth and maturation of ovarian follicles
				Testis seminiferous tubules	Germ-cell production (spermatogenesis)
			Interstitial cell stimulating or luteinizing hormone (ICSH, LH)	Ovary	Synergistically with FSH causing estrogen secretion, follicle maturation and ovulation, corpus luteum development in some species
				Testis Leydig cells	Stimulation of interstitial tissue, androgen secretion
			Luteotropic hormone (LTH, Prolactin, lactogenic hormone)	Corpus luteum	Stimulation and maintenance of functional activity with secretion of progesterone (only rat and possibly sheep)
				Mammary gland	Possibly favoring lactation
	Pars intermedia	Intermedin		Melanophore cells of amphibia and reptiles	Melanophore-expanding activity with resultant maintenance of skin color (in mammals, of negligible importance)
Neurohypophysis		Antidiuretic hormone (ADH, vasopressin)		Renal tubules (distal convoluted)	Regulation of water excretion by reabsorption of water, pressor effect only in high doses
		Oxytocic hormone		Mammary myoepithelium	Letdown of milk by contraction of myoepithelium
				Uterine myometrium	Contraction of uterine musculature to aid parturition, sperm transport, and cyclic activity

Source: V. A. Drill 1958. Pharmacology in Medicine. New York; McGraw-Hill. Used by permission.

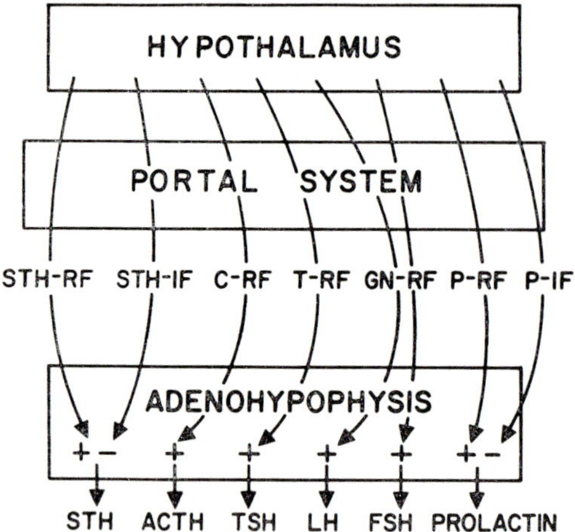

FIG. 31.2. The hypothalamic production of known releasing factors (RF) and inhibiting factors (IF) that reach the adenohypophysis via the portal system to influence the output of the six hormones.

ing link, the releasing factors (RF), seems to bring together these two great coordinating systems. (See Fig. 31.2.)

The hypothalamic releasing factors are physiological substances that will stimulate or inhibit the release of adenohypophyseal hormones. These "factors" by most definitions meet the requirements for a hormone and are sometimes referred to as hypothalamic releasing hormones.

We can now say with a considerable degree of accuracy that there are substances formed in the hypothalamus that pass via the hypophyseal portal system to influence the release of all six hormones from the adenohypophysis. Corticotrophin releasing factor (CRF) was the first releasing factor to be discovered. LH (luteinizing hormone) releasing factor and FSH (follicle-stimulating hormone) releasing factor are probably identical since they are not separable at the present time. This RF is referred to as GnRF, or gonadotropin releasing factor. TRF and SRF favor release of TSH and STH, respectively. (See Fig. 31.3.) SRF is sometimes referred to as GRF because STH is synonymous with growth hormone. Notice the difference between GnRF and GRF, a point of frequent confusion. The regulator of the release of prolactin is unusual in the mammal since it regulates the release of prolactin in a negative fashion and is referred to as prolactin inhibitory factor (PIF). The full significance of this prolactin inhibitory factor in the mammal is not fully understood. It is known, though, that in the pigeon and possibly other birds it is a "releasing factor" and causes the release of prolactin, which in turn causes the proliferation of the mucosa of the crop gland with the secretion of "crop milk." Why this control is reversed in the mammal is not known. (See Fig. 31.4.)

In addition to PIF influencing prolactin output, there is an inhibitory factor that negatively influences STH release. This inhibitory factor is called SIF, or somatostatin. There may be other undiscovered inhibitory factors controlling the release of the other pituitary hormones, but at this writing none is certain.

The identity of most releasing factors and the finding that they are small peptides led to chemical identification and synthesis of several. The chemical structure of SRF is still uncertain. The chemical struc-

TRF

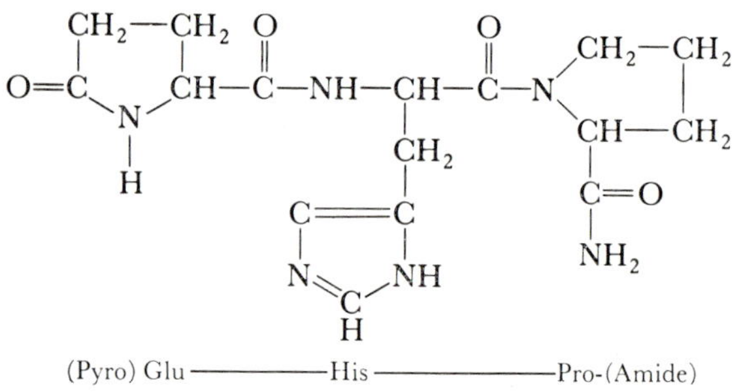

(Pyro) Glu——His——Pro-(Amide)

FIG. 31.3. Thyrotropin releasing factor (TRF). Amino acid sequence.

GnRF

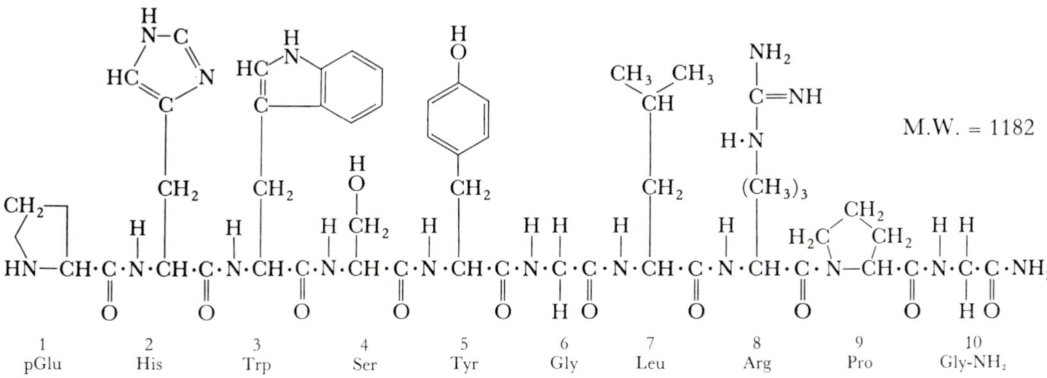

M.W. = 1182

HN—CH·C·N·CH·C·N·CH·C·N·CH·C·N·CH·C·N·C·C·N·CH·C·N·CH·C·N—CH·C·N·C·C·NH$_2$

1	2	3	4	5	6	7	8	9	10
pGlu	His	Trp	Ser	Tyr	Gly	Leu	Arg	Pro	Gly-NH$_2$

FIG. 31.4 Gonadotropin releasing factor (GnRF). Amino acid sequence of this decapeptide.

ture is known for CRF, TRF, and GnRF. The availability of these releasing factors and inhibitory factors undoubtedly will have an important impact on veterinary medicine since the control of these physiological processes in domestic animals is a long-awaited development. Thus far there does not appear to be species specificity for the releasing factors consequently that will simplify their use in animals.

The mechanism of action of the releasing factors is still uncertain, although it is known that it is an oxygen-requiring process, and cyclic adenosine monophosphate (cAMP) may be involved (see Fig. 31.5). After the administration of a releasing factor, there is a pituitary response in a matter of minutes. The circulating half-life of the releasing factors is very short, only a few minutes.

The control of production and release of the releasing factors by the hypothala-

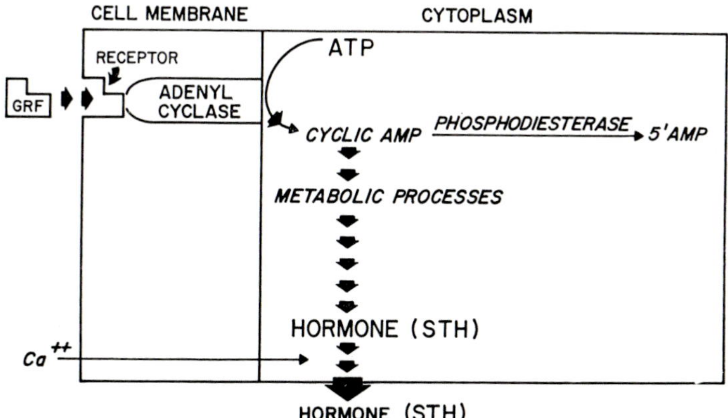

FIG. 31.5. Postulated action of GRF (SRF) on a somatotrope. In most tissues, adenyl cyclase is tightly bound to the plasma membrane. A hormone-specific receptor appropriate for the target tissue is linked to the adenyl cyclase. The enzyme catalyzes conversion of ATP to cyclic AMP. The latter is rapidly degraded by phosphodiesterase. Elevation of cyclic AMP levels in the tissue results in stimulation of metabolic processes in the cell, which leads to the expected physiological response by the target tissue. In the case of the somatotrope, this would include uptake of Ca^{++} by the cell and extrusion of STH from the cell. (From Ganong, W., and Martini, L., Frontiers in Neuroendocrinology, 1973, Oxford University Press)

mus is modified by a hormone feedback system from the target glands of the tropic hormones as described in Chapter 30. In addition to the feedback control, stimuli from the external environment also affect anterior pituitary hormone release. In seasonal breeding animals such as the ewe, bitch, or mare, the photoperiod must strongly influence the hypothalamus output of releasing factors. Many other external stimuli such as pain, emotional disturbance, restraint, anesthetics, sexual excitation, or milking influence the output of various releasing factors (Convey 1973).

Releasing factors are not approved for use in domestic animals at this writing but their approval should be forthcoming.

Somatotropin (STH)

Somatotropin or growth hormone is a complex protein that has been studied by many groups for several decades. There are species differences but they appear to be more similar than once thought and the molecular weight is approximately 22,000 for most species. The structure of human STH has been elucidated by Li and coworkers and has 188 amino acids with 2 disulfide bridges as shown in Fig. 31.6. There is species specificity for STH and most investigators attempt to use homologous hormone for experimental studies. Refractoriness develops with heterologous hormone, as well as other adverse effects from the injection of a foreign substance. The rat responds to most STH except fish STH. The human being responds only to human or monkey STH. Most domestic animals respond best to homologous STH and least to heterologous STH.

The complete protein molecule is not necessary for STH activity. There are particular peptide sequences that may be deleted without altering the biological potency. In fact, fragments of 38–40 amino acids have been found to be quite active and even nanopeptides have been found to have a low but important level of activity. These fragments are not species specific and may hold the greatest promise for

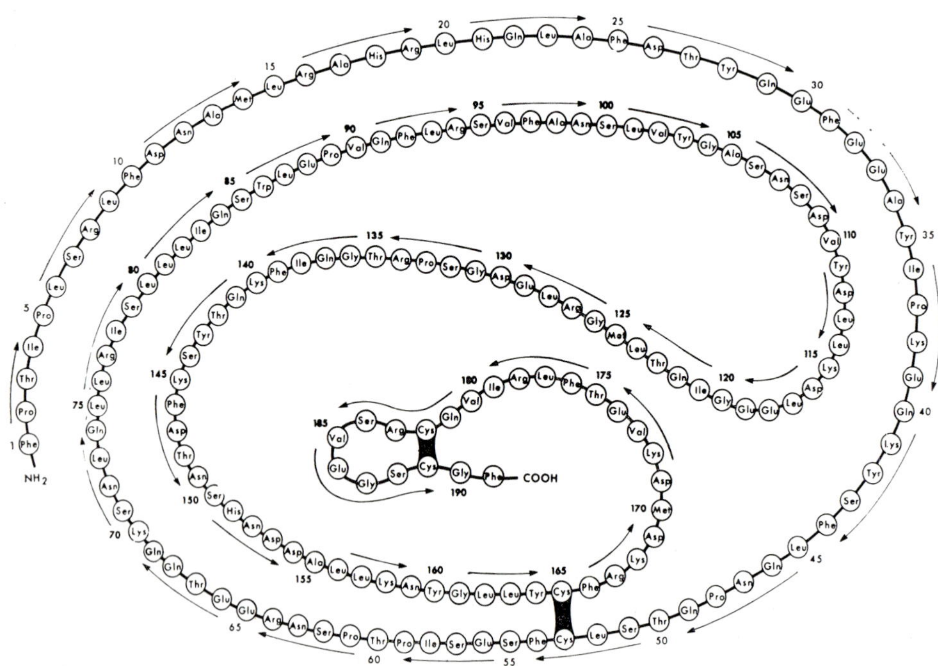

Fig. 31.6. The complete amino acid sequence of the human STH molecule. (From Li, C. H., Recent studies on the chemistry of human growth hormone, in M. Fontaine (ed.), La spécificité zoologique des hormones hypophysaires et de leurs activités. Paris, Centre National de la Recherche Scientifique, 1969)

growth stimulation in domestic animals since they will be easier and cheaper to synthesize.

Although the exact amino acid sequence is not presently known for growth hormone of species other than the human being, the carboxyl-terminal sequences of STH are known for several species. It is of interest that young birds that have been hypophysectomized do not respond to mammalian STH. To date STH has not been found in the avian species.

CONTROL OF OUTPUT

The control of STH output is somehow achieved by a balance between the growth hormone releasing factor (GRF) and growth hormone inhibiting factors (GIF, or somatostatin). Low blood glucose is believed to be the primary cause of GRF release, which in turn causes STH secretion. In addition, stress, high protein food intake, and sleep increase the levels of plasma STH. The amino acid arginine has a STH releasing effect, although its mechanism is not understood. Acromegaly follows elevated STH output, while dwarfism follows reduced STH output. Insulin, by lowering the blood glucose level, would cause an outpouring of STH, while high doses of glucocorticoids would elevate blood glucose and thereby decrease the circulating levels of STH. The physiological significance of somatostatin is yet to be determined, although it is known that it hinders STH secretion.

STH appears to be released at a rather similar rate throughout the life of the animal. Although skeletal growth ceases after puberty, STH has a biological role throughout life as an anabolic agent as well as a synergistic role by enhancing ACTH, TSH, LH, and FSH action on their target organs.

EFFECTS IN THE BODY

Somatotropin increases both the soft and osseous tissues of the body. Recent work indicates it has a profound effect on lactation. Any hormone that can promote such activity must act on many metabolic processes, and as the hormone becomes more readily available to researchers, these mechanisms will be more accurately determined.

Growth of the long bones continues so long as the epiphyseal lines do not close and in species such as the rat, where the epiphyseal lines do not close, giants can be created by prolonged administration of the hormone. In domestic animals, closure of epiphyseal lines soon after puberty signals the cessation of skeletal growth under normal conditions.

Protein metabolism is markedly influenced by STH. One of the most important ways that it affects protein metabolism is to increase the retention of nitrogen by the body. The loss of nitrogen into the urine as urea or other nitrogenous waste products is diminished, indicating retention within the body. In addition, another and possibly more *important effect of STH is to increase cell permeability to amino acids, thereby favoring a buildup of the muscle mass of the body.*

The effect of STH on carbohydrate metabolism is more indirect and vague, although it is known that it markedly influences carbohydrate metabolism. For example, the administration of STH to dogs, swine, and several other species will eventually induce a permanent diabetes mellitus. The mode of action may involve the elevation of blood sugar through some extra pancreatic mechanism. The high blood sugar level then stimulates the pancreatic islet cells to produce insulin until they are eventually exhausted and atrophy. It has been suggested that the mode of action of STH is to cause glucagon release, thereby elevating blood glucose.

It has long been known that the diabetes mellitus in the depancreatized dog can be ameliorated by hypophysectomizing the animal. This was first demonstrated by Professor Houssay and the depancreatized-hypophysectomized dog is referred to as the "Houssay dog." The way in which the Houssay dog is able to deal with the insulin deficiency most likely is by removing the hyperglycemic effect of STH.

In summary, it can be seen that STH favors economical use of proteins and carbohydrates, encouraging the body to retain these building blocks for tissue growth and development or for energy. The metabolism of these substances is extremely complicated, with many other hormones and factors involved in the process. Consequently, it is difficult to assign a specific action to STH in this scheme, but it can be concluded that STH is one of the important regulating factors of metabolism of carbohydrates, proteins, and fats. Thus the utility of STH throughout the life of the animal becomes clear. The constant level of STH production throughout life becomes rational because both the young growing animal and the adult have need for STH.

The lactation that often follows STH injection into an animal with lactiferous tissue is an area of current investigation. It appears that in the cow lactation can be induced in developed lactiferous tissue with STH more easily and with greater regularity than with the so-called lactogenic hormone (Cotes et al. 1949). Problems of contamination of these two pituitary hormones undoubtedly have complicated previous work. The anabolic effects of somatotropin in other parts of the body, along with its stimulating effect on lactiferous tissue, cause one to wonder if the so-called lactogenic hormone is a misnomer. Perhaps STH is the adenohypophyseal hormone most associated with lactation or STH and prolactin are synergistic.

Underproduction of STH in the immature animal results in underdevelopment referred to as pituitary dwarfism. Such an animal probably would show reduced activity in the other target organs of the pituitary (hypothyroidism, hypogonadism, hypoadrenocortical function). Pituitary dwarfs undoubtedly occur in domestic animals as a result of dysfunction of the pituitary gland or a destructive lesion thereof. Such domestic animals have difficulty surviving under farm conditions and are of little economic importance. Many studies have been made to determine if hypoproduction of STH caused the commonly occurring dwarfism of beef calves. Thus far no association has been established.

The effects of overproduction of STH depend to a great extent on the period of life of the animal in which this overproduction occurs. If the overproduction occurs before the epiphyseal lines close in the long bones, lengthening of the long bones and increased soft tissue deposition result in a "giant." This occasionally occurs in domestic animals. If excess production of STH occurs after the epiphyseal lines have closed, thickening of the membranous and long bones of the body results. This is termed "acromegaly." It is not observed often in domestic animals but it has been suggested that the conformation of the English bulldog is characteristic of an acromegalic condition.

Studies by Baird et al. (1952) indicated quite clearly that the rate of growth and the final size of swine may be selected for and against within a genetic line by retaining as breeding stock either the large animals and breeding therein or the small animals and breeding therein. This work points out that the genetic selection for body size in domestic animals may be related to the amount of STH that the animal is able to produce.

CLINICAL USE

There is little clinical use at the present time for somatotropin. The hormone that is available is expensive, species specific, and has some adverse side effects. Studies in swine (Doyle et al. 1956), dogs, and cats indicate that injection of STH frequently leads to the induction of diabetes mellitus and/or death of the animal. The islet of Langerhans cells are often damaged in injected animals. STH usage in food animals must be a frontier for future research. Its usage before puberty would result in large skeletal growth. STH after puberty would favor a lean animal possibly of great size without fat depots. Feed conversion may be enhanced since nitrogen loss should be minimized.

Synthesis of homologous STH may solve the species specificity and diabetes mellitus problems. Since synthetic STH or active fragments may be complex and expensive, use of GRF may be more feasible. If GIF is found to be a "physiological

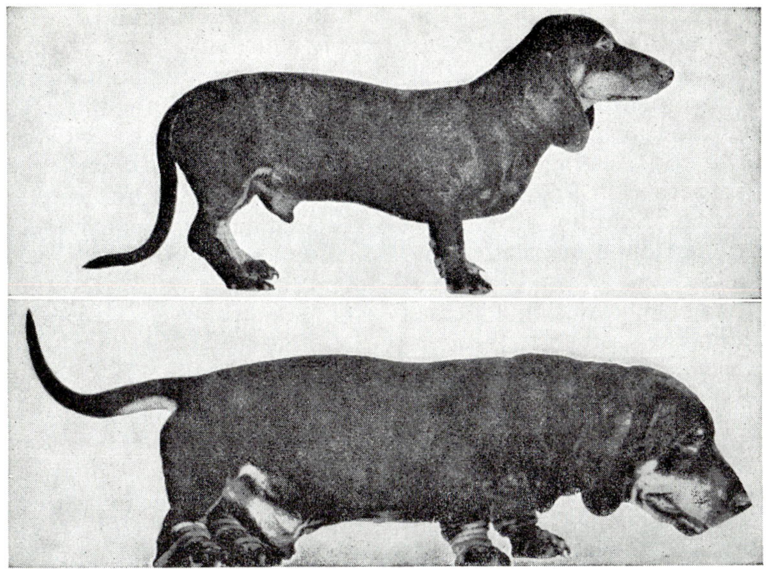

FIG. 31.7. Effect of chronic treatment with anterior pituitary extract in young dogs. Lower: male dachshund given daily intraperitoneal injections of pituitary extract containing growth hormone from 6th to 32nd week of life. Upper: littermate male, untreated. (From Evans et al., Growth and gonad-stimulating hormone of the anterior hypophysis. Berkeley, University of California Press, 1933)

brake" on STH production, an "inhibitor" of GIF may be the logical route. As more knowledge is gained, it is likely that STH will become an increasingly important hormone in the field of domestic animal production. There is no U.S.P. preparation of STH.

THYROTROPIC HORMONE (TSH)

The thyroid-stimulating hormone (TSH) or thyrotropic hormone is discussed in more detail in Chapter 33. Thyrotropic hormone is a glycoprotein with a molecular weight estimated to be 30,000. There is some species specificity to the hormone. TSH has morphological and functional effects on the thyroid. Functionally, the effect of TSH is to increase the activity of the chief cells of the thyroid gland. This activity involves three stages: (1) the uptake of iodide; (2) the production and release of thyroxin, or one of its analogs; and (3) the proteolysis of thyroglobulin. In human beings and the guinea pig, it appears that TSH excess can cause an increase in the retrobulbar fat, bringing about protrusion of the eyeballs. TSH causes hypertrophy of the chief cells as well as hyperplasia.

The functional level of the thyroid is dependent on stimulation by TSH. In the hypophysectomized animal, the thyroid functions at a very low level, consequently the basal metabolic rate (BMR) drops to minimal levels. It appears that TSH from the adenohypophysis and the thyroxin level from the thyroid gland exist in a state of mutual inhibition and stimulation (Fig. 30.6). A decrease in the level of circulating thyroid hormone results in the release of additional TSH. Conversely, an elevation of thyroid hormone causes inhibition of the output of TSH. This is the previously described "feedback" or "servomechanism" control. Formerly it was believed that the site of inhibition of thyroxin was the adenohypophysis proper; now it is recognized that most if not all this inhibition is *probably in the hypothalamus* and the inhibition is actually blocking the discharge of the releasing factor (TRF), which finds its way through the portal system into the adenohypophysis. In addition to this negative feedback mechanism, there is an effect manifested as a result of environmental temperature. This, too, is probably mediated through the hypothalamus since the temperature-regulating center is in close apposition and probably communicates with the site of releasing factor production. In any event, a lower environmental temperature or chilling of the animal either peripherally or internally causes release of TRF, then TSH, which leads to thyroxin formation, elevation of basal metabolic rate, and heat production to elevate body temperature.

Species differences in the concentration of anterior pituitary TSH have been found to be in the following increasing order: guinea pig, chick, cat, rabbit, human being, ox, sheep, pig, dog, mouse, and rat. This means the guinea pig and chick with their low concentration of TSH would have the most sensitive thyroid cells to TSH. They would be ideal assay animals for TSH.

CLINICAL USE

TSH (Dermathycin, Armathoid) is approved by the Food and Drug Administration (FDA) in the treatment of acanthosis nigricans in the dog. The dosage recommended is 1–2 units/day for 5 days. The efficacy of this therapy is still controversial and needs further study.

TSH (1 unit/3 lb) intramuscularly was used by Hoge et al. (1974) to determine thyroid responsiveness in the dog. Euthyroid dogs responded well in T_4 output within 8–12 hours, whereas hypothyroid dogs gave no T_4 response.

Adrenocorticotropic Hormone (ACTH)

Adrenocorticotropin (ACTH) is a peptide that in the sheep, pig, cow, and human being contains 39 amino acids in a straight chain molecule as determined by Li and co-workers at California. These four species have an identical sequence in the first 24 and last 7 amino acids but show minor differences in amino acid positions 25 through 32. It is in the first 24 amino acids that biological activity resides. The first 13 amino acids are similar to melanocyte-stimulating hormone (MSH, intermedin), which accounts for some overlapping of activity. Li has recently synthesized a polypeptide that contains one chain of 17 and one of 19 amino acids, which has properties similar to the naturally occurring 39 amino acid chain of the sheep. Schwayzer and Sieber synthesized ACTH that is identical to porcine ACTH in many ways. Although the main source of clinical ACTH remains abattoir pituitaries, a synthetic polypeptide containing 24 amino acids (Synacten, Ciba; Cortrosyn, Organon) is claimed to have all the therapeutic properties of natural ACTH.

The regulation of the output of ACTH appears to be intimately associated with the hypothalamus and a *servomechanism* exists similar in principle to the mechanism involved in thyroid function. Here the adrenal steroid acts on the hypothalamus, influencing the amount of CRF discharged. In addition, external stressful stimuli such as hemorrhage, temperature, toxins, and emotional states influence the release of ACTH by affecting the release of CRF. The hypophysectomized animal secretes enough corticoids to survive in a protected environment.

The primary physiological function of ACTH is to stimulate secretion by the adrenal cortex, especially cortisol and/or corticosterone. The adrenal cortex responds to ACTH morphologically by hypertrophy and functionally by an increased production of the glucocorticoids with lesser effects on the mineralocorticoids. It is only in the bird that ACTH is needed for aldosterone output. The specific action of ACTH in the adrenal gland appears to be the stimulation of cAMP production leading to the production of energy for corticoid biogenesis. The half-life of ACTH is only 6 minutes (in the rat it may be only 1 minute) but this can be obviated by the administration of an ACTH gel preparation. Such a preparation has a stimulating effect on the adrenal gland for approximately 12–24 hours, thereby reducing the frequency of injections. A U.S.P. unit of ACTH has the activity of 1 mg of the international standard. (See pages 669–71.)

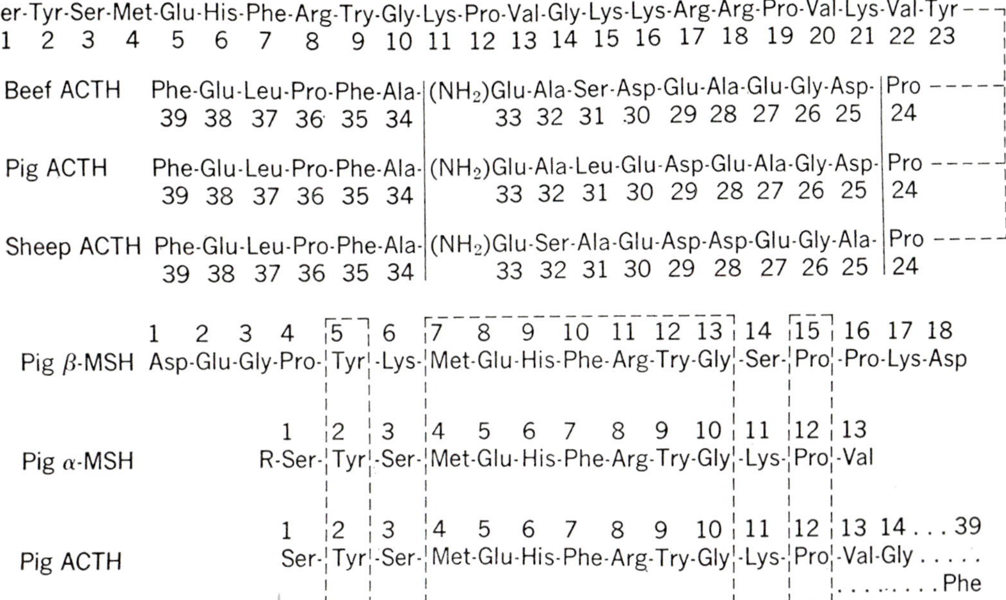

FIG. 31.8. Comparative structure of ACTH and MSH.

PITUITARY GONADOTROPINS

There are two hormones from the adenohypophysis that affect the gonads: FSH and LH (interstitial cell–stimulating hormone [ICSH]).

FOLLICLE-STIMULATING HORMONE (FSH)

FSH is a glycoprotein with a molecular weight of approximately 29,000 in the pig but 67,000 in the sheep and a 2- to 4-hour half-life. Its exact structure has not been determined. The pituitary output of FSH is under hypothalamic control, including a *feedback* mechanism involving the gonadal hormones. Rising estrogen levels from the follicle probably feed back to depress GnRF and then FSH output. Some investigators have suggested that testicular output of estrogens also feeds back to depress GnRF and then FSH output. In addition, environmental conditions such as changing seasons and daylight length must be mediated from some exteroceptor such as the eye to the hypothalamus, thus influencing GnRF output. The physiological effect of FSH in the hypophysectomized animal is to cause multiple follicle growth in the ovaries *without estrogen production* or ovulation; in the male the effect is a subtle one on the seminiferous tubules leading to spermatogenesis, providing androgen production by the Leydig cells has occurred. FSH does not stimulate Leydig cell production of androgen.

Hall does not believe that FSH alone causes estrogen output in the female. He also indicates that in the male the main function of FSH is to favor protein synthesis by acting on primary spermatocytes. ICSH is the hormone that causes steroid synthesis by the Leydig cells. Perhaps even estrogen output by the ovary is LH (ICSH) regulated.

The clinical use of pure pituitary FSH is limited in veterinary medicine because of the cost of the substance plus the fact that an economical source of an FSH-like hormone is available from the serum of pregnant mares. This is discussed later. There is no U.S.P. preparation of FSH but there is a FDA-approved product, F.S.H.-P. (Chromalloy Pharm).

LUTEINIZING (LH) OR INTERSTITIAL CELL–STIMULATING HORMONE (ICSH)

Interstitial cell–stimulating hormone or luteinizing hormone is the same hormone, the nomenclature reflecting the sex

TABLE 31.3. Comparative pituitary content of gonadotropic hormones

Species	Pituitary LH Content	Pituitary FSH Content	Relative Length of Estrus
Cattle	Highest	Lowest	Short, 14–18 hr (ovulation failure seldom a cause of infertility)
Sheep, pig	High	Intermediate	Intermediate, 24–35 hr for sheep, 2–3 days for pigs
Rabbit, rat	Intermediate	High	
Horse	Lowest	Highest	Long, 5–10 days (LH-like hormone often administered to terminate estrus and cause ovulation since ovulation failure often a cause of infertility)

of the animal concerned. LH is a glyprotein chemically different in the various species to the extent that sheep LH has a molecular weight of 40,000, whereas swine LH has a molecular weight of 30,000 and a half-life of 30 minutes. The pituitary content of LH is highest in cattle, sheep, and cats, and lowest in horses and human beings (Table 31.3).

The regulation of LH output from the pituitary gland is dependent on the hypothalamic control (GnRF), which in part is a feedback control mechanism involving the gonadal hormones. The normal effects of LH in the female are to stimulate the developing follicle toward maturation, estrogen production, and finally ovulation, provided FSH has already acted. Its role in corpus luteum function is presently uncertain in some species but LH is probably luteotropic in most domestic species.

In the male ICSH acts directly on the Leydig cells of the testicle, causing testosterone production, which in turn acts throughout the body. There is considerable clinical need for LH in veterinary medicine. The mare frequently fails to ovulate, and an injection of LH is quite effective. This may be supplied as a pituitary preparation such as unfractionated sheep's anterior pituitary (Vetrophin; Abbott) or by the administration of an LH-like hormone present in the urine of pregnant women (human chorionic gonadotropin).

Certain forms of nymphomania in cattle associated with large follicles or cysts can be corrected frequently by the administration of LH or LH-like hormone. This can be unfractionated sheep's anterior pituitary or human chorionic gonadotropin (HCG). Unfractionated sheep's anterior pituitary is a rich source of both FSH and LH and has considerable merit in the treatment of anestrus in any domestic animal. There is no U.S.P. preparation of LH, although there is a FDA-approved product (P.L.H.; Jen Sal Lab).

Sheep Pituitary Gonadotropin

The use of pure pituitary FSH or LH is not economically practical in veterinary medicine, but unfractionated sheep's anterior pituitary (Vetrophin; Abbott) as a source of both hormones has enjoyed a justifiable acceptance. Luteinization of ovarian cysts in 74 of 96 cows was induced by Casida et al. (1944) following the injection of unfractionated sheep's pituitary. Its use is preferred by many practitioners over human chorionic gonadotropin for cyst luteinization, although sheep's pituitary preparations are more expensive.

Sheep anterior pituitary preparations are of value in inducing ovulation in the mare or in stimulating the prepubertal, anestrous, or senile ovary of any species. It is preferred to pregnant mare serum (PMS) as an ovary stimulant except that it is costly. Its use may cause superovulation, multiple pregnancy, and antigenic reactions similar to but to a lesser degree than PMS. Similar precautions should be observed.

PREPARATIONS

Unfractionated sheep's anterior pituitary (Vetrophin) is assayed and each 5-ml vial contains hormonal activity equivalent to 5 mg of the respective reference standards for luteinizing hormone (NIH-LH-Sl) and follicle-stimulating hormone (NIH-FSH-Sl) supplied by the National Institutes of Health.

DOSAGE

Horses and cattle should be given 5 ml, containing 5 mg FSH and 5 mg LH. Smaller species should be given 1–5 mg, according to size. Intravenous administration is preferred but subcutaneous is satisfactory. Injection may be repeated in 2 or 3 weeks if necessary.

Luteotropic Hormone

Luteotropin (LTH), also called prolactin or lactogenic hormone, is presently under reconsideration insofar as its physiological function is concerned. This hormone appears to be a protein with a molecular weight of approximately 25,000. Hypophysectomy of a lactating animal will cause cessation of lactation. This and other facts led early workers to believe that the lactogenic hormone was of considerable importance in lactation. It now appears that STH is also considerably involved and may be complicating the results that the early lactogenic hormone studies obtained. The hormone stimulates the pigeon crop gland to hypertrophy and to secrete a caseous "crop milk," which is the usual means of assay (Riddle and Bates 1939). This hormone also appears to have a corpus luteum–stimulating effect, hence the name "luteotropin," at least in the mouse and rat and possibly the ferret or sheep but not the cow, guinea pig, human being, or rabbit. Its regulation of output and effects within the body remains obscure; consequently, clinical use is unknown. There is no U.S.P. preparation of luteotropin.

NONPITUITARY GONADOTROPINS

Gonadotropins whose sources are not the pituitary constitute a biological oddity. These gonadotropins are frequently referred to as anterior pituitarylike (APL) hormones. The two sources of most importance in veterinary medicine are pregnant mare serum gonadotropin (PMSG) and human chorionic gonadotropin (HCG), both of which are protein in nature, rather cheap in cost, and effective enough that their use is rather widespread in veterinary medicine.

Pregnant Mare Serum Gonadotropin

PMSG, or equine gonadotropin, is a glycoprotein that has a molecular weight of 68,000 and a half-life of 26 hours. The source of the hormone is the endometrial cups of the pregnant mare's uterus (Cole and Goss 1943). The hormone is in the blood of the pregnant mare between the 40th and 140th days of pregnancy, reaching a peak at approximately the 80th day.

PMSG activity is primarily like pituitary FSH but it does have some actions similar to pituitary LH. Therefore, PMSG is referred to as a FSH-like hormone. It has a long period of action due to the fact that it does not pass the renal filter and remains in the circulation of the injected animal or in the blood of the pregnant mare that has produced it. In the pregnant mare's own body, it acts on the maternal ovaries, causing follicular development and finally multiple ovulations, even though the mare is already pregnant. This leads to multiple corpora lutea formation. The gonads of the fetus likewise are stimulated since the hormone filters across the placenta from the maternal system.

Its pharmacologic use in veterinary medicine is widespread as an inexpensive means of inducing follicular growth in inactive ovaries of mature animals. There is some danger of overstimulation, and multiple ovulations can be induced. There is enough LH-like activity in the preparation to induce ovulation in most cases. Inactive ovaries that are dormant for various reasons may be stimulated into activity by PMSG.

In the cow, estrus and ovulation should occur within 2–5 days after a single subcutaneous injection. Superovulation may be induced in the recipient animal if sufficient PMSG is given. It is not advisable to breed the animal at this induced estrus since the monotocous animal may have multiple ova fertilized that may attempt to develop. Since regular cycles should follow, breeding at the next estrus is recommended to avoid superfetation. PMSG often is capable of inducing follicular development in prepubertal and senile ovaries.

The ovaries of the noncycling mare

are refractory to equine gonadotropin in midwinter during the period of natural ovarian inactivity. However, in the autumn and late winter, PMSG will produce estrus in 5–8 days, followed by ovulation if a follicle of adequate size is palpable in the ovary at the time of treatment.

Caution must be exercised in the use of this preparation because mare's serum is a foreign protein to other species, consequently an antigen-antibody reaction is elicited. Repeated administration of PMSG may bring about anaphylactic shock. In addition, response of the gonads may be of a decreasing order of magnitude due to antihormones produced against the early injections (Jainudren et al. 1966).

PREPARATIONS

PMSG is not accepted by the U.S.P. or N.N.D. but is standardized and expressed as rat units.

ADMINISTRATION

PMSG can be given intravenously, but subcutaneous injections are preferred. A single injection of the hormone seems to be as effective as the same quantity given in divided doses.

DOSAGE

The following doses are recommended: horses and cattle, 1000–2000 units; sheep, 100–500 units; swine, 200–800 units; dogs, 25–200 units; and cats, 25–100 units, administered by subcutaneous, intramuscular, or intravenous injection.

Human Chorionic Gonadotropin

Human Chorionic Gonadotropin, U.S.P., is a protein containing galactose and hexoseamine, with a molecular weight of 30,000 and a half-life of 8–12 hours. The hormone is chemically different from pituitary LH but its activity is primarily LH-like, with some effects similar to those caused by FSH.

The source of the hormone is the cytotrophoblasts of the chorionic villi of the human placenta. HCG appears in the urine a few weeks after conception, reaches a peak at approximately 50 days of pregnancy, and decreases thereafter to negligible quantities. This hormone is the basis for the Freidman pregnancy test, using the ovulating ability of the suspected pregnant woman's urine to cause ovulation in the rabbit. High levels of the hormone also occur in the urine of human beings if a hydatidiform mole or a chorionepithelioma is present. From the pharmocologic point of view, HCG provides an inexpensive hormone that mimics, to some extent, the effects of pituitary LH causing ovulation, or Leydig cell stimulation where increased androgen production is desired. In veterinary medicine HCG enjoys widespread use, in part due to its low cost, to cause ovulation in the mare at the time of breeding (Loy and Hughes 1965) and as the therapeutic agent to induce luteinization and possibly ovulation of cystic ovaries associated with nymphomania of cattle. Cryptorchidism of any species often responds to HCG therapy, provided the inguinal canal is patent and therapy commences early enough. The dog (500 units) and foal (1000 units), injected twice weekly intramuscularly for 4–6 weeks, often respond. Since cryptorchidism is genetically influenced, the treated male should not be used for breeding.

PREPARATIONS

The international unit of chorionic gonadotropin is 0.1 mg of the National Institutes of Health standard.

DOSAGE

The following doses are recommended: horse and cow, 2500 units intravenously to 10,000 units intramuscularly; sheep, 400–800 units; swine, 500–1000 units; dog, 100–500 units; and cat, 100–200 units. Intravenous administration is satisfactory when a prompt effect such as ovulation is desired, but the intramuscular route is more desirable when a prolonged effect such as Leydig cell stimulation is desired. Continued administration may be practiced, but antihormone production and anaphylactoid reactions may be elicited.

NEUROHYPOPHYSIS

The posterior lobe of the hypophysis is no longer thought to be an area of hormone formation but rather a storage and release area for hormones produced in the hypothalamus (the paired supraoptic and paraventricular nuclei). The hormones produced in the nuclei move down the axoplasm to the posterior lobe awaiting release. This establishes a profound relationship between the integrated nervous system and the humoral agents of the endocrine organs. Two chemically similar protein hormones are produced by these nuclei. One has a dual action, affecting the vascular system as well as the water reabsorption mechanism of the kidney, and is commonly referred to as "vasopressin" or "antidiuretic hormone." The other hormone has its primary action upon the smooth muscle of the mammary gland and the uterus and is referred to as "oxytocin."

Antidiuretic Hormone (Vasopressin)

Antidiuretic hormone (ADH) or vasopressin is a peptide containing 9 amino acids, 2 of which are sulfur linked (2 molecules of cysteine are united to form a single cystine molecule, which causes the hormone to contain only 8 *different* amino acids). A comparison of amino acid sequences is shown in Fig. 31.9.

There is a species difference in ADH composition since cattle, human, and most mammalian ADH contains arginine, while swine ADH contains lysine. Note the similarity in chemical structure between vasopressin and oxytocin (only two differences—isoleucine replaces phenylalanine and leucine replaces lysine or arginine). Although the chemical structure of ADH is now known (du Vigneaud et al. 1953a), the commercial source continues to be slaughterhouse material that is extracted for its ADH content. Synthetic vasopressin is available (Ferring, Malmo, Sweden).

Du Vigneaud and co-workers (1953b) not only determined the structure of oxytocin but synthesized the hormone, for which he was given the Nobel Prize. This

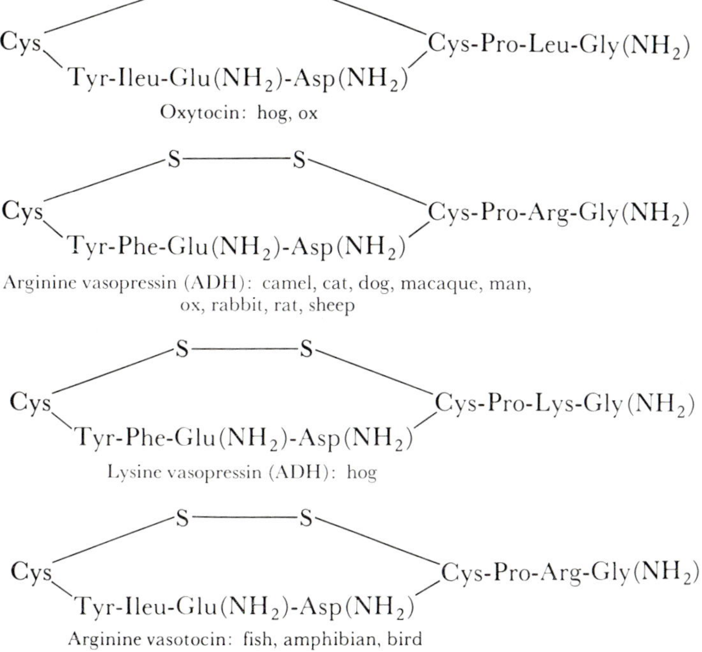

Fig. 31.9. A comparison of amino acid sequences of oxytocin and several vasopressins of various species.

marked the beginning of the identification and synthesis of the peptide hormones.

The output of ADH is directly related to the degree of hydration of the body. In fact, the osmoreceptors may be located in the supraoptic and paraventricular nuclei. Hydration of the body or injection of water into the blood going to the hypothalamus inhibits ADH release by favoring less water resorption from glomerular filtrate. This rids the body of the excess water. Dehydration of the body or injection of hypertonic electrolyte solutions into the hypothalamic artery favors ADH release, which in turn causes increased water resorption from the glomerular filtrate. The body water is increased and electrolytes are diluted; consequently, less urine is formed. Concentrated body fluids cause ADH release while dilute body fluids hinder ADH release. Other factors influence ADH release: pain favors ADH release, leading to less urine formation; ethyl alcohol inhibits ADH release, leading to its well-attested effect, diuresis.

EFFECTS IN THE BODY

Vasopressin, U.S.P., is commercially available, but its use as a *vasopressor agent* is very limited because its pressor effects are so much less than its effect as an antidiuretic agent. At a dosage hundreds of times larger than antidiuretic dosage, it does have pronounced pressor effects that may also lead to serious coronary constriction. The contractile mechanism of the capillaries is stimulated as well as gastrointestinal and uterine muscle, and a rather prolonged elevation of blood pressure follows. Its use as a pressor agent is discouraged because of the coronary effects and renal osmotic action. Sympathomimetic amines are available to produce peripheral vasoconstriction without these undesirable side effects. ADH possesses slight oxytocic activity such as milk ejection and myometrial stimulation, but oxytocin does not possess ADH properties. At physiologic levels, ADH does not affect electrolyte resorption.

The antidiuretic effect is pronounced, and a deficiency of the hormone leads to diabetes insipidus in the dog and cat (Pollack 1951). Experimental diabetes insipidus can be produced by a bilateral lesion of the neurohypophyseal tracts ventral to the supraoptic and tuberohypophyseal nuclei. Difficult parturition follows in some species. ADH acts on the distal convoluted tubule and collecting duct, bringing about increased water reabsorption by increasing the size of the pores or channels (Berliner et al. 1958). Conversely, experimental or natural diabetes insipidus results in lack of water resorption; therefore, polyuria (low specific gravity) ensues, which then causes polydipsia.

Talanti (1959) found decreased neurosecretory material in bitches suffering from a pyometra–diabetes insipidus complex. Further work is awaited to determine if this possible deficiency of ADH and oxytocin will explain the disease complex.

Asheim (1965) published an interesting paper wherein he suggests that the polyuria associated with the pyometra–diabetes insipidus complex has two stages in its pathogenesis. First, progesterone excess favors pyometra. Second, if *Escherichia coli* become established in the uterus, a toxin is formed that damages the renal tubules' ability to concentrate urine. Experimentally, the injection of *E. coli* toxin into healthy dogs causes polyuria.

CLINICAL USE

Diabetes insipidus, a condition wherein the posterior pituitary fails to release sufficient ADH to facilitate urine concentration and normal water retention by the animal, occurs occasionally in the dog and the cat. The increased thirst and urine volume should not be confused with diabetes mellitus, wherein the abnormal carbohydrate metabolism results in an increased urine volume of high specific gravity due to its glucose content.

PREPARATIONS

Once diabetes insipidus has been diagnosed, control can be instituted with *Vasopressin Injection,* U.S.P., or *Vasopressin Tannate Injection,* U.S.P. Since rather pure preparations of vasopressin are available, it is preferred to *Posterior Pituitary,* U.S.P., which contains oxytocin as well as ADH.

DOSAGE

Dosage must be calculated for the individual animal, with considerable caution exercised, because of the possible induction of coronary spasm and elevated blood pressure. The desired dosage for diuresis control is considerably less than the pressor dosage, hence a cautious approach should establish the dosage for the individual animal. Vasopressin tannate in oil is sufficiently long acting that an injection should maintain the animal 1–3 days. A trial dose of 2–10 units of *Vasopressin Injection,* U.S.P., could be used intramuscularly in the dog.

OXYTOCIN

Oxytocin is similar to ADH insofar as its origin and chemistry (Fig. 31.9) are concerned. Oxytocin does not possess pharmacological activities similar to ADH; instead it has specific effects on the smooth muscle of the uterus and the myoepithelial cells of the mammary gland. Its activity will be further discussed with other drugs that act on the uterus.

REFERENCES

Asheim, A. 1965. Pathogenesis of renal damage and polydipsia in dogs with pyometra. J Am Vet Med Assoc 147:736.

Baird, D. M.; Nalbandov, A. V.; and Norton, H. W. 1952. Some physiological causes of genetically different rates of growth in swine. J Anim Sci 11:292.

Berliner, R. W.; Levinski, N. G.; Davidson, D. G.; and Eden, M. 1958. Dilution and concentration of the urine and the action of antidiuretic hormone. Am J Med 24:730.

Casida, L. E.; McShan, W. H.; and Meyer, R. K. 1944. Effects of unfractionated pituitary extract upon cystic ovaries and nymphomania in cows. J Anim Sci 3:273.

Cole, H. H., and Goss, H. 1943. The source of equine gonadotropin. In Essays in Biology. Berkeley: Univ. of California Press.

Convey, E. M. 1973. Neuroendocrine relationships in farm animals: A review. J Anim Sci 37:745.

Cotes, P. M.; Crichton, J. A.; Folley, S. J.; and Young, F. G. 1949. Galactopoietic activity of purified anterior pituitary growth hormone. Nature 164:992.

Dockhorn, W., and Schutzler, H. 1973. Gonadotropin content of pregnant mares' serum with reference to the production of PMS gonadotropin. Monatsh Veterinaermed 28:220.

Doyle, L. P.; Turman, E. J.; and Andrews, F. N. 1956. Some pathological effects of anterior pituitary growth hormone preparations on swine. Am J Vet Res 17:174.

du Vigneaud, V.; Lawler, H.; Popenoe, C.; and Popenoe, E. A. 1953a. Enzymatic cleavage of glycinamide from vasopressin and a proposed structure for this pressor-antidiuretic hormone of the posterior pituitary. J Am Chem Soc 75:4880.

du Vigneaud, V.; Ressler, C.; Swan, J. M.; Roberts, C. W.; Katsoyannis, P. G.; and Gordon, S. 1953b. The synthesis of an octapeptide amide with the hormonal activity of oxytocin. J Am Chem Soc 75:4879.

Ginther, O. J., and Wentworth, B. C. 1974. Effect of a synthetic gonadotropin-releasing hormone on plasma concentrations of luteinizing hormone in ponies. Am J Vet Res 35:79.

Greig, W. A. 1963. Diabetes insipidus in the dog and cat. Proc 17th World Vet Congr, Hannover 2:1117.

Hoge, W. R.; Lund, J. E.; and Blakemore, J. C. 1974. Response to thyrotropin as a diagnostic aid for canine hypothyroidism. J Am Anim Hosp Assoc 10:167.

Jainudren, M. R.; Hafez, E. S. E.; Gollnick, P. D.; and Moustafa, L. A. 1966. Antigonadotropins in the serum of cows following repeated therapeutic pregnant mare serum injections. Am J Vet Res 27:669.

Jubb, K. V., and McEntee, K. 1955. Observations on the bovine pituitary gland. Cornell Vet 45:576.

Kaltenbach, C. C.; Dunn, T. G.; Kiser, T. E.; Corah, L. R.; Akbar, A. M.; and Niswender, G. D. 1974. Release of FSH and LH in beef heifers by synthetic gonadotrophin releasing hormone. J Anim Sci 38:357.

Li, C. H. 1958. In A. Neuberger, ed. Symposium on Protein Structure, p. 302. London: Methuen.

Loy, R. G., and Hughes, J. P. 1965. The effects of HCG on ovulation, length of estrus, and fertility in the mare. Cornell Vet 56:41.

McCann, S. M. 1962. A hypothalamic luteinizing-hormone-releasing factor. Am J Physiol 202:395.

Mahaux, J. 1939. Action de l'"hormone thyréotrope" sur le métabolisme basal de lapins normaux et de lapins ayant présente précédement une période d'inversion d'action de l'"hormone thyréotrope." C R Soc Biol 132(23–25):97.

Mason, N. R., and Savard, K. 1964. Specificity of gonadotropin stimulation of progesterone synthesis in bovine corpus luteum *in vitro*. Endocrinology 74:664.

Pollock, S. 1951. Diabetes inspidus of the dog. J Am Vet Med Assoc 118:12.

Riddle, O., and Bates, R. W. 1939. Sex and Internal Secretions, 2nd ed., p. 1088. Baltimore: Williams & Wilkins.

Roesel, O. F., and Neher, G. M. 1968. Experimental hypopituitarism in swine: Observations on clinical signs, growth and weights of organs. Am J Vet Res 29:1221.

Schally, A. V. 1973. Hypothalamic regulatory hormones. Science 179:341.

Talanti, S. 1959. Observations on pyometria of dogs with reference to hypothalamic hypophyseal neurosecretory system. Am J Vet Res 20:41.

Whitmore, H. L.; Wentworth, B. C.; and Ginther, O. J. 1973. Circulating concentrations of luteinizing hormone during estrous cycle of mares as determined by radioimmunoassay. Am J Vet Res 34:631.

Yousef, M. K.; Takahashi, Y.; Robertson, W. D.; Machlin, L. J.; and Johnson, H. D. 1969. Estimation of growth hormone secretion rate in cattle. J Anim Sci 29:341.

Zolman, J., and Convey, E. M. 1973. Gn-RH: Effect of serum FSH and androgens in bulls. J Anim Sci 37:334.

CHAPTER 32

HORMONES AFFECTING REPRODUCTION

LESLIE E. McDONALD

A consideration of all the hormones that affect reproduction would be quite inclusive. For organizational purposes, it has been necessary to consider some of the hormones under different headings because of their many effects in the body. For example, the pituitary and nonpituitary gonadotropins have been considered in the previous chapter, along with the other hormones produced by the adenohypophysis. Certainly an organized approach to reproduction would begin with the hypothalamus, then pituitary, since its production of the tropic hormones that act on the gonads is of extreme importance.

This chapter is concerned with the gonadal hormones, all of which are of a steroid nature and have multiple actions in the body, acting especially on the accessory sex organs and affecting the secondary sex characteristics. In addition, we must consider the agents acting on the uterus, including oxytocin—a hormone of the neurohypophysis having marked effects on uterine and mammary functions. Other hormones, such as thyroxin and adrenal corticoids, indirectly affect reproduction but are more appropriately considered in the following chapter concerned with hormones affecting metabolism.

The gonads of the male and female produce a limited number of steroids affecting sexual behavior, secondary sex characteristics, accessory sex organs, and reproduction in general. This is in contrast to the many steroids produced by the adrenal cortex under natural conditions.

Edgar Allen, in 1923, first determined estrogenic activity by use of the vaginal smear test, which was followed soon by the isolation of estrone from the urine of women by Doisy and Butenandt. Soon thereafter the structural configuration of this sex hormone was determined. Next Butenandt isolated androsterone from male urine in 1931 and then determined its steroid structure. In 1934 Butenandt isolated progesterone from the corpus luteum of sows, and this led to the discovery of its steroid structure by Slotta.

The gonadal hormones are closely related to the two main purposes of animal husbandry, namely, growth and reproduction. It is likely that considerable research effort will be expended in the near future to understand more fully these two processes insofar as their control by the gonadal hormones is concerned. This will be with a view toward hormone supplementation to bring about more effectively these two economically important and purposeful processes, growth and reproduction. The natural gonadal hormones of most concern include testosterone in the male and estradiol-17β and progesterone in the female. Various other synthetic or metabolized forms will be considered. These hormones are given group names as follows: androgens in the male and estrogens and progestins in the female.

MALE SEX HORMONES (ANDROGENS)

The male sex hormones have been grouped under the term androgen, although the biological actions are quite diverse, affecting such things as spermatogenesis, maleness, libido, body conformation, and metabolic effects such as water, nitrogen, and sodium metabolism.

The birth of endocrinology is sometimes credited to the experiments of Berthold who, in 1849, transplanted gonads into a capon, thereby preventing the occurrence of castration effects. He surmised that the transplanted testicle released some substance into the blood that maintained the maleness of the rooster. This aroused considerable interest by other investigators such as Brown-Sequard who, in 1889, as an established French physiologist, injected himself with testicular extracts, claiming rejuvenation. Others have claimed likewise even in modern times, but in most cases the injections were aqueous extracts that could not have contained the fat soluble steroids of the testis.

Chemistry

The main naturally produced and circulating androgen of all mammalian species appears to be testosterone, except in the rat in which biogenesis stopped at the androstenedione level (see Fig. 30.4). Many other substances, such as testosterone propionate, methyl testosterone, or testosterone cyclopentylpropionate, have marked androgenic activities and are the result of minor metabolic changes in the body or biochemical alterations in the laboratory (Fig. 32.1).

Source

The natural substance, testosterone, is produced by the interstitial or Leydig cells of the testicle under the stimulation of the interstitial cell-stimulating hormone (ICSH), also called the luteinizing hormone (LH), from the adenohypophysis. Testosterone was first isolated in crystalline form by Laqueur and co-workers in 1935, and this was soon followed by its structural determination and synthesis. Testosterone is 10 times as active as androsterone when measured by the common assay procedure involving the promotion of comb growth in the capon. To date no nonsteroid androgen has been found, in contrast to the estrogens. Testosterone, or some closely related androgenic substance, is known to be

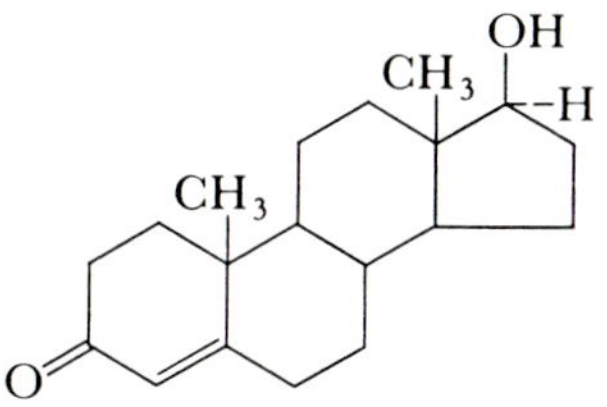

Testosterone

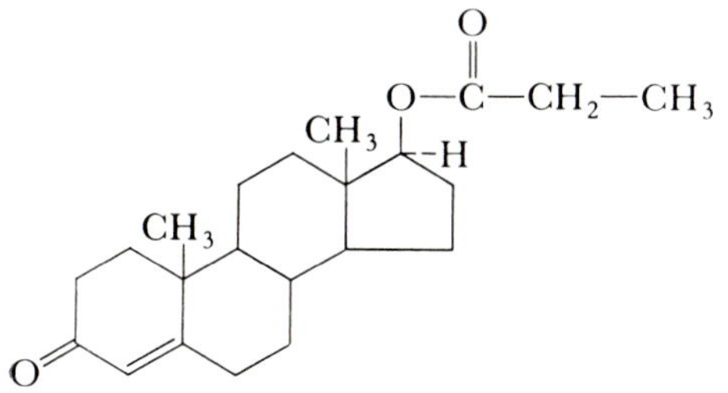

Testosterone Propionate

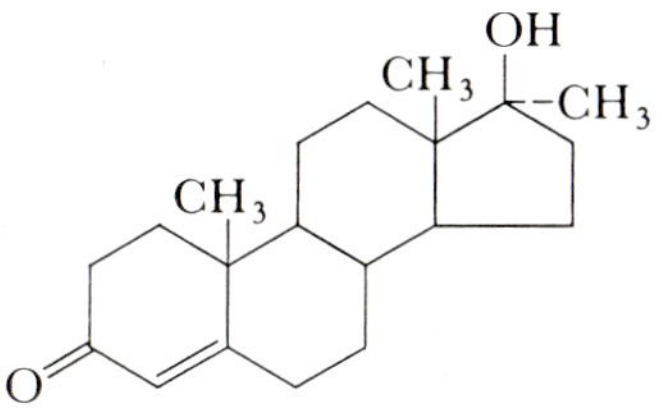

Methyltestosterone

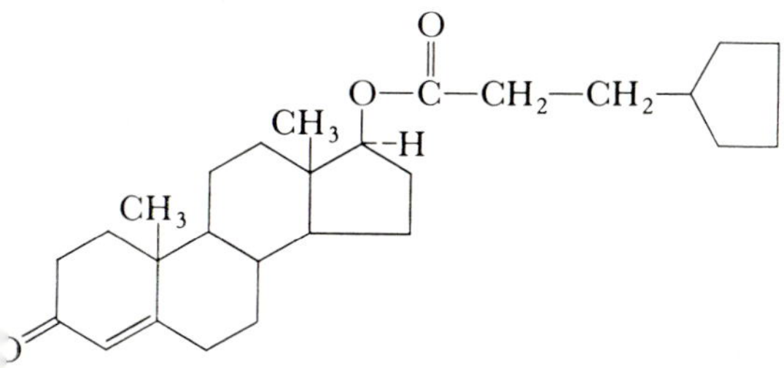

Testosterone Cyclopentylpropionate

Fig. 32.1.

produced by other tissues of the body such as the adrenal cortex, ovary, and placenta. Under normal conditions these sources are not of physiological importance. Many synthetic androgens are commercially available.

Regulation of Output

The work of Davidson and Sawyer (1961) clarifies considerably the regulation of gonadotropin output by the feedback mechanism of testosterone. It has generally been accepted that *the circulating level of testosterone acts in a feedback scheme on the hypothalamus, inhibiting output of gonadotropin releasing factor (GnRF)* (Figs. 31.1, 31.2), *which in turn reduces production and release of ICSH by the adenohypophysis, thereby regulating the amount of stimulation that the Leydig cells receive.* The work of Davidson and Sawyer (Fig. 32.2 and Table 32.1) indicates that in the male dog gonadotropin secretion is held in check by the action of androgen on the hypothalamus and that the latter site is a critical area involved in the negative feedback of androgen on pituitary function. Semen quality and prostate development deteriorated in those dogs that had implants of testosterone propionate in the median eminence region of the hypothalamus, whereas there

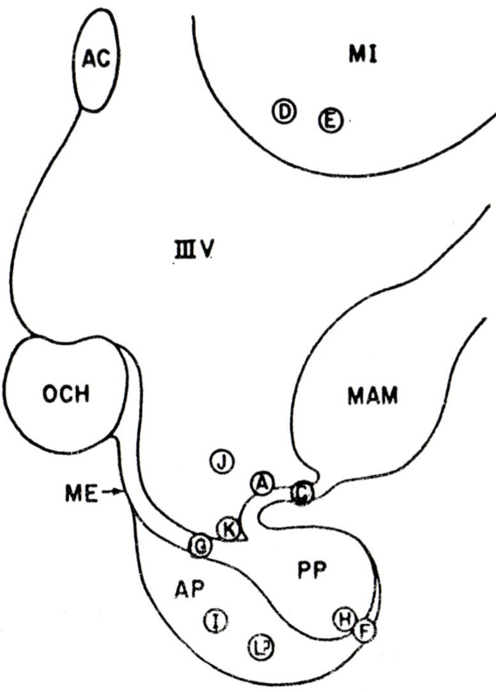

Fig. 32.2. Location of testosterone implants in dog brain and pituitary. Abbreviations: AC, anterior commissure; AP, anterior pituitary or pars distalis; MAM, mammillary body; ME, median eminence; MI, massa intermedia; OCH, optic chiasm; PP, posterior pituitary or infundibular process; III V, 3rd ventricle. (Davidson and Sawyer 1961)

TABLE 32.1. Effects of implanting testosterone propionate into brain or pituitary gland of the male dog

Group	Dog	Location of Implant	Testicular Wt (mg/kg body wt)	Testicular Histology	Prostatic Histology
I	A	Immediately above postmedian eminence	1,130	Moderately severe atrophy*	Atrophy
	C	Posterior tuber	711	Complete atrophy†	Atrophy
	G	Midmedian eminence	653	*Idem*	Atrophy
	K	Postmedian eminence	617	*Idem*	Atrophy
II	F	Pituitary	1,395	Normal	Normal
	H	Pituitary	1,550	Normal	Normal
	I	Pituitary	1,890	Normal	Normal
	L	Pituitary‡	1,080	Some tubular disorganization	Slight degeneration
III	D	Thalamus	1,480	Normal	Normal
	E	Thalamus	1,280	Normal	Normal
	J	Ventromedial area of hypothalamus	1,320	Normal	Normal

Source: Davidson and Sawyer 1961.
* Somewhat less atrophied than the condition in hypophysectomy.
† Similar to condition in hypophysectomy.
‡ Location of implant not verified postmortem.

was no decrease in semen quality or gonadal or prostatic development when the implants were located in the thalamus or pituitary itself. This study indicated quite clearly that the sensitive area for testosterone inhibition of gonadotropin output is in the lower hypothalamus. *ICSH, when released, stimulates the Leydig cells of the testicle to produce testosterone.*

Effects in the Body

The effects of testosterone or related androgens in the body must be divided into at least two main groups (Table 32.2). The first would include the effects of the hormone on the accessory organs such as the epididymis, vas deferens, prostate, urethra, etc. Also included would be the effects on the development of secondary sex characteristics of the animal such as masculine hair growth, masculine conformation and voice, and manner of sexual behavior. These are frequently referred to as the *androgenic* or *virilizing* or *masculinizing* effects of the hormone.

The second group would include the *anabolic effects* of the androgens and would include the retention of nitrogen, building of body tissues such as muscle mass, and favoring the building of dense bone.

Within the *first category of effects* would be the effect on the seminiferous tubules. Testosterone acts in conjunction with the follicle-stimulating hormone (FSH) to bring about spermatogenesis and the development of viable spermatozoa. The exact mechanism by which these two

TABLE 32.2. Classification of effects of testosterone

Androgenic or Virilizing or Masculinizing Effects	Anabolic Effects
Spermatogenesis	Nitrogen retention
Development of accessory sex organs	Protein sparing
—epididymis	Renotropic
—ductus deferens	Increased muscle mass
—prostate	Electrolyte retention (edema)
—seminal vesicles	Bone metabolism
Development of secondary sex characteristics	Erythropoiesis
—male body conformation	
—lowered voice	
—hair growth	
Libido or sex drive (?)	

hormones work synergistically is unknown, although it is recognized that FSH acts in some subtle way promoting the initiation of spermatogenesis. Following hypophysectomy, spermatogenesis can be maintained in some species only by the administration of physiological amounts of testosterone. This effect eventually wanes. It is probable that normal spermatogenesis requires the synergistic activities of FSH, ICSH, androgens, and possibly other hormones.

The development and integrity of the accessory sex organs are dependent almost entirely on testosterone. The secretions of the reproductive tract that make up the fluid component of semen are directly related to the presence and stimulation of testosterone. The development of secondary sex characteristics is a virilizing effect distinguishing the male from the female. This effect is partially the result of the anabolic processes that androgen enhances. The building of muscle mass; the development of heavy shoulders, crest, and hair coat; and increased development of the vocal cords leading to a lowered voice are all due to testosterone. Castration leads to regression of accessory sex organ development and fluid secretion and failure of further development of male conformation and appearance. The photographs in Fig. 32.3 demonstrate the effects of castration in the cockerel.

Libido stimulation is a moot problem. Prepuberal castration prevents libido development, and postpuberal castration causes regression of libido. Androgen administration to increase waning libido has been only partially successful. The dosage of androgen must be low to avoid the inhibition of gonadotropin release and the destruction of germinal epithelium.

The *anabolic effects* of testosterone are receiving increased attention. The mechanism by which testosterone causes retention of nitrogen is unknown. The effect is of considerable veterinary importance, however, because decreased nitrogen wastage and more efficient buildup of muscle mass are frequently desired. This is especially important in meat-producing animals during the growing period or during wasting disease associated with senility or debilitation in domestic animals, especially pet animals.

In addition to nitrogen retention, the androgens also cause retention of potassium and phosphorus, thereby affecting the electrolyte pattern to the extent that some edema can be created from the injudicious administration of the hormone. Physiological amounts of testosterone appear to favor the laying down of dense osseous tissue. In deficiency states (i.e., senility), demineralization may occur, which may be reversed by proper therapy. Physiological levels appear to favor dense bone and epiphyseal cartilage growth, whereas high doses at pharmacological levels may cause cessation of growth of the epiphyseal lines and premature closure.

Efforts have been made to select synthetic androgens that retain the anabolic effects but not the masculinizing effects. These will be discussed presently.

Metabolism and Excretion

The androgens are quite well absorbed from the gastrointestinal (GI) tract, but the liver and kidneys metabolize these substances quite rapidly. Testosterone and the other androgens are excreted in the urine of most animals as 17-ketosteroids. These excretory steroids represent for the most part those androgens that have arisen from the testes, but it must be kept in mind that the adrenal gland also produces steroids excreted as 17-ketosteroids. Therefore, the urinary level cannot always be interpreted to represent testicular testosterone production. The ruminant probably excretes some of its metabolized testosterone in the bile.

More sensitive and specific methods of hormone assay are being developed and the advent of the *competitive protein binding method* permits accurate determinations of plasma testosterone, cortisol, corticosterone, progesterone, aldosterone, estradiol, and most physiologically important steroids in nearly all species. The costs of these tests are declining and their clinical use may be feasible soon.

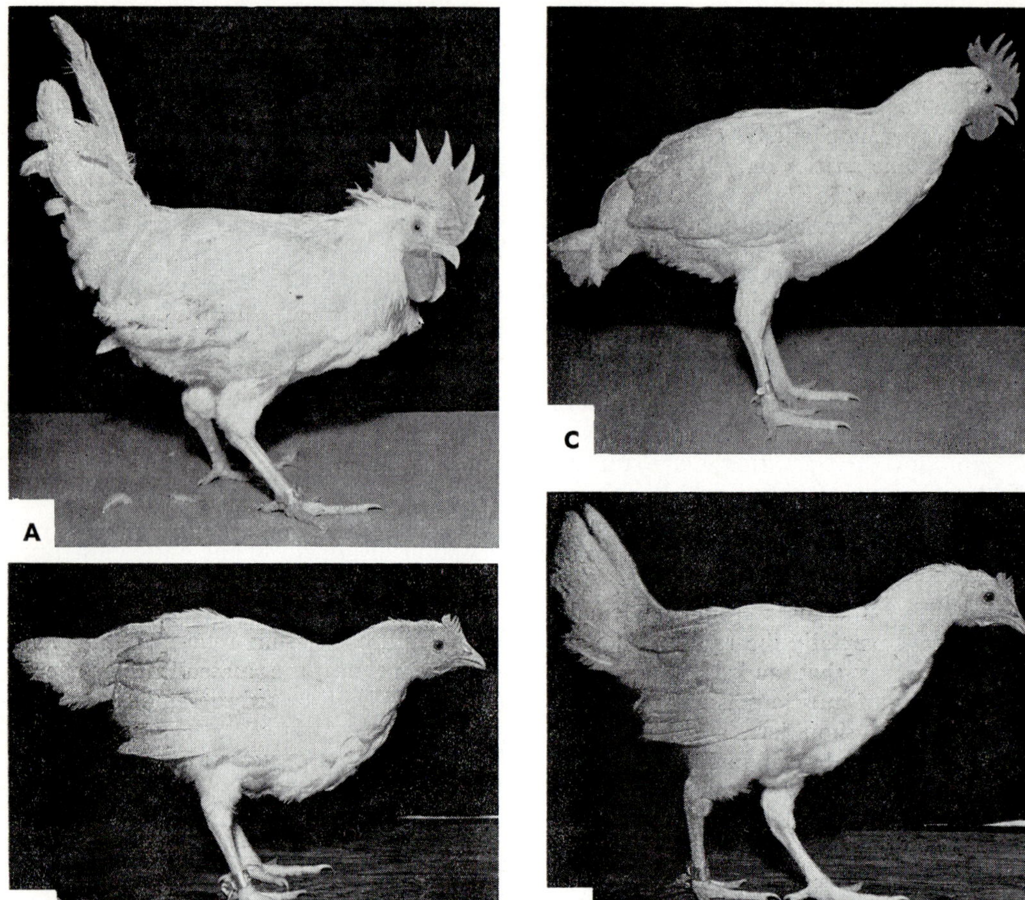

Fig. 32.3. The effect of sex hormones on the plumage of the White Leghorn. *A.* A normal cockerel. *B.* A capon produced by removal of the testes at the age of 4 weeks. *C.* Partial restoration of the secondary sex characters in a capon following the implantation of a pellet of testosterone. *D.* A capon produced by the implantation of a pellet of diethylstilbestrol into the subcutaneous tissues of the neck at the age of 4 weeks. (Courtesy of A. Grollman, Pharmacology and Therapeutics, 1962, Lea & Febiger, Philadephia)

Administration

Intramuscular administration of *Testosterone,* N.F., in oil will maintain a circulating level for 1–3 days. Implants of the hormone, or injection of microcrystals of testosterone in an aqueous solution that causes an implant to result, will maintain a level for 1–2 weeks. Esters such as *Testosterone Propionate,* U.S.P., have longer action than testosterone. *Methyltestosterone,* N.F., is active orally in simple-stomached animals, but the dosage must be increased 3 times the parenteral dosage of testosterone propionate.

clinical use

The treatment of infertility, hypogonadism, aspermia, or decreased libido in domestic animals has been rather unsatisfactory with any of the available androgens. Low or physiological levels of testosterone may increase libido and have a favorable effect on spermatogenesis, but doses above physiological levels block pituitary gonadotropin output, thereby causing spermatogenesis to cease. The dosage appears to be quite critical. High levels of testosterone have been used therapeutically in human beings to block spermatogenesis in infertile men, thereby preparing the seminiferous epithelium for the "rebound phenomena" when testosterone administration is stopped. Experiments by Meinecke and McDonald (1961) indicated that testosterone administration depresses spermatogenesis and withdrawal permits regeneration of the seminiferous epithelium, but there was no rebound in sperm production above control levels in normal bulls.

Prostatic cancer seems to be alleviated by removal of the source of androgen, therefore castration followed by administration of an estrogen gives subjective improvement to this androgen-dependent, accessory sex organ. Carcinoma of the mammary gland is frequently alleviated, temporarily at least, by castration and administration of testosterone. Hirsutism may then ensue.

Mammary gland function is primarily dependent on estrogen and progesterone, whereas androgen administration suppresses lactation. The administration of testosterone is indicated as a means of lactation suppression if other means are not satisfactory.

The administration of androgens to domestic farm animals to favor increased weight gains and efficiency is presently under experimental trial.

Androgen deficiency in the cryptorchid or prematurely castrated dog (Edgett 1943) and in the dog with Sertoli cell tumor, interstitial tumor, or seminomas (Brodey 1956) often results in bilateral alopecia. Testosterone therapy is often helpful.

There are other less established or clinically tested uses for androgens: for pseudopregnancy in the bitch, testosterone propionate or a combination of methyltestosterone and ethinyl estradiol for several weeks or until alleviation; for alopecia in the male dog or cat, any of the androgens; for cryptorchidism, only if no response to human chorionic gonadotropin (HCG); for urethral calculi of the sebaceous type in the castrated male cat, testosterone propionate, methyltestosterone, or testosterone implants.

Dosage

Testosterone Propionate, U.S.P., in oil should be given subcutaneously or intramuscularly 3 times weekly as follows: horse and bull, 100–300 mg; sheep, 25 mg; and dog, 5–20 mg. When *Testosterone,* N.F., is implanted subcutaneously, the following dosages are used every 60–90 days; horse and bull, 0.5–1 g; sheep, 100–250 mg; dog, 20–50 mg; and poultry, 10 mg. *Testosterone Cyclopentylpropionate,* U.S.P., route and dosage are similar to testosterone propionate, but only 1 injection is given every 7–14 days. *Methyltestosterone,* N.F., is given orally in the following dosages: dog, 10 mg; cat, 5 mg daily.

SYNTHETIC ANABOLIC STEROIDS

The activities of the male sex hormone may be divided into two categories: (1) the androgenic or masculinizing effects, which have been previously discussed, and (2) the anabolic (tissue building) effects. It is the latter effects that are gaining the most attention, and the greatest uses are found in clinical veterinary medicine. These synthetic anabolic steroids have a marked stimulatory effect on constructive metabolism that would be of use in the aging animal suffering from senility as well as the young animal that is recovering from a debilitating disease.

Some of the indications for the use of an anabolic steroid would include the wasting disease of old age wherein there are negative nitrogen and calcium balances leading to a loss of both the soft and hard tissues of the body. Such geriatric use is becoming more commonplace, particularly in pet animals. Use of the anabolic steroids in young animals or animals of any age is indicated to reverse tissue-depleting processes such as are often seen in canine distemper, malnutrition, heavy parasitism, or following glucocorticoid overdosage. Also benefit would occur during tissue repair periods such as postsurgery, delayed healing of soft or hard tissues, or following trauma. Another important use is the nonspecific stimulation of erythropoiesis. Although this erythropoietic activity is well established, the exact mechanism is unknown. Probably the site of action is on the kidney since that is the source of the erythropoietic factor in the dog. These anabolic steroids have been found useful in acquired aplastic anemia, myeloproliferative disorders, and lymphoma with associated nonregenerative anemia in cats and dogs. Approximately one-third of the dogs and cats suffering from nonregenerative anemia respond to anabolic steroids. Although one would question the value of these steroids in dogs suffering from anemia of renal failure, their use seems to be justified. Proper dietary reinforcement with additional protein and calcium is preferred in the treatment of all animals, along with the anabolic steroids.

Since estrogens have been shown to be so damaging to erythropoiesis in the dog, it is recommended that the anabolic steroids be used in the female dog even though the female sex hormone is anabolic in that sex.

Increased vigor and appetite have been reported from the use of the anabolic steroids. Some favorable effects have been seen in the hair coat, particularly in animals suffering from a deficiency of sex hormones. Prolonged or overdosage of the adrenal corticosteroids often induces tissue wasting, which becomes clinically important. The anabolic steroids may be an aid in reversing this condition.

The search for anabolic steroids has been particularly important in human medicine because of the need to avoid the masculinizing or virilizing effects seen from testosterone and its relatives. Although the synthetic compounds are never entirely devoid of these virilizing effects, this side effect is not as objectionable in domestic animals.

A number of anabolic steroids are available for veterinary use in other countries but in the United States only one, *Stanozolol,* N.F. (Winstrol-V, Winthrop), is approved by the Food and Drug Administration (FDA). Several anabolic steroids approved for human beings are in fairly widespread use in animal therapy in the United States, particularly oxymetholone. Table 32.3 shows the structure and dosage of several of the available anabolic steroids. Methyltestosterone use is discouraged because of its marked androgenic activity.

Toxicity

Since the anabolic steroids retain sodium and water, care will have to be exercised in their use in dogs with chronic interstitial nephritis. If the masculinizing effects become severe, dosage should be reduced or the drug discontinued.

The anabolic steroids appear to fill a need in clinical veterinary medicine and their uses are apt to increase, particularly in dogs and cats. Sufficient data are not available at the present time to guide their uses in larger domestic animals such as horses.

FEMALE SEX HORMONES

The ovarian follicle and the corpus luteum secrete female sex hormones necessary for normal development of the female reproductive tract: (1) the natural estrogens, which are derived from the ovarian follicle and the placenta; and (2) the progestational hormones, which are produced by the corpus luteum and the placenta. Estrogenic and progestational compounds have been synthesized in the laboratory and are widely used instead of the natural estrogens and progestins because of greater stability, economy, duration of action, and activity by the oral route.

Estrogens

NATURAL ESTROGENS

The naturally occurring estrogens are steroid compounds closely related chemically to the male sex hormones, the hormones of the adrenal cortex (Fig. 30.4), and to other steroids such as the cardiac glycosides, vitamin D, the bile acids, and the carcinogenic hydrocarbons. The principal female sex hormones in most species of animals are estradiol-17β, estrone, and estriol. Estradiol-17β is thought to be the initial

TABLE 32.3. Anabolic steroids

	Dosage	Comments
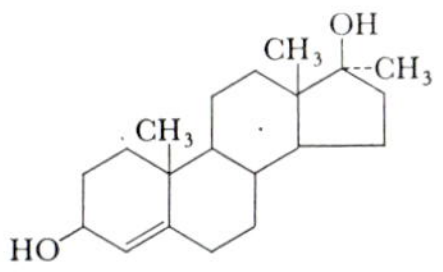 Methylandrostenediol	Calculate from human dose	Quite androgenic and seldom used
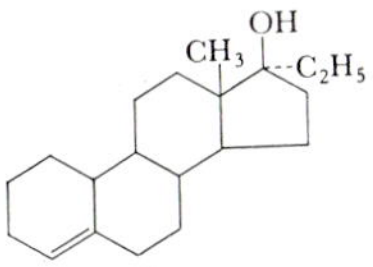 Ethylestrenol (Maxibolin, Organon)	Dogs: 0.05 mg/kg/day (up to 14 days)	
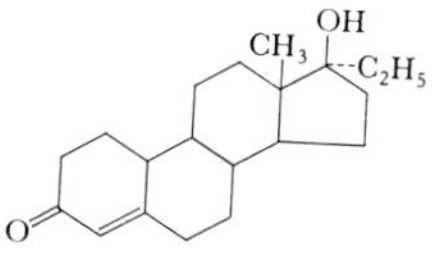 Norethandrolone, N.F.	Calculate from human dose	Some progestational effects
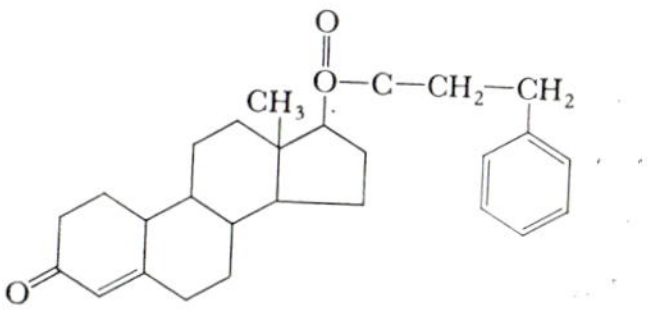 Nandrolone phenylpropionate, N.F.	H. + C.: 200–400 mg i.m./ 14 days Dog: 25–50 mg s.c./14 days Cat : 10–20 mg s.c./14 days	Available in Europe as Nandrolin and Laurabolin; some androgenic effects
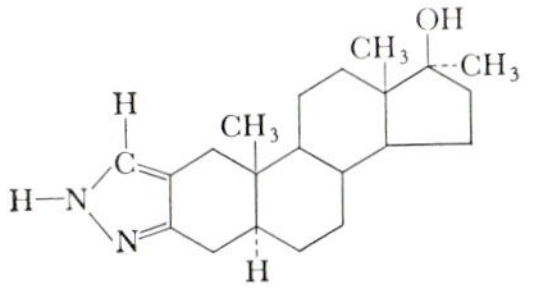 Stanozolol (methylandrostanol [3,2-o] pyrazole), N.F. (Winstrol-V, Winthrop)	Dogs: 0.25–3 mg/kg/day orally 2–10 mg/kg/week i.m.	Some androgenic effects
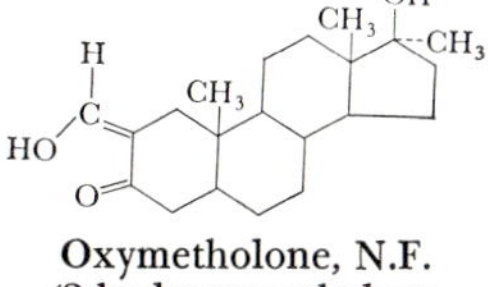 Oxymetholone, N.F. (2-hydroxymethylene methylandrostanolone)	Calculate from human dose	Some androgenic effects

compound secreted by the ovary. It is converted into estrone and estriol during the processes of metabolism. The adrenal cortex and corpus luteum produce some estrogens, and the placenta in late pregnancy produces large quantities of estrogens. Equine male urine and testes contain enormous quantities of estrogens.

Other natural estrogens are found in the urine of pregnant mares, i.e., equilin, hippulin, and equilenin. Natural estrogens are assayed as an international unit (I.U.) that equals 0.1 μg of standard estrone. A unit equals approximately one mouse unit; three mouse units equal one rat unit according to Doisy.

PROESTROGENS

Certain derivatives of triphenylethylene have no estrogenic activity until absorbed by the body and metabolically changed to an active form (Emmens 1941).

SYNTHETIC ESTROGENS

Several chemical compounds that exert the same biological action as the natural estrogens have been synthesized. The physiological effects of the synthetic estrogens are not different from the natural estrogens; *only the potency and duration of action may be different.* Notice how diethylstilbestrol lacks only one bond in rings B and C to complete the 4 rings of the steroid nucleus in Fig. 32.4. The most important of the synthetic estrogens and the the one first discovered is *Diethylstilbestrol,* U.S.P. (stilbestrol, DES).

Among the numerous derivatives of DES used clinically are *Hexestrol,* N.F., *Benzestrol,* N.F., and *Dienestrol,* N.F. The potency of the synthetic estrogens varies widely but may be as high as 3000 units/mg. The derivatives of DES produce a similar effect but are less potent and must be administered in much larger dosage.

REGULATION OF OUTPUT

The estrogens appear to be produced by the ovarian follicle after stimulation by FSH and some LH from the anterior pituitary. As the quantity of estrogen in the blood rises, it indirectly inhibits the production of FSH by the anterior pituitary. The exact route of pituitary FSH inhibition by estrogen involves depressing the hypothalamic GnRF much as androgen inhibits ICSH output in the male (see Table 32.1 and Fig. 32.3). The GnRF is a small polypeptide (Fig. 31.4). Thus an equilibrium (servomechanism or feedback) leading to balanced production of FSH and estrogen is established.

EFFECTS IN THE BODY

The estrogens stimulate and maintain the tissues of the tubular reproductive tract and the accessory reproductive organs, including duct growth of the mammary glands. Estrogens are necessary for the normal contractility of the uterus and for the response of that organ to oxytocin. In the absence of estrogen the estrous cycle disappears and the reproductive tract atrophies. The normal function and structure of the reproductive tract are reestablished by estrogen therapy. Estrogens increase the blood fat and calcium in the bird and apparently in some other species.

Estrogens stimulate the normal physiological processes of the female reproductive tract. Estrogens markedly increase the vascularity of these tissues, which results in increased secretions and endometrial function. Estrogens increase myometrial tone and normal spontaneous motility but not the extensive contractions that empty the uterus. Estrogens stimulate epithelial growth of the tubular genital organs and are often used in treating the vaginitis of senility. The estrogen-dominated uterus is more able to defend itself against invading microorganisms (McDonald et al. 1952). However, it must be emphasized that the above activities of estrogens are all within the bounds of normal physiological processes and that no estrogen, including DES, can stimulate excessive uterine contractions necessary to expel a retained placenta or other contents of the involved uterus.

The cow has a surprisingly low tolerance to estrogens. The daily administration of 600 rat units (R.U.) of estradiol produces behavioral estrus in ovariectomized heifers within 3 days. When the usual clinical dosages of estrogen are administered, a cow exhibits estrus promptly (12–48 hours) because of her sensitivity. However, the induced estrus is without ovulation so conception does not follow breeding during artificially induced estrus (Asdell et al. 1945).

In laboratory animals, administration of an estrogen in *low dosage* stimulates the release of gonadotropins by the anterior pituitary, which may reestablish the normal estrous cycle in an anestrous female. This process has not been demonstrated in domestic animals but there is empirical evidence that it may operate occasionally if low dosages are administered. This pro-

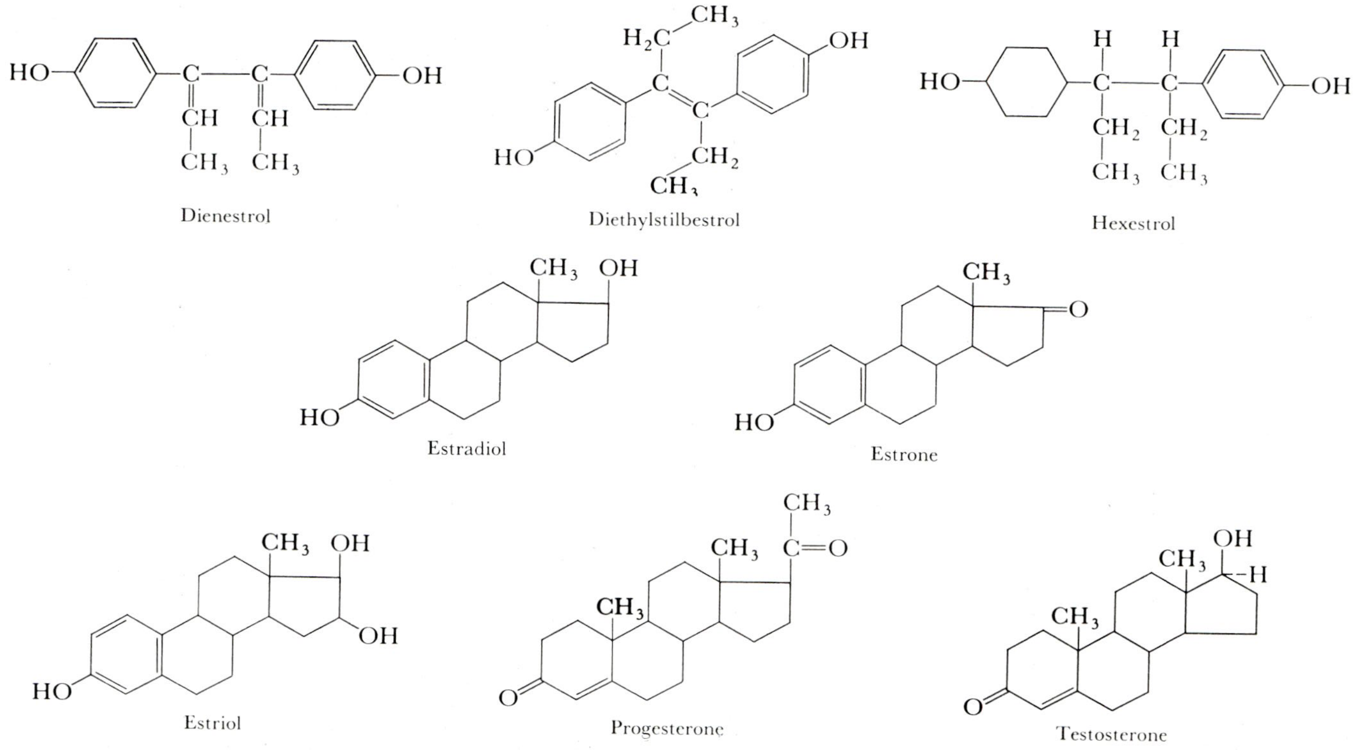

Dienestrol

Diethylstilbestrol

Hexestrol

Estradiol

Estrone

Estriol

Progesterone

Testosterone

Fig. 32.4. The structure of some hormones.

cedure has not been experimentally confirmed, hence it is not recommended. The administration of gonadotropic hormones is more reliable.

Duct growth in the mammary gland and uterus is stimulated by estrogen. This effect along with other stimulating effects on mitosis of epithelial tissue causes estrogen to be properly termed an epitheliotropic hormone.

The role of estrogens is especially important in ruminants because of the protein anabolic effect seen when a small amount of a synthetic nonsteroid estrogen, DES, is fed to fattening beef cattle. Subcutaneous implantation of this hormone also will bring about a marked anabolic effect. This favorable effect has been used for at least 20 years to enhance the ability of feedlot cattle to better use their nutrients. Approximately 10 mg of DES daily in the feed of a fattening steer will cause a 10% increase in weight gains at a 10% greater efficiency level. The exact mechanism of such stimulation is still unknown, although it is known that protein anabolism is enhanced along with some increase in water retention by the body. This favorable effect is only noticed when the animals are on a near-maximum intake of total digestible nutrients (TDN). Animals on lush pasture also get a favorable response to implants of DES.

TABLE 32.4. The effect of orally administered hormones on growth rate, feed consumption, and feed utilization of 2-year-old steers

	Lot I Control	Lot II Stilbestrol
		(10 mg)
No. per lot	10	10
Growth Rate		
Average initial weight, lb	875	875
Average final weight, lb	1,147	1,199
Total gain, lb	274	324*
Average daily gain, lb	2.33	2.64
Feed Consumption		
Ground corn, lb	11.6	12.6
Ground corn cobs, lb	9.2	9.4
Supplement A, lb	3.5	3.5
Mineral, lb	.03	.03
Feed Per Pound Gain		
Ground corn, lb	5.2	4.8
Ground corn cobs, lb	4.1	3.6
Supplement A, lb	1.6	1.3
Mineral, lb	.01	.01

Source: Perry, Beeson, Andrews, and Stobb 1955. Feedstuffs, Jan. 1.
* Highly significant difference.

Estrogen inhibits the growth of bones and favors ossification of the epiphyseal lines. This is why the female ceases to grow in size after puberty whereas the male, with a later puberty, will continue to grow for a longer period of time before androgens deter his skeletal growth.

Estrogen is properly termed an *epitheliotropic hormone* since vasostimulation and general health of the skin are favored. This is why the female has a softer, thinner, and more luxuriant skin than the male. Estrogen is a mitogenic hormone, especially of the epidermis and the epithelial lining of the tubular genital tract. This encourages straight tubular growth of the glands of the genital tract, especially the uterus. Vaginal cornification is caused by estrogen in the bitch and rat and to lesser degrees in other species.

Estrogen in *high doses* inhibits the pituitary output of gonadotropins. In high doses, nearly complete functional hypophysectomy can be induced. Both FSH and LH release are blocked. In low doses, though, some enhancement of FSH output and follicular growth occur. Moderate doses of estrogen similar to the levels during estrus favor output of LH.

Estrogen is properly termed a growth hormone of the genital tract, especially the myometrium, genital tract epithelium, and vascular system.

The psychic effect of estrogen must not be overlooked since it apparently affects the central nervous system (CNS), bringing about sexual receptivity in most species. There is some difficulty in determining which hormones are actually responsible for sexual receptivity in the various species. The cow is very responsive to estrogen and progesterone in the proper ratio, whereas the ewe needs some progesterone first to enhance the activity of estrogen. It has been reported that neither increases sexual receptivity in the human female but that an androgen may be more important in this species. Obviously, more work needs to be done in this area.

The effects of estrogen on the female reproductive organs consist first of a hyperemia followed by water and salt transudation and then hypertrophy. The edema of the tract associated with estrus is quite marked in domestic animals, consisting of swelling of the vulva and even a firmness of the uterus from the intercellular uptake of water. The myotropic effect of estrogen occurs quickly and spontaneous activity of the uterine myometrium begins with estrus. An estrogen-sensitized myometrium becomes very responsive to oxytocin. Prolonged treatment with high levels of estrogen will bring about uterine disturbances leading to hyperdevelopment of the glandular epithelium and glands and finally pyometra from excessive glandular secretion. Infertility of sheep has been reported in Australia when the animals grazed subterranean clover. The infertility was found to be due to the prolonged intake of a proestrogen, genistein, which after consumption is converted to an estrogen.

The pelvic structures are relaxed, the pubic symphysis softens, and the general perineal area enlarges under prolonged estrogen effects such as during pregnancy.

The *secondary sex characteristics* of the female are brought out by estrogen. These include changes in body conformation, hair growth, voice, mammary development, plumage, and beak color.

The estrogen-induced edema of the reproductive tract accounts for the edematous folds at the uterotubal junction that serve as valves to hold the zygotes in the oviduct for 3–5 days after ovulation in some species (Edgar and Asdell 1960). This may explain the success of the formerly empirical practice of administering estrogen to the ill-mated bitch for several days after copulation to prevent conception. This prolonged holding of the zygotes in the oviduct and/or the altered uterine environment favor degeneration.

ADMINISTRATION

The *natural estrogens* must be administered parenterally because they are partially destroyed following oral administration. They are slightly absorbed from the intact skin following local application. Natural estrogens are generally administered intramuscularly in aqueous or oil solutions. The oily vehicle prolongs the duration of action by delaying the tissue absorption. The benzoate and propionate esters of estrogen are used for intramuscular injection to delay the absorption and prolong the activity. When the aqueous solution of an estrogen is injected intravenously into the dog, about 90% of the dose disappears within a few minutes. Only a very small amount can be recovered from the urine.

The *synthetic estrogens* can be administered orally with results equal to those following intramuscular injection. However, in veterinary medicine most of the synthetic estrogens are administered parenterally. Oral administration of the synthetic estrogens for therapeutic uses is not recommended in ruminants because they are destroyed to some extent in the rumen.

The most widely used of the synthetic estrogens is DES. This compound is available as a suspension in oil or as the ester, *Diethylstibestrol Dipropionate,* N.F., which is poorly soluble in water but readily soluble in oils. An aqueous suspension of microcrystals of DES (Repositol) is available, and resorption of the water leaves a small implant that is effective 7–14 days.

METABOLISM AND EXCRETION

DES labeled with C^{14} was eliminated principally by the bile (64%–90%) following subcutaneous injection into the rat; some was excreted into the intestinal contents in other secretions; only 4% of the dose was recovered from the urine (Hanahan et al. 1951).

CLINICAL USE

The synthetic estrogens have nearly replaced the much more expensive natural estrogens in clinical use. DES has been used more widely than all other synthetic estrogens. It is emphasized again that DES has all the physiological properties of other natural or synthetic estrogens. For reasons of economy, DES may be used in veterinary practice whenever estrogen therapy is indicated.

DES does not stimulate the ovary and, therefore, is of no value for the induction of a normal and fertile estrus. It will induce an artificial estrus with the usual external manifestations but ovulation is lacking unless a follicle would have ruptured anyway. DES is of no value in cattle that show normal ovarian activity without manifesting estrus. Moderate-sized doses (15–25 mg) temporarily depress ovarian function in heifers and cows. A larger single dose or small repeated doses of DES cause hypoplasia of the ovaries. At the end of the estrogenic suppression, cystic follicles tend to occur.

DES has been administered intramuscularly (1 mg/lb) to prevent conception in dogs. Because of the work of Edgar and Asdell (1960) this practice is now logical. Treatment should occur within 2 days after breeding and the female should be kept from male dogs. (See Toxicity of DES.)

DES will correct urinary incontinence in the ovariectomized dog. It may also be of benefit in treating vaginitis that is found occasionally in ovariectomized dogs and that attracts male dogs. It has also been used to treat pseudopregnancy in the female dog, but with reservation (see Androgens).

Dermatitis of ovariectomized bitches may be due to a deficiency of estrogen, the epitheliotropic hormone. The dosage of estrogen administered must be low enough to avoid attracting male dogs but large enough to encourage epithelial vigor. Repositol DES (0.5–1.0 mg) once each 1–2 weeks may be followed by oral administration of DES (0.25–1.0 mg daily). Considerable individual variation of dosage should be anticipated.

DES has been used for innumerable other clinical conditions but never with consistent and unequivocal results. Moore (1946) concluded that DES is of no benefit in the treatment of retained placenta in the cow.

Relatively large amounts of DES implanted subcutaneously in virgin heifers or dry nonpregnant cows will initiate lactation in some cases, although generally the yield is relatively low. The maximum milk yield occurs about 2 months after implantation and the implant should be removed as soon as the peak of lactation is reached.

There is some danger of inducing abortion when large doses (100 mg) of DES are administered to pregnant cows. Abortion is frequently desired when range heifers are put in the feedlot. The administration of 50–100 mg of DES will usually cause abortion of fetuses up to 7 months of age. Likewise, enucleation of the corpus luteum before the 7th month of pregnancy will cause abortion (McDonald et al. 1954). Abortion from either cause is followed by retained placenta in late pregnancy.

Clinical claims of benefit are made for the use of DES in treatment of certain tumors of the prostate in dogs. Castration should accompany the estrogen therapy as a means of removing the androgen source since the prostate development is androgen dependent. DES for prolonged periods may induce mammary gland development or even lactation.

DOSAGE OF DES

The dosages of DES or diethylstilbestrol dipropionate in oil administered intramuscularly or subcutaneously are: horse and cow, 10–25 mg; sheep, 1–3 mg; swine, 3–10 mg; and dog, 0.2–5 mg.

Aqueous suspensions of DES microcrystals (Repositol) form implants after intramuscular injection, giving effects for 1 or 2 weeks and the dosages are: horse and cow, 50–100 mg; sheep and swine, 5–10 mg; dog and cat, 0.5–1.0 mg.

Pellets implanted subcutaneously release the hormone slowly for weeks or even months, simulating natural secretion. Dosage for the cow is 30 mg–1 g.

TOXICITY OF DES

DES in normal dosage is relatively free from toxic effects. Large and repeated doses may cause several undesirable effects. Large and prolonged doses in a cow may cause postparturient straining with prolapse of the vagina or even of the uterus. In pregnant cows abortion may be produced. Subcutaneous implantation of large doses of DES leads to changes in pelvic morphology, with fragility and fracture of the pelvis. Prolonged or excessive administration leads to ovarian suppression and hypoplasia, followed by the development of ovarian cysts. Feminization occurs in the male.

Evidence that large doses of an estrogen administered to a dog may cause anemia in various forms continues to accumulate. Some cases of aplastic anemia have been reported and often the anemia may lead to death (Tyslowitz and Dingemanse 1941; Steinberg 1970; Lowenstine et al. 1972). Estrogen therapy in the dog should never exceed 20 mg total dose and then several months should separate treatments. Estrogen therapy for long periods is discouraged in the dog because of this erythropoietic toxicity.

Estradiol-17β (0.05 mg/kg body weight, twice daily for 2 days) given to lactating cows, especially beyond the 4th month of lactation, encourages clinical mastitis in infected quarters. This dosage causes sexual receptivity, excitement, milk decline, and neutrophilia. Normal estrus does not favor mastitis (Guidry et al. 1975), although Frank and Pounden (1961) found some increase in mastitis incidence 3–9 days postestrous.

DES RESTRICTIONS IN FOOD ANIMALS

The use of DES in food-producing animals presents a special problem. The estrogens have been found to be carcinogenic at relatively low levels in certain laboratory animals. The United States food and drug laws restrict the marketing of meat from animals that have "detectable levels" of administered hormones because of this public health hazard. The detection methods are so sensitive that essentially all residues must be eliminated. At this writing no DES can be fed to cattle within 14 days before slaughter. Administration by other routes is also prohibited within the 14 days. Longer-acting forms of DES would have even longer withdrawal periods. In 1974 DES was temporarily banned in food-producing animals and the future may hold additional restrictions.

PROGESTINS

Maleness is primarily due to androgens, and femaleness is primarily due to estrogens. The remaining gonadal steroids come from the corpus luteum, and extracts from this organ are called *progestins*. The most common progestin is progesterone, which is the hormone mainly responsible for nidation and the maintenance of pregnancy. Corner and Allen first established that a hormone favoring gestation was present in the corpus luteum, but it was not until 1934 that the active principle was found to be primarily progesterone.

Marker's production of progesterone from sapogenins present in plants caused the price of progesterone to drop from \$80.00 to \$0.50/g during the last 35 years. This meant that progesterone therapy could be economically feasible in veterinary medicine. Since then, other progestins (6α-methyl-17α-acetoxyprogesterone) have been synthesized that are more potent than progesterone and are active by the oral route. The future surely holds more extensive use of this hormone in veterinary medicine.

The main source of progesterone is the luteal cells of the corpus luteum. Although progesterone has been isolated from the adrenal cortices and placentas of several animals, its main physiological source remains the corpus luteum. During late pregnancy the placenta may become a source of progesterone in some animals, although in the cow this does not appear to be the case.

The normal effects of progesterone are seen only after the target tissue has been subjected to a period of estrogen stimulation. This *priming by estrogen* leads to a synergistic effect. Progesterone acts on the uterus to cause quietening of the myometrium and a secretion of uterine milk by the endometrial glands. The uterine glands increase in depth but *especially in branching and tortuosity.* This coiling of the glands increases their functional capacity after the straight duct development has occurred under the influence of estrogen.

Large doses of progesterone inhibit gonadotropin output of the pituitary gland. In some cycling animals (cow group) this may be the regulator of the length of diestrus because as soon as the corpus luteum fails to secrete progesterone, a burst of FSH follows, which causes development of the follicles and proestrus.

Progesterone probably acts with estrogen in most species to bring about psychic estrus, or sexual receptivity. The ewe requires progesterone before a full response to estrogen can be seen. This may explain silent heat in the ewe during the first estrous cycle each breeding season in this seasonal breeding species. In the absence of some progesterone from the previous corpus luteum, the first surge of estrogen is unable to elicit heat. The influence of progesterone on lactation is important—it acts on the mammary glandular tissue much as it acts on the uterine glands.

The most dramatic role of progesterone probably occurs during *pregnancy.* As the name of the steroid implies, it *favors gestation,* at least in early pregnancy in all species. The early rise in progesterone following the development of the corpus luteum prepares the uterus for pregnancy at every cycle. Progesterone acts on the endometrium inhibiting myometrial activity and causing preparation for nidation regardless of whether or not a zygote is present.

Progesterone favors an economy of body metabolism and during pregnancy the female experiences a period of increased efficiency of nutrient utilization. Such an effect is favorable if the nutrient supply is limited or costly. But at the same time it must be borne in mind that this will favor obesity if permitted to excess. Appetite is encouraged during pregnancy, presumably due to the influence of progesterone, but there is a tendency toward less physical activity. The combination of these effects favors weight gain in the pregnant animal.

The psychic effects of progesterone favor maternal behavior in the female such as nest building. Progesterone in low doses favors ovulation in the cow, rat, rabbit, and bird. This is probably indirect through its effect on LH release.

The physiological half-life of progesterone is only *22–36 minutes* in the cow. This means that a constant secretion is essential to maintain the circulating level. This is a surprisingly short time when one considers its essentiality to maintain pregnancy.

CHEMISTRY

All substances thus far found to have

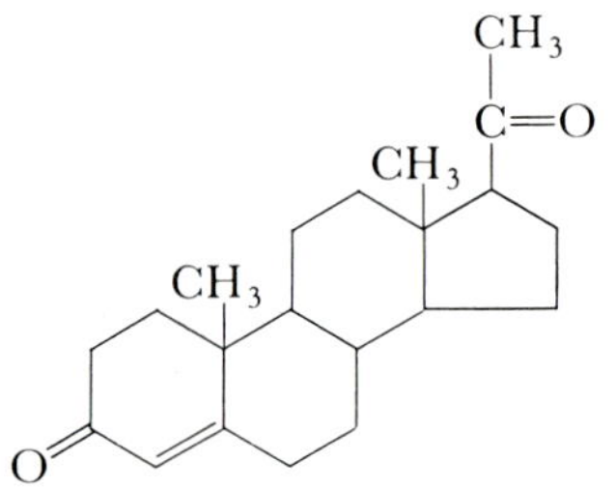

CH_3 $C{=}O$ CH_3 CH_3 O

Progesterone

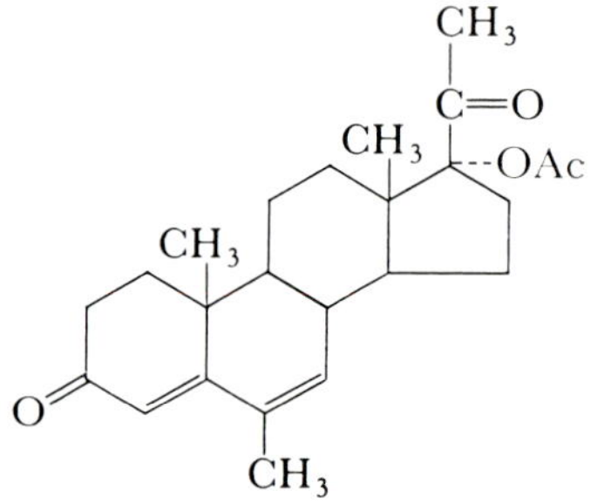

CH_3 $C{=}O$ CH_3 --OAc CH_3 O CH_3

Megestrol Acetate
(Ovaban, Schering)

FIG. 32.5.

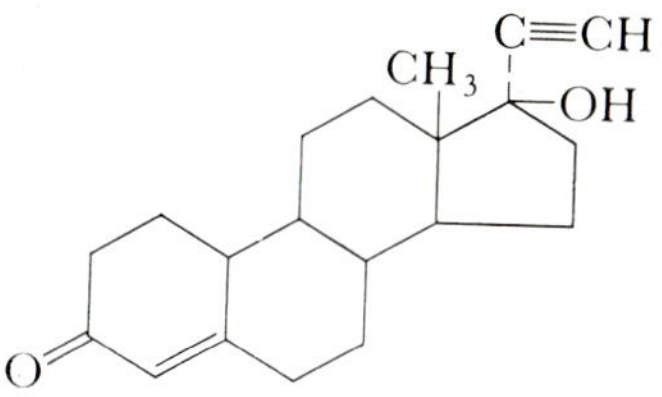

17 α-ethynyl-19-nortestosterone
(Norlutin)

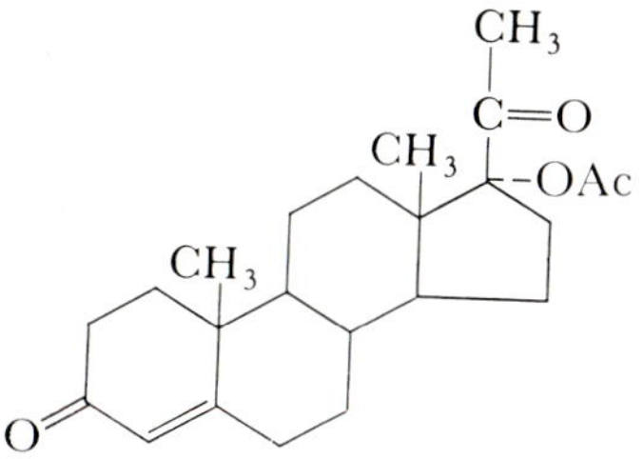

17α-acetoxyprogesterone
(Prodox)

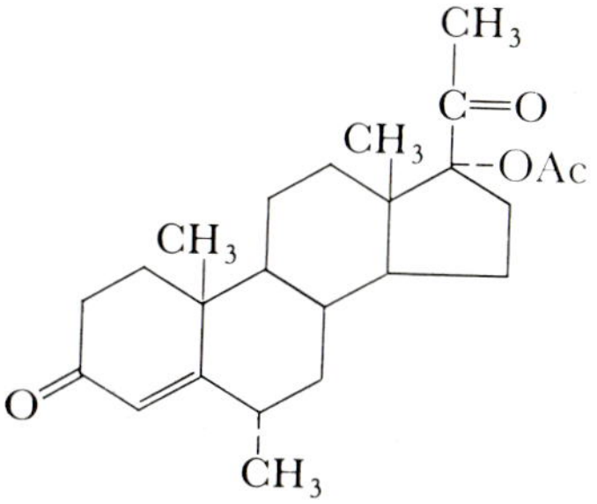

Medroxyprogesterone Acetate
(6α-methyl-17α-acetoxyprogesterone, Provera)

FIG. 32.6.

TABLE 32.5. Steroids present in bovine follicular fluid

Steroid	Concentration
	(μg/L)
Pregnenolone	3.3
Progesterone	233.0
20β-Hydroxypregn-4-en-3-one	23.0
17α-Hydroxyprogesterone	37.6
Androstenedione	31.5
Testosterone	22.1
Oestrone	5.4
Oestradiol-17β	94.0
Steroids that could not be detected	
Cortisol	< 5.0
19-Hydroxyandrostenedione	< 5.0
19-Norandrostenedione	< 5.0
*epi*Testosterone	< 5.0
17α:20β-Dihydroxypregn-4-en-3-one	< 5.0
6α-Hydroxyoestradiol-17β	< 5.0
Oestradiol-17α	< 10.0
17α-Hydroxypregnenolone	< 0.5
Dehydro*epi*androsterone	< 0.5

Source: Courtesy of R. Short 1962.

the effect of the naturally occurring hormone, progesterone, are steroid in nature. The structures of progesterone and several of the newer synthetic substances are shown in Figs. 32.5 and 32.6. The I.U. is 1 mg of progesterone.

SOURCE

The granulosa cells lining the developing follicle secrete progesterone even before ovulation, as shown in Table 32.5. Short (1962) found a surprisingly high level of progesterone and other progestins in the follicular fluid of the cow.

After ovulation, the luteal tissue proliferates to fill the cavity with functional luteal tissue that begins to produce progesterone at an increased rate. The circulating level of progesterone rises throughout the course of pregnancy or throughout most of the estrous cycle of the nonpregnant animal. As the placenta develops during pregnancy, increasing amounts of progesterone are elaborated by this organ. This appears to be nature's way of assuring adequate production of progesterone. In those animals in which the placenta becomes highly proficient in producing progesterone, the corpus luteum becomes less essential; i.e., in the horse, sheep, dog, and cat. Other animals such as the rabbit, pig, and goat remain dependent on the corpus luteum for progesterone throughout pregnancy.

The adrenal cortex also elaborates some progestins. Advances in the synthesis of progestins have led to the production of 17α-acetoxyprogesterone and others from plant sources that will likely replace progesterone as the therapeutic substance.

EFFECTS IN THE BODY

Progesterone acts on an already estrogen-primed uterus or mammary gland to bring about changes consistent with its function during pregnancy. The endometrium changes from a proliferative type to a secretory type and the myometrium hypertrophies further. The endometrial glands become tortuous, active, and begin to secrete a thick, nutritious material referred to as "uterine milk." The cervix and vagina secrete a thick, tenacious material that tends to occlude the cervix. Progesterone has an inhibiting effect on the spontaneous rhythmical myometrial contractions, leading to a more quiescent uterus during the luteal phase of the estrous cycle or pregnancy. This myometrial quieting may be due to intracellular shifting of K^+ and Na^+ in the myometrial cells. These events occur with each estrous cycle—the preparation of the uterus for possible nidation and pregnancy.

Glandular development in the mammary gland is similar to the glands of the endometrium. A definite lobuloalveolar system develops that is capable of secreting milk.

Progesterone has some sodium-retaining effect and other effects that substitute in part for the adrenal cortex. Adrenalectomized pregnant animals will live longer than adrenalectomized nonpregnant animals. Progesterone has a thermogenic effect in most species.

Progesterone administration appears to delay the onset of parturition in some species such as the rabbit, whereas in others such as the cow this does not seem to be the case (McDonald and Hays 1958).

Progesterone in rather high doses has the ability to prevent the development of follicles, thereby blocking ovulation in most animals and in the human female. This has led to the widespread use of and interest in the progestins as antifertility agents in women and to experimental work concerned with delaying estrus in domestic animals. This effect is likely manifested because progesterone, or other progestins, block pituitary gonadotropin release, thereby rendering the ovary inactive.

METABOLISM AND EXCRETION

Transport of estrogens (estradiol particularly) and the progestins (progesterone particularly) in the serum is similar for both the estrogens and the progestins. Both are weakly but extensively bound to albumin, which accounts for most of the circulating sex steroids. Of the remainder, progesterone is strongly bound to transcortin, while estrogen is weakly bound to the sex steroid binding globulin (SSBG). The relative importance of the above varies with species and is an area of current research activity.

Once the sex steroid reaches a target cell, it is released by the transporting protein and enters the target cell and performs its function. Once protein synthesis is induced, the target cell functions. For example, a glandular cell could secrete, mitosis could be encouraged in an epithelial cell, psychic estrus could be induced if the target cell was a particular neuron, or hypertrophy could be induced in a myometrial cell.

Progesterone is eliminated as various glucuronides in the urine of some species but in the bile of ruminant animals.

CLINICAL USE

Embryonic Death. Many clinicians have suspected that embryonic death in some animals may be due to a deficiency of progesterone. The hormone has been widely used with variable results in cows, mares, and other domestic animals. Woelffer (1953) reported favorable effects in reducing embryonic mortality of selected cases of cattle. Controlled work in cattle by Casida (1959) and in swine by Morrissette et al. (1963) indicate that only a portion of the naturally occurring embryonic deaths in these species can be corrected by the administration of a progestin. These results indicate that such therapy is not practicable for widespread use. Only in valuable and selected cases can it be recommended. *Progesterone in oil* should be given intramuscularly daily as follows: horse and cow, 50–100 mg; sheep, 10–15 mg; swine, 15–25 mg; and dog and cat, 2–5 mg.

Parturition Delay. Progesterone does not appear to be a satisfactory agent to delay parturition beyond the usual time in domestic animals. McDonald and Hays (1958) administered progesterone to cows during late gestation without affecting the parturition date. Others have found that parturition can be delayed in the rabbit by progesterone administration, but death of the fetuses usually occurs.

Nymphomania. Cattle with cystic ovaries showing nymphomaniac behavior are deficient in luteal tissue in most cases. The condition cannot be corrected by administration of progesterone since this is not the primary cause of the condition. The nymphomaniac behavior can be suppressed, only to return upon the cessation of progesterone administration. Progesterone is contraindicated in such cases.

Estrus Suppression. Considerable research has been done on blocking estrus in the bitch by the administration of progesterone or one of its analogs. The blockage of pituitary gonadotropins is successful and the ovary does not grow follicles. The bitch does not experience estrus while under the influence of exogenous progesterone. Insofar as control of the pituitary-ovarian axis is concerned, the procedure is satisfactory (Bryan 1960). In experimental cases, bitches have been kept on the progestin for several months and after discontinuance of the hormone there usually is no growth of ovarian follicles until the next season. Although the procedure is successful in controlling ovarian follicular growth, a serious problem develops in the uterus (Anderson et al. 1965; Pettit 1965) of the bitch and the queen (Thornton 1967). Recall that under the influence of progesterone during pregnancy, the endometrium and myometrium respond by hypertrophy, hyperplasia, and marked glandular development. The glandular development causes secretion of uterine fluid that ordinarily serves as nutritive material for the young zygotes. When the exogenous progesterone administration is continued for a long period, stimulation of the uterus causes glandular hyperplasia to the extent that the glands may become cystic. The uterus may become enlarged considerably with an accumulation of fluid. Progestins favor closure of the cervix similar to pregnancy; therefore, there is little if any cervical drainage of the uterine glandular secretions. The uterus may become infected (endometritis). Unfortunately, the use of progestins for the control of estrus in the bitch must be cautious.

Megestrol acetate (Ovaban, Schering) has been approved by the FDA for estrus suppression in the bitch. Treatment is recommended only if begun during the first 3 days of proestrus or during anestrus. The following doses are recommended: proestrus—1 mg/lb of body weight daily for 8 days; anestrus—0.25 mg/lb of body weight daily for 32 days.

Limited clinical trials indicate megestrol acetate may induce less cystic endometrial hyperplasia than other progestins. Vigilance should be exercised.

The use of orally administered or injected progestins may be indicated for a *few days only* to delay estrus in show stock or racing animals. Caution is stressed.

Estrus Synchronization. In the production of domestic animals, the control of the date of parturition would be an advance in the husbandry of these animals. For example, careful control of estrus would mean uniformity of age of the newborn. Labor associated with breeding or care of the newborn could be better programmed and there could be more efficient use of capital facilities. Likewise, if estrus can be controlled, one could delay estrus in the female during the racing season, during travel, or during livestock shows. The owners of pet animals, such as the cat and the bitch, may even wish to eliminate estrus. Artificial insemination of range beef cows would be enhanced since their remote locations preclude daily estrus checks and insemination. For these reasons considerable research has been done in the last two decades on the endocrine mechanisms that could be manipulated to control estrus and ovulation in the female. Added impetus has been given to this because of the importance of controlling or suppressing ovulation in the human female as a birth control mechanism.

The basic mechanism by which the

ovary is discouraged from growing follicles under natural conditions is by a blockade of FSH output by progesterone and possibly estrogen from the corpus luteum of the cycle, the corpus luteum of pregnancy, or possibly the placenta. Consequently, attention has been turned to the administration of these steroid hormones or their derivatives to mimic the natural effect of the corpus luteum. Progesterone has more depressive effects on follicular development than estrogen. Many of the preparations now on the market for human ovulation control contain a critical balance of these two hormones but in general the combination is progesterone dominant.

The use of progesteronelike compounds (progestins) to synchronize estrus in cattle has received a great deal of attention. In general, the administration of progestins has been fairly successful in holding follicular development in abeyance, but problems occur after the removal of the hormone. For example, the onset of the next estrus is spread over a period of up to 7 days. For purposes of artificial insemination this is not precise enough control. Another problem is that the conception rate in these newly ovulated animals is poor, sometimes running as low as 30% or 40% of those inseminated. Quite possibly exact control will be difficult because current information on the progesterone level in the cow indicates that after the progesterone level plummets on about day 16, the time before the onset of the next estrus varies a great deal. This means that there is not a definite period of time after the decrease of progesterone before the next estrus and ovulation. Most studies in cattle have involved the feeding of a progestin since this would be the most practical way in beef animals. Injections would be a problem in most cattle operations.

Another procedure that has been studied is the administration of follicle-stimulating hormones to cause the growth of follicles. Antihormones may develop. Multiple ovulation often occurs since dosage control is difficult.

Current experiments center on the use of PGF_{2a} to kill the corpus luteum (CL), possibly followed by the use of GnRF to more precisely time the onset of estrus. The current literature shows great promise and the student is referred to current journals for the latest findings. At this writing, these hormones are not approved by the FDA for commercial use but such is likely soon.

In the United Kingdom, a synthetic prostaglandin analog (fluprostenol, Equimate, ICI) has been approved for use in the mare. This PGF_{2a} appears to be quite effective, except for the first 5 days after ovulation, in killing the CL. Many feel that "the majority of nonpregnant mares which are not showing regular estrous cycles during the breeding season are in prolonged diestrus rather than anestrus" (Hughes et al. 1973). Consequently, PGF should be of value if the adverse side effects of some PGF can be eliminated, such as smooth muscle contraction of the GI and respiratory systems and sweating. Fluprostenol appears to meet these criteria. Estrus usually follows PGF_{2a} administration in 2–4 days, with ovulation and a conception rate similar to natural conditions. The recommended dosage is 250μg intramuscularly.

Sheep studies in Australia indicate a vaginal tampon containing a progestin is a good route of administration. Absorption of progesterone from the tampon holds the ovary in abeyance and on the designated day the tampons are removed. The results in sheep seem to be more favorable than in cattle. In most species the length of administration of the progestin is up to 3 weeks, which allows most of the animals in the herd to become synchronized (nonfunctional ovaries). Then withdrawal permits all ovaries to begin functioning simultaneously.

In swine a fairly effective antigonadotropin is methallibure (1α-methyl allythiocarbamoyl-2-methylthiocarbamoyl-hydrazine). When methallibure is administered orally at the rate of about 100 mg/day, beginning between days 7 and 18 of the estrous cycle and continuing 10–20 days, there is fairly successful inhibition of ovarian activity, heat, and ovulation. When methallibure is stopped, there is a fairly synchronized ovulation of the treated animals. The number of ovulations can be enhanced by the administration of pregnant mare's serum gonadotrophin (PMSG); a combination of PMSG and HCG gives a more timed ovulation (Christenson et al. 1973). This method of synchronizing estrus, enhancing ovulation, and timing ovulation is experimental but the relatively good fertility gives the technique potential.

Estrous synchronization is still in the experimental stages. Undoubtedly research will be continued because of the economic potential of the procedure.

SUPEROVULATION AND ZYGOTE TRANSFER

The success of artificial insemination in cattle has brought out the desirability of spreading the effects of the superior male by dividing a single ejaculate into many portions. Such success in multiplying the desirable genetic effects of the male has caused attention to be focused on the possibilities of spreading the superior genetic potential of some females. Under natural reproduction the female is quite limited in her ability to reproduce because of the time involved with pregnancy. In the case of the cow, a single calf is ordinarily delivered only once per year and her lifetime reproductive potential may be no greater than 8–15 calves even under the best conditions. Three-quarters of the year is devoted to pregnancy in the cow and any attempts to increase her potential should focus on this period. If the superior cow could serve purely as an egg donor, while an inferior cow could serve as the incubator, the potential of the superior animal could be enhanced. Such studies were first initiated by Heape in 1890 in England when he successfully transferred fertilized ova from 1 female rabbit to another during early pregnancy. These experiments were continued and were successful in the rat, mouse, rabbit, pig, sheep, goat, and within the last two decades in cows.

If 1 cow served merely as the donor animal, it would be possible for an egg to be shed approximately each 3 weeks, which would mean a potential of 16 or 17 eggs per year. This might be further enhanced if the ovary could be caused to shed several ova at each estrous period. It might also be possible to induce ovulation prior to the usual time of puberty, thereby extending the period of ovigenesis.

Superovulation procedures and zygote transfer trials have gained considerable attention, although the practical results have been limited in domestic animals. Some aspects of these interesting physiological experiments will be discussed.

Superovulation. Several procedures have been studied in an effort to cause superovulation of domestic animals. Generally these have centered on the use of FSH and the most practical source has been the use of PMSG. The administration of PMSG to the cow, ewe, mare, or sow will cause increased follicular growth, especially at the end of the estrous cycle or after corpus luteum removal. Dosage is critical because overstimulation of the ovaries can be induced. PMSG is especially high in follicle-stimulating activity, but it lacks ovulating capacity in most species. Consequently, the administration of the ovulating hormone, LH, is usually necessary. The most commonly available source of LH is HCG, which possesses many LH-like qualities. With the combination of these two hormones, superovulation usually can be induced, although the number of ova shed is difficult to control. Various efforts have been made to prime the donor with progesterone but with mixed results. In general, the use of homologous pituitary gonadotropins gives better results, but the supply of these hormones is limited. With the PMSG-HCG treatment, cows frequently ovulate as many as 10 or 12 ova and sows may shed as many as 30 ova. Since the ovaries apparently have an unlimited number of primordial follicles, there is little danger of exhaustion.

In vitro fertilization has been unsuccessful in most species with the exception of the rabbit. Consequently, it is best to breed or inseminate the superovulated female at the estrus accompanying superovulation. It is hoped the oviducts will contain these zygotes 3–6 days thereafter. There is some discrepancy in the success of transfer, depending on the time of recovery of the zygotes. In general, the earlier the zygotes are recovered from the donor, the greater the success of transfer. Once the zygotes have passed into the uterus, the success of transfer decreases.

At this point a word of discouragement must be given because the repeated use of PMSG causes an adverse reaction in the animal. There is an immunological basis for this reaction since PMSG is a foreign protein and an antigen-antibody reaction develops. During subsequent estrous cycles the ovarian response to PMSG injections becomes less and less as the antibody level rises. Eventually the response is so limited that the process has to be discontinued. In addition, serious anaphylactoid reactions may occur at the systemic level in the injected animal.

Zygote Recovery. In the early experimentation with domestic animals, the donor animal was usually sacrificed to obtain the tract for the flushing of the uterus and oviducts. This would not be practical since this would eliminate the donor animal. But it was hoped that the technique could be developed so that the donor's tract could be flushed and the zygotes recovered *in vivo.* At the present time this has been only moderately successful in domestic animals because of the small size of the zygotes and the remote location of the oviduct and uterus. Various vehicles for flushing and storage have been studied and homologous blood serum is one of the best fluids. The storage of rabbit eggs has been fairly successful under controlled conditions but storage of cow's zygotes has been discouraging.

Dr. Wilmut of England reported the birth of a calf in 1973 from a transferred blastocyst that had been frozen in liquid nitrogen for 6 days.

Uterine or Oviduct Deposition. Once the zygotes have been recovered, the problem centers on having a recipient synchronized with the donor. In most animals, and especially the cow, the recipient must be within 1 day of the same stage of the estrous cycle as the donor animal. The most successful transfer occurs when the zygotes are in the 4- to 32-cell stage, which means they have been recovered from the oviduct between the 2nd and 4th days after ovulation. Greater success follows the placing of zygotes into a recipient that is on the same day of the estrous cycle or 1 day advanced.

Since zygotes cannot be stored, considerable effort must be expended in achieving synchronization. This can be done by having enough recipient animals that one is available at all times. Another procedure would be to modify the cycle by the administration of a progestin. If estrous synchronization succeeds, this may be a lesser problem in the future.

A nonsurgical procedure for the transfer of the eggs in the cow involves passing a needle through the anterior dorsal wall of the vagina and depositing the zygote in the uterine lumen by transversing the peritoneal cavity. Surgical transfer in laboratory animals is successful by laparotomy and the deposition of the eggs by syringe into the oviduct or the uterus, depending on the stage of the zygotes.

In general, the success of superovulation and zygote transfer has been encouraging in the laboratory animals but limited in the domestic animals, especially the cow. The economic potential is greatest in the cow, but for unknown reasons success has been slow. The rather frequent success in such procedures in the sheep continued to encourage attempts in cattle. This is one of the most interesting aspects of reproductive physiology and it undoubtedly will continue to attract the attention of many investigators.

At this writing, many commercial organizations are entering the ova transfer field in cattle. Several things have prompted this in the seventies. The popularity and high value of certain exotic breeds of cattle recently introduced into the United States have lent financial encouragement. Also Rowson's group in Cambridge has developed a technique that may reach 70% success. Ultimately needed are (1) fertilized ova storage, (2) *in vitro* fertilization and culture, (3) nonsurgical collection and transfer, (4) precise synchronization techniques, (5) donor ovarian stimulation with careful control of numbers of ova shed and lack of ovarian refractoriness, (6) improved freezing techniques of ova or zygotes, and (7) cloning success.

The appearance of the prostaglandins may be an aid to synchronization, and GnRF may aid both synchronization and superovulation.

Many experiments have been conducted to see if zygotes of one species will develop in the uterus of another species. To date none has been successful although, as would be expected, the greatest success has occurred in closely related species such as the mouse and rat. In these species blastocysts will implant in the uterus of the opposite species. In fact, zygotes will begin developing in unusual places such as the peritoneal cavity, the anterior chamber of the eye, and beneath the capsule of the kidney or testes. Development does not continue beyond the early stages because implantation and nourishment are impaired.

PROSTAGLANDINS

Nobel Laureate von Euler, in 1934, coined the name prostaglandin (PG) for a substance found in human semen. Since 1960, considerable interest has been shown in this group of 20 carbon unsaturated fatty acids found in many mammalian tissues. The PGs are rapidly metabolized and are probably not hormones in the classical sense, but serve more as "local hormones" that act on tissue near the site of their formation. The trivial names of the PGs are by letter and subscript number as shown in Fig. 32.7 and include a wide variety of actions as follows: PGE_2 and $PGF_{2\alpha}$ (induction of labor, abortion, and destruction of the corpus luteum); PGA_1 (gastric secretion inhibition); PGE_1 and PGE_2 (bronchial dilation); PGA_1 (vasodilation and diuresis); and PGE_1 (inhibition of platelet aggregation).

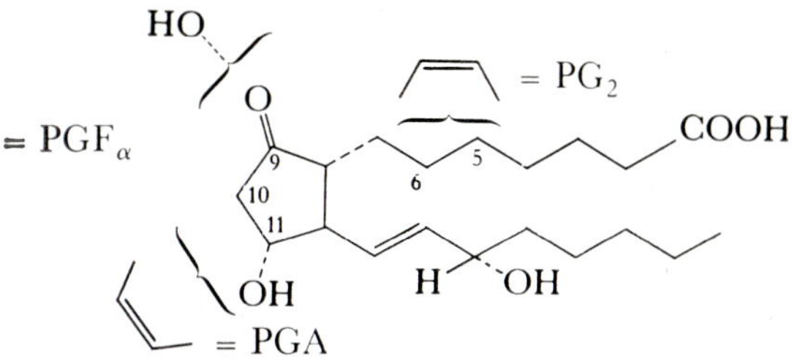

FIG. 32.7. Prostaglandin E_1. PG_2s have in addition a 5,6-*cis* double bond; PGFs have an α or β hydroxyl instead of oxo at carbon 9; PGAs are dehydrated analogs of PGEs with a 10,11 double bond in the ring.

In domestic animals the most important PG appears to be $PGF_{2\alpha}$. PGF is so named because it was found to be soluble in phosphate (spelled *fosfat* in Swedish) while PGE was found to be soluble in ether. At this writing consideration will be given primarily to the role of $PGF_{2\alpha}$ in animal reproduction.

Prostaglandins in Luteolysis

The elusive substance termed luteolysin, which is produced by the uterus when pregnancy has not occurred and finally causes regression of the corpus luteum, may be PG. Phariss and Wyngarden (1969) originally proposed that $PGF_{2\alpha}$ may cause luteolysis by constricting the utero-ovarian vessels causing ischemia and starvation of the luteal cells. McCracken (1971) cleverly proposed that the utero-ovarian transfer of PG could be by the countercurrent exchange mechanism, at least in the ewe, since the ovarian artery follows a tortuous closely adherent course along the utero-ovarian vein. In sheep, he found that the unilateral surgical separation of the ovarian artery from the vein led to a persistent corpus luteum, whereas infusion of labeled $PGF_{2\alpha}$ into the utero-ovarian vein led to radioactivity in the ovarian artery 30 times greater than that in systemic arterial blood. Other workers challenge this concept.

Abortion during early pregnancy and the induction of labor during late pregnancy have been demonstrated in most species with $PGF_{2\alpha}$. Abortion during the early periods of pregnancy is probably due to luteolysis since there is a sharp fall in progesterone production. Labor induction during late pregnancy may depend on the action of PGs on myometrium in addition to possible effects on the corpus luteum.

The ability of $PGF_{2\alpha}$ to induce luteolysis in cattle, sheep, mares, and other species has stimulated study of its use as a potential estrus control agent. The use of PGE and PGF to induce abortion or parturition is being investigated.

At the present time, a $PGF_{2\alpha}$ has been approved by the FDA for veterinary use in the United States in estrus control in the mare (Prostin F2 alpha, Upjohn). In the United Kingdom, a $PGF_{2\alpha}$ analog (Estrumate, ICI) is approved for bovine estrus control and another $PGF_{2\alpha}$ analog (Equimate, ICI) is approved for equine estrus control.

DRUGS ACTING ON THE UTERUS

No other musculature of the body undergoes such variation in size and response during the performance of its normal functions than does the uterus. The pattern and changes of uterine activity during the estrous cycle have been determined for several species of animals. In general, proestrus and estrus are characterized by slow, even contractions having a great amplitude. The contractions become more rapid but smaller during metestrus. During diestrus the contractions are feeble and small. When the estrogen concentration of the tissues is high, the uterus shows considerable motility. When the progesterone concentration is high and the estrogen level is low, the uterine motility is minimal.

One of the most confusing features in the study of the physiology and pharmacology of the uterus is the variation of response of the uterus to drug medication either *in situ* or *in vitro*. Not only has species variation been noted, but individual variation also has been recognized in the response of the uterus to specific drug medication. A variation in uterine response has also been noted according to the period of the estrous cycle or the gestational development. These variations and modifications have led to confusion. Certain fundamental factors, however, are gradually becoming apparent as they apply to most species of animals. Unfortunately, a dearth of information on the clinical effect of certain forms of drug therapy in domestic animals prevents a satisfactory discussion of uterine therapy. Clinical data available are largely the result of trial and error therapeutics, with little application of laboratory observations to domestic animals.

Posterior Pituitary Gland

The pituitary gland is a small but exceedingly important and complex endocrine structure located at the base of the brain. The numerous secretions and influences of the anterior pituitary lobe are considered in Chapters 30 and 31. The posterior lobe of the pituitary body secretes two active principles that cause (1) marked uterine contractions (oxytocic action); (2) myoepithelium contraction of the mammary gland and milk let-down (galactagogue effect); (3) an increase in arterial pressure (pressor effect); and (4) increased renal resorption of water (antidiuretic action). The oxytocic principle is responsible for the first two actions and will be considered in detail in this chapter. The last two effects are due to another polypeptide, vasopressin, or antidiuretic hormone, which was considered in Chapter 31.

Posterior Pituitary Preparations

Oliver and Shafer in 1895 found that injections of extracts of the posterior pituitary caused blood pressure to rise. Dale in 1906 reported posterior pituitary extracts increased uterine contraction. This led to its obstetric use as early as 1911. Posterior pituitary preparations then became commercially available and contained both the oxytocic and antidiuretic principles.

The use of posterior pituitary extracts increased in both human and veterinary medicine until the 1940s, when the two active principles became separately available commercially. Thereafter, clinicians sought either the antidiuretic hormone or oxytocic hormone separately since there is no indication for both substances. In fact, there is ample contraindication for their use simultaneously.

The administration of posterior pituitary extract for oxytocic activity frequently is accompanied by coronary constriction, cardiac ischemia, and momentary fall in blood pressure due to its vasopressin content. Fig. 32.8 demonstrates such a blood pressure decline that may be critical in clinical cases (Parsloe et al. 1950).

Although *Posterior Pituitary,* U.S.P., is available and standardized for its oxytocic activity, it is recommended that the clinician seek either *Oxytocin,* U.S.P., or *Vasopressin,* U.S.P. (antidiuretic hormone), for more specific effects as desired. Much of the veterinary usage and literature deals with the use of posterior pituitary extracts. Since its use is primarily for the oxytocic activity and the dosage is expressed in oxytocin units, it will be considered under oxytocin.

Oxytocin

CHEMISTRY

Du Vigneaud and co-workers (1953) determined the chemical structure of oxytocin and synthesized the octapeptide (Fig. 32.9). This was indeed a breakthrough in endocrine pharmacology.

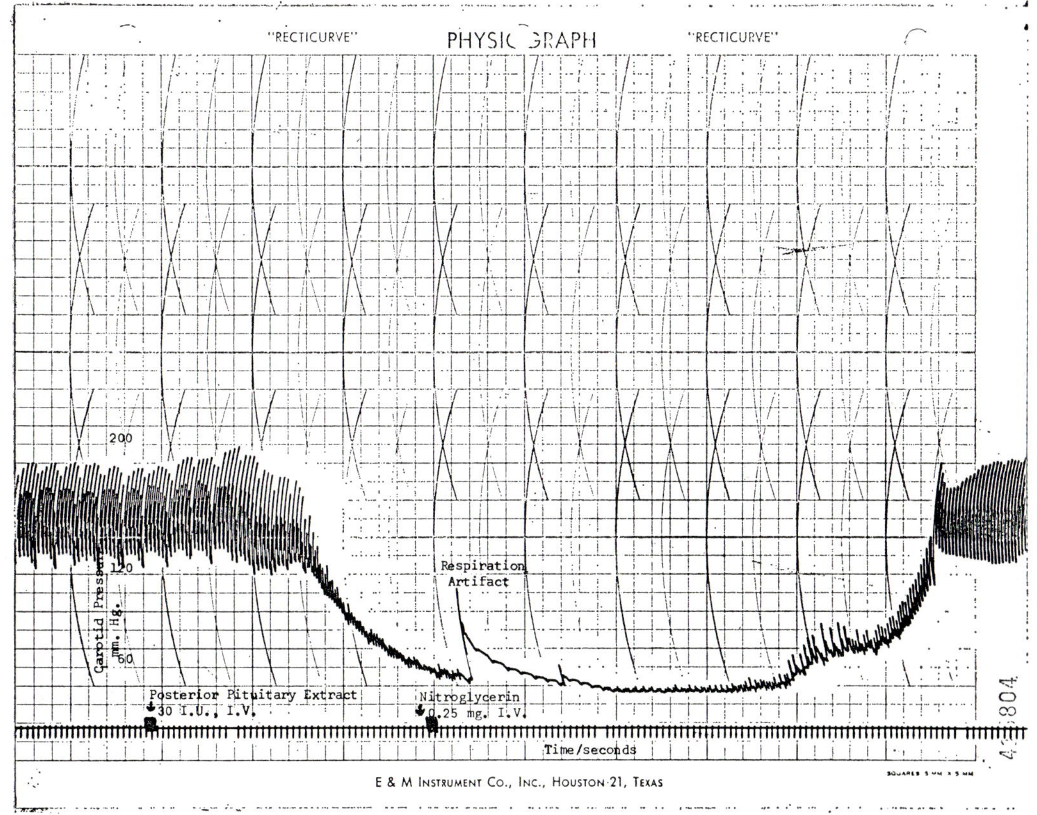

Fig. 32.8. Effect of posterior pituitary extract on blood pressure of a 50-lb dog (i.e., coronary constriction). Although the posterior pituitary extract is expressed in oxytocin units, this dose contained enough vasopressin (ADH) to cause severe coronary constriction and cardiac failure. If nitroglycerin had not been administered, death would have ensued in all probability. (Courtesy of M. C. Morrissette)

```
                              C6H4OH            C2H5
                                |                 |
              NH2              CH2              CH—CH3
               |                |                 |
        CH2—CH—CO—NH—CH—CO—NH—CH
      /                                              \
     S                                               CO
     |                                                |
     S                                               NH
      \                                              /
        CH2—CH—NH—CO—CH—NH—CO—CH—(CH2)2—CONH2
             |              |
            CO             CH2—CONH2
             |
      CH2——N
       |      \
       |       CH—CO—NH—CH—CO—NH—CH2—CONH2
      CH2—CH2/              |
                           CH2—CH(CH3)2
```

FIG. 32.9. Structural formula of oxytocin. Vasopressin or ADH of mammals other than swine differs from oxytocin in that phenylalanine and arginine replace isoleucine and leucine, respectively.

SOURCE

Oxytocin is produced in the area of the supraoptic and tuberohypophyseal nuclei of the hypothalamus, then stored and released from the neurohypophysis. Purified oxytocin prepared from slaughterhouse material is commercially available. Synthesized oxytocin is commercially available and is physiologically and chemically like natural oxytocin.

REGULATION OF OUTPUT

Release of oxytocin is dependent on a signal from the nervous system. Psychological stimuli or teat stimulation may be responsible when the galactagogue or milk let-down effect is desired. Genital tract stimulation, such as copulation, is sufficient to cause oxytocin release to aid in propulsion of semen through the tract.

EFFECTS IN THE BODY

The response of the uterus seems to be dependent on previous conditioning by estrogen and progesterone. Generally, *the response of the uterus to oxytocin is greatest when estrogen levels are high,* such as during estrus or proestrus and during late pregnancy. This makes "physiological sense" since the transport of semen at the time of estrus and copulation or labor contractions at term are beneficial to the animal.

Estrogen alone encourages spontaneous uterine motility whereas progesterone alone depresses spontaneous uterine motility. During pregnancy or the luteal phase of the estrous cycle, both hormones are present at various levels. Therefore, oxytocin can reinforce and further promote uterine motility in the estrogen-dominated uterus, but oxytocin is less able to stimulate motility in a uterus that is progesterone dominated.

There is considerable conflict in the literature concerning the action of oxytocin on the gravid versus the nongravid uterus, with some species differences appearing. This may, in part, be due to the following two experimental problems: (1) much of the older experimental work involved the use of posterior pituitary extracts containing both oxytocin and vasopressin, hence specific effects could not be separated, and (2) the pregnant uterus or the luteal phase uterus is under the influence of *both* estrogen and progesterone, therefore again specific effects could not be separated. Much of the older work needs to be repeated.

In most but not all species, the progesterone level drops before parturition. This indicates oxytocin can override the blockage of progesterone in some species at term or the sensitivity of the uterus to oxytocin rises at term as Fitzpatrick (1960) indicated in the cow. Fitzpatrick (1961) also found a marked increase in oxytocin release in the ewe at the time of parturition.

The uterine response to oxytocin increases throughout pregnancy. It is somewhat difficult to say whether this is entirely associated with the rising sensitization of the uterus to estrogen then oxytocin or whether it is due to a disappearance of the progesterone block. Nonetheless, most authorities agree that the uterus becomes critically sensitive to low but physiological concentrations of oxytocin prior to parturition. Recent work in several species indicates that there is a sudden release of oxytocin just before the final expulsion of the fetus. This has been particularly defined in the cow where Debackere and Peeters (1960) found that vaginal distention causes an increased release of oxytocin. Perhaps this is the final signal to cause the sudden release of oxytocin needed for complete expulsion of the fetus.

The importance of oxytocin is challenged, however, by the fact that a hypophysectomized animal can experience labor and delivery. Parturition may be achieved in such animals by other compensating forces such as spontaneous uterine contractions from the estrogen-dominated uterus or removal of the blocking effect of progesterone. Perhaps abdominal muscle contractions could assume an increased role in the hypophysectomized animal.

In summary, the effect of oxytocin on the uterus is to change the weak, spontaneous, irregular contractions of the estrogen-stimulated uterus into regular, forceful, slower, purposeful contractions. The effect of progesterone on oxytocin activity is unclear.

Oxytocin also causes contraction of the mammary myoepithelial tissue, causing milk let-down in the lactating animal. The physiological level of oxytocin that causes milk let-down in the cow also causes uterine contractions (Venable and McDonald 1958). Likewise, the level of oxytocin that copulation in the cow elicits for uterine contraction and semen transportation also causes milk let-down (Vandemark and Hays 1952).

Epinephrine at physiological levels markedly reduces the effect of oxytocin on the uterus or mammary gland. For this reason, the animal should not be aroused when complete oxytocin effect is desired to cause either milk let-down or uterine contractions.

Oxytocin has no known physiological function in the male.

CLINICAL USE

The role of oxytocin is further enhanced because oxytocin-induced labor is so similar to spontaneous labor that they are difficult to distinguish. *If the cervix is dilated,* administration of oxytocin will facilitate parturition. This is not practical in large domestic animals where physical delivery could be effected. But in small animals where physical intervention is difficult or impossible, such treatment might be considered. In the human being, an intravenous infusion of 2–4 mμ/minute will induce uterine contractions of similar magnitude to spontaneous labor (Caldeyro-Barcia and Sereno 1961). Cross (1958) induced delivery in the rabbit by a single intravenous injection of 100–200 mμ of oxytocin. Obviously, the cervix must be dilated or the induced contractions would cause fetal death or uterine damage.

The use of oxytocin in veterinary obstetrics should be encouraged, especially in small domestic animals, now that purified oxytocin is available. The slow intravenous drip is preferred but may not be practicable in farm animals. The intravenous or intramuscular routes are therefore justified. *When oxytocin is to be used as an aid to parturition, cervical dilation must be confirmed prior to administration so as to prevent rupture of the uterus.*

This use of oxytocin is especially helpful in the cat, bitch, and sow where manual manipulation is limited. At least the fetus may be forced into the pelvic canal where forceps can be applied. The cow, mare, and ewe lend themselves to manual manipulation, although some oxytocic aid may be helpful.

Oxytocin injections are recommended to induce contractions of the uterus after cesarean section, to aid expulsion of the placenta if the attachment is loosened, to aid the evacuation of uterine debris, and to aid postparturient uterine involution in all species.

Some veterinarians routinely inject 20–40 units of oxytocin intramuscularly in cases of dystocia in the sow. Some sows with uterine inertia that do not respond to the first dose may be re-treated 15 minutes later with a second dose. In most cases there is immediate uterine contraction that generally expels one or more pigs into the pelvis. It is important that the cervix be dilated in the sow before oxytocin is administered.

The use of oxytocin for its galactagogue effect is well established. Oxytocin has also been employed to stimulate letdown of milk in recently farrowed sows with agalactia. The same dose as above may stimulate the smooth muscles surrounding the alveoli of the mammary gland to expel the milk. Oxytocin does not appear to stimulate formation of milk by the mammary glands.

Oxytocin has also been employed to stimulate let-down of milk in cows exhibiting agalactia at parturition. Some first-calf heifers seem to have a poorly developed neurohormonal reflex mechanism for releasing milk following stimulation of the teats and udder by milking or suckling. An injection of 10 units of oxytocin parenterally is a suitable dose for a cow. This treatment is helpful when the udder is extremely edematous, painful, and swollen. The milk generally appears within a few minutes following the intravenous injection. Sometimes the injection needs to be repeated for several milkings. Oxytocin produces a slight temporary increase in the amount of milk and the percentage of butter fat (Knodt and Petersen 1944). This increase probably results from more complete evacuation of the udder.

Oxytocin has been recommended to evacuate the udder of the cow in mastitis treatment. Recent work does not find this use efficacious.

DOSAGE

Dosage schedules for intravenous or intramuscular injection are given in Table 32.6. Slow intravenous drip is preferred when possible for labor facilitation. By any route, low initial dosage is recommended and repeated administration is permissible.

CARBACHOL

The pharmacology of *Carbachol,* U.S.P. (Lentin), is discussed in Chapter 8. Although it enjoyed some usage in obstetrics in the past, the drug is seldom used. Oxytocin, the natural uterine muscle stimulant is the drug of choice.

TABLE 32.6. U.S.P. units of oxytocin

Animal	Obstetrics	Milk Letdown
Cat	5–10	1–10
Bitch	5–25	2–10
Ewe	30–50	5–20
Sow	30–50	5–20
Cow	75–100	10–20
Mare	75–150	10–20

REFERENCES

Allen, W. R., and Rowson, L. E. A. 1973. Control of the mare's estrous cycle by prostaglandins. J Reprod Fert 33:539.

Allen, W. R.; Stewart, F.; Cooper, M. J.; Crowhurst, R. C.; Simpson, D.; McEnery, R.; Greenwood, R.; Rossdale, P. D.; and Ricketts, S. 1974. Further studies on the use of synthetic PG analogues for inducing luteolysis in mares. Equine Vet J 6:31.

Anderson, R. K.; Gilmore, C. E.; and Schnelle, G. B. 1965. Utero-ovarian disorders associated with use of medroxyprogesterone in dogs. J Am Vet Med Assoc 146:1311.

Asdell, S. A.; De Alba, J.; and Roberts, S. J. 1945. The levels of ovarian hormones required to induce heat and other reactions in the ovariectomized cow. J Anim Sci 4:277.

Baker, R. D., and Rajamahendran, R. 1973. Induction of estrus, ovulation, and fertilization in prepuberal gilts by a single injection of PMSG, HCG, and PMSG:HCG combination. Can J Anim Sci 53:693.

Barker, C. A. V. 1967. Control of estrus in pigs fed I.C.I. compound 33828. Can Vet J 8:39.

Brodey, R. S. 1956. Multiple genital neoplasia (mast cell sarcoma, seminoma, and sertoli cell tumor) in a dog. J Am Vet Med Assoc 128:450.

Bryan, H. S. 1960. Utility of 17 α-acetoxyprogesterone in delaying estrus in the bitch. Proc Soc Exp Biol Med 105:23.

Caldeyro-Barcia, R., and Sereno, J. A. 1961. The reactivity of the human uterus to oxytocin throughout pregnancy. In R. Caldeyro-Barcia and H. Heller, eds. Oxytocin: Proceedings of Symposium on Oxytocin. Elmsford, N.Y.: Pergamon Press.

Casida, L. E. 1961. Present status of the repeat breeder cow problem. J Dairy Sci 44:2323.

Christenson, R. K.; Pope, C. E.; Zimmerman-Pope, V. A.; and Day, B. N. 1973. Synchronization of estrus and ovulation in superovulated gilts. J Anim Sci 36:914.

Cross, B. A. 1958. On the mechanism of labour in the rabbit. J Endocrinol 16:261.

Davidson, J. M., and Sawyer, C. H. 1961. Evidence for an hypothalamic focus of inhibition of gonadotrophin by androgen in the male. Proc Soc Exp Biol Med 107:4.

Debackere, M., and Peeters, G. 1960. The influence of vaginal distention on milk ejection and diuresis in the lactating cow. Arch Int Pharmacodyn 123:462.

du Vigneaud, V.; Ressler, C.; and Swan, J. M. 1953. The synthesis of an octapeptide amide with the hormonal activity of oxytocin. J Am Chem Soc 75:4879.

Edgar, D. G., and Asdell, S. A. 1960. The valve-like action of the utero-tubal junction of the ewe. J Endocrinol 21:315.

Edgett, J. A. 1943. Alopecia in a pomeranian due to hormonal disturbance. North Am Vet 24:675.

Emmens, C. W. 1941. Precursors of oestrogens. J Endocrinol 2:444.

Fitzpatrick, R. J. 1960. The reactivity of the ruminant uterus to posterior pituitary hormones. J Comp Pathol 70:36.

———. 1961. Hormones new and old. Vet Rec 73:111.

Frank, N. A., and Pounden, W. D. 1961. Prevalence of bovine mastitis during various stages of lactation. J Am Vet Med Assoc 138:184.

Ginther, O. J. 1967. Local utero-ovarian relationships. J Anim Sci 26:578.

Grollman, A. 1962. Pharmacology and Therapeutics, 5th ed. Philadelphia: Lea & Febiger.

Guidry, A. J.; Paape, M. J.; and Pearson, R. E. 1975. Effects of estrus and exogenous estrogen on mastitis in cows. Am J Vet Res 36:1555.

Hanahan, D. J.; Daskalakis, E. G.; Edwards, T.; Dauben, H. J., Jr.; and Meikle, R. W. 1951. Observations on metabolism of C^{14}-diethylstilbestrol. Arch Biochem Biophys 33:342.

Hughes, J. P.; Stabenfeldt, G. H.; and Evans, J. W. 1972. Clinical and endocrine aspects of the estrous cycle of the mare. Proc 18th Am Assoc Equine Pract 18:119.

Igarashi, M., and McCann, S. M. 1964. A hypothalamic follicle stimulating hormone-releasing factor. Endocrinology 74:446.

Inskeep, E. K. 1973. Potential uses of prostaglandins in control of reproductive cycles of domestic animals. J Anim Sci 36:1149.

Isachsen, N. O., and Lombard, F. A. 1960. Geriatric use of sex hormones in veterinary medicine. Vet Med 55:63.

Knodt, C. B., and Petersen, W. E. 1944. The effect of complete evacuation of the mammary gland by pitocin upon milk and fat production. J Dairy Sci 29:449.

Louis, T. M.; Hafs, H. D.; and Morrow, D. A. 1974. Intrauterine administration of prostaglandin F_2 in cows: Progesterone, estrogen, LH, estrus and ovulation. J Anim Sci 38:347.

Lowenstine, L. J.; Ling, G. V.; and Schalm, D. W. 1972. Exogenous estrogen toxicity in the dog. Calif Vet 26:14.

McCracken, J. A. 1971. Prostaglandin $F_{2\alpha}$ and corpus luteum regression. Ann NY Acad Sci 180:456.

McCracken, J. A.; Carlson, J. C.; Glew, M. E.; Goding, J. R.; Baird, D. T.; Green, K.; and Samuelsson, B. 1972. Prostaglandin $F_{2\alpha}$ identified as luteolytic hormone in the sheep. Nature [New Biol] 238:129.

McDonald, L. E., and Hays, R. L. 1958. The effects of prepartum administration of progesterone to the cow. Am J Vet Res 19:97.

McDonald, L. E.; Black, W. G.; McNutt, S. H.; and Casida, L. E. 1952. The response of the rabbit uterus to instillation of semen at different phases of the estrous cycle. Am J Vet Res 13:419.

McDonald, L. E.; McNutt, H. S.; and Nichols, R. E. 1954. Retained placenta-experimental production and prevention. Am J Vet Res 15:22.

Meinecke, C. F., and McDonald, L. E. 1961. The effects of exogenous testosterone on spermatogenesis of bulls. Am J Vet Res 22:209.

Mickelsen, W. D., and Degrofft, D. 1974. Prostaglandin as an estrus synchronizing agent in range cattle. Mod Vet Pract 55:289.

Moor, R. M., and Rowson, L. E. A. 1966. Local maintenance of the corpus luteum in sheep with embryos transferred to various isolated portions of the uterus. J Reprod Fertil 12:539.

Moore, G. R. 1946. Effects of stilbestrol on pyometra following retained fetal membranes. J Am Vet Med Assoc 108:153.

Morrisette, M. C.; McDonald, L. E.; Whatley, J. A.; and Morrison, R. D. 1963. Effect of progestins on embryonic mortality of swine. Am J Vet Res 24:317.

Newton, J. E. 1967. Effects of hormonal synchronization and PMS on breeding in ewes. Vet Res 81:422.

Norrish, J. G., and Burgess, T. D. 1968. Estrus control in swine through management and by the oral administration of megestrol acetate. Can Vet J 9:116.

Parsloe, C. P.; Morris, L. E.; and Orth, O. S. 1950. The relationship of various anesthetic agents to the action of pituitrin, pitressin and pitocin. Anesthesiology 11:76.

Pettit, G. D. 1965. Progesterone-induced pyometra in the bitch. Anim Hosp 1:151.

Pharriss, B. B., and Wyngarden, L. J. 1969. The effect of $PGF_{2}\alpha$, on the progestogen content of the ovaries from pseudopregnant rats. Proc Soc Exp Biol Med 130:92.

Polge, C., and Groves, T. W. 1968. Synchronization of ovulation and artificial insemination in pigs. Vet Rec 83:136.

Rowson, L. E. A., and Moor, R. M. 1966. Embryo transfer in the sheep: The significance of synchronizing oestrus in the donor and recipient animal. J Reprod Fertil 11:207.

Shaw, K. E., and Nichols, R. E. 1962. The influence of age upon the circulating 17-hydroxycorticosteroids of cattle subjected to blood sampling and exogenous adrenocorticotrophic hormone and hydrocortisone. Am J Vet Res 23:1217.

Short, R. V. 1959. Progesterone in blood. IV. Progesterone in the blood of mares. J Endocrinol 19:207.

———. 1962. Steroids present in the follicular fluid of the cow. J Endocrinol 23:410.

Steinberg, S. 1970. Aplastic anemia in a dog. J Am Vet Med Assoc 157:966.

Sugie, T. 1965. Successful transfer of a fertilizer bovine egg by non-surgical techniques. J Reprod Fertil 10:197.

Thornton, D. A. K. 1967. Uterine cystic hyperplasia in a Siamese cat following treatment with medroxyprogesterone. Vet Rec 80:380.

Tyslowitz, R., and Dingemanse, E. 1941. Effect of large doses of estrogen on the blood picture of dogs. Endocrinology 29: 817.

Venable, J. H., and McDonald, L. E. 1958. Postparturient bovine uterine motility—Normal and after experimentally produced retention of the fetal membranes. Am J Vet Res 71:308.

Woelffer, E. A. 1953. Use of progesterone to control habitual abortion in cattle. J Am Vet Med Assoc 122:505.

CHAPTER 33

HORMONES INFLUENCING METABOLISM

LESLIE E. McDONALD

THE ADRENAL CORTEX

The adrenal glands of the mammal are composite organs containing two embryologically and functionally different tissues —the medulla and the cortex. The medulla contains chromaffin tissue that produces epinephrine and norepinephrine, is not essential for life, and has been previously considered. The cortex is essential for life and affects many physiological processes in the body. Recognition of its essentiality dates to 1855 when Sir Thomas Addison found adrenal cortical insufficiency (Addison's disease). Hyperfunction of the adrenal cortex likewise causes a diseased state (Cushing's disease).

More than 50 steroids have been isolated from the adrenal cortex, and only a few are primarily responsible for the effects that the adrenal cortex exerts in the body. The steroids can be divided into the following three main groups based on their physiological activity: (1) the *glucocorticoids,* which affect predominantly carbohydrate and protein metabolism and exert an antiinflammatory effect (antiphlogistic); (2) the *mineralocorticoids,* which affect water and electrolyte metabolism; (3) the *adrenal sex hormones* (limited importance, whose activity was discussed previously).

Effects of the glucocorticoids are:

A. Carbohydrate and protein metabolism
   1. Increased gluconeogenesis
   2. Decreased peripheral utilization of glucose
   3. Antagonism to insulin
   4. Increased protein catabolism (antianabolism)

5. Reduced fat stores

B. Antiinflammatory effect
   1. Reduced circulating lymphocytes, eosinophils, and fixed lymphocytic tissue
   2. Reduction of degree of local inflammatory processes
   3. Possible adverse effect on immune body production

C. Inhibition of adrenocorticotropic hormone (ACTH) output

Effects of the mineralocorticoids are:
   1. Increased retention of sodium, chloride, and water
   2. Increased excretion of potassium, phosphorus, and calcium

Definite structural differences in the steroid molecule account for a predominance of either the glucocorticoid or mineralocorticoid effects as enumerated above (see Fig. 30.4). *Although there is an overlapping of physiological effects between the two groups,* for purposes of simplicity it is necessary to consider the two groups separately.

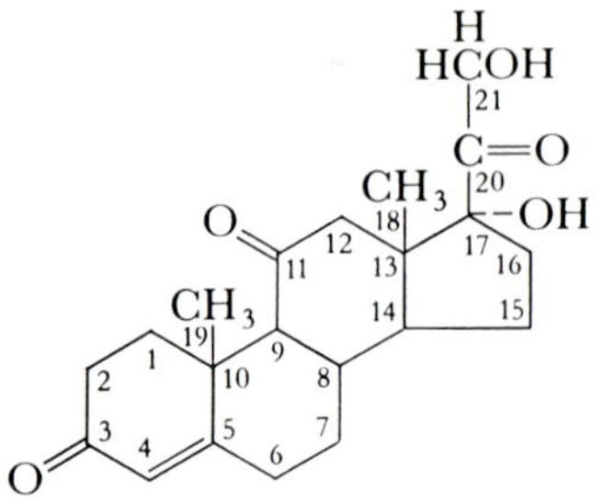

Cortisone
Compound E

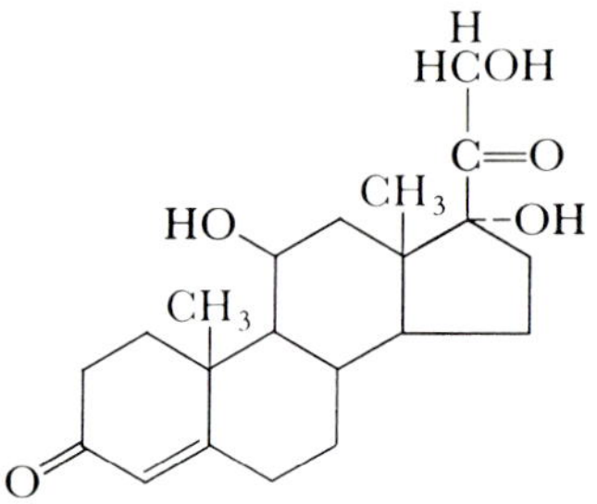

Hydrocortisone
Compound F
Cortisol

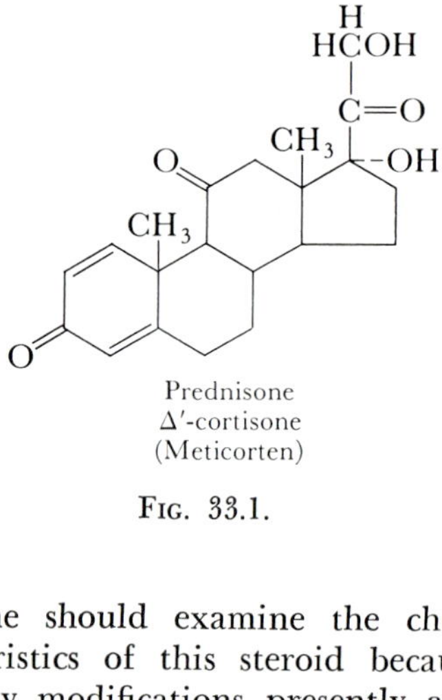

Prednisone
Δ'-cortisone
(Meticorten)

FIG. 33.1.

GLUCOCORTICOIDS (Figs. 33.1, 33.2)

Cortisol (hydrocortisone) and corticosterone are the principal glucocorticoids of the adrenal cortex. Cortisol predominates in the human being, pig, and dog but corticosterone predominates in the rabbit, mouse, and rat. The ruminant is intermediate since it secretes sizable amounts of both. Cortisone has been widely used in clinical medicine but it is not a naturally occurring substance of any significance since it is secreted in very small amounts by adrenal glands of mammals.

CHEMISTRY (STRUCTURE-FUNCTION RELATIONSHIP)

The reader is referred to Fig. 30.4 for a picture of the biogenesis of the adrenal steroids from acetate and cholesterol via progesterone, finally arriving at hydrocortisone or aldosterone as the major glucocorticoid and mineralocorticoid hormones, respectively.

Although hydrocortisone is the most common naturally occurring glucocorticoid, one should examine the chemical characteristics of this steroid because of the many modifications presently appearing on the market. The four-ring structure that constitutes the framework of all the adrenalcortical steroids is inactive biologically unless ketone groups are present at the 3rd and 20th carbon atoms. If the 21-hydroxy group is present, the effect is favorable, and esterfication of this 21-hydroxy group prolongs its pharmacologic action, although the potency is reduced.

Oxygenation of the 11th carbon atom

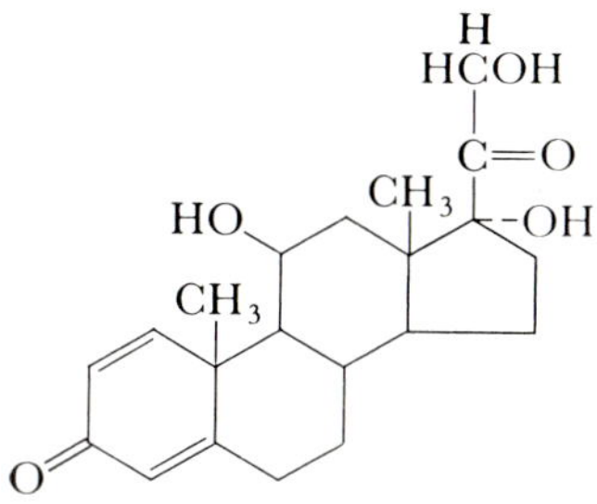

Prednisolone
Δ'-hydrocortisone
(Meticortelone)

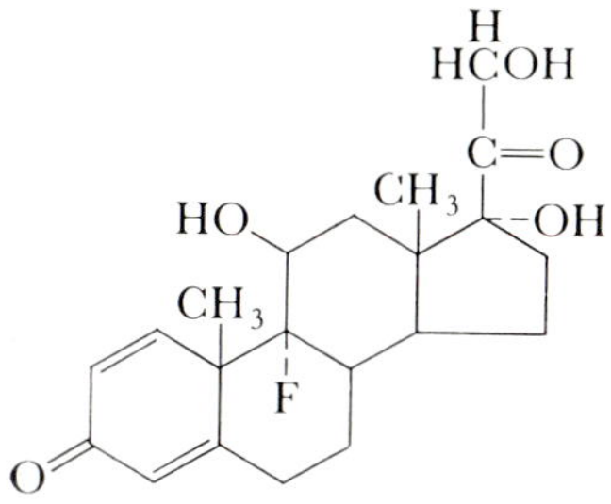

Fluoroprednisolone
(Predef)

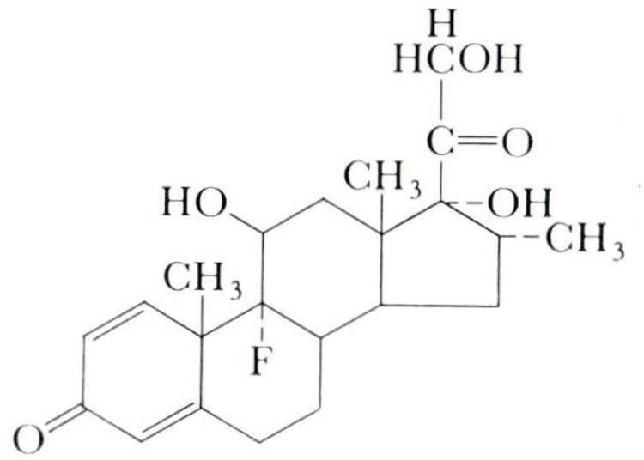

Dexamethasone
9 α-fluoro-16 α methylprednisolone

FIG. 33.2.

is important for activity. The 11-deoxy compounds have very little glucocorticoid activity (deoxycorticosterone). The 11-β hydroxy group (which hydrocortisone contains and is also present in synthetic hormones such as prednisolone and dexamethasone) decreases the mineralocorticoid or salt-retaining effects but is necessary for antiinflammatory activity. Hydroxylation of the 16th and 17th carbon atoms further strengthens the glucocorticoid activity.

Fluorination of the 6th, 9th, or 12th carbon atoms increases the potency of the glucocorticoid, but other halogens are less effective. In addition, dehydrogenation of the 1,2-methylene groups such as has been done in prednisone also increases the potency of the adrenal corticoids.

Methylation of the 6th or 16th carbon atom decreases the salt-retaining effects and slightly increases the glucocorticoid effects. Various combinations of the above alterations have created glucocorticoids that are extremely potent, less costly, and quite useful in veterinary medicine.

SOURCE

Although the adrenal cortices of slaughterhouse animals provided the substrate for early isolation, identification, and clinical trials of the adrenal steroids, this is no longer the source. All adrenal corticoids presently on the market for clinical use are produced synthetically in the laboratory. This contributes greatly to their decline in price, increased purity, and greater dependability.

FUNCTIONS OF GLUCOCORTICOIDS

Molecular Activity of Steroids. Considerable progress has been made in the past few years in understanding how steroid hormones act within the cell. According to O'Malley and Schrader (1976), there are at least six steps involved in steroid hormone action. This would apply to the adrenal corticosteroids as well as the sex steroids.

1. Entry of steroid hormone into target cell. Steroid hormones are lipid soluble and they diffuse through cell membranes to the cytoplasm without depending on a transport system.

2. Binding to specific receptor in target cell. A target cell has an inactive cytoplasmic receptor with a high affinity for a particular steroid that becomes an active site after binding.

3. Translocation to the nucleus. The steroid-receptor complex migrates into the nucleus where it attaches to a particular area of the chromosome.

4. Binding of steroid-receptor complex to nuclear acceptor site. Once bound, certain genes are then activated or de-repressed so new RNA can be formed.

5. Formation of new RNA. The

steroid receptor-nuclear complex forms mRNA, which then specifies which protein is to be made. These new proteins are important to the function of some cells and to replication of other cells. Once the mRNA has been produced, it could have an effect within the cell or it could be transported out of the cell for functions elsewhere.

6. Deinduction of the steroid. This could occur by metabolism if the steroid is modified to a nonactive form or it could be recycled.

From the above description it can be seen that a steroid molecule acts on a template, which is the chromosome, eventually becoming bound to a nuclear receptor that turns on the action of a particular gene. This process requires several hours, and after stimulation the effect would be realized only for a few hours unless a continuing supply of steroid acts on the target cell. Although the steroid hormone apparently enters most cells of the body, it is only the target cells that respond by making RNA since they alone have the cytoplasmic receptors for that particular steroid. Steroids having similar biological activity (i.e., the many estrogens) may share the same receptor sites.

PHARMACOLOGY OF CORTISOL

Cortisol, the important natural hormone from the adrenal cortex, affects a wide range of activities in the body, including electrolyte and water metabolism; metabolism of carbohydrates, proteins, and fats; and inflammatory processes. Cortisol also reduces certain formed elements of the blood such as lymphocytes and eosinophils, decreases growth, and inhibits wound healing.

Carbohydrate Metabolism. Cortisol increases gluconeogenesis and inhibits peripheral glucose utilization, which leads to an increase in tissue stores of glycogen, especially in the liver. *Hyperglycemia* and *glucosuria* (steroid diabetes) occur, which aggravate diabetes mellitus but may temporarily alleviate the hypoglycemia in the ketotic dairy cow.

Protein Metabolism. Cortisol causes catabolism of proteins leading to negative nitrogen balance and increased urinary elimination of nitrogen and uric acid. Anabolism of proteins is discouraged and, in fact, growth ceases in young animals, wounds heal more slowly, and there may be an inhibition of antibody production because of this antianabolic effect.

Cortisol causes the blood level of amino acids to rise, due to the increased breakdown of muscle protein. There is less transport of amino acids across all extrahepatic cell membranes but increased hepatic transport under the influence of cortisol. This mobilization of amino acids along with (1) conversion of amino acids to glucose (gluconeogenesis), (2) increased plasma and liver protein formation by the liver, and (3) increased deamination by the liver characterize the effects of cortisol. Most of this may simply depend on altered membrane permeability to amino acids favoring hepatic forces.

Fat Metabolism. The influence of adrenal corticoids on fat metabolism is not well understood. The induced gluconeogenesis does favor catabolism of fats, as well as shifting of the body stores of fats.

Water and Electrolyte Metabolism. The glucocorticoids exert lesser effects on water and electrolyte metabolism than the mineralocorticoids such as deoxycorticosterone and aldosterone. There is enough overlapping of effects of the glucocorticoids on mineral metabolism that the adrenalectomized animal can be kept alive by the administration of cortisol. Excessive administration of cortisol causes sodium retention and potassium diuresis. Continued high dosage of cortisol causes edema, hypochloremia, hypokalemia, and metabolic alkalosis. Potassium therapy alleviates this disorder and may be resorted to when clearly needed during prolonged cortisol therapy.

Endocrine System. When glucocorticoids are administered repeatedly at very high levels for several weeks or longer, the excess hormones may suppress the production of ACTH by the anterior pituitary and/or the release of corticotropin releasing factor (CRF). Such iatrogenic secondary adrenocortical insufficiency is fairly common in dogs on prolonged corticosteroid therapy for antiinflammatory or immunosuppressive purposes (Scott and Greene 1974). When ACTH is given in excess, the adrenal cortex hypertrophies.

Musculoskeletal System. Excessive therapy with glucocorticoids or hypercorticoidism of any sort causes muscular weakness as a result of potassium depletion. Muscular weakness is also observed with hypocorticoidism, but the mechanism is not understood.

Prolonged high dosage of the glucocorticoids and ACTH causes increased elimination of calcium, phosphorus, and nitrogen, which will produce or intensify osteoporosis and resultant fractures.

Antiinflammatory Effect. Glucocorticoids suppress the connective tissue response to injury, whether traumatic, anaphylactic, or infective. This antiinflammatory response arises from the ability of these hormones to suppress the activity of fibroblasts and granuloma formation. Glucocorticoids stabilize lysosomes in damaged tissue, thereby preventing lysosomal proteolytic enzymes from escaping to damage surrounding cells. This suppression of tissue response obviously interferes with host response to a bacterial infection. In addition, there are increased capillary tone and selective permeability that diminish plasma exudation into the tissues.

The exact mechanism is unknown, but the glucocorticoids obviously suppress the normal tissue response to injury and alleviate the symptoms of many conditions such as arthritis and allergy. The relief provided by these hormones is merely palliative and the syndrome may reappear when hormone therapy is terminated.

The same suppressive activity of the adrenocortical hormones can be used clinically in treating long-standing conditions such as pericardial, pleural, or peritoneal adhesions. Conversely, cortisol is of no value in the treatment of acute conditions such as histamine or anaphylactic shock. In the words of Hench (1952), an early and prominent worker in the field, the effect may be as follows:

> The hormone appears not to extinguish the fire or to act like a carpenter to repair the damage of the fire. Instead, it appears to "dampen the fire," or to provide, as it were, an asbestos suit behind which the patient, like some Biblical Shadrach, Meshach or Abednego, protects his tissues from the fire. If this protection is removed prematurely, before the fire has spent itself, the patient and his tissues will react again to the burning. But, if the protection is not discarded until the natural duration of the fire is over, the patient remains largely free of symptoms and apparently "well."

The normal day-to-day level of cortisol produced by the body is not enough to inhibit wound healing. The above-described events follow administration of large doses. These general body effects must be considered if systemic administration is for a localized area. Whenever possible, local or topical therapy is preferred.

Hematopoietic System. Glucocorticoids cause a marked reduction in circulating eosinophils. Prolonged therapy produces significant neutrophilic granulocytosis. Prolonged therapy is lympholytic; circulating lymphocytes decrease while lymph nodes, thymus, and spleen involute.

Antibody Production. Antibody production to some antigens may be crippled, which causes some veterinarians not to overlap immunization procedures with corticosteroid administration, unless absolutely necessary. The experimental information on this is not clear-cut (Enright et al. 1970; Gross et al. 1973). Generally it is best not to employ vaccination procedures while an animal is being treated with the corticoids.

The use of corticoids as immunosuppressive agents in tissue transplants is well documented in the human being. Rejection of foreign tissue such as skin grafts and heart and kidney transplants can be minimized in all mammals with corticoids. The immunological rejection system of foreign tissue can be corticoid suppressed but this would also enhance the entry of infectious agents and delay healing.

Vascular System. Evidence is accumulating to indicate that the glucocorticoids are necessary to sensitize the vascular system to the pressor action of epinephrine and norepinephrine. This may be especially true in the case of gram-negative bacterial endotoxin shock. Some researchers (Lillehei et al. 1964; Weil et al. 1964) believe dogs suffering from hemorrhagic or endotoxin shock respond well to large intravenous doses of glucocorticoids if they fail to respond to transfusions of blood or plasma. There is an increased splanchnic resistance, stagnant hypoxia, edema, and necrosis of the intestines in such shock.

Nonetheless, first therapy should involve expansion of extracellular fluid volume, antibiotics, and symptomatic relief. Thereafter, attention may be directed to corticoid therapy.

Other Actions. The glucocorticoids may increase the secretion of pepsin and hydrochloric acid. These hormones also exert an androgenic action that appears in both sexes following prolonged therapy. Hyaluronidase activity may be inhibited. Convulsive thresholds apparently are lowered.

Euphoria. Behavioral changes such as a feeling of well-being are frequently manifested following glucocorticoid therapy. This occurs despite such terminal conditions as cancer. Depressive states associated with other diseases may warrant such therapy provided corticoid therapy per se is not contraindicated.

NEWER SYNTHETIC GLUCOCORTICOIDS

The previous discussion of the pharmacology of cortisol in general holds with the weaker substance, cortisone. Chemically, cortisone has a ketone group at carbon atom 11 whereas cortisol has a hydroxyl group. Many synthetic glucocorticoids have been introduced, the antiinflammatory and gluconeogenic potencies of which are much greater than cortisol but in which the tendency to retain sodium is not increased correspondingly. Prednisone (cortisone with an additional double bond between carbon atoms 1 and 2) and prednisolone (cortisol with an additional double bond between carbon atoms 1 and 2) were the first to have enjoyed widespread use.

Considerable concern has been aroused over the use of these more potent corticoids in human patients because of the possible upset in sodium and potassium balance. Less emphasis has been placed on this aspect in veterinary medicine, and the work of Goetsch et al. (1959) indicates that Δ^1-9-α-fluorohydrocortisone (9-α-fluoroprednisolone) in the cow creates only minor sodium retention but a profound blood glucose elevation. Additional work by Neff et al. (1960) with the same hormone found some upset in phosphorus and potassium balance in the dairy cow, but again it was much less than has occurred in human beings, hence its widespread use in dairy cows as a gluconeogenic agent (see Fig. 33.3).

Caution should be exercised in the parenteral use of these extremely potent corticoids in the dog and cat until further work is done on their effect on mineral metabolism.

These corticoids are used topically in human medicine almost exclusively for their antiinflammatory and antiallergic effects, whereas in veterinary medicine the same hormones enjoy topical and parenteral antiinflammatory and antiallergic use but in addition are used parenterally to elevate blood glucose in the dairy cow suffering from ketosis. This is further discussed under the section dealing with ketosis treatment in the dairy cow.

From the pharmacologic aspect we are at a loss to explain how the glucocorticoids alleviate ketosis in the dairy cow. Granted that the induced gluconeogenesis elevates blood glucose levels to the normal range, one must also realize that there is a de-

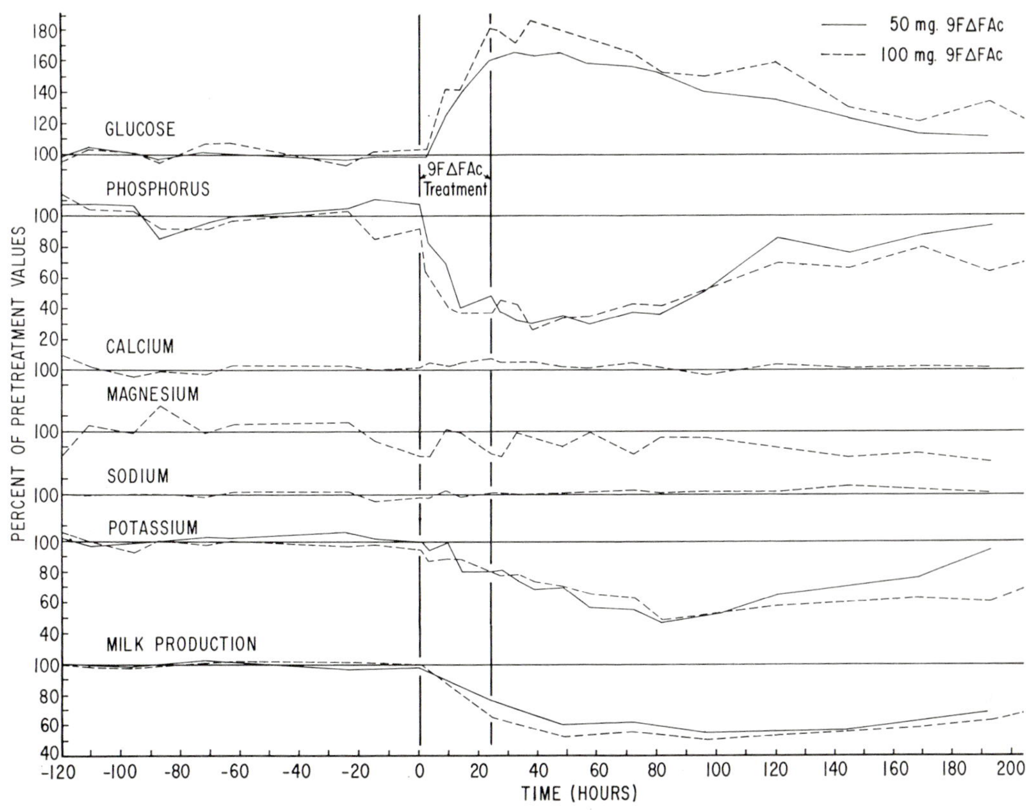

FIG. 33.3. Effect of high doses of FΔFAc i.m. on blood glucose, serum minerals, and milk production of normal dairy cows. 9-α-Fluoroprednisolone acetate, Predef [R]. (Neff et al. 1960)

creased peripheral utilization of glucose created at the same time. Perhaps the effect is due to the generalized catabolism of fat, carbohydrate, and protein stores serving as a sacrifice to elevate blood glucose, thereby allowing the cow to return to a normal metabolic pattern after the effects of the glucocorticoid have disappeared. If the glucocorticoids elevated blood glucose through enzyme induction, many hours to several days would elapse. The immediate glucose-elevating effect must be due to the decreased glucose utilization.

METABOLISM AND EXCRETION OF GLUCOCORTICOIDS

Circulating plasma steroids are in two forms. Upon adrenal secretion or injection of cortisol or presumably the injection of analogs, the molecule is (1) free but (2) soon becomes loosely attached to a specific serum protein (α-globulin) called *transcortin*. This binding is loose and reversible and its strength is inverse to the number of polar groups on the steroid molecule. A weakly polar steroid like estrone is tightly bound, whereas a highly polar steroid like cortisol is loosely bound. According to Lindner (1967), this binding of cortisol in ruminants is quite loose.

Cortisol is transported by the blood where it (1) reaches the hypothalamus and inhibits further output of ACTH-RF, (2) reaches the adenohypophysis to inhibit ACTH output, and (3) reaches the target tissue receptor site and becomes rather firmly attached and exerts its specific effects.

Normally, up to 75% of the plasma cortisol and corticosterone (plus analogs to varying degrees) is bound to transcortin. Another 10–15% is bound to albumen.

The remaining 10–15% of the cortisol and corticosterone is *unbound* and this is the *physiologically important* part because it is free to enter the cells and exert its effects. As the unbound form is metabolized by the target cells or conjugated by the liver for elimination, the transcortin bound portion is released to maintain the needed plasma level of unbound hormone.

Hypercortisolism (Cushing's disease) overloads the available transcortin, leading to unusually high plasma and urine levels of unbound cortisol and corticosterone.

Plasma protein deficiency may lead to a shortage of transcortin, whereas hyperestrogenism (i.e., pregnancy or injection) causes elevated transcortin. These deviations in transcortin levels only affect the bound levels and usually not the unbound physiologically active cortisol and corticosterone.

The half-life of cortisol is less than 2 hours, so it soon circulates back to the liver where it is conjugated mainly to glucuronic acid or less often to sulfuric acid. These are water-soluble substances ready for excretion in the urine (¾) or feces (¼). Ruminants favor the urine route.

The kidney tubules actively resorb 80–90% of the free cortisol but allow the conjugated forms to remain in the urine.

The body is less well adapted to metabolizing and eliminating the synthetic corticoids like prednisone—*hence their longer effect and increased potency. Probably the altered molecule is less likely to be attacked by the enzyme systems present.*

All the glucocorticoids are absorbed readily from the gastrointestinal tract. The onset of activity is prompt but the duration of action is short, especially in the simple-stomached animals where the medication must be provided in divided doses 3 or 4 times daily. A single daily oral dose of Δ^1-9-α-fluorohydrocortisone will elevate and maintain blood glucose in the cow (Goetsch et al. 1962). Parenteral administration of the glucocorticoids is commonly employed, with the intravenous route causing a prompt but short-lived effect.

The intramuscular route is most commonly employed. The duration of action of the corticoids, especially the acetate forms, is at least 24 hours, although the onset of action may be delayed several hours after intramuscular injection. The intramuscular and oral routes of administration are especially effective in sustaining the circulating level of the corticoids, thereby bringing about elevation of blood glucose and suppression of inflammatory reactions.

The topical application of corticoids for their antiinflammatory effect has enjoyed widespread use for nonspecific inflammatory conditions of the integument. Topical application does not raise the systemic level of the hormone appreciably; therefore, the very potent corticoids such as the fluorinated ones can be used topically without fear of upsetting sodium and potassium metabolism.

Cortisone acetate applied topically to the conjunctiva readily permeates the anterior chamber of the eye. The intraocular concentration drops rapidly within 24 hours after the end of therapy. Low but detectable levels of steroids are found in the vitreous humor. Cortisone acetate injected subconjunctivally produces a higher concentration within the eye more rapidly than does topical therapy. This route of administration is widely used in the treatment of inflammatory conditions of the eye since a more sustained level of corticoid can be maintained.

Intraarticular injection of corticoids for their antiinflammatory effect is widely practiced. In the usual dosages, systemic effects do not appear. This form of local application includes injection into tendon sheaths and bursa. Injections may be repeated 1–3 times weekly to maintain the effect.

CONTROL OF GLUCOCORTICOID SECRETION

The output of glucocorticoids by the adrenal cortex is at a minimal level in the absence of ACTH from the anterior pituitary. Evidence is quite conclusive that ACTH influences only the formation and release of the glucocorticoids, whereas the formation and release of the mineralocorticoids are under nonpituitary influence. One site of action of ACTH in the adrenal cortex is at the level of conversion of cholesterol to dihydroxycholesterol. Probably ACTH is also active at other levels in the biogenesis of cortisol. Nearly any stress on the animal will increase the production of ACTH, which then stimulates steroidogenesis.

Species differences in the ratios of cortisol to corticosterone are due to differences in the enzymatic systems involved in corticosteroid biosynthesis, this being principally the 17-hydroxylating enzyme activity. These differences between species are constant and unaltered by ACTH so long as it is homologous ACTH. An interesting experiment by Kass et al. (1954) showed that adrenal vein blood of rabbits contains corticosterone as the predominant steroid. Upon administration of porcine ACTH for 1 week, cortisol, as well as corticosterone, were found in the adrenal vein blood in a ratio of 1:2. When procine ACTH was administered for 21–28 days, cortisol predominated in the adrenal secretion, and the ratio of cortisol to corticosterone was 4:1.

The factors affecting the release of ACTH from the pituitary are multiple but it appears that a humoral substance, CRF, is released from the hypothalamus and carried by the portal system to the anterior pituitary effecting ACTH release.

Presently, four substances that cause release of ACTH have been isolated: vasopressin, α1, and α2-CRF, and β-CRF. Alpha$_1$-CRF is closely related to α-MSH (melanocyte-stimulating hormone), and may influence pigmentation in Addison's disease because in this disease α1-CRF output would have little or no brake. Although vasopressin (antidiuretic hormone, ADH) is not a RF, it may play a small role in adrenal cortical response to stress since McCann et al. (1966) found rats with hereditary diabetes insipidus, which lack vasopressin, less able to increase corticosterone output when stressed by ether, restraint, or bleeding than normal controls.

Many factors influence the hypothalamic release of CRF, such as impulses arising from sites of injury or burns in peripheral areas of the body, impulses arriving from the cortex of the brain, and other factors loosely termed "stressors." (See Fig. 33.4.) In addition, epinephrine levels arising from the adrenal medulla when the animal is frightened are sufficient to induce ACTH release. This has been established through infusion experiments of the adenohypophysis and possibly accounts for the rapid release of ACTH seen when an animal reacts to an unfavorable situation.

In addition, the effect of glucocorticoids acting directly on the adenohypophysis is part of a "servomechanism" and may be the effective scheme during normal day-to-day conditions. As the corticoid level rises, the output of ACTH is inhibited, and when the circulating level of glucocorticoids drops, the brake is released, allowing ACTH output. Others feel the servomechanism acts through the hypothalamus as part of the previously described CRF scheme. There is supporting evidence for both locations (adenohypophysis and hypothalamus) as sites for the negative feedback.

In addition to the effects of external factors (stressors) and negative feedback control on ACTH output, a third modulator is diurnal changes. This rhythm in glucocorticoid output is highest in the morning, having risen during sleep, and lowest in the afternoon and early evening (Bottoms et al. 1972). This would probably be reversed in the nocturnal species.

Mineralocorticoids

Following adrenalectomy, the specific cause of death is the depletion of sodium and the retention of potassium. This critical life-determining function of the adrenal cortex is due to aldosterone, which was not discovered as a specific substance until 1953. Aldosterone is a very potent substance (25–50x deoxycorticosterone) and its level in the adrenal gland or in the circulation is so low that it evaded detection for many years. In the meantime, the synthetic mineralocorticoid, deoxycorticosterone, was developed and used clinically.

The output of aldosterone by the adrenal cortex is not under control of the

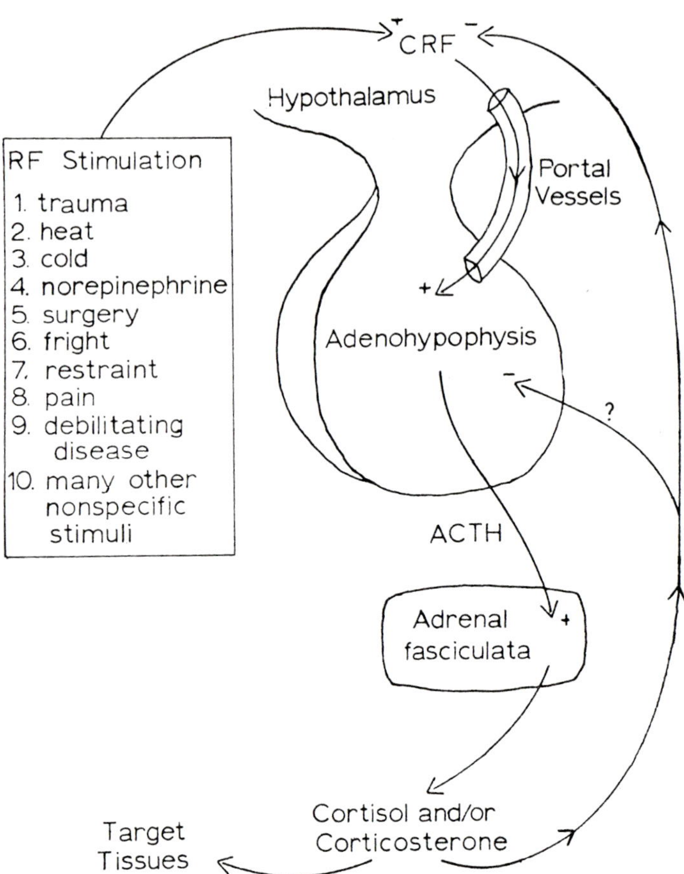

FIG. 33.4. The hypothalamic-adenohypophyseal control of adrenal output of cortisol/corticosterone and the feedback regulation. Also notice the other factors that favor corticotropin-releasing factor (CRF) output.

pituitary gland or ACTH. Davis (1962) has reviewed investigations on whether aldosterone secretion is under central control and concluded that a mechanism resides in the juxtaglomerular apparatus on the afferent arteriole of the kidney. (See Fig. 24.8.) A decrease in renal arterial pressure serves as a signal causing renin-angiotension release, which is carried to the zona glomerulosa causing aldosterone release. Aldosterone then acts on the renal tubules causing sodium retention which increases blood volume and blood pressure, these acting in a feedback scheme on the juxtaglomerular apparatus. The juxtaglomerular apparatus has been visualized as a stretch receptor by some and as an osmoreceptor by others (Fisher and Klein 1966).

The overproduction of aldosterone in domestic animals has not been clinically substantiated. In 1955 such a disease was first described in the human being and has been extended to several hundred patients. One of the first symptoms is muscular weakness, which is associated with excessive renal loss of potassium leading to hypokalemia. Usually there is a moderate hypernatremia and hypertension. In view of our discussion of the effects of aldosterone, one can readily see why the above-described symptoms would appear. The cause is usually an adrenalcortical tumor.

Clinical use of mineralocorticoids in veterinary medicine is limited to the treatment of chronic interstitial nephritis of the dog as described by Dickson and Ott (1955). These workers found that in such kidney failure a potassium intoxication occurs along with the uremia. Sodium also was depleted. The elimination of potassium can be aided by the administration of deoxycorticosterone acetate in a dosage of 2–5 mg intramuscularly for several days, along with supportive glucose, fluid therapy, and antibiotics if indicated.

Deoxycorticosterone is readily available and apparently just as good as aldosterone. It exerts its effect on the renal tubules, promoting reabsorption of sodium and loss of potassium. Aldosterone obviously exerts a powerful influence on water and electrolyte balance in health or disease. The old adage "where sodium goes, so goes water" merits attention. The role of aldosterone in relation to fluid balance and therapy is considered in another chapter.

Adrenocorticotropic Hormone (ACTH)

ACTH (Fig. 33.5) is produced by the basophilic cells of the anterior pituitary gland. It is a 39 amino acid polypeptide of low molecular weight and a biological activity of about 400 units/mg. ACTH produced commercially is extracted from the anterior pituitary glands of oxen and swine.

Because of more direct effect obtained by the administration of the glucocorticoids, ACTH is seldom used in practice.

ACTION

ACTH acts by stimulating the adrenal cortex, causing the production and release of glucocorticoids into the blood. This stimulus by ACTH is not vital because the adrenal cortex secretes sufficient hormones to maintain life in the hypophysectomized animal. The effectiveness of ACTH is entirely dependent on a responsive and functional adrenal cortex. The clinician must establish this before ACTH therapy is begun, otherwise corticoid therapy would be preferred. The use of ACTH clinically is declining in favor of the use of the synthetic corticoids.

Mechanism of ACTH Action. ACTH attaches to the receptors on the fasciculata cell surface and activates adenylate cyclase, which converts adenosine triphosphate (ATP) to cyclic AMP (Fig. 30.1), the "second messenger." cAMP then catalyzes the transfer of energy from ATP to form phosphorylated proteins (enzymes), which then enhance the rate-limiting step in steroidogenesis, i.e., cholesterol to pregnenolone (Fig. 30.4). In addition, ACTH causes growth of both zones, fasciculata (GC) and glomerulosa (MC). Steroids are not stored in the cortex, so most of the ACTH effect is on production and immediate release of the glucocorticoids from the fasciculata zone.

ABSORPTION

ACTH is absorbed readily following intramuscular injection. ACTH is partially destroyed by tissue enzymes at the site of intramuscular injection, but not sufficiently to prevent its administration by this route. Following intramuscular administration of ACTH solution (Wilson Laboratories, Chicago) to the dairy cow, Shaw and Nichols (1962) found increased secretion of 17-hydroxycorticosteroids within one-half hour that lasted more than 8 but less than 24 hours. Intramuscular hydrocortisone elevated plasma levels a similar length of time (Table 33.1).

ACTH is inactive orally because the polypeptides are rapidly destroyed by digestive enzymes.

EXCRETION

ACTH in aqueous solution disappears rapidly from the bloodstream following intravenous or intramuscular injection. Only small amounts of ACTH are excreted unchanged in the urine. The half-life of circulating ACTH is only 6 minutes.

PREPARATIONS

ACTH is available as *Corticotropin*, U.S.P., a lyophilized powdered tissue extract for dissolving in water at the time of injection. It is also available as a solution, *Corticotropin Injection,* U.S.P. One U.S.P. unit is identical with one International Unit (IU) and is defined as representing the specific adrenocorticotropic activity of 1 mg of the International Standard. ACTH is also available in a repository mixture containing 15% gelatin to delay absorption and thus prolong the action following

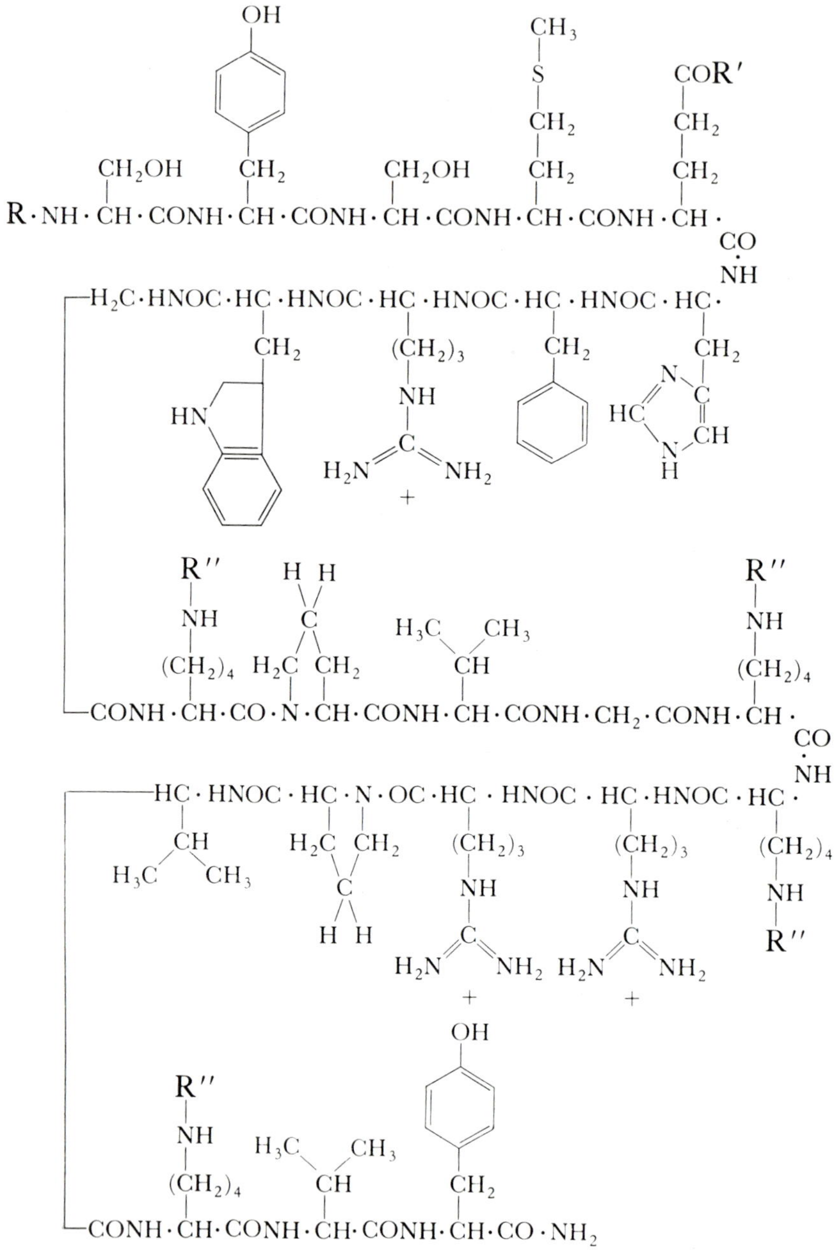

R·NH·CH·CONH·CH·CONH·CH·CONH·CH·CONH·CH·CO·NH (side chains: CH_2OH; CH_2–C$_6$H$_4$–OH; CH_2OH; $CH_2CH_2SCH_3$; CH_2CH_2COR')

—H_2C·HNOC·HC·HNOC·HC·HNOC·HC·HNOC·HC· (side chains: CH_2–indolyl; $(CH_2)_3$–NH–C(H_2N)=NH_2^+; CH_2–phenyl; CH_2–imidazolyl)

—CONH·CH·CO·N·CH·CONH·CH·CONH·CH_2·CONH·CH·CO·NH (side chains: $(CH_2)_4$–NH–R''; proline ring H_2C–C(H_2)–CH_2; CH(CH_3)$_2$; $(CH_2)_4$–NH–R'')

—HC·HNOC·HC·N·OC·HC·HNOC·HC·HNOC·HC· (side chains: CH(CH_3)$_2$; proline ring H_2C–C(H_2)–CH_2; $(CH_2)_3$–NH–C(H_2N)=NH_2^+; $(CH_2)_3$–NH–C(H_2N)=NH_2^+; $(CH_2)_4$–NH–R'')

—CONH·CH·CONH·CH·CONH·CH·CO·NH_2 (side chains: $(CH_2)_4$–NH–R''; CH(CH_3)$_2$; CH_2–C$_6$H$_4$–OH)

Corticotropin (ACTH)

FIG. 33.5.

TABLE 33.1. The effects of frequent blood sampling, intravenous adrenocorticotrophic hormone (ACTH), intramuscular ACTH, and intramuscular hydrocortisone on the plasma 17-hydroxycorticosteroid (μg/100 ml) of calves and cows

Time	Calves	Cows	Calves	Cows
	Blood Sampling Alone		Intravenous ACTH (100 I.U.)	
Pretreatment	90/4.67 ± 0.57	40/4.82 ± 0.58	90/4.67 ± 0.57	40/ 4.82 ± 0.58
½ hour later	11/5.61 ± 1.36	10/6.53 ± 0.90	15/6.15 ± 1.46	11/11.52 ± 2.10†
1 hour later	13/4.00 ± 1.12	10/5.69 ± 1.06	15/7.03 ± 1.41	11/11.09 ± 1.92†
2 hours later	14/5.03 ± 1.45	10/6.58 ± 1.05	14/7.53 ± 1.38†	11/11.16 ± 1.87†
4 hours later	14/3.25 ± 1.18	10/5.51 ± 0.84	15/3.70 ± 1.26	10/ 4.96 ± 1.41
24 hours later	14/4.23 ± 1.00	10/5.46 ± 0.71	14/3.82 ± 0.79	11/ 7.30 ± 1.53
	Intramuscular ACTH (200 I.U.)		Intramuscular Hydrocortisone (1 mg/kg of body wt.)	
Pretreatment	90/4.67 ± 0.57	40/ 4.82 ± 0.58	90/ 4.67 ± 0.57	40/ 4.82 ± 0.58
½ hour later	9/6.58 ± 2.08	10/10.57 ± 1.77†	9/15.15 ± 4.67†	10/28.94 ± 9.10†
1 hour later	9/8.57 ± 2.15*	10/10.33 ± 1.60†	9/11.88 ± 4.02†	10/15.25 ± 1.79†
2 hours later	9/9.71 ± 1.88†	10/15.02 ± 2.18†	9/11.48 ± 2.50†	10/24.59 ± 5.82†
4 hours later	9/9.59 ± 1.84†	10/13.76 ± 3.23†	9/ 8.44 ± 2.95*	10/12.22 ± 2.55†
8 hours later	9/8.69 ± 1.18*	10/14.09 ± 2.22†	9/ 5.36 ± 1.34	10/11.06 ± 2.10†
24 hours later	9/4.94 ± 1.58	10/ 6.43 ± 0.66	9/ 5.78 ± 1.98	10/ 7.28 ± 0.98

Source: Shaw and Nichols 1962.
Note: Numerator = number of samples; denominator = mean ± standard error.
* Significant at the 5% level.
† Highly significant at the 1% level.

intramuscular injection (*Repository Corticotropin Injection,* U.S.P.).

DOSAGE

	Horses and Cattle	*Dogs*
ACTH-gel U.S.P. units i.m. or subcutaneous	200–600	1/lb body wt
ACTH U.S.P. units i.v. or i.m. or subcutaneous	100–600	1/lb body wt

Therapy with ACTH or Glucocorticoids

SELECTION OF HORMONE

ACTH produces the same effect as the glucocorticoids and may be used whenever such therapy is indicated except in the presence of adrenal pathology or if the therapy is to be given orally or topically. Cortisol is about 20% more potent, weight for weight, than cortisone. Both drugs are effective orally or parenterally. Cortisol is the drug of choice for topical administration to the eye and skin and for intravenous or intrasynovial injection. Cortisone is effective in the eye but not on the skin.

Prednisone (Meticorten) and prednisolone (Meticortelone) are synthetic steroids. They appear to be 3–5 times as potent as cortisone or cortisol. (See Table 33.2.) At low dosages these new drugs do not produce salt retention or excessive potassium excretion in human beings, which is an

TABLE 33.2. Comparative activity of some glucocorticoids

Drug	Anti-inflammatory Activity	Gluconeogenic Activity	Sodium-retaining Activity
Cortisone	4	5	100
Hydrocortisone (cortisol)	5–6	7	100
Prednisone	20	20	80
Prednisolone	20	20	80
Methylprednisolone	25	25	Very weak
9-α-Fluoroprednisolone	50	80+	Weak in cattle, otherwise?
Dexamethasone	100+	100+	Very weak
Flumethasone	100+	100+	Very weak
Triamcinolone	100+	100+	Very weak

Source: Goetsch et al. 1959; Neff et al. 1960.

advantage over cortisone and cortisol. In other respects, the new synthetic steroids resemble the parent compounds. These drugs are also effective orally, intraocularly, and intraarticularly.

Development of even more potent glucocorticoids has led to methyprednisolone, 9-α-fluoroprednisolone (Predef), dexamethasone, and many others, which must surely confuse the clinician. Potency is now sufficiently high that cost per dose for large animals has been reduced. In addition, less mineralocorticoid effect is exerted while the antiinflammatory and gluconeogenic effects are potentiated. *Therefore, selection becomes a matter of personal choice based primarily on cost.* The cost per dose must be considered since much less of the newer potent hormones is required for effect.

CONTRAINDICATIONS

There are few contraindications to the use of ACTH or the glucocorticoids, but such conditions as late pregnancy, corneal ulcers, diabetes mellitus, hypertension, renal insufficiency, and decreased cardiac reserve must be considered cautiously. *Infectious conditions require special consideration because of dissemination.* It is the prolonged dosage that must be considered cautiously and the induction of Cushing's disease weighed against the value of the therapy. Muscle wasting in weak, thin animals and growth inhibition in young animals must be considered. A single dose would not be contraindicated anytime.

GENERAL PRINCIPLES

Considerable variation occurs in patient response to hormonal therapy, so dosage must be individualized. Adjustment of the initial maintenance dosage may be necessary. Frequent observation of the patient therefore is essential. Dosage is usually high in acute and normally brief processes and relatively low when prolonged medication is anticipated. In oral therapy the total daily dose should be divided into 3 or 4 doses per day in small animals. Single daily oral dosage of 100 mg of 9-α-fluoroprednisolone maintains elevation of blood glucose in the cow (Goetsch et al. 1962).

In prolonged medication, it is important to seek the minimal effective dosage to alleviate the condition. Larger doses for more than 3–4 days would cause systemic disturbances and possibly induce cortical involution.

Prolonged therapy with glucocorticoids at high dosages for several weeks may produce adrenal atrophy and cause decreased hormone production by the adrenal cortex. Abrupt termination of such therapy may result in a hypocortical state. Therefore, prolonged high dosage adrenocortical substitution therapy should be terminated by a gradual decrease in dosage over a period of 2 weeks or more. Normal cortical activity usually is restored within a few weeks. The administration of ACTH may help reestablish cortical function more promptly.

Such precautions are not necessary when prolonged corticosteroid therapy has been at low dosages similar to normal physiological levels. Likewise, high level dosage for 4 days or less probably does not seriously affect the pituitary-adrenal axis.

Alternate day therapy (ADT) of corticoids is often practiced to give the pituitary-adrenal axis opportunity to function. ADT is satisfactory in some chronic conditions.

IN THE DOG

Marshak et al. (1960) diligently recorded serum sodium and potassium before, during, and after corticoid therapy of spontaneous primary adrenocortical insufficiency in a dog. Anorexia, diarrhea, asthenia, polydipsia, hair loss, emesis, cardiovascular effects, eosinophilia, dehydration, anuria, azotemia, hyponatremia, and hyperkalemia characterized the disease. Cortisone, 1 mg/lb of body weight, dramatically reversed all abnormalities. The 27-lb dog was maintained thereafter on 0.125 mg 9-α-fluorohydrocortisone and 6.25 mg cortisone daily.

Various forms of *arthritis* have been treated in the dog with cortisone or hydrocortisone at a dosage approximating 1 mg/lb of body weight as the initial dose. Oral or intramuscular therapy is repeated daily and adjusted either upward or downward according to the apparent need of the patient. Clinical reports indicate that the majority of acute involvements give favorable responses but that most chronic affections do not. *Asthma* has been treated in dogs with cortisone at an initial dosage of 1 mg/lb of body weight orally or intramuscularly. This dosage is usually decreased for maintenance. *Eczema* of various types has been treated satisfactorily in some patients, but others do not respond well. Eczema characterized by pustular dermatitis often responds well to cortisone combined with a topical antibiotic such as polymycin, bacitracin, or neomycin. *Otitis externa* appears to respond moderately well to cortisone, especially if there is an abundance of granulation tissue. The treatment of *burns* has been difficult to evaluate clinically but from experimental data on hamsters it would appear that cortisone delays healing and markedly increases wound infection.

Limited information is available in veterinary medicine on the use of ACTH and the glucocorticoids in *inflammation of the eye of any species.* Most results have been favorable because of the marked antiinflammatory activity of these agents. Since the advent of synthetic corticosteroids, ACTH is seldom used. The glucocorticoids may be used orally, intramuscularly, or intravenously, and also locally as eye drops or ointment or by subconjunctival injection. *All topical ophthalmic preparations containing corticosteroids, with or without an antimicrobial agent, are contraindicated in the initial treatment of corneal ulcers. They should not be used until the infection is under control and corneal regeneration is well under way.*

Glucocorticoids can be used beneficially in controlling acute local inflammatory reactions in the eyes of dogs when not accompanied by suppuration. It seems to work especially well in controlling iritis. Cortisone tends to prevent an acute ocular inflammation from becoming chronic. Cortisone has been suspended in normal saline (1 to 4) and applied to the conjunctival sac at frequent intervals during the day. Cortisone has also been injected subconjunctivally in the anesthetized eye in a dose of 0.1–0.3 ml of a solution containing 25 mg/ml (Magrane 1951).

All inflammations of the inner eye should be treated by systemic therapy despite the traditional tendency to employ topical treatment.

Mast cell sarcoma may be temporarily alleviated by glucocorticoids, but enlargement follows later and fatal termination is invariable.

Canine *systemic lupus erythematosus* and other autoimmune diseases of dogs and cats often respond to steroid therapy. Dosage must be high (1 mg/lb/day) for 1–2 weeks then reduced to alternate-day therapy or even continual low dosage to maintain long-term remission. Complete recovery is seldom seen.

IN THE HORSE

Glucocorticoids have been used extensively in the horse for the treatment of various kinds of *lamenesses.* Most clinical evaluations of the therapy have been relatively favorable for the acute type of lameness, provided that adequate rest is permitted in conjunction with treatment. Chronic lameness does not respond well. Treatment has varied from a single period to as many as 4 periods of therapy at 2- or 3-day intervals. The dosage for injection into a tendon sheath, bursa, or joint capsule has varied from 50 to 250 mg of cortisone or cortisol. Acute *carpitis, tarsitis, gonitis,* and *metacarpalphalangeal arthritis* have given better responses than treatment of *navicular bursitis, coxitis,* and *bog spavin.* There are a few reports of success following the early treatment of *laminitis* in the horse with 50–150 units of ACTH injected intramuscularly. The response is claimed to be rapid and most satisfactory. Cortisol injected intravenously for immediate effect is also claimed to be beneficial in laminitis.

Ordinary procedure in the treatment of lameness in horses, characterized by a swollen bursa, sheath, or capsule, involves the sterile aspiration of excess fluid by hypodermic needle and syringe followed with injection of the hormone solution through the same needle with another syringe. If the aspirated fluid shows evidence of infection, an antibiotic such as penicillin or streptomycin is often injected along with the hormone.

IN OTHER SPECIES

In cattle, joint and tendon sheath enlargements have been treated occasionally in the same manner as in horses with a reasonable degree of success.

Cortisol or cortisone has been included in occasional chemotherapeutic liquid preparations for infusion into the *mastitic udder.* Little evidence is available to justify this inclusion, although there is some clinical opinion that the glucocorticoid decreases the swelling of the infected mammary gland. Inclusion of these steroid hormones has not provided any remarkable improvement in the clinical effectiveness of mastitis therapy. Swarbrick (1968) compared the efficacy of oxytetracycline with and without corticosteroids in intramammary infusion of field cases of mastitis. He concluded that the addition of corticosteroids had no beneficial effect and cannot be recommended.

The use of ACTH and the glucocorticoids in the therapy of *bovine ketosis* has received wide acclaim because of the glucocorticoids' gluconeogenic action. This raises the blood glucose level in this glucose-deficient condition. Peripherally though, the glucocorticoids inhibit glucose use. This also elevates blood glucose. Perhaps the condition is alleviated by eventually getting the glucose level high enough to permit the metabolic machinery to again begin normal function. Although the exact mechanism of corticoid effect in ketosis is unknown, the favorable effect is widely recognized.

Milk production is lowered in the ketotic cow after glucocorticoid injection. This effect lasts 3–5 days and the owner should be informed (Neff et al. 1960; Braun et al. 1970). Stöckle and Jockle (1971) did not observe a milk decline in well-fed healthy cows given glucocorticoids.

Dexamethasone (20 mg) given as a single intramuscular dose to cows from 235 to 280 days of pregnancy caused *parturition* within 2 days and *retained placenta* in nearly all treated cows (Adams 1969). The study did not include cows pregnant less than 235 days. *Caution must be exercised in the administration of any glucocorticoid to any pregnant animal* regardless of species or stage of pregnancy until more is known of this action.

In swine suffering from naturally occurring arthritis or chronic arthritis due to experimental *E. rhusiopathiae* infection, experimental intramuscular administration of cortisone (50–75 mg/day) enabled the animals to arise without assistance after 2 weeks of therapy. Previously they had been unable to get up. ACTH was of little benefit.

In the cat, glucocorticoid therapy is occasionally of benefit in relief of dermatitis. No doubt it might be beneficial in some other conditions also.

INDUCTION OF PARTURITION

The control of the time of parturition in farm animals, particularly those on the range such as beef cattle or sheep, would be an important management technique. The control of parturition within a few hours' period would permit veterinary and husbandry care to be concentrated, leading to the efficient use of facilities and personnel (providing no adverse effects were induced in the dam or the newborn). Control of the time of parturition would be an advantage in all species provided the above conditions could be met.

Oxytocin, PGF, and parasympathomimetic drugs have been used to induce myometrial contractions and labor in many species for several years. Oxytocin-induced labor is similar to spontaneous labor but the success of such parturition is dependent on a dilated cervix. If the cervix is not dilated, uterine rupture is possible in the large domestic animals. Once the cervix is dilated, it is more practical in most large domestic animals to effect delivery by physical means. In small animals in which physical intervention is difficult or impossible, such treatment might be considered. In the human being, an intravenous infusion of 2–4 mμ per minute of oxytocin will induce uterine contractions of a magnitude similar to that of spontaneous labor. Delivery can be induced in the rabbit by a single intravenous injection of 100–200 mμ of oxytocin. Obviously, even in small animals the cervix must be dilated or the induced contractions would cause fetal death or uterine damage.

After the report by Adams in 1969 that the synthetic glucocorticoids in large doses would induce parturition in cattle, sheep, and goats, many trials have been conducted. Parturition can be induced in a large percentage of the dams at or even preceding the expected date of parturition. An adverse side effect has been the frequent placental retention in cattle. The administration of 10–30 mg of dexamethasone intramuscularly in the cow within 2 weeks prior to the expected date of parturition usually causes delivery within 72 hours. The calves are somewhat weak, although survival is good, with the stronger calves being those delivered nearer the expected time of delivery. Retained placenta occurs in up to 90% of the treated cows and follow-up therapy for this pathological condition is necessary. The onset of milk production is somewhat slower than normal and the return of the uterus to the normal state is somewhat delayed compared to normal parturition, but the procedure has potential.

Estrogens, particularly diethylstilbestrol (DES, 50–100 mg intramuscularly), have been used during the first and second trimesters of pregnancy to cause abortion, particularly in feedlot heifers. However, during the second and third trimester, the efficacy of DES declines.

The mechanism of action of the corticosteroids in inducing parturition in the cow is quite likely due to its luteolytic effect, which causes a sharp drop in the progesterone level. Also there is a short but dramatic rise in estrogen. These events indicate that the administered corticosteroid acts much as would a signal from the fetal adrenal to induce parturition. The ewe does not appear to be responsive to corticosteroids before day 130 of gestation. During days 130–150, parturition can be induced by the corticosteroids, and placenta retention does not occur in the ewe. The mechanism of action in the ewe is probably not mediated through the corpus luteum (CL) since the CL is not essential in the final days of pregnancy. Instead, the corticosteroids probably mimic the effect of the fetal adrenal in inducing parturition.

In the mare induction of parturition with dexamethasone has been reported, although repeated administration of an extremely high dosage was necessary (100 mg daily for 4 days intramuscularly [Alm et al. 1974]).

PGE or PGF given intravenously induces premature parturition in the cow. PG has successfully terminated prolonged gestation in the cow although retained placenta occurs as in corticoid-induced parturition. PG has also shortened gestation in swine without adverse effects. Further work is needed to determine the ultimate value of PG for parturition induction in cows and sows. PGF_{2a} is an effective abortifacient in cats only after 40 days of gestation (0.5–1.0 mg PGF_{2a} tham salt/kg body wt subcutaneously for 2 days [Nachreiner and Marple 1975]), but preliminary studies in the dog have not been encouraging.

General Principles in Glucocorticoid Therapy

Seldom in the history of medicine and pharmacology has a group of drugs enjoyed such wide acclaim and usage after introduction as have the glucocorticoids and ACTH. As is the usual case with a new remedy, misuse and flagrant claims accompany their success. As a matter of caution it is well to keep in mind the following points:

1. ACTH is valueless unless a functional adrenal cortex is present. Prolonged high dosage of glucocorticoids may inhibit ACTH output to the extent that atrophy

TABLE 33.3. Glucocorticoid drugs

Name, Formula, and Preparations	Characteristics and Dosage
CORTISONE ACETATE (Cortone, Cortogen) Synthetic 17-hydroxy-11-dehydrocorticosterone-21-acetate Tablets, ophthalmic ointment and suspension, suspension for injection 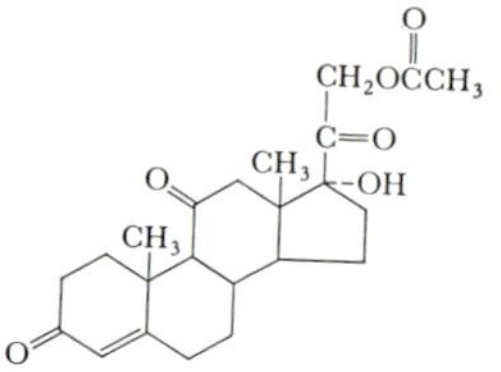	Used orally and i.m. for all generalized types of systemic glucocorticoid action. First compound introduced; now known not to be a natural body constituent and to act only after conversion to hydrocortisone. Least expensive. Ineffective topically. Dosage: Horse and cow, 1000–1500 mg daily i.m.; 50–250 mg within bursa, tendon sheath, or joint capsule of horse and cow. Dog, 1 mg/lb of body weight i.m. Divide in 3 or 4 doses if given orally. Subconjunctival 10–15 mg. *Caution:* Do not use high dosage in pregnant animals.
PREDNISONE (Deltra, Deltasone, Meticorten, Zenadrid, Hydeltrone-T.B.A., Paracort) Synthetic Δ 1,3-pregnadiene-17α,21-diol-3,11,20-trione; a dehydrogenated analog of cortisone Tablets, suspension for injection, ophthalmic ointment 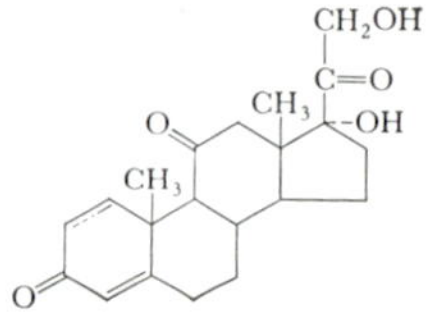	Less retention of electrolytes than cortisone; equally effective but just as likely to produce objectionable side actions. Sufficiently soluble to be nebulized. Dosage: Horse and cow, 100–300 mg daily i.m.; 50–250 mg within bursa, tendon sheath, or joint capsule of horse and cow. Dog, subconjunctival 1–2 mg. Orally or i.m., 0.25–1 mg/lb of body weight daily. *Caution:* Do not use high dosage in pregnant animals.
HYDROCORTISONE (Cortef, Cortril, Hycortole, Hydrocortone) Synthetic 17-hydroxycorticosterone; a replica of the compound naturally produced by the adrenal cortex in response to stimulation by corticotropin from the anterior pituitary Tablets, solution for injection, topical cream, lotion and ointment, oral suspension, vaginal tablets 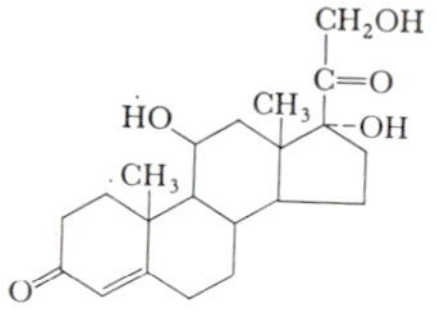	Used orally, i.m., i.v. for about the same effects, including adrenal cortical replacement, achievable with cortisone. Also used topically. Dosage: Same or slightly less than cortisone, *Caution:* Do not use high dosage in pregnant animals.
—ACETATE (same trade name as above, plus acetate)	Much used for intrasynovial injection and into aponeurotic or tendon cysts to promote a resolution without causing systemic effects; also topically. Intrasynovial injection, 5–10 mg for small joints or bursae to 250 mg for large joints. Topically in ointment; ophthalmologically in ointment or suspension. *Caution:* Do not use high dosage in pregnant animals.
PREDNISOLONE (Delta-Cortef, Hydeltra, Meticortelone, Meti-Derm, Paracortol) Synthetic Δ 1,4-pregnadiene-3,20-dione-11β,17α, 21-triol; a dehydrogenated analog of hydrocortisone Tablets, topical cream, suspension for injection	When given orally or parenterally has about the same effectiveness as prednisone; used topically in treating dermatoses without evidence of systemic effects; sufficiently soluble to be nebulized. Dosage: As for prednisone. *Caution:* Do not use high dosage for pregnant animals.

TABLE 33.3. ***(continued)***

Name, Formula, and Preparations	Characteristics and Dosage
–ACETATE (Sterane)	Same as above.
–SODIUM SUCCINATE (Solu-Delta-Cortef)	Salt form for i.v. or i.m. use.
–SODIUM PHOSPHATE (Prednis-A-Vet)	Usual uses plus i.v. for shock. Dosage: As for prednisone except larger for shock.
METHYLPREDNISOLONE (Medrol) Synthetic 6α-methylprednisolone; a slight chemical variant of prednisolone Tablets	Much like prednisolone in its effects but less retentive of electrolytes. Dosage: About two-thirds that of prednisolone. *Caution:* Do not use high dosage in pregnant animals.
–ACETATE (Depo-Medrol) Suspension for injection	May be used in certain dermatoses; may be injected intrasynovially and into soft tissues as well as injected i.m. for parenteral effects. *Caution:* Do not use high dosage in pregnant animals.
FLUOROPREDNISOLONE (Predef) Synthetic 9α-fluoroprednisolone; a fluorinated prednisolone Tablets, suspension for injection 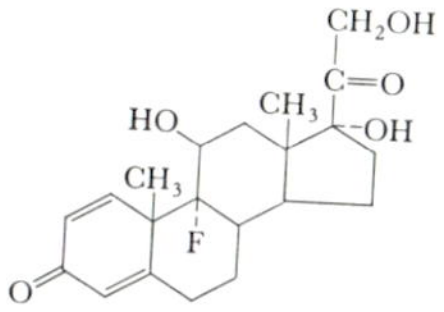	Slight mineralocorticoid effects in cow but unknown in other animals. Gluconeogenic agent in dairy cow. Dosage: Cow and horse, orally, 100 mg daily; i.m. 5–20 mg daily. *Caution:* Do not use high dosage in pregnant animals.
DEXAMETHASONE (Decadron, Deronil, Gammacorten, Azium) Synthetic 9α-fluoro-16α-methylprednisolone; basically resembles prednisolone Tablets, ophthalmic suspension, suspension for injection, powder 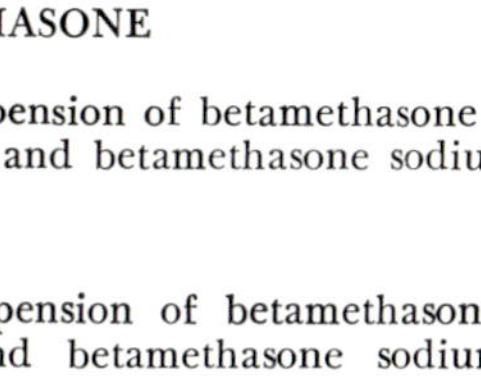	Effects probably about the same as achievable with other agents of the group that lack much electrolyte-retaining property, e.g., prednisone, prednisolone, methylprednisolone, and triamcinolone. Dosage: Cow, 5–20 mg daily i.m. or orally. Horse, 2.5–5 mg daily i.m. or 5–10 mg daily orally. Subsequent daily dose reduced. Dog and cat, 0.125–1 mg daily i.m. or orally. Subsequent daily dose reduced. *Caution:* Do not use high dosage in pregnant animals.
BETAMETHASONE (Betasone) Aqueous suspension of betamethasone dipropionate (5 mg/ml) and betamethasone sodium phosphate (2 mg/ml)	Used for dog pruritis; i.m. injection; effective for 3–6 weeks. Dosage: 0.25–0.50 ml/20 lb of body weight/i.m. every 3–6 weeks. *Caution:* Do not use high dosage in pregnant animals.
(Betavet) Aqueous suspension of betamethasone acetate (12 mg/ml) and betamethasone sodium phosphate (3.9 mg/ml)	Used for horse joint disease; intraarticular injection; effective up to 3 weeks. Dosage: 2.5–5 ml intraarticular every 1–3 weeks.

TABLE 33.3. ***(continued)***

Name, Formula, and Preparations	Characteristics and Dosage
TRIAMCINOLONE (Aristocort, Kenacort, Vetalog) Synthetic 9α-fluoro-16α-hydroxyprednisolone; a prednisolone derivative Tablets, suspension for injection, cream 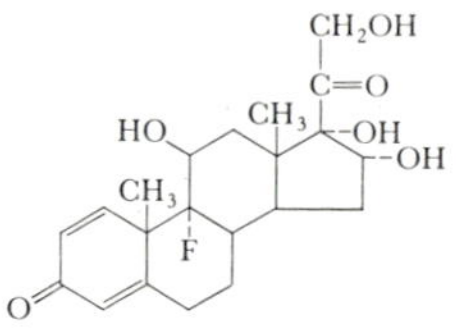	Probably the least electrolyte-retaining compound of the group, may even provoke diuresis and slight sodium loss in beginning of its use; otherwise equivalent to the others in systemic effects, perhaps less inclined to cause psychic stimulation; sometimes causes anorexia, weight loss, muscular weakness, hypoproteinemia, cutaneous erythema, dizziness, and sleepiness. Dosage: Cat and dog, 0.05–0.1 mg/lb of body weight orally or as a single i.m. or s.c. injection. Oral dosage should be reduced gradually within 2 weeks to maintenance levels of 0.01–0.02 mg/lb of body weight. By intraarticular or intrasynovial administration as a single injection of 1–3 mg, repeated if necessary after 3 or 4 days. Horse and cow, 12–30 mg by i.m. or s.c. injection; 6–30 mg as a single intraarticular or intrasynovial injection, repeated if necessary after 3 or 4 days. *Caution:* Do not use high dosage in pregnant animals.
FLUMETHASONE (Flucort, Anaprime, Methagon) Synthetic 6α, 9α-difluoro-16α-methylprednisolone Tablets, suspension for injection 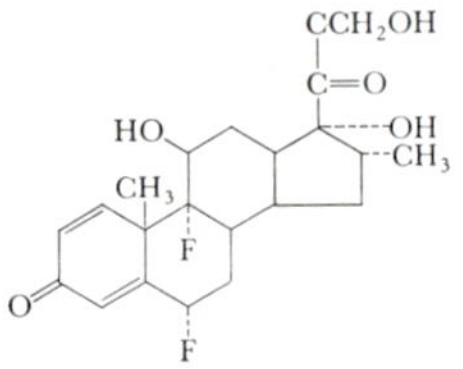	Probably the most potent glucocorticoid. Up to 700 times as potent as cortisol in rat liver glycogen deposition tests. Strong antiinflammatory effects; little mineralocorticoid effects. Indications: gluconeogenic or antiinflammatory. Dosage: Dog, 0.0625–0.25 mg daily i.m., oral, i.v., or s.c. Intraarticular to 1.0 mg. Cat, 0.03125–0.125 mg daily i.m., i.v., or s.c. Horse and cow, 1.25–5.0 mg daily i.v., i.m., or intraarticular. May be repeated. *Caution:* Do not use high dosage in pregnant animals.
FLUCINOLONE ACETONIDE (Synalor, Synsac, Synotic) Topical cream and solution 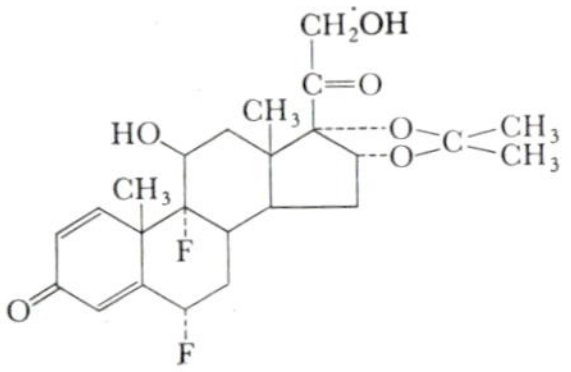	The acetonide group added to carbon atoms 16 and 17 reduced mineralocorticoid activity. Very active for topical use, e.g., dermatitis, otitis externa. Synsac is for anal sac injection.

of the adrenal cortex occurs and cessation of glucocorticoid administration finds the adrenal cortex nearly nonfunctional. Therefore, discontinuance of therapy may leave the animal in a hypocorticoid state. Steps should be taken to discontinue therapy slowly and in graded doses. Some clinicians recommend administering ACTH several days before corticoid discontinuance to stimulate the adrenal cortex to resume corticoid production. There is not general agreement on this practice.

Alternate day therapy of corticoids when required for long periods may be a better compromise that will allow ACTH surges and maintain cortex integrity.

Other disadvantages of ACTH are (compared to corticoids): ACTH must be administered parenterally, the resultant corticoid output is not predictable, the effect of ACTH is short, there is a lag of several hours for corticoid release, and ACTH is more expensive.

2. The antiinflammatory effects of the glucocorticoids do not cure any specific disease. This effect is palliative and some-

times temporary, although it may be quite dramatic and useful. Only in the case of Addison's disease does corticoid therapy represent replacement therapy specific for the disease.

3. *Special caution must be exercised in the use of the glucocorticoids if an infectious disease is present.* The antiinflammatory effect will promote dissemination of the infectious organisms throughout the body which may cause a fulminating infectious condition. The natural walling-off process in such chronic conditions as tuberculosis is destroyed by these hormones. On the other hand, if adequate antibiotic therapy is given that can specifically overwhelm the released organisms, a glucocorticoid is indicated. This procedure may permit an attack by the antibiotics on the specific organisms that would otherwise be impossible. The corticoids will suppress the usual fever seen when an infectious disease becomes systemic.

4. The antiinflammatory glucocorticoids are particularly valuable in chronic diseases occurring periodically and in the absence of a known cause such as arthritis, tendonitis, bursitis, conjunctivitis, and other forms of dermatitis. Local application should be used whenever possible since this would not affect the adrenal cortex proper.

5. Slow-healing wounds are not always undesirable. For example, corticoid-containing ointments may be applied topically to surgical and traumatic wounds of the prepuce in bulls to prevent rapid healing that would lead to stricture formation by proliferating connective tissue. Healing is delayed but strictures are thereby prevented.

6. *All topical ophthalmic preparations containing corticosteroids with or without an antimicrobial agent are contraindicated in the initial treatment of corneal ulcers. They should not be used until the infection is under control and corneal regeneration is well under way.*

7. Caution must be exercised in the use of high dosages of glucocorticoids in pregnant animals. (See previous discussion of work of Adams [1969] in the cow.)

8. *The euphoric effect may be a justifiable reason for use of the glucocorticoids.* Depressive states that affect pet animals and even the temperamental dairy cow may be relieved with the glucocorticoids.

9. A disease to be treated with a corticosteroid should be treated locally whenever possible rather than systemically. Even though some absorption may occur, the low systemic corticoid level preserves the integrity of the cortex while also maintaining a high local level of the drug.

10. Extravascular injections of synthetic esters of glucocorticoids have different absorption rates and duration of action. If a low but prolonged level is desired, the selection of injection would be different from that needed for a high but short therapy. The amount injected would also affect the level in either case. (See Table 33.4.)

11. The possible corticoid depressant effect on immune body production should be kept in mind when vaccination procedures are employed.

Adrenal Cortex Inhibitors

Hyperfunction of the adrenal cortex is rare, although Cushing's disease has been reported in the dog (Coffin and Munson 1953) and possibly mink. Adrenal blocking agents would have some clinical indication but the research potential is especially important. *o,p'*DDD, a relative of DDT, is 1,1-dichloro-2, 2-bis (*p*-chlorophenyl) ethane (Lysodren, Calif Biochem, or *o,p'*DDD, Aldrich Chem Co, Milwaukee) and has been found to suppress adrenal cortical activity in the dog (Schechter et al. 1973) but it is less successful in other species. Rats and monkeys are unaffected, but prolonged (1–2 months) administration of DDD to goats caused atrophy of the cortex and typical symptoms. Weber et al. (1958) found DDD

TABLE 33.4. Duration of action of steroid esters, extravascular injection

Absorption Period	Group
Minutes to hours	Succinate or phosphate
Days to weeks	Acetate or diacetate
Weeks	Acetonide or pivalate

caused transitory cytopathologenic effects on adrenal cortical cells of calves. Amphenone B (3,3-bis [*p*-aminophenyl] butane) also inhibits 17-ketosteroid production of the human being and dog. The mode of action of these compounds is unclear.

Metyrapone (Ciba) effectively blocks cortisol but not corticosterone production in young pigs (Stith and Bottoms 1972).

In the dog the dosage of *o,p'*DDD should be 50 mg/kg, given orally once a day until response or side effects, usually about 7 days (Schechter et al. 1973). Thereafter, once weekly may be necessary to keep cortisol depressed.

THYROID

The secretion of the thyroid gland, thyroxin, is not essential for life but is necessary for normal growth and reproduction in animals. Every cell of the body is a target of thyroxin. Many organ systems and body functions react when the circulating level of thyroxin changes. It is the purpose of this section to consider thyroid gland function and supplementation, the use of the various thyroid inhibitors, and iodine metabolism since it is vitally concerned with thyroid function.

Chemistry

The thyroid gland was described as an anatomic entity as early as 1656 by Wharton but it was not until 1915 that Kendall isolated the active substance, thyroxin. The chemical structure of thyroxin was established in 1926 by Harington. Since that time the building blocks have been determined and it is now believed that biogenesis begins with the iodination of tyrosine leading to the final substance, thyroxin (Fig. 33.6). Thyroxin or possibly triiodothyronine or diiodothyronine are the physiologically active circulating substances. The natural hormone is stored in the thyroid gland attached to a colloid as thyroglobulin, a protein with a molecular weight of approximately 680,000.

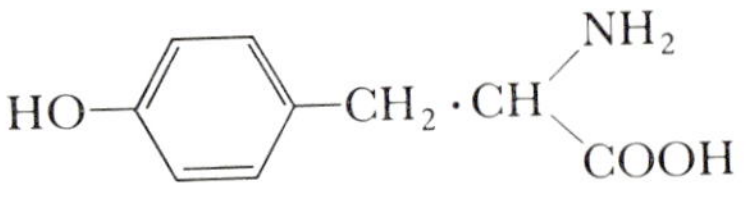

HO–C_6H_4–$CH_2 \cdot CH(NH_2)COOH$

Tyrosine

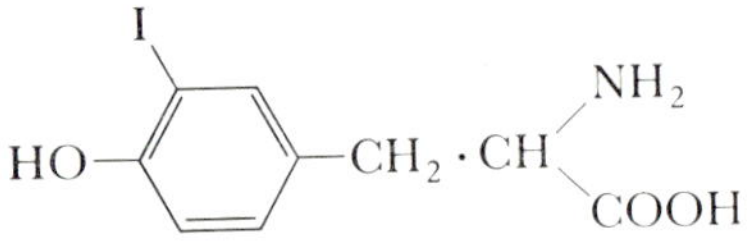

Monoiodotyrosine

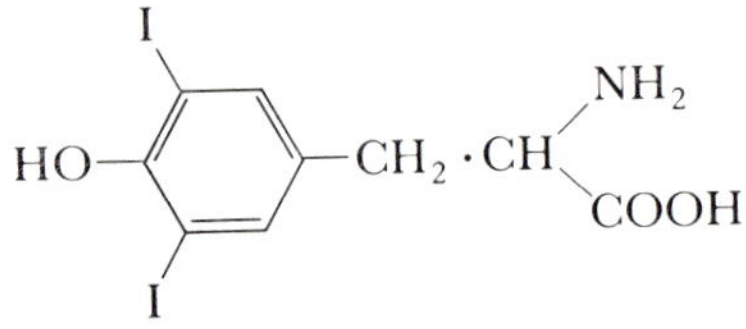

Diiodotyrosine

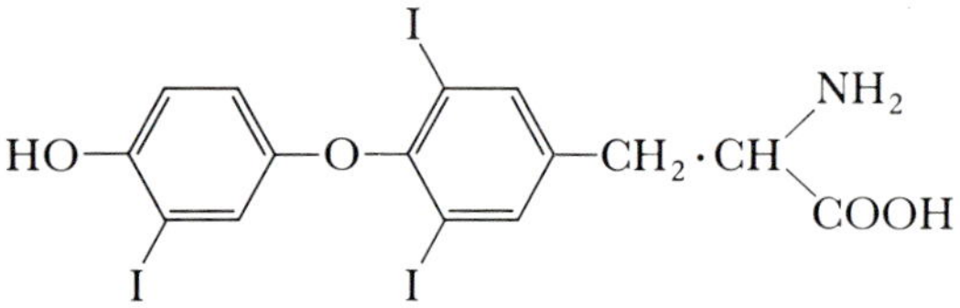

Triiodothyronine (T_3)

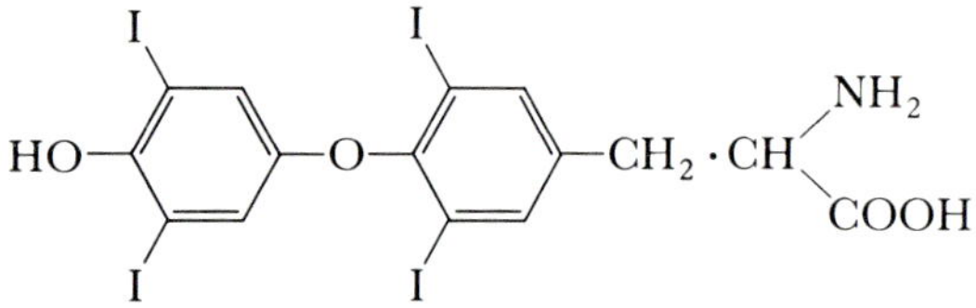

Thyroxin (T_4)

Fig. 33.6.

Source

With proper stimulation by the thyroid-stimulating hormone (TSH) plus adequate available iodine, the thyroid is able to produce thyroxin or one of its analogs for release into the blood or for storage within the thyroid gland. The best commercial source of the hormone is desiccated thyroid obtained from slaughterhouse animals. The powdered gland is standardized in terms of its iodine content and is usually satisfactory for substitution therapy. It is active by the oral route, which is unique for a hormone of a protein nature.

The thyroid gland has a terrific ability to take inorganic iodide from the circulating blood and concentrate it in the thyroid gland (iodide trapping). The next step consists of oxidation of the iodide to free iodine that is used in the formation of mono or diiodotyrosine. The coupling of 2 diiodotyrosines forms thyroxin. The hormone upon release becomes bound to the globulin or albumen of the plasma, which is referred to as the "protein bound iodine" (PBI) (Quinlan and Michaelson 1967). This PBI in the form of thyroxin or one of its analogs is the basis for the PBI determination test whereby the level of PBI correlates quite closely with thyroid function. Thyroxin does not circulate in the blood in its simple form since it is bound to serum proteins. The protein to which it is bound and the degree of binding varies from species to species. In the human being and many other species, it is bound primarily to α-globulin, whereas the rat and dog have thyroxin bound to albumen and α-globulin. The variation in the activity of triiodothyronine as compared to thyroxin appears to be dependent on the strength of the union between the respective hormone and serum protein. In the rat the strength of thyroxin binding to a serum protein is several times that of triiodothyronine; consequently, triiodothyronine is more active (available?) in the rat than thyroxin. In the chicken and duck thyroxin and triiodothyronine are bound equally by serum protein and their physiological activities are nearly equal. *Only the free hormone is able to diffuse into the cell and exert its effect.* Therefore, it appears that the strength of binding interferes with the passage of the hormone to the site of tissue activity, thereby determining which hormone is more effective in a particular species.

The ability of the thyroid to concentrate or trap iodide is demonstrated by the fact that the level of iodine within the thyroid is often several hundred times as high as the level of iodine in other body tissues. The iodination of tyrosine will occur *in vitro*; in fact, it has been found that many proteins will take up iodine *in vitro*. This forms the basis for the development of various iodinated proteins that are active in stimulating metabolism much as thyroxin does. The most commonly *in vitro* iodinated protein having thyroxinlike activity is casein, referred to as iodinated casein (Protomone). This unnatural thyroxinlike substance has been rather widely used in dairy cattle. Iodinated or thyroproteins have been fed to dairy cows to promote lactation (Table 33.5), but the increased milk yield is obtained with a marked loss of body weight and an increased feed consumption, so that the gains appear to be uneconomic as well as unphysiologic.

Regulation

The release, formation, and storage of thyroxin by the thyroid gland is primarily dependent on stimulation by TSH from the anterior pituitary. The thyroid gland will function at a minimal level in the absence of TSH as evidenced by the fact that the hypophysectomized animal does produce some thyroxin and the basal metabolic rate is about 60% of normal.

The hypothalamus exerts a continuous influence over pituitary release of TSH. The mediator from the hypothalamus to the pituitary is thyrotropin releasing factor (TRF). This humoral substance (TRF) travels through the portal system to the anterior pituitary. Certainly a servomechanism is in operation wherein thyroxin acts either on the hypothalamus influencing TRF release and/or directly on the anterior pituitary inhibiting further output of TSH. In addition, other effects such as temperature are mediated through the nervous system to the anterior pituitary affecting the output of TSH. (See Fig. 30.6.)

In summary, a low level of circulating thyroxin permits hypothalamic output of TRF to increase, which passes via the portal system to the adenohypophysis, causing release of TSH. Peripheral temperature receptors of the body are stimulated by cold and the impulse reaches the hypothalamus, causing TRF release. TRF then passes to the anterior pituitary gland by the portal system, causing TSH release. TSH goes to the thyroid gland, causing increased release of stored thyroxin or increased formation and release of thyroxin. The release of thyroxin from thyroglobu-

TABLE 33.5. Tabulation of hormonal adjuvants used in farm animal production

Product	Animal	Dosage	Mode of Administration	Limitations
Diethylstilbestrol*	Cattle, sheep	Not to exceed 10 mg/day for cattle and 2 mg/day for sheep	In feed	Beef cattle and lambs being finished for slaughter. Not to be fed within 14 days of slaughter. Not to be fed to breeding or dairy animals.
Diethylstilbestrol pellets*	Cattle, lambs	Cattle, 12–36 mg Lambs, 3 mg	Subcutaneous pellet implants Cattle, back side of ear near its base Lambs, may also be implanted in jaw	Beef cattle and lambs being finished for slaughter. Cattle: Administer 120 days before slaughter. Lambs: Administer 70 days before slaughter.
Diethylstilbestrol and testosterone paste*	Cattle	Testosterone, 120 mg Diethylstilbestrol, 24 mg	Subcutaneous injection of paste at back side of ear near its base	Not to be treated less than 60 days before marketing.
Testosterone propionate and estradiol benzoate	Heifers	Testosterone propionate, 200 mg Estradiol benzoate, 20 mg	Subcutaneous pellet implants at back side of ear near its base	Heifers weighing between 400 and 800 lb. Not to be used within 60 days of slaughter.
Progesterone and estradiol benzoate	Cattle, lambs	Lambs: progesterone, 25 mg; estradiol, 2.5 mg Steers: progesterone, 200 mg; estradiol benzoate, 20 mg	Subcutaneous pellet implants at back side of ear near its base	Lambs weighing between 60 and 85 lb. Steers between 400 and 1000 lb. Not to be used within 60 days of slaughter.
Dienestrol diacetate	Chickens	0.0023%–0.007% of total ration	In feed	Not to be fed for longer than 10 weeks. Discontinue feed at least 2 days before slaughter. Do not feed to laying hens.
Iodinated casein (thyroprotein)	Cattle, swine, ducks	Cows, 1–1.5 gm/100 lb of body weight Sows, 100 mg/lb of ration Ducks, 100–200 gm/ton of complete feed	In feed	Nursing sows: 3 days before farrowing and during lactation. Dairy cows: during lactation. Ducks: in the growing period only.
Estradiol monopalmitate paste	Chickens	10 mg	Subcutaneous injection of paste at base of skull	For roasting chickens not less than 5 weeks of age. Not to be used within 6 weeks of slaughter.

Source: Reprinted from National Academy of Sciences, 1966. National Research Council Publication 1415, p. 86.

* DES is under constant review by the FDA for use in food-producing animals. The reader is encouraged to check with the FDA for current approved usage.

lin is brought about by proteolytic enzyme activation. Thyroxin then passes through the epithelium of the chief cells and enters the circulation where it is bound to plasma protein and carried throughout the body.

Mechanism of Action

The mode of action of the thyroid hormone is poorly understood at the present time. A tremendous amount of research has been done on this but there is little agreement among workers on how the hormone acts at the cellular or subcellular level. One of the important effects of thyroxin is stimulation of oxygen utilization; consequently, there is a tendency to relate its mode of action to the increase in basal metabolic rate. To attempt to present the many points of view on the mode of action of thyroxin would be laborious and an unfruitful use of the student's time. Only a few concepts will be presented where there is some measure of agreement. It appears that an important function of thyroxin is on a cellular component, the mitochondrion. The administration of thyroxin until a hyperthyroid animal is produced causes an increased number of mitochondria per unit of body tissue. This results in an increased level of metabolic activity because there are *more mitochondria,* therefore more metabolic machinery per cell. In addition, thyroxin is known to cause a swelling of the mitochondria, which causes an *increased permeability of the mitochondrial membrane.* This increased permeability is thought to facilitate certain phosphorylation reactions. It has been found that in tissues from hyperthyroid animals the mitochondrial suspensions show a decrease in the formation of ATP from a given amount of oxygen utilization. Since mitochondria function as energy transducers to convert an electron flow into a chemical storage form of energy, ATP, it can be seen that the hyperthyroid animal would use more oxygen to produce a given amount of energy in the form of ATP. This is not necessarily advantageous to the animal but provides a possible explanation for the increased use of oxygen in the hyperthyroid animal. If the role of thyroxin is to alter the mitochondrial membrane permeability, it could be rationalized that more metabolites would be exposed to more enzymes that are present in the mitochondria.

Recent work indicates thyroxin may stimulate protein synthesis and the calorigenic action of thyroxin may be secondary to the energy requiring protein synthesis.

Effects in the Body

Thyroxin causes increased use of carbohydrates, increased protein metabolism as indicated by greater excretion of nitrogen, and greater oxidation of fats as indicated by loss in body weight. Several different drugs will increase the basal metabolic rate (BMR) but only thyroxin or desiccated thyroid provides relief from the clinical symptoms of thyroid deficiency. Apparently, the administration of thyroxin will increase the heart rate by lowering the threshold of response of the sympathetic nerves to the sympathomimetic secretions of the body.

Normal function of the central nervous system (CNS) is very dependent on the normal output of thyroxin. During periods when thyroxin levels are deficient, the CNS fails to function in the normal fashion and the animal is lethargic, dull, and stupid. The neurons are permanently damaged in the young growing animal by thyroxin deficiency. The neuronal dysfunction is reversible in the adult animal. On the other hand, excesses of thyroxin stimulate CNS activity to the extent that the animal is nervous, jumpy, irritable, and hyperactive. Likewise, oxygen utilization can be stimulated beyond normal levels by excess thyroxin administration or production.

Growth is dependent on many endocrine and other factors. Thyroid-deficient animals do not grow well, but it is thought that the action of thyroxin is "permissive" in that thyroxin is necessary to "permit" somatotropin and other factors to manifest their action.

METABOLISM AND EXCRETION

Thyroxin is slowly metabolized in the body, releasing the building blocks, iodine and tyrosine, back into the metabolic pool. The iodine may recirculate and be reutilized by the thyroid or it may be excreted by the liver in the bile and finally through the feces. Small amounts may appear in the urine. The half-life of circulating thyroxin is about 10 days.

CLINICAL USE

In the absence of sufficient thyroxin, many clinical symptoms appear because thyroxin affects all cells and organ systems of the body. For example, integument health is intimately associated with adequate thyroxin levels. CNS function, as well as the reproductive capacity, are closely associated with adequate thyroxin. In addition, growth and differentiation of the animal are intimately associated with thyroxin. For the most part, it is thought that thyroxin plays a permissive role in most of the functions of these organ systems. Only when adequate thyroxin is available are these organ systems permitted to carry out their normal functions.

Hyperfunction of the thyroid gland likewise brings on diseased states in domestic animals. Again, many organ systems and cells of the body are affected. One of the first symptoms to appear is the increased basal metabolic rate, which goes along with the increased activity, nervousness, and loss of weight. Table 33.6 summarizes some of the abnormalities, causes, and indicated therapy.

In the dog, hypothyroidism is a commonly occurring condition of considerable seriousness. The integument is most seriously affected although listlessness, inappetence, cold intolerance, and reproductive failure occur. Hair changes range from loss of hair to lack of luster. Skin changes range from apparent susceptibility to mites and bacteria and even lesions to simple scaliness. The first requisite to thyroid replacement therapy in the dog is recognition of the enormous dosage required compared to human beings or other species. Hightower et al. (1973) found that a 10-kg dog may require as much replacement therapy as a 70-kg human being. Twice-daily oral administration may also be necessary in the dog since plasma clearance of thyroxin in dogs is only 1 day compared to 6–8 days in human beings. Desiccated thyroid deteriorates on storage, so lack of response could be due to loss of activity.

Table 33.6 gives dosages and indications for thyroid replacement therapy.

Thyroprotein Effects on Lactation and Reproduction

Thyroprotein is a hormone-containing product produced by the iodination of casein under certain conditions. The active agent is thyroxin or an iodinated amino acid that has thyroxinlike properties. Thyroprotein is cheap, hence, it has been promoted as a way to increase the circulating level of thyroxin in the domestic animal. The cost is considerably less than the feeding or administration of desiccated thyroid gland.

EFFECTS ON LACTATION

The normal lactating dairy cow reaches a peak of production a few days or weeks after parturition and then begins a gradual but steady decline in lactation until the next parturition. A means of hindering or alleviating this declining rate of milk production has been of considerable concern to many investigators. The addition of thyroxin or thyroprotein to the diet of the lactating dairy cow has increased milk production from 15% to 20% above control animals, if a concomitant increase in energy intake was maintained. If additional feed is not given, the response is muted. Several reviews have been made of the work done in America and England on the economic feasibility of such practices and the National Research Council (Thomas 1953) released the following statement: "The available data suggest no definite economic advantage of feeding thyroprotein to dairy cows under most farm conditions. It appears more desirable for the dairyman who raises his own herd replacements to refrain from using thyroprotein, especially if the calf mortality ob-

TABLE 33.6. Summary of thyroid dysfunction and therapy

	Simple Goiter	Hypothyroidism		Hyperthyroidism
	Endemic goiter or colloid goiter	Cretinism	Myxedema	Thyrotoxicosis (Graves' disease)
Cause	Iodine deficiency leading only to enlargement of thyroid	Iodine deficiency in immature animal leading to exhaustion of thyroid gland, failure to grow, irreversible CNS dysfunction, mental dullness, dry brittle coat, thick skin, scaliness, dermatitis, possibly obesity; lethargy; hypercholesteremia	Iodine deficiency in mature animal leading to exhaustion of thyroid gland, failure to grow, reversible CNS dysfunction, mental dullness, dry brittle coat, thick skin, scaliness, dermatitis, possibly obesity; lethargy; hypercholesteremia	Excess production of thyroxin leading to nervousness, irritability, loss of body weight, polyphagia, cardiac irregularity
BMR	Low or normal	Low	Low	High
Treatment	Dietary iodine	Dietary iodine of no value if thyroid tissue completely exhausted. Desiccated Thyroid, U.S.P. Dog, 3–6 mg/lb/day (Borgman and Reineke 1950) or 0.5–1 mg iodinated casein/lb/day (Protamone, thyroprotein). Donovan and Venzke (1968) recommend Thyroid, U.S.P., for the dog at a dosage of 5–15 grains daily. Other species, 1–2 mg/kg/day orally. L-Thyroxin, U.S.P. Dog, up to 20–40 μg/kg orally in divided dose. Cattle, 50–100 mg/day orally. L-triiodothyronine (Liothyronine Na, U.S.P.) (Cytobin, Norden, Euthyroid, Warner-Chilcott) Dog, 1–5 μg/lb orally in divided dose. Cattle, up to 400 μg/day orally.	Dietary iodine of no value if thyroid tissue completely exhausted. Desiccated Thyroid, U.S.P. Dog, 3–6 mg/lb/day (Borgman and Reineke 1950) or 0.5–1 mg iodinated casein/lb/day (Protamone, thyroprotein). Donovan and Venzke (1968) recommend Thyroid, U.S.P., for the dog at a dosage of 5–15 grains daily. Other species, 1–2 mg/kg/day orally. L-Thyroxin, U.S.P. Dog, up to 20–40 μg/kg orally in divided dose. Cattle, 50–100 mg/day orally. L-triiodothyronine (Liothyronine Na, U.S.P.) (Cytobin, Norden, Euthyroid, Warner-Chilcott) Dog, 1–5 μg/lb orally in divided dose. Cattle, up to 400 μg/day orally.	*Antithyroid drugs* Methylthiouracil Dog, 50–100 mg/day (Ripps 1955) 2.5–5 mg/lb/day (Thorpe 1953) KI or NaI Dog, 2 mg/lb/day Thiouracil Dog, 6 mg/lb/day (Joshua 1953) Propylthiouracil Dog, 5 mg/lb orally 2× daily

servations are confirmed. It may, however, be advantageous to use thyroprotein in well-fed commercial herds in which maximum production per cow is emphasized or during periods of short milk supply, if permitted by law. It probably should not be fed for periods longer than 90 to 120 days and not during the first 50 days of lactation or in the terminal part of lactation."

Control cows will not consume as much feed as thyroprotein-fed cows, but if full feeding of control cows is permitted, frequently their milk production will approach the amount of thyroprotein-fed cows. The question actually becomes one of whether or not the extra cost and dangers associated with the administration of thyroprotein are adequately offset by the increase in milk production. This may vary from farm to farm and season to season along with the problem of establishing a higher milk production base at certain periods of the year, which is important in some milk-marketing zones.

Another problem that has been encountered is that sudden withdrawal of thyroprotein frequently causes milk production to drop below that of normal control animals. University of Tennessee investigators found gradual withdrawing of thyroprotein caused milk production to drop only to the expected level or to that of controls.

Some dairymen have experienced an increase in teat and other injuries and general excitability in the thyroprotein-fed herd. This is reasonable to expect. The overall seriousness of a problem will vary with a particular situation. During periods of extremely high environmental temperatures, there should be some caution exercised in the artificial induction of a hyperthyroid state. Obviously, heat tolerance of these animals would be reduced.

It appears that thyroprotein should not be fed to animals in their first lactation and that during later lactations it should be fed only during the declining days of lactation, withdrawal being at least 50 days before parturition.

The administration of thyroprotein to lactating sows has been recommended by some investigators. As in the cow, with additional energy intake, lactation would probably be increased, but one must keep in mind the adverse effects that may occur such as increased restlessness, nervousness, and possible damage to the piglets by the mother in a hyperthyroid condition. The experimental results are conflicting at the present time.

EFFECTS ON REPRODUCTION

Petersen, Spielman, and co-workers at the University of Minnesota reported in 1941 the effects of thyroidectomy on sexual behavior of the bovine. They found that thyroidectomy and the subsequent deficiency of thyroxin kept the calves from growing as fast as normally and the female never showed external estrus and the male never had libido. The libido or estrus could be returned by the feeding of fresh thyroid or dinitrophenol. Although libido was depressed in the male, there was no depression of spermatogenesis or fertility as judged from semen samples obtained by ampulla massage. Likewise, although the heifer did not show estrus, there were regular ovulations during "silent heat" and the ovum was fertilizable. Artificial insemination of these heifers with semen obtained from the thyroidectomized bulls resulted in normal pregnancies.

It has been assumed by some, although it has never been proved, that part of the seasonal variation in semen quality in bulls might be due to variations in the rate of thyroxin secretion as environmental temperatures change during the year. Other workers have incriminated high environmental temperatures and the accompanying anestrus of dairy cows with hypofunction of the thyroid gland.

In one artificial insemination program, Schultz and Davis (1946) fed thyroprotein to bulls for 30 days at the rate of 1 g/100 lb of body weight. Fertility improved in 5 of 7 bulls but only from a pretreatment rate of 51.7% to a posttreatment rate of 55.7%.

If bulls are in an iodine-deficient area, certainly the feeding of potassium iodide would be important and it has been reported by Knoop (1946) to improve spermatogenesis. More work is needed on the value of thyroprotein to improve libido and fertility of bulls. Some veterinarians believe thyroprotein is of value to the aged bull suffering from semen deterioration and lack of libido. However, the work of Spielman et al. (1945) indicates that thyroid supplementation is of value only if libido is deficient.

Lank (1958), in studies of anestrus of dairy cows in Louisiana, found that most of the infertility problem centered on the lack of recognition of estrus in the hot summer months since the cows were showing a "silent heat." Most of these animals were ovulating regularly, but under artificial insemination conditions they were not being detected by the herdsman. Supplementation with thyroxin or thyroprotein in these animals brought about normal manifestations of estrus and greatly improved the fertility in these herds. Again, one must consider the deleterious effects of hyperthyroidism during the seasons when heat tolerance is a problem.

Swanson and Boatman (1953) studied the effects of inducing hypothyroidism in the bull by feeding thiouracil. They recorded typical symptoms of hypothyroidism such as depression of spontaneous activity, roughness of hair coat, and susceptibility to cold. There was some depression of sperm cell concentration, motility, and livability and an increase in abnormally formed spermatozoa in 1 mature bull during a 91-day period of thiouracil treatment. The semen picture returned to normal on cessation of thiouracil feeding. A younger bull did not have a deterioration of the semen picture during treatment. He recorded no effects on libido, which is in contrast to what would be expected from the work of Spielman et al. (1945).

Antithyroid Drugs

An antithyroid drug may be defined as a drug that interferes with BMR by altering the synthesis, release, or peripheral action of the thyroid hormone. Cabbage has an antithyroid (goiterogenic) effect on rabbits (Webster and Chesney 1928) and sulfonamides depress thyroid activity in rats (Astwood et al. 1943).

The antithyroid drugs (thiourea, thiouracil, and their derivatives) have been used in meat-producing animals in an effort to increase the weight-gain efficiency, particularly to improve the "finish" of the animal for market by promoting fat deposition. This use of antithyroid drugs is still experimental and cannot be recommended in farm animal production yet (National Academy of Sciences–National Research Council 1959).

The use of antithyroid drugs is recommended in specific cases of thyroid hyperfunction. There is some species specificity in response to the drugs. Ripps (1955) found 50–100 mg of propylthiouracil sufficient to depress a hyperactive thyroid gland in the dog (Table 33.6).

A classification of antithyroid drugs and substances can be made according to mode of action.

- Inhibition of iodide trapping:
  - Thiocyanates (soybeans, cabbage)
  - Perchlorates
- Inhibition of thyroxin synthesis (iodination):
  - Thiouracil
  - Propylthiouracil
  - Methylthiouracil
  - Thiourea
  - Methimazole (Tapazole)
- Destruction of thyroid tissue:
  - I^{131} in large dosage
- Mode of action unknown:
  - Iodides in much higher dosage than dietary requirements.

Propylthiouracil is recommended in most species inasmuch as side effects are less than with thiouracil or methylthiouracil. Methimazole is much longer acting than propylthiouracil. These drugs cross the placenta and will render a fetus hypothyroid. (Fig. 33.7.)

Iodine

The minimum iodine requirement of various species of animals is unknown, but the daily amount of iodine required in the ration to prevent goiter in all species of animals is 0.001 mg/lb of body weight.

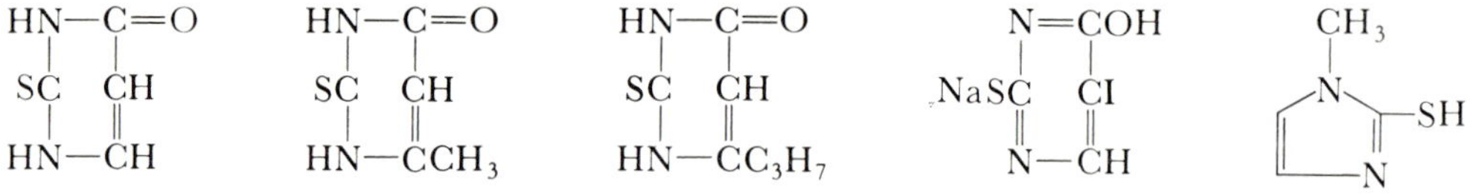

```
HN—C=O        HN—C=O         HN—C=O          N=COH           CH3
 |   |         |   |          |   |           |   |           |
SC   CH       SC   CH        SC   CH      NaSC   CI          N
 |   ||        |   ||         |   ||         ||   ||        /  \—SH
HN—CH         HN—CCH3        HN—CC3H7        N—CH          |    ||
                                                            \___N
```

Thiouracil — Methylthiouracil — Propylthiouracil — Sodium Iodothiouracil — Methimazole

FIG. 33.7.

Because most iodine deficiency in domestic animals is associated with pregnancy, the recommended minimal daily level of dietary iodine is increased to 0.002 mg/lb of body weight during pregnancy.

IODINE-DEFICIENT AREAS

Iodine deficiencies exist in certain areas of North America. In 1909 Marine and Lenhart studied the dog population around Cleveland, Ohio, on Lake Erie and showed that 90% of the dogs had hyperplastic thyroids. Several years ago thousands of hairless pigs were born annually in the area adjacent to Lake Superior and in Montana. Extensive losses have also been noted in lambs and colts. At one time it was almost impossible to raise horses in eastern British Columbia because of fetal mortality or early death of foals born weak and helpless to mares suffering from iodine deficiency.

Thyroid deficiencies recognized in animals occur largely in the newborn and are manifested by an enlarged thyroid gland, a lack of hair, generalized weakness, and fetal death at birth. Pups born of iodine-deficient mothers have enlarged thyroids and sometimes an enlarged thymus and spleen. Adult dogs suffering from iodine deficiency show poor hair coats, anemia, and sometimes deficient calcification of the bone.

The simple feeding of minute amounts of iodine as sodium or potassium iodide to the pregnant mother will avoid these conditions. With the more or less uniform incorporation of an iodine-containing salt and mineral mixtures fed to livestock the country over, fewer cases of iodine deficiency are now encountered among livestock. However, it is possible that obscure iodine deficiencies in livestock are passing unrecognized because the deficiency may cause only stillbirths and cretinous fetuses.

SOURCES OF IODINE

Most salt used by human beings and animals has been supplemented with a small but adequate amount of an iodide to prevent goiter or "big-neck" throughout the United States. Most dogs are fed scraps of human food and are well supplied with iodine because human beings generally use an excess amount of salt as a condiment. However, it is a good precautionary measure to add 1 or 2 drops of a potassium iodide solution or of tincture of iodine to the drinking water of pregnant dogs once or twice a week.

None of the common animal feedstuffs, except fish meal made of saltwater fish, provides significant amounts of iodine. Cod liver oil is a rich source of iodine as are sea plants, such as dried kelp. Organic iodine-containing compounds are in most instances no better sources of iodine than the cheaper inorganic iodides. The iodide salts are cheaper than the organic iodides and are absorbed equally as well.

Iodized salt readily loses its iodine content under some conditions of storage because of the catalytic action of impurities present. Some salts are processed by improved methods that stabilize the iodine. Iodized salt in mixed feeds is less subject to deterioration than in mineral mixtures because the iodine is stabilized by the proteins and unsaturated fats of the feed. Iodized salt can be prepared by adding 1 oz of potassium iodide to 600 lb of salt.

The thyroid gland has a large capacity for storing iodine so that this element needs to be supplied only at infrequent intervals, although daily administration in the feed may be more convenient.

RADIOACTIVE IODINE

Radioactive iodine, I^{131}, is the most commonly used isotope for diagnostic or therapeutic uses. I^{131} emits gamma and beta radiations and has a half-life of 8 days. This means that 99% of the radiant energy is expended within 56 days. The body tissues cannot distinguish this isotope from ordinary elemental iodine. The beta radiation is responsible for the destructive effects on tissues since the rays penetrate only 2.5 mm of tissue.

I^{131} AS A DIAGNOSTIC TOOL

Since I^{131} is taken up by the thyroid after administration at the same rate as ordinary iodine, this provides an ideal method to study iodine uptake rate that reflects thyroid function. This "trapping" of I^{131} by the thyroid can be measured by external application to the neck region of an isotope-counting device that detects the gamma radiation of the isotope coming from the thyroid. The gamma rays have high velocity and penetrability, thereby escaping from the body. Increased, decreased, or normal I^{131} uptake rate can be determined as well as the response of the thyroid to exogenous TSH. A failing thyroid gland that responds to TSH by increased uptake of I^{131} indicates pituitary TSH deficiency, whereas a failing thyroid that does not respond to TSH indicates primary thyroid dysfunction. Diseased states therefore can be clarified and proper therapy instituted.

These techniques have found wide application in human medicine and are being used somewhat in veterinary medicine (Kaneko et al. 1959; Goyings et al. 1962). The use of isotopes requires special training and equipment, hence the veterinary practitioner usually must seek aid from large veterinary hospitals or research groups. The paper by Kaneko et al. (1959) is recommended for additional background concerning the dog. For example, these workers confirmed earlier findings that the

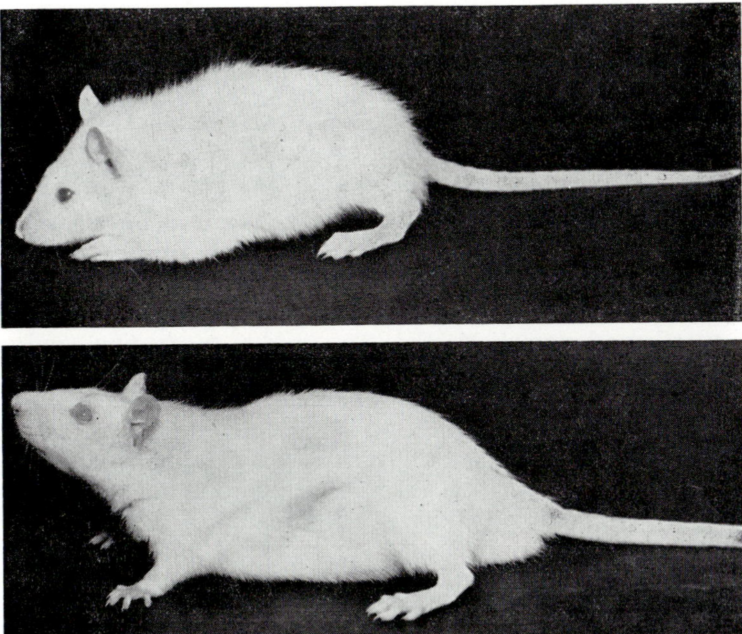

Fig. 33.8. The effect of radioactive iodine on the rat. The animal above received an injection of radioactive I^{131} at the age of 20 days. Destruction of the thyroid resulted in retardation of growth and the development of other signs of cretinism. The animal below shows its normal littermate control. (Courtesy of A. Grollman, Pharmacology and Therapeutics, 1962, Lea & Febiger, Philadelphia)

maximum uptake of I^{131} in the dog is approximately 72 hours postadministration, which is in contrast to human beings, with a maximum uptake at 24 hours.

I^{131} AS A THERAPEUTIC TOOL

The destructive effect of I^{131} emission of beta rays is greater in the thyroid than other tissues because of its greater concentration there and penetration of 2.5 mm of tissue. Heavy dosage of I^{131} can be used to destroy hyperactive thyroid tissue or thyroid carcinoma. Administration of TSH may be needed to encourage I^{131} uptake by the tumor. Danger of excessive destruction of thyroid tissue is not a problem since additive therapy with thyroxin could be instituted. This offers a more discrete means of removing thyroid tissue than by surgery plus the preservation of the parathyroid gland. Again, special training in the use of isotopes relegates their use to the larger institutions and research centers. The economic feasibility is also questionable.

PARATHYROID

The historical aspect of parathyroid physiology includes the unintentional removal of the parathyroid glands during thyroidectomies and subsequent death (first recorded by Raynard in 1834–1835). Sandstrom (1880) first described the parathyroid glands as separate organs, followed by Gley who in 1891 began to describe the symptoms of parathyroidectomy. MacCallum and Voegtlin (1909) first associated parathyroidectomy with serum calcium level. By 1925 extracts of the bovine parathyroid were prepared by Hanson and Collip and demonstrated to restore the calcium level of parathyroidectomized dogs suffering from tetany. Later work concerned the mode of action of the parathyroid hormone, attempting to determine whether its effect was on the kidney or on the osseous tissue of the body. The importance of vitamin D and the dietary level of calcium also entered the picture, creating a broad field involved with calcium-phosphate metabolism.

An excellent coverage of veterinary medical aspects of the parathyroid and other calcium-regulating hormones is presented by Capen (1975).

CHEMISTRY

Parathormone (PTH) is a low molecular weight polypeptide. Its structure is a single chain of 84 amino acids with a molecular weight of about 9500 (Brewer et al. 1974). Since the hormone is destroyed by proteolytic enzymes in the digestive tract, it must be administered parenterally. PTH is assayed by determining the amount necessary to raise the serum calcium of normal dogs after subcutaneous administration. A sensitive radioimmunoassay has been developed that can detect changes in blood PTH levels in response to fluctuating blood calcium levels. The pure hormone is so effective in elevating blood calcium and causing phosphate diuresis that we can now accept a single hormone as doing both rather than wondering if 2 hormones are involved. (See Fig. 33.9.)

PREPARATIONS

Parathyroid Injection, U.S.P. (parathyroid solution, parathyroid extract), is available. The usual source is bovine parathyroids, assayed according to the ability to raise the plasma calcium level of mature dogs. The dosage has not been established for domestic animals.

REGULATION OF OUTPUT

The production and/or release of parathyroid hormone from the gland appears to be dependent on the circulating level of calcium. Hypocalcemic blood transfused to the parathyroid gland of the dog causes an increased output of PTH. Restriction of dietary calcium in the dog, rabbit, and cow also causes hypertrophy of the parathyroid gland. Apparently parathyroid hormone output is decreased by hypercalcemia and when hypocalcemia develops there is an increased parathyroid hormone release to bring about an elevation of the serum calcium level, providing calcium is available. The pituitary gland does not regulate parathyroid function.

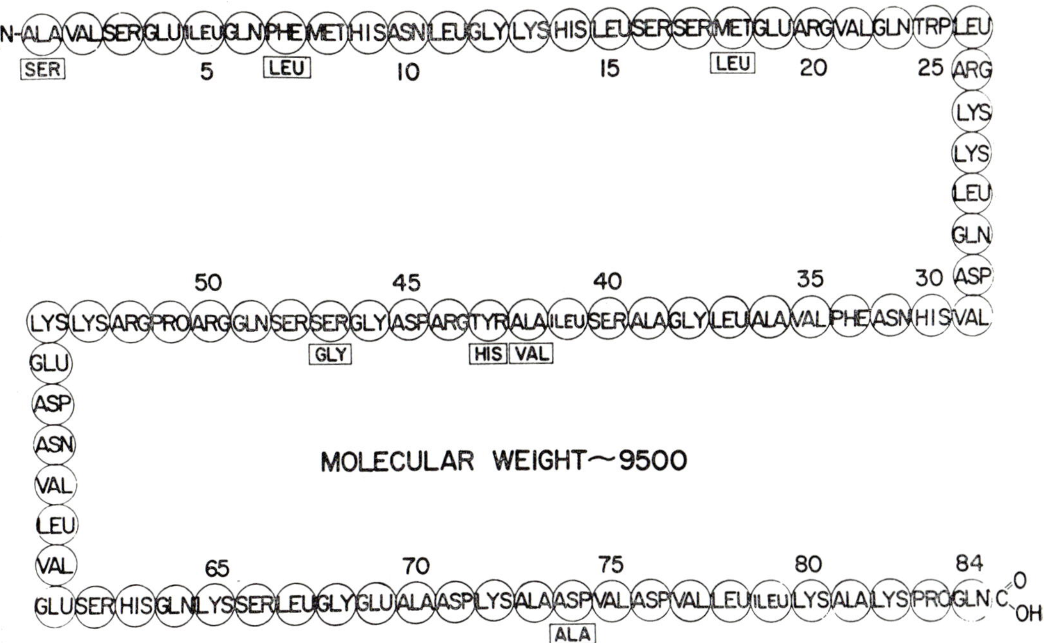

FIG. 33.9. Chemistry of bovine parathyroid hormone. The 7 differences in amino acid sequence between bovine and porcine PTH are indicated by the squares beneath the 1 to 84 PTH molecule. (Courtesy of C. C. Capen and Lea & Febiger, Philadelphia, from Veterinary Endocrinology and Reproduction, 2nd edition, 1975)

EFFECTS IN THE BODY

Calcium metabolism is dependent on several regulatory mechanisms in the body, including the parathyroid glands, calcitonin, vitamin D, and dietary calcium. It is difficult to consider any of these separately, and the reader is referred to the chapter on calcium metabolism as a background for consideration of the parathyroid gland. Approximately 10%–15% of the dietary calcium is absorbed by the gut if vitamin D is present to enhance its absorption by the intestinal mucosa. Of that which is absorbed and retained, 99% goes into the bones and teeth, leaving only 1% in the body fluids. A normal level of calcium is approximately 10 mg/100 ml of serum (5 mEq/L), one-half of which circulates as ionized calcium and the remaining one-half as a calcium proteinate. It is the ionized portion that is so important for proper functioning of the neuromuscular system, holding in abeyance symptoms such as tetany and convulsions that follow parathyroid removal. Tetany usually appears when serum calcium drops to 7 mg/100 ml of serum (3.5 mEq/L).

The threshold for electrical excitation of neurons is lowered when the ionized calcium level is decreased. This causes tetany to occur, which affects nearly all skeletal muscles of the body. Cardiac muscle is affected by changes in calcium in either direction and the disturbance is rather easily shown on the electrocardiograph. Smooth muscle responds to a calcium level change by inhibition of activity. The hypocalcemic tetany of skeletal muscles can be looked upon as a state of hyperexcitability of neurons and motor end-plates. The exact mode of action is not clearly understood but it is quite possible that the membrane permeability of the neurons is upset, thereby affecting sodium and potassium concentration and interfering with the normal processes of depolarization and repolarization.

Certain skeletal muscles seem to show hypocalcemic tetany sooner than others. In the cow this tends to be the muscles over the scapula but in the dog it tends to be the facial muscles and the muscles of the forelimbs. The terminal stage in the dog is a convulsion as shown in Fig. 33.10, whereas the terminal stage in the cow is muscle paralysis, including cardiac arrest.

Calcium balance is the difference between the calcium absorbed and the amount lost through the urine, feces, or milk. *Positive calcium balance* occurs during growth, pregnancy, or after calcium starvation. Hypervitaminosis D induces abnormally high absorption rates. *Negative balance* means a greater loss of calcium than intake such as in rickets, vitamin D deficiency, hyperparathyroidism, dietary calcium deficiency, or during lactation. The latter is especially important since the dairy cow is selected to lactate so profusely that she is in negative calcium balance throughout lactation. Since the declining phase of lactation is imposed on pregnancy, the problem is even more acute. Only during the 30- to 60-day dry period before parturition is the dairy cow able to replenish the calcium stores and enjoy a positive calcium balance. The cow's diet should reflect these demands. The situation is less critical in other domestic animals, including the beef cow, since milk production is limited to the needs of the suckling young.

Phosphorus metabolism is intimately associated with calcium metabolism. The normal inorganic phosphorus level of most animals is approximately 4 mg/100 ml of serum (2.3 mEq/L). The levels of serum calcium and phosphorus appear to be inversely related in the normal animal.

The role of PTH in regulating serum calcium and phosphate is far from being clear. It is difficult to give the student a concept that will facilitate an understanding of the clinical conditions without overwhelming him with reams of experimental data. At the risk of being arbitrary, some condensed version must be presented.

PTH probably affects many cells of the body but the following are certainly influenced: (1) bone (osteoclasts), (2) kidney (renal tubular cells), and (3) intestine (epithelial cells). The effects of PTH on each will be considered briefly.

Bone. Bone consists of approximately 65% calcium and phosphorus and 35% organic matrix. The mineral elements are deposited in the form of crystals much as would occur in a precipitation reaction. The crystals are oriented in such a way that favors strength of the bone and absorbs the stresses and strains applied during normal use. *Disuse of the body will cause a demineralization of the bones* or any part that is immobilized (fractured limbs, for example). Consequently, it behooves the animal body to receive daily exercise if at all possible. The bony skeleton is in a state of dynamic equilibrium, there being a constant deposition and resorption of calcium and phosphorus at all times. The skeleton is actually a mass of protein that has become heavily infiltrated with mineral crystals. The blood supply is fairly good but the nerve supply is rather poor. Many factors bear on the normal day-to-day function of the bone but the parathyroid is one of the dominant forces regulating the physiological processes involved.

Several points should be kept in mind when considering the effects of PTH on bone: PTH will elevate serum calcium even in a nephrectomized dog where renal phosphate diuresis could not occur; bone that is transplanted alongside the parathyroid is demineralized; PTH has a direct effect on bone even *in vitro*.

The exact site within the bone where PTH acts is on bone cells on endosteal surfaces and in the haversian cell envelope.

Kidney. Albright and Reifenstein (1948) were early investigators who claimed four events are induced by parathyroid hormone that form the basis for understanding its action. These events are in order of their occurrence: hyperphosphaturia, hypophosphatemia, hypercalcemia, and hypercalcuria. Parathyroidectomy causes these changes to occur in the opposite direction but in the same sequence. PTH acts rapidly (5–10 minutes) and directly on the renal tubules, causing *decreased* resorption of phosphorus and consequent phosphaturia. Also calcium resorption by the renal

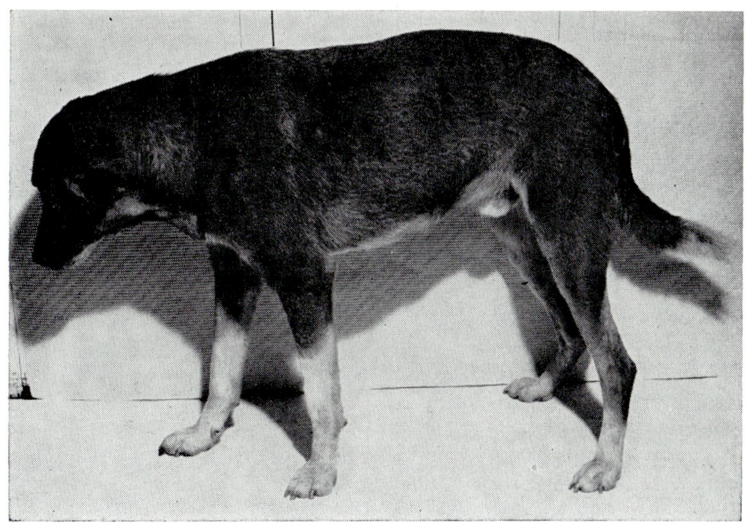

Fig. 33.10A. Effect of parathyroidectomy. Normal appearance immediately after parathyroidectomy. Serum calcium, 10.5 mg %; inorganic phosphate, 4.2 mg %.

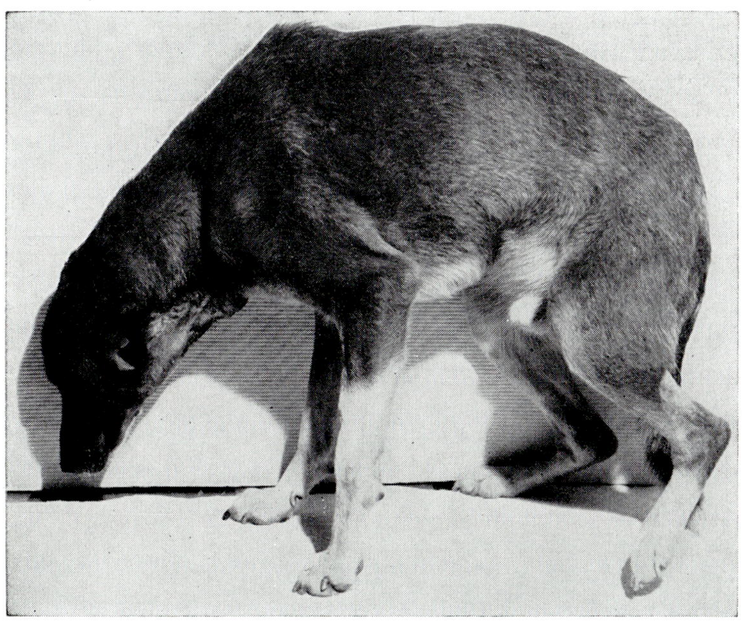

Fig. 10B. Effect of parathyroidectomy. Forty hours after parathyroidectomy, respiratory distress, difficult swallowing, skeletal muscle tetany, and incoordination. Serum calcium, 6.7 mg %; inorganic phosphate, 4.75 mg %.

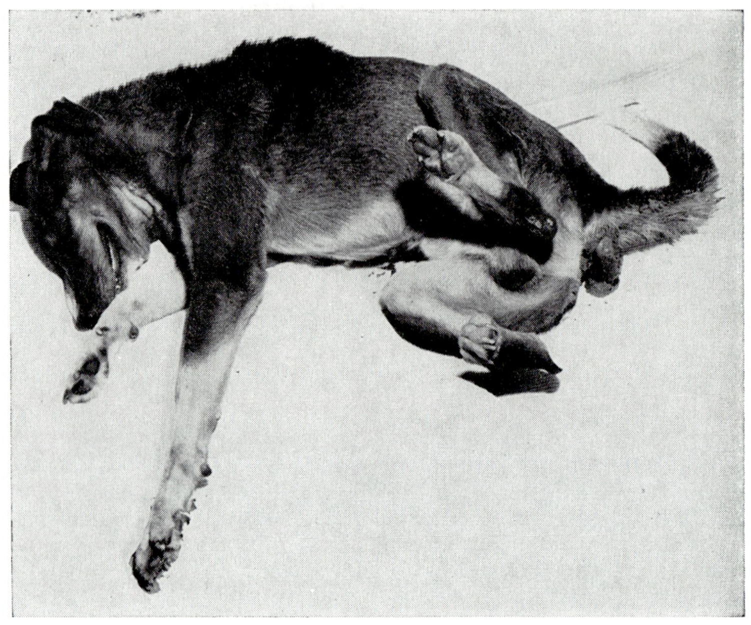

Fig. 33.10C. Effect of parathyroidectomy. Extreme tetany with death impending. Serum calcium, 5.2 mg % ; inorganic phosphate, 6.0 mg % .

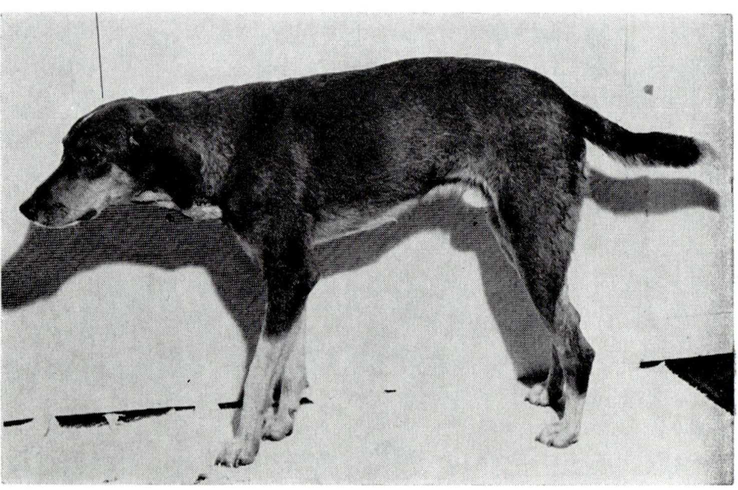

Fig. 33.10D. Effect of parathyroidectomy. Recovery after intravenous injection of 10 ml of 5% calcium gluconate.

tubules is favored by PTH at an important level.

PTH causes the kidney to convert 25-hydroxycholecalciferol to 1,25-dihydroxycholecalciferol, which is the major biologically active metabolite of cholecalciferol that acts on intestine and bone in calcium mobilization.

Intestine. PTH also acts on the intestinal mucosa to favor absorption of calcium. This can be demonstrated with an isolated loop of intestine from a previously injected rat donor.

It is obviously impossible with the present state of knowledge to support either theory entirely; it is quite likely that all systems are in effect at all times and that the parathyroid hormone acts several ways.

It seems puzzling that such a complex system is needed to control blood calcium level. Actually though, it can be rationalized somewhat because there is a "fine" response and a "coarse" response. The kidneys and intestinal mucosa respond quickly to PTH but in a limited capacity. Also these tissues are sensitive to small amounts of the hormone, *hence a control scheme for fine adjustments.* The response of bone is slow, insensitive, and of nearly unlimited capacity. The speed of the response may be related to the blood supply: the kidney and intestine with a good blood supply can respond quickly, *the bone with a sluggish blood supply can only respond slowly.* Therefore, by using these two types of responses the animal is able to have a fine control of calcium and phosphorus over a wider range of demands.

The effects of removal of the parathyroid gland in the simple-stomached animal are quite different from those of ruminants. The dog shows evidence of fine-muscle incoordination as early as 12–24 hours after removal, followed by inability to drink or eat, and finally tetany and death within 24–72 hours. Parathyroid tetany in the dog can be prevented to some extent by increased dietary levels of calcium such as cereals provide. The ruminant animal on a herbivorous diet has a dietary intake of calcium sufficient to prevent tetany in most animals following parathyroid removal, if the animal is not lactating or pregnant. Removal of the parathyroid glands that is not followed by tetany in nonruminants may be due to incomplete removal of the parathyroid tissue.

METABOLISM AND EXCRETION

Parenteral administration of parathyroid extracts is necessary since oral administration is ineffective. Subcutaneous or intramuscular injections bring about an elevated serum calcium level within 3–4 hours, reaching a peak at approximately 8–12 hours, and returning to control levels at 20–24 hours. This rate of metabolism and destruction indicates that injections must be given approximately each 12 hours to maintain an effect.

HYPOPARATHYROIDISM

Hypoparathyroidism is rarely recognized in domestic animals, although a few cases are seen in dogs, mainly the smaller breeds such as terriers and Schnauzers. Capen (1975) lists the possible pathogenic mechanisms of hypoparathyroidism:

- Congenital (agenesis, hypoplasia)
- Idiopathic (degeneration, parathyroiditis)
- Iatrogenic (neck surgery, irradiation)
- Metastatic neoplasms
- Trophic atrophy from hypercalcemia (excess vitamin D, ectopic PTH secretion, bone metastases)
- Failure to convert PRO-PTH to PTH
- Inability of target cells to respond
  - –lack of adenyl cyclase in bone and/or kidney
  - –pseudohypoparathyroidism

HYPOCALCEMIA

Hypoparathyroidism as a distinct clinical entity is seldom recognized in domestic animals. Hypocalcemia, however, is recognized as a distinct clinical symptom in the bitch, cat, and cow and is referred to as eclampsia in the bitch and cat and milk fever or hypocalcemic tetany in the cow. Since the parathyroid gland is so intimately associated with calcium metabolism, one is inclined to consider the parathyroid whenever disturbances of calcium metabolism occur. The hypocalcemic condition that develops following parturition in the bitch, cat, and cow is associated with a tremendous drain on the calcium stores of the body during lactation.

Boda and Cole (1953) were able to cause compensatory hypertrophy of the parathyroid glands in the cow by maintaining the animal on a calcium-deficient diet for approximately 1 month prior to delivery. The parathyroid compensatory hypertrophy rendered it capable of mobilizing sufficient calcium to prevent hypocalcemic tetany during the postparturient period when the demand for calcium rose, even though the animals were selected with a history for milk fever. In contrast to this, Jackson et al. (1962) found postparturient PTH injections to be valueless in preventing milk fever in the cow. Likewise, in the management of eclamsia of the bitch and cat, PTH injections are not usually indicated because of the latent effect of the hormone, as well as the fact that repeated injections elicit refractoriness to the hormone. The intravenous injection of calcium salts, or calcium gluconate, appears to be the most satisfactory method for immediate treatment for hypocalcemia in any species. This effect is short-lived as shown by Fig. 33.11.

Diets including sufficient available calcium and phosphorus are certainly important in the management of the pregnant and lactating animal. In addition, adequate supplies of vitamin D must be available in any species to facilitate the absorption of calcium by the intestinal mucosa. Hibbs and Pounden (1955) demonstrated that predelivery short-term feeding of 5,000,000–30,000,000 units of vitamin D daily to dairy cows prevented milk fever in animals with milk fever history. Serum calcium increased during therapy sufficiently to combat the postparturition drain on calcium reserves when lactation was initiated. Feeding of this amount of vitamin D for more than 7 days brought about detrimental calcification of the cardiovascular system. The problem is in predicting the date of delivery, thereby preventing long-term administration of the vitamin. Vitamin D acts by facilitating absorption of calcium by the intestinal mucosa.

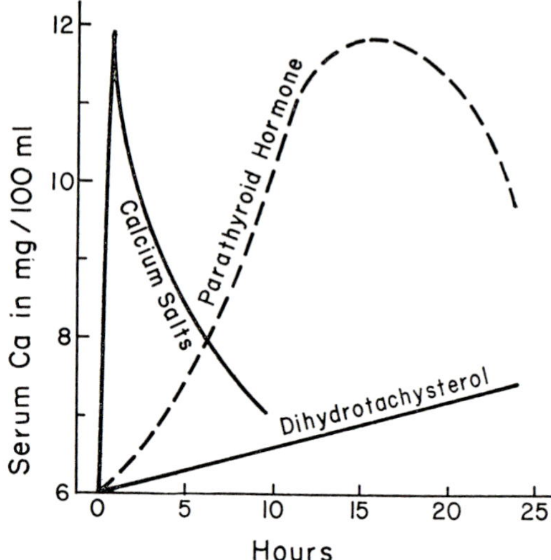

FIG. 33.11. The blood serum calcium response to various forms of therapy. Note the immediate rise and rapid decline in the calcium level following the intravenous injection of an inorganic calcium salt (5 ml of 5% calcium chloride); the slower rise but more prolonged effect following the hypodermic injection of 20 U.S.P. units of parathyroid extract; and the slow rise following the daily administration orally of 5 mg of dihydrotachysterol. Subject: human being. (Reproduced by permission of the publishers from Grollman's Essentials of Endocrinology, J. B. Lippincott Co., 1947)

Dihydrotachysterol (irradiated ergosterol) was administered to 3 dairy cows at the rate of 6 mg intramuscularly, and 1 cow received 12 mg orally (Lewis et al. 1953). The blood calcium level of these lactating postparturient dairy cows rose slightly, but more studies are needed before its use can be recommended. Its effect is thought to be similar to both parathyroid hormone (phosphate diuresis and bone calcium mobilization) and vitamin D (facilitates absorption of calcium by the intestinal mucosa).

Olson et al. (1973) gave 0.5–2.0 mg of 25-hydroxycholecalciferol intravenously to 11 parturient paresis cows and 6 recovered in 13 hours. They concluded that the prolonged recovery time precludes this treatment's usefulness. Olson et al. also used up to 8 mg intramuscularly before delivery as a preventative and reduced the incidence of hypocalcemic postparturient paresis about one-half. Due to selection, the dairy cow has a lactation system beyond the ability of the parathyroids to sufficiently mobilize calcium upon the initiation of lactation. Since hypocalcemia requires immediate correction, intravenous administration of calcium salts is preferred. Other measures such as administering dietary calcium, vitamin D, or dihydrotachysterol may be indicated after control of the acute deficiency of serum calcium in the cow, bitch, or cat. Therapy with parathyroid hormone is not recommended at the present time. *Parathyroid Injection,* U.S.P., is available.

HYPERPARATHYROIDISM
- Primary
  - adenoma
- Secondary
  - renal
  - nutritional

	Blood Ca	*Blood* P	*Urine* Ca	*Urine* P
PTH deficiency	↓	↑	↓	↓
PTH excess	↑	↓	↑	↑

Primary hyperparathyroidism has been recognized as a clinical entity in the dog. It may be due to an *adenoma* of the parathyroid. An adenoma of the parathyroid gland leads to *hyperplasia* and overproduction of PTH. The excessive PTH release may lead to excessive demineralization of bones, even leading to fractures and bone deformities. Chronic hyperparathyroidism can lead to kidney stone formation from the excessive calcium loss in the urine. Metastatic deposits of calcium may occur in soft tissues, including the kidney. Such renal damage may lead to hyperphosphatemia instead of the expected hypophosphatemia since the tubules are failing to excrete the phosphorus. Treatment is limited to surgical attempts to remove sufficient hyperactive tissue to reduce the level of hormone production to normal limits. This is obviously difficult. Radiation of the gland likewise is tedious.

Secondary hyperparathyroidism is secondary to (1) chronic *renal* disease or (2) chronic imbalance in the *nutritional* calcium-phosphorus intake.

Secondary hyperparathyroidism (renal) of dogs and cats is due to chronic renal dysfunction unrelated to the hyperparathyroidism. This renal failure leads to phosphate retention and then calcium depletion (reason unknown). During progressive development of renal lesions, the kidney becomes less and less able to excrete phosphate. The resulting elevations in plasma phosphate and altered calcium: phosphate ratio (low calcium) cause hyperactivity of the parathyroid. This causes demineralization of bone, resulting in further increases in plasma phosphate. Since the damaged kidney is unable to excrete phosphate adequately, plasma levels continue to rise. The chronic renal disease also interferes with 1,25-dihydroxycholecalciferol production.

Hypocalcemia then stimulates excessive PTH production and finally parathyroid hypertrophy. This condition is frequently referred to as "rubber jaw" or "osteitis fibrosa cystica" (more properly termed fibrous osteodystrophy), which is a chronic demineralization of the osseous tissue (Brodey 1954; Neilson and McSherry 1954; Storts and Koestner 1965). It is possible that these two manifestations are separate entities, although demineralization of the jaw is likely only part of the overall demineralization of the bones of the body seen in the generalized form.

Secondary hyperparathyroidism (nutritional) of horses, swine, cats, monkeys, fowl, and tigers occurs with a chronic imbalance of dietary calcium and phosphorus. A lameness sometimes develops in young fast-growing animals that are well fed. These animals have swollen joints, enlarged epiphyses, and an insidious shifting type lameness. Invariably, the diet of affected horses is one high in grain, which means an unusually high phosphorus intake. This leads to hyperphosphatemia

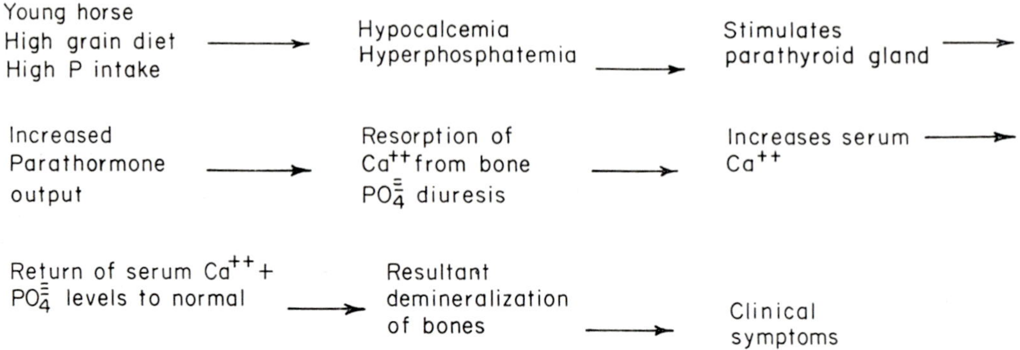

FIG. 33.12. Scheme of events leading to nutritional secondary hyperthyroidism in horses.

and hypocalcemia. Next, the low calcium stimulates PTH output, which causes resorption of bone calcium, thereby leading to demineralization and finally lameness.

In secondary nutritional hyperparathyroidism of nearly all species of animals, fibrous osteodystrophy is the main lesion along with parathyroid hypertrophy. The degree of bone demineralization and replacement of the bone compacta with fibrous tissue depends on the degree and duration of hyperparathyroidism. Such hyperparathyroidism can be induced by (1) reduced calcium intake, (2) excessive dietary phosphorus with normal calcium intake, or (3) a calcium deficiency and phosphorus overfeeding. Modern manipulation of animal diets by human beings is conducive to such dietary upsets.

DIAGNOSIS

There is a useful diagnostic point between primary and secondary hyperparathyroidism. In primary hyperparathyroidism, plasma calcium is in the hypercalcemic range whereas, in the secondary form, plasma calcium is usually in the low normal to subnormal range. The reason for this is that secondary hyperparathyroidism represents a compensatory mechanism to maintain calcium in the normal range despite the depressing effect of hyperphosphatemia on plasma calcium concentration. The solubility product may not explain the depressing effect of hyperphosphatemia on plasma calcium but the effect is an established observation regardless of the mechanism. Plasma phosphorus concentration would be expected to be elevated in secondary hyperparathyroidism and depressed in the primary form, but the daily and hourly fluctuations in the plasma concentration of this element distract from its diagnostic value, especially in borderline cases.

CALCITONIN (Thyrocalcitonin, CT)

There is another hormone that affects the blood calcium level. This is a fast-acting polypeptide composed of 32 amino acids with considerable species variability from the parafollicular cells of the thyroid gland called calcitonin (CT). It is released in response to hypercalcemia and causes a reduction in circulating calcium and often phosphorus. A particular parafollicular cell called the "C" or "light" cell has been located near the basement membrane of the thyroid follicle, which is believed to be the source of the hormone in mammals (Care and Keynes 1965). The hormone was first believed to come from the parathyroid gland. In birds and sharks and other submammals, CT appears to arise in the ultimobranchial body.

Klein et al. (1967) studied porcine CT in the rat and concluded that the primary way that the blood calcium is lowered is related to CT's ability to rapidly reduce bone resorption. The pig is a near ideal experimental animal for such studies since the thyroids are anatomically separate from the parathyroids. It appears that CT exerts a fine control by constantly being ready to lower blood calcium and avoid hypercalcemia.

CT's onset of action is rapid; it can lower serum calcium quickly. Likewise a slight hypercalcemia calls forth an immediate increase in radio immunoassayable CT.

C-cell neoplasms are quite common in bulls, less in cows, and infrequently in dogs and cats. CT levels are elevated, serum calcium is usually lowered, and bone changes often occur (Capen 1975).

INSULIN

The pancreas is an example of an endocrine and an exocrine gland being located in the same organ. The exocrine portion produces pancreatic enzymes that enter the digestive tract by way of the pancreatic ducts. The endocrine portion, the beta cells of the islets of Langerhans, secretes a hormone, insulin, which is of great importance to the metabolic scheme of the animal.

Human beings have suffered from a disease involving insulin deficiency, called diabetes mellitus, since the beginning of recorded time as found in the *Papyros Ebers*. In early writings it was referred to as "honey urine," and it was not until the eighteenth century that the sweetness of diabetic urine was identified as glucose. In the nineteenth century, advances were made to the point that in 1889 von Mering and Minkowski demonstrated that removal of the pancreas would produce the disease. Various attempts were made to isolate the active substance, but not until 1922 did Banting and Best finally isolate and purify insulin from the dog's pancreas. Rather crude preparations of insulin were immediately used in clinical medicine since the need was urgent for this life-preserving substance for the diabetic patient. Many adverse side effects occurred, including abscesses at the site of injection, but within a few years purified substances were available so that diabetes mellitus could be managed to some extent in human beings.

The story of the human conquest of this disease is much too interesting to deserve such a small consideration, so the reader is referred to more lengthy treatises on the subject. In recent years modified insulins have appeared on the market, the structure of insulin is now known (Sanger 1959), and work is proceeding on the development of orally active substances that may invalidate the need for hypodermic injections of the hormone.

The last 40 years have been characterized by intensive investigations into the mode of action of insulin. Some of the early work was clouded before a second hormone, glucagon, was crystallized in 1953 and found to come from the pancreas. Some of the confusing results undoubtedly were due to glucagon effects but the specific mode of action of insulin still remains somewhat unclear. Nearly all domestic species occasionally suffer from diabetes mellitus but the condition seems to be most commonly recognized in the dog.

Several hormones participate in the multihormonal control of carbohydrate metabolism, including insulin, glucagon, somatotropin, adrenal glucocorticoids, and epinephrine. The relative role of each of these hormones varies from species to species. The ruminant animal probably is not as dependent on the insulin-glucagon scheme as the nonruminant animal. This is associated with the fact that the ruminant animal is less dependent on blood glucose and more dependent on blood levels of volatile fatty acids as a source of energy. Nonetheless, blood glucose levels are important in all domestic animals and the roles of insulin and glucagon must be kept in mind. Insulin and glucagon are secreted directly into the hepatic portal system, hence the liver is the first organ subjected to the effects of these hormones before they are distributed to the peripheral areas of the body. This is quite different from the pharmacological case in which insulin is injected into the peripheral parts of the body and finds its way to the liver in a diluted form at a later time.

The blood glucose level in mammals is maintained within a very narrow range and fluctuations are kept at a minimum. In a nonruminant animal, a blood glucose level of about 80–100 mg/100 ml of blood is maintained with fluctuations of only 10%–20%. This minimal fluctuation could not be maintained if there were not precise control mechanisms, since the ingestion of a large carbohydrate meal, violent exercise, or starvation would certainly cause greater fluctuations. Therefore, the effect of insulin is to favor removal of glucose from the blood and its storage in the liver and other tissues as glycogen until needed. In contrast to this, glucagon causes the breakdown of liver glycogen to glucose, which then enters the blood to elevate blood glucose. From the above it is hoped that the student is impressed with the fact that the control of circulating levels of glucose and its metabolism is a very complex mechanism. One would be in error to look upon insulin as being all important. Instead, while considering the rather dramatic effects of insulin, it should be kept in mind that this is only one of many factors in play that maintain homeostasis of the carbohydrate pool.

Chemistry

Late in the last century the pancreas was strongly suspected of secreting a hormone and many attempts were made to isolate this substance from pancreatic tissue. These efforts were unsuccessful until Banting and Best hit upon the idea of inducing atrophy of the exocrine or acinar portion of the pancreas by ligating the pancreatic duct. This ligation caused pressure atrophy of the acinar tissue, thereby eliminating the pancreatic digestive enzymes that had been the cause of the destruction of the protein hormone, insulin. After this finding by Banting and Best, one of their co-workers, Collip, developed a method for extracting cattle pancreas that is now used in commercial insulin preparation.

Insulin was found to be a protein during the extraction trials. Abel was successful in crystallizing the hormone in 1926 but it was not until 1949 that Sanger and Tuppy found that insulin is 2 chains of amino acids, with 3 disulfide linkages. Sanger was awarded a Nobel prize for determining the specific chemical structure of insulin. The molecular weight of insulin is approximately 6000. The complete structure is shown in Fig. 33.13, along with the known variations of several species. Two other hormones, oxytocin and vasopressin, have a sequence of 6 amino acids enclosed by an S-S bridge much as is found in the A chain of insulin. It has been suggested that these hormones may use the S-S linkage in their interaction with a cell receptor site, which then leads to the action of the hormone at the cellular level. Heterologous insulin retains its activity for varying periods of time, although there is a tendency for an allergic reaction to occur in the human being to insulin from other species. The 2 chains contain 51 amino acids of which there are 17 different amino acids. The complexity of this molecule is better appreciated (as

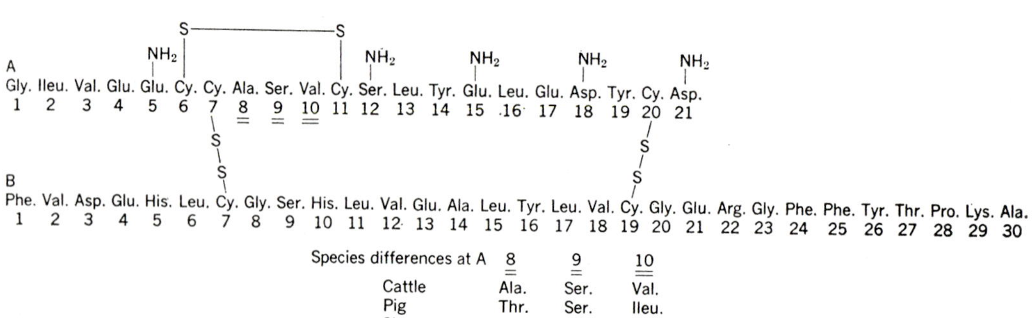

Fig. 33.13. Structure of insulin in various species.

well as Sanger's work) when one recalls that there are only 24 different amino acids known and 17 of these are present in insulin. Compare this with the fact that the English language has only 26 different letters, 2 more than the number of amino acids. Then a notion of the complexity of the protein puzzle can be seen. Since the sequence of the amino acids in insulin is critical, much as the letters in a word, the insulin-amino acid "word" or message can be appreciated.

SOURCE

Chemical extraction of the islet cells from slaughterhouse material continues to be the source of commercial insulin. These extraction techniques are quite well developed.

Merrifield and Katsoyannis in this country and others in Germany and China reported synthesis of bovine and sheep insulin in 1963 and 1965. This complicated set of 224 reactions has been automated by Merrifield (1963) so that synthetic insulin should become available. The purity of a synthetic hormone is always desirable and preferred to the extracted hormone.

The biological activity of insulin is dependent on the whole molecule, and minor modifications of the disulfide linkages will markedly reduce its activity. Insulin is assayed by two common methods: (1) determining the hypoglycemic effect of a standard compared with the unknown when administered to fasted rabbits or (2) finding the dose of the unknown that will produce hypoglycemic convulsions in mice when compared to a standard preparation.

Insulin becomes bound to target tissues much as do other hormones. It is difficult to wash insulin from a target tissue, especially muscle, after it becomes bound. This binding to the target tissue seems to be a necessary prerequisite for activity of most hormones.

REGULATION OF OUTPUT

A servomechanism controls the release of insulin from the islet cells. The normal stimulus for release of insulin is an elevation of blood glucose level acting directly on the islet cells.

Manns and Boda (1965) studied control of insulin secretion in sheep and found butyrate or a metabolite (but not acetate or propionate) promoted insulin secretion much in excess of that explainable by the hyperglycemia resulting from this compound. With increasing age (concomitant with decreased glucose tolerance), there appeared to be a reduction of insulin release to stimulation by glucose or butyrate.

EFFECTS IN THE BODY

The regulation and use of blood glucose is such an integral part of the overall metabolic scheme of the body that a discussion of insulin effects encompasses many areas. The fundamental mode of action of insulin remains somewhat disputed, although the most current and widely accepted theory rests on the fact that insulin is necessary for the transport of the glucose across the cell membrane and into the intracellular space where utilization can occur. It is postulated that a carrier system exists within the cell membrane that, when stimulated by insulin, favors the movement of glucose across the membrane into the intracellular space, subsequent phosphorylation, and entry into the usual glycolytic schemes. Hence, the elevated blood glucose level of the diabetic animal is due to the inability of the tissues of the body to utilize the glucose since it cannot enter the cell that is so desperately in need of glucose for energy generation.

Pancreatectomy produces acute diabetes mellitus in the dog. An early symptom of this disease is inability to use glucose for energy production or fat or glycogen synthesis. Because of this specific and primary disturbance in glucose use, the mechanism of action of insulin must be at the level of glucose utilization. For glucose to enter the glycolytic cycle and be used, two things must occur: (1) *it must enter the cell* and (2) *it must be phosphorylated by ATP* in the presence of hexokinase to form glucose-6-phosphate. The above processes occur in all tissues to some degree even in the absence of insulin. Insulin acts like other hormones since it only regulates the rate of a metabolic reaction. Some tissues of the body, especially nervous tissue and red blood cells, do not require insulin for the metabolism of glucose.

MECHANISM OF INSULIN ACTION

A single mechanism cannot explain the many diverse activities of insulin such as membrane transport, glycogen synthesis, protein metabolism, and lipolysis. These are mainly anabolic processes, which are a reverse of the cyclic adenosine monophosphate (cAMP) processes. Insulin decreases cAMP in adipose and liver cells. Also adenylate cyclase activity is inhibited by insulin in certain membrane preparations, which is the opposite effect of epinephrine, glucagon, or ACTH. Perhaps insulin acts by holding back the catabolic processes caused by cAMP and thereby favors glycogen synthesis.

Cells responding to insulin have receptors that are glycoprotein in nature. The binding is strong but the exact nature of the complex is not known. It is unfortunate that such important processes as glucose and amino acid transport across membranes are not better understood.

It is not within the scope of this discussion to include the management of diabetes mellitus. A consideration of the pharmacology of insulin, however, recognizes that insulin has the following effects: (1) blood glucose level decreases, (2) blood pyruvate and lactate increase, (3) inorganic phosphate decreases, and (4) potassium decreases. The first three of these are explained quite readily on the basis that increased glucose phosphoralation and utilization bring about these effects. Coincident to this, there would be a decrease in the ketone bodies that are present in the blood and urine and are detectable on the breath of a diabetic animal.

Preparations

Recent progress in purification of insulin allows a more uniform product. To prevent patient error, the unitage will soon be simplified with only 100 units/ml available.

Regular insulin is metabolized within a few hours so several long-acting forms are available (see Table 33.7). These preparations permit one injection a day to control diabetes after stabilization of the patient. The fast-acting preparations are available when needed in the acute patient.

Use in Diabetes Mellitus

Studies on human diabetes mellitus have shown a definite familial heredity predisposition to the condition. This predisposition, although hereditary, can possibly be manifested in several ways: an inherent gluconeogenic state such as hyperproduction of ACTH could lead to chronic hyperglycemia and finally islet cell exhaustion; a familial tendency toward high sugar diets could bring about the same chain of events leading to exhaustion of the islet cells; an abnormal nitrogen metabolism might produce an alloxanlike substance toxic to the beta cells; another possibility is that the enzyme insulinase may be present in abnormally high levels, thereby lowering prematurely the level of insulin. Others have suggested insulin inhibitors as being prevalent in the diabetic animal. Not enough work has been done in domestic animals to be able to classify the condition as to cause, although some familial canine diabetes is reported (Gershwin 1975).

In the dog diabetes mellitus is often a sequela to chronic pancreatitis, an infection of the acinar cells that may involve the islets. Although the pancreatitis may be controlled, permanent damage to the islet cells may remain (Anderson and Low 1965). In chronic diabetes mellitus, *the dog often develops cataracts.* The mechanism underlying this relationship is unknown.

Diabetes mellitus has been reported in the cow infrequently (Christensen and Schambye 1950) but more often in the dog and cat (Schlotthauer and Millar 1951; Roberts 1954). Hyperinsulinism due

TABLE 33.7. Properties of various preparations of insulin

Type	Preparation	Appearance	Protein Modifier	Approximate Time of Onset*	Approximate Duration of Action*	Compatible Mixed With
				(hours)	*(hours)*	
Fast-acting	*Insulin Injection,* U.S.P. (regular insulin)	Clear solution	None	1	6	All preparations
	Insulin Injection, U.S.P. "Insulin made from zinc-insulin crystals" (regular insulin)	Clear solution	None	1	8	All preparations
	Prompt Insulin Zinc Suspension, U.S.P. (Semilente insulin)	Cloudy suspension	None	1	14	Lente preparations
Intermediate-acting	*Isophane Insulin Suspension,* U.S.P. (NPH insulin, isophane insulin)	Cloudy suspension	Protamine	2	24	Insulin injection
	Insulin Zinc Suspension, U.S.P. (Lente insulin)	Cloudy suspension	None	2	24	Insulin injection, Semilente
	Globin Zinc Insulin Injection, U.S.P.	Clear solution	Globin	2	18	. . .
Long-acting	*Protamine Zinc Insulin Suspension,* U.S.P.	Cloudy suspension	Protamine	7	36	Insulin injection
	Extended Insulin Zinc Suspension, U.S.P. (Ultralente insulin)	Cloudy suspension	None	7	36	Insulin injection, Semilente

Source: Goodman and Gilman 1975.

* These figures are representative. The values may be expected to vary over a relatively wide range, depending on the dose and the individual patient.

to a tumor has been recognized in the dog (Cello and Kennedy 1957).

Most of the work concerning experimental diabetes mellitus has been done in the dog, and it is indeed unfortunate that the clinical management of naturally occurring diabetes mellitus in the dog is still in an unsettled state. The incidence of diabetes mellitus appears to be about 1 in each 1000 dogs but 5 times as frequent in the bitch (Krook et al. 1960), hence the occurrence is sufficient that most practitioners encounter the disease in their practices.

In the treatment of diabetes mellitus in the dog or cat, one must consider the dietary regime as well as the administration of insulin. Since the animal has difficulty using carbohydrates, the diet obviously must be minimal in carbohydates and high in protein. With impaired glucose utilization, there is altered fat metabolism to the extent that excess ketone bodies appear that lead to toxic manifestation or even coma. This coma is frequently referred to as diabetic coma (insufficient insulin and hyperglycemia) and must be differentiated from insulin shock (excess insulin and hypoglycemia), which also is a comatose state. Severe diabetes or coma must first be treated for acidosis and dehydration. Rapid-acting insulin is given as follows: dog, 1–2 units/kg; cat, 0.5 unit/kg with one-half intramuscularly and one-half intravenously (Schall 1972).

The diabetic animal experiences hyperglycemia, glucosuria, polydipsia, polyphagia, debilitation, ketosis leading to a ketotic breath, and finally polyuria, which contains detectable amounts of glucose. After management of the diet, the insulin injection must be adjusted to the needs of the individual patient. A trial dose for initial therapy with *Protamine Zinc Insulin,* U.S.P., in the dog would approximate 0.33–0.5 unit/lb of body weight/day subcutaneously. This dosage may need to be increased. With this therapy, the diabetic dog may approach its former physical condition and activity for an indefinite period of time.

Some difficulty has been experienced in preventing the hyperglycemia and glucosuria despite a marked clinical improvement in the general condition and activity of the dog treated with insulin. More extensive (twice weekly) use of appropriate laboratory tests to guide the therapy should reduce this difficulty to a minimum, although the economic factors became important at this stage.

Various attempts have been made to lengthen the action and eliminate the peaks and valleys of insulin activity. Table 33.7 serves as a guide in therapy.

ALLOXAN

Alloxan is a drug that will destroy the beta cells of the islets of Langerhans, causing permanent diabetes mellitus (Fig. 33.14). This drug is toxic and affects tissues other than the pancreas and the liver. It has been used in experimental studies and is very specific in causing destruction of the islet cells in the dog. Alloxan has greatly aided experimental studies of diabetes mellitus in the dog and other animals. The usual dosage in the dog is 100–200 mg/kg of body weight intravenously.

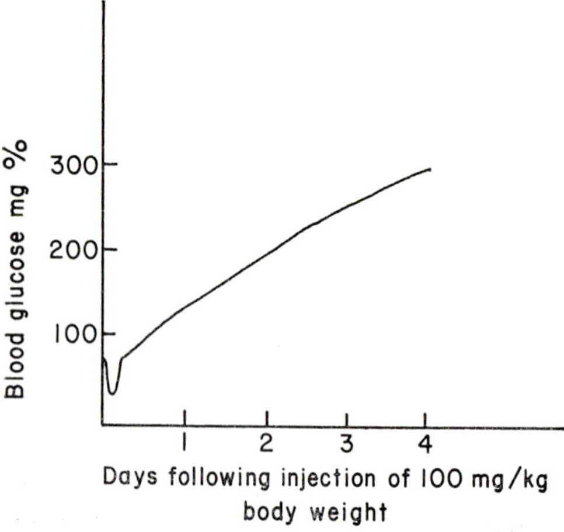

Fig. 33.14. Effect of alloxan on blood glucose level of the dog.

HYPOGLYCEMIC SULFONYLUREA SUBSTANCES

In early studies with some of the sulfonamides, it was found that a hypoglycemia developed. Subsequent studies established that several of the sulfonylureas could produce hypoglycemia in a normal animal but not in an animal with destroyed islet cells. The chemical structures of some of the most commonly used substances are shown in Fig. 33.15.

The mode of action of the sulfonylureas appears to be stimulation of the release of insulin from the beta cells. Obviously, for these hypoglycemic agents to be effective, the patient must have some functional islet cells capable of further stimulation. The most obvious advantage is the fact that they are orally active and their administration can be managed with ease.

These drugs have been of little value in canine diabetes treatment. Only the mildest cases have responded at all. Tolbutamide is hepatotoxic to the dog.

HYPERGLYCEMIC AGENTS (GLUCAGON)

Some of the early work using extracts from the pancreas, which supposedly contained only insulin, caused a hyperglycemia in the injected animal or at least interfered with the hypoglycemic effect expected from insulin. In time (1953) another hormone was found that comes from the alpha cells of the islets and is glycogenolytic. It is a polypeptide with 29 amino acids in a single chain (Fig. 33.16). Complete synthesis of the hormone was achieved at the Max Planck Institute in Munich.

The alpha cells are located throughout the pancreas along with the beta cells in most species; an exception is the dog, which does not have alpha cells in the uncinate process of the pancreas although beta cells are present. *The effect of glucagon is opposite to that of insulin.* The alpha cells are not subject to destruction by

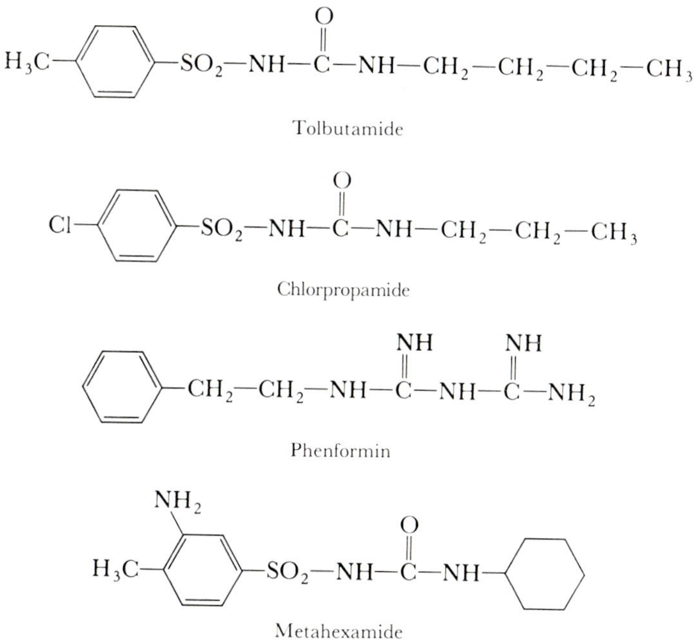

$H_3C{-}C_6H_4{-}SO_2{-}NH{-}C({=}O){-}NH{-}CH_2{-}CH_2{-}CH_2{-}CH_3$

Tolbutamide

$Cl{-}C_6H_4{-}SO_2{-}NH{-}C({=}O){-}NH{-}CH_2{-}CH_2{-}CH_3$

Chlorpropamide

$C_6H_5{-}CH_2{-}CH_2{-}NH{-}C({=}NH){-}NH{-}C({=}NH){-}NH_2$

Phenformin

$H_3C{-}C_6H_3(NH_2){-}SO_2{-}NH{-}C({=}O){-}NH{-}C_6H_{11}$

Metahexamide

Fig. 33.15.

alloxan. Although the effects of insulin are multifold, it appears that the mechanism of glucagon action is rather clear-cut in that it increases the activity of liver dephosphorylase kinase, which activates phosphorylase. Glucagon (or epinephrine) stimulates the production of 3′,5′-AMP (cyclic adenylic acid), which in turn favors the conversion of inactive to active phosphorylase, the limiting enzyme in glycogenolysis. The activation of phosphorylase favors glycogenolysis, thereby leading to an elevation of blood glucose. *This effect of glucagon is similiar to the effect elicited by epinephrine.* Glucagon has no effect on muscle phosphorylase; its effect is limited to hepatic glycogenolysis. Epinephrine acts both on hepatic tissue and muscle tissue.

Glucagon release is triggered by hypoglycemia. Critical and specific studies of glucagon are difficult because the alpha cells cannot be removed without removing the beta cells. This complicates the experiment because of the disturbed insulin balance. Much of our knowledge of glucagon is circumstantial and the exact role of glucagon in normal homeostasis remains to be established, although its presence in all animals favors its utility and causes one to believe that its full role is yet to be established.

Glucagon has been reported to be of value in treatment of circulatory shock. Clark et al. (1974) reviewed its usefulness in veterinary medicine.

Diabetes mellitus is usually more severe in the alloxan-treated than the pancreatectomized mammal; probably because the glucagon from the alpha cells continues to enhance glycogenolysis of the former.

PREPARATIONS

Glucagon for Injection, U.S.P., is available as a dry powder, the hydrochloride of glucagon, with separate diluent. Dosage has not been established in domestic animals, although 50 μg/kg intravenously have been suggested for cir-

his·ser·glu(NH_2)·gly·thr·phe·thr·ser·asp·tyr·ser·lys·tyr·leu·asp·ser·arg·arg·ala·glu(NH_2)·asp·phe·val·glu(NH_2)·try·leu·met·asp(NH_2)·thr

Fig. 33.16. Amino acid sequence of bovine glucagon. (Proposed by Behrens and Bromer 1958)

culatory shock, to be repeated at 30-minute intervals (Clark et al. 1974).

REFERENCES

Adams, W. M. 1969. The elective induction of labor and parturition in cattle. J Am Vet Med Assoc 154:261.

Albright, F., and Reifenstein, E. C., Jr. 1948. Parathyroid Glands and Metabolic Bone Disease, p. 393. Baltimore: Williams & Wilkins.

Alm, C. C.; Sullivan, J. J.; and First, N. L. 1974. Induction of premature parturition by parental administration of dexamethasone in the mare. J Am Vet Med Assoc 165:721.

Anderson, N. V., and Low, D. G. 1965. Diseases of the canine pancreas: A comparative summary of 103 cases. Anim Hosp 1:189.

Astwood, E. B.; Sullivan, J.; Bissell, A.; and Tyslowitz, R. 1943. Action of certain sulfonamides and of thiourea upon the function of the thyroid gland of the rat. Endocrinology 32:210.

Balazs, T. 1969. Effects of DDD and DDT on the production and metabolism of adrenocortical steroids in guinea pigs and dogs. Am J Vet Res 30:1535.

Beckman, H. 1961. Pharmacology: The Nature, Action and Use of Drugs, 2nd ed. Philadelphia: W. B. Saunders.

Behrens, O. K., and Bromer, W. W. 1958. Glucagon. In R. S. Harris and K. V. Thimann, eds. Vitamins and Hormones: Advances in Research and Application, vol. 16, p. 264. New York: Academic Press.

Boda, J. M., and Cole, H. H. 1953. The influence of dietary calcium and phosphorus on the incidence of milk fever in dairy cattle. J Dairy Sci 37:360.

Bonneau, N., and Reed, J. H. 1971. Adrenocortical insufficiency in a dog. Can Vet J 12:100.

Bottoms, G. D.; Roesel, O. F.; Rausch, F. D.; and Akins, E. L. 1972. Circadian variation in plasma cortisol and corticosterone in pigs and mares. Am J Vet Res 33:785.

Braun, R. K.; Bergman, E. N.; and Albert, T. F. 1970. Effects of various synthetic glucocorticoids on milk production and blood glucose and ketone body concentrations in normal ketotic cows. Am J Vet Med Assoc 157:941.

Brewer, H. B.; Fairwell, T.; Rittel, W.; Littledike, T.; and Arnaud, C. D. 1974. Recent studies on the chemistry of human, bovine and porcine parathyroid hormone. Am J Med 56:759.

Breznock, E. M., and McQueen, R. D. 1970. Adrenocortical function during aging in the dog. Am J Vet Res 31:1269.

Brodey, R. S. 1954. Renal osteitis fibrosa cystica in a wire-haired fox terrier. J Am Vet Med Assoc 124:275.

Brush, M. G. 1960. The effect of ACTH injections on plasma corticosteroid levels and milk yield in the cow. J Endocrinol 21:155.

Campbell, J. R., and Watts, C. 1973. Assessment of adrenal function in dogs. Br Vet J 129:134.

Capen, C. C. 1975. Parathyroid hormone, calcitonin, and cholecalciferol: The calcium regulating hormones. In L. E. McDonald, ed. Veterinary Endocrinology and Reproduction, 2nd ed. Philadelphia: Lea & Febiger.

Capen, C. C., and Koestner, A. 1967. Functional chromophobe adenomas of the canine adenohypophysis. Pathol Vet 4:326.

Care, A. D., and Keynes, W. M. 1965. The secretion of calcitonin by the parathyroid glands of the sheep. J Endocrinol 31:31.

Cello, R., and Kennedy, P. 1957. Hyperinsulinism in the dog due to pancreatic islet cell carcinoma. Cornell Vet 47:538.

Christensen, N. O., and Schambye, P. 1950. Diabetes mellitus in the cow. Nord Vet Med 2:863.

Clark, D. R.; Webb, T. J.; and McCrady, J. D. 1974. Physiologic actions and clinical usefulness of glucagon in veterinary medicine. Southwest Vet 27:255.

Coffin, D. L., and Munson, T. O. 1953. Endocrine diseases of the dog associated with hair loss. J Am Vet Med Assoc 123:402.

Colmano, G., and Gross, W. B. 1971. Effect of metyrapone and DDD on infectious diseases. Poult Sci 50:850.

Committee on Animal Nutrition, Agricultural Board. 1966. Hormonal Relationships and Applications in the Production of Meats, Milk, and Eggs [Suppl]. Publication 1415. Washington, D.C.: Academy of Sciences, National Research Council.

Davis, J. O. 1962. The control of aldosterone secretion. Physiologist 5:65.

Dickson, W. M., and Ott, R. L. 1955. Desoxycorticosterone in treatment of uremia of dogs. Vet Med 45:1.

Dickson, W. M.; Kainer, R. A.; and Gorham, J. R. 1954. Adrenogenital syndrome in a female mink. J Am Vet Med Assoc 125:45.

Donovan, E. F., and Venzke, W. G. 1968. Hypothyroidism in the dog. Norden News, pp. 14–17.

Enright, J. B.; Goggin, J. E.; Frye, F. L.; Franti, C. E.; and Behymer, D. E. 1970. Effect of corticosteroids on rabies virus infections in various animal species. J Am Vet Med Assoc 156:765.

Fisher, E. R., and Klein, H. Z. 1966. Effect of

sodium state on reactivity of renal juxtaglomerular cells and adrenal zona glomerulosa. Proc Soc Exp Biol Med 121:142.

Fox, J. G., and Beatty, J. O. 1973. Adrenal insufficiency in the dog: Two case reports. J Small Anim Pract 14:167.

Gershwin, L. J. 1975. Familial canine diabetes. J Am Vet Med Assoc 167:479.

Goetsch, D. D.; McDonald, L. E.; and Odell, G. 1959. The effects of four synthetic corticosteroids on leucocytes, blood glucose, and plasma sodium and potassium in the cow. Am J Vet Res 20:697.

———. 1962. Oral administration of 9 alpha-fluoroprednisolone to lactating dairy cows. Am J Vet Res 23:916.

Goodman, L. S., and Gilman, A. 1975. The Pharmacological Basis of Therapeutics, 5th ed., p. 1517. New York: Macmillian.

Goyings, L. S.; Reineke, E. P.; and Schirmer, R. G. 1962. Clinical diagnosis and therapy of hypothyroidism in dogs. J Am Vet Med Assoc 141:341.

Grollman, A. 1970. Pharmacology and Therapeutics, 7th ed. Philadelphia: Lea & Febiger.

Gross, W. B. 1972. Effect of social stress on occurrence of Marek's disease in chickens. Am J Vet Res 33:2275.

Gross, W. B., and Siegel, P. B. 1973. Effect of social stress and steroids on antibody production. Avian Dis 17:807.

Hall, W. W. 1972. Iatrogenic hyperadrenocorticism due to prolonged Azium therapy. Southwest Vet 26:62.

Hench, P. S. Quoted from Krantz, J. C., and Carr, C. J. 1961. Pharmacological Principles of Medical Practice, 5th ed., p. 1287. Baltimore: Williams & Wilkins.

Hibbs, J. W., and Pounden, W. D. 1955. Studies on milk fever in dairy cows. IV. Prevention by short-time prepartum feeding of massive doses of vitamin D. J Dairy Sci 38:65.

Hightower, D.; Kyzar, J. R.; Chester, D. K.; and Wright, E. M. 1973. Replacement therapy for induced hypothyroidism in dogs. J Am Vet Med Assoc 163:979.

Jackson, H. D.; Pappenhagen, A. R.; Goetsch. G. D.; and Noller, C. H.. 1962. Effect of parathyroid hormone on calcium and other plasma constituents of dairy cattle near parturition. J Dairy Sci 65:897.

Joshua, J. O. 1953. Three cases of thyroid tumour in dogs. Vet Rec 65:356.

Kaneko, J. J.; Tyler, W. S.; Wind, A.; and Cornelius, C. E. 1959. Clinical applications of the thyroidal I^{131} uptake test in the dog. J Am Vet Med Assoc 135:516.

Kass, E. H.; Hechter, O.; Macchi, I. A.; and Mow, T. W. 1954. Changes in patterns of secretion of corticosteroids in rabbits after prolonged treatment with ACTH. Proc Soc Exp Biol Med 85:583.

Katsoyannis, P. G. 1964. The synthesis of insulin chains and their combinations to biologically active material. Diabetes 13: 339.

Keeton, K. S.; Schechter, R. D.; and Schalm, O. W. 1972. Adrenocortical insufficiency in dogs. Mod Vet Pract 53:25.

Klein, D. C.; Morii, H.; and Talmage, R. V. 1967. Effect of thyrocalcitonin administered during peritoneal lavage, on removal of bone salts and their radioisotopes. Proc Soc Exp Biol Med 124:627.

Knoop, C. E. 1946. The effect of feeding potassium iodide and skim milk powder on spermatogenesis. J Dairy Sci 29:555.

Krook, L.; Larsson, S.; and Rooney, J. R. 1960. The interrelationship of diabetes mellitus, obesity, and pyometra in the dog. Am J Vet Res 21:120.

Lank, R. P. 1958. Personal communication.

Lewis, E.; Burrow, F.; and Burrow, H. 1953. The effect of dihydrotachysterol on bovine blood calcium, inorganic phosphate and sugar levels. Br Vet J 109:521.

Lillehei, R. C.; Langerbeam, J. K.; Block, J. H.; and Manax, W. V. 1964. The modern treatment of shock based on physiologic principles. Clin Pharmacol Ther 5:63.

Lindner, H. R. 1967. Comparative aspects of cortisol transport: Lack of firm binding to plasma proteins in domestic ruminants. J Endocrinol 28:301.

Lubberink, A. A. M. E.; Rijnberk, A.; der Kindren, P. J.; and Thijssen, J. H. H. 1971. Hyperfunction of the adrenal cortex: A review. Aust Vet J 47:504.

McCann, S. M.; Antunes-Rodrigues, J.; and Nallar, R. 1966. Pituitary-adrenal function in the absence of vasopressin. Endocrinology 79:1058.

Magrane, W. G. 1951. Cortisone in ophthalmology. North Am Vet 32:763.

Manns, J. G., and Boda, J. M. 1965. Control of insulin secretion in sheep: The effect of volatile fatty acids and glucose. Physiologist 8:227.

Marshak, R. R.; Webster, G. D., Jr.; and Skelley, J. F. 1960. Adrenocortical insufficiency. J Am Vet Med Assoc 136:274.

Merrifield, R. B. 1963. Solid phase peptide synthesis. I. The synthesis of a tetrapeptide. J Am Chem Soc 85:2149.

Moore, L. A. 1958. Thyroprotein for dairy cattle. J Dairy Sci 41:452.

Nachreiner, R. F., and Marple, D. N. 1975. Termination of pregnancy of cats with $PGF_{2\alpha}$. Prostaglandins 7:303.

Neff, A. W.; Connor, N. D.; and Bryan, H. S. 1960. Studies on 9-fluoroprednisolone acetate, a new synthetic corticosteroid for the treatment of bovine ketosis. J Dairy Sci 43:553.

Neilson, S. W., and McSherry, B. J. 1954. Renal hyperparathyroidism (rubber jaw syndrome) in a dog. J Am Vet Med Assoc 124:270.

Olson, W. G.; Jorgensen, N. A.; Bringe, A. N.; Schultz, L. H.; and DeLuca, H. F. 1973. 25-Hydroxycholecalciferol (25-OHD_3). I. Treatment of parturient paresis. J Dairy Sci 56:885.

O'Malley, B. W., and Schrader, W. T. 1976. The receptors of steroid hormones. Sci Am 234:32.

Peterson, W. E.; Spielman, A. A.; Pomeroy, B. S.; and Boyd, W. J. 1941. Effect of thyroidectomy upon sexual behavior of the male bovine. Proc Soc Exp Biol Med 46:16.

Quinlan, W., and Michaelson, S. M. 1967. Iodine-131 uptake and protein-bound iodine in normal adult beagles. Am J Vet Res 28:179.

Rijnberk, A.; der Kindren, P. J.; and Thijssen, J. H. H. 1968. Spontaneous hyperadrenocorticism in the dog. J Endocrinol 41:397.

Ripps, J. H. 1955. Graves' disease (hyperthyroidism) in the dog. North Am Vet 36:849.

Roberts, I. M. 1954. The diagnosis and treatment of diabetes mellitus in the dog. J Am Vet Med Assoc 124:443.

Sanger, F. 1959. Chemistry of insulin. Science 129:1340.

Schall, W. D. 1972. Fluid and electrolyte therapy of diabetic ketoacidosis. J Am Anim Hosp Assoc 8:206.

Schechter, R. D.; Stabenfeldt, G. H.; Gribble, D. H.; and Ling, G. V. 1973. Treatment of Cushing's syndrome in the dog with an adrenocorticolytic agent (*o,p'*DDD). J Am Vet Med Assoc 162:629.

Schlotthauer, C. F., and Millar, J. A. S. 1951. Diabetes mellitus in dogs and cats. J Am Vet Med Assoc 118:31.

Schultze, A. B., and Davis, H. P. 1946. The influence of feeding synthetic thyroprotein on fertility of bulls. J Dairy Sci 29:534.

Scott, D. W., and Greene, C. E. 1974. Iatrogenic secondary adrenocortical insufficiency in dogs. J Am Anim Assoc 10:555.

Shaw, K. E., and Nichols, R. C. 1962. The influence of age upon the circulating 17-hydroxycorticosteroids of cattle subjected to blood sampling and exogenous adrenocorticotrophic hormone and hydrocortisone. Am J Vet Res 23:1217.

Spielman, A. A.; Petersen, W. E.; Fitch, J. B.; and Pomeroy, B. S. 1945. General appearance, growth and reproduction of thyroidectomized bovine. J Dairy Sci 28:329.

Stith, R. D., and Bottoms, G. D. 1972. Effects of metyrapone on concentrations of cortisol and corticosterone in plasma of pigs. Am J Vet Res 33:963.

Stöckle, W., and Jockle, W. 1971. Corticosteroid-induced changes in plasma amino acids and thyroid activity in dairy cows treated early or late during lactation. J Dairy Sci 54:271.

Storts, R. W., and Koestner, A. 1965. Skeletal lesions associated with a dietary calcium and phosphorus imbalance in the pig. Am J Vet Res 26:280.

Swanson, E. W., and Boatman, J. P. 1953. The effect of thiouracil feeding upon seminal characteristics of dairy bulls. J Dairy Sci 36:246.

Swarbrick, O. 1968. Intramammary treatment of bovine mastitis. Vet Rec 82:2.

Thomas, J. W. 1953. The use of thyroprotein for milk production. Natl Res Counc Publ 266:47.

Thorpe, B. R. 1953. Thyroid enlargement in a dog, treated with iodine and methyl thiouracil. Aust Vet J 29:75.

Waisbren, B. A. 1964. Gram-negative shock and endotoxin shock. Am J Med 36:819.

Weber, A. F.; Bell, J. T.; and Sellers, A. F. 1958. Studies of the bovine adrenal gland. II. The histological and cytochemical effects of the administration of 1,1-dichloro-2,2-bis(*p*-chlorophenyl)ethane on the adrenal cortices of dairy calves. Am J Vet Res 21:51.

Webster, B., and Chesney, A. M. 1928. Endemic goiter in rabbits: Effect of administration of iodine. Bull Johns Hopkins Hosp 43:291.

Weil, M. H.; Shubin, H.; and Biddle, M. 1964. Shock caused by gram-negative microorganisms. Ann Intern Med 60:384.

S E C T I O N 9

Drugs Acting on the Digestive Tract

CHAPTER 34

DRUGS AFFECTING DIGESTION AND ABSORPTION

ROBERT W. PHILLIPS and LON D. LEWIS

FUNCTION OF THE DIGESTIVE SYSTEM

A knowledge of the function of the digestive system is an important prelude to the application of pharmacology and therapeutics. The secretory-absorptive surfaces of the gastrointestinal (GI) tract are the major site of absorption into the body. The concept of oral therapy to treat systemic conditions is based on the proper functioning of this absorptive system and the rapid movement of drugs into the body's vasculature. Conversely, much of the therapy of GI dysfunction, as well as the treatment of GI microbial and parasitic infestations, is based on the use of drugs that do not substantially cross this absorptive surface.

Proper digestive function is based on ingestion, maceration, and solubilization of a variety of dietary constituents. Solubilized particles are further degraded biochemically by either the host or its symbiotic organisms until they are sufficiently reduced in size to conveniently pass across the absorptive barrier into the body. These processes vary considerably in different domestic animals; however, the end products are in general similar.

Digestive function involves transport through the tract from mouth to anus, as well as across the epithelial boundary between the digestive tube and the interior of the body. The intestinal lumen is surrounded by but outside the body from a functional standpoint. Pharmacology as applied to digestive function generally involves an alteration in one of these transport functions.

APPETITE STIMULANTS

Partial or complete anorexia is a prominent occurrence with many diseases. Unfortunately, it occurs at a time when the animal may have increased nutritional requirements. Failure to treat the anorexia often prolongs or prevents recovery. Thus the stimulation of appetite is often desired in therapeutics. Currently, there is no single drug or group of drugs having this specific effect. Vitamins of the B complex, corticosteroids, and anabolic steroids have been advocated as appetite stimulants. Their effect, if any, is probably more related to making the animal feel better than it is to a specific effect upon appetite. For example, corticosteroids are capable of causing euphoria or a feeling of general well-being that may have a beneficial effect on appetite. The provision of small quantities of highly palatable food at frequent intervals is more likely to be helpful in restoring appetite than the use of appetite stimulants per se. Heating the food for carnivores is also helpful. Nux vomica, occasionally used as an appetite stimulant in ruminants and horses, is probably worthless for this purpose. If appetite stimulation is not successful, oral or parenteral alimentation is indicated.

DIGESTANTS

Digestants are drugs that promote the process of digestion in the GI tract. They are used in the treatment of conditions characterized by a lack of one or more of the substances that function in the digestion of foods in the alimentary tract. The digestants commonly used in veterinary medicine are digestive enzymes and choleretics.

Digestive Enzymes

Pancreatic extracts that simulate pancreatic exocrine secretions are of therapeutic benefit in cases of chronic pancreatitis where glandular function is diminished or destroyed. *Pancreatin,* N.F., obtained from hog pancreas, is the major ingredient of most commercial pancreatic enzyme preparations. Enteric-coated preparations (such as Panteric) to prevent destruction by pepsin in the stomach are generally thought to be better than noncoated preparations (Goodman and Gilman 1970). In a few instances enteric-coated preparations are the most effective in dogs with pancreatic insufficiency. These preparations are added to the food and must be provided with each meal for the life of the animal. Dosage is adjusted to obtain a normal stool. In addition, proper dietary control is essential. Low fat, low residue, highly digestible protein diets fed frequently in small portions are best. Fatty foods tend to curtail the enzymatic action of pancreatic extracts (Hill 1972). High fat diets may completely eliminate the beneficial effects of pancreatic extract supplementation in cases of pancreatic insufficiency. However, triglycerides containing 6–12 carbon atoms may be fed as an increased dietary energy source. Unlike the majority of fats containing 16 or 18 carbon atoms, the medium chain triglycerides are absorbed intact without requiring pancreatic lipolysis. Coconut oil is such a triglyceride and is readily accepted by dogs. It should be fed separately to prevent inhibition of the pancreatic extracts. Some cases of pancreatic insufficiency in the dog have not improved until medium chain triglycerides were fed (Hill 1972). Up to 25% of the dog's caloric requirements may be provided in this form. Supplementation greater than this will decrease the consumption of other nutrients to such a degree that deficiencies may result.

Choleretics

Choleretics are substances that stimulate hepatic bile secretion. The most effective choleretics are the natural bile salts and acids. Bile salts are the sodium and potassium salts of the bile acids. The bile acids, in turn, are formed by reaction of cholic acid with the amino acids taurine or glycine and are designated as taurocholic or glycocholic acid, respectively. Cholic acid is synthesized in the liver from cholesterol. The bile salts function to emulsify fat in the upper small intestine. This facilitates subsequent reactions with pancreatic lipase and thus enhances lipid absorption. In the absence of bile salts, only about 50% of the fat is absorbed and almost none of the fat-soluble vitamins. Bile salts used therapeutically have a dual action in directly promoting fat absorption and in stimulating biliary secretion after they have been absorbed.

Many bile preparations employed in therapy do not contain these natural bile salts; rather, they contain partially synthetic derivatives of the bile acids. The most important of these is an oxidation product of cholic acid, dehydrocholic acid. Dehydrocholic acid increases the volume of bile secretion to a much greater extent than do the natural bile salts, glycocholate and taurocholate. *Dehydrocholic Acid,* N.F., and ox bile extract are available in oral tablets and ampules containing 20% dehydrocholic acid. They are used therapeutically to replace endogenous bile salts when a deficiency is thought to exist because of fat malabsorption. Generally a 3-ml ampule is sufficient. However, this varies with the patient and dosage must be adjusted to obtain a normal stool. Overdosage will cause diarrhea. Proper dietary control is essential as in pancreatic exocrine deficiency. Low fat, highly digestible diets fed frequently in small portions are best. Proper dietary management may in some cases alleviate the need for choleretics.

ANTACIDS

Antacids are agents that neutralize or remove acid from the GI contents and are routinely used in human medicine to treat reflux esophagitis and to combat excess gastric acidity associated with peptic ulcers. There is little evidence that hyperacidity is of major concern in simple-stomached domestic animals, so analogous therapy is seldom required. Peptic ulcers, located in the pylorus and proximal duodenum, are occasionally reported in dogs (Murray et al. 1972). However, generally these seem to occur in association with other diseases and may not be related to gastric hyperacidity. Abomasal ulcers in ruminants are discussed in Chapter 36. These are not usually recognized until they result in perforations and peritonitis or extensive hemorrhage and shock. Both generally have very short courses, ending in death. Antacids may be indicated for nonperforating ulcers if the patient can be stabilized. However, there is no evidence that oral antacids after dilution in the rumen have any effect on abomasal acidity. The major use of antacids in veterinary medicine is in the treatment and prevention of GI acidosis from excessive concentrate intake.

Antacids may be systemic or nonsystemic. A systemic antacid is one capable of producing metabolic alkalosis. This occurs because of the absorption of any unneutralized anionic portion and because the cationic moiety does not form insoluble basic compounds in the intestine and is absorbed. Sodium bicarbonate is a prime example of a systemic antacid. The rapid liberation of carbon dioxide in the stomach following oral sodium bicarbonate may result in gastric distension and ulcer perforation. In conditions where sodium retention occurs, sodium bicarbonate may contribute to edema. For these reasons, sodium bicarbonate should not be used as an antacid. It is of value as a urine alkalinizer, if this is desired.

Nonsystemic antacids may be beneficial in cases of suspected gastric hyperacidity, gastritis, or GI acidosis. However, even the most effective antacids given in optimal amounts must be repeated every 1–2 hours to have a significant effect on the gastric pH (Fordtran and Collyns 1966). The major nonsystemic antacids, with regard to both use and effectiveness, are aluminum and magnesium hydroxide and calcium carbonate. Most antacids used in veterinary medicine contain one or more of these compounds, often in combination with various protectants, adsorbents, and astringents. One g of these compounds will neutralize 20–35 mEq of acid *in vitro.* In concentrations in which these compounds are present in the better commercially available antacid preparations, 0.5–1.0 ml/kg every 2–4 hours is required to significantly reduce gastric acidity (Fordtran et al. 1973).

Aluminum Hydroxide

Aluminum Hydroxide, U.S.P., is a good adsorbent and demulcent as well as a good antacid. The clinical significance of its adsorptive property is not clear, although it is used for this purpose in the treatment of intestinal toxemias. Its adsorbent properties greatly decrease tetracycline absorption (Waisbren and Hueckel 1950). Insoluble aluminum phosphates are formed in the intestine and excreted, thus decreasing phosphate absorption. Aluminum hydroxide may cause constipation, which is often circumvented by mixing it with magnesium salts in antacid preparations.

Magnesium Hydroxide

Magnesium Hydroxide, U.S.P. (milk of magnesia), and other magnesium salts have a cathartic effect. This results from soluble but unabsorbed magnesium compounds that remain in the intestine, thus retaining water. This effect is minimized by coadministering preparations that contain aluminum hydroxide or calcium carbonate, both of which have constipating effects. Magnesium hydroxide is a good antacid, having a prompt neutralizing effect with a prolonged action. One disadvantage as an antacid is that normally about 20% of the magnesium is absorbed. Ordinarily, the absorbed magnesium is rapidly excreted by the kidney. However, renal dysfunction and repeated administration can result in a dangerous degree of retention, causing neurological, neuromuscular, and cardiovascular impairment. Magnesium absorption is, however, desired in the prophylaxis of grass tetany of cattle (see Chapter 40). Magnesium oxide is generally used for this purpose rather than magnesium hydroxide. Magnesium oxide is also used as an antacid. Since it is converted in water to the hydroxide, its biological properties are the same as magnesium hydroxide. In the ruminant, it probably has ample time to react completely with water and, therefore, is as good an antacid as magnesium hydroxide. In the simple-stomached animal this is not true. Magnesium oxide is occasionally added as 2%–5% of the dry matter of feed for ruminants in an attempt to prevent or decrease GI acidosis due to high-concentrate rations. However, calcium carbonate, in these same amounts, is more commonly used, as discussed in Chapter 36.

Calcium Carbonate

Calcium carbonate (limestone) is an excellent antacid. Its effects are rapid in onset and prolonged in duration. Kirsner and Palmer (1940) found it to be the most effective antacid studied. However, other studies indicate that it is less beneficial clinically than other antacids (Baume and Hunt 1969). This may be due to calcium-induced gastric hypersecretion (Barreras 1970). All antacids increase gastric acid secretion. However, calcium carbonate is the only antacid that has been shown to cause an acid rebound, i.e., increased acid secretion outlasting the neutralizing effect (Fordtran 1968). Infrequently, hypercalcemia and hypercalciuria may follow the oral administration of calcium carbonate. Chronically, this may result in metastatic calcification (McMillan and Freeman 1965). Calcium salts also have a tendency to precipitate in the intestinal tract causing constipation and fecal concretions. This is usually alleviated by combining magnesium and calcium antacids.

With respect to antacid properties, preparations containing 2 or more antacids are no more effective than those containing only 1 antacid. As discussed above, there are other reasons for such combinations. In preparations for human patients, commercially available antacids vary markedly in their potency, with Maalox (aluminium and magnesium hydroxide) and Camalox (aluminum and magnesium hydroxide, and calcium carbonate) being the most effective of those tested both *in vivo* and *in vitro* (Fordtran et al. 1973). It may be expected that the same is true of veterinary preparations.

PROTECTANTS AND ADSORBENTS

These drugs represent two different approaches to the problem of decreasing absorption of unwanted substances or decreasing contact between possible irritants and the surface of the intestine. They have been used therapeutically for many years. Protectants act to protect the lining of the GI tract. They do this, it is believed, by coating or covering the mucous lining. This coating forms a protective layer between potentially toxic substances in the tract and the epithelial surface. The principal use for protectants is in the treatment of ulcerations or irritations of the bowel. Adsorbents are substances that bind with toxic agents and subsequently carry them out of the digestive tract. They are, therefore, used in cases of poisoning to decrease the rate of absorption. Many substances have both protectant and adsorbent qualities in varying degrees. The principal GI protectants are the insoluble salts of bismuth and magnesium, while the major adsorbents are aluminum silicates, pectin, and activated charcoal.

Bismuth and Magnesium Salts

A number of insoluble bismuth salts have been used for their protective action. Bismuth salicylate, subcarbonate, and subnitrate are the most common. The subnitrate has potential toxicity as the nitrite ion may accumulate, be absorbed, and cause methemoglobinemia. Its use should be discouraged. Magnesium trisilicate is an insoluble salt that is an effective GI adsorbent with moderate antacid activity. These salts are generally given to dogs and cats in doses of 1–5 mg/kg of body weight every 4–6 hours.

Aluminum Silicates

A number of natural clays have colloidal aluminum silicate as a base. When hydrated they first form a gel and, with the addition of more water, a sol. The most commonly used pharmaceutically are *Kaolin,* N.F., *Bentonite,* U.S.P., and *Fuller's earth.* These have slightly different physical characteristics but are essentially similar in their actions. They are believed to be adsorbent as well as protective. *Barium Sulfate,* U.S.P., which is used in radiology to visualize the GI tract, has some protective action and can be used for this purpose in doses of 20–60 ml per dog or cat, repeated every 4–6 hours.

Pectin

Pectin is a complex polysaccharide obtained from the rind of apples and citrus fruit. It is believed to have both protective and adsorbent qualities, particularly in combating bacterial enteritis. It can be dissolved in water to form an acidic colloidal solution. One percent pectin is often used in combination with 20% kaolin as an antidiarrheal preparation. Kirk (1971) recommends a dosage to dogs and cats of 20–60 ml of this kaolin-pectin combination per animal, repeated each time there is a bowel movement. He states, however, that it is of marginal effectiveness.

Activated Charcoal

Activated Charcoal, U.S.P., has primarily adsorbent properties. Because of its broad spectrum of adsorptive activity and its rapidity of action, *activated charcoal is one of the most valuable agents for the emergency treatment of certain cases of poisoning* (Holt and Holz 1963). One g of activated charcoal will adsorb the following substances in the amounts (mg) indicated in parentheses: mercuric chloride (1800), sulfanilamide (1000), strychnine nitrate (950), morphine hydrochloride (800), atropine sulfate (700), nicotine (700), salicylcic acid (550), phenol (400), phenobarbital (350), and alcohol (300) (Andersen 1946). It forms a stable complex with these substances that permits their evacuation from the body. In the common domestic species, 20–120 mg/kg of body weight of powdered activated charcoal are usually administered as a drench after mixing with water. An activated charcoal suspension may be used for gastric lavage in simple-stomached animals.

ASTRINGENTS

Astringents are substances that exert their effects by altering surface characteristics. They precipitate proteins but have so little penetrating ability that only the surface of the cells is affected. Consequently, the permeability of the cell is greatly reduced but the cell itself remains viable. Most GI astringents have a tannic acid base.

Tannic Acid

Tannic Acid, N.F., is formed from a number of glycosides or tannins that contain glucose and tannic acid in different combinations. The rate of hydrolysis of the glycosides and release of tannic acid varies with different plant sources. Astringent qualities are based on this release rate. The most common tannic acid is derived from nutgalls on oak trees. It is available as a powder that is readily soluble in water, glycerine, or alcohol. A solution of *Tannic Acid Glycerite,* N.F., which is 20% tannic acid and 1% sodium citrate in glycerin, is also available. Tannic acid is used in the leather industry where more prolonged application of stronger solutions results in protein precipitation and "tanning of the hide" into leather.

In the GI tract, in addition to reacting with mucous membrane proteins, tannic acid can form insoluble salts with some heavy metals, alkaloids, and glycosides, thus reducing their toxicity. However, there are many important alkaloids and heavy metals not precipitated by tannic acid. These include cocaine, nicotine, physostigmine, atropine, morphine, arsenic, antimony, and mercury. In addition, tannic acid interferes with the adsorbent action of activated charcoal (Picchioni et al. 1966). Tannic acid is not absorbed as such from the GI tract but is converted to gallic acid, which is nonastringent and is further metabolized following absorption. The major GI use of tannic acid is in the treatment of diarrhea. Several commercial antidiarrheal products contain tannic acid as one of the active ingredients. Although it has been reported to reduce the severity of diarrhea, its effectiveness in this regard is questionable (Goodman and Gilman 1970). It is most effective in the acid upper portions of the digestive tract and becomes less so in the more basic lower intestine.

Protected tannic acid and slow release glycosides have a prolonged astringent action in the lower intestine. These as well as tannic acid in the form of enemas and suppositories are not recommended because sufficient drug may be absorbed to induce liver damage (Goodman and Gilman 1970).

Tannic acid was at one time widely employed in the treatment of burns until it was found that it was absorbed and caused hepatic necrosis (Krezanoski 1966). Superior methods of burn therapy are available.

ORAL ELECTROLYTE FLUIDS

Fluid electrolyte therapy is indicated in many disease conditions as discussed in Section 7. Oral administration is the optimal route except in upper GI obstructions, displacements, and vomition. In extremely acute conditions, intestinal absorption may not be rapid enough to prevent death. Often animals with diarrhea will respond favorably to oral fluid administration. This might be anticipated in cases not caused by a decrease in intestinal absorption, such as *Escherichia coli* and *Vibrio cholera* endotoxin–induced diarrheas. However, oral fluids have been demonstrated to be quite effective even in cases of salmonellosis, a disease in which absorptive mechanisms have been shown to be disrupted (Powell et al. 1971a).

Many nutrients and electrolytes enhance the absorption of each other and therefore water, since its absorption is passive. Water absorption is dependent primarily on the development of osmotic gradients resulting from solute absorption. Maximum water absorption is obtained by facilitating solute absorption.

The solutes (1) glucose, (2) sodium, (3) bicarbonate, (4) neutral amino acids (other than glycine), and (5) glycine and imino amino acids have all been identified as facilitating the absorption of each other. For example, sodium and glucose will each double the rate of intestinal absorption of the other (Sladen and Dawson 1969; Saltzman et al. 1972). Solutions containing 118 mM sodium and 1% glucose (56 mM) have been shown to result in maximal intestinal absorption (Powell et al. 1971a). Bicarbonate also increases intestinal sodium absorption independent of the solution pH (Sladen and Dawson 1968). In fact, the jejunum is incapable of sodium absorption (from a 127 mM sodium solution) in the absence of luminal bicarbonate (Fordtran et al. 1968; Powell et al. 1971b). A concentration of at least 30 mM bicarbonate is required for maximum sodium and water absorption. In the intestines there appear to be separate systems for the active transport of (1) neutral (other than glycine), (2) basic, and (3) glycine and imino amino acids (Fitzgerald et al. 1971). The amino acids glycine, alanine, and leucine increase sodium and water absorption. This increase occurs linearly with increasing concentrations of the amino acids. Arginine, a basic amino acid, does not stimulate sodium and water absorption and at higher concentrations causes secretion (Hellier et al. 1973).

In conclusion, many conditions requiring fluid and electrolyte therapy may be successfully treated orally. Maximum intestinal water and electrolyte absorption may be expected from fluids containing 118 mM sodium; a minimum of 30 mM bicarbonate, and 1% glucose; plus glycine or imino amino acids; and at least one other neutral amino acid. Other electrolytes such as potassium and chloride may be added as needed. An osmolality as near isotonicity as possible, yet containing these ingredients, should be the goal. Solutes not absorbed from a hypertonic fluid will decrease absorption and cause a net secretion by osmotically pulling water into the intestinal lumen. Energy-supplying nutrients, such as carbohydrates and proteins, that are not absorbed may be utilized by intestinal organisms. This may result in bacterial overgrowth and increased intestinal fluid losses. These substances, therefore, should be added in the lowest concentrations necessary to give maximal enhancement of water and electrolyte absorption.

Oral-nutrient electrolyte fluids should be given a minimum of 2–3 times a day in the following amounts each time:

Calves, foals, and sheep: 1–2 L/animal
Lambs: 250–500 ml/animal
Cattle and horses: 6–10 L/animal
Dogs, cats and pigs: 150–250 ml/5 kg of body weight

Higher dosages and more frequent administration times should be used when dehydration and fluid losses are severe.

REFERENCES

Andersen, A. H. 1946. Experimental studies on the pharmacology of activated charcoal. I. Absorption power of charcoal in aqueous solutions. Acta Pharmacol Toxicol 2:69.

Barreras, J. F. 1970. Acid secretion after calcium carbonate in patients with duodenal ulcer. N Engl J Med 282:1402.

Baume, P. E., and Hunt, J. H. 1969. Failure of potent antacid therapy to hasten healing in chronic gastric ulcers. Aust Ann Med 18:113.

Fitzgerald, J. F.; Reiser, S.; and Christiansen, P. A. 1971. Developmental pattern of sugar and amino acid transport in postnatal rat small intestine. Pediatr Res 5:698.

Fordtran, J. S. 1968. Acid rebound. N Engl J Med 279:900.

Fordtran, J. S., and Collyns, J. A. H. 1966. Antacid pharmacology in duodenal ulcers. Effect of antacids on postcibal gastric acidity and peptic activity. N Engl J Med 274:921.

Fordtran, J. S.; Rector, F. C., Jr.; and Carter, N. W. 1968. The mechanism of sodium absorption in the human small intestine. J Clin Invest 47:884.

Fordtran, J. S.; Morawski, S. G.; and Richardson, C. T. 1973. *In vivo* and *in vitro* evolution of liquid antacids. N Engl J Med 288:923.

Goodman, L. S., and Gilman, A., eds. 1970. The Pharmacological Basis of Therapeutics, 4th ed., p. 981. New York: Macmillan.

Hellier, M. D.; Thirumalai, C.; and Holdsworth, C. D. 1973. The effect of amino acids and dipeptides on sodium and water absorption in man. Gut 14:41.

Hill, F. W. G. 1972. Malabsorption syndrome in the dog: A study of thirty-eight cases. J Small Anim Pract 13:575.

Holt, E. L., and Holz, P. H. 1963. The black bottle. J Pediatr 63:306.

Kirk, R. W. 1971. Vomiting and diarrhea: Pathophysiology and treatment. Proc Colo State Univ Ann Vet Conf.

Kirsner, J. B., and Palmer, W. L. 1940. The effect of various antacids upon hydrogen ion concentration of the gastric contents. Am J Dig Dis 7:85.

Krezanoski, J. Z. 1966. Tannic acid: Chemistry, analysis and toxicity. Radiology 87:655.

McMillan, D. E., and Freeman, R. B. 1965. The milk alkali syndrome: A study of the acute disorder with comments on the development of the chronic condition. Medicine 44:485.

Murray, M.; Robinson, P. B.; and McKeating, F. S. 1972. Peptic ulceration in the dog: A clinical-pathological study. Vet Rec 91: 445.

Picchioni, A. L.; Chin, L.; Verhulst, H. L.; and Dieterle, B. 1966. Activated charcoal versus "universal antidote" as an antidote for poisons. Toxicol Appl Pharmacol 8:447.

Powell, D. W.; Plotkin, G. R.; Solberg, L. I.; Catlin, D. H.; Maenza, R. M.; and Formal, S. B. 1971a. Experimental diarrhea. II. Glucose-stimulated sodium and water transport in rat salmonella enterocolitis. Gastroenterology 60:1065.

———. 1971b. Experimental diarrhea. III. Bicarbonate transport in rat salmonella enterocolitis. Gastroenterology 60:1076.

Saltzman, D. A.; Rector, F. C.; and Fordtran, J. S. 1972. The role of intraluminal sodium in glucose absorption *in vivo.* J Clin Invest 51:876.

Sladen, G. E., and Dawson, A. M. 1968. Effect of bicarbonate on sodium absorption by the human jejunum. Nature 218:267.

———. 1969. Inter-relationships between the absorption of glucose, sodium and water by the normal human jejunum. Clin Sci 36:119.

Waisbren, B. A., and Hueckel, J. S. 1950. Reduced absorption of Aureomycin caused by aluminum hydroxide gel. Proc Soc Exp Biol Med 73:73.

CHAPTER 35

DRUGS AFFECTING GASTROINTESTINAL MOTILITY AND INGESTA MOVEMENT

ROBERT W. PHILLIPS and LON D. LEWIS

EMETICS

Emesis or vomition is commonly seen only in carnivores and human beings. It is not considered to be a serious problem in swine, and rarely occurs in the larger herbivores. Emesis is a complicated reflex action. It involves strong contractions of the abdominal muscles and diaphragm as well as a sharp decrease in intrathoracic pressure, brought about by an inspiratory effort with a closed glottis. The pylorus contracts while the major portion of the stomach is relaxed during vomition and does not contribute actively to its own emptying.

Vomiting is controlled through the emetic center located in the lateral reticular formation of the medulla. It is activated by (1) some drugs, toxins, and metabolic factors acting centrally on the chemoreceptor trigger zone located in the floor of the fourth ventricle or (2) peripherally by irritation of the gastrointestinal (GI) tract, pharynx, peritoneum, mesenteric vasculature, and inner ear. Thus drugs and other factors affecting emesis may act either centrally or peripherally.

Medically, it may be desirable to either induce or inhibit vomiting. Emesis may be induced to empty the anterior portions of the digestive tract. This is usually desirable prior to the induction of general anesthesia and as a rapid means of eliminating orally ingested noncorrosive poisons.

Central Emetics

Although a number of drugs are capable of stimulating the emetic center centrally, the opium derivatives, particularly apomorphine, are the most commonly used (see Chapter 15 for a more complete description of the action of opiate drugs). In preanesthetic medication they have the additional advantage of causing central depression subsequent to evacuation of the digestive tract.

APOMORPHINE HYDROCHLORIDE

Apomorphine Hydrochloride, U.S.P.,

TABLE 35.1. Apomorphine administration in the dog

Route	Dosage	Minutes for Emesis
	(mg/kg)	
Intravenous	0.04	1–4
Subcutaneous	0.07	3–5
Intramuscular	0.07	3–5
Ocular*	0.25	5–12
Oral	0.25	5–12

* Drops or tablets in the conjunctival sac.

is a synthetic alkaloid derivative of morphine. It retains some of the depressant activity of the parent compound but in reduced amounts, while its emetic activity is enhanced. The principal effect of this drug is to stimulate directly the chemoreceptor trigger zone. Vomition generally occurs in 3–10 minutes following subcutaneous or conjunctival administration. It may occur as rapidly as 1 minute following intravenous administration. Sporadic or intermittent vomition may continue for a period about 5 times as long as the initial delay after administration. For example, if vomition was first seen in 4 minutes, it may occur sporadically for another 20 minutes.

Apomorphine can be administered by almost any route and cause vomition. Although more of the drug is required to produce emesis following oral dosage, this route of administration appears to produce as reliable an emetic effect as the more commonly employed parenteral routes (Harrison et al. 1972). Table 35.1 lists routes and dosage levels for apomorphine in the dog. Although apomorphine stimulates the vomition chemoreceptor trigger zone, it directly depresses the emetic center. Therefore, if the first dose does not produce emesis, subsequent doses are even less likely to do so.

Excessive doses of apomorphine have a depressant action upon the central nervous system (CNS) and produce respiratory depression. It is, therefore, contraindicated in the presence of existing central depression. In fact, the emetic center of a depressed animal often will not respond to the emetic action of apomorphine. Instead, the animal will become further depressed if the drug is administered. Obviously, then, apomorphine should not be used in conjunction with central depressants nor should dosage be repeated until all signs of depression have subsided. Nalorphine or levallorphan are the drugs of choice for apomorphine toxicity, as they are for other opiate derivatives (see Chapter 15).

XYLAZINE

Although apomorphine, like other opiate derivatives, is contraindicated in cats, a new sedative-analgesic, *xylazine* (Rompun), has recently been reported to be a predictable and safe emetic agent for cats. Maximum emetic effect is produced in the cat at 1 mg/kg after intramuscular injection. Sedation occurs, lasting 30–90 minutes, but analgesia is not noted at this dosage (Amend and Klavano 1973).

IPECAC

Ipecac, U.S.P. (syrup or powder), has been used as an emetic for many years. It has been shown to be safe and effective in cats (Yeary 1972). The syrup contains 7% ipecac in glycerin. Ipecac is a plant derivative and contains alkaloids that cause both gastric irritation and stimulation of the chemoreceptor center in the medulla, thus acting both peripherally and centrally on the vomiting center. In cats, 2.2–6.6 ml of the 7% ipecac in glycerin syrup/kg orally will produce vomition. The latency period decreases as the dose is increased. Vomition is caused by 2.2 ml/kg in 52 minutes while 6.6 ml/kg cause vomition in 12 minutes.

Local Emetics

A number of substances of varying reliability, availability, and safety can be used to induce emesis by irritating the GI mucosa or that of the pharyngeal region. In the case of poisoning with noncorrosive substances, a helpful procedure is administration of warm water by stomach tube, which dilutes the poison and may induce emesis. The addition of household detergent or soap to the water in quantities sufficient to make a good soapy solution enhances the possibility of vomition, particularly if given as a drench.

Copper sulfate solution will often produce emesis in dogs without damaging the GI tract. A single dose of copper sulfate is not sufficient to cause copper toxicity, due to its poor absorption. Fifty ml of a 1% solution have been recommended, with emesis occurring in about 10 minutes. Zinc sulfate solution at a similar level also has been used to produce vomition but is less reliable than copper sulfate.

A pinch of plain table salt or any neutral salt crystals placed in the pharyngeal region may induce emesis in dogs. This can be a practical technique for the pet owner at home in an emergency situation. The same can be said for a detergent solution that would be readily available in most households. Due to variability in their effect, other emetics such as ground mustard seed and tartar emetic are not in common use today.

ANTEMETICS

The most common use for antemetics in veterinary medicine is as a prophylactic measure for motion sickness in pets being transported, and occasionally antemetics are used in the treatment of chronic gastritis. Prolonged irritation of the gastric mucosa can lead to chronic vomition and serious electrolyte and fluid imbalances. Normally the chloride ion that is secreted by the gastric mucosa is reabsorbed in the small intestine. With prolonged vomition, chloride is lost and the animal develops a metabolic alkalosis. In addition, sodium and potassium deficiencies also develop because of losses in the vomitus and urine. Sodium and potassium bicarbonate are excreted in the urine as a result of renal compensation of the metabolic alkalosis. Isotonic sodium chloride fluids, with 20–25 mEq/L of potassium chloride added, should be given to replace these losses and restore normal body fluid, electrolyte, and acid-base balance. If there is renal shutdown and anuria, potassium should not be given until this is corrected.

In the case of nonspecific or undiagnosed vomition, it is preferable to determine the cause before applying palliative measures that may alter the symptomology and prevent a diagnosis of the true problem. The urge to treat these symptoms prior to diagnosis should be restrained for the long-term benefit of the patient.

Various agents have been used to counteract vomition caused by irritation or inflammation of the upper digestive tract. Protective agents include kaolin, pectin, and bismuth salts, as discussed in the previous chapter. They are generally of limited benefit. Gastric sedatives may be more effective. These include parasympatholytic drugs and local anesthetics administered orally. CNS sedatives such as barbiturates or chloral hydrate have also been advocated as potential depressants of the emetic center.

Antihistamines

The most effective of the centrally acting antemetics are certain of the antihistamine compounds (see Chapter 21 for a more complete description of the actions of antihistamines). Not all antihistamines possess antemetic activity. Those with specific antemetic activity do not directly depress the vomiting center. Some, such as diphenhydramine (Benadryl) and its active moiety, dimenhydramine (Dramamine), act on the chemoreceptor trigger zone and the vestibular apparatus of the inner ear. Others, such as chlorpromazine, a phenothiazine derivative, act centrally as well as peripherally against vomition induced by GI irritation. Benadryl is reported to be the most effective in human beings against emesis induced by opiate drugs or motion sickness (Moyer 1957). Antihistamines should be administered approximately 30 minutes prior to traveling. An oral dose of Benadryl (4–5 mg/kg) gives satisfactory antemetic activity for 4–6 hours with minimal sedation. Meclizine hydrochloride (Bonine), a piperazine type of antihistamine, is also an effective antemetic in the dog and human being. Meclizine will provide antemetic activity for 12–24 hours, causes minimal or no depression, and has no cumulative effect. The dosage for dogs weighing less than 20 kg is 25 mg daily. For larger dogs the dose is 50 mg.

Chlorpromazine is also used to combat motion sickness when, in addition to antemetic activity, tranquilization is desired. It has antemetic activity in the dog following parenteral or oral administration. Paradoxically, oral administration may induce vomition prior to its antemetic activity. The claim by manufacturers that chlorpromazine has antemetic action in the cat is questionable. It is known that chlorpromazine fails to inhibit apomorphine-induced emesis in the cat (Brand et al. 1954). For additional information see Chapter 17 on tranquilizers.

INTESTINAL MOTILITY INHIBITORS

Parasympatholytics

The major agents used to decrease intestinal motility are the parasympatholytics. These drugs, in addition to decreasing GI motility, will inhibit other parasympathetic activities, such as salivary and gastric secretions. They also reduce vagal tone on the cardiovascular system. The principal actions of the antimuscarinic or parasympatholytic drugs are covered in Chapter 8. Certain of the actions of some parasympatholytic drugs have been called antispasmodic in that they have a direct inhibitory action on the smooth muscle of the GI tract and reduce peristaltic activity. This particular action is a basis for the inclusion of pharmacologic agents such as the belladonna alkaloids, atropine and scopolamine, and a number of substituted and synthetic analogs, such as isopropamide and benzetimide in antidiarrheal therapy. It is generally believed that increased intestinal motility is associated with diarrhea. This common tenet is based on little evidence and undoubtedly is not true in many instances (Christensen 1971). Antispasmodics also are used routinely in horses for colic when it is suspected that there is an increase in intestinal motility. However, the more fundamental problem is intestinal stasis, and antispasmodics should be used with caution (Coffman and Garner 1972). For recommended dosage and usage of parasympatholytic drugs in treating digestive conditions, refer to Chapter 8.

Opiates

The opiate drugs, powdered *Opium*, U.S.P., and *Paregoric*, U.S.P., have been used for centuries for the treatment of diarrhea and dysentery. Paregoric is a 4% opium tincture in which there is also benzoic acid, camphor, and oil of anise. Opium is its only active ingredient. The usual dosage of paregoric in the dog is 1–3 ml and in the horse is 4–6 ml/100 kg of body weight. The use of opiate drugs as emetics was discussed previously in this chapter and more completely in Chapter 15. The effects of the opiates on the bowel may vary widely, depending on the species and the dosage. In general, opiates decrease gastric motility, greatly delay gastric emptying, markedly decrease large and small intestinal propulsive contractions, increase large intestinal tone to the point of spasm, and increase ileocecal valve and sphincter tone. These actions make the opiate drugs very effective agents for causing constipation and treating diarrhea and dysentery due to a number of causes. However, after their long-term usage, chronic diarrhea may occur, which will initially worsen upon opiate drug discontinuance (Cohen and Pops 1968).

Two drugs, methampyrone (Novin) and coecolysin bengen, used in veterinary medicine in the treatment of suspected cases of altered GI motility have recently been shown to have no effect in this regard (Gray and Yano 1975). Mention is made only because of their wide usage. Methampyrone is used in the treatment of colic in the horse and for GI spasm or hypermotility in several species. Coecolysin bengen, a commercial intestinal extract, was found to contain histamine as its only significant active ingredient.

CATHARTICS AND LAXATIVES

Cathartics and laxatives are drugs that promote defecation. The terms catharsis and laxative imply different intensities of drug effect. Cathartic effect implies a more fluid evacuation, whereas laxative effect suggests excretion of a soft, formed stool. Cathartics invariably increase the activity of the parasympathetic nervous system, either directly or reflexly. The increased intestinal motor activity promotes the more rapid passage of ingesta. This occurs directly with parasympathomimetic drugs. Others, such as the saline cathartics, act by increasing the bulk of ingesta in the intestinal tract, in which case increased distention increases parasympathetic activity and promotes defecation. A third possibility is to cause irritation to the mucosa, which results in a reflex enhancement of parasympathetic activity. Some cathartics may also alter electrolyte transport, although specific mechanisms have not been well delineated. Laxatives may also increase peristalsis, but to a milder degree than cathartics, or they may merely increase the hydration and softness of the stool. A drug designated as a cathartic can, and often should, be administered only in a dosage that will produce a laxative rather than a cathartic effect. Cathartics and laxatives are classified in Table 35.2 on the basis of their general mechanisms of action.

TABLE 35.2. Classification of cathartics and laxatives

Stimulant cathartics	Parasympathomimetics Castor oil Emodin (anthraquinones) Cascara sagrada Danthron
Saline cathartics	Magnesium salts Sodium sulfate (Glauber's salt)
Bulk-forming laxatives	Hydrophilic colloids Agar, tragacanth Acacia Plantago (Metamucil, Konsyl) Methylcellulose Bran
Emollient (lubricant) laxatives	Mineral oil Vegetable oils Surface-active agents Dioctyl sodium sulfosuccinate Dioctyl calcium sulfosuccinate (Surfak) Poloxalkol
Seldom used cathartics	Aloe, senna, rhubarb, podophyllum, phenophthalein, calomel (HgCl), croton oil

Cathartics and laxatives have a long history of use and misuse in human beings and animals. Purgative drugs were among the first to be recognized, and catharsis or purging was considered equivalent to cleansing the body. Many plant-derived, more irritant cathartics cannot be justifiably used today. Equally effective drugs with less toxic potential are available. The overall tendency in medical practice has been a decreasing use of cathartics. In cases of constipation or intestinal impaction, therapy of the underlying cause should be the prime consideration rather than treating the symptomology. However, symptomatic relief can be an important consideration and occasionally purging is desirable. A laxative effect may be extremely valuable in softening intestinal compaction and lubricating the feces so that stools may be passed with less straining.

Stimulant Cathartics

PARASYMPATHOMIMETIC DRUGS

Parasympathomimetic or cholinergic drugs directly stimulate the parasympathetic nervous system. Their overall action and uses are covered in more detail in Chapter 8. Considered as a group, their action on the GI tract is stimulatory. Salivary, gastric, and intestinal secretory rates are enhanced, as is motility. The net result is increased fluid in the intestinal tract and an increased rate of ingesta movement. As a result of these actions, there is a more rapid passage of a looser stool. Cholinergic drugs, therefore, have been widely used for their cathartic action. The principal cholinergic drugs used in veterinary pharmacology for their stimulatory effect on the GI tract are listed in Table 35.3. Intact innervation of the bowel is necessary for full parasympathomimetic action. These drugs should not be used when mechanical obstruction of the intestine is present or when the viability of the bowel is doubtful.

TABLE 35.3. Parasympathomimetic drugs used for their cathartic effect

Drug	Action
Carbachol, U.S.P., Lentin (carbamylcholine chloride)	Substituted choline ester
Neostigmine Bromide, U.S.P. (Prostigmin bromide)	Anticholinesterase
Physostigmine Salicylate, U.S.P. (eserine salicylate)	Anticholinesterase

Carbachol produces GI effects with minimum cardiovascular effects after subcutaneous or oral doses. The incidence and severity of toxic effects from carbachol are greatly increased after intravenous or intramuscular injections. Therefore, it should not be administered by these routes. In contrast to neostigmine, carbachol is effective for gastric atony in the absence of vagal innervation. It may also be of value in some cases of congenital megacolon. For this purpose, carbachol is given orally in small doses; the dose is gradually increased until optimum benefit is obtained. The recommended dosages for carbachol and neostigmine are presented in Chapter 8.

Neostigmine is often considered the drug of choice for facilitating transport and expulsion of intestinal contents in patients with nonobstructive paralytic ileus, particularly because side effects are minimal (bronchospasms, miosis, hypotension, etc.). It is preferred to physostigmine. Peristaltic activity commences 10–30 minutes after parenteral administration and 2–4 hours after oral administration. At one time pilocarpine was used to induce catharsis but it is now used primarily as a miotic agent.

IRRITANT CATHARTICS

The major irritant cathartics presently in use are castor oil and the emodin drugs. The principal action of these drugs is to irritate the intestinal mucosa, reflexly stimulating peristaltic activity. However, they may also act directly on the intestinal musculature, or even alter electrolyte and water transport causing increased intestinal secretion and decreased net absorption. The enhanced motor activity may be due in part to bowel distension. The net result is an increased rate of ingesta passage and a more fluid feces.

Many of the irritant cathartics are not in common use today, due to their drastic effects on the bowel. Equally effective and less dangerous products are available. Most of the highly active drugs are listed at the end of this chapter under the heading Seldom-used Cathartics.

Castor Oil, U.S.P., is the triglyceride of the unsaturated fatty acid ricinoleic acid ($C_{17}H_{32}OHCOOH$). It is obtained from the seeds of the castor bean *Ricinus communis.* It is a bland and soothing oil externally and can be used for topical application. Taken internally it is hydrolyzed by lipases in the small intestine to the free fatty acid. Ricinoleic acid is quite irritant and brings about rapid evacuation of the small and large intestines. Unlike the other irritant cathartics, which act primarily on the large intestine with a latency period of 6 hours, castor oil acts primarily on the small intestine, usually producing a more thorough catharsis. In small animals catharsis begins only 1–2 hours after giving castor oil, and soft feces are generally passed for 2–8 hours. The delay is dose dependent, larger doses yielding more immediate evacuation.

Castor oil has been used primarily in dogs and cats with some use in preruminant calves and foals. Larger doses may so completely empty the intestinal tract that defecation may not occur again for several days and constipation may result. A high bulk diet is recommended following its use. Castor oil is administered orally in the following amounts: cats, 3–15 ml; dogs, 5–25 ml; swine, 50–150 ml; calves and foals, 50–100 ml.

A portion of the ricinoleic acid, from castor oil digestion, is absorbed and metabolized in the body like other fatty acids. In lactating animals, after absorption a sufficient quantity may be secreted in the milk to cause a cathartic effect in the young. Castor beans also contain a toxic protein component, ricin, that is water soluble and not present in castor oil. Ricin has caused acute poisoning in children and pets.

EMODIN (ANTHRAQUINONE, ANTHRACENE) CATHARTICS

The emodin cathartics represent a group of natural and synthetic products in which the active ingredients are anthraquinone derivatives related to emodin (1,3,8,-trihydroxy-6-methyl-anthraquinone) whose structure is shown in Fig. 35.1.

In natural products emodin is present as inactive glycosides. Hydrolytic cleavage of the glycoside, releasing the active emodin, is necessary for cathartic action. The principal drugs in this group are cascara sagrada, danthron, and senna. Although these drugs possess many actions in common, their properties vary. This is due to both the rate of glycosidic hydrolysis and the presence of other constituents that may bind the active principle.

Very little hydrolysis occurs until the naturally occurring drugs reach the large intestine. Therefore, the emodin cathartics are slow to act. Generally defecation does not occur sooner than 6 hours following administration. Thus the emodin cathartics, in contrast to castor oil, exert their effect only on the lower portions of the digestive tract. They promote strong propulsive movements in the colon, resulting in defecation. As with castor oil, some of the active emodin may be absorbed and secreted in the milk, causing catharsis in the suckling young.

Cascara Sagrada, U.S.P., is an emodin cathartic drug native to western United States. It is obtained from the bark of the California buckthorn tree, *Rhamnus purshiana.* It was used as a cathartic by the American Indians. The active principle is

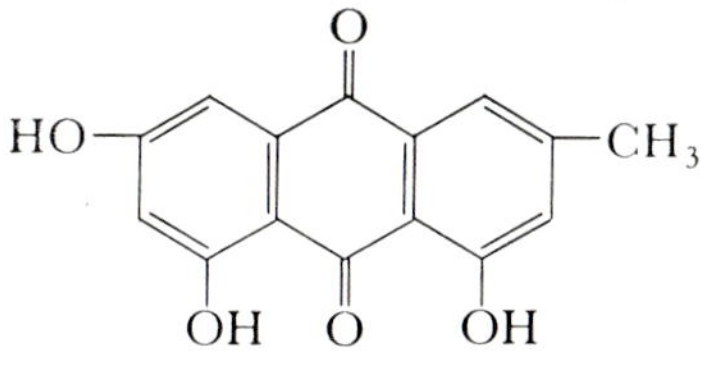

Emodin (trioxymethyl-anthraquinone)

FIG. 35.1.

emodin, which represents 1.4%–2% of the bark. The action of cascara sagrada is mild, usually causing a single soft or semifluid stool 6–10 hours after administration. It has the advantage of rarely causing colic. The drug is given as a pill or in a fluid extract. The suggested dosage of the pure drug is 0.2–0.5 g in the dog and 0.012–0.25 g in the cat.

Danthron, N.F. (Istizin, 1-8-dihydroxyanthraquinone), is a synthetic emodinlike free anthraquinone rather than a glycoside. In spite of the absence of the glycoside linkage, its pharmacological action is similar to natural anthraquinones. Danthron is a yellow crystalline powder with low solubility in water. Some of the drug is absorbed and subsequently excreted as a red dye in the urine. Dosages of danthron are: horses, 10–30 g; cattle, 20–45 g; foals and calves, 3–5 g; sheep, 4–6 g; and cats, 0.2–1 g.

SALINE CATHARTICS

The saline cathartics are soluble salts of poorly absorbed ions. Magnesium is the most commonly used cation. Sulfate, phosphate, tartrate, and citrate are all poorly absorbed anions. The basis for the action of saline cathartics is their slow and incomplete absorption and their ability to ionize. By remaining in the digestive tract they retain water by osmotic action. They do not need to be hypertonic to exert this effect. The increased bulk of intestinal contents reflexly stimulates peristaltic activity throughout the intestinal tract. In the colon the osmotic activity of the ions prevents the absorption of water and more hydrated feces are passed, generally within 3–6 hours after administration.

Saline cathartics have the advantage of being nonirritating to the GI mucosa, relatively inexpensive, and effective in simple-stomached animals. In ruminants saline cathartics are generally less effective and are ineffective in stimulating rumen motility. Some absorption of the component ions occurs and they may exert toxic effects in the systemic circulation. The amount absorbed greatly increases if the salts are not readily passed in the stools. Normally about 20% of the magnesium ions are absorbed from the intestinal tract. If renal function is normal, these ions are rapidly excreted. However, if renal function is impaired, the accumulation of magnesium in body fluids may cause CNS depression. In patients with congestive heart failure or renal dysfunction, sodium cathartics may cause edema and are, therefore, contraindicated. For these reasons, saline cathartics should never be used in patients with intestinal blockage of renal dysfunction.

Saline cathartics have been used as dry compounds in pill or capsule form, as hypertonic solutions, and as isotonic solutions. All three are effective in promoting cathartic action. The dry forms or hypertonic solutions may cause dehydration. This effect may be detrimental in some patients. Conversely, an equimolar quantity of the salt diluted to form an isotonic solution has the same degree of cathartic action without causing dehydration. The use of isotonic or slightly hypertonic solutions is a safer general practice. The difficulty with isotonic solutions is the total volume that must be administered.

A saline cathartic with two nonabsorbable ions is no more or less effective than a product with only one nonabsorbable ion. Relative effectiveness is based on several factors: (1) degree of ionization, (2) number of ions formed, and (3) degree of absorption. For example, if we compare magnesium sulfate (both ions being nonabsorbable) and sodium sulfate (sodium being readily absorbable) and assume complete ionization and equivalent absorption of sulfate ions from both salts, sodium sulfate will be a more effective cathartic. A 100 mM solution of Na_2SO_4 would have an osmolality of 300 mosm. Osmolality is the number of particles in solution. It would contain 200 mM of Na^+ and 100 mM of SO_4^{--}. Equivalent quantities of cations and anions, positive and negative charges, must remain in the gut. Therefore, even though Na^+ is readily absorbable, the presence of 200 mEq of the nonabsorbable SO_4^{--} anions (100 mM times a valence of 2) will prevent the absorption of 200 mEq of Na^+ (200 mM times a valence of 1). Thus 100 mM of Na_2SO_4 will provide 300 nonabsorbable mosm. In contrast, 100 mM of $MgSO_4$ would provide only 200 nonabsorbable mosm (100 mosm of Mg^{++} and 100 mosm of SO_4^{--}) and would be only two-thirds as effective as a cathartic.

Magnesium Sulfate, U.S.P. (Epsom salt), is a widely used saline cathartic. Although it has been used in capsule form, localized irritation of the gastric mucosa may cause vomition. Therefore, it is best administered as an isotonic or slightly hypertonic solution even though the large volume that this requires makes administration more difficult. In practice, solutions up to twice isotonicity will not seriously dehydrate the patient.

The dosages of magnesium sulfate commonly employed are: horses and cattle, 250–1000 g; foals and calves, 25–50 g; sheep and swine, 25–125 g; dogs, 5–25 g; cats, 2–5 g. An isotonic solution contains 34.4 g of $MgSO_4 \cdot 7H_2O/L$.

Milk of Magnesia, U.S.P. (magnesium hydroxide), is a 7%–8.5% aqueous suspension of magnesium hydroxide. It is somewhat slower in action than magnesium sulfate and is considered to be a mild cathartic. In addition, as discussed in Chapter 34, it is a good antacid. The use of milk of magnesia has been restricted to small animals and neonates of larger species. Human preparations are readily available.

Magnesium Oxide (MgO) and *Magnesium Carbonate* ($MgCO_3$) are slightly soluble magnesium cathartics. They are sometimes included in proprietary preparations for their cathartic action. They are more often used as antacids (see Chapter 34) than cathartics. Magnesium citrate solution is rarely used in veterinary medicine. Its chief advantage in human medicine is a pleasant taste, a factor unique in the magnesium cathartics, as most are quite bitter. It is relatively expensive when compared to other saline cathartics.

Sodium Sulfate, N.F. (Glauber's salt), is one of the cheapest yet most effective saline cathartics. It has the added advantage of being less toxic than magnesium cathartics following absorption. Sodium sulfate occurs as large odorless crystals with a very bitter taste. An isotonic solution contains 30 g/L but it is seldom used in such a dilute solution. A more practical approach is twice isotonicity or 60 g/L. Dosages in common use are: horses and cattle, 250–1000 g; foals and calves, 25–50 g; sheep and swine, 25–125 g; dogs, 5–25 g; cats, 2–5 g.

Bulk-forming Laxatives

The bulk-forming laxatives include various polysaccharides and cellulose derivatives that dissolve or swell in water to form a viscous solution that keeps the feces in a soft and hydrated condition. In addition, the indigestible, unabsorbable residue may stimulate peristalsis reflexly. The laxative effect is usually apparent within 12–24 hours, but the full effect is often not achieved until the 2nd or 3rd day of administration. The bulk laxatives may be useful to maintain soft stools and prevent straining when defecating. However, the lubricant laxatives are often preferred for this purpose. In cases of gross intestinal pathology, bulk laxatives may cause intestinal obstruction.

The bulk-forming laxatives include:

1. The hydrophilic semisynthetic cellulose derivatives, *Methylcellulose,* U.S.P., and *Sodium Carboxymethylcellulose,* U.S.P.
2. *Plantago seed preparations,* N.F. (psyllium seed).
3. *Agar,* U.S.P., is generally ineffective.
4. *Tragacanth,* U.S.P., may be a fairly effective bulk laxative but has been reported to cause allergic reactions in human beings.
5. *Wheat bran,* which is often fed to horses as a mild laxative and nutrient material, contains considerable fibrous matter that passes through the alimentary tract undigested. Mares approaching parturition often are fed moistened wheat bran to reduce straining. It may also be beneficial for this purpose following perianal surgery or following repair of vaginal or rectal prolapses, particularly in herbivores. However, lubricant laxatives would be preferred where administration is feasible. Moistening the bran increases its palatability and decreases its dustiness. It should not be fed to animals with intestinal ulceration or with partial or complete stenosis.

Emollient (Lubricant) Laxatives

The major lubricant laxatives are surface-active agents and oils that are not completely absorbed during their passage through the GI tract. These laxatives act to soften the feces without either direct or reflex stimulation of peristalsis. Consequently, their major usefulness is to keep the feces soft and prevent straining when defecating. They have particular value following repair of vaginal or rectal prolapses or perianal surgery when straining should be reduced.

Mineral Oil, U.S.P. (liquid petrolatum), is a mixture of liquid hydrocarbons obtained during the refining of crude oil. The oil is indigestible, nonmetabolizable, and absorbed only to a limited extent. Although it is effective in softening feces, it has the disadvantage of inhibiting the absorption of fat-soluble vitamins. With prolonged use, this may result in fat-soluble vitamin deficiencies. However, this does not preclude its use in correcting more acute problems. It has also been claimed, although not substantiated, that it may interfere with healing of postoperative wounds in the anorectal area and therefore should not be employed following surgery of these areas (Goodman and Gilman 1970). Suggested dosages of mineral oil are: horses and cattle, 250–1000 ml; sheep, 25–150 ml; swine, 25–300 ml; dogs, 5–30 ml; cats, 2–6 ml.

Cottonseed Oil, Corn Oil, Linseed Oil, and *Olive Oil,* U.S.P., can theoretically be used as intestinal laxatives for their lubricant action. They are all partially hydrolyzed and absorbed and must be given in excess of this amount to be effective. They are also more expensive to use than mineral oil. Since a substantial quantity is absorbed and used as an energy source, their prolonged use may result in obesity and nutritional deficiencies. Nutritional deficiencies may develop because the animal's energy requirements are satisfied by the oil and therefore the animal will stop eating before enough other nutrients have been ingested.

Raw linseed oil has been used as a laxative-cathartic, particularly in horses for impaction of the colon. The dosage is 500–750 ml. It acts as a lubricant and, in addition, has an irritant action on the intestinal mucosa when given in large amounts. *Boiled linseed oil must not be used* as it contains lead oxide introduced to enhance its qualities as a paint additive. Some raw linseed oil products used in the paint industry also contain toxic additives. Use of linseed oil in veterinary medicine is quite limited and should be discouraged unless one is sure that unwanted additives are absent.

The major surface-active agents used as lubricant laxatives are *Dioctyl Sodium Sulfosuccinate,* U.S.P.; *Dioctyl Calcium Sulfosuccinate,* N.F. (Surfak); and *Poloxalkol,* N.F. Only Surfak is widely used in veterinary medicine and therefore only it will be discussed. However, there is not much difference between the activity and uses of the 3 drugs.

Surfak is supplied in capsules or solutions containing 50 mg or 1.2% of the anionic surface-active agent dioctyl calcium sulfosuccinate. Surfak solution contains 5% of the saline cathartic sodium citrate. In addition to its use as a laxative, it is also recommended for the removal of excessive waxes from the ear canal. Oral administration produces a modest softening of the feces within 12–48 hours. This effect is attributed to its physical property of lowering surface tension, which is thought to facilitate penetration of the fecal mass by water and fats. It may also affect intestinal motor and secretory function, although this has not been substantiated (Lundholm and Svedmyr 1959; Lish 1961). Excessive doses produce anorexia, vomiting, diarrhea, and colic. The surface-active agents and mineral oil should not be mixed or administered together. The surface-active agent may enhance absorption of the oil, which if absorbed will produce a typical foreign-body reaction.

Seldom-used Cathartics

A number of once popular cathartic agents are rarely used today, although some may still be present in proprietary preparations. Aloe was at one time commonly used as a cathartic in horses. It is an emodin cathartic and one of the more irritating and vigorous preparations. Senna and rhubarb are emodin cathartics that are rarely used today.

A number of "resinous" cathartics were extensively used at one time. They include cambogia, podophyllum, jalap, colocynth, and bryonia. All act on the small intestine, are quite irritating, and produce profuse watery stools and considerable colic. Podophyllum is obtained from the roots of *Podophyllum peltatum,* commonly known as the mayapple or mandrake. It was used as a cathartic by the American Indians.

Croton oil, derived from the seeds of croton plants, is reputed to be the most potent of all cathartics. It is an oil that is hydrolyzed in the intestine to form crotonoleic acid. It is considerably more irritant than castor oil.

Phenolphthalein is a stable crystalline powder. It is occasionally used in human medicine as a cathartic but has been relatively ineffective in veterinary medicine.

Mercurous chloride (calomel) was commonly used as a cathartic but is seldom employed as such today. One problem associated with its use was slow absorption of highly toxic mercury into the bloodstream. Therefore, if it was ineffective as a cathartic and remained in the intestinal tract, it induced mercury poisoning.

REFERENCES

Amend, J. F., and Klavano, P. A. 1973. Xylazine, a new sedative-analgesic with predictable emetic properties in the cat. Vet Med Small Anim Clin 68:741.

Brand, E. D.; Harris, T. D.; Borison, H. L.; and Goodman, L. S. 1954. The antemetic activity of 10-(dimethylaminopropyl)-2-chlorophenothiazine (chlorpromazine) in the dog and cat. J Pharmacol Exp Ther 110:86.

Christensen, J. 1971. The controls of gastrointestinal movements: Some old and new views. N Engl J Med 285:85.

Coffman, J. R., and Garner, H. G. 1972. Acute abdominal diseases of the horse. J Am Vet Med Assoc 161:1195.

Cohen, R. W., and Pops, M. A. 1968. Paradoxical diarrhea with opiates. J Am Med Assoc 205:178.

Goodman, L. S., and Gilman, A., eds. 1970. The Pharmacological Basis of Therapeutics, 4th ed., p. 1028. New York: Macmillan.

Gray, G. W., and Yano, B. L. 1975. A study of the actions of methampyrone and a commercial intestinal extract preparation on intestinal motility. Am J Vet Res 36:201.

Harrison, W. A.; Lipe, W. A.; and Decker, W. J. 1972. Apomorphine induced emesis in the dog: Comparison of routes of administration. J Am Vet Med Assoc 160:85.

Lish, P. M. 1961. Some pharmacologic effects of dioctyl sodium sulfosuccinate on the gastrointestinal tract of the rat. Gastroenterology 41:580.

Lundholm, L., and Svedmyr, N. 1959, The influence of dioctyl sodium sulfosuccinate on the laxative action of some anthraquinone derivatives. Acta Pharmacol Toxicol 15:373.

Moyer, J. H. 1957. Effective antemetic agents. Med Clin North Am (March):405.

Yeary, R. 1972. Syrup of ipecac as an emetic in the cat. J Am Vet Med Assoc 161:1677.

CHAPTER 36

RUMINANT PHARMACOLOGY

ROBERT W. PHILLIPS and LON D. LEWIS

Earliest recorded history deals with the relationship of human beings to ruminants, and there is ample evidence that these ruminants were a major source of animal protein to our early ancestors. Cave drawings in southern Europe, painted 15,000–20,000 years ago in the Paleolithic period, indicate that as human society developed, several ruminant and semiruminant species were domesticated, a process that continues today.

The most widespread and economically successful domestications were the oxen, *Bos taurus,* and the sheep, *Ovis aries.* In certain areas of the world the goat, *Capra agagrius;* the reindeer, *Rangifer tarandus;* and the camel, *Camelus dromedarius,* play an integral part in the economy, supplying food, fiber, and transportation. Domestication has been followed by specialization and increasingly intensive efforts to maximize production either through rate of gain or quality and quantity of wool or milk produced. To achieve maximal production ruminants are encouraged to eat as much as they are capable of utilizing. This common practice, coupled with years of selective breeding for yield, has resulted in animals often balanced precariously on the edge of metabolic dysfunction. The veterinarian's job is to help the stockman maintain his animals in a high production state by prevention of these as well as other diseases. This requires knowledge of metabolism, nutrition, and normal ruminant function.

Ruminants, wild and domestic, have succeeded so well because their upper digestive tract is altered in such a way that they are able to use the energy in cellulose and hemicellulose, which are found in significant amounts in forages. The enzyme cellulase is responsible for the utilization of cellulose by breaking the beta glucopyranosyl bond between the glucose units. No vertebrate, including ruminants, produces cellulase. However, a number of microorganisms do. Herbivorous species, by having these cellulolytic microorganisms in their digestive tracts and being able to absorb and use the products of their digestion, are able to use cellulose for their bodily needs. In contrast, nonherbivores have no means of digesting and therefore utilizing cellulose. Ruminants have made optimal use of this system by having microbial fermentation prior to gastric digestion and the major absorptive surfaces of the small intestine. Not only are the microbial by-products utilized but bacterial and protozoal bodies are subsequently digested. In addition to permitting the ruminants to use cellulose as a nutrient source, the microbes produce large quantities of high-quality proteins as well as many water-soluble vitamins.

The horse and rabbit are notable examples of species in which cellulose fermentation occurs in the cecum after gastric digestion. Although it is believed that there is considerable absorption after cecal fermentation, there may be little utilization of the microbial bodies (Robinson and Slade 1974).

A second characteristic of ruminant species is regurgitation and remastication of partially digested food. This process, called rumination, results in a more complete use of ingested roughage by insuring that there is physical disruption of fibrous material. The processes involved in rumination are covered more thoroughly later.

Ruminants, then, are a diverse group of herbivores, with a specialized anterior digestive tract. They are capable of using cellulose through microbial fermentation and thus can be noncompetitive with human beings in regard to food supply. At the present time in much of the developed world, ruminants are fed high concentrate rations and thus compete with human beings. This, however, is a function of feeding practice, not digestive competence. Ruminants represent the major source of animal protein, milk and meat, for most peoples of the world and are the most important producers of animal fiber. They also serve as beasts of burden in many regions. This chapter is concerned with ruminant function and dysfunction and prophylaxis and therapy of these dysfunctions.

THE FORESTOMACH

The term forestomach refers to the reticulum, rumen, and omasum. These are nonglandular outpouchings of the true stomach or abomasum. In actuality the reticulorumen can be considered a single functional organ, although there are both histological and gross anatomical differences between the two compartments. Some ruminants, such as the camel, have no reticulum.

The following is a general description of the ruminant forestomach (Fig. 36.1). The esophagus, which is thin walled compared to nonruminants, empties into the reticulum at the cardia. There is no discrete cardiac sphincter, but there appear to be constrictions of the striated muscle of the esophagus that function as sphincters and prevent regurgitation. The reticulum is quite small compared to the rumen and connects freely and directly with it over the ruminoreticular fold, a muscular division capable of contraction. The cardia is adjacent to and connected

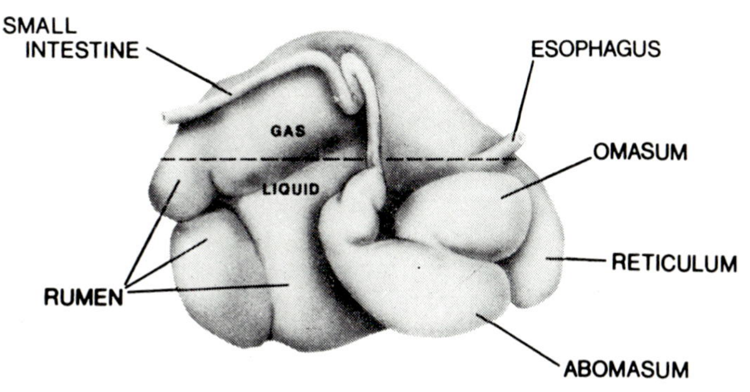

FIG. 36.1. Forestomach and abomasum of the ruminant.

with the esophageal groove. This transverse structure directly connects the esophagus and omasum. Its function in the young is to direct milk into the omasum, bypassing ruminal fermentation. The suckling reflex causes contraction of the muscles comprising the lips or edges of the groove. This forms a tube, in effect, an esophageal extension that can conduct milk directly into the omasum. Although the groove can close in the adult, it is not a normal function but the result of pharmacological levels of certain inorganic salts. In sheep 0.4 M $CuSO_4$ and in cattle 10% $NaHCO_3$ solutions are used to cause esophageal groove closure immediately prior to the administration of drugs or anthelmintics. This is done to cause dosing directly into the abomasum, thereby preventing drug dilution in the rumen contents. However, there is closure for less than 10 seconds after administration.

The rumen is a large elliptical organ. In the mature ruminant, when full, its contents comprise 15%–20% of the animal's weight. It is a wondrously complex and well-regulated continuous fermentation vat in which the following processes are simultaneously proceeding:

1. Mixing
2. Rumination
3. Fermentation of carbohydrates
4. Proteinolysis
5. Microbial growth
6. Protein synthesis
7. Vitamin synthesis
8. Absorption

Under normal dietary conditions, i.e., a diet high in roughage, the rumen contents are in several phases: (1) the lower phase, which is the most fluid and contains large amounts of liquid with partially digested food, particularly grains; (2) the middle phase, which is composed of food particles that have recently entered the rumen and are not yet impregnated with water, primarily the coarser forages; and (3) the upper gaseous phase, which is primarily carbon dioxide and methane that are continuously produced by microbial action (Fig. 36.1).

SALIVARY PRODUCTION

Ruminant salivary production is more voluminous than in nonruminant species. It can be as great as 100–200 L/day in an adult ox and up to 10 L/day in a sheep. Most of this flow is from the parotid salivary glands whose secretion is alkagenic in nature, i.e., they produce a very basic secretion. The parotid gland secretes continuously. Several of the smaller glands are also alkagenic. The submaxillary and sublingual are the major mucogenic glands. The primary mucoprotein of both sheep and cattle contains sialic acid, which is responsible for the viscous nature of the saliva.

Although there is continuous and copious salivary flow, it is increased during feeding. The mucogenic glands normally secrete only small amounts. Their secretion is greatly increased during feeding while the increase in the alkagenic glands is less. The mucogenic glands are not stimulated during rumination, although there is some increase in total salivary flow.

The control of parotid secretion rate has been extensively studied as the gland is readily accessible. Secretion rate is increased by the presence of coarse food near the cardia and the ruminoreticular fold. There are, in addition, receptors in the mouth and esophagus. Afferent pathways are via the vagus, glossopharyngeal, and lingual nerves. Almost all the efferent impulses travel via the glossopharyngeal nerve.

Saliva serves the same function in ruminants that it does in nonruminants, although no salivary amylase is present. In addition, the copious flow helps to keep rumen contents in a fluid state in spite of the considerable absorption that occurs. A second very important and unique function of saliva in the ruminant is the neutralization of organic acids formed during anaerobic fermentation. These acids, which are continuously formed from ingested carbohydrates, would greatly lower the rumen pH were it not for salivary secretion. The alkagenic secretion acts to buffer these acids and keeps the rumen pH near neutrality. It is generally in the range of 6–7 but may fall lower after a meal high in soluble carbohydrates.

As ruminants ingest food there is an initial mastication and ensalivation. The food is then formed into a discrete bolus by the tongue and palate. In the adult ox this bolus is approximately 2.5 cm in diameter and 7–10 cm in length. It is passed to the pharyngeal region by the tongue and thence into the esophagus. Esophageal peristalsis moves the bolus quickly through the cardia into the reticulorumen. Grains are not as discretely formed into boluses as forages, and the grain bolus tends to disintegrate and then sink. Heavy objects rapidly sink so that rocks, nails, wire, etc., tend to accumulate in the bottom of the reticulum. Because of this accumulation and the contractile movements of the reticulum, sharp metal objects may penetrate the reticular wall. This may result in localized or diffuse peritonitis and adhesions. When the penetration occurs anteriorally through the diaphragm, pericarditis and cardiac damage may occur.

RUMEN MOTILITY

Mixing

The reticulorumen has two basic types of muscular contractions believed to result in mixing, although no pattern of ingesta movement has been established. The rate and strength of these contractions are controlled by medullary centers via efferent vagal fibers. There are, in addition, vagal afferent fibers originating from stretch receptors in the rumen wall. The two sequences of movement have been termed A and B. The A sequence is initiated by a reticular contraction that moves posteriorly over the dorsum of the rumen and then ventrally through the posterior ventral blind sac and the ventral rumen. The B movement sequence is initiated in the posterior ventral blind sac, moves progressively up and forward over the dorsal rumen, and terminates in a contraction of the main ventral sac. These mixing movements normally occur 1 to 3 times per minute.

Rumination

In addition to the "mixing" movements, there is a second characteristic ruminal movement that results in regurgitation. It is a component of rumination and occurs when the animal is in a quiescent state, as neither regurgitation nor rumination occurs during excitation. This movement, although involuntary, is controlled and overridden by conscious activity. It proceeds in the following manner. A series of muscular contractions of the reticulum brings some of the coarse ruminal contents in the upper liquid phase into the area of the cardia. This is accomplished by raising the fluid level in this organ. These contractions are usually followed by the A sequence movement of the rumen. Simultaneously, there is an inspiratory effort with a closed glottis, and a quantity of ingesta is brought into the esophagus due to negative pressure. Reverse esophageal peristalsis carries it to the mouth where the fluid portion is squeezed out by compressing the ingesta between the tongue and palate. This fluid is immediately reswallowed. The solid components are thoroughly masticated, reinsalivated, formed into a bolus, and swallowed. At this point, the fibrous roughage has undergone an initial partial mastication, immersion in rumen fluid, some microbial degradation, and a thorough remastication. Its specific gravity is now greater and it tends to sink into the mass of the rumen contents instead of floating on top.

Eructation

The third type of ruminal movement is eructation. It is the expulsion of gas from the upper ruminal phase. Eructation is initiated by receptors sensitive to increased pressure. These are located in the dorsal rumen wall from which afferent vagal fibers arise. There are also eructation inhibitory fibers around the glottis that prevent eructation as long as ruminal contents surround the orifice. In initiating an eructation, a ruminal contraction starts in the dorsal sac of the rumen, goes forward, and down into the reticulum. The esophageal muscular constrictions are relaxed and gas passes up the esophagus (Dougherty 1968). Dysfunction of the eructation mechanism results in the condition known as ruminal bloat, which is covered later in this chapter.

RUMEN MICROBIAL LIFE AND ENVIRONMENT

The relationship between the ruminant and its microbial population is a true synergism. The ruminant provides an anaerobic environment with a constant temperature, pH, and nutrient supply. The anaerobic bacteria and protozoa in turn degrade cellulose and form volatile fatty acids, B vitamins, and bacterial and protozoal proteins. Members of the microbial community are continuously removed by passage into the omasum, abomasum, and small intestine where they are digested and absorbed. The ruminant, in effect, grows and harvests by a continuous system, a very high-quality nutrient supply. One may possibly conclude since protozoa are present and digested that the ruminant is a carnivore, not a herbivore. Perhaps omnivore would be a good term to use for the ruminant as well as for the domesticated dog as the latter is regularly fed large quantities of food having a plant origin.

Bacteria present in the rumen are diverse in their functions. Table 36.1 lists some predominant species, the substrate that they metabolize, and the end products of that metabolism. With high concentrate rations, rumen fluid may contain more than 1×10^{11} bacteria per ml with some species dividing approximately every 20 minutes under favorable conditions. As a result, the total rumen bacteria production in feedlot animals or in dairy cows is tremendous. Conversely, on poor rations or under fasting conditions, bacterial multiplication is slowed and the number of bacteria per ml may be less than 1×10^{8} or over a thousandfold less. When a ruminant's diet is altered, particularly toward higher concentrate or grain rations, which are high in soluble carbohydrates such as starch and low in cellulose, considerable time may be required for stabilization of the ruminal microbial population. Not only will total numbers increase but marked changes will occur in the kinds of bacteria present. If this ration change is made too rapidly, a clinical or subclinical ruminal acidosis may result. Acidosis is discussed in detail later.

Protozoa are less numerous than bacteria, 1×10^{6} per ml under normal conditions. They are primarily ciliates, although some flagellar types are usually

TABLE 36.1. Some ruminal bacteria, their substrates and products

Bacteria	Substrate	Products
Bacteroides spp.	Cellulose, cellobiose, starch, maltose, CO_2	Succinate, acetate, lactate, formate, ethanol
Butyrivibrio	Various carbohydrates	Butyrate, lactate, formate, ethanol
Streptococcus bovis	Starch, sugars	Lactate
Succinimonas amylolytica	Starch, maltose, CO_2	Succinate, acetate, propionate
Selenomonas ruminantium	Various carbohydrates	Acetate, propionate, CO_2
Eubacterium	Glucose, cellobiose	Butyrate, lactate, acetate, formate, CO_2, H_2
Ruminococcus	Cellulose, cellobiose, xylan, CO_2	Succinate, lactate, acetate, formate, H_2
Methanobacterium	CO_2, H_2, formate	CH_4, H_2O

Source: Adapted from Hungate 1968.

present. Protozoa, in general, utilize sugars, starch granules, and bacteria as nutrient sources and deposit ingested carbohydrates as glycogen within their bodies.

The rumen environment is anaerobic and there is a relative abundance of reducing equivalents, i.e., nearly all the nicotinamide adenine dinucleotide (NAD) present is reduced to NADH. Because of the lack of oxygen, ruminal microorganisms are unable to fully use ingested carbohydrates by metabolizing them completely to carbon dioxide and water. Therefore, end products of ruminal carbohydrate fermentation are carbon dioxide; water; methane; lactic acid; and the volatile fatty acids, acetic, propionic and butyric. Energy in the form of adenosine triphosphate (ATP) is needed by the microbial organisms to maintain cellular integrity and perform the functions of growth and multiplication. However, most ATP is derived from oxidation of reduced nucleotides in the cytochrome system, which requires the presence of available oxygen. Under anaerobic conditions, as found in the rumen, maximum use is made of the substrate phosphorylation that occurs during glycolysis and in the citric acid cycle. The excess hydrogen available from glycolysis and the citric acid cycle is used in the synthesis of volatile fatty acids and methane. These products are microbial waste and serve as a mechanism by which these organisms dispose of excess hydrogen. Methane serves well as a hydrogen sink or acceptor. Unfortunately, from the standpoint of energy conservation and utilization, methane is not significantly metabolized in ruminant tissues and is excreted by eructation. It has been estimated that in the adult cow as much as 25 L of methane per hour may be produced and lost. This can represent up to 10% of the animal's digestible energy. To prevent this loss, considerable interest has been focused in recent years on obtaining drugs that inhibit methane production or the methane-producing bacteria (Table 36.1). The other major hydrogen sinks used are pyruvate and acetate, which are transformed to propionate and butyrate, respectively. These compounds are readily used by ruminants after absorption.

RUMINANT PROTEIN METABOLISM

Another important property of ruminal microbes is their ability to convert nonprotein nitrogen (NPN) to amino acids and then to protein. This fact has been known and appreciated for many years and the ruminant with its microbial population is routinely used in modern agriculture to produce high-quality animal protein from inexpensive NPN sources. The most commonly and extensively used NPN source is urea ($NH_2{-}\overset{\overset{\displaystyle O}{\|}}{C}{-}NH_2$), although other NPN sources, such as biuret, and various industrial by-products are also used. Urea is added to the rumen by dietary supplementation and by the ruminantnant itself (see Fig. 36.5). Urea is reabsorbed from the renal tubules into the bloodstream and subsequently passes directly into the rumen from the blood vascular system or indirectly via salivary secretion. It has been estimated that in sheep 1.5 g of urea nitrogen may enter the rumen each day by these two means. To a certain extent, therefore, the ruminant provides its own NPN, formed as a result of normal urea cycle activity in the liver and conserved by renal reabsorption. The actual amount of renal reabsorption varies with the diet. On a percentage basis, much less urea is reabsorbed on a high-protein diet, although the total quantity is greater. Urea, after entering the rumen, is converted to ammonia and carbon dioxide by bacterial ureases. Ammonia is then used for amino acid synthesis by bacteria. Ammonia also will be absorbed from the rumen into the bloodstream. The rate and amount of ammonia absorption from the rumen depend on the rumen ammonia level, the rumen pH, and the dietary constituents present.

There are 22 amino acids. All are required by the cells and tissues of all animals. However, 12–14 can be synthesized in the body by the amination of keto acids. The remaining 8–10 amino acids must be present in the diet of nonherbivorous animals and are therefore called dietarily essential or the essential amino acids. In ruminants (other than the very young), ingested proteins or NPN sources are broken down to their constituent amino acids and ammonia. These compounds are interconverted by bacteria and protozoa to form the amino acids these organisms need for growth and multiplication. These are the same amino acids needed by the animal. Therefore, the ruminant has no dietary requirement for a specific amino acid, i.e., none is dietarily essential. However, adequate proteins must be ingested so that these amino acids may be produced by the ruminal organisms. The ruminant's protein diet is thus dependent more on what the rumen microorganisms have produced than on what the animal has eaten. Both bacterial and protozoal protein are well utilized by the host and have high biological value. Protozoa may be slightly more valuable (Hungate 1968). Biological value of a protein is determined from the amount of the most limiting essential amino acid present in that protein. Recently there has been concern over the adequacy of microbial protein for maximal production. Several investigators have reported that either methionine and/or lysine may be limiting (Mudd and Hooper 1973; Richardson and Hatfield 1975). Other research has demonstrated that microbial protein is sufficient. Which is correct depends on the diet, the ruminal environment and microbial populations, and the type of production being maximized. No overall recommendation can be made for the need to supplement ruminant diets with amino acids or proteins protected to bypass rumen fermentation. Such supplementation must be individualized.

An additional benefit the ruminal microbes provide is to synthesize B vitamins. Under most conditions this supply plus exogenous dietary B vitamin is ample for the ruminant's needs. Cobalt deficiency resulting in vitamin B_{12} deficiency represents a special case (see Ruminant Dysfunction and Chapter 41).

RUMINANT CARBOHYDRATE METABOLISM

The volatile fatty acids (VFA) and lactic acid are continuously absorbed from the rumen via the excellent blood supply in the rumen papillae. Absorption products are rapidly removed and carried by ruminal veins through the portal system to the liver. Although all three of the primary VFA, acetic, propionic, and butyric, are absorbed from the rumen, the mechanisms involved and their subsequent fate in the body are quite different, as illustrated in Fig. 36.2. It has been estimated that the VFA can contribute over 70% of the mature ruminant's daily energy needs. Both D- and L-lactic acid are formed by microbial fermentation. Unfortunately, however, ruminant tissue has little D-lactic dehydrogenase activity so that this metabolite may accumulate in the body after periods of rapid bacterial production, causing a metabolic acidosis.

Acetic Acid

Acetic acid is the VFA formed in the largest quantities. On a molar basis it represents 60%–65% of the absorbed VFA and undergoes only a minimal oxidation in the rumen wall. It is carried through the liver, with little utilization, being oxidized principally by skeletal muscle, mammary gland, or lipid deposits (Fig. 36.2). In addition, this exogenous acetate is the primary source of acetyl-CoA for lipid synthesis. Relatively small amounts of acetyl-CoA for lipid synthesis come from pyruvic decarboxylation. This represents a major difference between ruminant and nonruminant systems.

Propionic Acid

Some propionic acid is oxidized to lactic acid during absorption but most passes to the liver, which removes nearly all of it from the portal blood (Fig. 36.2). Its concentration in the systemic vascular

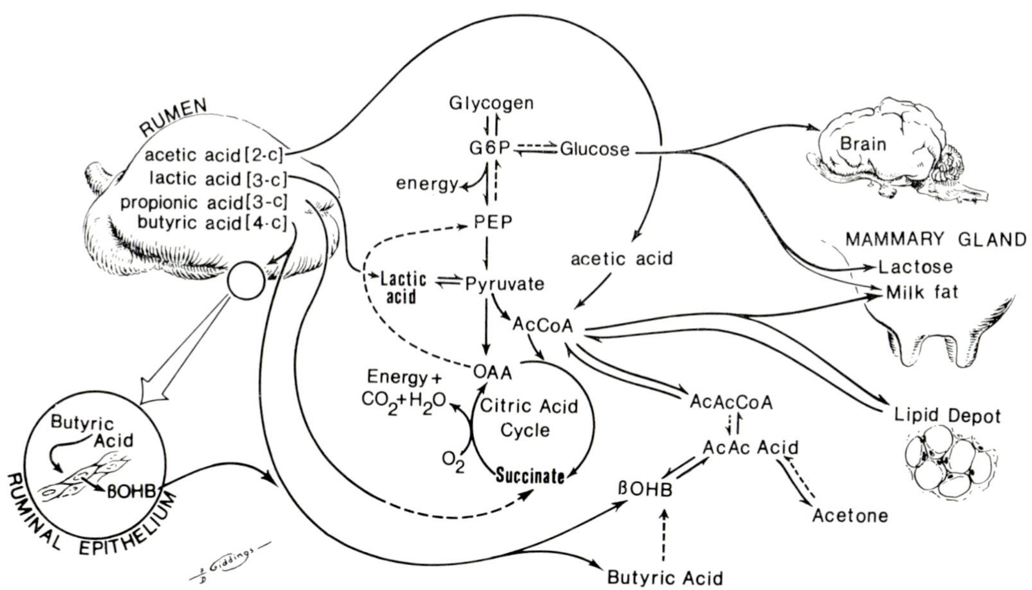

FIG. 36.2. Acetic, propionic, butyric, and lactic acid utilization in the ruminant.
→ = a reaction that can proceed in only one direction
⇌ = a reaction that can proceed in either direction
--- = a reaction that occurs primarily in the liver
— = a reaction that occurs in many tissues

system is therefore negligible. Propionic acid generally represents 20%–25% of the absorbed VFA. This proportion may be higher on concentrate rations and less on roughage rations. It is the most important substrate for hepatic glucose synthesis. The mechanism by which propionate is converted to glucose (Fig. 36.3) involves carbon dioxide fixation to form methylmalonyl-CoA, which is subsequently converted to succinyl-CoA. This step, catalyzed by methylmalonyl-CoA isomerase, requires vitamin B_{12} as a cofactor. Since ruminant microorganisms cannot synthesize vitamin B_{12} without dietary cobalt, a deficiency in this element can result in a starvation ketosis syndrome and hypoglycemia due to the inability of the ruminant to use available propionic acid.

Succinyl-CoA can subsequently be converted via citric acid cycle reactions to oxaloacetate (OAA) (Fig. 36.2). The essential gluconeogenic enzyme, phosphoenolpyruvate carboxykinase, converts this metabolite to phosphoenolpyruvic acid (PEP), which then passes by reverse glycolysis to glucose.

$$\text{Propionic Acid} + \text{HS}-\text{CoA} + \text{ATP} \xrightarrow{\text{Thiokinase}} \text{Propionyl CoA} + \text{AMP} + \text{PPi}$$

$$\text{Propionyl CoA} + CO_2 \xrightarrow[\text{Carboxylase}]{\boxed{\text{Biotin}}} \text{Methyl Malonyl CoA}$$

$$\text{Methyl Malonyl CoA} \xrightarrow[\text{Isomerase}]{\boxed{\text{Cobalamin}}} \text{Succinyl CoA}$$

FIG. 36.3. Metabolism of propionic acid.

The glucose is subsequently released from the liver for use in other tissues. In this process two molecules of propionic acid are converted to one molecule of glucose. Gluconeogenesis from propionic acid is essential for the ruminant since only small quantities of glucose are available following digestion. Other compounds, such as lactic acid, glycerol, and certain amino acids, are gluconeogenic but of lesser importance.

Butyric Acid

Butyric acid, which represents 10%–15% of the absorbed VFA, is metabolized in part to beta-hydroxybutyric acid (βOHB), a ketone body, by the rumen epithelium (Fig. 36.2). When the animal is on a low plane of nutrition, less VFA are formed and essentially all the absorbed butyrate is oxidized by the rumen wall to βOHB. As butyrate production and absorption increase, more butyrate is absorbed unchanged. Most of this butyrate is removed by the liver and oxidized to ketone bodies or to acetate.

RUMINANT DYSFUNCTIONS

When one considers the major noninfectious "dysfunctions" or diseases that affect domestic ruminants, two factors stand out:

1. Most diseases are related to sudden changes in diet, production, or environment, i.e., an induced stress.
2. Many of the diseases are more prevalent in animals with a high production potential.

Many of these ruminant diseases involve dysfunctions of organs other than the rumen. Some are related to excessive production, others to improper nutritional management, and many to combinations of these two factors. These factors result in metabolic dysfunctions and disease. In addition, other diseases are often associated with an initiating stress factor or combination of factors, such as transport, cold, humidity, fasting, and dehydration. Table 36.2 lists the most prevalent of these ruminant diseases, as well as the dietary state and initiating cause. It is outside the scope of this text to discuss all these disturbances in detail from the standpoint of pathogenesis and clinical and pathological manifestations. A brief summary will be presented, however, to emphasize their pharmacological and nutritional management with respect to both prevention and therapy. Parturient paresis is discussed in Chapter 40 and grass tetany and cobalt deficiency in Chapter 41.

The pattern for presentation will be first to cover those conditions that represent an initial ruminal dysfunction, for example, bloat and gastrointestinal (GI) acidosis. For convenience these will be termed primary rumen dysfunctions. The second group to be presented will be secondary rumen dysfunction, for example, ketosis. There is a great deal of overlap and no metabolic disease is restricted to one system.

Primary Dysfunctions

BLOAT, TYMPANITES

Bloat is an excessive accumulation of gas in the rumen. These gases are a normal product of rumen fermentation. Excessive ruminal gas production will not cause bloat unless there is a failure or inability to eructate this gas. Esophageal obstruction or any other factor preventing normal eructation, which was previously described, will result in the accumulation of free gas in the rumen, a nonfrothy bloat. This may occur in Hereford cattle as a result of a congenital condition perhaps due to anatomical alterations in the reticular area. In other chronic bloating animals, there may be an inability to eructate, due to a variety of undetermined causes or to inadequate salivary secretion. Nonfrothy bloat is the least common form of bloat encountered.

The most common form of bloat is due to excessive foaming of ruminal digesta. Gas becomes trapped in the foam and cannot be eructated. In addition, foam inhibits eructation (Johns 1965).

TABLE 36.2. **Metabolic and GI disorders of ruminants**

Condition	Animal	Ration	Physiologic State	Initiating Cause
Bloat	Cattle, sheep	High grain, legume	Varied, occurs on pasture or feedlot	Inability to eructate, may be associated with foam, excessive gas
Ruminal parakeratosis	Feedlot cattle, dairy cows	High grain	High grain over prolonged period	Presumed due to changing ruminal environment to high grain, low roughage ration
Ammonia (urea) toxicity	All ruminants	Excess nonprotein nitrogen	Varied	Rapid release of ruminal NH_3 and its absorption
Traumatic reticulitis	All	Any	Varied onset, often following parturition	Penetration of the reticulum by a sharp piece of metal previously ingested
GI acidosis	All ruminants	Sudden change to grain, low roughage	Grain overload	Excessive starch fermentation to organic and lactic acids
Liver abscesses	Feedlot cattle	High grain	High grain over prolonged period	Presumed associated with ruminal acidosis and increased number of bacteria penetrating vascular system across rumen epithelium
Abomasal displacement	Lactating dairy cow	High grain	Generally within 1 month of parturition	May be associated with GI acidosis, parturition, hypocalcemia, ketosis
Abomasal ulcers	Cattle	High grain, nursing calves	Lactation, feedlot, nursing	May be associated with GI acidosis and in calves "stress"
Abomasal impaction	Adult cattle	Often coarse roughage, inadequate water	Generally pregnant	Pyloric obstruction, abomasal adhesions
Polioencephalo malacia	Growing animals	Generally high grain	Often associated with higher concentrate ration	Increase of thiaminase activity in rumen, may be associated with gastrointestinal acidosis
Lactation ketosis	Dairy cow	High grain	Approaching peak milk production	Excessive glucose drain, lipid mobilization
Pregnancy ketosis (toxemia)	Ewe, rarely cow	Often inadequate	Terminal pregnancy	Excessive glucose drain, with inadequate intake
Transport tetany	Cows, ewes, feeder lambs	Fasting	Prolonged transportation or stress, increased during lactation	Dehydration, fasting, "stress"
Parturient paresis	Dairy cow	High calcium prepartum	Onset of lactation	Inability to mobilize body calcium stores rapidly
Grass tetany	Cow	Fresh spring grass	Lactating	Decreased magnesium absorption
Downer cow syndrome*	Adult cow	Any	Generally following parturition, also late pregnancy	Total body potassium deficit, hypocalcemia, hypophosphotemia, ketosis, cachexia
Wasting disease	All	Low in cobalt	Varied	Vitamin B_{12} deficiency; inability to support gluconeogenesis from propionic acid

* May also occur as a result of trauma, infectious conditions, and toxicities.

Frothy bloat is classified into two types; one is seen when legume pastures are grazed and the other occurs when high concentrate rations are fed, as in the feedlot. Both are similar in that excessive foaming of ruminal digesta is involved (Bartley 1965). Feedlot bloat occurs most frequently when cattle are on full feed and is associated with an increase in ruminal acidity. Major causes appear to be excessive concentrate intake and too fine feed particle size (Hironaka and Ching 1974). Legume bloat may occur when grazing either alfalfa or clover. Alfalfa is most often incriminated in North America, while clovers are more frequently associated with bloat in Australia and New Zealand.

A number of theories have been advanced to explain the occurrence of the stable gas bubbles causing frothy bloat. A few of the more prevalent suggestions are:

1. Increased bacterial slime, i.e., mucopolysaccharides capable of forming a stable froth.
2. An increase in ribonucleic acid (RNA) in the rumen as a result of destruction of protozoal cell bodies. RNA might increase viscosity and the tendency to bloat. A necessary corollary of this theory is a slow RNA turnover in rumen fluids.
3. A genetic tendency to bloat. Calves from "bloater" cows tend to produce less saliva than normal animals. Significance of this observation with regard to froth stabilization is not clear.
4. Saponins present in high concentration in legumes that are capable of stabilizing foams.

Numerous factors both prevent and enhance the coalescing of bubbles and the formation of a stable froth as depicted in Fig. 36.4. Extensive and varied approaches to the control of frothy bloat have been suggested. It seems likely that additional progress in prophylaxis and therapy will

A. Factors Increasing Bloat (Ruminal Froth)

1. Dietary Factors
   a. finely ground feeds
   b. plant pectins
   c. plant proteins
   d. plant saponins
2. Animal Factors
   a. genetic susceptibility
   b. salivary macromolecules
3. Ruminal Microbial Population Factors
   a. mucinolytic bacteria
   b. bacterial slime or mucopolysaccharides
   c. protozoal population

B. Factors Decreasing Bloat (Ruminal Froth)

1. Quantity of Saliva (particularly mucin)
2. Plant Tannins and Flavolans

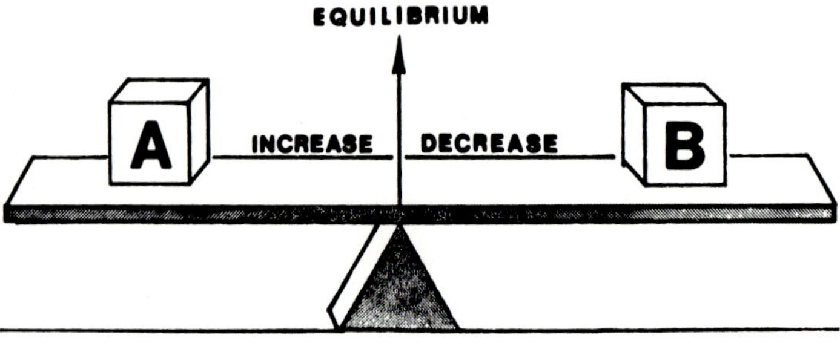

FIG. 36.4. Factors affecting froth stability in the rumen.

occur with enhanced understanding of the factors that lead to bloat.

Prophylaxis. Two of the more effective approaches to the prevention of bloat are (1) decreasing ruminal protozoa, specifically the holotrich protozoa, and (2) breaking down and preventing the formation of a stable foam in the rumen. In a recent study comparing three antibloat compounds, the most beneficial was $CuSO_4$ given orally at 4.4 g/100 kg to kill protozoa. An organic antiprotozoal agent, dioctyl sodium sulphosuccinate, and a surfactant, poloxalene, were also tested. All three decreased the incidence of bloat (Davis and Essig 1972). Some antiprotozoal agents, such as dimetridazole (1, 2-dimethyl-5-nitroimidazole), may decrease food intake, rumen fermentation, and milk production and are therefore of little value as a bloat prophylactic for dairy cattle even though they may decrease the incidence of bloat (Clarke et al. 1969).

The incidence of feedlot bloat may be decreased in three ways:

1. Increasing the feed particle size by adding 8% water to the grain a few hours before rolling it (Hironaka and Ching 1974).
2. Preventing ruminal acidity by maintaining no less than a 9:1 concentrate-roughage ratio in the diet after slowly adapting the animal to this high concentrate ratio.
3. Preventing excessive feed intake following a period of fasting, as often occurs during inclement weather. Animals should be reacclimated to full feed over a period of several days.

For legume bloat, procaine penicillin at a level of 100,000 units orally has been reported to decrease bloat without penicillin residues appearing in milk (Poole et al. 1967). However, continued use of antibiotics to prevent bloat has resulted in a decrease in its effectiveness. In addition, this practice may result in the development of penicillin-resistant organisms.

Several surface-active agents, such as silicone, poloxalene (Therabloat), and pluronic L64 (polyoxypropylene-polyoxyethylene), have been used in control of legume bloat. Initially, silicone appeared to be a good antibloat compound. In further studies it has not proved to be as beneficial as anticipated. For these agents to adequately control bloat, they must be administered on a regular or continuous basis as they are effective for only about 12 hours after intake (Essig and Shawyer 1968). Their addition to salt blocks, concentrates, and water has been used as an alternative to time-consuming daily drenching. If consumption is variable, as may occur particularly with salt blocks, these methods are less effective. A slow release capsule, containing a gel that releases a pluronic surface-active agent, has been reported to be effective for 50 days (Gyles 1970).

Seven percent poloxalene added to salt blocks has been beneficial but may not be completely effective (Essig and Shawyer 1968; Lippke et al. 1970). This is probably due to erratic salt and therefore poloxalene intake, since daily drenching with 25 g of poloxalene/animal has been reported to be quite effective in cattle (Bartley et al. 1967).

Pluronic L64 has been reported to greatly decrease or prevent legume bloat and, in addition, increase milk production. It may be added to the drinking water or given to cattle as a drench twice daily at a level of 7 ml/animal (Wright 1971). In a continuously filling water tank, initially enough pluronic L64 is added to make an 0.8%–1% solution, then an additional 3 ml/cow is added twice daily, or for very bloatogenic pastures, 6 ml/cow. The tank should be kept full by means of a float valve. In this manner the more the animals drink, the more dilute the drug; and the less they drink, the more concentrated, thus maintaining a more uniform intake (Phillips 1968).

Two additional prophylactic approaches to bloat control are selective breeding based on differing heritability to bloat susceptibility (Reid et al. 1972) and the development of bloat-free legumes.

Legumes containing flavolans are less bloatogenic. Flavolans form insoluble protein complexes and prevent foam production. A screening test for the presence of these substances in legumes has been developed. Using these techniques and plant hybridization, it may be possible to obtain bloat-free legumes by incorporating flavolans into existing bloat-inducing legume varieties (Jones et al. 1973).

Treatment. Free-gas bloat is treated by passing a stomach tube, allowing the gas to escape and, if it can be determined, correcting the cause. However, if bloating continues to reoccur, a small (1–2 cm) persistent rumen fistula can be made surgically in the anterior dorsal aspect of the left paralumbar fossa. Frothy bloat should be treated by drenching or administering by stomach tube 10 g of poloxalene/45 kg of body weight. This will generally result in relief within 15–30 minutes. Intraruminal injection of poloxalene will not give satisfactory results (Bartley et al. 1967).

RUMINAL PARAKERATOSIS

Parakeratosis is an increase in keratinized squamous epithelial cells on rumen papillae. It appears to be due to a lack of roughage and to feeding a finely ground diet. There may be decreased absorption and therefore decreased feed efficiency as the keratinization develops. A decrease in feed efficiency due to parakeratosis would be difficult to diagnose as it would occur in the latter stages of the feeding period. At this time, the efficiency of gain is less, due to increased fat deposition. Currently, it is not possible to separate these two processes under field conditions.

Prophylaxis. Addition of roughage to the diet of feedlot animals and increasing feed particle size, as previously described for the prevention of feedlot bloat, will prevent the occurrence of ruminal parakeratosis.

Treatment. There is no treatment as it is not easily recognized antemortem.

AMMONIA (UREA) TOXICITY

An increase in the blood ammonia levels is toxic for two reasons: (1) ammonia is a potent central nervous system (CNS) activity inhibitor and (2) it readily combines with alpha-ketoglutarate, which decreases available citric acid cycle intermediates, resulting in cerebral energy failure and encephalopathy. As shown in Fig. 36.5, an increase in blood ammonia may occur as a result of either excessive absorption from the GI tract or hepatic dysfunction resulting in decreased conversion of ammonia to urea. Excessive absorption from the GI tract occurs as a result of the excessive feeding of a non-protein nitrogen source such as urea. Urea fed at levels of 250 mg/kg is toxic and at 1 g/kg can be fatal for ruminants.

Ruminal bacteria convert urea to carbon dioxide and ammonia and then aminate keto acids to form microbial protein. Thus a nonprotein source of nitrogen is converted to a high-quality protein for subsequent digestion, absorption, and utilization by the animal. This decreases the amount of protein the animal must be fed and is the reason that these nonprotein nitrogen sources, which are a less expensive form of nitrogen than natural proteins, are incorporated into the ration. However, the production of microbial protein from these nonprotein nitrogen sources requires the presence of keto acids. Keto acids are formed primarily from starches and disaccharides from ingested concentrates or grains. Ruminal ammonia formation from urea occurs much faster than keto acids can be aminated. Thus an increase in ruminal ammonia level may occur as a result of either excessive urea intake or inadequate concentrate intake. When this occurs, ammonia is absorbed. If this absorption occurs faster than the liver is able to convert the ammonia to urea, the blood ammonia level increases and toxicity occurs. It should be emphasized that *ammonia is the toxic substance, not urea,* and that "urea toxicity" does not occur as a result of uremia. Uremia, a completely different condition, occurs as a result of renal dysfunction, not excessive urea intake or hepatic dysfunction.

A number of factors modify the de-

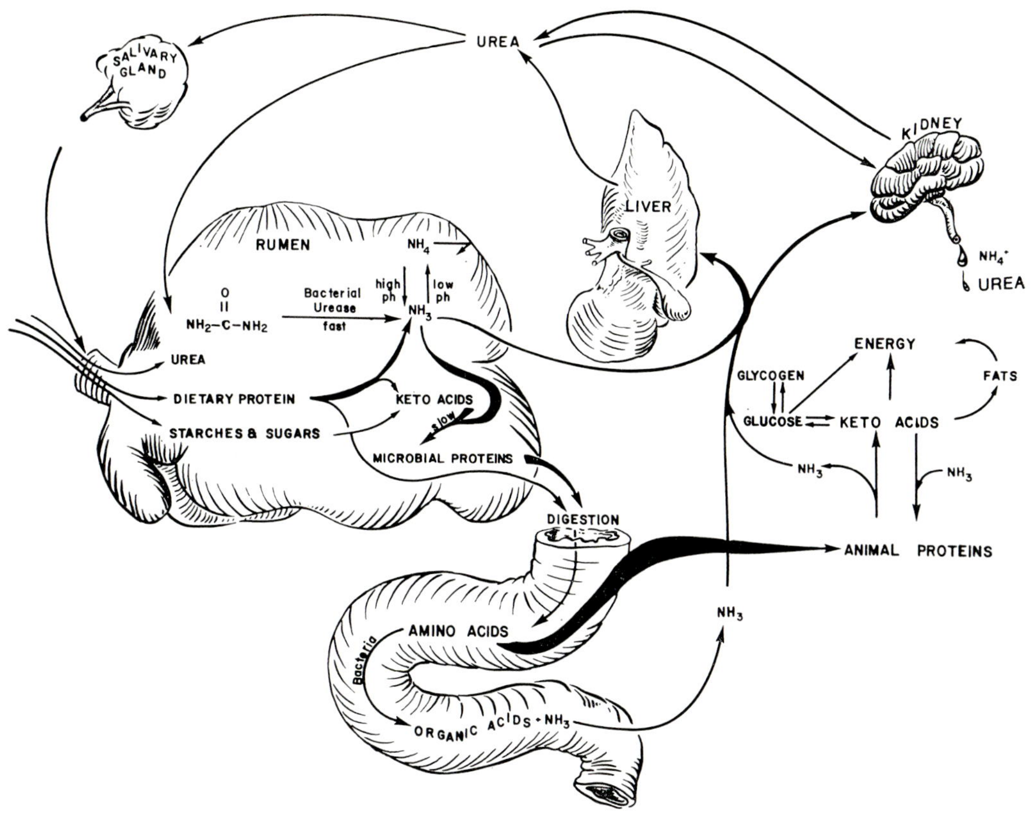

FIG. 36.5. Urea and ammonia utilization and excretion in the ruminant.

gree of toxicity of ingested ammonia-producing sources:

1. *The ammonia source.* Some ammonia-producing substances are broken down and thus release ammonia slower than others, e.g., isobutyl diurea (IBDU) and biuret (a condensation product formed when urea is heated). This permits more time for microbial protein synthesis and lessens the increase in rumen ammonia levels.

2. *Quantity of soluble carbohydrate available.* Readily fermented carbohydrate enhances bacterial growth and nitrogen uptake by microorganisms. It also lowers the rumen pH.

3. *Rumen pH.* The pK_a of the reaction $NH_4^+ \rightleftharpoons NH_3 + H^+$ is 9.02, (i.e., the pH at which there is 50% NH_4^+ and 50% NH_3). At a pH below 9, most of the ammonia will be present as the ammonium ion. Lipid-soluble ammonia readily crosses biological membranes while the ammonium ion does not. Therefore, ammonia will accumulate on the acidic side of a permeable biological membrane. The rumen is normally more acidic than the extracellular fluid (pH of 6–7 versus 7.4). However, ammonia is basic and will increase the rumen pH. If sufficient levels of ammonia are still present after this alkalinization, ammonia will be absorbed. Thus a low rumen pH is important in reducing ammonia absorption (Fig. 36.5). Following absorption and saturation of the body's ammonia-detoxifying mechanisms, ammonia in the blood will partition into the cells due to the lower intracellular pH (7.0) than that present in the blood (7.4).

4. *Ammonia detoxification.* Ruminants have a higher capacity to handle absorbed ammonia than do nonruminant species. This may be due to a greater

hepatic urea-synthesizing ability. However, an alternative hypothesis has recently been advanced (Lewis and Buttery 1973). Glutamate conversion to glutamine effectively removes ammonia from the blood. Ruminants have very high glutamine synthetase activity in several organs, particularly the spleen, the liver, and the brain (Lewis and Buttery 1973). This enzyme increases the amination of glutamate to glutamine effectively, creating an ammonia storage pool. Systemic ammonia levels are decreased until glutamate or glutamate precursors become depleted.

Prophylaxis. Nonprotein nitrogen added to the diet must be mixed thoroughly with the ration. There are several rules of thumb as to the amounts that may be added as given below and in Table 36.3.

1. Not more than one-third of the total nitrogen intake or 125 g of urea/kg of crude protein.
2. Not more than 1% of the total dry matter or 3% of the concentrate dry matter intake.

These are guidelines only, since, as previously discussed, several factors can modify the acceptable level of urea that may be fed. Dairy and beef cattle have been fed diets in which all the nitrogen was in a nonprotein nitrogen form without developing toxicity. However, this is not a practical nutritional regimen.

Slow release forms of urea appear to be effective as nitrogen sources and may be less toxic than urea. Feeding increased levels of concentrates with nonprotein nitrogen will enhance microbial protein synthesis and help to keep the rumen pH more acidic, thus decreasing ammonia absorption.

TABLE 36.3. Recommendations for urea supplementation for cattle

	Intake	
Roughage	Concentrate	Grams of urea/ animal/day
100% of ration	0	0
Free choice	1 kg	50
Minimum	Maximum	100

Therapy. Several approaches should be taken in the treatment of urea or ammonia toxicity:

1. Remove the offending source of nonprotein nitrogen from the diet.
2. Remove ammonia sources from the gut, using cathartics, enemas, and parasympathomimetics (see Chapter 35).
3. Decrease GI bacterial ammonia formation by giving oral antibiotics. Two to 4 mg of neomycin or 10–20 mg of chlortetracycline/kg of body weight every 6–8 hours may be used for this purpose.
4. Decrease ammonia absorption by acidifying the rumen. Two to 3 L of 5% acetic acid (vinegar)/100 kg of body weight by stomach tube with several L of water given every 6–8 hours may be used. Acidic enemas may also be used if necessary.
5. Increase hepatic ammonia detoxification and decrease CNS activity by giving phenobarbital intravenously (see Chapter 14).
6. Prevent ammonia-induced cerebral energy failure and increase hepatic ammonia detoxification by giving large quantities of glucose solutions, preferably by slow intravenous administration (1–2 L of 5% glucose/50 kg of body weight).

Steps 1–4 should be used in all cases of urea toxicity and steps 5 and 6 in severe cases.

TRAUMATIC RETICULITIS

The initiation of traumatic reticulitis resulting from the ingestion of sharp foreign objects and ruminoreticular movements was covered earlier in the chapter.

Prophylaxis. Better management practices should be instituted to decrease the opportunity for animals to ingest sharp metallic objects. Magnetic rods are used to capture metallic objects that are made of iron and prevent their penetration of the reticulum wall. One magnet should be given orally to each animal.

Treatment. Surgical removal of the penetrating objects may be necessary.

GASTROINTESTINAL ACIDOSIS

Different types of microorganisms are required to digest various forms of carbohydrates and other feedstuffs. If the diet is changed, the rumen microbial population must also change so that the necessary microorganisms will be present in sufficient numbers. It requires 3–6 weeks for this adaptation to be completed in the ruminant that has been changed from a high roughage to a high concentrate ration.

Rapid increases in dietary roughage are not harmful. Roughages are high in cellulose or crude fiber that cannot be digested until enough cellulase-containing microorganisms are present. In contrast, rapid increases in concentrates or grains in the diet can be detrimental. Concentrates are high in starch or readily available carbohydrate. These are rapidly broken down into products that can be harmful to the animal when present in large quantities.

The cause of GI acidosis is a rapid increase in the concentrate intake or decrease in the roughage intake, i.e., a rapid increase in the concentrate-roughage ratio. GI acidosis may develop not only when ruminants unaccustomed to concentrates suddenly consume a large quantity but also when the animal that has been on concentrates for several weeks receives a moderate increase. If an animal has been off feed for a day or more for any reason and is put directly back on feed, GI acidosis may develop. In addition, acidosis may occur when the proportion of roughage in the ration is lowered, even though the total concentrate intake is unchanged.

When the concentrate-roughage ratio is increased too rapidly, the following ruminal content changes are seen. Similar changes have been noted in the cecum (Allison et al. 1975). The readily soluble carbohydrates or starches in the concentrate are rapidly fermented to organic acids, thus lowering the pH from a normal of 7 to 6 or less. Gram-positive cocci, primarily *Streptococcus bovis,* increase. A lowering of the ruminal pH decreases rumen motility and appetite, which may cause the animal to go off feed. In addition, a lowered rumen pH decreases the production of acetic acid and increases the production of propionic acid. This change lowers the milk fat content (Annison 1973).

In more severe cases, the ruminal pH continues to fall. At a pH of 5 or less, lactobacilli predominate. Lactobacilli produce lactic acid, further decreasing the pH, often to less than 5. Normal ruminal flora and lactate-utilizing organisms are destroyed at this pH, and rumen motility is completely inhibited. In addition to the increase in ruminal fluid acidity, the osmolality is increased. It may reach 600–800 mosm/L. This occurs because of the breakdown of the large starch molecules into many smaller molecules.

The GI acidity and hypertonicity cause a gastroenteritis. Bacteria, primarily *Fusiformus necrophorus* and *Corynebacterium pyogenes,* and fungi may then invade. Deep ulcers may develop and perforate, causing local or diffuse peritonitis. In addition, these organisms having gained access to the body, may produce metastatic infections in other organs, particularly the liver, resulting in liver abscesses. Toxic products, such as histamine, tyramine, alcohol, thiaminase, and endotoxinlike products, may also be produced and absorbed. These absorbed toxins may cause cardiac, hepatic, CNS, and renal damage (Vestweber and Leipold 1974). The hepatic damage may decrease the body's ability to use lactic acid. The renal damage may cause uremia. The thiaminase may destroy thiamine, resulting in cerebral cortical necrosis or polioencephalomalacia. The absorbed histamine may cause a chronic laminitis (Ahrens 1967; Morrow et al. 1973) and decrease GI motility or tone, which may cause or at least predispose to abomasal displacements. Histamine will greatly decrease abomasal contractions. It has been observed that herds affected with a high incidence of abomasal displacements have been on rations with a high concentrate-roughage ratio.

The lactic acid produced in the rumen is absorbed. It is important to note that both the D and L isomers of lactic acid are produced in and absorbed from the rumen in equal proportions (Dunlop and Hammond 1965). D-lactic acid, however, is slowly metabolized by the liver and disappears from the blood very slowly as compared to L-lactic acid, which is normally the only form produced and metabolized in the body. A severe lactic acidosis with the total plasma lactate increased as much as 20–25 times normal (normal being 10–20 mg/100 ml) may occur. The blood pH may be decreased to as low as 7. Blood glucose and pyruvic acid levels may increase to 2–3 times normal. In the advanced stages of protracted acidosis, plasma calcium and magnesium levels may be decreased to less than one-half normal. In addition, diarrhea and dehydration occur due to the GI fluid hypertonicity (Huber 1971). The ruminal fluid becomes milky gray, has a sour smell, and has a pH of 6 or less. The urine becomes acidic, the specific gravity increases, and the quantity excreted decreases. In severe cases, recumbency, coma, and death can occur as early as 12–24 hours after the dietary insult.

Prophylaxis. The major means of preventing GI acidosis and all its many manifestations is proper nutritional management. Proper nutritional management of the dairy cow is given in Tables 36.4 and 36.5. In addition, prevention for all ruminants should include:

1. Gradual adaptation to an increased concentrate ration (Tremere et al. 1968). This may be accelerated by inoculation with fresh rumen contents from concentrate-adapted animals. Recent preliminary evidence indicates that the addition of a culture of lactate-utilizing organisms such as *Peptococcus asaccharolyticus* will protect roughage-adapted ruminants from rapid exposure to high grain rations (Huber 1975). Such a procedure may prove to be a valuable prophylactic approach.
2. Maintaining a minimum crude fiber content of 14% for fattening cattle and 17% for milking cows of the dry matter intake.
3. Frequent feeding (3–4 times a day) of a complete ration.
4. Feeding up to 5% of an alkalinizing agent as a buffer. Increasing the roughage by 5% instead of adding a buffer has been suggested as a beneficial alternative (Morrison 1973).

Treatment. Treatment of mild cases of ruminal acidosis may require nothing more than correcting the diet by increasing the crude fiber or roughage in the ration. In treating more severe cases, rumenotomy is undoubtedly the best treatment and generally the only treatment that will save an animal that is down or about to go down. It should include emptying the ru-

TABLE 36.4. Nutritional management of the nonlactating dairy cow*

Grass Hay†	Corn Silage‡	44% Protein Supplement	Concentrate Mix§ (grain + protein supplement)
	(kg of feed/600 kg cow/day)		
15	0	0	2.0–2.5
10	15	0.25	2.0–2.5
5	30	0.5	2.0–2.5
0	45	1.0	2.0–2.5

* A 50- to 60-day nonlactation period prior to parturition is necessary for maximum annual milk production. During this period feed any of the four rations listed above depending on the feed available. Limit the amount fed to that indicated. Allow free access to a calcium-free trace mineralized salt and add 2% monosodium phosphate to the concentrate mix. The amounts given represent feeds as they exist and *not* on an air dry or dry matter basis.

† Grass hay is preferred; if not available and 5 kg or more of alfalfa is fed, add 50% monosodium phosphate to the salt.

‡ Corn silage containing 65%–75% moisture and no urea. If 0.5% urea is added when the silage is made, protein supplement is needed only if feeding all silage, in which case feed 0.5 kg/cow/day.

§ Starting 1 week before parturition increase the concentrate fed 0.5 kg/cow/day so that the cow is on full feed, as given in Table 36.5, by 1 week postpartum.

TABLE 36.5. Nutritional management of the lactating dairy cow

Period	Amount of Roughage*		44% Protein Supplement in Concentrate Mix†	Concentrate-Milk Ratio‡
	Alfalfa hay	Corn silage		
First 10 weeks	1.0	0	26 ± 5%	1:4
	0.75	0.25	33 ± 5%	1:4
	0.50	0.50	40 ± 5%	1:4
	0.25	0.75	47 ± 5%	1:4
	0	1.0	54 ± 5%	1:4
Second 10 weeks	1.0	0	0	1:3
	0.75	0.25	6 ± 5%	1:3
	0.50	0.50	12 ± 5%	1:3
	0.25	0.75	18 ± 5%	1:3
	0	1.0	24 ± 5%	1:3
Rest of lactation	Same as second 10 weeks except for very low and very high producers. For cows producing per lactation period:			
	less than 5500 kg of milk			1:4
	more than 8000 kg of milk			1:2.5

* The amount of roughage (on an air or dry matter basis) fed equals the amount of concentrate fed. Depending on the roughage available, either alfalfa or silage may be fed, e.g., if corn silage is not available, use entirely alfalfa as the roughage or if both are available, both may be used in the amounts indicated. See example calculation below. Trace mineralized salt should be available free choice. If grass instead of alfalfa hay is fed, add 50% dicalcium phosphate or bone meal to the salt.

† Based on crude protein of 8%–9% in the silage and grain (corn) and 17% in the alfalfa. If a cereal grain other than corn is used, decrease the protein supplement in the concentrate mix 5%; if poor quality alfalfa or grass hay is fed, increase it 5%; and if 0.5% urea is added to the silage when it is made, decrease it 7%. This ration will provide 17%–18% crude protein in the ration during early lactation and 13%–14% thereafter.

‡ Feed 1 kg of concentrate mix (grain + protein supplement) for each 2.5–4 kg of milk produced/day as indicated by the C-M ratio. See example calculation below. Add 1%–2% dicalcium phosphate or bone meal plus 1% trace mineralized salt to the concentrate mix. If roughage is not green, add 3000–6000 I.U. of vitamin A/kg of concentrate.

Example Calculation:

Feeding ¾ alfalfa and ¼ corn silage (contains 70% moisture) as the roughage source to a cow producing 28 kg of milk/day during the first 10 weeks of lactation, feed the following:

1. Concentrate needed:
   (28 kg milk/day) × (1 kg concentrate/4 kg milk) = 7 kg concentrate/day
   The concentrate would contain ⅔ corn and ⅓ protein supplement.
2. Roughage needed:
   (a) Total amount is always the same as the amount of concentrate being fed, in this case 7 kg/day.
   (b) Alfalfa needed = (¾) × (7) or 5 kg/day
   The amount of moisture in hay can generally be ignored.
   (c) Silage needed = (¼) × (7) or 2 kg of silage dry matter/day
   In this example the corn silage contains 70% moisture, therefore 2/(1.0–0.7) or 7 kg of corn silage is needed.

men, rinsing, reemptying, and finally reinoculating with large quantities of fresh rumen contents from a healthy animal.

Sometimes the ruminal contents can be removed by lavage, particularly in the later stages of the disease after rumen contents have become liquified (Radostits and Magnuson 1971). If lavage is used, after pumping out all ruminal fluid possible,[1] extensive amounts of water should be flushed through the rumen and the rumen then reinoculated with fresh rumen contents from a nonaffected animal.

If it is not possible to remove the rumen contents by rumenotomy or lavage, or to obtain fresh rumen contents, it has been recommended to give orally at least 3 times a day 2–4 mg of neomycin, 10–20 mg of chlortetracyline, or 50 mg of chloramphenicol/kg of body weight (Dunlop 1970–71). An antibacterial agent specific

1. Pumps that will not clog are the PAL all-purpose pump from Peters and Russel, Inc., Springfield, Ohio, or the Marine Bilge pump, BM-124P, from Beckson Mfg., Bridgeport, Connecticut.

for gram-positive bacteria, such as erythromycin (10 mg/kg), may be more beneficial than broad-spectrum antibiotics (Johnson 1975). This therapy will have less effect on the normal ruminal gram-negative bacteria, yet will inhibit the gram-positive organisms responsible for producing the organic acids. Oral alkalinizing agents should not be given, since decreasing GI acidosis without decreasing lactic acid or histamine concentration will increase their absorption (Dirksen 1970; Dunlop 1970).

Regardless of the oral treatment used, or rumenotomy or lavage, supportive parenteral therapy should be instituted and is absolutely necessary in severe cases. It should include:

1. Antihistamines (see Chapter 21).
2. Thiamin (for dosage and routes see treatment for polioencephalomalacia later in this chapter).
3. A calcium-magnesium solution administered subcutaneously (250 ml of a 23% calcium gluconate + 6% magnesium solution) in advanced or prolonged stages of the disease.
4. Fluids intravenously
   a. Six to 10 L/100 kg of body weight.
   b. Ringer's bicarbonate with 50–75 mEq/L of additional bicarbonate and if not in shock 10 mEq/L of additional potassium.

In summary, GI acidosis is caused by a more rapid increase in the concentrate-roughage ratio than that to which the GI flora can adapt. The GI fluid osmolality and acidity increase, causing varying degrees of gastroenteritis. This results in subclinical to severe peracute symptoms that may be associated with or cause:

1. A low milk fat syndrome
2. Hypophagia
3. Laminitis
4. Liver abscesses
5. Displaced abomasum
6. Polioencephalomalacia
7. Feedlot bloat
8. Ulcers that may perforate, causing peritonitis
9. Shock, coma, and death caused by a lactic acidosis, diarrhea, and dehydration, which may occur as early at 12–24 hours after the dietary insult

Mild cases may be treated by merely correcting the diet. In more severe cases, the best treatment consists of emptying the rumen by rumenotomy, flushing, and reinoculating with fresh rumen contents and supportive parenteral therapy.

LIVER ABSCESS

Liver abscesses are commonly seen in feedlot animals at slaughter. Generally, they are not recognized as detrimental during the feeding period. Occasionally, one may rupture, leading to septicemia, peritonitis, and sudden death. Their major importance is due to condemnation of affected livers at slaughter, resulting in an economic loss.

Prophylaxis. The incidence of both liver abscesses and feedlot bloat appears to be closely related to GI acidosis and feed particle size. The same procedures described for the prevention of feedlot bloat and acidosis will assist in decreasing the incidence of liver abscesses. Low levels of antibiotics (70 mg/animal/day for cattle and 15 mg/animal/day for sheep of chlortetracycline, oxytetracycline, or zinc bacitracin) in the feed have for years been reported to decrease the incidence of liver abscesses. These antibiotics are routinely used because of their effect in increasing feed efficiency and rate of gain, usually about 5%–10% (Beeson 1969).

Treatment. Since the condition is not recognized upon antemortem examination, there is no treatment.

ABOMASAL DISPLACEMENT

Abomasal displacement has been recognized for the past 20 years and has apparently increased in incidence. It occurs most often in mature "middle-aged" dairy cows within 1 month after parturition. It appears to be caused by decreased abomasal tone. The abomasum in its normal state of tonicity would be extremely difficult to displace. The cause of the abomasal atony appears to be associated with (1) high concentrate feeding, which may increase abomasal gas production (Svendson 1970); (2) increased use of silage and haylage at the expense of coarse hay; (3) hypocalcemia with or without paresis (Hull and Waas 1973); (4) GI acidosis and its predisposing factors; and (5) an increase in histamine formation.

Prophylaxis. Proper nutritional management is the major means of preventing not only abomasal displacements but also parturient paresis, ketosis, and GI acidosis and all its manifestations. This management includes the frequent feeding of a complete ration (Whitlock 1973) and the proper feeding of the dairy cow as given in Tables 36.4 and 36.5.

A low calcium ration prior to parturition, as recommended in Table 36.4, stimulates increased parathyroid activity and efficiency of intestinal calcium absorption. This, in conjunction with a high calcium ration after parturition, assists in preventing or decreasing the severity of postparturient hypocalcemia and paresis (see Chapter 40). Since calcium is necessary for muscle tone and contraction, hypocalcemia may be partially responsible for abomasal atony and subsequent displacement. Increasing the concentrates in the ration prior to parturition (Table 36.4) allows the ruminal flora to adapt to the high concentrate ration needed for milk production following parturition. This assists in preventing subclinical or clinical GI acidosis. Acidosis decreases GI motility and tone and may be an initiating factor in causing abomasal displacements.

Treatment. Replacement of a left abomasal displacement may occasionally be accomplished by the following means. Cast the cow on the right side, roll her onto her back, and then gently rock her from one side to the other over a 90-degree arc for several minutes. Finally, place the animal on her left side, then at sternal recumbency, and then permit her to stand (Fox 1965). The reverse of this procedure may be tried for right abomasal displacement. If this procedure is not successful, or there is reoccurrence, surgical correction, abomasopexy, is required. Whether surgery is necessary or not, 250–500 ml of *Calcium Borogluconate,* U.S.P., should be given intravenously or subcutaneously. In addition, if dehydration is present, 20 L of isotonic, half NaCl plus half glucose with an additional 20–30 mEq/L of KCl added, should be administered intravenously over 4–8 hours. Ketosis is often present and should be treated as described later in this chapter.

ABOMASAL ULCERS

Abomasal ulcerative conditions probably occur more commonly than diagnosed. From 40% to 90% of all veal calves slaughtered have been reported to have ulcers that were apparently asymptomatic in the living animal (Shires 1974). Several herd outbreaks of perforating abomasal ulcers have been observed in beef calves following inclement weather. The diffuse peritonitis results in sudden death. Clinical and subclinical abomasal ulcers also occur in mature and aged cattle (Fox 1965; Aukema and Breukink 1974). Four clinical manifestations occur, depending on the extent of the involvement: (1) slight hemorrhage with some tarlike material mixed with the feces; (2) profuse hemorrhage, resulting in acute hemorrhagic shock and death within 2–10 hours; (3) perforation with circumscribed peritonitis closely resembling traumatic reticulitis; and (4) perforation with diffuse peritonitis, resulting in death within a few hours to a few days (Fox 1965).

The cause of abomasal ulcers is not known. Many cases are associated with abomasal atony, but it is not known whether this is a predisposing cause or a result. GI acidosis, as previously described, may be a predisposing or causative factor. Stress is known to increase gastric acid secretion via parasympathetic stimulation.

Prophylaxis. Absolute preventative measures are difficult since the etiology and predisposing factors are speculative. Preventing stress and GI acidosis, as previously described, may be beneficial.

Treatment. Anticholinergic drugs are commonly used to decrease gastric acid secretion in the treatment of ulcers in the human patient. However, they are not particularly effective in this regard and will also decrease GI motility and mucous secretion, both of which may be detrimental. Cimetidine, a drug undergoing human clinical trials, decreases gastric acid secretion by over 80% for 5 hours following oral administration of 400 mg, with no observed side effects. It may be of value in the treatment of ulcers but is not commercially available at this time (Richardson and Fordtran 1975). Cimetidine, an analog of metiamide, has its effect in the following manner. Vagal innervation and food stimulate gastric histamine secretion. Histamine in turn binds the H_2 receptor site on the parietal cell, which stimulates gastric acid secretion. Cimetidine and metiamide bind to this receptor site, thus blocking histamine-stimulated gastric acid secretion. Other antihistamines bind only the H_1 histamine receptor sites and therefore have no effect on gastric acid secretion.

If hemorrhage is considerable, Ringers' lactate (6–10 L/100 kg) or preferably blood (2 L/100 kg) should be administered intravenously. Anticoagulants may also be beneficial, as discussed in Chapter 22.

ABOMASAL IMPACTION

Although not a common condition, abomasal impactions are occasionally reported. They generally occur in pregnant beef cows on a coarse roughage diet with limited access to water (Fox 1965; Shires 1974). However, there are other causes such as foreign materials and lymphosarcoma, which obstruct the pylorus, or adhesions, which interefere with motility. Partial anorexia may be observed for several days. Fecal contents diminish and become hard. The rumen becomes distended since fluids are unable to pass the impacted abomasum.

Prophylaxis. Abomasal impaction when due to dietary causes may become a herd problem. Therefore, early correction of the ration may eliminate many cases. Where lush or at least green pasture is available, this is the best corrective ration.

Treatment. Treatment involves removal of the coarse ingesta by surgical or medical means. Laxatives and ruminatorics are ineffective since they do not reach the involved organ. Some success has been reported following the oral use of the surface-active agent dioctyl sodium sulfasuccinate (Shires 1974) (see Chapter 35). Intravenous maintenance fluids may be indicated to combat the dehydration resulting from ruminal fluid sequestration.[2]

POLIOENCEPHALOMALACIA (PEM) OR CEREBROCORTICAL NECROSIS

This metabolic disorder was first described in 1956 and has been reported from several countries where intensive agriculture is practiced. It affects both sheep and cattle, primarily after they have been in the feedlot 6–8 weeks and are on a high concentrate ration (Pierson and Jensen 1975a). However, it may also be seen following changes to lush pastures. In the last few years, the etiology has been clearly demonstrated to be a thiamin deficiency. The basic problem appears to be an increase in, or activation of, ruminal thiaminase so that both dietary and endogenous ruminal thiamin are destroyed. At this time the factors responsible for the increase in thiaminase activity have not been elucidated. *In vitro,* certain anthelmintics and tranquilizers can stimulate its activation (Roberts and Boyd 1974). However, development of PEM probably occurs over a longer time span than would generally be associated with administration of either of these drugs.

2. A maintenance fluid contains 5% glucose plus 20–30 mEq/L of sodium, potassium, chloride, and a bicarbonate equivalent (bicarbonate, acetate, or lactate).

Thiamin deficiency in ruminants, as seen with this condition, results in increased blood pyruvate levels and an inhibition of transketolase activity. Transketolases are thiamin-dependent enzymes. The affected animals show various neurological manifestations that are similar in nature to thiamin deficiency syndromes in nonruminant species.

Prophylaxis. The incidence of increased ruminal thiaminase activity is not predictable. Therefore, prophylactic measures are not currently in use. However, there is some indication that it may be related to subclinical GI acidosis. Preventing acidosis as previously described may decrease the incidence of PEM. Parenteral *Thiamin HCl,* U.S.P., can be used in herd outbreaks to decrease the incidence. The dosage for prophylaxis is the same as for treatment.

Treatment. PEM is treated with thiamin HCl given intramuscularly or intravenously. The recommended dosage in cattle is 1 g/animal and in sheep is 200–500 mg/animal. Repeated treatments at 2-day intervals may be required (Pierson and Jensen 1975a). This amount is probably excessive, as no control studies have been performed to establish a correct dosage. However, thiamin at many times these levels would not be toxic. A recent observation that additional nicotinic acid is necessary for complete restoration of *in vitro* thiamin activity would indicate that therapy using vitamin B complex, and not thiamin alone, may be more beneficial.

Secondary Dysfunctions

bovine or lactation ketosis (acetonemia)

Lactation ketosis is a disease complex affecting primarily high-producing dairy cows. It is typically seen from 1 to 6 weeks postpartum as milk production peaks. Most affected animals are in their peak production years (5–8), although it may occur at any age. Genetic and nutritional factors play an important role in the incidence of this disease. Improper nutritional management and genetic selection for high milk production have resulted in an increased incidence of lactation ketosis. However, a number of related factors can influence the incidence of ketosis in a given animal or herd. There have been a number of recent reviews of this topic. The most comprehensive reports are in a *Journal of Dairy Science Symposium* (Bergman 1971; Emery 1971; Fox 1971; Kronfeld 1971; Schultz 1971). They cover the topic from underlying phenomena to preventive management and clinical treatment.

Although a number of different types of lactation ketosis have been classified, they may be divided as follows:

Primary—spontaneous imbalance in carbohydrate and lipid metabolism as a result of high milk production.

Secondary—inappetence due to some other disease initiates the metabolic imbalance (analogous to fasting ketosis in many cases).

Primary ketosis usually develops slowly during the postpartum period as milk production is rapidly increasing. Milk production requires the synthesis of lactose, casein, and milk fats. During the first few weeks of lactation most dairy cows rely heavily on body reserves to support these activities, are in a negative nitrogen balance, and lose weight. Fig. 36.6 illustrates the metabolic flow necessary for milk production in the normal lactating cow. Protein metabolism, or casein synthesis, is omitted from this figure since most evidence indicates that it is not an important factor in ketosis (Schultz 1971). As illustrated in Fig. 36.2, milk fat is synthesized from acetic and butyric acids, which are absorbed from the rumen, with smaller contributions from the mobilization of body triglycerides (Bergman and Wolff 1971; Annison 1973). Milk lactose is formed from plasma glucose. Glucose is also required by mammary tissue to support milk fat synthesis. In addition, glucose is re-

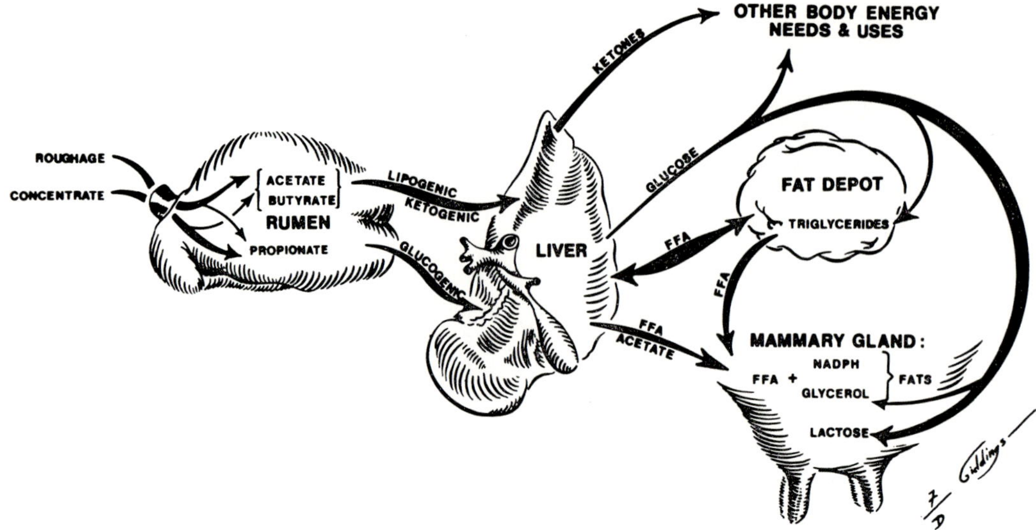

Fig. 36.6. Substrate flow in normal lactating cows.

quired for other body functions. However, in the ruminant, because of microbial fermentation in the rumen, little glucose normally reaches the intestine for absorption. Therefore, most plasma glucose must be synthesized from absorbed glucogenic precursors. Propionic acid is the major glucogenic precursor, although lactate, glycerol, and amino acids may also contribute (Bergman 1973).

It is important to note that no net glucose synthesis can occur from any compound that enters the metabolic pathways via acetyl-CoA (Fig. 36.2). This includes acetic and butyric acids, fats or fatty acids, and ketone bodies. Acetyl-CoA is a 2-carbon compound. Its major routes of metabolism are oxidation and lipid synthesis. During oxidation in the citric acid cycle, 2 molecules of carbon dioxide are given off for each molecule of acetyl-CoA that enters. Thus 2 carbon molecules enter the citric acid cycle via acetyl-CoA and 2 are given off as carbon dioxide, leaving none for the synthesis of any carbon-containing compound such as glucose.

If the demand for glucose exceeds the availability of glucogenic precursors, primary or secondary ketosis may develop. This may occur in the following situations:

1. High milk production or late pregnancy, which requires excessive amounts of glucose and lipids (primary ketosis) (Bergman 1971; Kronfeld 1973).

2. Inadequate intake (secondary ketosis).

3. Decreased glucogenic ability, such as with hepatic dysfunction (Baird et al. 1974) or cobalt deficiency (secondary ketosis). Cobalt is necessary for propionic acid utilization and therefore glucose synthesis from it.

4. Uncontrolled diabetes mellitus, due to a lack of available insulin for glucose transport into cells. This is not commonly considered to be a significant factor in lactation ketosis.

Several characteristics are associated with lactation ketosis. They include an increased mobilization of fat from adipose tissues, which results in an increase in hepatic ketone body production and hyperketonemia. Since the ketone bodies are acidic, a metabolic acidosis develops and the ketones are excreted in the milk and urine. The volatile ketone, acetone, may be excreted via the lungs. Hypoglycemia is commonly associated with lactation ketosis. However, occasionally hyperglycemia may occur. The reason for this is not clear. It may be due to decreased insulin secretion. Hypophagia and decreased milk production occur. Hypophagia worsens the situation by further decreasing the intake of glucogenic precursors.

Current theories of the genesis of ketosis are (1) an excess carbohydrate drain and hepatic inability to cope with increased substrate flow and lack of glucogenic precursors (Baird et al. 1974); (2) a deficiency in glucose formation due to a lack of oxaloacetate, a necessary intermediate in its formation (Krebs 1966); and (3) a deficiency of milk lipid precursors necessitating excessive fat mobilization. Hepatic metabolism of these lipids raises ketone production above the body's ability to use them (Bergman 1971; Kronfeld 1973). Fig. 36.7 illustrates some of the changes in metabolite flow that are commonly seen in ketotic cows compared to normal lactating cows (Fig. 36.6).

Prophylaxis. The continuous pressure to increase milk production to remain economically viable will undoubtedly insure that we will continue to overload our "milk factory's" metabolic system. Unfortunately, there is no absolute method available for prevention of lactation ketosis. However, proper nutritional management, as presented in Tables 36.4 and 36.5, will lessen the incidence of the disease. Dairy cows should be fed according to their milk production. Inadequate concentrate feeding results in a lack of glucogenic precursors and predisposes to ketosis (Fig. 36.7). However, too high a concentrate ration results in a decreased milk fat content, subclinical or clinical GI acidosis, and hypophagia. Hypophagia may then result in a secondary ketosis. Kronfeld and Emery (1970) have presented an easy-to-follow field method for determining if feed intake is adequate. A lactating dairy cow should receive 3 kg hay/100 kg of body weight/day and 1 kg of grain/3 kg of milk produced/day.

If ensilage is fed, it must be supplemented as indicated in Tables 36.4 and 36.5. Some ensilage is quite high in the ketogenic precursors, butyric and acetic acid, and low in glucogenic precursors. Thus, without supplementation with glu-

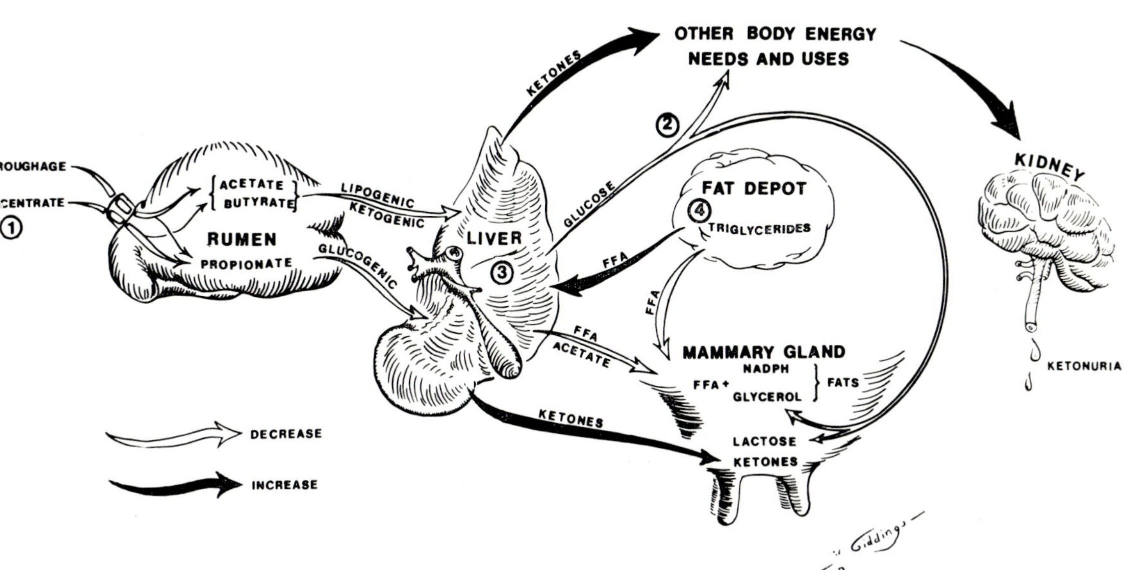

FIG. 36.7. Substrate flow in ketotic lactating cows. Points in prophylaxis and therapy.
(1) Increase glucogenic precursors (propylene glycol)
(2) Increase blood sugar level (glucose IV)
(3) Increase gluconeogenesis (glucocorticoids, ACTH)
(4) Inhibit free fatty acid release
(a) indirectly as a result of increased blood sugar
(b) directly (insulin, niacin)

cogenic precursors, this type of ensilage may predispose to ketosis.

During the nonlactation period, the feed intake must be restricted (Table 36.4). Failure to do this results in excessive fat deposits in the liver. Following parturition, a fatty liver–ketosis syndrome may occur. This may be due to a decrease in hepatic gluconeogenesis or increased lipid mobilization.

Early in lactation, stress and rapid increases in concentrate in the ration may cause the cow to go off feed. As indicated in Table 36.4, the grain should be increased by 0.5 kg/cow/day from 1 week before to 1 week after parturition. The cow should be on full feed by the 2nd week of lactation. If ketosis continues to occur, 125–250 g of either propylene glycol or sodium propionate/cow once or twice a day may be added to the grain ration during this period and for 1–2 months following parturition. Propylene glycol is preferred. These drugs support gluconeogenesis, usually increase milk production, and decrease the occurrence of clinical ketosis (Emery et al. 1964; Schultz 1971; Fisher et al. 1973). They are also a useful adjunct at this same level for supportive therapy.

Routine checks for urine or milk ketones may be used to detect subclinical cases for early treatment, thus preventing the clinical onset of the disease. Rothera's nitroprusside test (Fox 1971) or other easy-to-use commercial products are available. The urine will be positive before milk, as ketones are more concentrated in the urine. Thus urine can provide the earliest warning of impending ketosis. However, often heavily lactating cows have some increase in blood ketones and will give a positive urine test without developing ketosis or requiring prophylaxis or therapy. Therefore, the milk ketone test has been recommended as an indication of the need for prophylaxis (Schultz 1971).

Therapy. Many substances are used in the treatment of ketosis. Some of these are illustrated in Fig. 36.7. Glucose therapy is indicated since most cases are hypoglycemic, and since a cause of ketosis may be inadequate oxaloacetic acid for acetyl-CoA utilization in the citric acid cycle. Glucose is a good source of oxaloacetic acid. Five hundred ml of 50% *Dextrose,* U.S.P. (glucose), are generally given intravenously over a short period of time. This treatment will cause hyperglycemia and often glucosuria; relapses are common. More effective maintenance of the plasma glucose concentration is achieved with slow, 100–200 ml/hour, intravenous infusion of a 40% glucose solution (Roberts and Dye 1951). This procedure has been less used, but improved catherization capabilities for large animals make it more feasible.

Glucocorticoids or adrenocorticotropic hormones (ACTH) are commonly used. Their use, however, is controversial. Although they stimulate gluconeogenesis, they also increase fat and protein catabolism, which may be detrimental. For specific dosage recommendations and equivalences of the various preparations, see Section 8. Two hundred international units of protamine zinc insulin/cow given subcutaneously have also been recommended (Kronfeld and Emery 1970). Insulin decreases fat mobilization and therefore ketone body production. In addition, as previously discussed, some ketotic cows may be hyperglycemic, particularly in the latter stages of the disease, in which case insulin is indicated. All three of the preceding drugs, glucose, glucocorticoids, and insulin, can be used together and are particularly indicated for severe cases. Glucose by itself leads to a high number of relapses. Glucocorticoids by themselves may give unfavorable responses. Since hypoglycemia is present in most cases, insulin by itself is contraindicated.

Additional routine therapy should include oral glucogenic agents and vitamin B complex. Sodium propionate, glycerine, and propylene glycol or propanediol have been used as oral glucogenic agents. They are given at dosages of 125–250 g/cow twice a day for a minimum of 4 days. Sodium propionate, however, is unpalatable. Glycerine is expensive, very rapidly absorbed, converted to glucose, and metabolized; relapses may result. Propylene glycol is more palatable, less expensive, and more slowly converted to glucose via pyruvate and is the drug of choice. Little clinical data indicate the therapeutic benefit of the B vitamins. However, there is ample teleological evidence suggesting they may be beneficial. Cobalamine (B_{12}) is necessary for propionate conversion to glucose. Niacin inhibits free fatty acid release from adipose tissue and has been suggested as being beneficial in ketosis therapy (Schultz 1971; Waterman et al. 1972). Thiamin (B_1) as well as other B vitamins may be beneficial because of possible appetite stimulation and their necessity for metabolic activity. Because of these potential benefits and the lack of detrimental effects, the parenteral administration of vitamin B complex may be indicated.

In severe cases all the preceding treatments, glucose, glucocorticoids, insulin, propylene glycol, and vitamin B complex, are indicated. However, in less severe cases, showing only anorexia, decreased milk production, and ketone body excretion, only propylene glycol may be necessary or desired. In addition to these therapeutic regimes, several others have been advocated, depending to a large extent upon the particular case.

Recently, anabolic steroids have been recommended for the treatment of ketosis. A single intramuscular injection of 120 mg/cow of the synthetic compound trienbolone acetate was reported to quickly restore appetite, lower blood ketone levels, and promote recovery (Heitzman and Walker 1973). If the ketotic cow is hyperexcitable, as in the nervous form of ketosis, 15 g of chloral hydrate may be given orally twice a day. If a fatty liver is present, as indicated by an increase in the plasma lactate and pyruvate levels (Forenbacher 1967), liver biopsy, or history, it may be treated with substances that enhance fat mobilization from the liver. The fatty liver syndrome occurs in dairy cows that are overfed during the nonlactating period. The symptoms occur following parturition and are generally manifested as a persistently recumbent cow ("downer cow") that fails to respond to hypocalcemia and ketosis therapy. Liver biopsies reveal extreme hepatic lipidosis. Methionine, which enhances hepatic choline synthesis, and choline are lipotropic agents reported to be of benefit (Juslin 1965). Favorable response based on clinical impression and liver biopsies has been demonstrated following the administration of 25 g of choline chloride dissolved in 250 ml of sterile water given subcutaneously and repeated in 4 hours either subcutaneously or orally (Lewis and Price 1957; Knight 1975). It may be beneficial to follow this by feeding 30 g/cow/day of the hydroxy analog of methionine (Hydan) or methionine itself. Hydan is not destroyed by ruminal fermentation. It is absorbed and converted to methionine and subsequently to choline in the liver.

It is difficult to evaluate the efficacy of ketosis therapy. Over one-half of the cases of primary ketosis recover without treatment in 1–7 days. Successful treatment of secondary ketosis depends on the successful treatment of the initiating cause of the disease. In addition, extra handling and injections per se may initiate remission.

PREGNANCY TOXEMIA OR PREGNANCY KETOSIS

Pregnancy ketosis occurs in the latter stages of pregnancy in all ruminants. It is most common in the ewe, particularly when there is more than one fetus. Its occurrence is enhanced by poor nutrition and environmental and imposed stress, such as inclement weather and excessive handling. The fetus removes considerable quantities of glucose (Bergman 1963, 1973; Kronfeld 1966) and other nutrients from the ewe. Thus during the latter stages of pregnancy the ewe may be in negative energy balance with regard to her own tissues, particularly if she is receiving inadequate nutrition or is under stress. Blood glucose is lowered, initiating body fat mobilization and subsequently ketosis in the same manner as previously described for lactation ketosis.

The pathogenesis of pregnancy ketosis and lactation ketosis is similar in many

TABLE 36.6. Major differences between lactation ketosis and pregnancy ketosis

	Lactation Ketosis	Pregnancy Ketosis
Incidence	Usually individual	Often herd problem
Association with other conditions	Often secondary	Generally primary
Blood glucose, early	Decreased	Decreased
Blood glucose, late	Occasionally increased	Often increased
Acidosis	Usually mild	Usually severe
Renal failure	Does not occur	Often occurs in latter stages
Response to therapy	Good	Generally poor
Prophylactic nutritional control	Fair to good	Excellent
Without treatment	Most recover	Few survive

aspects and the two are often considered analogous, except for the time of occurrence. However, there are differences between the conditions as noted in Table 36.6. Pregnancy ketosis has been characterized as a hypoglycemic encephalopathy in which the neural changes become irreversible. This results in a poor response to therapy unless it is initiated early in the disease. Pregnancy ketosis is a fairly slowly developing disease whose course may be over 1 week. There is ample time for therapy if good husbandry is practiced.

Prophylaxis. Pregnancy ketosis is an excellent example of the adage "a gram of prevention is worth a kilogram of cure." Prevention of this disease is quite successful, while treatment is generally quite unsuccessful. Proper nutritional management, as given in Table 36.7 for the ewe or Tables 36.4 and 36.5 for the cow, is the key to the prevention of pregnancy ketosis. Both overfeeding and underfeeding must be avoided, since obesity and inadequate intake predispose to the disease. Ewes not on pasture should be driven one-half hour twice a day since insufficient exercise will predispose to pregnancy ketosis.

Treatment. Although pregnancy ketosis may be treated in the same manner as lactation ketosis, the response to therapy is usually quite poor. Two cases of pregnancy ketosis in obese cows due to adenohypophyseal insufficiency have been reported (Howard et al. 1968). These animals responded well to 100–200 units of adrenocorticotropin injected intramuscularly every few days until parturition. Generally, the only successful treatment is surgical removal of the fetus. During surgery an intravenous maintenance fluid containing 5% glucose plus 20–30 mEq/L of sodium, potassium, chloride, and a bicarbonate equivalent (bicarbonate, acetate, or lactate) should be given. If acidosis is present, the bicarbonate should be doubled. Approximately 10–12 L in the cow and 2–3 L in the ewe are necessary. Propylene glycol should be given orally twice a day for at least 4 days following surgery in dosages

TABLE 36.7. Nutritional management of the ewe

Period	Roughage	Concentrate
	(kg/ewe/day)	
Maintenance and first 3 months of pregnancy	1.5–2 kg hay or 3.5 kg ensilage	None ¼ kg protein supplement
Last 2 months of pregnancy	Same as maintenance	Same as maintenance plus ¼ kg of grain
Last 2 weeks of pregnancy	Same as maintenance	Same as maintenance plus 1 kg of grain
During lactation	Same as maintenance	1.3–1.5 kg grain
2 weeks before and 1 week after breeding	Same as maintenance	Same as maintenance plus ¼ kg grain

Note: At all times, 2 parts dicalcium phosphate or bone meal plus 2 parts iodized salt plus 1 part trace mineralized salt available free choice.

of 60 g/ewe/treatment and 125–250 g/cow/treatment. Once the disease has progressed to the point of severe neurological signs (recumbency and convulsions) the chances of recovery are quite small.

TRANSPORT TETANY

Transport tetany is a hypocalcemic condition of horses, cattle, and sheep characterized by a sudden onset of excitement, ataxia, recumbency, tetany, abortion, coma, and, without treatment, death within 2–3 days. It occurs most frequently in feedlot lambs within 4 days of transit (Pierson and Jensen 1975b) and in older ewes within 6 weeks before or after parturition (Asbury 1962). The factors playing a role in the pathogenesis of the disease are stress, hypophagia, and increased corticoid secretion. The mechanism by which clinical hypocalcemia occurs is not well established, although it is known that excess corticoids will increase renal calcium excretion and decrease intestinal calcium absorption. The absence of available feed and water during transit is a complicating factor. A similar condition may occur in older ewes on calcium-deficient diets or following stress, whether transport related or not. It is seen most commonly during hot, sultry weather. GI motility is decreased by the hypocalcemia and the rumen is often fluid filled. This has led to the misdiagnosis of water intoxication. With water intoxication there is cerebral edema, blindness, and often hemoglobinuria, none of which occurs in transport tetany. In pregnant ewes, it is differentiated from pregnancy ketosis by the absence of ketonuria and the acuteness of the condition.

Prophylaxis. The incidence of transport tetany can be greatly decreased by providing adequate food, water, and rest during and after transit. Exercise and handling should be restricted for several days following transit. Also, an ample quantity of good-quality alfalfa should be provided.

Treatment. Hypocalcemic tetany may be treated by intravenous or subcutaneous injections of calcium borogluconate (1 ml/kg). In feedlot lambs, although response to calcium is shown, this is often followed by relapse and death; repeated injections of calcium alone are of no value (Pierson and Jensen 1975b). Therefore, 30–40 ml of a maintenance fluid plus 1 ml of calcium borogluconate and 0.5 unit of insulin/kg of body weight given subcutaneously in several locations or slowly intravenously may be beneficial. The contents of a maintenance fluid have been described previously under abomasal impaction treatment. Insulin increases the effectiveness of treatment; if pyrexia is present, application of cold water is indicated (Pierson and Jensen 1975b).

REFERENCES

Ahrens, F. A. 1967. Histamine, lactic acid, and hypertonicity as factors in the development of rumenitis in cattle. Am J Vet Res 28: 1335.

Allison, M. J.; Robinson, I. M.; Dougherty, R. W.; and Bucklin, J. A. 1975. Grain overload in cattle and sheep: Changes in microbial population in the cecum and rumen. Am J Vet Res 36:181.

Annison, E. F. 1973. Studies on the low milk fat syndrome in the cow induced by low roughage diets. In J. M. Payne, K. G. Hibbitt, and B. F. Sansom, eds. Production Disease in Farm Animals. Baltimore: Williams & Wilkins.

Asbury, A. C. 1962. Hypocalcemia in ewes—A case report. J Am Vet Med Assoc 141:703.

Aukema, J. J., and Breukink, H. F. 1974. Abomasal ulcer in adult cattle with fatal hemorrhage. Cornell Vet 64:303.

Baird, G. D.; Heitzman, R. J.; Hibbitt, K. G.; and Hunter, G. D. 1974. Bovine ketosis. II. A review with recommendations for control and treatment. Br Vet J 130:318.

Bartley, E. E. 1965. An analysis of the bloat complex and progress toward its prevention. J Am Vet Med Assoc 147:1397.

Bartley, E. E.; Stiles, D. A.; Meyer, R. M.; Sceidy, S. F.; Clark, J. G.; and Bowen, F. W. 1967. Poloxalene for treatment of cattle with alfalfa bloat. J Am Vet Med Assoc 151:339.

Beeson, W. M. 1969. How beneficial are feed additives. J Am Vet Med Assoc 154:1214.

Bergman, E. N. 1963. Quantitative aspects of glucose metabolism in pregnant and nonpregnant sheep. Am J Physiol 204:147.

Bergman, E. N. 1971. Hyperketonemia-ketogenesis and ketone body metabolism. J Dairy Sci 54:936.

———. 1973. Glucose metabolism in ruminants as related to hypoglycemia and ketosis. Cornell Vet 63:342.

Bergman, E. N., and Wolff, J. E. 1971. Metabolism of volatile fatty acids by liver and portal-drained viscera in sheep. Am J Physiol 221:586.

Clarke, R. T. J.; Reid, C. S. W.; and Young, R. W. 1969. Bloat in cattle. NZ J Agric Res 12:446.

Davis, J. D., and Essig, H. W. 1972. Comparison of three bloat preventing compounds for cattle grazing clover. Can J Anim Sci 52:329.

Dirksen, G. 1970. Acidosis. In A. T. Phillipson, ed. Physiology of Digestion and Metabolism in the Ruminant, p. 612. Newcastle Eng.: Oriel Press.

Dougherty, R. W. 1968. Physiology of eructation in ruminants. In C. Code, ed. Handbook of Physiology, sec. 6, vol. 3. Baltimore: Williams & Wilkins.

Dunlop, R. H. 1970. A discussion of acidosis. In A. T. Phillipson, ed. Physiology of Digestion and Metabolism in the Ruminant, p. 626. Newcastle Eng.: Oriel Press.

———. 1970–71. Pathogenesis of ruminant lactic acidosis. Adv Vet Sci Comp Med 16: 259.

Dunlop, R. H., and Hammond, P. B. 1965. D-lactic acidosis of ruminants. Ann NY Acad Sci 119:1109.

Emery, R. S. 1971. Unifying conclusions. J Dairy Sci 54:974.

Emery, R. S.; Burg, N.; Brown, L. D.; and Blank, G. N. 1964. Detection, occurrence and prophylactic treatment of borderline ketosis with propylene glycol feeding. J Dairy Sci 47:1074.

Essig, H. W., and Shawyer, C. B. 1968. Methods of administration of poloxalene for control of bloat in beef cattle grazing ladino clover. J Anim Sci 27:1669.

Fisher, L. J.; Erfle, J. D.; Lodge, G. A.; and Sauer, F. D. 1973. Effect of propylene glycol or glycerol and composition and incidence of ketosis. Can J Anim Sci 53:289.

Forenbacher, S. 1967. Fatty degeneration of the liver in ketosis. Berl Munch Tieraerztl Wochenschr 80:4.

Fox, F. H. 1965. Abomasal disorders. J Am Vet Med Assoc 147:383.

———. 1971. Clinical diagnosis and treatment of ketosis. J Dairy Sci 54:974.

Gyles, A. 1970. A breakthrough in bloat control. J Agric Vict Dep Agric 68:156.

Heitzman, R. J., and Walker, M. S. 1973. The antiketogenic action of an anabolic steroid administered to ketotic cows. Res Vet Sci 15:70.

Hironaka, R., and Ching, K. J. 1974. Influence of feed particle size on feedlot cattle. Feedstuffs 29:36.

Howard, J. R.; Adams, W.; and Sloss, M. W. 1968. Adenohypophyseal insufficiency in two cows with pregnancy toxemia. J Am Vet Med Assoc 152:17.

Huber, T. L. 1971. Effect of acute indigestion on compartmental water volumes and osmolality in sheep. Am J Vet Res 32:887.

———. 1976. Physiology of systemic lactic acidosis. In M. S. Weinberg and A. L. Sheffner, eds. Buffers in Ruminant Physiology and Metabolism. New York: Church and Dwight.

Hull, B. L., and Wass, W. M. 1973. Abomasal displacement. II. Hypocalcemia as a contributing causative factor. Vet Med Small Anim Clin 68:412.

Hungate, R. E. 1968. Ruminal fermentation. In Handbook of Physiology, sec. 6, vol. 3. Baltimore: Williams & Wilkins.

Johns, A. T. 1965. Recent developments in bloat research. Vet Rev Annot 4:17.

Johnson, B. D. 1975. Personal communication.

Jones, W. T.; Anderson, L. B.; and Ross, M. D. 1973. XXXIX. Bloat in cattle. NZ J Agric Res 16:441.

Juslin, K. E. 1965. On the effect of choline chloride and cyanocobalamine on the liver of cows with parturient paresis. A preliminary report. Nord Vet Med 17:169.

Knight, A. P. 1975. Personal communication.

Krebs, H. A. 1966. Bovine ketosis. Vet Rec 78:187.

Kronfeld, D. S. 1966. The design of a therapeutic trial on bovine ketosis. J Am Vet Med Assoc 149:1610.

———. 1971. Hypoglycemia in ketotic cows. J Dairy Sci 54:949.

———. 1973. A lack of dietary fat relative to glucose precursors may cause ketosis or depress milk fat content. In J. M. Payne, K. G. Hibbitt, and B. F. Sansom, eds. Production Disease in Farm Animals, p. 136. Baltimore: Williams & Wilkins.

Kronfeld, D. S., and Emery, R. S. 1970. Acetonemia. In W. J. Gibbon, E. J. Catcott, and J. F. Smithcors, eds. Bovine Medicine and Surgery. Wheaton, Ill.: American Veterinary Publications.

Lewis, D., and Buttery, P. J. 1973. Ammonia toxicity in ruminants. In J. M. Payne, K. G. Hibbitt, and B. F. Sansom, eds. Production Disease in Farm Animals. Baltimore: Williams & Wilkins.

Lewis, E. F., and Price, E. K. 1957. The use of choline chloride as a lipotrophic agent in the treatment of bovine liver dysfunction. Br Vet J 113:242.

Lippke, H.; Vetter, R. L.; and Jacobson, N. L. 1970. Effect of poloxalene on performance of calves and lambs. J Anim Sci 31:1195.

Morrison, S. H. 1973. Nutrition in the lactating cow. Proc 6th Ann Conv Am Assoc Bovine Pract, p. 73.

Morrow, L. L.; Tumbleson, M. B.; Kinter, L. D.; Pfander, W. H.; and Preston, R. L. 1973. Laminitis in lambs injected with lactic acid. Am J Vet Res 34:1305.

Mudd, A. J., and Hooper, L. E. 1973. The limitation of amino acid supply to the dairy cow. In J. M. Payne, K. G. Hibbitt, and B. F. Sansom, eds. Production Disease in Farm Animals. Baltimore: Williams & Wilkins.

Phillips, D. S. M. 1968. The water intake of grazing cows and its effect on the intake of "Pluronic L-64" administered in the drinking water for the control of bloat. NZ J Agric Res 11:267.

Pierson, R. E., and Jensen, R. 1975a. Polioencephalomalacia in feedlot lambs. J Am Vet Med Assoc 166:257.

———. 1975b. Transport tetany of feedlot lambs. J Am Vet Med Assoc 166:260.

Poole, D. B. T.; Coulig, M. J.; and Cognat, M. 1967. The effect of penicillin in the prevention of bloat. Irish Vet J 22:190.

Radostits, O. M., and Magnuson, R. A. 1971. A modification of an old method for emptying the rumen of cattle. Can Vet J 12:150.

Reid, C. S. W.; Clarke, R. T. J.; Gurnsey, M. P.; Hungate, R. E.; and Macmillan, K. L. 1972. Breeding dairy cattle with reduced susceptibility to bloat. Proc NZ Soc Anim Prod 31:96.

Richardson, C. R., and Hatfield, E. E. 1975. Biological responses to abomasally infused amino acids. Fed Proc 35:902.

Richardson, C. T., and Fordtran, J. S. 1975. Effect of cimetidine, a new H_2 receptor antagonist, on food stimulated acid secretion in duodenal ulcer patients. Gastroenterology 68:972.

Roberts, G. W., and Boyd, J. W. 1974. Cerebrocortical necrosis in ruminants: Occurrence of thiaminase in the gut of normal and affected animals and its effect on thiamine status. J Comp Pathol 84:365.

Roberts, S. J., and Dye, J. A. 1951. The treatment of acetonemia in cattle by continuous intravenous injection of glucose. Cornell Vet 41:3.

Robinson, D. W., and Slade, L. M. 1974. The current status of knowledge on the nutrition of equines. J Anim Sci 39:1045.

Schultz, L. H. 1971. Management and nutritional aspects of ketosis. J Dairy Sci 54:962.

Shires, G. M. H. 1974. Diseases of metabolism and nutrition in cattle. Semin 118, Am Vet Med Assoc Ann Meet.

Svendson, P. E. 1970. Abomasal displacement in cattle. Nord Vet Med 22:571.

Tremere, A. W.; Merrill, W. G.; and Loosli, J. K. 1968. Adaptation to high concentrate feeding as related to acidosis and digestion disturbances in dairy heifers. J Dairy Sci 51:1065.

Vestweber, J. G. E., and Leipold, H. W. 1974. Experimentally induced bovine ruminant acidosis: Pathological changes. Am J Vet Res 35:1537.

Waterman, R.; Schwalm, J. W.; and Schultz, L. H. 1972. Nicotinic acid treatment of bovine ketosis: Effects on circulatory metabolites and inter-relationships. J Dairy Sci 55:1972.

Whitlock, R. H. 1973. Abomasal displacement: A disorder of throughput. In J. M. Payne, K. G. Hibbitt, and B. F. Sansom, eds. Production Disease in Farm Animals. Baltimore: Williams & Wilkins.

Wright, D. E. 1971. Effect of drenching with a "pluronic" on bloat and milk production. J Dairy Res 38:303.

SECTION 10

Nutritional Pharmacology

CHAPTER 37

INTRODUCTION

ROBERT W. PHILLIPS

Vitamins
Minerals
Food Processing
Disease Interaction

This section is concerned with the mineral and vitamin dietary constituents required for health and maximal growth and reproduction. Particularly in food animal medicine, obvious health is not the only requirement. Often animals can be "healthy" but not capable of producing up to their genetic potential because of deficiency, excess, or imbalance of one or more of the minor nutrients. These substances have extremely diverse actions in the body, ranging from structural to biochemical. The majority of the trace elements and vitamins act either directly as a constituent of a protein or indirectly as a cofactor stimulating enzyme activity.

Most of these nutrients are provided in sufficient but not excessive amounts under normal dietary regimes. Therefore, they are of less concern in a pharmacology text than they would be in a nutritional treatise. Calcium and phosphorus are the two elements most likely to be required in additional amounts, while vitamin A is the most commonly added organic micronutrient. The so-called trace elements are primarily cationic; their specific functions in the body have been a subject for intensive research in the past few years. An increased knowledge is now being translated into more effective nutritional supplementation and preventive therapeutics. Prevention of deficiencies and excesses rather than treatment of dietary imbalances should be the goal of veterinary medical practice. In the following chapters, heavy emphasis will be placed on techniques that can be employed to decrease the incidence of imbalances limiting the efficiency of animal protein production and the health of both food and pet animals.

Unless specifically stated to the contrary, all daily requirements are presented on the basis of current recommendations of the National Academy of Sciences, National Research Council Committee on Animal Nutrition. The specific publications entitled Nutrient Requirements of Swine, Beef Cattle, Dogs, etc., are regularly revised and present both normal requirements and feed compositions as well as photographic illustrations of deficiency syndromes. These publications are a valuable addition to the veterinarian's library. For a nominal fee they can be acquired from the Printing and Publishing Office, National Academy of Sciences, 2101 Constitution Ave., N.W., Washington, D.C. 20418.

VITAMINS

Vitamins are organic dietary essentials needed by animals. They have diverse actions and are considered as a group on the basis of being required in small amounts. The term "vitamin" originated with Casmir Funk in 1912 while he was working with thiamin (vitamin B_1), which he described as a "vital amine." Subsequently, the term has been shortened and it is known that not all vitamins contain amine groups.

The principal goal of vitamin prophylaxis and therapy is to provide a sufficient quantity of these metabolic essentials so that normal body functions can proceed. Plants and microbes normally synthesize vitamins or their precursors. Subsequent utilization of the plant or microbe by domestic animals provides the vitamin to the host.

One must assume that in the evolution of our domestic species they obtained a sufficient quantity of the vitamins from their normal food supplies. However, in our intensive agricultural system, we find that we must supplement diets with increased levels of vitamins. There are several reasons for this. Plants have been developed on the basis of their ability to form the major nutrients, total protein, and total carbohydrates per acre or per kg. Only recently, as our understanding of nutritional needs has become more advanced, have plant geneticists turned their attention to engineering increases in specific nutrients, such as high-lysine corn. To date, little attention has been given to altering the concentration of vitamins or trace minerals in plants. Processing and storage also may alter plant vitamin content. An additional facet of the need for vitamin supplementation of animals is that they are sometimes placed on a diet obtained from only a few sources, or even a single source, which may result in a deficiency. Our food-producing animals have been bred and are fed to maximize their productivity. "Maximum growth or lactation" may increase vitamin requirements. Fortunately, vitamin therapy is simplified in today's veterinary practice as all the vitamins are readily available in inexpensive forms. Their ubiquitous availability, coupled with a general lack of knowledge of requirements and deficiencies, and their low toxicity have resulted in indiscriminate use of vitamins. The rule of thumb seems to be: when in doubt, give vitamins. It can be considered, however, as a justifiable overprescription. Individual deficiencies are difficult to recognize in early stages and many of the manifestations are similar. To conduct the biochemical tests necessary to evaluate the vitamin status of an animal is both expensive and time-consuming. A more practical approach, when dealing with a sick animal that may have decreased its food intake, is to supplement with vitamins. This procedure, although generally justifiable, can be carried to excess.

Prophylaxis in herd management need not be so indiscriminate. Our knowledge of the vitamin needs to maintain health and of the vitamin levels in animal food is sufficient to permit a more judicious supplementation of normal animals.

MINERALS

Minerals represent the inorganic dietary essentials for health and productivity. They cannot, as in the case of some vitamins, be formed in the body. Minerals must be included in the diet either with the drinking water, as a constituent or contaminant of food, or as a supplement. The quantity of a given element that is present in a plant is dependent on the type of soil and concentration of that element in the soil, environmental conditions during growth, and the type of plant (Allaway 1975). The relationships between the various elements in animal nutrition and health may at times seem so complex as to be overwhelming (Schutte 1964). However, the major interactions and antagonisms have been elucidated.

With regard to supplementation of minerals, toxicities can occur or imbalances may develop from too liberal a supplementation with certain elements. However, the major problem in veterinary nutritional prophylaxis is not excesses but deficiencies. In range livestock, a mineral deficiency is often associated with the lack of a particular element in the soil or with the establishment of a single plant species that may not extract available elements from the soil. Single-source nutrients such as all corn to pigs or chickens will also result in mineral and vitamin deficiency if the diets are not supplemented. It is common practice to prophylactically supply additional elements to domestic food-producing animals. Ad libitum feeding of mineral mixes or a specific addition to a concentrate ration is used to provide the necessary elements.

Prepared pet foods are generally supplemented with minerals and vitamins but it is difficult to assess the quantities that may be available (Newberne 1974). Most of the principal pet food manufacturers are attempting to provide a healthful and nutritious product. Unless specific label suggestions recommend additional mineral or vitamin supplements, none need to be given to healthy animals.

Considerable controversy has been raised in recent years over all-meat diets and their capacity to provide a balanced input of the necessary elements. The overall value of all-meat diets for dogs and cats is still subject to debate.

FOOD PROCESSING

The effect of food processing on the vitamin and trace mineral content of the final product is important. Several of the vitamins are heat labile and may be destroyed during preparation. The concentration of some trace minerals, such as iron, may be increased during processing (Fritz 1973). Chelation may occur, which can markedly alter the bioavailablility of divalent cations.

Vitamin content tends to decrease with storage, particularly if there are oxidants present. Extra quantities of vitamin E or other antioxidants are often added to prevent excessive oxidation. Mineral mixes tend to destroy fat-soluble vitamins, especially vitamin E, so that premixing vitamin and minerals may decrease the quantity of vitamins available. Retinol, the precursor of vitamin A, is quite unstable so that it is usually added as the more stable acetate or palmitate ester.

DISEASE INTERACTION

An additional facet to consider with regard to vitamin and mineral therapeutics is the effect of deficiency or toxicity on the ability of the animal to combat other diseases or systemic infections. This area was recently reviewed (Newberne 1973). It is easy to show that infection or disease may result in decreased nutrition. The converse hypothesis that poor nutrition increases susceptibility to infectious disease is a general tenet.

The most significant interaction is between vitamin A deficiency and infection, but deficiencies of vitamin D and some components of the B complex are also reported to exacerbate infectious processes (Newberne 1973). The case is not as well defined for mineral elements, particularly trace minerals.

There is conflicting evidence concerning the role of iron in therapeutics. Plasma iron is reported to decrease during many systemic diseases. The hypothesis has been advanced that this is a homeostatic effect that may limit the multiplication of pathogenic organisms (Weinberg 1975). Conversely, low iron intake has been associated with an increase in respiratory disease.

Presumably more specific information will become available concerning the interaction of micronutrients and infectious disease processes. One unsolved problem is to separate the roles of the major nutrients, carbohydrates, proteins, and lipids from the roles of vitamins and minerals in disease susceptibility. Improved prophylactic and therapeutic nutrition can reduce the incidence and severity of disease processes.

REFERENCES

Allaway, W. H. 1975. The effect of soils and fertilizers on human and animal nutrition. Agric Inf Bull 378, USDA, Washington, D.C.

Fritz, J. C. 1973. Effect of processing on the availability and nutritional value of trace mineral elements. In Effect of Processing on the Nutritional Value of Feed. Washington, D.C.: National Academy of Sciences.

Newberne, P. M. 1973. The influence of nutrition response to infectious disease. In C. A. Brandly and C. B. Cornelius, eds. Advances in Veterinary Science and Comparative Medicine, vol. 17, p. 265. New York: Academic Press.

Newberne, P. M. 1974. Problems and opportunities in pet animal nutrition. Cornell Vet 64:159.

Schutte, K. H. 1964. The Biology of Trace Elements, 1st ed., p. 41. Philadelphia: J. P. Lippincott.

Weinberg, E. D. 1975. Nutritional immunity, host's attempt to withhold iron from microbial invaders. J Am Med Assoc 231:39.

CHAPTER 38

FAT-SOLUBLE VITAMINS

ROBERT W. PHILLIPS

Historically, a discussion of vitamins, be it nutritional, pharmacological, or biochemical, is based on separating these micronutrients on the basis of their solubility characteristics. Such a format will be followed here. Vitamin D, and to a certain extent vitamin A, could be considered hormones rather than vitamins, since the active form is synthesized in and released by the body as needed. However, they are usually considered vitamins.

There are four fat-soluble vitamins: A, D, E, and K.

VITAMIN A

Source and Occurrence

Vitamin A, retinol, is an organic alcohol formed in animal tissue from various plant carotenoids, a number of which have provitamin A activity. Vitamin A_2, dehydroretinol, is found in fish. The carotenoids vary in effectiveness as precursors of vitamin A. (See Fig. 38.1.) It is not possible to absolutely equate plant provitamin A activity with subsequent availability to the animal (Ullrey 1972).

In addition to differences in the effectiveness of carotenoid transformation to the active vitamin, the various species have a considerable range of ability to use the provitamins that are present (Tables 38.1 and 38.2). All green parts of plants have provitamin A activity; leaves have a higher concentration than stems. Legume hay is a richer source than grass hay. Considerable activity is lost during curing and storage of all roughage; provitamin A activity is close to zero within 6 months after harvest. Dehydrated alfalfa remains one of the better natural provitamin A sources. Yellow corn is the only concentrate containing significant amounts of provitamin A activity. Cereal grains contain negligible

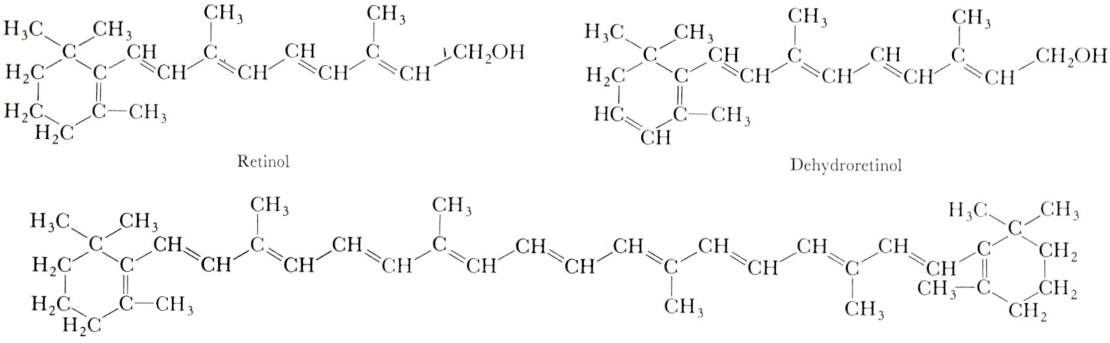

Retinol

Dehydroretinol

β-Carotene

FIG. 38.1.

TABLE 38.1. Conversion of vitamin A activity

Vitamin A should be quantified in terms of retinol equivalents (RE) or β-carotene equivalents (CE).

1 International Unit (I.U.)
of vitamin A = 1 U.S.P. unit
= retinol equivalent (vitamin A activity) of 0.300 μg of crystalline retinol or 0.550 μg of vitamin A palmitate.

∴ 1 μg RE = 3.33 I.U.
β-CE is the standard for provitamin A
1 β-CE = 0.5 μg RE
= 1.667 I.U.

TABLE 38.2. Species differences in β-carotene conversion to retinol and vitamin A requirements for growth and lactation

	Animal	% Conversion	Requirements: Retinol equivalent mg/kg feed	Requirements: β-Carotene equivalent mg/kg feed	Requirements: International Units/kg feed
Growth	Chicken	100	0.45	0.9	1500
Growth	Dog	50	1.50	6.0	5000
Growth	Pig	30	0.54	3.6	1800
Growth	Sheep	27	0.12	0.9	400
Growth	Horse	10	0.60	12.0	2000
Growth	Cattle	24	0.66	5.5	2200
	Lactating cow				
	Beef	24	1.16	9.7	3800
	Dairy	24	0.97	8.0	3200
	Pregnant ewe	27	0.22	1.6	750
	Laying hen	100	1.2	2.4	4000

Source: National Academy of Sciences, Nutrient Requirements of Domestic Animals: Poultry 1971; Dogs 1974; Swine 1973; Horses 1973; Beef Cattle 1970; Dairy Cattle 1971; Sheep 1968.

Note: % Conversion = the % of dietary β-carotene equivalent converted to retinol equivalents. To determine retinol equivalents (RE) from β-carotene equivalents (CE), RE = CE × % Conversion/2. The factor 2 represents the relative equivalence of 1 mg carotene and 1 mg retinol.

quantities. Animal fat products, particularly fish oils and liver, contain large amounts of vitamin A activity. Polar bear livers contain such high quantities that they are toxic if ingested by human beings. Today, pure vitamin A is synthesized commercially for supplementation and therapeutic use in medical practice.

The rate of absorption of all fat-soluble vitamins is dependent on other lipid constituents in the diet and on biliary and pancreatic secretions in the small intestine. Many carotenoids are believed to be destroyed in the rumen.

Chemistry

In an attempt to bring some degree of order to the problem of nomenclature and relative value, the various factors used to describe vitamin A activity are presented in Tables 38.1 and 38.2. The current recommendation of the American Institute of Nutrition (*Nomenclature Policy* 1974) is that vitamin A be quantified in terms of retinol equivalents in mg or μg. This is to replace International Units (I.U.) as a descriptive term. However, most of the current and recent literature is in either metric units of β carotene or I.U. of vitamin A. As with most changes of established nomenclature, the conversion will take some time to be complete.

The most important factors are that conversion of carotenoids to vitamin A is quite variable and that a vitamin A–sufficient diet for one species could require supplementation for another. Vitamin A equivalents in most published tables are presented as I.U. and mg of β carotene. These values may be derived by biochemical, physical, or biological assay. Most bioassays are conducted with rats, which have a high conversion of provitamin A carotenoid activity to retinol activity compared to domestic animals. *Such assays would overestimate their value to other animals.*

Both carotenoids and vitamin A lose potency with storage. Stability is decreased by heat, light, and oxidation. Mixing vitamin A supplements with mineral mixtures causes a rapid destruction of the vitamin. Up to 35% was destroyed after 2 hours of exposure to high humidity, sunlight, and moderate temperatures (Myburgh 1962). In general, green growing plants have a sufficient amount of vitamin A and vitamin A activity, and the value of cured roughages is directly proportional to the color. Green leafy alfalfa is a much better source than hay that has been bleached.

Function

Ingested provitamin A carotenoids are changed to vitamin A in the intestinal mucosal cells, not in the liver as was hypothesized several years ago. This does not preclude carotene–vitamin A conversions in other tissues; consequently, injected provitamin A carotenoids are biologically active. Vitamin A could be regarded as a hormone instead of a vitamin as it is secreted into the bloodstream, causing metabolic alterations in target tissues. The liver would act as an endocrine gland in this case (Wolf and DeLuca 1970).

Vitamin A maintains normal structure and function of epithelial cells. There appears to be a gradation of sensitivity of various epithelial surfaces to vitamin A. It acts to decrease keratinization and to stimulate production and differentiation of mucous-secreting cells. The lining of the gastrointestinal (GI) tract is quite sensitive to the presence or absence of vitamin A. Under normal dietary conditions, columnar mucous-secreting cells are formed. As deficiency develops, the epithelium progressively loses its mucous-secreting characteristics, becoming cuboidal and eventually stratified and keratinized. All epithelial surfaces have some sensitivity to the effects of vitamin A.

Another function of vitamin A is its well-defined role in the visual process. Vitamin A is converted to an aldehyde and combined with a protein, opsin, in the retina. The resultant compound, rhodopsin or visual purple, reacts with light, and in the process initiates the activation of visual neural pathways. Vitamin A is necessary for spermatogenesis in males and maintenance of pregnancy in females. Without sufficient vitamin A, fetus resorption occurs. One last defined function of vitamin A is to support osteoblastic activity and bone growth.

Deficiency

Vitamin A deficiency is manifest in all species by alterations of epithelial surfaces, bringing about increased keratinization and surface lesions. Mucus-secreting epithelia also become keratinized. These changes are seen in the respiratory, GI, and urogenital systems as well as the cornea of the eye. There are species differences with regard to the development of particular lesions but they are in general analogous. As keratinization proceeds and the epithelial surfaces lose their normal function, resistance to infection is decreased.

In cattle, sheep, horses, pigs, and dogs, night blindness occurs, followed by excessive lachrymation. Corneal keratinization and blindness are common in vitamin A deficiency. Anasarca occurs in vitamin A–deficient cattle. Marginal deficiencies result in decreased growth, a tendency toward diarrhea, a nasal discharge, dry scaly skin, and decreased resistance to infection. Such animals appear "unthrifty" but a specific diagnosis is difficult.

Reproductive efficiency is decreased due to both altered testicular function in the male and fetal resorption in the female. Offspring are often born weak, and retained placentas may occur in cattle. Blindness in neonates is caused by pressure necrosis of the optic nerve due to inadequate bone growth. In most species examined, there is an early increase in cerebrospinal fluid (CSF) pressure in vitamin A deficiency (Miller and Woolam 1958). Measurement of CSF pressure appears to be a reliable means of assessing vitamin A status. It has particular potential in herd health management programs. However, liver biopsy, for determination of vitamin A levels, is currently the most specific means of analyzing vitamin A status in cattle.

Prophylaxis and Therapy

Since vitamin A is one of the most limiting dietary essentials in domestic animals, supplementation is often necessary from a prophylactic standpoint.

Requirements are greatest during lactation and rapid growth. The potential for deficiency is maximized in food-producing animals when they are fed large quantities of concentrates, that are poor sources of vitamin A.

Vitamin A is added to animal feeds as vitamin A acetate or vitamin A palmitate. The esterification to the acid results in much greater stability. Natural product supplements such as fish oil are also used because of their dehydroretinol content. The quantity of retinol equivalent needed by animals is determined on the basis of their production rate and management program. It is beyond the scope of this book to detail the daily requirements of each species under varying conditions of maintenance, growth, lactation, and reproduction. The reader is referred to the respective National Academy of Science publications.

Prophylactic supplementation should be increased during pregnancy, lactation, and in neonates, as large stores are not present at birth. Fortunately, colostrum is a good source if the dam has had an adequate supply of vitamin A. Vitamin A is stored in the liver and it is possible for a 3- to 6-month supply to accumulate. This fact is of particular importance in grazing animals as ample supplies of the provitamins are available in the summer but only small quantities remain in winter grasses. Under natural conditions, herbivores must store enough vitamin A to last through the winter low-intake months and to sustain reproduction in the spring.

In addition, vitamin A needs increase in many diseases. Therapeutic use of vitamin A may be either oral or parenteral; both natural and synthetic sources are available. Single large doses are often given as a parenteral intramuscular injection to provide immediate benefit and to increase hepatic stores. Single injections may provide sufficient vitamin A activity for several months in spite of limited intake. A therapeutic dose to cattle may be as high as 600 mg RE (2×10^6 I.U.); however, doses greater than the liver storage capacity of approximately 2 mg/RE/kg of body weight (3000 I.U./lb) should not be given.

Preparations

Vitamin A, U.S.P., is available in natural fish oils and as a synthetic vitamin. Vitamin A acetate and vitamin A palmitate are the principal esters. Injectable and oral preparations may be obtained either singly or as multivitamin preparations. For injection, aqueous solutions should be used; oily solutions are reported to be of little benefit. Vitamin A is also available as a dietary supplement with various trace minerals, with trace minerals plus calcium and phosphate, and as a multivitamin, mineral, protein, and lipid supplement.

Toxicity

Vitamin A is one of the few vitamins that has toxic manifestations and this has caused sporadic problems. Vitamin A is readily available in high concentrations and the rationale of "if a little bit helps, give a lot" will continue to be followed. In hypervitaminosis, there is hyperesthesia and increased aging of epiphyseal cartilages. The epiphyseal junctions become particularly tender.

The toxic dose is quite large compared to prophylactic or therapeutic requirements (Hale et al. 1962; March et al. 1973). However, toxicity will occur if more than 4 times the storage capacity of the liver is administered. The signs of vitamin A toxicity resemble in many aspects the signs of vitamin A deficiency and include lethargy, colic, bone and joint pain, restlessness, brittle hoofs and nails, alopecia, and dry scaly skin.

VITAMIN D

Source and Occurrence

Vitamin D is the generic term for closely related steroids that have antirachitic activity. They are formed as provitamins in both plants and animals. The conversion of the provitamins by ultraviolet light is well established. The plant provitamin is ergocalciferol (vitamin D_2).

Green, growing plants contain only minute amounts of this vitamin. Most of it is formed in hay and grasses from ergosterol during the curing process. It is in higher concentration in the leaves than in the stem. Ergocalciferol has little biological activity in avian species, although it is effective in mammals. This is apparently due to more rapid excretion of vitamin D_2 so that its biological effect is minimized (Imrie et al. 1967). Cholecalciferol (vitamin D_3) is formed in animal tissue by the action of ultraviolet rays on 7-dehydrocholesterol, which is produced from cholesterol. The efficiency of conversion is dependent on several factors. A fair skin, light hair covering, nearness to the equator, and lack of cloud cover all promote conversion. The converse is also true in that animals with thick hair coats in northern latitudes do not obtain sufficient vitamin D from their own bodies. If they are inside or there is heavy cloud cover, the deficiency is intensified.

Artificial irradiation of plant and animal sterols provides much of today's vitamin D activity. Milk for human consumption is routinely irradiated to increase its vitamin D activity.

Chemistry

The chemical structures of ergosterol, ergocalciferol, and cholecalciferol are shown in Fig. 38.2. These compounds, although required for antirachitic activity, are not the biologically active form in the body but must undergo additional conversions. These conversions and their control have been the subject of intensive investigation in the past few years. Of particular importance has been the work of H. F. DeLuca and his colleagues at the University of Wisconsin. In a recent review a strong case was made that vitamin D should more correctly be considered as a hormone than as a catalytic vitamin (Omdahl and DeLuca 1973):

Unequivocal evidence is cited to demonstrate

Ergosterol

FIG. 38.2.

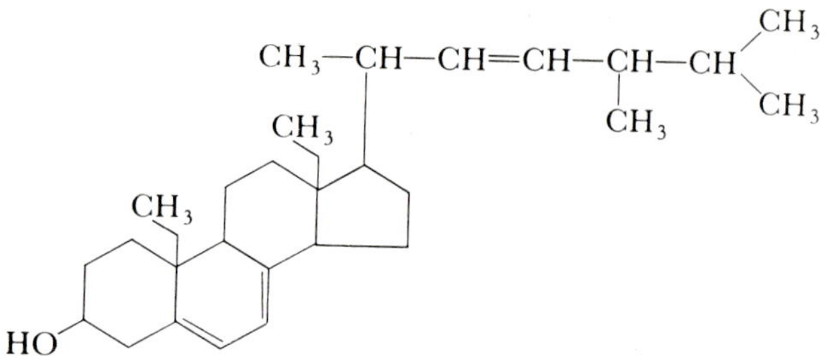

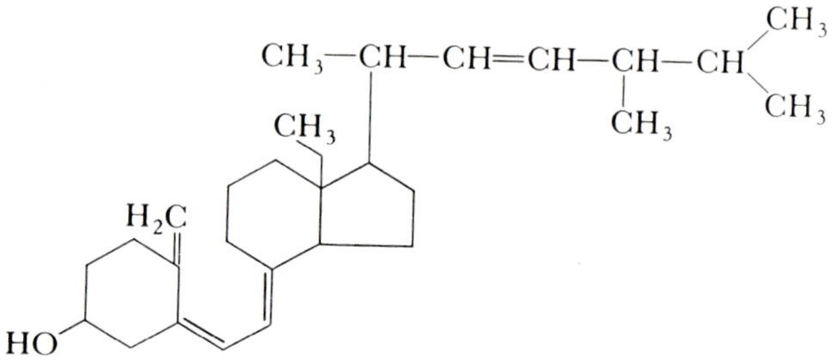

Vitamin D_2 (Ergocalciferol—in Plants)

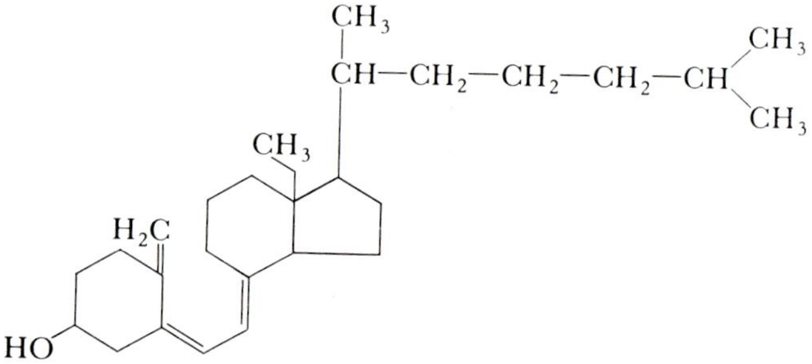

Vitamin D_3 (Cholecalciferol—in Animals)

that (1) vitamin D must first be metabolically altered before it functions; (2) functional metabolites of vitamin D are generated in organs other than their sites of action; (3) the rates of synthesis and secretion of these functional forms are feedback regulated; (4) this regulation is effected through humoral agents that probably involve the parathyroid hormone and possibly calcitonin; and (5) the final functional form of vitamin D that controls calcium movement from both intestine and bone is a major humoral substance responsible for regulating plasma calcium concentration. Vitamin D, therefore, must be considered not simply a catalytic material but one whose metabolism is dynamically interrelated with its functions in a complex system that plays a major role in the strict regulation of plasma calcium and phosphate concentrations.

FUNCTION

Vitamin D is absorbed and stored in all tissues of the body. High levels are found in liver and adipose tissue. As functional vitamin activity is required, vitamin D is converted to the 25-hydroxy derivative in the liver. Under the action of parathormone, 25-OHD_3 is converted to the final functional form 1,25-dihydroxycholecalciferol in the kidneys. This active form of vitamin D has two functions. One is to maintain the circulating level of calcium in the blood. To accomplish this, low blood calcium acts to release parathormone, which initiates vitamin D activation. Second, normal bone calcification requires vitamin D. It insures that Ca and

PO_4 are present in the blood in "supersaturated concentrations" so that bone may be formed.

The functions of vitamin D are accomplished by its action at three sites. First, to maintain the circulating level of the calcium ion in the blood, which is essential for many functions, vitamin D and parathormone together act to mobilize Ca and PO_4 from bone. This is a seemingly paradoxical situation since vitamin D has been used clinically for years to promote bone deposition and growth. A second major action is the activation of the intestinal epithelial cell transport system, which increases the absorption of Ca and PO_4. This function is obviously dependent on a sufficient dietary supply of available Ca and PO_4 (see Chapter 40 for details). In addition, vitamin D also affects renal tubule cells to bring about the reabsorption of phosphate and perhaps calcium. Fig. 38.3 summarizes the metabolic function of vitamin D in the body (Omdahl and DeLuca 1973).

Deficiency

Vitamin D deficiency, rickets, is commonly considered as a disease of growing animals. It is characterized by a low blood Ca and PO_4 concentration and a lack of normal ossification of cartilage. It appears as a thickening of the endochondral junctions, bowing of large bones, and stiffening and swelling of joints. Fractures occur more frequently. Rickets can be seen clinically in cattle, sheep, swine, dogs, and poultry. More acute forms of vitamin D–deficiency disease affect Ca and PO_4 mobilization; lactation paresis in sows and parturient paresis in cows are examples (Dobson and Ward 1974) (see calcium and phosphate metabolism in Chapter 40). In adult animals a deficiency of vitamin D is called osteomalacia. Daily requirements of vitamin D are presented in Table 38.3.

Prophylaxis and Therapy

To be effective, prophylactic and therapeutic measures may necessitate supplementation with calcium and phosphate.

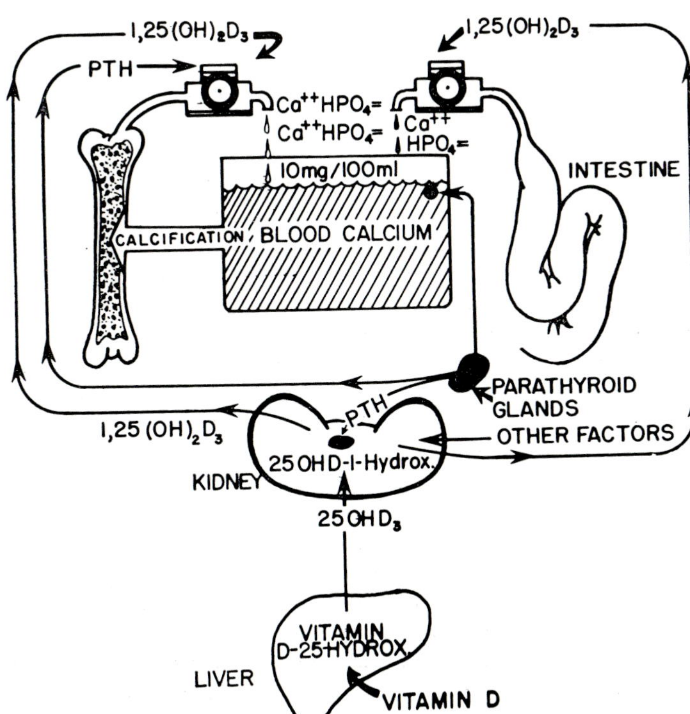

Fig. 38.3. Schematic designation of hormonal control loop for vitamin D metabolism and function. A drop below set point for serum calcium of 10 mg/100 ml prompts a proportional secretion of parathyroid hormone that acts to increase bone resorption and thus elevates serum calcium. Parathyroid hormone also directs metabolism of 25-OHD_3 to 1,25-$(OH)_2D_3$ in the kidney where "hormone" 1,25-$(OH)_2D_3$ acts both on bone and intestine to mobilize calcium from bone and intestinal contents. As serum calcium increases toward its set point, parathyroid hormone secretion is proportionately decreased. (Omdahl and DeLuca 1973).

TABLE 38.3. Vitamin D requirements for growth

Animal	I.U./kg Diet	I.U./kg Body Weight/Day
Dog	500	22.0
Sheep	70	6.0
Cattle	275	6.5
Pig	275	5.0
Horse	...	6.6
Chicken	200	14.0
Turkey	900	46.0

Note: 1 International Unit (I.U.) = 0.025 μg cholecalciferol.

Marginal deficiencies of vitamin D are hard to detect. They will most likely occur during winter months in young animals that have little opportunity for exposure to the sun. Fish meals and irradiated yeast may be used as a supplemental vitamin D source. Irradiated yeast supplies ergocalciferol, which has little effectiveness in avian species. Synthetic calf diets are routinely supplemented with vitamin D, 1400–1600 I.U./kg. Therapy for rickets has been suggested at a level of 10–20 times the daily requirement, alternate days for 1 week.

Preparations

As mentioned for vitamin A, a number of different preparations of vitamin D are available. Fish liver oils contain natural vitamin D. *Ergocalciferol,* U.S.P. (vitamin D_2), and *Cholecalciferol,* U.S.P. (vitamin D_3), are available in capsule and solution form. Many vitamin and vitamin-mineral mixtures contain vitamin D.

Toxicity

Overdoses of vitamin D decrease bone mineralization and cause calcification of some soft tissues due to excessive blood levels of calcium and phosphate. Toxicity tends to be chronic in nature as vitamin D is slowly metabolized. Toxicity is often more of a problem than vitamin D deficiency in oversupplemented pets.

VITAMIN E

Source and Occurrence

Vitamin E is the name given to a group of biologically active tocopherols. The principal naturally occurring active compound is *d*-α-tocopherol. Vitamin E is widely distributed in plant products. It is abundant in whole cereal grains and young green leafy plants. Alfalfa, including cured hay, is a good source of vitamin E.

Animal products are generally poor sources of vitamin E (except eggs from a hen on a high vitamin E intake). Plant oils have the highest content of natural products. Synthetic sources of vitamin E are available.

Function

A continuing controversy exists over the biological function of vitamin E, which was originally isolated as an essential for reproduction in rats. However, *this is not the case in other species.* The predominant role of vitamin E appears to be as an antioxidant. It functions in preventing lipid oxidation and prolonging the biological life of polyunsaturated fatty acids (PUFA). This action has been equated with stabilization of cell membranes since PUFA are important membrane constituents. More correctly, vitamin E prevents or slows the formation of free radicals and hyperperoxides from PUFA. The decrease in peroxide formation can be considered as having a stabilizing effect on cell membranes containing PUFA (Tappel 1974; Witting 1974). Other actions for vitamin E may be elucidated since simple antioxidant activity does not appear to explain all the changes occurring in deficient animals.

Pharmacologic levels of vitamin E have been reported to potentiate the body's immune mechanisms and increase resistance to bacterial and viral challenges (Heinzerlinger et al. 1974).

Relation with Selenium

There are a number of somewhat analogous pathological conditions in domestic animals that are degenerative in nature. They respond to either or both vitamin E and selenium. Most conditions are not absolutely cured or prevented by either agent alone. However, this is a difficult allegation to prove because most diets, except highly synthetic ones, contain traces of either vitamin E or selenium (Thompson and Scott 1969). The need for vitamin E dietary supplementation to prevent exudative diathesis is reduced when selenium is increased in the diet of chicks (Scott 1970). Yet Scott reported that selenium and vitamin E do not appear to be synergistic. See Chapter 41 for additional information on the role of selenium.

Hoekstra (1974) postulated a mechanism that can explain most of the interactions of vitamin E and selenium. It is presented in Fig. 38.4. Both micronutrients act to protect membrane lipids but in different fashions. Selenium works through glutathione and the glutathione peroxidase system to increase the destruction of peroxides, while vitamin E is believed to prevent the oxidation of unsaturated lipids.

Deficiency

Naturally occurring deficiencies are rare in adult animals. Most deficiency syndromes are associated with young animals from dams on vitamin E–deficient diets. Examples of diets that could be suspect are bleached hay and fish protein concentrates that contain large amounts of unsaturated fats and oil meals. Any feed that has significant quantities of unsaturated fats and is stored can be considered depleted of vitamin E and therefore potentially disease producing. Muscular dystrophy occurs in young rats, rabbits, poultry, dogs, pigs, cattle, sheep, and goats. In young ruminants and pigs, vitamin E deficiencies are seen in the first few weeks of life. The preliminary signs are stiffness and reluctance to move. Pale white areas of degeneration can be seen in skeletal muscles following necropsy. Heart lesions may be present. The disease is often associated with geographic areas where plants are selenium deficient. In poultry, vitamin E deficiency causes decreased hatchability of eggs due to embryonic death. Young chicks develop an encephalomalacia and exudative diathesis.

In carnivores or omnivores that receive a significant proportion of their diet from

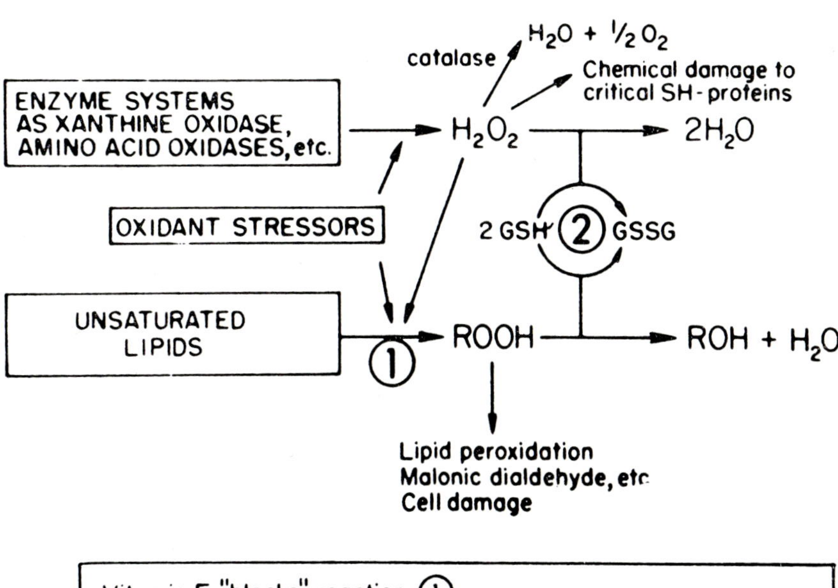

Fig. 38.4. Schematic representation of the postulated functions of selenium and vitamin E and mechanism of their relationship. (Hoekstra 1974)

TABLE 38.4. Recommended levels of vitamin E in diets for young animals

Animal	mg/kg Feed*
Calf	15–60
Chick	10
Pig	11
Poultry	10
Dog	50
Calf starter	300

* Some ration contents are listed in International Units (I.U.); 1 I.U. = 1 mg of *dl*-α-tocopherol acetate.

fish by-products, a condition of steatitis or yellow fat disease may develop. The deficiency is brought about by the high levels of unsaturated fats that destroy the naturally occurring vitamin E. Primary lesions are yellow brown pigment deposition in fat and inflammatory changes of adipose tissue.

Recommended vitamin E levels in diets for young animals are presented in Table 38.4. However, any diet that contains significant amounts of fish oils or other polyunsaturated oils may require additional vitamin E (Makdami et al. 1970). The use of synthetic antioxidants may decrease the vitamin E requirement.

Prophylaxis and Therapy

Most conditions that respond to vitamin E also respond to selenium so that combination therapy can be beneficial. Table 38.5 summarizes beneficial prophylactic responses for the major clinical diseases.

Wheat germ oil, which has a high vitamin E content, may be added to the diets of dogs and mink to protect against vitamin E deficiency. Similarly, supplementing the female of any species during gestation or egg laying in the case of poultry will insure that the offspring have an adequate supply of vitamin E. In selenium-deficient areas, combined selenium and vitamin E may be given orally or parenterally to the cow or ewe. An alternative method is to treat the offspring immediately after birth with selenium and vitamin E combinations. Recommended oral and parenteral dosages of vitamin E for young animals are given in Table 38.6. The decision concerning inclusion of selenium in the therapy should be made on the basis of geography and the level of selenium in the diet (see Chapter 41).

Therapy is beneficial if the disease has not progressed too far. When outbreaks of vitamin E deficiency occur, it is advisable to routinely supplement and/or add antioxidants to the feed as a prophylactic measure for all animals.

Preparations

Vitamin E, *dl-α-Tocopherol* and *dl-α-Tocopherol acetate,* U.S.P., is available for oral and parenteral use. It is often combined with selenium for both prophylactic and therapeutic administration. It is also available with vitamins A and D and in multivitamin supplements.

VITAMIN K

Source and Occurrence

Vitamin K, a quinone, is synthesized in significant and sufficient amounts in the digestive tract of all species but poultry. It is subsequently absorbed in the small intestine of ruminants and may be acquired by coprophagy or absorption from the

TABLE 38.5. Positive response of various diseases to vitamin E, selenium, and chemical antioxidants

Disease	Treatment Effect		
	Vitamin E	Selenium	Chemical antioxidants
White muscle disease (calves, lambs)	Yes	Yes	Partial
Hepatitis dietetica (swine, chicks)	Yes	Yes	No
Exudative diathesis and muscular dystrophy (chicks)	Yes	Partial	No
Yellow fat disease	Yes	No	Yes

TABLE 38.6. Treatment of vitamin E deficiencies in young animals*

Animal	Parenteral	Oral
Calf	25 mg/kg	40 mg/kg/day
Lamb	25 mg/kg	40 mg/kg/day
Pig	25 mg/kg	500 mg/pig/day
Dog	25 mg/kg	Up to 300 mg†
Cat	30 mg/kg	30 mg/kg
Mink	10–20 mg	2–5 mg/mink/day for 2 weeks
Poultry		300 mg/bird

* Vitamin E has a low toxicity; 2000 mg/kg prolonged administration were necessary to effect decreased growth (March et al. 1973).

† Single dose.

lower intestinal tract in other mammals. Green leafy plants and cured roughage are excellent sources of vitamin K. Fish meal and liver contain significant amounts.

Chemistry

Several natural and synthetic quinones have vitamin K activity. Menadione, a synthetic product, has more biological activity than the natural compounds. Vitamin K_1, a plant product, and vitamin K_2 from bacterial synthesis, as well as two synthetic compounds with vitamin K activity, are shown in Fig. 38.5.

Function

The primary function of vitamin K is to stimulate the production of prothrombin from a precursor protein (Suttie 1973). Prothrombin is an essential component of the blood coagulation process and is synthesized in the liver. Vitamin K is also involved with coagulation factors VII, IX, and X. Its specific role at the molecular level has not been established (Olson 1974).

Deficiency

Naturally occurring vitamin K deficiencies occur in poultry under intensive management practice where they do not obtain green plants. It is most often seen in younger birds. Symptoms are delayed clotting time and spontaneous hemorrhage.

Vitamin K may also become deficient with protracted liver disease and exposure to antivitamin K, such as dicoumarin from moldy sweet clover or the rodenticide, dicoumarol. These compounds interfere with prothrombin synthesis and eventually

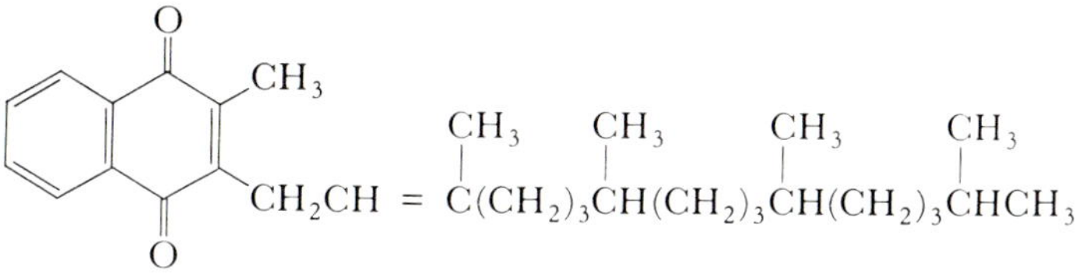

O, O, CH_3

$CH_2CH = C(CH_3)(CH_2)_3CH(CH_3)(CH_2)_3CH(CH_3)(CH_2)_3CH(CH_3)CH_3$

Vitamin K_1 (in plants)

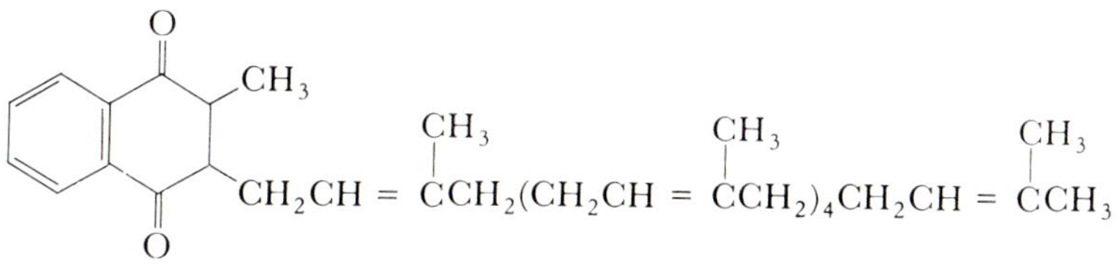

O, O, CH_3

$CH_2CH = C(CH_3)CH_2(CH_2CH = C(CH_3)CH_2)_4CH_2CH = C(CH_3)CH_3$

Vitamin K_2 (in bacteria)

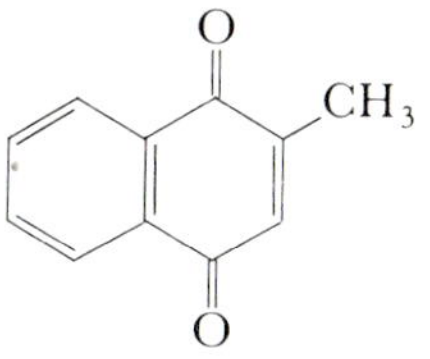

O, O, CH_3

Menadione

O, O, CH_3, SO_3Na

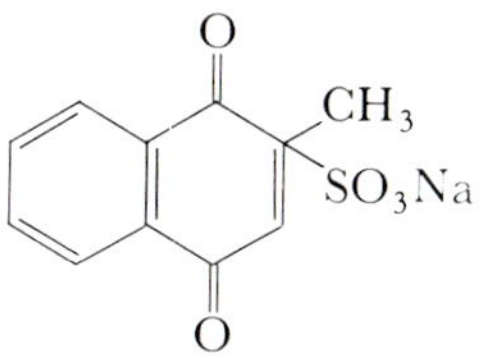

Menadione Sodium Bisulfite

Fig. 38.5.

blood clotting. These processes and their importance in anticoagulation therapy have been covered in Chapter 22.

PROPHYLAXIS AND THERAPY

In young, growing poultry vitamin K should be present in the rations at a level of 0.53 mg/kg for the chick and 0.7 mg/kg for the poult. If deficiencies develop, oral and injectable vitamin K preparations of both naturally occurring and synthetic vitamin K are available. *Phytonadione,* U.S.P. (K_1), also called phyllomenaquinone (preferred usage in nutrition) or phylloquinone, is the naturally occurring plant vitamin.

REFERENCES

Dobson, R. C., and Ward, G. 1974. Vitamin D physiology and its importance in dairy cattle: A review. J Dairy Sci 57:985.

Eaton, H. D.; Rousseau, J. E., Jr.; Hall, R. C., Jr.; Frier, H. I.; and Lucas, J. J. 1972. Reevaluation of the minimum vitamin A requirement of holstein male calves based upon elevated cerebrospinal fluid pressure. J Dairy Sci 55:232.

Hale, W. H.; Hubert, F., Jr.; Taylor, R. E.; Anderson, T. A.; and Taylor, B. 1962. Performance and tissue A levels in steers fed high levels of vitamin A. Am J Vet Res 23:992.

Harris, P. L., and Enbrene, N. D. 1963. Quantitative consideration of polyunsaturated fatty acid content of the diet upon the requirements for vitamin E. Am J Clin Nutr 13:385.

Hayes, K. C.; Nielsen, S. W.; and Rousseau, J. E. 1969. Vitamin E deficiency and fat stress in the dog. J Nutr 99:196.

Heinzerlinger, R. H.; Nockels, C. F.; Quarles, C. F.; and Tengerdy, R. P. 1974. Protection of chicks against *E. coli* infection by dietary supplementation with vitamin E. Proc Soc Exp Biol Med 146:279.

Hoekstra, W. 1974. In W. G. Hoekstra, J. W. Suttie, H. E. Ganther, and W. Mertz, eds. Trace Element Metabolism in Animals—2, Baltimore: University Park Press.

Imrie, M. H.; Neville, P. F.; Snellgrove, A. W.; and DeLuca, H. F. 1967. Metabolism of vitamin D_2 and D_3 in the rachitic chick. Arch Biochem Biophys 20:525.

Makdami, D. D.; Huber, J. T.; Sculthorpe, A. E.; and Michel, R. L. 1970. Vitamin E addition to milk replacers containing DCE-extracted fish protein concentrate. J Dairy Sci 53:675.

March, B. E.; Coates, V.; and Goudie, C. 1972. Delayed hatching time of chicks from hens fed excess vitamin A and from eggs injected with vitamin A. Poult Sci 51:891.

March, B. E.; Wong, E.; Seier, L.; Sim, J.; and Biely, J. 1973. Hypervitaminosis E in the chick. J Nutr 103:371.

Miller, J. W., and Woolam, D. H. M. 1958. Vitamins and cerebrospinal fluid. In G. E. W. Wolstenholme and C. M. O'Connor, eds. The Ciba Foundation Symposium on the Cerebrospinal Fluid, p. 168. Boston: Little Brown.

Myburgh, S. J. 1962. The stability of vitamin A in synthetic vitamin A concentrates (acetate or palmitate). I. In phosphatic stock licks with and without trace elements. Onderstepoort J Vet Res 29:269.

Nomenclature Policy. 1974. Generic description and trivial names for vitamins and related compounds. J Nutr 104:144.

Olson, R. E. 1974. New concepts relating to the mode of action of vitamin K. In Robert Harris et al., eds. Vitamins and Hormones: Advances in Research and Application, vol. 32, p. 483. New York: Academic Press.

Omdahl, J. L., and DeLuca, H. F. 1973. Regulation of vitamin D metabolism and function. Physiol Rev 53:327.

Scott, M. L. 1970. Studies on vitamin E and related factors in nutrition and metabolism. In H. F. DeLuca and J. W. Suttie, eds. The Fat Soluble Vitamins. Madison: Univ. of Wisconsin Press.

Suttie, J. W. 1973. Vitamin K and prothrombin synthesis. Nutr Rev 31:105.

Tappel, A. L. 1974. Selenium-glutathione peroxidase and vitamin E. Am J Clin Nutr 27:960.

Thompson, J. N., and Scott, M. L. 1969. Role of selenium in the nutrition of the chick. J Nutr 97:335.

Ullrey, D. E. 1972. Biological availability of fat-soluble vitamins: Vitamin A and carotene. J Anim Sci 35:648.

Witting, L. A. 1974. Vitamin E-polyunsaturated lipid relationship in diet and tissues. Am J Clin Nutr 27:952.

Wolf, G., and DeLuca, L. 1970. Recent studies on some metabolic functions of vitamin A. In H. F. DeLuca and J. W. Suttie, eds. The Fat Soluble Vitamins. Madison: Univ. of Wisconsin Press.

CHAPTER 39

WATER-SOLUBLE VITAMINS

ROBERT W. PHILLIPS

The water-soluble vitamins are a functionally diverse group of micronutrients required by all animals. Included in this classification are the B-complex vitamins and vitamin C. In most cases, the water-soluble vitamins are ingested as a natural dietary constituent or may be synthesized by gastrointestinal (GI) organisms. Most feeds contain adequate quantities of the water-soluble vitamins, particularly if they are not from a single source. Generally, prepared feeds, except those for mature ruminants, are supplemented with the vitamins deemed most likely to be deficient.

The assumption can be made that most domestic animals do not require additional prophylactic supplementation with these micronutrients. They are provided naturally in quantities sufficient to meet the animal's needs. In disease states where body metabolism is altered or in cases of prolonged inappetence or defects in intestinal absorption, multiple vitamin deficiencies may occur. Descriptions of individual deficiency syndromes can be found in animal nutrition textbooks. These usually are induced deficiencies, the result of feeding specialized or purified diets. Field or clinical deficiencies are rarely as clear cut and are often the result of multiple deficiency syndromes. These examples of unique and rarely observed pure deficiencies of individual vitamins do not represent important clinical therapeutic problems.

Most water-soluble vitamin therapy can be considered as prophylactic or supportive in nature. The B vitamins should be provided routinely to animals suffering from chronic diseases, prolonged inappetence, or diarrhea. The rationale for this approach is as follows:

1. The B-complex vitamins are not stored in the body to a great extent or for prolonged periods.
2. Decreased food intake and/or absorption will decrease the entry rate of these vitamins into the animal system.
3. Under disease conditions and altered metabolic function, vitamin stores may be depleted more rapidly.

4. It is almost impossible to recognize specific individual vitamin deficiencies or even to differentiate multivitamin imbalance from the effects of many diseases.

5. The water-soluble vitamins have a low toxicity.

6. The water-soluble vitamins are inexpensive.

The above factors provide justification for the common prophylactic use of vitamin therapy as an adjunct to more specific treatment of disease.

The goal of prophylaxis is to prevent disease and to inhibit exacerbation of existing pathology. In veterinary medicine it is not practical to assess the specific vitamin status in individual animals except in unusual cases. Specific vitamin assays are time-consuming and expensive. It is more costly to analyze for a vitamin than to administer it.

Parenteral multivitamin therapy, therefore, can be used to supplement other therapeutic regimes, particularly in chronic disease. There are many commercial multivitamin preparations available. The different products have varying ratios of the principal vitamins. Unfortunately, controlled studies are not available to permit assessment of maximally effective ratios.

Table 39.1 lists the common water-soluble vitamins and indicates their importance in initiating clinical disease conditions. Therapy with vitamins that are not responsible for specific clinical deficiency syndromes will not be presented here.

Ascorbic acid is a dietary requirement for primates, the guinea pig, and several exotic species. Its deficiency disease, scurvy, is unlikely to be of concern except to veterinarians dealing with primates or guinea pigs. There have been reports that vitamin C administration has beneficial effects in chronic disease malnutrition in the dog and that it increases the rate of soft tissue wound healing in the horse. The overall benefit of such therapy is difficult to assess due to a lack of controls. Normal healthy animals can apparently synthesize ascorbic acid in sufficient quantities for their functional needs.

VITAMIN DEFICIENCIES

Consider the four vitamins listed as potentially deficient in Table 39.1, thiamin, niacin, choline, and cobalamin. Field deficiencies of thiamin are associated with the presence of an enzyme, thiaminase, or other antivitamins. Thus excessive destruction of thiamin is the problem. Clinical deficiencies of niacin and choline are generally associated with the use of single-source proteins. Both are formed in mammalian tissue from dietary essential amino acids. Niacin may be formed from tryptophan, except by the cat, and choline from methionine. A deficiency of cobalamin is commonly associated with ruminants on

TABLE 39.1. Vitamins that may need to be supplemented when healthy animals are receiving "practical diets"

Vitamin	Dog	Pig	Horse	Sheep*	Ox*	Poultry
Thiamin	+	—	±	+	+	+
Riboflavin	—	—	—	—	—	—
Niacin†	+	±	—	—	—	+
Pantothenic acid	rare	rare	—	—	—	—
Folic acid	—	—	—	—	—	—
Choline	—	—	—	—	—	+‡
Biotin	—	—	—	—	—	+
Cobalamin	—	±	—	+§	+§	—
Ascorbic acid (vitamin C)	—	—	—	—	—	—

* Preruminant animals have dietary requirements but these are generally met by milk. Milk replacers are routinely supplemented.

† Dependent on the level of tryptophan in the diet.

‡ Linked with manganese deficiency in perosis and dependent on the level of methionine in the diet.

§ Dependent on the adequacy of cobalt in the diet (see Chapter 41).

low cobalt intakes. Biotin has been reported recently to be deficient in field cases of nutritional pathology in broiler chickens.

Therefore, clinically specific B vitamin deficiencies, where routine phophylaxis would be indicated, are rare. However, the therapeutic indications for the B vitamin, thiamin, are described below.

THIAMIN

Thiamin (thiamine, vitamin B_1, aneurin) was the first of the B-complex vitamins to be isolated and purified. It is a metabolic necessity for plants and animals. Thiamin is synthesized by plants and bacteria and has a ubiquitous distribution.

Source and Occurrence

Thiamin is present in most plant products. A high thiamin content is associated with green, leafy plants and protein. High-quality sun-cured hay retains much of its thiamin content. Whole cereal grains and certain milling by-products like wheat germ are rich sources. Processed flour is a poor source. Thiamin is heat labile and water soluble so that cooking may destroy much of the native vitamin. Brewer's yeast is the richest natural source. Since bacteria readily synthesize thiamin from organic precursors, the digestive tract and feces have fairly high levels. Sufficient thiamin is formed in the rumen and subsequently absorbed so that ruminants do not require an additional dietary source. In nonruminant species the combination of exogenous dietary thiamin and bacterial synthesis is sufficient to supply the animal's needs. Thiamin is absorbed from both large and small intestines. Due to the content of thiamin in the feces, animals that practice coprophagy either incidental to their usual food intake or as a conscious act will obtain added thiamin. Animals maintained in cages or on slats may be denied access to this normal dietary source and can become thiamin deficient.

Chemistry

The structure of thiamin pyrophosphate is shown in Fig. 39.1. It is stable in acidic solution but labile in heated basic solutions.

Function

Ingested thiamin is activated following absorption. The active form is thiamin pyrophosphate (TPP) or cocarboxylase, the coenzyme necessary for oxidative decarboxylation of α keto acids. From a metabolic standpoint, the critical or limiting enzymatic defect in thiamin deficiency is in the oxidative decarboxylation of pyruvic acid. This reaction is essential for the complete oxidation of glucose through the citric acid cycle. Tissues that are dependent on glucose or lactate-pyruvate for energy, such as the brain and heart, are particularly compromised in thiamin deficiency.

Thiamin is not stored to a great extent in the body of most animals, consequently deficiency syndromes occur in 2–4 weeks on thiamin-deficient diets. Pigs are an exception since they can store several months' supply of thiamin. Excess thiamin is readily eliminated by the kidneys.

Deficiency

Dietary thiamin deficiency is not a common clinical problem, although some animals could receive practical diets that are thiamin deficient, such as highly processed foods not supplemented with additional vitamins. Breeding flocks of tur-

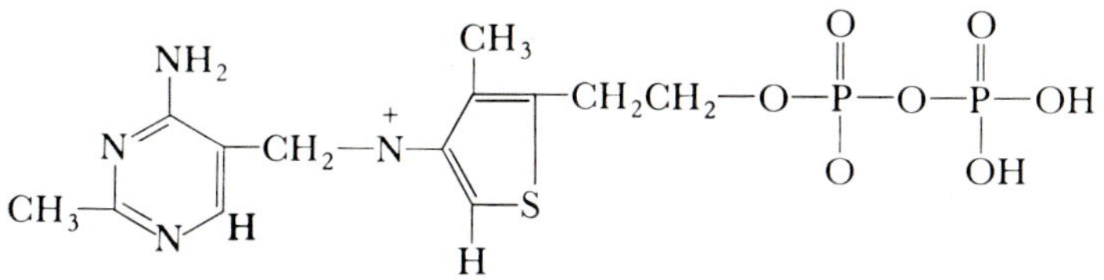

Thiamin Pyrophosphate
(Cocarboxylase)

Fig. 39.1.

keys and coturnix quail may have thiamin requirements in excess of those found in some practical diets (Charles et al. 1972). All animals that suffer from thiamin deficiency have increases in pyruvic and lactic acid in the blood as well as a decrease in the activity of the decarboxylase enzymes. The most common clinical signs are neuromuscular incoordination and tremors, followed by convulsions. Death is often due to cardiac failure. An excellent description of thiamin deficiency in chickens has been reported in conjunction with other induced vitamin syndromes (Gries and Scott 1972).

The principal cause of thiamin deficiency in animals is the presence of thiamin-destroying agents. These substances are widely distributed in nature (Somogyi 1973). In ruminants, polioencephalomalacia has been shown to be due to the appearance of an active thiaminase in the rumen. The disease occurs throughout the world and is associated with a dietary change to a higher concentrate level. Polioencephalomalacia was presented in more detail in Chapter 36. The origin of the thiaminase is not clearly established but is presumed to be produced by bacterial synthesis. It is not known how increased concentrate feeding triggers thiaminase production or activation.

Many plants contain an antithiamin phenolic acid derivative, highest in certain ferns, particularly bracken ferns. This plant antithiamin is not an enzymatic inhibitor of thiamin (Somogyi 1973). Instead, it undergoes an irreversible oxidation-reduction reaction with thiamin. Thiamin deficiency due to bracken fern ingestion is often seen in horses. Ingestion of the plant by laboratory animals will also result in thiamin deficiency. Fern poisoning in the United States is seen most frequently in the high rainfall coastal areas of Washington and Oregon. However, ferns containing the antithiamin compounds may be found elsewhere.

Symptoms of thiamin deficiency in the horse due to fern ingestion are similar to signs of thiamin deficiency in other animals, i.e., nervous incoordination, muscular tremors, posterior paralysis, and eventually convulsions with opisthotonus. In spite of the serious central nervous system (CNS) involvement, the ultimate cause of death is cardiac failure (Evans et al. 1951).

Carnivores may also receive an antithiamin compound if they ingest raw fish, especially the viscera. The disease, which is first manifested as a posterior paralysis, was initially recognized at a fox farm and is commonly known as Chastek's paralysis. Many freshwater and saltwater fish contain the antithiamin compound; it is highest in carp. The greatest antithiamin activity is in spleen, liver, intestines, and heart. The specific compound appears to be hemin, a partially degraded metabolite of hemoglobin. It acts to split thiamin at its methylene bridge. Any mammal that consumes large quantities of raw fish containing this hemin, without thiamin supplementation, will develop thiamin deficiency. Since the initial report in foxes, raw fish–induced thiamin deficiency has been recognized in dogs, cats, mink, and captive sea lions. Cooking destroys the activity of the thiamin antagonist. Thiamin deficiency is similar in all species; that induced by eating raw fish is no exception. Dogs, cats, and foxes show incoordination, a staggering gait, hyperirritability, convulsions, and death.

In addition to the thiamin antagonists from plants and fish viscera already mentioned, antithiamin compounds have been found in shellfish and are produced by some bacteria. This latter source may be relevant to the ruminal antithiamin compound whose origin is not established. There are commercial antithiamin compounds available. Amprolium, a coccidiostat for poultry and cattle, is a thiamin antagonist and its use can induce thiamin deficiency.

Daily Requirements

The daily dietary requirements for thiamin are met by most practical diets. Animals require more thiamin during pregnancy, lactation, and rapid growth but deficiencies are unlikely to occur unless thiamin antagonists are present. Processed, heat-treated food must have thiamin replaced.

Prophylaxis and Therapy

Unless animals are receiving a diet known to contain thiamin antagonists, prophylactic measures are not necessary. Bracken fern should not be heavily grazed nor should it be included in hay. Fish, especially carp to be fed to carnivores, should be cooked or fed at very low levels. Carp as 10% of the diet will induce the disease. Prophylactic parenteral administration of thiamin HCl to nonaffected ruminants may be of value in herd outbreaks of polioencephalomalacia.

Successful treatment of existing clinical deficiencies is dependent on the severity of the condition. Symptoms disappear rapidly unless irreversible damage to the CNS has occurred. Since most clinical thiamin deficiencies are due to dietary thiamin antagonists, feeding the vitamin may be of little benefit until the antivitamin has been cleared from the digestive tract. Parenteral administration of *Thiamin HCl,* U.S.P., is the preferred approach.

Recommended dosages vary widely and many represent excessive amounts of the vitamin. Since it has a low toxicity, a serious problem does not occur. Thiamin may be given intravenously, subcutaneously, or intramuscularly in the dosages shown in Table 39.2.

TABLE 39.2. Parenteral* thiamin therapy

Animal	Dosage
Horse	100–1000 mg
Ox	200–1000 mg
Calf	5–50 mg
Sheep	20–200 mg
Pig	5–100 mg
Dog	5–50 mg
Cat	1–20 mg
Poult	0.5–4 mg

* May be administered subcutaneously, intramuscularly, or intravenously, depending on the preparation.

NIACIN (NICOTINIC ACID, NICOTINAMIDE)

Niacin or its active form, nicotinamide, is a metabolic essential for all animals but is a dietary essential only under special conditions. In spite of this, niacin deficiency was a serious health problem for human beings in the early part of this century. With improper feeding, dogs may experience niacin deficiency.

Source and Occurrence

Niacin is found in high concentrations in yeast, liver, and peanuts. Other meats and meat products have fairly high levels (Kutsky 1973). Many grains contain niacin in a bound and unavailable form. A major source of niacin is the essential amino acid, tryptophan, which can be converted by most animals to niacin. Many animals can completely satisfy their niacin needs if sufficient quantities of tryptophan are present in the diet. It is reported that the cat is unable to make this conversion and therefore has a higher dietary niacin requirement (Scott 1964).

Chemistry

The structure of nicotinamide and its precursors, niacin and tryptophan, are shown in Fig. 39.2. The vitamin is a water-soluble crystalline powder. It is quite stable except in alkaline solutions (Kutsky 1973).

Function

Niacin is converted in the body to two similar coenzymes that are integral to hydrogen transfer in all major metabolic pathways, nicotinamide adenine dinucleotide (NAD) and nicotinamide adenine dinucleotide phosphate (NADP). These coenzymes were previously called diphosphopyridine nucleotide (DPN) and triphosphopyridine nucleotide (TPN), respectively. Although they are structurally similar, they serve different functions. NAD is more closely associated with the transfer of hydrogens to O_2 in completing oxidative metabolism. NAD, therefore, is closely related to hydrogen transfer in glycolysis and in the citric acid cycle. NADP is more commonly associated with hydrogen transfer in synthetic reactions in the body. For example, the first steps in the pentose phosphate pathway transfer hydrogens to

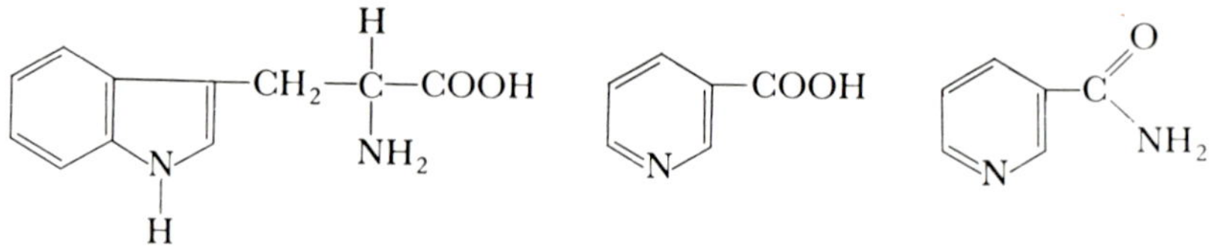

Tryptophan   Niacin (Nicotinic Acid)   Nicotinamide

Fig. 39.2.

NADP. Much of the stimulus for substrate flow through this path is the synthesis of lipids that requires NADPH.

Deficiency

Niacin is rarely deficient when "practical diets" are fed. When niacin deficiency occurs, it represents a good example of the dangers inherent in "single source" feeding. When human beings or nonherbivore domestic animals receive the majority of their food from corn, corn products, or certain other cereal grains, the deficiency syndrome will develop. Pellagra in human beings and black tongue in dogs are the classical diseases associated with niacin deficiency. In most species there are oral lesions affecting the mucosa that gives the blackened appearance and results in a thick saliva, malodorous breath, and ulcerative lesions. In addition, diarrhea and anemia are common as well as the usual signs of vitamin deficiency such as inappetence and poor growth.

Corn and the cereal grains contain fairly adequate quantities of niacin, but the vitamin is in a bound form and unavailable. In addition, corn and all the cereal grains are low in tryptophan. The combination of low tryptophan and unavailable dietary niacin results in a niacin deficiency. In current feeding practice in intensive agricultural situations, niacin or tryptophan should be added to high-concentrate diets of poultry and pigs.

Daily Requirements

Ruminants do not require an exogenous source of either niacin or tryptophan. They apparently receive a sufficient amount from ruminal synthesis. Horses also do not require either niacin or its amino acid precursor in their diets (Robinson and Slade 1974). Dogs develop the classical animal deficiency syndrome. The cure for pellagra in human beings, niacin and nicotinamide, was first shown to be effective in the dog (Elvehjem et al. 1937). Carnivores are unlikely to receive practical diets that are deficient in both niacin and tryptophan. The daily requirements of dogs and cats for niacin should be met easily by standard feeding practices so that supplementation is unnecessary. Swine and poultry often require additional niacin. The specific requirements vary with the type of production and the amount of precursor available.

Prophylaxis and Therapy

Swine and poultry on intensive production with high-concentrate cereal grains or corn should receive supplemental niacin, nicotinamide, or tryptophan. The assumption can be made that no niacin is available from cereal grains. Balanced diets that will insure sufficient niacin intake even on high grain rations can be formulated. Appropriate nutrient recommendations can be found in the National Academy Publications *Nutrient Requirements of Poultry*, 1971, and *Nutrient Requirements of Swine*, 1973. If niacin deficiency develops, it can be treated rapidly and effectively with oral or parenteral niacin or nicotinamide.

As mentioned in Chapter 36, a recent therapeutic use of niacin has been in the treatment of bovine ketosis. This therapy is based on its ability to decrease the release rate of free fatty acids from fat depots. Nicotinamide will not substitute for niacin in this action. Some care should be taken in intravenous administration of large quantities of niacin as some toxic side effects have been noted (Hayes and Hegsted 1973).

BIOTIN

A deficiency of biotin has been considered a curiosity since animals must receive an antivitamin, avidin, present in raw egg whites to develop a deficiency. Avidin is an albumin produced by the mucosa of the oviduct. It can bind biotin and render it unavailable. Quite recently a biotin deficiency has been linked with the clinical condition known as fatty liver and kidney syndrome (FLKS) (Payne 1975). FLKS has been recognized in broiler chickens that were fed wheat as a major dietary ingredient.

Prophylaxis and Therapy

For broiler chickens on high wheat intake, the diet should be supplemented with 75 μg biotin/kg of diet for prophylaxis. For therapy, a single dose of 100 μg biotin/chicken should be administered (Payne et al. 1974). Raw eggs in the diet of dogs will not improve the hair coat.

CHOLINE

Choline is in some ways analogous to niacin. Choline can be formed from an essential, although often limiting, amino acid precursor, methionine. Simple-stomached animals on high grain rations may develop choline deficiencies.

Source and Occurrence

Choline is in low concentration in cereal grains and corn but is relatively plentiful in other foods. Methionine can be considered a procholine molecule. Therefore, protein sources with high methionine content are valuable as sources of choline. Choline is a component of the phospholipid lecithin and is plentiful in many natural fats.

Chemistry

Choline is an important body metabolite. Its structure is shown in Fig. 39.3. Its formation from methionine involves several steps. Both methionine and choline can be considered as methyl donors.

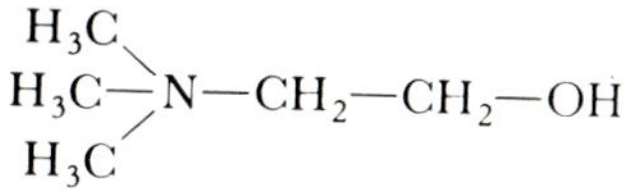

$$(H_3C)_3N{-}CH_2{-}CH_2{-}OH$$

Choline

Fig. 39.3.

Function

Choline is an integral part of the phospholipid lecithin. It is the base component of the neurohumor acetylcholine essential for all cholinergic neuromuscular transmission. Choline or methionine can partially replace each other in the diet; both may serve as sources of methyl groups (Griffith and Dyer 1968).

Deficiency

Choline deficiency, in addition to manganese deficiency, has long been associated with perosis in poultry (Wise et al. 1973). In the choline deficiency syndrome, fatty livers occur and a swelling and deformation of the tibiotarsal joints result in an uncoordinated gait. In sows, inadequate levels of choline may decrease reproductive efficiency. (NCR-42 Committee on Swine Nutrition 1973).

Daily Requirements

Most foods will meet the choline requirements of domestic animals. High grain diets with low fat intake may produce deficiencies.

Prophylaxis and Therapy

Proper ration formulation to insure adequate supplies of choline or its provitamins may be necessary for pigs and chickens on high-concentrate regimens. Choline deficiency is not generally recognized in other domestic animals. However, supplementation may be of benefit in the so-called fatty liver syndrome of dairy cows. See Chapter 36, under Bovine Ketosis, where in certain cases choline lipotropic action appears to be of therapeutic benefit. Twenty-five g of choline are administered subcutaneously in 250 ml of water, repeated in 4 hours if necessary.

REFERENCES

Bowland, J. P. 1973. Progress in swine nutrition for the veterinarian. Can Vet J 14:3.

Charles, O. W.; Roland, D. A.; and Edwards, H. M., Jr. 1972. Thiamine deficiency identification and treatment in commercial turkeys and coturnix quail. Poult Sci 51:419.

Elvehjem, C. A.; Madden, R. J.; Strong, F. M.; and Wooley, D. W. 1937. Relation of nicotinic acid and nicotinic acid amide to canine black tongue. J Am Chem Soc 59:1767.

Evans, E. T. R.; Evans, W. C.; and Roberts, H. E. 1951. Studies on bracken fern poisoning in the horse. Vet J 107:364, 399.

Gries, C. L., and Scott, M. L. 1972. The pathology of thiamin, riboflavin, pantothenic acid and niacin deficiencies in the chick. J Nutr 102:1269.

Griffith, W. H., and Dyer, H. M. 1968. Present knowledge of methyl groups in nutrition. Nutr Rev 26:1.

Hayes, K. C., and Hegsted, D. M. 1973. Toxicity of the vitamins. In Toxicants Occurring Naturally in Foods, 2nd ed. Washton, D.C.: National Academy of Sciences.

Kutsky, R. J. 1973. Handbook of Vitamins and Hormones. New York: Van Nostrand Reinhold.

NCR-42 Committee on Swine Nutrition. 1973. Effect of supplemental choline on reproductive performance of sows. J Anim Sci 37:281.

Payne, C. G. 1975. Biotin in poultry nutrition. Feedstuffs 47:923.

Payne, C. G.; Gilchrist, P.; Pearson, J. A.; and Hemsley, L. A. 1974. Involvement of biotin in the fatty liver and kidney syndrome of broilers. Br Poult Sci 15:489.

Robinson, D. W., and Slade, L. M. 1974. The current status of knowledge of the nutrition of equines. J Anim Sci 39:1045.

Scott, P. P. 1964. Nutritional requirements and deficiencies. In E. F. Catcott, ed. Feline Medicine and Surgery. Wheaton, Ill.: American Veterinary Publications.

Somogyi, J. C. 1973. Antivitamins. In Toxicants Occurring Naturally in Foods, 2nd ed., p. 234. Washington, D.C.: National Academy of Sciences.

Wise, D. R.; Jennings, A. R.; and Bostach, D. E. 1973. Perosis in turkeys. Res Vet Sci 14:167.

CHAPTER 40

CALCIUM AND PHOSPHORUS

ROBERT W. PHILLIPS

A consideration of calcium and phosphorus metabolism, as they relate to veterinary pharmacology and therapeutics, is complex. These two elements cannot be considered as unique entities separate from other elements, vitamins, and hormones. Vitamin D, in particular, is emerging as the primary controlling factor for calcium and phosphorus metabolism (Wasserman 1975). There have been several reviews relating to these two elements and their role in animal production and health (Jacobson et al. 1972; Dobson and Ward 1974; McBean and Speckmann 1974, Schryver et al. 1974, Wasserman 1975). An excellent review of calcium and phosphorus metabolism and the calcium-regulating hormones in animal disease is presented by Caspen (1975).

SOURCE AND OCCURRENCE

Calcium and phosphorus are universally distributed in soil and plants. They are essential for plant growth as well as for animal growth. They may vary in a given plant product with types of soil and fertilization, but several generalizations can be made. Hay contains more calcium than grain, and legume hay more than grass. Phosphorus is higher in grain than in hay. Many mineral supplements contain more calcium than phosphorus (Table 40.1).

The concentration of calcium and phosphorus in the crude diet is only one of the factors affecting the calcium-phosphorus status of animals from a health and production standpoint. An important limiting factor in animals that receive high levels of grains is the concentration of phytic acid and its salts. Phytic acid is inositol hexaphosphate and is shown in Fig. 40.1. Magnesium and calcium will bind to the phosphate radicals forming insoluble and unavailable complexes (Table 40.2). In general, phytic acid can be considered the only major feed ingredient that limits the avail-

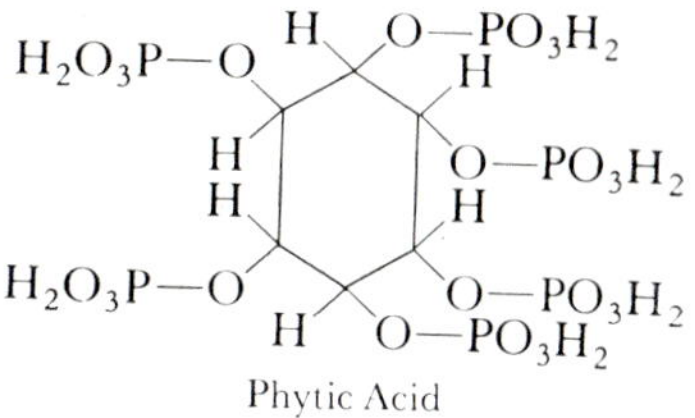

Phytic Acid

FIG. 40.1.

TABLE 40.1. Concentration of calcium and phosphorus in representative animal feeds and supplements

Source	Calcium	Digestibility*	Phosphorus	Digestibility*	Calcium-Phosphorus Ratio
	(g/kg)	*(%)*	*(g/kg)*	*(%)*	
Alfalfa hay	12.0	77	2.0	44	10.5†
Clover hay	11.5	77	2.2	44	9.1†
Timothy hay	3.6	70	1.6	46	3.4†
Corn silage	3.5	...	2.1	...	1.7
Barley	0.7	...	4.0	40	0.18
Corn	0.2	...	3.1	40	0.13
Wheat	0.5	...	4.0	40	0.16
Soybean seed	3.2	...	6.7	...	0.42
Sugar beet pulp	7.5	60	1.1	...	6.8
Citrus pulp	21.8	...	1.3	...	16.8
Dicalcium phosphate	231.3	74	186.5	58	1.6†
Monocalcium phosphate	170.0	...	210.0	58	0.8
Defluorinated phosphate	330.0	...	180.4	...	1.8
Bone meal	290.0	71	140.0	58	2.5†
Diamonium phosphate	0	...	200.0	...	...
Monosodium phosphate	0	...	220.0	...	...
Limestone ($CaCO_3$)	340.0	69	0	...	...
Oyster shells	350.0	...	0	...	...

* Schryver and Hintz 1975.
† Digestible calcium-phosphorus ratio.

ability of phosphorus, calcium, and magnesium. Specialized exceptions may occur such as forage oxalates or organic acids present in spring grasses (see Magnesium in Chapter 41). Most sources of calcium and phosphate are reasonably well utilized by all species (Table 40.1).

CALCIUM DISTRIBUTION AND FUNCTION

Calcium has a number of essential functions in the body. Predominant from a quantity standpoint is its role in providing structural stability as the major cation of bone crystalline hydroxyapatite. Hydroxyapatite is a complex molecule containing calcium phosphate and water, although other elements may be present in the bone crystalline structure. Calcium and phosphorus in bone are almost always in a ratio of 2:1.

Calcium has a wide variety of functions in addition to bone. One of the most basic and significant is its role in muscle contraction. Contractions are regulated by the calcium ion concentration in the sarcoplasm. The sarcoplasmic reticulum membranes contain an adenosine triphosphate (ATP)-dependent calcium pump mechanism that maintains a low calcium ion concentration in resting muscle. Upon stimulation, calcium is rapidly released from the terminal cisterna of the sarcoplasmic reticulum. The calcium binds to actin (thin filament) and promotes the formation of cross bridges between actin and myosin (thick filament), which causes them to be drawn to the center of the sarcomere. Grossly, this is seen as a shortening of the muscle. During relaxation, calcium ion is again sequestered within the sarcoplasmic reticulum and the cross bridges detach. Without calcium ions, this process will not proceed. The basic contraction phenome-

TABLE 40.2. Relative availability (%) of phosphorus from different sources

Source	Sheep	Cattle	Poultry	Swine
Dicalcium phosphate	100	100	100	100
Calcium phytate	66	50	50	35

Source: Peeler 1972.

non is associated with all voluntary movement as well as cardiac function and smooth muscle contraction. The molecular mechanisms of contraction are presented in detail in most physiology texts. On a lower order of magnitude than skeletal muscle, ciliary and flagellar contractions require the presence of calcium. At an even more microscopic level, there are intracellular contractile elements involved with the secretion of protein hormonal molecules. These contractile elements require calcium in order to function. Calcium is also required for neuromuscular excitability and transmission of nerve impulses. It is involved with the general phenomenon of membrane permeability and specifically activates certain enzyme systems. It is necessary for blood clotting. Calcium is required to be continually present and available for cells to function and for the organism to live.

Calcium level in the blood is maintained within rather narrow limits at 9–11 mg/100 ml (approximately 5 mEq/L) in most animals. Laying hens have higher concentrations. Approximately half of the blood calcium is in an ionized form. Most of the rest is bound to proteins and a small amount is complexed with other molecules. Calcium is in higher concentration in blood than in cells and it is primarily an extracellular ion. Magnesium, the other major divalent cation of the body, is primarily intracellular in nature (see Chapter 41).

PHOSPHORUS DISTRIBUTION AND FUNCTION

Approximately 80% of the body's phosphorus is deposited with calcium in bones and teeth. The rest, primarily in organic combination, is widely distributed. The single most fundamental phosphorus function is in the transfer of biological energy, particularly through ATP. The reversible binding of phosphate radicals is associated with the transfer of energy during the oxidation of hydrogen to form water. Although high-energy phosphates may be formed in other systems, oxidative phosphorylation is the route of importance. These high-energy phosphates have been referred to as the "common currency" of energy exchange in the body. Phosphates are also involved in the body's buffering capacity.

METABOLIC CONTROL

The control of calcium and phosphorus metabolism in the body is a very complex system. It involves intrinsic factors such as parathormone from the parathyroid gland and calcitonin from the C cells of the thyroid gland (Chapter 33). Vitamin D, however, is emerging as the more basic control factor in regulating calcium metabolism (Chapter 38). These three agents work in concert at the level of the intestinal tract, bone, and kidneys to continuously maintain the blood calcium and phosphorus levels and to bring about the deposition of bone. Fig. 40.2 illustrates many of the interactions that occur.

DIETARY EFFECTS

Most calcium is absorbed from the small intestine as shown for the horse in Fig. 40.3. Net phosphorus absorption may occur in the small intestine in some species but is primarily a function of the colon in horses (Fig. 40.4).

The rate at which calcium and phosphorus are absorbed is dependent on the form in which they are provided, calcium phytate and oxalate being less available. In addition, with increased age the ability to absorb calcium is decreased. However, the primary control is (1) related to the body's calcium rather than its phosphorus needs and (2) controlled by the active form of vitamin D (1,25-dihydroxycholecalciferol) that is generated in the kidney by the action of parathormone (Norman 1974). Calcium absorption is by active transport. Vitamin D also appears to have a direct effect on phosphorus absorption from the intestine. Excess dietary calcium and phos-

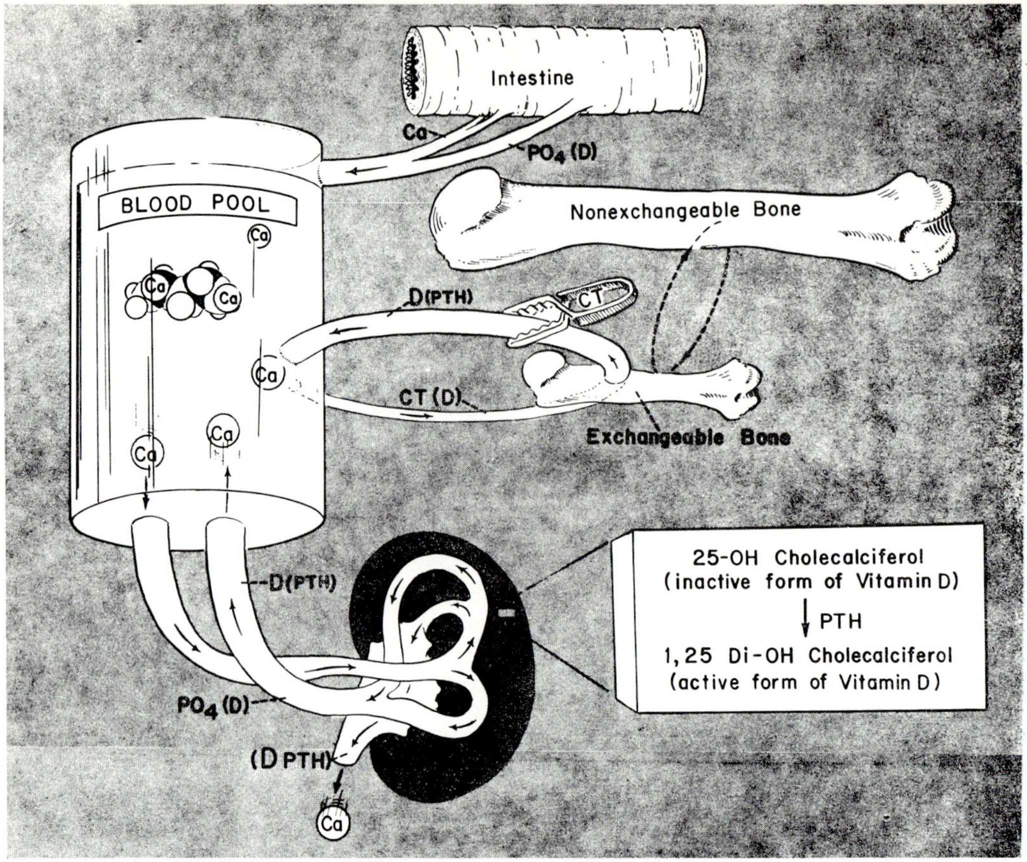

FIG. 40.2. The control of calcium and phosphorus metabolism in the body by parathormone, calcitonin, and vitamin D.

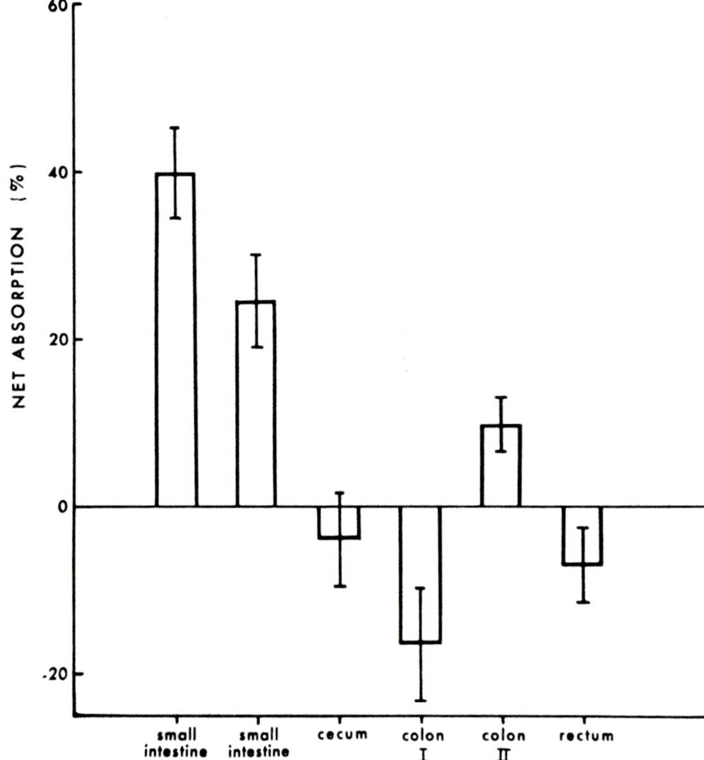

FIG. 40.3. Net fractional absorption of calcium from various regions of the intestine of the horse. The regions are the upper *(I)* and lower *(II)* portions of the small intestine, cecum, upper *(I)* and lower *(II)* parts of the large colon, and the small colon, including the rectum. Standard errors are shown. (Schryver et al. 1970)

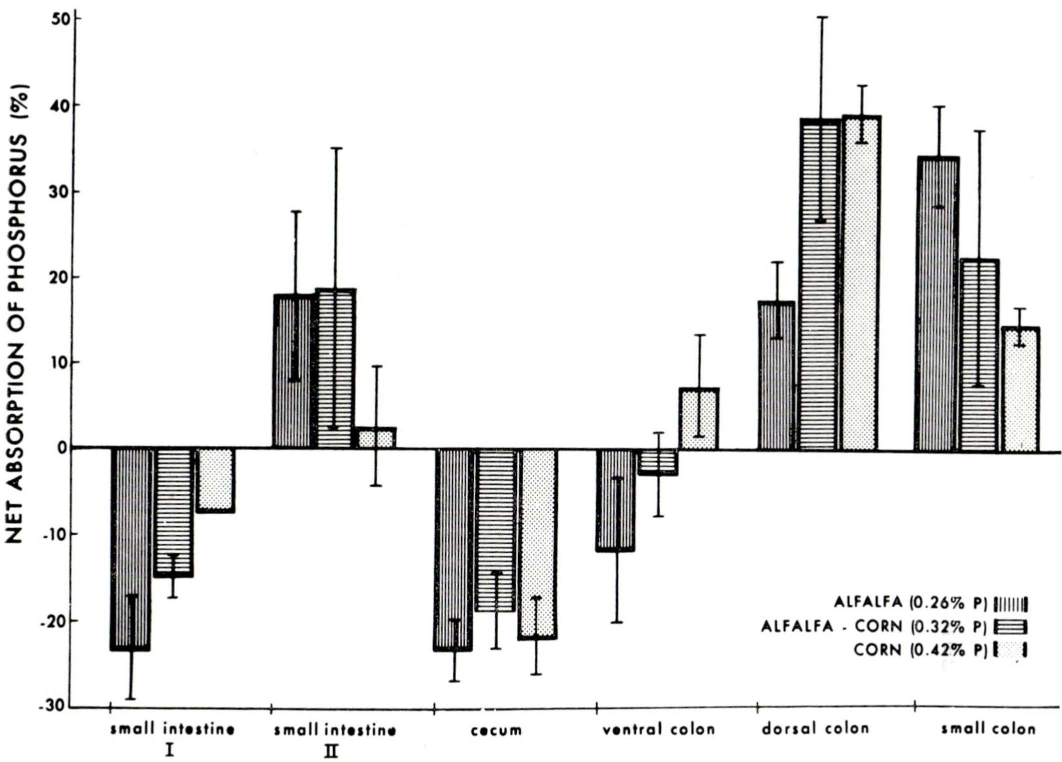

FIG. 40.4. Net percentage absorption of phosphorus that entered various regions of the intestine of ponies fed alfalfa, alfalfa-corn, or high corn diets. Each point is the mean of three (corn diet) or four (alfalfa, alfalfa-corn diets) observations. Standard errors are shown. (Schryver et al. 1972)

phorus are excreted directly in the feces.

Calcium in bone is present in an exchangeable and nonexchangeable form, although slow transfer can occur between these pools. Exchangeable and nonexchangeable pools do not represent absolute anatomical units but refer to relative availability. The exchangeable pool is much smaller (Fig. 40.2).

In growing animals calcium and phosphate are deposited in bone when their level is sufficiently high in blood. Vitamin D and parathormone increase calcium and phosphate levels in the blood and, therefore, enhance bone formation. The fact that this may be an indirect manifestation of these two modifiers is indicated parenthetically (Fig. 40.2).

The principal action of vitamin D on bone is to enhance resorption (Chapter 38). Calcitonin blocks calcium and phosphorus mobilization from bone and tends, therefore, to lower blood levels.

The kidneys activate vitamin D under the action of parathormone. Active vitamin D, in turn, appears to increase calcium and phosphorus reabsorption from the renal tubules, although the latter action may be indirect. Parathormone, on the other hand, causes a renal phosphate diuresis (Omdahl and DeLuca 1973). In some situations renal calcium excretion may be increased by vitamin D and parathormone, but the effect is due to the increased amount of calcium presented to the tubules as plasma levels increase.

REQUIREMENTS

The entire diet must be considered in evaluating the status of an animal with regard to calcium and phosphorus. In many

TABLE 40.3. Calcium-phosphorus requirement

Animal	Calcium g/kg Ration	Phosphorus g/kg Ration	Calcium-Phosphorus Ratio
Cattle			
Growing	3.9	3.1	1.26
Lactating beef	2.4	2.0	1.20
Lactating dairy (20–30 kg milk/day)	4.7	3.5	1.34
Horse			
Growing	4.4	3.0	1.47
Lactating	4.7	3.9	1.21
Adult, light work	2.5	2.0	1.25
Sheep			
Growing	2.0	1.8	1.11
Lactating	2.7	2.0	1.35
Swine			
Growing	6.5	5.0	1.30
Lactating	7.5	5.0	1.50
Dog			
Growing	11.0	9.0	1.22
Lactating	11.0	9.0	1.22
Chicken			
Growing	10.0	7.0	1.43
Laying	27.5*	6.0	4.58

* Calcium supplements are available free choice.

cases supplemental amounts of these elements are not necessary. For instance, legume hay should provide sufficient calcium and phosphorus for an adult horse (Tables 40.1, 40.3). The generalization may be made that the dietary calcium and phosphorus requirements are least for adults and greatest for lactating animals: adult $<$growing $<$lactating.

Table 40.3 summarizes calcium and phosphorus needs. For more specific information, refer to the current National Academy of Sciences publication for the species in question.

CALCIUM-PHOSPHORUS RATIO

In assessing the calcium and phosphorus status of an animal, quantity supplied by the diet in an available form is the most important consideration. Over the years frequent use has also been made of the calcium-phosphorus ratio (Ca-P). Table 40.1 lists this ratio for a few common mineral and nutrient sources. Varying Ca-PO_4 ratios have been recommended by different authors for domestic animals (Jacobson et al. 1972; Hedhammar et al. 1974; Schryver et al. 1974; Jordan et al. 1975). Most recommendations fall in the range 1:1 to 2:1. Ratios in that range should be adequate for most functional activities. However, the ratio alone is not sufficient. It must be related to the total requirement of both calcium and phosphorus. Laying poultry obviously require more calcium, due to the heavy calcium carbonate content of eggshell.

CLINICAL MANIFESTATIONS

There are a number of related clinical conditions resulting from alterations in calcium and phosphorus metabolism. Some may be due to frank deficiencies or excesses while others relate to vitamin-hormone imbalances and changes in production.

Deficiency

Two inherently different types of syndromes are associated with calcium or phosphorus imbalances. One is chronic in nature as exemplified by rickets in growing animals or osteomalacia in adults. Parturient paresis in milk cows is the most notable example of an acute imbalance seen in veterinary clinical medicine.

Parturient Paresis

Parturient paresis or milk fever is one of the metabolic diseases that has become more prevalent as agriculture has become specialized and intensified. It is characterized as a hypocalcemia and hypophosphatemia in milk cows during early lactation. The mechanisms that bring about parturient paresis are not completely elucidated (Kronfeld et al. 1973). A current concept is that the freshly parturient cow cannot mobilize sufficient bone calcium in spite of increased intestinal absorption. As mammary drain exceeds intestinal and renal absorption and the limited bone resorption, hypocalcemia occurs (Ramberg et al. 1970; Kronfeld 1971). The factors limiting bone resorption are subject to controversy. Some data indicate that the parathyroid gland is suppressed on high calcium intake and unable to respond rapidly to the increased calcium drain imposed by lactation (Black et al. 1973). Other workers have reported normal levels of parathormone and calcitonin at parturition (Mayer 1970). However, a portion of the plasma parathormone may be in an inactive state (Mayer et al. 1973). In addition, exogenous parathyroid extracts are of no benefit as a treatment for parturient paresis. The preponderance of the data at this time indicates that the problem is not the parathyroid gland.

It seems possible that the basic defect is related to some aspect of the vitamin D bone mobilizing system. This could occur either at the kidney, where 1,25-dihydroxycholecalciferol is formed under the action of parathormone, or in a delayed response to the activated vitamin D in bone. Whatever the cause, the hypocalcemic cow develops motor paralysis and may become unconscious. Hypophosphatemia, although present, is not considered as the prime defect. Occasionally, hyperglycemia has been reported in parturient paresis (Littledike et al. 1969).

PROPHYLAXIS

The basic dysfunction is a lag in the ability of the cow to mobilize bone calcium following parturition. An effective prophylactic approach is to place animals on a low calcium intake during the last two weeks of gestation so that their calcium mobilizing system is activated prior to the initiation of significant mammary drain (Kronfeld 1971; Goings et al. 1974; Jorgensen 1974). Effective suggested levels of "low calcium" intake vary from 100 g/cow/day to 8 g/450 kg/day. A level of 6–8 g/100 kg/day should prevent most cases of parturient paresis. The low intake will enhance the efficiency of calcium absorption and bone mobilization. Following parturition, dietary calcium levels should be increased to greater than 125 g/cow/day. Legume hays should be avoided in the prepartum period due to their high calcium content (Table 40.1).

Additional prophylactic measures include supplementation with oral or parenteral vitamin D and its analogs prior to parturition and supplemental calcium salts immediately following parturition. Intensive research in activated vitamin D and its analogs may well provide more effective prophylaxis (Schnoes and DeLuca 1974). Currently, vitamin D_3 may be used parenterally or orally, although hazards exist due to its potential toxic manifestations in high doses (Kronfeld 1971). Administration of 20–30 million units of vitamin D/day for 3–8 days prepartum effectively decreased the incidence of the disease and caused elevated blood calcium levels as shown in Fig. 40.5 (Hibbs and Pounden 1955). Prolonged administration of such large amounts of vitamin D may cause anorexia, decreased gastrointestinal motility, diuresis, and mineralization of the cardiovascular system. Relatively small amounts of the vitamin D analog, 25-hydroxycholecalciferol, prior to parturition have been reported to decrease the incidence of parturient paresis (Jorgensen 1974). Two hundred mg intravenously or 1–8 mg orally every 48 hours have been reasonably effective and do not appear to have the toxic side effects associated with vitamin D itself. Another analog, 1-α-hydroxy vitamin D_3, has also been reported to prevent parturient paresis when 100 μg were administered intravenously at least 24 hours prior

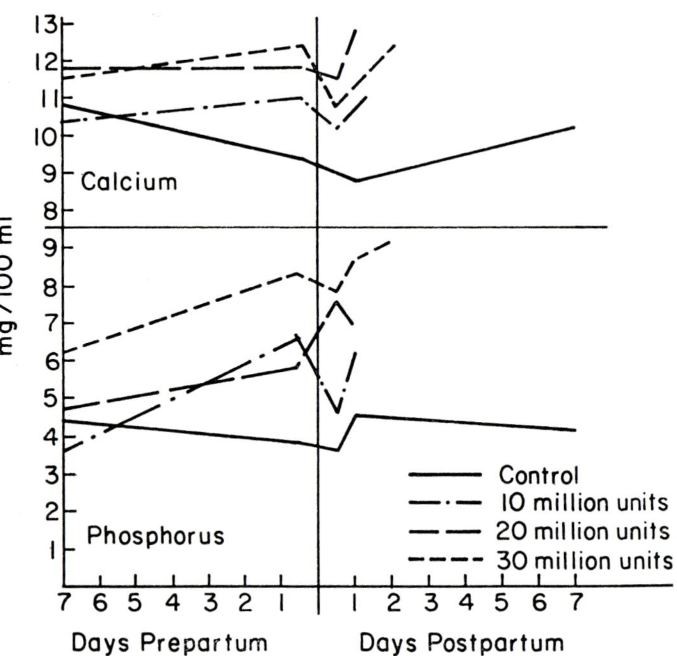

FIG. 40.5. The effect of various amounts of vitamin D fed 3–8 days before parturition on the blood serum calcium and phosphorus levels of parturient Jersey cows having two or more previous lactations. (Hibbs and Pounden 1955)

to predicted parturition and repeated every 48 hours (Marquardt et al. 1974). At this time neither of these analogs is commercially available or cleared for use in food-producing animals.

THERAPY

Even though prevention is the desired goal, short-term prepartum low-calcium diets are not always available or used for dairy cows; thus the disease will undoubtedly continue to be manifest. The oldest therapy is udder insufflation, which decreases the rate of milk formation. Therefore, the calcium drain is diminished on a temporary basis. Udder insufflation is not used extensively today. However, it can still be an effective means of therapy, and relapses are less frequent than with calcium therapy (Mayer et al. 1967).

The most common and effective therapy for parturient paresis is intravenous calcium ions. A number of other constituents have been suggested as additions to this therapy but their value has not been substantiated. Calcium gluconate, U.S.P., and calcium borogluconate are the most commonly used forms. The addition of boron markedly increases calcium solubility and stability of the product. The gluconate form causes less tissue irritation than calcium chloride. The concentrations of commercial calcium borogluconate solutions vary from 20% to 33%. Slow intravenous injection of 1 g calcium/50 kg of body weight is an adequate dosage for cattle and sheep suffering from hypocalcemia. If the calcium ion is injected too rapidly into the vascular system, a fatal heart block can develop.

Other parturient species can develop similar hypocalcemic conditions. Therapy is similar, modifications being more a function of size than of a change in philosophy. Although a more dilute solution of calcium is recommended, the same dosage can be used with small animals for parturient eclampsia. A 10% solution of calcium gluconate has been recommended for dogs and cats.

Other therapeutic forms of calcium have been suggested, many attempting to provide a slow release by a reversible binding of calcium with an organic constituent. The theoretical basis is to supply a slower release calcium ion that would provide a longer therapeutic effect with a decreased potential for cardiotoxicity.

Rickets

Young growing animals require adequate calcium, phosphorus, and active vitamin D for normal bone growth and calcification. True rickets is relatively uncommon since most animals receive adequate amounts of vitamin D (see Chapter 38).

A frank deficiency of calcium phosphate and/or calcium and phosphorus in the diet can cause nutritional secondary hyperparathyroidism often diagnosed as rickets. Hyperparathyroidism and hypoparathyroidism are discussed in Chapter 33.

Both the amounts of calcium and phosphorus in the diet and the ratio between these two elements are important. Other constituents of the diet may also modify mineral absorption and utilization. In a recent study with young rapidly growing Great Danes, it was shown that too rapid a growth due to an energy-rich diet resulted in bone dyscrasias even when mineral supplementation was believed to be adequate (Hedhammar et al. 1974).

REFERENCES

Beitz, D. C.; Burkhart, D. J.; and Jacobson, N. L. 1974. Effects of calcium to phosphorus ratio in the diet of dairy cows on incidence of parturient paresis. J Dairy Sci 57:49.

Black, H. E.; Capen, C. C.; and Arnaud, C. D. 1973. Ultrastructure of parathyroid glands and plasma immunoreactive parathyroid hormone in pregnant cows fed normal and high calcium diets. Lab Invest 29:173.

Capen, C. C. 1975. Parathyroid hormone, calcitonin, and cholecalciferol: The calcium regulating hormones. In L. E. McDonald, ed. Veterinary Endocrinology and Reproduction, 2nd ed., p. 62. Philadelphia: Lea & Febiger.

Dobson, R. C., and Ward, G. 1974. Vitamin D physiology and its importance in dairy cattle: A review. J Dairy Sci 57:985.

Goings, R. L.; Jacobson, N. L.; Beitz, D. C.; Littledyke, E. T.; and Wiggers, K. D. 1974. Prevention of parturient paresis by a prepartum calcium deficient diet. J Dairy Sci 57:1184.

Hedhammar, A.; Wu, F.-M.; Krook, L.; Schryver, H. F.; DeLahunta, A.; Whalen, J. P.; Kallfelz, F. A.; Nunez, E. A.; Hintz, H. F.; Sheffy, B. E.; and Ryan, G. D. 1974. Overnutrition and skeletal disease: An experimental study in growing Great Dane dogs. Cornell Vet 64, Suppl 5.

Hibbs, J. W., and Pounden, W. D. 1955. Studies on milk fever in dairy cows. IV. Prevention by short-time, prepartum feeding of massive doses of vitamin D. J Dairy Sci 38:65.

Jacobson, D. R.; Henken, R. W.; Button, F. S.; and Hatton, R. H. 1972. Mineral nutrition, calcium, phosphorus, magnesium and potassium interrelationships. J Dairy Sci 55:935.

Jordan, R. M.; Myers, V. S.; Bradford, Y.; and Spurrel, F. A. 1975. Effect of calcium and phosphorus levels on growth reproduction and bone development of ponies. J Anim Sci 40:78.

Jorgenson, N. A. 1974. Combating milk fever. J Dairy Sci 57:933.

Kronfeld, D. S. 1971. Parturient hypocalcemia in dairy cows. Adv Vet Sci Comp Med 15: 133.

Kronfeld, D. S.; Mayer, G. P.; and Ramberg, C. F. 1973. Calcium metabolism in dairy cows. In J. M. Payne, K. G. Hibbitt, and B. F. Sansom, eds. Production Disease in Farm Animals, p. 165. Baltimore: Williams & Wilkins.

Littledyke, E. T.; Whipp, S. C.; and Schroeder, L. 1969. Studies on parturient paresis. J Am Vet Med Assoc 155:1955.

McBean, L. D., and Speckmann, E. W. 1974. A recognition of the interrelationships of calcium with various dietary components. Am J Clin Nutr 27:603.

Marquardt, J. P.; Holick, M. F.; Horst, R. L.; Jorgenson, N. A.; and DeLuca, H. F. 1974. Efficacy of 1 α hydroxy Vitamin D_3 on prevention of parturient paresis. J Dairy Sci (Abstr) 57:606.

Mayer, G. P. 1970. The role of parathyroid hormone and thyrocalcitonin in parturient paresis. In J. J. B. Andersen, ed. Parturient Paresis, p. 177. New York: Academic Press.

Mayer, G. P.; Ramberg, C. F., Jun.; and Kronfeld, D. S. 1967. Udder insufflation and its physiological basis for treatment of parturient paresis. J Am Vet Med Assoc 151: 1673.

Mayer, G. P.; Habener, J. F.; and Potts, J. T. 1973. Significance of plasma immunoreactive parathyroid hormone in hypocalcemic cows. In J. M. Payne, K. G. Hibbitt, and B. F. Sansom, eds. Production Disease in Farm Animals, p. 217. Baltimore: Williams & Wilkins.

Norman, A. W. 1974. Hormone-like action of $1{,}25(OH)_2$-cholecalciferol. In Robert Harris et al., eds. Vitamin and Hormone Advances in Research and Application, vol. 32, p. 325. New York: Academic Press.

Omdahl, J. L., and DeLuca, H. F. 1973. Regulation of vitamin D metabolism and function. Physiol Rev 53:327.

Peeler, H. T. 1972. Biological availability of nutrients in feeds: Availability of major mineral ions. J Anim Sci 35:695.

Ramberg, C. F.; Mayer, G. P.; Kronfeld, D. S.; Phang, J. M.; and Berman, M. 1970. Calcium kinetics in cows during late pregnancy, parturition and early lactation. Am J Physiol 219:1167.

Robinson, D. W., and Slade, L. M. 1974. The current status of knowledge on the nutrition of equines. J Anim Sci 39:1045.

Schnoes, H. K., and DeLuca, H. F. 1974. Synthetic analogs of 1 α,25-dihydroxyvitamin D_3 and their biological activity. In Robert Harris et al., eds. Vitamin and Hormone Advances in Research and Application, vol. 32, p. 385. New York: Academic Press.

Schryver, H. F., and Hintz, H. F. 1975. Recent development in equine nutrition. Anim Nutr Health. April, p. 6.

Schryver, H. F.; Craig, P. H.; Hintz, H. F.; Hogue, D. E.; and Lowe, J. E. 1970. The site of calcium absorption in the horse. J Nutr 100:1127.

Schryver, H. F.; Hintz, H. F.; Craig, P. H.; Hogue, D. E.; and Lowe, J. E. 1972. Site of phosphorus absorption from the intestine of the horse. J Nutr 102:143.

Schryver, H. F.; Hintz, H. F.; and Lowe, J. E. 1974. Calcium and phosphorus in the nutrition of the horse. Cornell Vet 64:493.

Wasserman, R. H. 1975. Metabolism function and clinical aspects of vitamin D. Cornell Vet 65:3.

CHAPTER 41

TRACE ELEMENTS

ROBERT W. PHILLIPS

The trace elements of pharmacologic importance are those most likely to be deficient or excessive in the diet. Changing agricultural practices have led to increasingly intensive plant and animal husbandry that may alter availability of trace elements and their requirements by animals. As an example, increased fertilization and irrigation lead to both increased plant growth and increased leaching of well-drained soils. The former may cause direct changes in plant composition and the latter may deplete some microelements from the soil (Underwood 1972). These and other management and production techniques, such as maintaining swine on concrete throughout their lives, will alter the availability of trace elements to the animal and may result in deficiency syndromes in areas where they did not previously exist. Animals acquire trace elements naturally by oral ingestion of plants and also from soil contamination of herbage (Healy 1974).

Trace element interrelationships are very complex and there are many specific examples that might be cited to illustrate these interactions. One of the best defined is that between copper and molybdenum. Both of these elements may be deficient or present in toxic quantities and each reduces the absorption and utilization of the other. On molybdenum marginal soils, copper can cause a molybdenum deficiency, whereas copper is a therapeutic choice for animals having molybdenum toxicosis. Figure 41.1 diagrammatically represents a summation of some of the factors affecting the level of a particular trace element in the body. It does not include interactions between elements.

Prophylactically, the first concern is recognition of an actual or potential trace element deficiency or excess. For the most part, even frank deficiencies do not result in clear-cut pathognomonic signs. Since our goal is prevention, history, observation, intuition, and reason must be included with analytical determinations to develop appropriate programs of supplementation.

Specific diagnoses may be made on the basis of clinical signs but definitive information can also be gained by a knowledge of soil and plant elemental composition and the "nutritional" history of the region. The ultimate analysis should include tissue samples from the animal. Although blood sampling is a common method employed to determine functional status, it is of less value for some minor constituents that are primarily intracellular in nature. Biopsy of a representative number of ani-

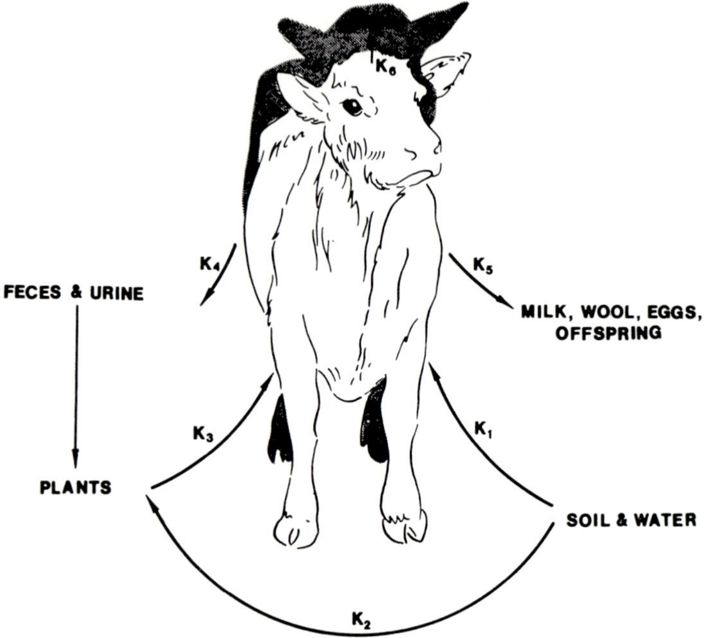

FIG. 41.1. Mineral fluxes in animals. The net retention of any mineral depends on a variety of input and output functions.

K_1 — Function of type of ground cover, intensity of grazing, moisture, form of elements in the soil.
K_2 — Function of form of elements in the soil, type of plants, ratio of elements in the soil, moisture, maturity of the plants.
K_3 — Function of palatability, digestibility, intensity of grazing.
K_4 — Function of digestibility, type of digestive tract, absorption, biliary excretion, quantity in the body, renal function, state of health, age.
K_5 — Function of intensity of production, type of production.
K_6 — Function of rate of growth.

mals or analysis of hair may provide more information.

Therapy or preventive supplementation can be tailored to the situation at hand. Table 41.1 lists some routes that have been successfully used to supplement trace element intake.

Not all forms of trace elements are equally available to the animal. Table 41.2 presents some of the forms that have been

TABLE 41.1. Supplementation of trace elements

Technique	Element	Use
Trace element fertilization of soil	Magnesium, copper, cobalt, selenium, iodine, zinc	Pasture, feed grains, roughage
Top dressing or spray of foliage	Magnesium, cobalt	Feed grains, roughage
Heavy, slow release pellets in the rumen	Magnesium, selenium, cobalt	Cattle, sheep
Trace mineral salt blocks	All elements	Range pasture
Incorporation in prepared diets	All elements	Feedlots, swine, poultry, horses, pets
Parenteral injection	Iron, magnesium, selenium, iodine, other elements except cobalt	

TABLE 41.2. Biological availability of oral trace elements

Element	Good	Poor
Iodine	Sodium and potassium iodide,* calcium iodate, potassium iodate, diiodothymol, pentacalciumorthoperiodate (PEOP)	Diiodosalicylic acid
Copper	Cupric sulfate,† cupric chloride, cupric carbonate, cupric nitrate	Cupric sulfide, oxide elemental copper
Cobalt	Cobalt carbonate,† cobalt chloride, cobalt nitrate, cobalt oxide,† cobalt sulfate	
Iron	Ferric chloride, ferric sulfate, ferrous sulfate, ferrous fumarate, ferrous ammonium sulfate	Ferric oxide, ferrous carbonate, ferric orthophosphate
Manganese	Manganese sulfate, manganese chloride, manganese carbonate, manganese dioxide, manganese potassium permanganate	Manganese silicate, rhodocrosite ($MnCO_3$ ore)
Magnesium	Magnesium oxide, magnesium chloride, magnesium carbonate, magnesium citrate, magnesium acetate, magnesium lactate, magnesium phosphate	Magnesium ore, magnesium silicate
Selenium	Sodium selenite, sodium selenate, elemental selenium	
Sulfur	Sulfur amino acids, sodium sulfate, calcium sulfate, sodium sulfide	Elemental sulfur
Zinc	Zinc chloride, zinc sulfate, zinc oxide, zinc proteinate, zinc carbonate	

Source: Ammerman and Muller 1972; Peeler 1972.
* May be unstable. †Commonly used form.

tested for bioavailability after oral ingestion.

In the following sections dealing with specific trace elements, all daily requirements, unless otherwise noted, are based on the most recent National Academy of Sciences publication, *Nutrient Requirements of Domestic Animals,* for that species in question and are not individually referenced. The reader is encouraged to refer to these publications for further information.

A number of trace elements have biological importance but are rarely incriminated in clinical veterinary medicine as being deficient or toxic. Some elements, for instance aluminum, are routinely found in plant and animal tissue but have no known function. Elements that are not of clinical concern are not presented here. The most complete current coverage of trace elements in animals is by Underwood (1971).

CHROMIUM

Metabolic Function and Chemistry

Chromium has been shown to be a dietary essential in several animals. It was first identified as the glucose tolerance factor (GTF), an organic form of trivalent chromium, present in brewer's yeast. Animals on chromium-free diets develop impaired glucose tolerance that is restored to normal upon the addition of chromium. The GTF appears to enhance the reaction between insulin and cellular membrane receptors, facilitating the action of insulin. Either trivalent or hexavalent chromium has been found to be biologically active. Chromium is also associated with a hepatic nucleoprotein and some ribonucleic acid (RNA), although the biological significance is unknown.

Source and Occurrence

Animal meats, grains, and Brewers' yeast contain chromium. Drinking water has variable amounts. Processing of feeds tends to remove chromium.

Requirements

No daily requirements have been established for domestic animals.

Prophylaxis and Therapeutics

To date, trivalent chromium has been used successfully to treat some cases of impaired glucose tolerance in adult diabetic human beings and undernourished children. Its value in veterinary therapeutics has not been established.

COBALT

Metabolic Function and Chemistry

The only established function of cobalt is as a component of vitamin B_{12} or cyanocobalamin. Nonruminants have not been shown to require elemental cobalt in their diets as they receive vitamin B_{12} preformed. The antianemic function of this vitamin is covered in Chapter 23.

Although cobalt as a component of B_{12} is necessary for erythropoiesis in ruminants, it has a broader role in metabolic utilization (see Chapter 36). Propionic acid, a major glucogenic rumen fermentation metabolite, is converted to glucose in the liver. One of the early steps involved in this conversion, methylmalonyl-CoA→ succinyl-CoA, is catalyzed by the enzyme methylmalonyl-CoA isomerase, which requires vitamin B_{12} as a cofactor. In the absence of cobalt, vitamin B_{12} is deficient and propionic acid cannot be utilized .

Source and Occurrence

Australia, New Zealand, and portions of Africa have cobalt-deficient areas. In North America cobalt deficiencies have been reported around the Great Lakes and in New England and Florida. In regions where cobalt is plentiful in the soil, it is provided to animals upon plant ingestion.

Deficiency

Ruminants in cobalt-deficient areas become weak and emaciated and show progressive inappetence and anemia. Under marginal deficiency conditions there is a decrease in production that is most noticeable in young animals in the spring when plant growth is most rapid. Cobalt is poorly absorbed from the digestive tract.

Requirements

A mature sheep requires 0.1 mg of cobalt daily. Feed that contains greater than 0.07 mg/kg cobalt on a dry matter basis is sufficient to prevent deficiency syndromes in sheep and cattle.

Prophylaxis and Therapeutics

In endemic areas top dressing of the soil with 100–150 g of $CoSO_4$/acre is generally sufficient to prevent deficiency. However, soil type can alter cobalt utilization by plants, thus an agronomist should be consulted to establish the suitability of this method.

Alternatively, cobalt oxide iron pellets have been placed in the reticulorumen to provide a slow release of cobalt. This method has two drawbacks: the pellet may be regurgitated and lost or it may be coated with calcium phosphate, which reduces cobalt availability. A steel core pellet covered with cobalt oxide–impregnated cotton gauze has been devised as a means of cobalt supplementation. As the cotton is digested by rumen microbes, cobalt is released. Calcium phosphate coating does not accrue (Connoly and Poole 1967).

Cobalt salts are sometimes included in trace mineral premixes and salt blocks. Cobalt salts can be added to loose salt at a ratio of 15 and 50 g/100 kg for sheep and cattle, respectively. With free choice supplementation, consumption may be inadequate. Cobalt may also be incorporated as a component of feed concentrates. For maximum production, cobalt should be provided as frequently as once per week. Therefore, oral drenching or B_{12} injections are not practical except to remedy frank deficiency syndromes. Cobalt is not effective parenterally since its active organic form must be synthesized in the rumen.

Toxicity

Cobalt is relatively nontoxic and toxicity is not recognized under natural conditions. Overdoses may result in depressed appetite, weight loss, and anemia, which is strangely analogous to the description of deficiency.

COPPER

Metabolic Function and Chemistry

Copper is an essential component of animal systems. It is directly involved in hematopoiesis (Chapter 23), connective tissue metabolism, myelin formation in newborn animals, pigmentation, and bone formation. Copper is an integral part of essential enzymes such as cytochrome oxidase and a number of the aromatic amino acid–metabolizing enzymes, i.e., tyrosinase, dopamine hydroxylase, and monoamine-oxidase. Recently it has been found that the cupreins, which are copper-containing proteins present in almost all aerobic cells, possess superoxide dismutase activity. A hypothesis has been developed that they function to protect tissues from oxygen toxicity instead of acting as copper storage or transport proteins as had been previously suggested (Frieden 1974).

Copper is, in general, poorly absorbed, with most of the absorption occurring in the upper small intestine. After absorption it is removed by the liver and the tissues for incorporation into protein. Much of the copper present in plasma is in the form of an α-globulin oxidase called ceruloplasmin. Measurement of ceruloplasmin is considered a better indication of copper status than the copper content of the blood.

Interactions

Copper has important interactions with molybdenum, zinc, iron, and calcium. All four of these latter elements can act to reduce copper availability. The reciprocal nature of Mo-Cu and Zn-Cu interaction has been clearly identified. High molybdenum soils may result in plant growth that causes copper deficiencies. Copper enzymes are necessary for adequate iron absorption.

Source and Occurrence

Most areas of the world have sufficient copper in the soil to prevent deficiency. In western Australia, lower areas of western Europe, and southeastern United States, particularly Florida, there are endemic deficiency regions. In addition, there are molybdenum toxicity areas in England, New Zealand, and western United States that may effectively cause copper deficiency.

Deficiency

Copper deficiency results in a depletion of circulating copper and hepatic stores. In most cases anemia is present and iron absorption is limited. In lambs, copper deficiency causes a disease, enzootic ataxia or swayback, in which there is spinal cord "demyelination" and cerebral necrosis. Similar conditions have been reported in goats and swine, but the most serious disease is seen in lambs. It has been associated with a decrease in cytochrome oxidase and impaired phospholipid synthesis. All animals except the pig show greater or lesser degrees of decreased hair pigmentation but sheep seem particularly sensitive. In addition, wool loses its crimp during periods of copper depletion. Copper plays a role in connective tissue metabolism, and both collagen in bone and elastin in arteries are defective when there is a copper deficiency. The defect is associated with a decrease in cross-linking between molecules so that the polymers do not have the requisite structural function (Hill et al. 1967).

Requirements

For most species copper levels in the diet of 5–8 mg/kg of dry matter are adequate to prevent deficiency. The only frank deficiency areas in the United States are in Florida and southeastern coastal regions. The requirement may be increased threefold to fourfold on high molybdenum soils. Milk is quite low in copper, and animals suckled without access to copper-containing feeds may need supplementation. Swine have been reported to respond favorably by increased production to high levels (150–250 mg/kg of feed) of elemental copper in the diet (Suttle and Mills 1966). The mechanisms are not well established. Calves do not respond similarly (Felsman et al. 1973).

Prophylaxis and Therapeutics

In deficient areas, copper in the form of cupric sulfate can be added to the salt at a rate of 0.5%. Soil fertilization with copper has been used in Australia and New Zealand but was ineffective in a high molybdenum area in Nevada in either reducing molybdenum or increasing copper content of feeds (Spencer et al. 1958). Treatment of pasture or crops with copper has not been extensively used in this country. It is likely that animals that are receiving concentrated diets and are not restricted to feed produced on copper-deficient soils will receive adequate copper. For this reason, poultry feeds rarely require supplemental copper.

If cattle and sheep on copper-deficient range or pasture are not receiving adequate copper, oral drenching with a soluble copper form will provide copper for several months. Single parenteral injections of organic copper forms such as Cu-Ca ethylenediaminetetraacetic acid (EDTA) or Cu methionate will alleviate deficiency signs.

Toxicity

As mentioned previously under Interactions, copper toxicity is dependent on dietary copper levels as well as the concentration of molybdenum, sulfur, iron, and zinc in the diet. Therefore, a single toxic level under field conditions cannot be determined.

Sheep, however, are most susceptible to copper toxicity; chronic copper poisoning occurs in several high-copper regions. It is characterized by a continuing accumulation of copper in the liver until a "breaking point" is reached. Copper is swiftly mobilized. A hemolytic crisis with icterus develops and there are hepatic necrosis and renal dysfunction.

FLUORINE

Metabolic Function and Chemistry

Several carefully controlled studies have provided evidence that fluorine may be an essential element. However, under practical field situations no deficiency has ever been noted in domestic animals. Thus our concern is related to fluorine's toxic manifestations. As in human beings, fluorine localizes in hard tissues such as bones and teeth.

Source and Occurrence

Fluorine occurrence is widespread. It is high in some livestock water and in nondefluorinated rock phosphate. It may be found in high concentrations on foliage surfaces but is rarely incorporated as a component of plants.

Deficiency

Fluorine deficiency is not a problem in domestic animals.

Requirements

No dietary supplementation is required.

Toxicity

Fluorine localizes in bones and teeth, causing enlargement and softening of mineral structures (fluorosis). It is generally of a chronic nature in domestic species. Poultry are least affected by high-fluorine levels. Therapy of chronic fluorosis is primarily directed at reducing intake by changing either water or dietary sources.

IODINE

Metabolic Function and Chemistry

The only known role for iodine in the body is as a component of the thyroid hormones, which have been covered in Chapter 33. Iodine is removed from the blood and incorporated into the organic form in the thyroid gland. Free iodine is negligible in the body.

Source and Occurrence

There are endemic iodine-deficient areas in all the major land masses of the world. In North America, the principal region is the so-called goiter belt, which extends from New England westward, surrounding the Great Lakes and covering the upper Midwest and the Pacific Northwest. Most of the rest of Canada and the United States can be considered iodine sufficient. Iodine may occur in either plants or water.

In plants it is generally higher in hay and roughage than in grains.

Deficiency

Iodine deficiency results in a deficiency of thyroid hormones, which in turn decreases all metabolic activities of the body (Chapter 33). The deficiency syndrome, goiter, is most commonly manifested in newborn or young growing animals.

Requirements

Exact daily requirements have not been ascertained for all animals. However, diets that contain 0.1–0.2 mg/kg of iodine are generally adequate. In most cases requirements are met by feeding iodized salt that contains 0.007% iodine. Lactating animals require an increased dietary supply as iodine is secreted in the milk.

Prophylaxis and Therapeutics

Iodized salt is the most practical and efficient prophylactic method of supplying iodine. Iodized salt should not be used to decrease consumption of concentrate feeds as too much iodine may be consumed. In exposed range conditions, sodium and potassium iodide are unstable and leach from the surface of the salt blocks. Recently some organic iodide salts have been shown to be both stable and biologically available to the animal (see Table 41.2). Miller and Swanson (1973) reported that ethylenediamine dihydroiodide (EDDI) was absorbed as efficiently as and had better tissue retention than an inorganic iodide form in lactating dairy cows.

Toxicity

Iodine in high quantities may be toxic. However, levels required for toxicity are above those that would be obtained under natural conditions. In growing calves and pigs, continual feeding of levels greater than 500 times recommended levels was required to induce obvious toxicity (Newton and Clawson 1974; Newton et al. 1974). For a discussion of toxicity of EDDI, see Chapter 61.

IRON

Metabolic Function and Chemistry

Metabolically, iron has evolved as an essential component of oxygen transport and oxidation systems. In a normal animal most of the iron present in the body at any time is in hemoglobin. The primary role of iron in veterinary pharmacology is in treating anemia. Primary coverage of this topic is in Chapter 23.

Source and Occurrence

Iron composes approximately 5% of the earth's crust and is in sufficient concentration in plant foods to provide for animal needs. Meat products, particularly liver, contain large amounts of iron.

Requirements

Specific daily requirements are not known for most adult domestic animals because deficiencies do not occur under normal feeding practices. Even though eggs contain large amounts of iron, high-producing laying hens do not require additional iron supplementation. Baby pigs and some other neonates maintained on milk require supplemental iron. Baby pigs' diets should contain at least 80 mg of iron/kg of diet. Dogs should receive 1.32 mg of iron/kg of body weight/week.

Prophylaxis and Therapeutics

Baby pigs are the only animals that routinely need to receive iron prophylactically. Since milk is a poor source, iron salts may be administered orally or parenteral iron dextran may be given. The fact that baby pigs are raised on concrete to reduce parasitic infestation increases their marginal iron deficiency state. Pigs raised on ground or with access to soil do not demonstrate the severe anemia problems associated with more intensive swine husbandry. Pigs raised on iron slats were reported not to require additional iron supplementation, so almost any iron form seems to be adequate in the prevention of baby pig anemia (Harmon et al. 1974).

Iron therapy associated with anemia is presented in Chapter 23.

Toxicity

Oral iron has a low toxicity, as body iron content is controlled by limiting absorption after body stores become adequate.

MAGNESIUM

Metabolic Function and Chemistry

Most of the body's magnesium, about 70%, is located in the crystalline structure of bone, with approximately 10% of this pool exchangeable with the more labile soft tissue magnesium. All cells contain magnesium.

From a distributional standpoint, magnesium is an intracellular ion and is an essential cofactor for many enzymes, particularly those involved in high-energy phosphate transfer. In excess, it induces neuromuscular paralysis, and in deficiency, hyperirritability. Magnesium is poorly absorbed from the gastrointestinal (GI) tract and quantities in excess of body needs are readily excreted via the kidneys.

Interaction

As potassium and nitrogen content of young grass increases, the availability of magnesium decreases.

Source and Occurrence

Most plants and plant components contain at least 1 g/kg of magnesium so that adequate intake generally occurs. Grass tetany, a hypomagnesemic condition in herbivores, is an exception. Legumes have a higher concentration than grasses.

Deficiency

Deficiency syndromes can be experimentally produced in any species, but it is a major clinical occurrence in herbivores, particularly cattle that are grazed on lush grass pastures or grain stubble fields.

Beef cattle that are producing milk are particularly susceptible since milk represents a significant additional drain of magnesium during critical periods. Rapid growth of grass occurs during early spring when lactation is also heavy. Dairy cows are less likely to be afflicted as they routinely receive concentrate or concentrate-mineral supplements during lactation. In

TABLE 41.3. Factors increasing the occurrence of grass tetany in grazing ruminants

Factors	Reference	Date
Animal		
Lactation	Merchon and Custer	1958
Pregnancy	Merchon and Custer	1958
All grass diet	Grunes et al.	1970
Low carbohydrate intake	Wilson et al.	1969
High NPN intake	Wilcox and Hoff	1974
Underfeeding	Allcroft and Burns	1968
Increasing age	Thomas	1965
High potassium intake	House and Van Campen	1971
Plant		
Rapid growth	Grunes et al.	1970
All grass or cereal grain pasture	Grunes	1973
Organic acids that complex magnesium	Bohman et al.	1969
	Stout et al.	1967
High nitrogen in plants	Wilcox and Hoff	1974
High potassium in plants	Hemingway et al.	1963
Soil		
High nitrogen fertilization	Grunes et al.	1970
	Wilcox and Hoff	1974
High potassium fertilization	Hemingway et al.	1963
Environmental		
Cool temperature	Wilcox and Hoff	1974

certain areas, grass tetany is seen in lactating ewes and in pregnant cattle and sheep.

The factors that result in grass tetany are complex and incompletely understood (Grunes 1973). Table 41.3 lists a number of conditions or circumstances that are commonly associated with the occurrence of grass tetany. Obviously, many are closely related, i.e., high potassium fertilization causes a high potassium content in plants that results in a high potassium intake. An interesting new hypothesis concerning the etiology of grass tetany and its relation to the rapid pasture growth phenomenon has been presented by Wilcox and Hoff (1974).

Requirements

Except for lactating animals, herbivorous and omnivorous species will obtain sufficient magnesium if the diet contains 0.6 g/kg of feed. This is adequately supplied by most sources. Lactating cows should receive a diet containing 2 g/kg of feed.

Prophylaxis and Therapeutics

Prophylaxis for grass tetany is based on increasing the magnesium intake of animals on grass pastures. Several methods are available. Fertilizing the soil with magnesium salts has been successful under some conditions. Levels of magnesite ore (principally MgO) have ranged from 50 to 2500 lb/acre. Results have been variable (Bartlett et al. 1954; Todd 1965). Heavier applications may be effective for several years. Soil fertilization of this magnitude would not be as feasible in large range operations. In addition, certain soil types are not improved by magnesium administration. An agronomist should be consulted before using this method.

Dusting or spraying MgO on the surface of foliage has been effective in some intensive pasture rotation systems. MgO, 30 lb/acre, can be applied every week as a dust. Mixing the MgO with water and bentonite (10% MgO, 1.5% bentonite) and spraying the pastures will increase magnesium retention on the leaves. These methods are practical only in intensive situations.

Many cases of grass tetany are seen in extensive management situations (Todd et al. 1966.) Additional oral supplementation is required. Feeding 50–60 g of MgO/cow/day for 2–4 weeks before putting on pasture and throughout the grass tetany season (spring) is recommended. Crash feeding programs begun after tetany appears in a herd are usually not adequate to curtail the disease. If pelleted supplements or protein blocks are used, add the following amounts of MgO:

lb of supplement fed/cow/day	lb of MgO needed/ton of supplement
2	100
3	70
4	50
5	40
6	35

More than 100 lb of MgO/ton of supplement decreases palatability. Therefore, at least 2 lb of supplement/day must be fed. MgO is preferred to $MgSO_4 \cdot 7H_2O$ (Epsom salts) because it is more palatable, cheaper, and contains 6 times more Mg/unit of weight. If supplements are not fed, mix salt 50–50 with MgO and feed no other salt or mineral. MgO in a supplement form is preferred to a salt mix.

Magnesium supplementation may also be provided by the use of magnesium "bullets." Variable results have been obtained due mostly to inadequate rates of magnesium release from the bullets. Loss of the bullets from the rumen has also been reported (Grunes 1973). The bullets are a metal magnesium alloy: 86% magnesium, 12% aluminum, 2% copper; 3″ in length, 1″ in diameter, and weighing 100 g. They release 1 g Mg/day. Two to 4 bullets/cow were effective in preventing hypomagnesemia (Richie and Hemingway 1968). Smaller 36-g bullets have been effectively used in sheep (Davey 1968). To prevent grass tetany, a daily or reasonably continual supply of available magnesium is required for animals on lush pastures, lush range conditions, or grain stubble, particularly wheat.

Animals suffering from hypomagnesemia may be treated parenterally by injecting 200 ml of a 20%–50% $MgSO_4$ solution subcutaneously to prevent relapse, followed by slow intravenous injection of 100–200 g of Ca-Mg borogluconate. This can be supplied by giving 500 ml of a 23% calcium borogluconate plus 6% $MgCl_2$ solution. The goal, however, is prophylaxis. Although it is difficult to prevent outbreaks of grass tetany, feeding MgO will greatly decrease the incidence.

Toxicity

Magnesium toxicity due to oral intake of magnesium is rare as magnesium is effectively excreted by the kidneys in addition to being poorly absorbed. Too rapid administration of magnesium salts intravenously can result in flaccid paralysis, anesthesia, bradycardia, and death by respiratory and cardiac arrest.

MANGANESE

Metabolic Function and Chemistry

The principal metabolic function of manganese is in the formation of the mucopolysaccharide chondroitin sulfate, which is an essential component of cartilage. Cartilage, in turn, is required for proper bone formation. The specific action of manganese is as a cofactor for the enzyme glycosyltransferase (Leach 1974). Manganese is a part of the enzyme pyruvic carboxylase and may serve as a cofactor for many other enzymes. However, other divalent cations may serve as efficient alternative activators for all but the glycosyltransferases (Leach 1974).

Source and Occurrence

Extremely variable levels of manganese are reported in most foods. Meat products are particularly low, with liver containing very little manganese compared to its concentration of some other trace elements and vitamins.

Deficiency

In domestic animals deficiencies of manganese are not recognized under practical conditions except in poultry. In growing birds this is seen as perosis or slipped tendon in which malformation of the tibial condyles allows the gastrocnemius tendon to be displaced. A number of other factors have also been associated with the perosis syndrome.

Requirements

Poultry diets should contain 55 mg of manganese/kg of feed.

Prophylaxis and Therapeutics

Birds require additional manganese supplementation, especially if they are receiving diets containing large amounts of corn or fish meal by-products as they are lower in manganese. It is unlikely that other species will require supplementation.

Toxicity

Manganese is one of the least toxic trace elements. It does not accumulate in body tissue with increased intake. This is due to rapid biliary excretion if excess manganese is injected. Poor absorption and rapid excretion into the gut decrease the potential toxicity of oral manganese. Urinary manganese excretion is limited.

MOLYBDENUM

Metabolic Function and Chemistry

Molybdenum is an essential component of the metalloenzyme xanthine oxidase, which converts the purine xanthine to uric acid prior to excretion.

Interaction

Molybdenum has a strong inverse interaction with copper and sulfur (see Copper).

Source and Occurrence

There is apparently sufficient molybdenum in all soils to provide plants and animals with an adequate supply.

Deficiency

Natural deficiencies of molybdenum have not been authenticated.

Daily Requirements

Daily requirements are not established but are presumably quite low.

Prophylaxis and Therapeutics

Prophylaxis relates to molybdenum toxicity, not deficiency, which is seen in cattle and sheep (see Toxicity). Therapeutic control is to remove animals from high molybdenum pastures or add supplemental copper to their diets; 1–2 g/animal/day of a copper salt are generally adequate to control the disease in adult cattle. Sheep should receive 0.25 g of copper sulfate/45 kg of body weight. High copper sulfate concentrate cubes may be used.

Toxicity

Molybdenum toxicity occurs in the British Isles, New Zealand, and areas of western United States. Cattle are the most commonly afflicted species, although toxicity has been seen in sheep. Horses and pigs are not usually affected by molybdenosis so that a practical prophylactic measure in high molybdenum areas would be to encourage the use of the less susceptible species. In cattle molybdenum toxicity is known as "teart"; high molybdenum areas are called teart soils and teart pastures. Cattle grazing teart pastures rapidly develop a profuse diarrhea, weight loss, and eventual death.

SELENIUM

Metabolic Function and Chemistry

Selenium is a dietary essential with a bad name. For years selenium's toxic manifestations have drawn more interest than its role in nutrition.

Selenium is absorbed from the upper intestinal tract and is distributed throughout the body. Nonruminants absorb a greater percentage of dietary selenium than ruminants, apparently because a portion of the selenium is reduced to an insoluble form in the rumen. Following absorption, excess selenium is excreted via the kidneys.

Selenium has been shown to be effective in prevention and treatment of a number of necrotizing diseases of domestic animals. It is necessary for growth and fertility and has an interaction with vitamin E that allows each to partially but not completely substitute for the other. Since both selenium and vitamin E have antioxidant properties, scientists have tried to relate their protective functions to this ability to prevent membrane damage. Hoekstra (1974) summarized work that established one function of selenium as a component of the enzyme glutathione reductase. He further postulated, as was presented in Chapter 38, that selenium and vitamin E work together to decrease lipid peroxidation (Fig. 38.4). Glutathione peroxidase functions to enhance the reaction of reduced glutathione (GSH) with hydrogen peroxide, which oxidizes the glutathione to GSSG and forms water. The result is less hydrogen peroxide available to cause lipid peroxidation. A decreased rate of lipid peroxidation lengthens the life of cellular membranes.

There may be other specific actions of selenium in the body, but this function can adequately explain many of the symptoms seen during deficiency states.

Interaction

Sulfur seems to exacerbate marginal selenium deficiencies. The effect is not strong enough to be of value in preventing toxicity.

Source and Occurrence

There are major geographic regions where either selenium toxicity or selenium deficiency occurs. Often they are adjoining areas. Fig. 41.2 is a map of the United States depicting major selenium deficiency and potential toxicity areas (Muth and Allaway 1963). The occurrence of selenium in plants is a function of the concentration of selenium in the soil and the presence of selenium accumulators, which are plants that make selenium more available.

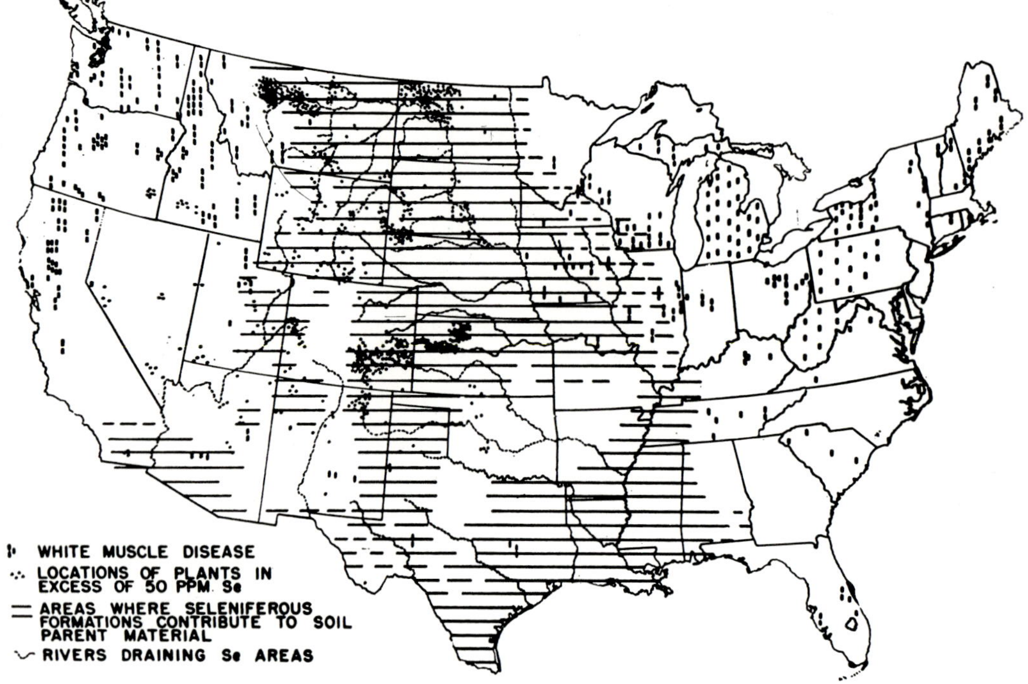

Fig. 41.2. The relationship of white muscle disease to the distribution of naturally occurring selenium in the United States. (Muth and Allaway 1963)

Changing swine management practices have increased the incidence of selenium deficiency in the Midwest. Confinement rearing of swine decreases their vitamin E intake and makes a marginal selenium deficiency more critical (Ullrey 1974).

Deficiency

Nutritional muscular dystrophy, white muscle disease (WMD), is seen in selenium-deficient young animals. Specific characteristics are degeneration of striated muscles in a bilaterally symmetrical fashion. The name "WMD" derives from the gross appearance of affected muscles that contain streaks of white. These are areas of noninflammatory necrosis. It is most severe and common in lambs but also occurs in calves, foals, and rabbits. Similar conditions are seen in swine and poultry but the disease has other manifestations and is not called WMD. In young pigs hepatosis dietetica is seen on selenium-deficient or tocopherol-deficient diets. Necrotic liver lesions are present in addition to muscle degeneration. In chicks the disease is called exudative diathesis and is characterized by edema, subcutaneous hemorrhages, progressive weakness, and death, as well as the more common muscle lesions. Decreased fertility and birth of dead or weak offspring may occur in all species.

Requirements

Dietary requirements for selenium vary somewhat with its form and with other components of the diet, such as vitamin E. In general, diets that contain 0.1 mg/kg are sufficient to prevent selenium deficiency. In selenium-deficient areas where crops or pasture may contain less than 0.05 mg/kg of selenium, it is necessary to supplement.

Prophylaxis and Therapeutics

Currently in the United States prophylactic supplementation of selenium is unsettled. Thus a number of factors must be considered in developing the most effective program for insuring optimum health and growth of domestic animals. There are legal considerations associated with dietary supplementation as only pigs and poultry can currently receive selenium in this form. Since selenium has toxic characteristics, it comes under Food and Drug Administration regulations. In February 1974, approval was given for its use in swine at a level of 0.1 mg/kg of diet (0.1 ppm). This is a level that is both adequate and safe (Ullrey 1974). Chickens and turkeys can also receive diets containing 0.1 mg/kg and 0.2 mg/kg, respectively. Although applications are pending, selenium cannot at this writing legally be added to the diets of other food-producing animals.

An interesting comparison has been made of tissue residues of selenium in domestic animals, depending on whether the selenium in the diet was native or supplemented (Allaway 1973). Allaway reported that native selenium resulted in much higher tissue residues than did supplemented selenium at equivalent dietary levels.

Depending on the species, the type of production, and legal restrictions, supplementation may be accomplished in several ways:

1. Selenium fertilization of soil
2. Selenium top dressing to plants
3. Addition of selenium to feeds
4. Oral drenching
5. Selenium pellets
6. Intramuscular injection

Selenium fertilization of marginal soils is effective but still experimental. For maximum benefit the selenium should be available to the plants for a long period but not so available that toxic levels accumulate (Allaway 1968). This practice may not be economically feasible on a large scale because selenium is not an abundant element. Fortunately, only small amounts of selenium need be added to substantially increase selenium concentrates in plants.

A sodium selenite solution has been used as a foliage spray to increase selenium concentration in plants. One ounce of selenium per acre was sufficient to raise plant concentration for several months (Grant 1965). This would be sufficient to raise levels during pregnancy when selenium is critical for grazing animals. Higher application levels resulted in some toxicity in this study.

Selenium is now being added to feeds for pigs and poultry in deficient areas at the levels previously given. Selenized salt preparations have been tried and can be effective in grazing herd situations (Paulson et al. 1968). However, quantitation of salt intake is difficult and variable. Individuals could develop toxicity or deficiency syndromes.

Oral administration of selenium salts to individual animals is effective but laborious. Selenium and selenium–vitamin E preparations are available.

The incorporation of elemental selenium with iron fillings as a pellet has proved quite effective in Australian experiments. The pellets were placed in the reticulorumen and provided a slow continuous release of biologically available selenium. This technique could be a valuable addition to prophylaxis as the rate at which selenium is made available is a function of its concentration in the pellet (Handreck and Godwin 1970).

Parenteral injection of selenium as a Se–vitamin E preparation is widely used as a prophylactic and therapeutic technique in endemic selenium-deficient areas. It has the advantage of rapid response and effective control of dosage. The disadvantage is that tissue levels may become high for a period following injection. Pigs given parenteral injections in the perinatal period did not have increased levels at slaughter age (Van Vleet et al. 1973). Intramuscular and subcutaneous injections of therapeutic levels of selenium may cause local irritation and necrosis (Herigstad et al. 1973; Herigstad and Whitehair 1974).

Toxicity

Toxic manifestations are not recognized below 5 mg/kg of diet. See Chapter 57 for a discussion of selenium toxicity.

SULFUR

Metabolic Function and Chemistry

Sulfur is necessary in the body in organic form, particularly in the sulfur-containing amino acids. Sulfur is also a constituent of coenzyme A, thiamin, biotin, and the mucopolysaccharides. The sulfur-containing amino acids have important functions in protein structure by forming disulfide bridges. Sulfhydryl groups are important in facilitating electron transfer either directly, as carriers, like glutathione, or by participating in catalysis. Fibrous proteins derive their structural characteristics from disulfide bridges.

Source and Occurrence

Sulfur and sulfur salts are widespread in water and soils. It has been estimated that drinking water provides 10%–45% of the daily sulfur requirements of ruminants and horses (*Nutrients and Toxic Substances* 1974). Rumen microorganisms can synthesize sulfur amino acids if inorganic sulfur is present, but nonruminants must rely on a primary source of preformed sulfur amino acid.

Deficiency

A deficiency of sulfur or sulfur-containing amino acids results in a limitation of growth and production. In severe cases inappetence is present, while in marginal deficiency there would be more subtle changes in growth.

Requirements

Nonprotein sulfur (NPS) is a necessary additive when ruminants or horses are fed urea or other nonprotein nitrogen (NPN) supplements. A direct relationship exists; as the level of NPN increases, so must the level of NPS. It would seem that the products produced by the ruminant contain more sulfur than those consumed (Garrigus 1970). A rule of thumb is that sulfur should be present at about 10% of the level of nitrogen. As sulfur, the ration should contain 2 g/kg of feed.

Prophylaxis and Therapeutics

The goal of prophylaxis for ruminants is to insure that diets containing large amounts of NPN also contain sulfur. The sulfur may be administered as elemental sulfur (the least usable form), as sulfates or other salts, and as organic sulfate such as the amino acid methionine. Methionine is the limiting substance in sulfur-deficient diets. In ruminants, preformed methionine should be supplied in a bound form or encapsulated to prevent ruminant breakdown but to allow digestion and absorption in the lower tract. The hydroxy analog of methionine (Hydan-DuPont), which is not destroyed by ruminal organisms but is absorbed and converted to methionine in the liver, may be fed at the rate of 30 g/cow/day for this purpose. Administering cysteine will lower the requirement for methionine.

Sulfur and sulfur amino acid metabolism is currently a very active research area. Several techniques are being evaluated to determine the best method of supplying usable sulfur to ruminants on NPN diets. It is hoped that the most effective and dependable of these methods will be sufficiently tested in the near future so that a more specific prophylactic regime can be presented. Some reports indicate that in nonruminants, particularly poultry, some dietary inorganic sulfur is converted to amino acid sulfur (Sasse and Baker 1974). The quantities are small and may relate to lower intestine absorption following microbial synthesis.

Toxicity

Under normal supplementation programs excess sulfur would be eliminated in the urine.

ZINC

Metabolic Function and Chemistry

Zinc is distributed throughout the body with high concentrations in muscle, hair, wool, male reproductive fluids, and the tapetum lucidum. It is a component of several enzymes, such as carbonic anhydrase and alkaline phosphatase. Zinc is essential for many normal functions in the body. Perhaps the most basic is RNA synthesis. Therefore, normal growth and repair are dependent on adequate zinc.

Interaction

Zinc interacts with several metallic ions. Iron and copper both reduce zinc absorption. Cadmium and zinc compete with each other.

Zinc is not well absorbed, but this depends on body needs. Excess levels of zinc are excreted via the pancreatic juice into the intestine. Zinc is present in most plant products. It is fairly high in milk and animal by-products, especially fish meal. Colostrum has a high zinc content. There are not wide geographic deficiencies of zinc as those that occur with selenium and iodine. Most concentrates contain marginal levels; sugar-beet products are particularly low.

Deficiency

Depressed growth and altered epithelial cell metabolism are the main signs of deficiency. Parakeratosis occurs in pigs and cattle on zinc-deficient diets. Parakeratosis is a hyperkeratinization of epithelial cells of skin and esophagus. Other keratinized tissue, i.e., hoofs, wool, feathers, and horns, are malformed. Wound healing is impaired in zinc deficiency as is reproduction. Both of these latter signs are indicative of the basic role of zinc in RNA synthesis.

Requirements

Dietary requirements vary with the species and the rest of the diet. For instance, phytic acid, which is high in soy beans, and calcium increase the need for zinc. Recommended levels in the diet are from 20 to 80 mg/kg of feed, depending on the species, growth rate, and type of production. Dairy cows, pigs, and poultry tend to have higher requirements than do beef animals or horses.

Prophylaxis and Therapeutics

Zinc should be added to concentrate rations as a precautionary measure. It can be accomplished by zinc salts in the salt mixture as well as incorporation in pelleted concentrates. Parakeratotic lesions may be treated superficially with ointments such as zinc oxide.

Toxicity

Zinc is relatively nontoxic. Dietary concentrations must be greater than 1 g/kg of feed to cause toxicity. Feed, however, is generally unpalatable when zinc concentrations are this high; most cases have been experimentally induced. Animals show inappetence and anemia. Changing the diet will remedy the condition.

TRACE MINERALS AND DISEASE

Digestive diseases or chronic conditions that result in prolonged dietary limitations may necessitate parenteral or oral therapy with trace minerals, as the availability of ingested minerals may not be sufficient. Requirements for this type of therapy are highly individualized and dependent on the species, age, and type of disease.

Infectious diseases that have either direct host invasion or endotoxin absorption also cause a decrease in plasma zinc and iron and an increase in plasma copper. Weinberg (1974) has suggested that these trace mineral alterations are part of the body's natural defense mechanisms and may act to limit bacterial multiplication. Fever increases the trace mineral response. If his theory is correct, supplementation with iron and zinc during acute infectious disease conditions would be contraindicated.

REFERENCES

Allaway, W. H. 1968. Agronomic controls over the environmental cycling of trace elements. Adv Agron 20:235.

———. 1973. Selenium in the food chain. Cornell Vet 63:151.

Allcroft, R., and Burns, K. N. 1968. Hypomagnesemia in cattle. NZ Vet J 16:109.

Almquist, H. J. 1970. Sulfur nutrition of nonruminant species. In O. H. Muth and J. E. Oldfield, eds. Symposium: Sulfur in Nutrition. Westport, Conn.: Avi Publishing.

Ammerman, C. B., and Miller, S. M. 1972. Biological availability of minor mineral ions: A review. J Anim Sci 35:681.

Bartlett, S.; Brown, B. B.; Joat, A. S.; Rowland, S. J.; Allcroft, R.; and Parr, W. H. 1954. The influence of fertilizer treatment of grassland on the incidence of hypomagnesemia in milking cows. Br Vet J 110:3.

Bohman, V. R.; Lesperance, A. L.; Harding, G. D.; and Grunes, D. L. 1969. Induction of experimental tetany in cattle. J Anim Sci 29:99.

Committee on Mineral Nutrition. 1973. Tracing and treating mineral disorders in dairy cattle. Center for Agricultural Publishing and Documentation. Wageningen, The Netherlands.

Connoly, J. F., and Poole, D. B. R. 1967. An experimental heavy pellet for prevention of cobalt deficiency in sheep. Ir J Agric Res 6:229.

Davey, L. A. 1968. Magnesium alloy bullets for grazing sheep. Vet Res 82:142.

Davies, E. B., and Watkinson, J. H. 1966. Uptake of native and applied selenium by pasture species. II. Effects of sulphate and of soil type and uptake of clover. NZ J Agric Res 9:641.

Felsman, R. J.; Wise, M. B.; Harvey, R. W.; and Barrick, E. R. 1973. Effect of added dietary levels of copper sulfate and an antibiotic on performance and certain blood constituents of calves. J Anim Sci 36:157.

Frieden, E. 1974. The biochemical evolution of the iron and copper proteins. In W. G. Hoekstra, J. W. Suttie, H. E. Ganther, and W. Mertz, eds. Trace Element Metabolism in Animals—2. Baltimore: University Park Press.

Garrigus, U. S. 1970. The need for sulfur in the diet of ruminants. In O. H. Muth and J. E. Oldfield, eds. Symposium: Sulfur in Nutrition. Westport, Conn.: Avi Publishing.

Grant, A. B. 1965. Pasture top dressing with selenium. NZ J Agric Res 8:681.

Grunes, D. L. 1973. Grass tetany of cattle and sheep. In Antiquality Components of Forages, p. 113. Madison, Wis.: Crop Science Society of America.

Grunes, D. L.; Stout, P. R.; and Brownell, J. R. 1970. Grass tetany of ruminants. Adv Agron 22:331.

Handreck, K. A., and Godwin, K. O. 1970. Distribution in the sheep of selenium derived from ^{75}Se-labelled ruminal pellets. Aust J Agric Res 21:71.

Harmon, B. G.; Cornelius, S. G.; Totsch, J.; Baker, D. H.; and Jensen, A. H. 1974. Oral iron dextran and iron from steel slats as hematinics for swine. J Anim Sci 39: 699.

Healy, W. B. 1974. Ingested soil as a source of elements to grazing animals. In W. G. Hoekstra, J. W. Suttie, H. E. Ganther, and W. Mertz, eds. Trace Element Metabolism in Animals—2. Baltimore: University Park Press.

Hemingway, R. G.; Ritchie, N. S.; Rutherford, A. R.; and Jolly, G. M. 1963. Effects of potassium fertilizers, age of ewe, and small magnesium supplementation on blood magnesium and calcium levels of lactating ewes. J Agric Sci 60:307.

Henken, R. W.; Vandersoll, J. H.; Sasse, B. A.; and Hibbs, J. W. 1971. Goitrogenic effects of a corn silage soybean meal supplemented ration. J Dairy Sci 54:85.

Herigstad, R. R., and Whitehair, C. K. 1974. Local and systemic effects of parenteral injection of sodium selenite in cattle and swine. Vet Med Small Anim Clin 69:1035.

Herigstad, R. R.; Whitehair, C. K.; and Olson, O.E. 1973. Inorganic and organic selenium toxicity in young swine: Comparison of pathologic change with those in swine with vitamin E-selenium deficiency. Am J Vet Res 34:1227.

Hill, C. H.; Starcher, B.; and Kim, C. 1967. Role of copper in the formation of elastin. Fed Proc 26:129.

Hoekstra, W. G. 1974. Biochemical role of selenium. In W. G. Hoekstra, J. W. Suttie, H. E. Ganther, and W. Mertz, eds. Trace Element Metabolism in Animals—2. Baltimore: University Park Press.

House, W. A., and Van Campen, D. R. 1971. Magnesium metabolism of sheep fed different levels of potassium and citric acid. J Nutr 101:1483.

Leach, R. M., Jr. 1967. Role of manganese in the synthesis of mucopolysaccharides. Fed Proc 26:118.

———. 1974. Biochemical role of manganese. In W. G. Hoekstra, J. W. Suttie, H. E. Ganther, and W. Mertz, eds. Trace Element Metabolism in Animals—2. Baltimore: University Park Press.

Merchon, M. M., and Custer, F. D. 1958. Tetany in cattle on winter rations. I. A clinical report. J Am Vet Med Assoc 132:396.

Miller, J. K., and Swanson, E. W. 1973. Metabolism of ethylenediaminedihydroiodide and sodium or potassium iodide by dairy cows. J Dairy Sci 56:378.

Muth, O. H., and Allaway, W. H. 1963. The relationship of white muscle disease to the distribution of naturally occurring selenium. J Am Vet Med Assoc 142:1379.

Newton, G. L., and Clawson, A. J. 1974. Iodine toxicity: Physiological effects of elevated dietary iodine on pigs. J Anim Sci 39:879.

Newton, G. L.; Barrick, E. R.; Harvey, R. W.; and Wise, M. B. 1974. Iodine toxicity. Physiological effects of elevated dietary iodine on calves. J Anim Sci 38:449.

Nutrients and Toxic Substances in Water for Livestock and Poultry. 1974. National Academy of Sciences, Washington, D.C.

Paulson, G. D.; Broderick, G. A.; Baumann, C. A.; and Pope, A. L. 1968. Effect of feeding sheep selenium fortified trace mineralized salt: Effect of tocopherol. J Anim Sci 27:195.

Peeler, H. T. 1972. Biological availability of major mineral ions. J Anim Sci 351:695.

Richie, N. S., and Hemingway, R. G. 1968. Magnesium alloy bullets for dairy cattle. Vet Rec 82:87.

Sasse, C. E., and Baker, D. H. 1974. Sulfur utilization by the chick with emphasis on the effect of inorganic sulfate on the cystine-methionine interrelationship. J Nutr 104:244.

Spencer, V. E.; Reading, R. E.; and Thran, L. W. 1958. Univ Nevada Agric Exp Sta Bull 202.

Stout, P. R.; Brownell, J. V.; and Burau, R. G. 1967. Occurrences of transaconitate in range forage species. Agron J 59:21.

Suttle, N. F., and Mills, C. F. 1966. Studies of toxicity of copper to pigs, effect of protein source and other dietary components on response to high and moderate intakes of copper. Br J Nutr 20:149.

Thomas, J. W. 1965. Mechanisms responsible for grass tetany. Proc Ga Nutr Conf for Feed, p. 14.

Todd, J. R. 1965. The influence of soil type on the effectiveness of single dressings of magnesia in raising pasture magnesium content and in controlling hypomagnesemia. Br Vet J 121:371.

Todd, J. R.; Scally, W. C. P.; and Ingram, J. M. 1966. Studies of the effectiveness of "free access" feeding of a magnesia-molasses mixture for the prevention of hypomagnesemia in dairy cows at pasture. Vet Rec 78:888.

Ullrey, D. E. 1974. The selenium-deficiency problem in animal agriculture. In W. G. Hoekstra, J. W. Suttie, H. E. Ganther, and W. Mertz, eds. Trace Element Metabolism in Animals—2. Baltimore: University Park Press.

Underwood, E. J. 1971. Trace Elements in Human and Animal Nutrition, 3rd ed., p. 469. New York: Academic Press.

Van Vleet, J. F.; Meyer, K. B.; and Olander, H. J. 1973. Control of selenium-vitamin E deficiency in growing swine by parenteral administration of selenium-vitamin E preparations to baby pigs or to pregnant sows and their baby pigs. J Am Vet Med Assoc 163:452.

Weinberg, E. D. 1974. Roles of temperature and trace metal metabolism in host-pathogen interactions. In W. G. Hoekstra, J. W. Suttie, H. E. Ganther, and W. Mertz, eds. Trace Element Metabolism in Animals—2. Baltimore: University Park Press.

Wilcox, G. E., and Hoff, J. E. 1974. Grass tetany: An hypothesis concerning its relationship with ammonium nutrition of spring grasses. J Dairy Sci 57:1085.

Wilson, G. F.; Reid, C. S. W.; Molloy, L. F.; Metson, A. J.; and Butler, G. W. 1969. Influence of starch and peanut oil supplementation on plasma magnesium, calcium and phosphorus levels in grazing dairy cows. NZ J Agric Res 12:410.

SECTION 11

Drugs Acting Locally on the Skin, Mucous Membranes, Eyes, and Ears

CHAPTER 42

TOPICAL AGENTS

NICHOLAS H. BOOTH

Many drug preparations are available for topical use in veterinary medicine. Generally, such preparations have specific therapeutic actions and are limited to specific sites of application such as the skin, mucous membranes, eyes, and ears. The terms used in the classification of these preparations indicate a physical type of drug action, i.e., emollient, demulcent, protectant, or absorbent. In addition, many of the preparations may also exert a chemical effect, including antiinflammatory, antimicrobial, and antifungal actions for treatment of ailments involving the skin, mucous membranes, eyes, and ears. Agents used topically to produce local anesthesia are discussed in Chapter 19.

EMOLLIENTS

Emollient materials are usually inert oily substances used to soothe irritated skin or mucous membrane. They are also of value in softening the skin. Active drug components such as antimicrobial agents that assist in reducing inflammation and promote healing are often incorporated into emollients.

Vegetable Oils

Olive Oil, U.S.P. (sweet oil), and other vegetable oils (cottonseed, corn, linseed, and theobroma) are among the most common oils used for emollient purposes. With the exception of oil of theobroma, all the above are liquids. Oil of theobroma (also referred to as cocoa butter) is a solid at room temperature but melts at body temperature. Such qualities make it useful as an inert base for suppository preparations. Castor oil is a bland and soothing oil sometimes used in emollient preparations. Only upon hydrolysis does castor oil have irritant or cathartic effects within the gastrointestinal (GI) tract.

Animal Fats

Anhydrous Lanolin, U.S.P. (wool fat), is the primary animal fat used in therapeutics for the incorporation of active medicinal agents into ointment form. Lanolin possesses excellent emollient qualities and permits the incorporation of 25%–30% of water in the mixture. At one time lard was extensively used as a vehicle for the incorporation of active medicinal agents in ointment preparations. Lard is not used as much as other emollients because it becomes rancid during storage.

Hydrocarbons

White Petrolatum, U.S.P., and *Liquid Petrolatum,* U.S.P. (mineral oil), are the major emollient hydrocarbons used in veterinary medicine. White petrolatum (vaseline) is an ointment base frequently used as a vehicle for medicinal agents. Mineral oil is used internally for cathartic purposes in animals (see Chapter 35).

Water-soluble Hydrocarbons

Polysorbate 80, U.S.P. ("Tween 80"), is a mixture of polyoxyethylene ethers of oleic acid esters of sorbitol. It is an oily, amber liquid that dissolves readily in water. Polysorbate 80 is used as an emollient-dispersing agent for oil-soluble preparations. Polyethylene glycols (carbowaxes) are water-soluble ointment bases at room temperature and liquids at a slightly higher temperature. Water-insoluble substances can be stirred into the carbowaxes while they solidify to produce a nonoily ointment.

DEMULCENTS

Demulcents are inert substances that soothe and relieve irritation primarily involving the mucous membranes. They may also be applied to the skin. Most of the demulcents are water-soluble compounds with a high molecular weight and are gums, mucilages, or starches. They tend to coat irritated or abraded tissue surfaces to protect the underlying cells from irritating contacts. A demulcent can be applied to the skin as a lotion or as a wet dressing. Demulcents can be applied to the mucous membranes as an electuary, a nebula, an enema, or a drench. They are often used as vehicles to mask the taste of obnoxious drugs and particularly to form more stable suspensions or emulsions of drugs in aqueous vehicles.

Acacia, U.S.P. (gum arabic), and *Tragacanth,* U.S.P. (gum tragacanth), are dried, gummy exudates from the appropriate plants. These gums readily dissolve in water to form mucilages. *Glycyrrhiza Extract,* U.S.P., and *Glycyrrhiza Syrup,* U.S.P., are demulcents derived from licorice root or the roots of the glycyrrhiza plant. Glycyrrhiza is also used as a flavoring or masking agent, especially for swine.

Glycerin, U.S.P., is extensively used as a vehicle for drugs applied to the skin. Glycerin in high concentration will absorb water and therefore is irritating and dehydrating to exposed tissue. The irritant action of glycerin accounts for its use in rectal suppositories.

PROTECTIVES AND ABSORBENTS

Certain insoluble, chemically inert, and finely ground substances are applied locally as mechanical protectives and absorbents. These materials prevent friction, reduce tissue irritation, and absorb toxins and exudative wastes.

Starch, U.S.P., and *Talc,* U.S.P., are relatively nonirritant powders employed as vehicles for the incorporation of added medicinal agents. These pharmaceutical preparations then become healing powders, which are applied to wounds. Many compounds such as *Zinc Oxide,* U.S.P., *Zinc Stearate,* U.S.P., and *Boric Acid,* N.F., have been employed as healing powders. *Calamine,* U.S.P., is a common healing powder (or lotion) composed of zinc oxide with ferric oxide impurities.

Zinc Stearate, U.S.P., clings to the tissues and sheds water, thus providing protection to the underlying tissue from watery discharges or irritant exudates. The indiscriminate and excessive use of zinc stearate on human infants has led to poisoning. A combination of equal parts of boric acid and calcium oxide has been used freely on wounds of large animals despite some probable irritation of the granulating tissues. These and other substances are incorporated into healing powders for the treatment of skin abrasions. These dry the area of application, absorb secretions, and provide unfavorable conditions for the growth of bacteria.

Collodion, U.S.P., is not an absorbent powder but does form a protective film over tissue. It is a solution of nitrated cellulose in a highly volatile solvent. When the collodion is applied to the skin, the solvent evaporates rapidly leaving a waterproof film that protects the underlying lesions. Other agents are sometimes incorporated into collodion.

ASTRINGENTS

Astringents are drugs that are used locally to precipitate proteins either externally or internally. These drugs do not penetrate deeply. Their precipitant action is exerted only on the surface cells and is relatively weak. After the action of an astringent drug upon the surface tissue cell, the permeability of the cell membrane is greatly reduced but the cell remains viable. Many germicidal preparations possess an astringent action even in high dilution. Astringent drugs include the salts of heavy metals such as silver, mercury, zinc, and aluminum.

Another group of astringent compounds is of vegetable origin. There is a wide variety of vegetable astringents, but nearly all these owe their activity to the presence of tannic acid. The principal vegetable astringents are tannic acid (gallotannic acid), gallic acid, kino, krameria, and rubus (blackberry).

WOUND-HEALING AGENTS

A number of preparations are available for the stimulation of wound healing. Many of these are formulated with two or more medicinal preparations in the form of solutions or ointments. Such drug combinations may contain an antimicrobial agent, antifungal compound, antiinflammatory steroid, local anesthetic agent, demulcent, or emollient as well as other preparations of importance in the promotion of wound healing.

Zinc Oxide Ointment

Of the zinc preparations, *Zinc Oxide Ointment,* U.S.P., is most popular as a topical protectant and astringent for treatment of superficial wounds; the ointment contains 20% zinc oxide. The drug has an important clinical use in the treatment of a wide variety of cutaneous diseases. Many dermatologic ointments, powders, pastes, and lotions contain zinc oxide. Several formulations of zinc oxide are described in the *United States Dispensatory.* No specific pharmacologic action can be ascribed to the action of zinc oxide on the skin. According to the *United States Dispensatory,* the popularity of zinc oxide for the treatment of cutaneous conditions may be attributed to four qualities: it is a protective, mildly astringent, possibly a weak antiseptic and it is nontoxic.

Zinc oxide ointment and healing powders containing the drug are generally applied to the affected skin 1–3 times daily for a few days. Although animals such as the cat and dog commonly lick the treated wounds, no toxic effects from the ingestion of zinc oxide have been observed.

Pancreatic Dornase

Pancreatic Dornase (Dornavac) is an enzyme preparation, desoxyribonuclease, that is extracted from the beef pancreas. The extract is lyophilized and sterilized in vials containing 100,000 units. Refrigeration of the enzyme is necessary to prevent deterioration. Following reconstitution with sterile water or with isotonic sodium chloride solution, the enzyme solution should be used immediately.

CLINICAL USE

Pancreatic dornase is useful topically for enzymatic debridement of wounds and infected tissues. It has been approved by the Food and Drug Administration (FDA) for use in most species. The recommended dosage is 50,000–100,000 units of the reconstituted enzyme solution alone or with an antibiotic. Pancreatic dornase may be administered as an irrigation or wet dressing or it may be injected into the infected tissue.

Flucinolone Acetonide-Dimethyl Sulfoxide (DMSO) Solution (Synsac)

This preparation has been approved by the FDA for use in the dog. Each ml of the solution contains 0.01% fluocinolone acetonide and 20% DMSO with propylene glycol.

CLINICAL USE

The drug preparation is useful for treatment of anal sac impaction in the dog.

It is also recommended to alleviate inflammation associated with the anal gland as well as to reduce the obnoxious odor of its secretions. One to 2 ml of the drug combination is instilled into each anal sac following expression of the anal sac contents. The total dosage per anal sac should not exceed 2 ml. Treatment may be required at 60-day intervals to maintain a relatively odor-free condition.

Trypsin-Peru Balsam-Castor Oil Liquid

This drug-aerosol combination has been approved by the FDA for use in most species. Each g of the aerosol preparation delivered to the wound site contains 0.12 mg of crystalline trypsin, 87 mg of peru balsam, and 788 mg of castor oil.

clinical use

This drug mixture is useful as an adjunct treatment of surface wounds. It enhances healing by assisting in the removal of necrotic tissue and exudate.

Neomycin Sulfate-9-Fluoroprednisolone Acetate and Tetracaine Hydrochloride Ointment (Neo-Predef with Tetracaine)

Each g of this ointment contains 5 mg of neomycin sulfate, 1 mg of 9-fluoroprednisolone acetate, and 5 mg of tetracaine hydrochloride.

clinical use

This drug preparation has been approved by the FDA for use in the horse, cat, and dog. In the dog, it is recommended for the treatment of anal gland infections. Its use in the horse, cat, and dog includes the application of the ointment as a dressing for minor cuts, lacerations, and abrasions. It may also be used following amputation of claws, dewclaws, and tails as well as after ear-trimming and castration procedures. Prior to use of the ointment on skin or mucous membranes, the area of treatment should be cleansed; a small quantity is then applied by gentle inunction 1–3 times daily. As soon as the desired clinical effect is obtained, the frequency of application may be reduced or discontinued.

precautions

Neomycin and tetracaine may produce hypersensitivity or allergy in animals. If this occurs, the medication should be discontinued. Therapy should be restricted to the period when local anesthesia is required to prevent or control self-inflicted mutilation.

Chlorhexidine Diacetate Ointment

A 1% concentration of chlorhexidine diacetate is available in ointment form for veterinary use. This drug preparation has been approved by the FDA for use as a topical antiseptic in the treatment of external wounds in the dog, cat, and horse. The affected area is cleansed prior to treatment and the ointment is applied once daily by gentle inunction. Chlorhexidine diacetate ointment must not be used in the food-producing animals.

Copper Naphthenate Solution

A preparation containing 37.5% copper naphthenate has been approved by the FDA in the treatment of wounds, foot rot, and ringworm in the horse, cow, pig, sheep, goat, and dog.

clinical use

Copper naphthenate solution is recommended once daily for drying superficial sores and necrotic material of wounds for subsequent removal as well as for cleaning open lesions and treatment of udder sores. Also, it is used in cattle for the treatment of heel cracks, hoof punctures, and dehorning wounds. Following dehorning, it is used by direct application to the wound with a swab. In the horse, the preparation is used in the treatment of thrush and scratches and for toughening spongy hooves. Its use in the dog includes the treatment of cracked skin over the elbows and toughening of the footpads.

For best effect, necrotic tissue should be removed as much as possible before the copper naphthenate is applied. In the event a scab is present, the preparation should be used once daily until the scab is easily removed. With removal of the scab, the drug is used every other day until healing occurs. In lactating dairy animals, copper naphthenate must not be used on the teats. Its use under this circumstance will result in the presence of violative levels of residues in the milk.

DERMATOLOGIC AND OTIC AGENTS

Every conceivable drug preparation has been concocted over the past several decades for the treatment of cutaneous diseases. The effectiveness of drugs in the treatment of various skin diseases has been a problem to evaluate because it is difficult to duplicate comparable clinical conditions with controls for experimental study. A number of preparations for use in the therapy of skin and ear conditions have incorporated compounds that have antimicrobial, antipruritic, antifungal, and antiinflammatory effects. An annotated description of most of these preparations, including the conditions of use and dosage, is available from the April 1, 1974, *Code of Federal Regulations,* Sections 135a. 2 through 135a. 52. Consequently, many combinations of drugs are available for clinical use in small animals for alleviating skin and ear diseases. Topical drug preparations for use in food-producing animals comparable to those available for use in small animals are nonexistent because of the problem of evaluating the potential hazard of tissue residues.

Undecylenic Acid

Undecylenic Acid, U.S.P. ($C_{11}H_{20}O_2$), is a fungistatic agent that is a normal constituent of sweat. It can also be prepared in the presence of a catalyst by heating castor oil in the absence of air, generally under hypobaric conditions.

The chemical is sometimes combined with zinc to form zinc undecylenate. Like undecylenic acid, this compound is a component of powders or ointments used in the treatment of fungus infections due to *Microsporum. Compound Undecylenic Acid Ointment,* U.S.P., contains both undecylenic acid (5%) and zinc undecylenate (20%). The efficacy of undecylenic acid compounds is questionable as a sole treatment of *Microsporum* infections in human beings (Harvey 1975). In veterinary medical usage, undecylenic acid is not used alone. It is combined with other drugs for the treatment of acute otitis externa in the cat (see description below).

Dexamethasone Acetate, Nitrofurathiazide, Griseofulvin, Undecylenic Acid, Tetracaine Hydrochloride Otic Suspension (Fulvidex Otic Suspension)

This otic suspension preparation contains in each ml 0.25 mg of dexamethasone acetate, 2 mg of nitrofurathiazide, 15 mg of griseofulvin, 10 mg of undecylenic acid, and 10 mg of tetracaine hydrochloride. It is approved by the FDA for use in the treatment of acute otitis externa in the cat.

CLINICAL USE

This drug suspension is instilled into the ear canal at the rate of 4–10 drops 2 or 3 times daily. Parenteral corticosteroids must not be administered during the use of this drug preparation.

Dimethyl Sulfoxide Solution

Dimethyl Sulfoxide (Domoso, DMSO) in a concentration of 90% is approved by the FDA for use in the dog and horse. The chemical occurs as a waste product from processing wood pulp. The molecule of DMSO is a pyramidal structure shown in Fig. 42.1. The sulfur-oxygen bond is quite polar, giving the liquid a high dielectric constant. DMSO is a clear liquid with a boiling point of 189° C at one atmosphere of pressure and has a specific gravity of 1.0958 at 25° C. It is a solvent for many aromatic and unsaturated hydrocarbons as well as organic nitrogen compounds and inorganic salts. Due to its hygroscopic characteristics, DMSO can absorb more than 70% of its weight of water from

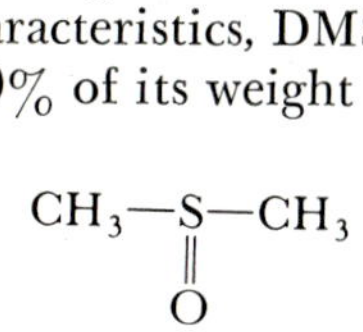

$$CH_3{-}\underset{\underset{\displaystyle O}{\|}}{S}{-}CH_3$$

Dimethyl Sulfoxide

Fig. 42.1.

air at 20° C and 65% relative humidity. Containers of DMSO should be tightly sealed to avoid dilution by the absorption of water from air.

PHARMACOLOGICAL CONSIDERATIONS

DMSO possesses some antiinflammatory, antimicrobial, and antifungal activity. However, of all the known pharmacological effects of the drug, the most important from a therapeutic aspect is its ability to absorb, penetrate, or pass through the skin following topical application. Soon after the topical application of DMSO to the skin, the drug reaches the systemic or internal regions of the body and can be detected in systemic secretions, excretions, or internal compartments of the body. Also, an obnoxious oyster or garlic odor is emitted from the breath in a matter of seconds after its application to the skin; the possible metabolites responsible for this odor are believed to be due to the formation of methyl disulfide and/or methyl sulfinic acid.

In the bovine, DMSO is metabolized and excreted in two principal metabolites, dimethyl sulfide and dimethyl sulfone (Tiews et al. 1975). This phenomenon is not at all surprising because dimethyl sulfone has been known to occur in cattle blood and adrenal glands. Dimethyl sulfide and dimethyl sulfone are normal constituents of cow's milk. Like milk, bovine meat always contains dimethyl sulfide and/or dimethyl sulfone in appreciable levels.

PENETRATION OF THE SKIN

DMSO produces a change in the permeability of the skin. The electrical potential difference, which normally exists across the skin, is decreased by the drug (Franz and Van Bruggen 1967). This effect appears to be due principally to an increased chloride conductance across the skin; there is little effect upon the rate of active sodium transport.

The morphologic characteristics of the skin and body membranes do not appear to be affected by DMSO. In its rapid penetration of membrane barriers, a number of compounds will move with it (Jacob et al. 1965). DMSO cannot pass rapidly through the nail or tooth enamel. Experimentally, it enhances the absorption of compounds through the intact urinary bladder of the dog such as heparin, salicylate, sulfadiazine, aminophylline, and other drugs. It increases the percutaneous absorption of fluocinolone acetonide by a fivefold factor, and for other compounds absorption may be enhanced by a factor of 25.

ANTIINFLAMMATORY AND ANALGESIC EFFECTS

DMSO has antiinflammatory characteristics by reducing the degree and extent of tissue inflammation. Also, some analgesic activity is produced by DMSO that may be attributable to the concentration of the drug at the site of inflammation where it apparently depresses the conduction of afferent nerve impulses from the inflamed area (Jacob et al. 1965). In addition, DMSO produces a thermal effect that may account for its significant alleviation of pain arising in muscles and joints (Bradham and Sample 1967). The temperature of the skin, subcutaneous tissue, and underlying muscle increases after the application of DMSO.

DISTRIBUTION, EXCRETION, AND FATE

Radiolabeled S^{35} studies have been conducted in small laboratory animals after the oral, intraperitoneal, and dermal administration of DMSO. The plasma radioactivity after an intraperitoneal dose is highest at 1 hour; the biological half-life is 5–6 hours (Jacob et al. 1965). Radioactivity levels in urine collected for 22 hours account for 60%–85% of an oral and intraperitoneal dose and 36%–50% of a dermal dose.

Cattle appear to metabolize and excrete DMSO rapidly and efficiently (Tiews et al. 1975). Excretion of DMSO by the urine attains peak levels within 6–12 hours and immediately thereafter declines rapidly with disappearance occurring in 12–28 hours after administration. Dimethyl sulfide elimination in exhaled air appears to parallel the disappearance of DMSO in the urine. Concurrently with the excretion of DMSO in the urine and dimethyl sulfide elimination in the exhaled air, the dimethyl sulfone level of the urine increases to a peak in the calf after 30–40 hours; it reaches a peak in adult cattle after 6–12 hours. Dimethyl sulfone, which is normally present in bovine urine (individual calf values prior to treatment averaged 8, 6, and 20 mg DMSO/L and cow values averaged 12 and 23 mg/L), returned to normal values within about 7 days in calves and as early as 3–5 days in cows (Tiews et al. 1975). Cattle are unlike small laboratory animals, dogs, monkeys, and human beings, with respect to DMSO metabolization and excretion. The only animal known to metabolize and excrete DMSO similarly to the bovine is the pig.

TOXICITY

DMSO has a low order of toxicity in single or in repeated dosages. No significant abnormalities in blood enzymes and other clinical diagnostic parameters have been seen in the dog given topical DMSO (1 g/kg) for 5 days weekly over a period of 18 months. In the unanesthetized cat, the LD50 of DMSO administered intravenously is of the order of 4 g/kg (Smith et al. 1967). However, anesthetized cats cannot tolerate dosages in excess of 0.4 g/kg; anesthetics appear to increase the lethal effects of DMSO. The LD50 in the unanesthetized dog is estimated at approximately 2.5 g/kg following intravenous administration. Toxic signs produced by DMSO include prostration, transient convulsions with opisthotonus, dyspnea, and marked pulmonary edema. Nonlethal dosages of the drug produce transient sedation and bloody urine.

SIDE EFFECTS AND CONTRAINDICATIONS

On occasion, an animal may develop transient erythema associated with local "burning" or irritation. If erythema or vesiculation of the skin occurs, it is considered self-limiting and reversible with no need to discontinue medication. Most cases of skin irritation do not increase in severity with continued use of DMSO. Only the medical grade of DMSO should be used in the treatment of animals because the technical or industrial grade preparations contain toxic impurities that can be carried through the skin. Also, DMSO must not be used on dogs or horses within a few days before or after treatment with or exposure to cholinesterase-inhibiting compounds.

DMSO should be used in accordance with the label instructions. It must not be used except in the dog and horse and only by topical application. It must not be used on animals intended for human consumption. Moreover, the drug is contraindicated in breeding animals. Developmental malformations or teratogenic effects have been observed in the pregnant hamster and chick embryo. Inasmuch as there is no information regarding the possible effect of topically applied DMSO upon breeding dogs and horses, it is not approved for use in breeding stock. Use of DMSO must not exceed 14 days. Prolonged use of DMSO, particularly at high dosages, produces lens changes in the eye of the dog and other animals (Rubin and Barnett 1967).

These and other studies were followed by an immediate order from the FDA to discontinue the clinical evaluation of DMSO in human beings. In recent years, however, clinical trials in human beings have resumed to determine the safety and efficacy of this so-called persecuted drug.

CLINICAL USE

In the Dog. The early clinical use of DMSO in the dog included its use in a number of inflammatory conditions (Knowles 1967). It is of particular benefit in the treatment of traumatic musculoskeletal injuries to reduce acute swelling in the racing greyhound (O'Brien 1965). In addition, contusion of the medial saphenous vein (referred to as a "jack") occurs commonly on the left rear limb on the medial side of the midshaft of the tibia. This injury occurs on turning to the left while racing. Also, in the greyhound the gracilis muscle is more susceptible to strain than other muscles. Such conditions may vary from a mild irritation to a complete rupture of the muscle ("dropped muscle"). According to O'Brien (1965), the recovery and return of normal function in the greyhound with these musculoskeletal disorders appear to be more rapid with a lessened incidence of scar tissue formation. Side effects consist of initial swelling of the treated area, which subsides in 24–36 hours; drying and scurfing of the treated skin may also occur.

DMSO is applied with cotton swabs, glass rods, daubers, and brushes; use of the bare hand to apply the drug is contraindicated. Rubber gloves are recommended. Massage of the affected region is unnecessary because of the rapid penetration and absorption of DMSO.

In the dog, DMSO is administered 3 or 4 times daily in a dosage not to exceed 20 ml/day. The amount of drug to be administered should be transferred to a suitable container with the original bottle being immediately recapped securely. Brushes should be rinsed with water and air-dried between applications. Bandages should not be used after the application of DMSO because there is a possibility that local irritation will be increased.

In the Horse. DMSO has been used topically in the horse for the rapid relief of pain and for the reduction of swelling and acute inflammation due to traumatic injuries. Its use in the treatment of musculoskeletal injuries and similar disorders has been reported (Teigland and Saurino 1967; Adkins 1972). The same precaution applies in the handling and use of DMSO described above for the dog.

The maximum recommended topical daily dose of DMSO in the horse is 100 ml divided equally into 2 or 3 applications. Total length of the therapy must not exceed 30 days in the horse. A gel preparation of DMSO is also available for use in the horse. The total daily dosage of the gel should not exceed 100 g. All other information on the frequency as well as the duration of use of the compound is identical to that of the DMSO solution. Acute swelling due to traumatic injury usually responds successfully to DMSO within 4–6 days.

In Exotic Species. DMSO has been used as a solvent for increasing the onset of action and rapidity of absorption of etorphine in the capture and restraint of wild animals (Wallach 1969). According to Wallach, the drug appears to offer little advantage because deep intramuscular injection of etorphine is still the most dependable method of administering etorphine to wild animals.

Triamcinolone Acetonide Cream

A concentration of 0.1% *Triamcinolone Acetonide,* U.S.P. (Vetalog Cream), is provided in the form of a cream as an antiinflammatory, antipruritic, and antiallergic agent for the topical treatment of dermatitis and summer eczema. This preparation is approved by the FDA for use only in the dog.

PRECAUTIONS AND CONTRAINDICATIONS

Triamcinolone acetonide cream must not be used in food animals. It is contraindicated for use in the eyes. Triamcinolone may be absorbed through the skin after topical application. In addition, systemic effects may occur following the animals' licking the cream from the skin. Signs of polydipsia, polyuria, and increased weight gain may occur following excessive absorption or licking of the cream, especially if it is used to cover large surface areas of the body or if it is used over long periods. In the event the skin condition is complicated by the presence of a bacterial infection, appropriate and concomitant use of antimicrobial agents will be necessary. If the bacterial infection cannot be immediately controlled or eliminated, the triamcinolone cream should be discontinued until the infection can be controlled.

CLINICAL USE

The triamcinolone acetonide cream is applied by inunction into the affected areas of the skin of the dog 2–4 times daily for 4–10 days.

Fluocinolone Acetonide Cream (Synalar Cream)

This preparation contains 0.025% fluocinolone acetonide and is approved by the FDA for topical use in the dog. It is recommended for the relief of pruritus and inflammation associated with acute and chronic dermatoses. Also, this drug preparation is used in the treatment of allergic and acute moist dermatitis as well as for the alleviation of superficial inflammatory conditions caused by chemical and physical abrasions and burns.

CLINICAL USE

A small quantity of the cream is rubbed into the affected region of the skin 2 or 3 times daily.

Fluocinolone Acetonide Solution (Synalar Solution)

The solution form of this preparation contains 0.01% fluocinolone acetonide in appropriate solvent bases. It is approved by the FDA for topical use in the dog and cat. Fluocinolone acetonide solution is recommended for the alleviation of pruritus and inflammatory conditions associated with otitis externa and certain acute and chronic dermatoses in both the dog and cat.

CLINICAL USE

For treatment of both the dog and cat, a small portion of the solution is applied to the affected areas 2 or 3 times daily.

Fluocinolone Acetonide Neomycin Sulfate Cream (Neo-Synalar Cream)

This topical preparation contains 0.025% fluocinolone acetonide and 0.5% neomycin sulfate. It has been approved by the FDA for use in the dog and cat.

CLINICAL USE

Fluocinolone and neomycin are recommended in the alleviation of pruritus and various dermatoses as well as in the treatment of allergic and acute moist dermatitis in the dog. Moreover, in both the dog and cat, it is recommended for the treatment of wound infections. The cream preparation is applied in small quantities 2 or 3 times daily to the affected areas.

Fluocinolone Acetonide, Dimethyl Sulfoxide Otic Solution (Synotic)

Each ml of this solution contains 0.01% of fluocinolone acetonide in 60% DMSO. It is approved by the FDA for use in the dog and recommended for the relief of pruritus as well as inflammation associated with acute and chronic otitis.

PRECAUTIONS

It is axiomatic that a generalized infection should not be treated with drug combinations containing corticosteroids unless supportive therapy with antimicrobial preparations is also included. An unfavorable response to this otic preparation may be attributable to the presence of a bacterial infection requiring identification by a sensitivity test. Once identification has been determined, an appropriate antimicrobial drug can be used. DMSO must not be used in breeding or pregnant animals because of the potential of embryonic malformations. The drug must not be used in the eyes. Care must be taken to prevent the preparation from coming in contact with the bare hands because DMSO will increase the absorption of the fluocinolone component through the skin.

CLINICAL USE

The ear canal should be cleaned prior to the instillation of 4–6 drops of the otic solution twice daily. Gentle massage of the ear should be performed following the instillation of the drug preparation. The total dosage used should not exceed 17 ml and therapy should be discontinued after 14 days.

Neomycin Sulfate-Thiabendazole-Dexamethasone Solution (Tresaderm)

This solution contains 3.2 mg of neomycin sulfate, 40 mg of thiabendazole, and 1 mg of dexamethasone in each ml. It has been approved by the FDA for use in the dog and cat. Conditions for the use of this preparation include the adjunctive treatment of bacterial, mycotic, and inflammatory dermatoses and otitis externa.

CLINICAL USE

Dermatoses involving areas other than the ears should be well moistened twice daily by the use of 2–4 drops per square inch of surface area. In the treatment of otitis externa, 5–15 drops of the drug are instilled into the ear twice daily. The total duration of the above treatments is restricted to a maximum of 7 days.

Neomycin Sulfate, Hydrocortisone Acetate, Tetracaine Hydrochloride Ear Ointment (Neo-Cortef with Tetracaine)

This drug combination contains 5 mg of neomycin sulfate, 5 mg of hydrocortisone acetate, and 5 mg of tetracaine hydrochloride in each g of ointment. It has been approved by the FDA for use in the dog and cat. The preparation is recommended for the treatment of acute otitis externa and, to a lesser extent, the chronic form of otitis externa.

PRECAUTIONS

Inasmuch as tetracaine and neomycin have the properties and potential to induce allergic hypersensitivity, caution should be taken to detect such clinical signs. In the event it is observed, use of the preparation should be discontinued. If the lesions fail to respond to the corticosteroid medication, the cause may be nonsusceptible organisms or the prolonged use of preparations containing antibiotics that favor the growth of other agents such as *Monilia*. If the response to the preparation is unfavorable within 2 or 3 days, the diagnosis should be reevaluated and appropriate therapeutic measures initiated.

CLINICAL USE

The ointment is placed in the external ear canal 1–3 times daily in the dog or cat.

Neomycin Sulfate, Prednisolone Acetate, Tetracaine Hydrochloride Eardrops

This otic preparation contains 5 mg of neomycin sulfate, 2.5 mg of prednisolone acetate, and 5 mg of tetracaine hydrochloride in each ml. The preparation has been approved by the FDA for use in the dog and cat. Indications and precautions for its use in the treatment of otitis externa are identical to those discussed for the neomycin sulfate, hydrocortisone acetate, and tetracaine hydrochloride ear ointment.

CLINICAL USE

The eardrops (2–6 drops) are placed in the external ear canal 2–3 times daily for the treatment of otitis externa in the dog and cat.

Chloramphenicol-Prednisolone-Tetracaine-Squalane Suspension

This topical preparation for use on the skin and in the ear contains 4.2 mg of chloramphenicol, 1.7 mg of prednisolone, 4.2 mg of tetracaine, and 0.21 ml of squalane in an oil base. It has been approved by the FDA for use in the dog and cat. The preparation is used in the treatment of acute otitis externa and pyodermas.

PRECAUTIONS

In vitro sensitivity tests prior to treatment are recommended. Severe infections should also be supplemented and supported by systemic treatment. This preparation must not be used in the eyes. Blood dyscrasias from the prolonged use of chloramphenicol may occur in the cat. Use of the preparation in food-producing animals is not sanctioned because of tissue residues.

CLINICAL USE

The suspension is applied 2–3 times daily or as required for not more than 7 days in the treatment of the dog and cat.

Cephalonium, Polymyxin B Sulfate, Flumethasone, Iodochlorhydroxyquin, Piperocaine Hydrochloride Topical-Otic Ointment (Toptic Ointment)

Each g of this topical preparation contains 10 mg of cephalonium, 5000 units of polymyxin B sulfate, 0.25 mg of flumethasone, 30 mg of iodochlorhydroxyquin, and 40 mg of piperocaine hydrochloride in an ointment base. The preparation is approved by the FDA for use in the dog and cat. It is recommended for cutaneous and otic use in the treatment of disorders complicated by bacterial, fungal, and yeast organisms.

SIDE EFFECTS

Long-term treatment may result in the development of hypersensitivity to the active components in the ointment. If this happens, treatment should be discontinued and reevaluated. In the event of corticosteroid overdosage, clinical signs may appear such as polydipsia, polyuria, gain in body weight, and delayed wound healing.

PRECAUTIONS AND CONTRAINDICATIONS

The ointment must not be used in conditions where corticosteroids are not indicated. Moreover, parenteral corticosteroids must not be administered during the course of treatment with this preparation. At high dosages, the incidence of osteoporosis may be increased, especially in older animals during the healing stages of a fractured bone. The antibiotic fractions in the ointment may result in the growth of nonsusceptible organisms. If nonsusceptible organisms (i.e., bacterial, fungal, or yeast) appear during treatment, the instituted therapy should be reevaluated and other clinical procedures initiated.

CLINICAL USE

The frequency of the topical application of the ointment is dependent on the severity of the skin or ear condition. For mild conditions, treatment may consist of once daily to twice weekly. In severe cases, the ointment is applied 1 or 2 times daily. The dose level of the ointment per treatment should not exceed 300 mg. As an aid in determining the weight of the ointment, a ⅛-inch diameter by a 2-inch long squirt from the tube is equivalent to about 100 mg. In the treatment of skin conditions, tissue debris should be removed prior to the treatment of encrusted lesions; the ointment is applied to the skin by lightly rubbing a thin layer on the infected area 1–2 times daily. For treatment of the ear, the ointment is used 1–2 times daily for not longer than 12 days.

Kanamycin Sulfate, Calcium Amphomycin, and Hydrocortisone Acetate (Kanfosone Otic Cream)

This drug preparation is a water-miscible ointment or cream base. Each g contains 5 mg of kanamycin sulfate, 5 mg of calcium amphomycin, and 10 mg of hydrocortisone acetate. The preparation is approved by the FDA for use in the dog and is recommended for the treatment of conditions associated with bacterial infections that are susceptible to kanamycin and/or amphomycin. Some of these conditions include acute otitis externa, furunculosis, folliculitis, pruritus, anal gland infections, erythema, decubital ulcer, superficial wounds, and superficial abscesses.

CLINICAL USE

Prior to the application of the ointment, the hair of the affected site should be clipped and the area should be cleaned to remove tissue debris. The ointment is then applied to the skin 2 times daily. For more severe and extensive lesions, the ointment may be applied more often. When improvement occurs following the initiation of treatment, the applications can be reduced to once daily. For the treatment of anal gland infections, the ointment should be instilled into the orifice of the gland rather than into any fistulous tract. In the event there is no response within 7 days from the use of this drug preparation, the diagnosis and treatment should be reassessed.

Nystatin, Neomycin, Thiostrepton, and Triamcinolone Acetonide Ointment (Panolog)

This ointment contains 100,000 units of nystatin, 2.5 mg neomycin sulfate, 2500 units of thiostrepton, and 1 mg of triamcinolone acetonide. It is approved by the FDA for use in the dog and cat. The preparation is recommended for local therapy as an antipruritic, antifungal, antibacterial, and antiinflammatory ointment for the topical treatment of dermal disorders. It is used in the treatment of acute and chronic otitis of different etiologies, in anal gland infections in the dog, and in the treatment of interdigital cysts in both the dog and cat. Moreover, it is recommended for dermatologic conditions complicated by bacterial or candidal infections. In addition, the ointment is used in the treatment of various forms of dermatitis (i.e., eczematous, seborrheic, and contact) and as an aid in the treatment of dermatitis due to parasitic infestation.

CLINICAL USE

In the treatment of otitis, the ear canal should be cleaned and all debris (impacted cerumen, foreign bodies, parasites) removed prior to the instillation of 3–5 drops of the ointment. For use in infected anal glands, the gland or cyst should be drained prior to infusion. In the treatment of other dermatologic conditions, the affected sites should be cleaned and all tissue debris removed, followed by an application of a thin film of ointment. The ointment should be applied once daily to only once a week for mild inflammations. For the more severe cases, the ointment may need to be applied 2–3 times daily. As improvement is noted, the frequency of the therapy may be reduced.

Nitrofurazone-Nifuroxime-Diperodon Hydrochloride Ear Solution

This ear solution contains on a weight-in-weight basis 0.2% nitrofurazone, 0.375% nifuroxime, and 2% diperodon hydrochloride. It is approved by the FDA for use in the dog and is recommended in the treatment of bacterial ear infections caused by organisms sensitive to nitrofurazone and/or nifuroxime.

CLINICAL USE

The preparation is used 2 or 3 times daily and should not be used longer than 14 days continuously. Hypersensitivity may occur requiring drug discontinuance in the treatment of ear infections.

Gentamicin Sulfate, Betamethasone Valerate Otic Solution (Gentocin)

Each cc of the solution contains gentamicin sulfate equivalent to 3 mg of gentamicin base and betamethasone valerate equivalent to 1 mg of betamethasone alcohol. The preparation is approved by the FDA for use in the dog and is recommended for the treatment of acute and chronic otitis externa caused by bacteria sensitive to gentamicin.

PRECAUTIONS AND CONTRAINDICATIONS

Sensitivity of pathogenic bacteria to antimicrobial agents should be determined before this preparation is administered. Topical antibiotics sometimes permit the enhanced growth of nonsusceptible bacteria, fungi, or yeasts. If this occurs, other courses of treatment must be initiated. The contraindications common to corticosteroids also apply to this preparation since the preparation contains betamethasone. For additional information, see Section 8 on corticosteroids. In the event hypersensitivity to any of the drug components develops, this preparation should be discontinued and other therapy initiated. The simultaneous administration of gentamicin with other drugs known to induce ototoxicity is not clinically acceptable.

CLINICAL USE

The solution is provided in a squeeze bottle for instillation of drops (3–8) into the ear canal 2 times daily for 7–14 days.

Neomycin Sulfate, 9-Fluoroprednisolone Acetate, Tetracaine Hydrochloride, and Myristyl-Gamma-Picolinium Chloride Topical Powder

This topical powder contains 5 mg of neomycin sulfate, 1 mg of 9-fluoroprednisolone acetate, 5 mg of tetracaine hydrochloride, and 0.2 mg of myristyl-gamma-picolinium chloride in each g. It is approved by the FDA for use in the horse, dog, and cat. The product is recommended in the treatment of certain ear and skin conditions as adjunctive therapy. Moreover, the preparation is indicated as a superficial dressing for cuts, wounds, lacerations, and abrasions. It may also be used as a dusting powder following amputation of claws, dewclaws, and tails or other surgical procedures. Additionally, the drug preparation may be used in the dog for the treatment of acute otitis externa, acute moist dermatitis, and interdigital dermatitis.

Squalane, Pyrethrins, and Piperonyl Butoxide

This product contains 25% squalane (hexamethyltetracosane), 0.05% pyrethrins, and 0.5% technical piperonyl butoxide. The preparation is approved by the FDA for use in the dog and cat for treatment of ear mites.

clinical use

Dosage levels recommended daily in each ear are as follows:

Species	*Body Weight (in lb)*	*Number of Drops*
Dog	5–15	4–5
	16–30	5–10
	over 30	10–15
Cat	5–15	4–5

The duration of treatment recommended is 7–10 days with repeated treatment in 2 weeks.

Oxytetracycline Hydrochloride and Hydrocortisone Spray

Each 3-oz container of the spray contains 300 mg of oxytetracycline hydrochloride and 100 mg of hydrocortisone so that a 1-second spray treatment will deliver about 2.5 mg of oxytetracycline and 0.8 mg of hydrocortisone. The preparation is approved by the FDA for use in the dog and cat. It is recommended for the alleviation of discomfort and continued therapy for many allergic, infectious, and traumatic skin conditions.

precautions

The product must not be sprayed into the eyes or on mucous membranes. It should be used in a well-ventilated area and inhalation of the spray should be avoided.

clinical use

The product is indicated in the treatment of superficial wounds, cuts, and abrasions as well as in the treatment of allergic dermatoses, including urticaria, eczema, and insect bites. Also, it is indicated in the treatment of infections associated with minor burns and wounds as well as in nonspecific cases of pruritus.

The product is sprayed onto the skin (hair clipped and cleansed) for 1–2 seconds by holding the container about 6 inches from the affected area. Use of the drug preparation in small quantities at frequent intervals (3 or 4 times daily) appears to provide the best results. Treatment is generally continued for 7–14 days.

Triethanolamine Polypeptide Oleate-Condensate Otic Solution

This otic preparation contains 10% triethanolamine polypeptide oleate-condensate in propylene glycol and chlorobutanol. The product is approved by the FDA for use in the dog and cat. It is used to assist in the removal of excess or impacted earwax.

clinical use

With the head of the animal in the tilted position, the ear canal is filled with the otic solution. For 15–30 minutes the canal is plugged with a pledget of cotton to prevent the instilled solution from draining out. Then the canal is gently washed or flushed with lukewarm water by the use of a soft rubber syringe. The procedure is repeated if necessary to remove all the earwax.

Cuprimyxin (Unitop)

This product is a topical cream containing 0.5% cuprimyxin (6-methoxy-1-phenazinol-5,10-dioxide, cupric complex). It is a new broad-spectrum antimicrobial agent consisting of a cupric complex of myxin, an antibiotic produced by a species of *Sorangium*. The drug has a broad spectrum of antibacterial and antifungal activity; the antifungal activity includes an effect against dermatophytes, *Trichophyton* and *Microsporum*, and against the yeast *Candida*.

PRECAUTIONS

If an adverse reaction occurs, the topical treatment should be discontinued. Caution should be exercised to avoid staining of clothing or household furnishings following the use of cuprimyxin. After its use on the skin, a change in color from dark green to pink is due to the release of free myxin from its copper complex.

CLINICAL USE

The topical cream is used on the affected area 2 times daily. If there is no clinical response within 7 days, the diagnosis and therapy should be reassessed. If a favorable response is noted and the treatment is successful, the therapy should be continued for an additional 3–5 days to prevent a possible relapse.

OPHTHALMIC AGENTS

There are numerous ophthalmic preparations for the treatment of eye conditions in small animals. In food-producing animals, there is a scarcity of preparations for use in therapy because of the difficulty pharmaceutical firms encounter in the evaluation of the potential hazards associated with the accumulation of minute tissue residues. Most of the resource information regarding ophthalmic preparations that is presented in this chapter originated from the April 1, 1974, *Code of Federal Regulations* covered by Sections 135a. 2 through 135a. 52.

Kanamycin Ophthalmic Ointment (Kantrim Ophthalmic Ointment)

The amount of kanamycin activity per g of ointment in this preparation is 3.5 mg. This ophthalmic preparation is approved by the FDA for use in the dog as a treatment for various eye infections involving kanamycin-sensitive microorganisms. The drug is recommended in conditions such as conjunctivitis, blepharitis, dacryocystitis, keratitis, and corneal ulcerations. Also, it is used as a prophylactic preparation in traumatic conditions, removal of foreign bodies, and intraocular surgery.

CLINICAL USE

A thin film of the ointment is applied to the affected eye 3–4 times daily or more frequently if it is necessary to achieve a satisfactory clinical response. It is advisable to continue the treatment for at least 48 hours after the eye appears normal.

Kanamycin Ophthalmic Aqueous Solution (Kantrim Ophthalmic Solution)

This aqueous solution contains a kanamycin activity of 10 mg/ml. Conditions for the use of this preparation are essentially identical to those described above for the ointment form of kanamycin. The preparation is approved by the FDA for use in the dog.

CLINICAL USE

A few drops (3–5) are instilled into the affected eye every 3 hours or more frequently if it is clinically prudent. The medication should be used as frequently as possible for the first 2 days. It should not be discontinued until at least 48 hours after the eye returns to normal.

Chloramphenicol Ophthalmic Solution

The concentration of chloramphenicol for ophthalmic use is 0.5%. The FDA has approved the use of this preparation in the dog and cat for the treatment of bacterial conjunctivitis caused by organisms susceptible to chloramphenicol.

PRECAUTIONS

The precautions connected with the use of preparations containing chloramphenicol have been previously covered and apply to this and similar products.

CLINICAL USE

Chloramphenicol drops (1 or 2) are instilled into the eye 4–6 times daily for the first 72 hours. The time period between applications may be increased after the first 2 days of treatment. Treatment should not be discontinued for at least 48 hours after the eye appears normal. The use of this preparation in the cat should not extend beyond 7 days.

Chloramphenicol Ophthalmic Ointment

This preparation contains chloramphenicol at the level of 10 mg/g (1%) of ointment. The product is approved by the FDA for use in the dog and cat. Conditions for its use are identical to those mentioned above for the aqueous form of chloramphenicol.

Chloramphenicol-Prednisolone Ophthalmic Ointment

Each g of this product contains 10 mg of chloramphenicol and 2 mg of prednisolone. The preparation is approved by the FDA for use in the dog and cat. Conditions for its use in the treatment of bacterial conjunctivitis and ocular inflammation are similar to those described above for the other ophthalmic preparations containing chloramphenicol. This preparation contains prednisolone, which is advantageous in the reduction of ocular inflammation associated with severe eye infections.

PRECAUTIONS

The general precautions previously discussed above for chloramphenicol apply to this product. In addition, ophthalmic preparations containing corticosteroids, with or without an antimicrobial agent, are contraindicated in the initial treatment phases of corneal ulcers. Corticosteroids should not be used until the infection is under control and corneal healing is well advanced.

CLINICAL USE

The ointment is applied in the eye 4–6 times daily for the first 72 hours. Therapy should not be discontinued for at least 48 hours after the eye appears normal. Use of this preparation in the cat should not proceed beyond 7 days.

Prednisolone Sodium Phosphate-Neomycin Sulfate Ophthalmic Ointment (Hydeltrone Ophthalmic Ointment)

This ophthalmic ointment contains prednisolone sodium phosphate equivalent to 2.5 mg of prednisolone 21-phosphate and 5 mg of neomycin sulfate in each g. The drug preparation is approved by the FDA for use in the cat and dog. It is recommended for use in ocular inflammations or infections limited to the conjunctiva or the anterior segment of the eye such as those associated with allergic reactions or gross irritants.

PRECAUTIONS

Precautions concerning the use of corticosteroids in the treatment of eye conditions have been previously discussed.

CLINICAL USE

A small amount of the ointment is expressed into the conjunctival sac 4 times a day at intervals of 1–8 hours for 7 days. In the event there is no improvement, the treatment should be reevaluated and other appropriate measures considered. However, if the response is favorable, the frequency of application may be reduced to 2 times daily. The total duration of treatment may require from a few days to several weeks.

Prednisolone Acetate, Sodium Sulfacetamide, Neomycin Ointment

This ophthalmic and otic ointment contains 5 mg of prednisolone acetate, 100 mg of sodium sulfacetamide, and 2.5 mg of neomycin sulfate in each g. The preparation is approved by the FDA for use in the dog and cat. It is recommended for treating external eye and ear infections caused by bacteria sensitive to neomycin or sulfacetamide and the inflammation, edema, and allergy that is often associated with these conditions.

PRECAUTIONS

The same general precautions previously mentioned for drug preparations containing corticosteroids and neomycin in this chapter also apply to this product.

CLINICAL USE

Use of the ointment for eye and ear conditions should be made frequently, 3–4 times daily. In chronic conditions, withdrawal of treatment is recommended by gradually decreasing the frequency of application.

Nystatin, Neomycin, Thiostrepton, and Triamcinolone Acetonide Ophthalmic Ointment (Panolog)

This liquefied ointment contains 100,000 units of nystatin, 2.5 mg of neomycin base, 2500 units of thiostrepton, and 1 mg of triamcinolone acetonide in each ml. The drug is approved by the FDA in cats, dogs, and cattle. In dogs and cats, the ointment is recommended for ophthalmic use as an antiinflammatory, antipruritic, antifungal *(Candida albicans)*, and antimicrobial agent for local therapy in conjunctivitis and keratitis. In cattle, it is recommended for infectious keratoconjunctivitis (pink eye).

clinical use

In the dog and cat, 1 drop of the ointment is instilled into the eye 2 or 3 times daily in the treatment of conjunctivitis and keratitis. If necessary, therapy may be continued for 2 weeks. For the treatment of bovine infectious keratoconjunctivitis, a small line of ointment is applied to the affected eyes once daily. If required, therapy may be continued for 2 weeks. The frequency of application of the drug is dependent on the severity of the condition. In the treatment of mild inflammatory conditions, a once daily to once weekly application of the drug may be used. In severe involvement of the eyes, the drug may need to be applied as often as 2–3 times daily. As improvement occurs, the frequency of the therapy may be decreased.

Neomycin Sulfate Ophthalmic Ointment

This ophthalmic preparation contains 5 mg of neomycin sulfate equivalent in activity to 3.5 mg of neomycin base per g of ointment. The preparation is approved by the FDA for use in the dog and cat in the treatment of superficial ocular infections confined to the conjunctival and anterior segments of the eye.

precautions

Supplemental systemic therapy is necessary in the presence of severe bacterial infections. Some animals may manifest a hypersensitivity to neomycin that may require discontinuance of the treatment. Moreover, long-term application of the drug may allow the growth of organisms not susceptible to neomycin.

clinical use

The ophthalmic ointment is applied 4 times daily.

Neomycin Sulfate and Polymyxin B Ophthalmic Solution (Optiprime Ophthalmic Solution)

This solution contains 5 mg of neomycin sulfate and 10,000 units of polymyxin B in each ml. It is approved by the FDA for use in the dog. The ophthalmic solution is recommended for the treatment of bacterial infections associated with conditions such as corneal injuries, superficial keratitis, conjunctivitis, keratoconjunctivitis and blepharitis.

contraindication

The product is contraindicated in clinical cases in which the microorganisms are insusceptible to the antibiotics of this preparation.

clinical use

The dosage level recommended for the eye is 1–2 drops every 6 hours. Successful treatment may require the use of this preparation for 7–10 days.

Flumethasone, Neomycin Sulfate, and Polymyxin B Sulfate Ophthalmic Solution (Anaprime)

This ophthalmic preparation contains 0.1 mg of flumethasone, 5 mg of neomycin sulfate, and 10,000 units of polymyxin B in each ml. The product is approved by the FDA for the dog. It is recommended for the treatment of inflammatory, edematous, and secondary infections associated with corneal injuries, conjunctivitis, keratitis, and other eye conditions.

PRECAUTIONS AND CONTRAINDICATIONS

The usual precautions and contraindications apply to this product because of its synthetic corticosteroid content. These have been previously discussed. Intraocular pressure should be determined periodically because corticosteroidal preparations have been known to cause an increase. This preparation is contraindicated in tuberculous lesions of the eye and acute stages of viral diseases of the conjunctiva and cornea, as well as fungal infections of the eye.

CLINICAL USE

The recommended dose of this preparation is 1–2 drops in each eye every 6 hours. Successful treatment may require 7–10 days.

TYLOSIN-NEOMYCIN EYE POWDER

This topical preparation contains 2% tylosin (as base), neomycin sulfate equivalent to 0.25% base, 1% piperocaine hydrochloride, 0.5% neutral acriflavine, and boric acid. It is approved by the FDA for treatment of infectious keratoconjunctivitis (pink eye) in cattle.

CLINICAL USE

The dusting powder is applied to the eyes once daily for up to 7 days. Animals should be protected from direct sunlight, flies, and dust. Due to the infectious nature of the disease, all animals in an affected herd with or without signs of the disease should receive at least 1 treatment.

ZINC BACITRACIN, POLYMYXIN B SULFATE, NEOMYCIN SULFATE, HYDROCORTISONE ACETATE OPHTHALMIC OINTMENT

This ointment preparation contains 400 units of zinc bacitracin, 5000 units of polymyxin B sulfate, 5 mg of neomycin sulfate, and 10 mg of hydrocortisone acetate in each g. It is approved by the FDA for use in the dog and cat in the treatment of acute or chronic conjunctivitis.

PRECAUTIONS AND CONTRAINDICATIONS

The usual precautions and contraindications apply to this product because of its corticosteroid content.

CLINICAL USE

A thin film of the ointment is applied over the corneal surface 3 or 4 times daily. Treatment is generally confined to 7 or 10 days.

ZINC BACITRACIN, POLYMYXIN B SULFATE, NEOMYCIN SULFATE OPHTHALMIC OINTMENT

This preparation contains 400 units of zinc bacitracin, 5 mg of neomycin sulfate, and 5000 units of polymyxin B sulfate in each g of ointment. The product is approved by the FDA for use in the dog and cat in the treatment of superficial bacterial infections of the conjunctiva.

CLINICAL USE

A thin film of the ointment is applied to the corneal surface 3 or 4 times daily. The duration of treatment is generally 7–10 days.

OXYTETRACYCLINE HYDROCHLORIDE, POLYMYXIN B SULFATE OPHTHALMIC OINTMENT

This ophthalmic preparation contains 5 mg of oxytetracycline and 10,000 units of polymyxin B in each g of the ointment. The drug preparation is approved by the FDA for use in the dog, cat, cow, sheep, and horse. It is recommended for the prophylaxis and local treatment of superficial ocular infections due to oxytetracycline- and polymyxin-susceptible organisms. Such infections include streptococci, rickettsiae, *E. coli,* and *A. aerogenes* (such as conjunctivitis, keratitis, pink eye, corneal ulcer, and blepharitis). Also, the ointment is indicated in ocular infections due to secondary bacterial complications associated with canine distemper.

PRECAUTIONS

Hypersensitivity or allergic reactions are sometimes noted. If these reactions are severe, treatment should be discontinued. If growth of nonsusceptible bacteria or fungi occurs, other therapeutic alternatives will need to be instituted.

REFERENCES

Adkins, J. 1972. Dimethyl sulfoxide (DMSO) and the equine practitioner. Southwest Vet 26:91.

Bradham, G. B., and Sample, J. J. 1967. The vascular and thermal effects of dimethyl sulfoxide. Ann NY Acad Sci 141:225.

Franz, T. J., and Van Bruggen, J. T. 1967. A possible mechanism of action of DMSO. Ann NY Acad Sci 141:302.

Harvey, S. C. 1975. Antiseptics and disinfectants; fungicides; ectoparasiticides. In L. S. Goodman and A. Gilman, eds. The Pharmacological Basis of Therapeutics, 5th ed., p. 1010. New York: Macmillan.

Jacob, S. W.; Herschler, R. J.; and Rosenbaum, E. E. 1965. Dimethyl sulfoxide (DMSO): Laboratory and clinical evaluation. J Am Vet Med Assoc 147:1350.

Knowles, R. P. 1967. Clinical experience with DMSO in small animal practice. Ann NY Acad Sci 141:478.

O'Brien, T. J. 1965. The use of DMSO in traumatic musculoskeletal injuries in racing greyhounds. J Am Anim Hosp Assoc 1:272.

Rubin, L. F., and Barnett, K. C. 1967. Ocular effects of oral and dermal application of dimethyl sulfoxide in animals. Ann NY Acad Sci 141:333.

Smith, E. R.; Hadidian, Z.; and Mason, M. M. 1967. The single- and repeated-dose toxicity of dimethyl sulfoxide. Ann NY Acad Sci 141:96.

Teigland, M. B., and Saurino, V. R. 1967. Clinical evaluation of dimethyl sulfoxide in equine applications. Ann NY Acad Sci 141:471.

Tiews, J.; Scharrer, E.; Harre, N.; and Flögel, L. 1975. Metabolism and excretion of dimethyl sulfoxide in cows and calves after topical and parenteral application. Ann NY Acad Sci 243:139.

Wallach, J. D. 1969. Etorphine (M-99), a new analgesic-immobilizing agent, and its antagonists. Vet Med Small Anim Clin 64:53.

CHAPTER 43

ANTITUSSIVE, EXPECTORANT, AND MUCOLYTIC AGENTS

NICHOLAS H. BOOTH

Antitussive agents are preparations used to relieve or suppress coughing. The cough is probably the most important mechanism of bronchial catharsis. Therefore, the objective of antitussive therapy is to decrease the severity and frequency of cough without the concomitant impairment of the evacuation of bronchopulmonary secretions (Sevelius et al. 1971).

Although a number of factors may be responsible for triggering a cough, it has been proposed that bronchoconstriction is the primary stimulus in its initiation (Salem and Aviado 1970a). The release of humoral agents such as serotonin, histamine, slow reacting substance (SRS), or other bronchoconstrictors may be involved in the mechanism. Bronchodilation apparently disrupts or interferes with the cough reflex by the inhibition of bronchoconstriction. An important pharmacologic action of most antitussive agents is their ability to produce bronchodilation. In the treatment of the asthmatic cough, the bronchodilator agents are most beneficial.

The cough may be described as useful or useless. The useful cough is a protective reflex and serves to raise secretions of the respiratory tract and thereby clears the respiratory passages. The useless cough is unproductive and due primarily to irritation of the respiratory passages. It may also lead to undesirable effects upon the circulatory and respiratory system (Bucher 1958). The undesirable effects generally result in an elevated intrathoracic pressure that may attain values as high as 300 mm Hg. An elevated intrathoracic pressure leads to a decline in the flow of blood to the right heart and results in a drop in cardiac output. Temporary loss of consciousness may result because of reduced cardiac output and flow of blood to the brain. In addition, an increase in the intrathoracic pressure may result in intrapulmonary rupture of the tissues, leading to emphysema. The useless cough may also aggravate pain and promote exhaustion. Severe paroxysmal coughing may result in postoperative ruptures or hemorrhages, and a chronic cough interferes with the patient's rest. For these and other reasons, relief of the useless cough, while constituting only symptomatic therapy, is still desirable.

Unfortunately, undue emphasis has been placed upon *relief* of the cough rather than upon eliminating its cause. The cough must be recognized as a *symptom*. Therefore, while antitussive agents may be beneficial in suppressing severe coughing so that the patient can get physical and mental rest, they generally do not correct the underlying disorder. Some clients, however, expect and want to administer these freely dispensed medicines at the slightest provocation.

NARCOTIC ANTITUSSIVE AGENTS

The principal narcotic drug of choice in this category is codeine. The antitussive action of codeine in animals and human beings has been well established. Codeine and other opiates are considered to remain among the most effective agents available for the suppression of the cough (Jaffe and Martin 1975).

Codeine Phosphate

Codeine Phosphate, U.S.P., or *Codeine Sulfate* is available in tablets of 15, 30, and 60 mg primarily for analgesic use. Liquid preparations of codeine are usually used to suppress the cough. *Terpin Hydrate and Codeine Elixir,* N.F., is also available and contains 10 mg of codeine in each 5 ml. The majority of codeine antitussive preparations contain this quantity of codeine, which is the limit for the nonprescription use of codeine.

The indication for an opiate in cough medicine is to depress a dry, irritating cough that has become chronic and extremely troublesome. Codeine phosphate is most commonly employed, although other opiates could be used. The opiates depress the cough center in the medulla so that it is less receptive to stimuli. Codeine phosphate is given preference over morphine sulfate for relief of a dry, irritating cough. It appears to be nearly as effective in depressing the cough center as morphine, and yet it is less depressant on other parts of the central nervous system (CNS). In addition, codeine is less depressant on the respiratory center and has less constipating action than morphine.

One hazard in the use of opiates as depressants of the cough center is the administration to a patient with a copious respiratory secretion. Opiates are definitely contraindicated in such a case because the secretions might accumulate in the lungs and the airways with disastrous results. Moreover, potent antitussive agents such as codeine and other opiates should not be given during aerosol therapy or during the application of nebulized mucolytic agents in the treatment of bronchitis or other respiratory complications. Inspissated exudates become liquified by the aerosol. If the cough reflex has been impaired by the administration of potent antitussive agents, the animal may drown in its secretions unless they are removed by oral or bronchoscopic suction (O'Brien and Todd 1971).

DOSAGE

Codeine is most commonly used in the dog. The dosage ranges from 10 to 65 mg administered subcutaneously. Orally, codeine phosphate is used in a cough medicine from 0.5 to 1 mg/lb of body weight 3–4 times daily. Far better results are obtained from repeated administration of smaller doses.

Although used less frequently in large animals, the recommended total dosages for codeine phosphate in the horse and cow are 0.2–2 g and for the pig 15–60 mg (Brander and Pugh 1971). For other species, information on the dosages of codeine is essentially unknown. Experimental studies in cats have shown that 0.25 mg/kg–4 mg/kg orally were effective as an antitussive agent (Salem and Aviado 1970b). Also, in the cat, intravenous dosages of codeine (0.1–1 mg/kg) depressed the cough reflex. In rabbits, the cough is partially suppressed by 3 mg/kg of codeine administered intravenously while 4 mg/kg suppress it completely. The intravenous antitussive doses of codeine phosphate in the guinea pig are reported to be 20–30 mg/kg. In the laboratory rat, an antitussive effect is achieved at 10 mg/kg.

Morphine Sulfate

As previously mentioned, codeine is the most frequently used opiate and is preferred over morphine. The contraindications in the use of morphine are essentially those described above for codeine.

DOSAGE

The subcutaneous dose of *Morphine Sulfate,* U.S.P., generally recommended in the dog is 5–30 mg.

Miscellaneous Opiates

Other opiate derivatives employed as antitussive agents are dihydrocodeinone,

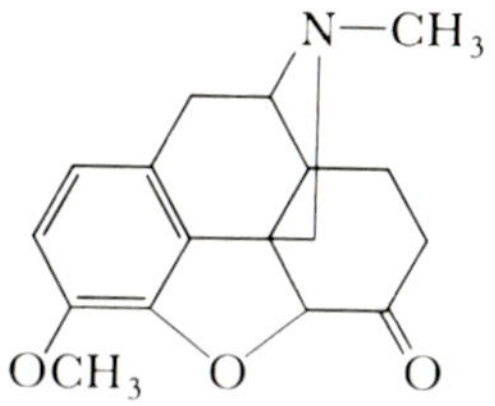

$N{-}CH_3$

OCH_3 O O

Dihydrocodeinone

FIG. 43.1.

noscapine, codoxime, and pholcodine. With the exception of dihydrocodeinone, which is only occasionally used in the dog, the other compounds have little or no importance in veterinary medicine. *Dihydrocodeinone Bitartrate,* N.F. (Hydrocodone), is chemically similar to codeine and is prepared by the hydrolysis of dihydrothebaine. (See Fig. 43.1.) Pharmacologically, it has an activity intermediate to that of codeine and morphine. Experimentally, the antitussive action of dihydrocodeinone is equivalent to that of codeine. An oral dose of 1 mg/kg of dihydrocodeinone suppresses a cough within one-half hour and lasts 2 hours in the unanesthetized dog. The effect of an oral dose of 1 mg/kg of codeine also is comparable to the effect of dihydrocodeinone.

CLINICAL USE

Dihydrocodeinone is recommended in the treatment of the harsh, dry, and nonproductive cough associated with bronchitis and bronchiectasis in the dog (Low 1964). It is also indicated for the alleviation of coughing associated with chronic pulmonary emphysema and in some stages of mitral valvular insufficiency in the older dog. A proprietary preparation (Hycodan) containing dihydrocodeinone and homatropine hydrobromide (2.5–5 mg) is recommended orally 2–4 times daily. In addition to the use of this drug combination to reduce coughing in cases associated with emphysema and mitral valvular insufficiency, ephedrine sulfate (10–20 mg) is administered every 4–6 hours to achieve bronchodilation (Low 1964).

NONNARCOTIC ANTITUSSIVE AGENTS

With the exception of dextromethorphan, there are few well-controlled clinical studies in human beings demonstrating the efficacy of many of the marketed nonnarcotic antitussives against pathological cough (Jaffe and Martin 1975). In veterinary medicine, a similar statement on efficacy probably can be made for most of the nonnarcotic antitussive drugs in current use. Extrapolation of experimental data obtained in small laboratory animals to the dog, cat, pig, cow, and other species presents a number of veterinary medical problems in the evaluation of these agents for safety and effectiveness.

DEXTROMETHORPHAN HYDROBROMIDE

Dextromethorphan Hydrobromide, N.F., has antitussive properties similar to those of codeine both with respect to potency and mechanism of action (Salem and Aviado 1970c). It is chemically related to opium but does not induce addiction like the opiates. Moreover, dextromethorphan seldom produces drowsiness or gastrointestinal (GI) disturbances as does codeine (Jaffe and Martin 1975).

In human beings, dextromethorphan is accepted as a safe and effective antitussive agent and is among the most extensively used components of cough preparations. All the information available on the antitussive effects of dextromethorphan in animals relates almost entirely to experimental rather than clinical experience.

Chemically, dextromethorphan is the dextro-rotatory isomer of 3-methoxy-*N*-methyl-morphine. Unlike the levo-rotatory isomer, the dextro isomer has no analgesic or addictive actions. The chemical structure of dextromethorphan is similar to that of morphine and related opiates. (See Fig. 43.2.)

EFFECT IN VARIOUS SPECIES

In the Dog. Experimentally, dextromethorphan compares favorably with codeine and other antitussive preparations in the suppression of cough in dogs. It has a rapid onset of action and essentially full effective-

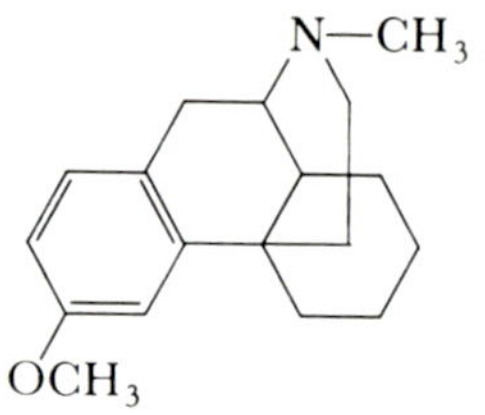

$N{-}CH_3$

OCH_3

Dextromethorphan

FIG. 43.2.

ness is attained in 30 minutes after oral administration of 0.5–16 mg/kg. The drug is effective in inhibiting postdistemper or postpneumonitis cough. Based on the experimental evidence of the effectiveness of dextromethorphan in the suppression of the cough, it appears that an oral dose of between 1 and 2 mg/kg administered 3 or 4 times daily would be a satisfactory therapeutic level.

In the Cat. Research studies have been conducted in the cat to determine the antitussive effects of dextromethorphan following experimentally induced pleurisy; a subcutaneous dose of 2 mg/kg of the drug is effective in suppression of the cough in pleuritic animals. Duration of action of the antitussive effect is about 6 hours. Following the administration of 4 mg/kg of the drug, the duration of action is 8 hours. By the intravenous route, dextromethorphan (2 mg/kg) has been reported to possess a greater antitussive effect in the cat than an intravenous dose of codeine (3.5 mg/kg). The antitussive effects of dextromethorphan by the oral route of administration have not been evaluated in the cat. Inasmuch as the drug is absorbed rapidly and is effective by the oral route in the dog, it should produce comparable effects by this route of administration in the cat.

In the Rabbit. In the anesthetized rabbit, dextromethorphan is reported to be effective in the suppression of cough following an oral dose of 100 mg/kg but not of 50 mg/kg. However, codeine is effective intravenously in the rabbit at only 4 mg/kg.

In the Chimpanzee. Dextromethorphan has been used experimentally with favorable results to suppress coughing due to common colds in the chimpanzee. Clinical signs of the common cold in the chimpanzee are similar to those in the human child. Based on the human dosage of dextromethorphan, 0.3–0.6 mg/kg orally 4 times daily would be expected to produce satisfactory antitussive effects in the chimpanzee.

TRIMEPRAZINE TARTRATE AND PREDNISOLONE (TEMARIL-P)

In human beings, trimeprazine was first used orally in the treatment of pruritis. Later clinical investigations revealed that trimeprazine possessed antihistaminic and antitussive properties in addition to sedative and tranquilizing action. Consequently, the drug became established in human medicine for the treatment of allergic skin as well as respiratory allergies, including bronchial asthma, rhinitis, and chronic cough.

In veterinary medicine, trimeprazine tartrate (5 mg) is combined with prednisolone (2 mg) in tablet form for oral administration in the dog. The dog is the only species in which this combination product (Temaril-P) has been approved for use by the FDA. Among its uses, the preparation is recommended as an adjunctive treatment in cough conditions associated with "kennel cough" and bronchitis. The oral dosage schedule for this drug was discussed in Chapter 17. *(Note: Drug withdrawn from market July 19, 1976.)*

DIPHENHYDRAMINE HYDROCHLORIDE

Antihistamines have some degree of antitussive action, particularly in coughs associated with histamine release in respiratory allergies. Each dose of most preparations of cough remedies contains from a twelfth to a half of the dose required for the alleviation of an allergic disorder. Although antihistamines are sometimes effective in relieving cough associated with bronchospasm, the drying effect is considered undesirable in some respiratory infections. In fact, some clinicians believe that the use of antihistamines in ordinary cough is contraindicated because they decrease pulmonary drainage.

An experimentally induced cough in the dog and cat has been reported to be blocked by *Diphenhydramine Hydrochloride,* U.S.P. (Benadryl). Compared to codeine, the subcutaneous administration of diphenhydramine in the dog is only about 0.4 as potent in elevating the threshold to coughing. Diphenhydramine as well as other antihistamines are combined with agents such as dextromethorphan, codeine, glyceryl guaiacolate, ephedrine, and other drugs having antitussive, bronchodilator, or expectorant effects.

Miscellaneous Nonnarcotic Antitussive Drugs

Other drugs reported to have antitussive action are *Carbetapentane Citrate,* N.F.; *Levopropoxyphen Napsylate,* N.F.; *Benzonatate,* N.F.; *oxolamine; caramiphen; and pipazethate.* These are used in human cough remedies. However, controlled clinical studies in human beings for most of these preparations are insufficient to determine whether they merit consideration as therapeutic alternatives to more thoroughly studied drugs (Jaffe and Martin 1975).

EXPECTORANTS

Expectorants are generally described as drugs that increase pulmonary secretions or sputum volume. They also assist in the removal of secretions or exudates from the respiratory tract and appear to enhance antitussive activity by virtue of increasing the output of respiratory tract secretions. In the presence of expectorants, especially in the acute inflammatory stage, the cough is less frequent but more productive. The viscosity of respiratory tract secretions may also be reduced by some of the expectorants to promote a more productive cough as well as to accelerate pulmonary drainage.

Stagnation of a thick, viscid mucus in the terminal bronchi is partly responsible for bronchial obstruction that destroys the bronchial mucosa with resultant bronchiectasis. Normally, the mucus of the terminal bronchi is more viscid than that secreted by the glands of the upper respiratory tract. As mucus from the lower parts of the respiratory tract is raised, it becomes diluted by the secretions of the upper tract. Normally, the physiologic dilution of the viscid secretions, so important to spontaneous pulmonary drainage, is an extremely slow one. Drugs may increase the secretions of the respiratory tract and promote the removal of viscid secretions. Bronchoscopic aspiration is employed in human beings to remove respiratory exudates. Although desirable, this technique would be difficult to employ in some species and is often impracticable. The mechanical drainage of secretions from the upper respiratory tract is promoted by the normal air currents of the respiratory exchange, by the action of the cilia of the respiratory epithelium, by the propulsive expiration of air while coughing, and by the action of expectorant drugs.

The expectorants may be classified in three main categories, i.e., sedative, stimulant, and anodyne expectorants.

Sedative Expectorants

Agents in this group actually have little, if any, antitussive activity. They stimulate the secretion of mucus that protects and reduces acute inflammatory conditions in the respiratory tract. When coughing occurs, it is more productive and effective but less frequent. Sedative expectorants are further subdivided into the saline, demulcent, and nauseant drugs.

saline expectorants

Expectorants of importance in this group include the ammonium and iodide salts. Ammonium chloride in an oral dose of 0.2 g/lb will increase the respiratory tract secretions by 88%, and ammonium carbonate in an oral dose of about 0.2 g/lb will increase the rate of secretion by 110% in experimental animals. In lower dosages, ammonium chloride does not stimulate the flow of respiratory secretions. The ammonium ion is believed to act by a reflex expectorant action arising from the stomach.

The ammonium ion, as present in ammonium chloride, will produce acute pulmonary edema when administered in toxic doses. Acidosis has been ruled out as a cause of lung edema. The syndrome of ammonium intoxication consists primarily of dyspnea, muscle fasciculations, and convulsions that terminate in acute pulmonary edema (Koenig and Koenig 1949).

Potassium iodide has been found to increase the respiratory tract secretions by about 150%. Ordinarily, iodides (sodium or potassium) are too irritating to use in the treatment of acute inflammatory conditions of the respiratory tract. Their use appears to be best confined to the later stages of bronchitis for purposes of liquefying or "loosening" tenacious secretions of the respiratory mucosa.

DEMULCENT EXPECTORANTS

The soothing, demulcent action of syrup is effective upon contact and may allay a mild irritation of the pharynx for 1–2 hours. Alone, syrup has no expectorant value. It does not increase the fluid secretions of the respiratory tract, but it may serve as a vehicle for an expectorant drug. An expectorant drug in syrup probably would begin to act about the time the effect of the syrup wears off.

NAUSEANT EXPECTORANTS

Antimony Potassium Tartrate, U.S.P. (tarter emetic), is also classified as a nauseant expectorant. It increases secretions of the respiratory tract by producing nausea, which serves to loosen a dry, harsh cough. The rationale for the continued use of this drug is subject to question. In human beings, it is considered to be too toxic to be used as an expectorant or emetic (Levine 1975).

Ipecac, U.S.P., administered orally at a dose of about 0.5 g/lb will increase the rate of respiratory secretions in cats by 143%. The drug apparently induces nausea that results in reflex secretions of the respiratory tract. Ipecac has toxic effects and is seldom used in veterinary medicine. Death has been occasionally noted by the author when it is administered to the cat.

STIMULANT EXPECTORANTS

Agents in this group tend to increase respiratory tract secretions and are used to stimulate or promote repair of chronic inflammatory processes. Many of the expectorants in this group are aromatic compounds that probably are eliminated in part by the respiratory mucosa.

The wood tar derivatives have long been employed for their stimulant expectorant action. Guaiacol administered in an oral dose of 2.5 ml/lb in cats will increase the volume of respiratory fluid by 78%. Guaiacol carbonate, 2.5 g/lb, results in an increase of 60%. Creosote in the same dosage increases respiratory tract fluids by 123% (Boyd and Lapp 1946). A water-soluble salt called potassium guaiacol sulfonate has been introduced as a substitute for the oil-soluble guaiacol and creosote. It is doubtful whether much real benefit has been derived from these drugs in animals because the dosages used in the therapy are below those given above.

When administered orally, guaiacol and creosote are absorbed and eliminated by various avenues, including respiratory secretion. Much of the drug is excreted in the urine as glucuronates or sulfates. Guaiacol and creosote probably are most effective in the treatment of a dry, chronically irritated membrane because they act by inducing hyperemia with increased secretion. Since guaiacol and creosote contain phenol derivatives, the administration of excessive amounts results in phenol poisoning. The guaiacol salts are relatively nontoxic.

Some volatile oils, such as oil of turpentine, oil of anise, oil of eucalyptus, oil of lemon, and oil of pine, will increase secretions of the respiratory tract by 1–3 times. They are used primarily as medicated vapor inhalations and by their slightly irritative effect induce hyperemia and repair.

Anodyne Expectorants

Camphorated Tincture of Opium, U.S.P. (paregoric), was found to increase respiratory tract secretions by 400%. It is believed to act by a reflex action through the GI tract, causing an elevation in output of fluid in the respiratory tract. In addition, paregoric has antitussive activity due to the presence of opium alkaloids such as morphine and codeine. Paregoric is seldom used because other preparations are more readily available and more convenient.

Miscellaneous Expectorants

steam

While steam is not a cough medicine, it does have an expectorant action. In fact, water applied in the form of steam or as a cool nebulized mist may be the best expectorant that can be employed in acute upper respiratory tract ailments. A nebulizer should be used that delivers an average particle size of 5 μ in order for it to penetrate the smaller bronchioles. The use of steam to increase the respiratory fluids has long been recognized as an extremely valuable clinical procedure in human beings. The warmth and moisture tend to liquefy the secretions already present and to induce hyperemia of the respiratory mucosa, which increases the volume but decreases the viscosity of the secretions. If unattended, the use of steam has some disadvantages in animal medicine. Steam vaporizers may elevate the ambient temperature sufficiently to cause heat stroke or may be turned over by the patient and cause burns (O'Brien and Todd 1971).

gases

Carbon dioxide gas has been recommended as an extremely efficient expectorant in patients with a thick tenacious secretion in the lower part of the respiratory tract. Carbon dioxide gas induces hyperemia of the involved bronchial mucosa, which results in a less viscous secretion that can be removed by the normal physiological processes. Carbon dioxide has been especially recommended because it reaches the lower recesses of the respiratory tract where the secretion is particularly tenacious and viscous.

One of the most important actions of carbon dioxide is to cause deeper and more active respiratory movements that aid in moving the respiratory secretion out of the tract. The administration of carbon dioxide gas in a 5% concentration could be accomplished easily in small animal medicine in gas chambers or by use of a tent for some large animals.

Oxygen acts as an antiexpectorant. It increases the viscosity and decreases the amount of the respiratory secretion by lowering the blood flow through the mucosa. The antiexpectorant action of oxygen may be neutralized during administration by the addition of 5% carbon dioxide and water vapor.

MUCOLYTIC AGENTS

In recent years, mucolytic agents have become available to loosen viscid or inspissated pulmonary secretions and to improve expectoration. These agents are administered by aerosol spray or mist that will deliver particles of 0.5–5 μ. Aerosol therapy is primarily used in small animals. It is used in patients with "kennel cough" (infectious tracheobronchitis) or other pulmonary conditions associated with obstruction due to mucus accumulation (Mulnix 1971).

In the proper use of mucolytic agents, some knowledge of the composition and nature of bronchial secretions is necessary. Normally, bronchial secretions are composed almost entirely of mucopolysaccharide fibers. In the presence of an infection, these fibers begin to break down and are replaced by deoxyribonucleic acid (DNA). DNA is present in purulent secretions as a result of cellular destruction and is not a component of normal mucus secretion. The viscosity of the secretion is subsequently increased due to the presence of DNA; lysis of a thick, tenacious secretion by leukocytic proteases is also inhibited by DNA. Flow of mucus and the expectoration or removal of these secretions are difficult when the rate of mucus production is excessive and when its viscosity interferes with normal ciliary function. Pulmonary infections often result in the excessive production of a viscous, purulent secretion or exudate.

Several mucolytic substances have been reported as being efficacious. However, most of them have been disappointingly ineffective or undesirable for clinical use (Lieberman 1970). Only those mucolytic agents, such as *N*-acetyl-L-cysteine and pancreatic dornase, that are most commonly employed in the treatment of pulmonic complications will be discussed in this chapter. For a more complete coverage of the mucolytic agents used experimentally as well as clinically, the reader is referred to Sheffner and Lish (1970).

Acetylcysteine

Chemically, *Acetylcysteine,* N.F. (Mucomyst, Respaire), is *N*-acetyl-L-cysteine and has a chemical structure as shown in Fig. 43.3. The chemical is a white crystalline powder having a molecular weight of 163 and a melting point of 109°–110° C. It is available in vials containing a 20% solution of acetylcysteine as the sodium salt.

Acetylcysteine is clinically effective on both purulent and nonpurulent (mucoid) pulmonary secretions. Mucolytic activity of the drug is dependent on its free sulfhydryl groups that interact with the disulfide bonds of mucoprotein; this interaction reduces the viscosity of the mucus. The activity of acetylcysteine is also dependent on a concentration of 10%–20% (dilution of the drug solution should be avoided) and a pH of 7–9. Aerosol devices that do not permit contact of the drug with rubber or metal parts of the equipment should be used to administer the drug solution. For most effective use of the drug, clinicians agree that intermittent positive pressure breathing is the only means of obtaining sufficient concentration of the aerosol into the small bronchioles and alveoli. In human beings, 1–2 cc of the drug solution can also be instilled into a tracheostomy, followed by immediate suction of the liquefied secretions (Lieberman 1970). Moreover, it can be administered through a bronchoscope or by bronchial lavage to liquefy accumulations of tenacious and thick mucus secretions.

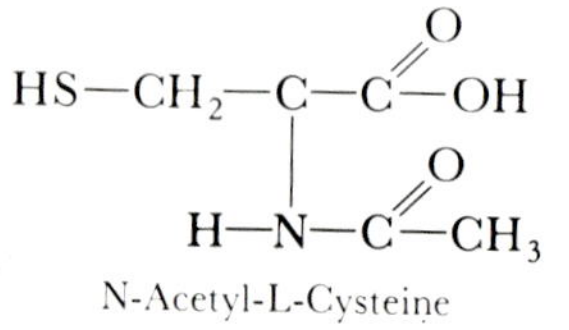

The human medical use of acetylcysteine occasionally leads to bronchospasm because of the unpleasant smell of the drug. Use of isoproterenol (0.25 ml of 1:200) or racemic epinephrine (2 mg) is recommended in combination with 3 cc of 10% or 20% acetylcysteine to prevent this undesirable effect. Antibiotics of the penicillin type and tetracycline are inactivated by acetylcysteine and should not be mixed together for aerosol administration (Lawson and Saggers 1965). When an antibiotic aerosol is required, the acetylcysteine aerosol is alternated with the antibiotic aerosol at 4-hour intervals. Antibiotics administered systemically are not inactivated by the inhalation of acetylcysteine. High concentrations of oxygen will rapidly inactivate acetylcysteine (Lawson and Saggers 1965). However, ethylenediaminetetraacetic acid (EDTA) is added to commercial preparations to prevent oxidation. Consequently, if oxygen therapy is required, there is no contraindication to the use of oxygen for nebulization. Use of acetylcysteine for long-term administration in a closed tent does not produce eye irritation in human beings.

```
                 O
                //
HS—CH2—C—C—OH
           |     O
           |    //
       H—N—C—CH3
```

N-Acetyl-L-Cysteine

Fig. 43.3.

Toxicity

The toxicity of acetylcysteine in a number of species has been studied. The oral LD50 in the dog and rat is 1 g/kg and 3 g/kg, respectively. Parenterally (intravenously or intraperitoneally), the LD50 for the dog is 700 mg/kg. This low level of toxicity of acetylcysteine indicates the very rapid rate of its conversion to the natural amino acid, L-cysteine. Hemograms and hepatic function tests have revealed no apparent abnormalities attributable to the drug (Sheffner and Lish 1970).

In the dog, rabbit, and rat, exposure to a chamber atmosphere produced by 30 seconds of nebulization of a 20% solution of acetylcysteine has been evaluated. These animals were exposed to this atmosphere for 15 minutes twice daily for 35 consecutive days. Also, additional groups of animals were exposed for 1 hour daily, 5 times a week for 12 weeks. No clinical or histopathological changes were found that could be associated with the exposure of the animals to acetylcysteine (Sheffner and Lish 1970).

CLINICAL USE

In small animals, aerosol therapy with acetylcysteine has given satisfactory results (Donovan 1967; O'Brien and Todd 1971). Animals are encouraged to exercise after aerosol treatment to promote or initiate coughing. Sharp percussion over both sides of the thorax may also induce coughing. Aerosol therapy for 2 or 3 days is necessary to obtain a favorable response. Therapy may be continued for 7 days, followed by reevaluation of the patient by radiographic and clinical examination. In the experience of O'Brien and Todd, the length of time for individual treatments is variable with a minimum of 30 minutes 2–3 times daily for chamber aerosol treatment.

Aerosol therapy may also be administered by the use of a face mask for 5 minutes 3 times daily and increased to 15 minutes 3 times daily with adaptation of the animal to the treatment (O'Brien and Todd 1971). These authors recommend the use of a DeVilbiss No. 40 or 841 nebulizer containing a minimum of 5 ml of acetylcysteine (10%–20%) and the administration of oxygen at a flow rate of 4–6 L/minute in the treatment of the dog.

Pancreatic Dornase (Dornavac)

This enzyme preparation has been discussed for topical use in Chapter 42. The drug product consists of purified deoxyribonuclease that is extracted from the beef pancreas. Pancreatic dornase is also an effective mucolytic agent. It depolymerizes DNA and is, therefore, useful in the liquefaction of purulent sputum (Lieberman 1970).

Pure solutions of DNA are viscid. Consequently, the presence of DNA in pulmonary secretions or sputum increases the viscosity. In addition, DNA reduces the spontaneous degradation of protein in purulent exudates or secretions by binding the protein and protecting it from leukocytic proteolytic enzyme activity, With the addition of pancreatic dornase to purulent secretions, there are both a breakdown of DNA and occurrence of proteolysis. There is good evidence showing that DNA also binds certain antibiotics, thus reducing their effectiveness. The destruction of DNA in viscid secretions suggests that antibiotics would have a greater effect in the presence of pancreatic dornase. It would appear that there is an advantage in using pancreatic dornase rather than acetylcysteine when pulmonary secretions or exudates are purulent (Lieberman 1970).

Antibiotics and bronchodilator agents can be added in appropriate concentrations to pancreatic dornase without inactivation. In human beings, the recommended nebulizing dose of pancreatic dornase is 200,000 units dissolved in 2 ml of either 10% propylene glycol or isotonic sodium chloride solution (Swinyard 1975). The evaluation of pancreatic dornase for clinical use in animals apparently has not been made. The only FDA-approved use of this preparation in animals is for topical use in the debridement of surface wounds.

OTHER AGENTS USED IN PULMONIC COMPLICATIONS

As indicated above, the drugs that have major importance and use as mucolytic agents are acetylcysteine and pancreatic dornase. The clinical effectiveness of other mucolytic compounds that are used in the treatment of pulmonic conditions has not been well established. Also, the value of detergent or wetting agents recommended for veterinary medical use as an adjunct in the treatment of bronchitis and other respiratory complications has not been clearly established.

Detergent or Wetting Agents

Detergent or wetting agents were advocated several years ago on the premise that their action would reduce surface tension and thus would enhance the loosening and removal of retained secretions in the pulmonary tract. *Alevaire* (superinone, 0.125%; glycerine, 5%; and sodium bicarbonate, 2%) and *Tergemist* (sodium-2-ethylhexyl sulfate, 0.125%; and potassium iodide, 0.1%) are commercial detergent and wetting agents available for this purpose (Sheffner and Lish 1970). Clinical evaluations have indicated both favorable and unfavorable responses following the use of these agents in the promotion of expectoration. Some clinicians have indicated that these drug preparations are no more effective than a water aerosol in the reduction of sputum viscosity.

Another product that has been employed as an aerosol treatment in small animals for respiratory complications is a streptokinase-streptodornase enzyme preparation (*Varidase*). It does not possess any particular advantage over the use of pancreatic dornase (see discussion above). The major clinical indications for streptokinase-streptodornase are in the treatment of traumatic and inflammatory conditions. It is recommended for the removal of blood clots and fibrinous or purulent exudates and in the treatment of chronic suppurating wounds that involve sinuses, bone infections, and other conditions requiring surgical debridement and drainage (Swinyard 1975).

Streptokinase-streptodornase must not be given by the intravenous route. It is injected into cavities and applied to surface wounds in the form of a jelly or solution. Drainage from cavities such as the sinuses should be established to accommodate drainage during the liquefying action of the enzyme preparation. In human beings, an initial dose of 200,000 units of streptokinase and 50,000 units of streptodornase in not less than 10 ml of isotonic saline chloride solution is recommended for the adjunct treatment of hemothorax or thoracic empyema (Swinyard 1975). Also, in human beings dosages of 10,000–15,000 units of streptokinase and 2500–3750 units of streptodornase in 2–3 ml of solution are indicated in the treatment of maxillary sinus empyema. Similar concentrations of the enzyme preparation are also recommended for debridement of surface wounds where wet dressings can be used.

REFERENCES

Boyd, E. M., and Lapp, M. S. 1946. On the expectorant action of parasympathomimetic drugs. J Pharmacol Exp Ther 87:24.

Brander, G. C., and Pugh, D. M. 1971. The respiratory system. Veterinary Applied Pharmacology and Therapeutics, 2nd ed., p. 64. Baltimore: Williams & Wilkins.

Bucher, K. 1958. Pathophysiology and pharmacology of cough. Pharmacol Rev 10:43.

Donovan, E. F. 1967. Nebulization therapy for canine cough. Mod Vet Pract 48:40.

Koenig, H., and Koenig, R. 1949. Production of acute pulmonary edema by ammonium salts. Proc Soc Exp Biol Med 70:375.

Jaffe, J. H., and Martin, W. R. 1975. Narcotic analgesics and antagonists. In L. S. Goodman and A. Gilman, eds. The Pharmacological Basis of Therapeutics, 5th ed., p. 245. New York: Macmillan.

Lawson, D., and Saggers, B. A. 1965. N.A.C. and antibiotics in cystic fibrosis. Br Med J 1:317.

Levine, W. G. 1975. Heavy metal antagonists. In L. S. Goodman and A. Gilman, eds. The Pharmacological Basis of Therapeutics, 5th ed., p. 929. New York: Macmillan.

Lieberman, J. 1970. The appropriate use of mucolytic agents. Am J Med 49:1.

Low, D. G. 1964. Cough. In R. W. Kirk, ed. Current Veterinary Therapy, 1st ed., p. 65. Philadelphia: W. B. Saunders.

Mulnix, J. A. 1971. Aerosol therapy. In R. W. Kirk, ed. Current Veterinary Therapy, 4th ed., p. 28. Philadelphia: W. B. Saunders.

O'Brien, J. A., and Todd, J. D. 1971. Bronchitis. In R. W. Kirk, ed. Current Veterinary Therapy, 4th ed., p. 138. Philadelphia: W. B. Saunders.

Salem, H., and Aviado, D. M., eds. 1970a. Physiology of the cough reflex. In Antitussive Agents, p. 235. Elmsford, N.Y.: Pergamon Press.

———. 1970b. Codeine. In Antitussive Agents, p. 301. Elmsford, N.Y.: Pergamon Press.

———. 1970c. Dextromethorphan. In Antitussive Agents, p. 383. Elmsford, N.Y.: Pergamon Press.

Sevelius, H.; McCoy, J. F.; and Colmore, J. P. 1971. Dose response to codeine in patients with chronic cough. Clin Pharmacol Ther 12:449.

Sheffner, A. L., and Lish, P. M. 1970. Acetylcysteine and other mucolytic agents. In H. Salem and D. M. Aviado, eds. Antitussive Agents, p. 785. Elmsford, N.Y.: Pergamon Press.

Swinyard, E. A. 1975. Surface-acting drugs. In L. S. Goodman and A. Gilman, eds. The Pharmacological Basis of Therapeutics, 5th ed., p. 955. New York: Macmillan.

SECTION 12

Gases of Therapeutic Value

CHAPTER 44

OXYGEN AND CARBON DIOXIDE

NICHOLAS H. BOOTH

"Oxygen is a double-edged sword; it not only promotes life, but it also destroys life" (Stewart 1972).

This chapter will discuss the therapeutic roles of oxygen and carbon dioxide as well as some of their toxic effects. No attempt will be made to cover the vast amount of biochemical and physiological information on these two gases. However, the reader may wish to refer to a physiology textbook (Tenney 1970), proceedings of a symposium (Ngai 1972), or other published information (Gillespie and Robinson 1971) for general review purposes.

OXYGEN

Oxygen, U.S.P., is indicated in a wide variety of clinical conditions whenever oxygen deprivation (hypoxia) is a potential threat to the life of an animal. Hypoxia, regardless of its origin, is a life-threatening condition that generally requires immediate medical attention. It may occur from respiratory depression or failure from the use of overdoses of anesthetics and narcotic analgesics. Obstruction of the airway by vomitus, exudates from pulmonary infections, edema of the glottis, edema from left ventricular failure, pulmonic parasites, tumors, and a tight lariat around the neck may all lead to a severe degree of hypoxia. Also, taking animals to high altitude in the mountains or by flight in an unpressurized airplane may result in the development of hypoxia. Animals that are severely anemic from exposure to certain infections or chemicals may also become severely hypoxic.

The ability of young animals to tolerate hypoxia for long periods compared to adult animals is well known. For example, the adult rabbit can tolerate an anoxic atmosphere of 100% nitrogen for only 1.5 minutes before death whereas the newborn rabbit can survive for as long as 27 minutes (Cohen 1972). A rabbit delivered by cesarean section several days before term can survive up to 44 minutes in a nitrogen atmosphere. In the adult dog, an acute occlusion of the cerebral circulation and the resultant hypoxia produce cessation of spontaneous respiration after only 20–30 seconds; in the 8- to 10-day-old puppy, this effect occurs in 5 minutes and in the newborn animal, in 27 minutes. Similar effects are observed in the cat and other species when they are subjected to hypoxic conditions.

Toxicity

In 1878, Paul Bert demonstrated the convulsive effects of oxygen in birds that were exposed to 15–20 atmospheres of air. He later showed that the same effects could be produced with one-fifth the pressure by using 100% oxygen. This led to the conclusion that the seizures were due to the tension of oxygen (P_{O_2}) and not to the total barometric pressure or the nitrogen content of air.

In the last decade, the level of clinical concern has increased with respect to the adverse complications that follow oxygen therapy in human beings (Morgan 1968). The increasing use of mechanical ventilatory devices for the prolonged administration of high concentrations of oxygen has contributed to this overall concern. Also, the knowledge that retrolental fibroplasia occurs in the premature infant as well as retinal damage in adults following the prolonged inhalation of high concentrations of oxygen has led to its more cautious use. In the dog, oxygen concentrations of less than 35% appear to have no adverse effect upon the retina of newborn animals. The first 21 days after birth is considered to be the most critical period for retinal damage in the dog from exposure to oxygen concentrations greater than 35%.

In animal studies, all warm-blooded species exposed to oxygen concentrations near 100% at atmospheric pressure eventually die (Morgan 1968). Upon postmortem examination, pneumonitis is observed. Unlike warm-blooded species, reptiles and amphibians can withstand pure oxygen for indefinite periods without the development of pneumonitis. They can also tolerate oxygen deprivation to a much greater degree than the mammalian species; for example, the turtle can tolerate anoxia produced by the inhalation of 100% nitrogen for several hours and a dose of cyanide 50 times greater than that toxic to the mammal.

Although the entire mechanism(s) of oxygen toxicity at the biochemical level is not entirely known, some of the gross manifestations typical of this entity can be identified. In the lungs the reaction to oxygen toxicity consists of an increase in pulmonary vascular resistance and alveolo-arterial diffusion gradient, decreased compliance, atelectasis, and alveolar transudation or edema. Inhalation of 100% oxygen at 1 atmosphere (i.e., 760 torr) produces toxic irritation that is detectable in 15–24 hours; the effects become pronounced in 1–3 days (Lambertsen 1966). At 2 atmospheres (i.e., 1,520 torr), severe pulmonary toxicity occurs within 10 hours.

Oxygen toxicity does not occur in human beings breathing 50% at 1 atmosphere of pressure or in those inhaling 100% at one-half an atmosphere for 24 hours or longer (Wollman and Smith 1975). The P_{O_2} for continuous clinical use has not been determined but it appears to be greater than 200 torr (i.e., less than one-third an atmosphere) in exposures of over 30 days. The principal etiologic factor in oxygen toxicity is the P_{O_2} rather than the concentration of the gas inspired. As previously mentioned, Paul Bert observed this phenomenon nearly a century ago.

Clinical Use

The principal objective underlying oxygen therapy is to prevent the complications associated with the development of hypoxemia. Oxygen is not a substitute for definitive treatment of the basic underlying cause and is given as temporary therapy to prevent tissue hypoxia. As with any therapeutic agent, the dose level of oxygen should be able to be determined since too much may be hazardous and too little may be insufficient.

Oxygen should be administered by mask or endotracheal tube whenever an animal is threatened by hypoxia or asphyxia. Oxygen chambers may also be employed (Gourley 1967), or an oxygen tent may be fabricated by running an oxygen line into a cage closed off with polyethylene (White 1971). Use of 100% oxygen is generally not necessary in most hypoxic conditions; inhalation of 30%–60% oxygen is considered adequate for most clinical usage (White 1971). According to White, the primary problem connected with oxygen therapy occurs when it is instituted in animals suffering from chronic respiratory disease or depression of the respiratory center by drugs. Inasmuch as *the respiratory cen-*

ter is stimulated by an oxygen lack or hypoxemia, the administration of high concentrations of oxygen will diminish the hypoxic stimulus that triggers an increased rate of respiration. This leads to a further hypoventilatory condition and the pileup of carbon dioxide (hypercarbia) along with a concomitant respiratory acidosis. Clinically, this is a well-established phenomenon in both animals and human beings. In the human usage of oxygen for treatment of chronic respiratory diseases, only inspired oxygen concentrations of 24%–38% are recommended. An oxygen therapy mask for cattle, which is an adaptation of the "Venti-mask" for human use, has been used to deliver an oxygen flow of 12 L/minute; this mask provides the same oxygen concentration (28%) that is often recommended for use in human beings (Weaver 1973).

ROLE IN ANESTHETIC AND RESUSCITATIVE PROCEDURES

The first step in preventing hypoxia is to establish an airway, preferably by the use of an endotracheal tube (Sattler 1971). When an emergency condition occurs such as cardiac arrest (Booth et al. 1958) or ventilatory failure during anesthesia, oxygen can be administered immediately. Oxygen is more effective and reliable in correcting hypoxia due to respiratory depression from anesthetic overdosage than is the use of analeptic agents. Emphasis on oxygen therapy in substitution for the analeptic drugs has increased with the introduction of the shorter-acting barbiturates and the increased use of inhalant anesthetics. By maintaining an animal in a state of good oxygenation, sufficient time is provided for the tissues to metabolize or eliminate the excess quantity of anesthetic.

When overdosage occurs inadvertently with the use of *inhalant anesthetics,* the anesthetic can be rapidly removed or "washed out" of the respiratory and circulatory systems by use of a breathing bag. Upon reduction of the concentration of the anesthetic, normal respiratory and circulatory functions are immediately reestablished (Booth et al. 1960). Approximately 10 minutes are necessary for gases to equilibrate between the patient and the breathing bag of a closed system when 100% oxygen and anesthetic gases are used (Sattler 1971). According to Sattler, a 2-L anesthesia or breathing bag soon may contain 1500 ml of nitrogen with little volume left for oxygen. The bag should be "dumped" several times in the first 10 minutes of anesthesia to empty the accumulated nitrogen or until the animal is essentially denitrogenized; use of larger bags often minimizes the influence of nitrogen pileup in concentrations that could be troublesome during anesthesia.

If manual or mechanical assist devices are not available for assisting respiration, oxygen can be administered simply by connecting a hose to an oxygen cylinder and flowmeter. The oxygen hose is in turn connected to a polyethylene or polyvinyl tube approximately 150 cm in length. The polyethylene or polyvinyl tubing is inserted inside an endotracheal catheter of the intubated animal to a point just above the tracheal bifurcation. Oxygen is empirically administered at a rate of 1 L/minute/10 lb of body weight. Experimentally, dogs made apneic with pentobarbital sodium have been oxygenated by this method for as long as 2 hours (Booth et al. 1958). This procedure is also useful in oxygenating dogs recovering from strychnine poisoning.

Chickens overanesthetized with pentobarbital sodium also can be readily resuscitated by inserting a polyethylene or polyvinyl tube directly into the trachea. An oxygen flow rate of 0.25–0.5 L/minute is sufficient to maintain oxygenation. The polyethylene or polyvinyl tube makes an inexpensive and rapid method of administering oxygen to many species when respiratory depression develops during the initiation of general anesthesia. This is especially true if an airway cannot be readily established with an endotracheal tube. In such an emergency the polyethylene or polyvinyl tube is inserted into a nostril of the animal (dog, cat, pig, goat) as far as the pharynx to administer oxygen. In animals suffering from apnea, ventilation is additionally enhanced by rhythmic and manual compression of the thorax.

Artificial resuscitation of larger animals, such as the cow or horse, poses greater physical difficulties. In the field, resuscitation can be employed in the horse by using an air bellows (Rankin et al. 1952). This method has been useful in correcting hypoxia induced by skeletal muscle relaxants (Booth and Rankin 1953). In the last decade, excellent advances have been made in the development of commercial equipment that is easily applied for the administration of oxygen and/or inhalant anesthetics in the large animal.

Oxygen should be administered with a minimum of delay when a hypoxic condition exists. Existence of an oxygen deficiency for only brief intervals of time produces irreversible histopathological changes in the brain. These changes have been identified experimentally in animals and have led to a general recognition of the danger of producing visual impairment and mental deficiencies in all types of patients by oxygen deprivation during surgical anesthesia. An oxygen lack is particularly detrimental to pregnant dogs and their fetuses. Experimental oxygen deprivation in dogs for brief periods during the last week of pregnancy induces parturition within a few hours. About 87% of the puppies born to these animals die within a few weeks of birth, and surviving puppies have convulsive seizures until 6 weeks of age (Fender et al. 1946).

Oxygen in a concentration of 100% can be bubbled into or mixed with the liquid anesthetics to hasten their volatilization without deleterious effect to the animal. Even when oxygen is used alone in this concentration and at 1 atmosphere of pressure for resuscitative purposes, it can be used safely up to 12 hours in animals over 1 month of age. If pure oxygen is administered beyond this period, oxygen toxicity or "oxygen burn" may result. This can lead to irritation and thickening of the alveolar membranes which reduce the proper diffusion of oxygen and carbon dioxide. Whenever oxygen is used in excess of 12 hours, the concentration should not exceed 70%. Ordinarily, concentrations achieved in practice seldom exceed 50%–60% unless a closed system is used. Other aspects of oxygen toxicity have been discussed above.

Although oxygen is not inflammable or explosive, it must be used prudently because it supports both of these conditions. For safety reasons, all gas cylinders should be properly secured on a carrier or else chained to a wall. If a cylinder should be upset, there is danger of the shutoff valve breaking off when it strikes the floor. This is especially true if the protective cap for the valve is not in place. Breaking the valve will cause the tank to jet dangerously about like a rocket as escape of the gas occurs. Lubricants or oil preparations are contraindicated on tank valves or other oxygen equipment.

HYPERBARIC OXYGEN THERAPY

Considerable interest in the use of oxygen at pressures greater than 1 atmosphere (i.e., greater than 760 torr) has evolved in the last decade. As early as 1878, Paul Bert conducted experimental studies in animals by compressing air to several atmospheres. Hyperbaric oxygenation has been recommended in the treatment of carbon monoxide poisoning because clearance of the toxic gas from hemoglobin is nearly twice as fast as the use of 95% oxygen and 5% carbon dioxide at 1 atmosphere of pressure. It has also been recommended in the treatment of barbiturate poisoning and for treatment of anaerobe infections such as tetanus, gas gangrene, or other clostridial diseases in human beings. Use of hyperbaric oxygen has been reported in the treatment of a *Clostridium tetani* infection in the dog (Lippincott and Harter 1963).

The application of hyperbaric oxygenation remains primarily in the experimental realm of clinical medicine (Hopkinson 1967). One serious drawback in its use is the problem related to oxygen toxicity. Toxicity has been reported in human beings after 6–96 minutes of exposure at 3.7 atmospheres of pressure. Treatment of patients for carbon monoxide poisoning with oxygen at 3 atmospheres of pressure has resulted in convulsive seizures. Most evidence to date appears to indicate that oxygen pressures greater than 2 atmospheres should not be used and then only for short periods of time. The use of inert gases such as helium to reduce hyperbaric oxygen toxicity as well as associated fire hazards has been studied.

CARBON DIOXIDE

Carbon Dioxide, U.S.P., produces the most powerful respiratory stimulation, yet it is structurally one of the simplest of drugs (Lambertsen 1966). Only its role in anesthesia and resuscitative procedures will be discussed in this chapter. Its use as an inhalant anesthetic, in euthanasia, and as a treatment for carbon monoxide poisoning have been discussed elsewhere in the text.

Role in Anesthetic and Resuscitative Procedures

Carbon dioxide (5%) mixed with oxygen was once considered to be of importance in stimulating a depressed respiratory center in anesthesia overdosages and following asphyxic conditions. The current philosophy in anesthesiology dictates that carbon dioxide should not be used in stimulating a depressed respiratory center. If the respiratory center is depressed or paralyzed by an overdose of anesthetic, the tension of metabolic carbon dioxide rises by virtue of the respiratory embarrassment. Consequently, the respiratory center is already subjected to an elevated tension of carbon dioxide. Under these circumstances an acidotic situation prevails. Administration of a carbon dioxide–oxygen mixture would only aggravate the severity of the acidosis already present. Complete heart block and arrest occur if the carbon dioxide acidosis is allowed to remain uncorrected.

It has been shown in the dog and rat that an increased carbon dioxide accumulation is contributory to inducing hepatic damage following chloroform administration. Hepatic injury is insignificant during chloroform anesthesia if hypercapnia and hypotension can be avoided (Morris 1960).

Although a carbon dioxide excess is known to be deleterious, the converse of this condition, a carbon dioxide deficiency, is also detrimental to the welfare of the animal. A deficiency is ordinarily produced by exuberant and vigorous artificial resuscitation using air or oxygen. Not infrequently the inexperienced individual will zealously resuscitate an animal to correct a hypoventilatory state and will unknowingly "wash out" the carbon dioxide to such a level that a hyperventilatory state exists. The hyperventilatory condition can be avoided by controlling the rate of ventilation or by momentarily stopping the artificial respiration altogether. The frequency of performing artificial respiration should be no greater than that required to correct cyanosis due to the hypoxia. Therefore, it is exceedingly important for the person conducting artificial resuscitation to be cognizant of the physiological role of carbon dioxide in maintaining the integrity of respiration, blood pH, and blood pressure. This means that the clinician must realize that both hypoxia and hypercapnia occur simultaneously whenever respiratory depression occurs during deep anesthesia. Furthermore, it is important to remember that both of these conditions must be corrected at the same time.

Physiologically, a deficiency of carbon dioxide results in alkalosis or an increased pH of the blood plasma. As mentioned above, this condition results from overventilation or hyperventilation during artificial resuscitation. Tone of the capillaries and veins is diminished, venous pressure drops, venous return to the heart is reduced, and cardiac output is drastically curtailed. If the hyperventilatory state continues, the heart ultimately goes into rigor and then into a complete standstill.

In human anesthesiology, vigorous ventilation of the patient with a mixture of oxygen and carbon dioxide to hasten anesthetic recovery at the termination of surgery is no longer encouraged because of the risk of provoking cardiac arrhythmias and ventricular fibrillation. In the dog, a sudden change from a high tension of carbon dioxide to room air is known to produce cardiac irregularities and ventricular fibrillation (Brown and Miller 1952).

In using closed-system anesthesia apparatus, it is necessary to provide a carbon dioxide absorber such as soda lime. During exhaustion of the soda lime, when it becomes converted from sodium and calcium hydroxides to sodium and calcium carbonates, carbon dioxide is no longer absorbed This results in accumulation of the asphyxic gas which eventually leads to a dangerous acidosis. The animal manifests a labored, gasping type of respiration concomitant with the rising carbon dioxide blood level. Since a labored or erratic type of respiration also occurs in Stage II (delirium or excitatory stage), it is easy to confuse the hypercapnic condition with this anesthetic stage. Consequently, the inexperienced person will increase the dose level of anesthesia to eliminate the Stage II respiration. Acidosis becomes increasingly severe with time and, if the asphyxic condition is not alleviated by replacing the exhausted soda lime, death occurs due to complete heart block and cardiac arrest. The color of the animal's mucous membrane remains normal even with the administration of oxygen under these circumstances. Only during the development of an oxygen lack, or hypoxia, does cyanosis manifest itself.

For optimal carbon dioxide absorption it is recommended that soda lime cannisters have an air space equal to or greater than the patient's tidal volume. The largest and probably the only air space concerned with air flow in absorbers is the void space (Brown 1958). The void space (air space) between the soda lime granules is dependent on the size of the granules and the tightness of the packing absorbed. The void space of soda lime with large particles is greater than the void space with a small particle size. Since the void space of soda lime is 45%–47% of the total absorber volume, a 1-L cannister filled with these preparations will accommodate a tidal air volume ranging from 450 to 470 ml. According to Jones (1961), a cannister holding 10 lb of soda lime is essential to accommodate the tidal volume (2–5 L) of a race horse. Moreover, the cannister should be cylindrical, with the length 1.5 times the diameter (Evans and Gray, cited by Jones 1961).

Soda lime will effectively absorb carbon dioxide for about 6 hours (Short 1974). It changes in color from white to blue or pink to bluish pink when the pH shifts from the alkaline to the acid side. If a partial change in the color of the soda lime occurs prior to the termination of anesthesia, the color will often return to normal when the anesthetic equipment is not in use. According to Short (1974), this does not indicate a rejuvenation of the soda lime but only a diminished carbon dioxide content. Soda lime should be changed frequently so that hypercarbia during anesthesia can be prevented. This is important because canalization of carbon dioxide–absorbing materials may also occur; if this happens, the carbon dioxide level in the inspired anesthetic mixture may be above normal before a color change of the absorber takes place (Sattler 1971).

REFERENCES

Booth, N. H., and Rankin, A. D. 1953. Studies on the pharmacodynamics of curare in the horse. I. Dosage and physiological activity of *d*-tubocurarine chloride. Am J Vet Res 14:51.

Booth, N. H.; Will, D. H.; Moss, L. C.; and Swenson, M. J. 1958. An electrical apparatus and its application in defibrillating the heart of the dog. J Am Vet Med Assoc 132:117.

Booth, N. H.; Rankin, A. D.; and Will, D. H. 1960. Simplified apparatus and method for administering oxygen and ether to the dog. J Am Vet Med Assoc 137:114.

Brown, E. B., Jr., and Miller, F. 1952. Ventricular fibrillation following a rapid fall in alveolar carbon dioxide concentration. Am J Physiol 169:56.

Brown, E. S. 1958. Voids, pores and total air space of carbon dioxide absorbents. Anesthesiology 19:1.

Cohen, P. J. 1972. The metabolic function of oxygen and biochemical lesions of hypoxia. Anesthesiology 37:148.

Fender, R. A.; Neff, W. B.; and Binger, G. 1946. Convulsions produced by fetal anoxia: Experimental study. Anesthesiology 7:10.

Gillespie, J. R., and Robinson, N. E. 1971. Clinical respiratory physiology. In R. W. Kirk, ed. Current Veterinary Therapy, 4th ed., p. 165. Philadelphia: W. B. Saunders.

Gourley, I. M. G. 1967. An environmental control unit for long term oxygen therapy in small animals. J Am Anim Hosp Assoc 3:181.

Hopkinson, W. I. 1967. Hyperbaric oxygen therapy. Vet Rec 80:40.

Jones, E. W. 1961. Equine anesthesia-maintenance by inhalation techniques. J Am Vet Med Assoc 139:785.

Lambertsen, C. J. 1966. Drugs and respiration. Ann Rev Pharmacol 6:327.

Lippincott, C. L., and Harter, W. L. 1963. Oxygen saturation under pressure as a treatment for tetanus in a dog. J Am Vet Med Assoc 142:872.

Morgan, A. P. 1968. The pulmonary toxicity of oxygen. Anesthesiology 29:570.

Morris, L. E. 1960. Comparison studies of hepatic function following anesthesia with the halogenated agents. Anesthesiology 21:109.

Ngai, S. H. 1972. Symposium on oxygen. Anesthesiology 37:99.

Rankin, A. D.; Booth, N. H.; and Sullivan, J. P. 1952. Artificial respiration in large animals. J Am Vet Med Assoc 120:196.

Sattler, F. P. 1971. Ventilation of the surgical patient. In R. W. Kirk, ed. Current Veterinary Therapy, 4th ed., p. 178. Philadelphia: W. B. Saunders.

Short, C. E. 1974. Technic and equipment for equine inhalation anesthesia. Mod Vet Pract 55:393.

Stewart, D. L. 1972. Oxygen and life. Anesthesiology 37:100.

Tenney, S. M. 1970. Respiration in mammals. In M. J. Swenson, ed. Dukes' Physiology of Domestic Animals, 8th ed., p. 293. Ithaca, N.Y.: Comstock.

Weaver, B. M. Q. 1973. An oxygen therapy mask for cattle. Vet Rec 92:133.

White, R. J. 1971. Acute respiratory failure. In R. W. Kirk, ed. Current Veterinary Therapy, 4th ed., p. 173. Philadelphia: W. B. Saunders.

Wollman, H., and Smith, T. C. 1975. The therapeutic gases: Oxygen, carbon dioxide and helium. In L. S. Goodman and A. Gilman, eds. The Pharmacological Basis of Therapeutics, 5th ed., p. 881. New York: Macmillan.

SECTION 13

Chemotherapy of Microbial, Fungal, and Viral Diseases

CHAPTER 45

ANTISEPTICS AND DISINFECTANTS

WILLIAM G. HUBER

Drugs used for topical application to animate and inanimate surfaces have numerous indispensable uses for the production of food-producing and companion animals. Although physicians express concern regarding indiscriminate use of germicidal drugs by laypersons, this problem does not seem to be obvious in the case of food-producing animals. The drugs serve generally as valuable aids, including disinfection of animal quarters, hospitals, and clinics. They serve also as sanitizing agents in food-processing establishments.

The emergence of drug-resistant microorganisms demands a thorough understanding of the principles and methods of antisepsis and disinfection. The advent of antibiotics, sulfonamides, and other antiinfective drugs has not obviated the need for utilizing good methods of sterilization, antisepsis, and disinfection. Antiseptics, disinfectants, and biocides deserve considerable attention. Careless use of certain systemic antiinfective drugs for topical or dermal application may preclude subsequent use for systemic therapy or inadvertently induce hypersensitization. In addition to therapeutic considerations, the local antiinfective drugs have other numerous applications. In the field of public health they are used to purify water, preserve foods, sterilize instruments and utensils, and reduce the spread of disease-producing organisms. The drugs are also included in many effective animal husbandry procedures to disinfect farrowing houses, maternity stalls, water and feed containers, etc.

As therapeutic agents, local antiinfective drugs may be used externally or internally. Internal application is restricted to mucous membranes and generally includes those drugs not absorbed. Antiseptics and disinfectants are applied to restricted areas to reduce the possibility of toxic reactions or tissue injury when applied to animal tissue.

A lack of agreement and desired uniformity exist in the terms used to discuss local antiinfective agents. It is often a question of the drugs' ability to kill the bacterium or merely attenuate its rate of growth and population. A *disinfectant* or *germi-*

cide is a substance used to destroy bacteria or other infective microorganisms. Disinfectants have *bactericidal* or germicidal activity and are usually applied to inanimate surfaces. An *antiseptic* substance does not kill microorganisms but inhibits reproduction or rate of growth. In the case of bacteria, this is described as *bacteriostatic* activity. Antiseptics are of value in treating local infections caused by microorganisms refractory to systemic chemotherapy.

The difference between an antiseptic and a disinfectant is usually a matter of reaction time, numbers of organisms, drug concentration, and temperature. Many disinfectants are chemicals destructive to bacterial protoplasm and, unless used discriminately, to host cell protoplasm as well.

Antiseptic substances generally are applied to tissues to suppress or prevent bacterial infection. The concentration of the antiseptic is usually low to avoid undesirable damage and tissue irritation. Increasing the concentration and potency of an antiseptic agent may irritate and perhaps kill normal host tissue as well as bacterial cells, thus interfering with normal growth of granulation tissue in the healing of wounds. Higher concentrations of some substances may be classified as irritants or caustics because of their destruction of tissue protoplasm. Conversely, some of the relatively mild substances possess no more than antiseptic or bacteriostatic activity. It is possible that a local antiinfective drug may have bactericidal, fungicidal, and viricidal activities.

A sanitizer is a compound that reduces the number of bacterial contaminants to populations judged safe by public health interpretations. Sterilization, however, refers to the complete destruction of all forms of life, primarily microorganisms, by chemical and/or physical processes. Germicides or biocides may be further defined by such terms as bactericide, fungicide, viricide, amebicide, or coccidiocide.

The term "local antiinfective drugs" includes antibiotics, sulfonamides, chemotherapeutic agents, disinfectants, antiseptics, and any other substances used having a static or cidal effect on animate or inanimate surfaces containing various types of microbial organisms.

HISTORY

Use of antiseptics and disinfectants was developed from the ancient Egyptian process of embalming. Embalming was developed to preserve the body for resurrection in the next world. The Egyptians and other ancient peoples used various concoctions such as volatile oils, oleoresins, wines, vinegars, honey, myrrh, and balsam. Wines and vinegars continued to be used through the Middle Ages for dressing wounds and preventing infection.

Chlorine, after its discovery in the Middle Ages, was widely used in a saturated aqueous solution as a deodorant and antiseptic substance. Chlorine was used in a Viennese hospital by Ignaz Semmelweis, a Hungarian obstetrician, in a practical demonstration of the beneficial action of antisepsis (1847–1849). Semmelweis was in charge of the charity ward which provided teaching material for medical students. The death rate from puerperal fever in this ward was many times greater than in other maternity wards of the hospital not used for teaching purposes. Semmelweis questioned this generally accepted fact and directed the medical students to wash their hands with soap and then with chlorine water after coming from the autopsy room and before assisting in the obstetrical delivery. The institution of this simple procedure reduced the death rate from puerperal fever in the obstetrical ward to that prevailing in the rest of the hospital. Semmelweis imediately called attention of the hospital administrators to his finding, but unfortunately they did not share his enthusiasm and belief in the results. He was soon dismissed from the hospital for criticizing the *status quo*. Semmelweis presented a brief report of his experiment in a medical journal.

A few years later, Louis Pasteur explained the origin of bacterial fermentation and the existence of infective agents as causes of disease. It remained for Joseph Lister to recognize the significance of the observations of Semmelweis, Pasteur, and others and to apply the principles to surgical techniques. In 1865, Lister announced the methods of sterilization of bandages, surgical dressings, and surgical instruments and of the antisepsis of wounds. By improvement of technique and methods, Lister introduced aseptic surgery. To achieve asepsis, he used carbolic acid and observed the general principle of cleanliness. Although early concentrations of carbolic acid were in excess and produced considerable tissue destruction, effective means were devised to reduce undesirable tissue reaction. In 1867, a published article by Lister appeared in Lancet describing a new method of treating compound fractures, abscesses, etc. Many agents have since been introduced for their antiseptic and disinfectant activity. Some of these will be discussed.

More highly selective, less toxic agents have replaced the older germicides and antiseptics for topical therapeutic application. A few of the newer agents have created problems dealing with acute allergic reactions and the development of resistant organisms. Due to a high degree of antigenicity, some of the antibiotics produce allergic manifestations. Thus sensitivity induced during a minor local or topical infection may obviate the use of antibiotics for systemic therapy at a later date. Bacterial resistance may develop in a similar manner. Thus it is important that infections that can be treated topically should be treated with antibiotics or chemotherapeutic agents not commonly used to treat major systemic infections.

PROPERTIES, ACTION, AND USE OF LOCAL ANTIINFECTIVE AGENTS

Many drugs are classified as antiseptics or disinfectants, each having characteristic advantages and disadvantages. A universally accepted antiseptic or disinfectant free of undesirable effects does not exist. Drugs may be classified on the basis of physical or chemical action resulting in the alteration of the protein portion of pathogenic organisms.

Properties of an Ideal Antiseptic

The properties of an antiseptic are more specific than those of a disinfectant. Characteristics of an ideal antiseptic include a wide spectrum of antibacterial activity, lack of irritation, low toxicity, high penetrability, activity in the presence of pus and necrotic tissue, noninterference with normal healing processes, cheapness, noncorrosiveness for certain types of surgical instruments, and color to define the areas to which it is applied.

Disinfectants, in addition to having some of the main characteristics of antiseptics, should also have the ability to penetrate crevices, cavities, and films of organic matter and to maintain lethal concentrations of the agent so that a *cidal* effect can be obtained in the presence of organic matter such as blood, soil, and fecal material. It is also desirable that the substance be compatible with soaps and other chemicals that are likely to be encountered when a disinfectant is used. A high degree of chemical stability is desired. Cost is also an important consideration if large amounts are needed.

Action

EFFECTIVENESS

The effectiveness of an antiseptic or disinfectant depends upon several factors, i.e., concentration, time, temperature of the antiseptic or disinfectant; susceptibility of the microbe; number of microbes present; and the nature of the medium in which the organisms are growing. Antibacterial activity of most antiseptics and disinfectants is directly proportional to the temperature within practical limits of the applied solutions. Frequently the bacterial medium may contain protein or other debris which may inhibit the antimicrobial action of the antiseptic or disinfectant drug.

MODE OF ACTION

The ways in which antiseptic and disinfectant substances act on pathogenic organisms vary considerably; however, the relationship between the lipophilicity of the microbe and the ability of the antiseptic or disinfectant to penetrate protoplasmic membranes is well established. Some dyes are adsorbed to the surface of the bacterial cell and form a thick layer of lethal substance that interferes with the normal physiological processes of the microbe. Some antiseptics and disinfectants, such as carbolic acid, enter the bacterial cell by simple diffusion. After an antimicrobial agent has entered the microbe, it may accumulate and then disrupt or interfere with vital metabolic enzyme systems. This occurs if the antimicrobial agent inactivates the enzyme or substrate by chemical combination. Antimetabolite inhibition of an enzyme usually results in a change of the oxidation-reduction potential that is unfavorable for normal enzyme activity. Surfactants (surface-acting agents) produce changes in the plasma membrane surrounding the pathogenic organism which alters the normal permeability characteristics; thus water diffuses inwardly until the cell is disrupted. Other local antiinfective drugs appear to agglutinate and precipitate bacterial cells by neutralization of cellular electrostatic charges.

TESTING ANTIBACTERIAL ACTIVITY

Testing the antibacterial activity of antiseptics and disinfectants has always been a problem. Only a portion of the antimicrobial agents has been properly standardized. Many of the available preparations have not been tested under the conditions of actual use. *In vitro* tests have been used most effectively to test disinfectants primarily for use on inanimate surfaces. The phenol coefficient, which is a ratio of the germicidal power of a drug or preparation being tested to that of phenol under identical *in vitro* conditions, has been the accepted test by the Food and Drug Administration (FDA). For example, if a new disinfectant, "A," has been found to have a phenol coefficient of 10, it has an activity 10 times greater than that of phenol under a similar set of circumstances. Although *in vitro* tests similar to the phenol coefficient are relatively simple and highly reproducible, they have limitations. For example, they do not detect a potential decrease in activity that may be associated with the presence of organic matter and other debris on the surface treated with the disinfectant. Recently, greater emphasis has been placed on clinical tests of the antiseptics, germicides, and disinfectants. One such method of evaluation is the serial basin hand-washing method. This method has specific application in the evaluation of antiseptics employed by surgeons in preoperative preparation.

Two types of information are desired when evaluating antiseptics: the ability of the drug to have an inhibitory or cidal effect on microorganisms and the safety of the drug to the tissue. A commonly employed test, representative of those designed to measure antimicrobial efficiency, is the estimation of the "degermation" of skin (Price 1957). Antiseptics are also tested against bacteria on abraded or incised skin of animals in attempting to determine "infection-prevention" activity.

TESTING VIRICIDAL ACTIVITY

Testing of viricidal drugs requires techniques different from those employed for determining bactericides. Standard techniques are not available for evaluating viricides. Inactivation of bacteriophages and reduction in infectivity of specific virus inocula for experimental animals are among the procedures used. Marked differences in susceptibility of viruses to different viricidal agents have been reported (Klein and De Forest 1963). It was noted that the difference depended primarily on whether the virus was lipophilic or hydrophilic and on the chemical nature of the disinfectant.

A test method using embryonating chicken eggs for evaluation of several types of disinfectants as viricides against vesicular stomatitis virus has been developed (Wright 1970). The test involved a virus recovery system which utilized a living host also susceptible to toxic effects of germicides. Thus it was found necessary to dilute the test germicide to decrease the direct toxic effect to the living host. An effective viricide was one that destroyed the viruses after 10 minutes of contact at 20° C.

The following compounds were effective viricides in this study: cresylic acid, 1%; phenol, 2.5%; chlorinated phenol, 0.2%; hydrochloric acid (pH 1.9), 0.4%; sodium orthophenylphenate, 2%; and sodium hypochlorite (commercial bleach), 0.645%. The following commonly used antiseptics and disinfectants were not found to have viricidal activity: quarternary ammonium compounds (alkyl dimethylbenzylammonium chlorides), 5%; ethyl alcohol, 70%–80%; and sodium hydroxide (pH 12.2), 10%.

Use of Antiseptics and Disinfectants

The presurgical use of antiseptics relates to their application to an operative area or their utility during the procedure to prepare the hands for aseptic surgery. It is not possible to sterilize the skin without destroying it although it is possible to reduce the number of bacteria present. Antisepsis of the hands is based on the concept of reducing the presence of bacteria.

Skin is irregularly pitted, ridged, and creased so that the epidermal surface is normally water-tight and forms an effective barrier against bacterial invasion. Bacteria can be found in large numbers on the skin surface attached to flakes of keratin, hair pits, sebaceous ducts, and foreign material adhering to the skin. Experiments have shown that transient organisms placed on the hands are nearly all removed (approximately 98%) by simple washing for 1 minute with soap under tap water. To remove the maximum number of organisms with certainty requires 7–8 minutes of scrubbing with brush, soap, and water. To prepare the hands for surgical operations, it is important that they be scrubbed thoroughly so as to remove all dirt, grease, and natural fats. If this is not done the antiseptic cannot make maximal contact with cutaneous bacteria. It has been demonstrated that approximately 7 minutes of conscientious washing with brush, soap, and water are required to remove all fats from the hands and arms.

Hand antiseptics should be both bacteriologically effective and harmless to the skin. Since the surgeon may use hand antiseptics several times a day, they should not be injurious to the skin of the hands and arms. Even with prolonged use, the antiseptics should not injure, irritate, or roughen the skin; penetrate the epidermis so as to be absorbed systemically; or produce a hypersensitivity.

Among several reasons why it is necessary to thoroughly scrub the hands even though the surgeon uses sterile gloves and gown, are: (1) it is almost impossible to gown and glove without serious breaks in aseptic technique and (2) hands that have not been thoroughly scrubbed soon develop abnormally large bacterial populations while the gloves are worn. Thus there is great opportunity for spillage of dangerous bacteria through any puncture or tear in the glove. Tears, puncture holes, and leaky patches in gloves occur quite frequently; it has been noted that 20% or more of the surgical gloves leak. Some hospital studies have reported even greater leakage in used gloves. Price (1966) stated: "The only effective way found thus far to prevent this troublesome increase and to maintain low counts is to wash the already degermed hands with pHisoHex immediately before putting on the gloves. Hexachlorophene soaps, quaternary ammonia compounds, and iodophores cannot be depended upon to accomplish that purpose."

A recommended routine procedure for preparing the hands is as follows: (1) trim and clean the fingernails; (2) scrub the hands and arms under warm water with nonmedicated soap or hexachlorophene soap and brush thoroughly for 7 minutes; (3) dry hands with a sterile towel; (4) rinse hands in 95% alcohol to remove remaining water; (5) wash the hands for a full 3 minutes in 70% alcohol, rubbing the skin thoroughly with gauze or washcloth; (6) lather the hands and arms with pHisoHex without a brush and rinse off with warm water; (7) dry the hands with a second sterile towel; and (8) put on gown and gloves.

It may not always be possible under some conditions of veterinary practice to have the necessary time and ideal antiseptics available. However, it should be remembered that cleanliness is of great importance in the use of this group of drugs since they have an indiscriminate affinity for extraneous protein which may decrease their germicidal effectiveness. In addition, dirt may form a physical barrier and prevent germicidal action. Under some farm conditions, if the water is extremely hard, the use of surfactants requires additional consideration. A thorough rinse with water is necessary to avoid the phenomenon of mutual antagonism that may result because of the physical or chemical incompatibilities of certain antiseptics and surfactants. Anionic surfactant soaps react chemically with cationic surfactants and negate the antiseptic activity of both drugs.

The problem of disinfecting the patient's skin for surgical procedures differs in several important aspects from hand disinfection. There is no opportunity for repeated periods of daily scrubbing the operative site as there is for the surgeon who scrubs and disinfects the hands many times each day. The skin microflora is protected by extraneous oils and natural fats. If they are not adequately removed prior to the application of the antiseptic, maximal protection cannot be achieved. The patient's skin will usually tolerate a single application of stronger and harsher antiseptic solutions than can the surgeon's hands, which must be scrubbed and disinfected repeatedly each day. It should be recognized that instantaneous disinfection by means of an antiseptic cannot be achieved. The longer an antiseptic acts, the more effective it will be. It has been noted that the use of gauze friction to apply the antiseptic is a more effective way of establishing contact between the bacteria and the bactericidal agent. Spray applications of aseptic solutions are not recommended since maximal contact is achieved by friction. After appropriate clipping and washing, the following standard method of preparing the field of operation is recommended: (1) wash with alcohol, (2) wash with benzalkonium, (3) wash with alcohol, (4) wash with benzalkonium, and (5) wash with alcohol. Price (1966) recommends this procedure, utilizing a 1:1000 tincture of benzalkonium containing a stain. Alcohol, either 70% ethyl alcohol (w/w) or 70% isopropyl alcohol (w/w), can be used. The alcohol not only removes soap which might interfere with the action of benzalkonium but also has its own antiseptic activity. Benzalkonium, under these conditions, has an antiseptic value equivalent to that of alcohol; the stain insures visual examination to show areas that have not received the antiseptic. Each step of the procedure should last for 3–5 minutes before going to the next one. This procedure does not interfere with subsequent healing of the incision.

Use of local antiinfective drugs, antiseptics, and disinfectants for treating local infections has become limited with the advent of systemic chemotherapeutic drugs. Some local infections respond more dramatically to chemotherapeutic drugs administered systemically than to topically applied antiseptics. The poor response to topically applied antiseptics or germicides may be related to poor penetrability for reaching the foci of infection and the reduction in potency of the antiseptic solution with body fluids and other debris in the infected area. Some limitations may be overcome by the appropriate choice of the antibacterial agent and surgical manipulations. However, it should be noted that the structure of the skin and the proliferation of scar tissue during repair processes facilitate the establishment of foci of bacteria and diminish the likelihood that the antiseptic material will have the opportunity to come into complete contact with all microorganisms. Antiseptics retain their usefulness for treating infections caused by organisms unaffected by systemic chemotherapeutic drugs through the development of drug resistance. Local antiinfective drugs are also occasionally employed in conjunction with systemic chemotherapeutic agents. Antiseptics and disinfectants are also useful to keep certain lesions from spreading.

Disinfectant preparations have been used on farms to control or prevent livestock diseases. Disinfection of farm lots, pens, and buildings with a hot 2% saponated cresol solution has been freely employed to control virulent infections following the death of an animal from an infectious disease. Disinfection procedures are required for prophylactic control of certain diseases and external parasitisms of animals imported into the United States. In addition, disinfectants are employed as therapeutic measures for certain skin diseases of animals.

Heat sterilization is more effective than chemical sterilization and should be used whenever possible. Moist heat is more effective than dry heat because of its greater penetration and faster action. Burning or incineration is always desirable for complete destruction of infected wound dressings or bedding. Because use of heat sterilization is limited by circumstances, there is considerable need for good disinfectants. Disinfection of the premises is most readily accomplished by the application of hot disinfectants.

TEAT DIPS AND DAIRY SANITIZERS

In the last decade, postmilking teat dips have been utilized both experimentally and clinically to assess their value to control bovine mastitis. The practice of dipping the teats in an antiseptic or germicidal solution following milking helps remove any residual amount of milk which may attract flies and provide nutrients for the proliferation of bacteria. Some germicide solutions help seal the teat orifice with an antiseptic material and inhibit bacterial introduction to the mammary gland. If abrasions or other lesions are encountered during milking, the application of antiseptic guards against the possibility of infection.

Several studies have been conducted using halogen disinfectants, surfactants, chlorhexidine, etc. Recent reports indicate the importance of the postmilking teat dip procedures in mastitis control. An approximate 50% reduction in new infections has been reported for some tests when the teats are dipped in various concentrations and forms of iodine. In some of the reported studies, valuable animal hygenic practices were also put into effect, including disinfection of teat cup clusters of milking machines and use of various antiseptics and germicides for washing the udder. Use of a teat dip as a preventive practice in dairy herds has generally resulted in the physical improvement of the udder (Huckle 1965). A few reports on the use of teat dips have not shown a beneficial response. Generally, aqueous solutions of teat dips have performed more effectively than those made with oil or organic solvent vehicles. Although postmilking teat dips of germicide solutions have been reported to help control the spread of mastitis, this practice has had little effect on the reduction of existent chronic mastitis in a given herd.

Antibacterial compounds as sanitizers as well as the application of steam and water at high temperatures have been used extensively to control bacterial populations in dairies and processing plants. The antimicrobial effectiveness of inorganic chlorine compounds such as calcium hypochlorite and sodium hypochlorite has been thoroughly demonstrated. The low cost and effectiveness of the hypochlorites have not provided an opportunistic potential for the development of replacement compounds. The high antimicrobial activity in varying water hardness at low or high temperatures have made the hypochlorites standards for comparative purposes.

A number of physical and biological factors are important in evaluating sanitizers: water hardness, solubility, pH, temperature, time, metal corrosiveness, and stability. Biological factors include ability to act against vegetative bacteria, spores, bacteriophage, fungi, and viruses and freedom of toxicity. The comprehensive review by Clegg (1967) is recommended for readers who desire additional information on the use of disinfectants and sanitizers in the dairy industry.

TYPES OF ANTISEPTICS AND DISINFECTANTS

Physical Agents

Two important physical agents are heat and light.

HEAT

Heat sterilization is an efficient and

convenient procedure. Moist heat has the advantage of penetrating clumps of organic matter and reaches surfaces not readily available to chemical disinfectants. Dry heat requires higher temperatures and longer exposure periods than does moist heat. Moist heat produces its germicidal effect by protein coagulation, whereas dry heat oxidizes or incinerates microorganisms.

Heating poultry litter to 65° C for 12 hours with floor and air heaters in experimental trials destroyed *Salmonella thompson*. This practice is presumed to inactivate other salmonella, viruses, fungi, and parasites present in poultry litter.

LIGHT

Ultraviolet light has antimicrobial activity. Small animal veterinary practitioners have employed the use of ultraviolet light in examination and operating rooms. In addition, ultraviolet light has been used by some clinicians in an attempt to control the epidemiologic problem of "kennel cough." Results have been inconsistent. Ultraviolet wavelengths of 2540–2800 angstrom units are most effective against gram-negative bacteria and nonsporulating bacteria, while staphylococci and streptococci as well as viruses are resistant.

The use of gamma rays has been studied for possible utilization as a means of disinfection. An exposure of 300,000 rads was bactericidal for pasteurellas whereas 1,500,000 rads were required for sporicidal activity for anthrax. Gamma irradiation has destroyed foot-and-mouth disease virus on infected carcasses; however, the high dosage affected the quality of meat.

Chemical Agents

Local antiinfective drugs may range from simple halogen atoms of chlorine and iodine to relatively complex organic dyes, organic halogens, and surfactants. Relationships between chemical analogs and biologic activity have been observed in a few groups, e.g., phenols. The chemical agents have many different types of action.

INORGANIC ACIDS

The strong mineral acids, hydrochloric or sulfuric, have been used to disinfect areas contaminated with excreta. Concentrations of 0.1–1 N have been used. Their corrosive action limits widespread usage.

Boric Acid, U.S.P., has a very weak germicidal activity. Its main attribute is that it does not irritate tissues and may be applied to delicate areas such as the cornea. Aqueous solutions greater than 2% may inhibit phagocytosis. When used clinically, boric acid in solution should be refrigerated to avoid phagocytocidal concentrations because at refrigerator temperatures it is only 1.95% soluble. As a mild antiseptic dusting powder, it serves as a relatively nonirritating drying substance which may be applied under splints. It may also be applied to eczematous areas of moist wounds.

ORGANIC ACIDS

Organic acids have limited application in the practice of veterinary medicine. *Salicylic Acid,* U.S.P., has low germicidal and fungicidal activity. It is mainly used with other drugs in dermatologic preparations for its keratolytic activity. *Benzoic Acid,* U.S.P., is a constituent of Whitfield's ointment, a preparation used for treating fungal infections. Other antifungal organic acids will be discussed later.

ALKALIES

Alkalies have been used as disinfectants since antiquity. The mechanism of action is related to hydroxyl ion concentration. A pH greater than 9 will inhibit most bacteria.

Lye (soda lye) contains approximately 94% sodium hydroxide and is widely used. It kills many common bacterial pathogens such as those causing fowl cholera and pullorum disease. Lye can be used to kill parasites of domestic animals while the parasites are separated from the host on inanimate objects. High concentrations of lye kill the spores of the anthrax bacillus but does not kill *Mycobacterium tuberculosis.*

Lye for disinfectant purposes should be applied as a 2% solution in hot or boiling water. For disinfection against anthrax, a 5% solution should be used. One lb lye to 5.5 gal water yields a 2% solution. The effectiveness of the lye solution can be increased by the addition of 2.5 lb water-slaked (not air-slaked) lime. The formation of whitewash increases the disinfectant value of the lye solution by delaying conversion of sodium hydroxide into sodium carbonate.

Concentrated lye is a caustic poison and must be handled with care. Solutions of lye must be disposed of properly to avoid injury to animals or man. Lye solutions are injurious to painted or varnished surfaces and to textiles if allowed to remain in contact very long. Lye does not injure bare wood, enamelware, earthenware, or common metals except aluminum. Containers of lye must be tightly closed to prevent conversion of sodium hydroxide to sodium carbonate by the carbon dioxide of the air.

Sodium carbonate and *trisodium phosphate* are used primarily as cleaning agents. The addition of 0.5% sodium hydroxide to the solution of these cleansing agents for general application will contribute considerable disinfectant action.

Lime, N.F. (calcium oxide [CaO], quicklime), occurs as an odorless, grayish white powder containing not less than 95% CaO. When CaO or quicklime is moistened with water, heat is generated and a white powder of $Ca(OH)_2$ (calcium hydroxide or slaked lime) is obtained. When lime is mixed with several parts of water, it is fully "slaked," i.e., the CaO is all converted to $Ca(OH)_2$, a compound similar to whitewash. Prolonged exposure of moistened lime converts to calcium carbonate, which is inert and worthless as a disinfectant. Lumps of lime sometimes explode when in contact with water; the lime dust in the air may get into the eyes and may be inhaled. Lime dust is very irritating.

Commercial lime is an inexpensive disinfectant and is commonly used in livestock pens and facilities. It may be applied as powder or in a thick mixture with water known as "milk of lime." Powdered lime (quicklime) may be scattered about yards and lots or swept over concrete floors as a general disinfectant. Care should be taken to avoid excess amounts of lime on concrete floors because it tends to dry the skin and hoofs of animals and sometimes causes dermal erosions, inviting infectious pododermatitis. The great advantages of lime as a disinfectant are its availability and cheapness. Lime does not destroy the spores of *Bacillus anthracis* or clostridia.

Calcium Hydroxide, U.S.P. (hydrated or air-slaked lime), occurs as a soft, white powder. When mixed with 4 volumes of water, an alkaline suspension or "milk of lime" results. Milk of lime has been used as a disinfectant for areas contaminated with excreta. It should be applied in liberal quantities and remain in contact with the excreta for at least 2 hours. Calcium hydroxide is now used in place of CaO in the preparation of lime water. Lime soaps formed by the reaction of $Ca(OH)_2$ with vegetable oils are adhesive and are sometimes used as an ointment base (lime liniment or "carron oil").

Calcium Hydroxide Solution, U.S.P. (lime water), contains not less than 0.14 g of $Ca(OH)_2$ in each 100 ml solution at 25° C. Calcium hydroxide is less soluble in hot water; it may be prepared by adding 3 g of $Ca(OH)_2$ to 1000 ml of cool distilled water. The mixture should be agitated vigorously for 1 hour.

It is important to keep the container of lime water carefully stoppered. When exposed to air, the lime water solution absorbs carbon dioxide and becomes covered with a pellicle of calcium carbonate. Successive pellicles will form and settle to the bottom until all the lime is precipitated.

The amount of $Ca(OH)_2$ in a solution of lime water is too small to be of value as an antacid. Lime water may have some value for gastritis in the dog and calf. It is claimed to decrease the size of the milk curd formed in the stomach of the newborn.

Sulfurated Lime Solution, N.F. (lime-sulfur solution), is a moderately alkaline, orange-colored liquid with an odor of hydrogen sulfide. It is produced by mixing air-slaked lime with sublimed sulfur and adding the mixture to water; the volume is reduced by boiling. The chemical reactions produce calcium disulfide, calcium penta-

$$CaO + H_2O \rightarrow Ca(OH)_2$$
$$3Ca(OH)_2 + 6S \rightarrow 2CaS_2 + CaS_2O_3 + 3H_2O$$
$$3Ca(OH)_2 + 12S \rightarrow 2CaS_5 + CaS_2O_3 + 3H_2O$$

FIG. 45.1.

sulfide, and calcium thiosulfate as shown in Fig. 45.1.

Sulfurated lime solution is used in veterinary medicine to control skin parasites.

Alkali Combinations. Alkalis are used extensively with various other disinfectants, especially in Europe and Russia. Such combinations include: (1) a mixture of 1% sodium hydroxide, 8% sodium hypochlorite, and 3%–5% formaldehyde (reported to inactivate transmissible gastroenteritis virus within 15 minutes) (Belak and Kisary 1974); (2) 2% calcinated sodium carbonate and 98% sodium chloride (for inactivation of foot-and-mouth disease virus on cattle hides) (Schjerning-Thiesen 1972); (3) an aqueous alkaline solution of hydrated lime and sodium hydroxide (for control of *Cryptococcus neoformans* in pigeon coops) (Walter and Coffee 1968); (4) sodium hydroxide and phenol (as a disinfectant at temperatures below freezing, i.e., —5°–0° C); (5) 2% sodium hydroxide and 2% cresol to inactivate hog cholera virus in excreta); (6) sodium hydroxide and potassium permanganate (for use against Talfan virus and porcine adenovirus type 2) (Derbyshire and Arkell 1971); and (7) a calcium hypochlorite mixture containing 2%–3% chlorine, 2% formol, and 2% sodium hydroxide at 60°–70° C (for disinfection of transport vehicles).

Care should be taken to avoid the use of excessive amounts of alkali mixtures since the compounds can cause excessive skin irritation resulting in skin and mucosal necrosis. Conditions favoring the formation of an irritating alkali dust should be avoided.

SURFACE-ACTIVE AGENTS (SURFACTANTS)

A surfactant is a chemical compound that lowers the surface tension of an aqueous solution. Emulsification is augmented by altering the wettable surface and reducing the wetting angle. Surfactants are widely used as wetting agents, detergents, and emulsifiers. Their major uses in veterinary medicine and animal production are as antiseptics and disinfectants.

There are three types of surfactants, based on the position of the hydrophobic (water repellent) moiety in the molecule: anionic, cationic, and, of lesser importance, nonionic. The cationic surfactants, in which a hydrophobic residue is balanced by a positively charged hydrophilic group (most usually a quaternary ammonium nucleus), are a very important group of bactericides. Several quaternary ammonium compounds have inactivated Newcastle disease and parainfluenza viruses (Kirchhoff 1968). Newcastle disease virus required a twofold increase in the concentration of the tested surfactants.

The quaternary ammonium compounds have also been used alone and in combination in an attempt to disinfect chicken and turkey eggs and reduce egg-transmitted infectious diseases (Mellor and Banwart 1965; Brown and Kolb 1974). Several quaternary ammonium compounds destroyed *Salmonella derby* growth when diluted according to manufacturers' instructions. Quaternary ammonium compounds used alone or with 3000 ppm tylosin tartrate were effective against *Pseudomonas, Arizona,* and *Alcoligenes* isolated from a hatchery. However, tylosin used alone at 3000 ppm was not lethal and neomycin at 2000 ppm killed only *Arizona.* Neomycin was antagonistic when added to the quaternary ammonium–tylosin tartrate combination.

It should be noted that surfactants are adsorbed to a significant degree by cotton, rubber, and porous materials, thus possibly reducing the effective concentration and antibacterial efficacy. Surfactants or detergents have been employed quite widely for cleaning surgical instruments and syringes. The detergents are in fact considered an essential adjunct for cleaning syringes (Darmady et al. 1965).

ANIONIC SURFACTANTS

Soaps. Soaps constitute the most significant

group of anionic detergents. Soaps have the general formula R — COONa. In aqueous solution, a soap dissociates to form sodium ions (Na^+) and fatty acid ions (R — COO^-). If the water contains a high concentration of calcium, the free calcium ion (Ca^{++}) reacts with 2 fatty acid ions to form a precipitate of hard calcium soap or "scum" on the surface of the water. Other substances, including cationic detergents, neutralize soap. The cation of the quaternary ammonium compounds combines with the anion of the soap, terminating the detergent activity of both compounds.

The soap molecule is dipolar. One end of the molecule is hydrophilic and the other lipophilic. When an aqueous solution of soap is applied to an oily or greasy surface, the soap molecules orient themselves diphasically so that one end of the molecule extends into the oil phase. This diphasic orientation of the soap molecules protects oil or fat droplets from coalescing. Soap may produce and maintain a discontinuity of phase between the water and fat particles.

Soaps are antibacterial against gram-positive and acid-fast organisms. The most important mechanism by which soap produces its beneficial effects is that of physical emulsification of the lipoidal secretions of the skin which contain bacteria; the bacteria become suspended in the lather and may be rinsed away. Although a large number of opportunist or transient bacteria are removed when the hands and arms are scrubbed with a brush, soap, and water, approximately 8% of the normal resident flora may remain. Some of the newer anionic surfactants have been used for scrubbing the skin because of greater disinfectant action and considerably less scum formation. With repeated use, they do not have the tendency to cause drying and cracking of the skin. In addition, the pH of many of the preparations is similar to that of the skin.

The antibacterial potency of soaps has been broadened by the inclusion of certain antiseptics. Potassium iodide has been added to soap and found to be effective against organisms resistant to soap. Hexachlorophene has been included in many of the older soaps as well as in some of the newer anionic surfactants. The anionic surfactant sodium octylphenoxyethyl ether sulfonate (Phisoderm, or if hexachlorophene has been added, pHisoHex) has found much use as a preoperative scrubbing agent. In addition to good antibacterial activity, good micelle formation is produced.

CATIONIC SURFACTANTS

Quaternary ammonium compounds are principal examples of cationic surfactants. The hydrophobic ion of the dissociated quaternary ammonium molecule carries a positive charge (see Fig. 45.2).

The hydrophobic ion of dissociated soap or anionic surfactant carries a negative charge. Each will neutralize the other; therefore, when a soap and a cationic surfactant, e.g., quaternary ammonium compound, are used in succession, a thorough rinsing must separate their applications.

Cationic surfactants, on an equal concentration basis, are more effective than anionic surfactants. Although surfactants have limited effect on viruses, they are effective against gram-negative and gram-positive bacteria. Gram-negative bacteria are susceptible to high concentrations. The cationic surfactants combine readily with proteins, fats, and some phosphates; thus they are of limited value in the presence of serum, blood, and other tissue debris. In general, cationic detergents do not possess viricidal, fungicidal, or sporicidal action.

Action. Cationic surfactants or detergents

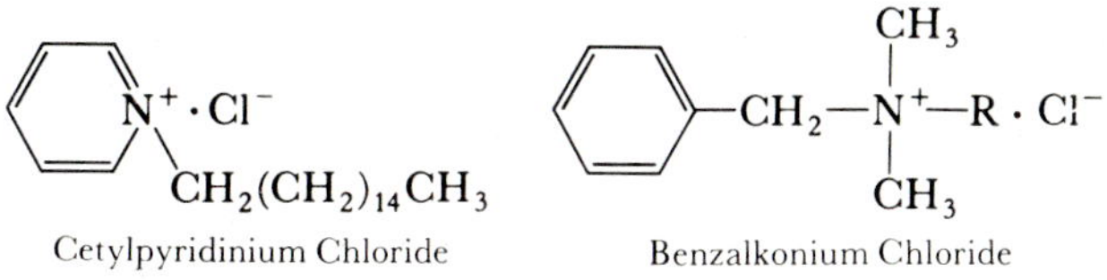

$N^+ \cdot Cl^-$ — $CH_2(CH_2)_{14}CH_3$

Cetylpyridinium Chloride

$C_6H_5\text{—}CH_2\text{—}N^+(CH_3)_2\text{—}R \cdot Cl^-$

Benzalkonium Chloride

FIG. 45.2.

are adsorbed to a high degree on the bacterial cell wall where they exert their antibacterial action. Most of the bacterial population are killed readily; the remaining bacteria show an increasing and surprising resistance. This phenomenon has been explained by the tendency for bacteria to agglutinate in an environment containing quaternary ammonium compounds. Bacteria on the inside of the agglutinated clumps are mechanically protected by a barrier and remain alive much longer than the more exposed bacteria.

Both the anionic and cationic surfactants denature proteins. At bactericidal and bacteriostatic concentrations, they decrease the surface tension and the permeability of the plasma membrane; thus the organism loses its ability to remain in equilibrium with its environment.

Undue reliance upon the quaternary ammonium compounds per se is undesirable because they tend to form a film on the skin under which the bacteria remain viable. The film is not readily broken and exerts little antibacterial action on its inner surface. The outer surface of the film acts against bacteria but it is of questionable action.

Uses. Quaternary ammonium compounds are applied to tissues in both aqueous and alcoholic solutions. The alcoholic solution or tincture may contain a variable amount of drug dissolved generally in 50% alcohol for surface antiseptis of the unbroken skin. The aqueous solution is used primarily for mucous membranes and denuded body surface or wounds. The unbroken skin of an occasional animal may be irritated slightly by these preparations.

The cationic detergents cannot be relied upon for sterilization of surgical instruments. They will, however, preserve the sterility of instruments previously sterilized. The quaternary ammonium compounds may be used as sanitizing rinses for eating and drinking utensils and for dairy equipment if organic matter has been mechanically cleaned from the objects. All soaps and other anionic detergents must be thoroughly removed before quaternary ammonium compounds are used. An increase in the temperature and the pH of the solution will increase the effectiveness of the quaternary ammonium compounds. They are not suitable for disinfection of premises because the large amount of organic debris present would immediately neutralize their antibacterial activity. The tendency for quaternary ammonium compounds to combine with milk solids is emphasized. If the milk equipment is cleansed thoroughly, these substances can be used effectively.

Quaternary ammonium compounds have been used for sanitizing egg shells since they have good germicidal activity at alkaline pH, have residual action, can be used at high temperature, and are less influenced by organic matter than other disinfectants (Ayres 1967). It has also been reported that quaternary ammonium compounds could eliminate salmonellae, the shell membrane system, and be very useful in the control of salmonellosis (Rizk et al. 1966).

Toxicity. As a rule, little toxicity is noted either from local application or accidental oral ingestion. A safety study was conducted in turkeys with a 20% solution of *n*-alkyldimethylbenzylammonium chlorides (Germex). In a 6-week experiment, doses up to 500 ppm active ingredient were given in the drinking water of growing turkey poults. The recommended concentration was approximately 65 ppm. The highest no-effect dose was about 200 ppm, which did not depress growth significantly ($P > 0.05$). More than 200 ppm gave some evidence of irritated oral mucosa and clinical signs of respiratory distress. The highest dose, 500 ppm, caused a 33% mortality between 6 and 17 days of medication (Reuber et al. 1970).

Preparations. *Benzalkonium Chloride,* U.S.P. (Zephiran chloride), is a mixture of alkyldimethylbenzylammonium chloride in which the alkyl radicals range from C_8H_{17} to $C_{18}H_{37}$. It may be used for general prophylactic disinfection of intact skin and mucous membranes and also for the treatment of superficial injuries and infected wounds. It will preserve the sterility of surgical instruments and rubber articles during storage. Sodium nitrite, 0.5%, can be added to solutions of benzalkonium chloride to prevent rusting of instruments. The tincture (1:100) may be used for preoperative disinfection of unbroken skin or for the treatment of wounds. Aqueous solutions of 1:2000–1:10,000 may be employed for the preoperative disinfection of mucous membranes and denuded skin, including irrigation of the eye, vagina, and other sensitive structures. Concentrations not to exceed 1:20,000 are recommended for irrigation of the urinary bladder and urethra. A saline irrigation may be used after benzalkonium irrigation. A 1:20,000 solution is also recommended for disinfection of catheters (Frederick 1963). Catheters and instruments were soaked for 15–30 minutes. A concentration of 1:1000 is recommended for storage of sterile instruments and rubber articles. A 10% aqueous solution of benzalkonium chloride (Roccal) is intended for general disinfection purposes.

The susceptibility of mycobacterial and nocardial species has been determined for benzalkonium chloride (Merkal and Thurston 1968). Mycobacteria isolated from lesions in man, cattle, pigs, and fowl were not sensitive to 0.1% benzalkonium chloride when exposed for 24 hours; however, the cationic surfactant was bactericidal for saprophytic mycobacteria and all tested strains of *Nocardia*. Benzalkonium chloride as Roccal inactivated several viral agents (e.g., distemper, rabies, fowl laryngotracheitis) after 10 minutes contact at 30° C (Armstrong and Froelich 1964).

The need for careful attention to labeled instructions and to establish a double check system for the application of any drug is illustrated by the following example (Serrano 1972). Cutaneous lesions characterized by depilation, necrosis, and ulceration as well as several unexpected deaths occurred in mice picked up with a forceps sterilized in benzalkonium. An investigation suggested an improper dilution of benzalkonium chloride for soaking the forceps. A single dermal application of 0.05 ml of 13% or 50% aqueous benzalkonium chloride produced death in 9 of 48 and 20 of 48 mice respectively. Survivors had the characteristic skin lesions.

Benzethonium Chloride, U.S.P. (Phemerol chloride), is a synthetic quaternary ammonium compound and occurs as odorless, colorless crystals with the same general characteristics as other quaternary ammonium compounds. Benzethonium is not effective against sporulating bacteria. It is used as a tincture in a concentration of 1:500 and in aqueous solution at a concentration of 1:1000. Ringworm in calves has been treated with twice-weekly applications of 1:1000 aqueous solutions of Phemerol applied to the area. Results have been variable.

Cetylpyridinium Chloride, N.N.D. (Ceepryn chloride), is a compound with characteristics similar to the previously mentioned quaternary ammonium compounds and is the monohydrate of the quaternary salt of pyridine and cetyl chloride. For preoperative scrubbing of the intact skin, a concentration of 1:100 in aqueous solution is used. A tincture of 1:500 may be applied to the skin. Concentrations of 1:5000 are desirable for delicate tissues. A combination of 0.25% cetylpyridinium acetate and 0.25% dequalinium acetate in 50% ethanol (Intersept) has been used as an aerosol foam.

Alcohols

The common aliphatic alcohols are good solvents, antiseptics, and disinfectants. Ethyl alcohol (ethanol) is traditionally the most common and widely used of the alcohols. Ethyl alcohol is also known as grain alcohol because it is produced from the fermentation of grains.

The use of isopropyl alcohol for external antisepsis and in drug manufacturing is increasing. The major advantage of the nonintoxicating isopropyl alcohol in the United States is its exemption from the special use tax which must be paid on ethyl alcohol and other intoxicating beverages. In addition, isopropyl alcohol is less expensive to produce than ethyl alcohol.

"Rubbing alcohol" is a crude distillate

TABLE 45.1. Germicidal effect of ethyl alcohol on *Staphylococcus albus**

Duration of Contact between Germicide and Bacteria	Concentration of Alcohol—% by Weight				
	30%	60%	70%	80%	99%
0 (control)	100.0	100.0	100.0	100.0	100.0
1 sec	80.2	59.5	27.1	29.9	61.9
10 sec	65.8	34.9	26.6	26.6	60.7
30 sec	50.2	18.4	21.2	34.1	48.7
1 min	49.8	9.3	18.6	14.9	46.8
5 min	42.2	12.2	21.7	24.4	26.2
10 min	24.6	13.5	23.4	20.1	41.8

Source: Price 1950.
* The numbers in the table indicate the % of test organisms surviving after contact with alcohol.

of alcohols that contains mostly isopropyl alcohol. This commercial product also contains small amounts of ethyl alcohol and several other alcohols. It is available in a 70% concentration suitable for general antiseptic and disinfectant purposes. Normal propyl alcohol also has considerable disinfectant power. Methyl alcohol is produced by the distillation of wood. It is a drastic poison and should be avoided under all circumstances. It is occasionally used as an industrial solvent. Methyl alcohol is oxidized in the body to release formaldehyde and formic acid, both of which are toxic.

ACTION

The alcohols have marked antibacterial action against the vegetative cells (see Table 45.1) but, like many disinfectants, they do not destroy bacterial spores. Ethyl alcohol is generally recognized by medical authorities as one of the best antiseptic and disinfectant substances available. Ethyl alcohol outstrips numerous other compounds in antibacterial action when applied locally to the tissues (see Figs. 45.3, 45.4).

Ethyl alcohol is commonly used in a dilution of 70% by weight or 78% by volume. During World War II, when a shortage of ethyl alcohol developed, isopropyl alcohol was used for antiseptic and disinfectant effects. It appears to be as satisfactory as ethyl alcohol for all external uses and is generally employed in the same concentrations as ethyl alcohol. Fifty percent isopropyl by weight is equivalent to 70% ethyl alcohol in its antibacterial action.

The structural activity relationships of aliphatic alcohols are notable; antibacterial action increases with the number of carbons up to a total of 8–10 in the molecule. The alcohols apparently produce their effects by denaturing soluble proteins and depressing surface tension. A critical concentration of alcohol providing the maximum antibacterial activity for all bacteria apparently cannot be stated because the susceptibility of some bacteria to alcohol varies.

The efficacy of ethanol as an antiseptic for preparation of the surgical site in dogs and cattle was investigated with a multiple point contactor (Price et al. 1968). Eight of 11 dogs demonstrated a 100% reduction in bacterial growth after ethanol (78% v/v) had been applied to the skin 2 minutes previously. Activity was comparable to *Iodine Tincture,* U.S.P. The bacterial skin flora of cows was reduced by ethanol more than fourfold; however, only 5 animals were used, and the results were not statistically significant.

LOCAL EFFECT

The brief irritant action of alcohol is noted when it is applied in high concentration to the skin and to mucous membranes. The unbroken skin may become slightly red and pruritic after a concentrated solution is applied. The irritation of alcohol results from the partial precipitation of the cellular proteins and from its dehydrating action. If the alcohol penetrates below the surface of the skin, it will destroy the cellular protoplasm until diluted by tissue fluids. If strong vapors of alcohol are inhaled, the irritation causes reflex closure of the glottis. A strong burning sensation

Fig. 45.3. Graph showing how the addition of iodine increases the antibacterial action of 70% ethyl alcohol upon the bacterial flora of the hands and arms. (Price 1951; by permission of Annals of Surgery, J. B. Lippincott Co., publishers)

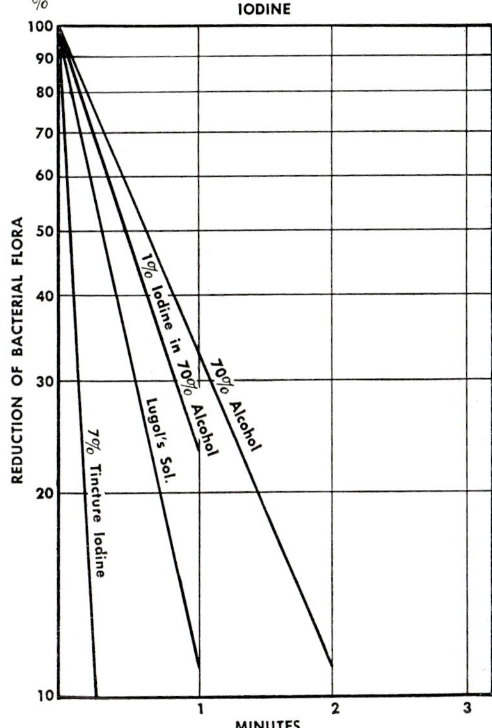

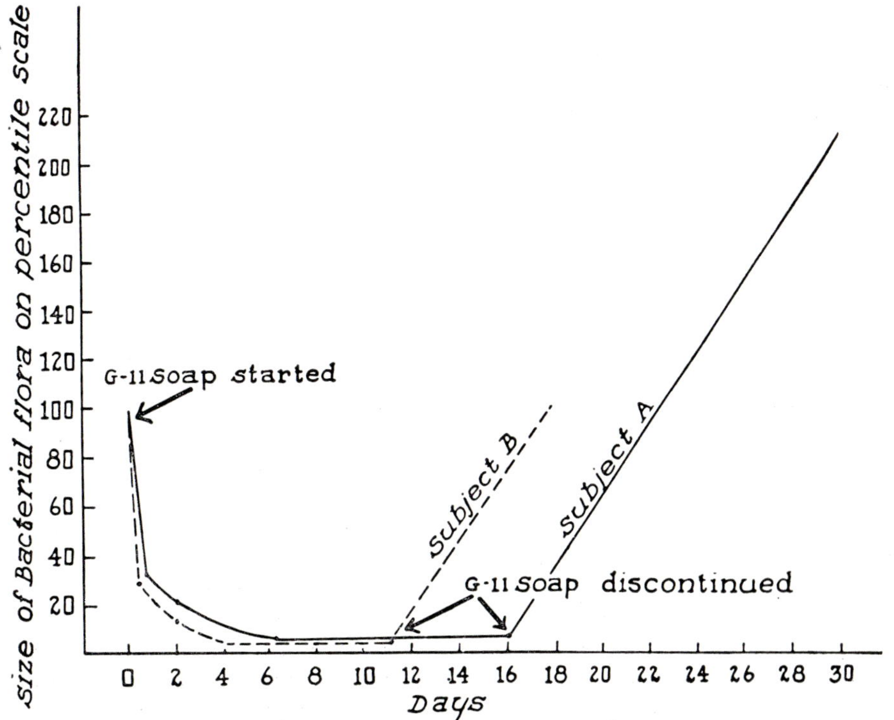

Fig. 45.4. Antibacterial action of hexachlorophene in soap (G-11) when used on successive days to wash the hands. (Price and Bonnett 1948; by permission of Annals of Surgery, J. B. Lippincott Co., publishers)

is noted in the throat, or in the stomach if the alcohol is introduced into that chamber.

High concentrations of alcohol (80%–95%) have been injected into nerves or ganglia to destroy the tissue and to provide relief from pain of the parts innervated. The pain is absent until restoration of the nerve fiber and normal transmission of impulses. Sometimes nerve destruction is permanent. The destruction arises from precipitation of the nerve cell proteins and from the solution of cellular lipids. Alcohol has been injected for the alleviation of pain in lame horses, and occasionally it has been injected epidurally in cattle to help correct chronic vaginal and/or rectal prolapse.

SYSTEMIC EFFECTS

Ethyl alcohol is rapidly absorbed from the digestive tract and affects the central nervous system (CNS) in particular. In human beings there is a loss of mental alertness but a marked increase in the sense of well-being, confidence, and usually in sociability. The individual loses considerable self-control and willpower, with a progressive loss of locomotor function. Consumption of large quantities of alcohol leads to deep sleep and eventually to total unconsciousness and a condition resembling anesthesia. Death frequently follows due to respiratory failure.

Occasionally the systemic effects of alcohol may be observed in animals that have ingested spoiled fermented feed containing various types of alcohols. The most prominent effect is ataxia. Occasionally an aggressive disposition may appear during the intoxication.

Because of the tendency of the human being under the influence of alcohol to exhibit a flushed face and to experience a sensation of warmth, alcohol was long viewed as a circulatory stimulant. Ethanol is absorbed and oxidized within the body as a form of energy when small amounts are consumed; however, if absorption exceeds the metabolic rate, ethanol toxemia results.

Alcohol is an important addition to other local antiinfective drugs because of its ability to solubilize fat and to exert a synergistic or additive effect when used in combination with other antiseptics or disinfectants. For example, a combination of 3% chloramine and 20% alcohol has been a very effective disinfectant, especially when it is used at below-freezing temperatures.

HALOGENS

Halogens owe their potent antibacterial effects to their ability to have a high affinity for protoplasm. The relative bacterial activities of the halogens in solutions free of organic matter are, in decreasing order, chlorine, bromine, and iodine. However, in the presence of organic matter iodine is the most active.

IODINE

Elementary iodine is available in crystalline form as dark, metallic, reddish brown scales. This material has a characteristic odor and rapidly iodizes most materials it contacts. Iodine dissolves poorly in water but is readily soluble in alcohol. It should be handled cautiously and not allowed to contact the unprotected skin. Iodine preparations are among the most commonly employed local antiinfective drugs. Metallic iodine and tinctures are too corrosive and expensive for general disinfectant usage. Iodine has been combined with surface-active agents to form iodophors. These compounds will be discussed later.

Antibacterial Action. Iodine apparently diffuses into the bacterial cell where its interference with vital metabolic reactions of the protoplasm results in the death of the cell. Bacterial spores and vegetative forms are killed by effective concentrations. Most bacteria are killed within 1 minute in a 50 ppm solution of iodine. Fifteen minutes are required to kill bacterial spores. Iodine in alcohol gives as pronounced an antibacterial action upon bacteria populating the unbroken skin as any antiseptic in common use. Ethyl alcohol, 70% by weight, is an excellent skin disinfectant. When iodine crystals are dissolved in alcohol, the antibacterial action of the combination is greater than the effect of alcohol alone (Fig. 45.3). Tincture of iodine (2%) is an excellent antiseptic compound. When applied to the skin, it produces a minimal irritation, spreads evenly, dries slowly, and in 3 minutes reduces the resident bacterial flora to less than 10% of its original population. Strong tincture of iodine (7%) has greater antibacterial action but is irritating. Strong tincture of iodine is still preferred by many large-animal practitioners for dermal application to food-producing animals exposed excessively to filth and bacterial contamination.

Clinical Uses. Tincture of iodine is used by surgeons and general practitioners for application before surgical incisions or hypodermic injections. It is sometimes used on wounds, but some practitioners hesitate to use it because of the possibility of delaying wound healing. Tincture of iodine has also been used in treatment of various skin diseases caused by fungi or ectoparasites.

Strong tincture of iodine is not intended for use on open wounds because it irritates and destroys tissue and thus delays wound healing. It acts as a powerful local irritant and is employed as a counterirritant for treatment of equine lameness. The strong tincture may be diluted with 1 or more parts of glycerin in order to decrease the intensity but prolong the irritative action when applied for counterirritation. It is important that it never be applied under a bandage unless severe counterirritation is desired. To leave the treated area bandaged may result in considerable tissue destruction. The strong tincture may be washed off the unbroken skin a few minutes after being applied to avoid blistering and intense irritation. If strong tincture of iodine is applied to a horse as a counterirritant, it is important that the head be tied in order to keep the animal from rubbing the irritant and blistering its nose and muzzle.

Preparations. *Iodine Tincture,* U.S.P., is a 2% solution of free iodine with 2.4% sodium iodide in 50% ethyl alcohol. Isopropyl alcohol is a satisfactory substitute. The iodine tincture produces a characteristic brown stain when applied to the skin. Single applications cause little irritation or damage to the skin. Other local antiinfective agents are better suited for application to the mucous membranes. Repeated applications of iodine tincture to the skin or mucous membranes cause blister formation and epithelial desquamation.

Strong Iodine Tincture, N.F., is an alcoholic solution containing 7 g of free iodine and 5 g of potassium iodide in each 100 ml of 85% ethyl alcohol. The potassium iodide stabilizes the solution by preventing conversion of the free iodine into hydrogen iodide and ethyl iodide, which tend to precipitate, and facilitates the spread of the solution and its adherence to the treated skin. In preparing the strong tincture, the potassium iodide should first be dissolved in water because of the low solubility of the salt in the hydroalcoholic solution. The iodine crystals can be added with alcohol.

Iodine is also employed in other preparations. *Iodine Solution,* N.F., contains about 2% free iodine and about 2.4% sodium iodide dissolved in aqueous solution. *Strong Iodine Solution,* U.S.P. (Lugol's solution), contains 5% free iodine and 10% potassium iodide in aqueous solution.

Iodoform, N.F. (CHI_3), was once widely used as a skin ointment, as an oily suspension in infected cavities or deep wounds, and in gelatin capsules for uterine infections. It has gradually fallen into disrepute, primarily because of its questionable activity. Iodoform with its characteristic penetrating odor is absorbed by the tissues and eliminated in the milk.

Iodophors. The discovery that polyvinylpyrrolidone and other surfactants could solubilize iodine and form germicidal compounds initiated the development of a new group of germicides and sanitizers. Iodophors (iodine bearers)—combinations of iodine with detergents, wetting agents, solubilizers, and other carriers—may contain iodine up to 30% of their weight, of which 70%–80% of the iodine may be released as available iodine when the solution is diluted (Davis 1962). Some iodine (20%–30%) may eventually be converted to inorganic iodide; however, this is not considered a severe limitation because of its germicidal action. Nonionic compounds are considered to be superior since anionic or cationic compounds are affected by the degree of water hardness and pH. Similar to chlorine, the effectiveness of iodine increases as the pH decreases; however, it is less sensitive to variation in pH than either chlorine or quaternary ammonium compounds. Iodophor solutions retain good bactericidal activity in the presence of organic matter as long as the pH does not go higher than 4.

Iodophors are considered safe, have very low toxicity, are almost free of odor, and have good stability. Iodophors may be categorized on the basis of their carrier, acidity, color, and odor. Most iodophors for skin disinfection have about 1% "available" iodine slowly released as the antibacterial agent (Price 1966). In addition, iodophor solutions are claimed to cleanse the skin at the same time the available iodine is exerting its antibacterial effect. Iodophors do not possess some of the undesirable properties of alcoholic and aqueous solutions of iodine, e.g., tissue irritation, allergic or toxic reactions, staining, or corrosiveness to certain metals.

Iodophors have been used as a valuable aid for mastitis control when incorporated in teat dips and antiseptics for washing the udder. Although the first acidic iodophors used for disinfecting purposes were found unsuitable because their use resulted in chapped teats, the application of less acidic iodophors did not have this adverse effect. Feagan et al. (1970) used an iodophor teat dip that provided 4600 ppm of iodine. After 1 week's use, the concentration dropped to 4000 ppm. They estimated the cost of the iodophor to be approximately 10 cents per day for a 50-cow herd. For teat dip usage, it appears that an iodophor with 1% available iodine is comparable to 0.2% chlorhexidine or a hypochlorite with 4% available chlorine (Schultze and Smith 1971; Natzke and Bray 1972).

Iodophors have also been used as dairy sanitizers. The best pH for antimicrobial activity is below 5, probably 3. At neutral or alkaline pH, antimicrobial activity is minimal; thus iodophors must be formulated as strong acid solutions to provide maximum effectiveness. Phosphoric acid is most often used for this purpose.

Iodine residues in milk have been studied in Sweden since 1970 (Iwarsson and Ekman 1973). An increased number of milk samples, individual and pooled or bulk, had been reported to have iodine concentrations of 300 μg/L and were classified as contaminated. An iodophor teat dip, yielding approximately 0.5% available iodine, was tested in 14 dairy herds. Total iodine concentrations in milk were determined during a control period and the postmilking teat dipping period. The average iodine concentration during the postmilking teat dipping increased 184 μg/L. The Swedish workers concluded that teat dipping with iodophors would increase the iodine content in milk.

A combination of an iodophor and phosphoric acid (Iosan) has been used as an antiseptic, disinfectant, and teat dip. Foot-and-mouth disease virus has been inactivated after a 1-hour exposure to 2%–3% Iosan. As a teat dip, a 33% concentration has been used; a reduction in the prevalence of acute and chronic mastitis, cow pox, and other cutaneous lesions of the udder was recorded in several dairy herds.

Povidone-Iodine, N.F. (Betadine, Isodine), is a water-soluble complex of iodine and polyvinylpyrrolidone used for general antiseptic purposes. Povidone-iodine retains the antimicrobial spectrum of iodine and does not have its disadvantages, e.g., irritation, toxicity, and ability to stain. Several veterinary preparations are available: aerosol spray, ointment, solution, and surgical scrub. All of these preparations provide from 0.5% to 1% titratable iodine. Although none of the four veterinary preparations are approved by the FDA for use in food-producing animals, the surgical scrub of povidone-iodine is approved for use on human beings. A 1:25 concentration killed *Brucella abortus* in 2 minutes. Undiluted povidone-iodine applied to the veterinarian's arms before recto-vaginal procedures effected a 1:5–1:10 concentration on the skin (Mansi and Lakin 1968).

Povidone-iodine has also been used in numerous surgical procedures in small animal and equine practice and as a therapeutic agent for various dermal and mucosal infections.

Another iodine preparation, iodotriethylene glycol, has been used as an aerosol prophylactically and therapeutically against avian infectious laryngotracheitis at concentrations of 160–300 mg of iodine/m^3.

CHLORINE

Solutions of chlorine in water have been available for many decades and have been used to cleanse wounds, arrest growth and development of bacteria, and treat necrotic tissues. Continuous or frequent irrigation of a wound with an aqueous solution of chlorine is now recognized as irritating and causing excessive granulation tissue in the wound. Chlorine is largely used for disinfection.

General Use. Chlorine disinfectants are powerful bleaching agents and tend to corrode metals. Their odor is very strong; for this reason they are not recommended for refrigerators, freezers, or any compartment where food is stored. Chlorine is widely used in dairies, creameries, and milk houses. Recommended concentration for disinfection is 800 ppm of available chlorine. Aqueous solutions of sodium hypochlorite are commonly employed to disinfect dairy equipment such as milk cans, bottles, and pipelines. In recommended concentrations, the hypochlorites effectively disinfect clean surfaces. A considerable residue of organic matter will combine with the chlorine solution and decrease its disinfectant action.

Preparations. *Sodium Hypochlorite Solution,* N.F., is a clear, aqueous solution containing 5% NaOCl. This solution decomposes on exposure to light. It can be used for irrigation of wounds if diluted 10 times; however, it dissolves not only necrotic tissue but also blood clots and healing may be delayed. Products very similar to this are used for laundering clothes and for disinfection of dairy equipment and milk utensils in general.

Calcium hypochlorite, containing 2%–5% chlorine and applied at a rate of 0.5 L/m^2, is a recommended disinfectant for many serious infectious diseases: anthrax, tetanus, tuberculosis, etc. Sodium hypochlorite is used in the same manner and has inactivated foot-and-mouth disease virus.

Organic Chlorides. Several organic chlorides have been used successfully because of the desirable property of not combining with organic materials as readily as the hypochlorites. Chlorine is weakly banded to nitrogen as the available halogen in organic chlorides with germicidal activity.

Chloramine-T, N.F. (Chlorazene) (Fig. 45.5), is a white crystalline powder having a slight odor of chlorine. It contains about 12% active chlorine and is readily soluble in water. The bactericidal action is caused by the release of chlorine and the formation of hypochlorous acid. Chloramine-T is less irritating, more stable, and more convenient to use than the hypochlorite solutions. It is excellent for use on dairy equipment, washing of bovine udders, milking machine cups, and numerous other dairy and livestock uses. Solutions of chloramine-T may be used to irrigate the accessible portion of the urinary system and for irrigation of wounds containing suppurative debris.

Chloramine-T was found to have the highest disinfectant activity on aerobic and

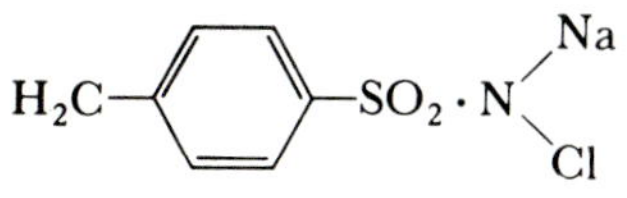

$$H_2C-C_6H_4-SO_2\cdot N\begin{matrix}Na\\Cl\end{matrix}$$

Chloramine-T

FIG. 45.5.

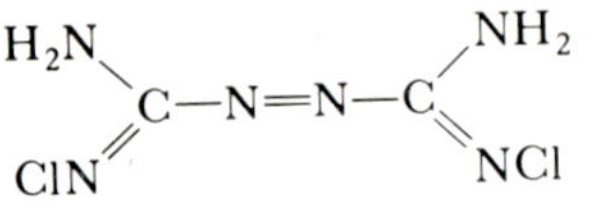

$$\begin{array}{ccc} H_2N & & NH_2 \\ & C{-}N{=}N{-}C & \\ ClN & & NCl \end{array}$$

Chloroaxodin

FIG. 45.6.

anaerobic bacteria when compared to a quaternary ammonium salt, caustic soda, and cationic detergents (Walkowiak and Alexandrowska 1969). A 0.5% solution was an effective disinfectant after a period of 30 minutes. Newcastle disease virus has been inactivated with a 1% solution. *Dichloramine-T* is similar to chloramine-T except that it contains about 29% active chlorine. Structurally dichloramine-T contains a second chlorine atom attached to the nitrogen atom. This compound is almost insoluble in water.

Chloroazodin, N.F. (Azochloramide) (Fig. 45.6), is a yellow crystalline powder containing 38% active chlorine. It has a faint chlorine odor, is slightly soluble in water, and is nonirritating to tissues. Therapeutic uses are similar to chloramine-T and dichloramine-T, but Azochloramide is claimed to be less inhibited by serum and organic matter.

Chlorinated lime (chloride of lime, bleaching powder) is a mixture of calcium hypochlorite and calcium chloride. It is a gray-white powder with a strong chlorine odor. Chlorinated lime yields 30% of its weight in available chlorine. It is highly irritant and must be handled carefully. It should be sorted in hermetically sealed containers because it deteriorates with loss of chlorine on exposure to air. Chlorinated lime should be handled only in well-ventilated rooms or outside because of the poisonous chlorine gas which it readily gives off. It is a practical and effective disinfectant for use on the farm to destroy disease organisms in organic matter and to promote the destruction of infected carcasses. For disinfection of premises and livestock quarters, it is important that the powdered chlorinated lime be sprinkled or dusted about in considerable excess to compensate for that inactivated by organic debris. Chlorinated lime is also a deodorant. A 5% solution inactivates Newcastle disease virus.

In an emergency, chlorinated lime can be used to disinfect water; however, it gives the water a disagreeable taste. For general household and farm use, 6 oz powdered chlorinated lime are mixed with 1 gal of water.

Iodine monochloride has the ability to penetrate the bacterial cell and accumulate in the cell wall and protoplasts. Bacterial death is presumed to be the result of malfunctioning enzyme systems and protein coagulation. A 1% solution of iodine monochloride kills *Clostridium perfringens* types C and D spores within 20 minutes and a 0.75% solution has been used as a disinfectant for washing the udders of dairy cattle. To disinfect inanimate substances, 10% solutions applied at the rate of 1 L/m^2 have been used.

Methyl bromide gas has been used as a disinfectant to destroy various microorganisms. When used at concentrations of 20–40 mg/L for 20 hours at 25° C, there is a significant reduction in the number of viable bacteria and some spores, e.g., *Aspergillus fumigatus.* At concentrations of 100 g/m^3 for 24 hours it has viricidal, bactericidal, and coccidiocidal activity. Methyl bromide has also been employed as a disinfectant for animal feeds and litter. Methyl bromide used at a concentration of 100 mg/hour/L inactivated sporulated and nonsporulated oocysts of *Eimeria tenella* and *acervulina* and at a concentration of 1 $kg/5.7\ m^3$ for 24 hours at 21° C or above killed several species of ticks, adults, larvae, and eggs.

COAL TAR DERIVATIVES

PHENOL

Phenol, U.S.P. (carbolic acid) (Fig. 45.7), was discovered in coal tar over 100 years ago and was first called carbolic acid. It was the first antiseptic to be used by Sir Joseph Lister in his introduction of aseptic surgery.

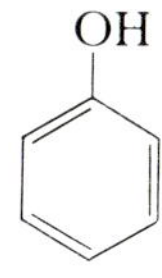

Phenol

FIG. 45.7.

CHEMISTRY

At room temperature, phenol is a colorless crystalline compound with a very characteristic odor. It melts at approximately 40° C. Aqueous solutions gradually darken on exposure to air and light.

ACTION

Phenol is a general protoplasmic poison. A 5% concentration is necessary to kill anthrax spores during an exposure of 48 hours. Most of the ordinary vegetative cells are readily killed by phenol. It is one of the best disinfectants for antitubercular activity. The addition of the chelating agent, ethylenediaminetetraacetic acid (EDTA), greatly enhances the bactericidal activity.

When applied to tissue, phenol exerts an antiseptic, irritant, anesthetic, or corrosive action, depending upon the concentration and the duration of exposure. Phenol coagulates proteins; it does not combine firmly with the proteins of the superficial cells but penetrates deeper in the tissues, in contrast to the metallic antiseptics (such as mercuric chloride) which do not escape from superficial protein coagulation.

Phenol may be extracted from the tissues by the use of alcohol following either intentional or accidental application. An alcohol bath or a dressing of alcohol applied to the affected area for several minutes will extract most of the phenol. Phenol has a much greater solubility in alcohol than in the aqueous tissue fluids and, therefore, diffuses out of the tissues. If the phenol has penetrated deeply, an oil dressing should be applied after two or three applications of alcohol. Phenol will also preferentially diffuse into the oil.

USES

Phenol has been used to cauterize infected areas, such as an infected umbilicus on a newborn animal. It has been applied to tissues in dilute solution for an antiseptic effect but it is generally considered too irritating. Phenol has been used in a concentration of 3%–4% for chemical sterilization of instruments. It has been occasionally used in ointments and other preparations for application to the skin to relieve itching.

Phenol is a good disinfectant but is expensive. A minimal concentration of 5% phenol in aqueous solution is used for disinfection of contaminated inanimate objects. This concentration is undesirably high for use on animal quarters. Concentrations in excess of 2% phenol are dangerous for all species, particularly cats, because of cutaneous absorption.

In summary, the advantages of phenol are reasonable effectiveness in destroying most of the common bacteria, slow inactivation by organic matter, availability, and the fact that a 5% solution sterilizes after contact for 1 hour without materially injuring metals or fabrics. Disadvantages of phenols are ineffectiveness against certain forms of bacteria, costliness, high toxicity, and a strong odor absorbed by foods.

CRESOL

Cresol, U.S.P. (cresylic acids, tricresol), is a colorless liquid; it develops a pink, then a yellowish, and finally a dark brown color after exposure to light and air. Cresol has a typical phenol odor and is soluble in water to about 2%. Commercial grades of cresol usually contain from 90% to 98% cresylic acids.

CHEMISTRY

The cresols are phenolic in nature but have a methyl group substituted for 1 hydrogen atom on the benzene ring. Cresol is composed of orthocresol, metacresol, and paracresol (Fig. 45.8) and the various isomers of each so that about 12 different isomeric compounds are known.

ACTION

Cresol is a general protoplasmic poison for bacterial and mammalian cells alike. Cresol is bactericidal against nearly all veg-

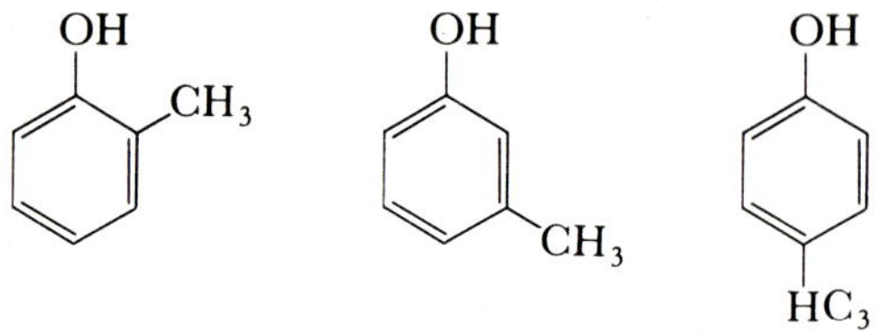

FIG. 45.8.

etative bacterial cells. It is effective against acid-fast bacteria but has limited viricidal action and no sporicidal activity. The antibacterial specificity of cresol closely parallels that of phenol. In contrast to other disinfectants, cresol retains its disinfectant action exceptionally well in the presence of organic matter.

Cresol is more bactericidal, but less caustic and less toxic than phenol. Nevertheless, it is irritant and even corrosive in concentrated form. Cresol is readily absorbed from the digestive tract or through the skin and produces acute or chronic poisoning. The same precautions should be practiced in handling cresol as are employed for phenol. Cresol has a stronger antibacterial action than phenol, so that a 2% solution of cresol may be regarded as equivalent to a 5% solution of phenol.

USES

The common grade of cresol is relatively inexpensive and efficient as a disinfectant. Cresol in a 2% solution is a satisfactory disinfectant for inanimate objects, e.g., stalls, gutters, excreta, truck boxes, railroad cars, yards, yard fences, and dirt floors.

Cresol is not readily soluble in water; therefore warm water should be used for preparing all solutions. Care must be taken to see that all the cresol is dissolved in water before the disinfectant solution is applied. Its low solubility is a serious disadvantage and has led to the manufacture of saponated cresol which forms a readily soluble solution for easier application.

PREPARATION

Saponated Cresol Solution, N.F., is a mixture of 50% cresol with about 35% soap in a hydroalcoholic diluent. Saponated cresol solution is a viscous, brown fluid that mixes readily with soft water in all proportions to form a soapy solution. It does not mix well with hard water. The saponated solution of cresol is generally used in a 2% concentration. A substitute for the saponated solution of cresol can be made by mixing *Cresol,* U.S.P., with ordinary green soap. The green soap will dissolve in an equal part of warm cresol, and the mixture is then stirred thoroughly with the remaining cresol.

The 2% saponated solution of cresol and especially the 2% nonsaponified solution of cresol in soft water should be applied as hot solutions for disinfecting animal quarters and premises. The easiest and most efficient method of application is with a pressure sprayer. The U.S. Agricultural Research Service requires a cresol disinfectant for the official disinfection of stock cars, boats, and yards in a fashion conforming to definite standards of application, composition, and solubility. The official regulations require the use of an acceptable cresol disinfectant diluted in the proportion of 4 oz in 1 gal water (3.15% solution of *Cresol,* U.S.P.). In addition to *Cresol,* U.S.P., and *Saponated Cresol Solution,* N.F., the U.S. Agricultural Research Service lists a number of proprietary cresylic disinfectants that have met required standards and can be used for official disinfection of livestock quarters and carriers.

Advantages in the use of the saponated cresol solution are: (1) equal volumes are more efficient and less expensive than phenol; (2) cresol will kill hog cholera virus; (3) the saponated solution of cresol is readily soluble; and (4) its soap content dissolves grease to permit complete contact with contaminated surfaces. Disadvantages of cresol are: (1) it cannot be used where human foods are stored because of the odor; (2) ordinary cresol is relatively insoluble in water, and even a saponated solution of cresol does not mix well with hard water; and (3) cresol is poisonous and must be handled carefully.

Other Coal Tar Derivatives

Sodium orthophenylphenate has been recognized as an official disinfectant primarily because it has been shown to be effective against germs of tuberculosis. Sodium orthophenylphenate is a light gray powder which must be stored in a closed container. It should be used as a hot 1% aqueous solution. It is suitable for use in dairy barns because it is free of objectionable odors. *Orthochlorophenol* emulsion (3%–5%) has demonstrated ovicidal activity for toxascaris and ascarids and has killed larvae and eggs of trichuris, *Metastrongylus* spp., *Oesophagostomum* spp., and *Strongyloides ransomi.*

A number of other coal tar derivatives such as *Resorcinol,* U.S.P., *Hexylresorcinol,* U.S.P., *Metacresylacetate,* N.N.D. (Cresatin), and *Thymol,* N.F., have been used for various purposes. *Chlorocresol-paraffin sulfonate* used in a 3% solution has a coccidiocidal effect on nonsporulated oocysts. *Hexachlorophenol* in a 1000 ppm aqueous solution inactivates foot-and-mouth disease virus. *o-Phenylphenol* inactivates African swine fever when used in a 1% spray.

Hexachlorophene, U.S.P. (Fig. 45.9), is a white, crystalline diphenol. It contains 6 chlorine ions. It is odorless and virtually insoluble in water but soluble in alkalis, alcohol, and acetone. The alkalinity of soap is sufficient to keep hexachlorophene in aqueous solution.

Hexachlorophene has been incorporated in solid and liquid soaps, detergent creams, and other vehicles for preooperative skin disinfection. It is active against many gram-positive bacteria but only a few gram-negative organisms. Hexachlorophene has a slow antibacterial action that parallels the degerming effect of ordinary soap during the first application. The action of hexachlorophene is attributed to the residue that remains on the skin after application. When antibacterial action is tested by a single application of the serial-basin hand washing technique (scrubbing the hands and arms for 5–10 minutes with hexachlorophene soap), the bacterial flora of the skin is reduced no more rapidly than by scrubbing with ordinary soap. Single washings or once-daily washings with hexachlorophene soap will not produce or maintain a low bacterial count on the skin because full regeneration of bacteria usually occurs within 24 hours. However, when hexachlorophene soap is used to wash the hands several times a day for 4 or more days, the resident bacterial flora is decreased to approximately 5% of its normal amount (Fig. 45.4). This low level of bacterial flora on the skin is maintained as long as the hexachlorophene soap is used frequently.

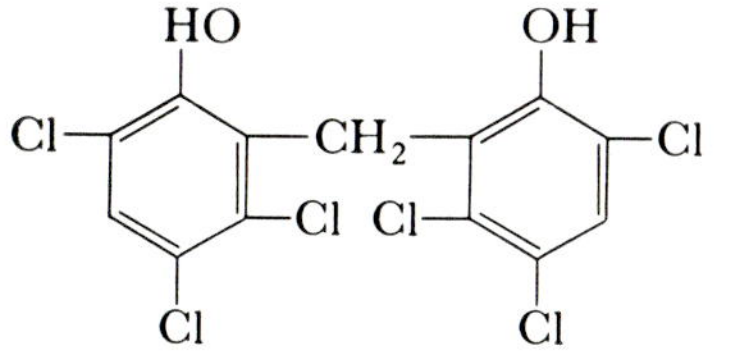

HO OH

Cl— —CH_2— —Cl

—Cl Cl—

Cl Cl

Hexachlorophene

Fig. 45.9.

Hexachlorophene is useful for preoperative skin disinfection of the surgeon's hands and arms, provided it can be used repeatedly. It is not used to reduce the bacterial flora of the operative site because it must be applied several times to have a good antibacterial action. Alcohol is an effective agent in reducing ordinary bacterial flora by a single application. Comparative studies indicate that the conventional 7-minute scrub, followed by a 3-minute wash in 70% alcohol, exerts considerably more antibacterial action than does a single wash with hexachlorophene soap.

Toxicity has been observed in dogs after they consumed soap containing hexachlorophene. The 24-hour oral single LD50 dose of hexachlorophene in dogs was 90 mg/kg of body weight (Koritz 1975). Signs of acute intoxication were attributable to the chemical action as an uncoupler of oxidative phosphorylation. Hyperthermia and hyperventilation were followed by depression and death at body temperatures of 108°–110° F, with a rapid onset of rigor mortis. Other signs included vomition, diarrhea, frequent micturition, dehydration, and respiratory alkalosis.

Pharmacokinetic parameters for a one-compartment open model were obtained by graphical treatment of plasma data following single intravenous and oral administration of hexachlorophene at 1, 5, and 100 mg/kg body weight. The half-life of absorption was estimated to be 0.6–1.4 hours and that of elimination to be 4–5.6 hours. The apparent volume of distribution was 34%–57% of body weight. Hexachlorophene was excreted into the bile and urine unchanged and as a glucoronide conjugate.

WOOD TAR DERIVATIVES

Wood tar is derived from the destructive distillation of pine and, occasionally, juniper wood. Further distillation of the initial crude tar or pitch yields several fractions, including turpentine and pine oil. Pine tar remains as a residue. The volatile pine oil contains various benzene derivatives, including phenols, creosol, toluene, and a mixture of methyl alcohol and acetone.

Wood tar derivatives have been applied to tissues more extensively than have coal tar derivatives since the wood tar derivatives are less irritant and toxic. Before the introduction of more specific therapy, the wood tar derivatives, e.g., guaiacol, were used widely for treatment of respiratory infections.

Preparations

Pine Tar, U.S.P., is a viscid, black-brown liquid. It is soluble in organic solvents but practically insoluble in water. When pine tar is distilled, it yields a volatile liquid portion (known as rectified tar oil) and a black pitch residue. The residue contains phenolic constituents, including benzene, phenol, creosol, and xylene.

Xylene has been demonstrated to be a good disinfectant for liquid manure when used at a concentration of 1000 ppm (Plummet and Plummet 1974). *Brucella abortus, Salmonella typhimurium, Pseudomonas aeruginosa, Escherichia coli, Staphylococcus aureus, Streptococcus faecalis,* and *Corynebacterium pyogenes* were killed when present in liquid manure. Four to 21 days were required for maximum disinfectant activity.

The antibacterial action of wood tar is due to its content of phenol derivatives. Currently, the primary use of wood tar in veterinary medicine is for the antiseptic bandaging of wounds of the hoof and horn. Pine tar applied to the hoof will keep it in good texture and reduce the chance of hoof cracks. It is also used in some preparations to treat various skin diseases and to repel biting insects.

Guaiacol, N.F., is the chief phenolic constituent of creosote and is generally available in liquid form, although it occurs as a crystalline solid also. Guaiacol has been employed as guaiacol carbonate and as the water-soluble *Potassium Guaiacol Sulfonate,* N.F. (soluble guaiacol), for expectorant and antitussive activity (see Chapter 43).

TOXICOLOGY OF COAL AND WOOD TAR DERIVATIVES

Local corrosive action of phenol, cresol, and related compounds upon the skin has been mentioned under the discussion of phenol.

Acute systemic poisoning from tar derivatives is occasionally seen in animals. It occurs more in cats than in any other species. Coal or wood tar derivatives must not be used on cats or on objects with which cats might have contact. Mink appear to be similarly affected. Excessive volatilization of coal tar disinfectants in heated, unventilated animal housing may cause severe or fatal respiratory distress and contact burns, e.g., skin and tail sloughs. Adequate ventilation promptly corrects the disorder. Chronic poisoning from wood or coal tar derivatives rarely occurs in animals. It usually results from prolonged absorption following repeated application of the tar derivative, either externally or internally.

Phenol is readily and rapidly absorbed from unbroken skin, wounds, and mucous membranes and is also easily absorbed following internal administration. Phenol compounds are excreted primarily in the urine as conjugated compounds. The vital functions and systems of the body are first stimulated and then depressed, leading to death by respiratory paralysis. The skeletal muscles show slight tremors which enlarge until convulsions are produced.

Chlorinated naphthalenes have been identified as causing bovine hyperkeratosis. The toxicity of the compounds is related to the extent of chlorination. Hexachloronaphthalene and heptachloronaphthalene are more toxic than dichloronaphthalene or trichloronaphthalene. These compounds have been added to some extreme pressure lubricants used in heavy machinery such as that employed for grinding feed for livestock. Small amounts of the lubricant may escape from moving parts of machinery while grinding or mixing feed and be ingested by cattle. As little as 25 g of a lubricant containing 2% hexachloronaphthalene is sufficient when ingested to produce hyperkeratosis in a 200-lb calf (Bell 1953). The chlorinated naphthalenes are obtained from other sources, such as a wood preservative used in Germany. The use of chlorinated naphthalenes has been severely curtailed around livestock and feed mixing equipment since it has been established as the etiologic agent of hyperkeratosis.

Treatment of systemic poisoning from phenolic compounds is symptomatic. Treatment with protein substances such as albumen and milk is indicated in an effort to bind the phenol. The protein should be followed by lavage to empty the stomach and intestine of monogastric animals. Oxygen and respiratory stimulants can be used to treat respiratory enhancement and failure.

HEAVY METALS

The toxic salts of heavy metals react with vital bacterial enzymes to form a complex with protein. This process, known as the oligodynamic effect, is detrimental to the bacterial cell.

Mercurials

ACTION

The antibacterial action of the mercurial compounds has been a controversial point since the introduction of mercuric bichloride by Koch in 1881. Numerous workers have demonstrated that the antibacterial action of the mercurial compounds on the vegetative bacterial cell is primarily bacteriostatic and only slowly bactericidal. Several common mercurial compounds do not kill pathogenic bacteria after being added to the culture medium. When a preparation of bacterial pathogen and a disinfecting concentration of a mercurial compound is injected into a susceptible laboratory animal, a high mortality occurs, indicating that growth is inhibited as long as the mercurial ion is neutralized by serum protein or by thioglycolate of the body tissues; however, as the antibacterial action of the mercurial ion decreases, bacterial growth is free to occur. Antibacterial action is related to the inhibition of essential enzyme activity and the ability of sulfhydryl groups to combine with the ions of inorganic and organic metallic compounds. Unfortunately, the antibacterial reactions are reversible.

The mercurials have little sporicidal activity. Live spores of *Clostridium tetani, Clostridium septicum,* and *Bacillus anthracis* are not killed by 24 hours of exposure to several of the organic and inorganic mercurial compounds.

USES

Mercurial compounds can be used on the skin for their bacteriostatic activity. However, the use of mercurials for surface antisepsis seems unwise when other agents are available that have a bactericidal action in addition to a bacteriostatic effect.

The organic or inorganic mercurials are also unsuitable for disinfection of inanimate objects because the organic debris promptly dissipates their action.

INORGANIC MERCURIALS

Mercuric Bichloride, U.S.P. (mercuric chloride, corrosive sublimate), is a white powdery substance readily soluble in water, giving a colorless solution. The lack of color has led to accidental cases of poisoning through confusion of the solution with water. Mercuric bichloride has sometimes been mistakenly employed for *mercurous chloride* (calomel), an archaic laxative, which is relatively insoluble and nontoxic.

Mercuric bichloride is bacteriostatic in very high dilutions *in vitro.* Its action *in vivo* is limited by protein and sulfur-containing compounds. It corrodes metal, coagulates protein, is nonsporicidal, and is toxic when taken internally or by injection.

The standard concentration employed for use has been 1:1000, which can be prepared by dissolving 1 standard tablet of mercuric bichloride (0.5 g) in 500 ml of water. These tablets are required to contain a coloring agent (usually methylene blue) and must be molded in a six-sided shape resembling a coffin to minimize accidental ingestion. The container of tablets must be identified with a label bearing the word poison.

ORGANIC MERCURIALS

These preparations were synthesized in the search for compounds that were less irritant and less toxic than the inorganic mercurials.

Merbromin, N.F. (Mercurochrome), is a combination of a mercury ion with a dye. It has been largely discarded because of its poor activity and penetrability. Its activity is greatly reduced by the presence of organic matter.

Thimerosal, N.F. (Merthiolate) (Fig. 45.10), contains approximately 49% mercury. The alcohol-acetone-water solution of thimerosal is usually colored with eosin and is an effective skin antiseptic when used in a concentration of 1:1000. It is incompatible with acids, salts of heavy metals, and iodine.

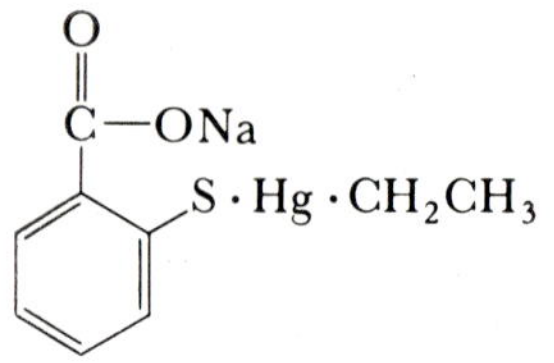

O
C—ONa
S · Hg · CH_2CH_3

Thimerosal

FIG. 45.10.

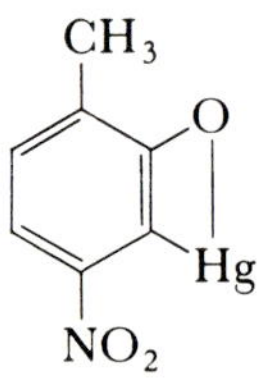

CH_3
O
Hg
NO_2

Nitromersol

FIG. 45.11.

Nitromersol, N.F. (Metaphen) (Fig. 45.11), is a combination of the mercury ion with the cresol radical. Nitromersol is insoluble in water unless the pH is strongly alkaline. It is commonly used as a tincture with 0.5% nitromersol in a solvent containing acetone (10%) and alcohol (50%).

Phenylmercuric Nitrate, N.F. (Merphenyl nitrate, basic) (Fig. 45.12), was one of the first organic mercurial compounds to be produced. Its action is apparently due to the phenylmercuric ion, which is free in solution. It is used as an ointment (1:1500) and as an aqueous solution (1:1500).

SILVER COMPOUNDS

Silver compounds are used in medicine to produce caustic, astringent, and antibacterial effects by the action of the free silver ion. The inorganic silver salts are highly ionized in aqueous solution and exhibit an astringent and caustic action. Colloidal silver preparations are less ionized and are employed for noncorrosive and nonirritant antiseptic action on sensitive tissues.

Silver compounds produce their germicidal effect by complex mechanisms. Metal-

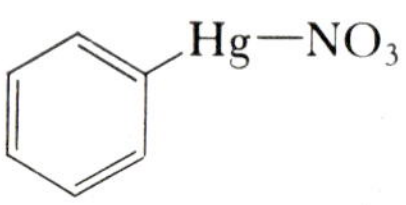

Hg—NO_3

Phenylmercuric Nitrate

FIG. 45.12.

lic silver has powerful oligodynamic action, whereas the simple silver salts ionize to liberate silver ions which immediately precipitate protein and produce an irritant effect. Organic silver preparations liberate silver ions slowly, thus producing a sustained effect.

INORGANIC SILVER SALTS

Silver Nitrate, U.S.P., is a white, crystalline, water-soluble salt that darkens on exposure to light. Aqueous solutions of 1:1000 are strongly antiseptic and somewhat irritant. Indolent ulcers are sometimes treated with this solution to stimulate healing. Silver nitrate may be used as a caustic, antiseptic, or astringent. *Toughened Silver Nitrate,* N.F., is a molded, pencil-shaped stick of silver nitrate called "lunar caustic" or "caustic pencil." The pencil is used for cauterization of small wounds, for treatment of ulcers, and for destruction of the keratinized horn or "nubbin" on the skull of young calves. The cauterized tissue is moistened before the silver nitrate pencil is applied. The cauterized tissue forms a dry scab over healthy tissue lying underneath. Care should be taken to keep calves from getting wet and from the possibility of a strong concentration of silver nitrate getting into the eye. The inorganic silver salts are readily neutralized by chlorides and organic debris. Silver nitrate has been used to cauterize the teat orifice of the dairy cow. This is done to remove constrictions or small amounts of granulation tissues which interfere with milking.

Silver lactate and *picrate* are also ionizable forms employed for the same uses as silver nitrate.

COLLOIDAL SILVER PREPARATIONS

These compounds are nonirritating, nonastringent, noncorrosive, and bacteriostatic. They contain considerable silver, but the metal is strongly attached to protein colloids so that only a slight degree of ionization occurs. They have the advantage of retaining much of their antiseptic activity in the presence of chloride or organic debris.

The colloidal silver compounds are generally used as mild antiseptics on mucous membranes. Although these compounds have limited use in veterinary medicine, they are used more for the antisepsis of the eye than for any other purpose. If applied repeatedly to the skin, they may produce a permanent bluish black discoloration (argyria); particles of colloidal silver deposited in the pores of the skin are reduced by sunlight. The collargol preparations contain about 75% metallic silver stabilized with denatured proteins. They are used in a concentration of 0.02%–1% solution.

ZINC SALTS

The *zinc salts,* e.g., sulfate, chloride, and oxide, are astringents, corrosives, and mild antiseptics. They are frequently used in powders, ointments, and lotions (see Chapter 42).

COPPER

Copper sulfate has astringent, germicidal, and fungicidal activities. In the United Kingdom its antibacterial effect is utilized as an approved feed additive for improving the rate of gain and feed efficiency of swine. It is not approved in the United States because of environmental concerns regarding bioconcentration in soil and surface water.

OXIDIZING AGENTS

Chemicals that release nascent oxygen are useful germicidal compounds. Nascent oxygen combines rapidly with all organic matter and is rendered inactive. It is active against some gram-negative and gram-positive aerobic bacteria. It briefly inhibits the growth of anaerobic organisms but does not destroy bacterial spores in concentrations that are nontoxic to tissues. The duration of germicidal action is very brief.

Hydrogen Peroxide Solution, U.S.P., is a colorless, aqueous solution containing 3% H_2O_2. Hydrogen peroxide liberates free oxygen readily, but the process is particularly rapid when the solution is in contact with mucous membranes or denuded surfaces that provide the enzyme catalase. When hydrogen peroxide is poured into a wound containing exudate, the effervescence of the peroxide in the recesses of the wound is beneficial in mechanically removing pus and cellular debris, as well as in providing limited germicidal activity. Hydrogen peroxide is valuable for cleaning and deodorizing infected tissue.

Potassium Permanganate, U.S.P., occurs as dark purple crystals which are soluble in water to the extent of 1 g in 15 ml. Potassium permanganate liberates oxygen on contact with organic matter. It is a strong oxidizing agent even in high dilution. Solutions of permanganate have a relatively strong antibacterial action although bacteria vary considerably in their susceptibility. Permanganate solutions do not penetrate deeply and have only a superficial action. Depending upon the concentration, solutions are bacteriostatic, astringent, irritant, or caustic. The normal color of an aqueous potassium permanganate solution is deep purple, but on standing it loses stability; if the solution turns a chocolate color, the preparation has lost most of its activity.

Potassium permanganate in a concentration of 0.1% (1:1000) or less may be applied to any of the tissues of the body as a deodorant or as an antiseptic irrigant for removal of exudates from the tissue. Generally, a lower concentration (1:3000) is preferred because of less irritation and resultant proliferation of granulation tissue in wounds. Potassium permanganate will stain.

Potassium permanganate has been recommended for treatment of poisoning with various alkaloids and other substances that can be oxidized. The theory has been that the permanganate would oxidize and thereby destroy the toxic action of the compound in the stomach before it was absorbed. However, permanganate also oxidizes the gastric mucosa, and it has not been shown that the permanganate attacks the alkaloids in preference to the protein-containing mucosal cells. Treatment with potassium permanganate certainly would be less reliable than use of a stomach tube or a gastrointestinal lavage for removal of the poisonous agent. A dilution of 1:5000 potassium permanganate has been used for irrigation of internal structures such as the urinary bladder.

Sodium Perborate, N.F., is a white, crystalline, stable powder. In aqueous solution, sodium perborate decomposes into sodium metaborate and hydrogen peroxide which in turn evolves oxygen. This preparation has been used extensively in the topical treatment of stomatitis, glossitis, and gingivitis. However, it should be used sparingly since repeated applications to mucous membranes may be irritating.

Metal peroxides are compounds in which the hydrogen of hydrogen peroxide has been replaced by metals such as zinc. The metallic peroxides liberate oxygen slowly for 24–48 hours. They differ in action according to their solubility and the alkalinity produced during the reaction. These compounds have not found extensive clinical application. *Medicinal Zinc Peroxide,* U.S.P., probably is the most common representative of this group. It consists of a mixture of zinc peroxide (45%), zinc carbonate, and zinc hydroxide.

DYE COMPOUNDS

Dyes have been employed as antibacterial agents since Ehrlich used them to stain and kill invading bacteria. Since the introduction of more specific chemotherapeutic agents, dyes have been used for their local antiseptic action. They have a remarkable specificity for various types of bacteria. The basic dyes are most active in the basic medium and are specific for gram-positive organisms, whereas the azo dyes which are most active in an acid medium are specific for gram-negative organisms.

Azo Dyes

The azo dyes contain the -N:N- linkage. *Scarlet Red,* N.F. (Biebrich scarlet R, medicinal scarlet red, Sudan IV), is nearly insoluble in water and therefore is used primarily as *Scarlet Red Ointment,* N.F. The latter is a 5% ointment used for stimulating the growth of epithelial cells associated with decubital sores, chronic ulcers, and wounds. *Scarlet Red Sulfonate,* N.N.D., is very similar to scarlet red. Also closely related is *dimazon.* The latter is used primarily as a dusting powder for similar indications. *Pyridium* is an azo dye that has been used as a urinary antiseptic. It is generally administered in a 1% solution by local irrigation of the urethra and the urinary bladder in treatment of cystitis. Many clinicians claim that the irrigation produces more relief by its local anesthetic action than by its antibacterial activity.

Acridine Derivatives

Most of the derivatives of acridine, a coal tar base, are yellow dyes that have been designated as "flavines." *Acriflavine,* N.F. (acriflavine base, neutral acriflavine, neutral Trypaflavine), is a reddish brown, water-soluble powder that was introduced by Ehrlich as a trypanocide. It is used for trichomoniasis in bulls by preputial application.

Acriflavine Hydrochloride, N.F. (Trypaflavine), is employed as a solution. It is slightly irritant due to the acid reaction. *Proflavine Sulfate,* N.F., is a closely related compound active against *Proteus* bacteria particularly and also against some other gram-positive and gram-negative bacteria. The antibacterial action of the dyes is weakened by the presence of serum. These dyes are relatively free from toxicity or irritation and do not inhibit phagocytosis. They are used in a concentration of 1:1000 in physiological saline applied by a cotton swab or as an irrigating fluid. Previous to the introduction of the sulfonamides and antibiotics, acriflavine, 1:1500, was an effective treatment for bovine mastitis.

The antibacterial effectiveness of acridine dyes are antagonized by hypochlorites and should not be used concurrently.

Triphenylmethane

The amino-derivatives of triphenylmethane are rosaniline and pararosaniline. The methyl derivatives constitute a series of basic dyes (*gentian violet, methyl violet, crystal violet,* and *brilliant green*) that are bactericidal for gram-positive bacteria. Gram-negative bacteria are resistant to these compounds.

Methylrosaniline Chloride, U.S.P., is soluble in water and antiseptic when applied to wounds, mucous membranes, burns, ulcerated areas, and moist eczema. *Methylrosaniline Chloride Solution,* U.S.P., a 1% solution in 10% alcohol and *Methylrosaniline Chloride Jelly,* N.F., are used for treatment of burns. Pyoktanin blue ointment made with zinc oxide and a petrolatum base has been widely used for skin lesions occurring around the hoofs, hocks, or shoulders ("shoulder gall") of horses. Pyoktanin in alcoholic solution also has been used for "shoulder gall" and "saddle sores."

Diagnostic Dyes

Fluorescein is a dye used for diagnosis of corneal lesions. A 2% aqueous solution of fluorescein with 3% sodium bicarbonate added will stain ulcerous areas of the cornea green. Only sterile preparations of fluorescein should be used in order to avoid the possibility of infection. A *Pseudomonas* infection of a dog's eye resulted from the use of contaminated fluorescein solutions (Cello and Lasmanis 1959). Fluorescein does not stain healthy tissue and may be applied daily to corneal ulcers in order to follow the course of the lesion. It does not irritate the cornea nor does it have antiseptic action.

Systemic administration of fluorescein has been used to diagnose intraocular inflammation. In the absence of inflammation, the intraocular chamber is clear, although the rest of the body becomes jaundiced within 24 hours. If the intraocular chamber is inflamed, as in iritis or glaucoma, the aqueous humor is colored a bright green. The oral dose for the dog is 0.5–4 g. For diagnosis of periodic ophthalmia in horses, 2 g injected intravenously will give a positive reaction within 5–10 minutes in the presence of disease. *Sodium fluorescein* has largely replaced fluorescein because no alkali is required to put it in solution.

Phenosulfonphthalein (phenol red) may be used to test kidney activity. Most of the dye will be excreted by tubular secretion and to a lesser extent by glomerular filtration. *Sulfobromophthalein sodium* (bromosulfophthalein) may be used by intravenous injection to determine the liver function.

OTHER AGENTS

Formaldehyde Solution, U.S.P., is an aqueous solution containing not less than 37% (usually 40%) formaldehyde gas with variable amounts of methyl alcohol to prevent polymerization. It is commonly known by the trade name of Formalin.

Formaldehyde (Fig. 45.13) is a colorless, markedly irritant and antibacterial gas but is not readily used in the gaseous state. Formaldehyde solution is bactericidal in concentrations of 1%–2% of the gas within a few minutes of exposure. A concentration of 4% by weight of formaldehyde gas in aqueous solution at body temperature will kill anthrax spores within 15 minutes. Formaldehyde solution will also kill the *Mycobacterium tuberculosis* and apparently most of the animal viruses.

Formalin is an excellent and reliable disinfectant. For general disinfection it is best diluted with water to a concentration of about 4% formaldehyde gas. Metal objects may be immersed in the solution for reasonable periods of time without corrosion.

Fumigation of a building may be carried out by placing 35 ml of commercial formaldehyde in a vessel for each 100 cubic feet of space. Potassium permanganate is then added in the proportion of 17.5 g/100 cu ft. A building fumigated in this manner and closed for 65 hours at a temperature of 70° F was found to be free of certain viruses, bacteria, and molds (Hundemann and Holbrook 1959).

A 4% aqueous solution of formaldehyde gas (Formalin diluted with 9 parts

$$H-\overset{\overset{O}{\|}}{C}-CH_2-CH_2-CH_2-\overset{\overset{O}{\|}}{C}-H$$

Formaldehyde

FIG. 45.13.

of water) is commonly used to preserve pathological specimens. Formaldehyde has been used in the production of certain biologics because of its ability to act as a preservative and its detoxifying properties. Such biologics are claimed to have retained their antigenic potency but to have lost their toxic activity. A 4% aqueous solution of formaldehyde may be used to destroy superficial tissue found in ulcerous lesions, malignant growths, and infections about the corium of the hoof and between the claws of the foot.

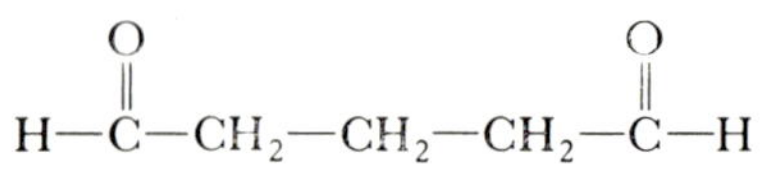

Formaldehyde is used (1) to treat sandy loam soil (5% solution at 20 L/m^2) to destroy anthrax spores and numerous other bacteria; (2) as an aerosol to kill the etiologic agent of avian infectious bronchitis; (3) to destroy avian mycoplasma organisms (40% solution at 15 ml/m^3); (4) to inactive laryngotracheitis and fowl pox and Newcastle viruses; and (5) to disinfect motor vehicles infected with foot-and-mouth disease virus with a 38%–40% formaldehyde aerosol at a temperature greater than 10° C and relative humidity of 60%–90%.

Formaldehyde flakes when mixed with poultry litter, 1%–3% (w/w), reduced mold, bacterial counts, and pH of the litter (Veloso et al. 1974).

As a disinfectant, formaldehyde solution has the following advantages: (1) it has a powerful germicidal action; (2) its action is not appreciably reduced by organic matter; (3) it has a low systemic toxicity although locally is quite corrosive; and (4) it is relatively noncorrosive to metals, paint, and fabric. Formaldehyde solution has certain disadvantages: (1) it gives off a penetrating and irritating gas; (2) prolonged exposure to the vapors must be avoided; and (3) contact with the solution kills the squamous epithelium so that all sensation is lost in the affected parts.

Glutaraldehyde, a saturated dialdehyde, has a high degree of sporicidal activity in alkaline solutions. Solutions of 1% and 2% glutaraldehyde destroy *Bacillus anthracis* spores more rapidly than 4% formaldehyde. Glutaraldehyde has a wide spectrum of antibacterial activity and is active in the presence of organic matter. It is an effective disinfectant for instruments, especially lensed instruments, e.g., cystoscopes, since it does not affect the lens cement. It is noncorrosive, its low surface tension permits easy penetration and washing, and it does not affect cutting edges.

Chlorhexidine hydrochloride (Nolvasan, Hibitane) is a synthetic compound; the chemical formula is 1,1′-hexamethylenebis[5-(*p*-chlorphenyl)biguanide] dihydrochloride. It is alkaline in reaction, slightly soluble in water, and relatively nontoxic. Chlorhexidine is active against a variety of gram-positive and gram-negative bacteria and other microorganisms. It is not appreciably inactivated by small quantities of organic matter such as blood, milk, pus, and tissue fluids. Chlorhexidine is available in a 2% solution, 1 g uterine tablets, 1% ointment, and a suspension containing 1 g chlorhexidine/28 ml of the vehicle. Chlorhexidine has been found useful in disinfection of contaminated equipment and premises, sanitizing udder cloths and milking equipment, and as a topical anti-infective agent for the treatment of wounds. It has been used in various postmilking teat dip studies. The concentration for this purpose ranges from 0.2% to 5% or higher. Sometimes it has been combined with other disinfectants, e.g., surfactants, dyes, and various vehicles such as glycerin. In most reports beneficial results were recorded as measured by the reduced prevalence of new mastitis cases and udder lesions.

Ethylene oxide and *propylene oxide* are gases which have been used for sterilizing laboratory animal feeds for germ-free and specific pathogen-free animals, inactivating viruses in litter and laboratory equipment, and decontaminating foodstuffs for human consumption. Ethylene oxide has been used at a rate of 2 kg/m^3 at a temperature of 25°–27° C with relative humidity of 69%–83% for 2 hours. A mixture of 1 part ethylene oxide and 2.5 parts methyl bromide has been used to inactive *Bacillus anthracis* spores.

Ethylene and propylene oxides are the gases most favored as industrial disinfectants to produce animal foodstuffs free of microbial contaminants, especially salmonellae. Propylene oxide has strong microbicidal properties but poor penetrability. Both propylene and ethylene oxides require dilution with inert gases for safety. Freon and carbon dioxide are used for this purpose. The flammability limits are approximately 2%–22% by volume. Mixing with inert gases can eliminate the flammability hazard. Greater than 800 mg/L are recommended for sterilization.

Polymeric biguanide (formulated with various emollients) is an antibacterial that has been used as a teat dip (Forse et al. 1970). The incorporation of glycerol appeared to control a serious outbreak of pseudo cow pox. Polymeric biguanide inactivated *Staphylococcus aureus* on the skin and appears to have residual action.

Carbon disulfide has been used as a disinfectant for animal quarters at the recommended concentration of 6% applied at the rate of 1–2 L/m^2. It has very limited activity for destroying nematode eggs under use conditions even though satisfactory *in vitro* activity has been observed.

β-Propiolactone, a heterocyclic ring compound, is a colorless, pungent liquid; its vapors have been used for antimicrobial activity, especially sporicidal activity. Best activity is achieved when the relative humidity is greater than 70%.

Hog cholera virus in excreta was killed when mixed with 0.15% propiolactone. Also, porcine enterovirus strain T80 was inactivated by propiolactone (1:2000) following contact for 3 hours at room temperature. Reports of propiolactone's carcinogenic activity and other undesirable physiologic properties have limited its development as a disinfectant. The hydrolysis product, *β-hydroxypropionic acid,* is noncarcinogenic and is safer to handle.

3,5-Dimethyl-1,3,5,2H-tetrahydrothiadiazine-2-thione or Dazomet is a soil fumigant that has demonstrated a lethal effect on salmonellae present in poultry litter (Simmons 1973). The granular form releases the active ingredient slowly and is safe for handling.

Stannous chloride with steam has been

used to treat pork carcasses in an effort to reduce surface bacteria. This combination effectively reduced the population of salmonellae and other bacteria and did not stain the carcasses.

Cottonseed oil has been used in broiler houses to control dust in an attempt to reduce the incidence of *Mycoplasma gallisepticum* infection (Griffin and Vardaman 1970). Dust control was achieved when cottonseed oil was applied at the rate of 0.3–0.6 L/m^2. No beneficial effect was noted on mycoplasmosis control.

GENERAL PRINCIPLES OF DISINFECTION

Since few disinfectants act instantly, ample time must be allowed for their bactericidal effect. As bactericidal agents, most disinfectants seem to act more effectively when applied in solution than as an emulsion, powder, aerosol, or gas because the solutions penetrate to a greater depth. The germicidal activity of disinfectant solutions is greater when they are heated. Hot solutions penetrate manure and other organic debris better than cold solutions.

It is extremely important to remove as much organic matter as practicable from the areas to be disinfected. Manure and debris should be moved to a place inaccessible to livestock and burned if possible. If the refuse cannot be burned, it should be thoroughly treated with a disinfectant.

The ultraviolet rays of direct sunlight are germicidal. The sun's rays and heat destroy most of the pathogenic bacteria in the excreta scattered on farmlands. However, the use of sunlight must be considered only as an accessory aid in the disinfection of animal quarters.

Heat is the most reliable of all agents for disinfection. Where practicable, contaminated materials should be burned. Moist heat is more satisfactory than dry heat because of greater penetration. Boiling in water for 10 minutes will destroy all ordinary disease germs, although it sometimes fails to kill the spores of *Bacillus anthracis* and of the clostridia. Disinfection with moist steam (in the autoclave) is the method most commonly employed in hospitals.

Disinfecting Animal Quarters and Transport Vehicles

The surfaces of buildings or vehicles should be cleaned. Manure and refuse should be removed, burned, or chemically disinfected. A reliable disinfectant should be sprayed on all surfaces. The spray should be applied as hot as possible and with sufficient force to drive the solution into all cracks and crevices.

The general methods of disinfection apply for the disinfection of vehicles. Disinfection of trucks immediately after unloading is of utmost importance in preventing the spread of infection upon departure of the vehicles. Two percent solutions of sodium hydroxide (soda lye, caustic soda), cresol, or saponated cresol solution in hot water are recommended.

Chemical Disinfection of the Hypodermic Syringe and Needle

STERILIZATION

In addition to sterilization of the hypodermic syringe by the autoclave and the hot air oven, dismantled syringes may be sterilized by boiling in antiseptic solutions for 15 minutes. The recommended solutions are: hydrated sodium carbonate, 2%, with or without the addition of 0.1% formaldehyde gas; a 2% solution of a recognized quaternary ammonium compound; and a 1:200,000 solution of phenylmercuric borate.

To prevent rusting of needles, sodium nitrite (0.5%) should be added to all of these solutions. The syringes should be rinsed with sterile distilled water before drawing in the solution to be injected. The rinsing protects against some incompatibility between the disinfectant and the medicament. No adverse reactions have been observed between the disinfectants and epinephrine; procaine; insulin; vitamins A, B, and C; penicillin; or certain hormones. Boiling hypodermic syringes and needles in water or immersion in 76% alcohol (v/v) does not kill certain bacterial spores. In fact, pathogenic spore-producing organisms have been found in alcohol.

STORAGE

When a syringe is to be employed for a series of operations in which the risk of contamination is slight, it is permissible to store the syringe in an antiseptic. Sterile syringes and needles may be stored in the following solutions: (1) 5% formaldehyde gas in 76.5% alcohol (v/v); (2) 5% quaternary ammonium compound with 0.5% sodium nitrite; (3) 2.5% formaldehyde gas with 0.5% liquefied phenol and 1.5% borax; and (4) 1:200,000 phenylmercuric borate with 0.5% sodium nitrite. The addition of 1.5% glycerin to all of these solutions aids in manipulating the syringes. The hypodermic syringe and needle should be immersed in the antiseptic solution for a minimum of 15 minutes. This procedure does not provide absolute sterilization. The syringe and needle must be rinsed thoroughly with sterile water or saline to remove the residual disinfectants that may react with the medications.

Frequently, veterinarians are in need of information on the viricidal activity of drugs.

A list of many disinfectants commonly used to inactivate viruses is as follows:

1. Newcastle disease virus: formaldehyde, Formalin, chloramine, chlorinated lime.

2. Fowl pox: formaldehyde, Formalin, methyl bromide, phenethyl alcohol.

3. Transmissible gastroenteritis virus: formaldehyde, mixture of sodium hydroxide (1%) and sodium hypochlorite (8%).

4. Foot-and-mouth disease virus: formaldehyde, sodium hydroxide, potassium permanganate, hexachlorophenol, sodium hypochlorite.

5. Marek's disease virus: formaldehyde, phenol, cresylic acid, chlorine-yielding compounds, sodium hydroxide.

6. Myxoviruses and arboviruses: phenethyl alcohol.

7. Infectious laryngotracheitis virus: benzalkonium chloride.

8. African swine fever: *o*-phenylphenol.

The conditions under which the above compounds were tested as viricides varied considerably, ranging from sealed chambers under pressure to crude livestock or poultry buildings. In most cases, the highest concentrations of the manufacturers' recommendations were used. The general principles for the effective use of bactericides, e.g., removal of organic matter, use of hot solutions, etc., are similar for the effective use of viricides.

Disinfectants are also used to help control parasite problems; a summary of the information published during the past 10 years is as follows:

1. Anticoccidial
   a. Methyl bromide (100 g/m^3 for 24 hours)
   b. Chlorocresol-paraffin sulfonate (3%) and carbon disulfide
2. Ovicidal
   a. Toxascaris and ascarids: orthochlorophenol (5%)
   b. Ascarids and parascaris: hot (75° C) sodium hydroxide (5%) or carbon disulfide
   c. *Metastrongylus* spp.: orthochlorophenol[1] (1%–3%)
   d. *Oesophagostomum* sp.: methyldithiocarbamate[1] (2%–5%)

REFERENCES

Armstrong, J. A., and Froelich, E. J. 1964. Inactivation of viruses by benzalkonium chloride. Appl Microbiol 12:132.

Ayres, J. C. 1967. Sanitation practices in egg handling and breaking plants and the application of several disinfectants for sanitizing eggs. J Appl Bact 30:106.

Belák, S., and Kisary, J. 1974. Viricidal effect of four disinfectants. Magy Allatorv Lapja 29:4.

Bell, W. B. 1953. The relative toxicity of chlorinated naphthalenes in experimentally

[1] Orthochlorophenol and methyldithiocarbamate also demonstrated larvicidal activity.

produced bovine hyperkeratosis (x-disease). Vet Med 48:135.

Brown, W. E., and Kolb, G. E. 1974. Antibiotic disinfection compatibility studies in solution used for dipping turkey hatching eggs. Poult Sci 53:10.

Cello, R. M., and Lasmanis, J. 1959. *Pseudomonas* infection of the eye of the dog resulting from the use of contaminated fluorescein solution. J Am Vet Med Assoc 132:297.

Clegg, L. F. L. 1967. Disinfectants in the dairy industry. J Appl Bacteriol 30:117.

Davis, J. G. 1962. Iodophors as detergent-sterilizers. J Appl Bacteriol 25:195.

Derbyshire, J. B., and Arkell, S. 1971. The activity of some chemical disinfectants against Talfan virus and porcine adenovirus type 2. Br Vet J 127:137.

Darmady, E. M.; Hughes, K. E. A.; Drewett, S. E.; Prince, D.; Tuke, W.; and Verdon, P. 1965. The cleaning of instruments and syringes. J Clin Pathol 18:6.

Feagan, J. T.; Hehir, A. F.; and White, B. R. 1970. The effectiveness in control of mastitis of iodine as a post-milking teat dip. Aust J Dairy Technol 25:87.

Forse, S. F.; Hall, R.; Jackson, P. S.; and Sandae, J. 1970. Evaluation of teat-dipping formulations containing a germicidal polymeric biguanide. Vet Rec 86:506.

Frederick, G. L. 1963. Note on prophylaxis of post-catheterization urinary tract infections. Can J Anim Sci 43:385.

Griffin, J. G., and Vardaman, T. H. 1970. Cottonseed oil spray for broiler houses: Effects on dust control, *Mycoplasma gallisepticum* spread and broiler performance. Poult Sci 49:1664.

Huckle, J. J. 1965. A new approach to mastitis control. Vet Med 60:532.

Hundemann, A. S., and Holbrook, A. A. 1959. A practical method for decontamination of microbiologic laboratories by the use of formaldehyde gas. J Am Vet Med Assoc 135:549.

Iwarsson, K., and Ekman, L. 1973. The effect of a post-milking teat dip on the iodine concentration of bulk herd milk. Acta Vet Scand 14:338.

Kirchhoff, H. 1968. Action of quaternary ammonium compounds on Newcastle disease and parainfluenza viruses. Dtsch Tieraerztl Wochenschr 75:160.

Klein, M., and De Forest, A. 1963. The inactivation of viruses by germicides. Chem Specialties Mfrs Assoc Proc 49:116.

Koritz, G. D. 1975. Personal communication.

Mansi, W., and Lakin, C. N. S. 1968. *In vitro* activity of povidone-iodine using *Brucella abortus* (Strain 19) as the test organism. Vet Rec 82:444.

Mellor, D. B., and Banwart, G. J. 1965. Recovery of *Salmonella derby* from inoculated egg shell surfaces following sanitizing. Poult Sci 44:1244.

Merkal, R. S., and Thurston, J. R. 1968. Susceptibilities of mycobacterial and nocardial species to benzalkonium chloride. Am J Vet Res 29:759.

Natzke, R. P., and Bray, D. R. 1972. Teat dip comparisons. J Dairy Sci 56:148.

Plummet, A. M., and Plummet, M. 1974. Destruction by xylene of various pathogenic bacteria in liquid manure of cattle. Ann Rech Vet 5:213.

Price, P. B. 1950. The meaning of bacteriostasis, bactericidal effect, and rate of disinfection. Ann NY Acad Sci 53:76.

———. 1951. Fallacy of a current surgical fad—The three-minute preoperative scrub with hexachlorophene soap. Ann Surg 134:476.

———. 1957. Antiseptics, Disinfectants, Fungicides, Chemical and Physical Sterilization. Philadelphia: Lea & Febiger.

———. 1966. Local antiseptics. In W. Model, ed. Drugs of Choice 1966–1967, p. 133. St. Louis: C. V. Mosby.

Price, P. B., and Bonnett, A. 1948. Antibacterial effects of G-5, G-11, and A-151, with special reference to their use in production of germicidal soap. Ann Surg 24:542.

Price, W. J.; Bowen, J. M.; and Wooley, R. E. 1968. Efficacy of ethyl alcohol in reducing canine and bovine cutaneous bacterial flora. J Am Vet Med Assoc 152:990.

Reuber, H. W.; Rude, T. A.; and Jorgenson, T. A. 1970. Safety evaluation of a quaternary ammonium sanitizer for turkey drinking water. Avian Dis 14:211.

Rizk, S. S.; Ayres, J. C.; and Kraft, A. A. 1966. Disinfection of eggs artificially inoculated with Salmonellae. Poult Sci 45:764.

Schjerning-Thiesen, K. 1972. The inactivating effect of a mixture of sodium chloride and sodium carbonate on foot-and-mouth disease virus on ox hides. Bull Off Int Epizoot 77:1125.

Schultze, W. D., and Smith, W. D. 1971. Effectiveness of postmilking teat dips. J Dairy Sci 55:426.

Serrano, L. J. 1972. Dermatitis and death in mice accidentally exposed to quaternary ammonium disinfectant. J Am Vet Med Assoc 161:652.

Simmons, G. C. 1973. Use of Dazomet as a

poultry litter fumigant for salmonellas. Aust Vet J 49:268.

Veloso, J. R.; Hamilton, P. B.; and Parkhurst, C. R. 1974. Use of formaldehyde flakes as an antimicrobial agent in built-up poultry litter. Poult Sci 53:78.

Walkowiak, E.; Alina, W.; and Aleksandrowska, I. 1969. Bactericidal activity of chloramine, sterinol, laurosept, and caustic soda in slaughter houses. Med Wer 71:176.

Walter, J. E., and Coffee, E. G. 1968. Control of *Cryptococcus neoformans* in pigeon coops by alkalinization. Am J Epidemiol 87:173.

Wright, H. S. 1970. Test method for determining the viricidal activity of disinfectants against vesicular stomatitis virus. Appl Microbiol 19:92.

CHAPTER 46

SULFONAMIDES

RICHARD F. BEVILL and
WILLIAM G. HUBER

The era of modern chemotherapy was ushered in following Gerhard Domagk's announcement in 1935 that Prontosil protected mice from experimental streptococcal infection. Events preceding the development of this drug began in 1910 when Paul Ehrlich synthesized arsphenamine, an antisyphilitic agent.

Ehrlich postulated the existence of chemoreceptors, developed a chemotherapeutic index, and modified chemical structures to obtain drugs having a selective toxicity for pathogens. In his work with arsonic acids, he recognized that the metabolic conversion of arsenic from the pentavalent to the trivalent state was a prerequisite to chemotherapeutic effectiveness and indicated the need for *in vivo* as well as *in vitro* drug testing.

Ehrlich, recognized as the Father of Chemotherapy, died in 1915. During the 20 years following his death, new mechanisms of drug action did not appear in the literature. His success in synthesizing chemotherapeutic dyes influenced the activities of a generation of chemists and bacteriologists since dyes remained the major class of chemicals examined for chemotherapeutic activity.

Several dyestuffs were tested in the period preceding the synthesis of Prontosil. In 1919, two investigators tested the coupling product of dihydrocupreine and *p*-aminobenzenesulfonamide. Unfortunately, this product lacked antibacterial activity, and its cleavage products were not investigated. Such studies could have led to the antibacterial activity of sulfanilamide 15 years prior to its discovery by French scientists. Although most investigators ignored Ehrlich's statements concerning the need for *in vivo* testing, Mietzsch, Klarer, and Domagk conducted *in vivo* tests on a large series of dyestuffs containing the sulfonamide (SO_2NH_2) group. During these investigations, the antibacterial activity of Prontosil, an azo dye containing the *p*-aminobenzenesulfonamide group, was demonstrated.

Later, scientists at the Pasteur Institute learned that Prontosil was excreted as a colorless product in the urine of animals receiving the dye. Subsequent studies revealed that acetylsulfanilamide was a major urinary excretion product of the dye. Previously, workers had demonstrated that aromatic amines were excreted as acetyl derivatives following their administration to animals. Pure sulfanilamide proved to be a potent antibacterial substance when administered to mice inoculated with otherwise lethal doses of bacteria.

The synthesis of sulfanilamide had been reported by Gelmo in 1908. Restrictive patents governing the production of Prontosil were essentially negated since production of the active portion of the drug was not protected by patent. During the next few years, over 5000 derivatives of sulfanilamide were synthesized and tested for antibacterial activity. Today, less than 30 of these compounds are used as clinically effective drugs.

Since their discovery, the sulfonamides have found varied use. Prior to the discovery of penicillin and other antibiotics, they were the mainstay of bacterial chemotherapy. Sulfonamides are still widely used for the treatment of diseases caused by sulfonamide-sensitive bacteria and as animal feed additives.

CHEMISTRY

Sulfanilamide, the amide of sulfanilic acid (*p*-aminobenzenesulfonic acid), and its derivatives are commonly known as sulfonamides or "sulfa drugs." As indicated in Fig. 46.1, the sulfonamide (SO_2NH_2) nitrogen has been designated N^1, and the amino nitrogen N^4.

Most antibacterial sulfonamides have been synthesized by chemical substitution at the N^1 position. Compounds resulting from substitution at N^4 have greatly reduced antibacterial activity when compared to their unsubstituted counterparts. However, certain N^4-substituted sulfonamides designed to provide antibacterial action within the lumen of the gastrointestinal tract are exceptions.

As a class, the sulfonamides are white crystalline powders that are relatively insoluble in water. They exhibit amphoteric behavior and form salts in strongly acidic or basic solutions. Their behavior as acids in basic solutions occurs as a result of proton donation at N^1. The pK_a for sufonamides of therapeutic interest ranges from 4.79 to 8.56. Although their action as bases in acidic solution is due to proton acceptance at N^4, it does not occur in the range of physiologic pH due to the weak basic character of the amino group. In general, sulfonamides behave as weak organic acids.

The sodium sulfonamide salts have greater water solubility than the parent compounds and are commonly included in commercial preparations. Sulfathiazole exemplifies the increased solubility one may expect when sodium salts are formed. The solubility of this drug in water is 300

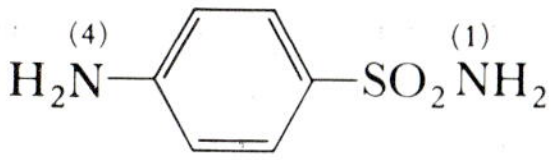

(4) H_2N—[benzene ring]—SO_2NH_2 (1)

Sulfanilamide

FIG. 46.1.

mg/100 ml whereas the solubility of the corresponding sodium salt is 40 g/100 ml. The N^4-acetylated sulfonamides, with the exception of those formed by the pyrimidine sulfonamides (sulfamerazine, sulfamethazine, sulfadiazine), are less soluble than their nonacetylated forms.

Lehr (1945) demonstrated that the solubility of a particular sulfonamide is not influenced by the presence of other sulfonamides in the same solution. Often referred to as the Law of Independent Solubility, this observation has important clinical implications which are discussed in detail later in the chapter.

The structural characteristics of sulfonamides in current use are illustrated in Fig. 46.2.

ANTIBACTERIAL ACTION

Experiments with sulfonamides *in vitro* have demonstrated they are bacteriostatic rather than bacteriocidal. When bacterial cultures whose growth has been inhibited by sulfonamides are transferred to a medium free of sulfonamides, bacterial cell division resumes. The bacteriostatic action of the sulfonamides is not immediately observed when the compounds are incorporated into the culture medium supporting sensitive bacterial populations. Several cell divisions may occur before bacteriostasis becomes evident. Similar patterns of growth inhibition were noted when diseased animals were treated. The time interval between sufonamide addition and bacteriostasis is often termed the "lag phase." During this interval, it appears that certain key metabolic intermediates required for bacterial cell growth and division are depleted as a result of sulfonamide action.

Woods (1940) and Fildes (1940) postulated that many chemotherapeutic agents produce their action through effects on essential bacterial metabolites. Woods noted that sulfanilamide was structurally similar to *p*-aminobenzoic acid (PABA) and postulated that it competed with PABA for a critical enzymatic site. Inhibition of bacterial growth resulted from reduced activity effected by the sulfonamide-bound enzyme.

Although other theories concerning the antibacterial activity of sulfonamides were advanced, the Woods-Fildes theory was strengthened by the discovery of folic acid, which contained PABA as a portion of its molecular structure. Further investigations revealed that the enzyme-catalyzed condensation of PABA and 2-amino-4-hydroxytetrahydropteridine, a necessary step in the synthesis of folic acid, was inhibited by the presence of sulfonamides. The competitive nature of this inhibition was demonstrated when increasing concentrations of PABA decreased the effect of sulfonamides.

Sulfonamide-sensitive bacteria are unable to utilize a preformed source of folic acid. Bacteria that do not require folic acid for growth or can utilize preformed folic acid are resistant to the antibacterial effects of sulfonamides.

Animals cells have an absolute requirement for preformed folic acid. The lack of folic acid synthesis in the animal host may explain the therapeutic success obtained with sulfonamides, since the drugs selectively inhibit bacterial synthesis of folic acid without producing concomitant effects in host tissue.

Role of Host Defense Mechanisms

The successful treatment of bacterial infections with sulfonamides is dependent on the presence of a sensitive bacterial population, adequate concentrations of the drug in blood and tissues to effect bacteriostasis, and the cellular and humoral defense mechanisms of the host. Active phagocytosis is required for the ultimate removal of infective organisms. Clinically, the sulfonamides have proved most effective when administered during the acute infective stages as bacterial cells are incorporating sizable quantities of exogenous nutrients into bacterial protoplasm. During this period, the cellular and humoral defense mechanisms of the host are mobilized and act in concert with the bacteriostatic action of sulfonamides. Sulfonamide therapy, in the presence of active sulfonamide bacteriostasis, is generally unproductive in

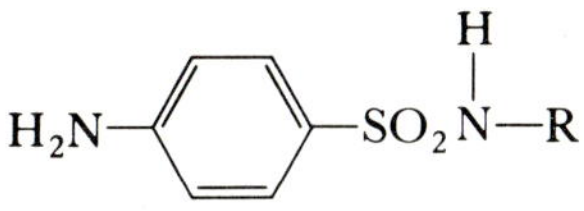

$H_2N-C_6H_4-SO_2N(H)-R$

(Parent Sulfonamide Nucleus)

SULFONAMIDE	R GROUP
SULFADIAZINE	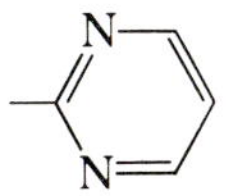 N, N
SULFAMERAZINE	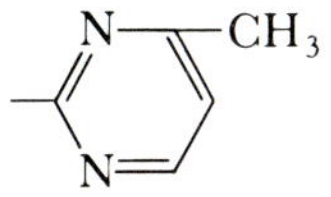 N, N, CH_3
SULFAMETHAZINE	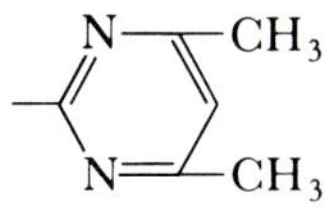 N, N, CH_3, CH_3
SULFABROMETHAZINE	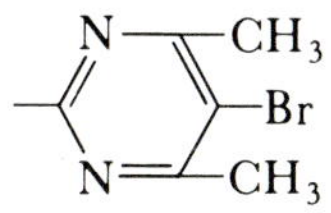 N, N, CH_3, Br, CH_3
SULFATHIAZOLE	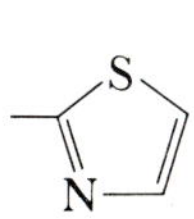 S, N
SULFISOXAZOLE	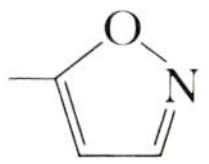 O, N
SULFADIMETHOXINE	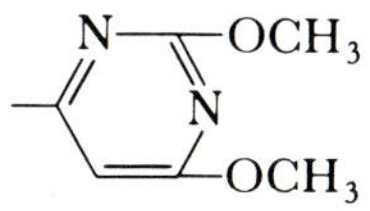 N, N, OCH_3, OCH_3
SULFAMETHOXYPYRIDAZINE	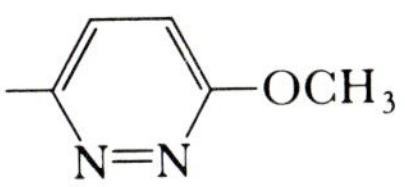 N=N, OCH_3
SULFAETHOXYPYRDAZINE	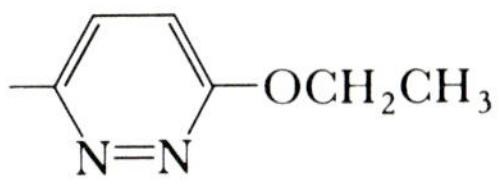 N=N, OCH_2CH_3
SULFACETAMIDE	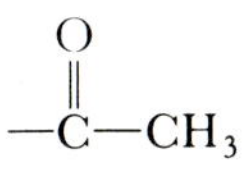 $-C(=O)-CH_3$

Fig. 46.2.

those situations (e.g., chronic disease states) in which phagocytosis occurs at a rate insufficient to clear inhibited bacterial cells from blood and tissue fluid.

Bacterial Resistance to Sulfonamides

Acquired bacterial resistance to sulfonamide action was reported a few years after the introduction of sulfanilamide. Numerous other reports indicate an initially sensitive organism could become resistant to sulfonamide action as a result of successive drug exposure.

Resistance may develop in a previously sensitive population as a result of enzyme adaptation, selection, or R factor–mediated infectious drug resistance. Resistance produced by enzyme adaptation occurs rapidly in the absence of cell division. In this situation, an alternate enzyme pathway is used by the bacterial cell. Resistance through selection is a slow process; it requires the selection of bacterial variants having enzymatic pathways that are distinctly different from their parents. R factor–mediated resistance, a recognized phenomenon of great concern, occurs through the transfer of extrachromosomal DNA between various gram negative organisms (Watanabe 1967). Regardless of the method of resistance development, the resultant alterations in enzyme activity cause an increased synthesis of PABA of sufficient magnitude to effectively antagonize the action of sulfonamides.

Acquired resistance to a specific sulfonamide is generally associated with cross resistance to all sulfonamides. Fortunately, this cross resistance does not extend to other classes of antimicrobial agents. Bacteria resistant to the actions of sulfonamides may be controlled with antibiotics. Recommended countermeasures to minimize the occurrence of acquired bacterial resistance include (Weinstein 1970):

1. Avoid promiscuous use of sulfonamides.
2. Initiate therapy with sulfonamides as early in the course of an acute infection as practicable.
3. Establish and maintain bacteriostatic concentrations of the drug in the animal host.

Correlation of *in vivo* and *in vitro* Sensitivity Testing

Tests to determine the relationship between the *in vivo* and *in vitro* activity of sulfonamides revealed little more than a crude qualitative correlation of the two (Niepp 1964). As a rule, *in vitro* tests give a general impression of the antibacterial spectrum but are not a satisfactory method of choosing the best dose for clinical use. In almost every instance, higher concentrations of sulfonamide are required for successful therapy of the host than are predicted by *in vitro* sensitivity tests. Some sulfonamides had marked *in vitro* antibacterial activity but were completely inactive when tested *in vivo* (Eisman et al. 1952).

Discrepancies between *in vitro* and *in vivo* tests are not surprising in view of the large number of variables encountered in either mode of testing. These include variability in the sensitivity of various test organisms, size of inoculum, and magnitude of the test dose. In general, the observed differences in the *in vivo* potency of sulfonamides against susceptible bacteria are not sufficiently great to warrant *in vitro* test of the organism against more than one sulfonamide. Once the susceptibility of the organism to sulfonamides has been established, rational selection of individual drugs should be based upon the unique pharmacological and toxicological properties of a given sulfonamide in the involved species.

SYNERGISTS OF SULFONAMIDE ACTIVITY

Tetrahydrofolic acid, the biologically active form of folic acid, plays an important role in bacterial purine and pyrimidine synthesis. The reduction of folic acid to tetrahydrofolic acid is catalyzed by tetrahydrofolic reductase. Certain 2,4-diaminopyrimidine (DAP) derivatives have a marked affinity for bacterial tetrahydrofolic reductase.

TABLE 46.1. Diseases treated with sulfonamides

Etiologic Agent	Disease
Actinobacillus lignieresi	Actinobacillosis
Actinomyces bovis	Actinomycoses
Coccidia	Coccidiosis
Corynebacterium pyogenes	Mastitis
Erlichia canis	Canine erlichiosis
Escherichia coli	Colibacillosis
Fusiformis necrophorus	Oral necrobacillosis, infectious foot rot, necrotic rhinitis
Haemophilus suis	Infectious polyarthritis
Klebsiella spp	Mastitis
Moraxella bovis	Infectious keratitis
Neorickettsia helminthoeca	Salmon poisoning
Pasteurella hemolytica	Pneumonia, mastitis
Pasteurella multocida	Respiratory infections
Salmonella spp	Salmonellosis
Staphylococcus aureus	Mastitis
Streptococcus equi	Strangles
Toxoplasma gondii	Toxoplasmosis

When trimethoprim or other DAP derivatives (e.g., *o*-methoprim) are administered with sulfonamides, they inhibit the formation (sulfonamides) and reduction (DAP) of bacterial folic acid. The sequential blockade effected by the drug combination produces an antibacterial action that is greater than the summated activities of the individual compounds. Combinations of sulfonamides and DAP derivatives are finding limited but ever-increasing uses in veterinary therapeutics. (See Table 46.1.)

ABSORPTION

The absorption of a sulfonamide, the passage of the drug from its site of administration to the blood, is governed by passive diffusion. The absorption rate of the solubilized drug is influenced by several factors, including the ionization state and lipophilicity of the drug, the vascularity of the absorption site, and the extent to which the drug is bound to material present at the site of administration. The absorptive process and the factors influencing its rate must be considered when sulfonamides are provided by oral, intramuscular, subcutaneous, or intraperitoneal routes of administration. Although sulfonamides may be absorbed following topical or intrauterine application, such uses are normally intended for local effect and their action is relatively independent of the absorptive process. When sulfonamides are administered intravenously, the total dose of drug is available for immediate distribution within the fluids and tissues of the animal.

Sulfonamides are commonly administered *per os*. In general, sulfonamides administered orally in solution or as a rapidly disintegrating bolus (solid dosage form) undergo rapid absorption from the gastrointestinal tract of monogastric and ruminant species. The so-called enteric sulfonamides (succinylsulfathiazole, phthalylsulfathiazole, and sulfaguanidine) are exceptions to the rule. The effects of age, dosage form, species, and environment on the absorption of sulfonamides following their oral administration have been noted. Sodium sulfathiazole was absorbed rapidly when it was administered to swine as an oral solution ($t_{1/2A} = 0.7$ hours). However, the drug was absorbed more slowly when administered to cattle ($t_{1/2A} = 10.3$ hours) and sheep ($t_{1/2A} = 26$ hours) in an identical manner (Koritz 1975).

When sulfathiazole was administered in a bolus to calves ranging in age from 1 to 16 weeks, the younger animals absorbed the drug more rapidly (Jones 1947).

Water deprivation and forced exercise influenced the absorption of sulfaethoxypyridazine from the gastrointestinal tract of calves (Heath and Teske 1973). Water deprivation decreased the absorption rate of the drug while forced exercise increased the rate of absorption.

The bioavailability and rate of absorption of sulfamethazine varied markedly when administered to healthy calves in several dosage forms. The drug was absorbed rapidly from oral solutions and rapidly disintegrating boluses but was absorbed more slowly when administered in a sustained release bolus. The dissolution of the sustained release bolus was the rate-limiting factor governing the absorption of sulfamethazine. The bioavailability of the drug in an oral solution, a rapidly disintegrating bolus, and a sustained release bolus was determined by comparing the relative area under the respective plasma concentration–time curves to that obtained when the drug was administered intravenously. The bioavailability of the drug in oral solution, rapidly disintegrating bolus, and sustained release bolus was 94%, 78%, and 43%, respectively (Dittert and Bourne 1975).

The absorption of sulfonamides by diseased animals may be quite different from that observed in healthy individuals of the same species. Experimental rumen stasis, produced with atropine, markedly reduced the absorption of sulfamethazine following its oral administration to sheep (Bischop et al. 1973).

The palatability of the preparation must be considered when administering sulfonamides in animals' drinking water. Although palatability has no direct effect on the processes governing drug absorption. it does influence water consumption and the amount of drug undergoing absorption at any given time. Unpalatable preparations will limit the amount of drug available for distribution and may be expected to produce subtherapeutic concentrations of the drug in blood and tissue fluids.

DISTRIBUTION

Once sulfonamides have been absorbed, they undergo rapid mixing in the bloodstream. The subsequent movement of these drugs into other biological fluids and tissues is influenced by the ionization state of the sulfonamide, the vascularity of specific tissues, the presence of specific barriers to sulfonamide diffusion, and the fraction of the administered dose bound to plasma proteins.

Distribution of sulfonamides into various tissues and fluids occurs as a result of passive diffusion. In the absence of active transport processes or ion-trapping phenomena, the concentration of sulfonamides in various fluids and tissues is a reflection of the rate at which the drug equilibrates between blood and other body components.

A variable fraction of a sulfonamide in blood is bound to plasma proteins, primarily albumin. Protein-bound sulfonamides are not bacteriostatic and do not pass from the blood to other extracellular fluids. However, the unbound drug fraction is freely diffusible. The ionization state of a sulfonamide has a profound influence upon further distribution once the drug has crossed the capillary endothelium. Unbound, nonionized drugs usually cross biological membranes more rapidly than their bound or ionized forms.

Eventually, a dynamic equilibrium is established between the sulfonamide in blood, other extracellular fluids, and intracellular fluids. The rate at which such an equilibrium is established is dependent upon the blood supply to specific tissues. Plasma-tissue equilibrium is established more rapidly in highly vascularized tissues. A consistent relationship exists between the concentration of a sulfonamide in plasma and that present in a specific tissue (Sharma 1975). Recent studies involving the intravenous administration of sulfathiazole to sheep reveal that the drug has a similar disappearance half-life in tissues and plasma (Bevill 1975). The parallelism exhibited by the plasma disappearance, urinary excretion, and tissue disappearance curves indicates the loss of drug from each tissue sampled was accurately reflected by the disappearance of the drug from plasma. The concentrations of sulfathiazole in tissues at specific postdosing times were consistently lower than those observed in plasma.

The blood-brain barrier is permeable to the nonionized fraction of unbound sulfonamides. As a result, the concentration of these compounds in cerebrospinal fluid is equivalent to the concentration of the unbound and nonionized drug in blood.

Sulfonamides are found in the milk of dairy cattle following their intravenous or oral administration but do not achieve sufficient concentrations in milk to be useful in the treatment of mastitis (Maclay and Slavin 1947). Sulfonamides are distributed between plasma and milk by passive diffusion of their unbound, nonionized forms (Sisodia and Stowe 1964).

Following the parenteral administration of sulfathiazole and sulfamethazine, the drugs were found in jejunal and colonic contents in concentrations approximating those present in blood (Dalgaard-Mikkelsen et al. 1953). Such behavior may be due to the passive diffusion of the drugs across the intestinal mucosa or to the limited secretion of the drug in intestinal juices or bile.

METABOLISM

Sulfonamides undergo numerous structural alterations during their sojourn in the animal body. Acetylation, oxidation, conjugation with sulfate or glucuronic acid, and the cleavage of their heterocyclic rings have been reported. The metabolism of sulfamethazine following its administration to cattle (Fig. 46.3) illustrates the varied processes involved in sulfonamide metabolism (Nielsen 1973).

The extent to which a sulfonamide is acetylated depends upon the drug administered as well as the recipient species. Ace-

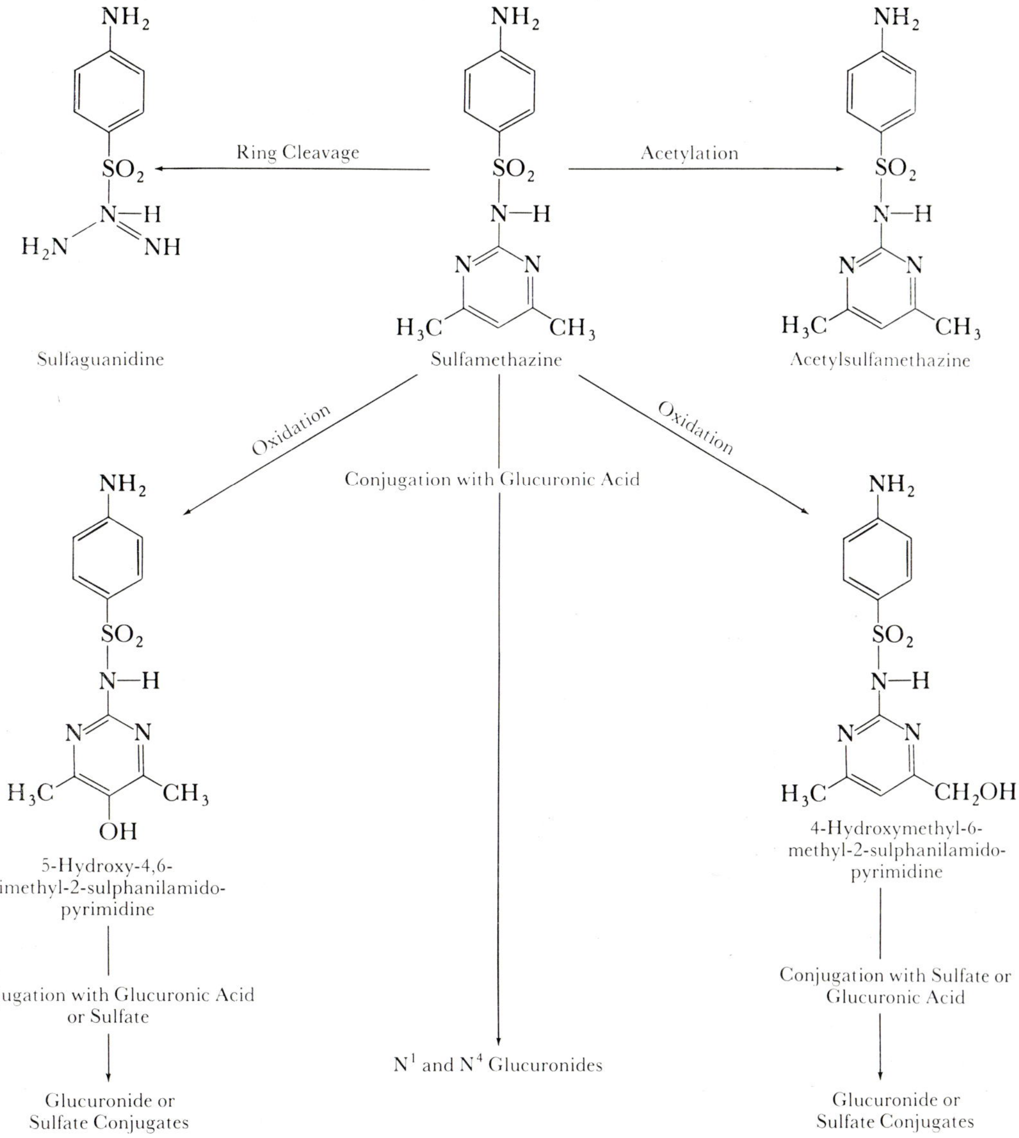

FIG. 46.3.

tylsulfathiazole is the principal metabolite found in the urine of swine, sheep, and cattle following enteral or parenteral administration of sulfathiazole. Sheep acetylate a lower percentage of the dose (10%) than do cattle (32%) or swine (39%). When sulfamethazine was administered intravenously to sheep, 8% of the dose was excreted in the urine as an acetylated metabolite, 24% as polar derivatives (glucuronide and sulfate conjugates), 18% as a hydroxylated derivative, and 22% as sulfamethazine.

When sulfamethazine was administered intravenously to cattle, the animals eliminated 11% of the dose in urine as N^4-acetylsulfamethazine. When the drug was administered orally to cattle, 25% of the dose appeared in the urine as N^4-acetylsulfamethazine. The increased acetylation which occurred following the oral administration of the drug may be related to the increased exposure of sulfamethazine to liver enzymes following absorption into the portal circulation.

The oxidation of the benzene and heterocyclic rings of sulfonamides is an important metabolic pathway in certain species. As illustrated in Fig. 46.3, the hydroxylation of the pyrimidine ring of sulfamethazine or its methyl substituents occurs when the drug is administered to cattle or sheep. Sheep eliminate 25% of an intravenous dose of sulfamethazine as 4-hydroxymethyl-6-methyl-2-sulfanilamidopyrimidine, while cattle eliminate 12% of an intravenous dose in this form. Swine are apparently unable to hydroxylate the drug, as no hydroxylated metabolites appear in swine urine following oral or intravenous administration of the compound.

Sulfonamides and their metabolites are often conjugated with glucuronic acid and sulfates. Conjugation commonly occurs at sites of previous hydroxylation (benzene ring, heterocyclic ring, or aliphatic constituents of heterocyclic rings) or at the N^1 or N^4 positions. The amount of drug eliminated in the urine as glucuronides or sulfates is dependent upon the sulfonamide administered and the species to which the drug is given.

Ring cleavage appears to be a metabolic pathway of minor importance in most animals as only small amounts of cleavage products are excreted in the urine.

The metabolism of sulfonamides is important because it affects the antibacterial activity and toxicity of the compounds. In general, the acetylated, hydroxylated, and conjugated forms of the sulfonamides exhibit a marked decrease in antibacterial activity when compared to their parent compounds. Acetylation reduces the solubility of a sulfonamide (the sulfapyrimidines are an exception) and increases the chance for renal damage by the compound. Usually, hydroxylated and conjugated metabolites are more soluble than the unchanged sulfonamide. These molecular forms are less likely to precipitate in renal tissues but represent a pathway where an antibacterially active drug can be removed more rapidly from the blood and tissues and excreted in urine.

EXCRETION

Following their absorption, distribution, and in some cases metabolic transformation, sulfonamides are eliminated in urine, feces, bile, milk, sweat, and tears. However, the kidney is the organ primarily involved in the excretion of these drugs. Thus the rate of sulfonamide excretion is determined primarily by the net consequences of glomerular filtration, renal tubular reabsorption, and active tubular secretion. All sulfonamides existing in an ultrafilterable state in plasma are filtered from the blood at the renal glomerulus. The rate of filtration is proportional to the concentration of unbound drug in the blood.

The renal tubular epithelium behaves as a lipoid boundary which permits the passive diffusion of nonionized sulfonamides or sulfonamide metabolites from the tubular lumen to the peritubular fluids and eventually to the blood. The amount of a sulfonamide available for reabsorption (nonionized form) by passive diffusion is dependent on the pH of fluids within the tubular lumen. Tubular fluids having a pH less than the pK_a of the sulfonamide favor the formation of nonionized forms and facilitate reabsorption of the drug. Tubular fluids having a pH greater than the pK_a of the sulfonamide favor drug ionization and decrease the amount of drug reabsorbed. The plasma disappearance half-life of certain sulfonamides administered to dogs, calves, and pigs was increased when the urine was acidified (Baggot 1968). The increased persistence of the drug in the body was attributed to renal processes of reabsorption which recycled filtered drug back into the blood. Increased rates of urine flow decrease the concentration of the nonionized diffusible drug in tubular fluid (dilution effect) and decrease the rate of sulfonamide reabsorption. Many long-acting sulfonamides are highly lipid soluble and undergo extensive reabsorption from the renal tubules.

Certain sulfonamides are secreted into renal tubular fluids by means of an active tubular secretory process (Dalgaard-Mikkelsen and Poulsen 1956). Saturation of the transport process occurs when elevated blood concentrations of sulfonamides exist. Substrate specificity within the transport system is dependent upon the SO_2N^- intramolecular sequence of the sulfonamide. Tubular secretion of sulfathiazole occurs in the horse; other reports indicate the drug evidences similar behavior in swine and cattle (Knudsen 1960). Acetylsulfathiazole undergoes tubular secretion in most species. Sulfamethomidene (Lee and Kaersgaard 1967), sulfamethazine, sulfadimethoxine, sulfamethoxazole (Jorgensen and Rasmussen 1972), and sulfamethylphenazole are also eliminated from the body of various species by an active tubular secretory process.

The importance of the kidney with regard to its influence on the duration of effective sulfonamide concentrations in body fluids cannot be overemphasized. Although all sulfonamides are filtered at the renal glomerulus, it is the degree of tubular reabsorption and/or tubular secretion that primarily influences the time course of drug action. During recent years, the primary thrust of sulfonamide development has been the production of heterocyclic sulfonamide derivatives having a high lipid solubility, which enhances their subsequent reabsorption from renal tubular fluids.

BLOOD CONCENTRATIONS

The efficacy of a sulfonamide can be correlated to some extent with the concentration of the drug in blood. Elevated blood concentrations of sulfonamides may produce toxic effects while lower concentrations may yield an unsatisfactory clinical response. Blood concentrations between 5 and 15 mg/dl are recognized as safe and efficacious. A crude correlation between sulfonamide blood concentration and therapeutic response has been demonstrated (Weinstein and Samet 1962). However, correlations were not observed consistently and the effectiveness of a sulfonamide depended on other factors including the intrinsic antibacterial activity of the drug, the degree of protein binding, the extent of drug metabolism, and the status of the host defense mechanisms.

Although the absolute value of sulfonamide blood concentrations as a means of predicting therapeutic response is subject to conjecture, no viable alternatives have been proposed. The concentration of a sulfonamide in blood is the net result of absorption, metabolism, distribution, and excretion. Minor variations in one or several of these processes can produce marked changes in sulfonamide blood concentration and the time course of drug action.

When comparing the relative effectiveness of two sulfonamides having equivalent antibacterial action, the duration of effective blood concentrations achieved with each drug should be given primary consideration. Sulfonamides having longer plasma disappearance half-lives are generally preferred to those having shorter half-lives.

ROUTES OF ADMINISTRATION

Oral

Sulfonamides are most commonly administered *per os*. A variety of dosage forms including tablets, boluses, solutions, feed premixes, and water-soluble powders are available.

The bitter taste of sulfonamides must be considered when the drugs are administered in drinking water. To increase the palatability of such preparations, various flavoring agents are often added to the water-sulfonamide mixture as a means of increasing water and drug consumption. Ambient temperature and the water requirement of a particular age or species of animal also must be considered when formulating the water-sulfonamide mixture.

Orally administered sulfonamides generally provide a minimum effective concentration of the drug in blood for a more protracted period of time than equivalent doses administered intravenously. The more prolonged minimal effective concentrations of blood sulfonamide observed after oral administration are the result of the sustained entry of the sulfonamide into blood from the gastrointestinal lumen and a reduction in the fraction of the total dose excreted during the first few hours following oral drug administration. In most instances, the rate of gastrointestinal absorption is sufficient to produce minimum effective concentrations of the drug in blood. However, the maximum concentration achieved following oral administration is somewhat less than that obtained when an equivalent dose of a sulfonamide is administered intravenously. Since the amount of drug excreted during any time period is directly proportional to the concentration of the drug in blood, a smaller fraction of the orally administered dose is excreted in the urine during the first few hours following drug administration. The fraction of the oral dose conserved as a result of reduced excretion during the early postdosing period is gradually absorbed from the gastrointestinal lumen and functions as a reservoir for blood sulfonamide replenishment.

The oral administration of sulfonamides to ruminants may produce changes in the rumen flora. Prolonged oral administration may produce vitamin K deficiency with attendant hemorrhage. Decreased cellulose digestion, glucose fermentation, and inappetence were noted when sulfonamides were given to ruminant animals by an oral route (Oyaert et al. 1951). Large-scale studies to evaluate the effect of orally administered sulfonamides on ruminant digestion have not been conducted. In light of present knowledge, the beneficial effect provided by the judicious use of orally administered sulfonamides far outweighs any detrimental effects that may accrue as a result of their action on rumen microorganisms.

Intravenous

The intravenous administration of sulfonamides should be reserved for the treatment of acute infection. When sulfonamides are administered intravenously, therapeutic blood concentrations are established immediately but the duration is shorter than administration via other routes. Immediately following the intravenous administration of certain sulfonamides, large amounts of drug are filtered at the glomerulus and favor the formation of crystals in the renal tubules. Sterile solutions of the sodium salts of sulfonamides are used for intravenous administration. Such solutions are alkaline and may produce irritation and necrosis if deposited perivascularly.

Continued intravenous use of sulfonamides is unwarranted. Once therapeutic concentrations have been established in blood, they should be maintained with oral dosage forms. Since all sulfonamides have a common mechanism of bacteriostatic action, the same drug given intravenously need not be utilized in the oral dosing regimen. Sulfonamides chosen to initiate therapy via the intravenous route should have an extended plasma half-life. Compounds such as sulfathiazole (elimination half-life of 1–2 hours) have no place in intravenous therapy since a high incidence of renal damage is commonly associated with intravenous doses as low as 32.5 mg/kg of body weight.

Intravenous preparations should be administered slowly as a means of reducing the occurrence of acute toxic reactions.

INTRAMUSCULAR

Strongly alkaline solutions of sodium sulfonamide salts produce tissue irritation and necrosis when administered intramuscularly or subcutaneously, although specific preparations of sulfonamides buffered to a neutral pH may be given by these routes. The absorption of sulfonamides from intramuscular sites is rapid, and therapeutic blood concentrations are usually established within 1 hour after drug administration.

INTRAPERITONEAL

Although sulfonamides are rapidly absorbed following intraperitoneal injection, this use should be avoided with highly alkaline solutions. In those circumstances where animal behavior prevents the oral or intravenous administration of sulfonamides, the intramuscular route of sulfonamide or antibiotic injection may be utilized.

INTRAUTERINE

Sulfonamides are often placed in the uterus in solutions or boluses to aid in the prophylaxis or treatment of genital infections. Often, urea is incorporated in these preparations as a sulfonamide adjuvant. High concentrations of urea increase the action of sulfonamides by increasing their solubility, by inhibiting their reaction with proteins, and by neutralizing certain antagonists of sulfonamide activity (Hawking and Lawrence 1951). The use of urea in such preparations is conjectural and open to further investigation.

The intrauterine use of sulfonamides may result in residues in meat and milk, and appropriate drug withdrawal periods should be observed. Miller noted that when solutions containing sulfamerazine, sulfacetamide, and sulfapyridine were infused into the uterus of dairy cows at the rate of 107 and 214 mg/kg of body weight, the drugs were detected in blood and milk for 24–48 hours thereafter (as cited by Seguin et al. 1974). The appearance of the drug in milk following its absorption from the uterus is in keeping with the observations of Rasmussen (1958) and Sisodia and Stowe (1964), who noted that the transfer of sulfonamide from plasma to milk occurred as a result of the passive diffusion of nonprotein bound, nonionized forms of the drug from blood to milk.

TOPICAL

The topical application of sulfonamides to control infections in wounds should be discouraged since blood, pus, and tissue breakdown products greatly decrease the antibacterial effectiveness of the drugs. In certain instances, topically applied sulfonamides may inhibit wound healing.

Solutions and ointments containing sulfacetamide have proved useful in the treatment of conjunctivitis produced by sulfonamide-sensitive organisms. High concentrations of this drug may be used, as it produces no irritation of the delicate tissues of the eye.

Mafenide (α-amino-*p*-toluenesulfonamide), when applied topically, has proved useful for the therapeutic management of burns.

ADVERSE REACTIONS TO SULFONAMIDES

Urinary tract disturbances may occur following administration of some sulfonamides. Crystalluria, hematuria, and urinary tract obstructions are the commonest sequelae. Renal crystallization of sulfonamides may occur as the marginally soluble sulfonamides (e.g., sulfathiazole, sulfanilamide) are concentrated within the renal tubular lumen. Concentration occurs as a result of the passive tubular reabsorption of water along osmotic gradients and in some cases as a result of renal tubular secretion of the drugs. As weak organic acids, sulfonamides are more soluble in alkaline than acidic solutions. When the urine pH decreases, the propensity of sulfonamides to precipitate increases. Decreased water consumption and aciduria increase the chances for crystallization. Rapidly excreted sulfonamides are more likely to produce crystalluria than those excreted more slowly, but the intrinsic solubility of individual sulfonamides and their metabolites influences crystallization. Acetyl derivatives, with the exception of those formed from the pyrimidine sulfonamides, are less soluble than their parent compounds. Glucuronic acid and sulfate conjugates are highly water soluble.

Judicious selection of sulfonamides having a long plasma half-life and a high intrinsic solubility will reduce the chances of renal damage. To maintain adequate hydration and insure adequate urine flow, water should be readily available to animals receiving sulfonamide therapy. Renal damage associated with the use of sulfonamides having low intrinsic urinary solubility can be reduced by using a mixture of two or three of these compounds. When several sulfonamides are administered concurrently, their antibacterial actions are summated but the urinary solubility of each sulfa remains unaffected by the presence of the others (Law of Independent Solubility). As a result, when multiple sulfonamides are administered, the concentration of each drug in urine is minimized, thus reducing the possibility of crystal formation, but the total sulfonamide blood concentration is of sufficient magnitude to achieve bacteriostasis (Lehr 1945).

Anorexia, depression, hematuria, crystalluria, renal colic, frequent attempts to urinate, and an elevation of blood urea nitrogen may be observed following the renal precipitation of sulfonamides. When urinary disturbances occur as a result of sulfonamide therapy, drug use should be discontinued. Fluids should be administered to those animals demonstrating urinary continence in an effort to increase urine production. Although sodium bicarbonate has been administered to increase urinary pH, base therapy must not be indiscriminately used for prophylaxis because it decreases the amount of drug available for tubular reabsorption and ultimate redistribution to blood and tissues. Fluid therapy for treatment of renal damage produced by sulfonamides is contraindicated in anuric animals due to the attendant risk of overhydration.

Acute Toxicity

Dogs receiving large doses (1 g/kg of body weight) of sulfanilamide exhibited increased salivation, vomition, diarrhea, hyperpnea, excitement, muscular weakness, ataxia, and spastic rigidity of the limbs. Similar signs were noted following the administration of sulfapyridine. In cats given large doses of sulfanilamide, spasticity of the limbs and dyspnea precede a state resembling anesthesia. Oral doses of 300–500 mg/kg of sulfamethoxypyridazine produced transient toxic symptoms in swine (Balintffy and Horvay 1964). Weakness, ataxia, and collapse occurred when intravenous doses of sulfabromethazine (140 mg/kg or greater) were administered to calves. Acute toxic effects, although rare, are most commonly associated with overdosage or too rapid rates of intravenous drug administration.

Chronic Toxic Effects

Disorders of the hematopoietic system have been observed following the use of sulfonamides for the treatment of animal disease. Vesicle hemorrhages and hepatic degeneration were associated with the administration of sulfamethazine to Aleutian mink (Nordstoga et al. 1970). Transient agranulocytosis and mild hemolytic anemia were observed in calves receiving sulfapyridine over a 5-day interval (Farquharson 1942). Depression of white cell counts, red cell counts, and hemoglobin concentrations has occurred when cattle were treated with sulfathiazole. Sulfanilamide may produce cyanosis (dogs) or jaundice (cattle) when administered for an extended period of time. Peripheral neuritis and involvement of the sciatic or brachial nerves may occur when sulfathiazole is administered to cattle. Myelin degeneration was observed in the spinal cord and peripheral nerves of cattle and chickens following sulfonamide administration. The condition occurred in cattle when the animals were given large intravenous doses of sulfaquinoxaline while chickens were affected after a long-term sulfanilamide feeding trial.

Decreased egg production, reduced weight gain, and the production of thin, rough-shelled eggs were observed when chickens were fed sulfanilamide as 0.3%–0.5% of their daily ration. Sulfamethylphenazole produced liver and kidney lesions in chicks when it was incorporated in their drinking water (0.3%–0.5%) for 15 days. When sulfaquinoxaline was fed to 16-week-old pullets and 30-week-old hens, a complete disappearance of granulocyte precursors was observed in the bone marrow of treated birds. The birds suffered from inappetence, severe anemia, agranulocytosis, and hydropericardium (Gylstorff and Tettenborn 1966). Chickens suffered mortalities of 1.1%, 4.5%, and 11% when sulfaquinoxaline was incorporated into their ration at concentrations of 0.0125%, 0.0174%, and 0.05%, respectively, for 4 weeks (Faddoul et al. 1967).

Hypoprothrombinemia has occurred following the administration of sulfaquinoxaline to chickens. The condition was prevented when elevated concentrations of vitamin K were incorporated in the ration.

Sulfaethoxypyridazine produced lens opacities in dogs receiving 30–150 mg/kg of the drug orally for a 14-week period (Ribelin et al. 1957). Thyroid hyperplasia progressed to nodularity or adenoma formation when rats were administered sulfamethoxazole in their diets. Withdrawal of the drug after 13 weeks of treatment resulted in an involution of the observed thyroid changes (Swarm et al. 1973).

SULFONAMIDES FOR THE TREATMENT OF SYSTEMIC INFECTIONS

Sulfathiazole is marketed as a crystalline, water-soluble salt. It may be administered in drinking water and is included in certain sulfonamide combinations intended for oral or intravenous administration. The intravenous use of sulfathiazole is not recommended because it is rapidly eliminated from plasma. Intravenous doses of 71.5 mg/kg of body weight routinely produced hematuria and crystalluria in cattle and sheep.

Following oral administration, sulfathiazole is absorbed rapidly by monogastric species but undergoes slow and variable absorption in ruminants. When administered as an oral bolus or in drinking water to cattle and sheep according to manufacturers' recommendations, blood concentrations seldom exceed 2 mg/dl. The drug is absorbed rapidly by swine when in a bolus or solution. Following its administration to swine in drinking water, erratic blood concentrations seldom exceeding 3 mg/dl, were observed (Bevill and Huber 1973). The erratic blood concentrations appeared to be due to variations in water consumption and the resultant variation in the amount of drug available for absorption. The addition of concentrated flavoring agents to sulfonamide-medicated water may improve palatability, increase water and drug consumption, and ultimately provide a more continuous concentration of the drug in blood.

Sulfamethazine, a pyrimidine sulfonamide, is absorbed rapidly following oral administration to swine, sheep, and cattle. The plasma disappearance half-life of the drug is 5 hours in cattle and sheep and 14–16 hours in swine. Intravenous doses of 107 mg/kg of body weight provide plasma concentrations of 5 mg/dl for at least 24 hours in all large domestic animals. The relatively slow excretion of sulfamethazine and the high degree of metabolite solubility reduce the occurrence of sulfonamide precipitation in the renal tubules.

The rapid absorption of the drug after oral administration and the relatively long sojourn of the drug in blood make sulfamethazine a fairly safe and effective drug for oral or parenteral administration. It is available in a wide variety of dosage forms including intravenous solutions, oral boluses, sustained release boluses, and crystalline powders. It is commonly marketed in its sodium salt form.

Sulfamerazine is a monomethylated pyrimidine sulfonamide. The drug is included commonly in triple sulfonamide mixtures intended for parenteral use. The absorption and excretion of sulfamerazine are similar to those described for sulfamethazine. This drug finds limited current use in veterinary therapeutics.

Sulfadiazine was the first pyrimidine sulfonamide tested for clinical use. When administered orally, it produced lower blood concentrations than equivalent doses of sulfamethazine or sulfamerazine. When administered intravenously, it has a plasma disappearance half-life approximating that of sulfamethazine. This compound finds infrequent veterinary use.

Sulfabromethazine is a brominated derivative of sulfamethazine. The drug has a lower solubility than sulfamethazine but oral doses of 198 mg/kg of body weight produced no detectable renal pathology when the drug was administered for 21 consecutive days. Intravenous doses of 66 mg/kg of body weight have produced transient reactions in some animals.

Sulfaethoxypyridazine is absorbed rapidly following oral administration to swine, sheep, and cattle. When administered intravenously, the plasma disappearance half-life of the drug is 15.6, 11, and 10 hours in swine, sheep, and cattle, respectively. Sheep excrete lower cumulative amounts of the drug and its metabolites in urine than do cattle or swine. Sulfaethoxypyridazine, its N^4-acetylated derivative, and an unidentified glucuronide conjugate constitute the principal urinary excretion products in cattle. The drug is extensively bound to plasma proteins. Similar urinary recoveries of the drug were noted following intravenous or oral administration (Linkheimer et al. 1965). Intravenous solutions and oral boluses containing sulfaethoxypyridazine have been approved by the Food and Drug Administration for use in cattle. Solutions of the drug intended for the medication of drinking water consumed by swine are currently marketed.

Sulfadimethoxine is absorbed rapidly following oral administration; peak blood concentrations are obtained within 4 hours after dosing. The plasma disappearance half-life of the drug in swine is 15.5 hours; it is 8.4, 9.64, and 11.3 hours in sheep, cattle, and horses, respectively. The relative volume of distribution of the drug approximates 35% of the body weight of cattle, swine, and horses. Sulfadimethoxine is marketed in several dosage forms including tablets; boluses (regular and sustained release); and solutions for intravenous, subcutaneous, and intramuscular administration. Crystalline preparations are available for medication of drinking water supplies. Unlike some sulfonamides, sulfadimethoxine is palatable when administered in drinking water (Hanson 1974).

Sulfamethoxypyridazine and *acetylsulfamethoxypyridazine* are currently available for oral use in dogs and cats. Following oral administration to dogs, sulfamethoxypyridazine is absorbed rapidly; peak blood concentrations may be expected by the eighth hour after dosing. Minimal effective concentrations are established within the first hour following oral drug administration.

Sulfachloropyrazine is marketed currently as a solution for the medication of drinking water supplied to chickens. The drug is absorbed rapidly from the alimentary tract of chickens.

Sulfachloropyridazine is eliminated rapidly from plasma following intravenous administration. Glomerular filtration and tubular secretion are involved in the excretory process. Tubular secretion of this drug is an important excretory route as renal clearance of the unbound drug in plasma is 6 times greater than that attributable to glomerular filtration (Edelbeck-Fredericksen and Rasmussen 1964).

Following intramuscular injection of the drug in swine, maximum blood concentrations were achieved in 30 minutes and maintained up to 3 hours postinjection (de Frenne 1962).

SULFONAMIDES FOR TOPICAL USE

Sulfacetamide is used primarily in the treatment of ophthalmic infections. High concentrations of the drug are nonirritating to the eye and surrounding tissues. Following ophthalmic application, elevated concentrations of the drug are found in the cornea, conjunctiva, aqueous humor, and iris. The compound is available as a 30% solution or a 10% ophthalmic ointment.

Mafenide (α-amino-*p*-toluenesulfonamide) has been used successfully in the management of burns. The drug produces an intense burning sensation when applied to denuded areas but will prevent the invasion of many gram-negative and gram-positive organisms in burned areas. Creams containing the drug should be applied to denuded areas twice daily because the drug is absorbed rapidly. The drug is a carbonic anhydrase inhibitor; hypochloremic acidosis has been reported following its use in human beings.

SULFONAMIDES USED IN THE TREATMENT OF URINARY TRACT INFECTIONS

Sulfisoxazole finds primary use in the treatment of urinary tract infections in the dog and cat. Following oral administration, the drug is absorbed rapidly and undergoes subsequent rapid excretion in the urine. The drug proved effective in controlling urinary tract infections caused by *Escherichia coli, Proteus vulgaris, Pseudomonas aeruginosa,* and gram-positive cocci.

SULFONAMIDES USED PRIMARILY FOR THEIR ACTION WITHIN THE GASTROINTESTINAL TRACT

Succinylsulfathiazole, phthalylsulfathiazole, and *sulfaguanidine* are a group of sulfonamides that are poorly absorbed following oral administration to domestic animals. Both the succinyl and phthalyl forms of sulfathiazole lack antibacterial activity *in vitro.* The compounds are hydrolyzed in the intestine to release succinic or phthalic acid and sulfathiazole; the latter is presumed to be the effective antibacterial agent. Although these agents greatly reduce the number of intestinal bacteria, they do not "sterilize" the digestive tract effectively. Their use as gastrointestinal "sterilants" prior to intestinal surgery offers no distinct advantage over proper surgical technique and skilled postoperative care (Weinstein 1970).

Sulfaguanidine is absorbed poorly when administered orally because it is consistently ionized at the pH of the gastrointestinal contents. It finds limited use in current veterinary therapy but was once used extensively for the treatment of enteric infections in domestic animals.

Sulfonamide dosage information is summarized in Table 46.2.

TABLE 46.2. Oral doses of sulfonamides (maximum treatment period 4 days)

Drug	Species	Dose		Dosing
		Initial	Maintenance	Interval
		(mg/lb)	*(mg/lb)*	*(hours)*
Sulfathiazole	Horse, calf	30	30	8
	Cow, sheep, pig, dog	30	30	4
Sulfamethazine	Domestic animals	25	25	12
Sulfamerazine	Domestic animals	30	30	12
Sulfadimethoxine	Dog	7–4	3–7	12
	Cattle	50	25	24
Sulfaethoxypyridazine	Cattle	25	25	24
	Pig	60	60	24
Sulfapyridine	Horse, cow, sheep	30	30	12
Sulfaguanidine	Domestic animals	120	60	24
Succinylsulfathiazole	Domestic animals	80	80	12

REFERENCES

Baggot, J. D. 1968. Influence of urinary pH on persistence of plasma levels of sulphonamides in dogs. Vet Rec 82:266.

Balintffy, I., and Horvay, S. 1964. Investigations with Quinoseptyl (sulphamethoxypyridazine), a long-acting sulphonamide. Magy Allatorv Lapja 19:175.

Bevill, R. F. 1975. Quarterly Report FDA 71–69 (Jan. 1, 1975–Mar. 31, 1975).

Bevill, R. F., and Huber, W. G. 1973. Quarterly Report FDA 71–69 (Jan. 1, 1973–Mar. 31, 1973).

Bischop, R. E.; Janzen, R. E.; Landals, D. C.; Manns, D. D.; McCartney, D. J.; Morean, O. A.; Pawlyshyn, V. P.; Scheinbein, A. J.; Scigliano, B. W.; and Taylor, K. L. 1973. Effects of rumen stasis on sulfamethazine blood levels after oral administration to sheep. Can J Vet Res 14:269.

Dalgaard-Mikkelsen, S., and Poulsen, E. 1956. Renal excretion of sulphathiazole and sulphadimidine in pigs. Acta Pharmacol Toxicol 12:233.

Dalgaard-Mikkelsen, S.; Poulsen, E.; and Simesen, B. 1953. Sulfadimidin og sulfathiazol til ungsvin. Nord Vet Med 5:965.

de Frenne, D. 1962. Untersuchungen über den Sulfonamideghalt in blute des Schweines nach verabreichung von Sulfamethylphenazol und Sufachloropyridazin. Inaug. dissertation, Hanover.

Dittert, L. W., and Bourne, D. W. A. 1975. Quarterly Report FDA 71–69 (Jan. 1, 1975–Mar. 31, 1975).

Edelbeck-Frederiksen, M. J., and Rasmussen, F. 1964. Mammary and renal excretion of sulphachloropyridazine in cows. Nord Vet Med 16:632.

Eisman, P. C.; Geftie, S. G.; Ligenzowski, F.; and Mayer, R. L. 1952. Chemotherapeutic activity of 6-sulfanilamido-2,4-dimethylpyrimidine (Elkosin). Proc Soc Exp Biol Med 80:493.

Faddoul, G. P.; Amato, S. V.; Sevoian, M.; and Fellows, G. W. 1967. Studies on intolerance to sulfaquinoxaline in chickens. Avian Dis 11:226.

Farquharson, J. 1942. The use of sulfonamides in the treatment of calf diphtheria. J Am Vet Med Assoc 101:88.

Fildes, P. 1940. The mechanism and antibacterial action of mercury. Br J Exp Pathol 21:67.

Gylstorff, I., and Tettenborn, D. 1966. Panmyelopathy induced by sulphaquinoxaline in fowls. Dtsch Tieraerztl Wochenschr 73: 420.

Hanson, L. J. 1974. Personal communication.

Hawking, F., and Lawrence, J. S. 1951. The Sulphonamides. New York: Grune & Stratton.

Heath, G. E., and Teske, R. H. 1973. Effect of water deprivation and forced exercise on blood concentrations of sulfaethoxypyridazine after its oral administration to calves. J Am Vet Med Assoc 162:749.

Jones, L. M. 1947. The chemotherapy of calf pneumonia. I. Some pharmacologic aspects of sulfonamide administration to normal calves. Am J Vet Res 8:1.

Jorgensen, S. T., and Rasmussen, F. 1972. Renal excretion of sulphanilamide, sulphadimidine, sulfadoxine, and sulfamethoxazole in goats. Nord Vet Med 24:601.

Knudsen, E. 1960. Renal clearance studies on the horse. II. Penicillin, sulfathiazole and sulfadimidine. Acta Vet Scand 1:188.

Kortiz, G. D. 1975. Ph.D. dissertation, Univ. of Illinois Library.

Lee, J., and Kaersgaard, P. 1967. Mammary and renal excretion of sulphamethomidine in cows. Nord Vet Med 19:578.

Lehr, D. 1945. Inhibition of drug precipitation in the urinary tract by the use of sulfonamide mixtures. I. Sulfathiazole-sulfadiazine mixture. Proc Soc Exp Biol Med 58:11.

Linkheimer, W. H.; Stolzenberg, S. J.; and Wozniak, L. A. 1965. The pharmacology of sulfaethoxypyridazine in the heifer. J Pharm Exp Ther 149:280.

Maclay, M. H., and Slavin, E. 1947. The absorption and excretion in dairy cows of sulphapyridine, sulphamerazine, sulphadiazine, sulphathiazole and sulphapyrazine. Vet Rec 59:313.

Nielsen, P. 1973. The metabolism of four sulfonamides in cows. Biochem J 136:1039.

Niepp, L. 1964. Antibacterial chemotherapy with sulfonamides. In R. J. Schnitzer and F. Hawkins, eds. Experimental Chemotherapy, vol. 2. New York: Academic Press.

Nordstoga, K.; Helgebostad, A.; Lottsgard, G.; and Storwoken, H. 1970. Vesicle hemorrhages in male Aleutian mink caused by hypersensitivity to sulphadimidine. Acta Vet Scand 11:481.

Oyaert, W.; Quin, J. I.; and Clark, R. 1951. Studies on alimentary tract of merino sheep in South Africa. XIX. The influence of sulfanilamide on the activity of the ruminal flora of sheep and cattle. Onderstepoort J Vet Res 25:59.

Rasmussen, F. 1958. Mammary excretion of sulfonamides. Acta Pharmacol Toxicol 15: 139.

Ribelin, W. E.; Owen, G.; Rubin, L. F.; Levinskas, G. J.; and Agersborg, H. P. K., Jr. 1967. Development of cataracts in dogs and rats from prolonged feeding of sulfaethoxypyridazine. Toxicol Appl Pharmacol 10:557.

Seguin, B. E.; Morrow, D. A.; and Oxender, W. D. 1974. Intrauterine therapy in the cow. J Am Vet Med Assoc 164:609.

Sharma, R. M. 1975. Ph.D. dissertation, Univ. of Illinois Library.

Sisodia, C. S., and Stowe, C. M. 1964. The mechanism of drug secretion into bovine milk. Ann NY Acad Sci 111:650.

Swarm, R. L.; Roberts, G. K. S.; Levy, A. C.; and Hines, L. R. 1973. Observations on the thyroid gland in rats following the administration of sulfamethoxazole and trimethoprim. Toxicol Appl Pharmacol 24: 351.

Watanabe, T. 1967. Infectious drug resistance. Sci Am 217(6):19.

Weinstein, L. 1970. The sulfonamides. In L. S. Goodman and A. Gilman, eds. The Pharmacological Basis of Therapeutics, 4th ed., p. 1177. New York: Macmillan.

Weinstein, L., and Samet, C. A. 1962. Sulfonamide blood levels and serum antibacterial activity. Arch Int Med 110:794.

Woods, D. D. 1940. The relation of *p*-aminobenzoic acid to the mechanism of the action of sulfonamide. Br J Exp Pathol 21: 74.

PENICILLINS

WILLIAM G. HUBER

HISTORY

In 1928, Alexander Fleming observed that a Penicillium mold contaminating a petri dish culture of staphylococcic colonies was surrounded by a clear zone free of growth. Fleming observed that the mold and the staphylococcic colonies had produced a state of antibiosis. It was suspected that the Penicillium mold elaborated an antibiotic substance that might be of benefit in combating staphylococcal infections. Fleming cultured the contaminating mold on a special medium and showed that the culture broth contained a potent antibacterial substance that was effective against a variety of gram-positive organisms. It was found to be relatively nontoxic to animals. Fleming named the substance penicillin. He was not able to isolate penicillin in active form nor produce a potent preparation; however, he demonstrated laboratory applications of penicillin and suggested that the purified extract might be injected into infected tissues to combat disease.

A British biochemist, Raistrick, extended Fleming's experiment on Penicillium. In 1930, he discovered that penicillin was an organic acid that could be extracted from an acidified culture medium by ether and that the compound was thermolabile. A decade later, Florey and his associates at Oxford isolated penicillin in the form of a brown, impure powder. They demonstrated that penicillin was the most powerful chemotherapeutic agent known at that time.

By 1941, great interest in penicillin had developed in the United States and the United Kingdom. Arrangements were made for the production of penicillin in the United States as a result of the awakened scientific interest in the clinical possibilities of this new drug as well as the impetus of expected casualties in World War II. The productive and investigative program was highly organized under a committee that functioned to coordinate the efforts in the United States with those in the United Kingdom. The experimental studies in industrial, academic, and government laboratories and hospitals were coordinated and summarized for the worldwide benefit of medical sciences.

Various strains of *Penicillium notatum* and *Penicillium chrysogenium* are used in the commercial production of penicillin. No new strain has been discovered that exceeds the penicillin-producing ability of the original Fleming mold for *surface* culture methods. The outstanding strain of penicillin-producing mold for the *submerged* culture method was discovered growing on a cantaloupe rind in a garbage can in Peoria, Illinois.

Soil-inhabiting organisms have been a potent source of antibiotic substances. Several hundred antibiotic agents have been isolated but relatively few have a favorable therapeutic index.

ROLE OF PHYSICAL AND CHEMICAL PROPERTIES

More than 30 penicillins have been identified. Some penicillins occur naturally, others are biosynthesized by altering culture media components as precursors.

Oxford workers used an arbitrary unit of potency to measure the concentration of penicillin. This unit became known as the Oxford Unit (O.U.) and has been accepted as the International Unit. The International Standard Unit for penicillin has been defined as that amount of activity present in 0.6 μg of the international pure crystalline standard sodium salt of penicillin G; 1 mg contains 1667 O.U.

Many different methods for assaying penicillin have been developed. The original assay method employed the cup-plate technique as demonstrated in Fig. 47.1. The penicillin was placed inside the cylinders in varying concentrations. The antibiotic diffused from the cylinder through the medium previously inoculated with the bacterium to be tested for susceptibility to the antibiotic; a zone of growth inhibition would show around the cylinder. If resistant, the bacterium grew over all of the medium. Later methods introduced for assay of penicillin have depended upon colormetric, titrimetric, polarographic, spectrophotometric, and iodometric methods.

The penicillin molecule contains a fused ring system, the β-lactam thiazolidine. The physical and chemical properties, especially solubilities, of penicillins are related to the structure of the acyl side chain and the cations to form salts.

Hydrolysis is the main cause of peni-

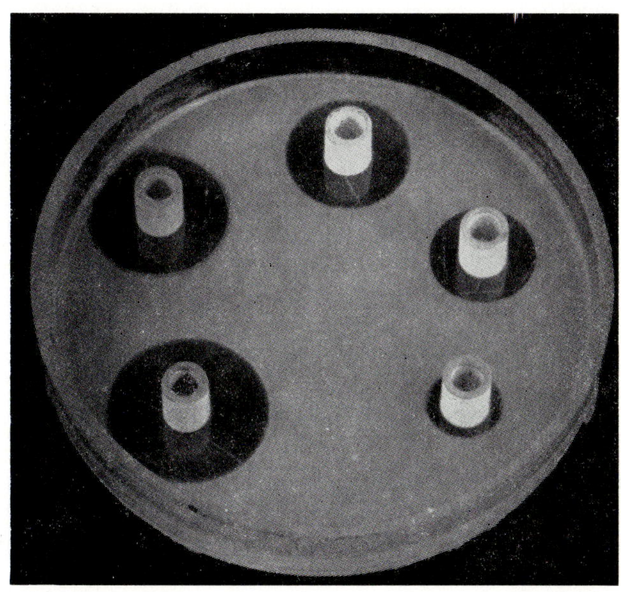

Fig. 47.1. An assay plate surface seeded with *Staphylococcus aureus*, which is lysed in the clear areas around the cylinders containing 0.25–4 units of penicillin per ml. (Garrod and Heatley 1944; courtesy of John Wright and Sons, Ltd.)

cillin degradation. Aqueous solutions of the sodium salts of sulfonamides rapidly inactivate penicillin because of their alkalinity. Penicillin is pharmaceutically compatible with a wide variety of therapeutic substances, provided the pH is favorable. A pH of 6–6.5 is optimal for stability of penicillin in aqueous solutions with a practical range of 5.5–7.5. Prolonged exposure of crystalline penicillin G to water promotes hydrolysis of the penicillin. Penicillin is incompatible with the ions of heavy metals, oxidizing agents, and strong concentrations of alcohol.

Some penicillins are rapidly hydrolyzed by gastric acid and are inactivated by penicillinase enzymes, the beta-lactamases and acylases. Gastric acid hydrolyzes the amide side chain and opens the lactam ring with the concomitant loss of antibacterial activity. Beta-lactamase is present as a natural substance in many microorganisms and as an antagonist to penicillin can produce resistance if present in sufficient quantities. Some of the newer semisynthetic penicillins have been structured to resist inactivation by acid hydrolysis and penicillinases. Currently, there are four groups of penicillins:

1. Natural penicillins (e.g., penicillin G)—are produced by mold cultures, then extracted and purified. These penicillins are rapidly hydrolyzed by gastric acid following oral administration.

2. Acid-resistant penicillins (e.g., phenoxymethyl or phenoxyethyl penicillin)—resist degradation by gastric acid; are routinely administered orally; have a phenoxy group attached to the alkyl group of the acyl moiety.

3. Penicillinase-resistant penicillins (e.g., oxacillin, nafcillin, methicillin, cloxacillin, dicloxacillin)—have a ring structure attached to the carbonyl carbon of the amide side chain. Substituents on the aromatic ring sterically protect the lactam ring from beta-lactamases.

4. Broad-spectrum penicillins (e.g., ampicillin, hetacillin)—have antibacterial activity against gram-positive and gram-negative bacteria. The antibacterial spectrum has been accomplished by structural changes in the acyl portion of the amide side chain.

ROUTES OF ADMINISTRATION

Parenteral

Penicillin can be injected intravenously without significant thrombophlebitis. Continuous intravenous infusion maintains a constant blood concentration. Most penicillin is administered by intermittent intramuscular injection; occasionally it is injected subcutaneously. Mercer et al. (1971) indicated that the subcutaneous route of administration of penicillin is better than intramuscular injection because while the pharmacokinetic parameters are comparable, the possibility of injection-site residues are minimized. If an immediate therapeutic effect is important, an intravenous injection is indicated (Fig. 47.2).

Oral

Penicillin suppresses bacterial metabolism in the digestive tract of herbivora and ordinarily is not administered orally for therapeutic purposes except in the very young or to specifically suppress bacterial fermentation in an attempt to prevent bloat.

Oral administration of penicillin is more applicable in human beings and small animals than in food-producing animals. Penicillin V (phenoxymethylpenicillin) and α-phenoxyethylpenicillin have been administered orally with beneficial results because they are stable in acid and pass through the stomach unchanged to the alkaline intestine, where they are well absorbed. Blood concentrations are higher and more sustained after oral administration than after an equivalent oral dose of penicillin G. The antibacterial spectrum of penicillin V is almost identical with that of penicillin G. Oxacillin, cloxacillin, dicloxacillin, and nafcillin also resist acid hydrolysis.

Topical

Penicillin has been applied topically or locally as a powder, solution, or oint-

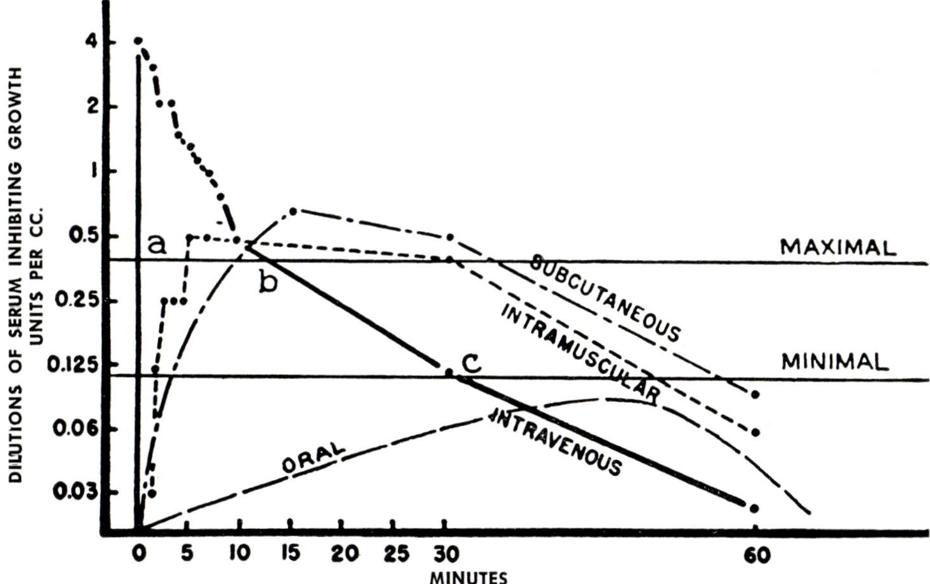

FIG. 47.2. A comparison of the antibacterial potencies of serum following the administration of 15,000 units of penicillin intravenously, subcutaneously, intramuscularly, or orally. (Fleming et al. 1944; modified by Salter 1952)

ment. In order to reduce the possibility of allergic reactions and development of bacterial resistance, penicillin should not be used topically until a bacteriologic diagnosis has been established and only if other nonsystemic antibacterial agents cannot be used. Penicillin G calcium is used in a nonirritating ointment base in the treatment of superficial infections of the eye. The application of penicillin by nebula, an aerosol, for upper respiratory infections remains of questionable value. Because of the possibility of unfavorable reactions on subsequent parenteral injections, other antibiotics or chemotherapeutic agents are better suited for topical application.

Intramammary Infusion

Penicillin is administered both intramammarily and systemically in the treatment of bovine mastitis. In addition to infusing the mammary gland via the teat canal, some cases of bovine mastitis require systemic treatment with antibiotics and/or sulfonamides.

Milk contaminated with antibiotics may cause public health problems as well as inhibit the process of making cheese. If milk is not discarded for the necessary period after penicillin has been infused intramammarily or administered parenterally, it is considered an adulterant. Traces of penicillin in milk and milk products sensitize susceptible human beings so that subsequent penicillin therapy may precipitate an allergic reaction.

The type of penicillin diluent or vehicle in mastitis infusion preparations is a factor in determining the time required for elimination of the antibiotic via the milk. The influence that antibiotic infusion vehicles have on the efficacy of mastitis treatments remains a controversial point. In general, penicillin in ointment or mineral oil vehicles persists longer in the bovine udder than penicillin administered in an aqueous vehicle; however, aqueous vehicles favor rapid release of the antibiotic to attain maximum therapeutic concentrations.

In 1960, the Food and Drug Administration established regulations to control antibiotic contamination of milk and milk products. Regulations require that milk from animals treated with antibiotic be discarded for 96 hours or whatever shorter period has been established to ensure that the milk is free of the drug. Bovine intramammary mastitis preparations are not to exceed 100,000 units of penicillin per infusion. Some individuals propose that larger volumes of vehicles should be used for larger doses so that milk-out times will not be unduly prolonged.

Individual ointment tubes and disposable plastic syringes containing penicillin for insertion in the teat canal have largely replaced the bougies and multiple-dose vials of penicillin for infusion. Individual tubes and plastic syringes are easy to use and avoid the danger of spreading infection. Each tube or syringe is fitted with a smooth, blunt infusion needle for convenient insertion into the streak canal of the teat.

DOSAGE

Most of the available data regarding the dosage of recent penicillins are obtained from laboratory measurements on normal animals. By arbitrarily selecting a blood concentration of penicillin as the minimal therapeutic concentration and establishing relationships to *in vitro* sensitivity testing, suggested dosages can be estimated. However, the arbitrary blood concentrations thought to be effective against the majority of bacterial invaders are subject to change because of variations in bacterial resistance.

Dosage of penicillin in the dog has always been higher than in larger animals. Originally, scarcity and cost prevented adequate dosage in the larger species. Differences in metabolic rates may also influence dosage requirements. Generally the minimal dose in the dog is 5000 units of penicillin G/lb of body weight, intramuscularly. In the presence of a virulent infection the dose should approach 10,000 units/lb. In general, a minimum dose of 10,000 units/lb should be given when repository types of penicillin are used. Increased dosage with procaine or benzathine penicillin beyond a certain point may prolong but not elevate serum penicillin concentrations.

The frequency of dosage depends upon a number of factors, including the type of penicillin and the vehicle. Generally the second dose should be administered at the following intervals: every 4 hours for sodium or potassium penicillin G, every 24 hours for procaine penicillin G in aqueous suspension, 48–72 hours for procaine penicillin G in oil with aluminum monostearate, and 5–7 days for benzathine penicillin G or a similar repository preparation.

There is a critical dose beyond which an increase in the amount of benzylpenicillins is not reflected with a proportional elevation in serum concentrations (English 1965). The critical dose for either crystalline potassium or sodium and procaine benzylpenicillin is 6000 units/kg of body weight, while the critical dose for the long-acting benzathine benzylpenicillin is 12,000 units/kg. English also proposed that the subcutaneous route is preferable to the intramuscular route in the cat and dog.

In the horse, cow, sheep, and swine, penicillin should be administered at a minimum dose of 5000 units/lb of body weight and repeated at suggested intervals. In severe infections, a dose of 10,000 units/lb should be used unhesitatingly. It is desirable to use procaine penicillin G in an aqueous suspension when treating horses because of the possibility of unfavorable reactions with the oil vehicle.

The importance of selecting the proper penicillin or combinations of penicillins to achieve optimal blood and tissue concentrations is shown in Fig. 47.2. Repeated treatments must be in accord with a logical sequence for obtaining optimal concentrations of penicillin.

In regard to the more recent penicillins, i.e., those that resist acid hydrolysis and penicillinase inactivation and those with a broad spectrum of antibacterial action, the approximate dosage ranges are listed with the individual drugs. It should be noted that some of these penicillins have not been widely used in veterinary medicine or animal production; thus the opportunity for clearly defined dosage ranges has not occurred in the United States.

ABSORPTION

Most penicillins are rapidly absorbed when injected in aqueous suspension intramuscularly or subcutaneously. Maximum blood concentrations result in 15–30 minutes. Intramuscular injection is the most common route of administration. Absorption of penicillin G from the gastrointestinal (GI) tract is incomplete and variable. It is necessary to administer 5 times the amount necessary for intramuscular injections to produce comparable concentrations in the blood because of inactivation by the gastric juice and the bacteria of the large intestine. Some of the newer penicillins are resistant to acid inactivation by the gastric juice and penicillinase.

Some absorption of penicillin may occur during the first few hours after intramammary infusion. Blood serum plays a significant role in the transfer of penicillin from treated to untreated quarters (Blobel 1960). Low concentrations of penicillin can be identified in blood taken from the subcutaneous abdominal vein of the cow for a short time following intramammary infusion of large amounts of penicillin. Part of the penicillin administered intramuscularly is excreted by way of the milk; therefore, milk from cows treated systemically should not be used for human consumption until the antibiotic is eliminated. The time required for milk-out will vary with the type of antibiotic preparation. This information will be provided on the label.

Mercer et al. (1974) demonstrated that penicillin formulated in aluminum monostearate was eliminated more slowly from infected quarters than from noninfected quarters. Penicillin blood concentrations were consistently higher when penicillin was infused in infected quarters than when infused in normal quarters.

Tissue concentrations of penicillin were lower and milk concentrations higher in mastitic quarters than in normal quarters (Edwards 1964). Penicillin was retained in the milk and tissue for 24 hours when an aqueous vehicle was used, 48 hours with an oil-water emulsion, and 72 hours with a vegetable and mineral oil vehicle.

Kidneys excrete crystalline penicillin rapidly. The problem of frequent administration of penicillin has been overcome by the utilization of slowly dissolving salts and/or slowly absorbed vehicles. The two salts most successful in this respect have been *Procaine Penicillin G,* U.S.P., and *Benzathine Penicillin G,* U.S.P.

The early introduction of sodium or potassium penicillin suspended in an inert oil prolonged the absorption of penicillin from the site of injection for approximately 18 hours. Incorporation of the poorly soluble procaine penicillin in oil prolonged the absorption for 24 or more hours. The addition of 2% aluminum monostearate to a suspension of penicillin in oil produced a gel with a high degree of water repellency which markedly slowed the absorption of procaine penicillin suspended in the medium.

A single intramuscular injection of 300,000 units of penicillin in oil with aluminum monostearate produces bacteriostatic concentrations in dogs for 96 hours (Table 47.1), which demonstrates the ability of the

TABLE 47.1. Effect of dosage form on average plasma penicillin concentration in dogs following a single intramuscular injection of 300,000 units of penicillin

Dosage Form		Average Plasma Penicillin Concentration *(units/ml)* at Different Hours Following Injection				
Penicillin salt	Vehicle	1 hour	8 hours	24 hours	72 hours	96 hours
Sodium	Water	22	0.06	.01		
Procaine	Water	2.7	2.5	.19	.03	
Procaine	Oil	3.8	1.7	.55	.02	
Procaine	Oil-monostearate	2.8	1.0	.51	.12	.09

Source: Miller et al. 1949.

vehicle or adjuvant to prolong the absorption of penicillin.

Although an oil vehicle will help produce longer blood concentrations, undesirable physical properties limit widespread usage. Horses may show unfavorable acute and chronic tissue reaction to the parenteral administration of an antibiotic in an oil vehicle.

Procaine penicillin G in a buffered aqueous suspension containing 300,000 units/ml is available for intramuscular injection. The absorption of penicillin from this preparation is prolonged. A small amount of the sodium or potassium salt of penicillin G may be added to establish a therapeutic concentration immediately following intramuscular injection because of its quicker rate of absorption.

Procaine Penicillin G, U.S.P., contains 1 molecule of procaine combined with 1 molecule of penicillin to give a compound with 41.5% procaine and a penicillin potency of 940 units/mg.

A search for repository or slowly absorbed salts of penicillin resulted in the introduction of esters of penicillin, so poorly soluble in the tissue fluid that absorption of a single intramuscular injection may be prolonged for 7 or more days. One such compound is *Benzathine Penicillin G,* U.S.P., a salt composed of 1 molecule of ammonium base and 2 molecules of penicillin G.

METABOLISM

The biological inactivation of penicillin G is not well understood. Penicillin G is not readily destroyed in the body; however, it can be inactivated in the GI tract by hydrochloric acid or by bacterial enzymes. Most of the penicillin in blood is in the plasma and less than 10% is found in the erythrocytes. Penicillin G is partially metabolized in the body by unknown mechanisms; however, approximately 90% of the drug is excreted unchanged. The distribution of penicillin is rapid but not uniform in various fluids and tissues.

DISTRIBUTION AND ELIMINATION

Experiments with S^{35}-labeled penicillin demonstrate that the concentration of penicillin is consistently higher in the kidneys than in other body tissues, although in the liver it is occasionally as high. The diffusion of penicillin into the tissues and fluids occurs as long as the unbound plasma concentration exceeds that of the tissues and fluids.

A specific blood concentration of penicillin that may allow diffusion of penicillin to lung, liver, or kidney tissue may not afford bactericidal concentrations to diffuse to other tissues such as the cornea or into joint fluids. The administration of potassium benzylpenicillin, 10,000 units/lb intramuscularly, produced a weak bacteriostatic effect in the aqueous humor of the dog (Rowley and Rubin 1969). Administration of 5000 units subconjunctivally produced a strong inhibitory concentration for 6.5 hours. The lowest rate of diffusion of penicillin into the central nervous system (CNS) occurs when the meninges are normal. The diffusion rate is increased when they are inflamed; however, the most effective way of administering penicillin in this condition is by the hazardous intrathecal injection. Penicillin may diffuse into an abscess following intramuscular injection. Penicillin diffuses across the placenta into the fetal circulation, reaching a peak concentration considerably below that of the maternal blood from 60 to 90 minutes after intramuscular injection into the dam. Penicillin G crossed the placenta very slowly and passed from dam to fetus more readily than from fetus to dam in a ruminant study (Kauffman et al. 1973). The placental transfer characteristics are consistent with the low lipid solubility and ionization constant. Therapeutic concentrations cannot be achieved in the fetus by administering routine doses to the dam.

Penicillin G is excreted primarily in the urine; 60%–100% of the dose is ordinarily recovered from the urine following injection of an aqueous solution. After the intramuscular injection of a therapeutic dose of sodium or potassium penicillin in aqueous solution, the greatest part of the penicillin is excreted in the urine within the first hour. Approximately 80% of the penicillin in the urine is excreted by the renal tubules and about 20% by glomerular filtration.

Penicillin may be eliminated in the milk. Thus it is mandatory that milk from treated dairy cows not be used for human consumption because of the possibility of inducing allergic reactions in susceptible human beings. If benzathine penicillin is injected intramuscularly, detectable amounts may be found in the milk for approximately 90 hours. Three million units of procaine penicillin administered intramuscularly to cattle produced penicillin residues in three posttreatment milkings, whereas 3 million units of benzathine penicillin produced penicillin residues in four posttreatment milkings (Jacobs and Hanselaar 1966).

The matter of residues and dry period intramammary infusions has been studied (Mol et al. 1970). If cows were infused with benzylpenicillin 60 days before parturition, residues did not appear in the milk; however, cows infused 30–45 days before parturition had penicillin residues in the milk which in some cases persisted for 14 days postcalving. Cloxacillin and oxacillin residues have persisted in the nonlactating bovine udder for at least 3 weeks postinfusion.

Milk has become contaminated with penicillin from the urine of treated stablemates (van Os and Goudswaard 1973). Milk samples from two cows appeared contaminated for unaccountable reasons; however, it was observed that the cutaneous areas around the udders contained large amounts of penicillin, apparently as a result of being in contact with the urine of a stablemate that had been parenterally treated.

The intrauterine administration of penicillin has produced penicillin concentrations in bovine milk. Concentrations of 0.1–11 units/ml were observed and were detectable for as long as 48 hours posttreatment (Uhlig 1973).

Mol (1968) reported that 90% of the milk residues were due to the use of intramammary infusion and the failure to observe drug withdrawal times and exclusion of milk from the treated quarter. The prevalence of milk residues was low, from 0.46% to 0.68%.

Efforts to overcome the rapid excretion of penicillin have been directed (1) at prolonging absorption from the site of injection and (2) at delaying excretion by the kidney. The greatest progress has been made in prolonging absorption of penicillin by use of sparingly soluble salts of penicillin and by slowly absorbed vehicles.

PHARMACODYNAMICS

Penicillins interfere with the development of the bacterial cell wall. The enzyme transpeptidase is inhibited and rendered inactive, thus removing its ability to form cross-linkage between two linear peptidoglycase strands.

Penicillins affect growing cells and have little effect on dormant bacteria, those in resting phase. Thus the administration of a bacteriostatic drug concomitantly with penicillin, essentially a bacterial drug, does not represent proper therapy since the bacteriostatic suppression may inhibit action of the penicillin. Penicillin is inert in mammalian systems because mammalian cells do not possess the type of rigid cell wall characteristic of bacteria.

The antibacterial action of penicillin is highest during the period of greatest bacterial multiplication. *In vivo* experiments in mice have demonstrated the peak of activity. When the mice were inoculated with highly virulent streptococci, the number of organisms increased rapidly within the first 9 hours but only slowly during the next 15 hours. When animals were treated with penicillin during the first period, no deaths occurred despite high mortality in the untreated mice. Treatment with the same dose of penicillin during the second period exerted a slow and irregular bactericidal action; the mortality rate was nearly as great as in the untreated controls. In order to cure the late-treated animals, therapy had to be continued for 6–8 days. The poor response of the second group was attributed to the fact that the bacteria were past their period of rapid growth when they are most susceptible to the action of penicillin.

In regard to pharmacologic compatibility, other antibiotics may act as synergistic or antagonistic agents when administered in combination with penicillin. Penicillin has a synergistic effect with streptomycin or gentamicin against *Listeria* (Moellering et al. 1972) and against *Pseudomonas* when used with cephalosporins (Sabath and Abraham 1964).

Antibiotics have been classified on the basis of their synergistic or antagonistic activity as follows:

Group I: Penicillin, streptomycin, bacitracin, and neomycin.

Group II: Bacteriostatic antibiotics, e.g., tetracyclines and chloramphenicol.

The antibiotics of group I have complementary effects and may be synergistic with other members of group I with regard to bactericidal effects. Those of group II may antagonize the cidal effect of penicillin and other members of group I.

If defense mechanisms are in optimal condition, the antagonistic or synergistic effects of combination antibiotic therapy are of little importance; if the animal is extremely debilitated and has limited defensive activity, these concepts become of vital importance. Combination antibiotic therapy should be used only after careful consideration of the effects of each antibiotic on the causative organism.

COMPOUNDS

Penicillin is markedly bactericidal to certain organisms during their growth phase. Penicillin G is specific in its action against gram-positive bacteria, but essentially ineffective against gram-negative organisms. However, ampicillin, carbenicillin, and hetacillin have antibacterial activity against gram-negative bacteria. Penicillin is active in the presence of blood, serum, and pus.

Microorganisms inhibited by less than 0.07 units of penicillin G/ml may be considered highly sensitive, e.g., *Clostridium perfringens, Clostridium tetani, Staphylococcus aureus, Streptococcus agalactiae,* and *Corynebacterium pyogenes.* Microorganisms not inhibited by more than 1 unit of penicillin G/ml are considered resistant or not susceptible. Most gram-negative bacilli, such as *Escherichia coli, Salmonella, Klebsiella, Shigella, Proteus,* and *Pseudomonas,* are highly resistant to penicillin G. When compared with the tetracyclines and other broad-spectrum antibiotics, penicillin G must be considered as having a relatively narrow but important antibacterial spectrum.

Penicillin G

Salts of *Penicillin G,* U.S.P. (Fig. 47.3), are most commonly used for parenteral administration. They are usually not administered orally because of the breakdown and inactivation by gastric acid. Procaine penicillin G in water or oil vehicle or an aqueous suspension of benzathine penicillin G are routinely administered intramuscularly. The dose ranges from 5000 to 10,000 units/lb of body weight.

Only the sodium or potassium salt of penicillin G should be administered intravenously since procaine could adversely affect the cardiac conduction mechanism. Preparations other than the sodium or potassium salts are usually suspensions rather than solutions.

The following preparations are available: benzathine penicillin G, penicillin G potassium, procaine penicillin G, and procaine penicillin G with aluminum monostearate.

In addition to single salts of penicillin G, combinations are also available so that the advantages of quick high blood concen-

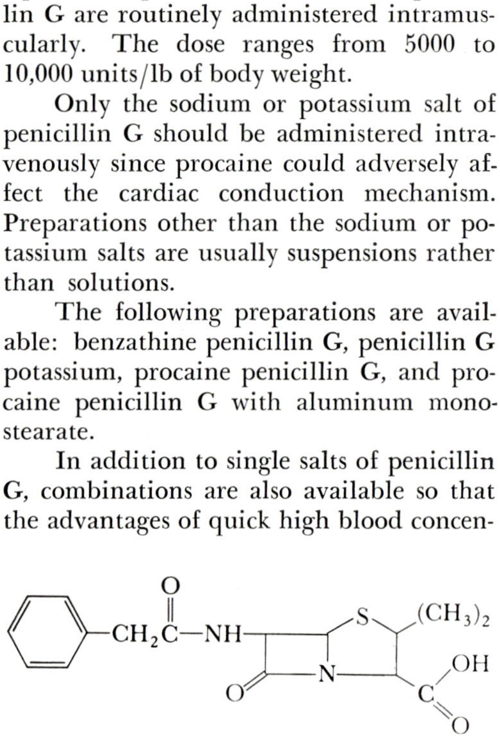

O ‖ —CH_2C—NH— S $(CH_3)_2$ N OH C O O

Penicillin G

Fig. 47.3.

trations can be combined with prolonged therapeutic concentrations, e.g., benzathine penicillin G combined with penicillin G potassium and procaine penicillin G; benzathine penicillin G and procaine penicillin G; procaine penicillin G and penicillin G sodium.

Phenoxymethyl Penicillin

Phenoxymethyl Penicillin, U.S.P. (Fig. 47.4), resists destruction by gastric acid and thus is administered orally. The antibacterial spectrum is comparable to penicillin G. Phenoxymethyl penicillin is available either as the potassium or benzathine salt. Doses of 1.5–2 mg of phenoxymethyl penicillin are administered 3–4 times daily for each lb of body weight. The recommended oral dose of phenoxymethyl penicillin in dogs is 20,000–30,000 units/kg of body weight every 6 hours (Roliński and Studnicki 1965).

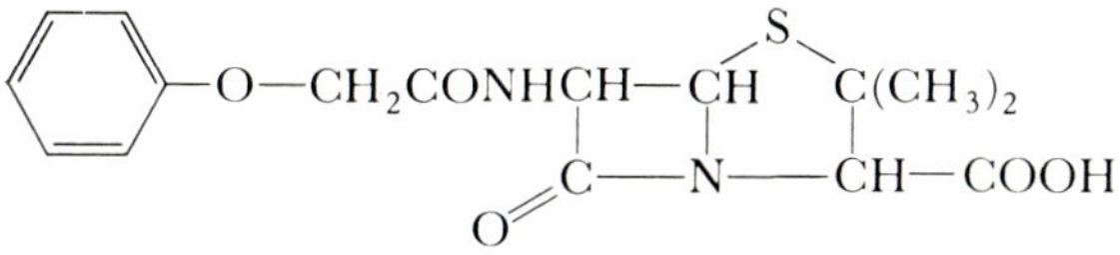

C_6H_5—O—CH_2CONHCH—CH—S—C$(CH_3)_2$; C(=O)—N—CH—COOH

Phenoxymethyl Penicillin

Fig. 47.4

Phenethicillin

Phenethicillin Potassium, N.F. (Fig. 47.5), is a semisynthetic homolog of phenoxymethyl and is quite resistant to gastric acid hydrolysis. It is used for oral administration and has activity comparable to penicillin G. The dosage of phenethicillin is similar to that of phenoxymethyl penicillin.

Methicillin

Methicillin Sodium, U.S.P. (Fig. 47.6),

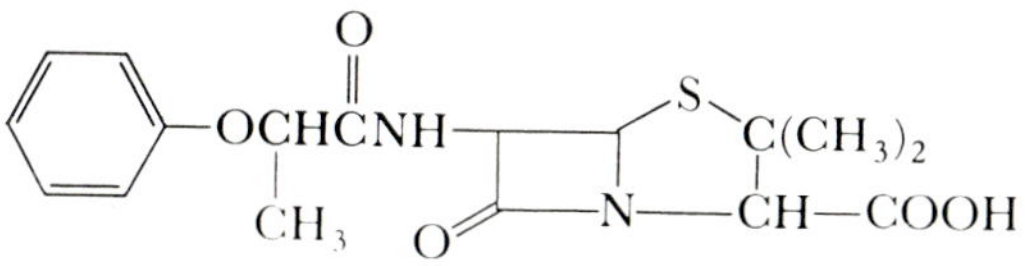

C_6H_5—OCH(CH_3)C(=O)NH— ; S ; C$(CH_3)_2$; O= —N—CH—COOH

Phenethicillin

Fig. 47.5

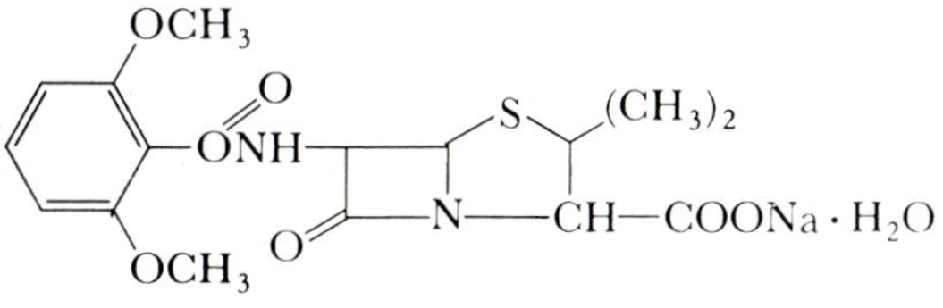

OCH_3, O, ONH—, S, $(CH_3)_2$, O, N—CH—COONa · H_2O, OCH_3

Methicillin Sodium

Fig. 47.6

is frequently used for penicillin G–resistant staphylococci. It is a water-soluble, penicillinase-resistant semisynthetic salt of penicillin. The drug produces therapeutic concentrations in the CNS. Methicillin sodium is easily eliminated in the urine; however, it is also found in the bile and other body fluids. Methicillin is a powerful inducer of penicillinase, and staphylococci may develop resistance by a nonpenicillinase mechanism.

Methicillin is used intravenously or intramuscularly and is usually well tolerated. Occasionally some pain may be observed following intramuscular injection. Care should be taken to decrease the dose in patients with reduced renal function, including the young, since a normal dose may persist beyond the desired period. Methicillin is primarily used as an antistaphylococcal drug.

Oxacillin

Sodium Oxacillin, U.S.P. (Fig. 47.7), is another semisynthetic penicillin that is highly resistant to penicillinase inactivation. The drug is well absorbed from the GI tract; 4–5 mg of sodium oxacillin are administered 4 times each day for each lb of body weight.

Cloxacillin

Sodium Cloxacillin, U.S.P., is oxacillin with a chlorine atom on the phenyl ring. It is administered at the same rate as sodium oxacillin.

Benzathine cloxacillin was infused in 5000 dairy cows during the dry period (Kingwill et al. 1967). Doses of 1 or 5 g were equally effective in controlling and preventing mastitis.

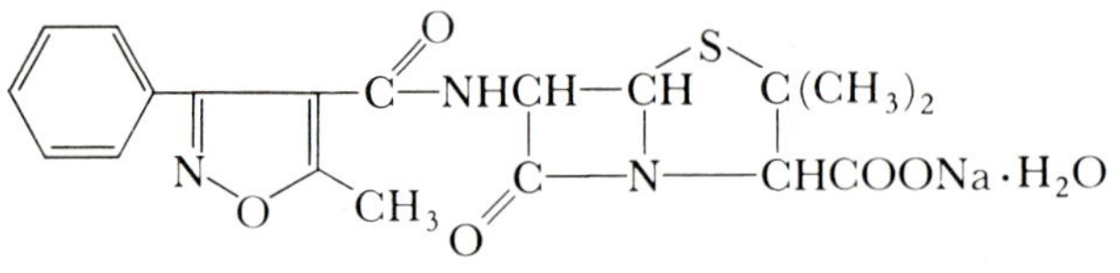

Sodium Oxacillin

FIG. 47.7

DICLOXACILLIN

If 2 chlorine atoms are substituted on the phenyl ring of sodium oxacillin, *sodium dicloxacillin* is formed. The substitution of the chlorine atoms is thought to improve the drug's stability and results in higher plasma concentrations.

All three penicillins—oxacillin, cloxacillin, and dicloxacillin—are administered orally and are primarily used for penicillin G–resistant organisms, e.g., staphylococci. Although they resist gastric acid inactivation, some inactivation occurs. Approximately 1 mg of sodium dicloxacillin is administered 4 times daily for each lb of body weight. The oral administration of dicloxacillin produced peak blood concentrations in dogs within 30–60 minutes after administration (Keefe and Christie 1973). These workers also reported that dicloxacillin was bactericidal for penicillin-resistant staphylococci and was rapidly distributed although the amount in the cerebrospinal fluid was limited. Doses of from 5 to 25 mg/lb of body weight were administered 2 or 3 times daily. Ninety-eight percent of the staphylococcal isolates were sensitive to dicloxacillin, whereas 54% were resistant to penicillin G.

NAFCILLIN

Sodium Nafcillin, U.S.P. (Fig. 47.8), is a semisynthetic penicillin resistant to penicillinase and acid hydrolysis. The drug can be administered orally and parenterally. Nafcillin has been used for penicillin G–resistant strains and is indicated in mixed infections caused by penicillin G–resistant staphylococci and streptococci. It is used as initial therapy if resistance is suspected but has yet to be established by *in vitro* tests.

Nafcillin has been effective for treating infections of the respiratory tract, soft tissues, skin, and suppurative osteomyelitis. Bile is nafcillin's route of excretion and some enterohepatic recycling occurs. Small amounts of nafcillin in synovial fluid have been detected after parenteral administration. Nafcillin may cause pain and irritation following intramuscular administration; thus care should be taken when treating small animals. It is administered 4–6 times daily at the rate of 3–5 mg/lb of body weight.

AMPICILLIN

Ampicillin, U.S.P. (Fig. 47.9), as well as hetacillin and carbenicillin, has a broader spectrum of antibacterial activity than the other penicillins. Ampicillin has antibacterial activity against the same gram-positive organisms sensitive to penicillin G and against gram-negative bacteria, including several pathogenic enteric organisms. Ampicillin has been used to treat infections caused by *Escherichia coli, Salmonella* spp., *Proteus* spp., and *Klebsiella.* It is not

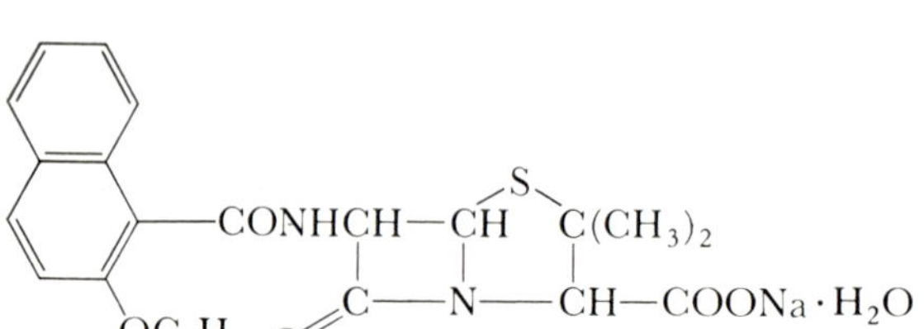

Sodium Nafcillin

FIG. 47.8

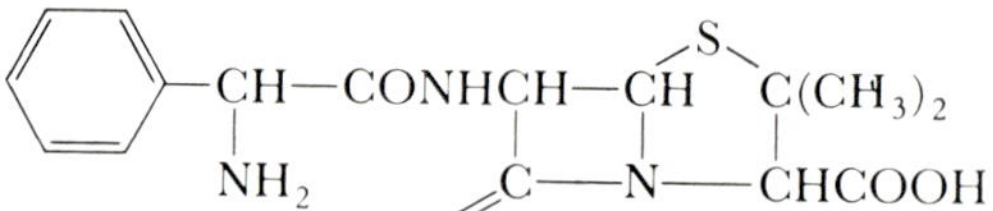

Ampicillin

FIG. 47.9

resistant to penicillinase and is similar to other penicillins in its hypersensitivity properties.

Ampicillin has been orally administered to dogs and cats at the rate of 5–10 mg/lb of body weight 2 or 3 times daily (Davis et al. 1972). Drug-related adverse reactions were reported for 5 of 266 dogs and 2 of 160 cats. Eighty-three percent of the animals treated had a beneficial response rated from excellent to good for animals suffering from bacterial infections.

Ampicillin has been used to treat bacterial infections in cattle (Keefe et al. 1972). A dose of 2–5 mg/lb of body weight (4.5–11 mg/kg) was administered parenterally once daily for 3 days. Clinical improvement was noted in 86% of the cases and no adverse effects were noted.

Ampicillin has comparatively few adverse properties, permitting it to be used preferentially over other agents such as chloramphenicol or tetracyclines when a broad-spectrum antibacterial drug is desired. It has been used as a treatment for urinary, respiratory, and GI infections and bacterial otitis. Since ampicillin is excreted in the bile it can be used to treat biliary tract infections. Superinfections caused by *Enterobacter, Pseudomonas,* or *Candida* have been noted during oral ampicillin therapy, necessitating a reduced dosage or substituting another antibacterial drug.

The oral dose of ampicillin is approximately 12 mg/kg of body weight 4 times daily.

HETACILLIN

Hetacillin is prepared by a reaction of ampicillin with acetone and when administered in an aqueous solution is rapidly converted back to ampicillin and acetone. Thus the spectrum of antibacterial activity is identical to that of ampicillin.

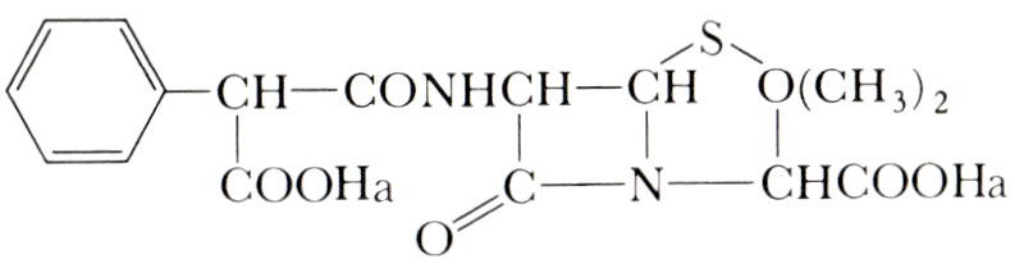

Carbenicillin

FIG. 47.10.

CARBENICILLIN

Carbenicillin (Fig. 47.10), a semisynthetic penicillin, was introduced first in England and then in the United States in 1970. Carbenicillin has a broad range of antibacterial activity which has been related to the carboxyl group substituted on the alpha carbon of the benzyl side chain.

Carbenicillin is not stable in acids nor does it resist penicillinases; thus it is administered parenterally because of poor oral absorption. It has been used for infections due to *Pseudomonas aeruginosa, Proteus* spp., and certain strains of *Escherichia coli.* A dose of 50–200 mg/kg has been divided for administration every 4–6 hours. Although carbenicillin is eliminated from the bovine mammary within 72 hours posttreatment, mastitis produced by *Pseudomonas aeruginosa* was not effectively treated; resistant organisms were recovered 24–48 hours postinfusion (Ziv et al. 1969).

Carbenicillin and gentamicin are synergistic against *Pseudomonas* infections (Rolinson and Sutherland 1968). This property helps improve carbenicillin's cost factor. Carbenicillin appears similar to other penicillins in regard to adverse effects, especially hypersensitivity.

AMOXICILLIN

Amoxicillin (α-amino-*p*-hydroxybenzylpenicillin) (Fig. 47.11) differs from ampicillin by the addition of a parahydroxy group. It has greater resistance to gastric juice than ampicillin. The biologic half-life of

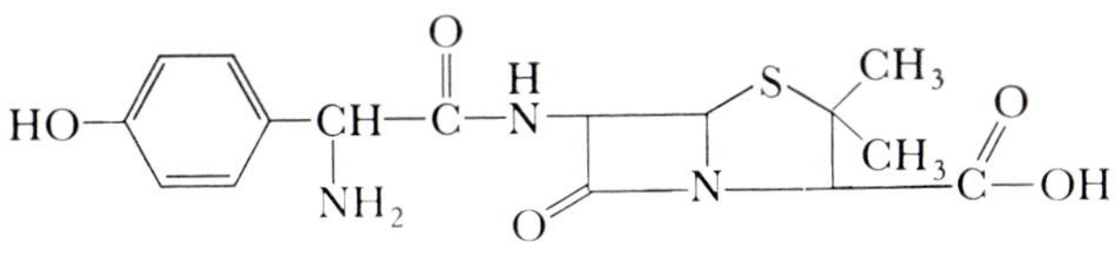

Amoxicillin

FIG. 47.11.

amoxicillin is 17 hours whereas ampicillin's half-life is 12 hours.

The antimicrobial activity of amoxicillin is similar to that of ampicillin. A number of strains and species of gram-negative enteric bacteria have cross-resistance for ampicillin and amoxicillin. Amoxicillin has been used to treat urinary tract infections as well as streptococcal infections of the upper respiratory tract and skin.

Apparently amoxicillin has more complete absorption than ampicillin, as demonstrated by a 70% urine recovery in 6 hours as compared to 40%–50% for ampicillin. Amoxicillin also induces greater serum concentrations.

Other ampicillinlike compounds are *epicillin* (aminocycloheradienylpenicillin), *azidocillin* (α-azidobenzylpenicillin), *cyclacillin* (aminocyclohexane penicillin), and *indanyl carbenicillin*. These penicillins may have future utility in veterinary medicine.

TOXICITY, RESISTANCE, AND PUBLIC HEALTH ASPECTS

In general, the direct toxic properties of penicillins are minimal; however, their ability to provoke hypersensitivity reactions in animals or human beings is a problem that requires consideration. These effects may occur with the naturally occurring biosynthetic or semisynthetic penicillins. Cross-reactions are common with the penicillins and in some instances with cephalosporins.

The prevalence of untoward effects, essentially hypersensitivity reactions, varies with the route of administration and the formulation. Injections of penicillin have caused the highest incidence of reactions while orally administered compounds have the smallest number of reactions. Hypersensitivity reactions to penicillin range from mild and transitory skin reactions to fatal anaphylactoid shock. Penicillin is considered to be one of the most common causes of drug allergy.

Veterinarians, physicians, nurses, and pharmacists have occasionally experienced contact dermatitis after handling penicillin preparations. Similarly, ill-advised use of topical applications of penicillin, including antimastitis medications, has resulted in the manifestations of penicillin reactions. Extremely small amounts of penicillin, its metabolites, or degradation product are sufficient to sensitize or provoke a hypersensitivity reaction in certain individuals.

A significant percentage of the human population, approximately 10%, show hypersensitivity reactions of penicillin. The source of initial exposure to penicillin may have been from a form of therapy or from the consumption of milk, milk products, or meat contaminated with penicillin, its metabolites, or degradation products. Of the antibiotics used for treating bovine mastitis, penicillin is a major concern because of its strong sensitizing properties. The broad-spectrum antibiotics are poor sensitizers and have not been implicated to the degree attained by penicillin.

The public health hazards of bovine mastitis treatments have stimulated the search for tests to determine the presence of adulterating antibiotics in milk destined for human consumption. The most widely used test is the *Bacillus subtilis* disc assay test as described in the tenth edition of the Handbook of Standard Methods of the American Public Health Association (Kosikowski 1961).

The clinician should be familiar with the milk-out times for the preparations administered or dispensed for use in dairy animals and must inform dairymen of the proper disposition of the milk obtained from treated animals.

Pharyngitis or "sore throat" has been noted in dogs after 4 days of penicillin therapy. Examination revealed an inflamed pharynx but no tonsillitis. When offered feed the dog may attempt to eat but stops because it is painful to swallow. Affected animals will lap water to maintain water intake and apparently soothe the irritated pharynx.

Acute allergic response to penicillin in the dog has been reported (Clarke 1960). A dog received a second injection of penicillin approximately 1 month after the first injection. Salivation, shivering, vomition, and urticaria appeared within 15 minutes after the second administration. The allergic response subsided in a few hours.

A Canadian survey was conducted to determine the prevalence of antibiotic reactions in cattle (Brisbane 1963). Forty-six practitioners reported 1200 adverse reactions in 1 year. The majority were anaphylactic reactions following the injection of penicillin or a penicillin-streptomycin combination. The highest prevalence of reactions was during the fall and winter months when large numbers of cattle were being transported and penicillin was extensively used prophylactically.

The author has observed acute allergic reactions in dairy cows that received an aqueous preparation of procaine penicillin G intramuscularly. The condition was characterized by labored breathing, salivation, and cutaneous edema of the head and perineal region. The condition lasted 2–3 hours, and parenteral administration of epinephrine appeared beneficial. These animals apparently became sensitized through previous intramammary infusions of penicillin mastitis medicaments.

If a penicillin preparation contains a carboxymethylcellulose adjuvant the probability of an anaphylactoid reaction in cattle is increased (Leemann et al. 1969). As little as 1 μg of carboxymethylcellulose produced anaphylactoid reactions after intradermal injections in cattle.

Dermatitis in animals apparently resulting from penicillin has been noted. Cutaneous plaques or wheals have been observed following penicillin therapy in white-haired horses with thin, sensitive skin. Local reactions such as muscle tenderness and edema occasionally occur at the site of injection. Fatal anaphylactic reactions are commonly observed in the chinchilla and guinea pig following antibiotic therapy. Occasionally, a similar reaction in a dog suggests that some dogs possess inherent antibiotic sensitivities.

It is well known that penicillin applied locally to the skin of some dogs causes sensitization reactions. The reaction tends to occur in dogs previously medicated internally with penicillin. The local allergic reaction is most evident in the eye of the dog. Soon after application of penicillin ointment, the conjunctiva becomes edematous and protrudes from its usual recessed position near the median canthus to form a border of swollen mucosal tissue at the median half of the eyeball. Such experiences indicate that if penicillin has been used for a systemic effect, it should not be applied topically. In order to avoid allergy and increased bacterial resistance to antibiotics, it is mandatory that the clinician decide which antibiotics should be reserved for exclusive systemic use.

In regard to its direct toxic properties, the LD50 of pure penicillin G administered intravenously to mice was 3,500,000 units/kg of body weight while that of the anesthetized cats was 500,000 units/kg.

The LD50 of procaine penicillin G administered intramuscularly to the chicken was found to be greater than 2,500,000 units/kg of body weight (Gray and Purmalis 1958). Intramuscular injections of 40,000 or more units of procaine penicillin G/kg to the chicken produced a watery diarrhea. It is apparent that penicillin has a large therapeutic index.

Penicillin contacting the CNS may cause stimulation, twitching, and convulsions. Convulsive responses in cats, dogs, monkeys, and human beings result from the injection of penicillin into the cerebral cortex. The convulsive threshold for the cat is about 1000 units of penicillin applied directly to the cerebral cortex. The maximum nonconvulsive dose of penicillin dissolved in water that should be injected into the cysterna magna of the dog is 10,000 units. Convulsions occur regularly in dogs when the critical level of 300 units of penicillin/ml of spinal fluid is exceeded. The central stimulation resulting from the application of penicillin to the CNS can be controlled readily by the intravenous administration of barbiturates.

Penicillin has produced fatal reactions in guinea pigs (Farrar and Kent 1965). After the administration of penicillin, a 10 millionfold increase in the number of cecal coliforms was observed. In some animals an even greater increase in the number of gram-negative rods was observed. The disease can be prevented by the oral administration of a nonabsorbable antibiotic with a coliform antibacterial spectrum. The condition is believed to be a bacterial superinfection with the attendant production of toxins.

The important aspects of bacterial resistance to antibacterial drugs have been presented in the sulfonamide chapter. Specifically, in regard to penicillin, many bacteria originally sensitive to penicillin are still susceptible. A study of the penicillin tolerance of some organisms infecting the bovine mammary gland showed that streptococci isolated from infected udders in a herd intensively treated with penicillin did not show unusual resistance to penicillin *in vitro*. However, staphylococci and enterococci from infected udders showed much greater tolerance to penicillin than the usual mastitis streptococci.

Strains of *Staphylococcus aureus* resistant to penicillin are isolated with increasing frequency. Three-fourths of the *Staphylococcus aureus* strains are highly resistant to penicillin (Finland 1955). Patients may acquire the penicillin-resistant organisms after admission to the clinic or hospital.

Emphasis needs to be placed upon avoiding the development and maintenance of an acquired resistance by staphylococci as a result of constant exposure to penicillin in hospitals and clinics. Penicillin-resistant staphylococci contaminate dust, utensils, instruments, and all surfaces, including the skin, wounds, etc.

Antibiotic-resistant staphylococci have become established in veterinary hospitals (Live and Nichols 1961). Veterinary hospitals may act as a source of organisms that become pathogenic for hospital attendants as well as hospitalized animals. Hospitalized animals may act as carriers of staphylococci, especially the epidemic strain, and may serve as reservoirs of bacteria for the human population. Hospitalized dogs had approximately a twofold increase in the number of antibiotic-resistant staphylococci when compared to outpatient-treated dogs.

Two main aspects of penicillin therapy must be considered: (1) the development of bacterial resistance and (2) the sensitizing ability of penicillin and its involvement as a public health hazard if proper precautions are not exercised.

The emergence of drug-resistant microorganisms is not a new phenomenon. In 1907 in Paul Ehrlich's laboratory, trypanosomes previously susceptible to the lethal action of the trypan dyes were found to have become resistant to these agents. It is apparent that when antibiotics and other antibacterial drugs are used promiscuously, resistant bacterial strains can be found in a significant portion of the population.

The medical and veterinary professions, as well as livestock and poultry producers, can benefit from the utilization of

TABLE 47.2. Diseases treated with penicillin

Etiologic Agent	Disease
Actinomyces bovis	Actinomycoses
Bacillus anthracis	Anthrax
Borrelia anserina	Avian spirochaetosis
Clostridium chauvoei	Blackleg
Clostridium hemolyticum	Bacillary hemoglobinuria
Clostridium novyi	Infectious necrotic hepatitis
Clostridium septicum	Malignant edema
Clostridium tetani	Tetanus
Corynebacterium equi	Corynebacterial pneumonia of foals
Corynebacterium pyogenes	Suppurative conditions, arthritis, mastitis, metritis
Corynebacterium pyogenes	Mastitis
Corynebacterium renale	Bovine pyelonephritis
Erysipelothrix insidiosa	Erysipelas
Fusiformis nodosus	Ovine foot rot
Leptospira spp.	Leptospirosis
Listeria monocytogenes	Listeriosis
Nanophyetus salmincola	Canine rickettsiosis
Nocardia spp.	Nocardiosis
Pasteurella multocida	Respiratory infections, fowl cholera, hemorrhagic septicemia
Salmonella spp.	Salmonellosis (penicillins with gram-negative activity, e.g., ampicillin, carbenicillin)
Staphylococcus hyicus	Exudative epidermitis
Staphylococcus hyos	Exudative epidermitis
Streptococcus agalactiae	Mastitis
Staphylococcus aureus	Mastitis, synovitis
Streptococcus dysgalactiae	Mastitis
Streptococcus equi	Strangles
Streptococcus uberis	Mastitis

practices, such as improving environmental hygiene, in order to help control infectious diseases. The practice of relying solely on antibacterial drugs to control bacterial disease losses should be avoided.

The problem of antibiotic contamination of milk requires that the dairyman, veterinarian, and milk processor be aware of the sensitizing ability of penicillin and the adherence to drug withdrawal times. In addition to having a good pharmacologic understanding of the antibiotic, the veterinarian must know the current state and federal regulations so he may serve both clients and the public.

ANTIBACTERIAL UTILITY

The antibacterial utility of the penicillins is presented in Table 47.2, which lists important diseases and their etiologic agents. Penicillins with gram-negative activity, e.g., ampicillin, hetacillin, and carbenicillin, have broader activity than the diseases listed in the table. The utilization of broad-spectrum penicillins will increase as they are used for diseases not traditionally treated with the gram-positive active penicillins.

REFERENCES

Blobel, H. 1960. Concentrations of penicillin in milk secretions and blood serum of cows following intramammary infusion of one or more quarters. J Am Vet Med Assoc 137:110.

Brisbane, W. P. 1963. Antibiotic reaction in cattle. Can Vet J 4:234.

Clarke, P. B. 1960. Acute allergic response to penicillin. Vet Rec 72:1054.

Davis, W. T.; Reynolds, W. A.; and Maplesden, D. C. 1972. Clinical efficacy of ampicillin capsules in dogs and cats. Vet Med Small Anim Clin 67:550.

Edwards, S. J. 1964. The diffusion and retention of penicillin after injection into the bovine udder. Vet Rec 76:545.

English, P. B. 1965. The therapeutic use of penicillin: The relationship between dose rate and plasma concentration after parenteral administration of benzylpenicillin (penicillin G). Vet Rec 77:810.

Farrar, W. E., and Kent, T. H. 1965. Enteritis and coliform bacteremia in guinea pigs given penicillin. Am J Pathol 47:629.

Finland, M. 1955. Changing patterns of resistance of bacteria to antimicrobial agents. N Engl J Med 252:570.

Fleming, A.; Young, M. Y.; Sughet, J.; and Rowe, A. J. 1944. Penicillin content of blood serum after doses of penicillin by various routes. Lancet 247.

Garrod, L. P., and Heatley, N. G. 1944. Bacteriological methods in connection with penicillin treatment. Br J Surg 32:117.

Gray, J. E., and Purmalis, A. 1958. The acute toxicity of procaine penicillin G and dihydrostreptomycin in the pigeon and the chicken. Avian Dis 2:187.

Jacobs, J., and Hanselaar, J. 1966. Antibiotic residues in milk of cows after parenteral administrations. Tijdschr Diergeneeskd 91:648.

Kauffman, R. E.; Baulus, B. M.; and Azarnoff, D. L. 1973. Placental transfer of penicillin G during constant rate infusion in the goat. Am J Obstet Gynecol 117:64.

Keefe, T. J., and Christie, G. J. 1973. Sodium dicloxacillin monohydrate: An anti-staphylococcus antibiotic. Vet Med Small Anim Clin 68:904.

Keefe, T. J.; Christie, G. J.; and Strum, P. W. 1972. Clinical efficacy of ampicillin trihydrate veterinary infection in cattle. Vet Med Small Anim Clin 67:1135.

Kingwill, R. G.; Neave, F. K.; Dodd, F. H.; and Wilson, C. D. 1967. Dry cow therapy. Vet Rec 81:199.

Kosikowski, F. V. 1961. An inquiring look at antibiotic residue control. J Dairy Sci 44:1554.

Leemann, W.; de Weck, A. L.; and Schneider, C. H. 1969. Hypersensitivity to carboxymethylcellulose as a cause of anaphylactic reactions to drugs in cattle. Nature 223:621.

Live, I., and Nichols, A. C. 1961. The animal hospital as a source of antibiotic-resistant staphylococci. J Infect Dis 108:195.

Mercer, H. D.; Rollins, L. D.; Garth, M. A.; and Carter, G. G. 1971. A residue study and comparison of penicillin and dihydrostreptomycin concentration after intramuscular and subcutaneous administration in cattle. J Am Vet Med Assoc 158:776.

Mercer, H. D.; Geleta, J. N.; and Carter, G. G. 1974. Absorption and excretion of penicillin G from the mastitic bovine udder. J Am Vet Med Assoc 164:613.

Miller, A. K.; Russo, H. F.; and Scheidy, S. F. 1949. Plasma penicillin concentrations following a single intramuscular injection of repository dosage forms in dogs. J Am Vet Med Assoc 115:97.

Moellering, R. C., Jr.; Medoff, G.; Leech, I.; Wennerstein, C.; and Kunz, L. J. 1972.

Antibiotic synergism against *Listeria monocytogenes*. Antimicrob Agents Chemother 1:30.

Mol, H. 1968. Occurrence of antibiotic residues in milk delivered to dairy factories. Tijdschr Diergeneeskd 93:579.

Mol, H.; Brandsma, S.; and Bukker-de-Koff, E. C. 1970. Effect of the length of the dry period on the occurrence of antibiotic residues in milk after penicillin treatment at the beginning of the dry period. Tijdschr Diergeneeskd 95:785.

Roliński, Z., and Studnicki, W. 1965. The blood concentration of penicillin in dogs after oral administration of phenoxymethylpenicillin. Med Vet 21:152.

Rolinson, G. N., and Sutherland, R. 1968. Carbenicillin, a new semisynthetic penicillin active against *Pseudomonas aeruginosa*. Antimicrob Agents Chemother 1967:609.

Rowley, R. A., and Rubin, L. F. 1969. Penetration of penicillin into the aqueous humour of the dog. Am J Vet Res 30:1945.

Sabath, L. D., and Abraham, E. P. 1964. Synergistic action of penicillins and cephalosporins against *Pseudomonas pyocyanea*. Nature 204:1066.

Salter, W. T. 1952. Textbook of Pharmacology. Philadelphia: W. B. Saunders.

Uhlig, A. 1973. Excretion of various penicillins in the milk after intrauterine administration to cows. Inaug. dissertation, Tieraerztl Fak Muenchen 332.

van Os, J. L., and Goudswaard, J. 1973. Contamination of milk with penicillin from the urine of treated cows. Tijdschr Diergeneeskd 98:547.

Ziv, G.; Rosenzuaig, A.; Risenberg-tirer, R.; Danieli, Y.; and Miller, I. 1969. Carbenicillin milk levels following intramammary treatment of bovine pseudomonas mastitis. Refu Vet 26:152.

CHAPTER 48

TETRACYCLINES

WILLIAM G. HUBER

The genus *Streptomyces,* belonging to Actinomycetales, is a rich source of antibiotics applicable in the control of bacterial diseases in animals and human beings. Streptomycin is produced by *Streptomyces griseus. Chlortetracycline,* U.S.P. (Aureomycin) is obtained from *Streptomyces aureofaciens; Oxytetracycline,* U.S.P. (Terramycin), is obtained from *Streptomyces rimosus.* Similarities of these two antibiotics noted in antibacterial and pharmacological studies were confirmed by the similarity of their chemical formulas; this parallelism led to the semisynthetic production of a third compound, the parent of the group, *Tetracycline,* U.S.P. (Achromycin, Panmycin, Polycycline, Tetracyn, etc.). The latter has also been isolated from a free-growing *Streptomyces.*

A mutant strain of *Streptomyces aureofaciens* has produced a metabolic product called demeclocycline (Declomycin). This demethylated tetracycline has been found to have an antibacterial spectrum similar to the other tetracyclines. Methacycline, doxycycline, and rolitetracycline have been more recently brought into medical use. Several other tetracycline compounds have also been noted to possess antibacterial activity. The generic name tetracycline is used to describe the entire group in addition to one specific compound. The tetracyclines are produced by fermentation processes or by chemical transformations of the natural products.

The tetracyclines are amphoteric compounds, forming salts with acids or bases; however, they crystallize in aqueous solutions of their salts unless stabilized by excess acid.

ANTIBACTERIAL SPECTRUM

The tetracyclines are called broad-spectrum antibiotics because they exhibit the wide range of antibacterial spectra of penicillin, streptomycin, and chloramphenicol (active against gram-positive and gram-negative bacteria). In addition, the tetracyclines will act against some pathogenic agents unaffected by other antibiotics, e.g., the rickettsiae (certain of the large viruses belonging to the psittacosis group in animals, the lymphogranuloma venereum group in human beings). They also have activity against mycoplasmas, spirochetes, and actinomyces. At high doses, some antiprotozoal activity has also been observed. The tetracycline antibiotics are relatively potent against most gram-positive bacteria, but less active against gram-negative organisms.

The tetracyclines affect rapidly growing organisms. *Considerably higher concentrations are required to kill the microorganism than to prevent multiplication.* The antibacterial activity of the tetracyclines is influenced to only a minor degree by the presence of serum, blood, and bacterial debris. The susceptibility of a particular microorganism to each of the tetracyclines is quite similar, although individual strain differences may be encountered.

Bacteria most susceptible to the tetracyclines are: beta hemolytic streptococci, nonhemolytic streptococci, clostridia, *Brucella, Hemophilus,* and *Klebsiella.* The moderately sensitive bacteria include: *Corynebacterium, Escherichia coli, Pasteurella, Salmonella,* and *Bacillus anthracis.* The relatively resistant bacteria include: *Proteus* spp., *Pseudomonas, Aerobacter aerogenes, Shigella, Streptococcus faecalis,* and many strains of staphylococci. Initially some staphylococci were moderately susceptible. Studies with chlortetracycline and *Mycoplasma hypopneumoniae* demonstrated that the antibiotic did not prevent the transmission of infection from treated to untreated pigs (Huhn 1971).

The activity of the tetracyclines against gram-negative microorganisms is similar to that of chloramphenicol or streptomycin. The tetracyclines are less effective than penicillin against most coccal bacteria, but more effective than streptomycin and chloramphenicol. Bacterial R^+ factor resistance to tetracyclines develops readily and persists for longer periods of time than many other antibiotics.

ADMINISTRATION AND ABSORPTION

Physical and Chemical Properties

The crystalline tetracycline bases are odorless, yellow, and slightly bitter. They are practically insoluble in distilled water but form soluble sodium and hydrochloride salts readily. In neutral aqueous solution, chlortetracycline loses most of its activity in 1 day and tetracycline in approximately 3 weeks. Oxytetracline dissolved in a propylene glycol–water solution has been found to be stable for relatively long periods. Aqueous solutions of tetracycline bases show greater instability with increases of pH and temperature. However, the bases and hydrochlorides are stable indefinitely as dried powders.

The hydrochloride salts are commonly used for oral administration and are usually encapsulated. Stable chelate complexes are formed with metals such as calcium, magnesium, and iron. It has been suggested that antibacterial activity may be related to the ability of tetracycline to remove essential metallic ions. Stable chelate complexes of tetracyclines and metallic ions, e.g., calcium or magnesium, will retard absorption from the gastrointestinal (GI) tract.

In general, the tetracyclines have an acid pH in aqueous solution and will lose potency when exposed to sunlight, air, or alkaline materials. Most tetracyclines are hygroscopic. The physical and chemical properties of the tetracyclines permit them to be available as parenterals, boluses, capsules, powders, feed additives, ointments, etc., for use in veterinary medicine and animal production. The pH of the GI tract and the pK_a of the tetracyclines enable these antibiotics to be absorbed and thus produce systemic antibacterial concentrations.

Routes of Administration

In herbivora, tetracyclines are administered parenterally, orally, and topically. Topical administration should be avoided if other suitable agents are available because of the sensitization and resistance risk. Initially, the normal bacterial fermentation of plant fiber in herbivorous animals is suppressed by the administration of tetracycline antibiotics. In carnivora, omnivora, and newborn herbivora, these drugs can be administered orally for therapeutic purposes with minimal side effects. Intravenous and intramuscular injections are common routes of administering tetracycline compounds in veterinary medicine. Special preparations of the tetracyclines buffered with sodium glycinate in powder form are available in sterile vials for intravenous injection. The preparations must be reconstituted prior to use. A solution of chlortetracycline will change from yellow to brown in approximately 1 hour.

For deep intramuscular injection, oxytetracycline hydrochloride is combined with 5% magnesium chloride and may be combined with 2% procaine hydrochloride to minimize postinjection discomfort at the site. Similar preparations of tetracycline also are injected intramuscularly, but chlortetracycline cannot be employed in these mixtures because it causes severe tissue irritation. Oxytetracycline is also available for parenteral administration in a propylene glycol-water vehicle with or without a local anesthetic.

Intrathecal injection of the intravenous preparations of tetracycline is extremely dangerous but can be employed in patients where a sufficient concentration in the cerebrospinal fluid cannot be attained by intravenous injection of any antibacterial agent. Intramammary infusion of the tetracycline antibiotics for treatment of mastitis is routinely employed in the cow, goat, and ewe.

Dosage

INTRAVENOUS

The suggested dosage for intravenous and intramuscular injection of the tetracycline antibiotics is 2–5 mg/lb of body weight daily. Intravenous injections are usually given once daily, but in acute illness administration of the daily dosage in divided doses at 12-hour intervals is more effective and reduces the likelihood of shock or toxemia from bacterial debris. Intravenous administration of tetracyclines is indicated if oral administration will produce digestive disturbances (e.g., bloat or vomition), if the patient is unable to retain an orally administered dose, or in severe acute diseases requiring effective therapeutic concentrations promptly.

INTRAMUSCULAR

Oxytetracycline hydrochloride in propylene glycol and water is commonly employed for deep intramuscular injection. Tetracycline is sometimes administered intramuscularly but is more irritating and may cause edema and inflammation at the site of injection. Chlortetracycline can be administered intramuscularly.

ORAL

The tetracycline antibiotics are administered orally to small animals at a dosage of 15–50 mg/lb of body weight/day, preferably divided into 2 or 3 doses. Chlortetracycline and oxytetracycline are also administered orally to large animals at subtherapeutic levels. Although they are primarily added to the feed to improve feed efficiency and gain, preventive and therapeutic disease claims are made.

Hens administered oxytetracycline had higher concentrations in the blood at 6 A.M. than at noon. It was suggested that the difference was due to difference in calcium absorption and the cycle of egg formation (Harms and Waldroup 1963).

LOCAL

A mammary infusion of 440 mg of the hydrochloride of any one of the tetracycline antibiotics has been used for treatment of bovine mastitis. An ophthalmic ointment containing 1 mg of tetracycline/g of ointment may be used on conjunctival membranes. The eye may also be treated with a buffered aqueous solution of tetracycline antibiotic containing 5 mg/ml.

INHALATION

Aerosols of tetracyclines have been administered to small pigs suffering from pneumonia. Fewer lesions and increased body weight were observed in the treated pigs. The procedure has been used for prophylactic effect. Until more research information is obtained and until suitable systems for mass medication are available, inhalation as a route of administration has limited clinical utility for antibacterial agents.

Recent pharmacokinetic studies have been conducted with oxytetracycline in horses and cattle (Pilloud 1973). It was concluded that currently used doses of oxytetracycline for these two species could be below the amounts needed for the successful treatment of infections caused by bacteria of average or low sensitivity.

Absorption

Following oral administration, the tetracyclines are absorbed readily from the stomach and the first part of the small intestine to give a peak plasma concentration in 2–4 hours in carnivorous animals. This blood level persists for 6 hours or longer, followed by a gradual drop until the drug is barely detectable at 24 hours; thus a 6-hour dosage interval is recommended. Calcium and magnesium ions in the GI tract will diminish absorption. Some of the drug is concentrated by the liver, excreted in the bile, and reabsorbed from the intestines so that a small amount persists in the blood for a long time after administration due to enterohepatic reabsorption.

The persistence of the tetracyclines in the blood following absorption is a surprising contrast to other antibiotics which are eliminated more rapidly. The recommended dosage of the tetracycline antibiotics produces significant plasma concentrations during most of the 24 hours post-administration. Plasma concentrations of tetracycline and oxytetracycline administered intramuscularly are detectable within 15 minutes, reach a peak within 1 hour, maintain significant blood concentrations for about 12 hours, and then decline to trace amounts approximately 24 hours after injection. Intramuscular and subcutaneous administration of some tetracyclines may produce severe tissue damage characterized by necrosis and polymorphonuclear infiltration. Oxytetracycline reconstituted with water or administered in a propylene glycol–water solvent produced the least tissue damage.

Preparations with local anesthetics are intended for intramuscular use and should not be administered intravenously because of the undesirable action local anesthetics may have on the cardiac conduction mechanism. Some absorption of chlortetracycline or oxytetracycline into the bloodstream occurs following intramammary infusion. The transfer of antibiotics from treated to nontreated quarters has been observed.

METABOLISM

The tetracyclines undergo metabolism to various degrees. The most frequently identified substance in urine, feces, and tissue is the parent tetracycline. As much as 30% of the tetracycline will be excreted unchanged in the feces.

The tetracyclines are reversibly bound to the plasma proteins and are widely distributed. The tetracyclines are cleared from the blood by the liver and high concentrations are achieved in the parenchyma and bile. Bile concentration may be 30 times that of blood; however, enterohepatic recirculation limits bile secretion and prolongs the maintenance of therapeutic concentrations. Oxytetracycline increased oxygen uptake in tissue metabolism studies in chickens (Stützel et al. 1964). Duodenum and thyroid gland oxygen uptake was increased as was labeled iodine uptake by the thyroid.

DISTRIBUTION AND ELIMINATION

Distribution

The tetracyclines diffuse throughout the body and are found in highest concentrations in the kidney, liver, spleen, and lung. They are also deposited at active sites of ossification. Sites of growth in the diaphysis and epiphysis can be identified by the fluorescence produced by tetracyclines. The concentration in fetal blood is approximately one-half that in the maternal blood.

The tetracyclines diffuse into the cerebrospinal fluid with difficulty but tetracycline somewhat more readily than chlortetracycline or oxytetracycline. The tetracyclines also pass through the bovine placenta and enter the fetal circulation. Since tetracyclines are also distributed to prostatic fluid, this group of antibiotics may be used to treat microbial diseases of the prostate gland of valuable breeding sires.

The tetracyclines may also be incorporated in egg shells (Ferguson et al. 1966). The eggs of chickens and turkeys contained chlortetracycline for 3 days following oral or parenteral administration.

Oxytetracycline serum concentrations were studied in horses (Teske et al. 1973). Intravenous administration was superior to intramuscular administration for maintenance of drug concentrations in serum. They reported biological half-lives for oxytetracycline administered intravenously and intramuscularly to be 15.7 and 10.5 hours, respectively.

Oxytetracycline concentrations in blood plasma of geese have been determined (Roliński 1967). Peak plasma concentrations of 3.4 μg/ml were achieved at 4 hours postadministration with a single oral dose of 50 mg/kg. At 24 hours postadministration, the plasma concentration declined to 0.8 μg/ml. An aqueous vehicle reduced the amount of time for peak concentrations of oxytetracycline to be achieved while an oil suspension vehicle prolonged the rate of absorption.

Chlortetracycline administered orally in a milk substitute at a daily dose of 8 mg/kg produced peak concentrations in 6–8 hours. The maximum concentration was 3 μg/ml of serum (Brüggemann et al. 1972). Undoubtedly, the presence of calcium and other ions in the milk substitute decreased absorption because of chlortetracycline's chelating action.

Elimination

The tetracyclines are excreted primarily by the kidneys. Approximately 25%–30% of a single dose of tetracycline can be found in the urine. The tetracycline serum half-lives are presented in Table 48.1.

Following oral administration, the highest concentration is found in the urine between 2 and 8 hours, but antibacterial activity can be detected for 3 days or more after therapy is discontinued. The urinary concentration of the tetracyclines depends upon the dose of drug and the urine volume. During a period of repeated medication, it usually reaches or exceeds 100 μg/ml, which is in excess of the amount required to inhibit growth of susceptible microorganisms present in urinary tract infections.

TABLE 48.1. Tetracycline serum half-lives

Drug	Hours*
Chlortetracycline	5.5
Tetracycline	8.5
Oxytetracycline	9.5
Methacycline	15.0
Demeclocycline	17.0
Minocycline	17.5
Doxycycline	19.5

* Approximate

Fecal elimination of tetracyclines occurs regardless of the route of administration. The amount eliminated following oral administration may reach 10% of the dose.

The tetracycline antibiotics are also eliminated in milk. The concentration of tetracycline in the milk is about one-half that of the maternal serum. No detectable concentrations of tetracycline antibiotic have been found in the serum of a suckling pig. Orally and parenterally administered tetracyclines are eliminated in bovine milk. Oxytetracycline administered parenterally at 2–4 mg/kg produced peak milk concentrations of 0.9–1.9 μg/ml in 6 hours (Høgh and Rasmussen 1964). Traces of the tetracycline were detected in the milk 48 hours postadministration. Chlortetracycline administered at a dose of 400 mg or higher to adult lactating cows produced detectable amounts in milk (Merkenschlager and Lösch 1967). Oxytetracycline was detected in the milk only if the cow received 2–12 g orally.

The incorporation of dyes to antimastitis preparations has been investigated as a visual means to estimate tetracycline elimination rates (Fritsche 1964; Feagen and Greffin 1965). The addition of green dye S to tetracycline antimastitis preparations had to be abandoned because the antibiotic continued to be excreted after the dye had been completely eliminated. However, Brilliant Blue F.C.F. dye has been eliminated at the same rate as oxytetracycline when used at a ratio of 0.25 g dye to 426 mg of oxytetracycline. In the United States, dye markers have not been approved by the Food and Drug Administration.

The effect of cooking on tetracycline residues in poultry tissues and eggs has been studied (Meredith et al. 1965). Tissue concentrations of oxytetracycline and chlortetracycline, produced after oral administration of 200–1000 ppm in the feed, were destroyed after roasting, frying, or autoclaving. However, poaching or scrambling eggs did not destroy all residues.

Tetracycline withdrawal times should be observed in food-producing animals as should all drug withdrawal times (see Chapter 63).

PHARMACODYNAMICS

The tetracyclines interfere with the bacterial protein synthesis of the rapidly growing and reproducing bacterial cell. The tetracyclines inhibit bacterial cellular metabolism by blocking the attachment of aminoacyl transfer RNA ribosomes, which interferes with protein synthesis. Only a small portion of the drug is irreversibly bound, and it appears that the reversibly bound antibiotic is responsible for the antibacterial action. Concentrations of chlortetracycline sufficient to inhibit bacterial growth will markedly reduce the conversion of glutamate into cell protein by the bacteria. Higher concentrations of chlortetracycline also interfere with the accumulation of glutamate within the cell.

R factor tetracycline resistance is caused by defective drug uptake by the bacteria. Tetracycline R factor–resistant bacteria have become efficient in excluding the drug and are resistant. A mutant of *Escherichia coli* has been shown to contain a defective uptake and binding system. The drug blocks protein synthesis by binding to the 50 S ribosomal subunit of the 70 S bacterial ribosome.

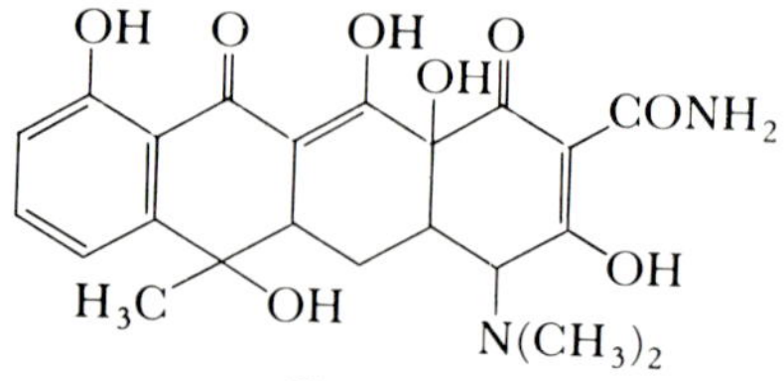

OH O OH O OH $CONH_2$ OH H_3C OH $N(CH_3)_2$

Tetracycline

Fig. 48.1.

COMPOUNDS

Tetracycline Hydrochloride, U.S.P. (Fig. 48.1), is an odorless, yellow crystalline powder that is freely soluble in water. A 1% solution in water has a pH of about 2.5. The powder is hygroscopic but moderately stable in air, although strong sunlight will darken it. It is destroyed by strongly alkaline solutions and by acid solutions below a pH of 2.

Tetracycline base, hydrochloride salt, and phosphate complex have the same spectrum of antibacterial activity as other tetracyclines.

Oxytetracycline Hydrochloride, U.S.P. (Terramycin) (Fig. 48.2), is a bitter, odorless, yellow crystalline powder that is freely soluble in water and organic solvents. A 1% solution in water has a pH of about 2.5. The powder is hygroscopic and moderately stable in the presence of light and moisture. It is rapidly destroyed by alkali and also by acid solutions below a pH of 2. Irrespective of the preparation or route of administration, oxytetracycline after absorption attains the pH of the blood and tissues so that the clinical efficacy of the various forms (hydrochloride, amphoteric base, sodium, salt) is about the same.

Oxytetracycline is the commonest in-

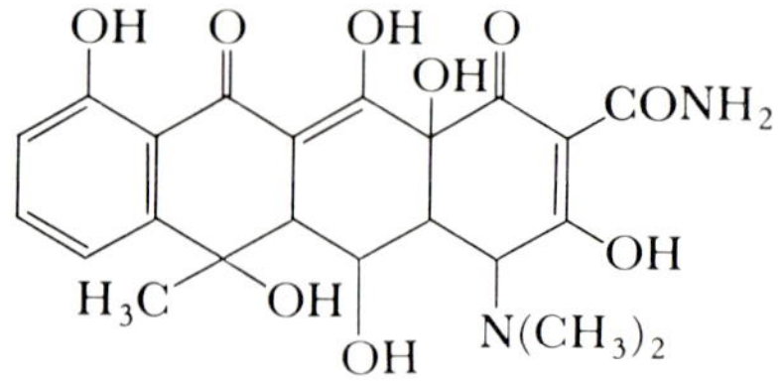

OH O OH O OH $CONH_2$ OH H_3C OH OH $N(CH_3)_2$

Oxytetracycline

Fig. 48.2.

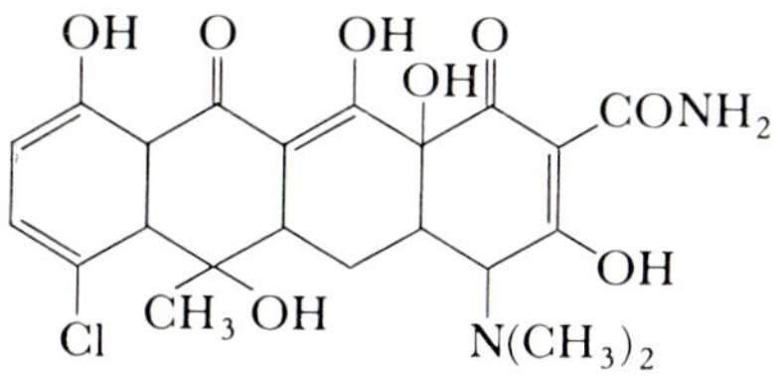

Chlortetracycline

Fig. 48.3.

tramuscularly administered tetracycline.

Chlortetracycline Hydrochloride, U.S.P. (Aureomycin) (Fig. 48.3), is a bitter, odorless, yellow crystalline powder that is sparingly soluble in water. It is stable in air, but deterioration is promoted by sunlight. A 0.5% solution in water has a pH of about 3.

Chlortetracycline's effectiveness is similar to that of the other tetracyclines. It should not be administered intramuscularly because of severe tissue irritation. The probability of hypersensitization may obviate topical use.

Demethylchlortetracycline, or 7-chloro-6-demethyltetracycline (Declomycin), is more stable in acid or alkali than the methylated corresponding compounds. This drug has not been used extensively for the treatment of animal diseases. It is administered orally to human beings. Efficacy appears comparable to other tetracyclines. In human beings, photosensitivity reactions appear more frequently than observed with other tetracyclines.

Other tetracyclines: doxycycline monohydrate (Vibramycin monohydrate), methacycline hydrochloride (Rondomycin), minocycline hydrochloride (Minocin), and rolitetracycline (Syntetrin) are tetracyclines of more recent vintage and may find utility in veterinary medicine. (See Fig. 48.4.)

Doxycycline is more completely absorbed and more slowly excreted than most other tetracyclines, thus it has a longer duration of action with attendant advantages of a smaller required dose and a less frequently administered maintenance dose. The serum half-life is 19–20 hours.

Methacycline is produced synthetically from oxytetracycline. Its safety and efficacy are comparable to other tetracyclines.

Minocycline is a semisynthetic tetracycline derivative. Minocycline does not share cross-resistance with other tetracyclines against certain strains of staphylococci. It appears to be more completely metabolized than other tetracyclines. If renal impairment exists, dosage should be reduced to avoid excessive systemic accumulation.

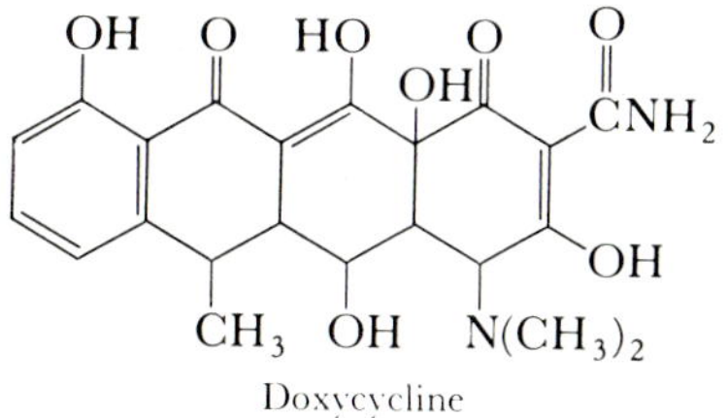

Doxycycline

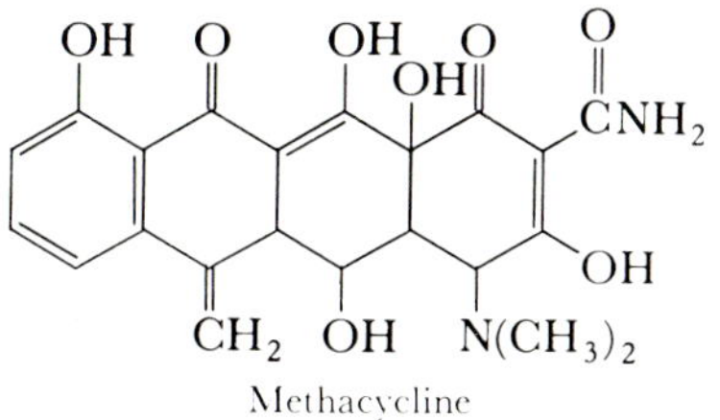

Methacycline

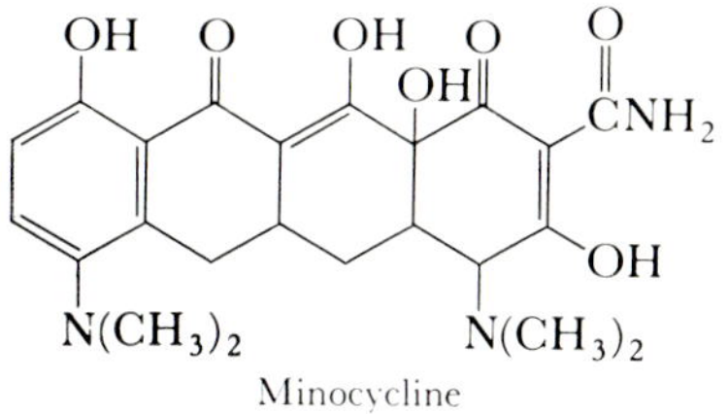

Minocycline

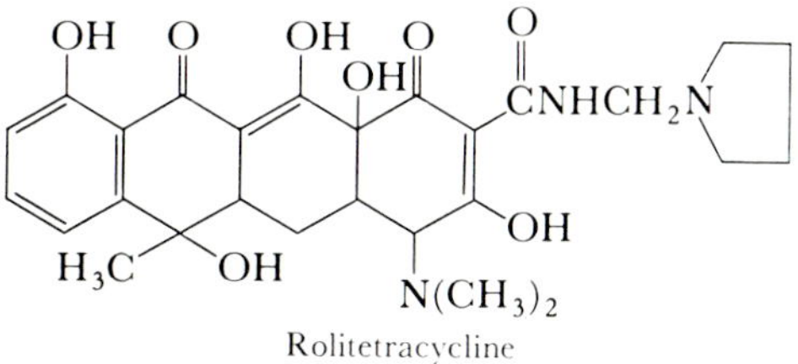

Rolitetracycline

Fig. 48.4.

TOXICITY

The tetracycline antibiotics are relatively nontoxic. The acute toxicity for intravenous tetracycline in mice, LD50, is between 150 and 180 mg/kg. Occasional vomition has been observed in dogs treated daily with intravenous injections of tetracycline of up to 30 mg/kg of body weight for 17 days. No loss of appetite or weight, evidence of renal inhibition, hematologic complications, or abnormal liver function were observed.

Dogs tolerate oxytetracycline hydrochloride intramuscularly in doses of 50–100 mg/kg/day. Oral doses of 75–465 mg/kg daily for as long as 8 weeks were tolerated in dogs without evidence of toxicity. Tetracyclines have been used in the presence of liver disease and renal pathology without untoward results. Sufficient tetracycline is excreted by the bile to suppress bacterial fermentation in herbivora, resulting in anorexia and occasionally diarrhea.

One of the complications following oral therapy is the alteration in the normal flora of microorganisms in the digestive tract. Such alteration is often followed by the disappearance of desirable microorganisms and the overgrowth of undesirable forms resistant to the antibiotics. Antifungal agents, e.g., nystatin, are frequently administered concurrently with the tetracyclines in an attempt to control overgrowth of undesirable fungi.

Digestive disturbances were observed in weaned beef calves fed a ration containing chlortetracycline and sulfamethazine (Woods et al. 1973). Acute tympanitis was observed in 11% of 46 animals receiving the medicated feed.

The role of antibiotics, specifically the tetracyclines, and immunologic responses has been investigated in food-producing animals. Daily oral doses of 1 g of chlortetracycline to young pigs resulted in reduced levels of antibodies in the blood serum. Similarly, chlortetracycline at 15 mg/kg suppressed immunity against an experimental infection of erysipelas (Lyashenko 1966). The increase in titre was slower and lower in chlortetracycline-medicated pigs than in nonmedicated pigs. It was concluded that tetracycline medication should not be used between 2 days before and 10 days after erysipelas vaccination. Similar studies in other species have suggested an immunosuppressive effect related to tetracycline. However, studies with oxytetracycline and crystal violet vaccination against swine fever did not demonstrate differences in immunologic responses between medicated and nonmedicated groups (Trumié et al. 1965).

The lack of a relationship among tetracycline, methoxyflurane anesthesia, and severe renal failure in dogs has been reported (Pedersoli and Jackson 1973). Although the administration of these two drugs has been reported to have a deleterious effect on renal function in human beings, renal pathology was not observed in dogs. Polyuria, which appeared 24 hours after the start of tetracycline therapy and disappeared after the last administration, was the only change noted.

The use of chlortetracycline for intramammary infusion in dairy cows during the dry period is contraindicated because of tissue irritation (Thompson and Leaver 1972). Chlortetracycline-treated cows failed to lactate after parturition and teat and udder damage were observed. The lesion was characterized as a chronic granuloma of predominantly fibrous tissue. Similar lesions and symptoms were observed in the udders of nonlactating, chlortetracycline-treated ewes.

Drug-related digestive disturbances have been observed in the horse with the postsurgical use of certain forms of tetracycline (Cook 1973). Oxytetracycline hydrochloride (2 mg/lb) produced acute postsurgical or postanesthetic colitis. It has been postulated that the intestinal flora of the horse is easily disturbed by biliary excretion of high doses of oxytetracycline. An abnormal bacterial flora was observed with a proliferation of *Clostridium perfringens* and possible toxin production.

Intraarticular injections of tetracycline or oxytetracycline have produced inflammatory responses and are contraindicated.

Turkeys fed a partially deficient vitamin A ration containing 500 g of chlortetracycline/ton of feed had a significantly greater number of *Candida albicans* lesions in the esophagus than turkeys on the same ration without chlortetracycline (Tripathy et al. 1967). The adverse antibacterial effect of chlortetracycline and other antibacterials should be considered when animals are exposed to fungal infections of the GI tract and appropriate antifungal therapy initiated. Adrenocortical hyperplasia and decreased thyroid follicular cell size were observed following intravenous injections of large therapeutic doses of oxytetracycline hydrochloride in goats (Davis et al. 1966).

RESISTANCE

The factors involved in acquired or inherent drug resistance, mutational and plasmid mediated, have been presented in the chapter on sulfonamides. However, since the tetracyclines are extensively used and have been reported to have a high prevalence in coliform multiresistant organisms, the veterinarian should consider dosage regimens very carefully and anticipate the likelihood of dealing with multiresistant organisms.

Resistance to members of the tetracycline group has been reported for some strains of the following bacteria: *Escherichia* spp., *Aerobacter* spp., *Salmonella choleraesius* var. *kunzendorf, Chlamydia psittaci, Salmonella typhimurium, Proteus* spp., beta hemolytic streptococci, *Staphylococcus aureus, Pseudomonas aeruginosa, Pasteurella multocida, Salmonella dublin, Klebsiella pneumoniae, Salmonella pullorum,* and *Salmonella gallinarum.*

Since it is not within the scope of this book to review in detail the many reports in the literature concerning antibacterial drug resistance in domestic animals, the reader may consult two reviews for an in-depth presentation of the subject (Smith 1971; Luther et al. 1974).

ANTIBACTERIAL UTILITY

The antibacterial utility of the tetracyclines is presented in Table 48.2, which lists the important diseases and their etio-

TABLE 48.2. Diseases treated with tetracycline antibiotics

Etiologic Agent	Disease
Actinobacillosis lignieresi	Actinobacillosis
Actinomyces bovis	Actinomycosis
Aerobacter aerogenes	Mastitis
Anaplasma marginale	Anaplasmosis
Bacillus anthracis	Anthrax
Borrelia anserina	Avian borreliosis
Brucella canis	Canine brucellosis
Clostridium chauvoei	Blackleg
Clostridium hemolyticum	Bacillary hemoglobinuria
Clostridium novyi	Infectious necrotic hepatitis
Clostridium perfringens B, C, D	Enterotoxemia
Clostridium septicum	Malignant edema
Clostridium tetani	Tetanus
Corynebacterium equi	Foal pneumonia
Corynebacterium pyogenes	Mastitis
Corynebacterium renale	Bovine pyelonephritis
Cowdria ruminantium	Heartwater disease
Dermatophilus congolensis	Cutaneous streptothricosis
Erysipelothrix insidiosa	Erysipelas
Escherichia coli	Mastitis, colibacillosis
Fusiformis necrophorus	Oral and hepatic necrobacilloses, infectious pododermatitis
Haemobartonella canis	Canine bartonellosis (tetracycline used concurrently with oxophenarsine)
Hemophilus spp.	Respiratory infections
Hemophilus suis	Infectious polyarthritis
Leptospira spp.	Leptospirosis
Listeria monocytogenes	Listeriosis
Moraxella bovis	Bovine infectious keratitis
Mycoplasma spp.	Mastitis, serositis-arthritis, agalactia
Mycoplasma hyopneumoniae	Porcine enzootic pneumonia
Nanophyetus salmincola	Canine rickettsiosis
Pasteurella anatipestifer	Pasteurellosis in pheasants
Pasteurella hemolytica	Mastitis, pasteurellosis
Pasteurella multocida	Pasteurellosis, fowl cholera, hemorrhagic septicemia
Salmonella abortus-ovis	Abortion
Shigella equirulis	Shigellosis of foals
Staphylococcus aureus	Mastitis, synovitis
Staphylococcus hyicus	Exudative epidermitis
Staphylococcus hyos	Exudative epidermitis
Streptococcus agalactiae	Mastitis
Streptococcus dysgalactiae	Mastitis
Streptococcus equi	Strangles
Streptococcus uberis	Mastitis
Vibrio fetus	Ovine vibriosis

logic agents that have been commonly treated with various tetracycline antibiotics. Symptomatology and diagnostic tests are not included since other appropriate texts are more suitable for greater detail. In regard to dosages, the reader should select the tetracycline formulation that will maximize the opportunity to attain systemic therapeutic concentrations. Information presented in this chapter, such as half-life, parenteral dosage forms of tetracyclines, and resistance, should provide the guidelines for determining the appropriate dosage regimen.

REFERENCES

Afunas'er, V. I. 1968. Antibiotic therapy by inhalation for pigs with pneumonia. Veterinariia 7:37.

Brüggemann, J.; Lösch, U.; and Knoll, G. 1972. The chlortetracycline concentration and its persistence in the serum of calves after oral administration. Z Tierphysiol 29:230.

Cook, W. R. 1973. Diarrhea in the horse associated with stress and tetracycline therapy. Vet Rec 93:15.

Davis, R. W.; Koenir, R. A.; and Flamboe, E. E. 1966. The effects of an oxytetracycline preparation on the thyroid gland: A preliminary report. Am J Vet Res 27:166.

Feagan, J. T., and Greffin, A. T. 1965. The use of Brilliant Blue FCF in tetracycline intramammary preparations. Aust J Dairy Tech 20:18.

Ferguson, T. N.; Smith, E. B.; and Couch, J. R. 1966. Distribution of chlortetracycline in turkey and chicken tissues. Fed Proc 25:688.

Fritsche, J. B. 1964. Staining of chloramphenicol and tetracycline hydrochloride for intramammary treatment in cattle with reference to drugs suspended in oily or fatty vehicles. Schweiz Arch Tierheilkd 106:285.

Harms, R. H., and Waldroup, P. W. 1963. Potentiation of Terramycin. III. Method of administering the antibiotic to laying hens. Avian Dis 7:467.

Høgh, P., and Rasmussen, F. 1964. Concentrations of oxytetracycline in blood plasma and milk after parenteral application of Terramycin in cows. Nord Vet Med 16:997.

Huhn, R. G. 1971. Swine enzootic pneumonia: Age susceptibility and treatment schemata. Can J Comp Med 35:77.

Luther, H. G.; Huber, W. G.; Siegel, D.; and Luther, H. G., Jr. 1974. Antibacterial feed additives: Residues and infectious drug resistance. In Proceedings of the Miles 1974 Symposium. Hamilton, Ontario: Nutrition Society of Canada.

Lyashenko, A. T. 1965. Influence of biomycin-supplemented feed on immunogenesis in pigs inoculated with erysipelas vaccine. Veterinariia 42:21.

———. 1966. Effect of feeding chlortetracycline on agglutinin formation in pigs vaccinated against erysipelas. Veterinariia 9:198.

Meredith, W. E.; Weiser, H. H.; and Winter, A. R. 1965. Chlortetracycline and oxytetracycline residues in poultry tissues and eggs. Appl Microbiol 13:86.

Merkenschlager, N., and Lösch, U. 1967. Excretion of tetracyclines in the milk of cows given food containing tetracyclines. Tieraerztl Umsch 22:423.

Pedersoli, W. N., and Jackson, J. A. 1973. Tetracycline, methoxyflurane anesthesia and severe renal failure in dogs. J Am Anim Hosp Assoc 9:57.

Pilloud, N. 1973. Pharmacokinetics, plasma protein binding and dosage of oxytetracycline in cattle and horses. Res Vet Sci 15(2):224.

Roliński, Z. 1967. Determination of oxytetracycline concentration in the blood of geese after oral and intramuscular administration of the antibiotic. Ann Univ Mariae Curie Sklodowska 21:127.

Smith, H. W. 1971. The effect of the use of antibacterial drugs on the emergence of drug-resistant bacteria in animals. Adv Vet Sci Comp Med 15:67.

Stützel, N.; Gaśpař, S. N.; Keměny, A.; and Baldizsár, H. 1964. Studies on the thyroid gland with radioiodine. V. The influence of feeding with antibiotics on the tissue metabolism of chickens. Acta Vet K 14:171.

Teske, R. H.; Rollins, L. D.; Condon, R. J.; and Curter, G. G. 1973. Serum oxytetracycline concentrations after intravenous and intramuscular administration in horses. J Am Vet Med Assoc 162(2):119.

Thompson, W. H., and Leaver, D. D. 1972. Udder lesions in cows associated with intramammary infusion of chlortetracycline preparations during the dry period. Aust Vet J 48:588.

Triputhy, S. B.; Kenzy, S. G.; and Mathey, W. J. 1967. Effects of vitamin A deficiency and high level chlortetracycline on experimental candidates of turkeys. Avian Dis 11:327.

Trumić, P.; Turubatavic, R.; Panjević, D.; and Grajzinger, N. 1965. Influence of dietary oxytetracycline supplements on immunity in pigs following crystal violet vaccination against swine fever. Acta Vet Bevgr 15:95.

Woods, G. T.; Mansfield, N. E.; and Cmarik, G. F. 1973. Effect of certain biologic and antibacterial agents on development of acute respiratory tract disease in weaned beef calves. J Am Vet Med Assoc 162:974.

CHAPTER 49

STREPTOMYCIN, CHLORAMPHENICOL, AND OTHER ANTIBACTERIAL AGENTS

WILLIAM G. HUBER

This chapter includes antibacterial drugs that have been used for long periods as well as those more recently made available for veterinary usage. Dihydrostreptomycin and streptomycin have found extensive use when administered in combination with various penicillins as a medication with broad-spectrum antibacterial activity. Chloramphenicol, although not approved for use in food-producing animals, was employed extensively before the availability of newer drugs in companion animal practice as a broad-spectrum antibiotic for organisms resistant to penicillin, dihydrostreptomycin, the tetracyclines, and other antibacterial agents.

Several other antibiotics have been isolated, identified, and used clinically. Some of the antibiotics discussed in this chapter are administered for their local effect because they are poorly absorbed from the gastrointestinal (GI) tract or because of inherent parenteral toxicity. Other antibiotics, e.g., chloramphenical, oleandomycin, as well as others, are administered parenterally for their systemic effect and are free of serious side effects.

Nonantibiotic chemicals, notably the nitrofuran derivatives, are also discussed. Most of the nitrofuran derivatives are poorly absorbed; thus their effect primarily occurs locally, such as in enteric infections or mastitis. Furaltadone, a nitrofuran derivative, is readily absorbed from the GI tract, resulting in therapeutic blood concentrations.

STREPTOMYCIN AND DIHYDROSTREPTOMYCIN

Chemical Properties and Administration

Streptomycin (Fig. 49.1) is a potent antibiotic isolated from *Streptomyces griseus* by Waksman and associates in 1943. Only certain strains of *S. griseus* produce the antibiotic. Streptomycin and dihydrostreptomycin are valuable therapeutic

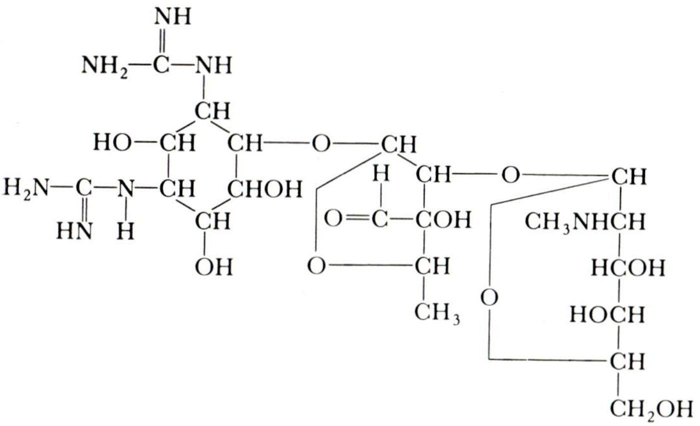

```
              NH
              ||
        NH2—C—NH
              |
             CH
           /    \
   HO—CH    CH——O——CH
       |     |          H  CH——O————CH
H2N—C—N—CH   CHOH        |   |         |
    ||   |    \   /    O=C—COH    CH3NHCH
    HN   H     CH          |          |
               |           |        HCOH
               OH      O———CH         |
                           |    O   HOCH
                          CH3         |
                                ——————CH
                                      |
                                    CH2OH
```

Streptomycin

Fig. 49.1.

agents because of their effectiveness against gram-negative bacteria. Also, they enhance the activity of other drugs that are only active against gram-positive bacteria.

Streptomycin is a glycoside hydrolyzed by acid into streptidine and streptobiosamine. The latter yields streptose and *N*-methyl-L-glycosamine. Streptomycin, a basic substance, is a white powder in the hydrochloride, sulfate, or double calcium chloride salts. The free base and the salts are freely soluble in water but insoluble in organic solvents. Streptomycin has been classified as an aminoglycoside.

Streptomycin Sulfate, U.S.P., can be reduced by catalytic hydrogenation. *Dihydrostreptomycin Sulfate,* U.S.P., has antibacterial activity comparable to that of streptomycin and apparently is more stable. Comments made about streptomycin will in most cases also be appropriate for dihydrostreptomycin and vice versa. Notable exceptions are evident in toxicologic activities.

Streptomycin and its salts are stable for at least 2 years at room temperature if stored in an unopened container. They are hygroscopic and readily take up moisture, which promotes disintegration. Dihydrostreptomycin salts are stable and are soluble in water. Streptomycin exhibits maximal antibacterial activity at a slightly alkaline pH.

Administration of streptomycin intramuscularly is the method of choice for treating systemic infections. Subcutaneous injections may also be employed. Intravenous injections of streptomycin (or dihydrostreptomycin) are not recommended because of the possibility of acute fatal toxicity, thrombophlebitis, shock, and rapid excretion. Intraperitoneal or intrapleural injections of a dilute solution may be used to supplement systemic therapy in treatment of peritonitis or empyema.

Oral administration of streptomycin or dihydrostreptomycin is satisfactory for treatment of enteric infections but unsatisfactory for treatment of systemic disease because it is poorly absorbed. A suspension or solution of streptomycin or dihydrostreptomycin may be administered intramammarily for treatment of mastitis.

The minimal therapeutic dose of streptomycin and dihydrostreptomycin base in mammals approximates 5 mg/lb of body weight intramuscularly at intervals of 8–12 hours. Chickens and turkeys have received 20–45 mg/lb of body weight.

Topical application is contraindicated because of poor absorption and a risk of sensitization and development of drug resistance.

Antibacterial Spectrum

Bacteria vary markedly in susceptibility to streptomycin. *In vitro* assessment generally indicates the susceptibilities of bacterial pathogens to the antibiotic. Streptomycin is particularly effective against *Pasteurella, Brucella, Hemophilus, Salmonella, Klebsiella, Shigella,* and *Mycobac-*

terium organisms. Dihydrostreptomycin is essentially equal to streptomycin in its antibacterial action.

Several factors influence the antibacterial potency of streptomycin. It is more effective in slightly alkaline than in acid pH; it is 20–80 times more active against gram-negative bacilli at a pH of 8 than at 5.8. For this reason, an alkalizing agent should be administered to carnivora and omnivora during streptomycin therapy for urinary tract infection. The increase in local acidity resulting from tissue damage may explain the failure of streptomycin to control bacteria in circumscribed tissue lesions.

Size of the inoculum and density of the bacterial population also influence the antibacterial activity of streptomycin. The rate of bacterial multiplication of susceptible bacteria varies inversely with the concentration. A larger therapeutic dose of the antibiotic is required when the susceptible bacterial disease is known to be highly contagious and when the exposure of the infective inoculum is large. Adequate initial dosage is essential for successful therapy. The intramuscular administration of dihydrostreptomycin to cattle at 25 mg/kg of body weight daily effectively reduces the shedding of leptospires in the urine (Stalheim 1969).

The other members of the aminoglycoside group, streptomycin, and dihydrostreptomycin are usually bactericidal for sensitive organisms, e.g., *Brucella, Pasteurella, Mycobacterium,* and *Shigella.* Cross resistance for streptomycin and/or dihydrostreptomycin and neomycin, gentamicin, and kanamycin may occur.

It appears that streptomycin is similar to penicillin in its ability to disturb the permeability of the bacterial cell membrane (Anand and Davis 1960; Anand et al. 1960). An increase in the outward permeability of nucleotides and amino acids was observed in studies with *Escherichia coli.* Inward permeability to citrate and streptomycin was also noted. It is apparent that the antibiotic does not alter the membrane directly but interferes with its development. Other investigators have suggested that streptomycin interferes with one or more of the cellular enzyme systems for bacterial cell division.

A synergism between penicillin and streptomycin may possibly occur from a dual effect on the bacterial cell membrane by disrupting the permeability barrier and aiding the entry of injurious substances. (See Fig. 49.2.)

Metabolism

Absorption of streptomycin from the GI tract is poor; dihydrostreptomycin is similarly absorbed. Two-thirds or more of a dose of streptomycin can be recovered in the feces. The dog may absorb 10% of the oral dose; however, only trace amounts of streptomycin are occasionally present in blood. The salts of dihydrostreptomycin seem to be less irritating to the digestive tract than those of streptomycin.

Streptomycin is absorbed rapidly after intramuscular injection. A peak concentration occurs in the blood within 1 hour after intramuscular injection. The rate of absorption of streptomycin following a subcutaneous injection or from serous cavities of the body may be slower than that following an intramuscular injection.

Fig. 49.3 illustrates the serum concentrations of dihydrostreptomycin produced in cattle following a single intramuscular injection of 5 or 7.5 mg/lb of body weight (Hammond 1953). Serum concentrations produced in sheep and horses parallel those obtained in cattle. A dose of 5 mg/lb injected intramuscularly in the dog produced a slightly lower serum concentration, i.e., 23 μg/ml at the end of the 1st hour and 6 μg/ml at the end of 4 hours (Venzke and Smith 1949).

In cattle, dihydrostreptomycin serum peaks were obtained 1 hour after intramuscular injection (Teske et al. 1972). Residues of dihydrostreptomycin were detected in the kidneys as long as 90 days after a single massive injection. Absorption of streptomycin from the mammary gland is limited. Following the infusion of 0.5 g/quarter, streptomycin is present in milk samples. Significant amounts are present in the urine.

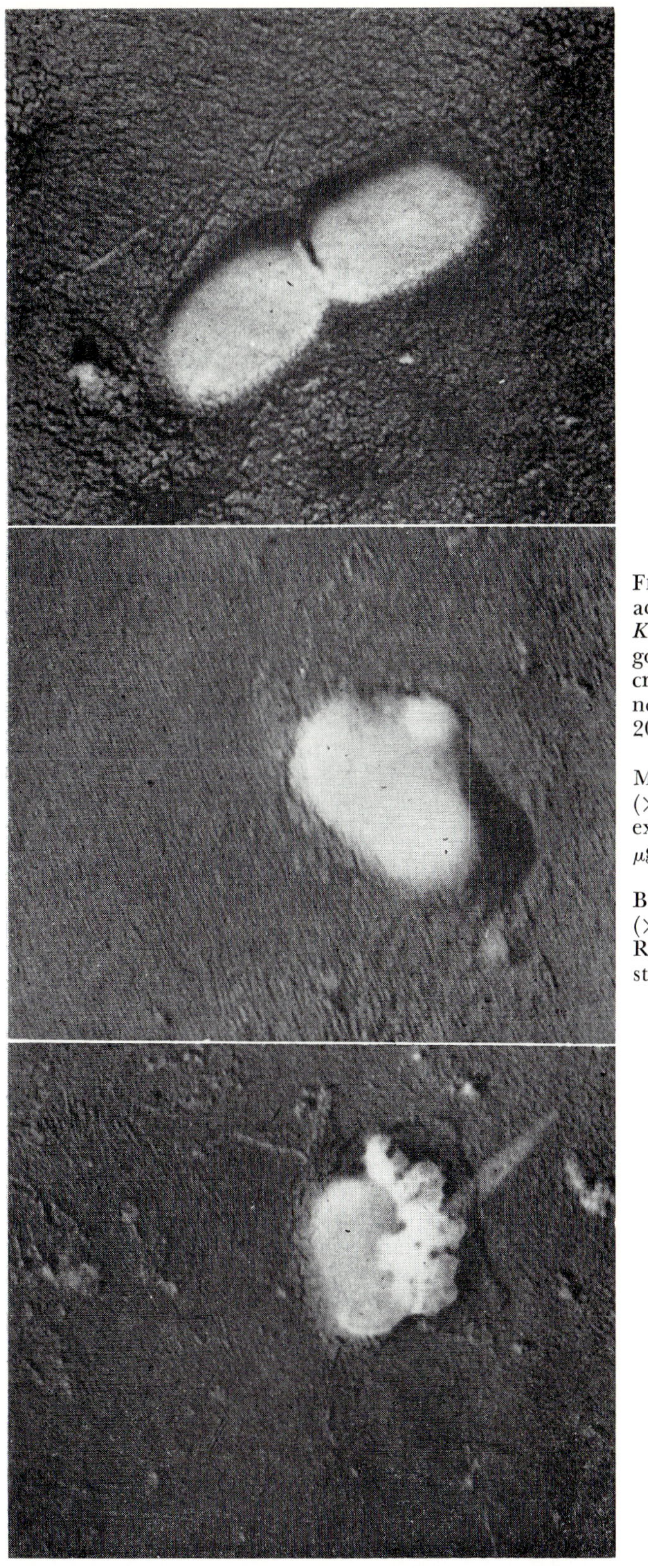

Fig. 49.2. The bactericidal action of streptomycin against *Klebsiella pneumoniae* shown gold-shadowed by electron microscope photographs. Above: normal cell division (×14,-200).

Middle: disintegration of cell (×16,400) after 18 hours of exposure to streptomycin (0.05 μg/ml of medium).

Below: further disintegration (×14,800). (Courtesy of G. R. Rake 1953, The Squibb Institute for Medical Research)

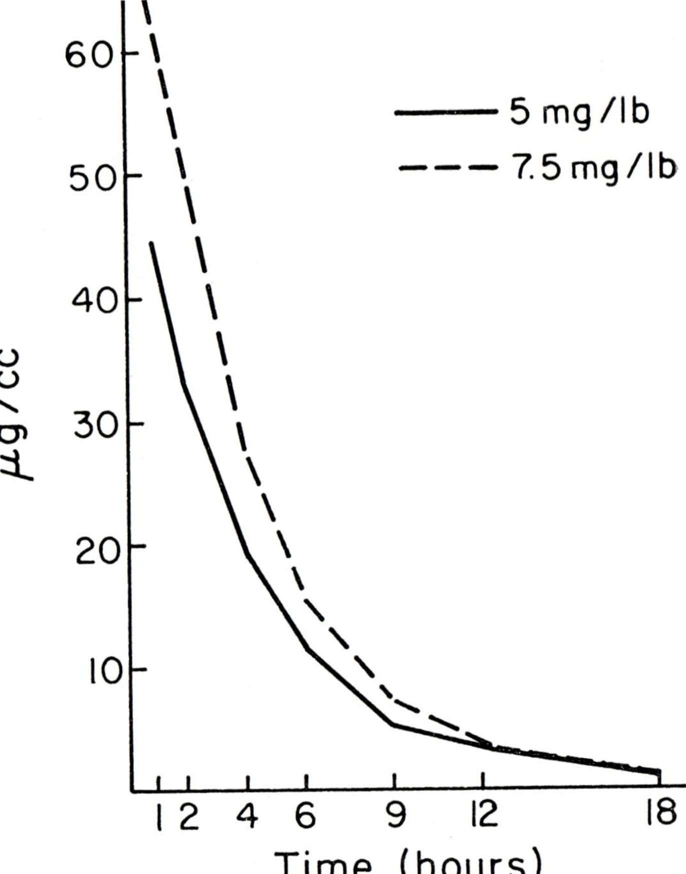

FIG. 49.3. Serum concentrations following the intramuscular injection of dihydrostreptomycin in cattle. (Hammond 1953)

Streptomycin and dihydrostreptomycin are rapidly distributed after parenteral administration. The drugs are present in the extracellular fluids and are apparently bound to the plasma proteins. The absorption half-life for dihydrostreptomycin in swine following intramuscular injection was reported to be 14 minutes based on 95% drug absorption at 1 hour (Mercer et al. 1971). Peak serum concentrations were achieved at 1 hour.

Suitable concentrations of streptomycin are attained in the fluids of body cavities after intramuscular injection. Large amounts also are noted in the bile. Moreover, it diffuses into the fetal blood and amniotic fluid after intramuscular injection. Dihydrostreptomycin attains a significant concentration in the skeletal tissues. Following parenteral administration, dihydrostreptomycin readily penetrates acute abscesses and diffuses well.

Following intramuscular injection, streptomycin is excreted primarily in the urine in about one-half its concentration in the blood. The normal kidney excretes about two-thirds of an intramuscular dose within 24 hours. Serum concentrations are prolonged when the renal clearance is defective. The excretion of streptomycin is decreased in renal insufficiency; if kidney function is severely impaired, little of the parenteral dose may be excreted in the urine. Also, the blood concentration may remain relatively constant.

Although most of the streptomycin administered parenterally appears in the urine, from 2% to 5% is excreted in bile. It also appears in the feces following parenteral or oral administration. Dihydrostreptomycin sulfate is eliminated in cows' milk soon after the intramuscular administration of 5, 10, or 20 mg/lb of body weight. Concentrations of the antibiotic range from 0.05 to 0.13 μg/ml of milk. In the various tissues, concentrations of dihydrostreptomycin are about the same as for streptomycin.

Toxicity and Resistance

ACUTE TOXICITY

As with most drugs, more pronounced toxic effects arise from intravenous injections and the least toxic effects occur following oral administration. The intravenous injection of streptomycin (100–200 mg/lb) in dogs causes an irreversible lowering of systemic arterial pressure, probably due to a depression of the vasomotor center. Respiration is paralyzed by large intravenous doses (75 mg/lb) of streptomycin.

Streptomycin was more toxic than dihydrostreptomycin to young pigs (Dewaele 1969). Paresis and depression appeared after the animals received intramuscular injections of streptomycin (100 mg/kg of body weight). All pigs died after receiving doses of 175 mg/kg. Interestingly, 6-day-old pigs tolerated dihydrostreptomycin (400 mg/kg) without untoward effects.

Signs of acute streptomycin poisoning following intravenous or subcutaneous injection include restlessness, nausea, labored respiration, loss of consciousness, and coma. Death appears to be due to respiratory failure and vasomotor depression; sometimes it may be avoided by artificial respiration administered promptly and maintained for a long time. Chickens and turkeys develop a severe respiratory depression and may become comatose. Streptomycin administered intramuscularly in ferrets at 170 and 250 mg/lb of body weight produced loss of consciousness and death (Ryan 1960). Dihydrostreptomycin sulfate administered intramuscularly in a dose greater than 150 mg/kg of body weight was fatal to pigeons (Bernau and Lüthgen 1970).

An intracisternal injection of a large dose of streptomycin in animals produces hyperexcitability with muscular tremors, followed by epileptiform convulsions within 30–60 minutes. The LD50 of dihydrostreptomycin base administered intramuscularly in 1-week-old and 4-week-old chicks is 338 mg/lb and 849 mg/lb of body weight, respectively (Huebner et al. 1956). In cats and dogs receiving streptomycin subcutaneously, the LD50 is 600 and 300 mg/kg, respectively. Since streptomycin has a weak neuromuscular blocking effect that enhances the action of other neuromuscular blocking drugs, it must be used with caution in patients receiving general anesthetics, magnesium preparations, and skeletal muscle relaxants.

CHRONIC NEUROTOXICITY

The most damaging toxicity of streptomycin is its action upon the vestibular and auditory mechanisms. Toxic effects develop after prolonged administration of large amounts of the drug. Impairment of auditory function results following administration of doses larger than those necessary to produce vestibular changes.

An obscure or latent disturbance of the vestibular apparatus in the dog or cat is not readily apparent clinically. Usually this effect can be demonstrated when an animal is forced to move in an unaccustomed manner, such as walking along a narrow board. Neurotoxicity is rarely observed in large animals because they are seldom treated for a prolonged time with high dosages.

The cat is very sensitive to the neurotoxic effects of streptomycin. A daily dose of 25–75 mg/lb will produce characteristic reactions within an average of 20 days. These neurotoxic effects involve posture and gait, ataxia first of the hind legs and then of the front legs, and a progressive loss of rotational nystagmus. Withdrawal of streptomycin results in a gradual disappearance of the symptoms and a complete but slow recovery of vestibular function.

If streptomycin sulfate and dihydrostreptomycin are administered to cats continuously, permanent damage of the vestibular end-organ occurs (McGee 1962). The lesion is limited to the inner ear. Impairment of vestibular function has been noted in dogs treated for cystitis following intramuscular injection of streptomycin in a dose of 20 mg/lb/day for 14 days (Venzke and Smith 1949).

If the correct therapeutic dose range is employed, the risk of neurotoxity from streptomycin is minimized. Generally, it is considered that neurotoxicity results only when the dosage administered is excessive for a prolonged period. The recognition that bacterial resistance develops during prolonged therapy has led to the reduction in duration of treatment. Consequently, there is little probability that neurotoxicity will develop during the usual course of streptomycin therapy.

Pure streptomycin is relatively nonirritating to the tissues unless it exceeds 20% concentration when injected subcutaneously or intramuscularly.

RESISTANCE

Bacteria have frequently shown a marked increase in their resistance to streptomycin during the course of therapy. Certain strains of bacteria have remarkable ability to modify their metabolic processes so they are no longer susceptible to the inhibitory action of streptomycin. Various laboratory workers have demonstrated that a bacterial organism, initially somewhat resistant to streptomycin, may become so adapted to the antibiotic by prolonged culture in streptomycin-containing media that it *cannot live without* streptomycin.

Clinicians are concerned with the ease with which pathogenic organisms become resistant to streptomycin. As a general policy, clinicians have attempted to control the infection as promptly as possible by the administration of adequate therapeutic doses of streptomycin. Additionally, strict adherence to the recommended intervals for maintenance therapy is important. In most cases, if the patient fails to respond favorably within 2 or 3 days, the use of streptomycin or dihydrostreptomycin should be discontinued. Bacteria that are resistant to streptomycin are also resistant to dihydrostreptomycin.

CHLORAMPHENICOL

Chloramphenicol, U.S.P. (Chloromycetin), is a crystalline antibiotic originally isolated from *Streptomyces venezuelae.*

Chemical Properties and Administration

The chemical structure of chloramphenicol (Fig. 49.4) has been determined and is produced synthetically. It is a white crystalline material with a bitter taste and considerable heat stability. It is also stable in neutral and acid solutions. Chloramphenicol is soluble in water, propylene glycol, and acetamide but is insoluble in vegetable oils.

Chloramphenicol palmitate is administered orally whereas chloramphenicol sodium succinate is administered intravenously or intramuscularly. Although the oral administration is preferred in some animals, chloramphenicol also may be given intramuscularly. Tablets and capsules are available. A topical preparation containing 1% chloramphenicol may be used for skin and ophthalmic infections (see Chapter 42).

In small animals, chloramphenicol is administered orally in a daily dose of 25–100 mg/lb of body weight divided into 3 or 4 doses. According to Watson (1972), an oral dose of 100 mg/kg administered twice daily provided reasonable blood concentrations in the greyhound, whereas an aqueous suspension of chloramphenicol administered intramuscularly at the manufacturer's recommended dose rate (i.e., 33 mg/kg/day) did not provide satisfactory plasma concentrations for adequate therapy. Topical application of an ointment containing 1%

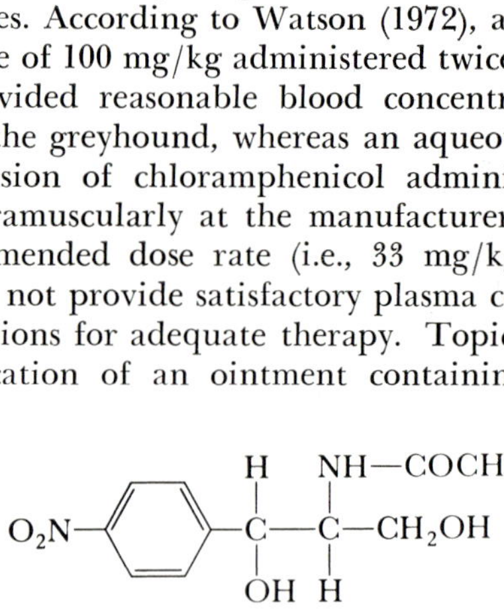

$$O_2N-C_6H_4-CH(OH)-CH(NH-COCHCl_2)-CH_2OH$$

Chloramphenicol

Fig. 49.4.

chloramphenicol on the corneas of healthy cats 3 times a day for 21 days did not produce adverse effects (Conner and Gupta 1973). Though traces of the drug were detected in the plasma and urine of the cats, no drug-related effect on the bone marrow or cellular elements of the peripheral blood was noted.

A dosage of chloramphenicol greater than 10 mg/kg (20–30 mg/kg) was necessary to produce concentrations of 5 or more μg/ml in blood of calves (Sisodia et al. 1973). The antibiotic was poorly absorbed after oral administration. Approximately 60% was bound to plasma proteins.

In small animals an intramuscular dose of 5–15 mg/lb of body weight may be used, depending upon the type and severity of the infection.

A single intramuscular injection of the sodium succinate ester of chloramphenicol at 50 mg/kg of body weight produced blood concentrations approximately 6 times greater than an equivalent dose of chloramphenicol dissolved in acetyldimethylamine propylene glycol (Ziv et al. 1973). Chloramphenicol concentrations in milk obtained from chronic but subclinical mastitic cows and ewes were approximately 50% of the corresponding serum concentrations. Milk concentrations of chloramphenicol in cows suffering from acute mastitis were only slightly higher than milk obtained from normal mammary glands.

Chloramphenicol is not approved by the Food and Drug Administration (FDA) for use in food-producing animals (see Section 16).

Antibacterial Spectrum

Chloramphenicol has a broad spectrum of activity against both gram-positive and gram-negative bacteria, rickettsia, and the psittacosis-lympho-granuloma group. Ostensibly, chloramphenicol is more active than streptomycin and many times more active than penicillin against gram-negative bacteria *in vitro*. The following bacteria are killed or inhibited *in vitro* by concentrations of chloramphenicol produced in urine and blood following administration of the recommended oral dosage: *Staphylococcus aureus, Streptococcus pyogenes, Shigella paradysenteria, Pseudomonas aeruginosa, Brucella* spp., *Aerobacter aerogenes, Pasteurella tularensis, Escherichia coli, Proteus vulgaris, Salmonella* spp., *Bacillus anthracis, Corynebacterium pyogenes, Erysipelothrix rhusiopathiae,* and *Klebsiella pneumoniae.*

Chloramphenicol has been useful for treating urinary tract infections caused by sensitive *Aerobacter aerogenes* and *Escherichia coli.* It has been successful for treating certain acute cases of salmonellosis. It may also be used to treat staphylococcal-coliform infections that have become resistant to other antibiotics. Chloramphenicol applied topically or systemically was reported as an efficacious antibiotic in the treatment of equine *Dermatophilus* infection (Pascoe 1972).

Bacterial resistance is related to usage. If widely used, bacterial resistance develops in a manner similar to that occurring from widespread use of other antibacterials. Pigs fed 20 ppm chloramphenicol had their sensitive coliforms completely replaced by resistant coliforms due to the presence of R factors (Bulling and Stephan 1971).

Metabolism

Chloramphenicol is readily absorbed in dogs following oral administration and is rapidly inactivated within the body by the formation of inactive nitro derivatives. The administration of 75 mg/lb/day divided into 3 or 4 doses will maintain a blood concentration of 5–10 μg/ml.

Plasma concentrations of chloramphenicol and kinetics of its disappearance from plasma after intravenous administration at a dose of 22 mg/kg of body weight were determined in dogs, cats, swine, goats, and ponies (Davis et al. 1972). The plasma half-life varied from 0.9 hours in ponies to 5.1 hours in cats. Apparent specific volumes of distribution varied from 1.02 L/kg in ponies to 2.36 L/kg in cats. The drug was bound to plasma proteins to a limited extent (30%–46%), and the extent of binding was independent of drug concentration.

Chloramphenicol was rapidly absorbed after intramuscular injection of chloramphenicol sodium succinate, but the dose of 22 mg/kg calculated as free base was insufficient to maintain therapeutic blood concentrations. Species differences have been observed in the absorption of chloramphenicol after the drug was administered orally. It was not detected in the plasma of goats following oral administration.

Chloramphenicol appears in most tissues within 0.5–1 hour after oral administration. It reaches the highest concentration in the liver, bile, and kidneys. Chloramphenicol apparently is present in the intracellular as well as the extracellular fluid. It is effective for use in eye infections since it readily penetrates ocular tissues. Chloramphenicol diffuses into the cerebrospinal and pleural fluids and diffuses across the placenta. It reaches a concentration in fetal blood of approximately 75% of that in the maternal blood 2 hours after administration.

Drinking water containing 40 ppm chloramphenicol was provided continuously for 5 days to laying hens to determine the extent of transmission of the drug into the eggs (Sisodia and Dunlop 1972a). Maximum residue levels of the antibiotic were achieved in the yolk 128 hours after medication was started. Residue levels of 0.33 ppm in the yolk and 0.17 ppm in the albumen were detected at the 80th hour of medication. After medication ceased, chloramphenicol disappeared from the albumen by the 76th hour but persisted in the yolk until at least the 108th hour.

Treatment of 7-week-old broiler chickens with drinking water containing 40 ppm of chloramphenicol for 5 days resulted in residues of approximately 0.2 ppm in the muscle, liver, skin, and fat; residues of the antibiotic also were detected in the kidney at a concentration of 0.6 ppm (Sisodia and Dunlop 1972b). Chloramphenicol was not detected after 48 hours in the muscle and liver or after 8 hours in the skin and fat. However, it was present in measurable concentrations of approximately 0.3 ppm in the kidney 72 hours after the medicated drinking water was removed.

Chloramphenicol is eliminated from the blood within 4–6 hours after intravenous injection and 12–16 hours after oral administration in dogs. During a 24-hour period of urinary excretion in the dog, about 55% of the total oral dose is recovered. Only 6.3% of the drug excreted is active chloramphenicol. The inactive form appears to be excreted largely by the renal tubules and the active form by the renal glomeruli. In the dog and rat, a large portion of the inactive metabolized drug is excreted in the bile as aromatic amines derived from chloramphenicol by reduction of the nitro group.

Toxicity

The toxic properties of chloramphenicol involve a few minor side effects. If administered for long periods the patient should be monitored for the possibility of serious hematopoietic disturbances. There is minimal danger of blood dyscrasia during an acute infection if the therapeutic dosage is determined carefully. Aplastic anemia has been observed in human beings after repeated administration.

Chloramphenicol administered orally to dogs at a dose of 100 mg/kg/day resulted in a decrease in bone marrow ferrochelatase activity of 5%–35% of the control values (Manyan and Yunis 1970). Drugs containing a benzene ring with an attached nitro or amino radical may depress the hematopoietic function of the bone marrow. Although aplastic anemia has resulted from the therapeutic use of chloramphenicol in human beings, the occurrence of blood dyscrasia in dogs from its use has not been established.

Chloramphenicol administered to the dog orally (45 mg/lb/day) for 2 years did not induce blood dyscrasia. Moreover, it did not depress hemoglobin or blood cell values and did not cause significant gross or histologic tissue abnormalities. However, the body weight gains were below normal. When the daily dose was increased to 115 mg/lb of body weight, anorexia, bone marrow hypocellularity, fatty livers, marked loss of weight, and high mortality were observed.

Allergic and adverse reactions, e.g., rashes, edema, urticaria, nausea, vomition, glossitis, stomatitis, and diarrhea, are observed infrequently. Most therapy with chloramphenicol in veterinary medicine is of short duration. It therefore seems unlikely that aplastic anemia would occur in domestic animals under usual conditions. In practically all other respects, chloramphenicol is free of undesirable drug reactions characterized by GI, neurotoxic, cutaneous, or allergic reactions.

Interactions of chloramphenicol may occur and the following should be noted: (1) avoid concomitant use with immunizing agents (anamnestic response); (2) chloramphenicol may lower prothrombin levels; (3) chloramphenicol inhibits the biotransformation of diphenylhydantoin, dicumarol, and other drugs metabolized by hepatic microsomal enzymes; and (4) chloramphenicol can prolong the duration of pentobarbital anesthesia in dogs and cats (Adams and Dixit 1970; Teske and Carter 1971).

OTHER ANTIBACTERIAL DRUGS

The aminoglycoside antibiotics share many pharmacologic properties and have similar antibacterial spectra and toxic effects. As discussed previously, streptomycin and dihydrostreptomycin are members of this group along with gentamicin and neomycin.

The only common characteristic of the remaining drugs to be considered in this chapter is their antibacterial activity; their morphologic, chemical, or pharmacologic categorizations are not applicable.

GENTAMICIN

Gentamicin Sulfate, U.S.P. (Fig. 49.5), an aminoglycoside, is isolated from *Micromonospora purpurea.* It is a mixture of three closely related antibacterial agents. Gentamicin sulfate is available for both parenteral and topical use; however, it is not given orally since very small amounts are absorbed from the GI tract.

Gentamicin is active against *Enterobacter aerogenes, Escherichia coli,* and *Klebsiella pneumoniae;* indol-positive and indol-negative *Proteus* species; *Pseudomo-*

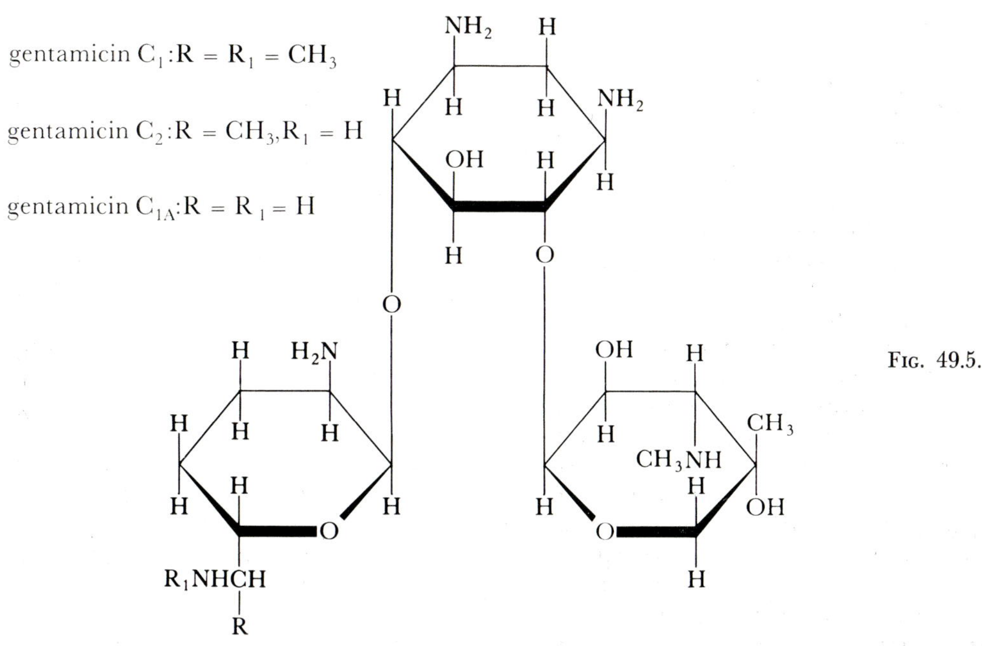

FIG. 49.5.

nas aeruginosa; some species of nonpigmented *Serratia;* and many species of *Salmonella* and *Shigella.*

Gentamicin is effective for treating *Pseudomonas aeruginosa* ocular infections (Favati and Marranghini 1968). It is administered by conjunctival instillation twice daily for 3 days. Systemic infections are treated with intramuscular injections of gentamicin (2 mg/kg) twice daily.

A solution of gentamicin sulfate was used for dipping turkey eggs in an effort to reduce *Mycoplasma* infections (Saif and Nestor 1972). Beneficial results were noted in a reduction of air sac lesions and the prevalence of *Mycoplasma* organisms. The dipping of turkey eggs in gentamicin also reduced the number of *Salmonella* isolations.

Turkey poults infected with *Paracolobactrum arizonae* were successfully treated with gentamicin (Solis and Barnett 1970). A dose of 2 mg/bird was effective for reducing mortality and for eliminating carriers.

An efficacy study with gentamicin and *tylosin* was conducted in specific pathogen-free (SPF) pigs that had received a suspension of *Vibrio coli* and *Treponema hyodysenteriae* (Harris et al. 1972). Gentamicin sulfate was administered in the drinking water of the pigs at a concentration of 50 or 100 mg/gal and compared to tylosin tartrate at a concentration of 2.5 g/gal for 3 days beginning with the onset of clinical symptoms. No deaths were observed in the 25 pigs receiving gentamicin; however, of 10 animals treated with tylosin, 2 deaths occurred.

Systemic administration of gentamicin sulfate should be restricted to severe infections caused by susceptible gram-negative bacteria. *In vitro* susceptibility of the bacterial infection is important because all strains of gram-negative organisms are not sensitive to the antibacterial action of gentamicin. In addition, when treating urinary tract infections, it is helpful to alkalize the urine, since the antibiotic is more effective in an alkaline medium.

Of the 479 strains of bacteria isolated from dogs and tested for sensitivity to gentamicin, 10% were found to be resistant. In the isolation of 63 strains of *Pseudomonas aeruginosa,* 10 strains were found to be resistant to gentamicin (Förster et al. 1969). Gentamicin has been successfully used for the treatment of canine otitis externa and urinary tract infections. The intrauterine infusion of gentamicin for equine endometritis was beneficial in 91 of 113 cases; of the 528 bacterial isolates obtained, almost all were sensitive to the antibiotic (Houdeshell and Hennessey 1972).

As with other systemic antibiotics, gentamicin probably should not be used topically because resistant organisms may develop which would obviate its use for systemic therapy. A topical preparation has been approved by the FDA for treatment of ear infections in the dog (see Chapter 42).

Gentamicin may impair renal function as well as damage the cochlear and vestibular portions of the eighth cranial nerve. Auditory impairment is maximal in the high frequency sound range; however, vestibular damage is observed more frequently. Patients with impaired renal function are most likely to manifest ototoxic disturbances; thus they should receive a reduced dosage and the interval between maintenance doses should be increased.

In cats, daily intramuscular injections of gentamicin of 20–80 mg/kg produced disturbances in vestibular function; after 7–25 days, mortality was observed (Vangelov 1973). A similar effect was not reported in rats.

Concentrations of gentamicin in serum may serve as a useful guide in the establishment of effective therapeutic levels. Therapeutic blood concentrations are usually in the range of 5–7 μg/ml, whereas serum concentrations in excess of 12 μg/ml are hazardous.

Gentamicin crosses the placenta and can induce renal impairment and ototoxicity in the fetus. Its use in pregnant animals is contraindicated. Gentamicin may interact with a number of drugs, e.g., it may produce neuromuscular paralysis and enhance the action of neuromuscular blocking drugs, general anesthetics, and the muscle relaxant properties of magnesium. Gentamicin also precipitates heparin and has the ability to inactivate carbenicillin.

CLINICAL USE

Gentamicin sulfate is approved by the FDA for treatment of urinary and respiratory tract infections in the dog and cat. It is administered intramuscularly or subcutaneously at a dosage rate of 2 mg/lb of body weight 2 times on the 1st day of treatment and only daily thereafter. If a favorable response is not noted after 7 days, other therapeutic measures should be considered.

KANAMYCIN

Kanamycin Sulfate, U.S.P. (Fig. 49.6) (Kantrex), is another aminoglycoside antibiotic. The drug has an antibacterial activity against *Escherichia coli,* some strains of *Enterobacter, Klebsiella, Mycobacterium, Proteus, Salmonella, Staphyloccus,* and *Vibrio.* Some *E. coli* and staphylococcal organisms develop resistance rapidly. Such resistance is cross-resistant to other drugs of the aminoglycoside group, e.g., neomycin, gentamicin, and streptomycin.

Kanamycin has been used to treat purulent conjunctivitis and keratoconjunctivitis in dogs and cats (Cunningham 1970). Complete remission occurred in 21 of 24 cases. *Staphylococci aureus* and *Staphylococcus epidermatis* were the most common isolates.

Kanamycin is used parenterally to treat infections caused by susceptible organisms; however, it is also used orally for the treatment of enteritis or to reduce the bacterial population in the GI tract. Limited absorption occurs after oral administration.

Kanamycin has been administered intramuscularly in cattle, sheep, dogs, and pigs (Andreini and Pignatelli 1972). It was readily absorbed from the injection site and doses of 5–12 mg/kg of body weight were recommended at 12-hour intervals. Milk samples were free of the antibiotic 36 hours after the last injection. Kanamycin residues persisted for the longest period in kidney tissue.

Use of kanamycin parenterally may cause permanent damage to the cochlear and vestibular portions of the eighth cranial nerve. Like other aminoglycoside antibiotics, kanamycin has a neuromuscular blocking action that enhances the effect of neuromuscular blocking drugs and general anesthetics. It should be used with extreme caution in patients receiving these drugs. *In vitro* studies support the theory that a calcium-kanamycin complex is involved in the neuromuscular blocking action of kanamycin (Crawford and Bowen 1971).

Kanamycin is approved for use in the dog and cat by the FDA. In general, the intramuscular dose of kanamycin is 15 mg/kg/day administered in 3 divided doses. The oral dose for systemic effect is 20–30 mg/kg/day administered in 3 or 4 divided doses. Young calves receiving an intramuscular injection of 10 mg/kg of kanamycin developed peak serum concentrations within 1 hour following administration. Therapeutic concentrations of the antibiotic persisted in the blood for 8 hours (Treppenhauer 1973). Also, in young calves subcutaneous injections of kanamycin pro-

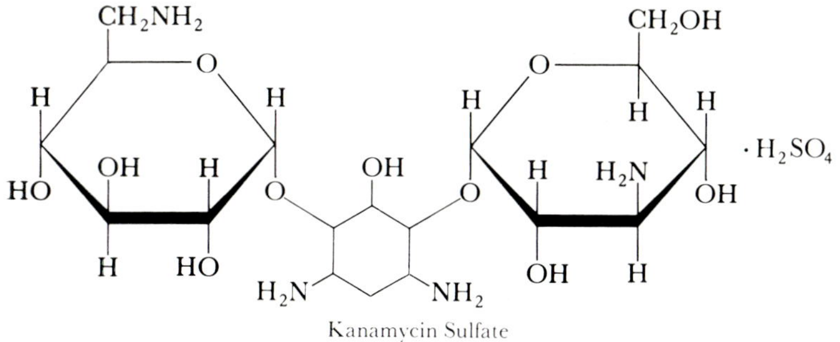

CH_2NH_2 CH_2OH HO OH H HO H_2N NH_2 OH H_2N H $\cdot H_2SO_4$

Kanamycin Sulfate

FIG. 49.6.

duced therapeutic concentrations in the serum for 12 hours. A dose of 3–5 mg/kg administered to heifers produced therapeutic serum concentrations which persisted for approximately 8 hours. An intramuscular injection of kanamycin sulfate (0.5–1 mg/kg) produced blood concentrations in chickens and pigs for 24 and 12 hours, respectively (Popoviciu et al. 1972).

Kanamycin sulfate is also available for topical treatment of bacterial infections associated with the skin and ears (see Section 11).

Neomycin

Neomycin Sulfate, U.S.P. (Fig. 49.7), an aminoglycoside antibiotic, was isolated from a soil organism, *Streptomyces fradiae* (Waksman and Lechevalier 1949). The organism elaborates a mixture of substances including an antifungal material (fradicin) and the neomycin complex which consists of components A, B, and C. Neomycin sulfate is a polybasic compound soluble in water but insoluble in organic solvents.

Although it is more toxic, neomycin is probably as efficacious as kanamycin. Both drugs are bactericidals. The antibacterial spectrum of neomycin is primarily against *Escherichia* and most species of *Enterobacter, Klebsiella, Salmonella, Shigella,* and *Proteus.* In veterinary medicine, neomycin has been used topically, orally, and parenterally. Usually, parenteral administration is limited to 1 or 2 injections because repeated administration may precipitate toxic reactions.

When neomycin is given orally, ototoxic and nephrotoxic effects may occcur. As with gentamicin and kanamycin, the nephrotoxicity may be reversible but the ototoxicity is usually irreversible. Deafness was produced in a 5-year-old female Labrador retriever after subcutaneous injections of 500 mg of neomycin for 5 days; the animal was undergoing treatment for hemorrhagic cystitis (Fowler 1968). As with other aminoglycoside antibiotics, neomycin is poorly absorbed from the GI tract or following topical application.

Neomycin also has a neuromuscular blocking action that enhances the neuromuscular blocking activity of skeletal muscle relaxants and general anesthetics. The effect of neomycin on skeletal muscle has been studied by Adams (1973); episodes of dyspnea and apnea were correlated with a decrease in muscle contraction. Administration of neostigmine or calcium chloride during respiratory depression and muscle depression rapidly reversed the antibiotic-induced neuromuscular paralysis.

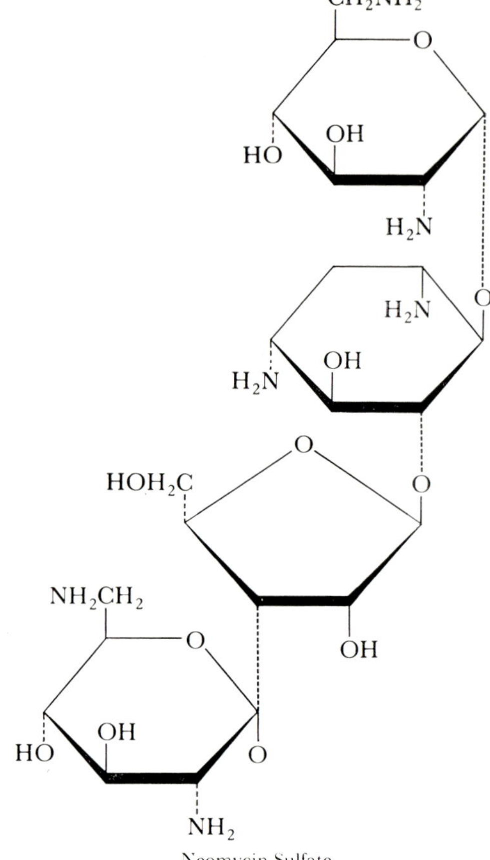

Neomycin Sulfate

Fig. 49.7.

When administered orally, the approximate dosage of neomycin is 100 mg/kg/day divided into 4 doses. If administered intramuscularly, the dose is 15 mg/kg/day divided into 4 doses. Although little neomycin is absorbed after oral administration, rapid absorption is noted following parenteral administration. LD50 values for neomycin in mice administered intravenously and orally are 14.8 mg/kg and 2880 mg/kg, respectively. Repeated administration of the antibiotic may cause nephrotoxic or ototoxic effects. No serious toxicity has been observed following oral or topical administration. Topical preparations of neomycin are discussed in Section 11. Oral preparations for the treatment of various enteric conditions may include kaolin, pectin, or methylcellulose.

Veterinary pharmaceutical forms of neomycin are available as boluses or liquids. Sterile solutions of neomycin (Biosol) containing 50 or 200 mg/ml are used for parenteral administration. A combination of neomycin and anticholinergic drug (Biosol-M) has been prepared for parenteral use. Each ml contains the equivalent of 140 mg of neomycin base and 2 mg of methscopolamine for the reduction of undesirable chlolinergic effects. Neomycin must not be used parenterally in food-producing animals because of the prolonged persistence of residues in edible tissues.

Erythromycin

Erythromycin, U.S.P. (Ilotycin, Gallimycin) (Fig. 49.8), is a macrolide (a large lactone ring) antibiotic produced by a strain of *Streptomyces erythreus,* a soilborne organism.

Erythromycin is an important and structurally complex member of the macrolide group of antibiotics (carbomycin, oleandomycin, spiramycin, etc.). It consists of two sugars, desosamine and cladinose, which are attached to erythronolide, a macrocyclic lactone. Erythromycin is readily soluble in some organic solvents but only slightly soluble in water (0.2%). Like streptomycin, erythromycin is more active at a pH of 8 than at neutrality and is unstable in an acid medium. Erythromycin is available in the form of estolate, ethylsuccinate, gluceptate, lactobionate, or stearate.

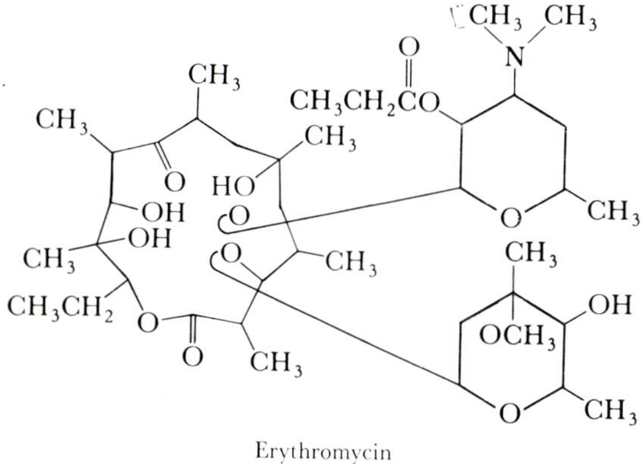

Erythromycin

Fig. 49.8.

Erythromycin is a selective antimicrobial drug and does not act upon as great a variety of bacteria as the tetracyclines. Erythromycin impedes protein synthesis *in vitro.* The following microorganisms are susceptible to the inhibitory action of erythromycin: *Streptococcus pyogenes, S. faecalis, Staphyloccus, Corynebacterium renale, C. pyogenes, Erysipelothrix rhusiopathiae, Bacillus anthracis, Pasteurella multocida, Hemophilus, Clostridia, Listeria,* and *Brucella suis.*

In general, erythromycin is effective against many gram-positive organisms. It is useful in the treatment of staphylococcal respiratory infections that are resistant to penicillin therapy. Clinical abuse of erythromycin can lead to the devlopment of resistant organisms.

Cross-resistance has been noted between erythromycin and oleandomycin. Erythromycin is primarily a bacteriostatic agent and does not have a bactericidal effect unless large amounts are administered.

Following oral administration, erythromycin is absorbed readily from the upper part of the small intestine and diffuses well throughout most tissues. Serum concentrations decline sharply within 4–6 hours after the drug is administered.

Erythromycin injected intramuscularly at a dose of 15 mg/kg of body weight has a plasma half-life of 8–9 hours and an average maximum blood concentration of 0.5 μg/ml. Two hours after administration, highest concentrations are detected in the liver, submaxillary glands, lungs, and kidneys. Only trace amounts of erythromycin are present in the brain or cerebrospinal fluid. Diffusion into the peritoneal and pleural fluids as well as across the placenta into the fetal circulation occurs readily so that therapeutically effective amounts of erythromycin are present. Erythromycin is present in prostatic fluid and semen in about one-third the concentration of that found in the blood.

Erythromycin is readily concentrated by the liver and eliminated in the bile in high concentrations. Excretion of these high concentrations of the active antibiotic in bile provides an adequate therapeutic level for many infections of the biliary tract. Depending upon the dose and frequency of administration, urinary excretion of erythromycin in a biologically active form is relatively constant. Elimination of erythromycin in relatively high concentrations in the feces may follow its oral administration. Gram-positive microorganisms are severely inhibited by the antibiotic in the feces; there is little effect upon gram-negative organisms.

The oral dose of erythromycin in nonherbivorous animals is about 3–4 mg/lb/day administered in 3 or 4 divided doses. *Erythromycin Stearate,* U.S.P., can also be administered orally using 2 or 3 mg/lb/day in 3 or 4 divided doses.

Erythromycin Lactobionate, U.S.P., may be administered parenterally at a dose of 1–2 mg/lb of body weight at intervals of 8–12 hours. The intravenous route is preferred over the intramuscular route of administration because pain and some tissue irritation is associated with the latter method of injection.

Infrequently, undesirable effects such as vomition and diarrhea are related to the oral administration of large doses of erythromycin. Erythromycin does not induce changes in the intestinal flora of the same magnitude as that produced by other antibiotics. Local or topical use is not favored because of occasional skin sensitivities.

Oleandomycin and Troleandomycin

Oleandomycin, N.F., is an antibiotic elaborated by strains of an actinomycete, *Streptomyces antibioticus. Oleandomycin phosphate,* a white crystalline powder, is a complex sugar molecule. It is slightly soluble in water and is soluble in most organic solvents. Aqueous solutions of oleandomycin are stable. An oleandomycin derivative, *Troleandomycin,* N.F. (Fig. 49.9), is used for oral administration because it is more rapidly and completely absorbed than the phosphate salt.

Both drugs are effective against certain gram-positive organisms, especially staphylococci and streptococci. Their antibacterial spectrum is similar to that of erythromycin, primarily an antistaphylococcal drug. Bacteria can acquire resistance to oleandomycin and troleandomycin; cross-resistance to erythromycin may occur.

Absorption is adequate following oral or parenteral administration of oleandomycin. It can be detected in the liver, kidney, spleen, heart, lungs, lymph nodes, pancreas, and bile. It does not penetrate the blood-brain barrier.

Oleandomycin phosphate or troleandomycin may be administered orally on the basis of 0.5–1 mg/lb of body weight 4 times daily. Also, it may be administered intravenously providing it is injected slowly;

Fig. 49.9.

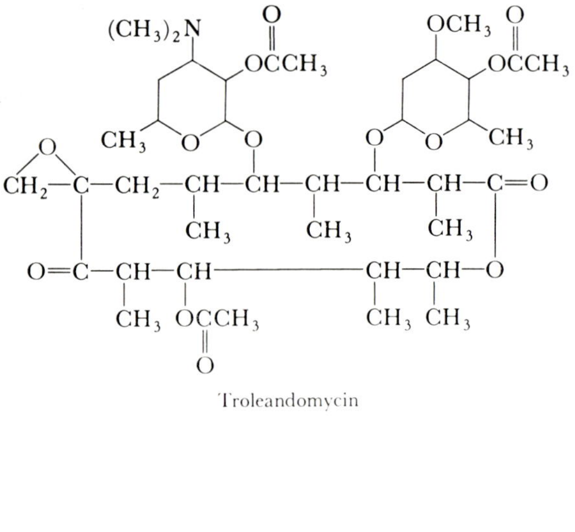

Troleandomycin

intramuscular administration is not desirable because of the pain and tissue irritation it induces.

The toxicity of oleandomycin is quite low. Minor undesirable effects such as cutaneous hypersensitivity or, rarely, diarrhea may occur.

POLYMYXINS: POLYMYXIN B AND COLISTIN

The polymyxins, *Polymyxin B Sulfate,* U.S.P., and *Colistin Sulfate,* U.S.P., do not possess broad clinical utility. Some of the polypeptide antibiotics possess limited bacterial activity and specific toxic actions must be recognized and anticipated. They should be employed parenterally with restraint for combatting infections generated by sensitive organisms. Some of the polypeptide antibiotics have serious toxic potentialities; however, they can be lifesaving because of their antibacterial specificity for certain microorganisms, especially those that are refractory to other therapeutic agents.

Polymyxin B and polymyxin E (colistin) are readily soluble in water or saline. The polymyxins are stable as acid salts for long periods and are readily destroyed by alkali. The unit of polymyxin is based on a theoretical potency of pure drug: 1 μg equals 10 units; 1 mg equals 10,000 units. The international unit of polymyxin B has been defined as the activity contained in 1.19×10^{-4} mg.

The polymyxins are highly selective in their antibacterial activity. They are 10–1000 times more active against gram-negative than gram-positive organisms. The following microorganisms are generally susceptible *in vitro* to 10 μg or less of polymyxin B/ml: *Aerobacter aerogenes, Escherichia coli, Hemophilus, Salmonella, Shigella, Pseudomonas aeruginosa, Pasteurella, Brucella, Vibrio,* and paracolon bacteria.

The polymyxins are very effective against *Pseudomonas aeruginosa.* This particular organism is a frequent pathogen in a variety of tissue infections. Resistance does not often develop in bacteria originally susceptible to polymyxin and colistin. Moreover, it does not develop rapidly in the presence of subinhibitory concentrations of polymyxin. Polymyxins are frequently combined with other antibiotics because cross-resistance does not develop in the bacteria and because they have a limited spectrum of antibacterial activity that can be supplemented by the addition of another drug. However, cross-resistance between colistin and polymyxin B is usually complete.

Polymyxins are strongly bactericidal. Antibacterial action of the polymyxins is dependent to some degree upon the inoculum or the number of bacteria present. Polymyxins are probably adsorbed onto the bacterial cell wall to combine with and disorganize structures responsible for the maintenance of osmotic equilibrium within the cell. As a result, the cell permeability is altered and cellular constituents, particularly purines and pyrimidines, escape from the cell protoplasm. Actual lysis of some susceptible bacterial cells may occur. Loss of soluble constituents from the bacterial cell is markedly similar to the action of quaternary ammonium cationic detergents. It is also possible that polymyxin B may attach to the polyphosphate groups on or near the cell surface. A competitive antagonism is known to exist between polymyxin and cations of the quaternary ammonium detergents for attachment to the cell.

Absorption of polymyxin from the GI tract is slow and limited so that ordinary oral doses do not produce detectable plasma concentrations. It is readily absorbed when injected subcutaneously or intramuscularly. Peak plasma concentrations are reached from 1 to 2 hours after injection; one-half of the peak concentration is present at 6 hours, and detectable amounts of polymyxin can be found in the plasma for 12 hours or more after injection.

Polymyxin is eliminated primarily through the kidneys. There is a tendency for tissue accumulation of polymyxin in renal insufficiency or following repeated administration of large doses. Little polymyxin is excreted by the kidney during the first 12 hours; ultimately, larger amounts are eliminated by this route. Urinary concentrations may reach 20–100 μg/ml after continued therapy. Renal elimination continues for 1–3 days after cessation of therapy. Approximately 60% of the administered dose can be recovered from the urine.

Polymyxin B is used widely in ointments containing 0.5–1 mg of antibiotic/g of ointment for topical application (see Chapter 42). A sterile aqueous solution of similar concentration is used for eyes infected with *Pseudomonas aeruginosa.* Polymyxin B is used in combination with neomycin and bacitracin or the tetracyclines for topical administration, especially for chronic otitis externa.

Polymyxin is seldom injected intramuscularly or by any parenteral route because of the possibility of nephrotoxicity. If systemic therapy is required, intramuscular injection is preferable over intravenous injection because the latter is more apt to produce renal toxicity. Intramuscular injection is indicated in severe urinary tract or systemic infections due to coliform bacteria or an organism such as *Pseudomonas aeruginosa.* Polymyxin B has a low degree of toxicity when administered parenterally in doses below 1.4 mg/lb of body weight.

Polymyxin B has been used orally in combination with bacitracin or neomycin for the preoperative suppression of intestinal flora or for susceptible intestinal infections. For suppression of fecal bacteria in small animals, the oral dose approximates 3 mg/lb/day given in 3 divided doses. If administered with another antibiotic (neomycin, bacitracin), one-half of the above amount may be adequate.

The intramuscular dose of polymyxin is approximately 1 mg/lb/day.

Polymyxin B injected intravenously in dogs at a dosage of 1–3 mg/kg depresses glomerular filtration and reduces urine volume. Following intramuscular injection, doses of 2.5 mg/kg/day for 2–6 weeks produces only a transient depression of tubular function in young dogs; it has no effect upon electrolyte excretion in the urine. Renal tubules from animals having the most marked functional disturbance revealed the presence of cloudy swelling of the tubular cells.

Both polymyxin B and colistin are nephrotoxic and must be used in reduced doses in patients with impaired renal function. Muscular weakness, paresis, or complete paralysis leading to respiratory arrest and death have been observed infrequently following the administration of these drugs with other neuromuscular agents.

Polymyxin B sulfate is available as Aerosporin or in powder form for parenteral use. It is also available in tablets.

Colistin (Fig. 49.10) is the generic name for an antibiotic obtained from *Bacillus colistinus.* Its antibacterial spectrum is characterized by bactericidal and bacteriostatic activity against gram-negative or-

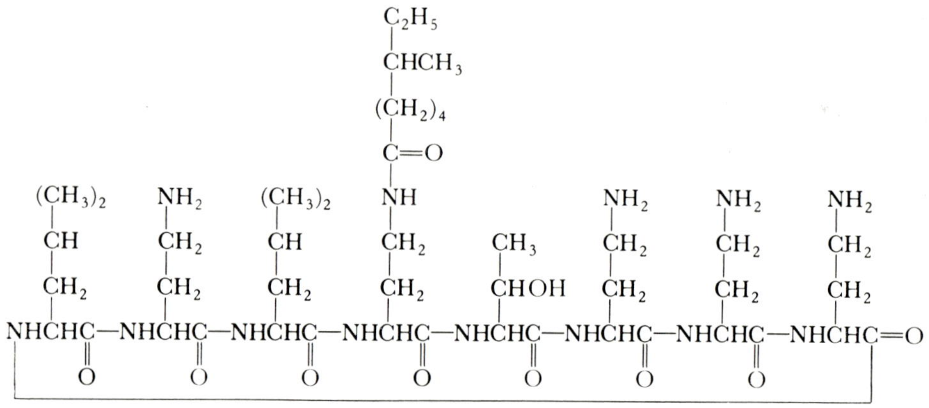

```
                                       C2H5
                                       |
                                       CHCH3
                                       |
                                      (CH2)4
                                       |
                                       C=O
                                       |
(CH3)2    NH2      (CH3)2              NH                 NH2      NH2      NH2
 |         |         |                 |                   |        |        |
 CH        CH2       CH                CH2       CH3       CH2      CH2      CH2
 |         |         |                 |         |         |        |        |
 CH2       CH2       CH2               CH2       CHOH      CH2      CH2      CH2
 |         |         |                 |         |         |        |        |
NHCHC—NHCHC—NHCHC—NHCHC—NHCHC—NHCHC—NHCHC—NHCHC=O
|    ‖      ‖      ‖      ‖      ‖      ‖      ‖      |
|    O      O      O      O      O      O      O      |
|_____________________________________________________|
```

Colistin

FIG. 49.10.

ganisms. It has been used to treat infections caused by *Shigella, Escherichia coli, Pseudomonas aeruginosa, Salmonella* organisms, and *Proteus vulgaris.* It is active against many gram-negative organisms. Although colistin has an antibacterial activity against *Pseudomonas aeruginosa,* gentamicin or carbenicillin is preferred in clinical usage.

Colistimethate sodium is effective in canine infections due to *E. coli, Pseudomonas aeruginosa, Klebsiella pneumoniae, Paracolobactrum* spp., and *Aerobacter aerogenes.* Infections caused by *Proteus* sp., *Streptococcus faecalis, Streptococcus pyogenes,* and *Staphylococcus aureus* were found to be resistant to the antibacterial action of colistimethate sodium (Mann and Bjotvedt 1964). Combinations of colistin with erythromycin, chloramphenicol, bacitracin, benzylpenicillin, tetracycline, novobiocin, or trimethoprim demonstrated a synergistic effect against 17 bacterial isolates that came from swine, including a *Bordetella bronchiseptica* strain.

Colistimethate sodium is the salt of the sulfamethyl derivative of colistin. The international standard for colistin has been established as 4.878×10^{-5} mg and is called the "international unit" (I.U.).

Blood urea nitrogen or serum creatinine tests should be determined for patients with acute renal failure or chronic nephropathies. Decreased urinary output and oliguria may be a sign of the onset of renal damage following therapeutic use of colistin.

The parenteral dose (intramuscular or intravenous) of colistimethate sodium is 2.5–5 mg/kg of body weight administered 3 times daily.

Colistin sulfate is the water-soluble salt of colistin. The drug is poorly absorbed from the GI tract, is relatively free of side effects, and is generally used in the treatment of susceptible gram-negative enteric infections.

Frequently, the polymyxins are in fixed combinations with other antibiotics such as bacitracin or neomycin. Fixed combinations may have value; however, if there are abrasions of the skin or mucous membranes, sufficient amounts of the drugs may be absorbed to cause system toxicity or hypersensitization.

Bacitracin

Bacitracin, U.S.P. (Fig. 49.11), was isolated from a strain of *Bacillus subtilus* in a contaminated wound of a patient named Tracy. Bacitracin is active against several kinds of bacteria found on the skin, i.e., hemolytic and nonhemolytic streptococci, coagulase-positive staphylococci, and some clostridia. Development of bacterial strains resistant to bacitracin is rare. The antibacterial spectrum is similar to that of penicillin; however, the inherent systemic toxicity of bacitracin restricts its widespread application.

Bacitracin methylenedisalicylate has the ability to inhibit the growth of *Streptococcus bovis.* This organism has been implicated in severe acidosis of cattle and sheep when they are fed an unrestricted high concentrate ration (Klatte and Thomas 1967). Although bacitracin has such an effect, it cannot be used specifically to inhibit the growth of *S. bovis* without inhibiting other rumen bacteria.

Bacitracin is a complex, labile polypeptide consisting of 5–10 components. It is a white powder that dissolves readily in water and is stable for approximately 4 weeks in an aqueous solution at a pH of 5–7. *Bacitracin Zinc,* U.S.P., and bacitracin methylenedisalicylate are more stable in the dry state than is bacitracin. Various forms of bacitracin have been used as feed additives for feed efficiency and gain purposes.

A great variety of ointments and solutions are available for topical application

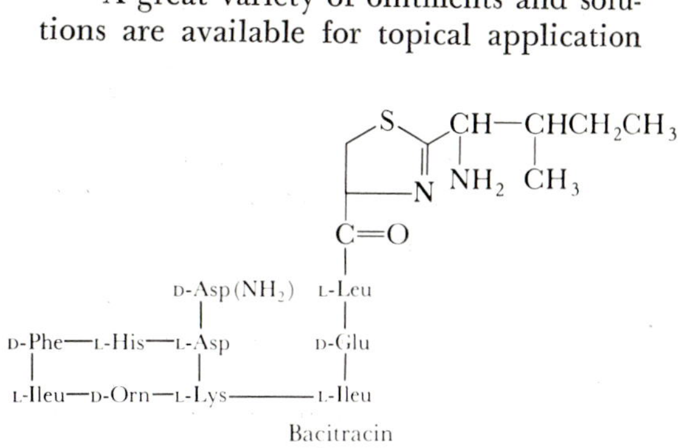

S, N, CH—CHCH$_2$CH$_3$, NH$_2$, CH$_3$, C=O

D-Asp(NH$_2$) L-Leu

D-Phe—L-His—L-Asp D-Glu

L-Ileu—D-Orn—L-Lys——L-Ileu

Bacitracin

Fig. 49.11.

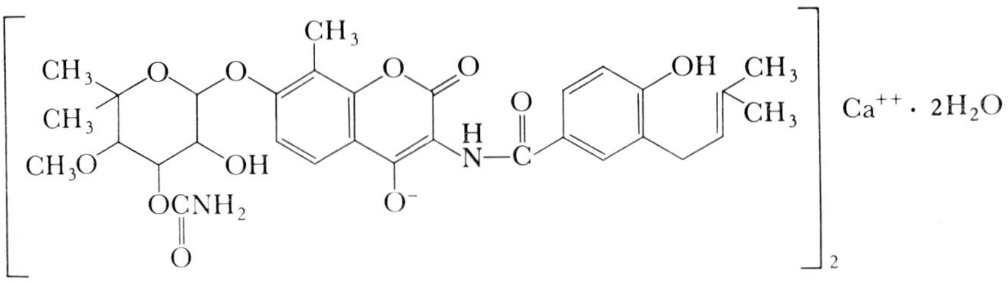

Novobiocin

Fig. 49.12.

(see Chapter 42). The concentration of bacitracin in these preparations ranges from 100 to 1000 units/g or ml. Bacitracin is commonly combined in these preparations with other poorly absorbed antibiotics (polymyxin B, neomycin) that act upon gram-negative bacteria. Absorption from the body surface is negligible and incidence of sensitization appears to be quite low. Bacitracin is useful when applied locally to combat gram-positive infections.

Bacitracin, bacitracin methylenedisalicylate, bacitracin manganese, and bacitracin zinc have been incorporated as additives in feed for various purposes of growth and disease control at a concentration from 1 to 100 g/ton of feed.

Novobiocin

Novobiocin, N.F. (calcium and sodium) (Albamycin) (Fig. 49.12), is a narrow-spectrum antibiotic with antibacterial activity against many gram-positive pathogens and some species of *Proteus* and *Pseudomonas.* It has also demonstrated activity against *Pasteurella multocida* (Hamdy and Blanchard 1970). Novobiocin in a concentration of 250–300 g/ton of feed or 1 g/gal of water resulted in a beneficial effect in turkeys by reducing the mortality produced by fowl cholera.

A synergistic effect occurred when novobiocin and a tetracycline were administered in combination (Calabi 1973). The frequency of adverse reactions relegates novobiocin to a role of secondary consideration. Skin rashes, blood dyscrasias, fever, irritation, nausea, vomition, and diarrhea have been observed following its administration. Novobiocin blocks the renal transport of drugs by specific inhibition at the peritubular site of the renal tubule and in this respect resembles probenecid (Fujimoto et al. 1973).

In a concentration of 200–350 g/ton of feed, the antibiotic has been used to control staphylococcal infections associated with breast blisters or synovitis in chickens and turkeys.

Spectinomycin

Spectinomycin dihydrochloride pentahydrate (Trobicin) (Fig. 49.13) is an aminocyclitol antibiotic produced by a strain of *Streptomyces spectabilis.* The antibiotic is active against gram-positive organisms and is frequently used for those organisms treated with penicillin G. No cross-resistance has been reported between spectinomycin and penicillin G. Spectinomycin is not bound appreciably by plasma proteins. It has been approved by the FDA for use in the chicken and turkey.

Spectinomycin has been used as a feed additive for pigs and chickens under certain conditions, i.e., in an attempt to control losses from *Mycoplasma gallisepticum* (PPLO) thought to cause chronic respiratory disease and for treating infections of

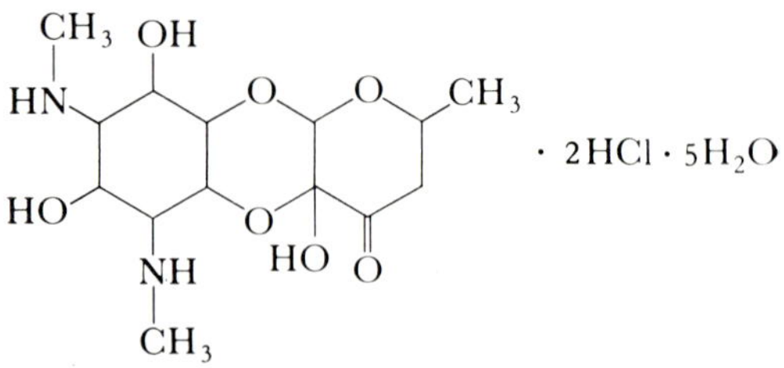

Spectinomycin

Fig. 49.13.

E. coli, Pasteurella multocida, and *Salmonella typhimurium.*

Clinically, spectinomycin has been used to control respiratory disease, *Salmonella typhimurium,* and fowl cholera in poultry. It is used in the treatment of 1- to 3-day-old turkey poults at the rate of 1–2 mg/poult in the prevention of mortality associated with *Arizona* group infection. Spectinomycin is also used at a rate of 5 mg/poult in the control of chronic respiratory disease associated with *E. coli.* In 1- to 3-day-old chicks, the antibiotic is administered at the rate of 2.5–5 mg/chick in the control of infections caused by *M. synoviae, S. infantis, S. typhimurium,* and *E. coli.* The drug is administered subcutaneously to both poults and chicks.

Spectinomycin has been used to treat coliform infections in swine and calves (Hardie 1973). In an oral dosage of 5–20 mg/lb, it has been used satisfactorily in the treatment of swine coliform infections. However, in calves suffering from acute respiratory infections from which *Pasteurella* organisms were isolated, administration of spectinomycin did not prove to be a satisfactory treatment.

An outbreak of *Salmonella dublin* infection in 5-week-old calves was successfully treated with spectinomycin administered subcutaneously at a dose of 10 mg/lb of body weight; this was followed by oral administration of the drug in a dose of 0.5 g for 5 days (Cook 1973). The calves had failed to respond to prior therapy with ampicillin, sulfadimidine, oxytetracycline, and chloramphenicol.

Strains of *Mycoplasma gallisepticum* and *Mycoplasma synoviae* became resistant to spectinomycin after 2 passages in media containing the antibiotic (Goren 1972). It is known that strains which become resistant to spectinomycin also show cross-resistance to tylosin. Even though *in vitro* results have not been promising, spectinomycin has been used in dogs in an oral dose of 10 mg/lb twice daily. It has also been administered parenterally and orally in chickens, pigs, and turkeys in dosages from 1 to 50 mg/animal, the dose dependent upon the age of the animal and route of administration.

The concentration of spectinomycin in the milk compared to serum exists in a ratio of 0.1:1 (Ziv and Sulman 1973b). Passage of spectinomycin into milk is limited by its high degree of ionization in serum and its low lipid solubility.

Lincomycin and Clindamycin

Lincomycin Hydrochloride, U.S.P. (Lincocin), is an antibacterial agent produced by *Streptomyces lincolnensis* var. *lincolnensis.* In addition, lincomycin (Fig. 49.14) has several semisynthetic derivatives: *clindamycin hydrochloride hydrate, clindamycin palmitate,* and *clindamycin phosphate.* All of these antibacterial agents have a limited spectrum very similar to that of erythromycin. They are active against gram-positive pathogens, including *Staphylococcus, Streptococcus, Clostridium tetani, Clostridium welchii,* several *Actinomyces* species, and some *Nocardia* species. This group of drugs also has some activity against certain strains of *Mycoplasma pneumoniae* (PPLO).

The combination of lincomycin and spectinomycin in a 1:2 ratio has greater activity against *Mycoplasma gallisepticum* and *Escherichia coli*–infected chickens than lincomycin, spectinomycin, or tylosin used alone (Hamdy and Blanchard 1970). A combination of lincomycin and spectinomycin administered in the drinking water was more effective than the drugs used individ-

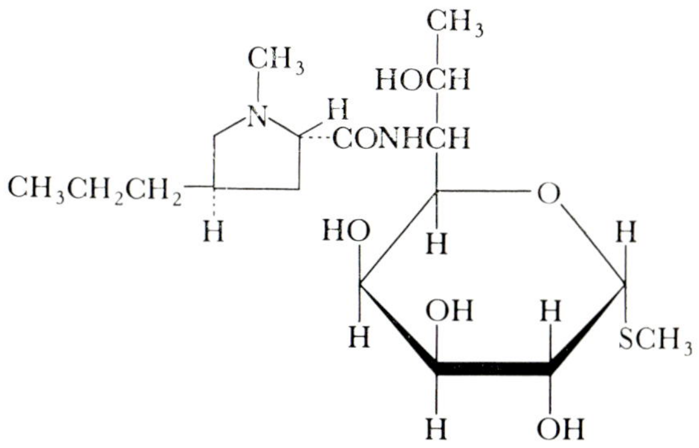

CH_3 HOCH CH_3 N H CONHCH $CH_3CH_2CH_2$ O H HO H H OH H H SCH_3 H OH

Lincomycin

Fig. 49.14.

ually. Also, this combination was more effective than tylosin in controlling air sacculitis of turkey poults.

Lincomycin and *Clindamycin Hydrochloride,* U.S.P., are particularly useful for treating susceptible infections resistant to the penicillins and erythromycin or in those patients that cannot tolerate penicillin or erythromycin. Clindamycin differs chemically from lincomycin by the substitution of a chlorine atom for a hydroxyl group. This substitution allows clindamycin to be absorbed better and the incidence of adverse effects is reduced. Drugs in this group can be administered orally, intramuscularly, or intravenously. Lincomycin is approved by the FDA for use in the dog, cat, and pig.

As might be expected, cross-resistance may occur between lincomycin and clindamycin; however, cross-resistance between these two drugs and other antibacterial agents has not been commonly encountered. An advantage of clindamycin over lincomycin is that the presence of food in the stomach does not appear to interfere with absorption.

Concentrations of lincomycin and clindamycin in the serum and milk of lactating ewes were evaluated following 2 intramuscular injections (Ziv and Sulman 1973a). The concentrations of the drugs in milk exceeded those noted at the peak serum concentration. Residues of the drugs persisted in the milk of the ewes 11 hours after treatment. In dairy cattle, a single intramuscular injection of lincomycin (10 mg/kg) revealed that the drug concentration in milk was 4–7 times higher than in blood plasma. Lincomycin is less bound to protein of milk than of blood plasma. The drug persists for 6–8 hours in cows' milk following a single intramuscular injection.

Pain, irritation, and induration occur following the intramuscular administration of lincomycin and clindamycin. Patients with impaired renal function should receive reduced dosages in conjunction with an increased period between successive maintenance therapy.

The acute and chronic toxicity of clindamycin was evaluated in dogs (Gray et al. 1972). Maximum daily dosages tolerated over a period of 1 year were between 300 and 600 mg/kg.

Lincomycin hydrochloride in a dose as small as 1/100 of that tolerated by rats and dogs produced diarrhea and death in rabbits (Gray and Lewis 1966). The extreme susceptibility of the rabbit to diarrhea produced by this and other antibiotics may be related to its vital dependence upon a very labile gram-positive bacterial flora in the cecum. Like the rabbit, a similar effect has been elicited by antibiotics in hamsters.

Lincomycin has been administered intramuscularly in swine in the treatment of arthritis and pneumonia involving the *Mycoplasma* species. It has also been used in cats and dogs for the treatment of infections produced by susceptible gram-positive organisms. The intramuscular dosage for cats and dogs is 5–10 mg/lb administered twice daily. In swine, lincomycin (5 mg/lb) is administered intramuscularly as a single dose for 5–6 days. The antibiotic must not be used within 48 hours of slaughter.

Thiostrepton

Thiostrepton is a polypeptide antibiotic produced by a strain of *Streptomyces aureus.* It is insoluble in water but soluble in various organic solvents. Thiostrepton is not absorbed from the intestinal tract. It is used primarily for its local antibacterial activity. Thiostrepton has antibacterial activity against gram-positive cocci and certain gram-negative microorganisms.

An ointment containing thiostrepton and various other drugs, e.g., an antibiotic, antifungal agent, adrenocorticosteroid derivative, is used for treatment of various dermatologic disorders in animals (see Chapter 42).

Tylosin

Tylosin (Tylan, Tylocine) is a macrolide antibiotic produced from a strain of *Streptomyces fradiae.* It has a structure similar to erythromycin; its empirical formula is $C_{45}H_{77}O_{17}$; and it has a molecular weight of 904. Tylosin is slightly soluble in water and is soluble in common organic solvents, e.g., ether, ethanol, and acetone. It is a weak base and forms water-soluble salts. Tylosin is not stable if the pH is less than 4; a degradation product, desmycosin, is formed at a lower pH. Desmycosin does not have antibacterial activity.

The antibacterial spectrum includes gram-positive organisms generally susceptible to the macrolide group of antibiotics. Organisms resistant to tylosin may also be cross-resistant to erythromycin. Tylosin is essentially a bacteriostatic agent. It has been used to treat chronic respiratory disease (CRD) of poultry and other infections caused by *Mycoplasma,* gram-positive bacteria, and some gram-negative bacteria.

Tylosin, in a concentration of 715 ppm, was used for dipping turkey eggs in an effort to control *Mycoplasma meleagridis* infections (Bigland 1970). Dipping the eggs in tylosin resulted in an 87% reduction in air sac lesions.

Mycoplasma gallisepticum is resistant to tylosin both *in vitro* and *in vivo* (Griffin 1969). The organism is also cross-resistant to spiramycin.

Use of tylosin has been assessed in the treatment of pleuropneumonia in naturally and experimentally infected goats (El Nasri 1964). Goats that had received tylosin intramuscularly in a dose of 3 mg/lb or 9 mg/lb of body weight daily for 5 days responded favorably compared to the untreated infected controls. Infected goats had marked lesions in lungs and lymph nodes whereas tissues of the treated animals appeared normal and no organisms were isolated.

Tylosin administered intramuscularly in a dose of 400 mg daily for 2 days controlled an abortion outbreak in ewes within 10 days after treatment (Baxter and Cripps 1967). The infectious organism involved in the abortion outbreak was sensitive to tylosin.

Concentrations of 1–2 g of tylosin/gal of drinking water have been used for the treatment of vibrionic dysentery in swine. An intramuscular injection of tylosin (8 mg/kg of body weight) has been used in the treatment of exudative dermatitis or greasy pig disease.

Tylosin is effective in experimental coccidial infections of poultry. A reduction in the number of *Eimeria tenella* oocysts shed as well as a reduction and prevention of mortality occurred following administration of tylosin at 400 or 800 g/ton of feed (Shumard 1965).

Absorption of tylosin occurs mainly in the intestine. While tylosin tartrate is readily absorbed, tylosin phosphate has limited absorption. Serum and milk concentrations have been determined by Ziv and Sulman (1973a) following the administration of tylosin in normal and mastitic cattle and sheep. In animals that had received an intramuscular or intravenous dose of 20 mg/kg of body weight, the concentration of tylosin in milk compared to serum was detected in a ratio of 5:1. The ratios were influenced by the pH of the milk.

The plasma half-life of tylosin in goats following an intramuscular injection of 15 mg/kg of body weight was 4–5 hours. An average concentration of the antibiotic in blood plasma (1.5 μg/ml) was attained in 2 hours.

Comparison of the duration of tylosin and erythromycin in blood following an oral dose (50 mg/kg) was evaluated in the pig (Grandadam et al. 1969). Erythromycin produced higher and more consistent concentrations. Both drugs achieved a maximum blood concentration 1 hour after administration.

Tylosin is excreted in the urine and bile. The LD50 of tylosin for the intravenous and intraperitoneal routes in mice and rats was demonstrated at 600 mg/kg of body weight; by the oral route, it was more than 5000 mg/kg (Anderson et al. 1965). Dogs tolerated an oral dose of 800 mg/kg. The oral administration of tylosin to dogs at a dose of 200 and 400 mg/kg/day for 2 years produced no visceral damage.

Dogs treated with tylosin in a dose of 5 mg/kg/day were more susceptible to the development of ventricular tachycardia and fibrillation during acute myocardial ischemia (Regan et al. 1969). For therapeutic purposes, tylosin is administered intramuscularly at a level of 1–2 mg/lb of body weight. Pain and local tissue irritation may occur following intramuscular injection.

Tylosin has been incorporated as a feed additive for swine, cattle, and chickens at doses ranging from 10 to 1000 g/ton in attempts to control diseases produced by tylosin-sensitive organisms. A regulatory tolerance of 0.2 ppm has been established for tylosin in edible animal tissues. No residues above the tolerance level were detected in tissues when tylosin was fed at 100, 200, or 500 g/ton (Kline and Waitt 1971).

Tyrothricin

Tyrothricin, N.F., is an antibacterial substance produced by *Bacillus brevis* and consists of gramicidin and tyrocidine. Tyrothricin is soluble in water but not soluble in alcohol and resists the action of pepsin and trypsin. It is active against gram-positive organisms, including streptococci and staphylococci. Tyrothricin causes lysis of susceptible bacteria by inhibiting growth through its depressive effect on enzymatic systems.

Tyrothricin has been used to treat bovine mastitis by intramammary infusion during the dry period and metritis by intrauterine infusion. It is irritating to the lactating mammary gland. Tyrothricin may be applied topically but its toxic properties prevent systemic administration. Topical application of tyrothricin to fresh wounds may cause hemolysis and hemorrhage.

Fusidic Acid

Fusidic acid (Fucidine) is an antibiotic used topically for staphylococcal and streptococcal infections of the skin and ear. It appears to have synergistic antibacterial activity with penicillin against certain organisms.

Carbadox

Chemically, *carbadox* (Mecadox) is a substituted quinoxaline 1,4-dioxide, methyl 3-(2-quinoxalvinylmethylene)carbazate N^1, N^4-dioxide. It is a yellow crystalline material insoluble in water and most organic solvents. The quinoxaline 1,4-dioxides as a class of compounds possess *in vitro* antibacterial activity.

TABLE 49.1. Activity of carbadox against gram-negative and gram-positive organisms

Organism	Minimum Inhibitory Concentration	PD50
	(μg/ml)	*(mg/kg)*
Gram-negative		
Escherichia coli	12.5–25	5.3–50
Pasteurella multocida	1.56	16
Salmonella choleraesuis	12.5	20
Salmonella typhimurium	12.5–50	2.5–51
Proteus vulgaris	25	50
Gram-positive		
Streptococcus pyogenes	25	125
Staphylococcus aureus	25	114

The mode of action of the quinoxaline 1,4-dioxide was investigated by incorporation of precursors of DNA, RNA, and protein synthesis in *Escherichia coli* using radioisotopic techniques. Data indicate that the activity of 2,3-dihydroxymethylquinoxaline-1,4-di-*N*-oxide is due to the inhibition of DNA synthesis.

Carbadox is active against a wide variety of organisms. Its activity is greater against gram-negative than gram-positive organisms (see Table 49.1).

No cross-resistance has been observed between carbadox and other antibiotics, e.g., the tetracyclines, streptomycin, or chloramphenicol (Kashiwazaki et al. 1972).

Carbadox is administered in a concentration of 50 g/ton of feed for prophylactic action against swine dysentery. The therapeutic action of carbadox at 50 g/ton has also been observed (Froe 1970). It is also used at 50 g/ton for control of bacterial swine enteritis caused by *Salmonella choleraesuis.* In the United States, it is not approved for use in swine weighing more than 75 lb and should not be fed within 10 weeks of slaughter. In other countries, withdrawal periods range from 4 to 10 weeks, depending upon government approval and feed system used.

Virginiamycin

Virginiamycin (Stafac) is an antibiotic mixture produced by *Streptomyces virginiae,* which was isolated from Belgian soil. It is composed of Factor M and Factor S, Factor M being predominant. Both factors are generally referred to as "peptolides."

The molecular formula for Factor M is $C_{28}H_{35}N_3O_7$ and $C_{43}H_{49}NO_{10}$ for Factor S.

Indications for the use of virginiamycin are: (1) in the treatment of dysentery in nonbreeding swine weighing over 120 lb (100 g/ton of feed for 2 weeks), (2) in the treatment and control of dysentery in pigs weighing up to 120 lb (100 g/ton of feed for 2 weeks and at 50 g/ton of feed thereafter), and (3) as an aid in control of dysentery in pigs weighing up to 120 lb and for animals with a history of dysentery where the symptoms have not developed (25 g/ton of feed).

Administered as a single oral dose, the maximum safe level of virginiamycin in the pig is greater than 800 mg/kg. Doses of virginiamycin up to 500 mg/kg were fed to pigs for 3 months with no adverse effects. Similarly, there were no adverse effects in pigs that had received medicated feed containing 10 g of virginiamycin/lb of body weight for 2 weeks.

Virginiamycin decreased the lactobacilli flora particularly in the anterior portions of the small intestine; however, a slight increase in the coliform and enterococcal bacteria was observed (Decuypere et al. 1973). Moreover, other anaerobes took the predominant place of the lactobacilli in the small intestine, and the clostridia were practically eliminated from the GI tract.

Single oral doses of virginiamycin up to 1500 mg/kg were given without ill effect to mice; also, doses up to 100 mg/kg were given daily to rats and dogs for 3 months without adverse effects. Virginiamycin administered in a concentration of 170.5 ppm in the feed of swine for 18 weeks demonstrated that residues greater than 1 ppm could not be detected in muscle, liver, fat, kidney, and skin (DiCuollo et al. 1973).

Nalidixic Acid

Nalidixic Acid, N.F. (NegGram) (Fig. 49.15), is an antibacterial drug with a narrow antibacterial spectrum. It is used primarily as a treatment for urinary infections. It has clinical activity against certain gram-negative bacteria, especially *Escherichia coli* and most species of *Proteus.* The treatment of infections caused by *Proteus* organisms is the most important indication since many strains are resistant to other agents. Nalidixic acid is much less active against other coliform bacteria such as *Enterobacter* and *Klebsiella.*

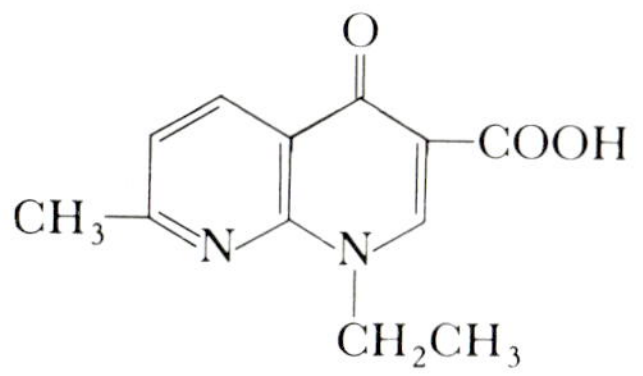

O
COOH
CH_3 N N
CH_2CH_3
Nalidixic Acid

Fig. 49.15.

The plasma half-life of nalidixic acid following a single oral dose was approximately 24 hours in 5- to 10-day-old calves (McChesney et al. 1969). In 7-day-old calves, a plasma half-life of 90 minutes was noted following intravenous administration; the drug appeared to be excreted in the bile and enterohepatic recycling may have occurred.

Bacteria sensitivity tests are helpful in determining when nalidixic acid should be used because the antibacterial spectrum is narrow. Low concentrations of naladixic acid in the blood and its binding by plasma proteins are disadvantages that make it clinically unsuitable for treating systemic infections. A combination of nalidixic acid and neomycin has been evaluated in calves for the treatment of dysentery due to *E. coli* infections (Vacirca and Sali 1970). The combination was more effective against all of the *E. coli* strains than when either drug was used alone.

Some organisms develop resistance to nalidixic acid quickly; it is useless as a therapeutic agent under these circumstances because therapy must be continued for 2 weeks or longer. No cross-resistance has appeared with nalidixic acid and other antibacterial drugs.

In veterinary medicine, it appears that

the use of nalidixic acid for treating urinary tract infections of dogs and cats should have merit. Although some studies have been conducted with nalidixic acid in the treatment of enteritis in calves, more definitive work is needed in the determination of the rate of resistance development.

The oral dose of nalidixic acid for the dog is approximately 50 mg/kg of body weight/day in 2–4 divided doses. This dosage is recommended for the treatment of urinary tract infections.

Methenamine

Methenamine, N.F. (Fig. 49.16), is another urinary antiseptic and provides its antibacterial activity by liberating formaldehyde in an acid medium. The amount of formaldehyde produced by hydrolysis will determine whether the effect is bacteriostatic or bactericidal. Caution must be taken to avoid excessive lowering of the urine pH because formaldehyde is irritating. It may be necessary to reduce the dosage to prevent a drug-induced nephritis or cystitis.

Methenamine has activity against a variety of gram-positive and gram-negative organisms including *Escherichia coli.* It should not be used as the sole therapeutic agent but in combination with other antibacterial agents. The drug is frequently administered to carnivores with large amounts of ascorbic acid, arginine hydrochloride, or methionine. Ammonium chloride may also be used to produce an acid urine.

Use of methenamine is often restricted to clinical cases that have become refractory to other antibacterial agents. Methenamine mandelate combines the antibacterial activity of methenamine with the weak antibacterial effects of mandelic acid. The preparation is effective only in acidic urine.

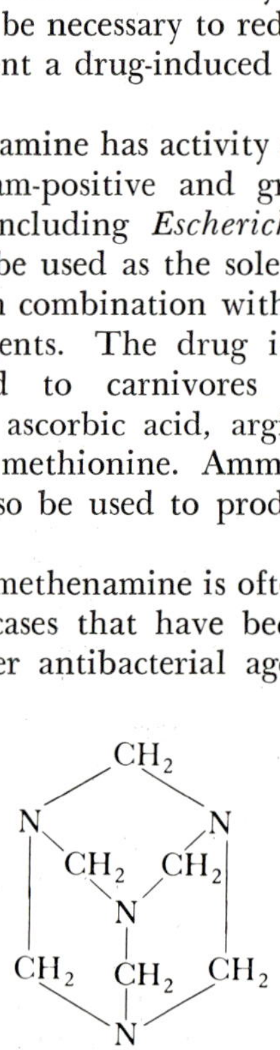

Methenamine compounds should not be used with sulfonamides because insoluble precipitates with formaldehyde may be formed.

In addition to the use of methenamine as a urinary antiseptic, veterinarians have administered the drug to sows for the control of pig scours caused by excessive consumption of milk by the nursing piglets. Formaldehyde is excreted in milk and reduces the milk intake of the piglets. The daily oral dose for dogs and cats ranges from 0.1 to 2 g in 2–4 divided doses, depending upon the size of the animal. The oral dose for sows ranges from 2 to 8 g and for horses from 8 to 15 g twice daily. In urinary tract infections, the sensitivity of the organism to several antibacterial agents should be determined to enable the correct course of antimicrobial therapy to be used with methenamine.

CH_2
N   N
CH_2 CH_2
N
CH_2 CH_2 CH_2
N

Methenamine

Fig. 49.16.

Cephalosporins

Cephalosporins, a group of semisynthetic antibacterial agents, are chemically related to penicillin. They contain the beta-lactam ring as part of the nucleus. A portion of the chemical nucleus is obtained from cephalosporin C, a substance elaborated by the fungus *Cephalosporium.* The cephalosporins interfere with cell wall synthesis by inactivating transpeptidase.

Cephalosporins are effective against most gram-positive cocci and some gram-negative organisms, primarily *Escherichia coli, Proteus mirabilis* and *Klebsiella.*

The cephalosporins are usually penicillinase resistant; however, they are sensitive to cephalosporinase, a substance comparable to beta-lactamase that is produced by gram-negative rods. Cross-resistance between cephalosporins and penicillins has been observed. In general, strains of *Staphylococcus aureus,* resistant to some penicillins, are also resistant to cephalosporins.

Cephalosporins are used to treat infections of the respiratory system, urinary

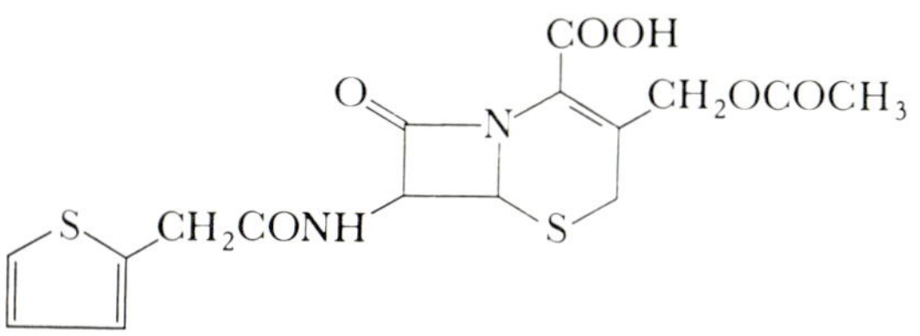

Cephalothin

FIG. 49.17.

tract, skin, and soft tissues, as well as diseases of the bones and joints.

Cephalothin Sodium, U.S.P. (Keflin), is a broad-spectrum antibiotic administered intramuscularly or intravenously. It is useful for treating urinary tract infections since high concentrations of the active drug are present in the urine. In addition, cephalothin has been employed successfully for treating peritonitis. (See Fig. 49.17.) Injections should be made deep into the muscle to minimize pain and irritation. Thrombophlebitis has been occasionally observed after intravenous administration.

Cephalosporins do not readily gain access to cerebrospinal fluid unless the anatomical structures are inflamed. Placental transfer occurs; however, it is believed that the drug can be used safely during pregnancy.

Cephaloridine, N.F., is a poorly absorbed cephalosporin and must be administered parenterally. A chief limiting factor is its potential nephrotoxicity. Thus it is recommended that the sensitivity of the causative organism be determined before therapy is initiated.

The drug has been used for severe respiratory and genitourinary infections of companion animals. *Proteus,* staphylococcal, and *Salmonella* infections have responded favorably to cephaloridine therapy. Intramuscular injections of 25 mg/kg twice daily have been used. Intramuscular and subcutaneous dosages approved by the FDA in the dog and cat are 5 mg/lb of body weight administered twice daily. Unless the therapy is reevaluated, the drug should not be administered in excess of 7 days.

Cephaloridine has been evaluated as an injectable antibiotic for treatment of bacterial infections in dogs and cats (Sampson et al. 1973). It was administered subcutaneously or intramuscularly in a dose of 1–20 mg/lb of body weight. Cephaloridine was effective in the treatment of infections of the respiratory, urinary, and enteric tracts. Infections of soft tissues were also effectively treated. Transient, adverse reactions were observed in 7%–8% of the dogs and cats.

Cephaloglycin dihydrate (Kafocin) and *cephalexin monohydrate* (Keflex) are two cephalosporins that can be administered orally. To date they are used mainly in human beings.

NITROFURAN DERIVATIVES

(Note: The FDA has proposed withdrawal of the nitrofurans from the market and has offered its manufacturers an opportunity for a hearing in late 1976.)

Nitrofuran derivatives are synthetic compounds that possess antimicrobial activity. They are substitution products of furan. The 5-nitro group is a requisite for antimicrobial activity. Nitrofuran derivatives have *in vitro* activity against an extensive range of gram-positive and gram-negative bacteria at concentrations ranging from 0.1 to 30 μg/ml. However, they are not active against all species of *Proteus* and rarely have activity against *Pseudomonas* species. Nitrofurans have the advantage that *in vivo* bacterial resistance appears to develop slowly and to a limited degree. (See Fig. 49.18.)

Nitrofurans are used primarily for their activity against gram-negative organisms but also have activity against some gram-positive bacteria. In addition, they have been employed as antifungal and antiprotozoal drugs.

The presence of blood, plasma, pus, and milk reduces the antibacterial activity of the nitrofurans. Depending upon the concentration used, they may be either bac-

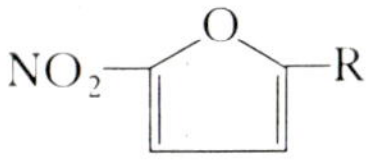

Nitrofuran

FIG. 49.18.

teriostatic or bactericidal. Bacterial resistance of the nitrofurans will develop but not to the same magnitude as other antiinfective drugs.

Although nitrofurans may inhibit an enzymatic oxidative process, the exact mechanism of action is unknown. Apparently, bacteriostatic activity results from a reversible inhibition of enzymes involved with the dissimilation of pyruvate.

Toxic and chemical properties of the nitrofurans have restricted their widespread usage as systemic antiinfective drugs. Vomition, diarrhea, GI bleeding, eosinophilia, ocular disturbances, peripheral neuritis, sensitization, and other undesirable effects have occurred following parenteral administration. Nitrofurans vary in their toxicity and solubility characteristics, limiting their clinical utility. Care should be exercised in treating chronic ulcerative skin lesions to avoid hypersensitivity.

Nitrofurazone, N.F. (Furacin) (5-nitro-2-furaldehyde semicarbazone), a yellow crystalline powder with no odor or taste, is heat stable and is slightly soluble in water.

Nitrofurazone has been used locally (see Chapter 42) but it is of little value as a systemic chemotherapeutic agent. Locally, it has been used to treat wounds and diseases of the skin, ear, eye, and reproductive tract. Nitrofurazone has found limited use alone or in combination with other agents in the treatment of bovine mastitis.

Nitrofurazone administered to dogs intravenously in a dose greater than 0.2 mg/lb of body weight produced adverse effects characterized by vomition and diarrhea (Thimmaiah 1970). Its use in so-called therapeutic doses in cockerels produced an adverse effect upon spermatogenesis, characterized by atrophy of the germinal testicular epithelium (Neuman et al. 1965).

In calves, orally administered nitrofurazone (3/mg/kg) resulted in paralysis of the hind limbs (Lister and Fisher 1970). When nitrofurazone was administered in a dose of 14 mg/kg for 3–5 weeks, hyperirritability and convulsions occurred. A dose of 7 mg/kg caused reduction of food intake but did not produce abnormal nervous system disturbances. The adverse effects were reversible when the drug was removed. Thiamine had no beneficial effect on counteracting these adverse effects.

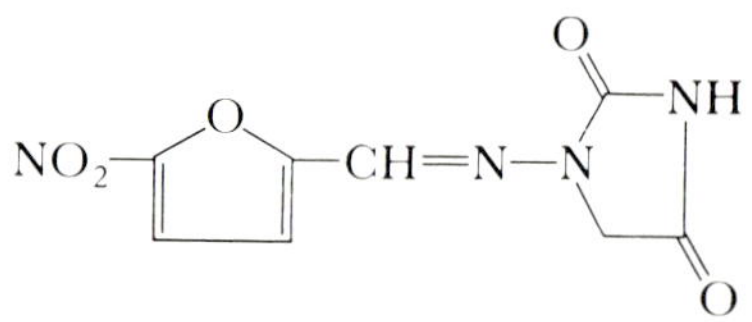

NO_2–(furan)–CH=N–N(hydantoin: C=O, NH, C=O)

Nitrofurantoin

FIG. 49.19.

Orally, nitrofurazone has been used as an aid in the prevention of infection by cecal and some species of intestinal coccidia in chickens (see Chapter 54). It has also been used for the treatment of swine enteritis. As a feed additive, doses have ranged from 50 to 500 g/ton of feed.

Nitrofurantoin, U.S.P. (Furadantin), *N*-(5-nitro-2-furfurylidene)-1-aminohydantoin (Fig. 49.19), is a bitter, yellow powder with a slight odor and is practically insoluble in water. Nitrofurantoin has a broad antibacterial action against gram-positive and gram-negative organisms. It affects *Escherichia coli, Staphylococcus aureus, S. albus, Streptococcus pyogenes,* and *Aerobacter aerogenes.* The following organisms are more resistant but sometimes can be eradicated from the urinary tract of carnivora: *Pseudomonas aeruginosa, Streptococcus faecalis,* and the *Proteus* spp.

Nitrofurantoin is absorbed rapidly and completely from the GI tract; it does not affect the intestinal bacterial flora to any significant degree. About 40% of the drug is eliminated in the urine; the remainder is catabolized. Concentrations excreted in the urine are bactericidal.

Nitrofurantoin is used as a urinary antiseptic in small animals. It can be administered orally, intravenously, or intramuscularly. It is often effective against severe urinary tract infections that are refractive to other antibacterial agents. Nitrofurantoin is concentrated in an acid urine. When the pH of the urine is reduced to about 5, the urine becomes supersaturated with nitrofurantoin without precipitation; this achieves a maximal antibacterial action in carnivora. In dogs, nitrofurantoin is ad-

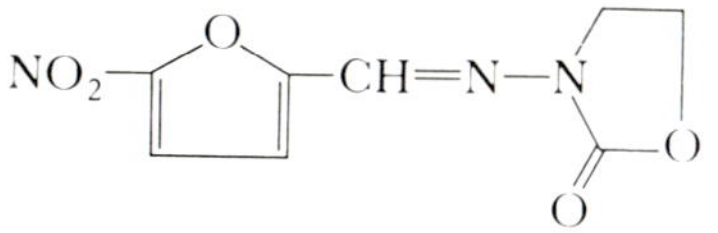

$$NO_2-\text{C}_4\text{H}_2\text{O}-CH{=}N-N\langle\text{oxazolidinone}\rangle$$

Furazolidone

FIG. 49.20.

ministered orally at 2 mg/lb 3 times a day and intramuscularly in a dose of 3.3 mg/kg twice daily. Doses of 10 mg/kg orally have been used daily in calves and horses.

Furazolidone, N.F. (Furoxone), *N*-(5-nitro-2-furfurylidene)-3-amino-2-oxazolidone (Fig. 49.20), is a yellow crystalline powder which can be mixed with feed. It is effective against the *Salmonella* spp. infecting the digestive tract. However, strains of *Salmonella gallinarum* have demonstrated *in vivo* resistance to furazolidone (Stuart et al. 1967). In a breeding flock outbreak of fowl typhoid, an increase in resistance was noted within a period of 39 days. Furazolidone has been administered to chickens, turkeys, and swine for the control of various infections of the digestive tract. It is used in the treatment of bacterial enteritis, dysentery, and giardiasis. Absorption is incomplete and traces of the drug appear in the urine. Furazolidone is active as an aid in preventing coccidiosis in chickens (see Chapter 54).

The mechanism of action of furazolidone is apparently through its ability to interfere with the acetylation of coenzyme A and possibly other enzyme systems.

Furazolidone (400 ppm) produced neurological symptoms when fed in combination with either Zoalene (1–5 ppm) or amprolium (125 ppm) (van Stratum et al. 1966). The simultaneous administration of furazolidone and dinitro-orthotoluamide (Zoalene) to broilers resulted in an adverse effect characterized by the loss of balance and abnormal posture. Zoalene was administered at a dosage of 30–40 g/100 kg of body weight; it was incorporated in the feed at a concentration of 0.0125%.

Furazolidone administered orally to horses in a dose of 4 mg/lb followed by 20 doses of 2 mg/lb at 8-hour intervals produced no serious adverse effect in yearling horses (Bryans et al. 1965). However, a dose of 8 mg/lb followed by 20 doses of 4 mg/lb produced inappetence.

Furazolidone has been used in feed additives for swine and poultry at concentrations ranging from 10 to 200 g/ton. Efficacy of the treatment is dependent upon identification of the sensitive pathogen(s) and the administration of a dose of the antibacterial agent that will exceed the minimum inhibitory concentration.

Furaltadone, N.N.D. (Altafur), has a medium spectrum of antibacterial activity and is readily absorbed from the GI tract. Metabolic distribution of the drug is unknown and relatively small amounts appear in the urine. Undesirable toxic effects have been observed in human beings following oral administration of furaltadone. The drug has been used intramammarily to treat bovine mastitis by administering 500 mg/quarter. It has also been used to treat strangles in the horse (Evers 1968). An intravenous dose of 6 mg/lb for 5 days reduced the severity of the systemic involvement and the length of illness.

Experimentally, furaltadone has been used successfully in the treatment of chickens infected with *Salmonella gallinarum* or *Salmonella typhimurium.* A concentration of 0.04% in the drinking water prevented mortality and did not permit a high carrier rate in survivors. Chickens experimentally infected with *Mycoplasma gallisepticum* had fewer and less extensive lesions following treatment with furaltadone than birds treated with tylosin (Matzer 1969). Furaltadone administered in the drinking water at 1 g/gal was effective in controlling artificially induced infectious synovitis in chickens (Olson 1967). Administration of the drug at 0.044% in the feed also prevented artificially induced infection.

Nifuraldezone (Furamazone), 5-nitro-2-furaldehyde semioxamazone, is a yellow crystalline substance with only slight solubility in water. It is administered orally with bismuth subsalicylate for the treatment of enteric diseases in calves. Relatively small amounts of nifuraldezone are absorbed from the GI tract; thus the drug does not attain systemic concentrations and must produce its action by contact with the microorganisms within the digestive tract. It has antibacterial action against certain gram-positive and gram-negative bacteria *in vitro* at concentrations of about 2 mg/100 cc.

An oral dose of 15 mg/kg twice daily is recommended in the treatment of digestive tract infections in calves.

TOXICOLOGY OF ANTIBIOTICS

Antibacterial drugs are an extremely useful group of compounds and represent an important and beneficial achievement for veterinary medicine. Comments on toxicology should be viewed with the utmost concern to maintain a proper perspective. As a group, the antibacterial agents are a safe group of compounds. Many are extremely safe and free of untoward effects. There is no doubt that the benefits resulting from the use of antibacterial drugs are much greater than the risks.

The acute adverse effects of antibiotics can be categorized on the basis of neuromuscular blocking effects, cardiovascular depressant effects, and the inhibition of drug metabolism. A review by Adams (1975) gives more detailed information. Mechanisms of the neuromuscular effects of various antibiotics have not been completely determined. The neomycin-streptomycin antibiotics have been studied for their actions inhibiting the release of acetylcholine from the motor nerve terminals and competitively blocking postsynaptic skeletal muscle receptors in a nondepolarizing "curarelike" manner that result in myoneuronal paralysis. The presynaptic and postsynaptic effects can be antagonized by cholinesterase inhibitors. The presynaptic effect can be reversed by the administration of calcium ions which may displace the antibiotics from the binding sites at the motor nerve terminal.

Some antibiotics have a synergistic effect with other drugs that alter neuromuscular function. General anesthetic agents and *d*-tubocurarine may enhance the neuromuscular blocking effects of various antibiotics. A summary of the neuromuscular blocking effects of various antibiotics is presented in Table 49.2.

The cardiovascular depressant effects of some antibiotics are summarized in Table 49.3. Experimental studies have demonstrated that some antibiotics have a direct cardiovascular effect in several species. Streptomycin, kanamycin, tetracycline, erythromycin, and colymycin produce a decrease in cardiac output, systemic arterial pressure, and myocardial contractile force in the anesthetized dog. Aminoglycosides may affect the peripheral vascular resistance and cause vasodilation.

The third effect antibiotics may have is their ability to inhibit hepatic microsomal enzymes that detoxify zenobiotics; e.g., chloramphenicol has been noted to increase the toxicity of such drugs as diphenylhydantoin and dicumarol.

The relationship between barbiturates and chloramphenicol in cats has been assessed. Studies demonstrate that the depressive effect of barbiturates is prolonged more than threefold by chloramphenicol

TABLE 49.2. Neuromuscular blocking effects of some commonly used antibiotics

Antibiotic	Neuromuscular Paralysis	
	Characteristics	Mechanism
Aminoglycosides Neomycin Streptomycin Dihydrostreptomycin Kanamycin Gentamicin	Nondepolarizing, flaccid	1. Competitive blockade of skeletal muscle nicotinic receptors 2. Inhibition of Ca^{++}-dependent release of acetylcholine from motor nerves
Tetracyclines	Flaccid	Unknown
Lincomycin	Flaccid	Unknown
Polymyxins	Flaccid	Unknown

TABLE 49.3. Cardiovascular depressant effects of some commonly used antibiotics

Antibiotic	Cardiovascular Depression	
	Characteristics	Mechanism
Aminoglycosides Neomycin Streptomycin Dihydrostreptomycin Kanamycin Gentamicin	Decreased cardiac output, hypotension, relative bradycardia	Myocardial depression, vascular effects
Tetracyclines	Decreased cardiac output	Myocardial depression, vascular effects
Lincomycin	Myocardial depression	Cardiac conductance disturbances
Chloramphenicol	Myocardial depression	Unknown

(see Chapter 13). Repeated administration of chlortetracycline inhibits hepatic drug metabolism, probably as a result of nonspecific inhibition of protein synthesis in the liver. Interestingly, griseofulvin has the opposite effect.

Most of the acute adverse effects of antibiotics have been noted clinically in human beings or experimentally in animals. Similar clinical reports in veterinary medicine are not readily available. It is important to point out that pathologic conditions contribute to the frequency of adverse effects, i.e., abnormalities of the cardiovascular and renal systems and the presence of infectious diseases. Adverse effects have been observed primarily in experimental animals that have received drugs concomittantly with other potent drugs. In most experimental studies, the dose of antibiotics required to demonstrate the potential for adverse effects in clinically healthy animals has been larger than those routinely used in therapy.

During surgical anesthesia, patients should be monitored as closely as possible for potential adverse reactions that might be falsely ascribed to anesthetic overdosage. Also, careful assessment should be made of possible drug idiosyncracies, allergic responses, shock, or other factors that may influence antibacterial therapy.

REFERENCES

Adams, H. R. 1973. Neuromuscular blocking effect of aminoglycoside antibiotics in nonhuman primates. J Am Vet Med Assoc 163:613.

———. 1975. Acute adverse effects of antibiotics. J Am Vet Med Assoc 166:983.

Adams, H. R., and Dixit, B. N. 1970. Prolongation of pentobarbital anesthesia by chloramphenicol in dogs and cats. J Am Vet Med Assoc 156:902.

Anand, N., and Davis, B. D. 1960. Effect of streptomycin on *Escherichia coli.* Nature 185:22.

Anand, N.; Davis, B. D.; and Armitage, A. K. 1960. Uptake of streptomycin by *Escherichia coli.* Nature 185:23.

Anderson, R. C.; Worth, H. M.; Small, R. M.; and Harris, P. N. 1965. Toxicological studies on tylosin: Its safety as a food additive. Toxicol Appl Pharmacol 7:478.

Andreini, G., and Pignattelli, P. 1972. Kanamycin blood levels and residues in domestic animals. Veterinariia 21:51.

Baxter, C. J., and Cripps, D. 1967. A treatment of vibrionic abortion in ewes. Vet Rec 80:440.

Bernau, U., and Lüthgen, W. 1970. Streptomycin in pigeons. Dtsch Tieraerztl Wochenschr 77:431.

Bigland, C. H. 1970. Experimental control of *Mycoplasma meleagridis* in turkeys by the dipping of eggs in tylosin and spiramycin. Can J Comp Med 34:26.

Bryans, J. T.; Moore, B. O.; and Crowe, M. W. 1965. Safety and efficacy of Furoxone in the treatment of equine salmonellosis. Vet Med Small Anim Clin 60:626.

Bulling, E., and Stephan, R. 1971. Effect of antibiotic supplements in nutritive doses on the development of resistance of the coliform gut flora in pigs. II. Spread of R-factors by the use of antibiotics in feed. Zentralbl Veterinaermed [A] 18B:449.

Calabi, O. 1973. Bactericidal synergism of novobiocin and tetracycline against *Pseudomonas pseudomallei.* J Med Microbiol 6:293.

Conner, G. H., and Gupta, B. N. 1973. Bone marrow, blood and assay levels following medication of cats with chloramphenicol ophthalmic ointment. Vet Med Small Anim Clin 68:895.

Cook, B. 1973. Successful treatment of an outbreak of *Salmonella dublin* infection in calves using spectinomycin. Vet Rec 93:80.

Crawford, L. M., and Bowen, J. M. 1971. Calcium binding as a property of kanamycin. Am J Vet Res 32:357.

Cunningham, G. R. 1970. Ophthalmic kanamycin in small animals. Vet Med Small Anim Clin 65:983.

Davis, L. E.; Neff, C. A.; Baggot, J. D.; and Powers, T. E. 1972. Pharmacokinetics of chloramphenicol in domesticated animals. Am J Vet Res 33:2259.

Decuypere, J.; Henderickx, H. K.; and Vervaeke, I. 1973. Influence of nutritional doses of virginiamycin and spiramycin on the quantitative and topographical composition of the gastro-intestinal flora of artificially reared piglets. Zentralbl Bakteriol [Orig B] 223A:348.

Dewaele, A. 1969. Comparative toxicity of streptomycin and dihydrostreptomycin for the young piglet. Ann Med Vet 113:368.

DiCuolo, C. J.; Miller, J. A.; and Miller, C. R. 1973. Tissue residue studies in swine treated with virginiamycin. J Agric Food Chem 21:818.

El Nasri, M. 1964. The effect of tylosin against experimental and natural infection with *Mycoplasma* in goats. Vet Rec 76:876.

Evers, W. 1968. Effect of furaltadone on strangles in horses. J Am Vet Med Assoc 152:1394.

Favati, V., and Marranghini, M. 1968. *Pseudomonas aeruginosa* infection in chinchillas. Treatment with a new antibiotic, gentamicin sulphate. Zooprofilassi 23:277.

Förster, D.; Müller, L. F.; and Dienemann, O. 1969. Test results and the first clinical observations on the use of gentamicin in dogs. Berl Munch Tieraerztl Wochenschr 82:264.

Fowler, N. G. 1968. The ototoxicity of neomycin in the dog. Vet Rec 82:267.

Froe, D. L. 1970. Mecadox for the treatment and control of swine dysentery. J Am Vet Med Assoc 156:1212.

Fujimoto, J. M.; Lech, J. J.; and Zamiatowski, R. 1973. A site of action of novobiocin in inhibiting renal tubular transport of drugs in the chicken. Biochem Pharmacol 22:971.

Goren, E. 1972. Effectiveness of spectinomycin against avian *Mycoplasma* cultures and cross-resistance with tylosin. Tijdschr Diergeneeskd 97:1185.

Grandadam, A.; Scheid, J. P.; Lacombe, A. M.; and Dreux, H. 1969. Comparison between the amounts of erythromycin and tylosin in the blood after oral administration to pigs. Recl Med Vet 145:1293.

Gray, J. E., and Lewis, C. 1966. Enigma of antibiotic-induced diarrhea in the laboratory rabbit. Toxicol Appl Pharmacol 8:342.

Gray, J. E.; Weaver, R. N.; Bollert, J. A.; and Feenstra, E. S. 1972. The oral toxicity of clindamycin in laboratory animals. Toxicol Appl Pharmacol 21:516.

Griffin, R. M. 1969. Antibiotic resistance to a strain of *Mycoplasma gallisepticum*. J Comp Pathol 79:33.

Hamdy, A. H., and Blanchard, C. J. 1969. Effect of lincomycin and spectinomycin water medication on chickens experimentally infected with *Mycoplasma gallisepticum* and *Escherichia coli*. Poult Sci 48:1703.

———. 1970. Effect of novobiocin on fowl cholera in turkeys. Avian Dis 14:770.

Hammond, P. B. 1953. Dihydrostreptomycin dose–serum level relationships in cattle. J Am Vet Med Assoc 122:203.

Hardie, H. 1973. Spectinomycin in veterinary practice. Vet Rec 92:123.

Harris, D. L.; Glock, R. D.; Dale, S. E.; and Ross, R. F. 1972. Efficacy of gentamicin sulfate for the treatment of swine dysentery. J Am Vet Med Assoc 161:1317.

Houdeshell, J. W., and Hennessey, P. W. 1972. Gentamicin in the treatment of equine metritis. Vet Med Small Anim Clin 67:1348.

Huebner, R. A.; Glassman, J. M.; Hudyma, G. M.; and Seifter, J. 1956. The toxic dose of dihydrostreptomycin in the fowl. Cornell Vet 46:219.

Kashiwazaki, M.; Mitani, K.; and Namioka, S. 1972. Sensitivity of faecal *Escherichia coli* from healthy pigs to carbadox. J Jpn Vet Med Assoc 25:615.

Klatte, F. J., and Thomas, R. D. 1967. Antibiotic effects on a lactic acid-producing rumen microorganism. J Anim Sci 26:922.

Kline, R. M., and Waitt, W. P. 1971. Tylosin residue analyses in swine tissue. J Assoc Off Anal Chem 54:112.

Lister, E. E., and Fisher, L. J. 1970. Establishment of the toxic level of nitrofurazone for young liquid-fed calves. J Dairy Sci 53:1490.

McChesney, E. W.; Conway, W. D.; Breamer, A. C.; and Koss, R. F. 1969. Metabolism of nalidixic acid in the calf: Effect of age. Toxicol Appl Pharmacol 14:138.

McGee, T. M. 1962. Streptomycin sulfate and dihydrostreptomycin toxicity: Behavioral and histopathologic studies. Arch Otolaryngol 75:295.

Mann, P. H., and Bjotvedt, G. 1964. Evaluation of colistin in the treatment of respiratory infections in dogs. Can J Comp Med 28:222.

Manyan, D. R., and Yunis, A. A. 1970. The effect of chloramphenicol treatment on ferrochelatase activity in dogs. Biochem Biophys Res Commun 41:926.

Matzer, N. 1969. Furaltadone and tylosin tartrate in the control of experimentally induced chronic respiratory disease complex in chickens. Poult Sci 48:701.

Mercer, H. D.; Righter, H. F.; and Carter, G. G. 1971. Serum concentrations of penicillin and dihydrostreptomycin after their parenteral administration in swine. J Am Vet Med Assoc 159:61.

Neuman, V.; Zendulka, M.; Sindelarova, K.; and Klimes, B. 1965. Effect of nitrofurazone on genital organs of male rats and cocks. Veterinarstvi 15:271.

Olson, N. O. 1967. Efficacy of furaltadone in drinking water or feed against an artificial infection of infectious synovitis in chickens. Avian Dis 11:120.

Pascoe, R. R. 1972. Further observations on *Dermatophilus* infections in horses. Aust Vet J 48:32.

Popoviciu, A.; Balaci, P.; and Tibrea, L. 1972. Study of kanamycin (in fowl and swine). Lucr Stiint Inst Agron Balcescu Ser C 15:237.

Rake, G. R. 1953. Squibb Institute for Medical Research.

Regan, T. J.; Passannante, A. J.; Oldewurtel, H. A.; and Khan, M. I. 1969. Ventricular arrhythmias related to antibiotic usage in dogs. Science 165:509.

Ryan, F. B. 1960. Acute streptomycin toxicity. Aust Vet J 36:329.

Saif, Y. M., and Nestor, K. E. 1972. Control of *Mycoplasma meleagridis* infection in turkey hatching eggs. Turk Res, p. 47.

Sampson, G. R.; Young, D. C.; Gregory, R. P.; and Rathmacher, R. P. 1973. Clinical evaluation of cephaloridine injectable antibiotic in dogs and cats. Vet Med Small Anim Clin 68:1302.

Shumard, R. F. 1965. Therapeutic effectiveness of tylosin in experimental coccidia infections in chickens. J Parasitol (Suppl) 51:54.

Sisodia, C. S., and Dunlop, R. H. 1972a. Chloramphenicol residue in eggs. Can Vet J 13: 279.

———. 1972b. Chloramphenicol residues in tissues of broiler chickens. Can Vet J 13: 263.

Sisodia, C. S.; Dunlop, R. H.; Gupta, V. S.; and Taksas, L. 1973. A pharmacologic study of chloramphenicol in cattle. Am J Vet Res 34:1147.

Solis, J., and Barnett, B. D. 1970. Effectiveness of gentamicin sulfate against *Paracolobactrum arizonae* infection of turkey poults. Poult Sci 49:1668.

Stalheim, O. H. V. 1969. Chemotherapy of renal leptospirosis in cattle. Am J Vet Res 30:1317.

Stuart, E. E.; Keenum, R. D.; and Bruins, H. W. 1967. The emergence of a furazolidone-resistant strain of *Salmonella gallinarum.* Avian Dis 11:139.

Teske, R. H., and Carter, G. G. 1971. Effect of chloramphenicol on pentobarbital-induced anesthesia in dogs. J Am Vet Med Assoc 159:777.

Teske, R. H.; Rollins, L. D.; and Carter, G. G. 1972. Penicillin and dihydrostreptomycin serum concentrations after administration in single and repeated doses to feeder steers. J Am Vet Med Assoc 160:873.

Thimmaiah, K. 1970. Effect of parenteral administration of Furacin (R) in dogs. Indian Vet J 47:429.

Treppenhauer, H. J. 1973. Comparative toxicological, bacteriological and pharmacokinetic studies on kanamycin. Dtsch Tieraerztl Wochenschr 80:473.

Vacirca, G., and Sali, G. 1970. First observations on the use of nalidixic acid and neomycin together in *Escherichia coli* infection of calves. Atti Soc Ital Buiatria 2:470.

Vangelov, S. 1973. Ototoxic effect of gentamicin on experimental animals and attempts to prevent it. Vet Med Nauki 10:83.

van Stratum, P. G. C.; Feron, V. J.; and Litjens, J. B. 1966. The effect of furazolidone on broiler chickens fed rations containing amprolium or Zoalene. III. Effect of 10 days' administration of 400 ppm furazolidone. Tijdschr Diergeneeskd 91:571.

Venzke, W. G., and Smith, C. R. 1949. Streptomycin in small animal medicine. In S. A. Waksman, ed. Streptomycin: Nature and Practical Applications, p. 580. Baltimore: Williams & Wilkins.

Waksman, S. A., and Lechevalier, H. A. 1949. Symposium on antibiotics: Neomycin production and antibiotic properties. J Clin Invest 28:934.

Watson, A. D. J. 1972. Chloramphenicol plasma levels in the dog: Multiple oral and intramuscular administration. J Small Anim Pract 13:153.

Ziv, G., and Sulman, F. G. 1973a. Penetration of lincomycin and clindamycin into milk in ewes. Br Vet J 129:83.

———. 1973b. Serum and milk concentrations of spectinomycin and tylosin in cows and ewes. Am J Vet Res 34:329.

Ziv, G.; Bogin, E.; and Sulman, F. G. 1973. Blood and milk levels of chloramphenicol in normal and mastitic cows and ewes after intramuscular administration of chloramphenicol and chloramphenicol sodium succinate. Zentralbl Veterinaermed [A] 20A (10):801.

CHAPTER 50

ANTIFUNGAL AND ANTIVIRAL AGENTS

WILLIAM G. HUBER

ANTIFUNGAL DRUGS

Fungal infections may be classified in two clinical groups: (1) dermatophytoses of the skin, hair, and nails (*Trichophyton* and *Microsporum* spp. infections) and candidiasis (moniliasis infections) of the moist skin or mucous membranes of the gastrointestinal (GI) tract and (2) systemic mycoses (histoplasmosis, aspergillosis).

Antifungal agents can be grouped according to their intended application, local or systemic. Antifungal agents used to treat superficial (dermatophytic) infections are usually applied topically and may contain keratolytic drugs. Keratolytic drugs facilitate surface contact of the antifungal agent and the fungus by removing a portion of the keratin. Some drugs have both fungicidal and keratolytic activity, e.g., resorcinol, salicylic acid.

Since some dermatophytic infections recover without treatment, it is of utmost importance that treatment does not create a lesion more severe than the fungal infection; drugs causing tissue irritation may interfere with the healing process. Chronic, low-grade fungal infections require judicious treatment because the chance of spontaneous recovery is very small.

Systemic administration of antifungal agents offers opportunities for treating both systemic and dermatophytic mycoses. Antifungal drugs, e.g., griseofulvin, administered orally are absorbed and incorporated in epithelial cells as they are formed. Keratin does not interfere with these absorbable drugs since griseofulvin-type drugs form a barrier below the keratin layer in the newly formed epithelial cells. If one treats topically, the use of keratolytic drugs for removing or diminishing the amount of keratin should be considered. In infections of heavily keratinzed areas, e.g., footpad, benzoic and salicylic acid ointment may help remove heavy layers of keratin and permit antifungal drug penetration to the base of the infection.

Since many antifungal drugs do not have antibacterial activity, maximal effort should be made to establish an etiologic diagnosis before treatment. Bacterial, fungal, or mixed infections, cannot always be established by evaluation of the clinical lesions. Before treating a dermatomycosis, the specific identity of the organism must be established since a single drug is not effective against both dermatophytes and *Candida* spp.

The veterinarian treating patients with dermatomycoses should constantly examine them for signs of sensitization or irritation related to medication.

Topical

ORGANIC ACIDS

Fatty acids (undecylenic, caprylic, propionic) have been used as fungistatic agents. Although the mechanism of action is not known they have been used to treat superficial mycoses.

Undecylenic Acid, U.S.P., is a yellow liquid with a characteristic sharp odor. The chemical formula is $CH_2{=}CH(CH_2)_8CO_2H$. It has a potent fungistatic activity for superficial fungal infections involving areas with very little hair and is available as a powder or in a 10% alcoholic solution. It has been used in combination with zinc undecylenate and salicylanilide for possibly improved efficacy.

Caprylic acid and *propionic acid* are two other fatty acids that have been used to treat dermatomycoses.

Benzoic Acid, U.S.P., is a white, odorless crystal. It is slightly soluble in water and is the main ingredient in *Whitfield's Ointment,* U.S.P., which contains 6% benzoic acid and 3% salicylic acid in a water–polyethylene glycol ointment base. It has both fungistatic and keratolytic activity and is used in treatment of dermatomycotic infections.

Salicylic Acid, U.S.P., is a white crystal and is slightly soluble in water. It has moderate fungistatic activity but is included in many topical antifungal preparations because of its good keratolytic ability. Its main application is in the treatment of chronic superficial dermatomycoses. Salicylic acid requires the presence of water to produce its keratolytic effect. Repeated applications may cause irritation.

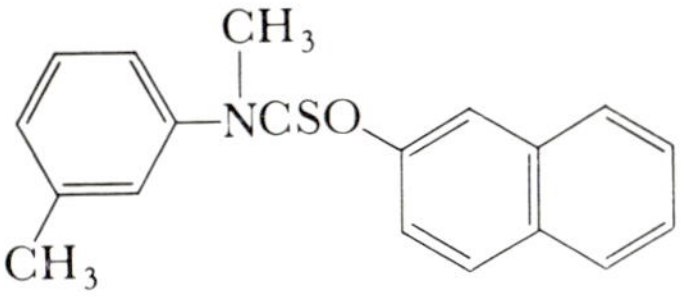

CH_3 / $-NCSO-$ / CH_3

Tolnaftate

Fig. 50.1.

TOLNAFTATE

Tolnaftate (Tinactin) (Fig. 50.1) is active against *Epidermophyton, Microsporum,* and *Trichophyton* infections. It does not have antibacterial activity nor is it active against candidal infections. Tolnaftate may be administered with griseofulvin for immediate topical effect. Tolnaftate is generally used as a 1% concentration.

CANDICIDIN

Candicidin is a fungistatic and fungicidal antibiotic obtained from *Streptomyces grisseus.* It is especially active against *Candida albicans* and is primarily used in moniliasis. Litwack (1966) reported that *in vitro* it was several times more effective than amphotericin B against *Candida albicans,* and more effective than nystatin against superficial dermatomycoses (ringworm).

HALOPROGIN

Haloprogin (Halotex) (Fig. 50.2) is a synthetic antifungal drug used to treat skin infections caused by *Trichophyton* spp. or *Microsporum canis.* A 1% cream is

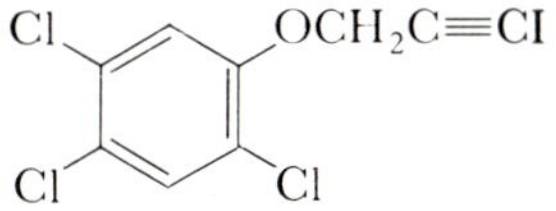

Cl / $OCH_2C{\equiv}CI$ / Cl / Cl

Haloprogin

Fig. 50.2.

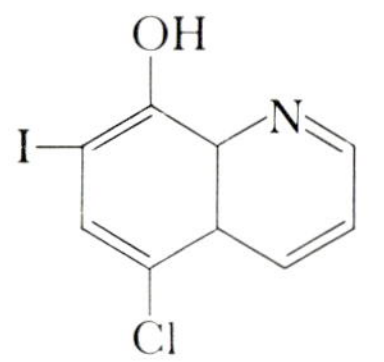

Iodochlorhydroxyquin

FIG. 50.3.

applied twice daily for 2 or 3 weeks. Care should be exercised to avoid contact with the eyes.

IODOCHLORHYDROXYQUIN

Iodochlorhydroxyquin (Vioform) (Fig. 50.3) has both antifungal and antibacterial activity and is useful in treating localized dermatophytic infections complicated by bacteria. A 3% cream, ointment, or powder may be used. Care should be taken to avoid contact with the eyes.

CUPRIMYXIN

Cuprimyxin (Unitop) (6-methoxy-1-phenazinol-5,10-dioxide, cupric complex) (Fig. 50.4) is a broad-spectrum antimicrobial agent developed for animal therapy. Cuprimyxin is a dark green crystalline material. After application, myxin is released from the copper complex and the color changes from green to pink. In addition to having antifungal activity against *Trichophyton, Microsporum,* and *Candida,* the drug has broad-spectrum antibacterial activity against gram-positive and gram-negative bacteria.

Cuprimyxin antimicrobial activity appears to be related to its ability to inhibit the synthesis of bacterial DNA and RNA. Care should be taken to avoid undesirable staining when applied to companion animals.

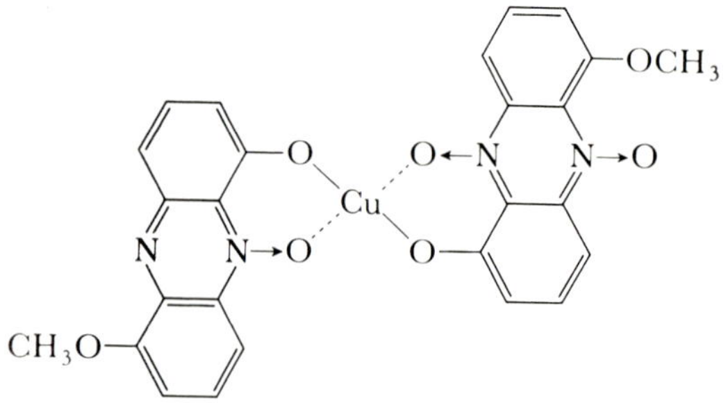

Cuprimyxin

FIG. 50.4.

THIABENDAZOLE

Thiabendazole, 2-(4-thiazolyl)benzimidazole (Fig. 50.5), has antifungal activity and has been reported to reduce aflatoxin formation in infected feeds (Robinson et al. 1969). Activity has been noted against species of *Blastomyces, Fusarium, Monilia, Penicillium,* and *Trichophyton.* Dermatophytic activity is not diminshed by the presence of serum.

Thiabendazole can be administered orally or topically. Some absorption takes place; the hydroxylated metabolite is eliminated primarly in urine and feces and to a lesser extent in milk.

Thiabendazole has a satisfactory margin of safety. The usual therapeutic dose for many species is 50 mg/kg. Most animals, especially ruminants, easily tolerate a dose 3–5 times greater than the therapeutic dose without serious adverse effects. No parasympathomimetic side effects have been reported.

As a fungicide, thiabendazole is thought to act by inhibiting transamination which is partially antagonized by exogenous pyridoxine and biotin. It also appears to act by interfering in the transfer of amino acids in protein synthesis (Allen and Gottlieb 1970).

OTHER AGENTS

Numerous antiseptics and disinfectants, e.g., phenols, iodine, mercurials, have antifungal properties in addition to their action on bacteria. These drugs should be used with care because they may injure normal tissue as well as have a toxic effect

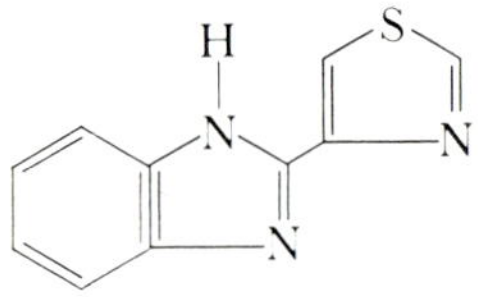

Thiabendazole

FIG. 50.5.

on the fungi. Primary irritant or contact dermatitis has been observed after some of these agents have been applied to inflamed skin.

Various dyes and dye combinations have been used as antifungal medications. *Carbol-Fuchsin Solution,* N.F., contains basic fuchsin 0.3%, phenol 4.5%, resorcinol 10%, acetone 5%, and ethyl alcohol 10%. An infected area should be washed with soap and water, dried, and the medication applied once or twice daily for 1 week. *Gentian violet* or *methylrosaniline chloride* has been used to treat fungal infections, e.g., candidiasis, either alone or in combination with other antimicrobial substances such as benzethonium chloride.

COMBINATIONS FOR TOPICAL ADMINISTRATION

Several preparations having antifungal, antibacterial, antiinflammatory, and anesthetic activity are available. Some fungal infections are mixed with bacteria and may not respond to treatment unless antibacterial activity is also present. However, it has been noted that some antibacterial agents and steroids help establish fungal infections such as cutaneous candidiasis (Wildfeuer 1973). The topical administration of *neomycin, hexachlorophene,* or *hydrocortisone* has accelerated the progression of candidia infections in rabbits. A similar effect of neomycin has been reported for other species. Preparations containing multiple active ingredients should be used selectively and not on a routine basis; they should not be used if irritation or sensitization is observed, because the veterinarian will not be able to identify the offending drug. The sensitizing or irritating ingredient may be found only by trial and error.

SYSTEMIC

Antifungal agents administered systemically consist primarily of antibiotics. Some agents have been used to treat fungal infections of the internal organs. Others have been administered for their effect in the GI tract or for their ability to enter cells that produce keratin.

The majority of commonly used antibacterial agents are contraindicated in fungal infections (Rheins et al. 1965). Neomycin and the tetracyclines have been observed to enhance *Candida* growth in keratitis.

GRISEOFULVIN

Griseofulvin (Fulvicin U/F, Grifulvin V) (Fig. 50.6) is an oral fungistatic antibiotic, colorless, slightly bitter, and is formed as a metabolic product of *Penicillium griseofulvin.*

After oral administration, griseofulvin is absorbed from the GI tract and deposited in new epithelial cells that make up the skin, hair, claws, and nails. Increasing the surface area of griseofulvin particles improves absorption. High dietary fat intake will also increase absorption. The concentration of griseofulvin in new cells of the epidermis affords fungistatic activity; thus fungi do not invade the new tissue. It is important that treatment be continued at least 1 week after disappearance of clinical signs.

Griseofulvin in a dimethyl sulfoxide vehicle has been applied topically to cats and guinea pigs infected with *Microsporum canis* (Levine et al. 1971). All animals responded favorably and were asymptomatic in 10 or less days. Dimethyl sulfoxide allowed griseofulvin penetration through the keratin layer.

Griseofulvin inhibits the growth of various species of *Microsporum, Epidermophyton,* and *Trichophyton.* It is ineffective against other fungi including *Candida* and bacteria. Thus it is imperative that the true pathogen be identified before griseofulvin is used.

Relatively large doses of griseofulvin have been administered without producing

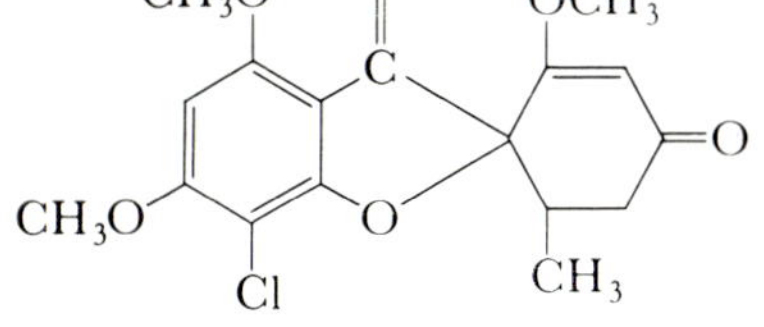

Griseofulvin

FIG. 50.6.

fatal reactions. It may interfere with spermatogenesis, but this effect has not been quantitated. Occasionally diarrhea and nausea are observed after oral administration of large doses.

Griseofulvin has been administered to horses at a dose of 100 mg/kg daily for 20 days without producing gross or microscopic lesions (Hiddleston 1970). The drug was well tolerated by mares receiving 10 mg/kg daily for alternate 30-day periods throughout pregnancy.

Griseofulvin is usually administered orally to dogs and cats at a dose of 7–20 mg/lb of body weight daily. Animals with fungal involvement of skin and hair should be treated for 3–4 weeks. Animals with infected nails or claws may require therapy for as long as 4 months.

Griseofulvin is commonly used for treatment of dermatomycoses in small animals. It is considered an efficacious drug for dermatophyte infections. Because of its low toxicity a 10-day dose has been administered as a single dose and repeated every 10 days (Muller 1968). Pharmacokinetic data to support this program of administration is not currently available.

The half-life of griseofulvin in canine plasma was found to be 47 minutes (Harris and Riegelman 1969). On the basis of a pharmacokinetic study, an oral dose of 90 mg/kg/day was proposed to maintain therapeutic concentrations. Increasing the dose severalfold did not change the pattern of elimination. Griseofulvin is mainly metabolized to 6-dimethylgriseofulvin and its glucuronide.

It has also been used in the prevention and treatment of ringworm in calves. Animals that became infected with *Trichophyton verrucosum* received griseofulvin orally for 3 weeks. At the end of 3 weeks, new hair had grown in the ringworm lesion. Histologic examination 2 weeks after the initial treatment did not reveal the presence of fungi.

Griseofulvin has been experimentally administered for the treatment of dermatomycoses in horses and cattle. Oral administration of 2.5–5 g, depending on body weight, has produced beneficial responses after 2 weeks of therapy in the cow, whereas the horse usually required 3–4 weeks of therapy.

Table 50.1 presents information regarding the doses of griseofulvin that produced a beneficial therapeutic or preventive effect. The ease of administering griseofulvin via feed, the success of dosage ranging from 10 to 30 mg/kg, and the duration of maintenance dosage from 7 to 35 days are significant characteristics of the drug that afford practical utilization.

Suggestions should be made to the owner of the pet or livestock regarding recurrence and poor hygenic conditions that contribute to fungal infections. Destruction of old bedding, adequate disinfection of quarters, close clipping of hair, and careful periodic examinations should reduce the incidence of reinfection.

Equine sporotrichosis *(Sporotrichum schencki)* was successfully treated with approximately 20–25 mg of griseofulvin/kg administered orally for 2 weeks and reducing the dose to approximately 10 mg/kg

TABLE 50.1. Griseofulvin dosage programs for ringworm

Animal	Dosage	Response	Reference
Calf	20–30 mg/kg, oral, >35 days	Therapeutic control	Nikiforov 1967
Silver fox	20 mg/kg, oral, 30 days	Prevention	Nikiforov 1967
Norwegian polar fox	20 mg/kg, oral, 20–35 days	Therapeutic control	Sarkhisov et al. 1968
Horse, donkey	10 mg/kg in feed, 7 days	Therapeutic control	Hiddleston 1970
Calf	10–16 mg/kg in milk or feed, 14–50 days	Prevention and therapeutic control	Horvath and Markoi 1970
Calf	20 mg/kg, oral, 15 days	Therapeutic control	Misra 1973
Rabbit	25 mg/kg, oral, 14 days	Therapeutic control	Hagen 1969

for an additional 46 days (Davis and Worthington 1964).

Griseofulvin has been tested as an agent to antagonize the action of ergotamine (Biggio et al. 1964). It facilitated a 90% reduction in ergotamine-induced necrosis and gangrene in the rat tail. It is possible that the drug may be utilized to treat ergotism, pending additional investigation.

NYSTATIN

Nystatin, U.S.P. (Mycostatin), is an antifungal antibiotic extracted from *Streptomyces nouresi.* It is insoluble in water and has a pale yellow color. Nystatin is administered orally in graduated units. U.S.P. standards require that 1 mg of the drug contain not less than 2000 units. Nystatin is poorly absorbed; its antifungal effect is excreted within the GI tract. It may also be applied topically. Its usefulness is limited to the treatment of candidal infections of the skin, mucous membranes, and GI tract. Nystatin is too toxic for parenteral use.

Nystatin has been used in the treatment and prevention of intestinal moniliasis. It has been dispersed in the drinking water of turkeys with sodium lauryl sulfate and, when used at concentrations of 62.5–250 ppm, was found beneficial in the treatment of crop mycosis (Wind and Yacowitz 1960). Nystatin has also been administered in combination with tetracycline for its prophylactic antifungal activity when tetracycline was used as an oral antibacterial agent.

Prolonged systemic antibiotic therapy was reported to facilitate the development of systemic candidiasis in calves (Mills and Levine 1967). Animals receiving antibacterial therapy for long periods must be closely monitored and examined for the possibility of fungal superinfections.

Nystatin inhibits or kills many species of fungi and yeasts. Its greatest effect is on yeastlike fungi in the growing stage. A concentration of 1 unit/ml is effective against *Candida albicans.* Nystatin is inactive against bacteria.

Nystatin may have some anticoccidial effect (Panfilova and Malakhova 1968). The daily oral administration of 20,000–30,000 units/chicken prevented mortality in 16-day-old chickens when infected with *Eimeria tenella* and *Eimeria maxima.*

Nystatin has been tested experimentally for preventive and therapeutic purposes against *Aspergillus fumigatus* with variable results. Nystatin aerosols were therapeutically active but oral administration was found to be inactive (Klimeš et al. 1964). Absorption from the GI tract is very limited.

Nystatin is available as an ointment for topical application and as a suspension and tablet. In addition to its action against *Candida albicans,* it has also demonstrated action against *Microsporum* spp.

The oral dose of nystatin for dogs is 10,000 units/lb of body weight daily.

AMPHOTERICIN B

Amphotericin B (Fungizone), a yellowish powder of low solubility, is an antibiotic isolated from strains of *Streptomyces nodosus.* Sodium desoxycholate has been added to make colloidal dispersions for intravenous injection. Blood concentrations of amphotericin B will persist for 18–24 hours after injection. Poor absorption obviates the use of oral administration.

Amphotericin B is useful for the treatment of systemic mycoses, e.g., histoplasmosis, blastomycosis, coccidiodomycosis. It has no activity against bacteria.

Amphotericin B has been used to treat canine histoplasmosis. The dose for dogs is approximately 1.8 mg/kg administered intravenously daily for 7 days. Treatment is discontinued for 7 days, then reinstituted for an additional 7 days. Blood urea nitrogen (BUN) determinations should be made during treatment. If BUN increases twofold over the pretreatment value, treatment should be stopped for approximately 7 days or until the BUN returns to normal.

In a study conducted in Kentucky, where histoplasmosis is endemic for both human beings and dogs, amphotericin B was administered intravenously at a total dose of 4 mg/kg of body weight divided into 10 doses and administered every 48 hours (Marx et al. 1970). *Histoplasma capsulatum* was isolated from 1 of 47 treated dogs and from 12 of 50 untreated dogs.

Amphotericin B has been used successfully to treat both canine histoplasmosis and blastomycosis by another program (Ausherman 1969). On day 1 the dog received intravenously 0.1 mg of amphotericin B/lb of body weight, on day 2, 0.15 mg/lb, and on day 3, 0.2 mg/lb. This last dose (0.2 mg/lb) was administered on alternate days until 10 doses had been administered. A BUN determination was made before each treatment and if the value was 1.5 times the normal, treatment was discontinued until normal values reappeared.

Amphotericin B has been injected subconjunctivally, 125 μg, for treatment of eyes infected with blastomycetes or *Histoplasma*.

The potential toxicity of amphotericin B restricts its widespread usage. The most serious undesirable effect is its ability to produce renal toxicity. Evidence of renal damage is noted by increased BUN and nonprotein nitrogen; decreased glomerular filtration, renal plasma flow, and creatinine clearance; and/or presence of granular and hyaline casts. Amphotericin B has an intravenous LD50 of 5 mg/kg for mice. Other undesirable effects are fever, nausea, emesis, anorexia, cellular and granular urine casts, hematuria, and proteinuria.

Amphotericin B has also been used for topical administration to treat candidiasis. It is normally applied 2–4 times daily for weeks but infections of the nails or claws (onchomycotic infections) often require treatment for several months.

A colloidal preparation of amphotericin B was reported to be approximately 8 times more effective for preventing crop mycosis caused by *C. albicans* in chickens than a colloidal preparation of nystatin (Kahn and Slocum 1966).

Amphotericin B has been administered intravenously to treat coccidioidomycosis. The dosage is administered on an incremental and alternate basis with doses comparable to those used for histoplasmosis.

ANTIVIRAL DRUGS

Before discussing antiviral drugs it is necessary to consider the properties of viruses from a biophysical, biological, and biochemical basis. Fundamental concepts must be explored in order to (1) assess the current therapeutic and prophylactic utility of antiviral drugs, (2) understand the pharmacodynamics of antiviral drugs, and (3) appreciate the problems and opportunities for developing new drugs.

The following presentation is based on the excellent review by Tilles (1974). For those who wish to pursue the subject in greater detail, the complete citation is found in the references.

The severest constraint limiting the utility of antiviral drugs is the concomitant toxicity to the mammalian host cells and the virus. A virus is an obligate intracellular invader that must parasitize the metabolic pathways of the host cells, whereas bacteria are more sensitive to attack since they have separate enzyme systems and subcellular particles different from their mammalian hosts. Drugs that are toxic for viruses are, in general, also toxic for mammalian cells. The therapeutic index for most commonly used antibacterial drugs is severalfold greater than the antiviral drugs.

Another antiviral drug constraint concerns the number of infectious particles per cell, or multiplicity. Multiplicity, or as in bacteriology—the inoculum effect, can determine if an antiviral agent will have a therapeutic or prophylactic effect. Most antiviral agents have less efficacy against a large number of infectious particles and greater efficacy against fewer infectious particles. Thus the antiviral agents have limited efficacy when the disease is symptomatic. However, such antiviral drugs may enjoy utility as chemoprophylactic agents.

The development of drug-resistant viruses must be considered since our current status of drug-resistant bacteria in veterinary medicine is characterized by therapeutic refractiveness and potential public health problems. Although it has been demonstrated that antiviral drug resistance can occur (Jawetz et al. 1970), drug resistance has not become a problem because of the limited utility of candidate antiviral drugs.

Structure, Classification, and Replicative Cycles of Viruses

There are two general types of viruses: DNA and RNA viruses. Animal DNA viruses have a double strand of DNA whereas animal RNA viruses usually have single-stranded RNA. Reoviruses and Colorado tick fever virus are exceptions. In addition, animal viruses may or may not have a lipid membrane or envelope. Thus it is convenient to classify viruses according to their nucleic acid and the presence of lipid membrane.

The replicative cycle for an RNA virus proceeds sequentially as follows:

(1) Attachment: the virus particle attaches to the host cell membrane.

(2) Viropexis: the virus penetrates the cell membrane.

(3) Uncoating: the protein coat of the virus opens and the viral nucleic acid is released in the host cell cytoplasm.

(4) Translation: polyribosomes form after viral RNA attaches to ribosomes and begin to translate the nucleic acid sequence into proteins.

(5) Complementary strand formation: the RNA-dependent RNA polymerase combines with a strand of input viral RNA to synthesize a complementary strand to the input RNA.

(6) Replicative form: the double-stranded form of the complementary strand serves as a template for viral RNA production.

(7) Transcription: a new single-stranded RNA is produced by two RNA polymerases. The new single-stranded RNA can serve as a message for protein synthesis, as a template for the production of more RNA, or become incorporated into mature virus.

(8) Assembly: the new RNA and structural protein combine or are assembled into a mature virus which is released from the cell.

The antiviral drugs act at the various steps in the formation of RNA viruses, e.g., amantadine acts at the penetration step as do neutralizing antibodies, interferon acts at the translation step and is thought to block replication of new RNA, guanidine will inhibit the initiation of RNA strands during transcription.

The replicative cycle of DNA viruses differs from that of RNA viruses after completion of the first three steps. The attachment, penetration, and uncoating steps are comparable for both the RNA and DNA viruses. There are differences among DNA viruses with regard to replicative cycles. Vaccinia virus is used in the following example.

Steps 1, 2, and 3 are analogous to the previous example for RNA viruses.

(4) Early transcription: a viral RNA message is transcribed from double-stranded DNA and forms an early polyribosome structure.

(5) Early translation: enzymes necessary to produce DNA are formed, e.g., "DNA polymerase," thymidine kinase, DNase.

(6) DNA replication: the new DNA (daughter DNA) is formed and is capable of being transcribed.

(7) Late transcription: daughter RNA is transcribed to late messenger RNA.

(8) Late translation: translation occurs on polyribosomes associated with late message. Structural proteins are formed for mature virus particles and "switch-off" protein.

(9) Assembly: the new DNA and structural protein are assembled on a newly formed membrane and ultimately the mature virus particle is released from the cell.

Interferon and isoprinosine can act on both RNA and DNA viruses. Interferon also inhibits the transcription of viruses that bring preformed polymerase into mammalian cells. Cytosine arabinoside, ioxuridine, and adenine arabinoside inhibit DNA production and act on the DNA replication step. The thiosemicarbazones act on the late translation step and rifampin appears to act immediately prior to assembly.

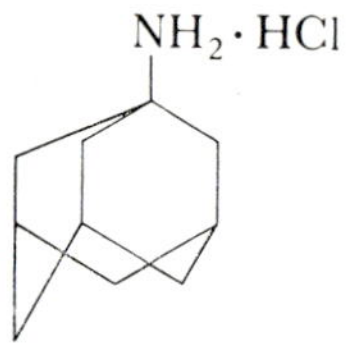

Amantadine

FIG. 50.7.

Candidate antiviral drugs are evaluated in three phases: (1) preclinical—the drug is evaluated in cell culture and animal models, (2) determination of safety and estimated dosage, and (3) objective—well-controlled trials to establish clinical efficacy.

DRUGS AND BIOLOGIC AGENTS

AMANTADINE

Amantadine, 1-adamantanamine hydrochloride (Fig. 50.7), prevents the penetration of several RNA membrane viruses, e.g., myxoviruses, paramyxovirus, in cell culture (Hoffmann et al. 1965). There is considerable variation in sensitivity among strains.

Amantadine is absorbed slowly but quite efficiently and has a half-life of 15 hours (Bleidner et al. 1965). Almost all of the drug is recovered in the urine following oral administration. The drug appears to have its greatest potential as a chemoprophylactic agent against sensitive strains of influenza virus. It is not able to overcome the viral multiplicity effect; however, its ability to reduce fever has been demonstrated.

IDOXURIDINE

Idoxuridine, 5-iodo-2′-deoxyuridine (IDU) (Fig. 50.8), is the most extensively tested halogenated pyrimidine nucleoside. It has the ability to incorporate bogus DNA and also inhibits the synthesis of DNA. In cell culture it has been effective against herpesvirus and poxvirus. Although IDU has been effective against corneal infections with herpesvirus or vaccinia in animals, its efficacy against systemic viral infection is not clearly established (Tomlinson and MacCallum 1970). The topical

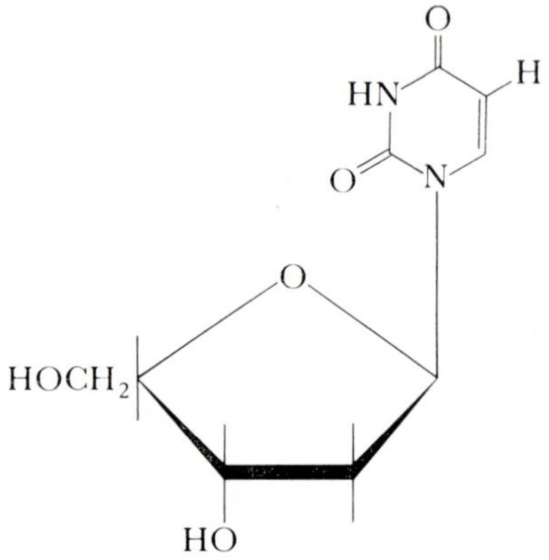

Idoxuridine

FIG. 50.8.

dose for herpetic keratitis is 12 times the maximal concentration achieved in the serum, which offers an explanation for the difference in topical and systemic efficacy.

IDU toxicity is noted most in those cells having a rapid turnover, e.g., mucosal, epidermal, cellular components of the blood (Calabresi 1961).

CYTOSINE ARABINOSIDE

Cytosine arabinoside, 1-β-D-arabinofuranosylcytosine (ara C) (Fig. 50.9), is an analog for cytosine deoxyribose. In cell culture ara C has activity against herpesvirus, poxvirus, vaccinia, and rabies (Underwood 1962). It has topical activity against herpesvirus hominis and vaccinia keratitis but systemic antiviral activity has not been established.

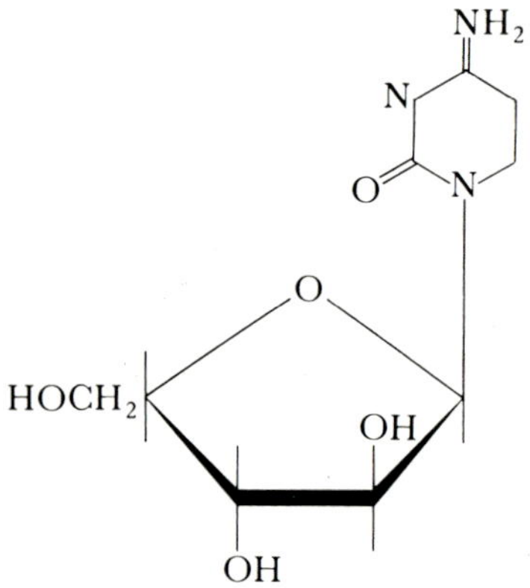

Cytosine Arabinose

FIG. 50.9.

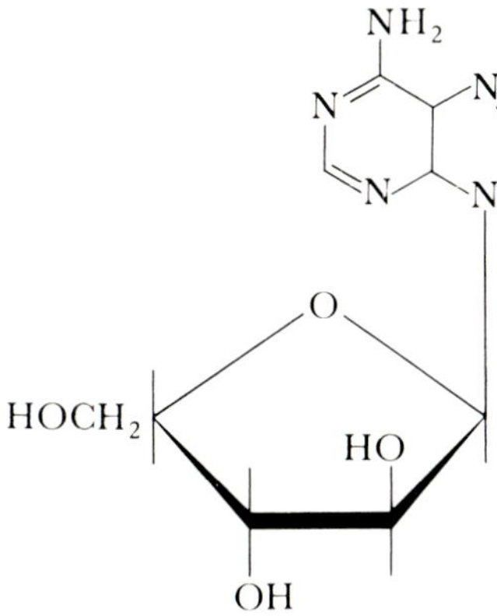

Adenine Arabinoside

FIG. 50.10.

ADENINE ARABINOSIDE

Adenine arabinoside, 1-β-D-arabinofuranosyladenine (ara A) (Fig. 50.10), differs from ara C by having adenine instead of cytosine. In experimental animals ara A has been found effective topically for herpesvirus hominis keratitis and systemically for encephalitis due to vaccinia and herpesvirus homivirus type 1 or 2 (Schabel 1968).

Ara A is deaminated to 1-β-D-arabinofuranosylhypoxanthine (ara Hx), which has comparable *in vivo* antiviral activity. Ara A may be more efficacious than ara C since ara A's deamination product, ara Hx, is also antiviral. Ara C is also deaminated; however, its deamination product is inactive.

METHISAZONE

Methisazone, N-methylisatin-3-thiosemicarbazone (Fig. 50.11), is considered the best antiviral candidate of the N-substituted analogs of isatin. The action of the thiosemicarbazones occurs late in the viral replicative cycle. Methisazone has demonstrated antiviral activity in cell culture against poxviruses and adenoviruses. In addition, it is active against mouse encephalitis caused by vaccinia and variola major viruses (Bauer and Sadler 1960).

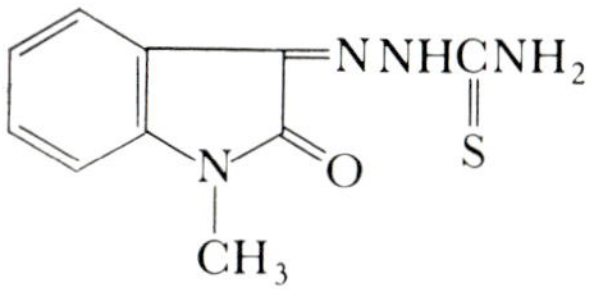

Methisazone

FIG. 50.11.

Methisazone must be given orally because of its low solubility. Little is known about its pharmacokinetics or efficacy as a chemotherapeutic agent.

INTERFERON

Interferon is a proteinaceous substance released from mammalian cells with the ability to cause other cells to resist a viral infection. Interferon is considered an important part of the natural defense mechanism. Considerable attention has been directed to the possibility of developing drugs capable of inducing interferon or using exogenous interferon to prevent or treat viral diseases. The antiviral activity of interferon is related to the production of a second protein. It has been demonstrated that the antiviral activity either inhibits the activity of RNA-dependent polymerases brought into the cell by a virus or attenuates ribosomes so they cannot read viral RNA. Interferon is phylogenetically related, species specific in its ability to protect cells from RNA and DNA viruses (Ho 1962). In animal experiments, topical or systemic viral infections are antagonized by interferon obtained from the same or related species (Finter 1966).

POLYRIBOINOSINIC ACID-POLYRIBOCYTIDYLIC ACID

Polyriboinosinic acid-polyribocytidylic acid (poly I • poly C) is the most studied inducer of interferon. It is the equal molar complex of synthetic homopolymers of nucleotides, inosinic acid, and cytidylic acid. Poly I · poly C will protect culture cells from a viral challenge. In larger amounts it will both protect cells and cause the release of interferon (Field et al. 1967). In animal studies, poly I · poly C is related to a rapid increase in interferon concentrations and a protective effect against local or systemic viral infections when administered topically or systemically, respectively. Dogs treated with poly I · poly C (0.2 mg/kg of body weight) survived an average of 2.3

days longer than controls when challenged with infectious canine hepatitis virus.

It has been noted that a hyporeactive state develops after parenteral administration and lasts several days during which there is no protection against the virus.

GAMMA GLOBULIN

Many preparations of *gamma globulin* are concentrated solutions of antibodies extracted from normal blood. Gamma globulin has been reported to be effective for preventing various viral infections in human beings, e.g., infectious hepatitis, measles, poliomyelitis, chicken pox. Gamma globulin has also been used as an adjunctive treatment for various bacterial infections that do not respond well to antibacterial therapy. Well-controlled studies would help determine the utility of gamma globulin in veterinary medicine.

In summary, considerable work must be done before the clinical efficacy of the antiviral drugs is optimally established. Antiviral drugs are clearly established for topical use in the treatment of herpetic keratitis (human beings); however, a suitable and reliable systemic antiviral drug for a specific disease entity has yet to be developed and established.

REFERENCES

Allen, P. M., and Gottlieb, D. 1970. Mechanism of action of the fungicide thiabendazole, 2-(4′-thiazolyl)benzimidazole. Appl Microbiol 20:919.

Ausherman, R. J. 1969. Canine histoplasmosis and blastomycosis therapy. Proc 36th Am Anim Hosp Assoc, p. 273.

Bauer, D. J., and Sadler, P. W. 1960. The structure activity relationships of the antiviral chemotherapeutic activity of isatin β-thiosemicarbazone. Br J Pharmacol Chemother 15:101.

Biggio, P.; Gessa, G. L.; and Pinetti, P. 1964. Protective action of griseofulvin against ischaemic necrosis of the tail caused by eryotamine in rats. Rass Med Sarda 16:55.

Bleidner, W. E.; Harmon, J. B.; Hewes, W. E.; Lynes, T. E.; and Hermann, E. C. 1965. Absorption, distribution and excretion of amantadine hydrochloride. J Pharmacol Exp Ther 150:484.

Calabresi, P. 1961. Regional protection with thymidine (TDR) during therapy with 5-iodo-2′-deoxyuridine (IUDR). Cancer Res 21:550.

Davis, H. H., and Worthington, W. E. 1964. Equine sporotrichosis. J Am Vet Med Assoc 145:692.

Field, A. K.; Tytell, A. A.; Lampson, G. P.; and Hilleman, M. R. 1967. Inducers of interferon and host resistance. II. Multistranded synthetic polynucleotide complexes. Proc Nat Acad Sci 58:1004.

Finter, N. B. 1966. Interferons, p. 232. New York: John Wiley & Sons.

Hagen, K. W. 1969. Ringworm in domestic rabbits: Oral treatment with griseofulvin. Anim Care 19:635.

Harris, P. A., and Riegelman, S. 1969. Metabolism of griseofulvin in dogs. J Pharm Sci 58(1):93.

Hiddleston, W. A. 1970. The use of griseofulvin mycellum in equine animals. Vet Res 87:119.

Ho, M. 1962. Medical progress interferons. N Engl J Med 266:1258.

Hoffmann, C. E.; Neumayer, E. M.; Haff, R. F.; and Goldsby, R. A. 1965. Mode of action of the antiviral activity of amantadine in tissue culture. J Bacteriol 90:623.

Horváth, Z., and Markói, B. 1970. Oral treatment of calf ringworm with griseofulvin. Magy Allatorv Lapja 25:345.

Jawetz, E.; Coleman, V. R.; Dawson, C. R.; and Thygeson, P. 1970. The dynamics of IUDR action in herpetic keratitis and the emergence of IUDR resistance *in vitro*. Ann NY Acad Sci 173(1):282.

Kahn, S. G., and Slocum, A. 1966. Water miscible amphotericin for the treatment of crop mycosis in chicks. Poult Sci 45:761.

Kliměs, B.; Novák, Z.; and Severa, K. 1964. Therapy of aspergillosis of chickens with fungicidin. Zentralbl Veterinaermed [B] 11:151.

Levine, H. B.; Cobb, J. M.; and Friedman, R. H. 1971. Griseofulvin in dimethyl sulfoxide: Penetration into guinea pig skin and clinical findings in feline ringworm. Sabouraudia 9:43.

Litwack, M. 1966. Candicidin therapy for mycotic dermatoses in dogs and cats. J Am Vet Med Assoc 148:23.

Marx, M. B.; Eastin, C. E.; Turner, C.; Smith, C. D.; Roeckel, I.; and Furcolow, M. L. 1970. The influence of amphotericin B upon histoplasma infection in dogs. Arch Environ Health 21:649.

Mills, Y. C. M., and Levine, H. B. 1967. Experimentally included immunity in the mycosis. Bacteriol Rev 31:35.

Misra, S. K. 1973. Comparative efficacy of Grisovin F.P., Ephytol and Multifugin against *Trichophyton verrucussum* Bodin, 1902 infection in cattle. Indian Vet J 50:290.

Muller, G. H. 1968. Griseofulvin in massive doses. J Am Vet Med Assoc 154:52.

Nikiforov, L. I. 1967. I. Antibiotics (trichotezin and griseofulvin) in the treatment and prophylaxis of bovine ringworm. II. Efficacy of trichotezin and griseofulvin in ringworm of fur animals. Byul Vses Inst Eksp Vet 2:112.

Panfilova, V. A., and Malakhova, T. J. 1968. Use of crude nystatin against coccidiosis of chicks. Veterinariia 2:74.

Rheins, M. S.; Suie, T.; and Van Winkle, M. G. 1965. Further investigation of the effects of antibiotics. Am J Ophthalmol 59:222.

Robinson, H. J.; Silber, R. H.; and Graessle, O. E. 1969. Thiabendazole: Toxicological, pharmacological and antifungal properties. Tex Rep Biol Med 27(Suppl 2):537.

Sarkhisov, A. Kh.; Nikiforov, L. J.; and Slugin, V. S. 1968. Ringworm caused by *Trichophyton flaviforme* in Norwegian polar foxes (Alopex lagopus) and its control. Krolikowod Zverovod 6:28.

Schabel, F. M., Jr. 1968. The antiviral activity of 9-β-D-arabinofuranosyladenine (ara-A). Chemotherapy 13:321.

Tilles, J. G. 1974. Antiviral agents. Annu Rev Pharmacol 14:469.

Tomlinson, A. H., and MacCallum, F. O. 1970. The effect of iodo-deoxyuridine on herpes simplex virus encephalitis in animals and man. Ann NY Acad Sci 173(1):20.

Underwood, G. E. 1962. Activity of 1-β-D-arabinofuranosylcytosine hydrochloride against herpes simplex keratitis. Proc Soc Exp Biol Med 111:660.

Wildfeuer, A. 1973. The treatment of cutaneous candidiasis in rabbits. Sabouraudia 11(1):4.

Wind, S., and Yacowitz, H. 1960. Use of mycostatin in the drinking water for treatment of crop mycosis in turkeys. Poult Sci 39:904.

SECTION 14

Chemotherapy of Parasitic Diseases

CHAPTER 51

INTRODUCTION

EDWARD L. ROBERSON

This chapter presents the general importance of parasitic diseases in veterinary medicine and how chemotherapeutic agents relate to the metabolism of parasites and to the host immunity initiated by parasitic organisms.

Following this introduction, the next four chapters are concerned with drugs used against specific groups of animal parasites. Discussion is given to compounds that are effective against internal parasitic nematodes (Chapter 52); cestodes and trematodes or tapeworms and flukes (Chapter 53); and protozoa, mainly the coccidia (Chapter 54). The use of pesticides against external parasites, i.e., arthropods, is covered in Chapter 55. The nematodes, cestodes, and trematodes collectively are called helminths. Drugs that are effective against any one or all three groups of parasites are termed *anthelmintics,* an elision of *anti* and *helminth.*

IMPORTANCE OF PARASITIC INFECTIONS

The prevalence of both internal and external parasitism in animals throughout the world has long required every possible effort, including chemotherapy, to attempt to balance the struggle in favor of human beings. These efforts have not always been successful as evidenced in certain parts of Africa where, in spite of present effective drugs and know-how, trypanosomiasis is so devastating to the bovine host that the economic production of beef and dairy cattle remains beyond present accomplishments. A similar imbalance in favor of the parasite existed until a decade ago between an intestinal nematode, *Nematodirus,* and sheep. This struggle took place in the United Kingdom and before the scales tilted thousands of lambs were lost each year because of these intestinal parasites. Not until certain epidemiological facts about the rather unique development of *Nematodirus* were unraveled, did we begin to gain the upper hand in this fight. It had long been recognized that *Nematodirus* like most other gastrointestinal (GI) parasites of sheep is transmitted directly and does not require an intermediate host. However, little attention was given in earlier years to a simple biological fact of the life cycle of *Nematodirus,* namely, that development of the parasite to its infective stage requires exposure to cold temperatures. Large numbers of *Nematodirus* eggs collecting on pastures throughout the spring, summer, and fall await the cold temperatures of winter and the subsequent favorable conditions of spring to hatch—all at one time. Newborn lambs with their immunologically incompetent systems are no match for the thousands of infective larvae ingested with pasture forage.

Knowledge of the climatic and biologic factors resulting in the sudden occurrence of massive numbers of *Nematodirus* infective larvae now allows sheep raisers in those parts of the world plagued with this nematode to minimize the exposure of lambs to parasites. Lessened exposure is accomplished both by the use of uncontaminated pastures for newborn and weaner lambs, when practical, and by the judicious use of anthelmintics both for the dam a month before parturition and for the lamb upon weaning.

The struggle between *Nematodirus* and agricultural efforts to raise a lamb crop profitably represents but one of numerous fights against the many internal and external parasites that plague food-producing and pet animals. It also illustrates the necessity of a complete knowledge of the biological intricacies of parasites if they are to be controlled. Equally important in the development of control programs is a knowledge of the immunological competence of animals for certain parasites and the relationship that antiparasitic drugs have to parasite immunity and to the total control program.

IMMUNITY TO PARASITES

Unlike bacterial organisms, metazoan and to some extent protozoan parasites do not elicit dramatic immune responses. There is in most cases no strong, fast-developing acquired immunity. In fact, for adult tapeworms, certain nematodes (e.g., the filarids), and flukes (e.g., *Fasciolia hepatica*), there is little evidence to suggest any protective immunity at all. On the other hand, some nematodes (e.g., cattle lungworm, *Dictyocaulus)* stimulate a marked immunity that prevents susceptibility to future challenges by the parasite. *Nematodirus* also elicits a similar response in sheep. These are primarily diseases of young or previously unexposed animals.

Development of resistance to parasites does not imply total resistance or the total absence of any parasites at all. A so-called parasite-resistant animal is one that maintains no more than a low worm burden even when faced with a fairly high level of exposure. In general, the numbers of new acquisitions of worms are balanced by the expulsion of an approximately equal number of resident worms so that with constant exposure a rather uniform parasite burden is maintained. Heavy exposure for these resistant animals does not dramatically alter the worm population.

The time necessary for development of a resistant state to nematodal parasites is generally quite long but varies according to the species of parasite. Resistance is longer in developing to most of the GI nematodes of ruminants than to either *Dictyocaulus* or *Nematodirus.* Young sheep exposed from birth to moderate levels of infection with *Trichostrongylus* develop a strong resistance to this intestinal parasite only after 6–9 months of exposure; once established, it is maintained for a long period in the absence of physiological or nutritional stresses. Resistance to the abomasal parasites, *Ostertagia* and *Haemonchus,* is both longer in developing (1 year–18 months) and more variable than that of *Trichostrongylus.* After resistance is established, rather constant exposure to infective larvae is necessary for maintenance of the resistant state. In the absence of continued exposure to *Haemonchus,* for example, it has been found that the level of resistance is lost in as few as 4 months.

In general, lambs or weaners and calves less than 6 months of age do not have the immune competence of a 9- to 12-month-old animal. There is convincing evidence that exposure of young animals to high numbers of infective larvae is not only liable to result in heavy worm burdens but also will likely impair the young animal's subsequent ability to develop a resistance to infection. In contrast, low levels of daily exposure to infective larvae over a period of months will allow for the gradual development of resistance in a well-nourished animal.

The eventual development of some level of natural resistance to parasites has prompted investigation into the possibility of artificial immunization. It is feasible to artificially immunize animals against only a few protozoan and metazoan parasites. Silverman (1970) reviews progress in this area. The problem in part stems from the incompetence of animals in very early life when protection is usually most needed. For example, sheep can be successfully vaccinated against *Haemonchus contortus* but lambs fail to become immunized (Urquhart et al. 1966). Vaccine production is also complicated by antigenic differences in various larval, immature, and adult stages of parasitic nematodes, all of which may occur in the host simultaneously. Also, many protozoa easily undergo antigenic variations within a single host, which serves to protect the organism against a specific immune response by the host. Despite the failures, some success with vaccines is gradually being made (Jarrett et al. 1960; Miller 1968), but until methods can be found that will confer an artificial protective immunity to a wide variety of parasites, drugs will play a highly important role in the control and treatment of parasitic infections.

ROLE OF ANTIPARASITIC DRUGS

The primary role of antiparasitic drugs is to reduce worm burdens to a tolerable level. Animals on pasture or in confined areas such as kennels are in environments that promote the direct transmission of parasites. The survival of directly transmitted parasites in the external environment is highly dependent on climatic conditions. The moderate temperatures and fairly consistent rainfall, occuring frequently in fall and spring in southeastern United States, are highly conducive to survival of strongyle parasites. These are the seasons when grazing animals acquire heavy worm burdens and are, consequently, the times when antiparasitic drugs are most needed. The frequency of administering anthelmintics during these seasons depends on the length of time the animals are exposed to high levels of infective larvae. A warm rainy fall insures high-level exposure for several months and treatment on a monthly basis is probably warranted. Little is to be gained from a single treatment unless the infection rate is low; otherwise reinfection can quickly restore worm burdens to pretreatment levels.

It is impossible to recommend general anthelmintic programs that are universally applicable. Environmental and epidemiological variations in different areas of this and other countries require that control programs, including the use of antiparasitic drugs, be tailored to the area as exactingly as possible.

Repeated application of antiparasitic drugs on a daily or monthly basis to reduce the parasite burden has some merit but must be weighed against the disadvantages of this approach. The addition of anticoccidial drugs to broiler feed for continuous control against outbreaks of coccidiosis is a common practice and is economically feasible in the broiler industry. Nevertheless, continuous use year after year has resulted in the mutagenic selection of strains of coccidia that are resistant to many of the earlier and even presently used anticoccidial drugs. The more recent use of different anticoccidials on a rotational basis between different broiler grow-outs, however, is helping to minimize the inducement of resistance.

Continuous feeding of antiparasitic drugs is not as widely practiced with livestock or pet animals as it is in the poultry industry, partially because of economics but also because of the fear of developing resistant strains of parasites. Inducement of drug resistance by medicating livestock and pets continuously should not be a problem in light of the increasing variety of effective drugs available today for rotational use in these animals.

Suggestions have been made that frequent weekly anthelmintic treatments may interfere with the development or maintenance of protection against parasites (Soulsby 1962; Gibson et al. 1970) by constantly eliminating the entire parasite population and thus the antigenic stimulus for resistance. It appears that intensive weekly treatment of grazing sheep with thiabendazole, may suppress infections to such an extent that development of resistance is delayed. Gordon (1973), however, doubts that seasonal or monthly use of anthelmintics interferes unduly with resistance. This is probably due to the fact that between monthly treatments reestablishment of infection, which serves as an antigenic stimulus, should be possible. Additionally, there is no evidence that continuous low-level feeding of small daily amounts of the anthelmintic, phenothiazine, interferes drastically with resistance in sheep and cattle. However, all worms are not eliminated by this method and the residual burden may serve antigenically to maintain an acquired level of resistance.

EFFECT OF DRUGS ON PARASITE METABOLISM

The mode of action of many of the early antiparasitic drugs is not known because tools for investigating the mechanisms were not available. It was considered enough simply to use the drug if it were effective against the parasite and not overly toxic to the host. A better understanding of mechanisms of antiparasitic drug action has come only with investigations into the biochemistry and physiological functions of parasites themselves. This area is still virtually untapped and much is yet to be learned. The present knowledge is at least beginning to broaden our understanding of how drugs expel parasites and, more importantly, it allows researchers to better formulate drugs that theoretically should be effective against specific biochemical pathways of parasites.

The present understanding of parasite physiology is extremely fragmentary and it is not within the scope of this book to review these facts. Reviews by Florkin and Scheer (1968, 1969), Saz (1970), Smith (1965, 1968), Smyth (1966, 1969), and von Brand (1966) should be consulted. The general concept will be presented that metazoan parasites possess morphological features—muscle systems, nervous systems, some semblance of circulatory and excretory systems, and sometimes a digestive system—not greatly unlike any other animal. Also, it is important to realize that physiological coordination of these systems is just as important to the well-being of the parasite as it is to higher animals. This involves enzymatic functions in the attainment of an energy source (usually anaerobic in parasites), the digestion of ingested or absorbed foods, the transmission of nerve impulses, and the general maintenance of the organism. Many of these biochemical functions are the same as those of higher animals; some are different; some differ also among various groups or even species of parasites. Acetylcholine, for example, a neurotransmitter in higher animals, serves the same purpose in most metazoan parasites. The enzyme acetylcholinesterase serves to destroy the neurotransmitter physiologically and thereby prevents overstimulation of the innervated smooth muscles and other effector sites. This enzyme occurs in many parasites as well as in animal hosts and is the target of organophosphorus drugs which are widely used as anthelmintics. The action of these drugs apparently is related to their binding acetylcholinesterase and preventing the enzyme's normal function of removing acetylcholine. Without regular control of this neurotransmitter, the effector site becomes malfunctioning due to constant stimulation by excess acetylcholine. Worms in the digestive tract, for example, no longer able to maintain their position in the ingesta or attachment to the mucosa, are swept along with the ingesta and pass in the feces.

The binding of acetylcholinesterase with organophosphorus drugs is reversible in some parasites due presumably to biochemical differences in the enzyme. If the bonding is easily uncoupled in a short time, the parasite probably will not be expelled. For this parasite the drug is essentially ineffective. It is in those parasites in which the bonding of enzyme and drug is more durable that efficacy of the drug is highest.

The question naturally arises as to what effect is put on the host by drugs that are active against biochemical reactions common to both the host and parasite. In the example of organophosphorus drugs used above, the host is very liable to experience effects of the drug since the animal's acetylcholinesterase may also be bound by the drug. It is the reversibility of enzyme bonding that determines the degree of toxicity of organophosphorus drugs to the host. In general, if the enzyme-drug complex in the host is easily reversible, the drug probably will have a sufficiently high margin of safety for use in that host; if the complex is poorly reversible, the drug will likely be too toxic.

Drugs Affecting the Parasite Neuromuscular System

The mode of action of certain other drugs is dependent on their affecting the parasite's neuromuscular system. Piperazine, long used against ascarid infections, has a curarelike effect on the neuromuscular junction of ascarids that results in a flaccid paralysis and expulsion of the worm. Piperazine's minimal activity on the neuromuscular junction of the mammalian host accounts for its wide margin of safety in animals and human beings.

In general, helminths are most vulnerable to biochemical interferences either with mechanisms essential for their motor activity (exemplified by piperazine and organophosphorus drugs) or with reactions that provide the generation of metabolic energy.

Drugs Affecting Energy Metabolism

Biochemical reactions involved in energy metabolism of parasites are frequent sites of drug action. Glucose uptake by the canine whipworm, *Trichuris vulpis,* is inhibited by dithiazanine, one of a group of antinematodal drugs known as cyanine dyes. Dithiazanine is also effective as a microfilaricide in the treatment of heartworm-infected dogs. Its action against heartworm microfilariae is assumed to be related also to the inhibition of glucose uptake.

Evidently, in a number of anaerobic helminths, e.g., *Ascaris,* the metabolic formation of high-energy bonds (adenosine triphosphate [ATP]) for muscular contraction is associated with the reduction of fumarate to succinate. The reaction serves to reoxidize nicotinamide adenine dinucleotide phosphate (NADPH) formed during glycolysis and generate ATP. The enzyme, fumarate reductase, necessary for the reduction of fumarate to succinate, appears to be the site of action of several antiparasitic drugs, including levamisole (*l*-tetramisole), which is effective against a wide variety of nematodes including *Ascaris* but not against cestodes, and bithionol and hexachlorophene, which are effective against the liver fluke, *Fasciola hepatica.* Basically, these drugs inhibit the fumarate reductase enzyme activity, thus blocking the generation of energy bonds (ATP) and resulting in muscular paralysis and eventual death of the parasite.

Several other anthelmintics of the phenolic type also interfere with the phosphorylation process (i.e., generation of ATP) in parasites but the biochemical means of action is not completely determined. The widely used anticestodal drugs niclosamide and dichlorophen are known to inhibit the incorporation of labeled phosphorus, ^{32}P, into ATP by the intact tapeworm, *Hymenolepis.* The inhibitory effect occurs in the mitochondria but the means of inhibition need further study. Although the nematode mitochondrial phosphorylation system is similar to that of cestodes, niclosamide and dichlorophen are not effective against nematodes, perhaps due to the inability of the drugs to penetrate the tissues of the intact nematode.

Drugs Affecting Parasite Reproduction

Little is known biochemically about protein synthesis and its relation to growth and egg production in parasites. Thus exact modes of action of drugs that affect this area of parasite metabolism remain unresolved. In general, however, drugs that act by inhibiting growth have greater activity against bacteria and those parasites such as protozoa that replicate at a rapid rate. In contrast, helminth parasites do not multiply within the host (except by egg production) and the growth of individual organisms is slow; thus helminth parasites are rather refractory to compounds that act by inhibiting growth.

Inhibition of egg production by helminths is, however, an important aspect of the activity of at least two of the widely used antinematodal drugs, thiabendazole and phenothiazine. In long-term, low-level feeding of these drugs to animals, parasites remaining in the digestive tract of the host are constantly inhibited in egg production. The practical significance of this action is the ultimate reduction in pasture contamination by helminth eggs—a control measure of important significance in cattle and sheep management.

Summary

The above discussion covers but a few drugs whose modes of action are known to be related to biochemical disfunctioning of some aspect of parasite metabolism. There are numerous other antiparasitic drugs for which the mode of action on the parasite and their biochemical effect on the host are unknown. In the following chapters, those aspects of drug action when known will be discussed briefly under the individual drugs.

PROPERTIES OF AN IDEAL ANTIPARASITIC DRUG

Several factors characterize an ideal antiparasitic drug. Specifically, those desirable properties are:

1. *Efficacy*—The drug must exhibit a high level of antiparasitic action when used under natural conditions. A drug has good efficacy if, for example, it eliminates 95% of a GI nematode burden from ruminants. Its efficacy is poor if it eliminates only 70% of these parasites.

In considering antinematodal drugs, it is important to know the percentage efficacy of the drug for immature and larval stages as well as for adult worms. The use of a drug effective only for the adult stage may need to be repeated one or more times in order to eliminate those adult worms that existed as unaffected larval stages at the time of initial treatment. An efficacy of 100% for all stages of the parasite is not necessarily the most desirable effect since this totally eliminates the source of antigenic stimulation by the organism and may weaken the animal's acquired resistance to the parasite.

2. *Wide therapeutic index*—The drug should be toxic to the parasite but have a good margin of safety for the host, i.e., a wide therapeutic index. This is a rather paradoxical situation since, as discussed earlier, the parasite and host share some of the same metabolic reactions against which many drugs are effective. In such cases, side effects are likely to occur in the host administered slightly above therapeutic doses. The organophosphorus anthelmintics and insecticides are generally poorly tolerated by the host because of the effect on the host's acetylcholinesterase as well as on that of the parasite. Drugs are generally much safer for the host when their mode of action involves biochemical pathways of the parasite not shared mutually with the host. Such appears to be the reason for the extreme safety of the thiabendazole-type anthelmintics.

3. *Ease of administration*—The route of administration of antiparasitic or other types of drugs is of practical importance. It may be more economical to use a drug that can be administered in the feed if facilities and personnel are not readily available for individual handling of the animals. Medication of the feed is the practical means of administering anticoccidial drugs to chickens which are raised by the thousands in a single building. Self-medication, although frequently used, is not as suitable for herds of larger livestock (swine, cattle, or sheep) being given a single 1-day treatment. This is because of variations in consumption rates. The smaller animals of a group are often bullied from the feeding trough and consequently receive less than a therapeutic dose of the drug while the more aggressive animals may receive a toxic dose. Oral administration of an individual dose assures greater dosage accuracy.

Subcutaneous injection is possible with only a few anthelmintic and antiprotozoan drugs. This route requires less time than administering compounds orally to large groups of animals.

4. *Residue*—The drug should not exceed certain Food and Drug Administration–approved limits of drug residue. Most antiparasitic drugs require specific withdrawal periods prior to slaughter; in the case of dairy animals, milk taken for a specified time after treatment should not be used for human consumption.

REFERENCES

Armour, J., and Urquhart, G. M. 1974. Clinical problems of preventive medicine: The control of helminthiasis in ruminants. Br Vet J 130:99.

Barber, H. J., and Berg, S. S. 1962. Structure and activity of antiprotozoan drugs. In L. G. Goodwin and R. H. Nimmo-Smith, eds. Drugs, Parasites and Hosts, p. 165. Boston: Little, Brown.

Florkin, M., and Sheer, B. T., eds. 1968. Porifera, coelenterata, and platyhelminthes. In Chemical Zoology, vol. 2. New York: Academic Press.

———. 1969. Echinodermata, nematoda and acanthocephala. In Chemical Zoology, vol. 3. New York: Academic Press.

Gibson, T. E.; Parfitt, J. W.; and Everett, G. 1970. The effect of anthelmintic treatment on the development of resistance to *Trichostrongylus colubriformis* in sheep. Res Vet Sci 11:138.

Gordon, H. McL. 1973. Epidemiology and control of gastrointestinal nematodes of ruminants. In C. A. Brandly and C. E. Cornelius, eds. Advances in Veterinary Science and Comparative Medicine, vol. 17, p. 395. New York: Academic Press.

Jarrett, W. F. H.; Jennings, F. W.; McIntyre, W. I. M.; Mulligan, W.; and Urquhart, G. M. 1960. Immunological studies on *Dictyocaulus viviparus* infection. Immunity produced by the administration of irradiated larvae. Immunology 3:145.

Miller, T. A. 1968. Development of an X-irradiated vaccine for ancylostomiasis: Current progress. Wellcome laboratories for experimental parasitology, Glasgow, Scotland.

Sanderson, B. E. 1970. The effects of anthelmintics on nematode metabolism. Comp Gen Pharmacol 1:135.

———. 1973. Anthelmintics in the study of helminth metabolism. In A. E. R. Taylor and R. Muller, eds. Chemotherapeutic Agents in the Study of Parasites, p. 53. Oxford: Blackwell Scientific Publications.

Saz, H. J. 1970. Comparative energy metabolisms of some parasitic helminths. J Parasitol 56:634.

Silverman, P. H. 1970. Vaccination: Progress and problems. In G. J. Jackson, R. Herman, and I. Singer, eds. Immunity to Parasitic Animals, vol. 2, p. 1165. New York: Appleton-Century-Crofts.

Smith, J. C. 1965. Bibliography on the metabolism of endoparasites exclusive of arthropods, 1951–62. Exp Parasitol 16:236.

———. 1968. Bibliography on the biochemistry of endoparasites. Exp Parasitol 22:352.

Smyth, J. D. 1966. The Physiology of Trematodes. London: Oliver and Boyd.

———. 1969. The Physiology of Cestodes. London: Oliver and Boyd.

Soulsby, E. J. L. 1962. The relation of immunity in helminth infections to anthelmintic treatment. In L. E. Goodwin and R. H. Nimmo-Smith, eds. Drugs, Parasites and Hosts, p. 62. A symposium on relation between chemotherapeutic drugs, infecting organisms and hosts. London: F. & A. Churchill.

Soulsby, E. J. L., ed. 1972. Immunity to Animal Parasites. New York: Academic Press.

Urquhart, G. M.; Jarrett, W. F. H.; Jennings, F. W.; McIntyre, W. I. M.; Mulligan, W.; and Sharp, N. C. C. 1966. Immunity to *Haemonchus contortus* infection failure of X-irradiated larvae to immunize young lambs. Am J Vet Res 27:1641.

von Brand, T. 1966. Biochemistry of Parasites. New York: Academic Press.

CHAPTER 52

ANTINEMATODAL DRUGS

EDWARD L. ROBERSON

Drugs used against animal nematodes in the early 1900s possessed a very limited range of activity. In attempting to control nematodal burdens, cupric sulfate, various arsenic compounds, and alkaloids, e.g., nicotine and oil of chenopodium, were frequently used but had very limited activity in the control of gastrointestinal (GI) parasitism and all too frequently were toxic to animals.

In 1938, the discovery of the anthelmintic properties of phenothiazine by Harwood and workers at the U.S. Bureau of Animal Industry gave the first dramatic advancement to antinematodal therapy for ruminants and horses. Since that time great strides toward the development of an ideal anthelmintic have been made, resulting in the present use of the so-called broad-spectrum drugs—imidazoles, tetrahydropyrimidines, and certain organophosphorus compounds—which constitute the major part of this chapter.

SIMPLE HETEROCYCLIC COMPOUNDS

PHENOTHIAZINE

Phenothiazine INN,[1] N.F. (Coopazine, Dr. Rogers' Products), was one of the early drugs with a fairly wide range of activity against GI nematodes. It was synthesized as early as 1885 but was not found to possess anthelmintic activity until 1938. In the following years it became extensively used in sheep, cattle, goats, horses, and

1. INN represents the proposed "International Nonproprietary Name."

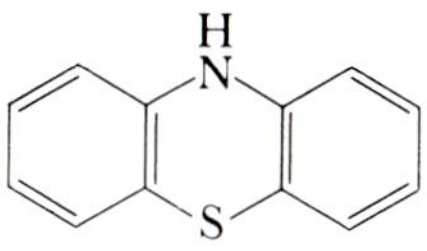

Phenothiazine

FIG. 52.1.

chickens. The advent of the truly broad-spectrum drugs in the 1960s has substantially reduced the use of phenothiazine but it is still one of the preferred anthelmintics for sheep and, because of the development of mixtures with other drugs for a broader spectrum, it remains widely used in horses. Its toxicity has limited its use in swine and altogether prevented its use in the dog, cat, and human being.

CHEMISTRY

Phenothiazine chemically is thiodiphenylamine INN, with the structural formula shown in Fig. 52.1.
The pure compound is a pale green-yellow powder. It is stable when dry but easily oxidizes when wet. It is very insoluble in water, soluble at approximately 1–800,000 parts.

ANTHELMINTIC SPECTRUM

Ruminants. Phenothiazine possesses particularly good anthelmintic efficacy (approaching 100%) against the large stomach worm *(Haemonchus)* and the nodular worm *(Oesophagostomum)* of sheep, goats, and cattle. Its efficacy for the smaller stomach worms *(Ostertagia* and *Trichostrongylus axei)* and the hookworm *(Bunostomum)* of ruminants is approximately 75%. Maximum dosages (20 g/100 lb body weight, not to exceed 80 g) are necessary to attain this level of *Bunostomum* removal. Phenothiazine has very limited activity, approximately 50%, against nematodes of the small intestine, i.e., *Cooperia, Nematodirus,* and *Trichostrongylus* spp.

The drug is not effective against parasitic larval stages or immature adult worms of any of the ruminant parasites except immature forms of *Haemonchus,* which are effectively removed. It has no activity against flukes or tapeworms. Some commercial products include a fasciolicide or lead arsenate as a taeniacide with phenothiazine.

Horse. Despite the greater sensitivity of horses than ruminants to phenothiazine poisoning, the drug is still widely used in the equine because of its excellent efficacy (nearly 100%) against the small strongyles *(Cyathostomum, Triodontophorus, Gyalocephalus,* and *Oesophagodontus).* Its effectiveness against large strongyles *(Strongylus* spp.) appears to vary directly with the size of the dose. Gibson (1950) reports that phenothiazine is nearly 100% effective against the large strongyles if, instead of the usual 3 g/100 lb of body weight, the dosage level is increased to 5 g/100 lb.

Phenothiazine is essentially ineffective against equine ascarids and has no activity against bots. For these reasons piperazine salts and carbon disulfide are added to phenothiazine in some commercial preparations (Parvex Plus) so as to eliminate ascarids and bots as well as strongyles in a single treatment. Improved efficacy against large strongyles can be accomplished without high doses of phenothiazine by combining the organophosphorus trichlorphon with phenothiazine (Equi-Verm). Another commercial product combines these two compounds plus piperazine in a single mixture (Dyrex T.F.).

Fowl. Phenothiazine has excellent efficacy for one parasite of chickens and turkeys, the cecal worm *(Heterakis gallinarum).* Its activity against ascarids in fowl is no greater than 50%. Piperazine and dibutyltin dilaureate are commercially added to phenothiazine (Wormal Tabs) to remove ascarids, tapeworms, and cecal worms.

FORMULATIONS AND ADMINISTRATION

The insolubility of phenothiazine in water dictates that it be formulated in a suspension. Colloidal aluminum silicate (bentonite) aids in keeping the drug in suspension; nevertheless, it should be shaken prior to dosing animals to insure even distribution.

Phenothiazine is also available as a powder for addition to feed or for incorporation in salt, mineral, or combined salt-mineral mixtures that are either added to the feed or made available to animals as salt licks. Powdered phenothiazine is generally used for prophylactic measures, i.e., continuous daily low-level medication, since its massive bulk limits the dosage level attainable via free choice feeding. In general, low-level medication is employed as an adjunct to a regular deworming program. Continuous low-level feeding of phenothiazine to sheep (approximately 0.5 g/animal/day) does not eliminate heavy worm burdens. Higher therapeutic doses of the drug should be used for this purpose. The principal advantage of prophylactic use of phenothiazine lies in its suppression of parasite repopulation of the pasture by parasite eggs passed in the feces. Egg production by female worms remaining in the host's digestive tract is depressed. Even a single therapeutic dose of phenothiazine will suppress the appearance of parasite eggs in the feces for approximately 3 weeks following therapy. When fed continuously, phenothiazine will progressively decontaminate the pastures by decreasing the number of viable parasite eggs shed in the feces and by killing parasite larvae as they hatch from the egg in feces on the pasture.

Oral drenching is the method by which phenothiazine is most often administered to ruminants that are exposed to moderate or heavy parasite burdens. The large bulk of drug required for anthelmintic activity can best be provided by drenching rather than by addition of the drug to the feed or its incorporation in salt-mineral mixes. Since spilling the suspension on the hair or wool results in a red discoloration, a drenching gun equipped with an esophageal nozzle is usually employed.

The frequency of drenching sheep with phenothiazine largely depends on the level of parasitism. The drug is not effective against larvae or most immature stages of GI parasites; thus worm burdens are quickly reestablished in animals that are grazing in heavily contaminated pastures. Monthly drenching, although laborious, is most desirable under these circumstances, especially if sheep cannot be moved to a less contaminated pasture. Sheep on moderately contaminated areas may require only once-a-season treatment if low-level phenothiazine feeding is also practiced. On farms with ample pasture and where the parasite burden of animals is low, pasture rotation and continuous low-level consumption of phenothiazine throughout the year may suppress and control GI parasites of sheep without therapeutic drenching.

In cattle, phenothiazine is used almost solely for drenching with a therapeutic dose. Prophylactic low-level dosing has had some application in dairy and feedlot cattle where addition of the drug to the feed is fairly practical but salt licks containing the drug have not proved beneficial. In the southern United States where parasitism is a constant problem, anthelmintic treatment of calves and yearlings is routinely done in the rainy fall season and again in the spring. Where the parasite population is heavy, the entire herd is treated in the fall, followed by a second treatment of the calves and yearlings in 21 days. In the northern states cattle are treated only when indicated.

In earlier years powdered phenothiazine was generally administered to horses in the feed (dry ground grain) on a continuous daily basis. There are reports of continuous dosing (up to 5 g/day) of individual animals for 5–10 years without untoward effects to the horse and without evidence of the development of parasite resistance. The advantages of this procedure are reducing egg production by female worms in the digestive tract, reducing hatchability of eggs passed in the medicated stools and, consequently, reducing pasture or paddock contamination with resulting lowered reinfection of the animal. Although this prophylactic procedure is still fairly widely practiced in the United Kingdom, it has given way to single dosing in the United States because of the formulation of phenothiazine in mixtures with other drugs requiring only single administration. For specific mixtures see the preceding section, Anthelmintic Spectrum. Mixtures containing phenothiazine may be administered to horses in feed or via stomach tube as a suspension.

Fowl are treated with a single dose of phenothiazine rather than continuous dosing. Pills or tablets provide the most accurate dose but administering them to individual birds is usually impractical. Therefore, addition of the drug to dry or wet mash feed for a 1-day treatment once a month is generally used to control cecal worm infections.

MODE OF ACTION

Approximately 50% of a dose of phenothiazine remains unabsorbed in the intestine and is responsible for the anthelmintic action. The drug is known to be ingested by parasites and also to be absorbed through the cuticle by at least some parasites. *Ascaridia galli,* in fact, has been shown to selectively absorb the drug, i.e., the parasite absorbs phenothiazine more rapidly and in greater quantities than the surrounding intestinal mucosa.

The exact means by which phenothiazine destroys worms is not known. It does not seem to be related to the quantity of drug absorbed by the worm. A resistant species of worm may absorb as much phenothiazine into its tissues as a susceptible species but show no signs of toxicity. These differences in susceptibility are likely related to differences in enzyme systems of the parasites.

PHARMACODYNAMICS

The manner of absorption of phenothiazine from the intestinal mucosa is debatable but it seems likely that the drug is converted to phenothiazine sulfoxide by cellular enzymes of the intestinal epithelium. In sheep, some phenothiazine is apparently absorbed directly without chemical change to the molecule. Once absorbed, phenothiazine sulfoxide is further oxidized in the liver principally to leucophenothiazone and leucothionol, two colorless substances which are excreted primarily in the urine. These excretory products, unfortunately, further oxidize in the atmosphere to brown-red dyes—phenothiazone and thionol. Not only the urine but also the milk is discolored for several days.

TOXICITY

The toxicity of phenothiazine varies not only among different host species but also among animals of a single species. Of the domestic animals, sheep, goats, and birds appear to be the most resistant to toxic effects of phenothiazine. Cattle are more susceptible, swine even more so, and horses are the most susceptible of the domestic animals in which the drug has been routinely used. Dogs and cats are easily poisoned by phenothiazine; therefore, it should never be used in these animals. The borderline susceptibility of hogs to phenothiazine and the limited efficacy of the compound to only nodular worms in this host has resulted in little use of the drug in swine.

Deaths among sheep due to phenothiazine toxicity are rare. Sheep in good condition tolerate single doses of 160 g or continuous dosing with 10 g daily for 49 days without side effects. Yet, a sheep in poor condition may die when administered a slightly greater than normal therapeutic dose.

Healthy cattle tolerate phenothiazine therapy well and withstand single large doses of 250 g of phenothiazine or 3 successive daily doses of 100 g without incidence. However, debilitated anemic cattle are considerably more susceptible to poisoning than healthy cattle or similarly debilitated sheep. An important toxic effect of the drug in debilitated animals is hemolysis of red blood cells, which compounds an existing anemia and may be fatal.

Cases of phenothiazine toxicity and deaths have been more numerous in horses than in other species of domestic animals. Most of these cases are among debilitated and anemic animals. Generally a toxic dose is above 50 g for an adult and above 30 g for a young horse; yet 28 g has been known to cause the death of a debilitated adult horse while 500 g has been tolerated by horses in good condition.

Toxic signs of phenothiazine poisoning in the horse include dullness, weakness, and anorexia and secondarily, oliguria, colic, constipation, fever, and rapid pulse. More exacting signs relating to hemolysis of red blood cells include icterus, anemia, and hemoglobinuria.

The treatment of phenothiazine toxicity in the horse is aimed primarily at replenishing the lost red blood cells by transfusing blood. An oil or saline cathartic should also be given to promote complete elimination of phenothiazine from the digestive tract.

Phenothiazine toxicity can be avoided in most instances by administering smaller doses of the drug to animals that are heavily parasitized and in poor condition. Not all worms will be eliminated by the smaller dose but with improved condition of the animal, a larger dose can be given to remove the remaining worms. Alternately, safer drugs such as the benzimidazoles may be used initially for animals in poor condition.

Phenothiazine is practically nontoxic in birds. The regular dose of 0.5 g has been administered daily to chickens for as long as 85 days without causing apparent ill effects (Nicholson and McCulloch 1942).

PHOTOSENSITIZATION

Photosensitization is a side effect that may accompany administration of phenothiazine when animals subsequently are exposed to bright sunlight. It is especially a problem in calves but sometimes occurs in goats and fowl and has been seen in Australian sheep. It apparently poses no problem in horses.

The physiological basis of photosensitization involves phenothiazine sulfoxide. When the dose of phenothiazine is high, not all of the oxidative substance, phenothiazine sulfoxide, is converted to phenothiazone by the liver. Calves evidently are less efficient at making this conversion than older cattle or sheep. Some of the nonconverted phenothiazine sulfoxide diffuses into the general circulation and ultimately into the aqueous humor of the eye. On exposure to ultraviolet rays, phenothiazine sulfoxide causes a photosensitization keratitis which is manifested by ulcerations of the cornea within 36 hours. Corneal ulceration with resulting blindness is especially enhanced in cattle administered the drug and subsequently exposed to bright sunlight reflected from snow-covered ground.

The nonpigmented areas of the skin may also show signs of photosensitization similar to sunburn—reddening, thickening of the ears and muzzle, with later development of scabs. Affected animals appear irritable, shaking the head and rubbing the ears.

Photosensitization following phenothiazine therapy can be prevented by keeping animals out of direct sunlight for 2–3 days. The condition is not seen in animals given continuous low-level prophylactic doses.

CONTRAINDICATIONS

As previously stated, phenothiazine poisoning most frequently occurs in cachectic animals. Use of the drug in animals that are weak, particularly anemic and emaciated animals, is strictly contraindicated. Animals known to be constipated should not be treated with phenothiazine since retention of the drug in the digestive tract and the resulting absorption of greater than normal quantities is liable to lead to drug poisoning.

The use of phenothiazine in pregnancy is contraindicated only during the last month of gestation. The drug causes no interference with conception or embryonic development, but Warwick et al. (1946) found a slight increase in the incidence of abortion in ewes when the drug was administered 3 weeks before the end of the gestation period.

OTHER DISADVANTAGES

Another disadvantage of phenothiazine administration is the pink coloration that metabolites of the drug give to the milk and urine. Although there is no harm in drinking the milk, its appearance does not allow its commercial use for human consumption. It can be used safely to feed other farm animals. Spoilage of the milk is actually retarded since the metabolites of phenothiazine are bacteriostatic. The pink discoloration of the milk lasts for 2–3 days following treatment.

The red coloring of the urine is a nuisance because the hair or wool of animals lying in the urine becomes permanently discolored. Spilling the phenothiazine suspension on the coat when dosing also results in permanent staining. These situations very likely result in an economic loss, especially to the sheep rancher. Dispersing animals immediately after treatment and use of sawdust or wood shavings on the animal's bedding help to prevent coat discoloration.

There is evidence of drug resistance by some strains of *Haemonchus* to phenothiazine when the drug is used over long periods of time. Drudge et al. (1957) found markedly reduced susceptibility by a strain of *H. contortus* in sheep that had had access to phenothiazine in salt continuously for 10 years. Similarly, other strains of phenothiazine-resistant *Haemonchus* are known to exist (Levine and Garrigus 1962). The present availability of a number of effective anthelmintics prevents the necessity of continued use of a single drug and should retard the development of drug-resistant strains of ruminant helminths.

DOSAGE

- Single dose treatment
  - Sheep and goat: weighing over 60 lb (27 kg) 25–30 g total; weighing 25–50 lb (11–23 kg), 12.5 g total
  - Cattle: 10 g/100 lb (45 kg) of body weight (maximum of 79 g, minimum of 10 g in small dairy calves)
  - Horse: 3 g/100 lb (45 kg) of body weight for small strongyles; 5 g/100 lb (45 kg) for large strongyles (split the dose and administer one-half on each of 2 days)
  - Chicken: 0.5 g/bird
    - Turkey: 1 g/bird
- Daily prophylactic treatment
  - Sheep and goat: 0.25–0.5 g/animal
  - Cattle: 0.5–5 g at a rate of 0.5 g/45 kg
  - Horse: adult 2–5 g; colt, 1 g

Piperazine and Its Derivatives

Piperazine was used in the early 1900s for treating human gout because of its excellence as a solvent for uric acid. Its anthelmintic activity was not recognized until the 1950s. Since then numerous derivatives, principally salts of piperazine, have been developed. All of the derivatives have similar efficacy: good for ascarid and nodular worm infections of all species of domestic animals, moderate for pinworm infections, and zero to variable for other veterinary helminths. Piperazine compounds have a wide margin of safety in all animals.

CHEMISTRY

Piperazine chemically is diethylenediamine. It is a simple ring structure (Fig. 52.2).

It is freely soluble in water and glycerol, less soluble in alcohol, and insoluble in ether. It is a strong base and consequently easily absorbs water and carbon dioxide; thus containers should be tightly closed and protected from light. In the presence of moisture, the hexahydrate of piperazine is formed, occurring as small colorless crystals which are very unstable and are soluble in water.

Stability of piperazine can be accomplished by use of its simple salts—piperazine adipate, citrate, phosphate, sulfate, tartrate, and hydrochloride—all of which are more stable than the piperazine base. All of these salts are white crystalline powders with a saline taste and are readily soluble in water except the insoluble phosphate and the colorless adipate which dissolves slowly to only a maximum of 5% in water.

A stable compound is also formed

```
      H2    H2
       \    /
        C—C
       /    \
  H—N        N—H
       \    /
        C—C
       /    \
      H2    H2
```

Piperazine (Diethylenediamine)

Fig. 52.2.

when piperazine is reacted with carbon disulfide to produce a polymer called the betaine of 1-piperazine carbodithiotic acid. This product is a gray, stable, tasteless wettable powder that is insoluble in water.

The antiparasitic activity of the various salts of piperazine depends almost solely on the piperazine base. The amount of base varies, of course, among different salts as reflected in the difference in the dosage level of each. The hexahydrate of piperazine contains 44% of the base. The dosages of the salts of piperazine are customarily expressed in terms of the hydrate equivalent, i.e., 100 mg of piperazine hydrate is approximately equivalent to 120 mg of piperazine adipate, to 125 mg of piperazine citrate, and to 104 mg of piperazine phosphate.

PHARMOCODYNAMICS

Piperazine and its simple salts are readily absorbed from the proximal region of the GI tract. Some of the piperazine base is metabolized in the tissues and the remainder (approximately 30%–40%) is excreted in the urine. Piperazine base is detectable in the urine as early as 30 minutes after the drug is administered; the excretion rate is maximal at 1–8 hours and urinary excretion is practically complete within 24 hours.

MODE OF ACTION

The anthelmintic activity of piperazine and its derivatives depends upon their anticholinergic action at the myoneural junction in worms, producing a neuromuscular block. Succinic acid production by the worm is also blocked. The end result is a narcotizing or paralytic effect. Worms lose their motility and thus their ability to maintain their position in the intestinal tract. They are passively swept along by intestinal peristalsis and voided live in the feces. If the drug is quickly voided by the host, e.g., when a purgative accompanies drug administration, the narcotized worm may regain its motility and reestablish its position in the gut. Purgation is consequently not generally advised when piperazine is being used.

Mature worms are more susceptible to the action of piperazine than are younger stages. Lumen-dwelling larvae and immature adults are sufficiently susceptible to be at least partially eliminated (Bikoryukov 1969). Larval stages in host tissues, especially larvae that are molting, are little affected by the drug; thus repeated treatments are generally indicated in 2 weeks for dogs and cats and 4 weeks for farm animals.

GENERAL TOXICITY

Experience over many years has confirmed the safety of piperazine. The oral LD50 of piperazine adipate in mice is 11.4 g/kg of body weight, which indicates a wide margin of safety. It is almost nontoxic under ordinary circumstances. Very young animals, e.g., 4-week-old calves, can be treated with the drug without ill effects.

Large oral doses occasionally produce emesis, diarrhea, and incoordination in cats and dogs. The latter neurologic sign may be related to the fact that the drug *in vitro* causes a 50% inhibition of oxidation by brain homogenate but no inhibition of oxidation by other tissues from laboratory animals (Osteux et al. 1971). There is little evidence of any direct ill effects of piperazine on the digestive tract (Cross et al. 1954). In fact, the drug is unique in being one of but a few compounds that can be safely administered to animals suffering from gastroenteritis.

Adult horses and foals tolerate 6–7 times the therapeutic dose of piperazine without any side effects. Four times the therapeutic dose of piperazine adipate in calves causes transitory diarrhea, tympany, and anorexia. Forced oral administration of 5 times the therapeutic dose of piperazine to swine results in semifluid feces and impaired appetite but has no lasting effects.

There are no known contraindications to the use of piperazine salts except in cases of long-standing renal or liver disease.

ANTHELMINTIC SPECTRUM

Dog and Cat. In domestic small animals several salts of piperazine as well as piperazine hexahydrate are used for the removal of ascarids. Virtually 100% efficacy occurs against both *Toxocara* and *Toxascaris* regardless of the piperazine compound. Acceptable efficacy also exists against the northern hookworm *(Uncinaria stenocephala),* but the efficacy of these compounds for the common *Ancylostoma caninum* is no greater than 75%. There is no activity against whipworms or tapeworms. Similar overall activity occurs in zoo canids and felines treated with piperazine salts.

Dogs and cats are usually dosed with tablets. Powder formulations for mixing with wet food also are commercially available. The latter apparently does not reduce the palatability of the food.

Horse. Piperazine salts in general give excellent efficacy against equine ascarids and some activity against strongyles and pinworms. The adipate salt of piperazine has been most widely used in horses but other piperazine compounds—citrate, phosphate, and carbodithiotic acid—are also effective. Nearly 100% of an ascarid burden is eliminated from foals, yearlings, or adult animals treated with any of the piperazine compounds. Repeated treatment of young animals at 10-week intervals is warranted in view of the 12-week patency period of *Parascaris equorum.*

Approximately 80% of mature pinworms *(Oxyuris equi)* are eliminated by piperazine adipate. There is little activity against the immature pinworms; thus retreatment in 3–4 weeks is necessary.

Among the equine strongyles, only one genus of small strongyles, *Trichonema,* is effectively removed by treatment with piperazine compounds. These drugs provide approximately 60% efficacy against *Strongylus vulgaris* and *Triodontophorus.* There is no activity against the other species of *Strongylus* or against stomach worms *(Habronema)* and tapeworms.

Piperazine is combined with other compounds to enhance the anthelmintic spectrum in horses. The addition of carbon disulfide (Parvex) provides activity against *Gastrophilus* bots in the equine stomach. The addition of phenothiazine to carbon disulfide and piperazine (Parvex Plus) enhances activity to a limited degree against equine strongyles. Trichlorfon, an organophosphorus compound, when combined with piperazine and phenothiazine (Dyrex T.F.), enhances elimination of both pinworms and ascarids. Trichlorfon additionally is effective against bots.

Piperazine compounds are usually administered to horses in bran mashes. If this method is unacceptable to the horse, the drug can be dissolved or suspended in a small quantity of water for administration by a stomach tube. Horses as young as 3 months of age can be given piperazine compounds without fear of toxic reactions.

Swine. Piperazine compounds have been used extensively in swine because of their excellent efficacy for the common ascarids and nodular worms that occur in this host. In the 1950s, sodium fluoride and cadmium salts, and earlier, oil of chenopodium, were the drugs of choice for treating ascarid infections of swine. These compounds have been supplanted essentially by piperazine over the past decade.

Approximately 100% of the lumen-dwelling stages of both ascarids and nodular worms can be eliminated by a single treatment with piperazine. Retreatment 2 months later may be necessary to remove worms that existed as histotropic stages during the initial treatment.

Piperazine preparations can be administered to swine via either the feed or drinking water. The citrate salt is most commonly used for a 1-day medication of the feed. The hexahydrate of piperazine is the compound of choice for application in the drinking water due to its suitability for storage in solution. The medicated feed or water should be consumed in an 8- to 12-hour period; therefore, withholding water or feed the previous night is beneficial.

Ruminants. Piperazine compounds are seldom used in cattle and sheep because their activity is limited in these hosts to nodular worms *(Oesophagostomum)* and additionally in the bovine to ascarids *(Neoascaris vitulorum).* Ascarid infections do not occur in sheep and occur only sporadically in calves in the southern and midwestern United States. Piperazine compounds have essentially no activity against the common abomasal and small intestinal nematodes of ruminants.

Administration of piperazine (usually citrate, adipate, or hexahydrate) to ruminants is either via the drinking water, suspension dosing, or by addition of the compound to dry or wet feed.

Chickens. *Ascaridia galli* is highly susceptible to the action of piperazine preparations. Chiefly the citrate and adipate salts have been used to control this parasite in chickens. The cecal worm *(Heterakis gallinarum)* is not effectively controlled by these drugs.

Piperazine compounds are usually administered to chickens in the feed or drinking water over a 2-day period, the citrate or adipate salts for feed and piperazine hexahydrate for drinking water.

DOSAGE

Dog and cat: 110 mg/kg of body weight (maximum of 250 mg for puppies under 2.5 kg and for cats and kittens)
Horse: 220–275 mg/kg of body weight (maximum of 80 g for an adult, 60 g for a yearling, and 30 g for a foal)
Cattle and swine: 275–440 mg/kg of body weight
Sheep and goat: 400–800 mg/kg of body weight
Poultry: 32 mg/kg of body weight (approximately 0.3 g for each adult bird) given in each of 2 successive feeds or in the drinking water for 2 days

BENZIMIDAZOLES

THIABENDAZOLE

The need for an anthelmintic with a wide range of antiparasitic action, a high degree of efficacy, a good margin of safety, and with versatility of administration prompted investigation of several hundred substituted benzimidazole compounds. The one compound that satisfied these requirements to an extraordinary degree was *Thiabendazole,* U.S.P. (Equizole, Omnizole, Thibenzole) (TBZ). Since the initial marketing of this product in the early 1960s, thiabendazole has been used extensively throughout the world for GI parasites of a range of hosts, i.e., sheep, cattle, goats, pigs, horses, birds, and human beings. For therapeutic use it can be given orally in a single dose; prophylactically it can be given at lower dosages in the feed or in mineral supplements for an extended period. Its wide range of antiparasitic activity qualifies it as a broad-spectrum drug and it additionally has larvicidal and ovicidal properties.

CHEMISTRY

TBZ is a stable white crystalline compound with no appreciable taste or odor. It is barely soluble in water (3.84% at pH 2.2) and only slightly soluble in alcohols, esters, and chlorinated hydrocarbons.

Its official nonproprietary name is thiabendazole INN and the chemical name is 2-(4-thiazolyl)benzimidazole INN. The structural formula of the drug is shown in Fig. 52.3.

PHARMACODYNAMICS

TBZ is rapidly absorbed from the digestive tract. It becomes distributed throughout most of the body tissues, its highest concentration in the blood occurring at 4–7 hours after administration.

It is quickly metabolized into 5-hydroxythiabendazole or, more likely, into the sulfate or glucuronide of the 5-hydroxy derivative. Excretion of these metabolites via the urine and feces is apparently complete within 3 days of administering a sin-

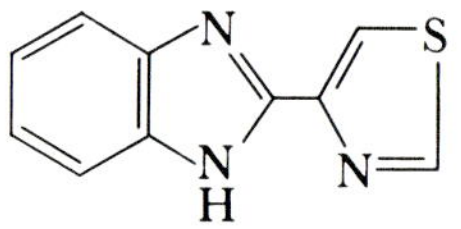

Thiabendazole

FIG. 52.3.

gle oral therapeutic dose. Less than 1% is excreted as TBZ.

MODE OF ACTION

The potency of TBZ coupled with its negligible mammalian toxicity has long suggested that the drug must interfere with a metabolic pathway essential to a number of helminths but of little to no importance to the host. Studies by Prichard (1970) have identified the enzyme fumarate reductase as the site of action of the drug. The fumurate reductase reaction is an essential component of fermentation, the process by which many parasitic helminths obtain their source of energy. The utilization of fermentation and anaerobic metabolism by parasites differs from principal metabolic pathways of their aerobic hosts. Consequently, drugs such as TBZ, which are active against components of metabolic pathways unique to the parasite, are generally well tolerated by the host.

Increasing concentrations of TBZ progressively decrease the rate of NADH oxidation in mitochondrial suspensions of *Haemonchus contortus,* which is susceptible to TBZ. NADH oxidation by similar suspensions of a strain of *H. contortus* resistant (tolerant) to thiabendazole is not inhibited by the drug.

The absorption of thiabendazole by parasites is probably through the cuticle. Evidence from *in vitro* studies (Davis et al. 1969) suggests that the absorption of the drug is by means of passive diffusion of the molecule through the lipid barrier of the nematode cuticle. This, of course, is not necessarily the case *in vivo.*

ANTHELMINTIC SPECTRUM

Sheep, Cattle, and Goats. The initial use of TBZ in the 1960s represented the greatest advancement in livestock anthelmintics since the advent of phenothiazine some 20 years earlier. The new drug was claimed by independent investigators to be superior to any anthelmintic for sheep nematodes. It still remains the antinematodal drug of choice for sheep and the one which new anthelmintics must equal or surpass.

TBZ has satisfactory to excellent efficacy against all the major GI nematodes of sheep, cattle, and goats except whipworms. At a dosage of 50 mg/kg in these three hosts it is especially efficacious for *Haemonchus, Trichostrongylus, Bunostomum, Chabertia, Oesophagostomum,* and *Strongyloides.* Several nematodes, i.e., *Ostertagia, Cooperia,* and *Nematodirus,* are less susceptible to the anthelmintic action of TBZ and occasional failures of the drug, especially in cattle, are usually associated with heavy burdens of these parasites. A higher dose, 100 mg/kg, usually gives satisfactory efficacy against *Cooperia* and *Nematodirus* and is more likely to give consistent results against *Ostertagia.* The drug becomes quite costly, however, at the higher dosage level. It is not sufficiently effective at practical dosage levels to be used against lungworm infections.

Horse. TBZ is over 90% effective in horses against mature large and small strongyles, *Trichostrongylus axei, Strongyloides westeri,* and mature *Oxyuris equi* at doses of 25–50 mg/kg. At these dosage levels the drug gives erratic activity against equine ascarids. A dose of 100 mg/kg will effectively remove ascarids (Drudge et al. 1962) but is costly. Piperazine is still the preferred drug for use against equine ascarids.

Immature equine strongyles apparently are not eliminated successfully by TBZ at the therapeutic dose of 44 mg/kg (Drudge 1964). Very high dosages of 440–500 mg/kg have been found to kill the somatic forms of *Strongylus vulgaris.* The cost of treatment with such large doses is prohibitive except perhaps in very valuable animals. TBZ has no activity against bots.

Pig. TBZ has its optimum efficacy in pigs against *Hyostrongylus rubidus, Strongyloides ransomi,* and *Oesophagostomum dentatum* but has very little activity against ascarids and whipworms. Dosages of 100 and even 50 mg/kg generally give better than 95% efficacy against the first three parasites. *Strongyloides* also can be effectively controlled in very young pigs. Leland et al. (1968), investigating different formulations and routes of administering the drug to baby pigs, suggested that a single intramuscular injection of a microaqueous formulation of TBZ be given to 1-day-old pigs; a dose of 100 mg/kg followed at 6 weeks of age by administering the drug in the feed for a 2-week period at a level of 0.1% was recommended. This therapeutic system is effective in controlling adult worms of *Strongyloides* in pigs and also inhibits the migration stages of the parasite. Young pigs readily accept the medicated feed whereas older animals initially reject it.

LARVICIDAL AND OVICIDAL ACTION

TBZ has its greatest action against mature worms but a high percentage of immature worms are also reported to be eliminated. The drug has larvicidal activity *in vitro* at dilutions as great as 10^{-5} μg/ml. *In vivo,* the immature worms eliminated by TBZ apparently are those that are lumen-dwelling rather than histotropic stages. *Ostertagia* larvae in abomasal nodules at the time of dosing, for example, are not affected appreciably by the drug.

There is also evidence that the drug possesses some degree of activity (not well delineated, however) against migrating larvae. Liver and lung pathology due to migrating larvae of *Ascaris suum* is reduced when pigs are given TBZ in the feed at concentrations of 0.01% or higher. Reduced levels of kidney worm infections following prophylactic feeding of the drug may be due to activity of the drug on the migrating larvae in addition to reduced numbers of the infective larvae. The early migratory larval stages as well as adult forms of *Trichinella spiralis* are known to be killed by TBZ and there is also some effect against the larvae that have already encysted in the musculature of hogs. The efficacy for the encysted stage is by no means complete but the drug has produced marked clinical improvement in some human cases of trichinosis and, in fact, is the only effective drug presently available for this disease in human beings.

TBZ also possesses ovicidal activity. Production of eggs by worms is inhibited within an hour of administration of the drug. Small daily doses of TBZ, like phenothiazine, sterilize the worms. This inhibition of egg production and the significant activity against lumen-dwelling immature worms (particularly the 4th stage) allows for transferring animals to clean paddocks after dosing, with reduced contamination of the new site.

PROPHYLACTIC USE

In Sheep. TBZ can be satisfactorily administered in the feed over an extended period at daily dosages lower than the single therapeutic dose. The cost of the drug limits widespread administration by this means; however, the ease of administration sometimes makes it more practical than drenching. Lambs given TBZ mixed with feed pellets to give the equivalent of 8 mg/kg/day for 4 weeks can be expected to lose most of their trichostrongylid infections and to have better weight gains than unmedicated controls.

In Dogs. Prophylactic use of TBZ is more efficacious for the parasites of dogs than is a single therapeutic dose. Fed to pups and dogs daily in the ration at a rate of 0.025% for 16 weeks, TBZ gives almost complete clearance of ascarids, hookworms, and whipworms and is highly effective in reducing the numbers of *Strongyloides stercoralis* (Yakstis et al. 1968). *Strongyloides* also is claimed to be controlled by TBZ in dosages of 55 mg/kg of body weight daily for 3 days each month (Georgi 1974). The drug is virtually ineffective against any of the canine parasites at a single therapeutic dosage of 100 mg/kg. Single dosages of 300 and 500 mg/kg are required to achieve 82% efficacy for ascarids and hookworms, respectively. At the latter dosage, marked vomition occurs.

In Birds. The gapeworm of fowl *(Syngamus trachea)* can be controlled by TBZ when it is incorporated in the diet at a level of 0.1% for 2–3 weeks. Generally the drug does not give satisfactory control of fowl ascarids and *Capillaria*.

SAFETY AND TOXICITY

TBZ has a high degree of safety for ruminants and horses, 20 times the therapeutic dose producing no appreciable side effects even in debilitated or very young animals. It is not irritating to the mucosae and skin and produces no photosensitization in animals when they are treated with the drug and subsequently exposed to ultraviolet light. No significant changes in blood pressure, hematologic values, or liver or renal function occur. In nonpregnant sheep, dosages as high as 800–1000 mg/kg are required to produce toxic depression and anorexia. Dosages of 1200 mg/kg may cause deaths in sheep.

There is no evidence of teratogenicity in rats but the drug is not so well tolerated by pregnant ewes since 4 times the therapeutic dose has been known to produce changes consistent with pregnancy toxemia in some ewes.

In dogs, a single dose of TBZ (200 mg/kg) administered orally results in vomition several hours later and induces inanition and leukopenia. Dogs that are continued on this daily dosage for as long as 2 years experience little disturbance except occasional attacks of vomition and the development of a moderate persistent anemia which seems to be associated with an increased rate of red cell destruction.

DOSAGE AND ADMINISTRATION

The oral route of administration is used in all animals treated with TBZ. The drug is available commercially both as a wettable powder and a suspension.

Sheep: 50–100 mg/kg of body weight
Cattle: 50–100 mg/kg of body weight
Horse: 50–100 mg/kg of body weight
Pig: 50 mg/kg of body weight

Other Benzimidazoles

Following the discovery of the anthelmintic effectiveness of thiabendazole in 1961, an extensive program was undertaken to structurally modify TBZ with an aim toward developing TBZ-related drugs with unique properties. Of several hundred synthesized compounds, those few selected for further development on the basis of overall safety and effectiveness included *cambendazole* INN, *fenbendazole, mebendazole* INN, and *parbendazole* INN. All four compounds are now commercially produced for anthelmintic use in various countries of the world. In the United States only cambendazole and mebendazole have Food and Drug Administration (FDA) approval at the present and are limited to use in horses. Both compounds are additionally effective against several parasites of fowl, and cambendazole is marketed in several foreign countries for use against GI parasites and lungworms of sheep and cattle. FDA approval for the use of fenbendazole and parbendazole against parasites of horses, cattle, sheep, and pigs is currently being sought in the United States.

CHEMISTRY

The four anthelmintics discussed in this section, like thiabendazole, are benzimidazoles. They differ structurally from TBZ in having a substitution on C-5 (Table 52.1). Cambendazole, fenbendazole, and parbendazole are white crystalline powders; mebendazole is an off-white to yellowish amorphous powder. All are insoluble to only slightly soluble in water; cambendazole and parbendazole are soluble in alcohols, mebendazole in formic acid, and fenbendazole in dimethylsulfoxide.

PHARMACODYNAMICS

Only limited amounts of a dose of any of the benzimidazoles are absorbed from the GI tract of the host. The limited absorption is probably related to the poor solubility of these drugs in water. Absorption of the limited quantity is generally rapid, peak plasma levels occurring within 2–4 hours after dosing with mebendazole, for example, or within 8–24 hours after dosing with parbendazole. Generally the plasma level is never greater than 1% of the dose administered.

The degree of metabolism of the benzimidazoles varies somewhat and is perhaps related to the substitution on C-5. Mebendazole is poorly metabolized and

TABLE 52.1. Names and formulas of benzimidazole anthelmintics

Compound	Trade Name	Chemical Name	Structural Formula
Thiabendazole	Equizole Omnizole Thibenzole	2-(4-Thiazolyl)benzimidazole INN	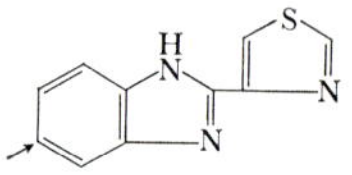
Cambendazole	Equiben Noviben Bonlam	Isopropyl 2-(4-thiazolyl)-5-benzimidazolecarbamate INN	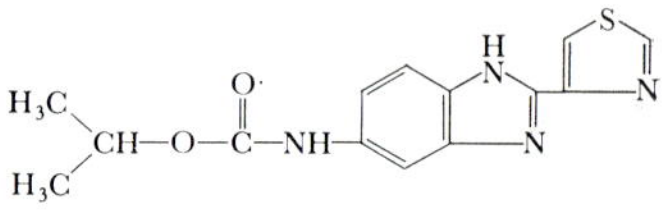
Fenbendazole	Panacur	Methyl-5(phenylthio)-2-benzimidazolecarbamate	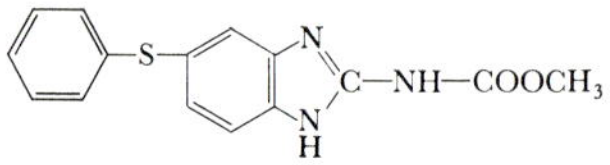
Mebendazole	Telmin	Methyl 5-benzoyl-2-benzimidazolecarbamate INN	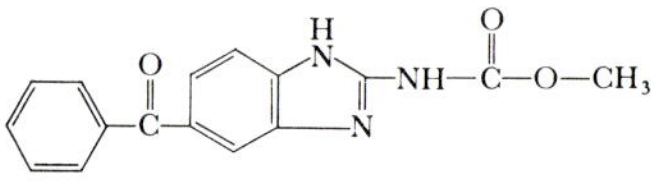
Parbendazole	Verminum Worm Guard Helmatac	Methyl 5-butyl-2-benzimidazolecarbamate INN	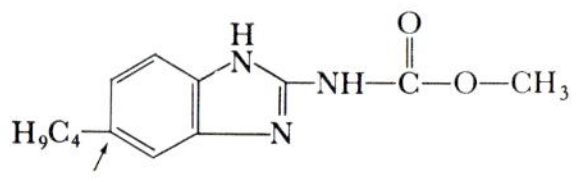

Note: ↗ denotes position of carbon 5.

most of it is excreted unchanged in the feces in 24–48 hours; between 5% and 10% is excreted in the urine; and only a small portion is excreted as the decarboxylated derivative of mebendazole. Cambendazole, on the other hand, is rapidly metabolized into a large number of degradation products. Less than 5% of the product excreted is actually intact cambendazole. Again the largest portion (approximately 75%) of the drug and its metabolites is excreted in the feces (the remainder in the urine) over a 48-hour period. Small amounts of the benzimidazoles are excreted for as long as 1 week after dosing. Residual quantities of these drugs are detectable in the tissues, especially the liver, at 2 weeks after dosing and occur in the range of 0.3 μg or less/g of tissue. Thus a withdrawal period before slaughter is necessary and the drug should not be administered to lactating animals whose milk is to be used for human consumption.

MODE OF ACTION

Among the substituted benzimidazoles it appears that mebendazole with relative certainty and probably also cambendazole and parbendazole act on nematodes by inhibiting the uptake of glucose. Normally glucose diffuses both passively and actively from the luminal fluid via the single-celled intestinal wall of the worm to its pseudocoelomic fluid. Evidence suggests that mebendazole interferes with the passive rather than active transport of glucose (Van den Bossche 1972). The lack of absorbed glucose causes a depletion of the worm's glycogen reserve and leaves it unable to produce the adenosine triphosphate (ATP) necessary for survival. Expulsion of the worm is slow, over a 2- to 3-day period after dosing. The glucose level in the mammalian host is evidently not affected by high doses of the benzimidazoles, judged by tests using mebendazole (Nollin and Van den Bossche 1973).

The substituted benzimidazoles and TBZ are assumed to have some common mode of action, at least to some degree, based in part upon the fact that a strain of *Haemonchus contortus,* which is resistant to cambendazole, mebendazole, and parbendazole, has also been found to be resistant to TBZ (Romanowski et al. 1975). As discussed earlier, the principal mode of activity of the substituted benzimidazoles appears to be inhibition of glucose transport and the stimulation of glycogen utilization in helminths. The principal activity of TBZ, on the other hand, is inhibition of the fumurate reductase mechanism. It has been found recently that the fumurate mechanism is also inhibited by cambendazole (Romanowski et al. 1975). Other substituted benzimidazoles when tested may also be found to share this common mode of activity with TBZ, which perhaps accounts for the cross-resistance of the *Haemonchus* strain to TBZ and the substituted benzimidazoles.

The extent to which the differences in the chemical structures of the substituted benzimidazoles and TBZ influence their mode of activity is not known. TBZ has neither a substitution in position 5 nor totally acts in the manner of the substituted benzimidazoles. It is generally recognized that simple structural modifications in drugs often result in differences in modes of action and, consequently, differences in anthelmintic spectra.

ANTHELMINTIC SPECTRUM

Horse. Three of the four substituted benzimidazoles (cambendazole, fenbendazole, and mebendazole), as well as the nonsubstituted TBZ, give comparable high activity (above 90%) against the large strongyles, small strongyles, mature *Oxyuris equi,* and the small pinworms *(Probstmayria vivipara).* Ascarids *(Parascaris equorum)* and immature *Oxyuris* are much more effectively eliminated by cambendazole, mebendazole, or fenbendazole than by TBZ (Enigk et al. 1974b; Drudge et al. 1975). Infections of *Strongyloides westeri* in young nursing foals are best treated with cambendazole, fenbendazole, or TBZ; however, higher than regular therapeutic doses are needed for satisfactory control. Results of treatment with mebendazole for *Strongyloides* are variable.

The benzimidazoles have little to no activity against several equine parasites. Cambendazole appears to have some activity against *Habronema muscae,* whereas the other drugs do not. None of the drugs appear to have any activity against the other equine stomach worms *(Draschia megastoma* and *Trichostrongylus axei),* against tapeworms *(Anoplocephala perfoliata* and *A. magna),* against lungworms *Dictyocaulus),* or against bots *(Gastrophilus intestinalis* and *G. nasalis).* Carbon disulfide can be safely administered in conjunction with any of the benzimidazoles for the control of bots.

Cattle and Sheep. One or more of the substituted benzimidazoles can be used to control lungworms of cattle and sheep and is markedly effective against the adult and many larval species of GI nematodes of these hosts. In particular, cambendazole and fenbendazole are effective for lungworm infections caused by *Dictyocaulus.* Cambendazole eliminates more than 90% of the adult infection and between 52% and 82% of the immature stages of *Dictyocaulus* in cattle (Baker et al. 1972). Fenbendazole gives even more satisfactory control of cattle lungworms. Ninety-nine percent of adults and 6- and 13-day-old larval stages of *Dictyocaulus* are eliminated by therapeutic doses of fenbendazole (Düwel 1974). Critical studies have not been reported relative to the effect of these drugs on lungworms of sheep.

All of the major GI parasites of ruminants *(Haemonchus, Ostertagia, Trichostrongylus, Cooperia, Nematodirus, Bunostomum, Chabertia, Oesophagostomum,* and *Strongyloides)* are eliminated by cambendazole, fenbendazole, or parbendazole. It is the adult form of these parasites that is most effectively expelled but immature stages are also eliminated to a high degree. Studies indicate that the majority of 3rd and 4th stage larvae of the GI parasites are eliminated by cambendazole. Parbendazole causes the death of 71% of 7-day-old *Ostertagia* larvae located in abomasal nodules; 96% of 14-day-old *Ostertagia* larvae are eliminated from cattle upon receiving a therapeutic dose. Activity of parbendazole against *Cooperia* and *Trichostrongylus* approaches 100% regardless of age of the larvae. Fenbendazole is also impressively effective against immature forms. More than 99% of the immature 5th stage of all major GI parasites of ruminants except

Cooperia (for which a critical study has not been reported) are eliminated by fenbendazole.

Fenbendazole is especially efficacious in its activity against the tissue stages of *Ostertagia,* which are difficult to attack therapeutically. Treatment with fenbendazole results in a 98% reduction of 3- and 10-day-old larval stages and a 94% reduction in 7-day-old larval stages of *Ostertagia* (Düwel et al. 1974). By contrast, tetramisole gives only a 40%–60% reduction; levamisole, a 36% reduction; and morantel, an 87% reduction in nodular stages of *Ostertagia.*

The substituted benzimidazoles have limited activity against tapeworms *(Moniezia)* of sheep and cattle. Their efficacy for ruminant whipworms is not well tested. Parbendazole apparently gives variable results against *Trichuris* in sheep and cattle.

None of the substituted benzimidazoles are presently approved by the FDA for use in cattle and sheep in the United States, but the success of these compounds in other countries and the rather extensive testing of some of them in the United States suggest their eventual acceptance here.

Swine. Three of the substituted benzimidazoles (cambendazole, fenbendazole, and parbendazole) are effectively used against the major GI parasites of swine. In general they are more potent than TBZ, especially against swine ascarids (Hoff et al. 1970), and are approximately equal to each other in efficacy for sexually mature adult forms of ascarids, stomach worms *(Hyostrongylus),* nodular worms *(Oesophagostomum),* and *Strongyloides.*

Efficacy for the adult forms of swine whipworms *(Trichuris suis)* is variable at regular therapeutic dosages. Parbendazole (20–50 mg/kg) expels 83%–97% of *T. suis* and fenbendazole (15 mg/kg) only 65%. Increasing the dosage of fenbendazole to 30 mg/kg improves the efficacy for *T. suis* to 96% but this is a 6-fold increase in the regular therapeutic dose of 5 mg/kg which, although completely safe, is more expensive and is probably only warranted in severe whipworm infections of swine. In such cases, however, dichlorvos may be more practical to use.

It is difficult to assess the comparative values of cambendazole, fenbendazole, and parbendazole against the larval and immature 5th stages of the GI parasites of swine since many reports on efficacy do not include this information. In general, however, a marked reduction in these stages of the parasites parallels the reduction in adult forms. Cambendazole is claimed to be more effective than TBZ against the young stages of *Strongyloides ransomi* (Enigk and Dey-Hazra 1971) and *Ascaris suum* (Hoff et al. 1970). Against the stomach worm *(Hyostrongylus),* parbendazole is approximately 50% efficient in eliminating the 14-day-old 5th stage immature forms while fenbendazole at doses of 6 mg/kg yields 99% efficacy for the 5th stage and approximately 75% efficacy for the younger 4th stage larvae (Enigk et al. 1974a). Fourth stage larvae and young 5th stage immature forms of *Oesophagostomum* of swine are also effectively reduced in numbers by 61% and 99%, respectively, when fenbendazole is administered to swine at the 6 mg/kg dosage. The value of other substituted benzimidazoles against young forms of the swine nodular worm is apparently not well established.

None of the benzimidazoles claim efficacy for the spirurid stomach worms or lungworms of swine.

Birds. Cambendazole and mebendazole can be used effectively against parasites of the GI and respiratory tracts of birds. Cambendazole eliminates 99% of the adult population of *Syngamus trachea* when administered to turkeys in the feed for 2 days at a dosage of 20 mg/kg/day. A higher dosage (50 mg/kg/day for 2 days) is required for the elimination of immature worms and 4th stage larvae. Cambendazole at a 0.05% level in the feed for 6 days is approximately equal to mebendazole in efficacy for *Syngamus* and is considered to be slightly better than TBZ and disophenol and 50% better than tetramisole (Enigk and Dey-Hazra 1970). Cambendazole at a dosage of 20 mg/kg/day for 2 days or mebendazole in a single dose of 50 mg/kg effectively eliminates ascarid and capillaria infections of birds.

OVICIDAL ACTIVITY

Studies on the culturability of parasite eggs in stools following treatment of the animals with substituted benzimidazoles suggest a strong ovicidal property of these drugs. These compounds have been found to be ovicidal for ruminant trichostrongylid eggs, swine stomachworm (*Hyostrongylus*) eggs, chicken ascarid eggs, and canine and human hookworm and whipworm eggs.

SAFETY AND TOXICITY

The substituted benzimidazoles, like the nonsubstituted TBZ, are extremely well tolerated by domestic and wild animals in general. All of this group of drugs are characteristically free of side effects at therapeutic doses even when administered to young, sick, or debilitated animals.

The tolerance to high doses of these drugs is varied but is generally very acceptable. Fenbendazole, for example, has been administered to sheep at 1000 times the therapeutic dose (5000 mg/kg) without producing clinical reactions. Cambendazole, on the other hand, may produce inappetence and listlessness in cattle at only 3 times the recommended dose. Cambendazole is, nevertheless, considered a safe drug as compared to organophosphates. A mild transient diarrhea in horses treated with cambendazole is seen only after exceeding dosages of 300 mg/kg. Mebendazole is tolerated in horses when given as a single dose equal to 40 times the therapeutic dose or as daily doses for 15 days at a total dose equal to 90 times the therapeutic dose. Parbendazole is tolerated in pigs at a dosage of 1000 mg/kg and mebendazole in chickens at a dosage of 2000 mg/kg.

An LD50 is not established for the substituted benzimidazoles in most of the domestic animals. Single doses of cambendazole (750–1000 mg/kg) are lethal for cattle, as is parbendazole (600 mg/kg) occasionally for sheep. The LD50 for mebendazole in horses is not known but in both dogs and guinea pigs this value is 640 mg/kg of body weight. LD50 values for fenbendazole in domestic animals have not been established. An acute toxic dose for sheep is estimated to be in excess of 500 mg/kg of body weight. The drug is extremely well tolerated. Attempts to cause fatalities by poisoning small laboratory animals have been unsuccessful because rats and mice tolerate the maximum quantities (10,000 mg/kg).

CONTRAINDICATIONS

Due to tissue and milk residues, slaughter clearance times are required and it is recommended that milk of treated animals not be used for human consumption. The slaughter clearance times for cattle or sheep treated with parbendazole are 5 and 6 days, respectively, and for those treated with cambendazole, 28 and 21 days.

In addition to slaughter clearance times the major contraindication for the use of some of the substituted benzimidazoles is during early pregnancy in sheep. Parbendazole and cambendazole exert a teratogenic effect when given to pregnant ewes during the 2nd–4th weeks of gestation. The greatest period of embryonic susceptibility to the drugs coincides with the time that normal embryonic limb development begins, i.e., around the 20th day of pregnancy. The principal malformations observed following treatment on the 21st–24th days of pregnancy have been rotational and flexing deformities of the limbs, overflexion of the carpal joints, and abnormalities of posture and gait. The incidences of malformed lambs born to ewes treated on the 21st and 24th days of gestation are 27% and 47% respectively. No abnormalities occur if the drugs are administered as early as the 10th or 14th days of pregnancy but treatment at this time does reduce the lambing rate (67% for drug-treated ewes versus 84% for nontreated controls). There is no restriction on the use of cambendazole in ewes following the 4th week of pregnancy. Manufacturers of parbendazole do not recommend its use at any time during pregnancy.

No teratogenic effect has been found

TABLE 52.2. Dosages of substituted benzimidazoles

Animal	Cambendazole	Fenbendazole	Mebendazole	Parbendazole
	(mg/kg of body weight)			
Horse	20	5	8.8	...
Cattle	25	5	...	30
Sheep	20	5	...	15–30
Pig	20–40	3–6	...	oral 25–50 in feed 20–30

in pregnant cattle treated with twice the therapeutic dose (50 mg/kg) of cambendazole on days 0, 20, 25, or 40 of gestation. It is, therefore, presently accepted for use in pregnant cattle; however, it is recommended that parbendazole not be used in either cattle or sheep at any time during pregnancy.

There are no known teratogenic effects of either mebendazole or fenbendazole. Repeated multiple therapeutic doses of fenbendazole in pregnant ewes and in laboratory animals have not shown ill effects. The only contraindication for the use of mebendazole in any horses (including pregnant mares) is that it should not be used in horses intended for human consumption.

All of the benzimidazoles are compatible with other drugs administered simultaneously. This represents a distinct advantage of the benzimidazoles over organophosphorus compounds. The latter drugs are generally incompatible with other organophosphorus drugs, insecticides, and other cholinesterase inhibitors.

ADMINISTRATION AND DOSAGE

The substituted benzimidazoles are administered only orally, generally as a suspension for drenching or a powder for administration in the feed. Additionally, a paste form of cambendazole is available for treating horses and cattle. Dosages are given in Table 52.2.

IMIDAZOTHIAZOLES

LEVAMISOLE

Levamisole INN (Levasole, Ripercol L, Tramisol) is a highly acceptable antinematodal drug because of its broad range of activity in a large number of hosts (sheep, cattle, pig, horse, chicken, dog, and cat). It is presently approved in the United States only for use in cattle, sheep, and swine. Two major advantages of levamisole over other drugs are: (1) it is effective against nematodes both of the lungs and of the GI tract and (2) it can be administered by subcutaneous injection. Also, it may be administered in the feed or by oral suspension. It has no activity against flukes, tapeworms, protozoa, bacteria, or fungi.

CHEMISTRY AND RELATION TO *dl*-TETRAMISOLE

Levamisole is the levo-isomer of *dl*-tetramisole. The latter drug was introduced as an anthelmintic in 1966 and is a racemic mixture of two optical isomers: S(—)tetramisole (= *l*-tetramisole = levamisole) rotates plane polarized light to the left; R(+)tetramisole (= *d*-tetramisole) rotates light to the right. (See Fig. 52.4.)

The mixture itself, known as tetramisole INN or *dl*-tetramisole (Nemicide, Nilverm, Ripercol), was extensively studied and soon marketed (1967) throughout the world as an anthelmintic for sheep, cattle, and various other hosts.

Following the marketing of the racemic mixture, pharmaceutical scientists were able to develop a process for separating the *dl*-tetramisole into its two isomers. Upon testing the two separated components it was found that the anthelmintic activity of the mixture rested almost solely with the *l*-isomer (levamisole); thus it was determined that the dosage could be cut in half by using the *l*-isomer alone. Reducing the dosage also increased the safety margin since equal high amounts of tetramisole or

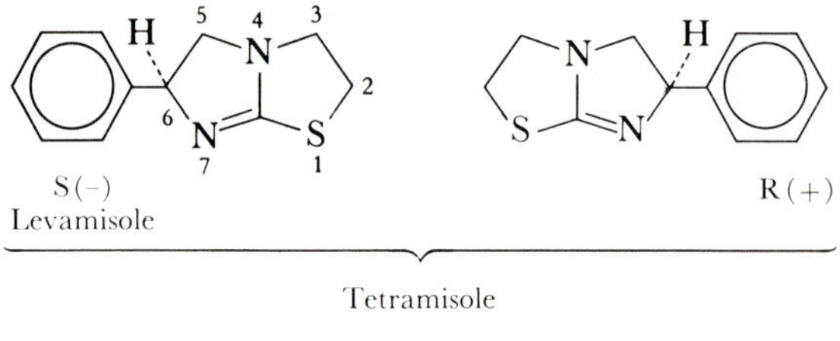

S(−) Levamisole   R(+)

Tetramisole

Fig. 52.4.

either of its components are of equal toxicity. Thus the compound available today in the United States and many other countries is levamisole rather than the parent tetramisole. Most of the attention in the following discussion will center on the *l*-isomer.

The chemical name of levamisole is (—)-2,3,5,6-tetrahydro-6-phenylimidazo[2,1-b]thiazol INN. The marketed form is either its hydrochloride (in bolus, drench, or injectable form) or its phosphate (also an injectable form). Levamisole hydrochloride, a white crystalline compound, is highly soluble in water. This solubility has allowed for the preparation of injectable solutions as well as a nonsettling drench.

MODE OF ACTION

Levamisole HCl has a paralyzing action on nematodes. Rapidly expelled worms are still alive in the feces; worms expelled later are decomposed and may not be apparent in the feces.

The paralytic action of levamisole on helminths is apparently related to an interference with the worm's energy supply. The drug blocks the metabolic pathway responsible for the formation of ATP. The blockage occurs at the site of fumarate reduction and succinate oxidation. Since ATP is the form in which cellular energy is stored, the lack of production of ATP and consequent interference with normal activity of cells result in paralysis and ultimately expulsion of the worm.

PHARMACODYNAMICS

The absorption and excretion of levamisole is rapid following oral administration of the radioactive-labeled drug to rats at a dosage of 15 mg/kg. Approximately 40% is excreted in the urine in 12 hours. Thereafter, urinary excretion decreases and only another 8% is eliminated over the next 8 days. Elimination in the feces over an 8-day period accounts for approximately 41% of the dose, the bulk of which passes in 12–24 hours. A small amount is expelled in respired gases, i.e., 0.2% of the dose during a 48-hour period immediately following dosing.

Tissue residues of the drug are not appreciable. Approximately 0.9% of the initial dose is found in the tissues (principally degradative and excretion organs like the liver and kidney) at 12–24 hours after dosing. By 7 days after dosing, levamisole is not detectable in the muscle, liver, kidney, fat, blood, or urine of rats or of other animals tested. On this basis, a 7-day slaughter clearance time has been set. The identified metabolites of levamisole are much less toxic than the parent compound; thus it is the parent drug that is sought in analysis of tissue samples.

The pharmacodynamic actions of levamisole (or tetramisole) in the host suggest that the drug exerts both muscarinic and nicotinic effects (Eyre 1970; Forbes 1972b; Van Nueten 1972). Signs (salivation, defecation, and respiratory distress due to smooth muscle contraction) of levamisole intoxication are like those of organophosphorus poisoning. Indeed, evidence suggests that some of the toxicity of this drug may be concerned with cholinesterase inhibition, leading to manifestations of the muscarinic action of acetylcholine, i.e., constriction of pupils and respiratory bronchioles, acceleration of motility of the digestive tract, slowing of the heart rate, etc.

Eyre's and Forbes' works suggest that levamisole additionally produces effects consistent with the nicotinic action of acetylcholine, i.e., initial stimulation but subsequent blocking of ganglionic transmission and skeletal neuromuscular transmission. The clinical signs of pronounced nicotinic action of acetylcholine are an initial rise in blood pressure, followed by a fall in arterial pressure and simultaneous respiratory paralysis. These nicotinic manifestations are only slightly represented in levamisole toxicosis; rather, it is the muscarinic manifestations of the drug that markedly predominate.

FORMULATIONS AND ADMINISTRATION

Levamisole is administered as a bolus, drench, feed additive, or injectable solution. The drug for drenching ruminants is marketed in powder form to which water can be added. Excess drench solution can be held for as long as 12 days without loss of anthelmintic activity.

Two formulations of levamisole HCl are prepared for administration in the feed of ruminants: one incorporates the drug in a pelleted ready-to-use dehydrated alfalfa carrier (the pellets should be mixed with one-half the regular daily ration and fed at one time); the second, a medicated premix containing 50% levamisole HCl, is made to be used by feed mills in manufacturing a worming supplement (0.8% levamisole HCl) for cattle and sheep. Feed should be withheld overnight. The following morning the medicated supplement can be mixed with one-half the daily ration.

Administration of levamisole HCl in the drinking water is used routinely only for swine and poultry. The drug intended for this use is marketed as a powder to which water is added. For treating swine, the medicated water is intended to be consumed in a 24-hour period at the rate of 1 gal/100 lb (3.8 L/45.4 kg) of body weight. Following mixing, the solution is stable up to 3 months if stored in a tightly capped bottle. For poultry, the medicated drinking water is prepared by calculating the total amount of tetramisole needed to provide a dosage of 40 mg/kg of body weight. This quantity is used to prepare an 0.01% (approximate) solution which should be consumed by the birds in 12 hours.

Levamisole has wide appeal as an injectable anthelmintic for cattle. Initially, an aqueous preparation of its hydrochloride was used either intramuscularly or subcutaneously in the lateral midneck region. The hydrochloride, however, proved to be irritating to tissues and resulted in moderate to severe reactions at the site of injection, especially when given intramuscularly. Recently the monobasic phosphoric acid salt ($-H_3PO_4$) of levamisole was found to be less irritating to the tissues. Nevertheless, some tissue reactions still occur following the injection of levamisole phosphate. Reactions are distinctly more frequent and more severe, for some unknown reason, in cattle nearing slaughter weight and condition. Thus levamisole phosphate solution is now recommended only for subcutaneous injection and only for stocker or feeder cattle.

ANTHELMINTIC SPECTRUM

Cattle and Sheep. The efficacy of levamisole HCl is essentially equal in ruminants regardless of whether the bolus, drench, pellet, or injectable formulation is used. The pellet formulation appears to be slightly less effective than the other preparations of the drug. The overall efficacy of the pellet for application in the feed is approximately 95% as compared with more than 98% for the other formulations. Adult stages of the major ruminant parasites of the abomasum *(Haemonchus, Ostertagia)*, the small intestine *(Cooperia, Trichostrongylus* spp., *Bunostomum)*, the large intestine *(Oesophagostomum, Trichuris)*, and the lungs *(Dictyocaulus)* are very satisfactorily removed by this broad-spectrum drug. Its efficacy for ruminant GI nematodes compares favorably with that of thiabendazole (TBZ) except that TBZ is far superior in eliminating *Strongyloides* and perhaps slightly superior in eliminating *Nematodirus* and *Trichostrongylus axei*. On the other hand, levamisole HCl is more than 96% effective for whipworms and is 98% effective for both mature and immature lungworms of ruminants, while TBZ has poor activity against both of these parasites. Levamisole HCl also is effective against TBZ-resistant strains of *Haemonchus* and *Trichostrongylus*.

Larval and immature stages of the GI parasites of ruminants are not so effectively removed by levamisole HCl as the mature stages. Approximately 33% and 53% of the lumen-dwelling immature forms of *Ostertagia* and *Haemonchus*, respectively, are eliminated from treated cattle. Immature forms of *Cooperia* are completely eliminated. Closely controlled studies of the effect of this or any other anthelmintic on the histotropic stages of GI parasites are quite difficult to accomplish and have not been done with levamisole HCl. A study using naturally infected animals with varying numbers of larval *Ostertagia* in the abomasal wall suggests approximately 25% reduction in histotropic *Ostertagia* following treatment with this drug (Presidente et al. 1971).

Swine. The convenient and most widely used method for deworming swine with levamisole HCl is to add the drug to the drinking water or feed. Whether using this FDA-approved method or administering the drug subcutaneously, in general, 90%–100% of ascarids *(Ascaris suum),* intestinal threadworms *(Strongyloides ransomi),* and lungworms (*Metastrongylus* spp.) are removed; efficacies most frequently approach 99%. The nodular worm (*Oesophagostomum* spp.) is also effectively expelled but the efficacies in separate studies range from 72%–99%. At present, levamisole HCl is approved in the United States only for the above parasites of swine. Insufficient data prevent FDA approval for its use against certain other swine parasites, namely *Hyostrongylus rubidus,* for which a reasonably high efficacy apparently exists (Probert et al. 1973). The drug has variable activity for swine whipworms and practically no activity for the kidney worm *(Stephanurus).*

Immature (11- to 13-day-old) stages of *A. suum* and *Metastrongylus* are as readily expelled by levamisole HCl as the adult forms of these parasites, but only approximately 64% of younger (5- to 7-day-old) ascarid stages are eliminated (Oakley 1974). The efficacy of the drug for larval or immature stages of other swine parasites is not well documented.

Chicken. Levamisole HCl administered to chickens in half the daily consumption of drinking water at a rate of either 36 or 48 mg/kg of body weight gives above 95% clearance of adult forms of *Ascaridia galli, Heterakis gallinarum,* and *Capillaria obsignata* and apparently eliminates a high percentage of the immature adults and larval stages of these parasites. At this dosage level the drug is palatable and without toxic signs in birds (Pankavich et al. 1973). Oral administration of levamisole HCl via the drinking water is also an effective means of eliminating the fowl eye worm *(Oxyspirura mansoni).* Additionally, the application of several drops of a 10% solution directly to the eye is nonirritating to the bird yet completely effective in killing the parasite in less than 1 hour.

Tetramisole is effective against the gapeworm *(Syngamus trachea).* Practically all worms will be expelled from the mouths of turkeys about 16 hours after they have access to the medicated water. The water should be prepared so as to provide 3.6 mg tetramisole/kg/day and continued for 3 days.

Dog. In dogs, more than 95% of both ascarids *(Toxocara* and *Toxascaris)* and hookworms *(Ancylostoma* and *Uncinaria)* are effectively removed following oral doses of 10 mg tetramisole/kg/day for 2 days or a single subcutaneous injection of 10 mg/kg. The drug is not effective for whipworms *(Trichuris vulpis)* and retreatment is sometimes necessary to eliminate heavy ascarid and hookworm burdens. Thienpont et al. (1968) reported establishing and maintaining a hookworm- and ascarid-free colony of several generations of beagles by giving bitches tetramisole (10 mg/kg) subcutaneously 2 weeks prior to parturition and by additionally giving bitches and pups the drug (20 mg/kg) orally 2 weeks after parturition.

The investigational use of levamisole HCl as a microfilaricide in heartworm *(Dirofilaria immitis)* infections of dogs is discussed under the section Drugs Used in Heartworm Disease in this chapter.

Cat. Lungworms *(Aelurostrongylus abstrusus)* of cats have resisted treatment by many drugs. Some success has been achieved in using tetramisole against this parasite. The very narrow toxic/therapeutic ratio requires that the cat be treated orally rather than subcutaneously. Cats dislike the taste of the drug and salivate profusely after treatment. Hamilton (1967) obtained measurable improvement in treated as compared with control cats given experimental lungworm infections. Repeated treatment was necessary. Hamilton scheduled a total of 6 treatments of varying dosages at 2-day intervals, i.e., 15 mg/kg of body weight on days 1, 3, and 5; 30 mg/kg on days 7 and 9; and a final dose of 60 mg/kg on day 11. Larval counts in the feces may be expected to drop to zero during the course of treatment but in the author's experience, the feces of at least one-half of the treated cats become positive for larvae again approximately 2 weeks after cessation of treatment. Nevertheless, even in these cats clinical improvement owing to the treatment apparently occurs. Clients should be warned that tetramisole is an investigational drug for cats and that deaths have occurred during its use. Hospitalization and possibly atropinization of the cat during the course of therapy is advisable.

Horse. In horses as in other animals levamisole HCl is particularly effective for ascarids and adult pinworms. *Parascaris equorum* is completely eliminated by oral dosages of 7.5–15 mg/kg (as a drench or in the food) or subcutaneous injections of 5–10 mg/kg. Lungworms *(Dictyocaulus)* of horses are also effectively eliminated (94%) by levamisole, especially when the drug is administered twice intramuscularly at a dosage of 5 mg/kg, 3–4 weeks apart.

Various large and small strongyles are not so effectively removed (range of 17%–85%) by levamisole even at dosages up to 40 mg/kg. The fact that dosages over 20 mg/kg have caused adverse effects and deaths plus the limited activity against large strongyles prevents the use of levamisole HCl in horses.

Zoo Animals. The anthelmintic activity of tetramisole or levamisole has been tried in a variety of zoo animals of which a few are mentioned here. In such animals critical trials involving the necropsy of treated animals to determine the remaining worm burdens are not possible; thus the percent efficacy is usually based on parasite egg counts in the stool. Such figures may or, more likely, may not reflect the actual worm burden of the host.

In the zebu, several major ruminant parasites *(Haemonchus, Bunostomum, Bosicola,* and *Cooperia)* are apparently effectively removed (90%–100%) by the administration of tetramisole (5 mg/kg) either orally or subcutaneously. Elephants ill from GI parasitism are reported to show clinical improvement following treatment with tetramisole (4.5–5 mg/kg).

The treatment of water and grass snakes harboring nematodal parasites *(Rhabdias)* of the lungs were judged successful on the basis of marked clinical improvement and the absence of larvae of the parasite in posttreatment stools (Zwart and Jansen 1969). Tetramisole was administered to the snakes intraperitoneally at a single dosage of 10 mg/kg.

SAFETY AND TOXICITY

Compared to TZB, tetramisole and its isolated active component, levamisole, have a much narrower safety range. Nevertheless, tetramisole itself has a safety margin variously estimated to be 2–6 times the therapeutic dose of 15 mg/kg and the safety factor of levamisole is about twice that of the parent compound since levamisole is equally as active against parasites in half the dosage.

Tetramisole is lethal to sheep at a dosage of 90 mg/kg. Signs suggestive of organophosphorus poisoning (salivation, lachrymation, head shaking, muscle tremors, mild excitability, etc.) occur in sheep at a dosage of 45 mg/kg. An occasional sheep dies even at dosages of only 30–50 mg/kg. Repeated daily doses of 20 mg/kg orally or 15 mg/kg subcutaneously in lambs cause no evidence of cumulative effect over a period of 1 month.

Side effects or death are more likely to occur when tetramisole is administered parenterally. The acute oral and subcutaneous LD50 in the mouse are 253 and 100 mg/kg of body weight, respectively. Cattle appear to be somewhat more tolerant of parenteral administration of the drug than sheep. In cattle, a 2-fold overdose of injectable levamisole phosphate may cause slight muzzle foam and licking of the lips in about two-thirds of the treated animals. These signs should disappear within an hour posttreatment.

Levamisole given to pigs at 3 times the recommended dose causes only occasional vomiting. Vomiting as well as coughing may be seen following therapeutic doses if the pigs are infected with mature lungworms. In such cases the reaction is due to expulsion of the worms and should terminate in several hours.

Chickens tolerate tetramisole (and presumably levamisole) very well. The LD50 for chickens is quite high, i.e., 2.75 g tetramisole/kg of body weight. Minimum toxic levels of the drug in chickens apparently have not been established but exceed 640 mg/kg. In geese, however, a dose of 300 mg/kg is known to be toxic. In chickens therapeutic dosages of levamisole HCl (36–40 mg/kg) cause no undesirable side effects and egg production, fertility, and hatchability are not adversely affected.

The narrow margin of safety of tetramisole in horses has not allowed for acceptance of this drug in equines. A single dose of 20 mg/kg may cause deaths; the therapeutic dose of 15 mg/kg is dangerously close to this figure. Levamisole can be administered at 8 mg/kg and thus is safer than tetramisole but its moderate efficacy for *Strongylus vulgaris* (63%) and small strongyles limits its usefulness as a broad-spectrum drug.

Dogs and cats are much more tolerant of oral than parenteral administration of tetramisole. When given to dogs orally, doses of 20 mg/kg are well tolerated and even 40 and 80 mg/kg are not fatal although vomiting occurs. When given subcutaneously, however, tetramisole at 40 mg/kg is fatal to dogs in 10–15 minutes. Even at 20 mg/kg subcutaneously, the drug causes severe reactions in dogs although they persist for only about 20 minutes. On the basis of these findings, the oral route of administering tetramisole is recommended for dogs and cats.

CONTRAINDICATIONS

Neither tetramisole nor levamisole should be administered within 72 hours of slaughtering swine or within 7 days of slaughtering cattle or sheep. Milk from dairy cows apparently is free of residues of levamisole or tetramisole within 48 hours but at present no withdrawal time for lactating dairy cows has been established by the FDA. Consequently, products containing these drugs should not be administered to lactating cattle that produce milk for human consumption. The drug is labeled, "Do not administer to dairy animals of breeding age."

Due to relatively frequent and pronounced tissue reactions of injectable levamisole, this method of administration is not recommended for cattle nearing slaughter condition and weight. It is recommended for cattle in stocker or feeder condition.

There are no specific contraindications in the administration of levamisole or tetramisole with other drugs. Some commercial preparations, in fact, combine two drugs for oral administration; e.g., Nilzan contains tetramisole and a fasciolicide, oxychlozanide.

DOSAGE

Tetramisole. In cattle, sheep, goats, and pigs, a dose of 15 mg/kg of body weight is recommended, but not to exceed a total of 4.5 g for cattle in a single oral or subcutaneous dose.

Levamisole. In cattle, sheep, goats, and pigs, a dose of 8 mg/kg of body weight is recommended in a single oral or subcutaneous dose.

TETRAHYDROPYRIMIDINES

PYRANTEL

Pyrantel INN (Banminth, Strongid) was introduced as a broad-spectrum anthelmintic in 1966, initially for use against GI parasites of sheep. It subsequently has come to be used in cattle, swine, horses,

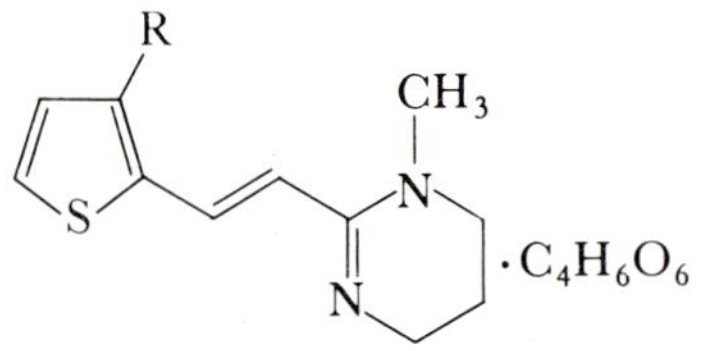

FIG. 52.5.

and dogs. Its FDA approval in the United States, however, is presently only for swine and horses.

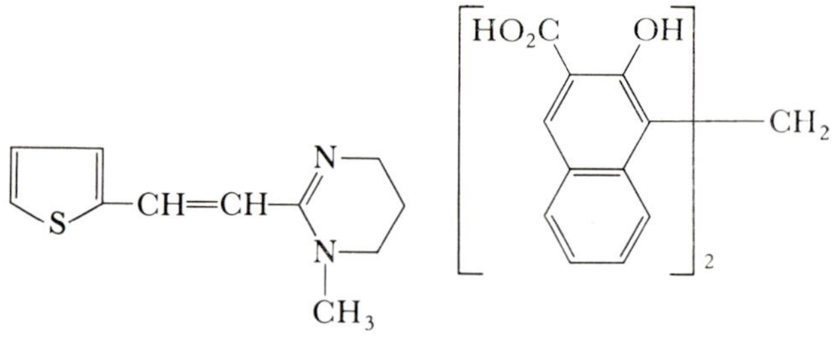

CHEMISTRY

Pyrantel is an imidazothiazole derivative. Its chemical formula is 1,4,5,6-tetrahydro-1-methyl-2-[*trans*-2-(2-thienyl)vinyl]-pyrimidine INN. It is prepared for commercial use as the tartrate or pamoate salt, the former being used principally as a veterinary anthelmintic and the latter for human usage. The structural formulas of the tartrate and pamoate salts of pyrantel and the methyl-substituted analog, morantel, are given in Fig. 52.5.

Pyrantel salts are relatively stable in the solid phase; aqueous solutions of the salts, however, upon exposure to light are subject to photoisomerization with resultant loss of potency. It is therefore recommended that the drug be used immediately after preparation of a drench suspension.

PHARMACODYNAMICS

Following oral administration, pyrantel tartrate is well absorbed in the pig, dog, and rat. There is less absorption of the drug by ruminants. Concentrations of radioactivity from the labeled drug is maximum in the plasma of the dog and pig at 2–3 hours after dosing but is highly variable in ruminants. The dog achieves the highest plasma levels (4.3 μg/ml).

The drug is quickly metabolized in the body, little of it surviving intact by the time it is excreted. Individual metabolites have not been identified but at least one-half of the metabolites are known to contain the *N*-methyl-1,3-propanediamine skeleton of the tetrahydropyrimidyl ring. This portion of the drug molecule evidently is more resistant to metabolic attack than the thiophene ring.

Urinary excretion of the drug is greatest in the dog and pig, accounting for about 40% of the dose in the dog and 34% in the pig, most of which is excreted as metabolites. The dog is the only species excreting more of the drug or its metabolites in the urine than in the feces. In ruminants, urinary excretion accounts for about 25% of the original dose, much of the remainder passing unchanged in the feces. In rats, urinary excretion of the drug is minor; bile is the major route of excretion of metabolites of the absorbed drug. The importance of excretion of the drug in the bile of other animals has not been investigated.

The pamoate salt of pyrantel is poorly soluble in water, which offers the advantage of reduced absorption of this salt from the gut and allowing the drug to reach and be effective against pinworms in the lower end of the large intestine. Formulations of the pamoate salt are especially beneficial for use against pinworm infections of the lower digestive tract of the human being and the equine.

The pharmacological effects of pyrantel tartrate on the host are similar to the effects of levamisole hydrochloride, diethylcarbamazine citrate (DEC), and morantel tartrate. All of these anthelmintics have biological properties that are shared with acetylcholine and act essentially by mimicking the effects of excessive amounts of this natural neurotransmitter. Acetylcholine in physiological amounts serves as a neurotransmitter by stimulating all autonomic ganglia, the adrenal medullas, the chemoreceptors of the carotid and aortic bodies, and the neuromuscular junction. In excess amounts of acetylcholine, however, these sites are paralyzed. It is this paralytic action that pyrantel, morantel, levamisole, and DEC have. It is similar to the paralytic effect caused by nicotine; thus the action of these anthelmintics is referred to as nicotinelike. In anesthetized dogs the use of these anthelmintics results in a precipitous pressor response and an enhancement of rate and depth of respiration. These effects are antagonized by hexamethonium and the pressor responses are nullified by the adrenergic blocking agent, phentolamine (Forbes 1972b).

MODE OF ACTION

Pyrantel tartrate is a depolarizing neuromuscular blocking agent in both nematodal parasites and the vertebrate host. The drug probably produces paralysis of worms by causing a contracture of the musculature similar to the contracture-inducing action of acetylcholine (Aubry et al. 1970). Pyrantel, as well as its analog morantel, although slower than acetylcholine in initiating the contracture, is 100 times more potent than acetylcholine. The effect of acetylcholine is easily reversible; that of pyrantel or morantel is not.

In contrast to the contractual action of pyrantel on *Ascaris* musculature, the action of piperazine results in relaxation. This suggests that the antagonistic actions of the two drugs may counterbalance each other. This is not the case, however, since simultaneous administration of the two drugs has shown no interference in the individual efficacies of each drug.

FORMULATION AND ADMINISTRATION

Both the tartrate and pamoate salts of pyrantel are used for treating horses. Pyrantel tartrate (Strongylid, Banminth) is generally administered dry in the feed rather than in solution to minimize the absorption of this highly soluble drug. A powder formulation containing 11.3% pyrantel tartrate is prepared for treating horses and ponies. A pelleted formulation containing 1.25% of the drug is prepared for use in colts and can also be used in horses and ponies. The amount of powder or pellet formulation necessary to yield a dosage of 12.5 mg/kg of body weight is mixed in an amount of feed normally consumed at one feeding.

The markedly less soluble pyrantel pamoate (Strongylid T) can be administered to horses or ponies by stomach tube or dose syringe as well as adding it to the feed. It is supplied commercially as a caramel flavored suspension and can be given directly by dose syringe or added to the grain ration. For administration by stomach tube the appropriate dose of pyrantel pamoate is mixed with the desired quantity of water and used immediately. Regardless of the method of administration, a dosage of 6.6 mg of the pyrantel base/kg of body weight should be used. The compound contains 34.6% base activity.

Fasting of horses prior to or following treatment with pyrantel is not necessary.

A powdered premix formulation containing 10.6% pyrantel tartrate is available for treating parasitic infections of swine via the feed. A dose of 22 mg/kg of body weight is used for a single therapeutic treatment. It is recommended that a sufficient quantity (i.e., 0.88 g of pyrantel tartrate/40 kg of body weight) of the powder formulation be added to 1 kg of meal ration (nonpelleted) after an overnight fast. Large quantities of medicated feed for the single therapeutic treatment can be prepared by adding 800 g of pyrantel tartrate to 1 ton of feed. A hog consuming 1 lb of the medicated feed/40 lb of body weight receives essentially a dosage of 22 mg/kg. The medicated feed is consumed by swine without reluctance. Drinking water should be available during the fasting and treatment periods.

The premix of pyrantel tartrate is also used to prepare medicated feeds that are employed mainly as a prophylactic measure against swine parasites. A 0.0106% medicated feed (96 g of pyrantel tartrate/ton of feed) can be fed to swine continuously as an aid in the prevention of migration and establishment of *Ascaris suum* and *Oeso-*

phagostomum infections. A 3-day use aids in the removal of existing ascarid burdens.

Pyrantel is administered to ruminants as a drench via a dosing gun. The drench is prepared by dissolving the powdered drug in water to make a 5% solution and administered in necessary quantity to yield a dose of 25 mg/kg of body weight.

ANTHELMINTIC SPECTRUM

Horse. In general, the activity of pyrantel on GI parasites of the horse and pony is independent of the method of administration (i.e., drench vs addition to the feed) and of the salt, whether it be the hydrochloride, tartrate, or pamoate of pyrantel (Lyons et al. 1974). The activity of each of the three salts is characterized by consistently high efficacies for *Parascaris equorum* (mature worms 86%–100%, immature worms 100%) *Strongylus vulgaris* (92%–100%), *Strongylus equinus* (100%), and the pinworm *(Probstmayria vivipara)* (93%–99%). Less effective and more variable activity of the three salts exists for *Strongylus edentatus* (42%–100%), small strongyles (69%–99%), immature *Oxyuris equi* (33%–100%), and mature *O. equi* (7%–100%). A specific study of one of the small strongyles, *Trichonema,* indicates that pyrantel is ineffective against histotropic stages although lumen-dwelling larval and immature worms are effectively removed.

Pyrantel is inactive to only slightly active against equine stomach worms *(Habronema muscae* and *Draschia megastoma),* tapeworms, and *Trichostrongylus axei.* It is also inactive against bots *(Gasterophilus* spp.) but can be administered simultaneously with carbon disulfide which is efficacious for bots. Simultaneous administration of the two drugs does not interfere with the singular activity of either compound.

Swine. Pyrantel tartrate is used in swine principally for its activity against infections of *Ascaris* and *Oesophagostomum.* When given in the feed at a dosage of 22 mg/kg of body weight it is effective against *Ascaris suum,* not only the adults but also histotropic stages and the infective ascarid larva following its hatching from the ingested egg and before penetrating the gut wall. Thus the drug provides prophylactic as well as therapeutic benefits against swine ascarids, especially when fed continuously at low levels (96 g of pyrantel tartrate/ton of feed). A single therapeutic dose of the drug is reported to be 99% effective for the lumen stages of *Oesophagostomum* and ineffective for swine whipworms.

In trials comparing the efficacies of single therapeutic doses of the principally used swine anthelmintics (haloxon, methyridine, pyrantel tartrate, tetramisole, TBZ, parbendazole, and dichlorvos) Plé and Abram (1971) maintained that parbendazole and dichlorvos yielded the highest efficacies against ascarid, nodular worm, and whipworm infections of swine.

Although pyrantel tartrate makes no label claims for activity against the swine stomach worm, *Hyostrongylus rubidus,* tests by Enigk et al. (1971) yielded efficacies of 96% for adult 24-day-old worms, 73% for immature 12-day-old worms, and 60% for 5-day-old larvae of this parasite.

Sheep and Cattle. Pyrantel tartrate is highly effective as a broad-spectrum anthelmintic for both sheep and cattle. Its use in lambs has been reported to result in slight to significantly increased weight gains over those of untreated controls or lambs treated with tetramisole, TBZ, methyridine, or bephenium hydroxynaphthoate. Specifically, pyrantel tartrate is quite effective in sheep, cattle, or goats against *Haemonchus contortus* (including the TBZ-resistant strains), *Ostertagia ostertagia* and *O. circumcinta, Trichostrongylus axei* and *T. colubriformis, Nematodirus battus* and *N. spathiger,* and *Cooperia* spp. Its activity against *Oesophagostomum* and *Chabertia* is usually but not consistently good.

The activity of pyrantel tartrate against the immature and larval stages of many of the above ruminant parasites is not known. It has been determined, however, that at the therapeutic dosage of 25 mg/kg the drug is more than 99% effective against 7-day-old, 81% effective against 14-day-old, and 94% effective against 21-day-old stages of *T. colubriformis* in sheep. It is less effective against these same stages of *T. colubriformis* in cattle. The drug is 100% effective for *N. battus* regardless of the stage of the parasite, i.e., 7, 14, or 21 days of age. Comparatively, methyridine gives similar high efficacies against these stages of *N. battus,* but halaxon has almost no efficacy against the young stages of this parasite and only approximately 35% efficacy against the adult worms.

Against *Ostertagia* infections, pyrantel, although highly effective against lumen-dwelling immature and mature worms, is only 42% effective against 7-day-old histotropic stages in sheep and markedly less effective against this same stage in cattle. Nevertheless, pryantel is preferred over methyridine or phenothiazine for the treatment of bovine ostertagiasis.

In addition to its therapeutic use in sheep, pyrantel tartrate can be used prophylactically in this host at a dosage of 3 mg/kg of body weight daily. Approximately 97% fewer GI worms occurred in sheep so treated than in untreated controls examined after a 50-day period.

Dog. Although not approved by the FDA for use in dogs, the pamoate or hydrochloride salts of pyrantel are highly effective (95%) for the common hookworms *(Ancylostoma caninum)* and ascarids *(Toxocara canis)* at single dosages of 6–25 and 5–7 mg/kg of body weight, respectively. Daily doses of the hydrochloride (2.5 mg/kg/day) for 30 days apparently prevented the establishment of hookworm and ascarid infections in dogs (Bradley and Conway 1970).

The hydrochloride and pamoate salts of pyrantel have limited efficacy against canine whipworms but these same salts of the meta-oxyphenyl analog of pyrantel, known as CP-14,445, have been investigated recently (Howes 1972). Especially the hydrochloride salt of this analog appears promising as an antiwhipworm compound.

SAFETY AND TOXICITY

In general, the salts of pyrantel are free of toxic effects in all hosts at dosages up to approximately 7 times the therapeutic dose. The oral LD50 of pyrantel tartrate in mice is 175 mg/kg and in rats 170 mg/kg. Dogs in chronic toxicity studies showed ill effects when administered the drug at 50 or more mg/kg/day for 3 months but no adverse effects when the dosage was reduced to 20 mg/kg/day for the same period.

Pyrantel is safe for horses and ponies of all ages including sucklings, weanlings, pregnant mares, and studs. At 20 times the recommended dose in horses, ponies, and foals pyrantel pamoate shows no adverse clinical effects or changes in blood cell values, serum cholinesterase, or glutamic oxalacetic transaminase.

Pyrantel tartrate is slightly less tolerated in horses than the pamoate salt. The tartrate salt (100 mg/kg) produced death in 1 of 3 horses. Toxic signs preceding death included a marked increase in respiration rate, profuse sweating, and incoordination. No signs of toxicity occurred following administration of 75 mg/kg.

Ataxia is seen in some cattle treated with a high dosage of pyrantel tartrate (200 mg/kg). The toxic dose of the drug in pigs is not known.

CONTRAINDICATIONS

Pyrantel is not recommended for use in severely debilitated animals presumably because its pharmacologic action (nicotine-like properties) is more pronounced in these hosts.

Withdrawal periods exist for swine and ruminants designated for human consumption. Due to lack of metabolism data in horses, the drug should not be used in horses intended for human consumption.

Because of its cholinergic properties, Forbes (1972a) suggests that administration of pyrantel together with other cholinergic drugs or substances with anticholinergic properties (e.g., organophosphorus compounds) may lead to potentiation of toxicity. Apparently no clinical evidence substantiates this claim (Smith 1973). Thus the labeling for pyrantel products indicates safety of pyrantel for simultaneous use with insecticides, tranquilizers, muscle relaxants, and central nervous system (CNS) depressants.

DOSAGE

Pyrantel tartrate
- Horse: 12.5 mg/kg of body weight
- Swine: 22 mg/kg of body weight
- Sheep, cattle, goat: 25 mg/kg of body weight

Pyrantel pamoate
- Horse: 6.6 mg (base)/kg of body weight

Morantel

Morantel INN (Banminth II) is the methyl ester analog of pyrantel. Principally the tartrate salt but also the fumarate salt is prepared for veterinary anthelmintic use. For the structural formula of morantel tartrate, see Fig. 52.5.

The salts of morantel have greater anthelmintic activity than the parent compound, pyrantel; their pharmacological properties are similar. The efficacies of both the tartrate and fumarate salts are quite good against the adult and immature stages of *Haemonchus, Ostertagia, Trichostrongylus, Cooperia,* and *Nematodirus* of ruminants. Morantel tartrate is marketed as an orally administered aqueous solution at a dosage of 10 mg/kg for sheep and 8.8 mg/kg for cattle. The fumarate salt is similarly administered to sheep at a dosage of 12.5 mg/kg.

Pharmacologically, morantel tartrate is a safer drug than pyrantel tartrate. The oral LD50 of pyrantel tartrate for mice is only 170 mg/kg while that of morantel tartrate is 5 g/kg. Chronic toxicity studies in sheep indicate that dosages up to 40 mg morantel tartrate/kg/day orally can be given for 60 days without untoward effects. The drug is absorbed rapidly from the abomasum and upper small intestine of sheep. Peak blood levels are reached 4–6 hours after administration. The drug is quickly metabolized, presumably in the liver, and 17% of the initial dose is excreted in the urine as metabolites within 96 hours after dosing; the remainder is excreted in the feces.

Since the recent introduction of morantel, its use as a ruminant anthelmintic and investigations of other potential uses have grown steadily in European countries. It is presently not approved for use in the United States.

ORGANOPHOSPHORUS COMPOUNDS

A number of organophosphorus compounds have come to be used as anthelmintics in the past decade. In general they have had their origin as pesticides and only subsequently have found use as anthelmintics. There are five such compounds widely used today: dichlorvos, trichlorfon, haloxon, naphthalophos, and crufomate. The first two are principally used against parasitic infections in horses, dogs, or pigs, the latter three against parasites of ruminants.

Mode of Action in Relation to Toxicity

Evidence now strongly supports the hypothesis that the main effect of organophosphorus compounds on animal parasites is an inhibition of nematodal cholinesterase, leading to an interference with neuromuscular transmission and consequent toxicity to the parasite (Knowles and Casida 1966). It is generally accepted that acetylcholine is involved in neural transmission in nematodes and that the enzyme cholinesterase, now identified in a number of nematodes, serves to destroy the transmitter, i.e., acetylcholine, as it does in other animal groups (Lee 1965). The cholinesterase of nematodes can be removed from its assumed physiological role by complexing with organophosphorus drugs in very dilute amounts. In the absence of the cholinesterase the unrestrained acetylcholine of the parasite presumably accumulates in unnatural quantities, which results in malfunctioning of the parasite's neuromuscular systems. These assumptions are made because a direct correlation is known to exist between the inhibition of the cholinesterase of certain parasites by organophosphorus drugs and the toxicity of the same drug for the parasite. From a large number of organophosphates tested in *Ascaris* by Knowles and Casida (1966), those drugs that were poisonous to the parasite were also inhibitors of the parasite's cholinesterase; the drugs that did not inhibit cholinesterase were not toxic.

The cholinesterases of host and parasite and those of different species of parasites vary in their susceptibility to organophosphorus drugs (Sanderson 1970, 1973). The cholinesterase of *Haemonchus contortus,* for example, forms an irreversible complex with the organophosphate haloxon, which evidently results in toxicity to the worm and eventual expulsion from treated cattle. The cholinesterase of ascarids, on the other hand, is not as susceptible to haloxon as that of *Haemonchus.* The ascarid cholinesterase is bound by haloxon but it is a reversible complex. The ascarid enzymatic activity recovers to near pretreatment levels within 32 hours after treatment with haloxon. Nevertheless, this is sufficient "stunning" time for the worms to be effectively expelled by peristalsis from the host's gut. A shorter stunning time evidently occurs when the drug is used against *Nematodirus* and *Oesophagostomum columbianum* since the efficacy of haloxon for these parasites is generally poor.

The degree of safety of organophosphates for the host is probably related to the lack of susceptibility of the host cholinesterase to the drug. The complex formed between sheep erythrocyte acetylcholinesterase and haloxon is quickly reversible, which probably accounts for the lack of toxicity of this drug in sheep given a therapeutic dose. On the other hand, haloxon is very toxic in geese and, indeed, the brain cholinesterase of geese is found to be irreversibly complexed by the drug. These findings illustrate the fact that the cholinesterase enzymes among mammalian hosts and certainly between host and nematode are not identical. In the development of organophosphorus anthelmintics, an attempt has been made to use this information to produce compounds with maximum effect against the parasite but minimum toxicity to the host.

General Efficacy

The range of activities of organophosphorus compounds in general cover the principal parasites of horses, pigs, and dogs satisfactorily but are somewhat restricted in activity against the parasites of ruminants. In ruminants, the organophosphates generally have satisfactory efficacy for nematodal parasites of the abomasum (especially *Haemonchus)* and small intestine but lack satisfactory efficacy for parasites of the bowel *(Oesophagostomum* and *Chabertia).* By contrast, the nonorganophosphorus broad-spectrum anthelmintics (benzimidazoles, tetramisole, and pyrimidines, i.e., pyrantel and morantel) are effective to various degrees against nematodes of both the lower and upper digestive tracts. Despite their somewhat restricted activity in ruminants, the organophosphates have become widely used in cattle and sheep because of their lower cost. In general, satisfactory control of ruminant parasites is obtained except in endemic areas of *Oesophagostomum* and *Chabertia* infections. Where the latter infections occur, it is generally recommended that following two consecutive treatments with organophosphorus compounds (e.g., haloxon or naphthalophos), cattle or sheep should be treated with a nonorganophosphorus broad-spectrum anthelmintic (Gordon 1973). In general it is advisable to alternate organophosphorus anthelmintics with anthelmintics of other classes to prevent the development of drug resistance by the parasites.

Precautions in Use

Certain precautions should be followed when using organophosphorus anthelmintics. These are discussed fully in the toxicology section of this book but are mentioned here briefly in conjunction with the use of organophosphates as anthelmintics. Generally, when treating animals with an organophosphate, the animals should not be treated simultaneously or within a few days with other cholinesterase-inhibiting drugs (eserine and prostigmin), pesticides, organophosphorus and carbamate insecticides, or muscle relaxants (e.g., succinylcholine). In cases where animals have been treated with an organophosphorus anthelmintic and a topical insecticide is needed, the insecticide should be limited to pyrethins, rotenone, or chlorinated hydrocarbon insecticides.

The margin of safety of organophosphorus anthelmintics is generally less than that of the broad-spectrum anthelmintics (benzimidazoles and pyrimidines); thus strict attention to dosage is necessary. This is important not only for the safety of the animal but also from the standpoint that higher than normal dosages may result in illegal residues of the drug in animal tissues and milk. Because of residues, organophosphorus drugs (except coumaphos) are not generally approved for use in lactating dairy animals. Also a withdrawal time of at least 7 days is generally required before slaughter. Additionally, the use of organophosphates within 30 days of parturition generally is not recommended, especially in the equine (Bello et al. 1974).

Toxic signs of organophosphorus poisoning include frequent defecation and urination plus vomition (especially in dogs and cats), watering of eyes, and muscular twitching. Subsequently, salivation, diarrhea, and muscular weakness occur. Toxic signs are more likely to develop in treated animals that are sick or in animals under stress, such as those just shipped, dehorned, castrated, or weaned within the preceding 3 weeks. The use of organophosphorus anthelmintics is usually contraindicated in such animals. When toxic signs occur, atropine sulfate or 2-PAM (pyridine-2-aldoxime) is usually antidotal. For further details on signs of organophosphorus poisoning and treatment refer to Toxicity under the individual drugs following and the general section on toxicology in this book.

Dichlorvos

Dichlorvos (Atgard, Equigard, Equigel, Task, Task Tabs, Worm-A-Cide) is unique among the organophosphorus anthelmintics in that it can be incorporated into polyvinyl chloride resin pellets. The volatile dichlorvos is released slowly from the undigestible pellets as they pass the length of the digestive tract. This allows for a therapeutic concentration against parasites all along the digestive tube. This slow release formulation of dichlorvos also is a safety factor for the host in that the normal host can detoxify the drug as it is absorbed over a 2- to 3-day period rather than having to detoxify a sudden concentrated dose not formulated in resin.

The compound is used as an anthelmintic principally in dogs, cats, swine, and horses. A chief advantage of dichlorvos over other broad-spectrum anthelmintics in dogs and swine is its efficacy against whipworms.

CHEMISTRY

Dichlorvos (or dichlorovos), abbreviated DDVP, chemically is *O,O*-dimethyl *O*-(2,2-dichlorovinyl) phosphate. It is a volatile substance that is easily destroyed by oxidizing agents and/or moisture (hydrolysis). It must be stored at temperatures below 80° F to assure proper shelf life. The compound is prepared by reacting trimethyl phosphite and chloral as shown in Fig. 52.6. Analogs of DDVP can be similarly prepared by the reaction of chloral with other trialkyl phosphites. DDVP and its analogs are called vinyl phosphates and are exemplified by the structure shown in Fig. 52.7. Vinyl phosphates are generally recognized for their in-

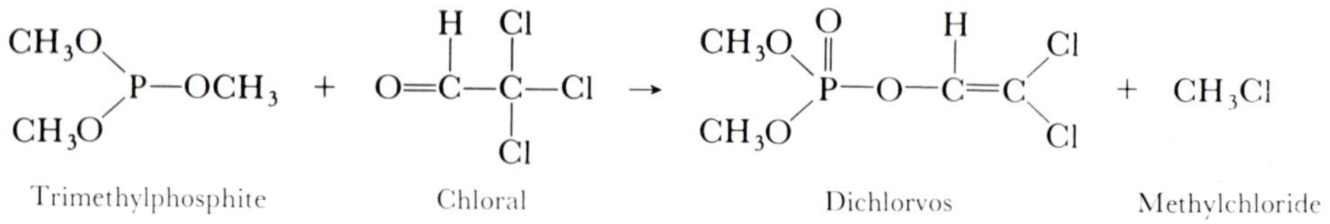

$$(CH_3O)_2P{-}OCH_3 \;+\; O{=}\overset{H}{C}{-}CCl_2{-}Cl \;\rightarrow\; (CH_3O)_2\overset{O}{\overset{\|}{P}}{-}O{-}\overset{H}{C}{=}CCl_2 \;+\; CH_3Cl$$

Trimethylphosphite · Chloral · Dichlorvos · Methylchloride

Fig. 52.6.

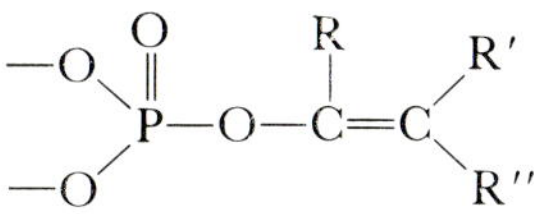

$$\begin{array}{l}-O\\-O\end{array}\!\!>\overset{O}{\overset{\|}{P}}-O-\overset{R}{\overset{|}{C}}=C\!<\!\begin{array}{l}R'\\R''\end{array}$$

FIG. 52.7.

secticidal properties; dichlorvos, additionally, has anthelmintic properties.

FORMULATIONS

The process of incorporating DDVP (or certain other liquids or soft polymers) into vinyl resins (usually polyvinyl chloride) is called plasticization. This plasticizing procedure allows for the preparation of stable slow-release formulations of DDVP in a plastic (resin) vehicle. The resin vehicle is cut into small pellets. When the pellets are ingested by an animal, the diffusion of the volatile DDVP from the pellets creates a concentration gradient of the drug. As the undigestible pellets traverse the GI tract from one site to another, DDVP continues to diffuse into the surrounding fluid system at a measurable rate (Hass 1970). This allows the drug to come into contact with helminths located throughout the digestive tract. The continual depletion of the drug gradually reduces the concentration gradient so that there is a correspondingly steady decrease in the diffusion rate. Pellets containing 20% DDVP formulated for a moderate release rate (Atgard V) will release approximately 48% of the incorporated DDVP in a 48-hour period as it traverses the digestive tract of swine. When passed in the feces (48–96 hours after ingestion), the pellets still contain approximately 45%–50% of the original quantity of DDVP. The DDVP continues to be released into the moisture associated with the fecal mass. Usually the concentration of the drug in the feces is sufficient to act as an effective insecticide against fecal fly larvae.

In general, plasticizing DDVP into a resin for administration to animals overcomes two principal difficulties associated with the properties of the drug itself. First, resin formulation markedly increases the safety margin of DDVP by allowing for the slow release of an otherwise excessively volatile and toxic drug. Second, the resin pellet protects the drug reservoir in the vehicle against slow hydrolytic degradation.

The geometry, size, and method of formulation (including coating or not coating) of the pellet plus the quantity of DDVP incorporated allow for a range of diffusion rates suitable for different host animals. The pellets formulated for dogs (Task), for example, are smaller in size so as to allow faster release of the drug in the short digestive tract of dogs as compared to the larger pellets (Atgard V) which have a moderate release rate in the longer digestive tract of swine.

ANTHELMINTIC SPECTRUM

Dog and Cat. DDVP causes total or nearly total expulsion of canine and/or feline hookworms (*Ancylostoma caninum, A. braziliensis, A. tubaeforme* and *Uncinaria stenocephala*), ascarids (*Toxocara canis, T. cati* and *Toxascaris leonina*), and the whipworm (*Trichuris vulpis*). In general, greater than 90% efficacy occurs with canine whipworm burdens of 1 to approximately 100 worms. When the burden exceeds 100 worms, the effectiveness of DDVP is reduced and retreatment is necessary.

There is little to no activity against the migrating larval forms of ascarids and hookworms or any efficacy for tapeworms. Residual DDVP from pellets passed in the stools of treated dogs is effective in reducing the numbers of developing infective larvae (Kalkofen 1971).

Swine. DDVP is the first broad-spectrum anthelmintic for use in swine. Collectively, different formulations of DDVP when administered at the recommended dosage level are effective in removing greater than 90% of the 4th stage larvae, juveniles, and mature adults of *Ascaris suum;* the swine nodular worm (*Oesophagostomum* spp.); the whipworm (*Trichuris suis*); and mature (but not immature) forms of two stomach worms (*Hyostrongylus rubidus* and *Ascarops strongylina*). It is not effective in the treatment of infestations due to the thorny-headed worm (*Macracanthorynchus hirudinaceus*) or *Strongyloides ransomi.*

There is little or no activity against larval forms migrating or buried in the intestinal mucosa. The hatchability of strongylid eggs passed in swine stools is not affected by the presence of the DDVP resin pellets; however, there is a detrimental effect upon a portion of the freshly hatched and free-living *Oesophagostomum* larvae.

Horse. DDVP is effectively used in horses against helminths and bots. It is 90%–100% effective against two of the three large strongyles (*Strongylus vulgaris* and *S. equinum*) as well as small strongyles, equine ascarids (*Parascaris equorum*), pinworms (*Oxyuris equi* and *Probstmayria vivipara*), and both migrating and sessile bots (*Gastrophilus intestinalis* and *G. nasalis*). Its efficacy against *S. edentatus* is approximately 75% (Drudge and Lyons 1972). Due to limited numbers of infections of the stomach worm, *Habronema* spp., among test animals treated with DDVP, the efficacy of the compound for this parasite is unknown.

Ruminants. Although its anthelmintic spectrum is fairly acceptable in cattle (Bris et al. 1968; Poeschel and Todd 1972) and sheep (Todd 1962), DDVP does not have FDA approval for use in ruminants due to a rather narrow safety margin.

Poultry. DDVP cannot be used in poultry because birds accumulate the resin pellets in their gizzards. The continuous release of the drug from a single locus can result in toxicity.

MODE OF ACTION

Like other organophosphorus compounds, DDVP inhibits cholinesterase enzymes, e.g., acetylcholinesterase, by phosphorylating the esteratic site. It is one of the most potent inhibitors of ascarid acetylcholinesterase both *in vitro* and *in vivo* and the drug has been known to be toxic to ascarids in minute amounts (Knowles and Casida 1966). The complexing of the parasite enzyme with the drug is thought to be associated with the toxicity to the worms and thus to be the mode of activity of DDVP.

PHARMACODYNAMICS

Studies indicate that following oral administration DDVP is rapidly absorbed from the host's digestive tract and is rapidly detoxified in the liver (Hass 1970). The pure nonplasticized compound evidently reaches toxic levels in the blood rather readily before detoxification can occur but formulation of DDVP in resin restricts the quantity of drug available for absorption from the host's digestive tract at any one time. Thus in the latter case, blood levels of DDVP are seldom high enough to produce toxic reactions.

The biochemistry of metabolism and detoxification of DDVP in the host is not known with certainty. The metabolite most likely to be formed initially is dichloroacetaldehyde (Robinson and Ziegler 1968). Other potential metabolites include dichloroethanol, dichloroacetic acid, desmethyl dichlorvos, and phosphorus-containing compounds. Almost none of these potential metabolites have actually been identified chemically, perhaps because of such rapid metabolic transformation. There is no evidence, however, that the metabolites are toxic. They do not persist as tissue residues and only trace levels are found in the milk of lactating mammals (Casida et al. 1962). Excretion is via the urine and feces and in the expired air as carbon dioxide.

There is no evidence that therapeutic doses of DDVP cause any interference with normal liver function. Levels of enzymes, e.g., serum glutamic pyruvic transaminase, serum glutamic oxalic transaminase, and serum alkaline phosphatase, are not altered by therapeutic administration of the drug except occasionally in greyhounds (Snow 1971). An increased level of serum enzymes in 1 of 10 treated dogs of this breed suggests liver damage, but no clinical signs of toxicity occurred in Snow's studies.

The principal effect of absorption of DDVP into the systemic circulation is the inhibition of the host's cholinesterase enzymes, especially inhibition of cholinesterase of the nervous system. The administration of the recommended dosage of DDVP to dogs causes a slight depression in red blood cell acetylcholinesterase and serum cholinesterase. These values return to normal in 5–10 days as the drug-enzyme complex reverses. The significance of depression of serum and red blood cell cholinesterase levels is not known since animals have been observed to live for long periods during chronic toxicologic studies with little or no detectable circulating cholinesterase activity. Other hematologic values are not affected by single or weekly repeated therapeutic doses of DDVP.

In greyhounds and horses, the drug-cholinesterase complex is apparently not so easily reversible. Snow (1971) reports considerable inhibition of both acetylcholinesterase and serum cholinesterases and a very slow return to pretreatment levels—3 weeks in greyhounds and 8 weeks in horses. However, there were no clinical signs of toxicity in these animals.

TOXICITY

The oral LD50 for drug grade DDVP (unformulated) and DDVP incorporated into pellets (formulated) is given in Table 52.3. The safety of the formulated product is in the range of 6–20 times greater than unformulated DDVP and is related to the fact that DDVP is released slowly, giving time for the drug to be detoxified normally before it accumulates to toxic levels. Only the formulated form of the drug is available commercially.

The incidence of side effects following therapeutic use of formulated DDVP is low and generally of short duration. Softening of stools may be expected to occur in approximately 4% of treated animals and milk emesis in 3% of the cats and 8% of the preweaned puppies given DDVP. Other signs of organophosphorus toxicity occur less frequently and usually are seen within 30 minutes of administration of a therapeutic dose. These side effects generally regress without treatment within 1–2 hours. The severity and duration of side effects are dose related.

TABLE 52.3. Acute toxicities of dichlorvos

Animal	Approximate Oral LD50 Unformulated	Approximate Oral LD50 Formulated	LD_1 Formulated
		(mg/kg)	
Swine	50–300	. . .	≃ 2500
Horse	50–316	800–1600	> 648
Dog (young adult)	28–45	387–1262	182–384
Puppy	. . .	244	99
Cat and kitten	. . .	84	55

In high enough doses, clinical signs of toxicity appear and are associated with interference of transmission of nerve impulses. This suggests that DDVP inhibits host acetylcholinesterase at the neuromuscular junction. The substrate acetylcholine evidently accumulates at the neuronal junctions with a resultant overstimulation of the motor and parasympathetic fibers. The extent of neuromuscular junction inhibition by dichlorvos with a therapeutic dose has not been determined and it may not be as severe as the inhibition of red cell acetylcholinesterase (Snow 1971).

Typical signs of cholinergic poisoning following the administration of high doses of DDVP include muscular fasciculations, retching, emesis, frequent defecation of watery stools, pupil contraction, secretion of tears, and labored breathing associated with constriction of the bronchioles. These signs represent excessive parasympathetic stimulation, which occurs as a result of excess acetylcholine in the absence of the drug-complexed enzyme, acetylcholinesterase.

The fatal effects of DDVP in rabbits, cats, and dogs are the result of the slow and long-term depression of peripheral blood pressure, bronchial spasm, and respiratory paralysis (Hass 1970).

The clinical signs of dichlorvos poisoning may be counteracted by administration of either an anticholinergic agent, e.g., atropine, or a cholinesterase reactivator, e.g., 2-PAM.

CONTRAINDICATIONS

DDVP should not be administered

within a few days of treatment of or exposure to other cholinesterase-inhibiting compounds, nor should it be given in conjunction with other anthelmintics, tranquilizers, muscle relaxants, or modified live-virus vaccines.

Due to the increased peristalsis following administration of DDVP, the drug should not be given to animals suffering from diarrhea or severe constipation, horses with colic, or dogs with mechanical blockage of the intestinal tract. Intestinal intussusception as a result of using the drug (Task) occurs very rarely in young dogs. The use of the lower dose tablet form (Task Tab) in puppies appears to circumvent this problem. Neither a puppy nor a kitten should be treated with the drug until it attains a weight of 1 lb (0.45 kg) and is at least 10 days of age.

The use of DDVP in dogs infected with heartworms *(Dirofilaria immitis)* is contraindicated. Evidently the blood level of the drug following a therapeutic dose is occasionally sufficiently high to cause migration of the parasite with resultant occlusion of the pulmonary artery or one of its branches. Dogs from endemic heartworm areas should be examined for the presence of *D. immitis* before administering DDVP.

Treatment with DDVP is not contraindicated during the breeding, gestation, or lactation of animals. In studies in which the drug was fed at high dosage levels to sows prior to breeding and throughout gestation, there were no adverse effects upon conception, embryonic development, litter mortality, or weaning performance of the pigs when these parameters were compared to those of nonmedicated control animals (Batte et al. 1969; Collins et al. 1971). Similar uncomplicated findings have been observed with dogs on continuous feeding experiments and with cats given twice weekly and horses bimonthly doses of DDVP throughout the breeding, gestation, and lactation periods. Prevention of the contamination of farrowing pens with swine parasite ova is best accomplished by treating sows 4 days before transferring them to the farrowing pens, followed by a second treatment 3 weeks later.

ADMINISTRATION

DDVP-plasticized pellets can be administered in the feed of swine, dogs, horses, and ruminants. Normally, the required dose is mixed with approximately one-third of the regular meal to insure complete consumption. For the treatment of dogs, the packeted pellets are mixed with canned dog food and for other animals, with grain, meal, or crumble-type feed.

DDVP is available in tablet form (Task Tabs) for the treatment of puppies and cats. Additionally, gelatin capsules containing the medicated pellets are available as an alternate method of treatment of dogs and ruminants. The compound is also prepared in a gel (Equigel) for the treatment of young foals that are not yet eating grain. The gel formulation is administered by a syringe onto the tongue of the foal. In reference to the dosages listed below, one-half of the single dose followed by the other half in 8–24 hours is as efficacious as the single full dose. The split dosage schedule is advisable in risk animals that are very old, heavily parasitized, anemic, or otherwise debilitated.

DDVP is normally administered to pigs as early as 5–6 weeks of age, i.e., just prior to sexual maturity of the worms against which the drug is effective. It can be used in dogs of any age but should not be used in puppies or kittens less than 10 days of age. The gel formulation of DDVP is designed for use against ascarids and bots (but not strongyles) in nursing foals older than 5 weeks. Efficacy and safety studies in foals less than 5 weeks of age have not been made.

DOSAGE, SINGLE TREATMENT

Horse: feed formulation, 31.2–40.7 mg/kg of body weight

Foal: gel formulation, 20 mg/kg of body weight for treatment of bots and ascarids; 10 mg/kg of body weight at 3- to 4-week intervals during fly season for control of bots

Swine: 11.2–21.6 mg/kg of body weight

Dog: 27–33 mg/kg of body weight

Puppy and cat: 11 mg/kg of body weight

Haloxon

Haloxon INN (Halox, Loxon) is probably the safest organophosphorus anthelmintic for use in ruminants. Its primary efficacy is against parasites of the abomasum and small intestine; it has only limited activity against parasites of the large bowel. It is approved by the FDA for use in sheep, cattle, and goats in the United States but is not for horses, pigs, and birds, although certain parasites are very satisfactorily controlled by the drug in these hosts.

CHEMISTRY

Chemically, haloxon is 3-chloro-7-hydroxy-4-methylcoumarin bis(2-chloroethyl) phosphate INN. The structural formula is given in Fig. 52.8. It is a white powder with virtually no odor. It is insoluble in water, slightly soluble in petroleum ether and vegetable oils, and highly soluble in acetone and chloroform.

FORMULATIONS

For general commercial use haloxon has been formulated as a wettable powder, a liquid suspension, and a paste. The drug is palatable and can be administered in the feed of horses, pigs, and poultry.

ANTHELMINTIC SPECTRUM

Sheep. In studies throughout the western world, exceptional efficacy of haloxon for adult (28-day-old) forms of *Haemonchus, Trichostrongylus, Cooperia,* and *Strongyloides* has been found when the drug is given to sheep at a dosage rate of 40 mg/kg of body weight. Its activity is somewhat less but still good against *Ostertagia, Bunostomum,* and one of the large bowel worms

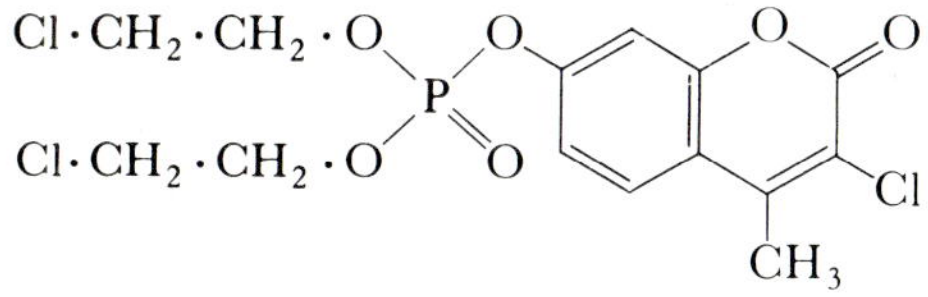

Haloxon

FIG. 52.8.

(Oesophagostomum venulosum). Its effect against *O. columbianum* is negligible. The activity against *Nematodirus* is variable and only slight activity occurs against *Chabertia* and *Trichuris.* Both pyrantel tartrate and methyridine are much more efficacious for *Nematodirus battus* infections in lambs than is haloxon (Gibson et al. 1969). Where control of nodular worms is needed, a mixture of piperazine with haloxon gives generally satisfactory results.

Haloxon is also larvicidal to varying degrees depending on the species and age of the parasite. At therapeutic dosages, 7- and 14-day-old *Haemonchus contortus, Cooperia curticei,* and *Trichostrongylus colubriformis* are almost completely eliminated while approximately 75% of 14-day-old worms and 44% of 7-day-old worms of *Ostertagia* spp. are eliminated.

Cattle. The activity of haloxon in cattle is similar to that in sheep, i.e., virtually complete control of *Haemonchus* and *Cooperia* (Baker and Douglas 1969; Benz 1972) and the ascarid, *Neoascaris.* The drug gives good, but not complete, efficacy against *Trichostrongylus, Ostertagia,* and *Oesophagostomum radiatum.* Again its activity against *Nematodirus* varies from good to mediocre. Its larvicidal activity is similar but overall somewhat less effective in cattle than in sheep.

Other Hosts. Although not approved by the FDA for use in swine, horses, or birds in the United States, haloxon has been found to be effective against certain parasites in these hosts. Approximately 100% of *Ascaris suum* and 50%–98% of *Oesophagostomum* spp. are removed from swine by a dosage of 35 mg/kg (Czipri 1970; Plé and Abram 1971). A higher dosage, 75 mg/kg, is necessary to give 75% efficacy for *Hyostrongylus.*

In horses, haloxon at a dosage rate of 60–75 mg/kg is satisfactorily effective against ascarids, pinworms, a number of species of small strongyles, and the large strongyle *(Strongylus vulgaris).* It is less effective (25%–42%) against *S. edentatus* and *S. equinus* (Cook 1973).

Domestic fowl, turkey, quail, and pigeons benefit from the use of haloxon against infections of *Capillaria obsignata* or *C. contorta* (but not *Hetarakis*). It is administered in the feed at the rate of 50–100 mg/kg of body weight. This dosage, however, is lethal for geese.

MODE OF ACTION

As appears to be true of other organophosphorus anthelmintics, haloxon acts on the neuromuscular system of the parasite by inhibiting cholinesterase. This apparently interferes with normal nervous transmission in nematodes, resulting in detachment from the wall of the digestive tract and expulsion by peristaltic movement of the host. The concentration of haloxon required to inhibit cholinesterase *in vitro* is extremely low, as little as 10^{-13} in the case of one parasite (Hart and Lee 1966).

For those parasites against which haloxon is highly efficacious, the nematodal cholinesterase-haloxon complex is apparently highly stable. This is true of the cholinesterase-haloxon complex of *Haemonchus,* which has been closely studied. The enzyme-haloxon complex of *Bunostomum,* however, is quite unstable and in fact is totally reversible in as little as 30 minutes. The failure of the drug against *Bunostomum* is attributed to the rapid recovery of the cholinesterase of the worm (Hart and Lee 1966). Any effects of haloxon inhibition are too short-lived to bring about removal of the worm.

Hart and Lee (1966) suggest that the lack of anthelmintic effect of haloxon against parasites of the lower digestive tract, i.e., *C. ovina, T. ovis,* and *O. columbianum,* is probably due to several factors: the resistance of their cholinesterases to inhibition, the long exposure to haloxon necessary for cholinesterase inhibition, and the small amount of drug that will reach the large bowel where these worms reside. The fact that *O. venulosum* (which also resides in the large bowel) is effectively removed by haloxon is associated with the fact that its cholinesterase is one of the most susceptible to inhibition by the drug.

PHARMACODYNAMICS

As are most anthelmintics, haloxon is readily absorbed from the gut, metabolized fairly rapidly, and excreted in the urine. The drug is hydrolyzed in the liver and plasma, evidently to nontoxic metabolites. The rapidity of hydrolysis of haloxon (and other halons) varies widely among individual sheep and is genetically determined, the higher rate of hydrolysis being due to the presence of one dominant allele that determines the presence or absence of an enzyme (A-esterase) necessary for rapid hydrolysis of the drug. In general, the incidence of ability to rapidly hydrolyze haloxon and similar compounds is between 20% and 30%. It is now established that those sheep rapidly hydrolyzing haloxon do not suffer ill effects from very high dosage levels (i.e., 3000 mg/kg) of the anthelmintic while toxic signs are seen in some sheep at one-tenth (300 mg/kg) the above dosage; the latter are slow hydrolyzers of haloxon.

SAFETY AND TOXICITY

Haloxon is probably the safest of the organophosphorus anthelmintics (Malone 1964). The relative freedom from toxic effects in the host (except certain birds) is probably due to the fact that mammals have cholinesterases that form unstable complexes with haloxon. Unlike closely related organophosphorus compounds, haloxon causes only slight depression of mammalian red cell cholinesterase, i.e., acetylcholinesterase. A therapeutic index of 3–4 for old ewes, 5–7 for young lambs, and approximately 5 for cattle has been confirmed among thousands of treated animals. The only side effect within these dosage ranges is an occasional transient anorexia.

At very large dosages (300–3000 mg/kg) of haloxon, toxic signs can be induced in some, but not all, sheep. These signs consist of anorexia, diarrhea, and death after several days. Some sheep and poultry show neurotoxicity in the form of posterior ataxia to bilateral posterior paresis at dosages above 353 mg/kg of body weight. Baker et al. (1970) have shown experimentally that sheep affected with neurotoxic signs at this dosage level do not possess the ability to rapidly hydrolyze the drug. Development of the neurotoxic signs occurred approximately 3 weeks after experimental administration of the high dosages of haloxon and resulted in death of 5 of the 7 sheep so affected. None of the sheep with the ability to rapidly hydrolyze haloxon developed neurotoxic signs and the depression of their red blood cell cholinesterase was less marked and the duration shorter than of the sheep that hydrolyzed haloxon slowly.

The extreme susceptibility of geese to haloxon poisoning is associated with the highly stable complex that haloxon forms with the cholinesterase in the nervous system of the goose.

Atropine is not an effective antidote to the toxic effects of haloxon. This suggests that cholinesterase inhibition in the host is not fully responsible for the toxic signs. Two-PAM serves as an effective antidote in geese but is not reported to be effective in other hosts.

CONTRAINDICATIONS

Haloxon, like other organophosphorus anthelmintics, should not be used simultaneously or within a few days of treatment with other cholinesterase-inhibiting drugs, pesticides, or chemicals, e.g., carbon tetrachloride.

The drug is intended for use in beef- and wool-producing animals and should not be used for treating dairy cattle or goats of breeding age or older because of milk residues. Dosing of sheep and beef cows during pregnancy and during the time of nursing the newborn has no adverse effect on parturition or the newborn. A 7-day preslaughter withdrawal period is required.

ADMINISTRATION AND DOSAGE

Haloxon is administered orally in bolus, drench, or paste form at a dosage rate of approximately 44 mg of active ingredient/kg of body weight to cattle and at a rate of 35–50 mg/kg to sheep and goats.

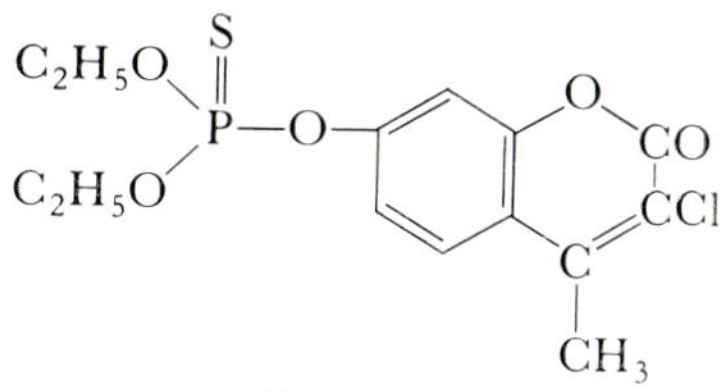

C_2H_5O, C_2H_5O, S, P—O—, O, CO, CCl, C, CH_3

Coumaphos

FIG. 52.9.

COUMAPHOS

Coumaphos (Asuntol, Baymix, Meldane), like many other organophosphates, was originally developed as a pesticide for the treatment of external parasites of livestock and later came to be used as an anthelmintic. It has an advantage over most other organophosphorus compounds in that it can be used in lactating animals without requiring the milk to be discarded after treatment.

Chemically, the compound is *O*-3-chloro-4-methyl-7-coumarinyl *O,O*-diethyl phosphorothioate INN. Its INN generic name is coumafos and its structural formula is given in Fig. 52.9.

ANTHELMINTIC SPECTRUM

Cattle and Sheep. Coumaphos is effective against the various species of adult *Haemonchus, Ostertagia, Trichostrongylus,* and *Cooperia.* Other parasites are irregularly affected.

Zoo Ruminants. Coumaphos likely has approximately the same anthelmintic spectrum in wild as in domesticated ruminants although critical studies have not been made. Whitetail deer, fallow deer, mule deer, elk, bison, and guanaco treated with coumaphos via the feed at a dosage of 2 mg/kg/day for 6 days tolerated the medication well and showed marked reduction in fecal egg counts (McWilliams et al. 1973).

Chickens. Coumaphos is efficacious for infections of *Capillaria obsignata* and markedly reduces the numbers of ascarids and cecal worms (Eleazer 1969). Naphthalophos gives better control of infections of *Capillaria contorta* than does coumaphos (Dawe et al. 1969). Coumaphos is designed for use in replacement pullets older than 8 weeks and in laying flocks.

TOXICITY

Coumaphos has a narrow range of safety, especially when it is administered as a drench rather than as a feed additive. The dose for drenching cattle, 15 mg/kg, is generally without side effects but deaths have occurred among cattle given doses of only 30 mg/kg. At a dosage of 20 mg/kg, mild signs of toxicity occur in cattle. In sheep, some toxic signs may be expected in a portion of cases even when the recommended dosage level for drenching is used.

Colored breeds of commercial layers are more sensitive to coumaphos medication than are white breeds. It is recommended, therefore, that colored layers not be treated while they are in production.

DOSAGE AND ADMINISTRATION

Beef and Dairy Cattle. Coumaphos is prepared as a feed supplement (Baymix) and applied as a top dressing over the daily ration at the rate of 2 mg/kg/day for 6 consecutive days. Additionally, a feed premix that can be mixed with the entire daily ration is available and should also be administered at the rate of 2 mg/kg/day for 6 days. The feed premix yields higher efficacies than the top dressing crumbles (Ciordia 1972a).

Drenching is the common means of administering coumaphos to beef cattle in Europe. The single dosage is 15 mg/kg of body weight. Greater anthelmintic activity occurs if the drench passes directly to the abomasum. The esophageal groove can be closed by premedication of the animal with sodium bicarbonate.

Sheep. Coumaphos (8 mg/kg of body weight) is given in a single drench. The esophageal groove should be closed by premedication of sheep with copper sulfate.

Chickens. Coumaphos is prepared as a feed premix (Meldane 2) for treating chickens via the ration. For replacement pullets, 40 ppm (0.004%) coumaphos-medicated feed is given for 10–14 days and for laying flocks, 30 ppm coumaphos-medicated feed is used for 14 days.

TRICHLORFON

Trichlorfon (Anthon, Dyrex, Freed) is another organophosphate used as an insecticide and pesticide for plants (Dylox) and livestock (Neguvon) as well as an anthelmintic for animals, principally the horse.

CHEMISTRY

The official nonproprietary name of trichlorfon is metrifonate INN, the chemical name, dimethyl (2,2,2-trichloro-1-hydroxyethyl)-phosphonate INN. Its structural formula is shown in Fig. 52.10.

FORMULATIONS AND ANTHELMINTIC SPECTRUM

Horse. Trichlorfon alone (Anthon, Dyrex) is administered to horses as a bolus or as granules mixed in a single day's ration. It is effective against bots *(Gastrophilus nasalis* and *G. intestinalis),* ascarids *(Parascaris equorum),* and pinworms *(Oxyuris equi).* The addition of piperazine and phenothiazine to trichlorfon (Dyrex T.F.) enhances the removal of ascarids and additionally eliminates small strongyles and *Strongylus vulgaris.* This mixture of drugs is administered to horses as a drench via stomach tube (i.e., tube formulation, T.F.).

Cutaneous habronemiasis is reported to be effectively treated with trichlorfon (Boyd and Bullard 1968; Joyce et al. 1972). In their studies, summer sores healed in approximately 30 days following a single intravenous treatment with trichlorfon (Neguvon) in a dose of 25 mg/kg of body weight given in 1 L of 5% dextrose or physiological saline solution. Half a grain (30 mg)

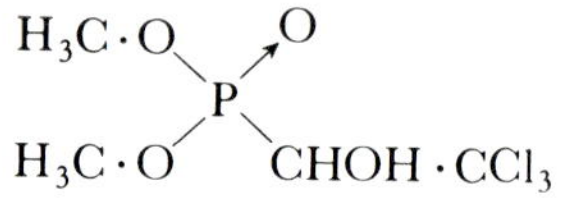

$$\begin{array}{c} H_3C\cdot O \quad\; O \\ \quad \diagdown \;\nearrow \\ P \\ \quad \diagup \;\diagdown \\ H_3C\cdot O \qquad CHOH\cdot CCl_3 \end{array}$$

Trichlorphon

FIG. 52.10.

of atropine sulfate was administered subcutaneously 20 minutes before administration of the organophosphate.

Laboratory Mice. Trichlorfon is used for the control of pinworm infections in mice. For this purpose it is available commercially for administration in the drinking water.

Dog. Trichlorfon (Freed) can be used systemically in dogs both for its anthelmintic and pesticidal properties. It is efficacious for the common nematodes of dogs, i.e., *Toxocara canis, Ancylostoma caninum,* and *Trichuris vulpis.* It also gives acceptable control of ticks and fleas and evidence suggests that it aids in the control of demodectic mange in approximately 70% of the treated cases. For all of these uses trichlorfon is administered to dogs orally in tablet form.

Fish. Trichlorfon (Masoten) is effective against anchorworms, gill flukes, and lice of goldfish and bait fish. A solution of the drug is applied to the surface of the fishpond. The drug should not be used for the treatment of fish intended for human consumption nor in streams or ponds that serve as a source of drinking water for human beings or animals.

Cattle and Sheep. Although not approved by the FDA for use in cattle and sheep, trichlorfon is effective against certain parasites of these hosts. It can be used in cattle against infections of *Haemonchus* spp. and *Oesophagostomum radiatum* in a single subcutaneous injection of 22 mg/kg of body weight (Gordon 1973). When given by mouth at 44–110 mg/kg it is effective not only against these parasites but also against mature *Ostertagia ostertagia, Trichostrongylus axei,* and *Neoascaris.* Its efficacy is poor against *Cooperia* spp. unless the oral medication is preceded by a dose of sodium bicarbonate (60 ml of 10% solution) to close the oesophageal groove. It is not effective against *Bunostomum* spp., *Chabertia* spp., or *Trichuris* spp.

At high dosages the efficacy of trichlorfon in sheep is similar to that in cattle but it approaches toxic levels; for this reason it is little used in sheep (Alexander 1969).

TOXICITY

Trichlorfon is a relatively safe organophosphate when used in those animals for which there is FDA approval, i.e., the horse, dog, and laboratory mouse. It is generally safe in cattle but mortalities occasionally occur. Its margin of safety in sheep is poor at the high dosages necessary for satisfactory efficacy against GI parasites.

The toxicity of trichlorfon is associated with the inhibition of cholinesterase. The drug is relatively quickly metabolized and recovery takes place in a few hours.

Atropine is an effective antidote. The dosage of atropine in the treatment of organophosphorus poisoning is 4–5 times its usual therapeutic dose.

DOSAGE

Horse: 44 mg/kg of body weight orally for nematodes and bots or one-half this dosage for bots only

Dog: 75 mg/kg of body weight orally for each of 3 treatments at 3- to 4-day intervals for control of nematodes and for as many treatments as desired for control of ectoparasites

Mice: 1669 mg active ingredient/1000 ml of drinking water

Fish: 0.25 ppm of active ingredient in the water

NAPHTHALOPHOS

Naphthalophos (Maretin, Rametin) is a medium-spectrum organophosphate used in sheep and cattle principally against parasites of the abomasum and small intestine. Generally, it is ineffective against parasites of the large bowel of ruminants.

CHEMISTRY

The official nonproprietary name of this drug is naftalofos INN. Its chemical name is *N*-hydroxynaphthalimide diethyl

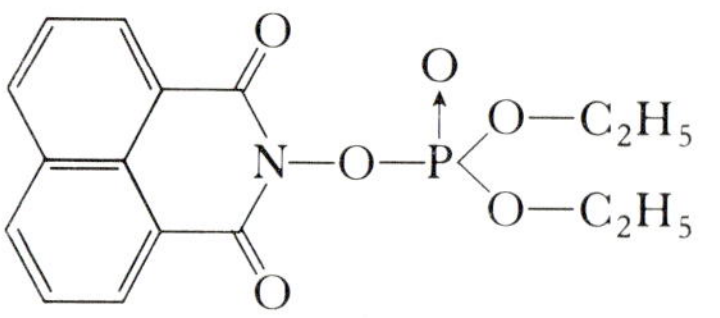

Naphthalophos

FIG. 52.11.

phosphate INN. The structural formula is shown in Fig. 52.11.

FORMULATIONS AND EFFICACY

Naphthalophos is commercially available as a bolus, drench, or feed additive. It appears to be slightly more efficacious when given as a bolus than as a drench and both of these formulations yield better results than the feed additive.

Sheep. Naphthalophos at 75 mg/kg is especially efficacious against 5th stage and adult *Haemonchus contortus, Ostertagia circumcincta, Trichostrongylus colubriformis,* and *Cooperia pectinata*. Younger parasitic stages are very little affected. The drug has greater than 80% efficacy for *Strongyloides papillosus* but gives erratic control of *Nematodirus* and is ineffective for *Oesophagostomum* and *Chabertia*. Its principal efficacy is for *Haemonchus,* against which it is 99%–100% effective in sheep even at reduced dosages of 25 mg/kg. Similar efficacies exist against these parasites of goats treated at the same dosage levels as sheep.

Cattle. The anthelmintic spectrum of naphthalophos in cattle is similar to its efficacy in sheep. As a drench at the rate of 50–75 mg/kg it removes practically all *Haemonchus* and generally more than 95% of adult *Cooperia* and *Trichostrongylus colubriformis* (Cox et al. 1967; Ciordia 1972b). It is less effective for *T. axei* (87%) and *Ostertagia ostertagia* (78%) and its efficacy for *Oesophagostomum radiatum* is variable (22%–100%). It may also be administered in the feed of cattle. Naphthalophos at a dosage of 10 mg/kg/day for 6 days is effective for *Haemonchus* and *Trichuris* but 20 mg/kg/day for 6 days is necessary to give satisfactory control of *Cooperia*.

Horse. *Parascaris* is satisfactorily eliminated from foals by naphthalophos at a dosage of 35 mg/kg but the spectrum of the drug for other equine parasites is limited.

Bird. Bobwhite quail can be treated with naphthalophos to eliminate infections of either *Capillaria contorta* or *C. obsignata* (Davis et al. 1969). The drug is administered in the feed (200 ppm) for 48 hours. It is not satisfactorily effective for *Heterakis gallinarum* at this dosage level.

TOXICITY

The margin of safety of naphthalophos is relatively narrow. Its LD50 in sheep is 300 mg/kg. The therapeutic dose, 50 mg/kg, and even 200 mg/kg, can be given orally to sheep without expecting deaths even though side effects including transient listlessness, loss of appetite, and increased salivation may be seen (Güralp and Dincer 1966). These signs disappear in 2–5 days without antidotal treatment. Even at the therapeutic dosage, diarrhea is often seen in sheep. If a therapeutic dose of 5 mg/kg is repeated daily for 10 days, subacute toxicity results in the death of approximately 40% of the sheep so treated. The administration of carbon tetrachloride concurrently or 7 days before or after administering naphthalophos does not enhance the toxicity for sheep (Hall 1965).

In cattle, toxic signs of naphthalophos poisoning begin to appear at dosages above 150 mg/kg of body weight but deaths are not expected with dosages up to 375 mg/kg. The LD50 for cattle is not known.

Naphthalophos has a very narrow margin of safety in chickens. A single dose of 50 mg/kg of body weight is fatal while a dosage as high as 25 mg/kg is required for satisfactory elimination of *Ascaridia* and *Heterakis* (Foxx and Hansen 1967).

DOSAGE

In sheep and cattle the recommended oral dose of naphthalophos is 50 mg/kg of body weight.

CRUFOMATE

The organophosphorus compound *cru-*

fomate INN (Ruelene) is used both as an anthelmintic and for warble fly control in cattle in Europe but does not have FDA approval for either of these purposes in the United States. The pour-on method of application used for fly control is of no anthelmintic value (Poole and Dooley 1972) but oral administration of crufomate to cattle at a dosage rate of 40 mg/kg yields greater than 95% efficacy for *Haemonchus* spp., *Cooperia* spp., *Bunostomum phlebotomum,* and *Trichuris discolor.* Its efficacy is approximately 70% and 80% for *Trichostrongylus axei* and *Oesophagostomum radiatum,* respectively (Costa et al. 1970).

MISCELLANEOUS ANTINEMATODAL COMPOUNDS

One or more intestinal nematodes of the dog and cat are treated successfully by drugs of unrelated structure and are included in this section. Ascarid infections, for example, can be treated with certain of the heterocyclic compounds (i.e., piperazine or its derivative, diethylcarbamazine) or with certain hydrocarbons (i.e., *n*-butyl chloride and toluene). The latter two drugs are discussed below; the piperazine compounds are covered elsewhere in this chapter. Hookworm infections of small animals are likewise susceptible to a variety of chemical compounds—disophenol, thenium clysolate, and tetrachloroethylene—as well as the antiascarid drugs *n*-butyl chloride and toluene. All of these drugs vary in chemical class. Similarly, two chemically unrelated drugs, phthalofyne and glycobiarsol, are highly effective for canine whipworms but are not effective for any other nematodes of small animals; they are discussed below. The two drugs DDVP and uredofos have a broad spectrum of activity in dogs and cats and are chemically related in that both are organophosphorus compounds. These drugs have activity against ascarids, hookworms, and whipworms. Uredofos (but not DDVP) additionally is highly active against tapeworms (*Taenia* and *Dipylidium*) of both the dog and cat. DDVP is discussed under Organophosphorus Compounds in this chapter.

n-Butyl Chloride

n-Butyl chloride (1-chlorobutane), a colorless liquid, can be administered in gelatin capsules to dogs and cats for the control of ascarid and hookworm infections. It is less efficacious for hookworms (60%) than for ascarids (98%) and has virtually no beneficial effect against whipworms unless administered at 3 times the ascarid dose, in which case approximately 50% of the whipworms are removed. Superior antiwhipworm drugs, however, have replaced the need of *n*-butyl chloride for the treatment of this parasite. The drug is still rather widely used as an over-the-counter product (e.g., Sergeants Capsules) for the treatment of ascarids and control of hookworm infections of young animals. It does not have satisfactory efficacy against parasites of other domestic animals.

n-Butyl chloride is essentially nontoxic to small animals when administered therapeutically. Vomition sometimes accompanies treatment but the drug does not produce the temporary depression associated with tetrachloroethylene or irritation of the intestinal mucosa caused by hexylresorcinol.

Overnight fasting and the use of a cathartic enhances worm expulsion but the latter practice is seldom employed by practitioners.

The recommended dosage of *n*-butyl chloride for ascarid and hookworm infections of small animals is:

Animal Weight	Dose
Under 2.25 kg (5 lb)	1 ml
2.25–4.5 kg	2 ml
4.5–9 kg	3 ml
9–18 kg	4 ml
Over 18 kg	5 ml

Toluene

Toluene (Methacide, Wurm Kaps), a hydrocarbon (methylbenzene) obtained from coal tars for use as an industrial solvent, has anthelmintic use against ascarids and hookworms of dogs and cats. Its efficacy for these parasites compares favorably or exceeds that of *n*-butyl chloride but toluene is the more toxic of the two (Enzie and Colglazier 1953). Therapeutic doses of toluene remove an average of more than 98% of the ascarids and 96% of the hookworms from both dogs and cats. Its efficacy for the canine whipworm (41%) is unsatisfactory.

For the most part, toluene is fairly well tolerated in therapeutic doses (0.1 cc/lb) although vomition occurs fairly commonly. Older animals tolerate 5 times the therapeutic dose of 0.1 ml/lb of body weight but show toxic signs of muscular tremors, unsteady gait, and vomition. Puppies and kittens experience toxicity more readily than older animals.

Combinations of toluene with certain other anthelmintics have had practical application in treating parasitic infections of small animals. Welter and Johnson (1963) found that the combination of toluene and *n*-butyl chloride (Nemantic) was synergistic in efficacy for hookworms and ascarids of the dog and cat, even at one-half the individual dose of each drug. Additionally, these two drugs when combined in dosages of suitable efficacy resulted in fewer toxic reactions (vomition, ataxia, dizziness) than therapeutic doses of either drug alone. Thus toluene in combination with *n*-butyl chloride has been more widely used for anthelmintic therapy of small animals than toluene alone.

Another toluene combination that has had widespread use, especially during the 1960s, employs an anticestodal drug, dichlorophen. The mixture of toluene and dichlorophen is marketed under various proprietary names, i.e., Vermiplex, Anaplex, or Paracide. Efficacy of the mixture is approximately 95% for ascarids, 82% for hookworms, and 70%–85% for *Taenia* and *Dipylidium* infections of the dog and cat.

Toluene is a liquid and is irritating to the digestive tract mucosa; thus a cathartic is not needed. Because it is also irritating to the oral mucosa, it is administered to small animals in gelatin capsules. The dosage of toluene for dogs, cats, puppies, or kittens is 0.1 ml/lb of body weight (0.22 ml/kg).

Tetrachloroethylene

Tetrachloroethylene (Nema, Tetracap), an unsaturated halogenated hydrocarbon, is a clear, colorless, volatile liquid; since its introduction in 1925, it has been used principally against hookworm infections of human beings, dogs, and cats. At one time it was used fairly extensively against GI parasites of ruminants. Its disadvantage in ruminants is the necessity of stimulating closure of the esophageal groove so that the medication is delivered directly to the abomasum rather than passing into the rumen which markedly reduces the effectiveness of the drug. After the advent of phenothiazine as a ruminant anthelmintic, little use has been made of the chlorinated hydrocarbons because phenothiazine is a superior anthelmintic and does not require closure of the esophageal groove. Tetrachloroethylene has continued to be used in small animals over the years but has been largely replaced by drugs that are less toxic and easier to administer.

Disadvantages of using tetrachloroethylene in small animals in general outweigh its effectiveness (98%) against hookworms. Animals to be treated must be on a fat-free diet for 48 hours before dosing since fats in the digestive tract at the time of medication increase the absorption of the drug and increase the frequency of toxic reactions. Excessive absorption of the drug will result in dizziness and incoordination and may cause liver damage and even death. No food or water should be allowed for 12–18 hours before and for 4 hours after dosing. The drug is contraindicated in tapeworm-infected animals since irritation of these worms may result in their balling up and occluding the digestive passage. It is also contraindicated in animals with distemper, febrile and debilitating diseases, e.g., nephritis, hepatitis, and enteritis, and should not be administered to nursing animals or those weighing less than 2 lb (approximately 1 kg).

The dosage of tetrachloroethylene in dogs and cats is 0.1 ml/lb (0.22 ml/kg) of body weight. The dose is administered orally in gelatin capsules.

Thenium

Thenium closylate INN (Canopar) has particular efficacy for hookworms of the dog but is only moderately active against ascarids unless combined with piperazine salts.

CHEMISTRY

Thenium is a colorless crystalline solid, almost insoluble in water (0.6% at 20° C), and possessing an extremely bitter taste. It is an analog of bephenium. Its chemical name is *N,N*-dimethyl-*N*-2-phenoxyethyl-*N*-2′-thenylammonium-*p*-chlorobenzenesulfonate. The structural formula is given in Fig. 52.12.

ANTHELMINTIC SPECTRUM

Thenium is 98% effective against adult and immature worms and 4th stage larvae of canine hookworms (Miller 1966). It is approximately 55% effective in eliminating 3rd stage larvae from the intestine.

The drug is moderately effective (up to 90%) for canine ascarids but less effective (50%–75%) for the feline ascarid *(Toxocara cati)*. It has little effect on *Trichuris vulpis* and none on the cestodes of dogs and cats.

TOXICITY

The only intolerance of the drug consists of vomiting in approximately 19% of the animals treated. Vomition does not impede the drug's action, as long as it takes place more than 2 hours after administration.

ADMINISTRATION AND DOSAGE

Thenium is administered orally, generally in tablet form, although it can be given by capsule or in the feed. Fasting or purgation is not necessary.

The dosage of thenium is not closely dictated by body weight since it is poorly absorbed from the intestinal tract of the host. Normally it is given as a 1-day treatment. Dogs weighing more than 10 lb (4.5 kg), regardless of total weight, are administered a single tablet of 500 mg base. For pups weighing 5–10 lb, it is safer and more effective to use one-fourth this dose in a 12-hour interval, i.e., 125 mg 2 times.

Ascarid infections are more effectively eliminated when a piperazine salt is administered concurrently with thenium in a dosage ratio of 2:1, i.e., 500 mg piperazine phosphate, for example, and 250 mg thenium base.

Disophenol

Disophenol (D.N.P., Ancylol, Syngamix) is an injectable antihookworm compound used for dogs and cats. Its special advantage is that it can be given without fasting to severely parasitized animals without causing stress and it can be used in very young puppies and kittens.

CHEMISTRY

Disophenol chemically is 2,6-diiodo-4-nitrophenol; the structural formula is shown in Fig. 52.13. The drug is supplied commercially as a 4.5% solution of disophenol (45 mg of disophenol/ml) in a water–polyethylene glycol vehicle for administration by subcutaneous injection.

MODE OF ACTION

Disophenol is rapidly absorbed from

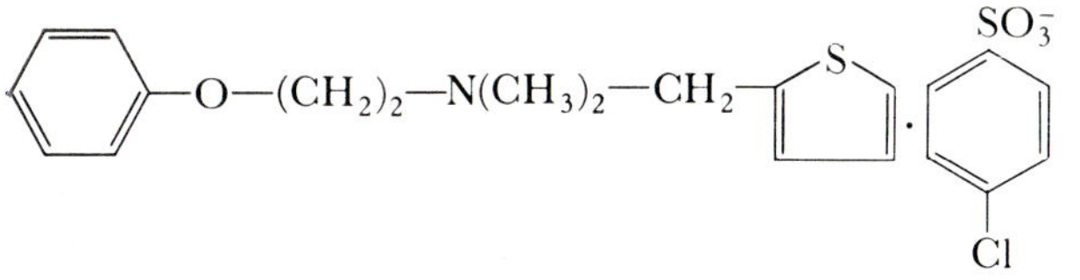

C_6H_5—O—$(CH_2)_2$—$N(CH_3)_2$—CH_2—(thienyl) · SO_3^-—C_6H_4—Cl

Thenium Closylate

Fig. 52.12.

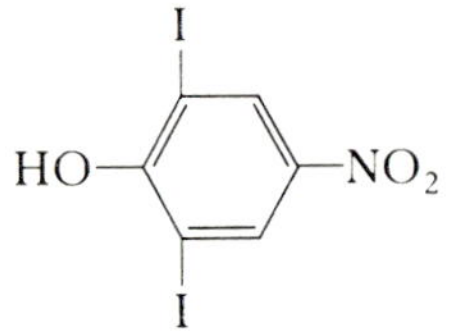

Disophenol

FIG. 52.13.

the digestive tract or from the site of parenteral injection and appears to accumulate in the plasma. Only a small portion of the dose is excreted in the urine during the first 24 hours following dosing. Regular therapeutic doses cause detectable increases in the heart rate, respiration rate, and body temperature.

The means by which disophenol exerts its anthelmintic action has not been determined. It is known that parasites, e.g., hookworms, are affected only after ingesting blood that contains the drug. Nonbloodsucking parasites are not affected by disophenol.

ADMINISTRATION AND ANTHELMINTIC ACTIVITY

Disophenol can be administered as a powder by mouth or parenterally (subcutaneous or intramuscular injections). The subcutaneous route is preferred for its ease of administration and general absence of pain that often accompanies intramuscular injections of the drug. Disophenol can be administered subcutaneously without fasting, which may be a distinct advantage to heavily parasitized animals that need prompt reduction of the worm burden.

A routine therapeutic dose of disophenol (10 mg/kg) given subcutaneously is reported to be nearly 100% effective in removing all species of canine hookworms (*Ancylostoma caninum, A. braziliense,* and *Uncinaria stenocephala)* (Wood et al. 1961), as well as *A. tubaeforme* of the cat. A lower dosage level of 7.5 mg/kg is equally effective as the 10 mg/kg level for the two canine species of *Ancylostoma* but gives variable results against *Uncinaria;* thus the higher dosage level is routinely used therapeutically. This level (10 mg/kg) is also reported to be effective against adult forms of *Spirocerca lupi* (Chhabra and Singh 1972).

Oral administration of the powder formulation or intramuscular injection of the solution of disophenol yields efficacies against canine hookworms similar to those obtained from subcutaneous administration of the drug.

Like other antihookworm drugs, disophenol does not eliminate histotropic larval forms of the parasite. Thus retreatment after 2 or more weeks may be necessary to remove these worms once they have matured and to reduce reinfections.

Disophenol has no appreciable efficacy against ascarids, whipworms, tapeworms, or lung flukes *(Paragonimus)* of dogs and cats.

Wild felids (black panthers, leopards, lions, and golden cats) are reported to have been treated effectively and safely with disophenol for infections of both *Ancylostoma* and *Gnathostoma* (Dutta et al. 1972). The dosage level is 6.6 mg/kg of body weight.

The gapeworm *(Syngamus trachea)* can be effectively removed (more than 90%) from turkey poults given disophenol. When the drug is administered to poults either in the feed for 5 days or in a single oral capsule dose, more than 90% of these worms are expelled from the trachea (Boisvenue 1963). Gapeworm infections traditionally have been treated by the inhalation of barium antimonyl tartrate dust (Link 1965). Although time consuming, the use of disophenol appears to be more practical than placing turkeys in dusting chambers (required when using the traditional drug).

TOXICITY

Disophenol has approximately a 3-fold margin of safety in the dog and cat. This margin is generally considered adequate for parenterally administered drugs for which precise amounts are given according to body weight. A 3-fold margin of safety for orally administered drugs is not as satisfactory since host differences in absorption from the digestive tract are more likely to result in toxicosis.

In general, at the recommended therapeutic dosage, disophenol is well tolerated by dogs and cats of all breeds and ages. Puppies as young as 2 days of age can be given the drug without ill effects except that occasional opacity of the lens is seen in puppies less than 4 months of age (Martin et al. 1972). Lenticular opacity in these cases is not severe and regresses within 7 days.

No side effects from therapeutic doses of disophenol are reported for pregnant animals, regardless of the stage of gestation, nor is it contraindicated in severely parasitized animals. One of its major advantages is its safety for use in heavily parasitized animals that need prompt removal of at least a portion of the worm burden without stress.

Signs of disophenol toxicosis in dogs are associated with an increased metabolic rate and include tachycardia, polypnea, hyperthermia, and early rigor mortis in fatal cases. Lenticular opacity of varying severity is likely to occur in adult as well as young dogs given higher than therapeutic doses of disophenol. There is perhaps some merit in treating toxic patients with antipyretics and ice baths (Penumarthy et al. 1975).

Other than vomiting, at the 2 highest dosage levels no toxic effects are seen in dogs given single subcutaneous doses of disophenol at levels of 7.5, 10, 15, or 30 mg/kg of body weight (Wood et al. 1961). Single doses equal to or greater than 36 mg/kg, however, are lethal to dogs.

There is at least one report of severe toxicosis in an Irish wolfhound that received the recommended 10 mg/kg dosage of disophenol subcutaneously. It is thought that vigorous muscular exercise and high ambient temperature were probable factors in the precipitation of this acute syndrome (Legendre 1973).

As determined in chronic toxicity studies, 1.6 times the recommended dose (i.e., 16.5 mg/kg) given subcutaneously once a week for 8 weeks is not toxic to dogs; yet, a lower dose of 7.5 mg/kg if repeated daily is lethal in 6 days. Toxicosis evidently occurs because of the accumulation of disophenol in the plasma. A rather sharp level of drug accumulation appears to be necessary for the development of toxic signs since slightly lower dosages, 5 mg/kg, have been repeated daily in dogs for as long as 60 days without adverse effects.

DOSAGE

Dog and cat: 0.22 ml (10 mg)/kg of body weight, i.e., 0.1 ml (4.5 mg)/lb (single subcutaneous injection)

Turkey poult: 3.5 mg/lb (7.7 mg/kg) of body weight/day (given in the feed for 5 days); 3.5 mg/lb (7.7 mg/kg) of body weight (single capsule dose)

PHTHALOFYNE

Phthalofyne (Whipcide) is marketed for the specific treatment of whipworm (*Trichuris vulpis*) infections in dogs. Clinical tricuriasis is uncommon but the prevalence of whipworm infections is quite high throughout most of the United States and many other countries.

CHEMISTRY

The accepted international generic name for this compound is ftalofyne INN. It is an ester of phthalic acid and has the chemical name 1-ethyl-1-methyl-2-propynyl hydrogen phthalate INN. The structural formula is shown in Fig. 52.14. Phthalofyne is unstable in strong alkali and relatively insoluble in water. Its sodium salt is highly soluble in water and is supplied commercially as a 50% solution for intravenous injection.

ADMINISTRATION AND EFFECTIVENESS

Phthalofyne can be administered orally

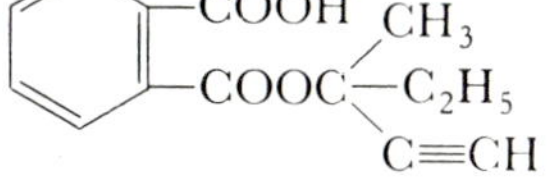

$C_6H_4(COOH)(COOC(CH_3)(C_2H_5)C{\equiv}CH)$

Phthalofyne

FIG. 52.14.

in tablet form or intravenously. The tablet formulation is routinely used for treating whipworm infections of dogs. Because of the greater toxic risk, the intravenous solution should be used only in those cases in which peroral treatment is either impractical or unfeasible. Slow administration of an intravenous dose over a period of 1–2 minutes reduces the chance of an adverse reaction. Also, feeding dogs 1 hour before administering phthalofyne intravenously helps to minimize side effects, as does giving 5–10 ml of a 50% solution of dextrose intravenously immediately after dosing. Inadvertent perivascular administration or leakage of phthalofyne causes cellulitis and results in necrosis.

The presence of food in the intestinal tract interferes with the anthelmintic action of orally administered phthalofyne; therefore, a 24-hour fast is required before oral dosing. In cases where this method produces vomiting, an alternate procedure is to administer 2 doses on the same day (morning and evening), each following a light meal. Each dose should be equal to the recommended single dose of phthalofyne.

Either oral or intravenous administration of phthalofyne yields approximately 95% efficacy against canine whipworms under experimental conditions (Burch 1954) and a slightly lower efficacy under practice conditions. Equal efficacy by the two routes of administration is obtained only if the intravenous dose of phthalofyne is about 1.25 times greater than the oral dose. The worms are expelled over a period of several days during which time the feces has an offensive musklike odor. The odor can be controlled by dosing with chlorophyll.

TOXICITY

Acute manifestations of phthalofyne toxicosis in mice are ataxia, stupor, and loss of righting reflex, followed by death in 48 hours from respiratory paralysis.

In the dog, toxic manifestations following intravenous injections of higher than therapeutic doses of the drug are similar to those described for mice and are preceded by vomiting. Actually, vomiting, ataxia, and drowsiness are seen in approximately 40% of dogs given a therapeutic dose of the drug intravenously and may last for several hours. Death occasionally occurs following intravenous administration of a therapeutic dose.

The occurrence of side effects is less frequent in dogs given the drug orally than in those given intravenous injections. Ataxia and drowsiness seldom occur in orally treated dogs; vomition, however, is fairly common. In dogs given higher than therapeutic oral doses, vomition is pronounced and may be beneficial in eliminating the excess dose.

Phthalofyne is contraindicated in dogs that have chronic nephritis, hepatitis, pancreatitis, or cardiac insufficiencies. Following phthalofyne therapy, if an anaphylactoidlike reaction, tetany, or collapse occurs, symptomatic treatment with oxygen, corticosteroids, and blood transfusions is indicated. There is no specific antidote for phthalofyne toxicosis.

DOSAGE

Oral: 200 mg/kg of body weight
Intravenous: 250 mg/kg of body weight

GLYCOBIARSOL

Glycobiarsol INN (Milibis-V, Viasept, Wintodon), like phthalofyne, is indicated for the treatment of whipworm *(Trichuris vulpis)* infections in dogs. Chemically, it is bismuth glycolylarsanilate. It is an odorless, tasteless powder with only slight solubility in water, which probably accounts for the small amount, about 2%, absorbed from the digestive tract.

ADMINISTRATION AND EFFECTIVENESS

Glycobiarsol is supplied commercially in tablets which can be either given orally or crushed and mixed in the feed. It is not necessary to fast or purge the animals prior to using the drug.

When given in the therapeutic dose of 220 mg/kg of body weight daily for 5 days, glycobiarsol can be expected to completely eliminate whipworms from at least 80% of the treated dogs and to reduce markedly the worm burdens in the remaining 20%. In obstinate cases, a second course of treatment should be given 2–4 weeks after the first. The drug has no activity against other intestinal helminths of the dog.

SIDE EFFECTS

In general, glycobiarsol is well tolerated and side effects other than occasional vomiting seldom occur in middle-aged dogs. Side effects are more likely to occur in young dogs less than 1 year of age or in very old dogs (Kibble 1969). Side effects in these cases usually consist of thirst, lethargy, and vomiting, and can be minimized by mixing the drug in the feed. Also, it is generally recommended that aged and debilitated dogs be given one-half the daily therapeutic dose for twice the period of time, i.e., 110 mg/kg of body weight for 10 days.

Apparently, massive single doses (2000, 5000 or 10,000 mg/kg) of glycobiarsol are tolerated with no greater toxic manifestations than the side effects mentioned above (Edwin 1964).

DOSAGE

The recommended dose of glycobiarsol in the dog is 220 mg/kg of body weight daily for 5 days.

UREDOFOS

Uredofos (Sansalid) is a newly developed broad-spectrum anthelmintic for use in dogs and cats. It is effective for tapeworms as well as ascarids, hookworms, and whipworms. It is discussed in detail under Anticestodal Drugs in the following chapter.

HYGROMYCIN B

Hygromycin B is an antibiotic produced by *Streptomyces hygroscopicus* and has some anthelmintic properties. It is added as a powder to the feed of swine and poultry for consumption over periods of several weeks. Especially *Ascaris suum* but also *Oesophagostomum* of swine can be controlled reasonably well by this method (Goldsby and Todd 1957). In chickens, continuous feeding of hygromycin B is effective against *Ascaridia galli, Capillaria obsignata,* and *Heterakis gallinarium* (Frazier 1959).

It is recommended that the antibiotic be fed to sows for 6 weeks prior to farrowing and during the nursing period. It should be supplied to weaned pigs throughout the period of ascarid susceptibility, i.e., until about 6 months of age. Better results are obtained by adding hygromycin B to the complete ration than by supplying it in a free choice protein supplement. A dose of 12 g hygromycin B/ton of total ration is recommended for swine. Evidence of impaired hearing, but no other toxic signs, exists in swine fed the antibiotic continuously.

For chickens, 8 g of hygromycin B/ton of feed provides effective control of the poultry nematodes. Somewhat better control is obtained from a combination of 7.2 g of hygromycin B/ton of feed plus enough phenothiazine to make a concentration of 0.05% in the total ration (Dixon et al. 1959). These levels of hygromycin B apparently cause no harmful effects to chickens or to egg production.

DRUGS USED IN HEARTWORM DISEASE

Heartworm disease of dogs results from parasitism by a filarial nematode *(Dirofilaria immitis)* that occupies the circulatory system—principally the right side of the heart, the pulmonary artery, and sometimes the posterior and anterior venae cavae. The parasite is transmitted to new hosts by mosquitoes, principally the salt marsh species which accounts for the high prevalence of canine infections in the Atlantic and Gulf coastal areas and along the Mississippi River waterways in the United States. The incidence of canine infections is presently increasing in the United States. Inland states such as Illinois, which had negligible infection rates 10 years ago, are now experiencing an increase in the incidence of heartworm infections.

The disease occurs throughout most of the world except the arctic and northern temperate areas. In Europe the warmer humid regions of southern France, the

Ibernian peninsula, and the Balkan countries are sites of greatest prevalence.

A thorough knowledge of the life cycle and pathogenesis of the heartworm is necessary in order to understand the rationale of sequential treatment for the adult worms, the microfilariae, and the infective stage.

Life Cycle

Adult *D. immitis* live principally in the right ventricle of the heart and in the conus of the pulmonary artery. Fertilized female worms expel motile young larvae (microfilariae) into the blood. The numbers of circulating microfilariae vary tremendously but are generally more numerous at night and are certainly more numerous in summer as compared with winter months. Their numbers, however, have no direct relationship to the numbers of adult worms in the animal. Microfilariae, which are picked up by any one of a large number of species of mosquitoes, can develop to the 3rd stage infective larvae (L_3) in a period of approximately 2 weeks. This development occurs in the Malphigian tubules of the mosquito. The infective larvae are transmitted to a definitive host when the mosquito subsequently feeds.

The development of the infective larva to an adult worm in the definitive host requires at least 6 and more likely 8 or 9 months. The initial development occurs in subcutaneous, subserosal, and adipose tissues of the dog. Here the L_3 molts to an L_4 in 2 weeks and the L_4 slowly develops to an L_5 (young immature adult) in approximately 2.5 months. It is the L_4 and especially the L_3 stages that are most susceptible to the preventive programs employing diethylcarbamazine (DEC) daily. The use of DEC is discussed in more detail under Preventive Programs later in the chapter.

Young immature worms pass into the bloodstream and take up residence in the heart and adjacent blood vessels where they grow and develop to sexual maturity in as little as 3 months. The immature adults like the mature adults are susceptible to the adulticidal drug, thiacetarsamide sodium.

Pathogenesis and Clinical Signs

Three manifestations of heartworm disease are recognized (Simpson and Jackson 1974). In many animals no clinical signs of disease are apparent. Such animals carry low burdens of worms, generally not more than 25, and are the best candidates for tolerating the arsenical treatment used to kill adult worms. In the second manifestation of heartworm disease (pneumonitis) little clinical evidence of disease is shown other than coughing. Villous endarteritis with resulting localized roughening of the luminal surface of vessels due to intimal hyperplasia is thought to be the initial step in the eventual production of a pneumonitis. Villous endarteritic lesions result at sites where adult worms are located and may be induced mechanically by the worms. These rough vascular lesions are ideal sites of thrombus formation. The thrombi upon dislodging pass to smaller branches of the pulmonary artery. These thromboemboli are believed to be the cause of pneumonitis and coughing, which may be the only clinical manifestation ever seen in a medium-sized dog with few to moderate (40) numbers of heartworms. In more severely parasitized dogs, pneumonitis with a resulting cough is often simply the initial step in what is recognized as the third manifestation, which is related to cardiovascular dysfunction and, terminally, to congestive cardiac failure.

Adult worms of *D. immitis* are large, 20–30 cm long by 1 mm wide; thus in their normal location in the right heart and its associated vessels, they can mechanically impede the proper closure of the cardiac and arterial valves, which permits valvular leakage during ventricular systole. In heavy infections, large numbers of worms may be clumped in the blood passageways to such an extent that they actually interfere with the flow of blood. These conditions serve to place a greater work demand upon the heart, but its ability to meet that demand is impaired. Compensatory myocardial hypertrophy gradually occurs; eventually the heart dilates beyond the point of adequate myocardial tension and cardiac output falls. The cardiac output cannot keep pace with the venous return; thus in this gradually developing cardiac failure syndrome there exists venous congestion of the abdominal organs (with resulting ascites) and lungs (manifested by shortness of breath and coughing) and pitting subcutaneous edema of the limbs. Animals that have advanced to this state are usually very cachectic and although death is inevitable without filaricidal treatment, no more than about 50% of the cases survive with treatment.

Infrequently, greater numbers of worms develop in the venae cavae than in the heart or pulmonary artery of dogs. This seems to occur mostly in young 3- to 5-year-old animals that have had little if any previous exposure to heartworms prior to receiving a massive infection of the parasite. Growth of large numbers of worms in the venae cavae restricts the blood flow on its return to the heart, resulting in congestion and impaired function of the liver and kidney.

The onset of clinical signs of this "venae cavae syndrome" develops suddenly overnight compared to the slow development of signs described for the three manifestations of average heartworm infections described above. An animal with no previous signs often suddenly stops eating, will not move, and appears very sick. In such animals, laboratory tests reveal hemoglobinuria, bilirubinuria, and an elevation in blood levels of both urea nitrogen (BUN) and a hepatic enzyme, serum glutamic pyruvic transaminase (SGPT), indicative of renal and hepatic damage (Jackson 1974b). The presence of hemoglobin in the urine is considered pathognomonic of the syndrome. Shock develops quickly in animals with the venae cavae syndrome and death usually occurs in 24–48 hours. Thus at least some of the occluding worms must be removed immediately. Because of the slow action of thiacetarsamide on the parasite (several days are required to kill worms), drug treatment is limited to use in early venae cavae syndrome cases that have not yet developed shock and in which the BUN has not exceeded 50 mg%. In these cases the usual therapeutic schedule of thiacetarsamide administration (described under Elimination of Adult Worms) is recommended. In the more advanced cases in which shock is evident and the BUN has exceeded 50 mg%, surgical intervention instead of chemotherapy is warranted. The technique described by Jackson (1974b) involves inserting forceps into the jugular vein in an effort to grasp worms located in the anterior and posterior venae cavae and right atrium of the heart.

Diagnosis

Diagnosis of heartworm infection is usually based upon finding microfilariae of the parasite in the peripheral blood. The microfilariae of *D. immitis* must be distinguished from blood microfilariae of another filarial parasite of dogs, *Dipetalonema reconditum*. Adults of the latter parasite are subcutaneous dwellers and are essentially nonpathogenic. Textbooks in parasitology should be consulted for information on the techniques used to recover and concentrate blood microfilariae and the basis for distinguishing the two species.

Approximately 5%–10% of the heartworm-infected dogs have no circulating microfilariae. Fertilization of the female worm by a male is necessary for the production of microfilariae. Occult infections, therefore, are due to the presence of only male or only female worms or the distant location of each sex in the circulatory system. In the absence of microfilariae a diagnosis must be made on the basis of signs of coughing and tiring after exercise and on radiographic signs indicating enlargement of the right heart and pulmonary artery.

Elimination of Adult Worms

The present procedure recommended by the AVMA Council on Veterinary Service (1973) for treatment of canine heartworm disease calls for eliminating the existing adult worms first, then eliminating the microfilariae, and subsequently placing dogs subject to reinfection on preventive medication. An arsenical, thiacetarsamide, is the only drug currently recommended for killing adult worms; however, it is relatively toxic to the host and must be administered with caution. Trivalent antimonial compounds, e.g., stibophen (Fuadin), were used in past years as adulticidal agents but were even more hepatotoxic and nephrotoxic than arsenicals and are not currently recommended.

THIACETARSAMIDE SODIUM

Thiacetarsamide sodium INN (Caparsolate sodium, Filaramide, Arsenamide) chemically consists of the disodium salt of *S,S*-diester of *p*-carbamoyldithiobenzenearsonous acid with mercaptoacetic acid INN. The structural formula is shown in Fig. 52.15.

Administration and Dosage. Since thiacetarsamide sodium is a hepatotoxic and nephrotoxic drug, proper functioning of the liver and kidneys must be attained before beginning treatment. Clinical pathological tests—urinalysis, BUN, complete blood count (CBC), and SGPT—are performed to monitor the condition of these organs before and during the course of the 2-day treatment.

The drug is administered intravenously. Caution must be exercised to avoid perivascular leakage since the drug is highly irritating to subcutaneous tissues, will result in marked local swelling, and may cause sloughing of the tissue. In the event of leakage or inadvertent perivascular administration, injecting steroids into the area will aid in reducing the inflammatory reaction.

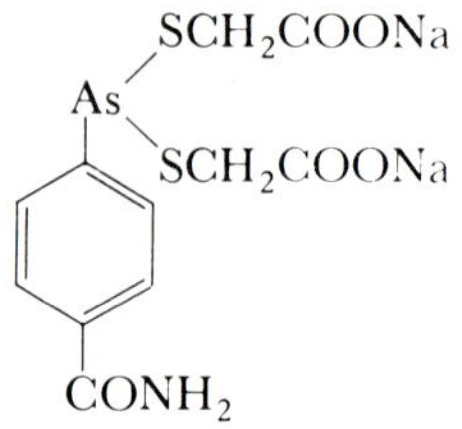

SCH_2COONa

As

SCH_2COONa

$CONH_2$

Thiacetarsamide Sodium

FIG. 52.15.

The recommended dosage schedule of thiacetarsamide sodium is 1 mg (0.1 ml)/lb of body weight (2.2 mg/kg) twice daily for 2 days. On this schedule, each dose provides 0.2 mg of elemental arsenic/lb of body weight. The dose should not be reduced for very large dogs (Jackson 1974a).

Splitting the daily dosage eliminates most of the toxic effects that were encountered in the past when only a single daily injection of 2 mg/lb was used. Feeding the dog an hour before each of the morning and afternoon injections is recommended. The dog's interest in eating provides some indication of its general condition. If the dog is eating well and there is no persistent vomition or indication of hepatic or renal damage (icterus or discoloring of the urine), the regimen of treatment is continued.

In cases of arsenic toxicity, evidenced principally by persistent vomition, icterus, or orange-colored urine, the treatment regimen should be stopped for a thorough reexamination of the animal including clinical pathology tests. If treatment has to be suspended, Jackson (1974) recommends waiting 6 weeks to begin the entire regimen again in order to prevent liver damage. Severe toxic reactions to thiacetarsamide sodium can be treated with dimercaprol (BAL). A dose of 4 mg/lb (0.45 kg)/day given in 4 divided doses usually gives relief.

Clinical Effectiveness. Following the 4 therapeutic injections of thiacetarsamide sodium, adult worms gradually die, usually within 5–7 days but occasionally not until 2 weeks. There is no effect on the circulating microfilariae. Dead or dying adult worms swept out of the heart by the blood flow lodge in the branches of the pulmonary artery, especially those of the diaphragmatic lobes. Here phagocytosis of the dead worms occurs during the next 2–3 months.

It is in the first month following treatment that the embolic shower of whole or partially phagocytized worms poses a distinct threat to the well-being of the animal. Absolute rest during the first 2 weeks (the most critical period) is necessary and only limited exercise should be allowed during the next 2 weeks. Increased body temperature and coughing indicate a pulmonary reaction to embolism.

The percentage of fatalities during or following thiacetarsamide therapy is directly related to the degree of clinical manifestation of heartworm disease. Hundreds of asymptomatic dogs are treated without a single loss. Among mildly symptomatic patients, approximately 3%–5% fatality is expected. The poorest risks are those dogs in which heartworm disease has advanced to the point of evident cachexia and abdominal ascites. Fifty percent mortality can be expected in this group during or immediately following therapy (Jackson 1974).

The occurrence of patent heartworm infections in cats is infrequent but occasional cases are observed in which elimination of the adult worms is needed. Only a few case reports on treating cats with thiacetarsamide sodium have been made. Jackson (1974) suggests the same dosage and schedule that is used for treating dogs.

Elimination of Microfilariae

The elimination of microfilariae is advisable for two principal reasons. First, this stage of the heartworm parasite is now known to cause glomerular damage in the kidney (Simpson et al. 1972). Second, the preventive drug, DEC, which is active against the infective 3rd stage larvae, is not safe for use in dogs until they are cleared of microfilariae.

It is advisable to wait 6 weeks between the time of treatment for adult worms and microfilariae. This time should allow improvement in the physical condition of the dog following the stressful use of the adulticidal thiacetarsamide sodium.

All of the drugs used to date as microfilaricides also have side effects. Fenthion (Talodex), once used extensively in the United States for its excellent efficacy against microfilariae, no longer has FDA approval because of an unacceptable number of toxic fatalities. Diethylcarbamazine, now used only as a preventive drug for heartworm infection, formerly was used but was unsuccessful in elimination of microfilariae. Severe reactions, some of which were fatal, prevent the use of this drug as a microfilaricide. Presently, the only microfilaricidal drug approved by the FDA is dithiazanine iodide. It is also potentially nephrotoxic and must be administered with caution.

An experimental drug that merits attention as a potential future microfilaricide is levamisole. It is currently approved in the United States for use against GI and pulmonary nematodes of cattle, sheep, and swine (see Levamisole in this chapter). Trials testing the efficacy of levamisole against heartworm microfilariae in dogs (Jackson 1972) indicate it is a satisfactory drug for this purpose. The present experimental dosage schedule is 5 mg/lb (0.45 kg) of active ingredient of levamisole in a single oral dose each day until the blood is free of microfilariae but not to exceed 15 daily treatments. Microfilariae are usually cleared between the 6th and 10th doses; therefore examination of the blood for remaining microfilariae should be made after the 6th dose.

Levamisole, like other microfilaricides, induces side effects. Vomiting frequently accompanies administration of this drug but can be controlled by giving atropine sulfate shortly before administration.

DITHIAZANINE IODIDE

Dithiazanine iodide INN (Dizan) is the only drug presently approved in the United States for use as a heartworm microfilaricide in dogs. Dithiazanine is a cyanine dye; its iodide salt, an intense blue-violet powder, is poorly soluble in water. The structural formula is shown in Fig. 52.16.

Administration and Dosage. Dithiazanine iodide is available as either a powder or tablet and is administered orally immediately after or during feeding.

The FDA-approved dosage is 3–5 mg/lb (6.6–11 mg/kg) of body weight daily for 7–10 days. Since vomiting and diarrhea are frequent side effects, the lowest dose (3 mg/lb) is recommended daily for 7 days.

FIG. 52.16.

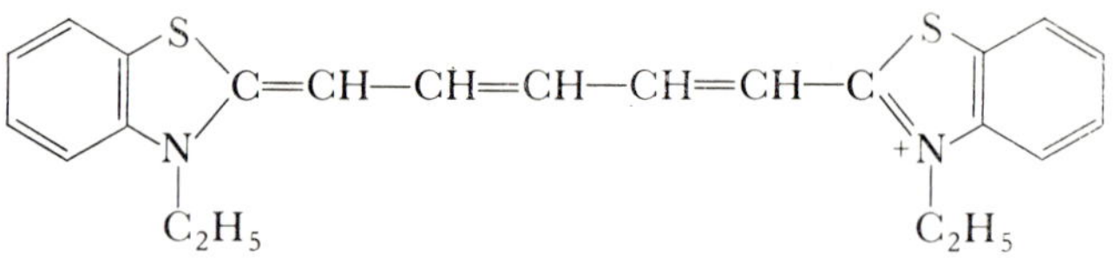

$$\text{C}_6\text{H}_4\text{(S)(N-C}_2\text{H}_5\text{)C=CH-CH=CH-CH=CH-C(S)(}^{+}\text{N-C}_2\text{H}_5\text{)C}_6\text{H}_4$$

[I]

Dithiazanine Iodide

Splitting the daily dosage and giving 1.5 mg/lb twice daily at feeding times helps to reduce the occurrence of side effects. If the animal is positive for circulating microfilariae after 7 days, the dosage may be increased to 5 mg/lb daily until the blood is negative for microfilariae or for no longer than 10 days. After the dog becomes negative for microfilariae, it can be started immediately on prophylactic treatment with DEC but should be checked in 3 months, and again at 6 months, for microfilaria from worms that may have escaped elimination at the time of treatment with the adulticide.

A small percentage of dogs treated with dithiazanine iodide do not become negative for microfilariae even after the full treatment. In these cases, as well as those in which treatment had to be discontinued because of side reactions, the optional use of the experimental levamisole may be of benefit; however, the latter drug has equally unsatisfactory side effects.

Mode of Action and Pharmacodynamics. The means by which dithiazanine iodide clears circulating microfilariae from the blood is not known. The microfilariae evidently lose motility, become trapped in capillary beds, and are eventually phagocytized by host cells. The drug is known to be detrimental to the development of microfilaria in the uteri of female worms. Studies in which dithiazanine iodide was administered at 3 or 5 mg/lb/day to dogs harboring adult worms revealed markedly reduced numbers of fully developed microfilariae, all of which were dead, in the uterus (Boisvenue 1974). These effects were not seen when a low dosage of 1 mg/kg/day was given.

The biochemical basis of action of dithiazanine iodide on helminths has been only partially determined. Studies with canine whipworms indicate that the drug causes an irreversible inhibition of glucose absorption, thus resulting in a marked reduction in free glucose and a consequent depletion in energy-rich phosphate bonds. Whether these physiological changes also occur in heartworm microfilariae exposed to the drug is not known.

Absorption of this blue-violet compound from the intestinal tract is minimal but is sufficient to cause a faint blue coloration of tissues. Since most of the drug remains unabsorbed in the ingesta, the stools and vomitus of dogs are blue-green to purple in color. Clients and veterinary practitioners alike esthetically object to this discoloration of excreta.

Toxicity. The sensitivity of different animals to dithiazanine iodide is highly variable. The acute oral LD50 of the drug in rats, for example, is 165–192 mg/kg while that in mice is only 4–16 mg/kg. Dogs are reported to tolerate a single high dose of 200 mg/kg but repeated daily doses of 12–20 mg/kg/day for 3–7 days are often poorly tolerated by dogs, causing vomiting, diarrhea, anorexia, and asthenia. A low percentage of dogs have been killed by the 20 mg/kg/day dosage in as few as 3 days.

Other Uses. Dithiazanine iodide has a broad spectrum of anthelmintic activity, being effective not only against heartworm microfilariae but also against the common intestinal nematodes of dogs (hookworms, ascarids, and whipworms), against *Strongyloides stercoralis,* and perhaps against *Spirocerca lupi.* It was used extensively in the early 1960s against the common intestinal parasites of dogs, the oral dosage being 20 mg/kg/day for 2–7 days. In general, 80% of the hookworm and ascarid burden is removed in 2–3 days, the remaining 20% gradually thereafter. Treatment is required for 5–7 days to eliminate the major part of the whipworm burden. With the subsequent discovery of other broad-spectrum anthelmintics, i.e., dichlorvos, which are effective in a single administration, the use of dithiazanine iodide for the treatment of common canine intestinal worms has markedly diminished.

Dithiazanine iodide is one of only a few drugs that can be used successfully against *Strongyloides stercoralis* infections of dogs. The recommended dosage schedule varies with authors. Worley and Thompson (1962) successfully cleared *Strongyloides* infections in dogs with daily oral administration of dithiazanine iodide (2.27 mg/lb or 5 mg/kg) for 10 consecutive days. Georgi (1974) recommends 10 mg/lb daily for 12 days. At the latter dose, vomiting and diarrhea are very likely to occur. Just as with dosing for clearance of microfilariae, splitting the daily dose, giving it twice a day during meals, should help to reduce the occurrence of side effects.

Evidently there is also some degree of clinical success following the use of dithiazanine iodide against the canine esophageal worm *(Spirocerca lupi)* (Tacal 1963). In the Philippines, where this infection is common, the drug has been used orally at the rate of 10 mg/lb/day for as few as 5 and as many as 52 days (average of 28 days) to eliminate the passing of *Spirocerca* eggs in the stool. Critical studies, including the necropsy of substantial numbers of experimental dogs following treatment with the drug, have not been performed. Thus the overall value of this method of treating spirocercosis is questionable.

Preventive Programs

Two approaches to the prevention of heartworm disease of dogs are currently in use. One is to give the adulticidal drug, thiacetarsamide sodium, at 6-month intervals. The regular therapeutic dose of 1 mg/lb (2.2 mg/kg) intravenously twice daily for 2 days is used. This approach is employed mostly in highly endemic areas where exposure is virtually assured. Given at 6-month intervals, the drug eliminates worms before a sufficient burden builds up to disease-inducing levels.

The second preventive approach, which is much more widely used, relies on the effectiveness of a larvicidal drug, DEC, which is detrimental in low daily doses to the infective 3rd stage and evidently the 4th stage larvae. This drug and its use as a heartworm preventive are further discussed below.

DIETHYLCARBAMAZINE CITRATE

Diethylcarbamazine Citrate INN, U.S.P. (Caricide, Dirocide), is a piperazine derivative. It is a colorless, odorless, crystalline solid, highly soluble in water, alcohol, and chloroform but insoluble in most organic solvents. It is stable under varied conditions of climate and moisture. The chemical name is 1-diethylcarbamoyl-4-methylpiperazine citrate; its structural formula is shown in Fig. 52.17.

Formulations and Administration. As a preventive for heartworm disease in dogs, DEC is prepared as either a syrup or tablet, both sold under the trade names Caricide or Dirocide. A powdered formulation of diethylcarbamazine base (Cypip) is also available, as is another syrup formulation (Styrid-Caricide), which contains not only DEC but also an ingredient effective against the 4th infective stage of hookworms. Each of the three formulations (syrup, tablet, or powder) is administered in either dry or wet feed or immediately after feeding each day throughout and for 2 months following the mosquito season. In warmer climates, e.g., in Florida, where the mosquito is prevalent all year, the medication should be administered daily without cessation for the lifetime of the dog.

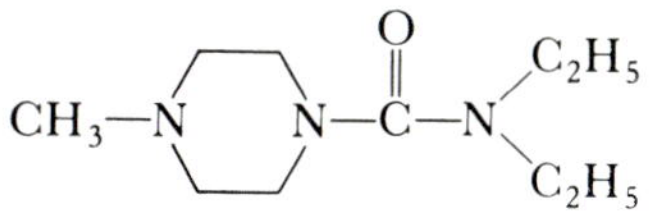

CH_3—N(piperazine ring)N—C(=O)—N(C_2H_5)(C_2H_5)

Diethylcarbamazine

Fig. 52.17.

Young pups can be started on a preventive program of daily intake of the drug as soon as they are weaned and eating well, i.e., about 8 weeks of age. An examination for microfilariae should be performed on a 6-month basis to detect the presence of worms that may have escaped destruction by the drug.

An infected dog must first be cleared of adult worms and microfilariae before starting it on DEC. The drug acts not only on infective larvae from the mosquito but also against microfilariae. One would expect this dual action to be a highly desirable characteristic. Unfortunately, however, an anaphylactic type reaction, sometimes fatal, occurs in a small percentage of dogs that are microfilariae-positive at the time the drug is given. Subjective estimates of the percentage of dogs undergoing shock following administration of the drug range from 0.3% to 5%. The reaction is fast in onset; in the fatal cases death occurs within a few hours after drug administration. The basis for this reaction is unknown but is thought to be immunologically based. Consequently, the use of DEC in microfilariae-positive dogs is strictly contraindicated.

Once a dog is cleared of adult worms with thiacetarsamide and of microfilariae with a microfilaricide, it can be started on prophylactic treatment with DEC.

Some dogs are incorrectly thought to be cleared of adult worms following the completion of microfilaricidal therapy, then microfilariae begin to appear in the blood again. If the dog has been placed on prophylactic treatment there should be no cause for alarm since reports of anaphylaxis are rare even though there is a gradual reappearance of microfilariae during use of DEC. The AVMA Council on Veterinary Services advises that all previously treated heartworm cases should be checked 3 months after the dog is started on DEC. If microfilariae are detected, the prophylactic program must be stopped until existing microfilariae are eliminated.

Dosage. DEC syrups and tablets used in a prophylactic heartworm schedule are administered daily at the rate of 3 mg/lb (0.45 kg) of body weight. The powder formulation (Cypip) is administered daily at the rate of 1.25 mg of base/lb of body weight.

Pharmacodynamics and Toxicity. Diethylcarbamazine is rapidly absorbed from the gut. The peak concentration in the blood occurs about 3 hours after oral administration and falls to zero in 48 hours. The drug is distributed to all organs and tissues except fat; neither the microfilariae nor adult heartworms concentrate the drug.

Excretion of DEC occurs almost entirely through the urine; 70% of the dose is eliminated in this manner within 24 hours of administration. Only 10%–25% of the drug is excreted unchanged; the remainder is excreted as 1 of 4 known metabolites, all of which contain the intact piperazine ring.

The rapid metabolism and excretion of DEC probably accounts for its low toxicity. It is relatively nontoxic and side effects usually do not occur at the low dosage (3 mg/lb) used for heartworm prevention. The greatest disadvantage of the drug is irritation to the gastric mucosa which occurs especially when high dosages (25–50 mg/lb) are used against ascarid infections of dogs and cats. In these cases, administration of the drug soon after the patient has eaten reduces the irritation and the occurrence of vomiting.

Other Uses. Low daily doses of DEC used as a prophylactic treatment for heartworm disease are also effective in preventing the establishment of canine ascarid infections. The addition of styrylpyridinium chloride to DEC (Styrid-Caricide) provides a means of preventing the establishment of hookworm infections as well.

Adult ascarids, however, are unaffected by low-level dosing of DEC. The adult ascarid burden of both dogs and cats can be eliminated by a single high oral dosage of 25–50 mg/lb. Tablets are generally used for this purpose and the treatment may be repeated in 10–20 days. DEC for treating canine and feline ascariasis is infrequently used since the less irritating piperazine salts are very effective for this purpose.

In sheep and especially in cattle, DEC has long been used for the treatment of lungworm infections caused by *Dictyocaulus*. Veterinarians in the United Kingdom, where heavy lungworm infections require some means of chemotherapy, have used this drug routinely at a dosage of 10 mg/lb (22 mg/kg) daily for 3 days. Intramuscular injection is the routine method of administration but equal efficacy apparently results when an initial intramuscular injection is followed by 2 orally administered doses. Immature worms are much more susceptible to the drug than are adult worms; thus the use of DEC is of greatest value when administered early in the infection.

REFERENCES

Alexander, F. 1969. An Introduction to Veterinary Pharmacology. Edinburgh and London: E. & S. Livingstone.

Aubry, M. L.; Cowell, P.; Davey, M. J.; and Shevde, S. 1970. Aspects of the pharmacology of a new anthelmintic: Pyrantel. Br J Pharmacol 38:332.

Baker, N. F., and Douglas, J. R. 1969. Anthelmintic activity of haloxon in calves with parasitic gastroenteritis. Am J Vet Res 30: 2233.

Baker, N. F.; Tucker, E. M.; Stormont, C.; and Fisk, R. A. 1970. Neurotoxicity of haloxon and its relationship to blood esterases of sheep. Am J Vet Res 31:865.

Baker, N. F.; Walters, G. T.; Hjerpe, C. A.; and Fisk, R. A. 1972. Experimental therapy of *Dictyocaulus viviparus* infection in cattle with cambendazole. Am J Vet Res 33:1127.

Batte, E. G.; Robison, O. W.; and Moncol, D. J. 1969. Influence of dichlorvos on swine reproduction and performance of offspring to weaning. J Am Vet Med Assoc 154:1397.

Bello, T. R.; Amborski, G. F.; and Torbert, B. J. 1974. Effects of organic phosphorus anthelmintics on blood cholinesterase values in horses and ponies. Am J Vet Res 35:73.

Benz, G. W. 1972. Anthelmintic activity of haloxon in calves. Am J Vet Res 33:1273.

Bikoryukov, A. A. 1969. Action of piperazine on larval and young *Ascaridia* in the gut of chicks. Sb Tr Vses Nauchn Issled Inst po Bolezn Ptits 3:209.

Boisvenue, R. J. 1963. Preliminary studies on the anthelmintic effects of 2,6-diiodo-4-nitrophenol against the gapeworm, *Syngamus trachea*. Am J Vet Res 24:1038.

———. 1974. Effectiveness of low doses of dithiazanine iodide on microfilariae of *Dirofilaria immitis* in dogs with established infections. In H. C. Morgan, ed. Proceedings of the Heartworm Symposium '74, p. 93. Bonner Springs, Kans.: V. M. Publishing.

Boyd, C. L., and Bullard, T. L. 1968. Organophosphate treatment of cutaneous habronemiasis in horses. J Am Vet Med Assoc 153:324.

Bradley, R. E., and Conway, D. P. 1970. Evaluation of pyrantel hydrochloride as an anthelmintic in dogs. Vet Med 65:767.

Bris, E. J.; Dyer, I. A.; Howes, A. D.; Schooley, M. A.; and Todd, A. C. 1968. Anthelmintic activity of 2,2-dichlorovinyl dimethyl phosphate in cattle. J Am Vet Med Assoc 152:175.

Burch, G. R. 1954. A new oral anthelmintic for canine whipworms. Vet Med 49:291.

Casida, J. E.; McBride, L.; and Niedermeir, R. P. 1962. Metabolism of 2,2-dichlorovinyl dimethyl phosphate in relation to residues in milk and mammalian tissues. J Agric Food Chem 10:370.

Chhabra, R. C., and Singh, K. S. 1972. Diagnosis, treatment and control of spirocercosis in dogs. Indian J Anim Sci 42:203.

Ciordia, H. 1972a. Activity of a feed premix and crumbles containing coumaphos in the control of gastrointestinal parasites of cattle. Am J Vet Res 33:623.

———. 1972b. Anthelmintic efficacy of Maretin in cattle. Proc Helminthol Soc Wash 39:16.

Collins, J. A.; Schooley, M. A.; and Singh, V. K. 1971. The effect of dietary dichlorvos on swine reproduction and viability of their offspring. Toxicol Appl Pharmacol 19:377.

Cook, T. F. 1973. The efficiency of a mixture of haloxon and trichlorfon against strongyles and bots in horses. NZ Vet J 21:157.

Costa, H. M. DeA.; Freitas, M. G.; and Guimaraes, M. P. 1970. Ruelene 8-DP in the treatment of gastro-intestinal helminthiasis of cattle. Pesqui Agropecu Bras 5:453.

Council on Veterinary Service. 1973. Procedures for the treatment and prevention of canine heartworm disease. J Am Vet Med Assoc 162:660.

Cox, D. D.; Mullee, M. T.; and Allen, A. D. 1967. Anthelmintic activity of two organic phosphorus compounds, coumaphos and naphthalophos, against gastrointestinal nematodes of cattle. Am J Vet Res 28:79.

Cross, B. G.; David, A.; and Vallance, D. K. 1954. Piperazine adipate: A new anthelmintic agent. II. Toxicological and pharmacological studies. J Pharm Pharmacol 6:711.

Czipri, D. A. 1970. The efficiency of haloxon against *Ascaris, Hyostrongylus* and *Oesophagostomum* in pigs. Vet Rec 86:306.

Davis, L. E.; Wescott, R. B.; and Musgrave, E. E. 1969. Influence of pH on uptake of thiabendazole by the nematode *Haemonchus contortus.* Am J Vet Res 30:1015.

Davis, R. B.; Good, R. E.; Tumlin, J. T.; and Brown, J. 1969. An effective anthelmintic in treatment of quail infected with *Capillaria contorta.* Avian Dis 13:690.

Dawe, D. L.; Brown, J.; Davis, R. B.; and Kellogg, F. E. 1969. Effectiveness of Maretin and Meldane as treatment for capillariasis in bobwhites. Avian Dis 13:662.

Dixon, J. M.; Johnson, W. A.; and Towers, B. A. 1959. Low level feeding of hygromycin B and phenothiazine for control of *Ascaridia galli* and *Heterakis gallinae* in broilers. Poult Sci 38:1199.

Douglas, J. R., and Baker, N. F. 1968. Chemotherapy of animal parasites. Annu Rev Pharmacol 8:213.

Drudge, J. H. 1964. New development in parasite control. Blood-Horse 87:132.

Drudge, J. H., and Lyons, E. T. 1972. Critical tests of a resin-pellet formulation of dichlorvos against internal parasites of the horse. Am J Vet Res 33:1365.

Drudge, J. H.; Leland, S. E., Jr.; and Wyant, Z. N. 1957. Strain variation in the response of sheep nematodes to the action of phenothiazine. II. Studies on pure infections of *Haemonchus contortus.* Am J Vet Res 18:137.

Drudge, J. H.; Szanto, J.; Wyant, Z. N.; and Elam, G. 1962. Critical tests on thiabendazole (MK-360) against parasites of the horse. J Parasitol (Suppl) 48:28.

Drudge, J. H.; Lyons, E. T.; and Tolliver, S. C. 1975. Critical and clinical test evaluations of mebendazole against internal parasites of the horse. Am J Vet Res 35:1409.

Dutta, B.; Chakravarty, A. K.; and Choudhury, T. 1972. Use of Ancylol against ancylostomiasis and gnathostomiasis in zoo animals. Orissa Vet J 7:27.

Düwel, D. 1974. The efficacy of fenbendazole in experimental nematodiasis of cattle. Meet 3rd Int Congr Parasitol, Munich, p. 1405.

Düwel, D.; Tiefenbach, B.; Kirsch, R.; and Dörrhöfer, H. 1974. Fenbendazole for the treatment of gastrointestinal parasitic infestations of sheep. Prakt Tieraerztl 8:425.

Edwin, J. P. 1964. The influence of glycobiarsol (Milibis) on *Trichuris vulpis.* Southwest Vet 17:218.

Eleazer, T. H. 1969. Coumaphos, a new anthelmintic for control of *Capillaria obsignata, Heterakis gallinarum* and *Ascaridia galli* in chickens. Avian Dis 13:228.

Enigk, K., and Dey-Hazra, A. 1970. Treatment of syngamosis in poultry. Dtsch Tieraerztl Wochenschr 77:609.

———. 1971. Therapy of *Strongyloides* infection in swine. Dtsch Tieraerztl Wochenschr 78:419.

Enigk, K.; Dey-Hazra, A.; and Gerlach, G. 1971. The therapy of *Hyostrongylus* infection of pigs. Dtsch Tieraerztl Wochenschr 78:569.

Enigk, K.; Dey-Hazra, A.; and Batke, J. 1974a. The efficacy of fenbendazol against gastrointestinal namatodes. Dtsch Tieraerztl Wochenschr 8:177.

———. 1974b. Treatment of helminthism in horses with fenbendazole. Prakt Tieraerztl 8:417.

Enzie, F. D., and Colglazier, M. L. 1953. Toluene (methylbenzene) for intestinal nematodes in dogs and cats. Vet Med Small Anim Pract 341:325.

Eyre, P. 1970. Some pharmacodynamic effects of the nematocides: Methyridine, tetramisole and pyrantel. J Pharm Pharmacol 22:26.

Forbes, L. S. 1972a. Some aspects of the pharmacology of pyrantel in the dog. NZ Vet J 20:83.

———. 1972b. Toxicological and pharmacological relations between levamisole, pyrantel and diethylcarbamazine and their significance in helminth chemotherapy. Southeast Asian J Trop Med Public Health 3:235.

Foxx, T. S., and Hansen, M. F. 1967. Action of naphthalophos and Yomesan against *Ascaridia galli* and *Heterakis gallinarum* in chickens. Avian Dis 11:680.

Frazier, M. N. 1959. Field trials with hygromycin as an anthelmintic in poultry. Avian Dis 3:478.

Georgi, J. R. 1974. Intestinal helminths. In R. W. Kirk, ed. Current Veterinary Therapy V. Small Animal Practice, p. 766. Philadelphia: W. B. Saunders.

Gibson, T. E. 1950. Critical tests of phenothiazine as an anthelmintic for horses. Vet Rec 62:341.

Gibson, T. E.; Everett, G.; and Mirzayans, A. 1969. A controlled test of methyridine, haloxon and pyrantel tartrate against *Nematodirus battus* in lambs. Res Vet Sci 10:307.

Goldsby, A. I., and Todd, A. C. 1957. Hygromycin, a broad-spectrum anthelmintic for swine. J Am Vet Med Assoc 131:471.

Gordon, H. McL. 1973. Anthelmintics—Ruminants and horses. In Course for Veterinarians on Parasitology and Epidemiology, No. 19, p. 319. Proc Univ Sydney, Post-Grad Comm Vet Sci.

Güralp, N., and Dincer, S. 1966. Koyunlardaki mide-barsak nematodlarinin tedavisinde maretin. Vet Fak Derg Ankara Univ 13:1.

Hall, C. A. 1965. Investigations into the safety of Rametin[R] (Bayer S 940 [9002]) when used as a sheep anthelmintic in Australia. Vet Med Rev, Leverkeusen 1:21.

Hamilton, J. M. 1967. The treatment of lungworm disease in the cat with tetramisole. J Small Anim Pract 8:325.

Hart, R. J., and Lee, R. M. 1966. Cholinesterase activities of various nematode parasites and their inhibition by the organophosphate anthelmintic haloxon. Exp Parasitol 18:332.

Hass, K. D. 1970. Dichlorvos—An organophosphate anthelmintic. In J. L. Rabinowitz and R. M. Myerson, eds. Topics in Medicinal Chemistry, vol. 3, p. 171. New York: John Wiley & Sons.

Hoff, D. R.; Fisher, M. H.; Bochis, R. J.; Lusi, A.; Waksmumski, F.; Egerton, J. R.; Yakstis, J. J.; Cuckler, A. C.; and Campbell, W. C. 1970. A new broad spectrum anthelmintic: 2-(4-thiazolyl)-5-*iso*propoxycarbonylaminobenzimidazole. Experientia 26: 550.

Howes, H. L., Jr. 1972. *Trans*-1,4,5,6-tetrahydro-2-(3-hydroxystyryl)-1-methylpyrimidine (CP-14,445), a new antiwhipworm agent. Proc Soc Exp Bio Med 139:394.

Jackson, R. F. 1972. Some new chemotherapeutic agents for dirofilariasis—A preliminary report. In R. E. Bradley and G. Pacheo, eds. Canine Heartworm Disease: The Current Knowledge, p. 129. Proc 2nd Univ of Fla Symp on Canine Heartworm Disease, Jacksonville, 1971.

———. 1974a. Treatment of the asymptomatic dog. In H. C. Morgan, ed. Proceedings of the Heartworm Symposium '74, p. 53. Bonner Springs, Kans.: V. M. Publishing.

———. 1974b. The venae cavae syndrome. In H. C. Morgan, ed. Proceedings of the Heartworm Symposium '74, p. 48. Bonner Springs, Kans.: V. M. Publishing.

Jackson, W. F. 1974. Management of the symptomatic patient. In H. C. Morgan, ed. Proceedings of the Heartworm Symposium '74, p. 56. Bonner Springs, Kans.: V. M. Publishing.

Joyce, J. R.; Hanselka, D. V.; and Boyd, C. L. 1972. Treatment of habronemiasis of the adnexa of the equine eye. Vet Med Small Anim Clin 67:1008.

Kalkofen, U. P. 1971. Effect of dichlorvos on eggs and larvae of *Ancylostoma caninum*. Am J Trop Med Hyg 20:436.

Kibble, R. M. 1969. Glycobiarsol for the control of *Trichuris vulpis* infection in the dog. Aust Vet J 45:387.

Knowles, C. O., and Casida, J. E. 1966. Mode of action of organophosphate anthelmintics. Cholinesterase inhibition in *Ascaris lumbricoides*. J Agric Food Chem 14:566.

Lee, D. L. 1965. The Physiology of Nematodes. San Francisco: W. H. Freeman.

Legendre, A. M. 1973. Disophenol toxicosis in a dog. J Am Vet Med Assoc 163:149.

Leland, S. E.; Combs, G. E.; and Wallace, L. J. 1968. Anthelmintic activity of thiabendazole and trichlorphon against migrating and adult *Strongyloides ransomi* in suckling and weanling pigs. Am J Vet Res 29:797.

Levine, N. D., and Garrigus, U. S. 1962. The effect of cu-nic and organophosphorus anthelmintics on phenothiazine-resistant *Haemonchus* in sheep. Am J Vet Res 22:489.

Link, R. P. 1965. Antinematodal drugs. In L. M. Jones, ed. Veterinary Pharmacology and Therapeutics, 3rd ed., p. 645. Ames: Iowa State Univ. Press.

Lyons, E. T.; Drudge, J. H.; and Tolliver, S. C. 1974. Critical tests of three salts of pyrantel against internal parasites of the horse. Am J Vet Res 35:1515.

McFarland, J. W. 1972. The chemotherapy of intestinal nematodes. In E. Jucker, ed. Progress in Drug Research, vol. 16, p. 157. Basel, Switzerland: Birkhäuser Verlog.

McWilliams, L. J.; Palmer, H. C.; and Good, R. E. 1973. A new anthelmintic for exotic ruminants. J Zoo Anim Med 4:12.

Malone, J. D. 1964. Toxicity of haloxon. Res Vet Sci 5:17.

Martin, C. L.; Christmas, R.; and Leipold, H. W. 1972. Formation of temporary cataracts in dogs given disophenol preparation. J Am Vet Med Assoc 161:294.

Miller, T. A. 1966. Anthelmintic activity of thenium *p*-chlorobenzenesulfonate against various stages of *Ancylostoma caninum* in young dogs. Am J Vet Res 27:54.

Nicholson, L. G., and McCullogh, E. C. 1942. Some effects of feeding phenothiazine to chickens in various amounts. J Am Vet Med Assoc 101:205.

Nollin, S. De., and Van den Bossche, H. 1973. Biochemical effects of mebendazole on *Trichinella spiralis* larvae. J Parasitol 59: 970.

Oakley, G. A. 1974. Activity of levamisole hydrochloride administered subcutaneously against *A. suum* infections in pigs. Vet Rec 95:190.

Osteux, R.; Lesieur-Demarguilly, I.; and Lesieur, D. 1971. Mode of action of piperazine on *Ascaris lumbricoides* var. *suum*. I. Study on respiration and antagonism between piperazine and both coenzyme A and adenosine triphosphate. Ann Pharm Fr 29:125.

Pankavich, J. A.; Poeschel, G. P.; Shor, A. L.; and Gallo, A. 1973. Evaluation of levamisole against experimental infections of *Ascaridia, Heterakis,* and *Capillaria* spp. in chickens. Am J Vet Res 34:501.

Penumarthy, L.; Dehme, F. W.; and Menhusen, M. J. 1975. Investigations of therapeutic measures for disophenol toxicosis in dogs. Am J Vet Res 36:1259.

Plé, V., and Abram, M. 1971. Comparison of the activity of seven anthelmintics used in pig. Rec Med Vet Ec Alfort 147:35.

Poeschel, G. P., and Todd, A. C. 1972. Controlled evaluation of formulated dichlorvos for use in cattle. Am J Vet Res 33:1071.

Poole, J. B., and Dooley, K. L. 1972. Anthelmintic efficacy of topically applied crufomate against gastrointestinal parasites in cattle. Am J Vet Res 33:1063.

Presidente, P. J. A.; Schlegel, M. W.; and Knapp, S. E. 1971. Efficacy of levamisole in alfalfa pellets against naturally occurring gastrointestinal nematode infections in calves. Am J Vet Res 32:1359.

Prichard, R. K. 1970. Mode of action of the anthelmintic thiabendazole in *Haemonchus contortus.* Nature 228:684.

———. 1973. The fumarate reductase reaction of *Haemonchus contortus* and the mode of action of some anthelmintics. Int J Parasitol 3:409.

Probert, A. J.; Smith, B. D. S.; and Herbert, I. V. 1973. The efficiency of orally and subcutaneously administered levamisole against mature and immature stages of *Hyostrongylus rubidus* (Hassal and Stiles 1892), the stomach worm of pigs. Vet Rec 93:302.

Robinson, L. R., and Ziegler, R. L. 1968. Clinical laboratory data derived from 102 *Macaca mulatta.* Lab Anim Care 18:50.

Romanowski, R. D.; Rhoads, M. L.; Colglazier, M. L.; and Kates, K. C. 1975. Effect of cambendazole, thiabendazole, and levamisole on fumarate reductase in cambendazole-resistant and -sensitive strains of *Haemonchus contortus.* J Parasitol 61:777.

Sanderson, B. E. 1970. The effects of anthelmintics on nematode metabolism. Comp Gen Pharmacol 1:135.

———. 1973. Anthelmintics in the study of helminth metabolism. In A. E. Taylor and R. Muller, eds. Chemotherapeutic Agents in the Study of Parasites, p. 53. London: Blackwell Scientific Publications.

Simpson, C. F., and Jackson, R. F. 1974. Pathophysiology of heartworm disease. In H. C. Morgan, ed. Proceedings of the Heartworm Symposium '74, p. 38. Bonner Springs, Kans.: V. M. Publishing.

Simpson, C. F.; Jackson, R. F.; and Bradley, R. E. 1972. Alterations of glomerular capillaries in canine heartworm disease. In R. E. Bradley and G. Pacheco, eds. Canine Heartworm Disease: The Current Knowledge, p. 39. Proc 2nd Univ of Fla Symp on Canine Heartworm Disease, Jacksonville, 1971.

Slack, R., and Nineham, A. W. 1968. Drugs in veterinary medicine. In R. Slack and A. W. Nineham, eds. Medical and Veterinary Chemicals, vol. 1, p. 200. Elmsford, N.Y.: Pergamon Press.

Smith, C. F. 1973. Some aspects of the pharmacology of pyrantel. NZ Vet J 21:52.

Snow, D. H. 1971. The effects of dichlorvos on several blood enzyme levels in the greyhound. Aust Vet J 47:468.

Standen, O. D. 1963. Chemotherapy of helminthic infections. In R. J. Schnitzer and F. Hawking, eds. Experimental Chemotherapy, vol. 1, p. 701. New York: Academic Press.

Tacal, J. V., Jr. 1963. Dithiazanine iodide treatment for canine spirocercosis. Mod Vet Pract 44:70.

Thienpont, D.; Vanparijs, O.; Spruyt, J.; and Marsboom, R. 1968. The anthelmintic activity of tetramisole in the dog. Vet Rec 83:369.

Todd, A. C. 1962. Comparison of three broad-spectrum anthelmintics in lambs. Vet Med 57:322.

Van den Bossche, H. 1972. Biochemical effects of the anthelmintic drug mebendazole. In H. Van den Bossche, ed. Comparative Biochemistry of Parasites, 1st ed., p. 139. Proc Int Symp, Belgium, 1971. New York: Academic Press.

Van Nueten, J. M. 1972. Pharmacological aspects of tetramisole. In H. Van den Bossche, ed. Comparative Biochemistry of Parasites, 1st ed., p. 101. Proc Int Symp, Belgium, 1971. New York: Academic Press.

Warwick, B. L.; Turk, R. D.; and Berry, R. O. 1946. Abortion in sheep following the administration of phenothiazine. J Am Vet Med Assoc 108:41.

Welter, C. J., and Johnson, D. R. 1963. Anthelmintic activity of *n*-butyl chloride and toluene combinations in dogs and cats. Vet Med 58:869.

Wood, I. B.; Pankavich, J. A.; Wallace, W. S.; Thorson, R. E.; Burkhart, R. L.; and Waletzky, E. 1961. Disophenol, an injectable anthelmintic for canine hookworms. J Am Vet Med Assoc 139:1101.

Worley, D. E., and Thompson, P. E. 1962.

Therapeutic effects of pyrvinium pamoate and dithiazanine iodide against experimental *Strongyloides stercoralis* infections in dogs. J Parasitol (Abstr) 48 (Sec 2) 2:27.

Yakstis, J. J.; Egerton, J. R.; Campbell, W. C.; and Cuckler, A. C. 1968. Use of thiabendazole—Medicated feed for prophylaxis of four common roundworm infections in dogs. J Parasitol 54:359.

Zwart, P., and Jansen, J., Jr. 1969. Treatment of lungworm in snakes with tetramisole. Vet Rec 84:374.

CHAPTER 53

ANTICESTODAL AND ANTITREMATODAL DRUGS

EDWARD L. ROBERSON

ANTICESTODAL DRUGS

Anticestodal (antitapeworm) drugs are referred to as *taeniacides* when they cause death of the tapeworm *in situ* and *taeniafuges* when they simply cause or facilitate tapeworm expulsion. Tapeworms maintain their position in the digestive tract by attachment of the scolex to the mucosa and by undulation.

Many of the older antitapeworm drugs are natural organic compounds which act as taeniafuges. These drugs, in general, paralyze the tapeworm at least temporarily. However, recovery from paralysis and reattachment are liable to occur before expulsion can take place. Thus purgation in conjunction with administration of the taeniafuge is generally required. This disadvantage of having to purge animals when using taenifuges plus the need for more highly efficacious anticestodal drugs has led to the synthesis of taeniacidal drugs which are simpler and more widely used today.

The aim of satisfactory treatment of tapeworm infections is the complete removal of the parasite. If the anticestodal drug simply causes destrobilization of the tapeworm, the intact scolex is likely to regenerate another body in less than 2 weeks. Thus examination of the animal's feces for tapeworm segments is advised at 14–21 days following the initial drug treatment.

Control of the intermediate host of tapeworms is necessary to prevent reinfection of the host following successful treatment for adult worms. Control of fleas and lice which vector *Dipylidium caninum* of dogs and cats can readily be accomplished. Also control of *Taenia* infections by preventing cats and dogs from ingesting rodents and lagomorphs, respectively, is within reason. But control of orbatid soil mites which vector ruminant and equine tapeworms is impractical at present.

NATURAL ORGANIC COMPOUNDS

COMPOUNDS OF HISTORIC INTEREST

The earliest anticestodal drugs used in human beings and sometimes in animals were of plant origin; e.g., a local remedy still used against cestodes in some countries is the ingestion of minced pumpkin seed. The active component in these seeds is cucurbitine, which appears to be totally lacking in toxicity even in debilitated patients and in children only 2–3 months of age. The relatively low efficacy of cucurbitine, 55% for *Taenia saginata* (Pawlowski and Chwirot 1970), has not warranted commercial promotion of this compound in either human or veterinary medicine.

The powdered rhizome of the male fern *(Dryopteris felix mas)* was used by Greek physicians for its anticestodal properties. Subsequently, ether extraction of the dried powdered rhizomes of the male fern was found to yield an oily residue, aspidium oleoresin, of which the principal active ingredient seems to be filicic acid. Aspidium oleoresin acts by paralyzing the muscles of the tapeworm; i.e., it is a taeniafuge that causes a temporary relaxation of the worm. A purge is necessary to ensure passage of the worms. It had been the best known and most commonly used anthelmintic for all species of human tapeworms until the advent of synthetic organic drugs in the 1950s.

Until recent years, another product of plant origin, kamala, was considered the drug of choice for removing the cat tapeworms *(Dipylidium caninum* and *Taenia tateniaformis).* Kamala is obtained from the glands and hairs covering the fruits of *Mallotus philippinensis,* a plant that is widespread in the Philippines and is found also in India, China, and Australia.

Kamala acts as a stimulant and then as a paralyzing agent both on the cestodes and on the host's intestinal muscle (Nurtaeva 1972). If the cestodes are washed after narcotization by a 1×10^{-3} concentration of kamala, they recover motility. At concentrations of 1×10^{-3} to 1×10^{-7}, kamala has been found to stimulate the intestinal muscles of rabbits and rats and then irreversibly paralyze them. Today it is virtually never used in veterinary medicine.

In earlier years, when other anticestodals were not available, nicotine sulfate was used in ruminants for removal of tapeworms. It was generally given in combination with copper sulfate. The efficacy for these two compounds for ruminant tapeworms and nematodes, respectively, was only about 50%. Newer, more efficient drugs have replaced their use today.

ARECOLINE AND ITS COMPOUNDS

Of the older anticestodals of natural origin, arecoline (Fig. 53.1) is still used today for the production of several anticestodal compounds that are useful in veterinary medicine, chiefly in dogs. Arecoline is an alkaloid obtained from the seeds of the betel nut palm *(Areca catechu),* which is grown in the Far East and South India. Arecoline itself is rather unstable; its derivatives (arecoline hydrobromide, arecoline-acetarsol, and arecoline carboxyphenylstilbonate), however, have a considerably longer shelf life and are in some places widely used against cestode infections of dogs and cats.

Arecoline Hydrobromide. *Arecoline Hydrobromide,* N.F., is a fine, white, bitter,

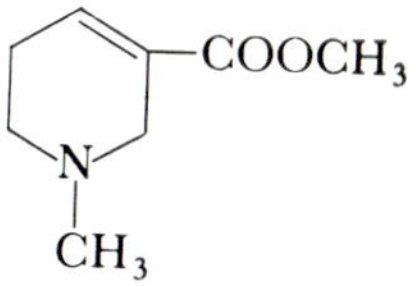

$-COOCH_3$

N

CH_3

Arecoline

FIG. 53.1.

crystalline material. It is relatively stable both when dry and when in aqueous solution. However, it should be stored in a light-resistant container.

Indications. Arecoline hydrobromide is effective against all tapeworms of dogs including *Echinococcus.* Laboratory-induced infections of *Taenia pisiformis, T. hydatigena, T. ovis, Multiceps multiceps,* and *Echinococcus granulosus* in dogs can be treated successfully with arecoline hydrobromide. In studies by Forbes (1964), the drug was given as a solution in gelatin capsules at a dosage of 2 mg/kg of body weight. The treatment removed all *Multiceps,* almost all *Taenia,* and 99% of the *Echinococcus* despite the fact that the *Echinococcus* that were expelled numbered in the thousands.

Until the advent of bunamidine, arecoline was the only substance satisfactory for the treatment of *Echinococcus* in dogs (Forbes 1966). It is effective against both nongravid and adult forms. *Echinococcus* infections in dogs in the Soviet Union have been markedly controlled by treatment with arecoline hydrobromide. This treatment campaign plus stringent laws against feeding sheep offal to dogs reduced the incidence of sheep hydatid from 40% to less than 10% from 1967 to 1970.

Mode of action. The anticestodal action of arecoline hydrobromide appears to be exerted both by paralyzing the worm until it looses its attachment to the intestinal mucosa and at the same time by stimulating increased peristalsis so that the detached worm is expelled. The drug causes only temporary paralysis of tapeworms. Worms are likely to recover and reattach if purgation has not occurred satisfactorily within approximately 2 hours following medication. In such cases, dogs should be given a saline enema to induce evacuation. The action of arecoline hydrobromide in causing purgation is a local one resulting from its cholinergic effects on the gastrointestinal (GI) muscle and the secretory glands (Forbes 1971).

Administration and pharmacodynamics. A 12- to 13-hour starvation period is optimum when arecoline hydrobromide is being used against canine cestodes (Nikitin et al. 1969). Administration of the drug in meat is recommended only where dosing with a pill is difficult.

Arecoline hydrobromide is administered orally but the formulation of the compound and dosing technique determine the presence and degree of toxic reactions. When the drug is administered in the form of enteric-coated tablets, it is absorbed from the gut, enters the portal circulation (Bell and Bennett 1970), and apparently is rapidly inactivated in the liver with minimal evidence of toxicity. However, when absorption occurs through the oral mucosa, as when administered in solution, systemic absorption is greater and signs of toxicity are 100-fold more likely to occur. In the United States, arecoline hydrobromide is almost always administered in the form of enteric-coated tablets which are intended to pass into the intestine before dissolving. If it is necessary to administer the drug in a solution, it should be given by syringe with an attached cannula which allows depositing the solution at the base of the tongue while the dog's head is held upward. This technique fairly well ensures rapid swallowing of the dose with minimal exposure of the drug to the oral mucosa.

The onset of catharsis in the dog occurs usually about 15 minutes after administration of arecoline hydrobromide in tablet form and lasts for 30–40 minutes. However, some dogs may not defecate for several hours. As previously indicated, catharsis is important since the tapeworms must be expelled during the approximately 2.5 hours they are paralyzed. More rapid onset of catharsis occurs when the drug is given orally in solution.

Dosage. For general use in dogs, a dosage of approximately 1 mg/kg of body weight is recommended (Batham 1946). With this dosage there is a minimum of discomfort and vomition and no unconsiousness is expected.

A dosage of 1.75 mg arecoline hydrobromide/kg of body weight has been used in dogs by many practitioners. With this dosage, one can expect greater discomfort to the dog, greater incidence of vomition, and occasional unconsciousness. No appreciable difference in the efficacy of arecoline hydrobromide for cestodes at dosage levels of 1 and 1.75 mg/kg has been shown.

Dosages of 3–4 mg/kg of body weight at intervals of 1.5 months have been used by Russians for treating working dogs in an effort to break the life cycle of *Multiceps* and *Echinococcus* and consequently reduce the mortality of sheep from coenuriasis and hydatid disease (Aminzhanov and Gel'diev 1972). The degree of toleration of these high dosages is not described.

Toxicity. Emesis and exaggerated catharsis with liquid feces occur in a low percentage of dogs given a therapeutic dose of arecoline hydrobromide. These reactions are mild and only transitory without particular discomfort to the dog. With larger doses, excessive vomition, diarrhea, and convulsions followed by unconsciousness occur in some dogs.

The toxic effect of administering 44 mg/kg of body weight has been tested in dogs. Although they showed signs of extreme discomfort and convulsions, there were no deaths.

The pharmacological antidote for arecoline hydrobromide is atropine sulfate, 0.044 mg/kg of body weight. Atropine does not appear to interfere with the paralyzing effect of arecoline hydrobromide on the parasite (Link 1965).

Arecoline hydrobromide is generally not used in cats because it is understood to cause excessive bronchial secretion, which may cause suffocation. Brander and Pugh (1971) observed that no scientific corroboration substantiated this claim.

Arecoline-Acetarsol. *Arecoline-acetarsol* (Drocarbil, Nemural) is the arecoline salt of 3-acetamido-4-hydroxyphenylarsonic acid. It is a white, tasteless, odorless powder, formulated into scored tablets for commercial use. Although soluble in water, it is unstable in solution and must be used shortly after dissolving.

Arecoline-acetarsol is used in both dogs and cats as an anticestodal for tapeworms *(Taenia* and *Dipylidium)* and as a laxative at lower doses. There is no claim for efficacy against *Echinococcus.* Following ingestion of the tablet, arecoline-acetarsol hydrolyzes in the stomach, releasing arecoline which is the active agent (Link 1965). Like arecoline hydrobromide, arecoline-acetarsol stimulates purgation which aids expulsion of the presumably narcotized tapeworms. Catharsis generally occurs within 25–40 minutes after administration. Should catharsis not occur within 3 hours, a saline cathartic or enema is indicated. The stimulation of peristalsis allows this drug to be used effectively as a laxative in both dogs and cats when one-half the anticestodal therapeutic dose is given.

Arecoline-acetarsol is generally well tolerated. Vomition occasionally occurs. Rarely, adverse reactions include salivation, restlessness, ataxia, and labored breathing. Puppies less than 3 months of age and cats less than 1 year should not be treated with arecoline-acetarsol. It is also contraindicated in animals having febrile conditions, intestinal disturbances, or severe cardiac or circulatory disturbances. Atropine is an antidote.

Dosage. The dosage of arecoline-acetarsol for anticestodal therapy in both dogs and adult cats is 18 mg/8 lb (4.9 mg/kg) of body weight. For dogs, the drug is best given with a piece of meat in the morning about 1 hour following a light meal. For cats, it is recommended that arecoline-acetarsol be given in milk 3 hours after a principal meal.

For its laxative effect, the drug can be used in both dogs and cats at a dosage of 18 mg/15 lb (2.6 mg/kg) of body weight; as a purgative, a dosage of 18 mg/10 lb (4 mg/kg) of body weight is recommended.

Arecoline Carboxyphenylstilbonate. *Arecoline carboxyphenylstilbonate* (Anthelin) is used in dogs for the removal of tapeworms *(Taenia* and *Dipylidium).* It is available in tablet form and should be administered orally at a dosage level of 4.7 mg/lb (10.3 mg/kg) of body weight up to a maximum dose of 211.5 mg of drug for dogs weighing 45 lb (20.5 kg) or over. Only milk should be fed during the 24 hours prior to treatment. Like other arecoline derivatives, catharsis generally occurs and is desired. If catharsis does not occur within 3 hours, an enema will facilitate passage of worms. The treatment can be repeated in 1 week if indicated.

Signs of toxicity include depression, nausea, vomiting, and colic. Should toxicity occur, dogs should be fed within 1 hour after administering the drug; otherwise a regular meal should be given 4–8 hours after medication. Toxicity is more likely to occur in sick or undernourished dogs; therefore arecoline carboxyphenylstilbonate is contraindicated in these animals.

Inorganic Compounds

Tin compounds (mixtures of metallic tin with its oxide or chloride of dibutyltin dilaurate) were used rather extensively a decade ago as anticestodals for humans but only infrequently for domestic animals. The anticestodal activity of tin compounds is thought to depend on the coating of the tapeworm cuticle with a thin layer of tin particles which renders the strobila susceptible to digestion (Harant et al. 1957). The efficacy of tin preparations in human cestodiasis is judged to be in the range of 72%–98%. The necessity that tin compounds be given once/day over a period of several days and the variable frequency of side effects now limit their use in human beings since newer less toxic taeniacides of probable greater efficacy are available (Davis 1973).

There is little work to substantiate recommending tin compounds for use in domesticated animals. Poultry tapeworms, especially species of *Davainea* and *Raillietina,* have been successfully treated with single oral dosages of dibutyltin dilaurate (Butynorate) at a level of 35 mg/kg of body weight. Satisfactory results are also reported for the use of tin compounds against *Dipylidium* in dogs.

Lead arsenate ($PbHAsO_4$) has been used throughout the world to treat *Moniezia* infections in lambs, calves, and kids. It was first used as an insecticidal spray for orchard fruit parasites. The value of this drug as an anticestodal was recognized when it was observed that sheep eating grass from beneath lead arsenate-treated trees subsequently expelled large numbers of tapeworms. Controlled tests show almost 100% efficacy of lead arsenate for *Moniezia* in feeder lambs and almost equally high efficacy for this parasite in calves and kids (Link 1965). It is not effective, however, against the fringed tapeworm (*Thysanosoma*).

Lead arsenate is thought to be hydrolyzed in the digestive tract to its respective forms, lead and arsenic. The lead is probably converted to lead oxide and the pentavalent arsenic to its more toxic trivalent form (Link 1965).

A single dose of 1 g of lead arsenate is required for highest efficacy against *Moniezia* in lambs over 2 months of age and in calves over 3 months. A dose of 0.5 g/head is recommended for calves under 3 months of age and for kids. The dose is generally administered in capsules without fasting. Lambs under 2 months of age should not be treated. Taeniasis is a disease of young animals; consequently, rarely is treatment for tapeworms indicated after ruminants reach 6 months of age.

The margin of safety of lead arsenate is markedly low. Daily doses of 2 g have killed sheep in only 2 days and daily doses of 1 g were fatal to sheep after 6 days. The signs of severe toxicity in animals include profuse diarrhea, oliguria, extreme weakness, and increased capillary permeability resulting in a marked drop in arterial pressure and resultant shock. If the recommended dosage is strictly adhered to, toxicity is not likely to develop in ruminants. This compound, however, should never be used in poultry.

Synthetic Organic Compounds

salts of bunamidine

Synthesis of salts of bunamidine and subsequent testing in the 1960s led to the identification of three compounds that possessed exceptional anticestodal properties. One of these, bunamidine hydrochloride, is widely used presently in the United Kingdom and the United States against tapeworms of dogs and cats. The second, bunamidine hydroxynapththoate, is used against *Moniezia* infections in sheep and goats. The third salt of bunamidine, bunamidine *p*-toluene sulfonate, is active against *Taenia pisiformis* of dogs but marked vomition (Hatton 1967) probably accounts for the limited development of this compound for use as an anticestodal.

Bunamidine Hydrochloride. *Chemistry.* The compound *bunamidine hydrochloride* (Scolaban) chemically is *N,N*-dibutyl-4-hexyloxynaphthamidine hydrochloride; the structural formula is shown in Fig. 53.2. It is a white, odorless, crystalline solid, soluble in methanol and hot water. Its melting point is 208°–211° C.

Anticestodal spectrum. Bunamidine hydrochloride in a single dose has high efficacy against all tapeworms of the dog and cat including adult forms of *Echinococcus granulosus.* There are differences of opinion as to the need for a second treatment at 48 hours to remove the immature worms of *E. granulosus.* Andersen et al. (1975) have found no particular advantage of dual over single treatment since each regimen yielded between 86% and 99% efficacy for immature *E. granulosus* in their studies. The drug does not have labeled indication for *E. granulosus* in the United States at this time. It is also highly effective for *Moniezia expansa* but is not marketed in the United States for sheep. Efficacy is reduced if the drug is administered at any time other than when the animal's stomach is empty. This compound has limited efficacy also for ascarids of both dogs and cats but other drugs adequately eliminate these worms.

Mode of action. All of the bunamidine

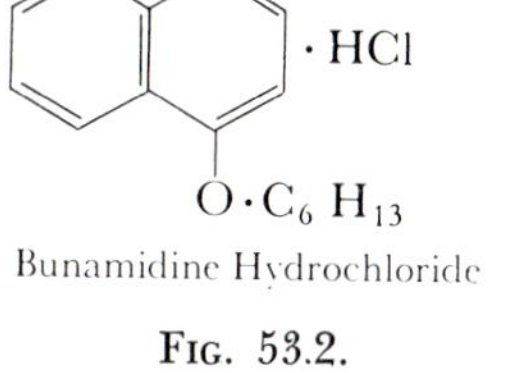

$$HN{=}C\cdot N\cdot(C_4H_9)_2$$

$$\cdot HCl$$

$$O\cdot C_6H_{13}$$

Bunamidine Hydrochloride

Fig. 53.2.

salts act as taeniacides. Tapeworms are digested in the host's gut. The physiological mechanism of destroying the tapeworm is not known. In cases in which the scolex *in situ* is covered by mucus (as may occur with enteric pathology), disintegration of the protected scolex evidently does not occur and the efficacy is reduced. The drug does not cause purging.

Administration, pharmocodynamics, and toxicity. Commercially available bunamidine hydrochloride is administered orally in compression-coated tablet form. The tablets disintegrate quickly in the stomach and the drug is immediately available for action against tapeworms located in the duodenal area of the small intestine.

Tablets of bunamidine hydrochloride should not be crushed or dissolved in liquid prior to administration since irritation of the oral mucous membranes occurs. Additionally, oral absorption evidently results in greater levels of the drug in general circulation and, consequently, a greater danger of toxic effects than when absorption is strictly from the gut. The drug is thought to be absorbed from the gut by the normal liver, with very little of the bunamidine hydrochloride getting past the liver into general circulation (Fastier 1972).

Although oral administration of bunamidine hydrochloride in tablets is relatively safe for dogs, intravenous administration of the drug into general circulation is highly toxic. Even small dosages, i.e., 5 mg/kg, when given intravenously may be fatal and a dosage of 1–2 mg/kg produces a marked fall in arterial pressure (Bills et al. 1970). Similar doses when administered orally by tablet generally do not result in reduced blood pressure.

Fatalities following routine oral administration of the tablet formulation of bunamidine hydrochloride occasionally occur. In fatal cases on which postmortem examinations have been performed, liver damage has often been found. Additionally, dosing dogs with 50 mg (normal therapeutic level) or 200 mg/kg at a 2-day interval results in increases in serum glutamic pyruvic transaminase (GPT) and alkaline phosphatase levels, indicating liver damage due to treatment (Menrath et al. 1973). Blood glucose and blood lactate levels were not consistently altered in these studies. The existence of hepatic disease at the time of administration of the drug, however, may allow for accumulation of higher levels of bunamidine hydrochloride or its metabolites in general circulation. However, liver damage is not thought to be the usual cause of death.

Ventricular fibrillation has been implicated as a mechanism of death in fatal cases of bunamidine hydrochloride treatment. This concept has been supported both experimentally and from field observations (Fastier 1972). A typical field case history involves sudden death during exercise of the dog within several to 24 hours following administration of the drug. Indeed, it is probably significant that the death rate for country working-type dogs in New Zealand is 3 times higher than that of town dogs following routine use of bunamidine hydrochloride. These observations of death following excitement are similar to the situation where death occurs when animals are injected with adrenaline subsequent to administration of chloroform or amarin. Fortunately, the propensity for bunamidine hydrochloride to give rise to ventricular fibrillation seems to be much less than that of these drugs. It should be emphasized that the incidence of sudden death following routine administration of bunamidine hydrochloride as an anticestodal is extremely low (1 dog in about 2000).

The most likely side effects from using bunamidine hydrochloride in dogs and cats is occasional emesis and/or transient diarrhea. Of 55 stray animals tested by Burrows and Lillis (1966), 9% experienced vomition and a few had loose stools within 24 hours following administration of the drug. In the author's experience, this percentage of vomition and loose stools is approximately what is expected in a group of stray animals becoming acclimated to confinement and a regular diet. Other workers, however, have associated both vomition and loose stools directly to use of the drug and it seems to be a valid, though only slightly important, criticism of the compound.

Reduced spermatogenesis has been found in dogs but not in cats at 4 days and up to 28 days following administration of the maximum recommended dosage (50 mg) of bunamidine hydrochloride.

Bunamidine hydrochloride can be administered to bitches at all stages of pregnancy. No ill effects have been experienced in animals so treated nor in their litters.

Dosage. A single dose of bunamidine hydrochloride at 25–50 mg/kg of body weight is recommended for dogs and cats after a 3- to 4-hour fast. The animal may be fed 3 hours after treatment.

Bunamidine Hydroxynaphthoate. The hydroxynaphthoate of bunamidine (Buban) is a pale yellow crystalline solid, insoluble in water, but soluble at 20° C in 35 parts of alcohol.

The drug is marketed in the United Kingdom for use against *Moniezia expansa* and *M. benedeni* in sheep and goats. Separate studies have indicated that bunamidine hydroxynaphthoate has an efficacy range of 83%–100% for these parasites. It was somewhat less efficacious (83%) than niclosamide (100%) against *M. expansa* in a comparative study in goats. However, the goats were dosed on a full stomach and the efficacy of bunamidine hydroxynaphthoate is likely to have been greater had the goats been fasted.

The drug appears to be quite safe for sheep and goats. Pregnant goats given the recommended dosage and kids given twice the recommended dosage suffer no ill effects. Mild scouring can be expected in kids given 3 times the recommended dosage. In the United Kingdom, a single dose is given to sheep and goats during the spring or summer followed by a second dose in the autumn if reinfection occurs. The dose is given as an oral drench, 25–50 mg/kg of body weight.

Bunamidine hydroxynaphthoate has been tried as an anticestodal in dogs. It was relatively inactive against *Taenia pisiformis* when given on an empty stomach but was highly effective (4-fold increase) against both *T. pisiformis* and *T. hydatigena* when administered in food at 25 mg/kg (Hatton 1967). This contrasts with the results obtained with the hydrochloride of bunamidine, which tends to have reduced efficacy when administered on a full or partially full stomach. Bunamidine hydroxynaphthoate in single doses appears to produce only negligible side effects in dogs, i.e., diarrhea in some cases. Incorporation of bunamidine hydroxynaphthoate into a prepared food for continuous (up to 4 days) daily treatment of dogs infected with *Echinococcus* and *Taenia* has proved efficacious but impractical due to problems associated with palatability and excessive vomition (Gemmell and Oudemans 1974).

NICLOSAMIDE

Chemistry. *Niclosamide* INN (Yomesan, Mansonil), known as phenasal in the Soviet Union, has the chemical formula 2′,5-dichloro-4′-nitrosalicylanilide INN; its structural formula is shown in Fig. 53.3. It is a yellow-white tasteless powder that is virtually insoluble in water but is soluble at 20° C in 150 parts of alcohol.

Indications. Niclosamide, since the early 1960s, has increased in use throughout the world for tapeworm infections of domestic animals and human beings. It is marketed in the United States for use only in dogs and cats among domestic animals and has Food and Drug Administration (FDA) approval for the removal of *Dipylidium caninum, Taenia pisiformis, T. hydatigena,* and *T. taeniaformis.* Most studies indicate poor efficacy of niclosamide for *Echinococcus* infections of dogs. In the author's experience, niclosamide is distinctly less effective against *Dipylidium* infections in dogs than is bunamidine hydrochloride or diuredosan. Sharp et al. (1973) found disappointing efficacy of niclosamide (18%) against canine *Dipylidium;* but relatively good efficacies against *Dipylidium* were obtained with Anthelin (87%) and Nemural (75%).

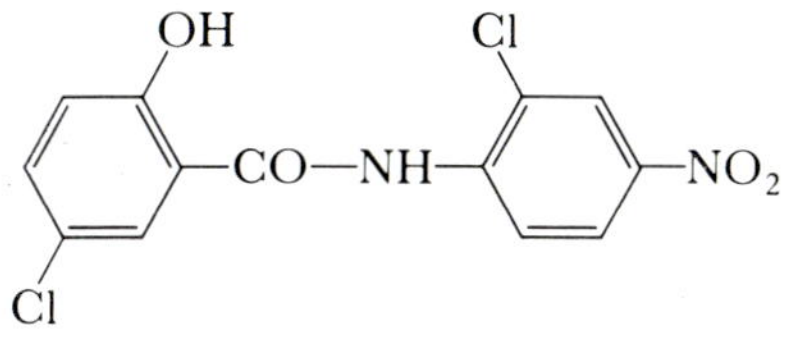

Niclosamide appears to be widely used in other countries not only for tapeworms of dogs and cats but also for *Moniezia* infections of cattle, sheep, and goats. It is highly effective against the fringed tapeworm (*Thysanosoma)* found in cattle, sheep, and deer in the United States and South America. Experimentally, niclosamide (phenasal) has been used successfully against anoplocephalid infections *(Anoplocephala magna, A. perfoliata,* and *Paranoplocephala mamillana)* of horses and cestode infections *(Bothriocephalus)* of certain fish (carp) in the Soviet Union.

OH, Cl — [benzene ring]—CO—NH—[benzene ring]—NO_2 — Cl

Niclosamide

FIG. 53.3.

Mode of Action. Niclosamide is a taeniacidal drug. The dead tapeworm is subject to digestion before passing from the host. Therefore, identification of proglottids and scolices in the stools of treated patients generally is not possible.

The cestocidal activity of niclosamide is due to the inhibition of absorption of glucose by the tapeworm and to the uncoupling of the oxidative phosphorylation process in the mitochondia of cestodes. The resultant blocking of the Krebs cycle leads to accumulation of lactic acid which kills the tapeworm. The glycogen content in tissues of *Hymenolepis nana* decreases substantially following treatment of infected mice with the drug. It is also thought that overstimulation of adenosine triphosphatase (ATPase) activity of the mitochondria may be related to the cestodal action of niclosamide (Pütter 1970).

Pharmacodynamics. Niclosamide is poorly absorbed from the host's GI tract which perhaps accounts for its low toxicity. The small quantities absorbed are transformed into an inactive metabolite, aminoniclosamide, which has virtually no pharmacodynamic action.

Administration and Dosage. Niclosamide is administered orally in tablet form to dogs and cats at a dosage of 100–157 mg/kg of body weight. It is usually administered to ruminants as a drench at a dosage of 50 mg/kg for cattle and at 100 mg/kg for sheep and goats. An overnight fast is recommended for all animals prior to treatment.

In the Soviet Union, it is also administered for convenience in the feed of ruminants at a dosage of 70 mg/kg of body weight. The efficacy of the drug as a feed additive, however, is less than that obtained by drenching, i.e., approximately 85% versus 100%, respectively.

Safety and Toxicity. Niclosamide has a wide margin of safety. Single overdoses up to 40 times the therapeutic dose in cattle and sheep have been found to be nontoxic (Prieto 1971). The limits of safety of the drug in dogs and cats is not well established. Twice the recommended dose in either of these hosts causes no ill effects except possibly transient softness of the feces. Five times the recommended dose in dogs results in slight focal dystrophy of the liver and the appearance of an exudate in the kidney glomeruli (Sosipatrova and Leushin 1971).

Contraindications. There are no known contraindications to the use of niclosamide. This advantage plus its wide margin of safety and its reputation for excellence in the removal of *Taenia* spp. in human beings has accounted for its widespread use as a taeniacide in human and veterinary medicine. It has been used during all phases of pregnancy and in debilitated patients without ill effects.

Use with Other Drugs. Niclosamide can be administered in conjunction with several other drugs; tests have shown no apparent complications. For example, niclosamide and tetramisole can be administered simultaneously to calves and lambs for concurrent tapeworm and nematode treatment. A dose of 3 g niclosamide and 0.5 g tetramisole is used for lambs and 6 g niclosamide and 1 g tetramisole for calves.

The effectiveness of niclosamide for tapeworms of mice is enhanced when it is given in conjunction with cucurbitine or procaine. Niclosamide at 450–590 mg/kg of body weight is approximately 50% more potent for *Hymenolepis nana* infections of mice when given simultaneously with 500 mg/kg of cucurbitine or 120 mg/kg of procaine (Krotov and Rusak 1972). The latter two drugs are ineffective against the parasite when given alone.

Derivatives of Niclosamide. A number of compounds (notably salts and esters) have been prepared from niclosamide (phenasal), principally by the Russians. The lithium, potassium, tin, and magnesium salts of niclosamide are approximately equal in activity against *Hymenolepis nana* of mice but are less active and slightly more toxic than niclosamide. However, the sodium salt, while virtually equal in toxicity to niclosamide, is twice as active (Nurtaeva et al. 1973).

Of particular importance among the derivatives of phenasal is the piperazine salt of phenasal, *phenolsulfonphthalein* (PSP), which in single doses is 1.5–3 times more effective against *M. expansa* in lambs and *H. nana* in mice than its parent compound. The salt is also effective against oxyurids (pinworms) in mice while phenasal is not. PSP has given 100% cure rates at 100 mg/kg of body weight individually or at 200 mg/kg in group feeding against *Moniezia* spp. in sheep. This drug appears to be gaining wide acceptance in the Soviet Union. The exact mode of action of PSP is not known but *in vitro* concentrations of 0.01 mg/ml produce irreversible spasmodic contracture of *Moniezia* proglottids followed by complete cessation of activity. Following 1–12 hours of exposure to this concentration, cell degeneration and necrosis in all three tegument layers are seen in young proglottids and in the outer and median tegument layers of mature proglottids.

DICHLOROPHEN

Dichlorophen INN (Di-phenthane-70, Teniatol), in addition to its bactericidal and fungicidal properties, has been used as a taeniacide in veterinary medicine for many years.

Dichlorophen is similar to niclosamide in certain properties. Both are phenol derivatives. Chemically, dichlorophen is 2,2′-methylenebis(4-chlorophenol) INN; it is a creamy white powder that is almost insoluble in water. Like niclosamides, the insolubility of dichlorophen in water limits the amount of absorption from the GI tract and probably accounts for its relatively low toxicity. The two drugs are presumed to have similar modes of action, i.e., uncoupling of the oxidative phosphorylation process in the tapeworm. Following its death, the tapeworm is digested and nothing recognizable or only partially disintegrated segments can be seen in the stool.

The anticestodal range of dichlorophen includes efficacy against *Taenia* and *Dipylidium* in the dog and cat and limited efficacy against *Moniezia expansa* of sheep. Its effect on *Echinococcus* in dogs and *Thysanosoma* in sheep is variable; thus dichlorophen is not the drug of choice for removal of these two genera of tapeworms.

Administration and Dosage. Dichlorophen can be administered in either tablet or suspension and is best given after an overnight fast. No purgation is needed. Dosages of dichlorophen are recommended as follows:

Dog: 0.3 g/kg of body weight
Cat: 0.1–0.2 g/kg of body weight
Sheep: 0.5 g/2.5 kg of body weight
(adults 5–15 g; lambs 2–4 g)

Combination with Other Drugs. Despite certain disadvantages of the drug, namely, frequent vomition, colic, diarrhea, and bulky dosage, dichlorophen still has rather wide use as an anticestodal in small animal practice principally because it is combined with certain nematodal drugs to formulate several proprietary mixtures. Such mixtures have a convenience advantage in that both nematodes and cestodes can be treated simultaneously. Notable among these mixtures is the combination of dichlorophen with toluene (Vermiplex, Anaplex, Paracide), employed for dogs and cats. Tests of this combination in dogs by Blair (1949) resulted in removal of 95% of the ascarids, 82% of the hookworms, 72% of the *Taenia,* and 85% of the *Dipylidium* tapeworms. The efficacy for tapeworms in these tests may have been less than the percentages given above since no reported search was made following treatment for destrobilated scolices that may have remained attached to the intestinal mucosa. A wide margin of safety is claimed for the combination, the toxic dose being 10 times the therapeutic dose. Six daily treatments have been employed by Hollister (1967) at less than single dose levels without undesirable side effects.

HEXACHLOROPHENE

Although the principal anthelmintic use of *hexachlorophene* INN is for liver flukes in sheep and cattle (see Antitrematodal Drugs in this chapter), it also has limited use as an anticestodal drug in these two hosts and in poultry and dogs. In controlled trials by Vibe et al. (1971) in the Soviet Union, hexachlorophene at a dose of 2 g/head apparently gave 100% clearance of two genera of tapeworms (*Avitellina* and *Thysaniezia*) in 84 sheep within a 6-day period following treatment. There appear to be no specific studies, however, of the efficacy of this compound for the common western tapeworm (*Moniezia*) of cattle and sheep.

In the Soviet Union and Bulgaria, efficacy studies were conducted in the dog with hexachlorophene. Tests indicated that 90%–100% of the treated dogs were completely cleared of heavy burdens of *Echinococcus granulosus* and *Taenia multiceps* when the drug was administered in a single dosage of 15 mg/kg of body weight. The only side effect with this dosage was vomiting, usually once, in some animals. The drug is ineffective for *Echinococcus* at 10 mg/kg. It produces undesirable side effects (vomition, leucocytosis, and protein in the urine) in dogs at single dosages of 20–25 mg/kg of body weight. Repeated treatment within a few days of an initial treatment with this drug should not be made since 11% of a group of dogs died following dual treatment with 7–15 mg/kg at a 24-hour interval (Enchev et al. 1972).

The principal anticestodal use of hexachlorophene in the United States has been for the control of chicken tapeworms, especially *Raillietina cesticillus*. A single oral dosage of 30–60 mg/kg of body weight after an overnight fast removes most of these tapeworms. Up to a 30% drop in egg production may be expected following treatment. Combinations of hexachlorophene and nicotine sulfate or phenothiazine makes it possible to deworm poultry for both tapeworms and ascarids simultaneously. These drug combinations are usually added to the feed.

RESORANTEL

In recent years a new anticestodal drug, *resorantel* INN (Terenol), for ruminants has received much attention and is now commercially available in parts of Europe and the Soviet Union. It is a hydroxybenzanilide, chemically named 4′-bromo-γ-resorcylanilide INN. Resorantel is highly effective, 95%–100%, against *Moniezia* spp. in both sheep and cattle at drench dosages of 65 mg/kg of body weight. Field trials with large numbers of lambs have shown improved weight gains following removal of the tapeworm burdens.

An additional advantage of resorantel is its use against rumen flukes *(Paramphistomum)*, for which it appears to be approximately 90% effective in sheep and cattle against adult and immature forms (see Paramphistomiasis in this chapter).

Little is known presently about the pharmacodynamics of resorantel. It is excreted rapidly and serum levels of the drug are undetectable at 48 hours after treatment. Three days after treatment, the total body residue is less than 0.1% of the dose administered. Minimal blood changes seen in sheep given 3 times the therapeutic dose are rapidly reversible. Side effects of therapeutic doses are limited to slight diarrhea in an occasional animal for 36 hours following treatment. It is well tolerated even in sheep treated 2–3 days before lambing.

The mode of action of resorantel is evidently related to a block in the final stages of glucose degradation and hence an impaired energy metabolism of the cestode. Tapeworms exposed to the drug show a decrease in ATP, adenosine diphosphate (ADP), and glycogen concentrations and a simultaneous increase in adenosine monophosphate (AMP) and pyruvate levels.

BITHIONOL

Bithionol, N.F., INN (Bithin, Lorothidol), possesses bacteriostatic and antifungal as well as anthelmintic properties.

Chemistry. Bithionol is a phenolic compound; its chemical formula is 2,2′-thiobis (4,6-dichlorophenol) INN, and the structural formula is shown in Fig. 53.4. It is a white crystalline solid with a faint phenolic odor and is almost completely insoluble in water.

Indications and Effectiveness. Bithionol is used for the treatment of tapeworm infections of dogs, cats, and poultry and for tapeworm and rumen fluke infections of sheep, cattle, and goats. In dogs and cats, bithionol is highly effective for *Taenia* spp. but less effective for *Dipylidium caninum*. Among fowl, chickens can be treated with bithionol for the removal of several common cestodes including *Rail-*

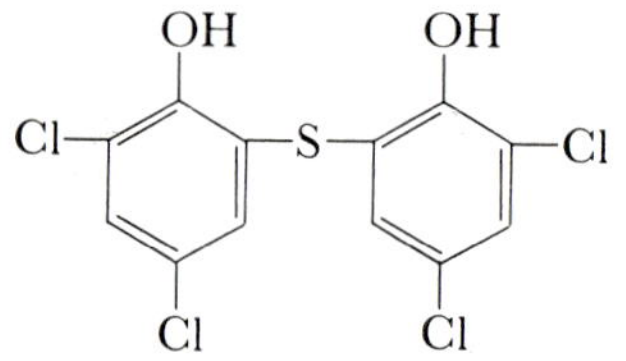

OH OH
Cl– –S– –Cl
Cl Cl

Bithionol

FIG. 53.4.

lietina cesticillus, R. tetragona, and *Choanotaenia.* Most tapeworms of geese are effectively removed by the drug. In ruminants, the efficacy of bithionol for tapeworms (*Moniezia* spp. and *Thysanosoma)* is generally good. The drug seems to be less effective in removing *Thysanosoma* from adult sheep than from lambs. Bithionol is completely effective against adult flukes of the genus *Paramphistomum,* which attach to the rumen wall, and is approximately 87% effective against the immature forms of this parasite which are found migrating in the walls of the abomasum and upper small intestine (see Paramphistomiasis).

Mode of Action. Bithionol treatment of adult worms *in vivo* decreases glycolytic and oxidative metabolism. Specifically, succinate oxidation is inhibited (Hamajima 1973). Although the exact mode of action of bithionol is not known, it is suggested that its action may depend on phenolic OH groups acting as acceptors of hydrogen which otherwise would enter into reactions associated with succinate oxidation. The interference of these reactions perhaps deprives the fluke of the necessary quantity of energy for maintenance of life.

Pharmacodynamics. Bithionol is evidently absorbed to a limited degree from the host's digestive tract and is detected in the blood and especially in the bile in which it is excreted from the body. Peak concentrations of bithionol are found in the bile within 2 hours following treatment. Blood concentrations of the drug are significantly lower than those found in bile.

Bithionol has a cholinomimetic effect on the intestinal tract of the host and thus stimulates purgation.

Toxicity. Bithionol is well tolerated by dogs, cats, sheep, cattle, goats, chickens, and geese. Occasional emesis in dogs and infrequent transient diarrhea in all species of hosts may result from administering therapeutic doses of the drug. These effects become enhanced but not serious when 5 times the therapeutic dose is given to sheep. Toxicity is moderately to markedly enhanced when bithionol is administered in combination with carbon tetrachloride, sodium antimonyl tartrate, emetine hydrochloride, hexachloroethane, or hexachloroparaxylene.

Administration and Dosage. An oral dose of approximately 200 mg/kg of body weight is used for dogs, cats, sheep, and goats. Acceptable efficacy for tapeworms in fowl requires a higher dose, i.e., 600 mg/kg for geese in a single treatment and 2 dosages, 4 days apart, of 200 mg/kg for chickens. The drug is administered to fowl in the feed and to other animals in gelatin capsules, tablets, or boluses.

Derivatives of Bithionol. A sulfinyl derivative of bithionol, bithionol sulfoxide, has anticestodal properties approximately equal to bithionol in dogs and sheep but the additional advantage of a lower therapeutic dosage (60 mg/kg). The worms are expelled intact. It has not been tested sufficiently in cats, cattle, or fowl to be recommended for use as an anticestodal drug in these species.

The major advantage of bithionol sulfoxide over its parent compound is its excellent efficacy for liver flukes of both sheep and cattle (see Antitrematodal Drugs).

UREDOFOS

Uredofos (Sansalid) is a new drug developed for broad anthelmintic use against both cestodes and nematodes (see Antinematodal Drugs in this chapter) of dogs and cats. It is not marketed in any country but application for use in the United States is being considered by the FDA.

Chemistry. The chemical name of uredofos is diethyl-[thio[-*o*-[3-(*p*-tolylsulfonyl)-ureido] -phenyl] -carbamoyl] -phosphoramidate. It is a colorless drug, dispensed in tablet form.

Mode of Action. The specific mode of action of uredofos on intestinal helminths is not known. Some evidence suggests that the drug is a cholinesterase inhibitor but this is not confirmed. Tapeworms are partially to completely disintegrated by the drug so there is little to no evidence of them in stools.

Pharmacodynamics and Toxicity. Approximately 21% of a therapeutic oral dose (50 mg/kg) in dogs is excreted in the urine and the remainder in the feces.

The drug is well tolerated by both cats and dogs. Physiological parameters (i.e., hematological, biochemical, renal function) are unaltered in cats administered 5 times the therapeutic dose at weekly intervals for a month. Dogs given similar high repeated doses may develop a slight increase in serum glutamic oxaloacetic acid transaminase (SGOT) levels. The oral LD50 range in dogs is between 1000 and 1500 mg/kg of body weight.

Adverse effects may occur in approximately 1 out of 10 treated dogs. These effects include soft to loose stools, diarrhea, nausea, or vomition. In the author's experience, these effects are not serious and may be attributed as readily to the effect of heavy parasitism as to the drug. No adverse effects have been noted in cats undergoing clinical trials.

Contraindications. At present, contraindications for this drug have not been demonstrated. Dosage levels of 55 or 175 mg/kg, administered weekly for 4 weeks, do not affect spermatogenesis in dogs. Repeated administration of 55 mg/kg to beagle bitches at 1- to 2-week intervals during ova implantation and throughout pregnancy has caused no fetal abnormalities. The drug has been used also in heartworm-positive dogs without evidence of adverse effects. Neither adult heartworms nor microfilaria are killed by therapeutic use of the drug for intestinal parasites.

Dosage and Clinical Use. A single oral dose of 50 mg/kg of body weight in dogs following an overnight fast has given 100% clearance of tapeworms *(Dipylidium caninum* and *Taenia* spp.) and more than 96% average clearance of ascarids *(Toxocara canis)* and hookworms *(Ancylostoma caninum* and *Uncinaria stenocephala)* in large numbers of test dogs. Whipworm infections of dogs are not effectively eliminated by a single dosage of the drug even at 100 mg/kg but 2 doses of 50 mg/kg each at 24-hour intervals are markedly effective (98.5%) against whipworms.

The dosage used in cats is also 50 mg/kg. The average for combined mean efficacies of natural and experimentally infected cats is 96% for ascarids, 97% for hookworms, and 83% for tapeworms.

Anticestodal Drugs for Horses

Horses in the United States are not routinely treated for cestode infections. This is partially because infections of the two more common equine tapeworms *(Anoplocephala perfoliata* and *A. magna)* are generally light. An additional and probably more important reason, however, is the limited reasearch aimed at developing anticestodal drugs for the horse. Consequently, there is no specifically labeled product available in the United States for removing equine cestodes. Limited tests have shown niclosamide at 88 mg/kg of body weight, dichlorophen at 20 mg/kg, or bithionol at 7 mg/kg to be effective and safe in horses.

ANTITREMATODAL DRUGS

Among the trematodal diseases of domestic animals, fascioliasis, caused by *Fasciola hepatica,* is the most common throughout the world and of greatest economic importance. Most of this section on antitrematodal drugs will be devoted to those compounds used in the treatment of infections of *F. hepatica.* Following the discussion on fascioliasis, brief attention will be given to the treatment of infections caused by rumen flukes *(Paramphistomum* spp.) in cattle and sheep and by lung flukes *(Paragonimus* spp.) in dogs and cats.

Fascioliasis

Sheep, and to a much smaller degree, cattle, can be seriously affected by liver-dwelling trematodes *(Fasciola hepatica)* in southern and western United States, United Kingdom, Australia, and some tropical regions of the world. Sheep in the United Kingdom have suffered three major outbreaks of acute and chronic fascioliasis since World War II. The disease in the United States is generally more chronic and often subclinical in nature.

Both the immature and mature flukes damage the host's liver. Following ingestion by sheep or cattle during grazing, the encysted metacercaria ruptures from its cyst, penetrates the wall of the small intestine, traverses the peritoneal cavity, and penetrates the liver capsule within 4 days of infection. During the next several weeks the young immature flukes tunnel through the liver tissues, feeding and increasing rapidly in size. The extensive damage and resultant hemorrhaging of the liver will often result in clinical signs of acute fascioliasis within 6–8 weeks after infection. Deaths often occur at this point. Among survivors, during the 8th week of infection the flukes begin to penetrate the main bile ducts, where they attain sexual maturity approximately 10–12 weeks after infection. It is at this stage that the flukes are most susceptible (or perhaps most accessible) to fasciolicidal drugs.

The adult flukes, often in pairs, lodge within a bile canal, causing hyperplasia and progressive occlusion. Heavily infected areas may become walled off from the rest of the liver by connective tissue. Such areas become progressively less penetrable by therapeutic agents and, consequently, more difficult to treat.

The seriousness of *F. hepatica* infections in sheep is enhanced because of the fluke's probable role of disseminating enteric bacteria *(Clostridium novyi)* throughout the liver during migration. The resultant infectious necrotic hepatitis (black disease) can be quite serious. A vaccine against *C. novyi,* however, is helpful in controlling black disease.

DRUGS EFFECTIVE AGAINST ADULT FLUKES

Since the introduction of carbon tetrachloride for the treatment of helminth infections of animals in the 1920s, numerous other compounds have been investigated for efficacy against *F. hepatica* in sheep. Some have proved to be efficacious, as has carbon tetrachloride.

On the basis of chemical structure, the fasciolicidal drugs can be separated into three groups: (1) the halogenated hydrocarbons (carbon tetrachloride, hexachloroethane, tetrachlorodifluoroethane, and hexachloroparaxylene); (2) the bisphenolic compounds (hexachlorophene, bithionol sulfoxide, the bromsalans, oxyclozanide, and clioxanide); and (3) the nitrophenolic compounds (disophenol, niclofolan, and nitroxinil). A common feature of the drugs of each group is the presence of halogen atoms. Whether the halogen atom presents a common mechanism for fasciolicidal activity of all these drugs is not known but is suggested to be unlikely (Fowler 1971).

The efficacy of the fasciolicidal drugs has been invariably directed toward adult flukes. Immature flukes in the liver parenchyma have largely if not wholly escaped the therapeutic action of these drugs until the introduction of diamphenethide in 1971. The latter drug has its greatest efficacy against the very young flukes; it eliminates the void left by other fasciolicides. The therapeutic effectiveness of diamphenethide diminishes as the flukes age.

It is not feasible in this section to give proper attention to all of the rather equally important fasciolicides; thus details will be given for only single examples of an adulticidal and a larvicidal drug. For the latter, diamphenethide is obviously the choice. For the former, carbon tetrachloride will be discussed because of its longstanding and recently renewed parenteral use against adult *F. hepatica.* Other drugs with principal use against the adult fluke will be discussed briefly.

Carbon Tetrachloride. *Carbon tetrachloride* (CCl_4) was the first truly effective remedy to be introduced for the treatment of fascioliasis. Its effectiveness against GI nematodes was recognized by Hall of the U.S. Bureau of Animal Industry in 1921.

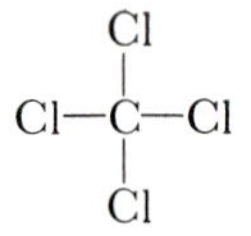

$$\begin{array}{c} Cl \\ | \\ Cl{-}C{-}Cl \\ | \\ Cl \end{array}$$

Carbon Tetrachloride

FIG. 53.5.

Subsequently, veterinary researchers in both Germany and North Wales found it to be effective against *F. hepatica* in sheep.

Chemistry. Carbon tetrachloride (Fig. 53.5) is produced by the chlorination of carbon disulfide or by the reaction of the disulfide with sulfur monochloride. Its principal use is as an industrial solvent. It is a volatile colorless liquid, soluble in organic solvents, but relatively insoluble in water. It has a burning taste and its odor is similar to chloroform.

Indications. Carbon tetrachloride has been used to treat a variety of parasitic infections in both large and small animals. Its principal anthelmintic use today is in the treatment of fascioliasis in sheep. In general, it is equally as effective against adult flukes (i.e., over 10 weeks of age) as any other fasciolicide and is economical. Its lack of activity against immature flukes is a major drawback. A second drawback is its marked toxicity to the mammalian liver. This toxicity almost precludes its use in cattle. It is sufficiently well tolerated in sheep, however, and has had extensive use in this host. Pigs, horses, and cats are not suitable hosts for treatment with this drug.

In addition to use against *F. hepatica,* CCl_4 was used in earlier years against ascarid infections of chickens and dogs and against blood-sucking nematodes including *Ancylostoma* in dogs and cats, *Haemonchus* and *Bunostomum* in cattle and sheep, and strongyles in horses. Other more effective drugs, however, have now replaced its use against these nematodes. Due to the toxicity of CCl_4 in cattle, hexachloroethane has replaced it as a treatment for liver fluke infections in this host.

Pharmacodynamics. Following oral administration, CCl_4 passes through the stomach unchanged and is absorbed to a limited extent from the intestine at a slow rate. Prolongation of the absorptive period (by split or repeated small dosages rather than a single dose) increases the toxicity of the drug. Following a therapeutic oral dose (180 mg/kg) in sheep, the concentration of CCl_4 measures approximately 21 ppm in the blood and 65 ppm in the bile within 12 hours of administration.

Elimination of the absorbed drug occurs through expired air and via the kidneys and especially the liver. Increased respiration, as may occur in sheep stressed by heat, allows for more rapid elimination of CCl_4 and thus less toxicity. Conversely, CCl_4 poisoning is increased by exposure to temperatures below normal (Kondos and McClymont 1966) because elimination of the drug by expiration is slowed.

Metabolism of CCl_4 evidently occurs in the liver, particularly in the microsomes, and the metabolites are excreted in the bile and urine.

Mode of action. The normal blood and bile levels of CCl_4 following oral administration of a therapeutic dose to sheep are 21 and 65 ppm, respectively. Both levels are far from the required level of 500 ppm for *in vitro* toxicity to the fluke. It is generally accepted now that CCl_4 exerts its anthelmintic action indirectly, either via one or more unknown metabolites (Fowler 1971) or by inducing the formation of toxic substances in the liver. In favor of the latter, Posthuma and Vaatstra (1971) have demonstrated the presence of methylsterols, lethal to the liver fluke, in the livers of rabbits treated with CCl_4. Methylsterols are thought to be intermediates in the biosynthesis of cholesterol. Because of the accumulation of methylsterols in the livers, bile, and urine of CCl_4-treated animals, it is assumed that the drug blocks cholesterol synthesis at a point that allows the buildup of the toxic methylsterols. This suggests that the fluke suffers the consequences of a defect (brought about by CCl_4) in the cholesterol biosynthesis of the host.

Whatever the mode of action of this drug, histological examinations of flukes from CCl_4-treated animals suggest that the toxic principal penetrates the fluke both orally and via its integument. The lethal effect seems to be associated with an interference with the secretory and enzymatic activity of the gut epithelium.

Toxicity. Carbon tetrachloride is toxic to all mammals but especially to swine, in which this drug should never be used. The susceptibility of cattle to CCl_4 requires that extreme caution be used when administering the drug to this host. Among farm mammals, sheep tolerate the drug with least toxicity; yet the idiosyncratic susceptibility of sheep invariably results in some losses. In birds, the drug is essentially nontoxic.

Both acute and delayed toxic effects may occur following the administration of CCl_4. The predominant signs of acute poisoning are the result of depression of the central nervous system (CNS) with resultant drowsiness, diarrhea, incoordination in movement, and perhaps cardiovascular collapse in 12–24 hours. This normally occurs only at dosages that considerably exceed the therapeutic dose.

The expected delayed toxicity of the drug following therapeutic dosing is related to liver damage. The absorption of small amounts of CCl_4 produces fatty degeneration of the liver; larger amounts may produce hepatic cell necrosis, the extent of which can be judged by increases in plasma enzyme levels (Harvey and Hoe 1971). Hepatotoxicity, if extensive, may be fatal during the succeeding 1–2 weeks. If enough normal tissue remains to sustain life, the damaged liver cells undergo complete resolution and normal function returns within approximately 8 days.

Restoration of normal liver structure can be hastened by certain compounds that enhance protein synthesis. These include orotic acid and methylthiouracil (Metacil). When either of these compounds is given to sheep 5 days prior to administration of CCl_4 and 5 days afterward, restoration of normal liver structure is significantly more rapid than in sheep given CCl_4 alone. Although beneficial, it is not a practical procedure.

Factors affecting toxicity and contraindications. Factors that either reduce or exacerbate the toxicity of CCl_4 have been recognized and should be considered when using this drug. As mentioned earlier, cold weather reduces the respiration rate so that elimination of the volatile CCl_4 through expired air is slowed and toxicity is increased. Therefore, in the winter months it is advisable to shelter animals for several days during treatment with CCl_4.

Lambs less than 5 months of age should not be treated with CCl_4 at any time of the year, nor should ewes while they are suckling lambs or immediately after weaning.

Diet affects susceptibility to the toxicity of CCl_4. In general, protein-deficient diets increase resistance to CCl_4 intoxication. Experimentally, sheep on a diet of 6.4% crude protein show little evidence of hepatotoxicity following treatment with CCl_4, whereas sheep on a high-protein (15.5%) diet suffer a significantly higher level of liver damage (Hunt 1971). The exact reasons are unexplained. High-fat diets (which increase the total amount of CCl_4 absorbed) and diets containing clover and kale, crushed beet tops, lucerne, mangolds, or stinkwort are contraindicated. Feeding solely on pasture or hay (without concentrates) during the week of drenching and feeding calcium supplement for a week before drenching is preferred. Sheep in high or fat condition and those in very poor condition do not tolerate dosing with CCl_4 as well as those in intermediate condition.

Concurrent treatment of mammals with CCl_4 and certain drugs, notably DDT and sodium phenobarbital, markedly increases susceptibility (approximately 10-fold) to CCl_4 toxicity. Birds, on the other hand, are not affected by simultaneous use of these products. It is thought that DDT and sodium phenobarbital stimulate greater microsomal enzyme activity in mammals (but not in birds), resulting in enhanced metabolism of CCl_4 and increased quantities of toxic metabolic products (Fowler 1971).

Several compounds have been shown

to reduce the toxicity of CCl_4 when administered simultaneously with the drug. A dose of 5 mg of selenium given orally about 20 minutes before CCl_4 administration reduces susceptibility of sheep to CCl_4 toxicity (Kondos and McClymont 1967). Similar protection from liver damage and toxicity occurs when carbon disulfide is given orally at 0.05 ml/kg of body weight either prior to or at the time of CCl_4 administration.

Flocks of sheep vary in their susceptibility to CCl_4 toxicity. It is advisable to try the drug on a few of the worst and best animals in the flock a week before treating the entire flock.

Treatment of the toxic reaction. If signs of toxic reaction (depression, diarrhea, incoordination) occur, a gastric saline lavage helps to prevent further absorption of the drug from the intestine. The delayed toxic effects upon the liver can be suppressed to some degree by dextrose solution given intravenously in large amounts. Intravenous calcium therapy with calcium borogluconate produces variable response but is probably worthwhile.

Dosage and administration. Dosages of CCl_4 are recommended as follows:

Sheep: orally, 1–3 ml

Dog: orally, 1–5 ml at the rate of 0.1–0.2 ml/kg

Poultry: orally, 1–5 ml

Carbon tetrachloride can be administered either orally or parenterally to sheep. It is frequently administered in capsules or as a drench when mixed in 300–600 ml of liquid paraffin. The first method is preferred because the drug has anesthetic properties similar to chloroform. Although fasting is not required, dosing is usually carried out early in the morning before the sheep are fed.

Parenteral administration of CCl_4 has been used with greater frequency in sheep and cattle during the past 15 years. Solutions of the drug in liquid paraffin containing butyl alcohol as a local anesthetic can be administered either subcutaneously or intramuscularly. Some necrosis at the site of injection often occurs. A maximum parenteral dose of 4 ml of CCl_4 in sheep and 30 ml in cattle is needed for satisfactory efficacy. The parenteral dosage rate in cattle is 1 ml/9 kg of body weight.

In dogs, the drug is usually administered in soft gelatin capsules.

Hexachloroethane. Other simple chlorinated hydrocarbons, e.g., *hexachloroethane* (Fig. 53.6), were developed as anthelmintics subsequent to the initial use of CCl_4 in the 1920s. Hexachloroethane was found to be less toxic than CCl_4 in cattle and has been used extensively against all species of *Fasciola* in this host. The drug is also effective against *Haemonchus* spp. and *Trichostrongylus axei* but not against intestinal nematodes of ruminants. Like CCl_4, it is to some degree hepatotoxic and its activity against *F. hepatica* is limited to adult flukes. Retreatment at approximately monthly intervals during the snail season is necessary.

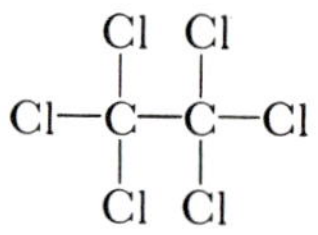

```
   Cl  Cl
   |   |
Cl—C———C—Cl
   |   |
   Cl  Cl
```

Hexachloroethane

FIG. 53.6.

In general, as with CCl_4, a correlation between toxicity of hexachloroethane and certain types of feed occurs so use of the drug requires dietary precautions. These limitations and the occurrence of its somewhat frequent side effects in both cattle and sheep have resulted in decreased use of hexachloroethane in favor of newer drugs when the latter are available.

Oral dosages recommended in sheep and cattle are 8–15 g/head and 15–100 g (at the rate of 10 g/50 kg), respectively.

Tetrachlorodifluoroethane. *Tetrachlorodifluoroethane* (Freon 112, Frigen 112) (Fig. 53.7), a halogenated hydrocarbon used as

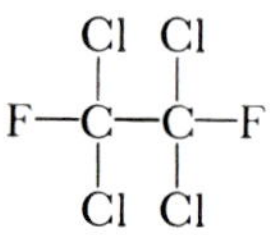

```
  Cl  Cl
  |   |
F—C———C—F
  |   |
  Cl  Cl
```

Tetrachlorodifluoroethane

FIG. 53.7.

an industrial refrigerant, was found by Dimidov (a Russian) in 1955 to have fasciolicidal properties. Numerous tests have confirmed its efficacy for adult forms (but not immature forms) of *F. hepatica* and its tolerance in sheep. Unpleasant to severe toxic reactions plus inadequate efficacy for liver flukes in cattle preclude its use in this host. An oral dose of 300 mg/kg has been employed in sheep.

Hexachloroparaxylene. The chemical name of *hexachloroparaxylene* (Bitriben, Hetol) is 1,4-bis(trichloromethyl)benzene; its structural formula is shown in Fig. 53.8. Hexachloroparaxylene, often referred to under the Russian common name chloxyle, is a chlorinated derivative of benzene. Since its initial use in 1958 as a fasciolicide, numerous tests have confirmed its high efficacy for *F. hepatica* and its rather excellent tolerance in sheep, which withstand 4 times the minimum therapeutic dose of 150 mg/kg without blood dyscrasia or other side effects. These properties rank it superior to both carbon tetrachloride and hexachloroethane for use as a fasciolicide in sheep. Like the latter drugs, however, it is only effective for adult flukes.

In cattle, the tolerance of hexachloroparaxylene and its efficacy for liver flukes are slightly less acceptable than in sheep. Transient side effects may occur following treatment with the drug when certain plants (notably sugar beets, turnips, and turnip leaves) are included in the diet. Additionally, in older cattle, increased doses up to 225 mg/kg are required for satisfactory efficacy.

Hexachloroparaxylene is compatible with phenothiazine. Mixtures of these two compounds are used for simultaneous treatment of liver flukes and GI nematodes in ruminants.

Oral dosages recommended in sheep and cattle are 150 mg/kg and 125–135 mg/kg, respectively.

Cl Cl
Cl—C—⟨benzene⟩—C—Cl
Cl Cl

Hexachloroparaxylene

FIG. 53.8.

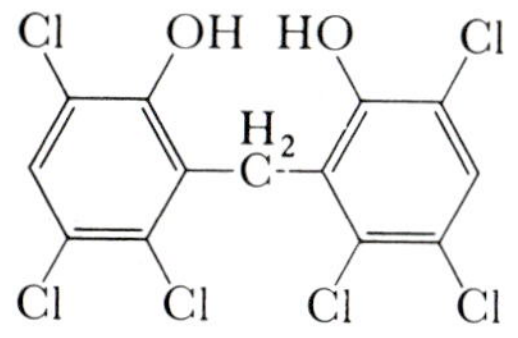

Hexachlorophene. *Hexachlorophene* INN (Coopaphene, Distodin, Fasciophene) has the chemical name 2,2′-methylenebis-(3,4,6-trichlorophenol) INN; the structural formula is shown in Fig. 53.9. Until it was outlawed, hexachlorophene was used extensively as an antibacterial agent in soaps, cosmetics, and antiseptic solutions and as a broad-spectrum fungicide and bactericide on food crops. It also has anthelmintic efficacy which has allowed for its use in the treatment of ruminant and human liver flukes and ruminant and canine cestodes (see Anticestodal Drugs).

Studies supporting the efficacy of hexachlorophene for liver flukes of sheep and cattle have been carried out in fairly recent years in Europe and the Soviet Union. In general, a very high efficacy (approaching 100%) is obtained with this drug against mature (at least 12-week-old) forms of both *F. hepatica* and *F. gigantica* in sheep and cattle. Hexachlorophene is not effective, however, in removing immature flukes (less than 8 weeks of age) from the liver parenchyma where they are bathed in blood. Actually, both immature and mature forms are equally susceptible to hexachlorophene but the activity of the drug is greater in the presence of bile than in blood. This is due, at least in part, to protein binding of the drug in blood and consequent reduced availability to the immature forms. Additionally, hexachlorophene is excreted from the host's circulatory system into the bile as a metabolite, glucuronide, which has high activity against the fluke, specifically against the adult forms since they occupy the bile ducts.

At 25 mg/kg of body weight, an oral

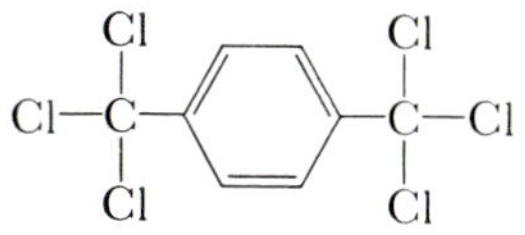

Cl OH HO Cl
H_2
C
Cl Cl Cl Cl

Hexachlorophene

FIG. 53.9.

dose of hexachlorophene in either sheep or cattle seems to cause no toxicity. Its chemotherapeutic range is narrow; exact dosing is necessary, especially in cattle. Overdosing may produce nervous symptoms such as excitability or depression (possibly followed by death) and impairment of vision which may be permanent. Subcutaneous injection of the drug has been used therapeutically (25 mg/kg) but is more likely to result in the toxic signs described above than is an orally administerd therapeutic dose.

Bithionol Sulfoxide. The chemical name of *bithionol sulfoxide* is 2,2′-sulphinyl-bis-(4,6-dichlorophenol), the Russian generic name being sulfene.

In addition to its anticestodal properties (see Anticestodal Drugs), bithionol sulfoxide is effective against liver flukes of domesticated ruminants. Efficacies of greater than 90% can generally be expected when the drug is used against *F. hepatica.*

Like most fasciolicides, it is distinctly more effective for adult than for immature flukes.

The therapeutic dose of bithionol sulfoxide for sheep and cattle is 60 mg/kg of body weight. It is administered to ruminants in boluses or in the feed. No toxic effects have been noted at double the therapeutic dosage. Dosages of 425 mg/kg in lambs cause congestion and transient necrotic changes in the liver and kidneys.

Combinations of bithionol sulfoxide with certain other fasciolicides are safe and effective against *F. hepatica.* A combination of bithionol sulfoxide at 30 mg/kg and hexachlorophene at 5 mg/kg of body weight in both cattle and sheep has been found to be 100% effective against mature *F. hepatica* (over 11 weeks old). The combination, like its individual constituents, is relatively less effective the younger the fluke. It is ineffective against flukes aged 6 weeks or less. Thus retreatment may be necessary in 4–6 weeks when fluke eggs again begin to be shed in the stools.

The Bromsalans: Dibromsalan and Tribromsalan. The chemical name of *dibromsalan* INN is 5-bromosalicylic acid-4′-bromoanilide and that of *tribromsalan* INN is 3,5-dibromosalicylic acid-4′-bromoanilide. The structural formulas are shown in Fig. 53.10 (dibromsalan) and Fig. 53.11 (tribromsalan).

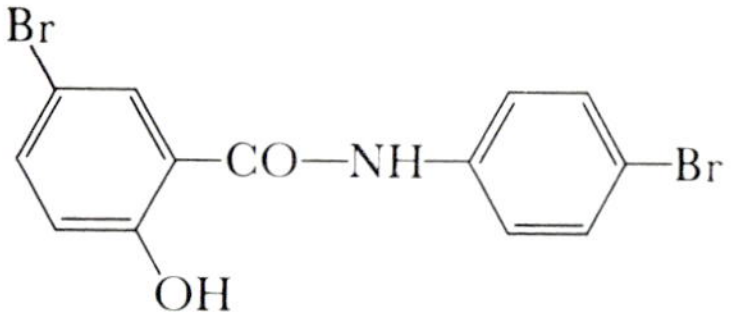

Dibromsalan

Fig. 53.10.

These two bisphenolic compounds have been used since the 1960s as mixtures for the treatment of *F. hepatica* infections. Commercially available Hilomid contains a mixture of dibromsalan and tribromsalan in a 1:1 ratio; Diaphene contains a 1:3 ratio. These commercial mixtures have approximately the same efficacy for adult flukes (greater than 12 weeks of age) as other fasciolicides. An advantage of the bromsalans over the halogenated hydrocarbons and several bisphenolic and nitrophenolic compounds is their near 100% efficacy for juvenile flukes (6- to 12-week range). These mixtures have a narrow but adequate chemotherapeutic index of approximately 3 in sheep, the minimum curative dose being 30 mg/kg and the maximum tolerated dose 90 mg/kg. Oral dosages used in sheep for adult and juvenile flukes are 30 mg/kg and 60 mg/kg, respectively.

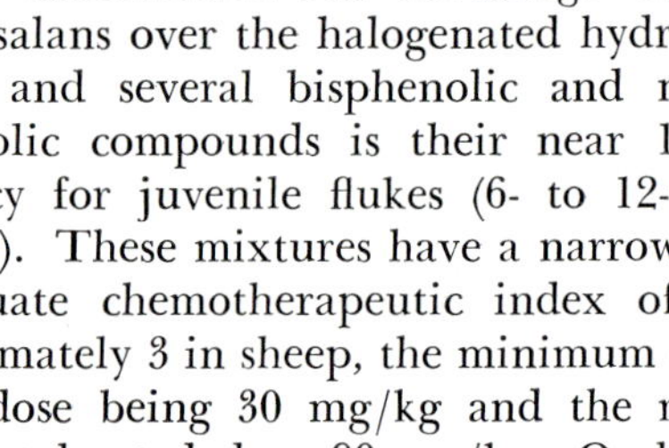

Tribromsalan

Fig. 53.11.

Oxyclozanide. *Oxyclozanide* INN (Zanil) was introduced for its fasciolicidal activity in 1966. It is a white crystalline substance with the chemical name 3,3′,5,5′,6-pentachloro-2′-hydroxysalicylanilide INN. The

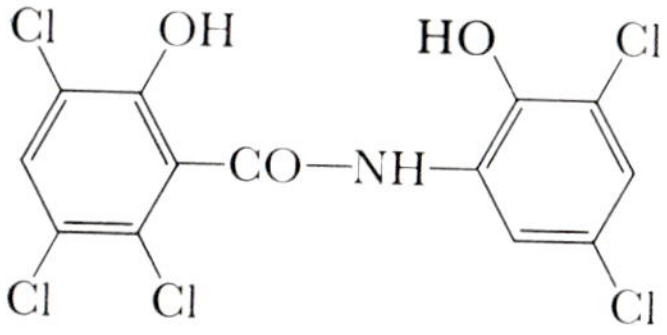

Oxyclozanide

FIG. 53.12.

structural formula is shown in Fig. 53.12. It is virtually insoluble in water. It is formulated, however, as an aqueous suspension of 10-μ particle size for oral dosing of sheep and cattle. Following absorption, oxyclozanide reaches highest concentrations in the liver, kidney, and intestines and is excreted as an active glucuronide metabolite into the bile.

Its mode of action is not known with certainty. However, like other salicylanilides and substituted phenols, oxyclozanide is an uncoupler of oxidative phosphorylation. Corbett and Goose (1971) have evidence that this interference by oxyclozanide, nitroxinil, and hexachlorophene is lethal to *F. hepatica*. *In vivo,* only adult flukes are affected. These drugs are not effective against immature flukes perhaps because of protein binding of the drugs in blood, which bathes the immature flukes in the liver parenchyma (O'Brien 1970).

The efficacy of oxyclozanide for adult liver flukes is approximately equal to that of carbon tetrachloride, hexachloroethane, and hexachlorophene and it has the advantage of low toxicity. Its chemotherapeutic index is approximately 4. It can be used at therapeutic dosages in debilitated and pregnant animals without side effects. There are no special dietary requirements for animals being treated with the drug. Detectable amounts of oxyclozanide (as well as niclofolan) pass in the milk, thus treatment of lactating animals is contraindicated.

The maximum tolerated dosage of oxyclozanide in both sheep and cattle is approximately 60 mg/kg of body weight. Dosages of 25 mg/kg may produce minor side effects including softening of feces, increased frequency of defecation, slight depression, and inappetence, but not death except perhaps in animals with extensive chronic liver damage. In sheep and cattle, recommended oral dosages are 15 mg/kg and 10–15 mg/kg, respectively.

Clioxanide. *Clioxanide* INN (Tremerad), with the chemical name 4′-chloro-2-hydroxy-3,5-diiodobenzanilide acetate INN, is very effective against adult and immature *F. hepatica.* The mature flukes (12 weeks or older) are effectively removed by dosages of 15 mg/kg with a safety index of 6.7 in sheep (Gibson 1969). Unfortunately, progressively higher dosages of the drug, with resulting reduced safety, are necessary for the effective removal of younger flukes. Dosages of 40 mg/kg (safety index of 2.5) are necessary for satisfactory efficacy against 6-week-old flukes and 135 mg/kg (safety margin of only 0.7) for 4-week-old flukes. Some deaths from toxicity in sheep may be expected when using dosage levels of either 40 mg/kg or 135 mg/kg, especially the latter, even though the approximate LD50 in sheep is as high as 414 mg/kg.

The signs of acute toxicity usually develop 2–3 days after administration and take the form of progressive malaise, pyrexia, respiratory distress, incoordination leading to ataxia, recumbency, and death (O'Brien 1970). In general, the increased toxicity of clioxanide at high dosages has resulted in field uses of not more than 40 mg/kg. At these lower levels it appears to be safe for use in pregnant, parturient, and lactating ewes (Pearson et al. 1970). It can be safely given concurrently with the antinematodal drug, thiabenazole. Presidente et al. (1972), in the United States, have used clioxanide against *F. hepatica* in calves and found efficacies of 88.5%, 94.9%, and 95.5% against mature flukes when dosing different groups of calves with 12.5, 25, and 50 mg/kg, respectively.

Clioxanide is significantly more active if, following oral dosing, it passes first to the rumen rather than directly to the abomasum. In regular treatment (4–9 ml) for mature flukes in sheep, the small size of the dose generally allows it to pass into the rumen. The larger volumes necessary for treating acute fascioliasis (caused by younger flukes) pass to the rumen only approximately 50% of the time. Thus the flock efficacy of larger volumes of the drug is markedly reduced. Except in cases when intraruminal injection of large doses of the drug is feasible, the use of clioxanide against acute fascioliasis has given way to the newer larvicidal compounds, diamphenethide and rafoxanide.

Niclofolan. *Niclofolan* INN (Bilevon M, Bilevon R) is a nitro-substituted analog of hexachlorophene. Its alternate generic name, menichlopholan, is used in Europe. Its chemical formula is 4,4′-dichloro-6,6′-dinitro-*o,o*-biphenol INN.

Niclofolan is effective against mature forms of *F. hepatica* in sheep, cattle, and pigs at safe dosage levels. It is also effective against immature forms but progressively higher dosages, limited by safety, are required for younger flukes. In sheep (host in which the drug is most used), 2.7 mg/kg will remove 12-week-old (mature) flukes in chronic infections with a safety index of 4.4; 6 mg/kg will remove 6-week-old (immature) flukes with a safety margin of 2; and 8 mg/kg is required to move 4-week-old immature forms with a safety margin of only 1.5 (Gibson 1969). Side effects are not expected in sheep treated at dosages of 4 mg/kg or less but do occur with dosages of 6 mg/kg. Side effects include fever, tachypnea, and sweating; these last for 2–3 days and occasionally result in death.

In cattle, niclofolan is effective against mature *F. hepatica* at dosages of 3 mg/kg of body weight and is well tolerated in heifers over 6 months of age and in pregnant and diseased cattle. Dosages of 16–20 mg/kg, necessary for removal of immature forms, produce toxic signs similar to those mentioned above for sheep.

Niclofolan, like oxyclozanide, is excreted in the milk of cattle for 5–8 days posttreatment at concentrations up to 0.1 ppm. This milk should not be used for human consumption since the limits of these substances in consumable milk is 0.01 ppm.

Fascioliasis in pigs rarely occurs but in endemic areas it sometimes requires therapeutic attention. Niclofolan is effective for mature flukes in pigs and is well tolerated at a dosage of 3–5 mg/kg of body weight.

Although niclofolan can be administered subcutaneously in sheep, it is usually administered orally and passes into the rumen. The drug is known to be metabolized to some degree in the rumen of cattle; this reduces its efficacy (Zarnowski 1967). Administration of sodium chloride with niclofolan prevents the drug from passing into the rumen by causing reflex closure of the sulcus oesophageus. However, the use of sodium chloride increases the incidence of toxic side effects, so this practice is not widely employed.

Nitroxynil. *Nitroxynil* (Trodax), whose INN generic name is nitroxinil, has the chemical name 4-hydroxy-3-iodo-5-nitrobenzonitrile INN. The structural formula is shown in Fig. 53.13.

Nitroxynil has been developed in the United Kingdom since the late 1960s as an injectable fasciolicide for both sheep and cattle. It can be administered orally but is more effective when administered either subcutaneously or intramuscularly. The latter two methods of administration give approximately equal efficacy for liver flukes but the subcutaneous route has become the method of choice in practice. It is injected in the side of the neck of cattle and at any convenient site in sheep. The ease of subcutaneous administration gives nitroxynil an advantage over other fasciolicides that must be administered orally. This compound stains wool or hair yellow; thus care must be exercised to avoid spilling. Local tolerance at the site of injection is satisfactory although transitory inflammatory swellings are occasionally observed in cattle.

Nitroxynil is effective against mature

I

HO— —CN

O_2N

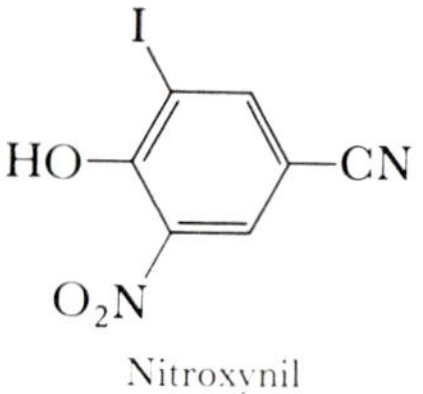

Nitroxynil

Fig. 53.13.

flukes of both species of *Fasciola,* i.e., *F. hepatica* and *F. gigantica,* in both sheep and cattle and can be used to treat haemonchosis in these hosts. At therapeutic dosages of 10 mg/kg of body weight, the drug is very well tolerated and has high activity against mature liver flukes of either species and, perhaps, useful activity against immature flukes in that mortality due to acute fascioliasis is arrested following treatment at this dosage level. Approximately 30% of the 6-week-old flukes and greater percentages of younger flukes are not removed by the 10 mg/kg dose. Higher dosages which would be more efficacious for immature flukes are not recommended because of the host's increased susceptibility to the drug.

The maximum tolerated dose of 40 mg nitroxynil/kg body weight in sheep and calves causes marked increases in heart, respiration, and metabolic rates. The mechanism by which the drug exerts its pharmacological and toxic effects has not been investigated. However, the nature of the toxic signs suggests that it may act by uncoupling oxidative phosphorylation in the cells.

Nitroxynil is slowly eliminated from the body via the urine and feces over a period of 31 days. Animals should not be slaughtered for human consumption within that period. The drug is also passed in the milk and therefore should not be administered to lactating cows.

In compatibility studies with other drugs, nitroxynil was found to be safe when administered concurrently with antinematodal drugs, e.g., phenothiazine, thiabendazole, naphthalophos, and tetramisole. Ill effects do not occur when nitroxynil is administered at the time of clostridial vaccination or at the time of dipping in an organophosphorus preparation. Several tests now indicate that pigs can be safely and effectively treated for fascioliasis with nitroxynil using a subcutaneous dose of 10 mg/kg of body weight. In sheep and cattle, a subcutaneous injection of the active constituent (10 mg/kg) is recommended.

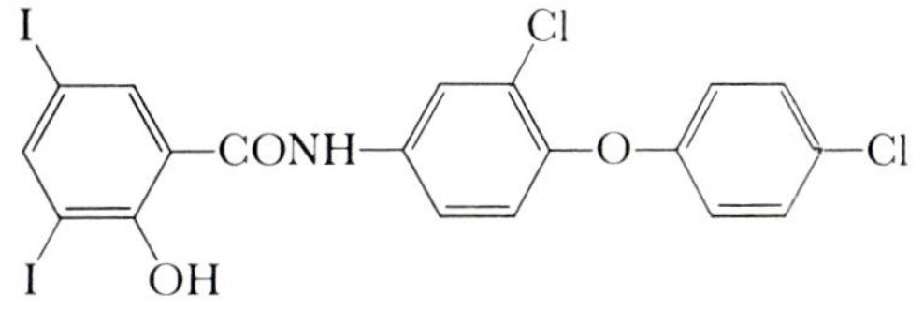

I, I, OH, —CONH—, Cl, —O—, —Cl

Rafoxanide

FIG. 53.14.

Rafoxanide. *Chemistry.* Chemically, *rafoxanide* INN (Flukanide, Ranide) is a halogenated salicylanilide. Its chemical formula is 3′-chloro-4′(*p*-chlorophenoxy)-3, 5-diiodosalicylanilide INN; its structural formula is shown in Fig. 53.14. It is an off-white crystalline powder and is commercially formulated for use as a bolus or drenching suspension.

Indications and effectiveness. Rafoxanide was developed in 1969 and subsequently has had extensive testing and recent commercial use for fascioliasis and haemonchosis in sheep and cattle in the United Kingdom, Europe, Australia, Brazil, and South Africa. Its principal use is as an adulticide for both *F. hepatica* and *F. gigantica* but it also has respectable efficacy for immature flukes. With a single therapeutic dose (7.5 mg/kg) in sheep, Armour and Corba (1970) and Annen (1973) have determined the efficacy of rafoxanide for various age forms of *F. hepatica* as follows: almost 100% for 12-week-old (mature) flukes, 86%–99% for 6-week-old (immature) flukes, and 50% up to 98% for 4-week-old flukes. Similar efficacies against *F. hepatica* in cattle are found at the same dosage level. The rather reliable efficacy for 4- and 6-week-old flukes gives this drug an advantage over strictly adulticidal drugs in the treatment of acute fascioliasis. Repeat treatment is necessary at 3-week intervals to eliminate maturing flukes that escape being killed at earlier treatment times.

Treatment of sheep infected with *F. gigantica* gives better than 99% efficacy for 8-, 10-, and 12-week-old flukes but only approximately 50% efficacy for 6-week-old forms (Boray et al. 1973).

Rafoxanide is also indicated in the treatment of haemonchosis and sheep nasal bots. Greater than 96% efficacy for adult

Haemonchus spp. in cattle and for both adult and immature forms of this parasite in sheep is claimed. It appears also to be highly effective (98%) against all parasitic larval stages of the sheep nasal bot.

Pharmacodynamics and mode of action. Following oral dosing, rafoxanide is absorbed, presumably from the small intestine, into the bloodstream. Peak plasma levels occur between 24 and 48 hours. The drug is not metabolized to any detectable degree by cattle or sheep. Its biologic half-life varies from 5 to 10 days in sheep. Following a single oral dose of 15 mg/kg in cattle, no residue of the compound is detectable in edible tissues at 28 days post-dosing.

The mode of action of rafoxanide apparently is not known.

Toxicity and contraindications. Rafoxanide has a safety index of approximately 5. Although the therapeutic dose in cattle and sheep is 7.5 mg/kg, no untoward effects have been seen when using single doses of 58 mg/kg in cattle or 45 mg/kg in sheep. At a dosage of 80 mg/kg, inappetence and diarrhea occur in cattle and, although not reported, would be expected to occur in sheep. Dosages above 45 mg/kg cause ocular pathological changes (equatorial cataracts and optic nerve degeneration) in sheep. These changes may lead to blindness. In cattle, blindness is an inconsistent toxic effect when a single dose of 125 mg/kg is administered. A LD50 of rafoxanide for either sheep or cattle has not been determined. The LD50 of this compound for the rat is approximately 2300 mg/kg.

In general, rafoxanide at therapeutic dosages can be used in cattle and sheep of all ages under commonly encountered conditions without hazard. It has been used simultaneously with organophosphate and arsenical dips without adverse effects.

The use of rafoxanide is contraindicated in lactating animals whose milk or milk products are to be used for human consumption and in animals intended for slaughter within 28 days. An oral dose of the drug (7.5 mg/kg) is recommended in the treatment of both sheep and cattle.

Combination with thiabendazole. Rafoxanide is combined with thiabendazole in a commercial product, Ranizole, for the simultaneous treatment of liver flukes and GI nematodes of sheep and cattle. The combination does not appear to alter the safety factor of either drug; that of thiabendazole is very high, thus the safety of the combination is limited by the lower margin of safety of rafoxanide as described under Toxicity above.

DRUGS WITH PRINCIPAL ACTIVITY AGAINST IMMATURE FLUKES

Diamphenethide. *Diamphenethide* (Coriban) is unique among the fasciolicides available today in that it possesses exceptionally high activity against the youngest immature stages of the liver fluke (*F. hepatica*). Its activity decreases with aging of the fluke. This is in direct contrast to other currently used fasciolicides which tend to be less active against younger flukes. The development of diamphenethide has finally opened the door for a potential prophylactic program against liver fluke disease in sheep.

Chemistry. In 1971, diamphenethide was selected from among several hundred related compounds for its fasciolicidal activity. Chemically it is β,β'-bis-(4-acetamidophenyloxy)ethyl ether; the structural formula is shown in Fig. 53.15.

Pharmacodynamics. Following oral administration, diamphenethide is absorbed into the blood and is distributed throughout the body. At 3 days after dosing, its concentration is greatest in the liver and gall bladder, especially in the gall bladder contents. It should be noted that these are the sites occupied by flukes. At 7 days after dosing, concentrations of the drug in these sites are reduced approximately 10-fold to a range of only 0.1–0.5 ppm, while low concentrations in the musculature are approximately 0.02 ppm. In the United Kingdom, where the drug is currently used, animals for human consumption are permitted to be slaughtered 7 days after treatment.

Mode of action. The efficacy of diamphenethide appears to depend upon deacylation of the drug by liver enzymes (deacy-

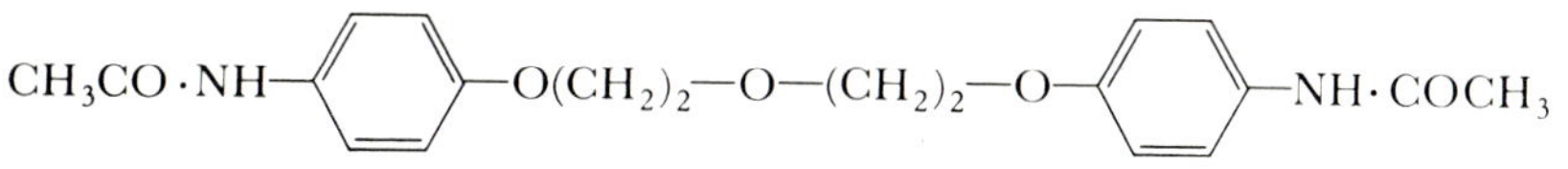

$$CH_3CO \cdot NH - C_6H_4 - O(CH_2)_2 - O - (CH_2)_2 - O - C_6H_4 - NH \cdot COCH_3$$

Diamphenethide

FIG. 53.15.

lases) to an amine metabolite (Harfenist 1973) which is active against the parasite. Diamphenethide is not active against liver flukes *in vitro* unless incubated in the presence of enzymatically functional liver cells. The locally high concentrations of the amine metabolite formed in the liver parenchyma cause rapid killing of immature flukes which are also located in the parenchyma until they are at least 7 weeks of age. It is thought that the metabolite is also rapidly destroyed in the liver. Small amounts of the metabolite may escape into the bloodstream but become diluted. Therefore, the efficacy of the metabolite for mature flukes located in the bile ducts is reduced since the quantity of active substance reaching the mature flukes is small. The safety of this drug for the host can be explained on the basis of destruction of the toxic metabolite by the liver and dilution in the blood so that only small quantities of the substance reach other tissues of the body.

Treatment of acute fascioliasis. Diamphenethide is used for the treatment of acute fascioliasis resulting from the activity of immature forms of *F. hepatica* in the liver parenchyma of sheep. It possesses an activity of almost 100% against flukes of from 1 day to 9 weeks of age at a dosage level of 100 mg/kg (Rowlands 1973).

The activity of diamphenethide for 10-week-old newly matured flukes diminishes to 78% and the efficacy for flukes 12 weeks of age or older is 70% or less. Thus a single treatment normally eliminates all of the young flukes but leaves at least 30% of the mature flukes which will continue to shed eggs and, consequently, contaminate pastures. The effects of concurrent or subsequent use of an adulticidal drug with diamphenethide seems feasible but apparently has not yet been reported.

Prophylaxis. The fundamental prerequisites of successful prophylaxis for fascioliasis include elimination of the existing fluke population *en toto;* arresting the contamination of pastures with fluke eggs; and prevention of the development of acute, chronic, or subclinical fascioliasis. The ideal fasciolicide for accomplishing all these prerequisites of necessity would need to be highly efficacious for all parasitic stages of *F. hepatica.* Of the current drugs, rafoxanide, with an efficacy that spans 4-week-old to adult flukes, and diamphenethide, which is effective against 1-day-old to 10-week-old flukes, most closely approach the ideal fasciolicide and therefore offer the best chance for chemoprophylaxis of fascioliasis.

The value of rafoxanide as a prophylaxis of fascioliasis has already been demonstrated in West Scotland (Armour and Corba 1972). The drenching of ewes twice (in the spring and early summer) at an interval of 6 weeks kept the test pastures virtually clear of fluke eggs over the vital period of snail breeding and infection by miracidia. Two further treatments in the fall, 6 weeks apart, reduced infection in the ewes to negligible proportions in the winter. Armour and Corba (1972) have proposed that treatments with diamphenethide, which is significantly more efficacious for the very young flukes than is rafoxanide, at 8-week intervals (twice in the spring and twice in the fall) should provide excellent control of fascioliasis. Whether this is indeed the case, has yet to be demonstrated.

Toxicity. The usual oral dose of 100 mg diamphenethide/kg of body weight in sheep is apparently safe. A single oral dose 4 times the therapeutic dose (400 mg/kg) produces no toxic signs. At higher dosages, toxic effects include temporary impairment of vision and loss of wool. Pastured sheep are less susceptible to toxic effects than housed sheep. At a dosage of 1600 mg/kg, diamphenethide produces a low incidence of mortality. An acute LD50 value for sheep has apparently not been established.

Contraindications. There appear to be no significant contraindications for the use of diamphenethide. No teratogenic effects or adverse effects on fertility have been noted among pregnant ewes dosed with 200 mg/kg once weekly on 2, 3, or 4 consecutive occasions during the 21-week gestation period, nor have ill effects been noted on the fertility of ewes and rams dosed with the drug during the mating period.

Administration and dosage. Diamphenethide is commercially prepared as a ready-to-use suspension for oral administration to sheep in a single dose of 100 mg/kg of body weight.

Paramphistomiasis

Rumen fluke (*Paramphistomum* spp.) infections are common throughout the world in cattle and sheep. The adult fluke, attached to the rumen wall, is of little consequence to the health of the animal. Large numbers of the immature stages, however, during migration in the duodenal wall can be seriously pathogenic in young, previously uninfected sheep or cattle. Animals that exhibit severe anorexia, increased intake of water, and watery fetid diarrhea require immediate treatment to avoid losses due to death and reduced production.

In general, intestinal paramphistomiasis responds well to treatment with one of several drugs that are effective for liver fluke and/or cestode infections in ruminants. In sheep, two fasciolicides (tetrachloroethane and niclofolan) and the anticestodal drug (niclosamide) independently give satisfactory efficacy against the immature migrating stages of *Paramphistomum* spp. and marked improvement in the clinical condition of weaners following treatment. Niclosamide at 90 mg/kg of body weight provides consistently high efficacy (almost 100%) against the immature flukes; the efficacy of niclofolan at 6 mg/kg is more variable (Boray 1969).

Resorantel and bithionol are used effectively for the treatment of intestinal paramphistomiasis in both sheep and cattle. Various efficacy studies using resorantel indicate 84%–100% clearance of both the adult and immature (20- to 30-day-old) forms of *Paramphistomum* at therapeutic dosages of 65 mg/kg of body weight. In parts of Europe and the Soviet Union, resorantel is commercially available for the treatment of paramphistomiasis as well as tapeworm infections in cattle and sheep (see Anticestodal Drugs). Of the trematodes, only *Paramphistomum* appears to be affected by resorantel since the efficacy for *Fasciola hepatica, F. gigantica,* and *Stilesia hepatica* is nil (Gaenssler and Reinecke 1970). The drug is very well tolerated by both sheep and cattle.

Bithionol is approximately 87% effective against immature forms of *Paramphistomum* spp. in the intestinal and abomasal walls and is 100% effective for mature flukes in the rumen. The compound is administered orally in 2 doses of 70 mg/kg of body weight each at a 48-hour interval.

Paragonimiasis

Lung fluke infection by *Paragonimus* spp. is occasionally diagnosed in the dog and cat in the Americas and Far East. Currently no drug is available for totally satisfactory treatment. Bithionol has limited efficacy for lung flukes but appears to be the only drug that can be recommmended for use in treating paragonimiasis in dogs and cats. Its efficacy is variable, ranging from 85% down to only 15% reduction in worm burdens in some individuals (Yokogawa et al. 1961). The oral dosage of bithionol for both dogs and cats is 100 mg/kg of body weight every other day for a total of 10–15 treatments. A decrease in numbers of fluke eggs in the stools generally begins after the 2nd or 3rd treatment and may progress to zero during the course of treatment. Surviving flukes, whose reproductive system is temporarily nonproductive as a result of drug action, begin to shed eggs again within approximately 1–2 weeks of the termination of treatment.

REFERENCES

Aminzhanov, M., and Gel'diev, M. 1972. Control of coenuriasis and hydatid in sheep. Veterinariia 49:66.

Andersen, F. L.; Loveless, R. M.; and Jensen, L. A. 1975. Efficacy of bunamidine hydrochloride against immature and mature stages of *Echinococcus granulosus*. Am J Vet Res 36:673.

Annen, J. M. 1973. Investigations of the efficacy and acceptability of rafoxanide and diamphenethide in the treatment of acute and chronic fascioliasis of sheep, with consideration of clinical and biochemical changes. Inaug. dissertation, Zurich Univ., Switzerland.

Armour, J., and Corba, J. 1970. The anthelmintic activity of rafoxanide against immature *Fasciola hepatica* in sheep. Vet Rec 87:213.

———. 1972. The anthelmintic efficiency of diamphenethide against *Fasciola hepatica* in sheep. Vet Rec 91:211.

Batham, E. J. 1946. Testing arecoline hydrobromide as an anthelmintic for hydatid worms in dogs. Parasitology 37:185.

Bell, M. E., and Bennett, E. W. 1970. Effects of arecoline on dogs: Influence of route of administration. Proc Univ Otago Med Sch 48:3.

Bills, G. N. B.; Sharard, A.; and Fastier, F. N. 1970. Possible role of the liver in bunamidine toxicity. Proc Univ Otago Med Sch 48:59.

Blair, H. E. 1949. Vermiplex, a new anthelmintic for dogs. North Am Vet 30:306.

Boray, J. C. 1969. The anthelmintic efficiency of niclosamide and menichlopholan in the treatment of intestinal paramphistomosis in sheep. Aust Vet J 45:133.

Boray, J. C.; Wolff, K.; and Trepp, H. C. 1973. Testing of new fasciolicides. I. Efficacy and toxicity of rafoxanide in sheep experimentally infected with *Fasciola hepatica* and *F. gigantica*. Schweiz Arch Tierheilkd 115:367.

Brander, G. C., and Pugh, D. M. 1971. Veterinary Applied Pharmacology and Therapeutics, 2nd ed., p. 403. Baltimore: Williams & Wilkins.

Burrows, R. B., and Lillis, W. G. 1966. Treatment of canine and feline tapeworm infections with bunamidine hydrochloride. Am J Vet Res 27:1381.

Corbett, J. R., and Goose, J. 1971. The biochemical mode of action of the fasciolicides nitroxynil, hexachlorophene, and oxyclozanide. Biochem J 121:41.

de Carneri, I., and Vita, G. 1973. Drugs used in cestode diseases. In R. Cavier and F. Hawking, eds. Chemotherapy of Helminthiasis, vol. 1, p. 145. Elmsford, N.Y.: Pergamon Press.

Davis, A. 1973. Drug Treatment in Intestinal Helminthiases, p. 95. Geneva: World Health Organization.

Enchev, S.; Veselinova, A.; and Bratanov, V. 1972. Morphological changes in the parenchyma of organs of dogs treated with hexachlorophene. Vet Med Nauki 9:27.

Fastier, F. N. 1972. Pharmacological aspects of bunamidine dosing of dogs. NZ Vet J 20:148.

Forbes, L. S. 1964. The use of arecoline hydrobromide in the treatment of taeniid infections in dogs. An Trop Med Parasitol 58:116.

———. 1966. Anthelminthics in the control of hydatid infections. In Proceedings of the 1st International Congress on Parasitology, Rome, 1964, vol. 2, p. 770.

———. 1971. Anthelminthic toxicity, administration technique and routes of absorption. Aust Vet J 47:601.

Fowler, J. S. L. 1971. Toxicity of carbon tetrachloride and other fasciocidal drugs in sheep and chickens. Br Vet J 127:304.

Gaenssler, J. G., and Reinecke, R. K. 1970. The anthelmintic efficacy of resorantel. J S Afr Vet Assoc 41:211.

Gemmell, M. A., and Oudemans, G. 1974. Treatment of *Echinococcus granulosus* and *Taenia hydatigena* in dogs with bunamidine hydroxynaphthoate in a prepared food. Res Vet Sci 16:85.

Gibson, T. E. 1969. Advances in veterinary anthelmintic medication. Adv Parasitol 7:349.

Hamajima, F. 1973. Studies on metabolism of lung fluke genus *Paragonimus*. VII. Action of bithionol on glycolytic and oxidative metabolism of adult worms. Exp Parasitol 34:1.

Harant, H.; Castel, P.; and Gras, G. 1957. Elimination d'*Hymenolepis fraterna* de la souris et du rat par le dilaurate et le dichlorure d'etain di-n-octyle. Bull Soc Pathol Exot 50:427.

Harfenist, M. 1973. Diamphenethide—A new fasciolicide active against immature parasites. Pestic Sci 4:871.

Harvey, D. G., and Hoe, C. M. 1971. The application of some liver function tests to sheep dosed with carbon tetrachloride and hexachlorophene. Vet Rec 88:562.

Hatton, C. J. 1967. Efficiency of bunamidine salts against tapeworms. Vet Rec 81:104.

Hollister, J. T. 1967. Treatment for tapeworms in dogs. Vet Med Small Anim Clin 62:990.

Hunt, E. R. 1971. Hepatotoxicity of carbon

tetrachloride in sheep. I. The influence of diet. Aust Vet J 47:272.

Keeling, J. E. D. 1968. The chemotherapy of cestode infections. In A. Goldin, F. Hawking, and R. Schnitzer, eds. Advances in Chemotherapy, vol. 3, p. 107. New York: Academic Press.

Kondos, A. C., and McClymont, G. L. 1966. Pharmacology and toxicology of carbon tetrachloride in the sheep. III. Effect of cold and heat stress on toxicity and rates of elimination. Aust J Agric Res 17:363.

———. 1967. Pharmacology and toxicology of carbon tetrachloride in the sheep. IV. Reduction and augmentation of toxicity by selenium. Aust J Agric Res 18:667.

Krotov, A. I., and Rusak, L. V. 1972. Experimental study of the efficacy of combinations of phenasal with cucurbitine and Novocain in hymenolepidid infection of white mice. Med Parazitol (Mosk) 41:417.

Lammler, G. 1968. Chemotherapy of trematode infections. In A. Goldin, F. Hawking, and R. Schnitzer, eds. Advances in Chemotherapy, vol. 3, p. 153. New York: Academic Press.

Link, R. P. 1965. Anticestodal drugs. In L. M. Jones, ed. Veterinary Pharmacology and Therapeutics, 3rd ed., p. 652. Ames: Iowa State Univ. Press.

Menrath, R. L. E.; Sharard, A.; Gray, K. W.; and Cameron, C. W. 1973. Toxicity of bunamidine. II. Metabolic effects. NZ Vet J 21:212.

Nikitin, V. F.; Kondrat'ev, V. P.; and Redzhepov, A. R. 1969. Determination of the right duration of starvation diet before arecoline treatment of dogs. Byull Vses Inst Gel'mintol KI Skryabina 3:74.

Nurtaeva, K. S. 1972. Experimental study of kamala and its combination with phenasal. Med Parazitol (Mosk) 41:741.

Nurtaeva, K. S.; Bekhill, A. F.; and Vorob'eva, Z. G. 1973. Metallic salts of phenasal and their anthelmintic activity. Med Parazitol (Mosk) 42:86.

O'Brien, J. J. 1970. Toxicological aspects of some modern anthelmintics. Aust Vet J 46:297.

Pawlowski, Z., and Chwirot, E. 1970. Nebenwirkungen bei der Behandlung von Taeniarhynchosen. I. Beobachtungen bei 2014 aubulanten Patienten. In V Internationaler Kongress fur Infektionskrankheiten, Vienna, Austria, p. 277.

Pearson, I. G.; Whitlock, H. V.; DeGoosh, C. P.; Farrington, K. J.; Jones, R. C.; and Haigh, J. A. 1970. Clioxanide, a new anthelmintic against *Fasciola hepatica* and *Haemonchus contortus* in sheep. Aust Vet J 46:480.

Posthuma, D., and Vaatstra, W. J. 1971. Changes in rabbit liver sterol patterns after administration of carbon tetrachloride in doses effective against *Fasciola hepatica*, the liver fluke. Biochem Pharmacol 20: 1133.

Presidente, P. J. A.; Knapp, S. E.; Schlegel, M. W.; and Armstrong, J. N. 1972. Anthelmintic efficacy of clioxanide against experimentally induced *Fasciola hepatica* infections in calves. Am J Vet Res 33:1593.

Prieto, R. 1971. Efficacia de la niclosamida en el tratamiento de la monieziosis en bovinos y ovinos jóvenes. Rvta Cub Cienc Vet 2:75.

Pütter, J. 1970. Mode of action of the cesticidal drug niclosamide. I. Effect on enzyme systems. Arzneim Forsch 20:203.

Rowlands, D. ap T. 1973. Diamphenethide—A drug offering a fresh approach to the treatment of liver fluke disease in sheep. Pestic Sci 4:883.

Sharp, M. L.; Sepesi, J.; and Collins, J. A. 1973. A comparative critical assay on canine anthelmintics. Vet Med Small Anim Clin 68:131.

Slack, R., and Nineham, A. W. 1968. Medical and Veterinary Chemicals, vol. 1, pt. 2, p. 217. Elmsford, N.Y.: Pergamon Press.

Sosipatrova, L. A., and Leushin, N. V. 1971. Histological changes in dogs following administration of phenasal. Byull Vses Inst Gel'mintol KI Skryabina 5:119.

Vibe, P. P.; Sultankulov, T. D.; and Mozalev, N. S. 1971. Testing the efficacy of phenasal and hexachlorophene on *Avitellina* and *Thysaniezia* infections (Moscow). Izdatel'stvo "KOLOS," p. 80.

Yokogawa, M.; Yoshimura, H.; Sano, M.; Okura, T.; Tsuji, M.; Takizawa, A.; Harada, Y.; and Kihata, M. 1961. Chemotherapy of paragonimiasis with bithionol. I. Experimental chemotherapy on the animal infected with *Paragonimus westermani* or *P. ohirai*. Jpn J Parasitol 10:302.

Zarnowski, E. 1967. The importance of reflex of sulcus oesophageus in preoral administration of drugs. Acta Parasitol Pol 15:1.

CHAPTER 54

ANTIPROTOZOAN DRUGS

EDWARD L. ROBERSON

AVIAN COCCIDIOSIS

Nine species of *Eimeria* are known to infect the digestive tract of chickens; at least seven infect turkeys; and still others infect geese, ducks, and wild birds. The degree of pathogenesis caused by each species of *Eimeria* varies. Among chickens, for example, only six of the nine species are thought to be of economic importance. Roughly in order of decreasing severity, these six are *E. tenella, E. necatrix, E. brunetti, E. acervulina, E. mivati,* and *E. maxima.* Among these, *E. tenella* and *E. necatrix* can give rise to spectacular outbreaks of disease, with appreciable blood loss and mortality. The other four economically important species are more insidious in their attack.

Coccidiosis has been estimated to cost the U.S. poultry industry in excess of 50 million dollars annually (Edgar 1971). Such losses are not so much due to dramatic coccidial outbreaks and mortalities but primarily to impaired feed conversion, depressed growth, and downgrading at processing. Despite such losses, the U.S. poultry industry is a multibillion dollar business due partly to the extensive use of anticoccidials for controlling avian coccidiosis.

History of Anticoccidials

The control of coccidiosis in poultry was attempted prior to the 1940s by using various kinds of alchemic recipes, skimmed

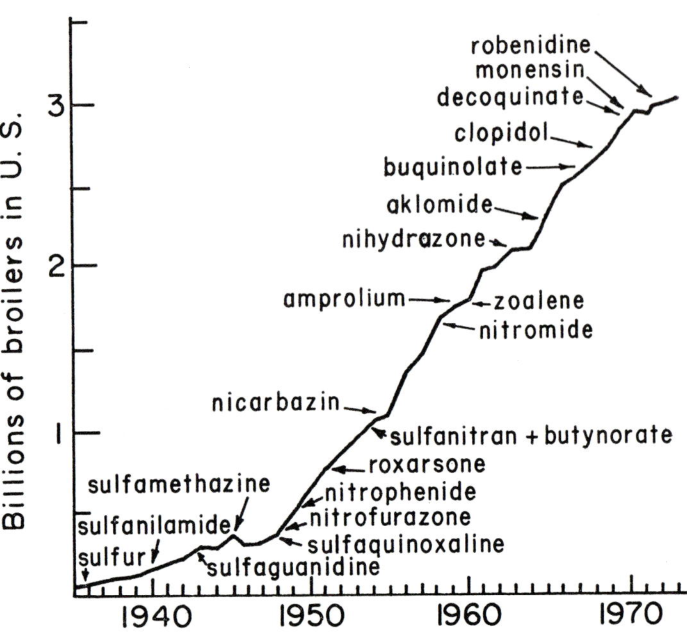

Fig. 54.1. Year of introduction of representative anticoccidials superimposed upon a graph showing increases in U.S. broiler production. Source of the broiler production data is the Marketing Division of the U.S. Department of Agriculture. (Reid 1975)

milk, vinegar, and flowers of sulfur. The discovery in the early 1940s that the sulfonamides had potent anticoccidial activity transformed the treatment of avian coccidiosis.

With the remarkable growth of the poultry industry in the past 35 years has come a steady procession of chemical agents used to combat coccidiosis (Fig. 54.1). The increasingly greater confinement rearing of broilers (2000–20,000 birds/house) has tremendously enhanced the opportunity for coccidial outbreaks and thus necessitated a continuous search for more efficient anticoccidials. In general, the early anticoccidials were limited in activity, whereas in recent years, wide-spectrum drugs effective against several to most species of chicken coccidia have been introduced.

Today, a chicken weighing 3 lb can be produced in less than 7 weeks with a little over 6 lb of feed. This attests to the innovations of the poultry industry; in the 1940s, 15 lb of feed over a 15-week period were required to produce a 3-lb chicken. At least a part of this success is due to the extensive use of chemical agents to combat coccidiosis.

Present Use of Anticoccidials

broilers

Anticoccidials are almost universally used now in starter rations for meat-type birds being raised under confinement (floor-pen management). The aim of the broiler industry is to produce as much chicken meat as possible in the shortest time possible and with the least possible expenditure of feed. Under these conditions, it is not feasible to depend on immunity of the birds to coccidiosis. Acquiring protective levels of immunity necessitates exposure to the organism, which invariably involves at least a temporary setback in growth and feed conversion. Such setbacks are rarely overcome in the short life of broilers. Thus establishment of immunity in these birds is not considered. Rather, the objective is to achieve total continual prevention from or suppression of coccidiosis. Therefore, anticoccidials generally are used prophylactically throughout the entire growing period of broilers. Premarketing withdrawal of medication is required for about two-thirds of the available anticoccidials. These are classified as 1- to 10-day "withdrawal" types. Early withdrawal, however, poses a threat to what are probably highly susceptible birds (McDougald and Reid 1971). Thus growers often substitute a "no withdrawal" anticoccidial for the withdrawal product during the final days before marketing.

LAYER AND REPLACEMENT FLOCKS

The use of anticoccidials in layer flocks of chickens, whether they are breeders or producers of eggs for human consumption, is not as universal as in broilers. With these long-lived birds, an effort is generally made toward establishing natural immunity against coccidiosis for both safety and economic reasons. A temporary setback in the growth of such birds is of less long-range significance provided the coccidial infection is not so severe as to cause permanent damage or death.

Agreement has not been reached on the best way to establish coccidial immunity and at the same time protect layers and replacement birds from heavy exposure and consequent clinical illness. Three general types of coccidiosis control programs are being used to rear layer and replacement flocks (Reid 1966).

1. The most widely employed program consists of using a preventative anticoccidial in the feed (at lower than broiler levels) for 6–22 weeks after which medication is discontinued. This level may be reduced stepwise as the bird gets older and gradually develops a protective level of immunity. Most producers discontinue use of anticoccidials after 14 weeks. The use of low levels of anticoccidials in this manner is aimed at allowing the birds to experience a "controlled" infection with coccidial organisms sufficiently severe to stimulate an immune response but insufficient to cause death or permanent disability. The continuous exposure of birds to viable oocysts of *Eimeria* depends upon the fact that at low levels the drugs, which otherwise are coccidiocidal (killing) or coccidiostatic (arresting development), are not accomplishing these functions completely. Therefore, sufficient numbers of organisms complete the cycle, thereby allowing for continual exposure to new generations of oocysts. A disadvantage of this approach is that it is precisely this use of suboptimal levels of anticoccidials that is most likely to enhance development of drug-resistant lines (Ryley and Betts 1973).

2. A second program followed by a few producers uses no preventive anticoccidial during the growing period of layers. Treatment is introduced when and if coccidiosis breaks out in the flock. In larger houses for growing birds, an outbreak is a progressive thing. Initially, only a small percentage of the birds will be so severely affected as to lead to death or require culling. If the flock can be treated at this time by using compounds that act against the later stages of the cycle, e.g., sulfonamides, it should be possible to salvage most of the flock and at the same time allow immunity to develop.

3. A third program is planned immunization. It accomplishes immunization by exposing 3-day-old chicks to measured quantities of four to seven species of viable oocysts in the feed or drinking water. Such suspensions of oocysts are commercially available as CocciVac. The mild infection initiated by the vaccine produces some immunity and introduces a natural cycling of the organism which reinforces immunity. A prophylactic level of an anticoccidial is used to prevent loss from accidental overexposure.

Resistance to Anticoccidials: "Shuttle" and "Switch" Programs

The continued use of an anticoccidial may result in selection and survival of drug-resistant strains. After extended use, resistant strains have been encountered for all anticoccidials. Fewer resistant strains have been found with some products than with others. Resistance to a particular drug is not recognized suddenly because of dramatic increases in mortality and severity of lesions. Rather, resistance generally becomes suspected because of accumulated decreases in weight gains and feed conversion.

Principally because of potential resistance, it has become an increasingly common practice in the broiler industry to use two or more anticoccidials, not concurrently but sequentially, at various intervals. A change from one anticoccidial to another in a single grow-out is referred to as a "shuttle program," whereas a change of anticoccidials between two grow-outs is termed a "switch program." The need for frequent switching is sometimes overemphasized by competitive marketing. Reid (1972a) maintains that since oocysts may survive for several months in the soil, rotation more often than once every 6 months may be self-defeating.

When switching, it is necessary that the new product have a different mode of action from the previous drug, i.e., it is preferred that one product affect the sporozoite stage of the parasite while the other affect the first generation merozoite. If both drugs act specifically against the same stage, there probably is no advantage in switching. Apparently no danger to chickens results from any possible switch from one anticoccidial to another with the possible exception of sulfonamides (Reid 1972). Sulfonamide toxicity has occurred when switching partially grown chickens from an anticoccidial containing no sulfonamide to one containing either sulfanitran or sulfaquinoxaline.

ANTICOCCIDIALS FOR USE IN CHICKENS

Fig. 54.2 presents a diagrammatic review of the life cycle stages of avian coccidia as represented by *E. tenella.* There are two asexual cycles, which require collectively 4.5 days for completion; a sexual cycle of 2 days; and oocyst sporulation outside the host, which requires another 1 or more days. In order to be effective against *E. tenella* (or in general, against any species of avian coccidia since all species have es-

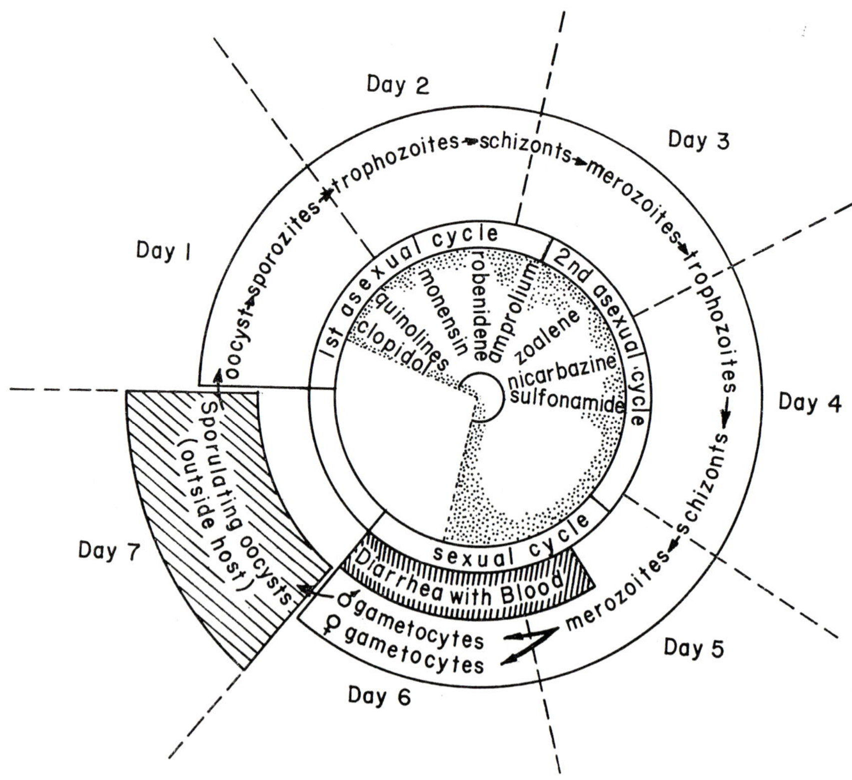

FIG. 54.2. Time of peak activity of representative anticoccidials against *Eimeria tenella.* (Reid 1975)

sentially similar cycles), anticoccidials must be used prophylactically instead of therapeutically. Few anticoccidials continue strong activity into day 5 or 6 during the sexual cycle. By the time signs of anorexia and hemorrhage appear on day 4 or 5, initiating anticoccidial treatment will provide little protection.

For most anticoccidials, the time in the life cycle against which the drug is active is known. All anticoccidials show their greatest efficacy against the first or second asexual cycle; none primarily inhibit the sexual stages of the cycle. Only a few anticoccidials have been studied sufficiently to identify the chemical metabolic pathway by which the drug blocks the specific stage of the parasite.

The following brief discussion lists anticoccidials in their chemical groups in order of day of peak activity beginning with day 1. Most of the compounds have Food and Drug Administration (FDA) approval in the United States for use in poultry feeds.

Clopidol

Clopidol INN (Coyden), 3,5-dichloro-2, 6-dimethyl-4-pyridinol, is also called metichlorpindol or clopindol. It is the only member of its class (the pyridinols) having useful anticoccidial properties. It is most active against the sporozoite stage of *Eimeria*. Thus clopidol needs to be in the feed of chickens on the day of exposure to coccidial oocysts to produce full anticoccidial potential. In general, a specific anticoccidial must be added to the feed at least 24 hours before its day of peak activity against the cycle if it is to be beneficial. The day of peak activity for clopidol is designated as day 1 of the coccidian cycle.

Clopidol is more coccidiostatic than coccidiocidal. Its coccidiostatic activity may hold the sporozoite undeveloped in an epithelial or host macrophage cell for as long as 60 days, i.e., long after the cycle normally would have been completed. If the drug is withdrawn during this static state, latent coccidiosis may appear as the parasite resumes development. Field cases of latent coccidiosis, however, are quite rare.

No appreciable immunity is developed by chickens exposed to coccidia while consuming feed containing clopidol. The drug is generally administered at 125 ppm in the feed.

Quinolones

Hundreds of quinolones have been synthesized. A number of them have shown activity of one sort or another against various groups of parasites. *Buquinolate* INN (Bonaid), *decoquinate* INN (Deccox), and *nequinate* (Statyl) have shown good efficacy against all species of chicken coccidia.

All the quinolones are virtually insoluble in water, which limits absorption. Since activity is influenced by the degree of absorption, the quinolones are micronized into a fine particle size of approximately 1.8 μm. Still, absorption by the host is minimal which probably accounts for the remarkable freedom from toxicity. Ryley and Betts (1973) were unable to induce toxicity with nequinate in any animal examined other than by intravenous injection with suspensions sufficient to cause blockage of the circulation. Tissue residues of quinolones are very low, the greatest concentrations occurring in the liver.

Most classes of anticoccidials are not able to give complete control of oocyst production. The lack of complete elimination of oocysts enhances the potential for development of drug-resistant strains of coccidia. The quinolones, as a class, are no exception and, in fact, seem to have a greater tendency than many other groups in allowing drug-resistant strains to develop. Thus their usefulness as chicken anticoccidials is now limited.

All the quinolones are chemical analogs and act on the sporozoite stage of the life cycle. The sporozoite is evidently able to penetrate the host intestinal cell, but further development is prevented. Thus the day of maximum activity of these compounds is day 1 of the cycle. These drugs must be in the feed on the day of exposure to coccidia to give maximum advantage.

A delay of 24 hours between exposure of chickens to a lethal challenge of coccidia and the subsequent addition of quinolones to the feed markedly reduces protection for the birds.

The biochemical basis for anticoccidial activity by the quinolones is not known. Several antibacterial quinolones are known to interfere with deoxyribonucleic acid (DNA) synthesis at the thymidine synthetase step. None of the antibacterial quinolones show anticoccidial activity (and vice versa); thus a different mode of biochemical action that is effective against coccidia may exist for quinolones.

ROXARSONE

Roxarsone INN (3-Nitro) is an organic arsenical with the chemical formula 3-nitro-4-hydroxyphenylarsonic acid. It was known to possess anticoccidial activity as early as 1944 but its acceptance by the poultry industry has been due primarily to improved growth, feed conversion, and pigmentation by broilers being fed rations containing the compound. At least 50% of the broiler industry uses roxarsone at the present time as a growth promoter (Reid 1974). Similar growth-promoting and anticoccidial activities are attributed to arsanilic acid.

The anticoccidial activity of roxarsone is directed against the sporozoite stage. There is at least some interference with cell invasion. No subsequent stages of the cycle, however, are adversely affected by the drug. Thus peak activity of roxarsone occurs on the 1st day of infection; it is recommended that the drug be in the feed at least 12–24 hours prior to anticipated exposure to coccidia to obtain maximum efficacy. In the United States, the FDA no longer approves roxarsone for anticoccidial activity but it is approved for use in chicken and turkey feeds because of its growth promotion and pigmentation properties. A number of other anticoccidials that also contain roxarsone or arsanilic acid are approved for use in feeds.

MONENSIN

Like other antibiotics, *monensin* INN (Coban) is a fermentation product; it is the first antibiotic, however, developed and marketed exclusively as an anticoccidial. Other antibiotics such as the tetracyclines and spiramycin have some degree of anticoccidial activity but monensin appears to be the only natural product having useful activity in quantities that are realistic for incorporation into feed. It is a metabolite produced during the growth of *Streptomyces cinnamonensis*. The structural formula is shown in Fig. 54.3.

Despite relatively unimpressive results in laboratory trials, monensin has given excellent results against all species of chicken coccidia in floor-pen trials which more closely simulate field conditions. It has been extensively used in the United States since receiving FDA approval in 1974 and to date there is no evidence of parasite resistance. Twenty-two serial passages of *E. tenella* and 20 passages of *E. acervulina* conducted in the presence of monensin have not lead to any decrease in drug sensitivity. Additionally, sufficient coccidial development takes place in the presence of monensin to allow immunity to develop in all species except *E. necatrix*. Due to incomplete suppression of oocyst production,

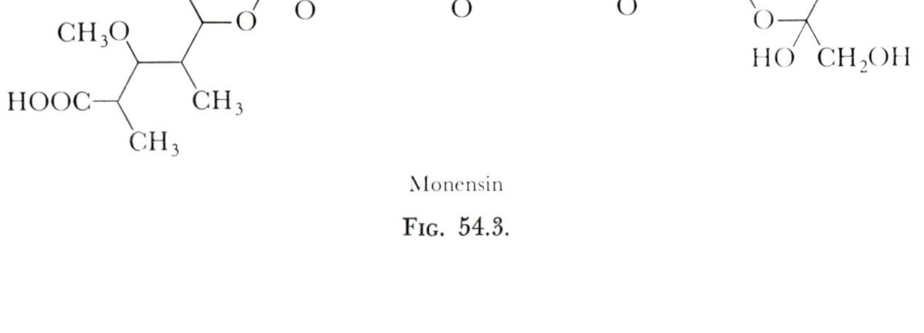

Monensin

FIG. 54.3.

resistant strains of coccidia are liable to develop eventually.

Anticoccidial activity of monensin is largely confined to the first 2 days of the cycle. The tropozoite (the stage harbored by the host cell following sporozoite penetration) and, perhaps, the first generation schizont are the stages attacked. The drug is able to form complexes with sodium and potassium ions in the developing parasite. The significance of this to the mode of action of monensin is not clear. It has been shown, however, that the monensin-cation complex specifically inhibits the transport of potassium ions into rat liver mitochondria. As a result, certain mitochondrial functions, including substrate oxidations and adenosine triphosphate (ATP) hydrolysis, are inhibited. Ryley and Betts (1973) suggest it is possible, although not proved, that coccidial mitochondria may be more susceptible than those of the host to these inhibitions, and this may explain the anticoccidial activity of the compound.

Robenidine

A guanidine derivative, *robenidine* (Robenz), is an FDA-approved (January 1973) anticoccidial. Its chemical name is 1,3-bis(parachlorobenzylidene amino)-guanidine hydrochloride. Its structural formula is shown in Fig. 54.4.

The early efficacy studies with robenidine, using the compound at 66 ppm in the diet, indicated high prophylactic protection against eight species of chicken coccidia. In addition, field strains that had shown some degree of resistance to one or more of the older anticoccidials were effectively suppressed by this drug. In comparative studies, robenidine at 66 ppm was as effective as or more effective than 125 ppm

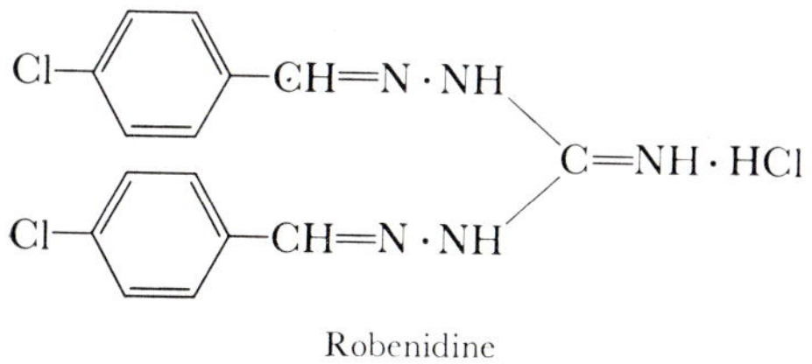

Cl—C₆H₄—CH=N·NH
C=NH·HCl
Cl—C₆H₄—CH=N·NH

Robenidine

Fig. 54.4.

clopidol against the six most pathogenic species of chicken coccidia.

The maximum activity of robenidine is during day 2 of the life cycle of *E. tenella*. The drug allows intracellular development to take place up to the first generation multinucleate schizont, but differentiation of merozoites to form a mature schizont is prevented. At this point degeneration begins but some parasites apparently can survive for as long as 14 days in the presence of the drug and still continue development upon withdrawal of medication.

An undesirable property of robenidine is the unpleasant taste it imparts to the flesh of broiler birds fed diets containing 66 ppm of the drug until slaughter. The taste is also imparted to the eggs of layers when fed at the level of 66 ppm. By no means is all of the human population able to detect the unpleasant taste; the ability to do so seems to be genetically linked. Both the United States and the United Kingdom have eliminated the taste problem by reducing the incorporation level of robenidine to 33 ppm and by withdrawing the drug 7 days before slaughter. At the new level of 33 ppm, oocyst production is not so effectively suppressed as at 66 ppm; thus the possibility for emergence of resistant coccidial strains is more acute.

Amprolium

Amprolium INN (Amprol) is an acidic white crystalline powder, practically odorless, and slightly hygroscopic. Chemically, it is 1-[(4-amino-2-propyl-5-pyrimidinyl)-methyl]-2-picolinium chloride hydrochloride.

It decomposes slowly when mixed with broiler rations, showing an average loss of 8% when stored at room temperature for 60 days. It is compatible with vitamins, antibiotics, minerals, and other ingredients commonly used in poultry rations.

Amprolium at 125 ppm in broiler diets has given acceptable activity against *E. tenella* and *E. acervulina* but relatively unacceptable control against *E. necatrix, E. brunetti, E. maxima,* and *E. mivati.* Total suppression of oocyst production is not at-

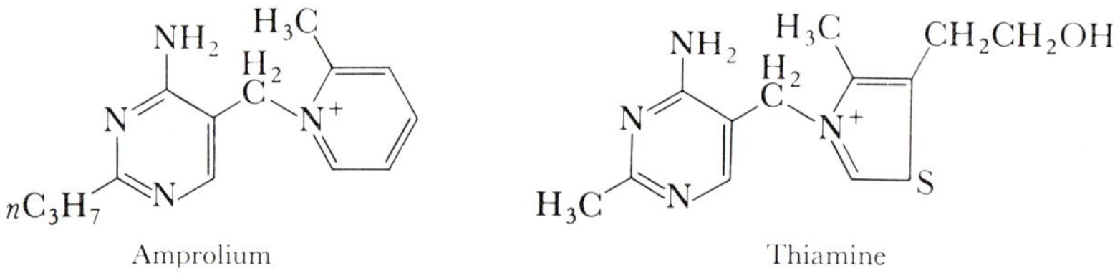

Amprolium

Thiamine

FIG. 54.5.

tained at this level of medication. Nevertheless, the fact that there is no withdrawal period on amprolium diets free of antibiotics allows for rather extensive use of this anticoccidial in the poultry industry today. Besides roxarsone, amprolium is the only anticoccidial approved as a feed additive for use in laying birds. As a preventative, it can be administered continuously to layers at 0.0125% of the feed. For treatment of moderate or severe outbreaks among layers, it is fed for a 2-week period at either 0.0125% or 0.025%, respectively.

The mode of action of amprolium depends on its ability to substitute for thiamine in the metabolism of the parasite. This occurs because of the close structural similarity of the two compounds (Fig. 54.5). Thiamine deficiency in the host may occur at high incorporation rates of amprolium but is reversible by the addition of thiamine to the diet. Anticoccidial activity of the drug may also be annulled by thiamine.

Other similar thiamine antagonists (*beclotiamine* and *dimethialium*) have been developed as anticoccidials by the Japanese. The latter two drugs are not approved for use in the United States.

Amprolium evidently shows peak activity early in day 3 of the life cycle of *E. tenella*. It is reported to act chiefly upon the first generation schizont, preventing differentiation of the merozoites. Evidence suggests that it also suppresses to some degree the sexual stages (gametogony) and sporozoites.

COMBINATION WITH OTHER ANTICOCCIDIALS

Unsatisfactory efficacy of amprolium against several intestinal species of chicken coccidia has led to the development of mixtures of anticoccidials to achieve wider-spectrum control. One such combination is amprolium and sulfaquinoxaline (SQ), used widely in the United Kingdom. With this mixture, amprolium gives control of cecal species and SQ control of intestinal species of coccidia.

Amprolium plus ethopabate (Amprol Plus) and amprolium, ethopabate, plus SQ (Pancoxin) are successful combinations used respectively in the United States and the United Kingdom. *Ethopabate* is a substituted benzoic acid having anticoccidial activity against a number of strains of *E. maxima, E. brunetti,* and other intestinal species. Its lack of activity against the cecal species *(E. tenella)* is compensated for by the activity of amprolium against this species. The mode of action of ethopabate, like sulfonamides and pyrimidines, is the blockage of tetrahydrofolic acid synthesis. Its peak activity is listed as day 4 of the cycle, evidently affecting the second asexual generation, although this is not known with certainty.

DINITOLMIDE

The nitrobenzamide anticoccidials are represented by *nitromide* (Unistat-2), *aklomide* (Aklomix), and *dinitolmide* INN (Zoalene, Zoamix). Subsequent to initial marketing, each of these compounds has appeared in combinations with sulfanitran and roxarsone. All three compounds, but especially dinitolmide, have had worldwide use as chicken anticoccidials.

The chemical name of dinitolmide is 3,5-dinitro-*o*-toluamide; its structural formula is shown in Fig. 54.6.

Dinitolmide is therapeutically active against *E. necatrix, E. tenella, E. brunetti, E. acervulina,* and *E. maxima* of chickens. *E. necatrix,* the most pathogenic species of intestinal coccidia, appears to be highly susceptible to dinitolmide medication. The

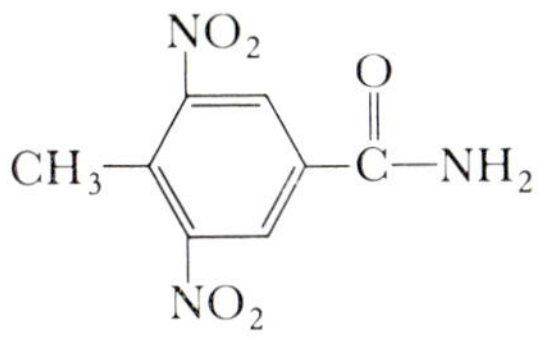

NO_2, O, CH_3, C—NH_2, NO_2

Zoalene

FIG. 54.6.

therapeutic dosage in the feed is twice the prophylactic dosage, i.e., 0.025% and 0.0125% of the total ration, respectively.

Peak activity of dinitolmide is directed against the asexual merozoite stage of the coccidian cycle, i.e., during the early part of the 3rd day of infection. If dinitolmide is begun at 48 hours postinfection in the feed or at 60 hours postinfection in the water and continued for a period of 36 hours, test infections of *E. tenella* and *E. necatrix* are completely controlled. Withdrawal of dinitolmide, however, on an experimental basis is known to result in latent coccidiosis 5–6 days after withdrawal.

NICARBAZIN

Nicarbazin (Nicarb) is an equimolecular complex of 4,4′-dinitrocarbanilide (DNC) and 2-hydroxy-4,6-dimethylpyrimidine (HDP). The two components are absorbed separately from the chicken digestive tract. DNC is absorbed more rapidly but disappears more slowly from the tissues than HDP. Two days are required for tissue clearance of nicarbazin following feeding of a 0.015% level to chickens for 7 days.

Nicarbazin is effective prophylactically against cecal *(E. tenella)* and intestinal *(E. acervulina, E. maxima, E. necatrix,* and *E. brunetti)* coccidiosis in chickens. The absence of lesions while employing this drug has enhanced its popularity in the poultry industry. A level of 0.0125% nicarbazin is used in starter mash or pellets. This level may be reduced to 0.01% when shifting to a growing ration. Despite continuous feeding of either of these levels, massive natural exposure to infective oocysts is liable to cause an outbreak of coccidiosis, in which case treatment with more potent coccidiostats, i.e., sulfonamides or sulfonamide derivatives, is advisable.

The day of peak activity of nicarbazin has been designated as early in day 4. The life cycle stage most seriously suppressed is the second generation schizont. There is less activity against other stages. The suppression by nicarbazin appears to be more coccidiocidal than coccidiostatic in nature but the biochemical mode of action is not known.

A 4-day withdrawal of nicarbazin is required before broilers are marketed. The drug does not have FDA approval for laying birds in production.

SULFONAMIDES

The sulfonamides were the first synthetic anticoccidials used successfully in coccidiosis treatment (1940–1948). The original drugs or their derivatives have been used widely for prophylaxis and treatment of coccidiosis of chickens, other food-producing animals, and pet animals.

Relative to avian coccidia, the sulfonamides are much more effective against intestinal than against cecal species of coccidia. In order to control cecal species, high concentrations of sulfonamides, e.g., *sulfadimidine* INN (*Sulfamethazine,* U.S.P.) or *sulfaquinoxaline,* for 2 days out of a 5-day period are necessary. Such high levels are not economically feasible, are sometimes toxic, and are sometimes associated with a hemorrhagic syndrome. The poor control of *E. tenella* at acceptable dosage levels plus the advent of more satisfactory anticoccidials have essentially resulted in abandoning the use of SQ or sulfadimidine alone.

Two newer sulfonamides, *Sulfadimethoxine,* N.F. (Agribon), and *sulfachloropyrazine* (Esb_3), are less toxic than sulfadimidine or SQ and have been recommended for therapeutic use in avian coccidial outbreaks. A 3-day course of treatment using 0.03% Esb_3 in the drinking water is the commercial recommendation for outbreaks of avian coccidiosis in the United Kingdom. Sulfadimethoxine, N^1(2,6-dimethoxy-4-pyrimidinyl)-sulfanilamide, can also be used prophylactically at an FDA-approved level of 0.0125% for continuous feeding of broilers. It must be withdrawn 2 days before slaughter and cannot be fed to chickens over 16 weeks of age.

General agreement exists among investigators that sulfonamides produce maximum effects against the second generation schizont of the several species of avian coccidia studied. Sulfaquinoxaline additionally causes some degree of damage against sporozoites and first generation schizonts of *E. tenella*. Peak activity of the sulfonamides is day 4 of the cycle; therefore, access to sulfonamide anticoccidials as late as the 2nd or in some cases even the 3rd day following exposure to infective oocysts provides control of avian coccidiosis. The fact that the peak activity of sulfonamides is late in the cycle, as compared to peak activities of other compounds, is the reason sulfonamides are often effectively used when clinical signs of a coccidial outbreak begin to show up within a population of birds. The second generation schizont seems to be especially important in the development of coccidial immunity. Since this stage develops to some degree during continuous sulfonamide feeding, natural immunity eventually develops in chickens on a sulfonamide prophylactic program.

The biochemical basis of activity of the sulfonamides is associated with their interference with the paraaminobenzoic acid (PABA) and/or folic acid pathways. PABA and folic acid are particularly important in the synthesis of large amounts of nuclear material during development of the coccidial second generation schizont. Blockage of the PABA and folic acid pathways by sulfonamides prevents proper development of the schizont.

SIMPLE AND POTENTIATED MIXTURES

The most significant advancement in the use of sulfonamides in the poultry industry has been the development of sulfonamide-containing mixtures (Table 54.1). The activities of components of the mixtures have been found to be additive (simple mixtures) or, in some cases, actually enhanced (potentiated mixtures).

The components of simple mixtures are generally inadequate anticoccidials on their own. When mixed together, substantially better control of mortality and weight gain are accomplished because of an additive effect. For example, Polystat contains two anticoccidials, sulfanitran and dinsed. Several of the simple mixtures, including Polystat, also contain the growth-promoting arsenical, roxarsone.

Potentiation of anticoccidial activity seems most pronounced with drugs that independently interfere with various parts of the PABA–folic acid pathway (Ryley 1972). Both sulfaquinoxaline and *Pyrimethamine, U.S.P.*, are folic acid antagonists. The synergistic mixture (Whitsyn) of these two

TABLE 54.1. Sulfonamide-containing mixtures for use as anticoccidials

Trade Name	Components	Anticoccidial Use	Administration
Simple mixtures			
Pancoxin	Sulfaquinoxaline + amprolium + ethopabate	Prophylactic	Feed
Supracox	Sulfaquinoxaline + amprolium + ethopabate + pyrimethamine	Prophylactic	Feed
Polystat	Sulfanitran + butynorate + dinsed + roxarsone	Prophylactic	Feed
Unistat	Sulfanitran + nitromide + roxarsone	Prophylactic	Feed
Novastat	Sulfanitran + aklomide	Prophylactic	Feed
Novastat-W	Sulfanitran + aklomide	Treatment	Water
Novastat-3	Sulfanitran + aklomide + rosarsone	Prophylactic	Feed
Potentiated mixtures			
Whitsyn-S	Sulfaquinoxaline + pyrimethamine	Prophylactic or treatment	Feed or water
Darvisul	Sulfaquinoxaline (80 ppm) + diaveridine (10 ppm)	Prophylactic	Water
Saquadil	Sulfaquinoxaline (62.5 ppm) + diaveridine (55 ppm)	Treatment	Water
Rofenaid	Sulfadimethoxine (125 ppm) + ormetoprim (75 ppm)	Prophylactic	Feed

components is highly efficacious both prophylactically and therapeutically for avian coccidia. Pyrimethamine, however, is potentially a very toxic compound and is best restricted to short-term treatment procedures (Ryley and Betts 1973). A less toxic folic acid antagonist is *diaveridine* INN which has good anticoccidial efficacy against *E. tenella.* Its combination with SQ at either 10 or 55 ppm diaveridine yields, respectively, prophylactic and therapeutic mixtures for use against avian coccidia.

A more recent potentiated sulfonamide mixture for coccidial prophylaxis is Rofenaid which consists of sulfadimethoxine and ormetoprim. The latter compound is a close analog of diaveridine. Rofenaid has antibacterial as well as anticoccidial properties. *E. brunetti* is especially susceptible to the mixture. Additionally, acceptable control of *E. tenella, E. necatrix, E. acervulina, E. maxima,* and *E. mivati* with regard to mortality, growth, and feed conversion in chickens has been shown. Development of coccidial immunity occurs while birds are on continuous Rofenaid feeding.

COCCIDIOSIS IN TURKEYS

Of nine species of turkey coccidia, three are recognized as pathogenic. *Eimeria meleagrimitis, E. adenoeides,* and *E. gallopavonis* are highly pathogenic for poults under 5 weeks of age. In older poults, none of these species cause any signs other than weight loss over the short period of the infection. This is perhaps due to age resistance.

Anticoccidials are not used as extensively in turkeys as in chickens. This is due in part to range versus confinement rearing of turkeys. Concentration of birds markedly enhances the opportunity for overdoses of coccidial oocysts. The turkey industry presently is tending toward more confinement rearing, in which case the necessity for using anticoccidials on a preventative and/or therapeutic basis in 3- to 8-week old poults will increase.

In general, turkeys respond to the anticoccidials used in chickens. Drugs currently used in the United States for treatment of coccidial outbreaks in turkeys include 0.05% SQ, 0.025% sulfadimethoxine plus 0.006%–0.024% amprolium, 0.2% sulfamethazine, and 0.03% Esb_3.

These compounds generally are administered therapeutically in the drinking water for a designated number of days. Turkeys drink water containing amprolium and SQ sufficiently well to obtain therapeutic levels of the drug, but are reluctant to drink water containing sulfamethazine.

Preventative coccidial programs for turkeys are more widely used in the eastern, midwestern, and south central parts of the United States than in the southeastern and western areas (Reid 1972b). In the latter areas, preventative programs are more restricted to isolated farms or endemic areas of coccidial outbreaks. Compounds currently approved by the FDA as feed additives for preventative programs in turkeys include amprolium (0.0125%–0.025%), SQ (0.0175%), butynorate (0.0375%), and Zoalene (0.0125%). Anticoccidial mixtures approved for turkeys include Polystat (0.02% butynorate, 0.03% sulfanitran, 0.02% dinsed, 0.0025%–0.005% roxarsone) and Rofenaid (sulfadimethoxine, ormetoprim). Additionally, two mixtures are available that contain antihistomonal as well as anticoccidial agents. One of them combines the antihistomonal drug, *Carbarsone,* N.F., with Zoalene. The second combines the antihistomonal drug ipronidazole and an antibiotic, ormetoprim, with sulfadimethoxine.

Recent floor-pen trials have indicated that monensin provides rather dramatic protection against coccidiosis in turkeys (Anderson et al. 1975). Mixed species of *E. adenoeides, E. gallopavonis,* and *E. meleagrimitis* caused no deaths among turkeys continuously fed 60, 80, or 10 ppm monensin, while 75% of the similarly challenged but unmedicated controls died. Weight gains for medicated challenged birds were within 92% of gains recorded for unmedicated unchallenged controls. Weight gains of challenged birds receiving no medication averaged only 29%. These trials suggest that monensin will be satisfactory, prophylactically, against turkey coccidiosis.

BOVINE COCCIDIOSIS

Although 15 species have been described as occurring in cattle worldwide, only 2 species *(Eimeria bovis* and *E. zuernii)* are known to regularly cause clinical coccidiosis accompanied by bloody diarrhea with resultant anemia, dehydration, anorexia, and loss of condition. Severe cases of coccidiosis most often occur in calves. Yearling cattle that have been severely affected by coccidiosis when 2 months of age may be as much as 43.2 kg (95 lbs) lighter in weight than uninfected controls (Fitzgerald and Mansfield 1969).

Older cattle are more resistant to clinical coccidiosis due either to age resistance and/or to acquired immunity. Nevertheless, previously unexposed older animals are susceptible to heavy doses of infective oocysts, more especially *E. zuernii* than *E. bovis* (Hammond 1964). Additionally, so-called immune cattle carry low-level infections and seed premises with oocysts. In confinement rearing, as is more likely with dairy than with beef cattle, the chance of heavy exposure is much greater.

Use of Anticoccidials

Before the early 1960s, little attention was given to specific treatment of bovine coccidiosis. Veterinary practitioners employed supportive therapy in the form of antibiotics, sulfonamides, astringents, antidiarrhetics, and fluids.

Since 1960, relatively more but still inadequate attention has been given to therapy and prevention of bovine coccidiosis. Many of the drugs marketed for avian coccidiosis have been tested against bovine coccidia. None has given positive results except amprolium and, more recently, monensin. Amprolium (Corid) has FDA approval as an anticoccidial in cattle and calves. It has a wide margin of safety and can be administered in the feed, in drinking water, or as a drench at either preventive (5 mg/kg/day for 21 days) or therapeutic (10 mg/kg/day for 5 days) levels. Low dosages of amprolium at 1 mg/kg for 5 days or high dosages up to 143 mg/kg for fewer than 5 days are generally ineffective against coccidia in calves. Studies by Slater et al. (1970) indicate that the site of action of amprolium in bovine coccidia is the first generation schizont.

The avian anticoccidial, monensin, is not approved by the FDA for use in cattle but experimental trials with this compound have shown efficient control of *Eimeria bovis* in calves (Fitzgerald and Mansfield 1973). In their studies, 0.25, 1, or 2 mg monensin/kg of body weight incorporated in pelleted feed and fed twice daily for 33 days protected 10-week-old holstein-friesian calves against clinical signs of coccidiosis following heavy challenge. The 1 mg/kg dosage (0.006% concentration in the feed) was the most suitable level tested with regard to palatability, weight gain, and prevention of light infections. The higher level (2 mg/kg) was reluctantly consumed due to poor palatability and resulted in erratic prevention of infection. The marked reduction in total serum protein levels seen in unmedicated infected controls was not observed in treated animals. No evidence of toxic reaction to monensin was observed at any level studied.

Diiodohydroxyquinoline, U.S.P. (Zoaquin), has recently been marketed in the United Kingdom for treatment of coccidiosis in cattle. It is administered orally in 5-g tablets for each 500 lb of body weight daily for 2–3 days.

Sulfonamides are still used to treat bovine coccidial infections. They are only partially effective because diarrhea is not prevented. However, the severity of the disease is reduced. Sulfamethazine, *Sulfamerazine,* U.S.P., INN, or SQ each appear to be most effective when administered continuously between the 13th and 17th days of experimental coccidial infections.

OVINE AND CAPRINE COCCIDIOSIS

Although coccidiosis is not a problem in range sheep, it rather frequently becomes a clinical disease during feedlot confinement. The clinical condition, which generally appears 12 days to 3 weeks after arrival at the feedlot, resembles that of cattle and in general can be similarly treated. No drugs are specifically approved by the FDA as ovine anticoccidials but a number of compounds have proved beneficial during coccidial outbreaks in sheep.

Sulfaguanidine, N.F., has given satisfactory prophylactic control of coccidiosis when lambs were fed 0.2% sulfaguanidine continuously (or were administered 3 g/lamb/day) for 20 days beginning 1 day after administration of an infective dose of 500,000 oocysts (Christensen and Foster 1943). It is important that the sulfaguanidine, or other sulfonamides, be administered early in the infection. If sulfaguanidine therapy is begun only after clinical signs appear, it is of little value in reducing the severity of the infection.

Studies by Shelton (1969) indicate that SQ at 2.5 or 4 g/head can be safely administered to goats in combination with either phenothiazine, thiabendazole, or haloxon anthelmintics. At 6 g alone, SQ was highly toxic and resulted in deaths of 5 of 18 goats. *Nitrofurazone*[1] has also given satisfactory control of coccidiosis in both lambs and goat kids. It is mixed with sugar and administered daily for 7 days at a dosage of 70.4 mg/kg of body weight.

Avian anticoccidials found to be efficacious for ovine coccidiosis include amprolium, amprolium plus ethopabate, and monensin. Amprolium protects lambs against severe clinical disease when administered at a dosage rate of 55 mg/kg twice daily for 19 days beginning 1 day prior to heavy oocyst exposure (Hammond et al. 1967). The same dosage when limited to 14 days gives only moderate protection. However, a 14-day treatment period of amprolium at 62.5 mg/kg of body weight plus ethopabate at 3.2 mg/kg administered via the drinking water is reported to enhance weight gains and reduce oocyst counts in naturally parasitized lambs (Ross 1968). Similar dosage levels of amprolium and periods of treatment have prevented clinical coccidiosis in goats.

Monensin, a coccidiostatic antibiotic used against avian coccidiosis, has been experimentally tested recently against several species of *Eimeria* in 3-month-old lambs (Bergstrom and Maki 1974). The compound was administered at the rate of 33 mg/kg of feed (1.6 mg/kg of body weight daily) for periods of either 28 or 44 days. A slight palatability problem evidently occurred upon initial access to the monensin-medicated food as evidenced by poorer food consumption by medicated lambs compared with nontreated controls during the 1st week. Subsequently, treated lambs consumed the medicated food without reluctance, gained more rapidly, and had an 11% greater feed efficiency than nonmedicated control lambs. Clinical signs of diarrhea and slight loss of body weight were observed in control groups but were prevented in treated groups. Oocyst counts dropped markedly to very low numbers during the course of treatment but following withdrawal of the drug rose again to the pretreatment level, suggesting that monensin at this dosage level in lambs is more coccidiostatic than coccidiocidal. No toxic effects were attributed to monensin in lambs.

[1] See Note on nitrofurans on p. 965.

SWINE COCCIDIOSIS

Although coccidia are rather common in swine, coccidiosis is not an important disease in temperate parts of the world. Consequently, little attention has been given to its treatment in swine. It has been found that sulfaguanidine, when administered for 3 days at the beginning of oocyst discharge, reduced the numbers of oocysts produced. Prophylactic feeding of sulfaguanidine at the rate of 0.22 mg/kg of body weight during the period of infection has been found to prevent clinical signs and suppress the fecal discharge of oocysts. Perhaps other anticoccidials, e.g., amprolium, would have a therapeutic advantage in swine coccidiosis but trials to test this evidently have not been performed.

CANINE COCCIDIOSIS

As it is with other confined animals, coccidiosis is probably the most formidable parasitic disease of kenneled puppies. The oocysts are easily spread from one animal to another. Even under the most stringent sanitary measures, coccidial outbreaks still occasionally occur among confined puppies. Puppies under stress, as during shipping, seem especially prone to develop clinical coccidiosis.

The difficulty of preventing coccidial outbreaks has prompted some kennel veterinarians to use an avian anticoccidial, amprolium (Amprol), on a regular preventative basis (Smart 1974). Prior to shipping, pups are given either water or food to which this compound has been added. The medicated water is prepared by adding 1 oz (30 ml) of 9.6% amprolium solution to 1 gal (3.8 L) of drinking water. The medicated food is prepared by adding one-fourth teaspoonful (about 1.25 g) of 20% amprolium powder to sufficient meal to feed four pups daily. Either the medicated food or medicated water, but not both, is the sole source of food or water for the pups for a period of 7 days just prior to shipping.

As an additional preventative measure, bitches are given water medicated with amprolium, as above, as the only source of water for a period of 10 days prior to whelping.

Since amprolium is a thiamine inhibitor, 1 or 2 pups out of 1000 may be expected to show nervous signs of thiamine deficiency. In such deficiency cases, pups are administered thiamine, injectable calcium gluconate, and fluids.

The conventional method of treating clinical coccidiosis in the canine includes symptomatic treatment plus the use of a sulfonamide. Sulfadimethoxine is recommended. It is given either orally or parenterally at the rate of 55 mg/kg of body weight daily in either single or divided doses for 21 days. The stage of the coccidian cycle affected by this compound in the canine has not been closely studied.

RABBIT COCCIDIOSIS

Coccidiosis is the most serious parasitic disease of colonized rabbits. The bile duct epithelium is parasitized by *Eimeria stiedae.* The intestinal epithelium is parasitized by several species of *Eimeria,* some of which are pathogenic and some nonpathogenic.

Prophylaxis

The sulfonamides have been used for both prophylactic and therapeutic control of rabbit coccidiosis. Prophylactic measures are generally necessary in facilities where young rabbits are raised. Several sulfonamides, when added to either the feed or water, have efficacy against hepatic and intestinal coccidia. These drugs in general reduce the severity of coccidial infections, reduce mortality, reduce oocyst production, and evidently allow for some degree of immunity to develop so that rabbits are at least somewhat better able to cope with subsequent challenges. One sulfonamide that has shown beneficial prophylactic use in rabbitries is 0.1% Esb_3. It is administered in the drinking water for 1 month, i.e., from weaning at 1 month of age until the rabbits are 2 months old. Also, SQ or sulfamerazine administered continuously in the drinking water for a period of 3–4 weeks and at a concentration of 0.02% will prevent the development of hepatic coccidiosis in rabbits heavily infected with *E. stiedae.* Additionally, 1% sulfamethazine mixed in the feed is reported to prevent fatal hepatic coccidiosis even if administration of the medicated feed is delayed as many as 10 days after challenge with a fatal dose of *E. stiedae* oocysts.

Treatment

A number of different therapeutic regimens have been tried and recommended for treating natural outbreaks of coccidiosis in weaned rabbits. Among older programs is the use of SQ or sulfamerazine, each at 0.03% in the drinking water for 10 days.

Newer sulfonamides that are beneficial in treating rabbit coccidiosis include sulfadimethoxine and *formosulfathiazole.* Of the two, sulfadimethoxine has received greater attention; several programs of treatment using this drug have been recommended. At oral doses of 75 mg/kg of body weight, it can be given on an intermittent schedule of 3 cycles, each cycle consisting of 3 days on medication followed by 7 days off medication. Another schedule employs sulfadimethoxine at a higher dosage of 200 mg/kg for the 1st day of oral treatment followed by 4 days of medication at 100 mg/kg. Sulfadimethoxine can also be administered in the food or drinking water. When given by food or water, sulfadimethoxine is mixed with diaveridine at a ratio of 3:1. The mixture is added to the feed at the rate of 100–125 mg/100 g of food and to water at the rate of 100 mg/gal (3.8 L) of drinking water. Recommendations call for giving the medicated food for 3 days or medicated water for 8 days.

The therapeutic use of formosulfathiazole calls for mixing the drug in the feed so as to give a dose of 375 mg/kg of body weight daily. The medicated food is fed for 4–7 days. Best results seem to occur if the period of therapy is begun on approximately the 7th day of infection.

Russian workers (Reshetnyak et al. 1970) have reported highly satisfactory therapeutic control of outbreaks of coccidiosis in rabbits using metronidazole (Flagyl). The Russian common name of this compound is trichopol. It is marketed in the Western Hemisphere for use against human infections of vaginal trichomonads and hepatic amoebae. Rabbits with spontaneous coccidiosis have shown reduction in clinical signs and in both intestinal and hepatic lesions following treatment with metronidazole. In the studies of Reshetnyak et al., the drug was administered orally at a daily dosage of 40 mg/kg for 3 days. Each rabbit also received a daily subcutaneous injection of 1% metronidazole at a dosage of 20 mg/kg. No toxic signs were observed. Although of value perhaps for treating small numbers of rabbits, this therapeutic procedure seems impractical in a large rabbitry.

CANINE GIARDIASIS

Giardia canis commonly has been associated with diarrhetic stools in dogs, especially in puppies. Typical stools in which the trophozoite as well as the cysts are found are soft to loose, light colored, and occasionally mixed with mucus and blood. Increased defecation and tenesmus are generally consistent signs. Canine giardiasis has been reported in a large number of surveys from throughout the United States and Canada as well as South America.

Two compounds appear to be particularly beneficial in the treatment of canine giardiasis. These are quinacrine hydrochloride and metronidazole.

Quinacrine Hydrochloride

CHEMISTRY

Quinacrine Hydrochloride, U.S.P. (Atabrine, Atebrin), also known as mepacrine hydrochloride INN, is chemically 6-chloro-9-(4-[diethylamino]-1-methylbutylamino)-2-methoxyacridine dihydrochloride INN. It contains approximately 80% quinacrine base.

It is a bright yellow, odorless crystalline powder with a bitter taste. It dissolves in water at the ratio of 1:35. It is soluble in alcohol but almost insoluble in acetone or chloroform.

ADMINISTRATION AND PHARMACODYNAMICS

Quinacrine hydrochloride is usually administered orally in tablet form. If the oral route cannot be used, it can be given intravenously or intramuscularly, preferably the latter.

The compound is readily absorbed from the gastrointestinal (GI) tract and from intramuscular sites of injection. Severe diarrhea does not interfere with absorption.

Quinacrine hydrochloride is widely distributed in tissues throughout the body. With repeated daily administration, the drug accumulates in the tissues, particularly the liver, spleen, lungs, and adrenal glands. It can cross the placental barrier. Its degradation in the body is not well known.

The compound is eliminated slowly, primarily in the urine which may become distinctly yellow in color following the 3rd day of continuous administration. Detectable amounts of the drug occur in the urine for at least 2 months after therapy is discontinued. Only negligible amounts are excreted in body secretions, i.e., milk, sweat, saliva, and bile.

INDICATIONS AND DOSAGE

Quinacrine hydrochloride is used in veterinary medicine to treat giardiasis of dogs. An effective dose in large breeds of dogs is 200 mg/dog 3 times on the 1st day and twice during each of the subsequent 6 days. In smaller breeds, 100 mg administered twice on the 1st day and once daily for each of the next 6 days is recommended. In puppies, a schedule of 50 mg twice a day for 6 days has been used successfully. Concurrent administration of sodium bicarbonate aids in preventing vomition.

Quinacrine hydrochloride is also used in dogs to restore auricular fibrillation to a normal sinus rhythm. The dose for this purpose is 2.64 mg/kg of body weight intravenously. *Quinine* and *quinidine* have similar restorative activity on the heart. The latter drugs are more toxic, however, than is quinacrine hydrochloride.

The use of quinacrine hydrochloride in human medicine is principally as a suppressive drug against malaria.

TOXICITY

The single acute lethal dose of quinacrine in the dog is approximately 300 mg/kg of body weight. On a continuous daily basis for 15–27 days, 110 mg/kg is fatal to dogs. Therapeutic doses sometimes cause vomition and, less frequently, disturbances of motor and psychomotor activity in dogs, cats, and rabbits (Choquette 1940).

METRONIDAZOLE

CHEMISTRY

Metronidazole, U.S.P., INN (Flagyl) has the chemical name 1-(β-hydroxyethyl)-2-methyl-5-nitroimidazole; the structural formula is shown in Fig. 54.7.

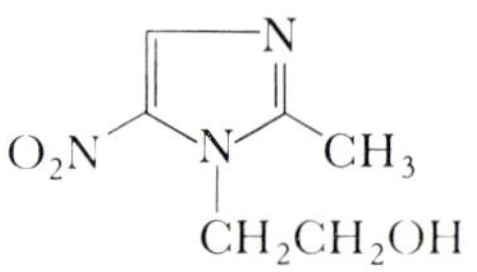

It is a white to pale yellow crystalline powder, odorless, stable in air, but darkens on exposure to light and melts between 159° and 163° C. It is only slightly soluble

O_2N — N — CH_3 ; N ; CH_2CH_2OH

Metronidazole

FIG. 54.7.

in water and ethanol, hence must be administered orally.

INDICATIONS

The success of metronidazole in treating human infections of giardiasis, vaginal and oral trichomoniasis, and hepatic and intestinal amoebiasis has lead to investigations of its potential use against certain protozoan diseases of domestic animals. These are principally bovine trichomoniasis, rabbit coccidiosis, and canine giardiasis. The response to treatment of giardiasis in the dog is usually dramatic. Diarrhea associated with the disease may be expected to stop in 2–3 days during a 5-day period of medication.

PHARMACODYNAMICS

Metronidazole is well absorbed after oral administration. In adult human beings given a single therapeutic dose of 200 mg 3 times daily, a peak serum level of 8 μg/ml is reached in 8 hours (i.e., 4 hours after the second dose). Fifty percent of the drug is excreted in the urine of human beings in 24 hours, most of which is unchanged. The rate of urinary excretion of the drug following 24 hours varies markedly. The compound is at least partly metabolized in the body. Following high dosages, metabolites of the drug may darken the urine.

TOXICITY AND CONTRAINDICATIONS

In general, metronidazole is not very toxic for dogs. Adult dogs tolerate oral doses of 100 mg/kg/day for a month without toxicity. Higher dosages may produce neurological disturbances characterized by tremor, weakness, muscle spasticity, and ataxia.

Serious blood dyscrasia has not been recorded in human beings during medication with this drug. In an appreciable proportion of treated patients, a moderate leukopenia has been observed. The white cell count returns to normal, however, following completion of the course of medication.

Metronidazole probably should not be administered during pregnancy or to nursing bitches. There is not sufficient data at this time to warrant recommending its use during pregnancy or lactation. The drug is known to pass rapidly into fetal circulation and is excreted in breast milk. In female pregnant rats, no teratogenic effect has been observed following administrations of 250 mg/kg/day for 1–12 days or 100 mg/kg/day for 40 days. Administration of the latter dose to male rats in excess of 60 days results in some degree of testicular damage with disturbance of spermatogenesis. These parameters have not been extensively studied in dogs. However, during several years of treatment of human trichomoniasis in both males and females, the drug has not been found to cause fetal abnormalities or quantitative or qualitative changes in sperm (Michaels 1968).

ADMINISTRATION AND DOSAGE

Metronidazole is administered orally. The effective dosage for treatment of canine giardiasis is 50 mg/kg/day for 5 days.

Bovine trichomoniasis *(Trichomonas foetus)* in experimentally infected bulls has been successfully treated with metronidazole either by intravenous injections of 75 mg/kg (3 times at 12-hour intervals) or by topical administration of a 5% ointment plus a urethral douche containing 30 ml of a 1% solution of the drug (Gasparini et al. 1963).

BABESIOSIS

Babesiosis is a tick-borne protozoal disease of the host's erythrocytes. The disease is characterized by fever, anemia, and icterus. Two or more species of *Babesia* are independently responsible for producing the disease in each of several hosts: in dogs, *B. canis* and *B. gibsoni;* in horses, *B. equi* and *B. caballi;* and in cattle, *B. bigemina, B. argentina, B. divergens,* and *B. bovis (B. berbera).* In endemic areas of bovine babesiosis, indigenous animals seldom show clinical signs but introduced cattle are very susceptible. Survivors of an acute infection become carriers.

Distribution

The disease occurs in tropical and subtropical parts of the world. Canine babesiosis has been reported from the United States as well as India, Ceylon, Egypt, Malaysia, and Korea (Ruff et al. 1973). Both *B. equi* and *B. caballi* of horses have been introduced into the United States via Florida, probably from Cuba, in 1958–1960 (Ristic 1972). The tropical horse tick *(Dermacentor nitens)* has vectored the disease throughout southern Florida. Bovine babesiosis caused by *B. bigemina* was eradicated from the United States in the early 1930s. This species, however, still plagues cattle in many parts of the world including southern Europe, Central and South America, Africa, and Australia. *B. bovis* occurs essentially in southern Europe and *B. divergens* in northern Europe. *B. argentina* causes bovine babesiosis in Argentina and Central and South America.

Vector Control

Although chemotherapy as discussed below is extremely important in the attempted eradication of babesiosis in various parts of the world, the benefits of concurrent tick control cannot be overemphasized. The natural transmission of *Babesia* spp. depends on ticks, and eradication of the disease can be accomplished by an adequate tick control program. Taylor (1973) suggests that the effort to eradicate equine babesiosis in Florida should be based primarily on control of vector ticks and secondarily on chemotherapy since none of the available antibabesial drugs are completely safe for horses or reliable for sterilizing *B. equi* infections. Vector control, however, is generally quite difficult. In many countries tick control programs cannot be implemented for various reasons. Thus attention is still directed primarily toward chemotherapy and, in some countries, vaccination.

Antibabesial Drugs

older drugs

A number of drugs have been used to treat babesiosis in different hosts. Some of the earlier used drugs are briefly discussed below.

Trypan Blue. An azo dye, *trypan blue* was first used in babesiosis of dogs in 1909. Its use in other hosts soon became established. It is effective primarily against the larger species of *Babesia,* namely *B. canis* in dogs, *B. caballi* in horses, and *B. bigemina* in cattle. It is best used as a 1% solution at the rate of 5–10 ml for the dog and 50–100 ml for cattle in a single dose. It must be given intravenously. In the event of inadvertent perivascular administration or leakage from the vein, tissue sloughing occurs. This disadvantage plus the objectionable discoloration of the flesh of treated patients and the frequency of relapses following treatment have resulted in infrequent use of trypan blue for babesiosis for the past 40 years.

Quinuronium Derivatives. *Quinuronium* (6,6′-di[*N*-methylquinolyl]urea dimethosulfate) is essentially the active component of a number of commercial antibabesials: Acaprin, Babesan, Pirevan, Piroparv, and Piroplasmin. These drugs are superior to trypan blue in effectiveness against the large babesias *(B. canis, B. bigemina,* and *B. caballi).* They have some value also against the small babesias *(B. bovis* and *B. argentina)* and were used extensively until the discovery of the aromatic diamidines in the 1940s. Single doses of the quinuronium drugs are administered subcutaneously at the rate of 0.6–1 mg/kg in horses, 1 mg/kg in cattle, or 0.25 mg/kg in dogs. There is no danger of tissue sloughing following subcutaneous injections of these drugs.

This group of potent drugs inhibits cholinesterase and affects the parasympathetic nervous system. Alarming reactions are likely to occur, including salivation, sweating, copious urination, diarrhea, panting, and even collapse and death (Riek 1968). Adrenaline and atropine are antidotal. The margin between the toxic and therapeutic doses is quite small and has resulted in the continued search for safer drugs.

Acridine Derivatives. Several antibabesial drugs have been derived from acridine dye and dispensed commercially as Acriflavin, Flavin, Euflavin, and Gonacrine. In earlier years these were the drugs of choice for treating infections of *B. equi.* They were administered intravenously at a dosage of 4.4 ml of a 5% solution/100 kg of body weight. The acridine derivatives have negligible systemic effects.

aromatic diamidines and carbanilides

A number of diamidino compounds and carbanilides have been tested against babesial infections in various hosts. The most successful of these are listed in Table 54.2.

Pharmacodynamics. The pharmacodynamics of the human drug pentamidine is rather representative of the diamidines. Following parenteral injection, pentamidine shows transient blood levels. It accumulates for months in the liver and kidneys and will enter fetal circulation. Very small amounts accumulate in the central nervous system (CNS), remaining for

TABLE 54.2. Diamidine and carbanilide antibabesial drugs

Generic Name	Trade Name	Chemical Name
Imidocarb	Imizol	3,3′-Bis(2-imidazolin-2-yl)carbanilide
Amicarbalide INN	Diampron	3,3′-Diamidinocarbanilide diisethionate
Diminazene INN	Berenil	4,4′-Diamidinodiazoaminobenzene diaceturate
Phenamidine	Ganaseg	4,4′-Diamidinodiphenyl ether

months. The cumulative effect of the diamidines allows them to be used prophylactically with varying degrees of success.

Data on imidocarb suggests that this drug may be concentrated in and resorbed unchanged from the kidney and that it is detoxified (metabolized) in the liver.

Mode of Action. Very little is known about the mechanism of action of any of the antibabesial drugs. It appears that imidocarb acts directly on the parasite, causing an alteration in number and size of nuclei and in morphology (vacuolation) of the cytoplasm (Beveridge 1969).

The antiparasitic activity of the aromatic diamidines may be related to interference with aerobic glycolysis as well as interference with synthesis of DNA in the parasite. All of these drugs give rise to hypoglycemia in the treated host. *Babesia* spp., as well as many other parasites like trypanosomes, depend upon the host's glucose for aerobic glycolysis. Specifically, the mechanism of trypanocidal action of *pentamidine* INN is said to depend upon the drug's inhibition of aerobic glycolysis and denaturing of nucleoproteins of the parasite (Seneca 1971), the relative importance of which is not known.

Selective blocking of kinetoplast DNA replication appears to be the mode of activity of at least one of the diamidines, i.e., *diminazene*. The activity of this drug against trypanosomes has been extensively studied by Newton (1972). Diminazene is rapidly and irreversibly bound by the trypanosome's DNA-containing organelles, first in the kinetoplast and subsequently in the nucleus. The ratio of binding is 1 molecule of diminazene for every 4–5 DNA nucleotides. Further studies strongly suggest that the drug-DNA complex inhibits kinetoplast DNA synthesis. The exact relation of this to death of the trypanosomes is not known, nor is the significance of nuclear DNA binding of the drug. Thus many questions are still unanswered relative to the activity of the diamidines; practically no studies of this nature have been conducted with babesial organisms.

Prophylactic Use. Interest in the diamidino compounds and carbanilides has not only centered around their use in the treatment of clinical babesiosis but also their use as prophylactic drugs. An acceptable prophylactic effect depends on long residual activity, so the drug should be administered to the animal before exposure to *Babesia*. Prophylaxis is of distinct advantage for several reasons. Protection against *Babesia* infection is needed when susceptible cattle are being moved from a tick-free and *Babesia*-free country through an infected area. Vaccination has been used under these circumstances but this is somewhat hazardous and a safer procedure is needed. Indeed, a prophylactic drug is also of interest because of its possible use in controlled immunization programs. Todorovic et al. (1973) have proposed that application of a prophylactic drug and exposure of cattle to ticks infected with *Babesia* might help in the development of natural immunity without hazardous losses.

Of the babesicidal drugs, *amicarbalide* and especially *imidocarb* have shown prophylactic properties against *Babesia* spp. in mice, rats, and cattle. The other drugs show hardly any such effect. A single subcutaneous or intramuscular injection of the dihydrochloride salt of imidocarb at a dosage level of 2 mg/kg of body weight protects cattle against challenge with *B. argentina, B. bigemina,* or *B. divergens* even when challenge is made as late as 1 month after administration of the drug (Callow and McGregor 1970). It appears that animals under imidocarb protection are able to mount an immune reaction to *Babesia* spp. when a natural infection is acquired. Not all workers (Roy-Smith 1971) agree that imidocarb is satisfactorily protective against *B. bigemina;* however, different results may occur because different strains of *Babesia* spp. with different drug resistances may have been used. Prophylactic activity of amicarbalide has not been as encouraging in field trials in cattle as that of imidocarb. Cattle are partially susceptible to *B. bigemina* within 1 week of treatment with amicarbalide at 7 mg/kg and fully susceptible within 2–3 weeks (Callow and McGregor 1970).

Evidence of some benefit from the use of a prophylactic babesicide in immunization programs has been shown. In Australia and Israel, mass immunization schemes have been developed. These programs depend upon the inoculation of small doses of blood from carrier animals. Standardization of the pathogenicity of the inocula is difficult and invariably it is necessary to treat some of the animals that react severely. Limited use of imidocarb during vaccination programs has not only protected against disease but also it appears that the drug does not inhibit the development of immunity in vaccinated animals. Amicarbalide, as an adjunct to the immunization of cattle by vaccination, has similar but less dramatic prophylactic properties.

Therapeutic Uses. The newer antibabesials (aromatic diamidines and carbanilides) are all effective in suppressing the parasitemia (i.e., numbers of babesial organisms in the blood). However, Beveridge (1969) has found that imidocarb has a lower ED50 (the dose required to reduce the parasitemia by 50% compared with nonmedicated controls) than amicarbalide, diminazene, or quinuronium in mice infected with *B. rodhaini* (Table 54.3). Additionally, the margin of safety of imidocarb is greater than other drugs against *B. rodhaini* in mice as measured by the values obtained from dividing the LD50 by the ED50. Whether these values remain relatively unchanged in other hosts, e.g., dogs, cattle, and horses, is not known.

TABLE 54.3. The effect and toxicity of antibabesial drugs on *B. rodhaini* in mice

Drug	ED50	LD50	LD50/ED50
	(mg/kg)	*(mg/kg)*	
Imidocarb	0.22	107	485
Amicarbalide	0.93	168	172
Diminazene	7.37	539	70
Quinuronium	0.33	8	25

Source: Modified from Beveridge 1969. (Used with permission.)

Note: Dose levels refer in every case to the salt of the preparations: imidocarb dihydrochloride, amicarbalide diisethionate, diminazene diaceturate and quinuronium sulfate.

In cattle. The dihydrochloride salt of imidocarb has demonstrated high activity in arresting the parasitemia and suppressing the development of anemia in clinical bovine babesiosis. It has proved effective against all species of *Babesia* in the bovine at a dosage of 1 mg/kg administered either intramuscularly or subcutaneously. Furthermore, at slightly higher than therapeutic dosages, i.e., 2 mg/kg, the infection can be sterilized. These dosages are calculated on the actual amount of salt used, 82 mg base being equivalent to 100 mg dihydrochloride.

The prophylactic activity of imidocarb gives it a distinct advantage over other babesicidal drugs, the dosage for prophylactic use being 2 mg/kg of body weight.

Amicarbalide is effective in reducing the parasitemia and mortality when administered to cattle during infections of either *B. bigemia, B. argentina,* or *B. bovis.* It can be given either subcutaneously or intramuscularly. In some cases, infection may be expected to recur. If treatment is delayed after the 4th day of fever, the drug is not effective in destroying the parasites in the end capillaries of the brain and cerebral basesiasis is liable to develop.

The standard therapeutic dose of amicarbalide in cattle is 5 mg/kg of body weight. A double dose, i.e., 10 mg/kg, is used in peracute cases in adult cattle. If hemaglobinuria persists beyond 24 hours following treatment, the treatment should be repeated.

The activity of diminazene varies against different species of *Babesia* in cattle. The drug rapidly clears *B. bigemina* from the blood when a therapeutic dose of 3.5 mg/kg is given subcutaneously or intramuscularly. In contrast, only partial clearance of *B. divergens* and *B. bovis* occurs. Diminazene seems to exert a restrained activity against the latter two species. Parasites can be found in the blood up to 4 days after treatment, indicating the drug causes inhibition of multiplication of the parasites rather than their destruction. Therapeutic use of diminazene in clinically affected cattle does reduce the severity of babesiosis. The elevated body temperature will generally drop within 24–48 hours following treatment, and mortality is reduced.

Diminazene does not give satisfactory results when used prophylactically against subsequent challenge with *Babesia* spp. It has been used successfully on a prophylactic basis against certain African trypanosomes of cattle.

In horses. Generally, *B. caballi* is much more responsive to chemotherapy than *B. equi.* Horses infected with either species of *Babesia* respond clinically to treatment with amicarbalide, diminazene, phenamidine, or imidocarb but only *B. caballi* infections are successfully sterilized by these drugs. Even repeated administration of large dosages of these compounds cannot be relied upon for the eradication of *B. equi* and are usually toxic.

Dosages of diamidino compounds and carbanilides in all animals, but especially horses, must be controlled very closely. The therapeutic dose of amicarbalide generally recommended for horses is 8.8 mg/kg given intramuscularly for 2 consecutive days. Similarly, diminazene is recommended at 5 mg/kg intramuscularly on 2 consecutive days. Imidocarb dihydrochloride can be administered to horses intramuscularly, subcutaneously, or intravenously at a dosage of 2.2 mg/kg for 2 consecutive days to treat *B. caballi.* Four intramuscular injections of imidocarb dihydrochloride (4 mg/kg) at 72-hour intervals are necessary to treat infections of *B. equi* (Frerich et al. 1973). The 72-hour interval is safer and gives better therapeutic results for *B. equi* than 24-hour intervals of treatment. *Phenamidine* is used at a dosage of 8.8 mg/kg on 2 consecutive days for treating *B. caballi* and for 4–5 consecutive days to treat *B. equi.* The latter regimen may be hazardous, especially in debilitated animals with liver damage. Phenamidine is given intramuscularly in multiple sites.

In dogs. As is true of the two species of *Babesia* in horses, the larger sized species *(B. canis)* in dogs is more readily controlled by chemotherapy than the smaller *B. gibsoni.* Both diminazene and phenamidine are reported to give clinical cures in cases of babesiosis caused by either species. Complete elimination of *B. gibsoni,* however, is not accomplished by any current drugs (Ruff et al. 1973). The therapeutic dose of diminazene in the dog is a single intramuscular or subcutaneous injection of 3.5 mg/kg of body weight; that of phenamidine is 15 mg/kg (i.e., 0.3 ml of 5% solution/kg) injected subcutaneously on each of 2 consecutive days.

Toxicity. All of the antibabesial drugs, including the aromatic diamidines and carbanilides, are potentially toxic. Multiple therapeutic doses of diminazene or phenamidine in healthy dogs produce severe nervous signs and prominent hemorrhagic and malacic lesions of the cerebellum, midbrain, and thalamus. Degenerative fatty changes occur in the liver, kidneys, myocardium, and muscles of some dogs so treated. In cattle given multiple doses of diminazene or phenamidine, the fatty degeneration is more severe but only mild nervous signs are seen. The severe brain lesions of dogs are not found in cattle.

The pharmacological effects of amicarbalide in horses have been studied by Taylor et al. (1972). Doses equal to twice the therapeutic dose cause a significant increase in serum glutamic oxalacetic transaminase, sorbitol dehydrogenase, and serum urea nitrogen. Doses equal to 5 times the therapeutic dose result in death. Massive necrosis of the liver and kidney tubules is found at necropsy.

Imidocarb is considered to be less toxic than other antibabesials but is by no means a totally safe drug. An LD50 has not been firmly established in any of the domestic animals. Studies suggest that in donkeys the LD50 is less than 4 intramuscular doses of 2 mg/kg at 24-hour intervals. Intravenous injections of the compound (even at low dosages of 1 mg/kg) are acutely toxic and this method of administration is not advised (Wood 1971).

There is little difference in toxicity when imidocarb is given by the intramuscular versus the subcutaneous route. Mortalities among cattle are not expected to occur at dosages up to 10 mg/kg of body weight when the drug is given intramuscularly or subcutaneously. At low dosages of 1 mg/kg, there are few or no signs of toxicity. At 2 mg/kg, approximately one-half the treated cattle may be expected to show transient signs of an anticholinesterase effect, i.e., coughing, muscular tremors, salivation, and colic. Recovery is generally within an hour of treatment. At 3 or 5 mg/kg, the above signs, though still transient, become progressively more marked. At 10 mg/kg, as indicated above, some fatalities begin to occur. Tolerance levels in other hosts are similar to those described for cattle.

Local reactions at the site of injection of imidocarb are seldom seen when low dosages of 1 mg/kg are used. At higher dosages (5 mg/kg), local irritation is more frequent and of longer duration, especially following subcutaneous injections.

Drug Resistance. Evidently babesial organisms can develop resistance to the antibabesial drugs. Experimentally, several resistant strains of *B. rodhaini* in mice have been developed for diminazene, amicarbalide, and imidocarb. Each specific drug-resistant strain showed some cross-resistance to the other two drugs and also to phenamidine and quinuronium. The extent of drug resistance in therapeutic and prophylactic use of these drugs in the field is not known.

ANAPLASMOSIS

In tropical and subtropical areas of the world, anaplasmosis is one of the most severe hemotrophic diseases of cattle and to a large measure has hampered the development of the livestock industry. Two approaches, vaccination and chemotherapy, have been aimed at controlling the disease in cattle.

Vaccination

Efforts toward vaccinating have included the administration of controlled amounts of virulent organisms or, more recently, killed organisms. The use of virulent organisms is based on the concept that it is necessary to infect an animal in order to protect it. This procedure cannot be well controlled and may result in severe losses. An additional disadvantage is the fact that it establishes an animal as a carrier. Thus immunization with virulent organisms is used only in enzootic areas such as tropical South America and Africa; it is contraindicated in the United States where efforts toward eradication seem feasible (Kuttler and Zaraza 1970).

Use of a killed vaccine (Anaplaz) in the United States has reduced the severity of anaplasmosis in cattle and cut death losses. It does not prevent the disease. Furthermore, there have been some deaths among newborn calves whose dams have been administered the vaccine. The vaccine is of bovine blood origin. If the constituent blood of the vaccine is foreign to the dam, her immunological response results in the production of antibodies which are passed to the calf in the dam's colostrum. Depending on the blood type of the sire, the calf's erythrocytes may be agglutinated by the antibodies the calf has ingested from its mother's milk. Thus the isoimmunohemolytic disease of neonatal calves has been a limiting factor in use of the killed vaccine of bovine origin. This disadvantage has directed recent attention toward growing *Anaplasma marginale* in blood-free culture; results of these investigations are not yet available.

Chemotherapy

Chemotherapy is important in the attempted control of anaplasmosis for several reasons. First, the use of virulent vaccinations are generally accompanied by some losses which can be minimized by prompt treatment of animals that develop clinical anaplasmosis following exposure to the vaccine. Second, a complete sterile immunity has never been demonstrated in cattle following the infection. A premunition type immunity exists following the infection because animals are carriers of low numbers of the organism. The carrier state, however, serves to propagate the spread of the organism. Thus the need exists for a compound that not only will provide therapeutic relief of clinical signs but also will prevent the carrier state of cattle. Of the many drugs (arsenicals, antimony derivatives, antimalarials, dyes) tested against *A. marginale* in cattle, only three types, i.e., the tetracyclines, dithiosemicarbazones, and imidocarb, are therapeutically effective and only two of these, the tetracyclines and imidocarb, eliminate the carrier state.

TETRACYCLINES

Tetracycline, U.S.P., INN, *Chlortetracycline,* N.F., INN, and *Oxytetracycline,* N.F., INN are equally effective in the treatment of clinical anaplasmosis. These antibiotics have been used against *Anaplasma* infections since the early 1950s. Early use of the tetracyclines in the disease, i.e., before hemoglobin values fall below 4 mg%, generally allows for 100% survival as compared with approximately 85% survival when therapy is delayed (Miller 1956). The standard treatment for anaplasmosis with antibiotics consists of at least 1 intramuscular injection of tetracycline (6.6–11 mg/kg). Additionally, the slow transfusion of 2–4 L of blood is recommended.

The carrier state of *Anaplasma* can be eliminated by the tetracyclines. To do so, chlortetracycline must be administered orally each day for 60 days at a dosage of 2.2 mg/kg or for 90 days at a dosage of 1.1 mg/kg. This procedure is both time-consuming and expensive; thus the use of tetracyclines for eliminating the carrier state is limited.

DITHIOSEMICARBAZONES

Tests of 22 dithiosemicarbazones in 1965 led to the selection of 1 of these compounds for its activity against *A. marginale.* The compound selected was α-ethoxyethylglyoxal dithiosemicarbazone (gloxazone, Contrapar). A single intravenous injection at the rate of 5 mg/kg is as effective as the tetracyclines in initial suppression of multiplication of the parasite and protection against death losses. However, the suppression of parasitemia in cattle treated with the dithiosemicarbazone is only temporary since some degree of parasitic relapse almost invariably occurs within 3–4 weeks of treatment. The relapse is usually milder than the primary infection seen in untreated animals; therefore the severity of infections can be reduced by therapeutic use of the drug. In general, it has been used to reduce losses in areas where premunition with virulent *A. marginale* is the method of choice for prophylaxis. The therapeutic dose of gloxazone is 5–10 mg/kg intravenously.

As indicated previously, sterilization of infections of *A. marginale* does not occur following therapy with this compound. Repeated dosages of 5 mg/kg daily for 10 days appear to eliminate the carrier state but are also 100% fatal (Kuttler and Adams 1970).

IMIDOCARB

Originally developed for its activity against *Babesia* spp. (see Antibabesial Drugs in this chapter), imidocarb (the dihydrochloride salt) has recently been found to be effective both in the treatment of anaplasmosis and in the elimination of the carrier state. Therapeutically, it is at least as effective as tetracycline and dithiosemicarbazone and has a distinct economic advantage over tetracycline. Imidocarb is given therapeutically in a single subcutaneous dose of 1.5 mg/kg. Oral administration is ineffective.

To eliminate the carrier state of animals, 2 or 3 doses of imidocarb at higher than therapeutic levels are required. Two intramuscular or subcutaneous doses, each 5 mg/kg, 14 days apart are effective. Also 3 injections of imidocarb (4, 5, or 6 mg/kg) at 24-hour intervals are effective.

The low cost of imidocarb plus its effectiveness in the treatment of anaplasmosis and elimination of the carrier state will undoubtedly result in its expanded use in the next several years.

REFERENCES

Anderson, W. I.; Reid, W. M.; and McDougald, L. R. 1975. Personal communication.

Bergstrom, R. C., and Maki, L. R. 1974. Effect of monensin in young crossbred lambs with naturally occurring coccidiosis. J Am Vet Med Assoc 165:228.

Beveridge, E. 1969. Babesicidal effect of basically substituted carbanilides. II. Imidocarb in rats and mice: Toxicity and activity against *Babesia rodhaini.* Res Vet Sci 10:534.

Callow, L. L., and McGregor, W. 1970. The effect of imidocarb against *Babesia argentina* and *Babesia bigemina* infections of cattle. Aust Vet J 46:195.

Choquette, L. P. E. 1940. Canine giardiasis and its treatment with Atebrin. Can J Comp Med 14:230.

Christensen, J. F., and Foster, A. O. 1943. Further studies with sulfaguanidine in the control of ovine coccidiosis. Vet Med 38:144.

Edgar, S. A. 1971. The past, present and future of coccidiosis control in poultry. Vet Med Rev 2/3:349.

Fitzgerald, P. R., and Mansfield, M. E. 1969. Economic significance of coccidiosis in calves. J Parasitol (abstr) 55:39.

———. 1973. Efficacy of monensin against bovine coccidiosis in young holsteinfriesian calves. J Protozool 20:121.

Frerichs, W. M.; Allen, P. C.; and Holbrook, A. A. 1973. Equine piroplasmosis *(Babesia equi)*: Therapeutic trials of imidocarb dihydrochloride in horses and donkeys. Vet Rec 93:73.

Gasparini, G.; Vaghi, M.; and Tardani, A. 1963. Treatment of bovine trichomoniasis with metronidazole (8823 R.P.). Vet Rec 75:940.

Hammond, D. M. 1964. Coccidiosis of cattle. 30th Faculty Honor Lecture, Utah State Univ., Logan.

Hammond, D. M.; Kuta, J. E.; and Miner, M. L. 1967. Amprolium for control of experimental coccidiosis in lambs. Cornell Vet 57:611.

Joyner, L. P., and Brocklesby, D. W. 1973. Chemotherapy of anaplasmosis, babsesiasis, and theileriasis. Adv Pharmacol Chemother 11:321.

Kuttler, K. L., and Adams, L. G. 1970. Comparative efficacy of oxytetracycline and a dithiosemicarbazone in eliminating *Anaplasma marginale* infection in splenectomized calves. Res Vet Sci 11:339.

Kuttler, K. L., and Zaraza, H. 1970. A preliminary evaluation of a dithiosemicarbazone for the treatment of anaplasmosis. Res Vet Sci 11:334.

McDougald, L. R., and Reid, W. M. 1971. Susceptibility of broilers to coccidiosis following early coccidiostat withdrawal. Poult Sci 50:1164.

Michaels, R. M. 1968. Chemotherapy of trichomoniasis. Adv Chemother 3:39.

Miller, J. F. 1956. The prevention and treatment of anaplasmosis. Ann NY Acad Sci 64:49.

Newton, B. A. 1972. Recent studies on the mechanism of action of Berenil (diminazene) and related compounds. In H. Van den Bossche, ed. Comparative Biochemistry of Parasites, p. 127. New York: Academic Press.

Reid, W. M. 1966. Relationship between layer flock immunity to six species of coccidia and the use of coccidiostats. In Proceedings of the 13th World's Poultry Congress, Kiev, USSR, p. 453.

———. 1972a. Anticoccidials used in the poultry industry: Time of action against the coccidial life cycle. Folia Vet Lat 2:641.

———. 1972b. Protozoa. In M. S. Hofstad, ed. Diseases of Poultry, 6th ed., p. 983. Ames: Iowa State Univ. Press.

———. 1974. Anticoccidials: Differences in day of peak activity against *Eimeria tenella.* In Proceedings of the Symposium on Coccidia and Related Organisms, Guelph, Ontario, 1973, p. 119. Guelph: Univ. of Guelph.

———. 1975. Progress in the control of coccidiosis with anticoccidials and planned immunization. Am J Vet Res 36:593.

Reshetnyak, V. Z.; Bartenev, V. S.; and Rubanov, A. A. 1970. Trichopol (metronidazole), an effective drug against coccidiosis in rabbits. Veterinariia 3:75.

Riek, R. F. 1968. Babesiosis. In D. Weinman and M. Ristic, eds. Infectious Blood Diseases of Man and Animals, vol. 2, p. 219. New York: Academic Press.

Ristic, M. 1972. Protozoal diseases. In E. J. Catcott and J. F. Smithcors, eds. Equine Medicine and Surgery, 2nd ed., p. 137. Wheaton, Ill.: American Veterinary Publications.

Ross, D. B. 1968. Successful treatment of coccidiosis in lambs. Vet Rec 83:189.

Roy-Smith, F. 1971. The prophylactic effects of imidocarb against *Babesia argentina* and *Babesia bigemina* infections in cattle. Aust Vet J 47:418.

Ruff, M. D.; Fowler, J. L.; Fernau, R. C.; and Matsuda, K. 1973. Action of certain antiprotozoal compounds against *Babesia gibsoni* in dogs. Am J Vet Res 34:641.

Ryley, J. F. 1972. Cytochemistry, physiology, and biochemistry. In D. M. Hammond, ed. The Coccidia, p. 145. Baltimore: University Park Press.

Ryley, J. F., and Betts, M. J. 1973. Chemotherapy of chicken coccidiosis. Adv Pharmacol Chemother 11:221.

Seneca, H. 1971. Biological Basis of Chemotherapy of Infections and Infestations, p. 979. Philadelphia: F. A. Davis.

Shelton, M. 1969. Coccidiosis in Angora goats. Texas A & M Univ Res Rep on Sheep and Angora Goat, Wool and Mohair. Pr-2635, p. 11.

Slater, R. L.; Hammond, D. M.; and Miner, M. L. 1970, *Eimeria bovis*: Development in calves treated with thiamine metabolic antagonist (amprolium) in feed. Trans Am Microsc Soc 89:55.

Smart, J. H. 1974. General management and prophylactic procedures for commercial kennels or puppy farms. In R. W. Kirk, ed. Current Veterinary Therapy V, p. 56. Philadelphia: W. B. Saunders.

Taylor, W. M. 1973. Chemotherapy of equine piroplasmosis. In J. T. Bryans and H. Gerber, eds. Equine Infectious Diseases III, p. 476. Basel, Switzerland: S. Karger.

Taylor, W. M.; Simpson, C. F.; and Martin, F. G. 1972. Certain aspects of toxicity of an amicarbalide formulation to ponies. Am J Vet Res 33:533.

Todorovic, R. A. 1974. Bovine babesiasis: Its diagnosis and control. Am J Vet Res 35:1045.

Todorovic, R. A.; Vizcaino, O. G.; Gonzalez, E. F.; and Adams, L. G. 1973. Chemoprophylaxis (imidocarb) against *Babesia bigemina* and *Babesia argentina* infections. Am J Vet Res 34:1153.

Wood, J. C. 1971. The activity of imidocarb against *Babesia* infections of cattle. Ir Vet J 25:254.

CHAPTER 55

EXTERNAL PARASITE CONTROL

MAXCY P. NOLAN and
EDWARD L. ROBERSON

Domestic animals are attacked by many different arthropod parasites. Flies, mites, lice, ticks, bots, grubs, etc., cost livestock producers and pet owners large sums of money. In the United States, more than $500,000,000 annually are lost in livestock production to parasites. Pests of domestic animals (1) predispose animals to diseases, (2) cause anemia (due to blood loss), (3) reduce weight gains, (4) reduce feed efficiency, (5) transmit several important animal diseases (encephalitis of horses, anaplasmosis of cattle, heartworm of dogs, etc.), and (6) irritate animals, thereby reducing the pleasure derived from pets. The following discussion presents the more common pests attacking different types of domestic animals, the damage they cause, and recommended treatments. An understanding of the biology of the pests to be controlled is necessary for effective, economical, and safe pest control. When control involves the use of pesticides, caution must be exercised to prevent contaminating human beings, their food supply, and their environment.

PESTICIDE TOXICITY

Pests can weaken animals, thereby causing unthriftiness, disease, and death. Pesticides, therefore, are used to protect animals from parasitic arthropods; however, all pesticides are poisons and can be toxic to warm-blooded as well as cold-blooded animals. For this reason, recommended pesticides must be applied properly to prevent injury to animals.

Individual animals sometimes readily show toxicity to certain pesticides and materials contained in pesticide formulations. Applicators should be aware of signs of pesticide toxicity. Poisoning is usually exhibited as excessive salivation, lacrimation, defecation, urination, and muscle twitching. The skin of some animals, especially the horse, is extremely sensitive to various pesticide formulations and may show urtication or hyperemia, suggestive of toxicity. Should this happen, the pesticide should be removed as quickly as possible by washing the animal's coat. Sensitive animals should not be retreated with this drug or should be treated only with pesticide formulations nontoxic to the animal.

Animals under stress or that will be put under stress should not be treated unless extreme caution is exercised. Pesticides should not be applied in combination with other pesticides or with certain other drugs unless so stated on the label. Details relative to the toxicity of different types of pesticides (carbamates, organophosphorus compounds, chlorinated hydrocarbons, etc.) are presented in Section 15.

RESIDUE POTENTIAL OF PESTICIDES

Many domestic animals are raised for the human food products they produce. Consequently, it is extremely important that pesticide residues not be allowed to accumulate in illegal amounts in edible tissues. Only approved insecticides should be applied to animals that are being finished for slaughter or are producing edible products such as milk. Some insecticides are eliminated slowly from animal tissues, others quickly. For this reason, it is important to adhere strictly to recommended intervals between the time of application and the time of slaughter or use of eggs and milk for human food. Label directions for pesticides must be followed carefully. Failure to do so may be dangerous to human health. Violators of the recommended procedures are subject to legal prosecution and to confiscation of their animals.

Section 16 should be consulted for discussion of residue potential for the various chemical types of pesticides.

PESTICIDE FORMULATIONS

The formulation of pesticides to be used must be taken into consideration when treating agricultural animals. *Sprays* and *dips* generally are suited for treating most animals except when temperatures are below freezing. *Pour-on* and *dust* formulations are recommended when treating animals in freezing temperatures because they do not add excessive amounts of moisture to the animal's coat. Treating animals under extremely hot, humid weather conditions is contraindicated because of enhancing the possibility of toxic reactions. Any formulation of pesticides applied under such weather conditions may be hazardous.

Ready-to-use *oil sprays* are applied so as to treat the external hair coat and not the skin. For example, 1–2 oz (30–60 ml) of ready-to-use oil-based pesticides are normally applied to beef and dairy cattle as light mist sprays on the hair coat. Oils increase pesticide absorption through the skin and easily allow toxic levels to be reached.

Pesticides may also be administered to livestock as *feed additives.* Those absorbed from the digestive tract *(systemic insecticides)* are highly effective against most blood-sucking ectoparasites. Systemic insecticides as well as those insecticides not absorbed from the digestive tract are effective against equine bots. These compounds, when passed in the feces, are also effective against larval or pupal development of numerous flies which lay their eggs in fecal material. The administration of insecticides via the feed is highly practical; consequently this technique is being used with increasing frequency for arthropod pest control.

Application Techniques

When treating farm animals for external parasites, it is important that insecticides be applied so that contact with the parasites will occur. The selection of an insecticide delivery system will depend upon the animal to be treated and the pest to be controlled. For example, when treating animals for lice, mites, and ticks, the depth of coat penetration is normally very important. Pressure of 100–200 lb/in.^{2} (psi) should be used when applying pesticides for control of these pests. Pesticides kill only the mites and lice, not their eggs; thus retreatment is needed to control newly hatched parasitic arthropods unless the compound used has residual or ovicidal activity.

Spray treatment against cattle grubs (*Hypoderma* spp.) should be applied in such a manner that the skin, not just the hair of the animal, becomes thoroughly wet. Spray pressures of 200–400 psi are recommended, depending on the thickness of the hair coat. Treatment is administered following completion of the egg-laying season of heel flies, i.e., after approximately February in the southern United States and October in the more northern states.

Power sprayers, knapsack sprayers, compressed air sprayers, and rubbing devices such as backrubbers and facerubbers are satisfactory for applying liquid insecticides to large animals. Rubbing devices usually consist of a pesticide reservoir and a material on which animals rub that acts as a wick to pull the insecticide from the reservoir. Homemade rubbing devices normally consist of burlap bags rolled around chains or wire. The insecticide is poured on the burlap bag to keep it charged. Automatic sprayers are used to apply liquid insecticides to animals on a frequent basis, most commonly to dairy animals as they exit milking parlors.

Dusts may be used for control of some external parasites. They may be applied by hand or in suspended self-treatment dust bags, power dusters, or electrostatic power dusters. The latter devices charge dust particles and thereby enhance their adhesion to objects on which the insecticide is applied.

Systemic insecticides are those that gain access to the host's circulatory system and are distributed throughout the animal's body. They can be applied as pour-ons, spot-ons, sprays, feed additives, and in dipping vats. Absorption of the drug through the skin or from the digestive tract accounts for the systemic presence of these drugs. Systemic insecticides, namely the organophosphorus compounds, are used especially for their effectiveness against grubs, horn flies, and lice.

Dosage

Even when animals are healthy, their age and size are important considerations when applying pesticides. The application of many insecticides is based on the estimated body weight of the animal. Systemic insecticides and ready-to-use oil sprays must be applied in exact amounts for adequate control of pests and prevention of injury to animals. Many other insecticides are applied to the skin to the point of run off. The dosage of medication applied in this manner is not exacting; such compounds should have a wide safety margin. Young animals, especially those under 6 months of age, cannot be treated with all the pesticides used on adult animals. Labels on the pesticide packaging should be consulted for contraindicated use in young animals.

Many pests on animals can be controlled with very small quantities of pesticides applied to specific areas on the infested animal; e.g., when treating maggot-infested wounds, only the wound and immediate surrounding area are treated.

When treating livestock for fly control, it is usually more efficient to treat animals daily with small quantities of pesticides. If rubbing devices such as backrubbers and dust bags are placed where animals cannot avoid them, they will treat themselves daily with small amounts of insecticides, thus obtaining good pest control with less material. The pesticide and method of application should be selected on the basis of providing adequate, economical, and safe control of ectoparasites with the least excitability to the animal and a minimum of contamination of the environment.

CONTROL OF BEEF CATTLE PESTS

Horn Fly

Among the ectoparasites of cattle, the horn fly *(Haematobia irritans)* is the most important fly pest in the United States, where its prevalence is well established. Endemic to Europe, the horn fly was accidentally introduced into the United States, being first reported in New Jersey by Riley and Smith in 1887. Populations of these small flies, which appear on cattle in early spring and remain on them until frost in the fall, may reach levels of 3000/animal to as high as 20,000 on herd bulls. Adult flies remain on the cattle most of the day and night, feeding intermittently as many as 20 times each day. They remove large quantities of blood from the host and annoy the animals enough to interfere with normal grazing and resting. Laake (1946) reported weight gains were lowered by 30–70 lb/animal in untreated as compared to treated herds. Treatment of these pests requires direct application of insecticides to the cattle rather than treatment of the premises.

Fortunately, a number of insecticides including the systemics are very effective against horn flies. In most areas, this insect has not developed a resistance to most insecticides. The recommended insecticides are effectively applied by many different techniques. Since the horn fly remains on cattle almost constantly and travels only short distances to infest other cattle, insecticide deposits are usually effective.

RECOMMENDED INSECTICIDES

Self-treatment rubbing devices such as backrubbers, facerubbers, and dust bags are especially effective against horn flies. When cattle are forced to use these devices, better control is obtained. In most herds, good horn fly control will be realized if rubbing devices are located at sites convenient to the cattle. Infested animals tormented by horn flies will visit these devices regularly. The small quantity of insecticide that is deposited on the animal during each visit provides excellent control. Backrubbers are available commercially or may be constructed of chain, cable, or wire wrapped with burlap. Dust bags are available commercially or can be made with doubled burlap bags. Dust bags must be suspended where cattle have access to them, preferably in a dusting station that provides protection from the weather.

Backrubbers should be located convenient to cattle and kept charged with an insecticide plus oil mixture. Compounds containing 1% coumaphos, Ciovap (crotoxyphos plus dichlorvos), ronnel, or stirofos; 1.5% dioxathion; 2% malathion; or 5% methoxychlor or toxaphene are recommended and are equally effective. The oil (usually #2 diesel fuel) retards excessive evaporation of the insecticide and enhances adherence of the compound to the animal's coat.

Dust bags should contain dust formulations of 3% crotoxyphos or stirofos, 1% or 5% coumaphos, 10% methoxychlor, or 5% phosmet.

Sprays can be applied with power sprayers. Pressure above 100 psi is recommended to thoroughly penetrate the hair coat. Aqueous solutions containing 0.06% coumaphos; 0.15% dioxathion; 0.25% phosmet; 0.375% crufomate; 0.5% Ciovap, ronnel, malathion, methoxychlor, or toxaphene; or 1% trichlorfon or dichlorvos emulsifiable concentrate should be applied so as to thoroughly cover the animal's body. Usually, 1 gal (3.8 L) of spray is recommended for each mature cow.

Dust formulations containing 3% crotoxyphos, 10% methoxychlor, or 5% toxaphene applied by hand or power dusters are also effective insecticides for horn fly control.

Pour-on systemic insecticides such as crufomate, ronnel, and phosmet can be applied with a minimum of equipment. Proper treatment is best assured by putting the cattle through a squeeze chute.

Feed additives containing 6% ronnel in loose mineral mixture or 5.5% ronnel in either a block or loose mineral mix are fed free choice during the horn fly season. The 6% formulation is fed at the rate of 0.20 lb/100 lb (.09 kg/45 kg) of body weight/month and the 5.5% formulation at a rate of 0.25 lb/100 lb of body weight/month.

Dips offer thorough coverage of animals and are made using coumaphos 0.06% or 0.25%, crufomate 0.25%, dioxathion 0.15%, or toxaphene 0.5%. Crufomate and coumaphos are the insecticides most often used against horn flies because of their additional control of cattle grubs.

Stable Fly, Horse Fly, Deer or Yellow Fly, and Mosquito

These blood-sucking flies can travel fairly long distances to infest animals. This is especially true of stable flies, which can cover distances up to 70 miles in 2 days. Most control measures are applied to the animal because it is usually not feasible to treat the breeding sites of these insects.

In addition to those insecticide sprays and dusts recommended for horn fly control, ready-to-use oil or water sprays containing 1% dichlorvos or Ciovap or 0.1% pyrethrins plus 1% synergist offer temporary control. Ready-to-use oil sprays are applied at the rate of 1–2 oz (30–60 ml) and water sprays at the rate of 0.5–2 quarts (0.47–1.9 L) daily/animal. Treatment of the animal is usually continued daily throughout the fly pest season. Additionally, the treatment of barn walls aids in reducing stable fly populations since these flies rest on walls subsequent to feeding on the animal.

Face Fly

The face fly, although only recently introduced from Europe, has spread rapidly throughout most of the United States. It often becomes a major pest of cattle in newly infested areas. A relative of the house fly, it feeds on secretions of the facial moist areas, e.g., eyes, nostrils, of cattle and horses. This characteristic makes the face fly difficult to control and allows it to contribute to the spread of pinkeye, eye worm (*Thelazia* spp.), and other eye ailments. It is not a blood-sucking insect.

Effective control is difficult. Best results are realized by using methods that allow frequent applications of insecticides to the animal's face. Dust bags that are kept dry and located where cattle will use them daily offer some relief. Dust bags should be charged with 3% stirofos or crotoxyphos, 5% coumaphos, or 10% methoxychlor. Ready-to-use oil sprays containing pyrethrins, dichlorvos, or Ciovap as recommended for stable flies are temporarily effective. Daily treatment is needed for best results.

Lice

Blood-sucking and chewing types of lice are common on cattle. Heavy populations build up in a short time on untreated animals especially during cold months. Heavily infested animals appear in poor condition and have large areas rubbed free of hair, with the remaining hair coat rough and matted in appearance. Heavy infestations of sucking lice cause marked anemia. A small number of cattle in a herd tend to be more heavily infested than the majority of the herd. These animals, called "carriers," act as a reinfestation focus for the other animals.

Sprays should be applied to wet the skin of the animal, not just the hair coat. Thus the spray should be under a pressure of 100–200 psi. Coumaphos 0.06%; dioxathion 0.15%; crufomate or ronnel 0.25%; lindane 0.03%; or toxaphene, methoxychlor, or malathion 0.5% is recommended.

Dusts of 3% crotoxyphos, 1% lindane, 4%–5% malathion, 10% methoxychlor, or 5% toxaphene are effective against cattle lice.

Pour-on solutions are being used increasingly by beef producers for lice control. Little equipment is required and during the colder months this method is better than complete wetting of the animal. Several insecticides are approved in the United States for application as pour-on solutions.

These include 4% ready-to-use coumaphos, 6% ronnel, 8% ready-to-use trichlorfon, 6%–8% crufomate and 13.4% ready-to-use crufomate, 3% ready-to-use fenthion, and 13.2% ready-to-use famphur.

Dips offer thorough coverage of beef cattle but should be used only during the warmer seasons. A dipping solution containing 0.06% coumaphos, 0.03% lindane, 0.5% toxaphene, 0.15% dioxathion, or 0.25% crufomate is effective against lice.

Tick

Ticks are serious external parasites of beef cattle. They are most bothersome where cattle are allowed to roam in wooded areas. Ear ticks are especially difficult to control due to their location on the host. Application of the pesticide must be directed toward thorough coverage of the ear and surrounding area. In general, ticks can be controlled by spraying, dusting, or dipping animals using the following pesticides.

Sprays should be applied so as to penetrate the hair coat thoroughly. Coumaphos 0.125%, toxaphene or malathion 0.5%, ronnel 0.75%, Ciovap 0.25%, dioxathion 0.15%, lindane 0.03%–0.05%, or methoxychlor 0.05% is recommended.

Dips include coumaphos 0.125%, dioxathion 0.15%, lindane 0.03%, and toxaphene 0.5%.

Dusts are especially effective for ear ticks. These include coumaphos and ronnel 5%, lindane 1%, and malathion 4%–5%.

Cattle Grub

For most effective grub control, cattle should be treated with an approved animal systemic insecticide. Best results will be obtained by treating infested cattle during migration of the grubs through the tissues of the animal. Treatment should be administered immediately following completion of egg-laying activity by the adult heel fly and at least 6 weeks before the expected appearance of the grubs in the animal's back. Cattle treated when large numbers of grubs are present in the esophagus or spinal canal may develop complications because of localized edema and swelling in sites where larvae are killed. This is followed by the release of toxic substances into the surrounding sensitized tissues. Swelling in the area of the spinal cord may result in paralysis. In the area of the esophagus, swelling may exert pressure on the trachea, causing its partial occlusion and consequent respiratory distress. These conditions are referred to as the host-parasite reaction syndrome (HPR). Treatment either before or after the period during which the grubs are in the esophagus or spinal canal will avoid the HPR syndrome.

Spray pressures of 200–400 psi are recommended depending on the thickness of the animal's hair coat. A gallon (3.8 L) of spray/mature animal should be applied so as to wet the animal thoroughly. Coumaphos 0.37%–0.5%, crufomate 0.375%, phosmet 0.25%, or trichlorfon 1% is effective against cattle grubs when used in sprays.

Pour-on solutions for cattle grub control are effective and easily administered. A calibrated applicator should be used for pouring the solution along the backline. Pour-on insecticides that may be used include fenthion 3%, coumaphos 4%, and trichlorfon 8%; each preparation is used at the dosage level of 0.5 fluid oz/100 lb (15 ml/45 kg) of body weight. Additionally, phosmet 4%, crufomate 8%, or famphur 13.2% may be applied at 1 fluid oz/100 lb (30 ml/45 kg) of body weight up to 800 lb (360 kg) or 13.4% crufomate may be used at a dosage level of 1 fluid oz/100 lb (30 ml/45 kg) of body weight up to 1000 lb (450 kg).

Spot-on ready-to-use 20% fenthion may be applied with a topical syringe adapted for this purpose at the rate of 4 cc/300 lb (135 kg) of body weight up to 1200 lb (540 kg).

Feed additives include ronnel 5.5% (mineral block or granules) fed free choice at 0.25 lb/100 lb (0.11 kg/45 kg) of body weight for at least 75 days. Additionally, ronnel 6% mineral feed supplement or mineral salt mix will control cattle grubs.

Dips for the control of cattle grubs include coumaphos and crufomate, each at 0.25%.

Cattle Mite

Cattle mites can be controlled using dips containing 0.5% toxaphene or 0.06% lindane. Infested cattle should be dipped twice, 10–14 days apart.

CONTROL OF DAIRY CATTLE PESTS

External parasites and cattle grubs attacking dairy cattle are the same as those that attack beef cattle. Normally, the stable fly *(Stomoxys calcitrans)* is the most serious external parasite of dairy cattle because of the abundance of breeding sites around dairies. House flies pose a serious problem because they are capable of contaminating milk.

Treating lactating dairy cattle requires extreme caution because illegal pesticide residues cannot be allowed in milk.

Recommended Insecticides

Crotoxyphos, Ciovap, coumaphos, dichlorvos, ronnel, malathion, methoxychlor, pyrethrins, and famphur presently have FDA approval for application to lactating dairy cattle for the control of various external pests. In addition, trichlorfon, crufomate, and famphur may be applied to nonlactating dairy cattle.

Stable Fly

Control is difficult to obtain due to the fly's habit of being in contact with the animal only during feeding. Otherwise, it rests on barn walls, fences, trees, and other convenient objects near cattle. Insecticides carefully applied to these resting areas can provide some control. Stable flies usually breed in manure that has been mixed with plant material such as straw, silage, or hay. Removal of these breeding sites is helpful in reducing the fly population.

When applying insecticides to cattle, particular attention should be given to treating the legs, lower portion of the sides, and belly of the animal. These areas of the body are most often infested. Frequent applications will be necessary because insecticide deposits are easily diluted or washed away.

Insecticide sprays containing 0.05%–1% crotoxyphos, 0.5%–1% Ciovap, or 0.1% pyrethrins plus 1% synergist (piperonyl butoxide) may be applied as wetting sprays (up to 2 quarts [1.9 L]/mature animal). Low volume oil- and water-based sprays containing 2% crotoxyphos, 1% dichlorvos, or 0.75% pyrethrins plus 0.75% synergist may be applied at 1–2 ounces (30–60 ml)/animal/day.

Horn Fly

This common external parasite of dairy cattle breeds in fresh cattle manure. Because of the adult fly's habit of remaining on the animal for extended periods, control is relatively easily accomplished by applying insecticides directly to the animal. In addition to the sprays recommended for stable fly control, crotoxyphos 3% dust, malathion 4% or 5% dust, or methoxychlor 50% wettable powder may be applied to the backline, poll, neck, and upper portions of the sides. Self-treatment dust bags containing 3% crotoxyphos dust or 1% or 5% coumaphos dust, when located where cattle use them daily, will provide excellent control. Backrubbers and facerubbers charged with 1% crotoxyphos, Ciovap, coumaphos, or ronnel also provide an easy method of applying effective insecticides for horn fly control.

Face Fly

These persistent flies are most often found feeding on secretions around the natural openings on the animal's face. Some face flies can also be found on the back and sides of animals; however, they cause the most irritation to the cow when feeding on its face. In addition, they are capable of transmitting the causative organism of pinkeye.

Face fly control is very difficult to obtain because of the persistent population of these pests and the fact that insecticides do not readily adhere to the animal's face. The insecticide that does adhere is easily rubbed off when the animal is grazing in tall grass or it may be washed from the muzzle when the animal drinks water. Very limited control of face flies can be obtained with sprays containing crotoxyphos, Ciovap, pyrethrins, or dichlorvos applied to animals daily as they exit the milking parlor. Also, self-treatment dust bags, backrubbers, and facerubbers containing these compounds and located where cattle have easy access to them will reduce the number of face flies.

Cattle Louse

Lice on dairy cattle are most abundant during the cold months when the hair coat becomes thick and long and the skin is relatively dry of oil. During these months, all growth stages of lice are on the animal.

Penetration of the hair on infested animals is essential if effective lice control is to be obtained. Most of the insecticides recommended for fly control will also control lice; however, those formulations recommended for lice control are usually less concentrated and consequently require greater quantities to provide thorough treatment. Wetting sprays containing 0.05%–1.0% crotoxyphos, 0.25%–1% Ciovap, 0.03% coumaphos, or 0.025% pyrethrins plus 0.25% synergist are effective. The higher concentrations are applied at the rate of 1–2 pints (0.47–0.95 L)/animal, whereas the lower concentrations may be applied up to 1 gal (3.8 L)/mature animal.

Cattle Grub

No insecticidal treatment has been recommended for cattle grub control on lactating dairy cattle. Systemic insecticides may be applied as sprays or pour-ons for treating nonlactating or dry cattle. Systemic sprays contain coumaphos, trichlorfon, or crufomate. Pour-on systemics contain coumaphos, trichlorfon, crufomate, or famphur. It is important to adhere strictly to the required waiting period between application and freshening of dairy animals because of the potential for residues of these compounds occurring in the milk.

House Fly

Cow manure in dairy operations is an excellent breeding ground for house flies. Sanitation is basic in any house fly control program. Insecticides are used to supplement basic sanitation practices. Residual (contact) and bait sprays should be applied to surfaces where flies congregate. Fenthion, crotoxyphos, Ciovap, dimethoate, naled, malathion, methoxychlor, stirofos, Ravap, ronnel, or dichlorvos may be applied as a wet spray to surfaces in the dairy, i.e., floors, manure, etc. These residual sprays should be applied to the point of runoff (1 gal [3.8 L]/500–1000 sq ft). Space sprays (fogs or mists) containing naled, pyrethrins, or dichlorvos may be applied as contact sprays when adult flies are present. Dry sugar baits impregnated with naled or dichlorvos may be scattered on floors and other areas throughout the dairy where flies congregate but away from the animals.

CONTROL OF SWINE PESTS

Swine are usually infested with a limited number of arthropod ectoparasites, principally lice and mange mites. These parasites suck blood and cause irritation and itching resulting in reduced weight gains.

Hog Louse

The hog louse is the most common external parasite of swine. Lice are blood suckers. The tormented hog scratches vigorously on any convenient object, resulting in excoriation, thickening, and soreness of the skin. Infested animals are restless, less profitable, and more susceptible to disease.

A number of insecticides are recommended for use as sprays to control hog lice. Thorough applications are necessary. Most applications should be made to the point of runoff, usually 1–2 qt (0.95–1.9 L)/mature animal. An application of Ciovap 0.025%–0.5%; coumaphos 0.06%; dioxathion 0.15%; lindane, malathion, or methoxychlor 0.05%; ronnel 0.25%; or toxaphene 0.5% is recommended. In addition, dusts containing 3% crotoxyphos, 1% lindane, 4%–5% malathion, 50% methoxychlor, or 5% toxaphene may be applied as an overall body treatment. Ronnel 5% granules applied to swine bedding at the rate of 0.5 lb/100 ft^2 (227 g/9 m^2) of bedding is an effective and easy method of controlling swine lice.

Hog Mange Mite

Although mange is a problem in swine, it is not subject to quarantine and compulsory treatment like mange infestations in cattle, sheep, and goats. Lindane, malathion, and toxaphene are effective miticides for use on swine. Infested animals must be treated thoroughly. It is likely that a second application will be needed after 2–3 weeks. Young animals should not be treated with sprays or dips containing more than 0.03% lindane.

CONTROL OF HORSE PESTS

Horses are infested with a number of mite, tick, and insect parasites. Many of these parasites are found in large numbers and can be annoying and debilitating to the host. In addition, because of the blood-sucking habit of a number of these parasites, disease transmission can occur. To prevent disease transmission, irritation, and even death loss, it is necessary to treat horses with insecticide.

Horse Bot

Horse bot larvae cause considerable irritation to the lining of the stomach and small intestine and may cause colic or other gastric ailments. Systemic insecticides for the control of bots are generally administered to horses in the feed or via a stomach tube. The available drugs that will remove a high percentage of bots from the digestive tract are carbon disulfide, trichlorfon, and dichlorvos. Bot medication is usually administered 30 days after a killing frost and repeated in midwinter. More frequent treatment for bots is advocated if infection is heavy.

Frequent grooming of horses is an important bot preventative measure. Visible eggs which are cemented to the horse's hair by the adult *Gastrophilus* fly are not easily removed by brushing; however, the eggs can be induced to hatch by applying warm water to affected areas of the horse's coat. The hatched larvae can then be washed away.

Ticks, Lice, and Mites

Horses are parasitized by a variety of ticks, lice, and mites that suck blood, burrow in the skin, feed on body fluids, and in general cause irritation to horses. Of special interest is the fact that certain ticks of horses may carry diseases from animal to animal.

Horses have been treated with insecticides for the control of ticks, lice, and mites in several ways. These methods of application include whole-body sprays, dips, and dusts and topical applications to the dermis and ears. Thorough treatment of the infested areas is required. This is especially true when ticks infest the ears or when mites infest localized patches on the animal's skin. Coumaphos, malathion, carbaryl, dioxathion, methoxychlor, and lindane effectively control ticks, lice, and mites. Concentrations of these insecticides should be similar to those recommended for beef cattle.

Flies

Horses are parasitized by a number of blood-sucking (biting) flies that are of particular importance because they not only cause considerable annoyance to horses but also transmit diseases such as equine encephalomyelitis and infectious equine anemia (swamp fever). In addition, horses are annoyed by face flies, which do not bite. Flies normally cause most concern during the warmer months of the year. During these months, control is especially difficult because animals perspire more heavily and frequent grooming removes insecticide deposits. Light applications of recommended insecticides applied frequently usually give the best results. Horses may be treated with insecticides in dips, whole-body sprays, or fine mist sprays; as toxicants or repellents in aerosols; or as sponge-on, smear-on, or wipe-on applications for the control of biting flies. Coumaphos, malathion, carbaryl, dioxathion, methoxychlor, pyrethrins, dichlorvos, or stirofos is recommended for horses. Concentrations should be similar to those recommended for beef cattle.

CONTROL OF SHEEP AND GOAT PESTS

Sheep and goats are parasitized by a variety of arthropods that suck blood, live on skin debris and hair or wool, invade tissues, and even live in the nasal chambers and sinuses. Control of arthropod parasites is essential to the health and productivity of the animals.

Sheep and Goat Lice

Sheep and goats are parasitized by a variety of both biting and blood-sucking lice. Biting lice live on skin debris and may create intense dermal irritation which causes the animals to rub and bite the wool or mohair, resulting in a fleece or coat that becomes matted, ragged, torn, and greatly reduced in value. Sucking lice adversely affect sheep and goats because of blood loss and skin excoriations which are susceptible to bacterial infections. In general, lice cause reduction in the amount and quality of wool or mohair and heavy infestations may lead to reduced weight gains and loss of vitality of the animal.

A number of techniques have been utilized to apply insecticides to the external surfaces of sheep and goats for the control of lice. Insecticidal formulations for this purpose include dips, sprays, pour-ons (spot-ons), and dusts. Crotoxyphos 0.1%–1% spray, Ciovap 0.25%–1% spray, coumaphos 0.06% spray or dip, dioxathion 0.15% spray or dip, lindane 0.05% spray, malathion and methoxychlor 0.05% spray or dip, ronnel 0.25% spray or dip, rotenone 0.25% spray and 0.5%–1% dust, and toxaphene 0.25% dip and 0.5% spray are recommended insecticides for use on sheep and goats. Dioxathion, lindane, malathion, methoxychlor, ronnel, or toxaphene should not be applied to milk goats.

Sheep Ked

The sheep ked is a wingless blood-sucking fly that spends its life in the fleece of sheep and may infest goats pastured with sheep. Sheep keds cause a reduction in market value of leather, decrease carcass weights, lessen wool growth, and, in general, are a prime cause of the sheep skin condition called "cockle." General methods for the control of this parasite are to treat sheep dermally with insecticides.

Dips, sprays, or dusts containing a suitable insecticide applied soon after shearing are generally recommended as practical methods for controlling sheep keds. One thorough treatment will suffice to virtually eradicate the parasite for the season. Coumaphos 0.5% or diazinon 2% may be applied by power dusters. Small numbers of animals may be hand dusted with 4%–5% malathion dust. High-pressure sprays (high-gallonage) should contain 0.125% coumaphos, 0.03% diazinon, 0.5% toxaphene or malathion, 0.25% ronnel, or 0.15% dioxathion. Low-pressure sprays (low-gallonage) should contain 0.06% diazinon or 0.5% ronnel. Dips may also be used and should contain 0.125% dioxathion or 0.25% toxaphene.

Scab and Mange Mites

Both sheep and goats are parasitized by several species of mange and scab mites that burrow and tunnel in the outer layer of skin causing considerable irritation. Animals bite, scratch, and rub the infested areas, often causing the loss of wool or mohair. Scab or mange mites cause a decrease in the quantity and and quality of wool or mohair, loss of weight, and general unthriftiness. Fine wool varieties of sheep usually are more seriously infested than coarse wool varieties.

The most common and effective method of treatment is dipping. Some control can be realized by using high-pressure (high-gallonage) whole-body sprays. It is extremely important that the treatment be thorough and complete to assure that all lesions are treated. Dips containing 0.5% toxaphene or lime sulfur are effective.

Screwworm and Fleeceworm

Both sheep and goats are attacked by

screwworms, larvae of *Cochliomyia (Callitroga) hominivorax,* which invade living tissues. This species has not been completely eradicated in southwestern United States and Mexico. Sheep and sometimes goats are also attacked by other wound-infesting larvae (fleeceworms) that live on the skin of these animals or in their fleece or mohair. Fleeceworms rarely invade living tissue but live in damp wool or mohair that is soiled with urine or feces. The infested area may become irritated, denuded of wool or mohair, and eventually invaded by secondary infections of bacteria.

Sheep and goats may be treated for control of screwworms and fleeceworms by dipping, spraying, or dusting. Dips or sprays (high-pressure and high-gallonage spray) containing 0.125% coumaphos, 0.15% dioxathion, 0.5% ronnel, or 0.03% diazinon may be used. Hand treatments include the use of 5% ronnel smear or ronnel-pressurized livestock spray. Special care should be taken to treat the infested area thoroughly.

Sheep Nose Bot

The larvae of the sheep nose bot fly live in the passages, sinuses, and mucous surfaces of the nasal and sinus chambers of sheep and occasionally goats. During warm weather, female bot flies deposit living larvae onto and in the nostrils of sheep. Infestations of larvae can cause irritation to the nasal chambers. Sheep characteristically try to prevent flies from larvipositing by burying theirs heads in the earth, shaking their heads, and stomping their feet.

Among several systemic insecticides, crufomate and fenthion are effective in ridding sheep of head bots. However, neither of these two compounds nor any other drug is currently approved by the Food and Drug Administration (FDA) for use against nose bots in sheep.

CONTROL OF POULTRY PESTS

Poultry, including chickens, turkeys, and a number of domestic fowl, are infested with a variety of arthropod ectoparasites that live on the skin of the birds, chew skin debris and feathers, and suck blood; this decreases growth rates, lessens egg production, and may lead to debilitation and death of heavily infested birds. It is usually necessary to treat poultry with insecticides to prevent massive buildup of populations of these ectoparasites. In addition, poultry houses are the source of a variety of flies; they are a considerable nuisance and must be controlled.

Specific Pests

LICE

Poultry are infested with a number of species of biting lice that live on the skin and feathers of the host.

FOWL MITES

Fowl mites suck blood and spend their entire life on poultry or in poultry houses. Mites can be controlled by applying insecticides to the birds, litter, or nests.

TURKEY CHIGGER

In certain areas of the southern United States, turkeys on range are infested with chiggers. The chiggers cause downgrading of processed turkey carcasses because it is necessary to trim the lesions they cause. The chiggers can be effectively eliminated with insecticides prior to marketing the turkeys but 3 or 4 weeks are required for healing the lesions.

FOWL TICK

Both male and female ticks (also called bluebugs) feed on chickens at night and subsequently seek shelter in cracks and crevices where the female deposits eggs. Ticks are effectively controlled by treatment of either the birds or the premises.

FLEA

Chickens are infested with the sticktight (southern chicken) flea. These are usually first noticed as black rings around the legs of young birds or black spots on wattles or combs. The blood-sucking action of fleas reduces growth rate and egg production.

RECOMMENDED INSECTICIDES

Several insecticidal dusts are available for the control of poultry pests. Dusts include 0.5% coumaphos, 4% or 5% malathion, 3% stirofos, and 5% carbaryl. These insecticides may be applied directly to the birds or to the litter or in self-treatment dust boxes. Additionally, 50% stirofos may be used on the litter or in self-treatment dust boxes but *should not* be applied directly to the bird. Sprays also may be used. Penetration of the feathers around the vent is essential. Directed sprays should be applied using 100–125 psi. When spraying poultry houses, the spray should be forced into cracks and crevices. Recommended sprays include 0.25% coumaphos, 0.3% naled, and 0.5% malathion, stirofos, and carbaryl. When treating turkey ranges for chigger control, the insecticide should be broadcast on the range in water. Either malathion, 0.05 lb (227 g) active ingredient, or chlorpyrifos, 4 lb (1.8 g) active ingredient, in 100–150 gal of water/acre (380–570 L of water/0.4 ha) gives adequate coverage.

HOUSE FLY

In caged layer operations, the chicken manure found under cages is a favorable location for house fly breeding. Removing manure twice weekly will prevent adult house fly emergence in most cases. When insecticides are needed, one of the following is effective: residual or bait sprays, 1.0% stirofos; contact sprays, 0.3% or 1% naled, 0.1%–1.25% pyrethrins plus 1%–12.5% piperonyl butoxide, or 0.5% dichlorvos; larvicide sprays, 1% dimethoate, 0.3% naled or Supona, 1.0% stirofos or Ravap, or 0.5% dichlorvos; dry sugar baits, naled, trichlorfon, or dichlorvos.

CONTROL OF DOG AND CAT PESTS

Three groups of external parasites commonly infest dogs and cats, i.e., fleas, ticks, and mites. Additionally, chewing and sucking lice are occasional pests of small animals in the United States. All of these pests can incite a dermatitis which is sometimes complicated by secondary bacterial infection and is sometimes allergic in nature (e.g., fleas). Also, tick infestations may lead to tick paralysis. In addition to these direct assaults, external parasites also transmit internal parasites *(Dipylidium caninum* and *Dipetalonema)* to dogs and/or cats.

RECOMMENDED INSECTICIDES

SHAMPOOS

A basic aid to the treatment of dermatological problems associated with ectoparasites of the dog and cat is thorough cleaning of the skin and hair. Some commercial shampoos for this purpose contain insecticides that help to reduce the ectoparasite population of fleas, lice, ticks, and mites. Such shampoos usually contain pyrethrins (Fleaban, Fleatol) or sulfur (Sebbafon) which are safe for both cats and dogs. Additional shampoos for dogs only often contain benzene hexachloride or an organophosphorus insecticide (Dermaton). After shampooing, the animal should be allowed to dry without toweling to provide residual activity. The residual activity of insecticides in shampoos is not as prolonged as that of dips and dusts. Thus shampooing is an initial step toward ectoparasite control and needs to be followed by dipping, dusting, spraying, or the application of a flea collar or tag.

DIPS

Dipping probably offers the best means of ectoparasite control for dogs but is less frequently used for cats. Dipping has the advantage of thorough coverage of the skin and coat with an insecticide. The head can be submerged to allow the insecticide access to parasites, especially ticks and mites, that are located on the ears or around the eyes. The eyes should be protected with a bland ointment before dipping. Where the dog is likely to be picking up additional ticks or fleas from heavily infested premises, repeated dipping at weekly intervals for 4–6 weeks is necessary. Sarcoptic mites of dogs and notoedric mites of cats do not normally leave their host; thus the premises do not provide a source of reinfestation.

Nevertheless, repeated weekly dipping of infested animals is necessary in order to eventually eliminate the mites.

Several insecticides are effectively used in dips to control fleas, ticks, or lice of dogs. Pyrethrins plus piperonyl butoxide is frequently used as are organophosphorus compounds (Dermaton, Co-Nav). Also effective is a concentrated mixture of 16% malathion, 2% lindane, and 0.75% captan which is available commercially as Zema-Dip. Two fluid oz (60 ml) of the concentrate is diluted in 1 gal (3.8 L) of water. Similarly, a commercial preparation, Tick-Rid, that contains 5% diazinon, 69% metholated napthelenes, and 16% ronnel when diluted with water offers an excellent insecticidal dip for dogs. The hydrocarbon chlordane is highly effective against ectoparasites and was once widely used as an insecticidal dip for dogs. It is no longer available for this purpose as a result of Environmental Protection Agency (EPA) restrictions which attempt to limit the increasing levels of insecticidal hydrocarbons in the environment.

Numerous clinical observations substantiate the belief that cats experience more toxicity from insecticides than other species of domestic animals. This susceptibility may be an inherent characteristic of cats but it more likely results from the greater tendency of these animals to lick their fur, with resulting ingestion of toxic levels of applied insecticides. This seems especially true following the wetting of a cat's fur by sprays or dips; thus many of the insecticidal dips used for dogs are not safe for cats. Lime sulfur dips can be safely and effectively used as a 2.5% solution to treat notoedric mange as well as lice, ticks, and fleas. Dipping can be repeated weekly for at least 3 weeks.

DUSTING POWDERS

Heavy infestations of fleas, ticks, and lice on cats are generally controlled by dusting with insecticidal powders. Dusts containing pyrethrins 0.06% plus piperonyl butoxide 0.48%, carbaryl 3% (Sevin), or rotenone 0.75% have FDA approval for use on cats and dogs. Additionally, a higher level of carbaryl dust (5%) is available for dogs.

Dusting powders are especially satisfactory for the control of lice which are generally easily killed and develop little to no resistance to insecticides. Powders also provide satisfactory control of fleas and ticks for short intervals and are especially useful for light or infrequent infestations of these parasites. With heavy infestations of fleas or ticks, dips offer more satisfactory control of these pests on dogs but dusting is most commonly employed for cats.

Most of the insecticides available as powders are also available in aerosol sprays for cats and dogs. Malathion is added to some of these sprays as a treatment for flies, mosquitoes, and gnats. In general, spraying frightens most animals and is less satisfactory than dusting or sponging the animals for flea and tick control.

FLEA AND TICK COLLARS AND TAGS

The introduction of insecticide-impregnated collars and tags since 1965 has provided an effective and widely used method of tick and especially flea control for dogs and cats. Collars fitted to the neck and tags that hang as a medallion from a neck strap are made of a polyvinyl resin from which vapors of the impregnated insecticide are slowly released over 2–3 months. Thus a continuous insecticidal environment exists around the wearer.

The insecticides presently used in collars and tags include dichlorvos, lindane, fospirate, naled, and propoxur. The first four insecticides principally provide control of fleas, while propoxur gives satisfactory tick and flea control. Dichlorvos has been the longest and most extensively used insecticide for the control of fleas. Collars commercially available for dogs and cats contain 8.9% and 4.65% dichlorvos, respectively, and tags for both dogs and cats contain approximately 20% dichlorvos. Lindane-impregnated collars may also be used on both dogs and cats. The range of active ingredient is 0.54%–1.46% and

0.12%–0.61% lindane in dog and cat collars, respectively. Collars containing 15% fospirate or 0.4% propoxur are approved for use only on dogs.

Flea collar dermatitis has occurred around the neck of some dogs and cats while wearing dichlorvos-impregnated collars. Elsea et al. (1970) found that a polyvinyl collar, whether containing an insecticide or not, if tightly fitting is liable to initiate a dermatitis at the site of skin contact and that loosening the collar usually alleviates the dermatitis. Nevertheless, these studies indicate that the insecticide in collars contributes to some extent to the irritation. Thus airing of collars for several days prior to use to dissipate potency, applying collars loosely, and cutting off any excess length help to minimize the chance of a collar-associated dermatitis.

Some controversy has existed in recent years over the concern that the wearing of dichlorvos-impregnated collars may potentiate barbiturate anesthesia if the collars are not removed 2 weeks prior to anesthesia (Smith 1968; Schnelle 1969, 1970). Two well-planned studies, one with purebred beagles (Young et al. 1970) and one using dogs of mixed breeding (Elsea et al. 1970), were designed to study this problem. In both studies, the depth and duration of barbiturate anesthesia were not significantly different between dogs wearing placebo (control) collars and those wearing dichlorvos-impregnated collars up to the time of anesthesia. Return of basic physiologic functions (toe-pinch reflex, jaw muscle tones, palpebral reflex) following anesthesia was as rapid in test as in control dogs. The only hepatic or haematologic differences between test and control dogs in these studies was the temporary depression in plasma and red blood cell cholinesterase levels of test dogs, which is common in animals exposed to organophosphates.

REFERENCES

Elsea, J.; Cloyd, G. D.; Gilbert, D. L.; Perkinson, E.; and Ward, J. W. 1970. Barbiturate anesthesia in dogs wearing collars containing dichlorvos. J Am Vet Med Assoc 157:2068.

Laake, E. W. 1946. DDT for the control of horn fly in Kansas. J Econ Entomol 39:65.

Smith, H. 1968. Safety of chemically impregnated devices questioned. J Am Vet Med Assoc (letter) 153:1264.

Schnelle, G. 1969. Flea collar safety. J Am Vet Assoc (letter) 154:137.

———. 1970. Flea collar safety. J Am Vet Assoc (letter) 156:393.

Young, R.; Johnson, L. G.; and Brown, L. J. 1970. Effects of pentobarbital sodium on the sleeping time of dogs wearing placebo or dichlorvos-containing flea control collars. Vet Med Small Anim Clin 65:609.

SECTION 15

Veterinary Toxicology

CHAPTER 56

INTRODUCTION

ROGER C. HATCH

Everything is poisonous. If dosage and route of entry into the living organism are not restricted, then no substance on earth is completely free of toxic effects. This fact generates problems in any attempt to capsulize medical toxicology for lucid presentation in a pharmacology-toxicology textbook.

One of the problems is to determine where pharmacology leaves off and toxicology begins. The two subjects blend together at all levels of biologic inquiry, i.e., biophysical, biochemical, subcellular, cellular, tissue, organ, and whole organism levels. Traditionally, this problem is resolved by dividing medical toxicology into its two major components: drug toxicology, which deals with deleterious effects of therapeutic agents; and, "just plain toxicology," which deals with deleterious effects of nearly everything else!

Another problem is to decide how many agents to discuss. In pharmacology we are tempted to discuss nearly every drug in a given drug classification because the professional person must have knowledge of more than one drug to use in treatment of a condition. Moreover, new drugs seem to appear faster than older ones become obsolete. In veterinary "nondrug toxicology" we need only discuss those agents our clients are likely to have on the premises. A guiding principle here is the knowledge that if animals have access to chemicals, then those animals may ingest the chemicals out of curiosity. Another guideline is the fact that use of chemicals also predisposes to misuse of chemicals and exposure of animals on the premises. Use of guidelines such as these, tempered with knowledge of the kinds of agents for which veterinary toxicology testing service laboratories are asked to analyze animal tissues, allows compilation of a list of poisons most important to the practicing veterinarian.

This list, which is dissected in the following chapters, is considered by the author to be the heart of veterinary toxicology in North America. The agents are presented in depth suitable to the needs of a professional and in length conforming to space limitations. Information not presented can be found in one of the more encylopedic texts of pharmacology and toxicology mentioned in the reference lists.

Having constructed a list of poisons relevant to veterinary practice, the main problem in presentation is how to classify them. Although poisons vary greatly in chemical form, they also overlap each other in clinical signs, lesions, organ or system affected, and even aspects of mechanism of action. Moreover, there are variations in response to different poisons based on age, sex, species, breed, dosage of poison, duration of intake of poison, and other factors including climate. These overlaps and variations cause most classification schemes to fail. The largest number of poisons may fall into the "miscellaneous" category. Alternately, a given poison can fall into several categories. This confuses students and toxicologists alike.

If poisons are classified according to some combination of major clinical manifestations plus mechanism by which those manifestations are produced, then toxicology becomes more orderly, or at least less disorderly. It is hoped that this type of classification system, imperfect as it is, will help the student grasp the essentials of the entire subject of veterinary toxicology.

TERMS AND DEFINITIONS

Toxicology is the study of poisonous (toxic) substances. This study includes sources of poisons; chemical and physical properties; toxicity (LD50, LD100, MLD); factors that affect toxicity, toxicodynamics, mechanism of action, clinical signs, postmortem findings, and histopathology; diagnosis and differential diagnosis; principles of treatment; and analytical procedures. In addition, toxicology includes study of special effects of toxicants such as carcinogenesis, immunosuppression, behavior development abnormalities, genetic abnormalities, interaction with other agents, teratogenic effects, reproductive effects, and ecological effects. Thus toxicology is every bit as complex as pharmacology and just as fascinating as pharmacology once the student learns where the exciting frontiers of these sciences lie in veterinary practice and in research.

A *poison* is any substance that causes deleterious effects in a living organism. A synonym for poison is *toxicant*. The latter term is often preferable because it sounds more professional and is less accusatory of certain substances such as food additives or pesticides which cause no deleterious effects when properly used. In verbal communication, nearly all practitioners and toxicologists naturally use the term poison or poisoning when sick or dead animals are the focus of attention. In this situation it is pompous to grapple with one's vocabulary to find the most professional and delicate word when everybody involved is thinking "poisoning." To tell a client that his cow ingested a toxicant, is intoxicated, or is suffering a toxicosis might elicit from him a suspicious glance, when any fool can plainly see the cow was just plain poisoned! The point here is not to let one's vocabulary get in the way of communication.

Toxins are special kinds of poisons. They are produced by living organisms and are generally not well defined chemically. Toxins from certain plants are called *phytotoxins*. Toxins from bacteria are called *bacterial toxins* and may be further categorized into *endotoxins* (found within bacterial cells) or *exotoxins* (elaborated from bacterial cells). Toxins from certain fungi are called *mycotoxins*. Toxins from lower animals *(zootoxins)* are likely to have the genus name as prefix (e.g., bufotoxin from the toad *Bufo* sp.). If the zootoxin is transmitted by bite or sting, it is called a *venom*. After a toxin has been thoroughly characterized and its chemical structure determined, it is often renamed according to its chemical structure. Thus there is a host of toxic alkaloids, glycosides, polypeptides, amines, and other substances found in living organisms.

All poisonous substances are not equally toxic. Some substances, such as water, must be administered in large quantity before toxicosis results. Other substances, such as botulinum toxin, need be present only in microgram (μg) quantities in the body in order to kill the animal. Some authors have tried to define degrees of toxicity by assigning arbitrary dosage values corresponding to extremely toxic, highly toxic, moderately toxic, slightly toxic, practically nontoxic, and relatively harmless designations. It is difficult to ask students to learn these arbitrary values because the values do not correspond to actual dosage of toxicants animals receive in the field, and the values do not reflect the duration of exposure or the myriad of factors that modify body response to toxicants. In other words, a "slightly toxic" substance under one set of conditions may be extremely toxic, or under other conditions relatively harmless. Toxicity of compounds, then, exists as a spectrum of dosage values (or LD50 values). This is not to say the toxicity of all substances overlap as conditions change. Certainly, some chemicals are much more dangerous than others. The point is, relative toxicity is best learned during study of individual agents.

Intoxication may be acute or chronic. Acute intoxication results from a relatively large intake of toxicant over a period of minutes, hours, or a few days. Illness is usually severe. Onset of death is rapid, sometimes sudden and unobserved. Chronic intoxication occurs when relatively small quantities of toxicant are ingested or absorbed by the body over a period of several days, weeks, months, or years. Onset of illness is gradual, often appearing first as a decline in feed intake or weight gains. Clinical signs gradually worsen, giving time for medical treatment. Death, therefore, may not occur. In veterinary practice, most poisoning cases are acute; therefore treatment must be swift and sure.

Presence of a chemical in feed or in the body does not necessarily mean the feed is poisonous or the animal is poisoned. There is a *no-effect level* for most toxicants, defined as the largest dosage that will be without deleterious effects over a given period of time. Also, guidelines of permissible residues in food intended for human consumption have been established; some toxicants have a zero tolerance level in food. The chapter on drug residues provides useful detail in these regards.

Presence of a chemical on the premises does not necessarily mean animals were poisoned by that chemical. The veterinarian can determine by inspection whether animals had access to the chemical and whether they ingested any of it. In other words, for each chemical found on the premises, a certain level of probability exists that the chemical caused the toxicosis being investigated. This probability is the basis of the term *hazard,* which refers to the likelihood of poisoning by a particular toxicant. Thus warfarin may be a dangerous chemical to have on the premises, but if the warfarin is kept locked in a room to which animals have no access, then the chemical is not a hazard to livestock.

TOXICODYNAMICS

Toxicodynamics refers to the manner in which a toxicant is absorbed and distributed in the body (including carrier states such as being bound to plasma protein or erythrocytes). The term also refers to interaction between poison molecules and their target substances. The term "receptor" is used with caution in toxicology because most nontherapeutic chemical agents do not have specific antidotes that could be said to act by displacing the poison from some stereoselective active site. Also, little is known about the nature of target substances of most poisons, and in many cases it is not known what biochemical upset is most to blame for death due to poisoning. Nevertheless, it is true that nontherapeutic chemicals do interact with various biochemical systems in a dose-dependent fashion and that clinical signs and lesions are referable to the biochemical systems affected and also are characteristic for the particular poison of interest. Thus toxicodynamics also includes kinetics of interaction between toxicant and cellular or subcellular materials (i.e., membranes and enzymes) and persistence of active (unbound) toxicant in the bloodstream. In addition, toxicodynamics refers to entry and exit of toxic agents from storage sites such as body fat and bone. Finally, toxicodynamics includes the manner and rate of elimination of toxicant from the body.

It can be seen that toxicodynamics is to toxicology what pharmacodynamics is to pharmacology and that there is no great difference between the sojourn of toxicants and of drugs in the body. Thus reference to Section 2 of this book will provide information on principles of toxicodynamics. Information on toxicodynamics of specific poisons will be given in the following chapters whenever the information has special bearing on toxicity, mechanism of action, or treatment.

METABOLISM

Metabolism, or more correctly, metabolic inactivation or activation of poisons, involves the same organs and enzyme systems as does metabolism of drugs. The subject will not be discussed again in these chapters except for specific toxicants for which the metabolic scheme is specially relevant to toxicity, mechanism of action, or treatment.

FACTORS AFFECTING TOXICITY

Factors that affect toxicity of a substance need not be memorized even though toxicology examinations frequently ask the student to list 10 or 20 such factors. It is only biological common sense to recognize that illness or death due to poisoning is the net result of the operation of variables such as route of entry into the bloodstream, physical state of the toxicant (e.g., finely divided particles dissolve more readily than chunks of toxicant and are then absorbed faster by the body), vehicle in which the toxicant is dissolved or suspended (e.g., oils facilitate skin penetration by some agents but may retard intestinal absorption of others), dosage form (solid, liquid, suspension, solution, gas, or vapor), and alkalinity or acidity of the gastrointestinal (GI) tract (in which rate of absorption of a toxicant may be directly related to the proportion of nonionized molecules of toxicant present). Additional variables are dosage of toxicant, duration of exposure, and past experience of the animal with the toxicant (i.e., presence of acute or chronic forms of tolerance or presence of toxicant in storage depots or bound to blood, tissue cells, or plasma protein). Other variables include rate of metabolic inactivation, rate of elimination from the body, presence of other substances or drugs, and relative health and nutritional state of the animal. Still other variables are degree of crowding and other stress factors such as shipping, climate changes, and handling practices. Then, there are the variables of breed, species, age, sex, and reproductive state. Doubtless the student can think of other variables that might influence toxicity of a compound.

When all of these influencing factors are accounted for or controlled in an experiment, a "uniform" group of animals will still manifest some variability in response to a toxicant or any other treatment. This variability (called *individual variation*) exists because each individual animal is biochemically different from every other animal. This is true even of littermates and identical twins. Individual variation contributes to *biological variation,* i.e., variability of response due to operation of unknown and uncontrollable factors in an experimental group. Biological variation, together with animal sampling error and measurement error, can combine with a large number of recognized variables mentioned above to cause great variation in response of animals to toxic substances. The veterinarian who does not realize this fact will become very frustrated when he attempts to learn exactly how toxic an agent is in a given species or exactly what concentration of toxic agent in a tissue or blood sample is of diagnostic significance.

PRINCIPLES AND CONCEPTS

Of various general principles and concepts in toxicology, perhaps the most important is the fact that completely harmless substances do not exist. Given the right route of entry into the body and the right dosage rate, any substance can be poisonous. Animals generally become poisoned by ingesting the toxicant of interest, although toxicants can also penetrate skin and mucous membranes, be inhaled, or be injected by syringe. Once in the body, poisons do not as a rule act at their site of entry but are transported by the bloodstream to their target organs. The blood concentration of a toxicant may or may not correlate with severity of clinical signs. Occasionally, clinical manifestations may be severe but blood concentration of the toxicant very small. This is because the toxicant has been deposited in storage depots and body tissues in which the poison is acting or else the toxicant has already done its damage and been eliminated from the body. On other occasions, clinical manifestations may be mild but blood concentration of toxicant very large. This is because the toxicant binds to serum proteins or blood cells or it has not yet been fully distributed in the body. Also, the animal may be unusually resistant to a large dosage of the toxicant due to the operation of factors already mentioned.

It is fortunate for veterinarians and their clients that animals do not commit suicide or intentionally poison themselves! Thus in veterinary practice, every case of animal poisoning has a human factor of some type. This human factor is usually accidental, or at most a matter of ignorance, unconcern, or misuse or improper storage and handling of chemical agents. Sometimes pets or livestock are poisoned maliciously. Malicious poisoning is a growing problem in urban and suburban areas but is difficult to substantiate because the guilty party is usually not observed in the act of exposing animals to a poison. Moreover, malicious intent is difficult to prove.

Occasionally the veterinarian is asked whether a pasture freshly sprayed with a chemical is safe for grazing. Since it is impossible to guarantee that an unsprayed pasture is absolutely safe for grazing under all conditions, laws of probability would cause the sprayed pasture to be considered less safe than the unsprayed pasture. In practice, the veterinarian should never pronounce a sprayed pasture absolutely safe for grazing. Instead, he should recommend that the pasture not be grazed until one or more hard rains have fallen. Then grazing should begin with only a few animals. Alternately, the forage can be tested to determine spray residue or nitrate accumulation. Then the approximate intake of toxicants can be calculated from knowledge of how much forage each animal is likely to eat. The safety of the pasture can then be estimated, but the estimate should be expressed as such and should not overlook the fact that individual animals differ in response to a given toxicant. Truly, the question: "Is my pasture safe for grazing?" is most difficult to answer in a simple, straightforward way. The client might just as well ask whether he can safely drive his car that day! The veterinarian may wish to avoid the consequences of wrong advice about the sprayed pasture by simply referring the client to the instruction label of the spray product used. Alternately, since the problem is also one of agriculture and husbandry, the county agriculture agent or the local college department of animal science may be consulted by the client.

Sometimes the veterinarian is asked whether a batch of moldy feed, grain, silage, or hay is safe to feed to animals. Farmers have been feeding moldy feed to livestock ever since farming began. Molds are present everywhere, and the molding of feedstuffs cannot always be prevented. Many farmers will assert they never had a problem arise after giving moldy feed to their livestock, although most modern farmers avoid using feed that is badly molded. If the veterinarian says it is safe to give moldy feeds to animals, the statement may be regretted. It is now recognized that many molds can, under the right environmental conditions, produce highly toxic metabolites (mycotoxins). How is the veterinarian to know that the environmental conditions conducive to mycotoxin production did not occur sometime in the previous several months? Moldy feedstuffs should *never* be pronounced absolutely safe for livestock. Likewise, growing plants that are molded should never be called absolutely safe, because mycotoxins or toxic metabolites of the infected plant can be present in the living plant too.

A large batch of moldy feed or grain does pose an economic problem because the farmer may not be able to stand the cost of replacement feed. He may ask whether the moldy feed can be diluted with other feed or fed to some other species. It is not appropriate for a veterinarian to encourage such alternatives. Mycotoxins can be very potent and dilution may not eliminate the hazard. Other species can be more susceptible to the toxins as well as less susceptible.

ARITHMETIC

Arithmetic problems in toxicology, as far as the practicing veterinarian is concerned, are confined mainly to interpretation of toxicologic test reports; estimation of dosage of toxicant an animal has consumed in feed, water, or forage containing the toxicant in known concentration; and calculation of concentration of chemicals per ton of feed based on feed analysis figures. Other calculations such as dosage of antidotes and preparation of solutions, sprays, or dips in given percent concentrations are performed using high school arithmetic.

It is important to remember 1 part per million (ppm) concentration of toxicant in feed, water, or body tissue = 1 mg/kg = 0.0001% = 1 μg/g. Parts per billion (ppb) may have significance in measurement of tissue residues, but such trace concentrations are seldom meaningful in cases of poisoning encountered in veterinary practice. It is also important to remember 1 g of chemical per ton of feed = 1.1 ppm.

In order to estimate dosage of toxicant ingested in feed, the veterinarian must know the concentration of toxicant in the feed (from analysis or by reading the feed label), how much feed the animal has consumed (a variable figure best provided by the client), and weight of the animal in kg. From this information, dosage in mg/kg can be calculated and compared with published LD50, LD100, or MLD values. The main difficulty here is finding such values for the species of interest. Toxicity data are abundant for rats and mice but sometimes hard to find for other species.

TESTING AND TEST REPORTS

Toxicologic testing, from the veterinarian's viewpoint, involves shipment of samples to a testing laboratory, interpreting the laboratory report, and instituting therapeutic or prophylactic measures based on the report. From the viewpoint of the testing laboratory, the operation often involves a combination of problems and obstacles. Samples may be poorly packaged, unidentified, mixed together in one unlabeled container, unrefrigerated, and insufficient for testing. Requested tests may be nonspecific or all-encompassing. The case history may be absent. Samples may be the wrong kind for a given poison, or the samples may be fixed in formalin. There may be too many different kinds of samples or only one kind. The requested test is sometimes not within the current capability of the laboratory. Test results are sometimes expected the following day. The veterinarian is sometimes unable to interpret the significance of test results and he hopes the laboratory can diagnose the case for him.

Details for proper submission of samples should be obtained from the toxicology laboratory. In general, samples should be packaged or bottled unfixed in separate containers properly labeled as to sample and case number. The samples should be frozen (except blood or serum which is refrigerated) and shipped by express. Included with the samples should be a form (provided by most laboratories) on which pertinent information about the case is presented. History, clinical signs, and necropsy findings should be included. The veterinarian must tell the laboratory what poisons to test for because a comprehensive test for all poisons is not possible in most laboratories.

Quantity and kind of sample to send for toxicologic testing vary a little from one laboratory to another. Generally, the preferred samples are feed or suspect bait (100 g), stomach or rumen contents or vomitus (100 g), rumen juice (200 ml), liver (50–100 g), and kidney (50–100 g). With halogenated hydrocarbon toxicants, omental or perirenal fat (100 g) should be sent. Other samples that can be tested are fresh whole blood (10–25 ml, unhemolyzed), blood serum or plasma (10–25 ml), milk (50–100 ml), feces (50 g), urine (50–100 ml), and water (200 ml). Selection of samples should be based on the need to know that potentially toxic concentrations of toxicant are present in the suspect feed or bait (establishing the source of the toxicant), in the GI tract (establishing that the toxicant was ingested), and in at least one body tissue (establishing that the toxicant was absorbed by the body). If the animal is still alive, these needs can be met by obtaining suspect feed or bait; feces or vomitus; and blood, serum, milk, or urine. A toxicant may be found in one tissue and not in others; therefore at least two different tissues or biological fluids should be submitted for testing.

The toxicology testing laboratory will report its findings within a few days or weeks, depending on the complexity of tests required and the work load of the laboratory. Thus the veterinarian should not expect test results prior to instituting treatment.

Test results are generally reported as ppm expressed on the wet weight basis. Most toxicologists will not comment on the significance of test results except in a general way because they have not talked with the client, observed the sick animals, done the necropsies, or seen how the surviving animals responded to antidotal measures. Also, most toxicologists are not clinicians or practicing veterinarians (although some may have been) and should not be expected to perform long distance differential diagnosis.

DIAGNOSIS OF POISONING

Dr. R. W. Hughes (formerly at Purdue University) used to mimic the old-time country practitioner who supposedly impressed his client by expounding, "That old cow must've either been poisoned or got a virus, 'cause she sure didn't respond to antibiotics." Obviously, failure of a sick animal to respond to antibiotic treatment is no way to diagnose poisoning, viral disease, or anything else! In fact, "poisoning" is no diagnosis at all.

The proper way to diagnose poisoning by a specific agent is the same procedure used to diagnose nearly any other condition, i.e., by use of the process of elimination. A *tentative* diagnosis can be made after obtaining a detailed history, observing and examining sick animals, and noting lesions at autopsy. Questioning of the client should be accompanied by an inspection of the premises to locate possible sources of toxic chemicals or plants. Examination of sick animals cannot be done from the other side of a fence. It is important to actually touch the animals; ausculate the lungs, heart, and rumen; determine body temperature; and examine mucous membranes. Sometimes a single petechial hemorrhage in conjunctival, oral, or vulvar mucosa can be a valuable clue to the nature of the illness. Similarly, necropsy of dead animals cannot be approached too gingerly. One literally must get his nose into the carcass to detect small lesions on adrenal glands or to detect the characteristic but fleeting odor of cyanide or ammonia in the rumen.

Diagnosis of a poisoning becomes *presumptive* when more is learned about the illness; when a source of toxicants appears to be accessible to the animals and there is evidence that actual access occurred; and when the history, clinical signs, and lesions are consistent with poisoning by the suspected agent. In addition, response to specific antidotal measures may help to provide the presumptive diagnosis. Lack of response to an antidote does not, however, rule out a given poison as the cause of the illness because no antidote is 100% effective under all conditions, or the antidote may have been given too late.

Diagnosis of poisoning may be *confirmed* by laboratory test results providing the right samples were selected and were preserved and shipped properly. Sometimes testing will indicate little or no toxicant present even though poisoning did occur by that agent. This may be due to sampling error, metabolic disposition of toxicant, or extreme sensitivity of the animal to the toxicant. Thus a negative or very small test figure may obviate a confirmed diagnosis but does not necessarily compromise the tentative and presumptive diagnoses.

Similarly, testing may sometimes indicate a seemingly significant amount of a toxicant, but the animals may not have been poisoned by that toxicant. This is because the toxicant may also be a natural substance in the body (e.g., nitrate, urea, ammonia) or the animal may have been particularly resistant to the toxicant. Thus a test result may appear to contradict the tentative and presumptive diagnoses. A meticulous review of the case may, however, indicate that the initial (sometimes hasty) tentative and presumptive diagnoses were wrong!

Test results, then, are not always as indisputable as their mystique might infer. Diagnosis of poisoning must always be a synthesis of history, clinical signs, lesions, test results, response to therapy, and professional judgment based on knowledge and experience with toxicology problems.

TREATMENT PRINCIPLES

Treatment principles in cases of poisoning are not much different than principles of treatment of any other disease. Treatment is aimed at elimination of toxicant from its region of absorption (i.e., skin, stomach, intestinal tract), reduction in rate of absorption or reabsorption from the enterohepatic-biliary cycle, blockade of the actions of the toxicant using specific or nonspecific antidotes, and hastening metabolic inactivation and excretion of the toxicant. In addition, treatment is given to combat side effects, i.e., excitation, convulsions, fever, dehydration, diarrhea, or other manifestations. The animal is made as comfortable as possible. Antibiotic treatment may be given prophylactically along with a corticosteroid and possibly a tranquilizer to provide sedation and eliminate harmful effects of stress. Multiple vitamins may also be administered. Animals are observed closely until recovery. The source of the toxicant is eliminated. Therapy for specific toxicoses will be mentioned in the following chapters.

FUTURE OF VETERINARY TOXICOLOGY

The future of veterinary toxicology is very bright if one can take any comfort in the knowledge that animals will continue to be poisoned by more and different chemicals. The general field of comparative toxicology is particularly suited to the veterinarian's training and is likely to need many more veterinary toxicologists in the near future. Many employers advertise specifically for D.V.M.-toxicologists. There is a general shortage of veterinary toxicologists and toxicologists with orientation to animals.

This is not to say that veterinary pharmacologists are not needed too. The study of drug actions in animals is perhaps better done by a pharmacologist with veterinary qualifications than by anybody else.

If, however, students are not excited by the prospect of studying how chemical agents make sick animals well, then perhaps they will be interested in studying how chemical agents make well animals sick! Both of these areas of endeavor have held the author's fascination for many years; both areas require constant replenishment with bright new minds.

CHAPTER 57

POISONS CAUSING RESPIRATORY INSUFFICIENCY

ROGER C. HATCH

POISONS HINDERING OXYGEN UPTAKE FROM PULMONARY ALVEOLI

Alpha-Naphthyl Thiourea (ANTU)

USE

ANTU is employed as a rodenticide. According to Berg (1974), it is a specific control for the adult Norway rat, is less toxic to other rat species, is relatively safe for domestic animals, and induces vomiting in dogs. The preceding statement is somewhat misleading. Although the LD50 of ANTU is very small in Norway rats compared with other species (see below), the substance can easily be a hazard to other animals under conditions of use. Moreover, ANTU may not cause immediate vomiting (a lifesaving reflex with many poisons) if the animal has food in its stomach.

SOURCE

Baited dumps and other rat-infested areas or buildings are sources for ANTU poisoning. ANTU is usually mixed in 1%–3% concentration with meat, sausage, bread, dogfood, or other foodstuff. The poisoned baits are placed in scattered locations in rat-infested areas. Ideally, only the rats eat the bait; all leftover baits are retrieved to prevent accidental poisoning of other animals that may frequent the baited area. Unfortunately, these other animals do not know that the baits are intended only for rats. The baits can be sought out by a dog, cat, pig, skunk, or other carnivore and consumed in quantity in spite of elaborate precautions to prevent this. Moreover, poisoned baits are not always retrieved after baiting. The baits then begin to stink and may attract animals that would not otherwise have entered the baited area. This is also true of baits containing any other rodenticide.

PROPERTIES OF TOXICOLOGIC IMPORTANCE.

ANTU powder is gray or blue-gray, insoluble in water, and free of detectable offensive taste or odor. Rats that have survived ANTU poisoning (up to 10% of the exposed population) can apparently sense the poison and will avoid it subsequently for 4 months or longer. Similar avoidance phenomena occur with other rodenticides such as inorganic arsenic, barium carbonate, squill, zinc phophide, and sodium fluoroacetate (Sollmann 1957). ANTU is a potent emetic, being irritant to the gastric mucosa and possibly having a central emetic action also (Clarke and Clarke 1967). Emesis can prevent poisoning in animals that can vomit, particularly if the gastric mucosa is not protected by food. Onset of ANTU poisoning in rats is 12–25 minutes. Thus the rats are apt to die in or near the baited premises before they have time to carry poisoned bait back to their nests. Properties of ANTU, when compared with those of warfarin, have led to near abandonment of ANTU as a rodenticide. Still, ANTU is used often enough to cause occasional incidents of poisoning in dogs or other carnivores. In addition, ANTU could possibly be involved in malicious poisoning of pets or livestock.

TOXICITY

Species differ markedly in susceptibility to ANTU; the rat is most susceptible. Published acute oral LD50 values in mg/kg of body weight are: rat, 2.5–6.25; dog, 10–40; pig, 25–50; horse, 30–80; cat, 75–100; ruminant, more than 50; and fowl, 2500–5000 (Clarke and Clarke 1967; Radeleff 1970). Other factors affecting toxicity of ANTU include age (old dogs are more susceptible than young ones), amount of food in the stomach of animals that can vomit, and particle size of ANTU (50- to 100-μ particles are more toxic than 5-μ particles). In addition, animals can become tolerant to ANTU over a period of time if they eat small quantities. This tolerance takes several weeks to disappear (Sollmann 1957).

TOXICODYNAMIC CONSIDERATIONS

ANTU is rapidly absorbed from the gut and can cause illness in dogs in less than an hour. Death occurs within 6–48 hours, but survival for 12 hours may indicate possible recovery. Thus ANTU is probably metabolized rapidly or quickly eliminated from the body (see Analysis).

MECHANISM OF ACTION

ANTU prevents effective uptake of oxygen from pulmonary alveoli by causing massive pulmonary edema and transudation of fluid into air passages. The transudate is agitated to a froth by the intense respiratory efforts of the animal; this froth further blocks the pulmonary tree. The animal actually drowns in its own body fluids. The cause of the pulmonary edema is an increase in permeability of lung capillaries. Apparently lymph production in the lung exceeds the capacity of the lung to drain lymph.

The cause of this increase in lymph production is not known positively. The heart muscle, cardiac output, and systemic arterial blood pressure are not to blame (Sollmann 1957). It is possible that ANTU causes pulmonary edema by inhibiting a sulfhydryl-containing enzyme (e.g., an enzyme involved in membrane transport of electrolytes or nutrients) because a similar pulmonary edema is produced by the sulfhydryl inhibitors alloxan, iodoacetamide, and oxophenarsine. Moreover, the pulmonary hypertension produced by these agents is inhibited by sulfhydryl-containing agents such as dimercaprol (BAL), 1-thiosorbitol, and cysteine. Furthermore, there seems to be a competitive antagonism of this pulmonary hypertension by nontoxic thiourea derivatives. The degree of competitive inhibition is not directly related to the antithyroid activity of these agents (Sollmann 1957).

Selectivity of ANTU for lung capillaries would seem to exclude inhibition of a presumably ubiquitous sulfhydryl enzyme as the primary mechanism by which the poison causes pulmonary edema. Reasonably, an enzyme involved in membrane transport in lung capillary cells, for example, should also be present in capillary cells in other organs (organs that do not develop massive edema in poisoned animals). This kind of reasoning leads to the suspicion that ANTU may not act in the lung at all but in some area that controls pulmonary fluid dynamics (vasomotion). The brain becomes highly suspect in this regard. Evidence for possible neural involvement in the production of pulmonary edema by ANTU includes pulmonary hypertension, hyperglycemia, hepatic glycogenolysis, and failure of glycogen deposition in the liver. In addition, the pulmonary edema produced by thiosemicarbizide (a related substance) is prevented by sympatholytic drugs, cervical spinal transection, central nervous depressants, and antihistaminic drugs. Pulmonary edema is not seen in heart-lung preparations perfused with thiosemicarbizide (Sollmann 1957).

The seemingly contradictory evidence for pulmonary sulfhydryl enzyme inhibition versus central nervous malfunction in the production of pulmonary edema by ANTU could be resolved not by disregarding either kind of evidence but by postulating that both mechanisms could be correct if we visualize the sulfhydryl enzyme(s) to be located in the central nervous system (CNS) and functioning within a neural system that regulates diameter of arteries and other vessels in the lungs.

Whether ANTU actually acts by any of the basic mechanisms discussed above awaits further research.

CLINICAL SIGNS

Clinical signs consist of vomiting, labored breathing that gets progressively worse, and cyanosis. Auscultation of the chest reveals bubbly respiratory sounds and muffled, rapid heartbeats. Thoracic percussion results in a solid sound rather than the characteristic deep thump of an air-filled cavity. The animal may prefer to sit, in order to breathe better. Developing anoxemia causes weakness and incoordination that progress to prostration. Prostrate animals may cough, snort, gag, and swallow due to fluid leakage into the bronchi. As asphyxiation proceeds, coma ensues and terminal clonic convulsive movements may occur.

LESIONS

At necropsy cyanosis and dark colored arterial blood are observed. The lungs are heavy, very edematous, and the bronchi contain blood-tinged fluid and froth. Fluid is also present in the chest cavity. There is hyperemia of tracheal, bronchial, and gastrointestinal (GI) mucosas and of the liver and kidneys. If terminal convulsions were severe, or if dyspnea was particularly severe, there may be scattered petechial or ecchymotic hemorrhages on the heart or on the surface of the lungs or other organs, but these "agonal" hemorrhages would not form a characteristic pattern of distribution. Histopathological findings are consistent with the gross pathological findings.

DIFFERENTIAL DIAGNOSIS

Fulminating pulmonary edema with pleural effusion and absence of marked signs and lesions of disease in other organs is very characteristic of ANTU poisoning. If serious doubt exists that ANTU was the cause of poisoning, the veterinarian may wish to consider inhaled irritants (e.g., hydrogen sulfide, ammonia, nitrogen oxides, sulfur oxides, ozone, chlorine, or other gases, vapors, fumes, or dusts), organophosphate pesticides, polychlorinated biphenyls, cardioactive glycosides, and other chemicals such as hydrazine, thiourea, alloxan, iodoacetamide, oxophenarsine, thiosemicarbizide, and phenylthiocarbamide. Actual drowning should be ruled out, along with anaphylaxis, snakebite, and peracute infectious diseases.

TREATMENT

There is no reliable way to treat ANTU poisoning. Logic would dictate use of an emetic (apomorphine) or gastric lavage to remove ANTU from the stomach. The animal may be sedated or anesthetized with a barbiturate in order to reduce tissue oxygen demand and to reduce dyspnea and the production of foam in the bronchioles. The animal may be placed on an incline so that fluids can escape from the bronchi. An electrically heated warming board used for this purpose also serves to maintain body temperature. The chest may be compressed periodically to facilitate drainage. Oxygen may be administered under positive pressure. A 10% silicone aerosol may possibly be administered in order to break some of the foam in the bronchi (Hammond 1965).

It is possible that the barbiturate may slow the pulmonary edema process and that administration of a sulfhydryl-containing drug (BAL, cysteine, 1-thiosorbitol, or *n*-amyl mercaptan) may compete successfully with the postulated sulfhydryl enzyme(s) supposedly inhibited by ANTU and so "tie up" some of the available ANTU in a nontoxic complex. Additional steps to reduce the pulmonary edema may be administration of an alpha-adrenolytic agent (to dilate pulmonary vessels and relieve pulmonary arterial hypertension) and administration of an osmotic diuretic (50% glucose or 50% mannitol) to expel some body water and promote redistribution of water from the lungs to other tissues.

Atropine methylnitrate may be given in small doses (0.02–0.05 mg/kg) as premedication for barbiturate anesthesia, but atropine should not be expected to "dry up" the pulmonary edema. Atropine does dry up secretions mediated by muscarinic cholinergic receptors, but it does not mend leaky capillaries or prevent transudation. Atropine sulfate should not be given because it can readily enter the brain and it may prolong barbiturate anesthesia (Hatch 1967, 1972a). Atropine sulfate may also interfere with central nervous mechanisms being manipulated by other drug therapy.

Although the above measures are theoretically sound, none have been proved in clinical practice. No treatment is likely to help an animal that is already comatose.

ANALYSIS

ANTU is most readily detected in vomitus or stomach contents. Tissues and blood may be found to contain ANTU, but all these samples must be obtained within 24 hours of onset of illness. Tissues obtained later than this may no longer contain detectable concentrations of the poison. ANTU is not a normal biochemical constituent of the body; therefore, any concentration of ANTU detected in the tissues is of diagnostic significance if the history, clinical signs, and lesions are compatible with ANTU poisoning.

Hydrogen Sulfide Gas (small concentrations)

Concentrations of hydrogen sulfide gas (H_2S) that do not cause immediate death can cause dyspnea, cyanosis, and severe pulmonary edema. Death is the result of tissue hypoxia due to the pulmonary edema and also to the ability of H_2S to inhibit cellular respiration. Hydrogen sulfide is discussed in detail later in this chapter.

Ammonia Gas and Ammonium Compounds

USE

Ammonia (NH_3) and ammonium compounds are used primarily as fertilizers. Ammonia gas is injected directly into the soil. Ammonium nitrate, carbonate, phosphate, and other salts or combinations thereof may be applied to soils in liquid solutions.

SOURCE

Ammonia gas used as a fertilizer is not likely to be a toxicologic hazard because it is stored in tanks and injected directly into the soil, from which little ammonia escapes. Ammonium compounds used as fertilizers are a toxicologic hazard when livestock have access to residues or pools of solution on a pasture. In this regard, ammonium nitrate is probably the most worrisome of the ammonium compounds, not because of its capability of producing ammonia toxicity, but because it can easily produce nitrite poisoning (see Nitrite, Methylene Blue). Other ammonium compounds are discussed elsewhere (Clarke and Clarke 1967; see also Urea, Chapter 59).

The feeding of nonprotein nitrogen supplements can cause a form of ammonia poisoning in ruminants in which clinical signs relate mainly to the GI tract (see Urea, Chapter 59).

Toxic concentrations of ammonia can be liberated from decomposing manure that is confined to a slurry pit or chicken house. Animals or birds confined to the same area may then inhale the gas. This is the concern in this chapter.

PROPERTIES OF TOXICOLOGIC IMPORTANCE

Ammonia gas has a characteristic sharp, cloying, repellent odor. There is a certain degree of olfactory accommodation to small concentrations of the gas; an ammoniacal odor may be detected by the farmer when he first enters an area but not subsequently. Ammonia is heavier than air and can therefore flow downhill from slurry pits or chicken houses into barns and houses. This is also true of other toxic gases from slurry pits and silos. Ammonia readily associates with hydroxyl ions in fluids coating mucous membranes and is considered to be both irritant and caustic.

TOXICITY

Constant exposure of guinea pigs to a 0.02% concentration of NH_3 in air can cause lesions. Two weeks' exposure of chicks to a 0.2% NH_3 concentration can cause severe keratoconjunctivitis (Clarke and Clarke 1967). Human beings can detect 15 ppm of NH_3 in air and their eyes burn at 25–35 ppm. Corneal damage can occur in broilers at concentrations of 60–75 ppm, but incidence of respiratory disease may increase at a 50 ppm concentration. Egg production is reduced at a NH_3 concentration of 20 ppm (Buck et al. 1973). From these figures it might be inferred that animals and birds should not be chronically exposed to NH_3 concentrations that a human being can detect and that NH_3 concentrations sufficient to burn human eyes are likely to cause ocular and pulmonary lesions in animals and birds.

TOXICODYNAMIC CONSIDERATIONS

Besides being convertible to a strong irritant on mucous membranes, NH_3 can enter the bloodstream via the lungs and cause alkalosis and compensatory acidosis. It can also be carried to tissue cells in which it may inhibit the citric acid cycle (See Urea, Chapter 59).

MECHANISM OF ACTION

Keratoconjunctival lesions, tearing, sniffing, coughing, or sneezing are due to the irritant property of NH_3. Increased susceptibility to respiratory disease may also be due to the direct irritant effects of NH_3 on pulmonary epithelium. Severe pulmonary edema and lung congestion due to inhalation of large concentrations of NH_3 are attributed to an increase in permeability of lung capillaries. This is said to be due to a neurally-mediated adrenergic mechanism (Clarke and Clarke 1967). One wonders if NH_3 might act on a part of the same mechanism affected by ANTU in the production of pulmonary edema. Other aspects of NH_3 toxicosis are discussed under Chlorinated Hydrocarbon Pesticides and Fluoroacetate in Chapter 58 and Urea in Chapter 59.

CLINICAL SIGNS

Clinical signs include reddened mucous membranes, lacrimation, coughing, sneezing, decreased egg production in birds, nasal discharge (serous to mucous), and dyspnea due to pulmonary edema. Fluid sounds may be detected in the lungs. Death may result partly from asphyxia and partly from electrolyte and cellular metabolic actions of NH_3. Terminal signs include cyanosis, possible violent struggling and bellowing (as in urea toxicosis), and clonic convulsions.

LESIONS

Large concentrations of NH_3 produce pulmonary edema and congestion, congestion in other organs, cyanosis, and scattered hemorrhages in various organs, e.g., lung, liver, kidney, and heart.

DIFFERENTIAL DIAGNOSIS

See ANTU. The odor of NH_3 on the premises may make the diagnosis obvious. Slurry pits can also liberate lethal amounts of hydrogen sulfide (rotten egg odor). This gas may mimic or complicate NH_3 toxicosis, or vice versa.

TREATMENT

Removal of the source of NH_3 is essential. Animal quarters must be kept clean and well ventilated. Soothing ointments may be applied to animals' eyes. Antibiotics may prevent secondary bacterial infections. Fresh air is a good treatment for the dyspnea. If pulmonary edema is severe, some of the procedures discussed under ANTU poisoning may be useful. If the animal manifests severe colic, violent behavior, or other signs similiar to urea toxicosis (these can occur in poisoning by inorganic salts of ammonia), then measures discussed under urea toxicosis can be instituted. It must be remembered, however, that poisoning due to inhalation of a large concentration of NH_3 is not exactly the same as poisoning from ingestion of compounds of ammonia.

ANALYSIS

Analyses are not routinely made with inhaled gases.

Nitrogen Oxide Gases

USE

One of the nitrogen oxides, nitrous oxide (N_2O), is used as an inhalant general anesthetic. Its toxic properties have already been discussed. Other gaseous oxides of nitrogen have no medical or agricultural uses but they can be a toxicologic hazard.

SOURCE

Nitrogen dioxide (NO_2, not to be confused with the NO_2^- ion of nitrite toxicosis) and nitrogen tetroxide (N_2O_4) gases are produced by incomplete reduction of nitrates. This can occur during the fermentation process in silos and could possibly occur within the rumen of cattle. Forage rich in nitrate favors the production of toxic nitrogen oxide gases. Forage nitrate concentrations depend on environmental conditions during the growing season, nitrate fertilization or overfertilization, and, possibly, the use of 2,4-D herbicide, which can cause many plants to accumulate nitrate.

PROPERTIES OF TOXICOLOGIC IMPORTANCE

Nitrogen dioxide is reddish brown. Nitrogen tetroxide is colorless. The two gases readily convert to one another, but the relative amount of NO_2 is increased at lower temperatures. The mixture, seen leaking from silos, is yellow or yellowish brown. The gases are about as dense as air and can therefore flow into animal quarters or houses. In water, the gases form nitric acid (HNO_3) and nitric oxide (NO). Alkali converts the gases to nitrates and nitrites. The gas mixture has an irritating, chlorinelike odor. In smogs, sunlight converts nitrogen oxides and oxygen to NO_2 and ozone. Ozone may then contribute to smog-induced lung damage such as emphysema (Freeman et al. 1973; Freeman et al. 1974; Kavet and Brain 1974; Penha and Werthamer 1974; Werthamer et al. 1974).

TOXICITY

Textbooks generally discuss NO_2 toxicosis, but not the toxicity of N_2O_4. In reality, both gases exist in chemical equilibrium and both contribute to the production of toxicosis. Thus published information on toxicity of NO_2 really applies to the mixture NO_2–N_2O_4. In human beings, a condition known as "silo filler's disease" (bronchiolitis obliterans) results from inhalation of NO_2–N_2O_4. The disease is nearly always fatal (Ebert 1967). A concentration of 100 ppm in air is dangerous for human beings, even for a short time; 200 ppm may be fatal (Stecher 1968). Silos may easily contain 100–150 ppm; concentrations as high as 100,000 ppm have been measured in some silos. The safety limit for prolonged exposure in human beings is 1 ppm. A concentration of 8–12 ppm administered to rabbits for 12 weeks killed about one-half the animals. Animals have been acutely exposed to 25 ppm without ill effect, but long exposure to only a few ppm can lower resistance to respiratory infections (Buck et al. 1973). Exposure of swine to 250–310 ppm total nitrogen oxides from a silo for 10 minutes caused death in 21–72 minutes (Giddens et al. 1970).

Animal quarters that develop the irritant odor of NO_2–N_2O_4, or that contain a yellowish haze in the air must *not* be entered, even to save the animals. It makes no sense to commit suicide in order to save some doomed animals! Instead, the quarters should be quickly ventilated (by the fire department if necessary). Then the animals can be removed safely, and all exposed people can be sent to a physician.

Silage from a silo giving off nitrogen oxide gases should not be fed to animals. They may be poisoned even if they are not actually breathing the gas mixture. Also, the silage may be dangerously high in nitrate concentration, which may cause nitrite toxicosis.

TOXICODYNAMIC CONSIDERATIONS

Nitrogen dioxide–nitrogen tetroxide gases can form nitric acid upon contact with mucous membranes. In addition, either the acid or the gases may penetrate pulmonary epithelial cells and cause cellular damage.

MECHANISM OF ACTION

Initial coughing, lacrimation, and reddening of mucous membranes may be due to the direct irritant effect of HNO_3 formed from the gases. These signs may subside quickly if the animal is removed from the contaminated area. However, this will not prevent lung lesions. Progressively severe dyspnea is due to inhibition of oxygen uptake from pulmonary alveoli. The reason for this is probably a combination of severe pulmonary edema, damage to alveolar membranes by the direct (denaturant?) irritant effect of the HNO_3 formed from the gases, peroxidation of pulmonary lipids, plus the presence of lesions. The exact means by which these lung lesions are produced is not known. The delayed onset of pulmonary edema (several hours after exposure) suggests that the edema may be caused by some toxic byproduct of a chemical reaction between NO_2–N_2O_4 (or HNO_3 or NO) and cellular constituents.

CLINICAL SIGNS

In cattle, first coughing, panting or irregular respiration, reddening of mucous membranes, lacrimation, and salivation are observed. Then food and water intake is decreased, leading to wasting and dehydration. Dyspnea becomes severe as pulmonary edema develops. Fluid sounds may be auscultated in the lungs. Fever is also noted. Death of anoxemia occurs 3–25 days after exposure. Cattle exposed to small concentrations of the gases over a period of time may require longer to die. In these animals, signs of respiratory distress are intensified by development of bacterial pneumonia and other lung lesions (Buck et al. 1973). In swine, acute toxicosis is manifested by sneezing, coughing, attempts to avoid the gas, hyperpnea, dyspnea, open-mouth breathing, ataxia, and death in as few as 21 minutes (Giddens et al. 1970).

LESIONS

Pulmonary edema, hyperemia, and hemorrhage occur. Also, fibrin deposits, infarcts, and emphysema may be present in the lungs. Bronchioles may be inflamed and contain granulation tissue. In addition, cyanosis, methemoglobinemia, necrosis of skeletal muscle, and dark red kidneys are manifested. In human beings, the pulmonary lesions resemble miliary tuberculosis in radiographs (Ebert 1967).

DIFFERENTIAL DIAGNOSIS

See ANTU. A history of exposure to nitrogen oxide gases makes the diagnosis clear.

TREATMENT

Fresh air will not save animals exposed to large concentrations of NO_2–N_2O_4. Apparently, once the gases are inhaled, they set off a sequence of events that invariably leads to pulmonary edema and other lesions in both human beings and animals. Some of the treatment measures discussed under ANTU poisoning could be tried, but success would be doubtful.

ANALYSIS

No analyses are made for NO_2–N_2O_4. Methemoglobinemia would not likely be a reliable index of severity of poisoning.

CHRONIC TOXICOSIS

Trace amounts of NO_2 breathed over a long time have caused pulmonary lesions in experimental animals. These lesions and their pathogenesis have been described by Kavet and Brain (1974).

Sulfur Oxide Gases

SOURCE

Sulfur dioxide (SO_2) and sulfur trioxide (SO_3) are industrial atmospheric effluents. Heavy smogs are likely to contain these gases in combination with sulfuric acid and other pollutants.

PROPERTIES OF TOXICOLOGIC IMPORTANCE

The gases are sharply irritant to mucous membranes because of their ability to form sulfurous and sulfuric acids on contact with water. There is no easily describable odor. Rather, the gases evoke coughing, choking, breath holding, and a feeling of suffocation when inhaled.

TOXICITY

The acute lethal concentration of SO_2 for rats is 1000 ppm in air. In human beings, SO_3 causes coughing and choking at a concentration of 1 ppm (Stecher 1968).

Sulfur dioxide concentrations of 500–600 ppm are fatal for cats within 30–60 minutes and 600–800 ppm kill mice, guinea pigs, and dogs in 10 minutes to 6 hours. Continuous exposure of mice and guinea pigs to 65 ppm of SO_2 causes acute gastric distension in 9 days in one-third of the animals. Exposure to 300 ppm causes multiple hemorrhagic gastric ulcers and some gastric perforations in mice and guinea pigs within 3 days (Sollmann 1957). It should be noted that these high concentrations of sulfur oxides are not really breathable and will be avoided by animals if possible.

Animals confined to areas near smelters may become poisoned by SO_2 as may animals confined near power plants or factories burning large amounts of coal, particularly if it is a high-sulfur coal and the antipollution controls are lax. Exposure of grazing animals to a SO_2 concentration of 500 ppm for 1 hour is dangerous. Pigs exposed to SO_2 at 5–40 ppm for 8 hours can become poisoned (Clarke and Clarke 1967).

According to Buck et al. (1973), forage damaged by SO_2 may be safe for dairy cattle, but forage containing 1700–2500 ppm sulfuric acid (formed from SO_2) is toxic for grazing livestock. Moreover, acute exposure to 5 ppm SO_2 causes irritation of mucous membranes, while pulmonary hemorrhage and emphysema can occur within a day after 8 hours' exposure to 40 ppm SO_2. Exposure of pigs to 40 ppm SO_2 for 8 hours can cause pulmonary fibrosis as a delayed effect within 160 days. Sulfuric acid mist (present in smogs) is more toxic than SO_2; a 22 ppm concentration kills guinea pigs after 3 hours' exposure.

TOXICODYNAMIC CONSIDERATIONS

The sulfur oxides form sulfurous and sulfuric acids upon contact with moist mucous membranes.

MECHANISM OF ACTION

The sulfurous and sulfuric acids formed from sulfur oxides are irritant and caustic to mucous membranes. Clinical signs and postmortem findings are attributable to these direct effects. Mucosal irritation also causes reflex bronchoconstriction, which is apparently mediated by vagal efferent nerve fibers. Atropine is reported capable of preventing this bronchoconstriction (Kavet and Brain 1974).

CLINICAL SIGNS

Clinical signs include reddening of mucous membranes, lacrimation, salivation, and coughing. Respiration may first be irregular, then dyspneic if the gas concentration is high enough. Severe dyspnea develops due to bronchoconstriction, pulmonary edema, hemorrhage, and emphysema. Death is due to anoxemia which results from inadequate oxygen uptake from the damaged, edematous lungs.

LESIONS

At necropsy, cyanosis, pulmonary edema, hyperemia, emphysema, atelectasis, and hemorrhages are observed. External mucous membranes may show signs of irritation. Secondary bacterial pneumonia may be seen in animals exposed to sulfur oxides for prolonged periods. Pulmonary fibrosis may exist several months after a single exposure.

DIFFERENTIAL DIAGNOSIS

See ANTU. There is usually a history of exposure to SO_2 and SO_3. Smogs and effluents containing sulfur compounds may also contain toxic amounts of hydrogen sulfide (rotten egg odor). This gas may mimic or complicate sulfur oxide gas toxicosis, or vice versa.

TREATMENT

Animals must be removed from the contaminated area. Fresh air may help prevent severe consequences of small exposures but little can be done for animals exposed to large concentrations of sulfur oxide gases. Some of the measures given for ANTU poisoning may be tried as an alternative to doing nothing.

Other Irritant Gases, Vapors, Fumes, Dusts

A variety of irritants can be inhaled by animals and human beings. Generally these agents cause clinical signs related to respiratory irritation, pulmonary edema or other lung damage, and consequent insufficient uptake of oxygen from pulmonary alveoli.

Chlorine gas in industrial effluents or liberated from bleaching and disinfectant compounds can form hydrochloric acid on contact with the moisture of mucous membranes. Other lung irritants may include ozone, solvent vapors, fumes and smokes from burning rubbish or toxic plants, mold spores, and a variety of chemical dusts (Kilburn 1974).

In all cases treatment is aimed at alleviating the respiratory distress and preventing secondary bacterial infection. The prognosis is always guarded.

Petroleum Products

USE

Petroleum products are used mainly as lubricants and fuels.

SOURCE

Every farm and household has various petroleum distillates in the form of gasoline, kerosene, lubricating oils, and fuel oil or diesel oil. Crude petroleum may be found on rangelands after drilling operations. Oil spills can occur anywhere oil is transported. Sometimes petroleum products are used as vehicles for insecticides or they are applied directly to the skin for control of ectoparasites. Very often, open containers of oil, kerosene, gasoline, or used crankcase oil (drained from tractors) are left on the premises within easy access of curious animals. Cattle in particular are apt to taste materials left in the barnyard and have been known to drink the entire amount of oil drained from a tractor engine.

PROPERTIES OF TOXICOLOGIC IMPORTANCE

Petroleum products are irritant to mucous membranes. Their oily nature makes them difficult to remove from skin and mucous membranes and impossible to remove from internal membranes such as pulmonary epithelium. Additionally, many petroleum products contain toxic materials. Crude petroleum that is rich in low-temperature distillates such as gasoline, kerosene, and naphtha (so-called sweet crude), is more toxic than petroleum containing a lot of sulfur but less of the low-temperature distillates (sour crude). Gasoline containing tetraethyllead (leaded gas) is more dangerous than unleaded gas (see Lead, Chapter 58). Crankcase oil can contain large amounts of lead derived from internal combustion of leaded gasoline. Some oils purchased several years ago and still being used on the premises may contain chlorinated naphthalenes. These chemicals are very stable and can cause bovine hyperkeratosis (see Chlorinated Naphthalenes, Chapter 60).

TOXICITY

The minimum lethal doses of sweet crude oil, sour crude oil, and kerosene are 48, 74, and 56 ml/kg of body weight, respectively, in cattle given these products over a 7-day period (Rowe et al. 1973). The intratracheal LD50 of kerosene is 140 times lower than the oral LD50 (Gerarde 1971). A single dose of 560 ml of tractor oil/100 lb of body weight had no effect in cows, but a dose of 900 ml/100 lb killed cows in 32 days (Clarke and Clarke 1967). It would be expected that intratracheal administration (mimicking aspiration) would result in much smaller lethal doses of tractor oil in cattle.

Animals other than cattle can also be poisoned by petroleum products, but these animals are probably less apt to drink oil or kerosene out of curiosity. Cats and dogs may get doused with oil or gasoline and become poisoned by absorption of toxic hydrocarbons or lead through the skin and by swallowing the oil while attempting to lick it from the fur or hair. Waterfowl that become covered with oil are unable to fly or float properly. They may either drown or ingest lethal amounts of oil in attempting to clean their feathers.

TOXICODYNAMIC CONSIDERATIONS

Once an oily substance is aspirated into the lungs, it cannot be eliminated readily by the body's normal defense mechanisms (coughing, ciliary action).

MECHANISM OF ACTION

Ingestion of irritant oils leads to vomition (or abnormal eructation in ruminants). This leads to aspiration of oily stomach contents into the trachea and bronchi. The irritant oil–stomach contents–microbial mixture then acts as a foreign body in the lungs and causes aspiration pneumonia. Respiratory difficulty develops when the pneumonia renders large areas of lung tissue unable to function in respiratory exchange. Death is due to anoxemia and possible toxemia from bacterial infection of the lungs. If the oil contains a large amount of lead, the animal may die of acute lead poisoning rather than aspiration pneumonia. If gasoline or naphtha is the ingested material, some of the clinical signs may also reflect GI damage, liver and kidney damage, and CNS damage. Ingestion of leaded gasoline is likely to kill by causing acute lead poisoning and damage to vital organs rather than aspiration pneumonia, although both lead poisoning and pneumonia could develop in some animals.

CLINICAL SIGNS

Perhaps the most consistent signs are those of aspiration pneumonia. The animal manifests shivering, apparent incoordination, anorexia, weight loss, fever, abnormal lung sounds, coughing, dyspnea, and possibly oil in the feces. The breath may smell of oil or kerosene. Presence of low-temperature hydrocarbon distillates may cause signs of CNS damage. Lead poisoning signs may coexist with signs of respiratory distress if the oil or gasoline contains lead. Pneumonia becomes more and more severe, and the animal or bird dies of anoxemic anoxia.

LESIONS

At autopsy lesions typical of aspiration pneumonia, possible pleuritis, and possible hydrothorax are observed. Oil may be found in the bronchi. Ulcers or raised yellow-green plaques may exist on the ventral mucosa of the trachea. Oil may be found in the GI tract.

DIFFERENTIAL DIAGNOSIS

Pneumonia due to inhalation of oil should be differentiated from other pneumonias. The history of exposure plus the presence of oil in the lungs or GI tract make the diagnosis obvious enough.

TREATMENT

The condition is treated as any other type of aspiration pneumonia. In early cases the GI tract should be emptied, taking care to keep stomach contents out of the trachea. Oil on the body surfaces must be removed. This is done with soap and water and may require 2 or 3 lathers. Cats and dogs may be restrained with ketamine (cats) or xylazine (dogs) to expedite the bathing and lavage procedures, Emetics should not be used because of the danger of further aspiration of stomach contents. Lead poisoning, if present, is treated as discussed under that topic. The prognosis is considered grave, due to the persistence of oil in the lungs.

ANALYSIS

GI contents can be suspended in water and shaken; petroleum products will float to the surface. Precise identification of the product is not within the analytical capability of most veterinary toxicology testing laboratories because petroleum products are very complex mixtures of hydrocarbons. The toxicologist can likely differentiate gasoline, kerosene, fuel oil, used crankcase oil, motor oil, and petroleum, but so can the practicing veterinarian.

OXYGEN-DISPLACING AGENTS

This is a group of gases which, when inhaled in large concentration, displace oxygen from pulmonary alveoli and cause death primarily by oxygen deprivation. They are not important poisons in veterinary practice but deserve mention when we discuss agents preventing oxygen uptake from the lungs. Some of the agents are helium, nitrogen, nitrous oxide, carbon dioxide, methane, ethylene, propylene, and butylenes. Central nervous depression is produced by some of these compounds at normal nitrous oxide, carbon dioxide) or elevated (nitrogen) atmospheric pressures.

POISONS HINDERING OXYGEN TRANSPORT TO TISSUES

NITRITE, METHYLENE BLUE

USE

Methylene blue is used to treat acute nitrite toxicosis. It is included here because, due to its redox properties, it can also enhance nitrite toxicosis if overdosed (see Treatment).

Organic nitrites are used in human medicine as vasodilator-hypotensive agents. Examples are amyl nitrite and octyl nitrite. Inorganic nitrite is used as a food additive and a machine oil additive. These example uses of nitrites are not usually related to outbreaks of nitrite toxicosis in veterinary practice. Rather, nitrite toxicosis arises from the use or presence of excess nitrates.

Nitrates are widely used in fertilizers; this use may be linked with nitrite toxicosis. Other uses of nitrates that might be of interest include the addition to milk to prevent fermentation in the making of cheese (the whey then contains *nitrite*) and the manufacture of dynamite (containing ammonium nitrate). Some pickling brines may contain nitrate. Organic nitrates (nitroglycerin, "polynitrates") are used as vasodilator-hypotensive agents. Animals may conceivably ingest any of these materials.

SOURCE

Nitrates are naturally present in soils, groundwater, forages, silages, row crops, weeds, animal tissues, and excreta. This ubiquity is due to participation of nitrates in the nitrogen cycle: Atmospheric nitrogen → Microbial fixation as nitrate in soils → Incorporation into plant protein → Incorporation into animal protein → Plant and animal tissue metabolic waste and degradation to nitrate, urea, or ammonia→ Microbial conversion to nitrate, nitrite, or ammonia → Liberation of nitrogen into the atmosphere. Nitrite poisoning problems usually arise when animals consume plants, feed, or water containing excessive amounts of nitrate or when animals ingest nitrate fertilizer spills or residues. Animals may also ingest nitrite directly—whenever feed or water rich in nitrate has undergone microbial decomposition. This can occur in moist haystacks, farm ponds, silages, pig swills, water troughs, and whey. Nitrite is also administered intravenously, along with sodium thiosulfate, in the treatment of cyanide poisoning. Overzealousness in this therapy can result in nitrite toxicosis.

The question arises as to how plants and drinking water happen to contain toxic amounts of nitrate in the first place. The answer is: excess nitrates in soil are accumulated by plants and also washed into wells and ponds. Nitrate concentration by plants is enhanced by rains adequate for uptake; low soil pH; low soil molybdenum, sulfur, or phosphorus; low (55° F) soil temperature; soil aeration; drought; insufficient light to maintain proper activity rate of the enzyme nitrate reductase; and use of 2,4-D or other phenoxyacetic acid herbicides. Nitrate accumulation in ponds and wells is due to increased water runoff from nitrate-rich soils or direct contamination with nitrates and nitrites.

The next question concerns the sources of nitrate that cause elevation of soil and water nitrate concentrations. These include fertilizers; animal wastes; sewage; decaying organic matter; silo juices; industrial effluents; and geologic sources such as limestone, calcites, caves, and playa deposits (Clarke and Clarke 1967; Buck et al. 1973; Ridder and Oehme 1974).

The question: Which plants accumulate nitrate? is purposely left to the end of this discussion of sources of nitrates. Lists of such plants have been published by Kingsbury (1964) and Clarke and Clarke (1967). The lists include many crops and weeds and are so extensive that it seems prudent to warn that *any* plant may be suspected of containing large concentrations of nitrate under the right conditions, particularly if the plant is abundant on the premises where nitrite poisoning has been associated with consumption of the plant. This is a roundabout way of saying, do not exclude a plant as a possible cause of nitrite poisoning just because the plant's name does not appear on a list of "known" nitrate accumulators. Maybe the plant is an "unknown" nitrate accumulator! And do not be too hasty in eliminating a plant on the grounds that it is a poisonous plant and not normally eaten by livestock. Animals will eat poisonous plants if no better forage is available or if the plants have been rendered more succulent by 2,4-D type herbicides. In this case, the resulting toxicosis may be a confusion of clinical signs and lesions of both the plant poison and the excess nitrate.

PROPERTIES OF TOXICOLOGIC IMPORTANCE

Nitrates are water-soluble and therefore easily carried from feedlots, pigpens, silos, and fertilizer residues into the soil and thence into plants, wells, and ponds. Nitrates and nitrites are sources of toxic nitrogen oxide gases in silos (see Nitrogen Oxide Gases). Nitrate fertilizers are salty: this may lead to their ingestion by animals. The most important property of nitrates is their ease of microbial conversion to nitrite.

TOXICITY

In cattle (the usual victims) the acute

oral MLD of nitrate may be as small as 500 mg/kg of body weight, or 2% of the diet Radeleff (1970). The acute oral MLD of sodium nitrate is 650–750 mg/kg and that of sodium nitrite is 150–170 mg/kg (Clarke and Clarke 1967). Potassium nitrate at 1000 mg/kg is lethal. The acute oral LD50 of nitrate is 1000 mg/kg (Buck et al. 1973; Ridder and Oehme 1974).

In sheep a total oral dose of 454 g of nitrate may cause toxicosis under certain circumstances but not under others. The acute oral lethal dose of potassium nitrate is 1000 mg/kg of body weight (Clarke and Clarke 1967). If nitrite (40–60 mg/kg) is administered intraruminally to sheep, death occurs. If the same amount of nitrite is fed to sheep, no adverse effects are seen. Apparently, rumen flora can degrade nitrite fast enough to prevent poisoning in some cases (Sinclair and Jones 1967).

In experimental horses an oral dose of 1000 mg/kg of body weight of potassium nitrate caused illness but not death (Clarke and Clarke 1967). Nitrate has been associated with the death of horses under field conditions, however.

In swine the acute oral MLD of sodium nitrite is 70–75 mg/kg of body weight (Clarke and Clarke 1967). The toxic level is given at 88 mg/kg of body weight of nitrite (Ridder and Oehme 1974). It may be difficult to poison pigs with nitrates because of rapid passage of ingesta through the intestinal tract, rapid conversion of nitrate to ammonia, and because porcine hemoglobin is rather slowly oxidized by nitrite ion. However, pigs can be poisoned if their feed or water contains excess nitrites. Workers at Purdue University (London et al. 1967) were able to make pigs ill with acute oral doses of 12.2–19.8 mg/kg of body weight of potassium nitrite and to kill pigs with doses of 21.3 mg/kg or more. Clinical signs of poisoning were noted when 20% of the hemoglobin was converted to methemoglobin; death occurred (90–150 minutes after dosage) when 76%–82% of the hemoglobin was so converted.

In dogs and rats no effects are produced by feeding nitrate at 2% and 1% of the ration, respectively (Ridder and Oehme 1974).

Chronic poisoning by nitrates apparently does occur on certain farms under certain conditions, but workers have not been able to produce a well-defined chronic nitrate toxicosis experimentally. Ridder and Oehme (1974) hint that they are seeing signs of hypovitaminosis A and E and thyroid deficiency signs in livestock exposed to excess concentrations of nitrate in drinking water, but at this writing those workers have not positively stated they can produce a reproducible chronic nitrate toxicosis. Meanwhile, there is controversy that chronic nitrate toxicosis exists. The controversy is apparently between those who have seen the condition (see Clinical Signs) and those who have not.

The toxicity of nitrates is enhanced by a number of factors: large total intake of nitrate over a short period of time; lack of prior exposure to nitrates; poor feeding practices and nutritional status; poor rumen function; rapid eating by a partly starved animal; hypovitaminosis A; poor quality carbohydrate diet, leading to poor microbial detoxification of nitrite in the rumen; change in ruminal pH; deficiency of molybdenum, copper, or iron in the rumen; prior conversion of nitrate to nitrite in the feed or water (nitrite is 6–10 times as toxic as nitrate); and presence of anemia, methemoglobinemia, or any chemical or disease that can diminish hemoglobin concentration or erythrocyte numbers. Very young animals are more susceptible to nitrite toxicosis than are adult animals. Animals suffering from acute nitrite toxicosis can be killed by the heroic use of methylene blue or by intravenous administration of sodium nitrite in the mistaken belief that the animals are suffering from cyanide poisoning.

TOXICODYNAMIC CONSIDERATIONS

Nitrite formed in the GI tract is rapidly absorbed into the bloodstream. Some nitrate is also absorbed and can probably undergo reduction to nitrite in various tissues. Once in the bloodstream, nitrite ion is in direct contact with arterial walls and erythrocytes. The ion acts directly upon vascular smooth muscle and easily enters the erythrocytes in exchange for chloride ion (Sollmann 1957). Nitrite can also pass the placental barrier and enter fetal erythrocytes. Fetal hemoglobin is especially sensitive to nitrite. In dogs, sheep, and ponies the biological half-life of blood nitrate is 44.7, 4.2, and 4.8 hours, respectively. Comparable figures for nitrite are 0.5, 0.48, and 0.57 hours. Only small amounts of nitrate or nitrite are bound to plasma proteins (Schneider and Yeary 1975).

MECHANISM OF ACTION

Acute poisoning is a result of two actions of nitrite ion. One action is to directly relax smooth muscle, particularly vascular smooth muscle. The exact mechanism of smooth muscle relaxation is not known. The action has been termed "nonspecific" (Nickerson 1970), although Needleman and Johnson (1973) give evidence that the receptor for organic nitrates (which are thought to act the same way as inorganic nitrate and nitrite in causing vasodilation) may involve a sulfhydryl group. In any event, the physiological changes brought about by vasodilatory actions of nitrite ion include pulmonary arterial, central venous, and systemic arterial hypotension and decreased cardiac output. These changes probably contribute to tissue oxygen starvation brought about by the second (and major) action of nitrite ion.

The second action of nitrite ion is to interact with hemoglobin. One molecule of nitrite interacts with 2 molecules of hemoglobin (Sollmann 1957). The interaction is an oxidation of normal ferrous hemoglobin (Fe-II) to ferric hemoglobin (Fe-III), which is called methemoglobin. Simultaneously, nitrite is reduced to nitroso (NO), the role of which in nitrite poisoning is not clear. Given time, methemoglobin will be converted back to ferrous hemoglobin by two reducing enzyme systems in the blood: NAD–dependent diaphorase I and NADP–dependent diaphorase II. Unfortunately, time is not always available. The problem is, methemoglobin cannot carry oxygen. If 20%–40% of the hemoglobin exists as methemoglobin (depending on species and degree of activity of the animal), clinical signs of anoxia develop. These signs worsen as more methemoglobin is formed. Death of anoxemia occurs when 80%–90% of the hemoglobin exists as methemoglobin (but death can occur in active animals with only 50%–60% methemoglobin).

Chronic nitrite poisoning is poorly understood. In well-nourished animals it may not occur at all. Abortions and fetal resorptions attributed to nitrite are probably a result of fetal death due to fetal methemoglobinemia; the fetus is more susceptible than the dam to nitrite and anoxemia. Other actions of subacute concentrations of nitrite may cause signs of hypovitaminosis A and E, thyroid dysfunction, poor conception rate, and decreased weight gains (Ridder and Oehme 1974). Participation of nitrosohemoglobin cannot be ruled out in chronic nitrite poisoning.

CLINICAL SIGNS

Onset of signs is in 0.5–4 hours or more. Initially, there may be frequent urination, vomiting, diarrhea, and colic if the nitrate is concentrated enough. Then prominent signs of respiratory insufficiency such as dyspnea, cyanosis, rapid and weak pulse, and weakness are evident. Exertion causes exacerbation of these signs. There are trembling, collapse, coma, and possible terminal clonic convulsions. Death occurs within a day, sometimes within hours. Signs of chronic poisoning may be those mentioned previously or possibly a several-day onset of respiratory signs due to methemoglobinemia.

LESIONS

Methemoglobin is chocolate brown, so the blood may be some shade of red-brown to brown and the tissues may be stained brown. Brown blood is not apparent in every case of nitrite poisoning, however. Various organs manifest congestion due to the vasodilatory effects of nitrite. Organ surfaces have petechial and ecchymotic hemorrhages. Mucous membranes are cyanotic.

DIFFERENTIAL DIAGNOSIS

Outstanding signs of respiratory distress without evidence of lung lesions should always suggest a defect in oxygen-carrying capacity of the blood or a defect in ability of tissue cells to utilize oxygen. Simple suffocation by oxygen-displacing gases can usually be ruled out on the basis of probability alone. Agents inhibiting oxygen utilization by tissue cells (cyanide, hydrogen sulfide) cause the venous blood to become bright red (from cyanide) or dark (from hydrogen sulfide) not chocolate brown.

Many compounds can cause a defect in oxygen-carrying capacity of the blood. *Carbon monoxide* does this by changing hemoglobin into carboxyhemoglobin, which is bright red, not brown. *Hemolytic agents* do this by rupturing erythrocytes. The hemolysis can be detected by inspection of fresh plasma, not old serum, which may be red due to other factors. Some hemolytic agents are listed under Chlorate. *Hemorrhage inducers* also impair oxygen distribution to tissues. These agents cause evidence of massive hemorrhage and increased capillary permeability. Some of the agents are listed under Warfarin. *Hypotensive agents* can mimic nitrite poisoning, but the history and the absence of brown blood help eliminate these. Such agents cause pooling of blood in the viscera so that insufficient blood is available for participation in oxygen transport. Some of these compounds are given under Zinc Phosphide. Circulatory shock from other causes should also be ruled out. *Cardiac poisons* can hinder oxygen transport by causing weak or abnormal heartbeats; tissues are not perfused with enough oxygenated blood. Again, brown blood is not found in these cases, and cardiac irregularities not found in nitrite poisoning are present. The responsible agents are usually such drugs as digitoxin, magnesium sulfate, or calcium gluconate or plant poisons from Japanese yew, monkshood, oleander, or lily-of-the-valley, but could also be toad poison (bufotoxin) or certain chemicals such as fluoroacetate in herbivores, cobalt, or potassium ion. *Methemoglobin producers other than nitrite or methylene blue* are numerous but are less likely to be the cause of a given case of methemoglobinemia in veterinary practice. The compounds produce brown blood and all of the other acute signs of nitrite poisoning. Some are also hemolytic. The compounds include chlorate, aniline dyes, nitrobenzenes, acetanilid, acetaminophen, acetophenetidin, bromate, iodate, hydroquinone, organic nitrates, beta-napthylamine, *p*-aminophenol, methyl *p*-aminophenol, pyrogallol, toluidine, bismuth subnitrate, sulfonamides, trinitrotoluene, phenylhydrazine, ascorbic acid, ferricyanide ion, copper-II ion, alloxan, and other oxidizing chemicals.

Diagnosis of nitrite poisoning, or nearly any other methemoglobinemia, can be facilitated if one observes a positive response to specific treatment (see below).

TREATMENT

Acute poisoning (methemoglobinemia) is treated by slow intravenous injection of a 1% w/v solution of methylene blue in isotonic saline, given at the rate of 8.8 mg/kg of body weight (cattle, sheep) or 4.4 mg/kg (other species). The dosage can be repeated carefully if clinical response is not satisfactory in 15–30 minutes. In the bloodstream, the oxidizing agent methylene blue is converted by an $NADPH_2$-dependent system to the reducing agent leucomethylene blue. Leucomethylene blue then reduces methemoglobin to hemoglobin, which can carry oxygen. The leucomethylene blue is oxidizd back to methylene blue in this reaction but can be reconverted to leucomethylene blue as long as there is sufficient $NADPH_2$. This $NADPH_2$ system might be saturated if there is too much methylene blue, with the result that excess methylene blue may directly oxidize hemoglobin to more methemoglobin. Sheehy and Way (1974) deny that excess methylene blue can cause methemoglobin formation. Unfortunately, the basis for this denial consists mainly of reports that are subject to methodological criticism (Stossel and Jennings 1966; Rentsch and Wittekind 1967).

Blood transfusion and oxygen therapy

may speed recovery from nitrite poisoning. In mice, combined methylene blue and oxygen give better protection against nitrite lethality than either methylene blue or oxygen alone (Sheehy and Way 1974). Other measures include saline purgatives to empty the GI tract, mineral oil to soothe GI linings, and oral administration of a broad-spectrum antibiotic in 3–5 gal of cold water to inhibit microbial conversion of nitrate to nitrite.

If hypotension is a serious complication, shock therapy can be instituted. The only warning here would be that alpha-adrenergic stimulants (advocated by those who want to "get the pressure up") also increase tissue oxygen demand and alpha-adrenolytic agents (advocated by those who want to "get the tissues perfused") also cause hypotension. These agents should not be used unless adequate hemoglobin is present to carry oxygen to the vital organs. Then they should be used carefully.

Chronic nitrite poisoning is treated by dietary supplementation with vitamins A, D, and E and additional iodized salt and trace minerals, taking care to provide plenty of water at all times in order to avoid "salt poisoning." Too much iodized salt may cause iodism or other complications discussed under Ethylenediamine Dihydroiodide (Chapter 61).

The source of nitrate or nitrite must be found and eliminated or fenced away from livestock.

ANALYSIS

Well water containing more than 10 ppm nitrate is considered hazardous for human beings (Sollmann 1957) although the U.S. Public Health Service Drinking Water Standards set 45 ppm as the maximum safe concentration in rural wells. Drinking water containing 500 ppm (Ridder and Oehme 1974) or more than 1500 ppm (Buck et al. 1973) of nitrate is associated with acute nitrite poisoning in ruminants.

In plants, 0.5% nitrate is the maximum safe concentration; a 1% concentration may be toxic (Radeleff 1970). Kingsbury (1964) says that sublethal nitrate poisoning may occur in livestock that ingest plants containing 0.5%–1.5% potassium nitrate (dry weight basis) and that potassium nitrate concentrations above 1.5% may be lethal. Nitrate concentrations above 1% (dry weight) in forage are believed to cause acute toxicosis (Buck et al. 1973). The author has observed that fresh pasture grass containing elevated concentrations of nitrate may also contain enough nitrite to be of concern in possible instances of chronic nitrite toxicosis. Perhaps the enzyme nitrate reductase is responsible for the presence of nitrite in this situation. In any case, plants should be tested for nitrite as well as nitrate whenever the plants are suspected of causing nitrite poisoning. Nitrates from different sources (water, forage, feed) can be additive in their toxic effects. Application of 2,4-D to plants can cause nitrates to accumulate to 4.5%, expressed as potassium nitrate on a dry weight basis (Clarke and Clarke 1967), or to 10%–30% nitrate (Radeleff 1970).

In hay the safe concentration of potassium nitrate is 1.5%, but hay containing 2% may kill sheep in 6–10 weeks (Clarke and Clarke 1967). In feed, acute nitrite poisoning in ruminants may occur at a nitrate concentration of 0.5% (Ridder and Oehme 1974).

Nitrates and nitrites are normal constituents of the body; their concentrations will vary depending on the type of tissue and its state of preservation. Generally, fresh serum or plasma should not contain more than 25 ppm nitrate or 0.75 ppm nitrite in normal ruminants (Buck et al. 1973).

Fresh unclotted blood can be tested for methemoglobin concentration. Normal human blood contains only 1%–3% methemoglobin. Blood from grazing animals may contain varying amounts of methemoglobin, but nitrite toxicosis is generally associated with methemoglobin concentrations ranging from 20%–40% (sublethal concentration) to 50%–90% (lethal concentration).

The biologic half-life of nitrite is only about 0.5 hour in dogs, sheep, and ponies.

Also, methemoglobin can increase or decrease in concentration due to causes other than nitrite (Schneider and Yeary 1975). Thus blood samples should be obtained and refrigerated promptly.

Interpretation of test results for nitrate, nitrite, or methemoglobin rests on thorough knowledge of history, clinical signs, lesions, and response to therapy.

Carbon Monoxide

Carbon monoxide (CO) is produced during incomplete combustion of any organic material. It is an important component of polluted air in large cities, being discharged into the atmosphere in large amounts in industrial areas and engine exhausts.

Much has been written about CO. It is discussed in detail in textbooks of biochemistry, physiology, pharmacology, and medicine. A recent conference may be of interest (Coburn 1970). Lethal effects of the gas are well known. Animal euthanasia has been performed with it.

Confined animals may be poisoned accidentally by CO emitted from engines, space heaters, or fires. Such instances are not common in veterinary practice, but occasionally a dog or cat has been killed in the back seat of an automobile that was left running, or cattle or chickens were killed in a closed barn in which a tractor was idling.

The veterinarian seldom treats CO poisoning because the animals are usually dead. Carbon monoxide combines with hemoglobin to form carboxyhemoglobin, which cannot carry oxygen. This reaction is very efficient. In addition, carboxyhemoglobin interferes with the release of whatever oxygen is carried by normal hemoglobin (Goldsmith and Landaw 1968). Animals die of anoxemia before treatment can be instituted. In dead animals, the blood is bright red and mucous membranes are a healthy pink because carboxyhemoglobin is bright red and because the animals hyperventilate themselves before death. There are no significant lesions in acute cases. Chronic cases are discussed by Buck et al. (1973).

Should the veterinarian actually see the poisoned animals before they die, treatment consists of oxygen or 5% carbon dioxide (CO_2) in oxygen administered with positive pressure plus blood transfusion. Oxygen is given in order to saturate the plasma water and to displace CO from hemoglobin. The latter is not easy because CO has about 200 times more affinity for hemoglobin than does oxygen. Blood is given in order to provide the animal with some normal hemoglobin. Recovery occurs quickly or not at all depending on severity and duration of toxicosis and mental and physical prowess of the veterinarian.

Chlorate

USE

Chlorate is used as a herbicide and defoliant in the form of a spray or dry salt.

SOURCE

Animals may eat foliage sprayed with sodium or potassium chlorate. Lumps of chlorate spilled on the ground may also be eaten. Chlorate may be misidentified and used in place of salt in mixing feed.

PROPERTIES OF TOXICOLOGIC IMPORTANCE

Chlorate salts look like common sodium chloride. Animals may eat or drink chlorate because of the salty taste. Chlorate is a strong oxidizing agent and can cause fire or explosion if mixed with organic matter, sulfuric acid, sulfur, sulfide, sulfite, hypophosphite, phosphorus, or reduced iron.

TOXICITY

In human beings, toxicosis and possible death result from ingestion of 5 g, more or less, of potassium chlorate (Esplin 1970). In horses, 250 g is lethal (about 500 mg/kg). Calves have ingested 260 and 525 mg/kg of body weight without ill effect, but as little as 60 mg/kg eaten daily for 3 days can cause illness and prostration in cows. Larger dosages cause hemoglobinuria and methemoglobinemia in cows; a dosage of 1000 mg/kg of body weight is lethal (Radeleff 1970; Buck et al. 1973). In sheep, 1.5–2.5 g/kg of body weight is lethal; in poultry a lethal dose is 5 g/kg (Clarke and

Clarke 1967). In dogs the acute oral MLD of sodium chlorate is about 2 g/kg. Lethality may be greater in dogs with chronic interstitial nephritis (Sheahan et al. 1971). Daily dosage of dogs with sodium chlorate (300 or more mg/kg of body weight) caused illness and death. A dog freely drank sufficient 2% sodium chlorate solution to kill himself in 24 hours (Heywood et al. 1972). In rats the oral LD50 is 1.2 g/kg of body weight (Buck et al. 1973).

TOXICODYNAMIC CONSIDERATIONS

Chlorate is rapidly absorbed from the gut. In the body, chlorate does not readily give up its oxygen; therefore it continues to exert its damaging effects as long as it is present. It is excreted largely unchanged.

MECHANISM OF ACTION

Chlorate has a triple mechanism of action. It is directly irritant to the GI tract. It oxidizes hemoglobin to methemoglobin. This action is slower than that of nitrite ion, but chlorate is not inactivated or used up in the process. Rather, it continues to form methemoglobin for as long as it is present in the bloodstream. The exact mechanism by which chlorate interacts with hemoglobin is not known. The third mechanism is to cause severe hemolysis by some action on erythrocyte membranes. The combination of methemoglobinemia and hemolysis drastically reduces the oxygen-carrying capacity of the blood, and the animal dies of anoxemia.

CLINICAL SIGNS

The clinical signs are similar to those of nitrite poisoning, but GI signs (vomiting, staggering, diarrhea, colic) may be predominant in the early stages of toxicosis. There is also hematuria.

LESIONS

The lesions are similar to those caused by nitrite poisoning but more GI damage occurs. Dark, "tarry" blood may be seen exuding from body orifices.

DIFFERENTIAL DIAGNOSIS

Nitrite toxicosis should be ruled out, if possible, by careful inspection of the premises and by a detailed history. The blood will continue to turn brown after death due to chlorate but not in death due to nitrite. Other methemoglobin formers may be considered (see Nitrite, Methylene Blue).

There are a number of other hemolytic agents, including copper, bromate, iodate, arsine gas, dimethyl sulfate, dimethyl sulfoxide (DMSO), dinitrophenol, naphthalene, mephenesin, nitrofurantoin, phenylhydrazine, sulfonamides, *N*-propyl disulfide (in wild onions), gossypol (in cottonseed, cottonseed meal), and certain snake venoms. Hemolytic anemia or hemorrhage due to microorganisms and parasites may also be listed here.

In human beings a large number of drugs may cause a hemolytic crisis if the individual has a genetic deficiency of erythrocyte glucose-6-phosphate dehydrogenase (G-6-PD) or a defect in erythrocyte glutathione synthesis or reduction. Some of these drugs are antimalarials, sulfonamides, methylene blue, vitamin K, acetylsalicylic acid, nitrofurans, quinidine, probenecid, acetanilid, acetophenetidin, and chloramphenicol. Many other drugs can produce hemolysis in G-6-PD-deficient people who also have a viral or bacterial infection. A number of drugs can cause hemolysis due to antigen-antibody interaction (Beutler 1969). These remarks are made here because the human being is not a unique animal in all respects. Animals too could be genetically or immunologically prone to chemically induced hemolysis. Sheep that have as much as 30% of normal erythrocytic glutathione concentrations are not especially sensitive to chemical hemolysis, however (Agar et al. 1975).

Chlorate poisoning should also be differentiated from CO poisoning, poisoning by hemorrhage inducers (listed under Warfarin), poisoning by hypotensive agents (listed under Zinc Phosphide), and poisoning by cardiac poisons (listed under Nitrite; see also cardiac drugs in Index). All of these agents may cause signs of respiratory insufficiency without outstanding lesions of the lungs, but none produces chocolate brown blood.

TREATMENT

See Nitrite, Methylene Blue. Chlorate poisoning is considered more severe and more resistant to therapy than nitrite poisoning. Animals may die in spite of treatment. Some texts just say there is no treatment. It is best, however, to apply rigorous treatment for methemoglobinemia-hemolysis shock rather than just stand there and watch an animal die. Who knows, perhaps the animal will survive!

ANALYSIS

Chlorate is not a normal constituent of the body. Its presence in blood, urine, or tissues (determined analytically) indicates chlorate poisoning if the history, clinical signs, lesions, and response to therapy are consistent with this diagnosis. Chlorate can be found in dog urine for at least 20 hours after ingestion of sodium chlorate (Sheahan et al. 1971).

COPPER

The complex interrelationship between copper (Cu) and other elements such as molybdenum or sulfur has been discussed elsewhere in this text. It is important here, however, to stress and elaborate upon the aspect of this relationship that is most relevant to practical veterinary toxicology, namely copper poisoning.

SOURCE

Animals may ingest excess copper from sprayed foliage, pasture grass (which may accumulate up to 200 ppm of copper from the soil), salt licks, dietary supplements, contaminated forage in the vicinity of mines or smelters, water from copper pipes, copper sulfate spills, ponds treated with copper sulfate for its algicidal property, or foot baths containing copper sulfate. Copper sulfate may also be administered orally as an anthelmintic. Administration of copper sulfate to poultry for control of intestinal parasites causes the elimination of large concentrations of copper in the droppings. Chicken manure is considered to be a good source of nonprotein nitrogen for ruminants and may be mixed with silage or other feed. If the manure contains excessive concentrations of copper, the silage or feed can cause copper poisoning in animals that eat it.

Molybdenum deficiency causes signs and lesions of copper toxicosis. This phenomenon is discussed earlier in this text and also by Buck et al. (1973).

PROPERTIES OF TOXICOLOGIC IMPORTANCE

Copper sulfate is caustic. Acute poisoning is largely due to this property. Copper exists in the +2 (cupric, divalent) and the +1 (cuprous, monovalent) oxidation states. The oxidation state may be relevant to binding of copper ion in the tissues, mechanism of toxic action, and treatment with chelating agents.

TOXICITY

In sheep the toxic oral dose of copper sulfate is 20 mg Cu/kg of body weight (less for lambs). As little as 50 ppm of copper in feed pellets can poison sheep, as can ingestion of 25 mg Cu/day for 8 months. In cattle the toxic oral dose is about 200 mg Cu/kg of body weight.

In calves, as little as 100 ppm of copper in the ration can dangerously elevate the concentration in the liver; a ration containing 250 ppm of copper is fatal. Young (1- to 2-month-old) calves have been killed by subcutaneous injection of 0.8–3.6 mg Cu/kg of body weight given as the cupric-bis-8-hydroxyquinoline-5-7-disulfonic acid salt of tetradiethylamine. Copper glycinate is absorbed more slowly and may not be this toxic for calves.

In pigs, oral intake of 250–400 ppm of copper is toxic eventually and 1000 ppm is considered lethal.

In chicks, 325 ppm of copper in the diet can cause signs of toxicosis, although if the copper is present as copper oxide, chicks may tolerate 500 ppm without ill effect.

For detail see Hammond (1965), Clarke and Clarke (1967), and Mylrea and Byrne (1974).

Age and species are obvious factors that influence copper toxicity. In addition, a number of factors can precipitate copper toxicosis. These include a decrease in the plane of nutrition, fasting, physical activity, stress, molybdenum deficiency, and ingestion of hepatotoxins such as pyrrolizidine alkaloids from ragwort (*Senecio* spp.) (Clarke and Clarke 1967; Buck et al. 1973).

TOXICODYNAMIC CONSIDERATIONS

Copper is absorbed from the intestine and it then enters a carrier state in the blood, being in the erythrocytes as well as the serum. The liver removes most of the copper from the blood, but other soft tissues store some copper too. Copper is apparently tightly bound to high-affinity sites other than essential enzymes in the lysosomes, mitochondria, and nucleus (Lal et al. 1974).

Copper is not stored to the same degree by the liver of all species. The liver excretes copper in the bile, but there is reabsorption in the intestine.

MECHANISM OF ACTION

The exact mechanism by which copper causes various signs and lesions is not known. A sequence of events can be postulated, based on some observed facts and a little reasoning.

It is known that the liver (and other tissues) cannot store an infinite amount of copper. It is also known that it takes large concentrations of copper to inhibit essential metabolic enzymes (Lal et al. 1974). Presumably, enzyme inhibition may occur as cells become saturated with copper.

Inhibition of vital enzymes may lead to liver malfunction, and this may initiate liver necrosis and inability of the liver to excrete and store more copper. As a result, there are increases in serum glutamic oxaloacetic acid transaminase (SGOT), lactic dehydrogenase (LDH), plasma arginase, and plasma bilirubin and a decrease in liver function that may occur days or weeks before death (Clarke and Clarke 1967; Buck et al. 1973). Other evidence of biochemical imbalance in the liver includes ultrastructural changes in mitochondria, endoplasmic reticulum, Golgi apparatus, and sinusoidal borders. Also, the histochemical distribution of acid phosphatase is altered (Smith et al. 1972).

The liver then releases large amounts of copper into the bloodstream. The copper enters erythrocytes and is also excreted in large amount in the urine 24 hours before the oncoming hemolytic crisis (Clarke and Clarke 1967). Erythrocytes cannot release copper easily; therefore the concentration of copper becomes large in the erythrocytes (McCosker 1968).

Inside the erythrocytes, normal ferrous hemoglobin is converted to methemoglobin by the copper-II ion. As much as 35% of the hemoglobin may be so converted in sheep (Clarke and Clarke 1967). This is a significant but not an extraordinary concentration of methemoglobin. Another peculiar thing happens in the erythrocytes just prior to the hemolytic crisis. The erythrocyte concentration of glutathione (GSH) drops suddenly (Thompson and Todd 1974) (see Selenium for a list of functions of GSH).

Copper-II, in oxidizing hemoglobin to methemoglobin, is reduced to copper-I. In the monovalent state, copper would be capable of strong interaction with a sulfhydryl group such as that of GSH (Burger 1973). The author speculates that this interaction, or a similar interaction with enzymes of the GSH system, may be responsible for decreased erythrocyte GSH concentrations. Whether or not this is so, it is possible that the erythrocytes become very fragile (susceptible to lysis by osmotic or chemical forces) *because of* the decrease in GSH concentration.

Just before the hemolytic crisis there is a marked increase in packed cell volume due to a decrease in blood volume, an increase in erythrocyte size, and possibly an increase in number of erythrocytes (McCosker 1968). Also, liver and kidney copper concentration and kidney iron concentration are increased. Cytoplasmic inclusions appear in renal proximal tubules, but kidney function is not yet impaired (Gopinath et al. 1974).

Osmotic changes caused by the increased packed cell volume, coupled with precipitating factors (mentioned under Toxicity), then cause sudden and massive lysis of erythrocytes—the hemolytic crisis. This crisis is said to be absent in nonruminants, perhaps because they store less copper than ruminants (Clarke and Clarke 1967).

During the hemolytic crisis the kidneys fail due to clogging of renal tubules with hemoglobin and to renal tubular and glomerular necrosis brought about by excessive amounts of copper in the kidneys (Gopinath et al. 1974). The hemolytic crisis is accompanied by an elevated plasma creatinine phosphokinase (CPK) concentration indicative of damage to the skeletal muscles. This damage is thought to be due to anoxia and some factor released during hemolysis (Thompson and Todd 1974).

Brain lesions seen in some sheep that die of copper poisoning could be due to increases in blood urea and ammonia concentrations (Hooper 1972), the release of some factor during the hemolytic crisis, or an alteration of glial transport mechanisms by a late-occurring inhibition of adenosine triphosphatase (ATPase) caused by metabolic changes in the glia (Howell et al. 1974).

If animals survive the hemolytic crisis, they may then die of uremia (Thompson and Todd 1974).

The above sequence of events is for so-called chronic copper poisoning, the usual form of copper toxicosis. The term "chronic" is misleading. Ingestion of copper can be chronic but onset of toxicosis is acute, due to sudden release of copper from the liver.

Acute copper poisoning, in which animals ingest a large amount of copper salt at one time, is a type of caustic poisoning (see Chapter 59) and is treated accordingly.

CLINICAL SIGNS

In sheep (the species in which chronic copper poisoning is most prevalent) there is a rather sudden onset of weakness and trembling (exhaustion), anorexia, hemoglobinuria, jaundice, and bloody nasal discharge. Signs of respiratory insufficiency (dyspnea, panting) and shock (tachycardia, weak pulse, cold extremities) are to be expected. Death occurs 1–4 days after onset of clinical signs (Clarke and Clarke 1967; Buck et al. 1973). Other ruminants respond about the same way to chronic ingestion of copper.

In 1- to 2-month-old calves injected subcutaneously with an organocopper complex, there is an abrupt to several-day onset of signs. The calves manifest cessation of nursing, gathering about water sources, dehydration, and harsh haircoat. Fluid sounds in the chest and abdomen and jaundice are also evident. In the final 12–24 hours extreme thirst, depression, and sternal recumbency with head extended occur. Death comes quietly within 1–12 days of the injection of copper (Mylrea and Byrne 1974).

In nonruminants such as swine, the respiratory signs are not prominent because there is no hemolytic crisis. Jaundice is the main clinical sign (Buck et al. 1973).

LESIONS

In sheep, icterus, hemolysis, methemoglobinemia, and congestion of the abomasum and intestines are evident. The liver is enlarged, yellow or orange, and friable. The gall bladder is distended and contains thick greenish bile. The kidneys are enlarged, hemorrhagic, and friable. The spleen is enlarged and dark brown to black (the so-called blackberry jam spleen that is seen in some hemolytic diseases such as anthrax). Excess fluid is present in the body cavities and pericardial sac. The heart may contain hemorrhages and the lungs may be edematous. The musculature may be rather dark due to methemoglobin and metmyoglobin or to muscle necrosis. Microscopically, lesions are consistent with gross findings. Liver cells are vacuolated and necrotic. Kidneys manifest tubular and glomerular necrosis and clogging of tubules with hemoglobin. Tubule cells contain large amounts of cytoplasmic inclusions of hemoglobin. The brain may manifest spongy degeneration and astrocyte damage (Clarke and Clarke 1967; Gopinath et al. 1974; Thompson and Todd 1974).

Lesions in 1- to 2-month-old calves poisoned by an injection of organocopper complex occur in a progression that depends on how long the calf lived. If death occurred early, the lesions consist of liver necrosis and hemorrhage, perirenal edema (see Ethylene Glycol for other causes of perirenal edema), renal tubular necrosis, and congestion of the intestines. After a few days, damage to liver and kidneys may be less severe. Instead, there are hemoglobinuria, excess red-colored fluid in the body cavities and pericardial sac, and kidneys that are pale to brown. After several more days, extensive hemorrhages, jaundice, hemoglobinuria, and fluid in the body cavities occur, with only minor damage to the liver and kidneys (Mylrea and Byrne 1974).

DIFFERENTIAL DIAGNOSIS

Chronic copper poisoning should be suspected in ruminants (especially sheep) that manifest a sudden onset of hemoglobinuria, jaundice, and signs of shock and respiratory distress unaccompanied by many signs of acute abdominal distress or gastroenteritis.

Other conditions that may mimic this toxicosis include hemolytic diseases, hepatitis, and poisoning by other hemolytic agents listed under Chlorate.

TREATMENT

The dithiol-containing chelator BAL (see Inorganic Arsenic, Chapter 59) would be expected to complex monovalent copper and hasten the elimination of copper in the urine of affected animals; however, this chelator does not (Clarke and Clarke 1967). Maybe the chelator is unable to compete successfully with GSH or other sulfhydryl-containing compounds or enzymes in the body. Research with other chelating agents has yet to be done. The chelator ethylenediamine tetraacetate (EDTA) (see Lead, Chapter 58) has a high affinity for divalent copper *in vitro* (Burger 1973) and may be capable of removing divalent copper from the animal body *if* the chelator can "break" the very strong attachment between copper and its binding sites in liver and other tissue cells. However, EDTA apparently does not enter erythrocytes.

In animals that have not yet manifested the hemolytic crisis, it seems logical to administer GSH and its precursors, cysteine, glycine, and glutamine (slowly and in dilute solution intravenously), and thereby prevent the sudden drop in GSH concentration that occurs in erythrocytes just prior to the hemolytic crisis. This therapy has not been tried.

It also seems logical to administer isotonic glucose or sodium chloride to precrisis animals in order to minimize hemoconcentration and thereby decrease the severity of osmotic and chemical influences on fragile erythrocyte membranes. This rationale has not been used either.

In addition, no reports have mentioned the possibility of treating the methemoglobinemia that precedes (and could be an integral part of) the chemical events leading to the hemolytic crisis.

One might also attempt to trap copper in the intestine (with charcoal for instance) and help prevent reabsorption of copper excreted in the bile. This treatment has not been mentioned in the literature.

In fact, despite the prevalence of copper toxicosis, especially in Australia where sheep are an agricultural mainstay, no one has come forth with a specific *treatment* for animals that are developing overt copper toxicosis. Instead, animals in high-risk areas are subjected to *preventative* measures.

To prevent copper toxicosis from becoming overt, sheep are given a daily oral dosage of ammonium molybdate (50–500 mg total) plus sodium sulfate (0.3–1 g total) for 3 weeks. This mixture balances the excess copper ingested and prevents accumulation of too much copper in the liver. The mixture is of no value in treating copper toxicosis once it has developed. Other preventative measures may include application of molybdenum to pastures or the use of mineral mixes containing molybdenum (Buck et al. 1973). Molybdenum cannot be mixed with ruminant feeds according to existing U.S. regulations.

Symptomatic treatment may save some animals poisoned by copper, but the prognosis is grave once the hemolytic crisis occurs.

ANALYSIS

In sheep, copper toxicosis is associated with concentrations greater than 500 ppm in the liver (dry weight basis) (Clarke and Clarke 1967) or 150 ppm wet weight. Kidney tissue contains more than 15 ppm (wet weight); blood contains copper concentrations that are much in excess of the normal level of 0.75–1.35 ppm (Buck et al. 1973).

In adult horses the normal concentration of copper in the liver (mean ± standard deviation) is 31 ± 16 ppm; in the equine fetus the normal value is 317 ± 153 ppm; and in foals the normal value is 219 ± 196 ppm (dry weight basis) (Egan and Murrin 1973).

Calves that died after a single subcutaneous injection of 0.8–3.6 mg Cu as an organic complex had 290–1190 (mean 558) ppm of copper in the liver, 15–97 (mean 39) ppm in the kidneys, and 1–3.2 ppm in the plasma (dry weight basis) (Mylrea and Byrne 1974). Livers of pigs poisoned by copper may contain 750–6000 ppm of copper on a dry weight basis (Clarke and Clarke 1967).

Copper is a normal constituent of tissues and blood. Diagnosis of chronic copper poisoning, therefore, depends on finding markedly elevated concentrations of copper in the tissues of animals having the history, clinical signs, and lesions of copper toxicosis. The diagnosis is generally no problem in high-risk regions or when the feed or forage contains excess copper and deficient molybdenum.

IRON

USE

Iron (Fe) is used as an antianemic agent, primarily in baby pigs.

SOURCE

Sources of iron poisoning are injectable iron-carbohydrate complexes (iron-dextran, -dextrin, -polysaccharide, -sorbitol) or orally administered iron salts such as ferrous sulfate, chloride, glutamate, lactate, fumarate, or carbonate; ferric sulfate, citrate, or ammonium citrate; or ferric phosphate with sodium citrate. Any of these dosage forms can cause systemic reactions.

PROPERTIES OF TOXICOLOGIC IMPORTANCE

Iron is poorly absorbed from the GI tract. Absorption is under physiological control and depends on the amount of iron already in the body. A large oral dosage of iron can damage the process of control of iron absorption. Iron can precipitate phosphate in the GI tract. In intestinal mucosal cells, iron can form ferritin, a sodium-iron-albumin complex containing 6% iron.

TOXICITY

All animals are susceptible to iron poisoning, but the condition is usually seen in baby pigs. A normal dose (100–150 mg total) of injectable iron complex ordinarily has no adverse effect. Occasionally, however, a pig will manifest an anaphylactoidlike reaction and sudden death occurs.

Dietary concentrations of 5000 ppm iron in baby pig rations can cause stunting and rickets.

Iron toxicosis may develop with oral dosages of iron larger than 150 mg/kg of body weight (Buck et al. 1973). Another source (Clarke and Clarke 1967) gives the toxic dose of ferrous sulfate in young pigs as 0.6 mg/kg of body weight, expressed as Fe. This figure is questionable because the usual therapeutic dose of ferrous sulfate in pigs is 0.5–2 g (total dose) (Jones 1965). In the individual animal, iron toxicity varies directly with the amount of iron already in the body.

TOXICODYNAMIC CONSIDERATIONS

Excess iron in the circulation is not readily eliminated because there is no mechanism for excretion. The iron interacts with cellular oxidative enzymes and also forms the vasodepressor substance ferritin.

MECHANISM OF ACTION

Anaphylactoidlike reaction to injectable iron complexes is an adverse reaction characteristic of several kinds of drugs and biologics, particularly when given inadvertently by the intravenous or intraarterial route.

True iron toxicosis is due to: (1) direct damage of GI linings and subsequent absorption of iron in excess of the body's needs; (2) direct damage to the liver (perhaps by inhibition of oxidative enzymes) with resulting metabolic acidosis; (3) hypotension and increased capillary permeability, likely due to direct vasodilatory effects of ferritin; and (4) interference with blood coagulation. These mechanisms interact and underlie the clinical signs of severe shock. Death is due to inadequate perfusion of vital organs with blood.

CLINICAL SIGNS

Acute anaphylactoidlike reaction to injected iron complexes may occur within minutes of injection. The pig may first stagger, then collapse, manifesting cyanosis, dyspnea, and other signs of shock.

Signs of poisoning by orally administered iron salts include emesis, bloody diarrhea, paleness, and weakness and then prostration, cyanosis, and other signs of circulatory collapse.

LESIONS

In anaphylactoidlike reactions, cyanosis, congestion of major organs, and swelling at the site of injection are apparent, with perhaps some agonal hemorrhages on the heart.

Iron toxicosis is characterized by hepatic necrosis, organ congestion, and edema and possibly yellow-brown discoloration of tissues.

DIFFERENTIAL DIAGNOSIS

A history of treatment with iron preparations and the appearance of shocklike signs and lesions make the diagnosis fairly obvious. Other agents capable of causing hemorrhages are listed under Warfarin. Agents capable of causing hypotension (shock) are listed under Zinc Phosphide. Shocklike signs can also be produced by methemoglobin formers and hemolytic agents (see Nitrite and Chlorate). Probability of poisoning by these various chemicals is not great in baby pigs. Similarly, poisoning by other hepatotoxins (see Chapter 59) is of low incidence in baby pigs.

TREATMENT

Anaphylactoid type reactions may be treated with antihistamines, oxygen, and nursing care, but usually the pig does not live long enough for a veterinarian to get to the farm and institute treatment.

Iron toxicosis is a severe illness. Its treatment is hindered by the presence of hepatic necrosis, hemorrhage, and shock. Orally administered milk of magnesia can precipitate iron, as the hydroxide, in the gut. Shock may be treated by standard methods. In dogs, circulating iron can be trapped in a chemical complex (chelated) by slow intravenous drip (0.75 mg/kg of body weight/minute) of desferrioxamine (Desferal), but this agent is hypotensive and neither its dosage nor its efficacy has been established in animals under practical conditions. Experiments in rats show that 2,3-dihydroxybenzoic acid may prove to be a useful iron chelator. It apparently acts on a different "pool" of body iron than desferrioxamine (Graziano et al. 1974). Overall, iron toxicosis carries a grave prognosis.

ANALYSIS

In dogs, serum iron concentration varies normally from 1–2 ppm (fasting state) to 3 or 5.5 ppm at 3–4 hours after an oral dosage of ferrous chloride (Sollmann 1957). Another source (Buck et al. 1973) gives 1–9 ppm as normal plasma iron concentrations in the dog. In children, iron toxicosis can occur at serum iron concentrations of about 5 ppm, but larger concentrations have been measured. Presumably, iron toxicosis in baby pigs could be associated with serum iron concentrations of 5 ppm or greater. Analytical results should be interpreted with care because serum and tissue iron concentrations can vary under different conditions.

WARFARIN AND CONGENERS

USE

Warfarin and its congeners have anticoagulant effects that make them useful as rodenticides. This group of agents includes warfarin (Warfarin), pindone (Pival), diphacinone (Diphacin), chlorophacinone (Drat, Rozol), coumafuryl (Fumarin), naphthylindandione (Radione), coumatetralyl (Endox, Racumin), and other synthetic coumarin and indandione derivatives.

The compounds are generally sold as 0.5% powders for mixing with bait material in a 1:19 proportion (0.025% final concentration). The compounds are also present in prepared baits sold as household and barnyard rat poisons. Some of the compounds are mixed with a sulfonamide that is said to inhibit microbial synthesis of vitamin K in the intestine of the rat. Whether this action actually influences effectiveness of the rodenticide under practical conditions is difficult to ascertain.

A number of coumarin and indandione derivatives are used as oral anticoagulant medications in human medicine.

SOURCE

Animals can be poisoned if they eat residues of the rodenticides that are spilled or stored in insecure places where leakage can occur. Generally, poisoning occurs when animals ingest baits intended for rats and mice. Swine, dogs, and cats can be poisoned by eating rats or mice that were killed by these compounds. Warfarin and related compounds are readily available to the general public. Baits are not always secure from family pets or children. Moreover, warfarin and other rodenticides may be hidden in meat or sausage and purposely left in yards to poison animals maliciously.

PROPERTIES OF TOXICOLOGIC IMPORTANCE

Warfarin and congeners are odorless and tasteless; therefore they do not tend to induce bait shyness in the rodent population. The poisons act slowly, over a period of about a week; therefore the baits are carried to nesting places for consumption by other rodents. Rats and mice may die in inaccessible locations, thus giving the premises a distinctive odor.

TOXICITY

The anticoagulant rodenticides are most toxic when ingested daily over a period of 5–7 days. Single-dose toxicity may be 5–100 times the multiple-dose toxicity, depending on the species. Rats and mice are very susceptible to warfarin. They die after ingesting 1 mg/kg of body weight/day for 5 days (or 50–150 mg/kg in a single dose). Fowl are most resistant to warfarin. Birds would have to eat one-half their body weight of feed containing 0.1 mg warfarin/kg of feed in order to be poisoned. Horses are resistant to warfarin, but toxicity data are lacking. Ruminants can tolerate a lot of warfarin; death occurs at a dosage of 200 mg/kg of body weight/day for 12 days. Dogs and cats are sensitive to warfarin. A single dose of 20–50 mg/kg can kill dogs (5–50 mg/kg for cats). Dogs and cats may die if they ingest 0.2 mg/kg/day for a prolonged period, or 1–5 mg/kg/day for 5–15 days. Pigs are more susceptible to warfarin than are rats and mice. Ingestion of 0.05–0.4 mg/kg of body weight/day for 7 days can kill pigs (Clarke and Clarke 1967; Buck et al. 1973).

Anticoagulant rodenticides other than warfarin have roughly the same overall toxicity as warfarin in the different species.

Factors that may enhance toxicity of anticoagulant rodenticides include: (1) deficiency of vitamin K due to prolonged oral antibiotic or sulfonamide therapy or to high dietary fat concentration; (2) liver abnormalities or other lesions in tissues that produce blood-clotting factors; (3) presence of other poisons that increase capillary permeability or cause clotting disorders, hemorrhage, anemia, hemolysis, or methemoglobinemia; (4) restraint, motor activity, or excitement; (5) presence of drugs (phenylbutazone, oxyphenbutazone, diphenylhydantoin, salicylates) that displace the anticoagulant from plasma albumin; (6) administration of adrenocorticotropic hormone (ACTH), steroids, or thyroxin, which may increase receptor site affinity for the anticoagulant; (7) trauma, including surgical procedures, in animals known to have been exposed to an anticoagulant rodenticide; (8) renal insufficiency; and (9) fever. In addition, newborn animals and extremely debilitated animals are extra sensitive to anticoagulant rodenticides, while lactating animals and animals given lactogenic hormone may be resistant (Levine 1970).

TOXICODYNAMIC CONSIDERATIONS

Anticoagulant rodenticides are absorbed slowly but fairly completely from the intestinal tract. In the bloodstream, these compounds are bound to a large extent to plasma albumin. The bound poison is not active, but the extent of binding can be decreased by other drugs and possibly by substances (e.g., fatty acids) released during stress. ACTH and adrenal steroids, also released during stress, may enhance the interaction between warfarin and its receptor in the liver. Compounds (e.g., barbiturates, chlorinated hydrocarbon pesticides) that are capable of inducing synthesis of enzymes in the liver can cause faster biodegradation of coumarin derivatives.

MECHANISM OF ACTION

Animals poisoned by warfarin and other anticoagulant rodenticides die of tissue hypoxia resulting from massive internal bleeding. The bleeding is due to increased capillary permeability and decreased blood coagulability. The exact cause of capillary damage is not known, but its presence is evidenced by the fact that hemorrhages occur in tissues not subjected to much mechanical stress.

The coagulation defect is the result of decreased blood concentrations of the coagulation proteins factor II (prothrombin), factor VII (proconvertin, autoprothrombin I), factor IX (Christmas factor, autoprothrombin II, PTC), and factor X (Stuart factor, autoprothrombin III). These coagulation factors are decreased because their synthesis in the liver has been inhibited. Biosynthesis of these particular proteins is inhibited because each one requires adequate activity of vitamin K for biosynthesis, but the rodenticide interferes with the normal function of vitamin K. Chemical structural features common to vitamin K and the anticoagulant rodenticides suggest that the rodenticides may act by competing with vitamin K for some receptor site involved in synthesis of the coagulation factors. This proposal is supported by the fact that large doses of vitamin K antagonize the coagulation defect and allow eventual restoration of normal blood concentrations of factors II, VII, IX, and X. Caldwell et al. (1974) suggest that warfarin and congeners may inhibit the cyclic interconversion between active vitamin K and the inactive phylloquinone epoxide by inhibiting the epoxidase step.

It is not known exactly how vitamin K and its antagonists act to alter biosynthesis of clotting proteins. Warfarin does not inhibit incorporation of amino acids into proteins *in vitro,* nor does vitamin K-induced synthesis of clotting factors cease when protein synthesis inhibitors such as dactinomycin or puromycin are present. Thus it is possible that coumarin derivatives hinder *transport* of vitamin K to its site of activity. In other words, the "receptor" for vitamin K and the K-antagonist rodenticides could be some stereoselective molecule that carries vitamin K to its target apoenzymes (Levine 1970). On the other hand, Ciaccio (1971) relates that dactinomycin (an inhibitor of RNA synthesis) does not prevent vitamin K–induced synthesis of clotting factors, but puromycin and other inhibitors of protein synthesis *do* inhibit the K effect. The inference is that vitamin K, and presumably the K antagonists, acts within the pathway of protein synthesis at a point subsequent to transcription of the genetic code to messenger RNA. This appears to be the favored view as to the relative location and general mechanism of vitamin K activity. Current research (Nelsestuen et al. 1974; Suttie et al. 1974) indicates that the molecular function of vitamin K is postribosomal "modification" of factors II, VII, IX, and X. This modification is apparently a sort of final "touch-up" of the protein molecules—probably a carboxylation step that renders the proteins physiologically active. Presumably this carboxylation is catalyzed by enzymes that can be inhibited directly or indirectly by the anticoagulant rodenticides (e.g., by inhibition of vitamin K–dependent carboxylating enzymes or by inhibition of the vitamin K–regenerative epoxidase system). From the evidence at hand, however, the author cannot state categorically that warfarin and congeners do not also inhibit a *transport* molecule for vitamin K.

Very small concentrations of a coumarin derivative can inhibit hepatic mitochondrial electron transport enzymes and uncouple oxidative phosphorylation *in vitro* (Levine 1970). These observations (which can also be made for a number of other drugs and poisons) seem to confuse the issue of molecular mechanism of action of anticoagulant rodenticides, but the confusion can be eased by the realization that such actions, if very pronounced *in vivo,* would have widespread and profound metabolic effects not seen in warfarin poisoning. Still, it is not prudent to completely disregard these observations from experiments done *in vitro.* Rather, we could say that the relevance of the observations with regard to poisoning by anticoagulant rodenticides has not been established.

As to initiation of hemorrhage, the normal movement of muscles (skeletal, smooth, and cardiac) and organs due to body locomotion is sufficient to cause damaged capillaries to leak blood. Hemorrhages may also occur spontaneously in organs of little movement. The bleeding continues because a mechanism of natural hemostasis no longer exists.

Additional details about warfarin and other coumarin type anticoagulants can be found in the review by Deckert (1974), which covers historical aspects, chemistry, modes of action, absorption and metabolic fate, and factors affecting anticoagulant response.

CLINICAL SIGNS

Clinical signs relate to massive hemorrhage and include bloody discharge from body orifices, visible hematomas under skin and around joints, purpura, dyspnea, weakness, and signs of shock. Death may occur unobserved. Abortion may occur in cattle.

LESIONS

Massive hemorrhage is the general characteristic. The hemorrhages can occur in any location in the body. Usually blood is found in the GI tract, thorax, mediastinal space, joint tissues, subcutaneous tissues, abdominal cavity, locomotor muscles, and heart. Hepatic necrosis (due to tissue hypoxia) may be seen in subacute cases. Icterus might be seen if the postmortem interval was long enough for autolysis of blood to occur in mucous membranes.

DIFFERENTIAL DIAGNOSIS

The severity and extent of hemorrhage is often sufficient to rule out other poisons that cause hemorrhage. Some of these poisons are inorganic arsenic, lead, mercury, iron, zinc phosphide, ricin (from castor beans), saponins (from coffee weed), monocrotaline (from crotalaria), gossypol (from cottonseed), a factor in bracken fern that causes hemorrhage in ruminants, a factor in tung oil trees, mold toxins (aflatoxins, rubratoxins, T-2 toxin), and rattlesnake venom. Anaphylactic reactions should be ruled out, as should infectious disease, radiation sickness, thrombocytopenia, and severe trauma.

Widespread hemorrhage is characteristic of *dicoumarol.* This substance may be present in spoiled sweet clover hay. It acts the same way as warfarin and indandiones. Deficiency of vitamin K can also mimic warfarin poisoning, particularly in swine and poultry. A detailed history should enable exclusion of dicoumarol or hypovitaminosis K. Other anticoagulants (e.g., heparin) can cause massive hemorrhage if administered in large dosages intravenously, but this is an unlikely circumstance in veterinary practice. Hypervitaminosis A can cause hemorrhaging due to an antivitamin K action, but vitamin A poisoning is not a likely event in veterinary practice.

TREATMENT

The injured capillaries cannot be mended but other measures may save the animal. Restraint and handling should be minimized. A sedative or tranquilizer may be of assistance in restraint, calming the animal and reducing locomotion, which decreases tissue oxygen demand. Oxygen may be given, but manual "pumping" of the chest is not advisable. Dyspnea may be relieved by thoracentesis. Clotting factors should be provided in the form of a blood transfusion (20 ml/kg, one-half injected quickly). Warfarin should be antagonized with a slow intravenous injection of vitamin K_1. Dogs and cats are given 5 mg/kg of body weight. This dosage is repeated for 2 more days, using the intramuscular route. Larger animals are given 0.5–1 mg/kg and oral vitamin K_1 should be administered daily for 4–6 days. The vitamin will not evoke a sudden dramatic cure; rather, the bleeding tendency will gradually abate as clotting factors begin to be synthesized by the liver. Menadione (vitamin K_3) is not as effective as vitamin K_1 in treatment of warfarin toxicosis. Residual defects such as lameness or central nervous signs due to localized hemorrhages may disappear with the gradual resorption of extravasated blood. Liver damage may be compensated by regeneration of hepatic cells.

ANALYSIS

Warfarin is not a natural constituent of the body, nor are the other anticoagulant rodenticides. Therefore any concentration of these rodenticides in fresh plasma, liver, kidney, or spleen is diagnostically significant if the history, clinical signs, and lesions are consistent with poisoning by these agents. Positive response to vitamin K_1 therapy helps confirm the diagnosis. Lack of response to vitamin K_1 does not necessarily mean that an anticoagulant rodenticide was not the cause of poisoning; therapy may have been instituted too late to save the animal or the amount of rodenticide ingested may have been quite large. Warfarin metabolites may be detected in urine for several days after ingestion of the rodenticide.

ZINC PHOSPHIDE

USE

Zinc phosphide (Zn_3P_2) is a rodenticide used for control of rats, mice, ground squirrels, and prairie dogs. A 2.5% or 5% concentration is mixed with an appropriate bait such as meat, moist grain mash, moist oatmeal, sugar, or bread mash.

SOURCE

Baits intended for rodents may be eaten by other animals or birds. Malicious poisoning with Zn_3P_2 may also occur.

PROPERTIES OF TOXICOLOGIC IMPORTANCE

Zinc phosphide is a gray powder with a carbide (acetylene) odor that is somewhat disagreeable to people but not to rodents. The powder is stable when dry but slowly decomposes in moist air or bait so that its potency is lost in about 2 weeks. Under acid conditions the compound liberates phosphine gas (PH_3), which is spontaneously flammable and also toxic. This reaction is violent with concentrated acids and other oxidizing agents.

TOXICITY

Acute poisoning is due to the PH_3 liberated from Zn_3P_2 in the stomach and upper intestine. In rats the acute oral LD50 of Zn_3P_2 is 45.7 mg/kg of body weight (Stecher 1968). Poultry are killed by 20–30 mg/kg, and other species succumb to 20–40 mg/kg (Clarke and Clarke 1967). Gastric hydrogen chloride (HCl) enhances toxicity of Zn_3P_2. Dogs may eat 300 mg/kg of body weight of Zn_3P_2 on an empty stomach and survive, but the presence of food (or bait) stimulates gastric HCl secretion and greatly increases susceptibility to poisoning (Buck et al. 1973). Chronic poisoning is probably due to both Zn_3P_2 and PH_3.

TOXICODYNAMIC CONSIDERATIONS

Both Zn_3P_2 and PH_3 are absorbed from the GI tract.

MECHANISM OF ACTION

Zinc phosphide is directly irritant to the gut. This action causes emesis, a life-saving response, in animals that can vomit. The irritant action is probably partly to blame for gastroenteritis seen at autopsy.

Acute toxicosis is due to absorbed PH_3, not to zinc or phosphorus. In human beings, symptoms of PH_3 inhalation include dyspnea, syncope, hypotension, bradycardia, nausea and vomiting, convulsions or paralysis, coma, and asphyxia. The postmortem lesions are lung congestion and edema, thrombosis, and hemolysis (Sollmann 1957). These symptoms and lesions, considering their rapidity of onset, are suggestive of some kind of direct damage to membranes of blood vessels and erythrocytes. In animals too, signs and lesions reflect cardiovascular collapse (see below). Death is likely a result of tissue hypoxia.

In animals surviving for more than a few hours, liver and kidney damage may occur. This is thought to be due to direct effects of Zn_3P_2.

CLINICAL SIGNS

Signs of poisoning begin in less than an hour and consist of anorexia, lethargy, vomiting of blood, increase in rate and depth of respiration, stertorous respiration, abdominal pain, bloat (in cattle), ataxia, weakness, prostration, dyspnea, gasping, struggling, convulsions or hyperesthesia, coma, and death in 3–48 hours (Buck et al. 1973).

LESIONS

Pulmonary congestion and edema, pleural effusion and subpleural hemorrhages, congestion of the liver and kidneys, and gastroenteritis (perhaps hemorrhagic), are manifested with possibly the odor of acetylene in the stomach. The liver may manifest yellow mottling in animals that lived long enough for liver damage to occur.

DIFFERENTIAL DIAGNOSIS

The signs and lesions are fairly indicative of Zn_3P_2 poisoning in animals that die suddenly after exposure to that compound. If the history is incomplete and no odor of acetylene is present about the animal, then the veterinarian may need to consider other hypotensive agents. Some of these are acetanilid, anesthetics, salicylates, corrosives, allergens, iron, lead, mercury, nitrites, nitrates, and rattlesnake venom. Hemorrhage inducers (listed under Warfarin) and agents that cause pulmonary edema (listed under ANTU) should be eliminated. Certain cardiac poisons cause hypotension, but these do not cause hemorrhage or lung edema of the magnitude seen in Zn_3P_2 poisoning.

TREATMENT

There is no specific antidote for Zn_3P_2 or PH_3. The GI tract should be emptied as best as possible by lavage with 5% sodium bicarbonate. This solution will also limit acid hydrolysis of Zn_3P_2. Acidosis may be treated with calcium gluconate and one-sixth molar sodium lactate. Respiratory difficulty may be treated as described under ANTU. Shock may be treated by routine measures. Liver and kidney damage may be minimized by intravenous 5% glucose. The prognosis is considered grave. The veterinarian should not feel responsible if the animal dies in spite of rigorous therapy. In most instances the animal is dead before the veterinarian is able to institute therapy.

ANALYSIS

There is no routine test for PH_3, but its presence may be detected by its acetylene odor in stomach contents. Stomach contents, liver, and kidney can be tested for Zn_3P_2. The chemical is not normally in tissues; thus its presence is indicative of poisoning if the history, signs, and lesions are compatible with Zn_3P_2 poisoning.

CADMIUM

Acute and subacute poisoning by cadmium is unlikely in animals because cadmium-coated metals are not widely used in homes and about farms. Salts such as cadmium succinate, chloride, and sebacate may be used as turf fungicides. Cadmium sulfate may be used as a fungicide on the bark of apple and pear trees. These uses do not expose many animals to toxic amounts of cadmium. Moreover, the emetic properties of cadmium protect several species from the poison.

Chronic poisoning by cadmium may be another matter. The metal is an atmospheric, soil, and water pollutant in the vicinity of smelting and other industrial operations. It is conceivable that livestock could be poisoned by chronic ingestion of cadmium, although this has not been a problem to date.

In experimental animals, chronic ingestion of cadmium causes (among other things) a microcytic hypochromic anemia. Associated with the anemia is cardiomegaly, growth retardation, bone marrow hyperplasia, and, presumably, signs of inadequate oxygenation of vital tissues. Renal and hepatic damage may also be present.

The anemia caused by cadmium responds to iron therapy. It is thought that cadmium somehow interferes with iron metabolism (Sansi and Pond 1974; Stowe et al. 1974).

Chelating agents such as BAL and ethylenediamine tetraacetate (EDTA) have not proved useful in treating cadmium toxicosis in animals. In fact, these chelators can increase its renal toxicity.

For a detailed discussion on cadmium, see Friberg et al. (1974) and the reviews cited by Fassett (1975).

T-2 Mold Toxin

SOURCE

Moldy corn is probably the major source of T-2 toxin although other stored feeds that are moldy could also be a source. The mold thought to be the major producer of T-2 is *Fusarium tricinctum,* but T-2 or other toxins may also be isolated from species of *Trichoderma, Gliocladium, Trichothecium, Myrothecium, Nigospora, Epicoccum, Alternaria, Penicillium,* and other *Fusarium* species that may infest corn. These storage fungi are ubiquitous and not all strains are toxigenic. However, if corn is late-maturing or of high moisture content and stored in cribs exposed to temperature changes, then cold temperatures and alternate freezing and thawing can cause normally harmless molds to grow and elaborate lethal toxins. The toxin of interest here is T-2 toxin. It is discussed in detail by Bamburg and Strong (1971).

PROPERTIES OF TOXICOLOGIC IMPORTANCE

T-2 toxin is 3-hydroxy,4,15-diacetoxy-8-(3-methylbutyloxy)-12,13-epoxy-delta^9 trichothecene. This compound is a direct irritant of skin and mucous membranes. It is soluble in organic solvents and fats and can penetrate skin to cause toxicosis and death in laboratory animals. The toxin is resistant to heat and is indefinitely persistent in feed.

TOXICITY

In swine and rats the acute oral LD50 of T-2 toxin is about 4 mg/kg of body weight (Smalley 1973). The LD50 of other trichothecene toxins varies from 1 to 1000 mg/kg or more (Lillehoj 1973). More than one mold or mold toxin may be present in moldy feed, depending on factors such as temperature, humidity, moisture content of the feed, type of feed, duration of incubation, and degree of aerobiasis. Thus moldy feeds from different sources can be expected to vary in toxicity. Toxicity will also vary with the species. T-2 is teratogenic in mice (Stanford et al. 1975).

TOXICODYNAMIC CONSIDERATIONS

T-2 toxin is absorbed in the small intestine of the rat (Smalley 1973).

MECHANISM OF ACTION

The irritant property of T-2 toxin is probably the cause of skin and mucosal lesions. In addition, T-2 toxin causes increased capillary permeability and a clotting defect of the blood (Smalley 1973). The exact mechanism by which the toxin acts may relate to inhibition of protein synthesis (Cundliffe et al. 1974). Death is probably due to tissue hypoxia resulting from shock due to severe hemorrhage and toxemia. Toxemia could be a result of liver and kidney damage and/or absorption of bacterial toxins from the GI tract. Much of this is speculative; other factors may contribute to death of the animal. Animals may take several weeks to die. On the other hand, oral administration of T-2 toxin extract from moldy corn can kill rats in only 3 hours (Smalley 1973).

CLINICAL SIGNS

Clinical signs include anorexia or refusal of the moldy corn, hypothermia, digestive disorders and diarrhea, lack of growth, and general unthriftiness. Later in the course of the disease (perhaps days, weeks, or months) extensive hemorrhages occur in various organs, with possible external evidence of this such as bloody diarrhea, hematuria, and shock. The oral mucosa and skin patches may be sloughing away and bleeding, due to the direct irritant property of T-2 toxin. The clinical signs (Smalley 1973) have been likened to those seen in alimentary toxic aleukia (ATA) in human beings (Pier 1973). ATA is also caused by toxins from species of *Fusarium;* ATA toxins have produced severe hemorrhagic phenomena and sloughing of skin and mucous membranes in various animals (Newberne 1974).

LESIONS

At necropsy, necrosis of skin, oral mucosa, intestines, and liver may be manifested. There may also be extensive hemorrhages in various organs such as the stomach, heart, intestines, lungs, urinary bladder, and kidneys (Pier 1973; Smalley 1973).

DIFFERENTIAL DIAGNOSIS

T-2 toxin poisoning may be difficult to differentiate from poisoning due to other mold toxins such as aflatoxins and rubratoxins. All of these produce nonspecific early signs and all produce hemorrhages and liver and kidney damage. However, mucosal and skin sloughing is characteristic of T-2 type toxins. Laboratory tests will help confirm the diagnosis. While awaiting test results, the veterinarian should attempt to exclude other causes of severe hemorrhaging and organ damage such as infectious disease, corrosives, and hemorrhage-inducing agents (listed under Warfarin). Hepatotoxic agents (Chapter 59) and photosensitizing plants (Chapter 60) might be excluded on the basis of the smaller, more limited amount of hemorrhage produced by these materials, but they should not be overlooked as possible contributing factors to mold toxicosis. Extensive "detective work" and testing may be needed before T-2 toxin, or any other mold toxin, can be incriminated as the sole cause of death in cases of "moldy feed poisoning."

TREATMENT

There is no specific treatment for T-2 or any other mold toxicosis. Animals are treated "symptomatically" for GI signs, skin and oral lesions, toxemia, and shock. The prognosis is grave in severely ill animals. Surviving animals must not be fed any more of the moldy feed, and the premises should be inspected thoroughly for plants or chemicals that could be contributing to mold toxicosis.

ANALYSIS

Corn containing T-2 toxin (about 2 mg/kg dry weight) has caused 20% lethality in dairy cattle fed the corn over a 5-month period (Smalley 1973). Smaller concentrations of toxin would be expected to be dangerous. At present, precise quantitative analysis of T-2 toxin is not available in most laboratories. Extracts of moldy corn produce a characteristic reaction when applied to the skin of laboratory animals if T-2 toxin is present (Chung et al. 1974). *Fusarium tricinctum* or other toxigenic molds may be cultured from the feed, but isolation per se does not mean the feed is toxic, because molds can be isolated from feeds at any time. No analytical method is available at present to detect trichothecene toxins in animal tissues.

Plant Poisons

A number of plant poisons are capable

of causing signs of respiratory insufficiency by hindering in some way the transport of oxygen to tissues.

Hemolytic agents include *N*-propyl disulfide (from wild onion—*Allium* sp.) and gossypol (from cottonseed—*Gossypium* sp.).

Hemorrhage inducers include monocrotaline (from rattlebox—*Crotalaria* sp.), dicoumarol (from spoiled sweet clover hay—*Melilotus* sp.), unidentified principles in bracken fern (*Pteridium* sp.) and male fern (*Dryopteris* sp.) that cause hemorrhage in ruminants, and lobeline (from Indian tobacco—*Lobelia* sp.).

Hypotensive agents include veratramine and related alkaloids from false hellebore (*Veratrum* sp.), death camas (*Zygadenus* sp.), and staggergrass (*Amaianthium* sp.).

Cardiac poisons include aconitine (from monkshood—*Aconitum* sp.), nerioside, oleandroside, and odoroside (from oleander—*Nerium* sp.), and taxine (from Japanese yew—*Taxus* sp.).

Methemoglobin formation by nitrite derived from nitrate in plants should also be mentioned here (see Nitrite).

This list of plant poisons is not exhaustive. Moreover, some plant poisons can cause GI hemorrhages or shocklike signs that are associated more strongly with signs of acute abdominal distress than with respiratory insufficiency. Such poisons (see Chapter 59) are difficult to classify exactly, but they may be considered in differential diagnosis of plant poisoning.

Geographic location will eliminate many plants during differential diagnosis of plant poisoning. All of the poisonous plants do not grow in every region of the country. Even so, one should not be too eager to disregard seemingly "foreign" plants. Animals can eat a plant in one locale and become ill in another, after shipping. Also, prepared feed products shipped from one region may be contaminated by poisonous plants or seeds from the region and cause poisoning in animals in another region in which the plant does not grow.

Kingsbury's (1964) excellent text should be consulted for more detail on plants, plant poisons, and treatment of plant poisoning.

Snake Venoms

Poisonous snakes in North America include rattlesnakes (*Crotalus* sp., *Sistrus* sp.), cottonmouths and copperheads (*Agkistrodon* sp.) of the family Crotalidae, and coral snakes (*Micruoides* sp.) of the family Elapidae.

Coral snakes are very timid and have small mouths and small teeth. They live only in the southern United States and points farther south. Animals are not likely to be bitten by coral snakes. Cottonmouths not only live in more southerly regions, but they prefer swamps and marshes. The probability of animal poisoning by cottonmouths is low, and depends on whether the animal encountered the snake while hunting or wandering in a southern swamp. Rattlesnakes and copperheads are more ubiquitous; animals may encounter these nearly anywhere during the warm months.

Farm animals are relatively large. Therefore venom absorbed from a snakebite is diluted considerably in the body and is less apt to be lethal in horses and cattle than in smaller species. Still, a large rattlesnake can kill a large horse or cow, and smaller snakes can kill sheep or swine. Cats are not frequently bitten because they look where they are going and do not attempt to play with or otherwise antagonize an angry snake. Dogs, on the other hand, do not have keen eyesight and do not look closely at the terrain they are traversing. They may be bitten after blundering into a snake or during attempts to play with, investigate, or follow a snake. Dogs are usually bitten on the head, neck, or shoulder.

All North American poisonous snakes have venoms that cause clinical signs of respiratory insufficiency due to defects produced in transport of oxygen to tissues. Rattlesnakes are the most dangerous in this regard; the large timber rattlers and diamondback rattlers are the most lethal of the rattlesnakes. Rattlesnake venoms cause a combination of massive local swelling and tissue damage, hypotension, bradycardia or tachycardia, localized and generalized hemorrhage, hemoconcentration, hemolysis, pooling of blood in the viscera, and myocardial damage with ventricular arrhythmias. Copperhead venom causes mainly hypotension. Cottonmouth venom causes mainly hypotension and bradycardia. Coral snake venom causes hypotension, bradycardia, direct myocardial depression, and in addition, respiratory difficulty by neuromuscular blockade and by direct depression of skeletal muscle.

TREATMENT

The local area should be isolated by a tourniquet if possible. An ice pack may be applied to reduce swelling and absorption of venom. Incision and suction may not be tolerated by the animal and may do no good if there is much swelling. Massive swelling and tissue necrosis may be prevented by infiltration of the area of the bite with the calcium chelator EDTA, because much of the local damage from Crotalidae venoms is due to venom enzymes that are calcium dependent. Shock should be treated by blood transfusion, oxygen, and glucocorticoid. Specific (if possible) or polyvalent antivenin (1 to several vials depending on clinical response) should be given by intravenous drip. The antivenins are horse sera, so it may be necessary to administer epinephrine, antihistamine, and more corticosteroid to combat possible serum reactions. The animal should be kept warm and quiet. Antibiotics may be given to prevent bacterial infections. Total recovery may take weeks.

The prognosis is always guarded with snakebite cases; severe envenomation, indicated by extensive swelling and coma, carries a grave prognosis.

The student should refer to Brown (1973) for more detail. In veterinary practice, when more detail is needed about snakebites, the information is needed immediately.

POISONS INHIBITING OXYGEN UTILIZATION BY TISSUE CELLS

Hydrogen Sulfide Gas

SOURCE

Hydrogen sulfide (H_2S) (along with NH_3, CO_2, and methane [CH_4]) is liberated from slurry pits, sewage, and other organic matter containing sulfur. It is a toxic product of ingested sulfur and intestinal microbial putrefaction. The gas is found in some smogs and industrial effluents or may be liberated in coal pits, gas wells, or sulfur springs. It is formed in the rumen and intestines from sulfate. The author has seen a case in which a large amount of H_2S was present in bovine rumen contents that also contained a large amount of pyrite sand from a creek bottom. Excess lead was also present in this case, so that the relationship between death of the animal and the presence of pyritic sand and hydrogen sulfide in the rumen was not clear. Pyrites do contain sulfur, which could be liberated as H_2S in acidic rumen contents.

PROPERTIES OF TOXICOLOGIC IMPORTANCE

Hydrogen sulfide gas has an odor of rotten eggs (more correctly, rotten eggs have the odor of H_2S). The gas is flammable; it is perceptible in air at a concentration of 0.002 ppm. Lethal concentrations do not smell much stronger than sublethal concentrations because the gas paralyzes the olfactory nerves. The gas is irritating to mucous membranes, partly because of its own acidity in solution and partly because of formation of sodium sulfide on contact with moist tissues. Hydrogen sulfide can penetrate the skin and cause toxicosis in people exposed to large concentrations over a long period (Sollmann 1957). The gas reacts with silver, iron, lead, and other metals to form black or dark colored compounds in the GI tract and maybe in tissues as well.

TOXICITY

The speed of onset of acute H_2S poisoning and the potency of H_2S are almost the same as for cyanide gas; H_2S is no less dangerous than hydrogen cyanide (HCN). Thus a "rotten egg" odor about the premises is not a laughing matter. It is decidedly unsafe to enter a building or area that has a strong odor of H_2S.

Human beings can easily detect H_2S at air concentrations of 0.005–0.1 ppm. Twenty ppm cause ocular irritation, 50 ppm severe symptoms, and 1000 ppm rapid unconsciousness and death in about 1 hour (Thienes and Haley 1972).

In animals, sudden exposure to H_2S concentrations in the neighborhood of 400 ppm may be quickly fatal. Such concentrations can occur in barns or stables exposed to the gases emitted from a slurry tank, especially when the tank is agitated (Clarke and Clarke 1967; Buck et al. 1973).

Ammonia, CH_4, and CO_2 are also liberated from slurry tanks. The latter two gases are relatively harmless. Hydrogen sulfide is the most dangerous sewage gas, but NH_3 may mimic or complicate H_2S poisoning (see Ammonia). In smogs, other irritant materials may synergize with H_2S.

TOXICODYNAMIC CONSIDERATIONS

Besides being irritant to mucous membranes, H_2S is readily absorbed through the skin, lungs, and digestive tract lining. In the bloodstream the gas is converted to alkali sulfides. The hydrosulfide radical (presumably the agent responsible for systemic lesions) is excreted by the lungs and in the urine. Part of the sulfide is oxidized to sulfate and thiosulfate and excreted in the urine. Some of the sulfide may be "trapped" by natural disulfides (e.g., glutathione) in the bloodstream (Smith and Abbanat 1966). Some sulfide is also excreted as iron sulfide in the feces (Thienes and Haley 1972).

MECHANISM OF ACTION

Hydrogen sulfide does two things: it directly irritates mucous membranes, including respiratory linings, and it inhibits cellular respiration. Direct irritation is likely the major cause of pulmonary edema, hyperemia, and dyspnea seen in animals that do not die outright. Thus H_2S was classified under the previous section of this chapter as one of the agents capable of causing interference with oxygen uptake from pulmonary alveoli. The exact means by which it produces pulmonary edema is not known, but it is not reasonable to attribute the edema to some unique mechanism set apart from the means by which any other irritant increases permeability of lung capillaries.

Sudden death from inhalation of large concentrations of H_2S is due to inhibition of cellular respiration in vital tissues, particularly the brain. Undoubtedly, this inhibition also occurs to some extent in animals exposed to smaller concentrations; therefore H_2S is properly classified along with cyanide as an agent capable of preventing oxygen utilization by cells.

The detailed molecular mechanism of inhibition of cellular respiration by H_2S has not been elucidated as clearly as it has for HCN. Apparently both inhibit cytochrome oxidase, thus inhibiting the electron-transport system. However, the *way* in which the two poisons inhibit cytochrome oxidase differs. Cyanide does it by complexing with ferric iron sites of the cytochrome complex. Hydrogen sulfide may also do this, but in addition may cleave vital disulfide bonds necessary for activity of cytochrome oxidase (Smith and Abbanat 1966). The result is inability of tissue cells to utilize oxygen, no matter how much oxygen is present in the bloodstream. It is known that artificial respiration does not save animals poisoned acutely by either H_2S or HCN.

Hydrogen sulfide turns the blood dark and imparts a greenish or greenish-purple discoloration to tissues. The mechanism here is not known but may explain why the blood is not bright red like it is in HCN poisoning. Perhaps the dark coloration is due to the formation of metal sulfide salts.

CLINICAL SIGNS

If exposure is not too great, coughing, lacrimation, mucous nasal discharge, dyspnea, depression, fluid sounds in the lungs, and terminal cyanosis and possible convulsions may occur. Large concentrations of

H_2S may cause sudden collapse, cyanosis, dyspnea, anoxic convulsions, and rapid death.

LESIONS

There may be pulmonary edema and edema of the intestines and brain. The blood is dark and fails to clot. Hemorrhages may occur in various organs. Liver and kidney may manifest degenerative changes. The tissues may be dark or discolored. In acute cases there may be few lesions except some agonal hemorrhages on heart and lungs. The carcass may have a definite odor of H_2S. If the source of H_2S was ingested, then the GI contents may be dark gray or black and smell of raw sewage. This finding should be given particular importance in a fresh carcass.

DIFFERENTIAL DIAGNOSIS

If pulmonary edema and other lesions indicative of lung irritation and organ degeneration are present, infectious disease should be ruled out first. Other agents that cause such lesions are listed under ANTU. The odor of H_2S and the color of the blood and tissues, taken with a history of exposure to H_2S, should make the diagnosis clear. Acute poisoning is usually associated with known exposure to H_2S.

TREATMENT

If exposure was not too severe, measures discussed under ANTU may be of benefit. The source of H_2S must be eliminated. There is no specific antidote for H_2S although two interesting observations may have therapeutic implications: (1) The hydrated sulfide radical can be complexed to some degree by methemoglobin, suggesting that the treatment for cyanide toxicosis could be partly effective for H_2S. (2) The hydrated sulfide anion can interact with disulfides such as oxidized glutathione (Smith and Abbanat 1966).

ANALYSIS

Hydrogen sulfide has an unmistakable odor. Its presence in a fresh carcass is indicative of H_2S poisoning if the history, clinical signs, and lesions are consistent with such a diagnosis. It should be remembered that the intestinal tract will normally contain a small amount of H_2S, but not enough to produce black gut contents and sewerlike odor under normal conditions.

CYANIDE

SOURCE

Cyanide poisoning in animals is generally a result of ingestion of certain plants that are stunted, wilted, trampled, frost damaged, or treated with 2,4-D. These plants contain glycosides (so-called cyanogenic glycosides) that can liberate toxic amounts of HCN by an enzymatic hydrolysis initiated in some way after damage to the plant. In the stomach, HCN from the plant is readily absorbed; the cyanogenic glycoside can continue to be hydrolyzed (microbially or by acid hydrolysis) to liberate more HCN.

Plants most often incriminated in HCN poisoning of farm animals are wild cherry (*Prunus* spp.), which contains the glycoside amygdalin, and the various tall grasses such as sudan grass, Johnson grass, and sorghums (*Sorghum* spp.), which contain the glycoside dhurrin. Other plants that have cyanogenic potential in their foliage are catclaw, bahia, mountain mahogany, florestina, fowl mannagrass, velvet grass, hydrangea, flax, bird's-foot trefoil, lima bean, cultivated cherry, apple, apricot, peach, poison suckleya, white clover, arrowgrass, vetch seed, elderberry, and corn. See Kingsbury (1964) for more detail.

Cyanide is used as a fumigant and cyanide compounds are used as rodenticides. The fertilizer calcium cyanimide may be a source of cyanide for animals.

Inorganic salts of cyanide do not necessarily cause signs of cyanide poisoning. Thiocyanates, or thiocyanate glycosides found in rape seed, brussels sprouts, rutabaga, kohlrabi, mustard, kale, broccoli, cabbage, turnip (*Brassica* spp.), soybean (*Glycine* sp.), or flax (*Linum* sp.) may be goitrogenic (Kingsbury 1964). Cyanates and thiocyanates can also cause CNS and endocrine effects (Cerami et al. 1973; Graziano et al.

1973; Smith 1973; Shaw et al. 1974), but these are of little veterinary significance.

PROPERTIES OF TOXICOLOGIC IMPORTANCE

Hydrogen cyanide is a volatile gas that is irritant to mucous membranes. It has a characteristic odor usually described as an odor of bitter almond. Most of us have never smelled bitter almond. To some people, the odor is ammoniacal; others disagree. Actually, the odor is *exactly* like HCN! The student should find out what HCN smells like. Cyanide in plant tissues will disappear into the air rather quickly as the foliage dries. Thus foliage samples are frozen for shipping to the analytical laboratory. Cyanide in rumen contents will also disappear (or continue to rise if there is much glycoside present) soon after removal from the animal. The CN^- radical forms complexes with a number of other chemicals (e.g., in tissues) and has a strong affinity for cobalt.

TOXICITY

The acute oral MLD of HCN and its alkali salts is about the same in all species, i.e., 2–2.3 mg HCN/kg of body weight. Cyanogenic plants vary in toxicity. Plants that are young and growing contain more glycoside. Factors that increase the likelihood of HCN poisoning from ingestion of cyanogenic plants include: (1) large amounts of free HCN and cyanogenic glycoside in the plant; (2) rapid ingestion; (3) ingestion of a large amount of the plant; and (4) ruminal pH and microflora that continue to hydrolyze the glycoside. Rapid intake of plant material equivalent to about 4 mg HCN/kg of body weight is considered to be a lethal amount of plant material. Gastric HCl destroys the plant enzyme that hydrolyzes the cyanogenic glycosides, but acid hydrolysis can occur to some extent. Ruminants are more susceptible to cyanogenic plants than are horses and swine. Sheep are somewhat less susceptible than cattle, and some breeds of cattle may be less susceptible than others (Clarke and Clarke 1967).

In human beings (with reference to fumigating operations), exposure to 150 ppm of HCN for 30–60 minutes may cause death. Death will result from a few minutes' exposure to 300 ppm (Stecher 1968). These values probably also hold for animals.

TOXICODYNAMIC CONSIDERATIONS

Cyanide is rapidly absorbed from the GI tract or lungs. In the bloodstream, thiosulfate reacts with the CN^- radical to form thiocyanate, which is relatively harmless and is excreted in the urine. The reaction is catalyzed by the enzyme *rhodanese*. Ready stores of thiosulfate can be depleted in this detoxification reaction. Cyanide can also be inactivated in the bloodstream by complexation with the ferric iron of methemoglobin. However, there is not normally much methemoglobin present in the bloodstream. Some HCN is eliminated by exhalation from the lungs.

MECHANISM OF ACTION

The CN^- radical complexes with the ferric iron of cytochrome oxidase. Thus the electron transport system is inhibited and cells die from lack of usable oxygen. This action occurs despite large concentrations of oxygen in the bloodstream. All tissues are affected, but death is due primarily to tissue anoxia in the brain. Cardiovascular collapse seen in cyanide poisoning is probably secondary to tissue anoxia in brain, heart, and blood vessels and to electrolyte disturbances created by tissue anoxia. It has been shown that cyanide decreases myocardial intracellular potassium and increases extracellular potassium concentrations in the cat (Karzel et al. 1974).

CLINICAL SIGNS

Animals may be found dead. If several animals in a herd have eaten cyanogenic plants, clinical signs may vary from mild tachypnea and apparent anxiety to severe panting, gasping, and behavioral alarm. Other signs include salivation, muscle tremors, lacrimation, urination and defecation, severe colic, emesis, prostration, bright red mucous membranes due to hyperoxygenation of the blood, clonic convulsions, mydriasis, and rapid death. The heart rate becomes progressively slower and the heart stops a few minutes after cessation of respiration. Similar signs occur in all species.

Consciousness is apparently not lost until the animal actually collapses. This may be many minutes or even hours after ingestion of cyanogenic plants, although cyanide poisoning is generally considered to be of extremely rapid onset. The author has injected potassium cyanide (KCN) solution intracardially into a pig in order to judge the onset of unconsciousness and death. Collapse was rapid, but the animal was responsive to external stimuli during the early part of the 4–5 minutes required for death to occur.

Occasionally, animals may die without manifesting clinical signs (Clarke and Clarke 1967), although a trained observer could probably record several signs if he were watching closely.

LESIONS

Mucous membranes are a healthy pink and the blood is cherry red and may not clot. The red color is due to hyperoxygenation that occurs while the animal is dying. There may be agonal hemorrhages on the heart. The GI tract and lungs may have congestion and petechial hemorrhages. The stomach contents may be identifiable as plant material that does not belong there; the contents may smell faintly of cyanide. The odor may be fleeting, partly because gaseous HCN leaves the exposed stomach contents rapidly, partly because our olfactory mechanism can adapt to the odor of HCN, and partly because the odor may be masked by other odors present.

DIFFERENTIAL DIAGNOSIS

The acute onset, bright red mucous membranes and blood, and the odor of cyanide are indicative of cyanide poisoning. Carbon monoxide causes bright red blood, but the probability of poisoning by this agent is low. Hydrogen sulfide causes rapid death by inhibition of cytochrome oxidase, but the blood and tissues will be dark and the carcass may smell of H_2S. Nitrite can cause rapid death with few lesions, but the blood will likely be brown. Urea may cause rapid death without many lesions, but urea causes severe colic and nervous and behavioral signs and generates an odor of ammonia in the rumen. Many other poisons can kill animals without the client actually seeing sick animals. A detailed history and thorough inspection of the premises will usually rule out most other poisons and leave the veterinarian with the idea that cyanogenic plants were the cause of death. A recent frost or pruning of trees is often associated with cyanide poisoning.

TREATMENT

The major objectives are to get CN^- off of the ferric iron of cytochrome oxidase and to replace or augment the available thiosulfate in the bloodstream. These objectives are accomplished by giving intravenous injections of sodium nitrite and sodium thiosulfate. Sodium nitrite (15–25 mg/kg of body weight) changes some of the (ferrous) hemoglobin to (ferric) methemoglobin. Methemoglobin then competes with ferric cytochrome oxidase for CN^- and regenerates cytochrome oxidase while forming cyanmethemoglobin. *This treatment should not be repeated because of the danger of producing nitrite toxicosis.*

Sodium thiosulfate (1.25 g/kg) reacts with CN^- in the bloodstream, or CN^- liberated from cyanmethemoglobin, and forms thiocyanate, which is excreted. Additional thiosulfate can be given if necessary.

In addition to giving excess thiosulfate, a large dosage of hydroxocobalamin (vitamin B-12_a) or aquocobalamin (B-12_b) may be given. The cobalt in these preparations may complex additional cyanide in the circulation (Friedberg and Shukla 1975). Cobalt chloride and cobalt EDTA have been used to prevent cyanide toxicosis (Hillman and Bardhan 1974; Isom and Way 1974) but such treatments may cause cobalt toxicosis (hypertension, cardiac arrhythmias, possible cardiac fibrillation) under field conditions. The author has tested a balanced solution of cobalt chloride, EDTA, and methionine and found the mixture less effective than combined sodium nitrite–sodium thiosulfate in the protection of mice against KCN lethality. Similar results are reported for dicobalt EDTA (Kelocyanor) (Frankenberg and Sörbo 1975).

Other measures include cooling, diluting, and acidifying the rumen contents by giving the cow 1 gal (3.8 L) of vinegar in 3–5 gal of cold water to slow microbial hydrolysis of cyanogenic glycoside. Mineral oil can be administered to soothe irritated GI linings.

If the animal survives a day, no further treatment will likely be needed.

ANALYSIS

Plant material containing 200 ppm or more of HCN is potentially toxic. A small amount of cyanide is normally present in rumen contents. Tissues that are degenerating may contain cyanide in traces. Cyanide poisoning may be indicated if fresh rumen contents contain more than 10 ppm HCN or if fresh liver contains 1.4 ppm or more (Clarke and Clarke 1967). History, clinical signs, lesions, and responses to specific therapy should be used to support the final diagnosis.

POISONS MARKEDLY INCREASING TISSUE OXYGEN DEMAND

Chlorophenols, Nitrophenols

USE

Pentachlorophenol (PCP) and sodium pentachlorophenate are common wood preservatives, while compounds such as dinitrophenol (commonly abbreviated DNP), 2-*sec*-butyl-4,6-dinitrophenol (DNBP), and 2-methyl-4,6-dinitrophenol (dinitro-orthocresol, DNOC) are used as insecticides (dormant insects), fungicides, acaricides, and herbicides. Disophenol (2,6-diiodo-4-nitrophenol, which has a trade name DNP), is used as an injectable for the control of hookworms in dogs and gapeworms in turkeys and game birds.

SOURCE

Animals may be poisoned by licking wood that is treated with chlorophenols. In addition, animals may inhale toxic amounts of PCP from treated walls in sheds or barns, even if the chemical was applied months or years ago. The vapors can also penetrate the intact skin, although this route of exposure is more important with direct contact with the chemicals in the group. Spills of chlorophenols and nitrophenols or recently sprayed foliage can be ingested by animals. Water supplies may be contaminated by the rinsing of spray apparatus or by rain water runoff from sprayed areas. "Empty" containers of these compounds may be licked out by curious animals. DNP can cause poisoning in dogs after only a therapeutic dosage under some conditions (see Toxicity; Legendre 1973).

PROPERTIES OF TOXICOLOGIC IMPORTANCE

Chlorophenols and nitrophenols are generally not very water-soluble. They are soluble in oils and organic solvents and can readily penetrate intact skin. PCP is volatile and can give off toxic vapors in sufficient concentration to kill animals confined in small quarters with wooden walls treated with the chemical. This is especially true at high ambient temperatures.

TOXICITY

Some acute oral LD50 values (mg/kg of body weight) in rats are: PCP, 50–200; sodium pentachlorophenate, 100–210; DNBP, 40–60; DNOC, 20–50; and DNP, 0.027–0.1 (Buck et al. 1973; Berg 1974). A dog was poisoned by a therapeutic dose of 10 mg disophenol/kg of body weight (Legendre 1973), but it was hot outside that day and the dog was very active (see below).

The acute oral minimum lethal dose of PCP (mg/kg of body weight) in some other species is: dog, 70; guinea pig, 100; sheep, 120; and calf, 140. Adult ruminants may tolerate more ingested PCP than calves or nonruminants, due to a protective effect of rumen microorganisms. Sheep can become thin and unthrifty if fed 28–56 mg PCP/kg of body weight/day. Calves can die if they ingest 35–50 mg/kg/day over a period of time. For fish the maximum nontoxic concentration of PCP in water is 0.2–0.6 ppm; death occurs at 1 ppm (Sollmann 1957; Clarke and Clarke 1967; Buck et al. 1973).

The acute oral LD50 of DNOC in mice, guinea pigs, rabbits, and dogs is about 50 mg/kg of body weight. In pigs the acute oral lethal dose of DNOC is 50–100 mg/kg. Dosage of sheep with 25 mg/kg/day causes toxicosis in 2–4 days. The alkylamine salts of DNOC are much less toxic to sheep. Again, adult ruminants can eat more DNOC than nonruminants (Clarke and Clarke 1967; Radeleff 1970).

Several factors affect the toxicity of chlorophenols and nitrophenols. Toxicity is enhanced by high ambient temperature, physical activity, poor condition, oily or organic solvent vehicles, prior exposures, and hyperthyroid states. Toxicity is diminished by cold temperatures, antithyroid drugs, and the presence of body fat, which is the major substrate for the metabolic stimulant effects of these compounds (Sollmann 1957; Clarke and Clarke 1967).

TOXICODYNAMIC CONSIDERATIONS

Chlorophenols and nitrophenols are eliminated slowly from the body, thus necessitating several days of treatment.

MECHANISM OF ACTION

These compounds quickly and markedly increase metabolic rate. This is accomplished by a biochemical disconnection of oxidation and phosphorylation, without direct effects on cellular respiration. The result is that aerobic oxidation proceeds at an increasing rate, producing a lot of heat but little high-energy phosphates such as ATP. The exact molecular mechanisms of the metabolic stimulant effects of chlorophenols and nitrophenols are not known. The toxic mechanism resides within tissue cells and is not mediated by hormones or nerves (Clarke and Clarke 1967; Astwood 1970). Death results when the animal is unable to obtain enough oxygen to meet tissue oxygen demands. Fever also contributes to the cause of death.

CLINICAL SIGNS

Onset and duration of toxicosis may be so fast that no signs are seen. If animals are still alive, they appear severely overheated and manifest fever, tachycardia, deep panting or dyspnea, lethargy, stumbling or incoordination, possible sweating, thirst, oliguria, weakness, cyanosis, collapse, terminal convulsions, and rapid death. Less severely affected animals may not die but just manifest hyperthermia and signs of oxygen deficiency. GI signs can be expected if the poison was ingested. Abortion may occur.

LESIONS

Rigor mortis occurs quickly after death. The dinitrophenols are yellow dyes and may impart a yellow-green color to the tissues and urine and to external surfaces contacted by the chemicals. There may be cyanosis. Parenchymatous organs may manifest degenerative changes consistent with oxygen starvation and high body temperature. Agonal hemorrhages may be found on the heart and lungs. The blood would be expected to be dark, due to antemortem deprivation of oxygen by oxygen-hungry tissues. Gastroenteritis may be present if the poison was ingested.

DIFFERENTIAL DIAGNOSIS

A history of exposure to a chlorophenol or nitrophenol compound, signs of rapid overheating and respiratory distress, and lesions like fast rigor mortis, dark blood, and yellow tissues (with nitrophenols) should allow a presumptive diagnosis. Actual heatstroke may have to be ruled out.

If exposure to these chemicals is not obvious in the history or after examination of the premises, other poisons that cause respiratory insufficiency may be considered. Of primary interest might be nitrite (which causes brown blood, no fever), carbon monoxide (bright red blood, no fever), cyanide (bright red blood, usually no fever), and pesticides (marked neuromuscular signs, autonomic manifestations). Peracute infectious disease should also be ruled out.

TREATMENT

Some texts say there is no treatment

for poisoning by chlorophenols and nitrophenols. Actually, much can be done that may save the animal if it is not already moribund. Oxygen should be provided immediately to satisfy tissue oxygen demand. Concurrently, body temperature should be lowered by cold water rinsing, ice packs, or ethanol spraying. An intramuscular dosage of a phenothiazine tranquilizer may facilitate handling, help reduce tissue oxygen demand by reducing exertion, reduce complications of stress, and allow more rapid cooling by the poikilothermic side effect of these drugs. However, sedatives should not be given to a depressed or comatose animal.

If the poison was absorbed through skin contact, a soap and water bath is required, taking care that gloves are used to avoid absorbing poison from the skin and hair of the animal. If the poison was ingested, a saline purgative such as magnesium sulfate should be given, or a gastric lavage with 5% sodium bicarbonate. Metabolic acidosis and dehydration should be treated with fluids and electrolytes. If fever is refractory to cold therapy, an antithyroid drug such as sodium methylthiouracil given intravenously may rapidly reduce the metabolic rate, but this has not been tried in veterinary practice.

If the animal survives for 24 hours, the chances for complete recovery are fair, but there can be secondary bacterial infection predisposed by liver, kidney, and intestinal damage from the irritant, anoxic, heat, and stress effects of the poison. Prophylactic use of corticosteroids, antibiotics, and multiple vitamins may be indicated at the discretion of the veterinarian. For references on therapy see Sollmann (1957), Clarke and Clarke (1967), Astwood (1970), Hayes (1971), and Legendre (1973).

ANALYSIS

Chlorophenols and nitrophenols do not normally belong in animal tissues and body fluids. In the absence of data on correlation between tissue residues and clinical illness, it must be concluded that any concentration of these agents in animal tissues and body fluids could be diagnostically meaningful if the history, clinical signs, and lesions are consistent with poisoning by these agents. Buck et al. (1973) have presented some data indicating that some species can tolerate certain oral dosages of PCP without much ill effect. The same dosages could be fatal, however, if the various factors that enhance toxicity of such compounds (see Toxicity) are operating. No "safe" dosage of chlorophenols and nitrophenols exists; the figures of Buck et al. were not meant to imply a "safe" dosage of PCP.

Other Metabolic Stimulants

Any compound capable of accelerating tissue oxygen demand beyond oxygen availability could be placed in this category. Such compounds are generally drugs and are discussed elsewhere. It is worth naming some of the drugs here, however. They include thyroxin and other thyroid stimulants, epinephrine and other sympathomimetic agents, nearly all analeptic drugs, and all convulsant compounds. Respiratory inadequacy is most likely to develop with these drugs if there is some defect in the animal's respiratory mechanism or some lesion or obstruction in the lungs or bronchi.

Fever can develop whenever the heat of physical activity or convulsions exceeds the capacity of heat-dissipating mechanisms. When fever is superimposed on tissue oxygen starvation, the prognosis is guarded and the treatment should always include cooling measures in addition to oxygen therapy and (if possible) the antidote for the offending drug. Antipyretic drugs are generally ineffective and too slow-acting for emergency treatment of chemical-induced fevers, although sedatives or phenothiazine tranquilizers may be useful adjuncts to therapy (see Treatment, Chlorophenols, Nitrophenols).

POISONS DEPRESSING THE RESPIRATORY CENTERS

Metaldehyde

USE

Metaldehyde is used as a snail and slug

killer as well as a solid fuel for certain kinds of camp stoves.

SOURCE

Animals generally obtain metaldehyde-treated baits from areas baited for the control of molluscan crop pests. The bait may also be spilled or insecurely stored so as to allow access by animals.

PROPERTIES OF TOXICOLOGIC IMPORTANCE

Metaldehyde is a polycyclic condensation product (polymer) of acetaldehyde; it has the empirical formula $(C_2H_4O)_n$. It is a flammable, white, crystalline or powdery material that sublimes at about 112° F but decomposes slowly above 80° F, with partial generation of acetaldehyde. Metaldehyde is poorly soluble in water, sparingly soluble in alcohol and ether, and soluble in benzene and chloroform.

TOXICITY

The acute oral LD50 of metaldehyde in rats is 630–690 mg/kg of body weight. In dogs it is 210–1000 mg/kg. The acute oral lethal dose (not LD50) in some species (in mg/kg) is: guinea pig, 400–700; rabbit, 1250; duck, 500; chicken, 2000; and human being, 100. Illness can occur with smaller dosages than these (Clarke and Clarke 1967; Berg 1974; Verschuuren et al. 1975). The lethal dose of metaldehyde can vary greatly in a given species. This could be related to the rate of degradation and the quantity of toxic fragments of the polymer. It is not known what role acetaldehyde may have in metaldehyde toxicity. The LD50 of acetaldehyde in rats is 1900 mg/kg of body weight, a value that is 3 times larger than the LD50 of metaldehyde in that species.

TOXICODYNAMIC CONSIDERATIONS

Metaldehyde is readily absorbed from the GI tract, probably as different sized fragments of the acetaldehyde polymer. Some acetaldehyde is undoubtedly absorbed also. These substances readily cross the blood-brain barrier, as evidenced by their effect on level of consciousness.

MECHANISM OF ACTION

Metaldehyde or its fragments cause central nervous depression (or in some cases excitation) by some unknown mechanism. In addition, the substance has irritant properties that may cause gastroenteritis, liver damage, brain damage, and other lesions. Death is generally due to overdepression of vital medullary respiratory and vasomotor control centers, just as with the general anesthetics. The animal may recover from the initial narcosis and then die a few days later of hepatic insufficiency.

CLINICAL SIGNS

In dogs (the species most often poisoned), emesis, depression, incoordination, hyperpnea, tachycardia, prostration, and cyanosis occur. Some dogs may manifest salivation, hyperesthesia, tremors, fever (102°–107° F), and continuous convulsions with opisthotonos prior to death. If the dog does not die of respiratory depression, it may die in a few days of liver malfunction. In cats the signs are similar to those in dogs, but nystagmus is often seen. In sheep, staggering and incoordination, head pressing, hyperpnea, salivation, fever (108° to more than 110° F), recumbency, cyanosis, and paddling convulsions are manifested. Poultry demonstrate excitability, tremors, muscle spasms, diarrhea, dyspnea, and polypnea (Clarke and Clarke 1967; Buck et al. 1973; Udall 1973; Simmons and Scott 1974).

LESIONS

The above references state that lesions found in dogs killed by metaldehyde include congestion of the liver, kidney, and lung; interstitial hemorrhages in the lung; and degeneration of the liver and of brain "ganglion cells." A formaldehydelike (acetaldehyde) odor may be present in the stomach contents. In sheep the lesions include subcutaneous edema of the neck, pale and friable liver, froth in the trachea and bronchi, petechial hemorrhages in the urinary bladder and lungs, ecchymotic hemorrhages in the heart and the mucosa of the small intestine, blood in the intestinal lumen, and a rumen pH of about 6.

DIFFERENTIAL DIAGNOSIS

Metaldehyde poisoning is not very common, even in dogs. Thus the appearance of excitatory or convulsant signs accompanied by respiratory and neuromuscular signs with salivation and fever might suggest poisoning by lead, chlorinated hydrocarbon pesticides, or a number of other agents discussed in Chapter 58. Generally, however, the dog manifests behavioral and respiratory depression. The overall picture may resemble ethylene glycol toxicosis, even to the extent of apparent recovery and later relapse. In metaldehyde poisoning an acetaldehyde odor may be noted in the vomitus or stomach contents; a test of these samples will reveal the presence of aldehydes. Moreover, oxalate crystals do not appear in the renal tubules of animals poisoned by metaldehyde, as happens in animals poisoned by ethylene glycol. Also, the relapse phenomenon in metaldehyde toxicosis is hepatogenous, whereas in ethylene glycol poisoning it is due to renal failure. Still, it may be difficult to differentiate metaldehyde and ethylene glycol poisoning without tests. Hopefully, the history may indicate exposure to metaldehyde.

TREATMENT

Since we do not know exactly how metaldehyde kills animals, there is no specific antidote. Excitement or convulsions can be treated with sedatives or anesthetics. Respiratory and behavior depression can be treated with oxygen and stimulants. Fever can be controlled by cold water rinsing. The GI tract should be emptied by lavage, emetics, or a saline purgative. Liver damage can be treated with intravenously administered 5% glucose in saline (Udall 1973). Dogs that are markedly depressed to begin with may die in spite of vigorous therapy.

ANALYSIS

The presence of aldehydes in vomitus or stomach contents is indicative of metaldehyde poisoning in animals that have signs and lesions described above. Quantitative analysis of the aldehydes is not a useful indicator of severity of poisoning because the rate of liberation of aldehydes from metaldehyde and the absorption of toxic fragments of the polymer by the animal will vary. Also, we do not know exactly which fragments of metaldehyde polymer are toxic.

Alcohols

Most alcohols are central nervous depressants; the outstanding signs of poisoning by them would be hypnosis, narcosis, or a state of anesthesia followed by cyanosis, signs of shock, and respiratory arrest due to overdepression of the medullary respiratory centers.

Animals could ingest or be given ethanol (in whiskey, as a vehicle for other drugs, or in the treatment of ethylene glycol toxicosis), methanol (wood alcohol), or isopropanol (rubbing alcohol). Generally, the treatment of these toxicoses consists of artificial respiration, nursing care, and (except when ethylene glycol is present) stimulants. Sometimes, as with methanol, there may be irreversible brain damage or blindness.

Dihydric alcohols (see Ethylene Glycol) have a central depressant component but there are complicating signs and lesions due to metabolites of these alcohols. Moreover, the different dihydric and ester-containing monohydric alcohols differ among themselves regarding toxicity, signs, lesions, and possible mechanisms of action (Sollmann 1957).

POISONS HAVING MULTIPLE ACTIONS ON RESPIRATORY EFFICIENCY

Selenium

USE

Selenium (Se) is used in medicated shampoos for the treatment of some types of dermatitis. The element is also an essential trace nutrient and is administered along with vitamin E in the treatment and prevention of selenium-deficiency states in animals and fowl.

SOURCE

Although poisoning can occur from improper use of selenium-containing shampoos or injectables, the usual source for poisoning of livestock is forage or feed that comes from soils rich in selenium. Soils containing cretaceous rock are rich in selenium, particularly if such soils are not excessively leached out by rain. The selenium is present in inorganic and organic forms. A number of plants can accumulate selenium from the soil. They grow mainly in the dryer portions of the United States such as the Great Plains and western states where conditions favor retention of selenium in the topsoil or surface rock. The *obligate accumulators,* known as selenium-indicator plants, require selenium for growth. Such plants include species of *Astragalus* (poison vetch), *Stanleya* (prince's plume), *Oonopsis* (golden weed), and *Xylorrhiza* (woody aster). These plants may contain as much as 15,000 ppm of selenium. The *facultative accumulators* do not require selenium, but they may take the element up from the soil under the right conditions. Selenium concentration in facultative accumulators may be one-tenth the concentration found in obligate accumulators growing in the same soil. Examples of facultative accumulators that can cause selenium toxicosis are species of *Aster* (aster), *Atriplex* (saltbush), *Castilleja* (paint brush), *Comandra* (bastard toadflax), *Grayia* (hopsage), *Grindelia* (gumweeds), *Gutierrezia* (snakeweed), *Machaeranthera* (tansy aster), *Penstemon* (beard tongue), and *Sideranthus* (ironweed). The *passive accumulators* of selenium may contain a hundredth the selenium concentration of obligate accumulators growing in the same soil. This is still a potentially toxic concentration. Passive accumulation occurs simply because the soil contains selenium, not because the plant takes the element up preferentially. Many plants can accumulate selenium passively. Crop plants such as corn, wheat, oats, barley, grass, and hay, as well as other plants, can do this. Selenium poisoning can occur in any part of the country if toxic feeds are shipped there from seleniferous regions. For detail on selenium in plants, see Kingsbury (1964).

PROPERTIES OF TOXICOLOGIC IMPORTANCE

The metalloid selenium is in Group VI of the Periodic Chart of the Elements. It has 3 major oxidation states, +6 (selenate), +4 (selenite), and —2 (selenide). Selenium has chemical and physical properties similar to those of sulfur and tellurium, which are also in Group VI. In addition, selenium and arsenic are neighbors in the Periodic Chart; they also have some chemical and physical similarities.

Selenium (—2) is capable of combining with a number of metals and is often found in nature in the sulfide ores of heavy metals. Selenium (+4) combines with halogens (except iodine), hydrogen, and the sulfhydryl group of glutathione. These chemical interactions may have direct bearing on the toxic mechanisms of selenium (see Mechanism of Action).

Selenium is an essential micronutrient required for prevention of several disease states of cellular degeneration and cell membrane damage in animals and fowl. The element may function in this regard as an intracellular antioxidant. The exact mechanism here is not known, but may relate to prevention of peroxide accumulation through reduction of peroxides by glutathione in the presence of the selenium-containing enzyme glutathione peroxidase (Hafeman et al. 1974; Stadtman 1974). Alternately or concomitantly, an oxidation-reduction role for selenium may exist in heart and skeletal muscles in which a low molecular weight selenoprotein containing a heme component similar to cytochrome C has been isolated (Stadtman 1974). The reason for stating this here is that the redox properties of selenium are physiologically important and identifiable in the body and (as with other redox systems) an oversupply of one of the reactants (i.e., selenium) may have undesirable effects on the system's equilibrium.

Like other metalloids and metals, selenium is directly irritant to mucous membranes. This property may also be important in selenium toxicosis.

TOXICITY

The toxicity ranking of selenium in various forms is: organoselenium of plants and grains 2 × > selenate (+6) = selenite (+4) > selenide (—2) > synthetic organoselenium compounds. Elemental selenium is relatively nontoxic.

The acute oral minimum lethal dose of selenium as selenate or selenite in several species (mg/kg of body weight) is: horse, 3.3; cow, 10; pig, 17; and cat, rabbit, and rat, 1.5–3. Death occurs in a few minutes in dogs given 4 mg selenate or selenite/kg orally. Pigs can die in 24–48 hours if given 1 mg selenite/kg of body weight in combination with vitamin E. Pigs from selenium-deficient farms are more susceptible than normal pigs to this form of acute toxicosis; the calculated 48 hour LD50 of selenite in combination with vitamin E is 1.4 mg Se/kg in normal pigs and 0.9–1 mg Se/kg in pigs from selenium-deficient farms. Calves can die in as few as 2 hours after parenteral injection of about 0.5 mg Se/kg of body weight. Other calves may die weeks later from the same dose.

Chronic poisoning can occur with dietary organic selenium concentrations of 7 ppm (swine), 8 ppm (cattle), 10 ppm (sheep), and 15 ppm (poultry), expressed as Se. There is no minimum toxic level of dietary selenium; even 2 ppm in the diet can cause weight loss in rats under prolonged exposure. Forage or grain containing 25 ppm or greater can cause acute toxicosis in herbivorous species.

Toxicity data were obtained from Sollmann (1957), Clarke and Clarke (1967), Radeleff (1970), Shortridge et al. (1971), Allaway (1973), Buck et al. (1973), and Van Fleet et al. (1974).

Selenium can cause acute, subacute, or chronic toxicosis, or no toxicosis at all, depending on a number of factors. Toxicosis is favored by selenium deficiency (swine), large or rapid intake of selenium, intake of selenium in organic combinations found in plants, presence of other toxins in the plant, poor health or condition of the animal, slow elimination of selenium, previous exposures to selenium, and individual and species susceptibility. Toxicity is reduced by a high-protein diet and by ingestion of other elements that might complex selenium in the gut (e.g., arsenic or iron). Seleniferous plants have a bad odor and may not be eaten by discriminating or native species unless better forage is not available.

TOXICODYNAMIC CONSIDERATIONS

Selenium is readily absorbed from the gut and distributed throughout the body, particularly to the liver, kidneys, and spleen. Chronic exposure results in large concentrations in hair and hoof. Selenium can cross the placental barrier of mammals and also enter avian eggs, causing fetal malformations and embryotoxic effects. Selenium does not penetrate intact skin but may penetrate abraded or diseased skin.

Absorbed organic selenium (e.g., selenomethionine) may be oxidized from the —2 state (selenide) to the +4 state (selenite) within the body. Inorganic selenate (+6) may be reduced to selenite, whereas absorbed inorganic selenite seems to require no change in oxidation state. Selenite, from whatever original form, may then substitute for sulfur in the synthesis of amino acids and thence protein. Additionally, selenite may be complexed or bonded by glutathione and then excreted as trimethyl selonium ion in the urine, metal selenides or elemental selenium in the feces, and volatile methyl selenides in exhaled air. From 25% to 70% of subtoxic amounts of dietary selenium may be eliminated within 2 days of ingestion. Added detail on metabolism and excretion of selenium is presented by Allaway (1973). It is emphasized that we do not really know much about selenium toxicodynamics. What we do know is based on isolated experiments in different species.

MECHANISM OF ACTION

Acute or subacute GI signs and lesions probably result in part from the irritant nature of selenium in large concentrations.

Selenium has a number of biochemical effects in the body, including:

1. Replacement of sulfur in amino acids such as cysteine and methionine (Al-

laway 1973; Stadtman 1974), with possible later synthesis of abnormal structural and enzyme proteins. This may also explain the hoof and hair defects of chronic selenosis, although this is speculative.

2. Decrease in ATP synthesis in chronic cases, possibly due to inhibition of sulfhydryl-containing enzymes such as succinic and other dehydrogenases (Buck et al. 1973). Oxygen utilization is decreased in liver, kidney, and brain but not in muscle tissue *in vitro.* Fetal oxidation processes are also suppressed (Sollmann 1957; Buck et al. 1973).

3. Interference with metabolism of vitamins A and C. The latter vitamin is diminished in tissues, possibly due to enhanced oxidation by ascorbic oxidases (see below). Administration of vitamin C does not protect against selenium toxicosis (Sollmann 1957).

4. Inhibition of cell oxidations in a manner related to item 2 above, but possibly by interfering with the heme-containing selenoprotein found in muscle tissue of selenium-treated animals (Stadtman 1974).

5. A dramatic reduction in tissue glutathione (GSH) concentration. This could be brought about by direct complexation of 2 molecules of GSH for every selenite ion, decreased synthesis or regeneration of GSH due to inhibition of some sulfhydryl enzyme or perhaps to competition between selenium and sulfur in the regeneration or synthesis of GSH, stimulation of liver and erythrocyte GSH-peroxidase activity (a selenium-containing enzyme), or some combination of these mechanisms (Hafeman et al. 1974; Stadtman 1974). None of the above biochemical effects of selenium have been causally related to signs and lesions of selenium poisoning.

The effect of selenium on tissue GSH concentration is particularly intriguing. Animal tissues normally contain 300–2000 ppm of GSH. This amount of GSH could easily be depleted by concentrations (up to 25 ppm) of selenium found in tissues of animals killed by selenium. Some functions of GSH in tissues include:

1. Acting as a hydrogen donor to restore enzyme and hemoglobin sulfhydryl groups to the active reduced state (Hatch 1972b; Beutler 1975). During this type of reaction, 2 GSH molecules interact with each other by forming a disulfide bond. The products are oxidized GSH (GSSG) plus 2 hydrogens. GSSG can accept hydrogen from other redox systems or enzymes. In fact, GSH is normally regenerated from GSSG by a specific $NADH_2$-dependent GSH reductase. The required $NADH_2$ comes from NAD plus glucose-6-phosphate (G-6-P), catalyzed by glucose-6-phosphate dehydrogenase (G-6-PD). Enzymes in this sequence and proximal to G-6-P in the glycolytic pathway could theoretically be inhibited by selenium.

2. Helping to prevent the accumulation of toxic peroxides. Two molecules of GSH can form 2 of water plus 1 of GSSG when reacted with H_2O_2 in the presence of the selenium-containing enzyme GSH peroxidase. Exogenous selenium can enhance the activity of GSH peroxidase, thus favoring depletion of tissue GSH stores (Rotruck et al. 1972; Stadtman 1974).

3. Serving as sulfhydryl-regenerating agent in the pentose phosphate pathway (Hatch 1972b; Agar and O'Shea 1975).

4. Supplying γ-glutamyl groups for carrying amino acids across cell membranes. Resynthesis of GSH for this function is catalyzed by enzymes that could be inhibited by selenium (Meister 1973, 1975).

5. Destruction of insulin. GSH is a major participant in cleavage of disulfide bonds in the insulin molecule although other mechanisms for insulin degradation are also operable (Travis and Sayers 1970). Selenosis is not manifested as hyperinsulinism.

6. Protection of tissue ascorbate against oxidation by ascorbic oxidase or copper (Sollmann 1957).

7. Detoxification of selenium. GSH probably participates in the enzymatic formation of dimethyl selenide and GSH selenopersulfide (Allaway 1973). Other metals may also be detoxified by GSH.

8. Detoxification of tissue-damaging metabolic intermediates of a number of compounds including simple and polycyclic phenols that arise from the arene oxides of

simple and polycyclic aromatic hydrocarbons. GSH is bound nonenzymatically to these phenols (Jerina and Daly 1974).

9. Enzymatic conjugation (and mercapturic acid formation) with arene oxides of halobenzenes, or with the *trans*-dihydrodiol derivatives of the arene oxides of aromatic hydrocarbons, or with drug (e.g., acetaminophen) metabolites. Tissue damage by these substances is thereby prevented (Reid et al. 1973; Jerina and Daly 1974; Gillette et al. 1974; Mitchell et al. 1974).

10. Detoxification of tissue-damaging metabolites of certain chlorinated hydrocarbons (e.g., carbon tetrachloride, chloroform) by two mechanisms: decreasing the covalent bonding of toxic intermediates to cellular macromolecules and preventing microsomal lipid peroxidation (an antioxidant action) by interacting with free peroxides (see item 2 above) (Brown et al. 1974; Gillette et al. 1974).

11. Enzymatic conjugation (and mercapturic acid formation) with the sulfoxide metabolites of certain compounds (e.g., thiocarbamate herbicides). Perhaps the low toxicity of these herbicides relates to carbamoylation of GSH or other tissue thiols by the herbicide sulfoxide (Lay et al., 1975).

It can be anticipated that any agent capable of interfering with GSH metabolism could have profound effects on metabolic and detoxification processes throughout the body. Cell membrane integrity might well be the first thing to suffer under these circumstances. In human beings, erythrocyte membranes are very susceptible to damage by drugs when there is a deficiency of G-6-PD or of GSH synthesis in the cells (see Chlorate).

None of this discussion has elucidated the exact mechanism of tissue damage and death in selenium poisoning. Death of acute and subacute selenosis is generally attributed to respiratory insufficiency resulting from pulmonary edema and hemorrhage. In chronic selenosis, death may not occur directly from any metabolic lesions although the animal may be so weak, lame, blind, and emaciated as to die of thirst and starvation.

CLINICAL SIGNS

Selenosis occurs in acute, subacute, and chronic forms, depending on the amount and form of selenium ingested and the duration of exposure. Acute selenosis in ruminants is manifested in a few hours to a few days by signs such as colic, bloat, dark watery diarrhea, polyuria, fever (103°–105° F), mydriasis, uncertain gait, peculiar rooted-to-one-spot stance with head and ears lowered, fast and weak pulse, pale or cyanotic mucous membranes, dyspnea with fluid sounds in the lungs and blood-tinged froth exuding from the nares, prostration, and death in hours or a day. In swine, acute selenosis is characterized by anorexia, emesis, diarrhea, lethargy, unsteady gait, weakness and paresis, dyspnea, prostration, coma, and death in 1–2 days. Horses are not generally victims of selenosis because they avoid malodorous selenium-containing plants. However, horses would be expected to manifest similar signs of acute selenosis as described above.

A subacute to chronic form of selenosis has been called "blind staggers" by ranchers and stockmen, but the animal may not be blind and may not stagger. In a first stage, cattle manifest poor appetite; they wander aimlessly, circling, disregarding obstacles, and stumbling over them or walking through them. Respiration and temperature are normal. In the second stage, in addition to stage 1 activity, an animal manifests depression, incoordination, and foreleg weakness causing the animal to go down on its knees. Anorexia is complete. In the third stage, colic, subnormal temperature, emaciation, swollen inflamed eyelids, clouded corneas, near-blindness, paresis including the muscles of swallowing, dyspnea and tachypnea, coma, and death in hours occur. These signs in other animals are about the same as in cattle, but the stages of toxicosis are not well defined.

Chronic selenosis has been called "alkali disease" but it has nothing to do with the drinking of alkali water as formerly thought. This form of selenosis is mentioned again in Chapter 60 because of the lameness and hoof and hair abnormalities it causes. However, long-term ingestion of selenium also causes partial blindness, paresis, incoordination, emaciation, lethargy, and peripheral circulatory insufficiency; some of these signs are consistent with the lesions of other forms of selenosis.

For detail see Clarke and Clarke (1967), Radeleff (1970), Buck et al. (1973), and Van Fleet et al. (1974).

LESIONS

The overall impression at necropsy is one of congested organs and leaky blood vessels that caused edema, transudates, and hemorrhages. These lesions are prominent in the lungs but are also present in the liver, kidney, spleen, gut, heart, and brain. Thoracic, pericardial, and abdominal cavities may contain excess fluid. Hemorrhagic enteritis may be present and the gut contents may smell of rotten garlic (hydrogen selenide). If the animal lived long enough, softening and necrosis in various organs or even fibrosis may be manifested. The carcass may be emaciated (Clarke and Clarke 1967; Shortridge et al. 1971; Buck et al. 1973; Van Fleet et al. 1974). Smith et al. (1972) attribute much of the organ pathology to a primary cardiac insufficiency brought about by myocardial necrosis, but they attribute hemorrhages to direct toxic actions of selenium. Of course, even the myocardial lesions are probably due to direct toxic actions of selenium on myocardial vascular endothelium and on myocardial cells themselves.

DIFFERENTIAL DIAGNOSIS

Usually, diagnosing selenosis is no problem. If grazing stock had access to known seleniferous plants and later developed the typical signs and lesions described above, selenium was likely at fault. It is important to remember that selenium poisoning generally occurs in the arid, selenium-containing regions of the country. A test for selenium in forage, grain, stomach contents, and animal tissues, blood, or urine can confirm the diagnosis. Diseases that might be confused with acute or subacute selenosis include pneumonia, anthrax, infectious hepatitis, enterotoxemia, and pasteurellosis. Conditions that mimic aspects of chronic selenosis include freezing, ergotism, molybdenosis, fluorosis, and laminitis. Several other poisons can cause edema and hemorrhages, but not generally in so many organs in the same animal. The odor of rotten garlic or rotten horseradish in a fresh carcass is suggestive of acute or subacute selenosis, but the absence of such an odor does not rule out selenosis because the volatile selenides may escape quickly or cause olfactory accommodation.

TREATMENT

Treatment measures include removal of the source of selenium, elimination of selenium from the gut with saline purgatives such as magnesium sulfate, and providing symptomatic care such as oxygen therapy and treatment for circulatory shock. A high-protein diet is known to reduce the toxicity of selenium, but of course the animals have to eat in order for this to work. In chronic cases the feeding of salt containing arsenic (40 ppm) or a ration containing arsanilic acid (50–100 ppm) may benefit, but the mechanism for the toxicity-lowering effect of arsenicals in selenium toxicosis is not known. Arsenic also inhibits enzyme sulfhydryl groups and can cause vascular lesions if fed in excess. Thus arsenic feeding appears to make no sense, even though it seems to benefit some animals chronically poisoned by selenium.

Vitamin E is contraindicated because of its synergism with selenium (see Toxicity).

Attempts to strengthen the animal with a tonic dose of strychnine or neostigmine may help temporarily, but this kind of therapy (i.e., using one dangerous substance to treat symptoms of another) is open to criticism. This can also be said for treatment with arsenic. In chicks, selenium toxicosis has been reversed by feeding mercury, copper, or cadmium (Hill 1974), but such therapy is not recommended at present.

Actually, once the lesions of selenosis are well established, no treatment can heal them. But this may not always be so in the future. Ideally, one would want to be able to eliminate excess selenium from the body by some combination of acceleration of selenium detoxication plus chelation therapy and to restore vascular endothelial membrane integrity by correction of the biochemical lesions responsible for the loss of membrane integrity.

The sulfhydryl-containing chelator BAL is not effective in treating selenosis. It alleviates liver damage but worsens kidney damage. Other chelators, however, may prove useful in the future. In the chemical analysis of selenium, some special chelators are used. These include 1,2- and 2,3-diaminonaphthalene, 3,3′-diaminobenzidine, *o*-phenylenediamine, 4-nitro-*o*-phenylenediamine, and diaminochrysazine (Olson 1973; Shimoishi 1973; Young and Christian 1973; Brown 1975). It is possible that these or other *o*-diamines having the appropriate intermolecular distance between amine groups could be safe and effective chelators of selenium *in vivo*.

As for a way to speed detoxication of selenium and to partly restore vascular endothelial membrane integrity, it is possible that these aims could be met by parenteral administration of GSH and its precursor amino acids (glutamic acid, cysteine, glycine) plus sufficient glucose to provide excess substrate for generation of energy and $NADH_2$. This kind of treatment has not been tried.

ANALYSIS

Animal tissues normally contain only traces of selenium. Ingested selenium is excreted within a few days as long as the animal is healthy. Adult animals that die of selenosis generally have the following concentrations (in ppm) of selenium in the tissues: blood, 1–4 in chronic cases and up to 25 in acute cases; liver and kidney, 4–25; and urine, 0.1–8. Milk from poisoned cows may contain toxic amounts (3 ppm) of selenium. In chronic selenosis, bovine hoof and hair may contain selenium at 5–20 and 5–10 ppm, respectively, while equine hoof and hair may contain 11–45 and 11 ppm, respectively (Buck et al. 1973). In calves dying 48–72 hours after parenteral injection of about 0.5 mg Se/kg of body weight, liver and kidney may contain 1.5–3.1 ppm of selenium, but calves that take 30 days to die from the same dose of selenium may have only 0.76–0.89 ppm in these tissues (Shortridge et al. 1971).

These concentrations of selenium are of diagnostic significance if the history, signs, and lesions are compatible with selenium poisoning.

Ethylene Glycol

USE

Ethylene glycol is used mainly as an antifreeze additive in the coolant system of vehicle engines. Other substances that may contain ethylene glycol are hydraulic brake fluid, paints, and inks. Although ethylene glycol is a good solvent, vehicle, and hygroscopic liquid, its toxic properties have precluded its use in medicines intended for internal use.

SOURCE

Animals usually obtain ethylene glycol by drinking water drained from the radiator of a tractor, truck, or auto engine or by drinking the antifreeze directly from open containers.

PROPERTIES OF TOXICOLOGIC IMPORTANCE

Ethylene glycol has a sweet taste and looks like water. Thus it is attractive to some animals. The antifreeze product may be colored so that adult people will not mistake it for water or a soft drink, but this safety precaution does not deter animals (and children) from drinking it. Moreover, water drained from a radiator may dilute the color and also contain rust so the appearance is one of rusty or dirty water. Animals don't mind that either!

Ethylene glycol is 1,2-ethanediol ($HOCH_2CH_2OH$), a dihydric alcohol. It is miscible with water, other alcohols, glycerol, acetic acid, and short-chain aldehydes and ketones, but nearly insoluble in benzene, chlorinated hydrocarbon solvents, ethers, and oils. Thus attempts to remove it from the GI tract should rely on its water miscibility in spite of its slightly oily characteristics.

TOXICITY

The acute oral LD50 of ethylene glycol in rats and mice is 5.8 and 12 ml/kg of body weight, respectively, and is said to vary in small species from 3 to 13 ml/kg. The acute oral minimum lethal dose in ml/kg of body weight is: cat, 1–2.5; adult human being, 1.4 (but some people may survive 4 times this amount); dog, 4–5; and fowl, 7–8 (pigeons and geese are more resistant than other fowl) (Clarke and Clarke 1967; Forney and Harger 1971; Buck et al. 1973; Moriarty and McDonald 1974; Mundy et al. 1974; Penumarthy and Oehme 1975).

Obviously, it does not take much ethylene glycol to kill animals. Even the residue in an "empty" container might poison a cat or dog.

Toxicity is enhanced by kidney and liver disease, poor condition, and insufficient water supply. Animals that can vomit will do so after ingesting ethylene glycol. This may favor survival, although the substance is rapidly absorbed and the animal may die in spite of (and partly as a result of) severe and prolonged emesis. Possibly age and species variations in liver alcohol dehydrogenase activity may influence toxicity of ethylene glycol also.

Whether the toxicity of ethylene glycol is due to the substance itself or to one or more metabolic products has been debated (see below).

TOXICODYNAMIC CONSIDERATIONS

Ethylene glycol is rapidly absorbed from the GI tract and distributed throughout the body. Clinical signs of toxicosis may be due partly to ethylene glycol itself because it is more toxic in species (like the cat) that excrete the most oxalate and unchanged ethylene glycol in the urine and less toxic in species that can metabolize the substance to CO_2 and H_2O.

Ethylene glycol is degraded in the liver by alcohol dehydrogenase and other enzymes. The metabolic products are glyoxylate (formylformic acid), glycoaldehyde, glycolate (hydroxyacetic acid), oxalic acid, formic acid, glycine, CO_2, and H_2O. Several of these substances are toxic and probably contribute to the overall condition of ethylene glycol toxicosis. For more detail, refer to review material given by Sanyer et al. (1973), Moriarty and McDonald (1974), Penumarthy and Oehme (1975), and Van Stee et al. (1975).

Part of the oxalic acid formed from ethylene glycol reacts with blood calcium to form calcium oxalate which, if urine volume is small or if the amount of oxalic acid is relatively large, crystallizes in the renal tubules, causing nephrotic signs and lesions (see Clinical Signs, Lesions).

MECHANISM OF ACTION

Veterinarians used to think ethylene glycol toxicosis was due entirely to renal failure that resulted from blockage of renal tubules by calcium oxalate crystals. Actually, renal blockage occurs relatively late in the condition and may not always be so complete as to cause death from renal blockage alone.

The initial vomiting seen in dogs and cats is probably due in part to direct irritant effects of ethylene glycol on the gastric mucosa and the medullary chemoreceptor trigger zone. The early signs of depression, incoordination, and collapse are probably due to a direct depressant action of ethylene glycol and/or some of its metabolites in the brain. It is well known that alcohols are central depressants.

Acidosis is produced by ethylene glycol, although it is doubtful this is due directly to acid products of ethylene glycol itself because the blood is capable of neutralizing a large amount of exogenous and endogenous acids. The acidosis may be a result of some biochemical-respiratory effect of ethylene glycol or its metabolites. Glyoxylate may be the most toxic metabolite (Sanyer et al. 1973; Penumarthy and Oehme 1975); it is capable of inhibiting the citric acid cycle.

Along with metabolic acidosis, an increase and a later decrease in blood P_{O_2}, a decrease in body temperature, and increases in blood potassium, phosphate, urea, and creatinine are manifested. Blood calcium concentration decreases (Beckett and Shields 1971; Sanyer et al. 1973; Van Stee et al. 1975). None of these changes provides much insight into the exact mechanism by which ethylene glycol kills animals. We have to say that early death is probably due to direct depressant effects on the respiratory centers, complicated by muscle paralysis, metabolic acidosis, and other possible metabolic lesions. Delayed death is a result of uremia and subsequent cardiac arrest due to hyperkalemia and hypocalcemia. Convulsions, when they occur, are thought to be due to the deposition of calcium oxalate crystals in blood vessel walls and perivascular spaces in the brain.

CLINICAL SIGNS

Clinical signs are about the same in all species and occur in two phases. In the early or acute phase of poisoning (within 0.5–6 hours of ingestion of ethylene glycol) initial apprehension and vomiting occur. Rapid progression to depression, ataxia, weakness, flaccid paralysis beginning caudally, and decreased reflex responsiveness follow. There is also tachypnea and progressive hypothermia. Possible terminal clonic convulsions, then coma and death occur in a few hours or half a day.

It is possible for an animal to survive the acute phase and appear to recover. However, metabolic lesions are still present and calcium oxalate crystals are forming in the renal tubules. The net result of these processes is renal failure. This may become apparent 24 hours after ingestion of ethylene glycol. The clinical signs of this second phase of toxicosis include emesis, dehydration, weight loss, thirst, weakness, hematuria or anuria, ataxia, possible clonic convulsions, coma, and death in 1–3 days. In swine the chronic phase of poisoning is characterized by reluctance to move, fluid sounds in chest and abdomen, muffled heart sounds, and sternal recumbency, all being signs of fluid accumulation in the chest and peritoneal cavities.

LESIONS

Postmortem examination reveals congestion of all tissues, hemorrhagic gastritis or enteritis, pulmonary edema, a heart that is dilated and flaccid, and kidneys that are pale and streaked with gray or yellow, especially at the corticomedullary junction. Renal changes are most prominent in animals that survived the longest. Microscopically, pale yellow crystals of calcium oxalate are observed in the renal tubules; the tubules are distended and manifest flattened epithelial cells and varying degrees of degeneration, from hydropic changes to necrosis. The amount of renal degeneration does not necessarily correspond to the amount of calcium oxalate crystals present. In the brain, oxalate crystals can be found in and around blood vessel walls.

In swine, in addition to the above lesions, hydrothorax, ascites, edema of the abdominal wall, perirenal edema and edema of the terminal colon, lateral ligaments of the bladder, and mesometrium may be manifested. Petechial and ecchymotic hemorrhages may be found in the kidneys.

For detail on clinical signs and lesions, see Clarke and Clarke (1967), Beckett and Shields (1971), Osweiler and Eness (1972), Buck et al. (1973), Sanyer et al. (1973), Penumarthy and Oehme (1975), and Van Stee et al. (1975).

DIFFERENTIAL DIAGNOSIS

Antifreeze is often drained from coolant systems in late spring and added to coolant systems in late fall. Animals that manifest depressive and paralytic signs and then appear to recover only to develop uremia and die should be suspected of having ingested ethylene glycol, especially if there is a history of antifreeze manipulations on the premises.

Metaldehyde can cause signs and lesions similar to those of ethylene glycol in dogs. The differential diagnosis of these two agents is discussed under Metaldehyde.

A variety of diseases are accompanied by renal failure. These should be excluded by careful questioning and by examination of urine sediment and blood films. In ethylene glycol poisoning the urine contains many oxalate crystals; hematologic studies are not indicative of acute infectious disease.

Gross lesions of ethylene glycol poisoning are not pathognomonic of the condition. Even in swine the lesions of perirenal edema and other edematous changes may be produced by *Amaranthus retroflexus* (pigweed), *Solanum nigrum* (black nightshade), *Quercus* spp. (oaks), and mycotoxins such as those of *Penicillium viridicatum*. These materials do not, however, cause the accumulation of excess calcium oxalate crystals in the kidneys.

A number of plants contain sufficient concentrations of soluble oxalates to cause deposition of oxalate crystals in the kidneys plus other signs similar to those of ethylene glycol poisoning. These plants include *Beta* spp. (beet), *Halogeton* spp. (halogeton), *Oxalis* spp. (sorrell), *Portulaca oleracea* (purslane), *Rheum* spp. (rhubarb), *Rumex* spp. (dock), *Salsola* spp. (Russian thistle), and *Sarcobatus vermiculatus* (greasewood) (Kingsbury 1964). While these plants must be considered in the differential diagnosis of conditions involving oxalate nephrosis in horses and ruminants, it must be remembered that dogs and cats (species usually poisoned by ethylene glycol) do not graze on oxalate-containing plants!

Ethylene glycol toxicosis can occur in any species, however, and the veterinarian should not be surprised to be called upon to treat horses, cattle, calves, sheep, or swine for "antifreeze poisoning."

TREATMENT

The treatment of ethylene glycol toxicosis is mainly symptomatic. Emesis can be controlled with an antiemetic phenothiazine tranquilizer or antihistaminic. The stomach should be washed out with 5% sodium bicarbonate solution, taking care to prevent aspiration of stomach washings. Acidosis can be treated with sodium bicarbonate given intravenously. Convulsions can be controlled with small doses of an ultrashort-acting barbiturate (cat) or a short-acting barbiturate (other species). Stimulants are not recommended because they may induce convulsions and aggravate the acidosis or have no useful effect on respiration.

Uremia should be treated by standard methods such as peritoneal dialysis. Oxalate crystals in the kidneys are not easily removed. Bicarbonate administration may favor renal excretion of sodium and citrate, urinary alkalization, and combination of urinary citrate with calcium. This could reduce the available amount of calcium for the formation of calcium oxalate crystals but may also predispose to early cardiac arrest by aggravation of the existing state of hyperkalemia and hypocalcemia.

One target for more specific treatment of ethylene glycol toxicosis is alcohol dehydrogenase. If this enzyme could be inhibited, the formation of toxic metabolites of ethylene glycol might be decreased. Ethanol competes very well with ethylene glycol for the enzyme. Ethanol has been used (with bicarbonate) in the treatment of experimental ethylene glycol toxicosis in dogs (Sanyer et al. 1973) and cats (Penumarthy and Oehme 1975). The treatment is most successful in animals when dosages of ethylene glycol are small and when treatment is begun 4 hours after administration. Less success is achieved in animals given larger dosages of ethylene glycol and treated 6 hours later. It is doubtful that ethanol can save very many animals in practice because the amount of ethylene glycol ingested is not known (it could be several fatal doses), the animals are not presented for treatment early enough, or they die too soon to be transported to the veterinarian.

For those wishing to use the ethanol treatment, the dosage of ethanol in dogs is 5.5 ml/kg of body weight given intravenously as a 20% solution in isotonic saline every 4–6 hours for about 40 hours or more. With each administration of ethanol, bicarbonate is given intraperitoneally as a 5% solution in saline at the dosage rate of 8 ml/kg of body weight. The bicarbonate is meant to combat acidosis and could just as well be given in a more controlled way by intravenous administration.

In cats, ethanol-bicarbonate therapy consists of intraperitoneal injection of 5 ml of 20% ethanol in isotonic saline plus 6 ml of 5% sodium bicarbonate in isotonic saline/kg of body weight every 6–8 hours for about 56 hours or longer.

Hypnotic effects of ethanol may complicate matters, but these effects are less pronounced with each dose of ethanol.

Another inhibitor of alcohol dehydrogenase is pyrazole. Van Stee (1975) has shown that a large proportion of experimental dogs may survive 10–12.5 ml ethylene glycol/kg of body weight if they are treated within 6 hours with a regimen of sodium bicarbonate, B-complex vitamins, vitamin C, hydrocortisone, 5% glucose in water, and pyrazole. The pyrazole is administered intravenously at the rate of 0.9 mmol/kg of body weight initially, and then 0.5 mmol/kg at 6 and 30 hours thereafter. Van Stee points out that inhibition of aldehyde dehydrogenase (by disulfiram or by *n*-butyraldoxime) could possibly be a useful adjunct in the treatment of ethylene glycol toxicosis because this enzyme is probably involved in the production of toxic metabolites of ethylene glycol.

The prognosis for full recovery from ethylene glycol toxicosis is always guarded no matter what treatment is given. According to the study by Van Stee (1975), the prognosis may be grave if at 30 hours postexposure, acidosis, hypothermia, hypocalcemia, hyperphosphatemia, or rapidly rising BUN or serum creatinine concentration still exists.

ANALYSIS

Blood can be analyzed for ethylene glycol. Normally, no ethylene glycol is present in the bloodstream. Thus a positive test is diagnostically significant if a typical history, signs, and lesions of ethylene glycol toxicosis are manifested.

PLANT POISONS AFFECTING RESPIRATION BY UNKNOWN MECHANISMS

Lupinine and other alkaloids in lupines (*Lupinus* spp.) cause a variety of clinical signs in different species, i.e., signs that may mimic those of heavy metal or pesticide poisoning. Severe dyspnea or heavy breathing is characteristic of lupinosis, which is seen mainly in sheep.

Certain of the locoweeds (*Astragalus* spp.) do not produce true locoism at all, but a condition typified by paralytic manifestations; severe panting, dyspnea, or excitement; and possibly sudden death due to asphyxia. The causative plants are called "timber milk vetch" by local ranchers. The toxic principle could be a mineral, but this is only speculative at present.

Cocklebur sprouts (*Xanthium* sp.) contain hydroquinone. This substance causes a spectrum of clinical signs (usually in pigs) that can mimic those of other GI irritants. Dyspnea is a noticeable sign in cocklebur sprout poisoning, however.

Other plant poisons that can cause signs of respiratory insufficiency include coniine (from poison hemlock—*Conium* sp.), nicotine (from tobacco—*Nicotiana* spp.), isoquinoline alkaloids (from Dutchman's breeches and squirrel corn—*Dicentra* spp.), unknown principles in box (*Buxus* spp.), various principles from plants mentioned previously in this chapter, and nearly any other principle capable of causing central nervous stimulation, depression, or abdominal pain. See Kingsbury (1964) for more detail.

Obviously, respiratory insufficiency can be a secondary sign with a variety of poisons and is intimately associated with death from any cause. Thus the diagnostic significance of respiratory or circulatory insufficiency signs such as dyspnea or shock should be judged from a knowledge of the condition of the animal and the nature of other signs or complicating factors. No artificial classification of poisons, such as the one used herein, should be used as the sole basis of differential diagnosis of agents that can cause respiratory failure However, such a classification can be a useful guide.

REFERENCES

Agar, N. S., and O'Shea, T. 1975. Erythrocyte metabolism in normal and glutathione-deficient sheep. Am J Vet Res 36:953.

Agar, N. S.; Roberts, J.; and Sheedy, J. 1975. Certain features of erythrocytes of normal and glutathione-deficient sheep. Am J Vet Res 36:949.

Allaway, W. H. 1973. Selenium in the food chain. Cornell Vet 63:151.

Astwood, E. B. 1970. Thyroid and antithyroid drugs. In L. S. Goodman and A. Gilman, eds. The Pharmacological Basis of Therapeutics, 4th ed. New York: Macmillan.

Bamburg, J. R., and Strong, F. M. 1971. 12, 13-Epoxytrichothecenes. In S. Kadis, A. Ciegler, and S. J. Ajl, eds. Microbial Toxins, vol. 7. New York: Academic Press.

Beckett, S. D., and Shields, R. P. 1971. Treatment of acute ethylene glycol (antifreeze) toxicosis in the dog. J Am Vet Med Assoc 158:472.

Berg, G. L., ed. 1974. Farm Chemicals Handbook 1974. Willoughby, Ohio: Meister.

Beutler, E. 1969. Drug-induced hemolytic anemia. Pharmacol Rev 21:73.

———. 1975. Disorders in glutathione metabolism. Life Sci 16:1499.

Brown, B. R., Jr.; Sipes, I. G.; and Sagalyn, A. M. 1974. Mechanisms of acute hepatic toxicity: Chloroform, halothane, and glutathione. Anesthesiology 41:554.

Brown, J. H. 1973. Toxicology and Pharmacology of Venoms from Poisonous Snakes. Springfield, Ill.: Charles C Thomas.

Brown, R. S. 1975. Spectrophotometric determination of selenium (IV) with diaminochrysazine. Anal Chim Acta 74:441.

Buck, W. B.; Osweiler, G. D.; and Van Gelder, G. A. 1973. Clinical and Diagnostic Veterinary Toxicology. Dubuque, Iowa: Kendall/Hunt.

Burger, K. 1973. Organic Reagents in Metal Analysis. Elmsford, N.Y.: Pergamon Press.

Caldwell, P. T.; Ren, P.; and Bell, R. G. 1974. Warfarin and metabolism of vitamin K_1. Biochem Pharmacol 23:3353.

Cerami, A.; Allen, T. A.; Graziano, J. H.; de Furia, F. G.; Manning, J. M.; and Gillette, P. N. 1973. Pharmacology of cyanate. I. General effects on experimental animals. J Pharm Pharmacol 185:653.

Chung, C. W.; Trucksess, M. W.; Giles, A. L., Jr.; and Friedman, L. 1974. Rabbit skin test for estimation of T-2 toxin and other skin-irritating toxins in contaminated corn. J Assoc Off Anal Chem 57:1121.

Ciaccio, E. I. 1971. The vitamins. In J. R. DiPalma, ed. Drill's Pharmacology in Medicine, 4th ed. New York: McGraw-Hill.

Clarke, E. G. C., and Clarke, M. L. 1967. Garner's Veterinary Toxicology, 3rd ed. Baltimore: Williams & Wilkins.

Coburn, R. F., ed. 1970. Biological Effects of Carbon Monoxide, vol. 174. N.Y. Academy of Sciences.

Cundliffe, E.; Cannon, M.; and Davis, J. 1974. Mechanism of inhibition of eukaryotic protein synthesis by trichothecene fungal toxins. Proc Natl Acad Sci USA 71:30.

Deckert, F. W. 1974. Coumarin anticoagulants: A review of some current research areas. South Med J 67:1191.

Ebert, R. V. 1967. Acute diseases of the bronchi. In P. B. Beeson and W. McDermott, eds. Textbook of Medicine, 12th ed. Philadelphia: W. B. Saunders.

Egan, D. A., and Murrin, M. P. 1973. Copper concentration and distribution in the livers of equine fetuses, neonates and foals. Res Vet Sci 15:147.

Esplin, D. W. 1970. Antiseptics and disinfectants; fungicides; ectoparasiticides. In L. S. Goodman and A. Gilman, eds. The Pharmacological Basis of Therapeutics, 4th ed. New York: Macmillan.

Fassett, D. W. 1975. Cadmium: Biological effects and occurrence in the environment. Annu Rev Pharmacol 15:425.

Forney, R. B., and Harger, R. N. 1971. The alcohols. In J. R. DiPalma, ed. Drill's Pharmacology in Medicine, 4th ed. New York: McGraw-Hill.

Frankenberg, L., and Sörbo, B. 1975. Effect of cyanide antidotes on the metabolic conversion of cyanide to thiocyanate. Arch Toxicol 33:81.

Freeman, G.; Stephens, R. J.; Coffin, D. L.; and Stara, J. F. 1973. Changes in dogs' lungs after long-terms exposure to ozone. Arch Environ Health 26:209.

Freeman, G.; Juhos, L. T.; Furiosi, N. J.; Mussenden, R.; Stephens, R. J.; and Evans, M. J. 1974. Pathology of pulmonary disease from exposure to interdependent ambient gases (nitrogen dioxide and ozone). Arch Environ Health 29:203.

Friberg, L.; Piscator, M.; Nordberg, G. F.; and Kjellström, T. 1974. Cadmium in the Environment, 2nd ed. Cleveland: CRC Press.

Friedberg, K. D., and Shukla, U. R. 1975. The effciency of aquocobalamine as an antidote in cyanide poisoning when given alone or combined with sodium thiosulfate. Arch Toxicol 33:103.

Gerarde, H. W. 1971. Noxious gases and vapors. II. Hydrocarbon mixtures. In J. R. DiPalma, ed. Drill's Pharmacology in Medicine, 4th ed. New York: McGraw-Hill.

Giddens, W. E., Jr.; Whitehair, C. K.; and Sleight, S. D. 1970. Nitrogen dioxide (silo gas) poisoning in pigs. Am J Vet Res 31:1779.

Gillette, J. R.; Mitchell, J. R.; and Brodie, B. B. 1974. Biochemical mechanisms of drug toxicity. Annu Rev Pharmacol 14:271.

Goldsmith, J. R., and Landaw, S. A. 1968. Carbon monoxide and human health. Science 162:1352.

Gopinath, C.; Hall, G. A.; and Howell, J. M. 1974. The effect of chronic copper poisoning on the kidneys of sheep. Res Vet Sci 16:57.

Graziano, J. H.; Thornton, Y. S.; Leong, J. K.; and Cerami, A. 1973. Pharmacology of cyanate. II. Effects on the endocrine system. J Pharmacol Exp Ther 185:667.

Graziano, J. H.; Grady, R. W.; and Cerami, A. 1974. The identification of 2,3-dihydroxybenzoic acid as a potentially useful iron-chelating drug. J Pharmacol Exp Ther 190:570.

Hafeman, D. G.; Sunde, R. A.; and Hoekstra, W. G. 1974. Effect of dietary selenium on erythrocyte and liver glutathione peroxidase in the rat. J Nutr 104:580.

Hammond, P. B. 1965. Rodenticides. In L. M. Jones, ed. Veterinary Pharmacology and Therapeutics, 3rd ed. Ames: Iowa State Univ. Press.

Hatch, R. C. 1967. Restraint, preanesthetic medication, and postanesthetic medication of dogs with chlorpromazine and atropine. J Am Vet Med Assoc 150:27.

———. 1972a. Effect of autonomic blocking agents on development of acute tolerance to thiopental in dogs. Am J Vet Res 33:365.

———. 1972b. Interaction of barbital with glutathione and adenine *in vitro*: Relevance to barbiturate anesthesia. Am J Vet Res 33:1263.

Hayes, W. J., Jr. 1971. Insecticides, rodenticides, and other economic poisons. In J. R. DiPalma, ed. Drill's Pharmacology in Medicine, 4th ed. New York: McGraw-Hill.

Heywood, R.; Sortwell, R. J.; Kelly, P. J.; and Street, A. E. 1972. Toxicity of sodium chlorate to the dog. Vet Rec 90:416.

Hill, C. H. 1974. Reversal of selenium toxicity in chicks by mercury, copper and cadmium. J Nutr 104:593.

Hillman, B., and Bardhan, K. D. 1974. The use of dicobalt edetate (Kelocyanor) in cyanide poisoning. Postgrad Med J 50:171.

Hooper, P. T. 1972. Spongy degeneration in the brain in relation to hepatic disease and ammonia toxicity in domestic animals. Vet Rec 90:37.

Howell, J. M.; Blakemore, W. F.; Gopinath, C.; and Hall, G. A. 1974. Chronic copper poisoning and changes in the central nervous system of sheep. Acta Neuropathol (Berl) 29:9.

Isom, G., and Way, J. L. 1973. Cyanide intoxication: Protection with cobaltous chloride. Toxicol Appl Pharmacol 24:449.

Jerina, D. M., and Daly, J. W. 1974. Arene oxides: A new aspect of drug metabolism. Science 185:573.

Jones, L. M., ed. 1965. Veterinary Pharmacology and Therapeutics, 3rd ed. Ames: Iowa State Univ. Press.

Karzel, K.; Tauberger, G.; and Ayertey, E. K. 1974. Elektrolytgehalt des Blutes sowie der Herz- und Skelettmuskulatur bei der akuten experimentellen Cyanidvergiftung. Arch Int Pharmacodyn Ther 209:259.

Kavet, R. I., and Brain, J. D. 1974. Reaction of the lung to air pollutant exposure. Life Sci 15:849.

Kilburn, K. H., ed. 1974. Pulmonary Reactions to Organic Materials. vol. 221. New York: N.Y. Academy of Sciences.

Kingsbury, J. M. 1964. Poisonous Plants of the United States and Canada. Englewood Cliffs, N.J.: Prentice-Hall.

Lal, S.; Papeschi, R.; Duncan, R. J. S.; and Sourkes, T. L. 1974. Effect of copper loading on various tissue enzymes and brain monoamines in the rat. Toxicol Appl Pharmacol 28:395.

Lay, M.-M.; Hubbell, J. P.; and Casida, J. E. 1975. Dichloroacetamide antidotes for thiocarbamate herbicides: Mode of action. Science 189:287.

Legendre, A. M. 1973. Disophenol toxicosis in a dog. J Am Vet Med Assoc 163:149.

Levine, W. G. 1970. Anticoagulants. In L. S. Goodman and A. Gilman, eds. The Pharmacological Basis of Therapeutics, 4th ed. New York: Macmillan.

Lillehoj, E. B. 1973. Feed sources and conditions conducive to production of aflatoxin, ochratoxin, *Fusarium* toxins, and zearalenone. J Am Vet Med Assoc 163:1281.

London, W. T.; Henderson, W.; and Cross, R. F. 1967. An attempt to produce chronic nitrite toxicosis in swine. J Am Vet Med Assoc 150:398.

McCosker, P. J. 1968. Observations on blood copper in the sheep. II. Chronic copper poisoning. Res Vet Sci 9:103.

Meister, A. 1973. On the enzymology of amino acid transport. Science 180:33.

———. 1975. Function of glutathione in kidney via the γ-glutamyl cycle. Med Clin North Am 1:649.

Mitchell, J. R.; Thorgeirsson, S. S.; Potter, W. Z.; Jollow, D. J.; and Keiser, H. 1974. Acetaminophen-induced hepatic injury: Protective role of glutathione in man and rationale for therapy. Clin Pharmacol Ther 16:676.

Moriarty, R. W., and McDonald, R. H., Jr. 1974. The spectrum of ethylene glycol poisoning. Clin Toxicol 7:583.

Mundy, R. L.; Hall, L. M.; and Teague, R. S. 1974. Pyrazole as an antidote for ethylene glycol poisoning. Toxicol Appl Pharmacol 28:320.

Mylrea, P. J., and Byrne, D. T. 1974. An outbreak of acute copper poisoning in calves. Aust Vet J 50:169.

Needleman, P., and Johnson, E. M., Jr. 1973. Mechanism of tolerance development to organic nitrates. J Pharmacol Exp Ther 184:709.

Nelsestuen, G. L.; Zytkoviez, T. H.; and Howard, J. B. 1974. The mode of action of vitamin K: Identification of γ-carboxyglutamic acid as a component of prothrombin. J Biol Chem 249:6347.

Newberne, P. M. 1974. The new world of mycotoxins—Animal and human health. Clin Toxicol 7:161.

Nickerson, M. 1970. Vasodilator drugs. In L. S. Goodman and A. Gilman, eds. The Pharmacological Basis of Therapeutics, 4th ed. New York: Macmillan.

Olson, O. E. 1973. Simplified spectrophotometric analysis of plants for selenium. J Assoc Off Anal Chem 56:1073.

Osweiler, G. D., and Eness, P. G. 1972. Ethylene glycol poisoning in swine. J Am Vet Med Assoc 160:746.

Penha, P. D., and Werthamer, S. 1974. Pulmonary lesions induced by long-term exposure to ozone. II. Ultrastructure observations of proliferative and regressive lesions. Arch Environ Health 29:282.

Penumarthy, L., and Oehme, F. W. 1975. Treatment of ethylene glycol toxicosis in cats. Am J Vet Res 36:209.

Pier, A. C. 1973. An overview of the mycotoxicoses of domestic animals. J Am Vet Med Assoc 163:1259.

Radeleff, R. D. 1970. Veterinary Toxicology, 2nd ed. Philadelphia: Lea & Febiger.

Reid. W. D.; Krishna. G.; Gillette, J. R.; and Brodie, B. B. 1973. Biochemical mechanism of hepatic necrosis induced by aromatic hydrocarbons. Pharmacology 10:193.

Rentsch, G., and Wittekind, D. 1967. Methylene blue and erythrocytes in the living animal. Contribution to the toxicology of methylene blue and formation of heinz bodies. Toxicol Appl Pharmacol 11:81.

Ridder, W. E., and Oehme, F. W. 1974. Nitrates as an environmental, animal, and human hazard. Clin Toxicol 7:145.

Rotruck, J. T.; Pope, A. L.; Ganther, H. E.; and Hoekstra, W. G. 1972. Prevention of oxidative damage to rat erythrocytes by dietary selenium. J Nutr 102:689.

Rowe, L. D.; Dollahite, J. W.; and Camp, B. J. 1973. Toxicity of two crude oils and of kerosene to cattle. J Am Vet Med Assoc 162:61.

Sansi, K. A. O., and Pond, W. G. 1974. Pathology of dietary cadmium toxicity in growing rats and the protective effect of injected iron. Nutr Rep Int 9:407.

Sanyer, J. L.; Oehme, F. W.; and McGavin, M. D. 1973. Systematic treatment of ethylene glycol toxicosis in dogs. Am J Vet Res 34:527.

Schneider, N. R., and Yeary, R. A. 1975. Nitrite and nitrate pharmacokinetics in the dog, sheep, and pony. Am J Vet Res 36:941.

Shaw, C.-M.; Papayannopoulou, T.; and Stamatoyannopoulos, G. 1974. Neuropathology of cyanate toxicity in rhesus monkeys. Pharmacology 12:166.

Sheahan, B. J.; Pugh, D. M.; and Winstanley, E. W. 1971. Experimental sodium chlorate poisoning in dogs. Res Vet Sci 12:387.

Sheehy, M. H., and Way, J. L. 1974. Nitrite intoxication: Protection with methylene blue and oxygen. Toxicol Appl Pharmacol 30:221.

Shimoishi, Y. 1973. The determination of selenium in sea water by gas chromatography with electron-capture detection. Anal Chim Acta 64:465.

Shortridge, E. H.; O'Hara, P. J.; and Marshall, P. M. 1971. Acute selenium poisoning in cattle. NZ Vet J 19:47.

Simmons, J. R., and Scott, W. A. 1974. An outbreak of metaldehyde poisoning in sheep. Vet Rec 95:211.

Sinclair, K. B., and Jones, D. I. H. 1967. Nitrite toxicity in sheep. Res Vet Sci 8:65.

Smalley, E. B. 1973. T-2 toxin. J Am Vet Med Assoc 163:1278.

Smith, H. A.; Jones, T. C.; and Hunt, R. D. 1972. Veterinary Pathology, 4th ed. Philadelphia: Lea & Febiger.

Smith, R. P. 1973. Cyanate and thiocyanate: Acute toxicity. Proc Soc Exp Biol Med 142:1041.

Smith, R. P., and Abbanat, R. A. 1966. Protective effect of oxidized glutathione in acute sulfide poisoning. Toxicol Appl Pharmacol 9:209.

Sollmann, T. 1957. A Manual of Pharmacology and Its Application to Therapeutics and Toxicology, 8th ed. Philadelphia: W. B. Saunders.

Stadtman, T. C. 1974. Selenium biochemistry. Science 183:915.

Stanford, G. K.; Hood, R. D.; and Hayes, A. W. 1975. Effect of prenatal administration of T-2 toxin to mice. Res Commun Chem Pathol Pharmacol 10:743.

Stecher, P. G., ed. 1968. The Merck Index, 8th ed. Rahway, N.J.: Merck.

Stossel, T. P., and Jennings, R. B. 1966. Failure of methylene blue to produce methemoglobinemia *in vivo*. Am J Clin Pathol 45:600.

Stowe, H. D.; Goyer, R. A.; Medley, P.; and Cates, M. 1974. Influence of dietary pyridoxine on cadmium toxicity in rats. Arch Environ Health 28:209.

Suttie, J. W.; Grant, G. A.; Esmon, C. T.; and Shah, D. V. 1974. Postribosomal function of vitamin K in prothrombin synthesis. Mayo Clin Proc 49:933.

Thienes, C. H., and Haley, T. J. 1972. Clinical Toxicology, 5th ed. Philadelphia: Lea & Febiger.

Thompson, R. H., and Todd, J. R. 1974. Muscle damage in chronic copper poisoning of sheep. Res Vet Sci 16:97.

Travis, R. H., and Sayers, G. 1970. Insulin and oral hypoglycemic drugs. In L. S. Goodman and A. Gilman, eds. The Pharmacological Basis of Therapeutics, 4th ed. New York: Macmillan.

Udall, N. D. 1973. The toxicity of the molluscicides metaldehyde and methiocarb to dogs. Vet Rec 93:420.

Van Fleet, J. F.; Meyer, K. B.; and Olander, H. J. 1974. Acute selenium toxicosis induced in baby pigs by parenteral administration of selenium-vitamin E preparations. J Am Vet Med Assoc 165:543.

Van Stee, E. W.; Harris, A. M.; Horton, M. L.; and Back, K. C. 1975. The treatment of ethylene glycol toxicosis with pyrazole. J Pharmacol Exp Ther 192:251.

Verschuuren, H. G.; Kroes, R.; Den Tonkelaar, E. M.; Berkvens, J. M.; Helleman, P. W.; and Van Esch, G. J. 1975. Long-term toxicity and reproduction studies with metaldehyde in rats. Toxicology 4:97.

Werthamer, S.; Penha, P. D.; and Amaral, L. 1974. Pulmonary lesions induced by chronic exposure to ozone. I. Biochemical alterations. Arch Environ Health 29:164.

Young, J. W., and Christian, G. D. 1973. Gas-chromatographic determination of selenium. Anal Chim Acta 65:127.

CHAPTER 58

POISONS CAUSING NERVOUS STIMULATION OR DEPRESSION

ROGER C. HATCH

POISONS DIRECTLY DAMAGING THE BRAIN OR SPINAL CORD

Salt (Water Deprivation)

USE

Salt is an essential nutrient. It is also added to rations to increase or decrease palatability, depending on how much ration the animals are meant to eat.

SOURCE

Salt is normally present at about 0.5%–1% concentration in feeds. Large amounts of salt may be fed in mash made with brine or whey, in garbage, or in improperly compounded feeds. Salt licks, or free-choice trace mineralized salt are a source of salt, and the drinking water may also contain salt. In addition, there may be other sources of sodium (e.g., drug salts) that can precipitate toxicosis.

PROPERTIES OF TOXICOLOGIC IMPORTANCE

One obvious property of salt is its taste, which is attractive to animals. Another property is the relatively mild irritant effect of salt on mucous membranes; i.e., animals can ingest large amounts of salt without manifesting nausea, vomiting, or other external signs of gastric irritation. Such signs can develop, however, if enough salt is consumed in a short period.

TOXICITY

Swine and poultry are most susceptible to so-called salt poisoning, but other species can also develop toxicosis. The acute oral lethal dose of salt is about 2.2 g/kg of body weight in horses, cattle, and swine; 6 g/kg in sheep; and 4 g/kg in dogs (Buck et al. 1973). These numbers are misleading, however, for they are affected by two major factors: (1) degree of salt hunger, i.e., a salt-hungry animal will consume large amounts of salt and tend to overdose itself, and (2) availability of drinking water. If animals have free access to sufficient water, large concentrations (up to 13% of the ration of swine) can be tolerated without apparent ill effect. Thus the very term "salt poisoning" is a misnomer, although the term is still in general use to designate a condition that is presently considered to be *water deprivation–induced sodium toxicosis.* This nomenclature too is questionable because sodium may be involved only by the coincidence that it is a major feed constituent involved in maintenance of tissue water balance.

TOXICODYNAMIC CONSIDERATIONS

Salt is rapidly absorbed from the intestinal tract and distributed throughout the body. Sodium and chloride ions have a number of essential functions in the body. One major function, which is attributed more to sodium than to chloride ion, is maintenance of proper water balance between cells and interstitial spaces. If dietary intake of salt is large, the excess of absorbed sodium is normally excreted rapidly by the kidneys, as long as there is enough water present to accompany the sodium ions osmotically into the urine. The animal normally increases water consumption to provide the water necessary for sodium excretion. If the animal does *not* increase water consumption in response to the thirst generated by excess sodium (hypertonicity of blood), the excess sodium in the blood can initiate a sequence of events that culminates in toxicosis.

MECHANISM OF ACTION

The exact molecular mechanisms of salt poisoning are still being debated. A logical chain of events might be as follows:

1. Ingestion of excess salt. "Excess" means nearly any concentration of salt under conditions of water deprivation or water insufficiency in hot or windy conditions or in active animals. Under these circumstances the animal body loses rather large amounts of water by sensible and insensible routes of elimination.

2. Mild irritation of gastrointestinal (GI) linings, causing vague digestive signs. Also, the presence of a large concentration of salt in the gut may cause diarrhea by acting as a saline cathartic. Animals that later become dehydrated may absorb some water from the colon and rectum and thus manifest constipation.

3. Absorption of salt from the intestine, with resulting hypertonicity of blood.

4. Extreme thirst due to activation of osmoreceptor mechanisms in the brain.

5. At the same time there might be shrinkage of kidney tubule cells due to osmotic attraction of water from the tubule cells into the blood. This would cause widening of urine and blood channels in the kidney (Sollmann 1957) and enhance the next effect.

6. Polyuria of a transient nature due to initial excretion of salt in the urine. Water would accompany the salt by osmotic attraction, but this effect would soon be limited by the increasing osmotic pressure of the blood.

7. Simultaneously, the excess salt in the bloodstream would tend to shrink capillary vascular endothelial cells in the brain and meninges, thus opening wide the perivascular spaces of Virchow-Robin (Rapoport 1970; Rapoport et al. 1971; Rapoport et al. 1972; Rapoport and Thompson 1973). This effect would be expected to be very prominent in the brain and meninges because of the large blood supply (vascularity) of these structures. Other organs would also be expected to manifest shrinkage of capillary endothelial cells.

8. Salt would escape from the blood into secretions (e.g., saliva, mucosal secretions) and into serosal fluids. Water would accompany this salt (by osmosis) and cause the hypersalivation, nasal secretions, hydropericardium, hydrothorax, and ascites

seen in salt poisoning. Damage to capillary endothelium would enhance these fluid accumulations.

9. Shrinkage of capillary endothelial cells would increase capillary permeability and allow water to escape from the blood into the interstitial spaces. This edema would predominate in the brain because of the rich vascular supply to this organ, but some edema would also be expected to occur in other organs and tissues.

10. Sodium would be distributed in large concentrations throughout the body, but the cerebrospinal fluid (CSF) would be expected to contain a larger concentration of sodium than the plasma because of the rich blood supply to the brain and because of the pronounced increase in brain capillary permeability mentioned above. It has been shown that CSF sodium concentration *is* higher than plasma sodium concentration in pigs that die of salt poisoning (Osweiler and Hurd 1974).

11. The excess sodium in the CSF would also diffuse into brain cells, thus making them hypertonic with respect to CSF. Water would then enter the brain cells and overhydrate them. The cerebral edema of salt poisoning would be due to leakage of water from damaged capillaries and also to osmotic attraction of water into CSF and brain cells.

12. Pronounced signs of nervous derangement seen in salt poisoning are probably due mainly to overhydration of brain cells. Similar signs can be produced in dogs by overhydration of brain cells by force-feeding water (Sollmann 1957), by using urea infusion to cause cerebral edema (Hammond 1965), or by hydration of rat or mouse brain cells by intraperitoneal injection of water or isosmolar glucose solution (Swinyard 1969; and previous work by this well-known worker in the field of anticonvulsant screening).

Some of the neurological signs seen in salt poisoning could be due to physical damage to neurons or synapses caused by the tearing apart of brain tissues by fluid accumulations. The malacia and necrosis seen in the brain of some animals could be due to circulatory disruption by this physical damage.

In the above presentation, sodium starts out to be the major offender in salt poisoning but the actual clinical signs and most of the lesions are due to *water.* Thus although the pathogenesis of salt poisoning has not been confirmed experimentally, it might be prudent to play down sodium in naming the toxicosis caused by ingestion of excess salt. Perhaps the condition should be called *water deprivation–induced sodium–dependent water toxicosis,* or more simply, *sodium-water toxicosis.*

Once developed, brain cell overhydration due to attraction of water into cells by sodium is considered almost irreversible. This may be due to the fact that sodium extrusion from excitable cells requires energy. This energy may be unavailable because sodium may inhibit cellular glycolysis (Hammond 1965; Buck et al. 1973). Death from salt poisoning is probably due to combined metabolic lesions in vital organs (from overhydration and antiglycolytic effects of sodium) and physical damage from edema fluids in the brain.

One peculiar lesion of salt poisoning is seen only in pigs. It consists of the filling of cerebral and meningeal perivascular spaces with eosinophils (so-called eosinophilic meningoencephalitis). This lesion, though pathognomonic of salt poisoning in pigs, has not been explained. Since the lesion occurs only in pigs, the author sees no reason to attribute special importance to it in the pathogenesis of salt poisoning in animals. It is conceivable that the physical damage done to brain tissue surrounding the Virchow-Robin spaces triggers the release of a chemical factor that is peculiar to the porcine species and that eosinophils then enter the perivascular spaces through the distended capillary pores by a process of chemotaxis. Later on the eosinophils disappear from the perivascular spaces, perhaps because the chemotactic substance ceases to be liberated or is washed out or diluted in the edema process. Certainly, chemotaxis is not some unusual phenomenon, for it occurs throughout the body whenever leucocytes are needed in tissues (e.g., in inflammation). What is unusual about the leucocyte lesion in salt poisoning of pigs is that the leucocytes are eosinophils and are confined to the perivascular spaces of the brain and meninges.

CLINICAL SIGNS

Signs attributable to excess salt in the GI tract include anorexia, diarrhea, possible vomiting, and colic. Excess salt in the bloodstream may cause hypersalivation, thirst, polyuria, nasal discharge, and possible constipation. Excess water in the pericardium and body cavities may cause muffling of normal sounds ausculated from the chest or abdomen. There may be fluid sounds in the lungs. Cerebral edema and brain cell overhydration may cause a variety of signs, depending on severity of the condition. These include initial hypersensitivity or excitement, shivering, tremors, muscle twitching, normal body temperature, blindness, deafness, unresponsiveness to stimuli or environment, refusal of water or inability to drink, wandering about, stumbling, circling, pivoting, walking backwards, pushing against objects, standing with back arched and hind legs forward while swaying weakly, prostration, intermittent clonic-tonic opisthotonic seizures, paddling of limbs, coma, and death in a few hours or a few days. These signs are about the same for most species, although poultry tend to manifest weakness and paralysis rather than motor excitation phenomena (Clarke and Clarke 1967; Radeleff 1970; Smith et al. 1972; Buck et al. 1973).

LESIONS

At postmortem examination, gastric congestion or inflammation with pinpoint ulceration, dark fluid feces or dry feces, tissue and organ edema, fluid in body cavities and pericardium, and a prominent cerebral edema with possible malacia or early necrosis may be observed. Under the microscope, the brain manifests vascular endothelial proliferation, distended perivascular spaces (possibly filled with eosinophils in the pig), vacuolization and disruption of the area between cortex and white matter, and histiocytosis in subcortical white matter. In chicks the liver is congested. If the chicks were poisoned by salty mash, edema of various tissues predominates. If the chicks were poisoned by salty water, urate nephritis may predominate (see references cited above).

DIFFERENTIAL DIAGNOSIS

The history of salt (or sodium compound) ingestion and relative water scarcity or deprivation, taken with the encephalitic signs and postmortem findings, should indicate salt poisoning, particularly in pigs. Clinical signs may be confused with infectious diseases, but clinical pathological and microbiological tests should rule these out. Signs may also be similar to those produced by lead and other heavy metals (with which GI signs may be severe), chlorinated hydrocarbon pesticides (which generally cause fever and no thirst), or organophosphate pesticides (which cause parasympathomimetic signs). Anything that damages the brain can cause encephalitic signs. Thus the veterinarian may wish to give some consideration to trauma, tumor, vitamin deficiency, or heat stroke. Other agents that can cause signs of nervous stimulation include solvents, carbon monoxide, asphyxiants, penicillin overdose (in baby pigs), cyanide, metaldehyde, nicotine, tranquilizer overdose, ergot mold toxins, fluoride, and a variety of plant poisons listed in this chapter.

TREATMENT

The ideal treatment for salt poisoning would be to "pull" sodium out of brain cells, CSF, and tissues so that sodium and water could enter the blood and be excreted in the urine. Once the excess sodium was eliminated from the body, most of the clinical signs and lesions would disappear (theoretically). Unfortunately, no such treatment exists. Giving a strongly natriuretic diuretic would not likely reverse the sodium-inhibited glycolytic cycle and enable sodium to be pumped out of brain cells. Giving water in large amounts would likely kill the animal by producing more cerebral edema (remember, the brain cells and CSF are hypertonic with respect to the blood). Anticonvulsant medication would not correct the cause of the convulsions.

If the animal is ambulatory, it may recover by itself if it is provided with drinking water. The probability of recovery may be 50% or less. If the animal is recumbent and convulsing, little can be done.

ANALYSIS

Pig feed containing 2.5% salt can cause death if water is restricted. With cattle, intake of salt in feed can safely amount to 900 g total/day or drinking water can contain up to 0.9%–1.1% salt, but the two sources of salt are additive in potential toxicity. If feed is salty, then water should not be salty. Sheep can safely ingest 1% salt in the ration if provided adequate salt-free water. For sheep, drinking water may contain up to 0.9%–1.7% salt, but the feed must not contain salt. For horses, drinking water can contain up to 0.5%–0.9% salt if the ration is relatively salt-free. With adult chickens the dry ration can be fatal if it contains 20%–30% salt, but ducks may become ill and manifest decreased growth, decreased fertility, and decreased egg hatchability if dry feed contains 2% salt. For chicks the maximum safe concentration of salt in drinking water is 0.25%. Wet mash can be rapidly fatal for chicks if it contains 5%–10% salt.

Generally speaking, any concentration of salt in feed or water could be diagnostically meaningful if the history, clinical signs, and lesions are compatible with salt poisoning. In pigs the diagnosis can be reinforced if CSF contains a larger concentration of sodium than plasma, if sodium chloride exceeds 0.51%, 0.26%, or 0.165% in stomach, small intestine, and large intestine, respectively, or if liver chloride concentration exceeds 0.33%–0.35%. In ruminants a chloride concentration larger than 0.36% in the small intestine may be of diagnostic significance.

For references, see Hammond (1965), Clarke and Clarke (1967), Smith et al. (1972), and Osweiler and Hurd (1974).

ORGANOMERCURIALS IN DOGS, CATS, AND CALVES

Now that seed grains are no longer dressed with mercurial antifungal compounds, mercury poisoning in farm animals is not so common. Yet, environmental pollution problems are widespread and mercury is present in some industrial wastes. Thus the potential for poisoning of animals by mercury has not disappeared.

Animals may ingest toxic amounts of mercury if they drink polluted water or eat meat or processed food from animals in which mercury (Hg) has accumulated as methylmercury or other alkylmercury compounds.

Central nervous stimulation is seen in dogs, cats, and calves poisoned by organomercurials. Other species (adult cattle, swine, fowl) manifest central nervous depression. Sheep manifest GI signs (see Chapter 59).

In dogs and cats the toxic dosage of methylmercury is 0.4–1 mg Hg/kg of body weight when consumed in multiple feedings over a period of 10–90 days, a cumulative dosage of 10–20 mg/kg. In cats, 2 or 3 mg of ethylmercury or diethylmercury compounds/kg/day cause clinical signs in 2–3 weeks and death in 2 more weeks (Buck et al. 1973). Methylmercury fed to cats at a dosage rate of 0.25 mg Hg/kg/day, either as the pure compound or in methylmercury-contaminated fish, causes marked clinical signs in 55–96 days, when total dosage of mercury is 14–24 mg/kg (Charbonneau et al. 1974).

In calves the toxic dosage of methylmercury is about 0.4 mg Hg/kg of body weight when fed over a period of 35 days, a total dosage of 11.7 mg Hg/kg (Herigstad et al. 1972). In another experiment, this time with an ethylmercurial compound, it took 36 days for a calf to become ill when given a daily dosage of the compound at the rate of 4.72 mg Hg/kg of body weight (Oliver and Platonow 1960).

Clinical signs of alkylmercury poisoning in dogs, cats, and calves are similar to those seen in rats, primates, and human beings. The signs seen in a dog were blindness, convulsions, and involuntary chewing movements every 30 seconds, but the electroencephalogram was normal (Kahrs 1968). In cats the signs are (in sequence) posterior weakness and incoordination, gradual onset of ataxia (cerebellar "zigzag" type, with sudden head movements) and hind leg rigidity, compensatory widening of stance, high-step gait, and intention tremors. Further signs are loss of the righting reflex and inability to land on the feet when jumping; occurrence of tonic-clonic convulsions that are signaled by a glassy stare of the eyes; followed by vocalization, hypersalivation, and urinary incontinence. Vision and other senses are impaired if cats convulse intermittently for more than 1 day, but hearing and segmental reflexes are not lost (Charbonneau et al. 1974). Electroencephalogram patterns change 2–3 weeks before onset of neurological signs in cats fed 0.25 mg methylmercury/kg of body weight. Blood mercury concentration is correlated with onset and severity of poisoning and ranges from 12.7 (electroencephalogram changes) to 16.3 ppm (Willes et al. 1975).

Clinical signs in calves given organomercurials over a period of several days or weeks include sudden onset of ataxia and incoordination; body swaying; stumbling; stilted gait; side-to-side head movements; twitching of eyelid, ear, and neck muscles; hypersensitivity to external stimuli; normal to subnormal temperature; good appetite but inability to secure and swallow food; salivation; tremors; GI signs; electrocardiogram changes; possible head-pressing (see Lead); possible visual defect; recumbency; paddling of the limbs; and clonic or tonic convulsions with opisthotonos, coma, and death (Oliver and Platonow 1960; Herigstad et al. 1972).

Postmortem findings in the dog include irregular reduction in size of dorsal gyri of the cerebellum, with widening of sulci and subdural space. Microscopically, diffuse astrogliosis in cerebral cortex, demyelination of corticospinal pathways, and degenerative changes in neurons of cerebral cortex and subcortical nuclei occur (Kahrs 1968). In cats, lesions include gray discoloration of the leptomeninges and microscopic changes such as disintegration of visual, auditory, and other sensory neurons of the cerebral cortex; proliferation of microglia; and loss of granular cells and Purkinje cells of the dorsal cerebellum, with proliferation of Bergman glial cells. No lesions occur in the spinal cord, peripheral nerve, kidneys, or other organs. The signs and lesions in cats appear when mercury concentrations in ppm (wet weight) are: blood, 14–17; cerebral cortex, 17–18; cerebellum, 27–29; spinal cord, 8–10; sciatic nerve, 8–10; liver, 72–74; kidney, 37; and gastrocnemius muscle, 22–24 (Charbonneau et al. 1974).

The lesions of organomercurial poisoning in calves are mainly microscopic and consist of degeneration and reduction in number of cerebellar Purkinje cells, with edema or hemorrhages in the cerebellar cortex and gliosis in the molecular and granular layers. There may be neuronal degeneration, gliosis, and focal malacia in the cerebrum. The spinal cord manifests edema and hemorrhage in myelin sheaths in the dorsal horn area. Degenerative changes may occur in myocardial fibers and cardiac Purkinje fibers. The kidneys may manifest focal to diffuse toxic nephrosis in the proximal convoluted tubules. Grossly pale areas of skeletal muscle manifest fragmented, hyalinized, necrotic fibers under the microscope. Hematologic changes are minimal and nonspecific (Oliver and Platonow 1960; Herigstad et al. 1972). In the study by Oliver and Platonow, concentrations of mercury in the kidney cortex at time of death ranged from 30 (highest dosage) to 107 ppm (lowest dosage). In the liver, concentrations of mercury were 46–108 ppm. Other tissues had variable and lesser amounts of mercury. Herigstad et al. found that in calves the concentration of mercury in body hair was the best index of exposure to methylmercury compounds.

Alkylmercurials would seem to kill dogs, cats, and calves by destroying cerebral and cerebellar neurons (but see also Organomercurials in Adult Cattle, Swine, and Fowl). The exact mechanism for this cell destruction is not known. Chang and Hartman (1972) confirm the findings of Steinwall and Olsson (1969) that small concentrations of mercurials damage the blood-brain barrier of rats. It is postulated that neuronal damage may result from a combination of direct toxic effects of blood solutes normally excluded from the brain and failure of mercury-inhibited or mercury-damaged blood-brain barrier transport mechanisms to supply neurons with essential amino acids and other metabolites. Taking this postulate a bit further, it seems that a defect in protein synthesis could be the initial biochemical lesion in neurons poisoned by organomercurials. In dogs given a large dosage of methylmercury, protein synthesis by brain cells is inhibited *before* there are any neurological signs. Also, clinical signs in poisoned animals are accompanied by structural changes in neuronal ribosomes, the sites of protein synthesis (Clarkson 1972). As to the *cause* of a defect in protein synthesis, perhaps the report of Kasuya (1975) is relevant. He finds that the membrane-stabilizing effects of vitamin E protect cultured cerebellar cells of newborn rats against methylmercury and ethylmercury. Possibly, the organomercurials disrupt membranes of subcellular structures such as lysosomes and ribosomes, thus affecting protein synthesis and cell integrity.

The ability of mercury ion to complex with sulfhydryl or disulfide groups may or may not be a basis for interference with enzyme-mediated brain barrier transport mechanisms for amino acids or for interference with protein synthesis. Organomercurials can liberate some mercury ions in the body, but the toxicity of methylmercury and ethylmercury is not believed to be a primary result of the action of mercury ions (Clarkson 1972).

It is well known that alkylmercurials can cross the placental barrier. Recent reports (Bryce-Smith 1972; Zenick 1974; Olson and Boush 1975) indicate that if pregnant cats, mice, and rats are given ethylmercurials or methylmercurials during gestation, the offspring may have a behavioral or learning defect. In rats (Zenick 1974) the learning disability persists "permanently" in the absence of detectable mercury in the brain. This bit of behavioral toxicology is mentioned here because of the possible implications in training and behavior of dogs and cats. A puppy's ancestors may all have been magnificent, steady, working or hunting dogs. But if the bitch was exposed to alkylmercurials during pregnancy, the puppy might have subtle brain damage that could make him untrainable. Similar speculations can be made about exposure to lead during pregnancy (see Lead).

There is no satisfactory treatment of alkylmercury poisoning. The lesions in the brain are considered to be irreversible. Attempts at chelation therapy using a competitive sulfhydryl-containing compound such as BAL have been of doubtful value, perhaps because mercurials may bind to a 2-point receptor in the body, i.e., a sulfhydryl group plus some other adjacent group that could prevent chelation of the metal (Clarkson 1972). New chelating agents specific for mercury (phthalyltetrathioacetic acid, glutaraldehyde-butanedithiol polymer) are effective in mice poisoned by methylmercury (Jones and Harbison 1975). These agents may also prove useful in treatment of alkylmercury toxicosis in other species.

Other observations that could have some therapeutic implications include: (1) the chelator mercaptodextran facilitates excretion of already mobilized mercury in mice (Aaseth 1973); (2) small amounts of dietary selenium enhance mercury-binding to blood cells and other tissues of rats and protect against methylmercury neurotoxicosis (Potter and Matrone 1974); (3) in rats, antithyroid drugs or thyroparathyroidectomy protect against acute toxicosis from diphenylmercury or dimethylmercury (Szabo et al. 1974); and (4) spironolactone complexes with mercury and facilitates its uptake by rat erythrocytes, a possible basis for the protective effect of spironolactone in mercury toxicosis (Kushlan et al. 1975).

Organomercurials in Adult Cattle, Swine, and Fowl

Methylmercurials and ethylmercurials cause brain damage that results in central nervous excitatory signs in dogs, cats, calves, rats, primates, and human beings. However, in adult cattle, swine, and to a lesser extent fowl, the clinical signs of organomercurial toxicosis are associated with central nervous depression. In sheep, organomercurials produce mainly GI signs (Chapter 59). Possibly, some of these species differences in response are due to differences in organomercurial compounds, but this explanation is not totally acceptable because studies have been done in several species with the same organomercurial. It appears that a given organomercurial can produce a different spectrum of pathologic changes in different species, and even in adult cattle versus calves.

The toxic dose of organomercurials is as small as 0.24 mg Hg/kg of body weight/day for 199 days in swine (Charlton 1974). The single-dose acute oral LD50 of organomercurial in swine is about 13.4 mg Hg/kg. In adult cattle the toxic dose of organomercurial is about 1 mg Hg/kg of body weight/day (Buck et al. 1973). In turkeys the toxic dose is about 1.3 mg Hg/kg/day (Palmer et al. 1973).

In adult cattle the clinical signs of chronic organomercurial toxicosis are anorexia; weight loss; weakness; depression; incoordination; facial muscle spasms; salivation; lacrimation; frequent (possibly bloody) urination; diarrhea (possibly bloody); colic; loose teeth; fever; enlarged lymph nodes; cardiac irregularities; mucosal paleness or hemorrhages; epistaxis; respiratory signs such as cough, nasal discharge, and dyspnea; and skin manifestations like eczema, itchiness, pustules, ulcers, hyperkeratinization, and depilation of the tailhead. Convulsions are rare. The animal becomes recumbent and may die a few weeks after mercury ingestion began, or there may be a 3- to 6-month recovery (Buck et al. 1973; Palmer et al. 1973). Death is more likely if a very high body temperature and many hemorrhagic and skin signs are manifested.

In swine the signs of acute organomercury poisoning are similar to those of chronic poisoning, but more GI signs exist and death comes more rapidly. The signs include anorexia, weight loss, weakness, depression, incoordination, compulsive hypermotility, tremors, muscle twitching, stiff gait, staggering, swaying, reluctance to move after episodes of aimless walking, paddling in recumbency, and hump-backed postural abnormalities (acute cases) and blindness, posterior paralysis, and possible wall climbing (chronic cases) (see Lead). Also, salivation, diarrhea, coughing, red spots on the skin, hyperkeratinization, ventral wall cyanosis, fever, thirst, vomiting, petechial hemorrhages in mucous membranes, polyuria, hematuria, and bloody stools may be manifested. With swine, the nervous and behavioral signs are much more pronounced than in adult cattle (Clarke and Clarke 1967; Loosmore et al. 1967; Kahrs 1968; Curley et al. 1971; Piper et al. 1971; Charlton 1974).

In turkeys, organomercurials cause weakness, ataxia, incoordination, and pale wattles. Convulsions are not common (Palmer et al. 1973). Chickens manifest more obvious depression than do turkeys.

Tissue concentrations of mercury from animals fatally poisoned by methylmercury and ethylmercury compounds vary considerably. In adult cattle the liver may contain 0–74.5 ppm and the kidney 2–112 ppm (Buck et al. 1973; Palmer et al. 1973). In acutely poisoned swine the liver may contain 2.7–125 ppm and the kidney cortex 3.6–105 ppm (Piper et al. 1971). In chronically poisoned swine the liver may contain 48–72 ppm and the kidney cortex 44–107 ppm (Charlton 1974). In chronically poisoned turkeys the liver may contain 5.8–59 ppm and the kidneys 9.7–39.5 ppm (Palmer et al. 1973). Other tissues and body fluids in these species contain variable and generally smaller concentrations of mercury. So-called normal tissue concentrations (in ppm) of mercury in animals and birds are: brain, 0.1; kidney, 2.75; liver, 0.3; muscle, 0.15; and large intestine, 0.05 (Buck et al. 1973). Some overlap exists between "normal" and small tissue concentrations of mercury that might be found in some animals poisoned by organomercurials. This phenomenon of overlap is also seen with other metals such as lead and arsenic and serves to illustrate why quotation marks are used about the phrase "diagnostically significant concentration." Sometimes even large concentrations of these metals in tissues may not be "diagnostic," depending on duration of intake, accumulation and tolerance, and individual susceptibility to poisoning.

In attempting to explain species and age differences in clinical signs of organomercurial poisoning, we can cite differences in the organomercury compound involved, but (as already mentioned) this explanation is not a confident one. The lesions of organomercury toxicosis are different in adult cattle versus calves. Adult cattle manifest minimal brain damage (cerebral congestion and possible focal hemorrhages). Stomatitis, enlarged and pale kidneys, enlarged lymph nodes, bronchopneumonia, enteritis (possibly hemorrhagic), and multiple petechial hemorrhages on the heart and in serosas and mucosal surfaces are also seen. Microscopically, subacute interstitial nephritis, subacute catarrhal bronchitis, enlarged splenic follicles, and hepatic focal necrosis also exist (Buck et al. 1973; Palmer et al. 1973). This spectrum of lesions is different from the one in calves in which somatic lesions are minimal and microscopic lesions in the brain are marked. It appears that organomercurials kill adult cattle by some mechanism other than brain cell destruction.

Just to complicate things further, organomercurials produce several lesions in the nervous system of swine. Grossly, the cerebral gyri may be decreased in size and the cortex may be thin. Microscopically, the brain may manifest neuronal degeneration and gliosis. These lesions could be due to cerebral ischemia, because there may also be cerebrovascular lesions such as focal cellular accumulations around vessel wall adventitia, hyalinization of muscle layers of vessel walls, and occasionally necrosis of the media of some meningeal arterioles. In the peripheral nervous system there are neuronal axonal degeneration leading to Wallerian degeneration of sensory fibers and neuronal degeneration in dorsal root ganglia. Other lesions in swine include colonic ulcers or necrosis and sloughing of the entire colonic mucosa; petechial hemorrhages in urinary bladder, larynx, kidney surfaces, and lymph nodes; and renal congestion or degeneration. Microscopically, renal tubular degeneration and some degeneration in liver lobules are manifested (Kahrs 1968; Loosmore et al. 1967; Buck et al. 1973; Charlton 1974).

The variable signs and lesions of organomercury poisoning in different species do not help us to understand how the metal acts. Brain damage may be a big factor in the cause of death in dogs, cats, calves, swine, rats, primates, and human beings, but *cellular metabolic lesions may underlie the toxicosis in all species.* That such metabolic lesions should be expressed so differently in different species is inconvenient and seems to indicate a great deal of biochemical difference among species and even among different-aged animals of the same species.

Neurotoxic mechanisms of organomercurial toxicosis were discussed for dogs, cats, and calves. Such mechanisms may also apply to adult cattle, swine, and fowl. In addition, we must consider other mechanisms. Organomercurials are not thought to act by release of mercury ion, but by metabolic actions of their own such as inhibition of sulfhydryl or disulfide groups. Maybe glutathione is an important determinant of mercury toxicity because renal glutathione concentration is directly correlated with mercury concentration in kidneys of rats given methylmercury (Richardson and Murphy 1975). For information about glutathione, see Selenium, Chapter 57. In rats given mercuric chloride, renal cell death is preceded by a sequence of ultrastructural changes involving the ribosomes, cytoplasmic membranes, and nuclear chromatin. Mitochondrial damage occurs only as the cells begin to die. Inhibition of mitochondrial function is probably not the cause of cell death with mercury derived from mercuric chloride (Ganote et al. 1974).

Treatment of organomercury toxicosis, as discussed for dogs, cats, and calves, is not very successful using the common chelating agents, but other chemicals may prove to be of therapeutic value.

Hexachlorophene

USE

Hexachlorophene is used as a germicide in soaps, shampoos, and disinfectant solutions; as an antitrematodal agent in ruminants; as a soil and plant fungicide; and as a plant bactericide and acaricide.

SOURCE

Dogs and cats may be exposed by percutaneous absorption of hexachlorophene from medicated soaps and shampoos. Dogs may eat soap containing hexachlorophene. Ruminants may be overdosed with the chemical during treatment of fascioliasis. Herbivores may ingest sprayed foliage, spilled spray concentrate, contaminated water, or concentrate in "empty" containers. Dairy cattle may absorb hexachlorophene from antiseptic solutions used to cleanse the udder, or calves may ingest the compound if they are watered from contaminated buckets.

PROPERTIES OF TOXICOLOGIC IMPORTANCE

Hexachlorophene is a phenol. Specifically, it is 2,2′-methylenebis(3,4,6-trichlorophenol). The compound is insoluble in water but soluble in aliphatic organic solvents. It is fairly stable in the environment, as might be inferred from its use as a soil and foliage spray. Residues of hexachlorophene remain on the skin and continue to exert antibacterial actions. These residues can also be continuously absorbed or licked from the skin.

TOXICITY

The acute oral LD50 of hexachlorophene is (in mg/kg of body weight): male rat, 66; female rat, 56 (other studies in rats may report values of 126–320 for hexachlorophene and 900 for its sodium salt); weanling rat, 120; mouse, 80–187; ruminant, 30–60; and puppy (2- to 3-week-old), 15–30. Adult dogs are killed by single oral doses of 36–50 mg/kg (Kimbrough 1973; Scott et al. 1973; Edds and Simpson 1974). Sheep tolerate 1 dose of hexachlorophene (20 mg/kg) but a 2nd or 3rd dose the next 1 or 2 days can be fatal (Hall and Reid 1974). Calves can become ill if they drink from improperly rinsed buckets that formerly contained hexachlorophene solution used for udder washing.

Compounds (e.g., dieldrin, polychlorinated biphenyls) that induce hepatic oxidative enzymes can markedly decrease hexachlorophene toxicity in rats (Jones et al. 1974). In rats, hexachlorophene is more toxic at 10–13 days of age (the critical period for development of myelin in the brain) than in younger or older rats (Ulsamer et al. 1975).

TOXICODYNAMIC CONSIDERATIONS

Hexachlorophene is readily absorbed from the skin and intestinal tract. It is metabolized in the body and excreted mainly in the feces. A small amount appears in the urine. Most of the compound is eliminated from the body in several days.

MECHANISM OF ACTION

Some biochemical actions of hexachlorophene include uncoupling of oxidative phosphorylation with resulting hyperthermia (Kimbrough 1973) and inhibition of cytochrome oxidase, lactic dehydrogenase, and succinoxidases of liver, kidney, and heart cells (Scott et al. 1973). The compound may also directly damage cell membranes (Hall and Reid 1974). It is not known whether any of these actions are causally related to the clinical signs and lesions of hexachlorophene poisoning. In developing rats, hexachlorophene (10 mg/kg/day) does not seem to affect brain adenosine triphosphate (ATP), phospholipid, sterol, protein, or DNA or RNA concentrations (Ulsamer et al. 1975).

Electron microscopic examination of the cerebral white matter of hexachlorophene-poisoned rats reveals that the myelin vacuolization that gives rise to status spongiosis is due to "a split in the interperiod line of the myelin seat" (Kimbrough

1973) or to "the separation of the myelin lamellae at the intraperiod line" (Towfighi et al. 1974). Such observations do not tell us the biochemical basis of the myelin defect. Hexachlorophene causes osmotic swelling of erythrocyte membranes by altering their permeability to sodium and potassium (Miller and Buhler 1974), but whether a similar action on neural membranes could initiate the severe central and peripheral nerve demyelination and axonal degeneration described by several authors is not known.

CLINICAL SIGNS

In puppies, onset of shaking, shivering, jaw stretching and chewing, body writhing, whining, tonic-clonic opisthotonic convulsions involving the forelegs mainly, and coma is rapid and death comes in a few hours. Some pups may recover (Edds and Simpson 1974).

In cats, early lassitude, weakness, hindlimb ataxia, impaired righting reflex, patellar hyperreflexia (and later hyporeflexia), anuria, and complete flaccid paralysis are manifested (Kimbrough 1973).

Sheep manifest dullness, incoordination, and death (Hall and Reid 1974). Also hyperexcitability, convulsions, and sudden respiratory failure occur. Calves manifest muscle tremors, stiffness, tottering gait, and tetanic spasms (Edds and Simpson 1974).

LESIONS

The important lesion is status spongiosus and edema in the cerebral white matter of all species (Kimbrough 1973; Edds and Simpson 1974; Hall and Reid 1974). This lesion appears first in larger myelinated fibers, especially those of the optic tracts. Optic nerves may be severely compressed and atrophic due to increased cerebrospinal fluid pressure and stricture by the unyielding optic foramina. The vacuolar lesion also occurs in myelinated fibers of the rest of the brain, spinal cord, and peripheral nerves, but less severe lesions occur in the periphery. Towfighi et al. (1974) present a detailed study of these lesions.

Some liver and kidney damage and visceral focal hemorrhage also occur, especially in pups.

DIFFERENTIAL DIAGNOSIS

Probability is on the side of the practitioner because hexachlorophene poisoning is not as common as other toxicoses that may mimic it. There is usually a history of exposure to hexachlorophene. If a fairly rapid onset of nervous signs, convulsions, and fever are also manifested, but no locomotor, behavioral, or autonomic signs to speak of, hexachlorophene is the probable cause of toxicosis. The lesions and laboratory tests help establish the diagnosis.

Cerebral status spongiosus is not unique to hexachlorophene. Similar focal or diffuse lesions may be produced by ammonium salts, organic tin fungicides, lead, copper, aflatoxin, pyrrolizidine alkaloids from *Senecio* spp., *Echium* spp., and *Crotalaria* spp., and viral encephalopathy such as canine distemper. Moreover, liver damage associated with fascioliasis, facial eczema syndrome, anemia, and congestive heart failure may cause hyperammonemia and subsequent spongy degenerative changes in the brain (Hooper 1972). These diverse hepatotoxic encephalopathies can be differentiated from hexachlorophene toxicosis on the basis of detailed history, clinical signs, gross lesions, laboratory tests, and thorough histopathologic examination.

TREATMENT

No specific treatment for hexachlorophene poisoning is known. Fever can be controlled by cold water rinsing. Convulsions in dogs may not be controllable with barbiturates (Edds and Simpson 1974), but attempts should be made to alleviate convulsions with depressants if the animal is to be saved. Gastric lavage or saline cathartic therapy is indicated. Fluid therapy may help speed elimination of the poison. If brain damage is not too severe, animals may recover and the brain lesions may regress.

ANALYSIS

Hexachlorophene is not a normal constituent of the body. If the substance is found in feces, vomitus, or stomach contents and blood or tissues, and if the history, signs, and lesions are those of hexachlorophene poisoning, the diagnosis is confirmed.

Equine Leucoencephalomalacia
Mold Toxin

Equine leucoencephalomalacia (moldy corn poisoning, cornstalk disease) has been reviewed by Wilson et al. (1973). The condition mimics viral encephalitis clinically, but postmortem examination usually reveals focal or generalized areas of liquifaction necrosis in cerebral white matter. Necrotic lesions can also be found in the thalamus, brainstem, and cerebellum and hemorrhage may be prominent in all necrotic areas of the brain. The lesions are pathognomonic of moldy corn poisoning and are produced by an unidentified toxin associated with the pink to red colored storage mold *Fusarium moniliforme.* This mold is normally present in stored corn, and the corn might be fed to animals without ill effect. However, if the corn has a high moisture content when stored, and if it is then exposed to cold temperatures, *Fusarium* molds can produce toxic metabolites.

It is not known why the toxin produced by *F. moniliforme* causes cerebral liquifaction necrosis only in Equidae. Perhaps this is due to a species difference in effective dosage of the toxin, for there is no compelling reason to regard horse brains as unique organs that make them particularly susceptible to the toxin of *F. moniliforme.* The toxin is thought to act by damaging cerebral blood vessels. Such a mechanism, if true, should also occur in cerebral blood vessels of other species if enough toxin is consumed. On the other hand, Equidae are different from other species in several ways, one of which is the digestive system and diet. It is conceivable that *F. moniliforme* metabolites may undergo chemical changes to toxic metabolites in the equine digestive tract or liver, but not in the digestive tract or liver of other species. The toxin(s) may then cause brain damage not by some exclusive predeliction for cerebral blood vessels (to the exclusion of all other blood vessels in the body) but perhaps by some special affinity for the myelin that makes up so much of the bulk of cerebral white matter. This is all sheer speculation, however, and the exact mechanism of action of *F. moniliforme* toxin in horses remains to be determined.

There is no treatment for moldy corn poisoning in horses; it is considered unsafe to feed moldy corn to horses or to any other species.

Plant Poisons

Plant poisons that can cause depression and incoordination and other neurotoxic signs by a direct damaging effect on the central nervous system (CNS) include locoine from locoweeds (*Oxytropis* spp., *Astragalus* spp.), which causes Golgi degeneration; unknown chemicals in sensitive fern (*Onochea* spp.), which cause cerebral edema, gliosis, and neuronal degeneration; and neurolathyrogenic compounds in sweet peas (*Lathyrus* spp.), which cause a number of spinal and brain lesions. The review of Barrow et al. (1974) on lathyrism is of special interest. Detail on neurotoxic plants can be found in Kingsbury (1964).

POISONS ACTING ON KNOWN RECEPTOR SITES

Organophosphate Pesticides

USE

Organophosphates are used as contact insecticides and acaricides; animal systemic/topical insecticides and parasiticides; plant systemic insecticides; soil nematocides, fungicides, herbicides, and defoliants; rodenticides; insecticide synergists; and insect repellents and chemosterilants. Not all of the compounds have all of these uses, but members of several classes of organophosphates do have multiple uses. The major *classes* of organophosphates are phosphates, phosphorothionates, phosphorothiolothionates, phosphorothiolates, phosphoramidates, pyrophosphates, phosphonates, and phosphoramides (see Eto 1974 for a more complete classification).

The veterinarian should know the names of commonly used organophosphates in order to know what a client is talking about when asked what pesticides are in use on the premises. Some of these are listed under Toxicity.

If the name given by the client does not identify a compound as an organophosphate, the product label should be carefully studied. The label may not come right out and say, "This Product is an Organophosphate Compound"; but the *chemical name* may say it. Chemical names of organophosphate pesticides generally contain all or part of the name of the chemical class of the compound (see *classes* above). Thus a product label indicating a major ingredient is diethyl *S*-(ethylthiomethyl)phosphorothiolothionate tells the veterinarian that the ingredient is an organophosphate. One need not necessarily know a brand name (Thimet), or the common name (phorate). Should the veterinarian's memory of various classes of organophosphorus compounds dim, the nature of the product can likely be guessed if the chemical name is complex, obviously an organic compound, and if the name contains the word *phosphate* or the partial words *phos, phoro, phosphor,* or some other derivative of the word phosphorus. Proper identification of the kind of pesticide is very important. Animals poisoned by an organophosphate may manifest signs very similar to those of other toxicoses, and it is indefensible to treat an animal for a condition it does not have when it could be saved with antidotes that are specific for organophosphate toxicosis.

SOURCE

Widely used chemicals such as organophosphates may become causes of animal poisoning in a variety of ways. Feeds may be contaminated at the processing plant or during shipping, storage, or handling on the farm. Feed crops may be dusted with insecticide, or the harvested crop may be accidentally contaminated. Animal premises may be sprayed or dusted or animals may be directly dusted or painted with too much pesticide. Systemic antiparasitic compounds may be overdosed or they may have additive or synergistic effects with other pesticides to which animals have been exposed. Drinking water may be contaminated by spillage or by rinsing out of spray tanks and hoses. Sometimes the source of pesticide contamination cannot be found. Perhaps the source is a confined spill in a large pasture or orchard or perhaps pesticide granules have been spilled and the portions not eaten by livestock have washed away. Empty pesticide containers are never really empty; animals can be poisoned if they are fed or watered with these containers or if they have access to dumps where chemical containers are discarded.

PROPERTIES OF TOXICOLOGIC IMPORTANCE

Most organophosphates are not very persistent in the environment and dissipate in 2–4 weeks. Exceptions are fensulfothion, prophos, and trichloronate (which may persist in soil for more than 4 weeks) and chlorfenvinphos, phospholan, dichlorfenthion, and oxydisulfoton (which persist more than 36 weeks in soil).

Organophosphates are poorly soluble in water. Thus they must be used as dusts, wettable powders, or emulsions. Improper formulation of a pesticide-vehicle mixture can lead to underexposure or overexposure of animals to the pesticide. These compounds are soluble in organic solvents and also in fats and oils. Therefore, the compounds can penetrate into waxy coatings of leaves or fruits or be absorbed directly through the skin of human beings and animals. Oily vehicles or organic solvents can facilitate passage of organophosphate pesticide through the skin.

TOXICITY

Buck et al. (1973) have done an admirable job tabulating the oral and dermal toxicity values of many pesticides in a variety of species of different ages.

In adult cattle the minimum toxic oral

dosage of organophosphate pesticides varies from 1 to 125 mg/kg of body weight; the minimum toxic dermal concentration varies from 0.5% to 3%, but these figures are not sacred. The literature is not complete with regard to animal toxicity of organophosphates; even if it were, the toxicity values would not be reliable because of the number of factors that influence toxicity of these chemicals under different conditions of use. It is these factors, not actual numbers, that warrant discussion here.

A number of *physicochemical factors* affect toxicity of organophosphate pesticides. Toxicity of these compounds decreases as they are degraded by sun, water, microbes, alkali, or metal ions such as iron or copper. Increase in toxicity may occur by storage activation, in which highly toxic isomers of certain pesticides are formed spontaneously in polar solvents or water. The phosphorothionates and phosphorothiolothionates are notable in this regard and can partly isomerize to the corresponding thiolates and dithiolates, which are more toxic than the original compounds. This reaction is speeded by heat. Examples of compounds that can undergo this kind of storage activation are parathion, malathion, fenitrothion, fenthion, Abate, chloropyrifos, diazinon, carbophenothion, ethion, coumaphos, dimethoate, demeton, and methyl demeton. Technical grade organophosphates are often more toxic than the pure compound due to heat-induced isomerizations of the kind mentioned above. The isomerization can continue when the pesticide is diluted and stored. Another kind of storage activation is chemical alteration to a more toxic pesticide. Thus trichlorfon can change to dichlorvos in solutions of pH 7–8. The storage activation phenomena are good reasons to use only freshly prepared suspensions, emulsions, or solutions.

Ambient temperature is another physicochemical factor that affects toxicity of organophosphates. High temperature increases toxicity of parathion in mice; low temperature increases toxicity of malathion in rats; volatility of certain fumigant compounds such as dichlorvos is greater at higher temperatures, thus increasing the inhalation hazard. Another physicochemical factor is the nature of the vehicle in which the pesticide is dispersed. Vehicles containing a "sticking agent" can cause pesticides to adhere to animals as well as plant foliage. Moreover, vehicles that are organic solvents or oils can carry pesticide through the skin and cause toxicosis.

Biological factors also influence toxicity of organophosphates. Species is very important here. Cattle are more sensitive than sheep to dimethoate, ronnel, cruformate, and phosmet; more sensitive than swine to phorate; and more resistant than many other species to parathion. Brahman cattle are more sensitive than other European cattle to famphur, dioxathion, and crotoxyphos. Swine and horses are less sensitive than cattle to cruformate. Dogs are very resistant to chlorfenvinphos and fairly resistant to cruformate and ronnel. Rats are highly sensitive to chlorfenvinphos. Mice are more sensitive than rats or guinea pigs to fenthion. Methyl azinphos (azinphosmethyl) is more toxic to mice, pigs, and cats than to guinea pigs. Many of these species differences are caused by differences in enzymatic activation or degradation of various pesticides.

Age of the animal is another biological factor that alters toxicity of organophosphate pesticides. Compounds that do not require enzymatic activation are more toxic in very young animals, in which the enzymes of pesticide degradation are deficient. Compounds that require enzymatic activation are not so toxic for very young animals because the enzymes of activation are deficient during the early weeks of life.

Sex of the animal can also alter toxicity of organophosphates. Brahman bulls are more sensitive than Brahman or Hereford heifers to dioxathion. Adult male rats are more resistant than females to the organophosphates that are degraded by liver microsomal enzymes, less resistant than females to the organophosphates that are activated by liver enzymes, and equally susceptible as females to organophosphates that are not metabolized in the body.

The presence of other chemicals can

alter organophosphate toxicity. Combined effects of two organophosphates can either be synergistic (malathion plus EPN, coumaphos, or trichlorfon; acethion or dimethoate plus EPN; methyl azinphos plus trichlorfon; Narlene plus EPN) or antagonistic (malathion plus parathion or methyl azinphos; EPN plus trichlorfon or *cis*-mevinphos; carbophenothion plus trichlorfon). Drugs that have neuromuscular blocking properties may possibly enhance organophosphate toxicity or vice versa. Such drugs include inhalant anesthetics, magnesium ion, antibiotics (streptomycin, dihydrostreptomycin, neomycin, kanamycin, gentamycin, polymyxin-B, and others), and the depolarizing and nondepolarizing neuromuscular blocking agents. Drugs that compete with organophosphates for target esterases may also enhance organophosphate toxicity or vice versa. These drugs include succinylcholine, phenothiazine, and procaine. Methylmercury enhances anticholinesterase activity of parathion in quail (Dieter and Ludke 1975). A number of central nervous depressants can enhance parathion toxicity in rats (Weiss and Orzel 1967). Any drug that interferes with muscle function can be expected to interact unfavorably with organophosphates. In addition, any other pesticide that causes clinical signs similar to those of organophosphates (e.g., the chlorinated hydrocarbons) may synergize unfavorably with organophosphates. In fact, *any chemical* that causes toxicosis can theoretically cause more severe toxicosis in the presence of an organophosphate, and *any disease* can be considered capable of enhancing organophosphate pesticide toxicity. Furthermore, any agent capable of inducing hepatic enzymes (e.g., phenobarbital, chlorinated hydrocarbon pesticides, polychlorinated biphenyls, and others) may either increase, decrease, or fail to alter organophosphate toxicity, depending on the organophosphate, species of interest, or age of the animal.

With so many factors operating to determine the toxicity of organophosphates, it is no wonder that confusion abounds in this matter! Still, it is possible to classify the organophosphate pesticides roughly according to their acute oral LD50 in rats. Such a classification is given in Tables 58.1 and 58.2 and may help to group the com-

TABLE 58.1. Relatively safe organophosphates (Rat acute oral LD50 > 500 mg/kg of body weight)

Common Name	Trade Name	LD50 *(mg/kg)*
tetrachlorvinphos	Gardona	4000
abate	Abate	1000–4000
phostex	Phostex	2500
iodofenphos	Alfacron	2100
merphos	Folex	1270
menazon	Sayfos	900–1950
ronnel	Ectoral	906–1750
propyl thiopyrophosphate	Aspon	900–1700
malathion	Cythion	347–1375
tribufon	Butonate	1100
acethion	Acethion	800–1100
narlene	Narlene	1000
cruformate	Ruelene	660–1000
acephate	Ortran	945
chlorthion	Chlorthion	880
fenitrothion	Sumithion	740–870
cyanophos	Cyanox	580–860
trichlorfon	Neguvon	390–630
formothion	Aflix	330–530

TABLE 58.2. Relatively hazardous organophosphates (Rat acute oral LD50 < 20 mg/kg of body weight)

Common Name	Trade Name	LD50 *(mg/kg)*
amiton	Citram	0.5–7
dimefox	Terra-systam	1–5
phorate	Thimet	1–9
fensulfothion	Dasanit	2–10
disulfoton	Disyston	2–12
demeton	Systox	2–30
cyanthoate	Tartan	3–4
parathion	Thiophos	3–6
mevinphos	Phosdrin	3–7
oxydisulfoton	Disyston-S	3.5
sulfotep	Bladafum	5
thionazin	Nemafos	5–12
dialifor	Torak	5–97
carbophenothion	Trithion	6–32
EPN	EPN	7–24
fonofos	Dyfonate	8–16
methyl azinphos	Gusathion	8–18
methyl parathion	Parathion-methyl	9
phosfolan	Cyolane	9
prothoate	Fostion	10
methyl oxydemeton	Metasystox-R	10–70
phosphamidon	Dimecron	11–27
coroxon	Coroxon	12
ethyl azinphos	Gusathion-A	12.5
ethion	Nialate	13
phenamiphos	Nemacur	15–19
dioxathion	Delnav	19

pounds according to degree of potential danger to other species.

Between the extremes of relatively safe and relatively hazardous organophosphates lie a large number of compounds that may tend toward one extreme or the other or just lie in the middle. Examples of compounds that tend to be close to the hazardous group are schradan, dichlorvos, monocrotophos, dicrotophos, and methidathion. Compounds that tend toward the safer group include naled, dicapthon, bromophos, and phenkapton. It is emphasized that this classification is for *rats* treated under laboratory conditions, not for domestic animals in field conditions. It should also be emphasized that regardless of what may be the supposed toxic dosage of organophosphate in a given species, the occurrence of clinical signs of organophosphate poisoning in animals exposed to these compounds automatically indicates that the dosage received was too large, no matter how small it was!

Additional detail on toxicity of organophosphates can be found in Clarke and Clarke (1967), Gaines (1969), Radeleff (1970), Buck et al. (1973), Kahn (1973), Berg (1974), and Eto 1974). Palmer and Schlinke (1973b) report the toxicity of merphos (Folex), a cotton defoliant, in cattle and sheep. Tucker and Haegele (1971) give LD50 values of some organophosphates and carbamates in six species of birds.

Because of its use as a fumigant insecticide in hang-up strips and in flea collars for pets and because of its increasing use as a systemic antiparasitic agent, dichlorvos (Vapona, DDVP) has stimulated research on safety of this compound in human beings and animals. Papers by Walker and Stevenson (1968), Cavagna et al. (1969), Hughes and Lang (1973), Snow (1973), Snow and Watson (1973), Leary et al. (1974), and Blair et al. (1975) can be consulted for detail on this compound. More detail on toxicity of antiparasitic organophosphorous compounds can be found in Section 14.

TOXICODYNAMIC CONSIDERATIONS

Following absorption from the GI tract, skin, or lungs, organophosphate pesticides are distributed throughout the body. They do not accumulate in any particular tissue. Most of the compounds are not potent inhibitors of esterases until they are activated in the liver, mainly by microsomal oxidative enzymes. The *phosphate* class and the *phosphorothiolate* class of organophosphates do *not* require this activation and can inhibit esterases immediately upon entry into the bloodstream. Examples of these immediately active compounds are the phosphates: dichlorvos, naled, chlorfenvinphos, tetrachlorvinphos, and propophos and the phosphorothiolates: acetofos, cyanthoate, PTMD (Danifos), and DMCP (Fujithion) (Eto 1974).

Some organophosphates are transformed to quaternary compounds in the body. They cannot enter the brain very easily. Such compounds are *phosphoramidates,* e.g., amidothioate and methamidophos (Monitor) (Kahn 1973).

Interaction of organophosphates with esterases (the main basis for the acute toxicity of these chemicals) is only one way in which the body attempts to detoxify organophosphates. In the liver, and to some extent in other tissues, a variety of enzymes may attack the pesticides at rates dependent upon class of pesticide, species, and age of the animal. For details on metabolism of organophosphates, see Eto (1974). Water-soluble metabolites may be formed very quickly and the pesticide excreted rapidly in the urine. The rate of degradation of pesticide may be so fast as to preclude the appearance of clinical signs of poisoning; this fact may be reflected in extremely large LD50 values for certain pesticides in certain species, although the LD50 is also influenced by rate of activation, route of entry into the body, and various factors already discussed (see Toxicity; see also Section 2).

When an animal is chronically exposed to small amounts of an organophosphate pesticide, the animal may develop *tolerance* to the pesticide. Tolerance (ability to withstand exposure to larger and larger concentrations of pesticide) is due to induction by the pesticide of hepatic microsomal oxidative enzymes, continual synthesis of esterases, physiological adaptation to decreased esterase levels, and adaptation of cholinergic receptors to the presence of excessive amounts of acetylcholine (Kahn 1973). Enzymes that detoxify organophosphates can also be induced by other chemicals that are detoxified by the same enzymes. Thus a *cross-tolerance* may develop between some organophosphates and compounds such as the chlorinated hydrocarbons. However, it should be emphasized that neither tolerance nor cross-tolerance is operable for all organophosphates, and we should not shrug off the importance of chronic low-level exposure of animals to these agents. It should also be emphasized that those organophosphates that require activation in the body in order to be good inhibitors of esterases can also induce the enzymes of activation, thus resulting in a *decreased resistance* to the pesticide over a period of time.

In the individual animal the clinical effects of a given organophosphate compound will be a *net effect* of the operation of a dynamic equilibrium between the complex mechanisms of pesticide absorption, activation, enzyme induction/activity, tolerance, detoxification rate, and excretion rate. These mechanisms underlie many of the factors that influence toxicity of organophosphates. The diversity of chemical structures among organophosphate pesticides makes it difficult to predict what effects a given compound may have under a prescribed set of conditions. Sometimes the clinical manifestations of a particular organophosphate are not even logically consistent with the mechanism of action of this group of pesticides.

MECHANISM OF ACTION

Acute toxicosis (the most common occurrence) is due to an irreversible inhibition of acetylcholinesterase (ACh-E) wherever acetylcholine (ACh) functions as a transmitter substance. The molecular mechanism of ACh-E inhibition has already been discussed elsewhere in this text. The result of ACh-E inhibition is accumulation of ACh in neuromuscular junctions, parasympathetic postganglionic terminals in smooth muscle, cardiac muscle, and glands, all autonomic ganglia, and in cholinergic synapses within the CNS. Thus all muscarinic and nicotinic cholinergic receptors are overstimulated by the ACh, which would normally be destroyed if ACh-E were not inhibited. If this overstimulation is intense enough, ACh receptors may become blocked, just as if a depolarizing type of neuromuscular or ganglion blocking agent had been administered. Usually, however, complete blockage of all cholinergic receptors is not produced, and the clinical signs (at least the early ones) reflect hyperfunction of these receptors.

If exposure is not too severe, animals may not die. ACh-E is not likely to be inhibited 100% and the enzyme is constantly being synthesized by neurons. Nevertheless, several days or weeks may be required for complete recovery from a sublethal dosage of pesticide.

Lethal amounts of organophosphates cause death by a combination of effects of muscarinic, nicotinic, and central cholinergic overstimulation and/or receptor paralysis. Thus hypotension, bradycardia, bronchoconstriction and bronchial fluid accumulation, inability of tonically rigid (or flaccid-paralytic) respiratory muscles to work properly, cyanosis, and central respiratory depression are manifested. The animal dies of asphyxia. From this it would seem that organophosphates should be classified under poisons causing outstanding signs of respiratory insufficiency. Indeed, the terminal signs would demand such reclassification; the reader may wish to pause here and put an appropriate notation in Chapter 57. In practice, however, the outstanding clinical signs seen in herd outbreaks and in ambulatory animals are generally those of behavioral, motor, and muscle stimulation. Respiratory failure is characteristic of death by any cause and is secondary to the stimulatory and paralytic effects of ACh. So, organophosphate pesticides are rightly classified as agents causing signs of nervous stimulation by acting on a known receptor, the receptor being the esteratic site of ACh-E.

Organophosphates interact with esterases other than the ACh-E of neuroeffector junctions and synapses. Type A esterases (arylesterases) hydrolyze organophosphates but *are not* inhibited in the process. These esterases help detoxify the pesticides. Type B esterases, of which ACh-E is a member, also include carboxyesterases and cholinesterases that *are* inhibited by organophosphates. Of the type B esterases, ACh-E is located in erythrocytes as well as cholinergic neuroeffector junctions and synapses; cholinesterase (also called pseudocholinesterase) is located in serum, pancreas, heart, and liver; carboxyesterases (aliesterases) are located in the liver (Eto 1974). The functional significance of esterases other than ACh-E is not known except that they do hydrolyze esters other than ACh. Inhibition of pseudocholinesterase by organophosphates can prevent hydrolysis of drugs such as succinylcholine or procaine and its congeners, thus leading to adverse reactions or (possibly) prolonged blood levels of these drugs. Inhibition of serum and liver esterases may serve to "tie up" some organophosphate, thus decreasing the amount of pesticide available for inhibition of ACh-E. The role of various serum and liver esterases in the pathogenesis of acute organophosphate toxicosis remains to be determined.

There are other forms of organophosphate toxicosis besides the classical acute toxicosis already described. *Delayed neurotoxicity* (Buck et al. 1973; Kahn 1973; Eto 1974) may occur days or weeks after minimal exposure. The species most sensitive to delayed neurotoxic effects of organophosphates are human being, chicken, calf, cat, lamb, and rabbit. Other species such as rat, dog, and monkey are more resistant. Chickens are insensitive prior to 55 days of age. The lesion of delayed neurotoxicity is a degeneration of motor nerve axons, beginning at the periphery and then following the motor nerves into the spinal cord and up spinocerebellar, vestibulospinal, and other tracts. Demyelination of affected axons occurs after the axon degenerates and clinical signs appear. The mechanism by which organophosphates destroy motor axons is not known. On the basis of structure-activity studies, it is postulated that a neurotoxic complex is formed when certain organophosphates bind to the active site of an esterase (Eto 1974; Johnson 1974). This esterase (presumably located within motor neurons) has been characterized by its ability to hydrolyze phenyl phenylacetate and by its inhibition by neurotoxic organophosphates but not by nonneurotoxic ones. Brown and Sharma (1975) postulate that delayed neurotoxicity may be due to inhibition of neural membrane ATPases, with resulting interference in the ability of neurons to obtain sufficient energy for their needs. Organophosphates capable of causing delayed neurotoxicity are listed below:

- tri-*o*-cresyl phosphate (TOCP), a plasticizer, oil additive, lubricant, and solvent; not an insecticide
- tri-*p*-ethylphenyl phosphate (TPEP), not an insecticide
- di-isopropylfluorophosphate (DFP), mainly an experimental compound, also used in ophthalmic medicine
- haloxon, carbophenothion, and related di-2-chloroethyl phosphates
- EPN and related phosphonate esters
- butifos (DEF), a defoliant, and related compounds such as merphos (Folex)
- DMPA (Zytron), a herbicide, and related compounds
- mipafox (Isopestox), no longer used

A number of other organophosphates can cause paralytic effects in atropinized hens (this is how neurotoxicity is detected), but these effects occur within 24 hours of exposure and the hens recover in about a month. The compounds listed below may or may not act by the same neurotoxic mechanisms as those listed above (Gaines 1969):

Abate	ethion
azinphosmethyl	fenthion
chloropyrifos	malathion
coumaphos	menazon
crotoxyphos	methyl parathion

cruformate
dicapthon
dioxathion
disulfoton
methyl carbophenothion
phorate
ronnel

Organophosphates may also cause *myopathy.* This is a necrosis of skeletal muscle that might occur in acutely poisoned animals. In dogs given dichlorvos orally or intravenously, skeletal muscle necrosis is thought to be secondary to the severe fasciculations, hemorrhages, and metabolic disturbances produced in muscle as a result of ACh-E inhibition (Snow 1973). In rats, parathion, paraoxon, phospholene, and "probably all cholinesterase inhibitors seem capable of producing skeletal necrosis by allowing excessive ACh stimulation of muscle" (Kibler 1973). In rats, parathion causes skeletal muscle necrosis after only 1 dosage. Therefore, muscle necrosis may contribute to failure of respiratory muscles during acute toxicosis (Kibler 1973).

Some organophosphates may be *teratogenic.* Such compounds include *cis*-dicrotophos and homologs, phosphamidon, mevinphos, dichlorvos, DEF, DEF-phosphate, and parathion—all capable of producing deformed chicks when injected into eggs. The teratogenic effect is not due to ACh-E inhibition, but may be due to inhibition of other cholinesterases (Eto 1974). In rats 11 days pregnant, intraperitoneal injection of parathion, dichlorvos, diazinon, apholate, or tepa causes fetal malformations, resorptions, or decreased fetal or placental weights (Eto 1974).

Other effects of organophosphates may relate to toxicosis. These chemicals can inhibit a large number of enzymes other than esterases; they can also cause release of adrenal steroids and catecholamines.

CLINICAL SIGNS

Signs of muscarinic cholinergic overstimulation include profuse salivation; lacrimation; serous or seromucous nasal discharge; increased respiratory sounds due to bronchoconstriction and excess bronchial secretions; pronounced GI sounds, colic, and diarrhea due to increased GI motility; bradycardia; pupil constriction; sweating; coughing; vomiting; and frequent urination. These parasympathetic signs usually begin appearing first. Signs of nicotinic cholinergic overstimulation appear soon after onset of the muscarinic signs and include muscle fasciculations, tremors, twitching, spasms, and hypertonicity causing a stiff gait or rigid stance. Central nervous signs attributable to ACh accumulation include apparent anxiety, restlessness, and hyperactivity that may or may not proceed to clonic or clonic-tonic convulsive activity.

Not all animals manifest all of these signs, not all organophosphates produce the same sequence of signs in the same time span, and not all species react the same way to a given organophosphate. However, in a herd outbreak or group situation the overall impressions will likely be similar to the signs given above.

As the toxicosis proceeds, overstimulation of nicotinic cholinergic receptors may cause a depolarizing type neuromuscular blockade with resulting muscular paralysis. In addition, similar depolarizing type paralyses may occur in central nervous pathways involved in regulation of respiration, vasomotion, behavior, and level of consciousness. The result may be a fairly rapid onset of central nervous depression, prostration, coma, dyspnea, cyanosis, and death due to respiratory failure.

Clinical signs associated with individual organophosphates are given by Clarke and Clarke (1967) and Radeleff (1970).

Should animals survive acute poisoning, a neurotoxic reaction might ensue, depending on the organophosphate compound and species involved. This manifests itself as muscle weakness and ataxia, especially in the rear limbs. The condition could progress to the point that the animal could not stand or recline upright and therefore would be unable to eat or drink. Depending on the organophosphate compound, this condition could either be irreversible (due to axonal degeneration/demyelination) or slowly reversible within weeks (see Mechanism of Action).

LESIONS

Sometimes lesions are not manifested

in animals that die quickly of organophosphate poisoning. In animals that take several hours to die, pulmonary edema and congestion, cyanosis, agonal hemorrhages on the heart, hemorrhages in other organs or in skeletal muscle, congestion and edema in various organs including the brain, and possibly patches of necrosis in skeletal muscle may occur. If death is delayed for days or weeks, the carcass is dehydrated and emaciated. If delayed neurotoxicity has occurred, peripheral and spinal motor neurons may manifest degeneration and demyelination.

DIFFERENTIAL DIAGNOSIS

If the history indicates exposure to an organophosphate, and if the clinical signs, lesions, and response to specific therapy are consistent with poisoning by an organophosphate, chances are that an organophosphate caused the toxicosis. Alternatively, a carbamate pesticide may have been at fault since carbamate pesticides are also inhibitors of ACh-E. Should the history be inadequate, and should specific therapy for organophosphate/carbamate poisoning fail, there could be a diagnostic dilemma that may only be resolved by laboratory tests.

The dilemma is due to these facts: some organophosphates produce illness that does not respond very dramatically to specific therapy (see Treatment); a variety of other conditions can mimic organophosphate poisoning; and some organophosphates (e.g., cruformate, coumaphos) may not even cause typical organophosphate poisoning (Buck et al. 1973). Thus the veterinarian may be treating an animal unsuccessfully for what appears to be organophosphate poisoning but *is not,* what appears to be organophosphate poisoning and *is,* or what appears to be some other condition but is really organophosphate poisoning!

In practice, the veterinarian is usually able to exclude most of the conditions that cause respiratory insufficiency (Chapter 57), incoordination and depression (this chapter), and acute abdominal distress (Chapter 59), but there may be some trouble excluding agents that cause nervous stimulation. Often, the main concern is differentiation of organophosphate toxicosis from chlorinated hydrocarbon toxicosis. Signs and lesions of the two conditions overlap considerably. As a rule, however, the chlorinated hydrocarbons do not cause a spectrum of parasympathetic signs, and they produce more severe excitant and convulsant effects accompanied by elevation of body temperature.

TREATMENT

Many of the central and peripheral effects of organophosphates can be blocked with the muscarinic cholinolytic agent atropine sulfate. The dosage required is 0.2–0.5 mg/kg of body weight, one-fourth given intravenously and the rest intramuscularly or subcutaneously. Atropine tends to wear off because of receptor competition by ACh. Therefore, it is necessary to repeat the dosage at 3- to 6-hour intervals for a day or more. Adequate atropinization exists when the pupils are dilated, salivation ceases, and the animal appears to be recovering. Overdosage of atropine sulfate can cause behavioral excitation, hypermotility, and signs of delirium. These effects might make the animal worse or lead to its death. Although atropine sulfate can cause marked improvement in the condition of an animal poisoned by an organophosphate, the drug does not block the nicotinic cholinergic effects of the pesticide. Therefore, the animal will continue to shiver, twitch, or be still (or paralyzed) even after atropinization. A nicotinic-cholinergic blocking agent would seem to be indicated, but in fact is *contraindicated* because of the danger of precipitating or worsening paralysis of respiratory muscles. Thus tubocurarine or gallium triethiodide should *not* be administered. Neither should any other muscle relaxant.

If muscle fasciculations, twitching, spasms, and rigidity are severe, or if the animal is becoming paralyzed, the nicotinic cholinergic signs should be countered by careful administration of one of the cholinesterase-reactivating *oximes.* Examples of these drugs, in order of increasing potency as reactivators of human ACh-E, are:

diacetylmonoxime (DAM); monoisonitrosoacetone (MINA); salts of *N*-methyl-2-pyridinium aldoxime, e.g., 2-pyridine aldoxime methiodide (2-PAM, pralidoxime, Protopam), 2-pyridine aldoxime methchloride (2-PAM chloride, pralidoxime chloride, Protopam chloride), and 2-pyridine aldoxime methanesulfonate (P2S); trimedoxime bromide (TMB-4); and obidoxime chloride (Toxogonin) (Sim 1971). Of these oximes, 2-PAM chloride is probably the drug of choice because it is highly soluble and fairly stable in water, it has few side effects and is widely used for treatment of organophosphate toxicosis in human beings, and it is readily available in pharmacies and hospitals when emergencies arise. The agents P2S and obidoxime are used in Europe.

Sim (1971) has discussed the pharmacology and toxicology of cholinesterase-reactivating oximes. Of main concern in the present discussion is administration and mechanism of action. Oximes work best in the presence of atropine sulfate and therefore should be given to the animal after atropine has been administered. The dossage of atropine may require reduction when oximes are to be used. The dosage of 2-PAM chloride in small animals is 20–50 mg/kg of body weight given as a 10% solution intramuscularly or by slow intravenous injection. The dosage can be repeated as needed. In large animals the dosage of 2-PAM chloride is 25–50 mg/kg of body weight given as a 20% solution during a 6-minute intravenous injection or a maximum dosage of 100 mg/kg by intravenous drip (Szabuniewicz et al. 1971). The treatment can be repeated if signs of toxicosis reappear.

Care must be used in administration of oximes. The drugs do not quickly antagonize signs of poisoning because molecular structure of a particular organophosphate may hinder rapid access of the oxime to the phosphorylated esteratic site of ACh-E; because the esterase-reactivation process is an equilibrium reaction that takes time; and because the treatment may be delayed. The delay may allow time for phosphorylated esterases to become "aged." This aging process, first noticed *in vitro,* is a spontaneous partial dealkylation of the pesticide, causing the phosphorylated esteratic site of ACh-E to acquire a negative charge. This charge makes the site refractory to dephosphorylation by oximes. The rate of aging of phosphorylated esterases depends on many factors, including kind of organophosphate. Methyl, secondary alkyl, and benzyl groups are more likely to split away from phosphorylated esterases than are some other groups. In any event, some treatment failures may be due to the fact that much of the phosphorylated esterases have aged. Thus treatment with oximes has more chance of success if started immediately.

In addition, oximes may not work at all against certain organophosphates (e.g., schradan), may work slowly against pesticides still being absorbed and/or activated in the body, and may tend to increase the toxicosis by virtue of their own anti-ACh-E activity when given in large amounts. The acute intravenous LD50 of 2-PAM chloride in mice is 115 mg/kg of body weight, in dogs 190 mg/kg, and in rabbits 95 mg/kg. Signs of 2-PAM toxicosis in dogs include restlessness, weakness of neck muscles, ataxia, hyperventilation, vomiting, generalized muscle weakness, prostration, intermittent convulsions, respiratory arrest, and death (Sim 1971).

Oximes work by two mechanisms: they react directly with the organophosphate and form a relatively nontoxic complex that can be excreted in the urine and they remove the organophosphate from ACh-E, thus reactivating (dephosphorylating) the enzyme. In this latter reaction (assuming the phosphorylated esterases have not aged appreciably as described above) the oxime is capable of breaking the bond (by nucleophilic attack) between the esteratic site of ACh-E and the phosphoryl group of the pesticide. In doing so, the oxime becomes phosphorylated and ACh-E is liberated (disinhibited). The pesticide-oxime conjugate is then metabolized in the liver and the breakdown products are excreted in the urine.

Other treatment measures in cases of

organophosphate toxicosis are: oxygen therapy if cyanosis and dyspnea are prominent; removal of the source of pesticide; bathing the animal with detergent and water if exposure was by way of the skin; oral administration of mineral oil to retard absorption of pesticide from the gut and to help eliminate the pesticide from the GI tract; keeping the animal quiet and comfortable (without the use of narcotics, tranquilizers, or sedatives); and administration of supportive therapy such as fluids, electrolytes, and multiple vitamins. The animal may require 2–3 days to recover from acute toxicosis.

Should a neurotoxic reaction appear during or after treatment, there is no specific antidote. The animal might survive if given intensive nursing care, but the condition of muscular weakness or prostration may last for weeks. If the pesticide is one that causes degeneration and demyelination of peripheral and spinal motor neurons, euthanasia may be the best treatment. Care must be taken, however, to determine that a condition of muscular weakness is actually a neurotoxic reaction and not some prolonged weakness due to anti-ACh-E activity of slowly absorbed or slowly activated pesticide or incomplete dephosphorylation of ACh-E by oximes. As long as the animal can eat and drink, it is worthwhile to wait and see if muscle weakness is going to abate over a period of days or weeks. In other words, it is not advisable, although perhaps it is economical, to kill an animal that may eventually recover from organophosphate toxicosis.

ANALYSIS

Organophosphates do not stay in tissues very long after the animal is exposed. The liver breaks them down. Fresh tissues *can* be tested for the presence of organophosphates, but test results may be negative. Similarly, blood, urine, and milk may be negative.

Whole blood ACh-E activity is an index of exposure to organophosphates. If blood ACh-E activity is less than 25% of normal, one can assume exposure to excess organophosphate or other cholinesterase inhibitor. Normal whole blood ACh-E activity expressed in terms of change in pH (by a modified Michel method) in various species is: horse, 0.2–0.65; cattle, 0.3–0.75; sheep, 0.1–0.3; goat, 0.04–0.24; and dog, 0.43 mean value (Buck et al. 1973).

Tests for organophosphates are tedious and require sophisticated equipment and techniques and highly trained personnel. Such tests are expensive. Some laboratories charge the veterinarian $15–$20 for each sample tested; the total charge for testing several feeds or suspect materials involved in a case of poisoning may be prohibitive. Other laboratories do not charge for testing services.

Response to specific therapy remains a valuable diagnostic aid but should be supported with a blood ACh-E determination. There are no "normal levels" of organophosphate pesticides in feeds or animal tissues. If the pesticide is present in material to which typically-ill animals were exposed, chances are that the material was to blame for the toxicosis.

Carbamate Pesticides

USE

These compounds are used for the same general purposes as the organophosphates.

SOURCE

Animals may ingest carbamate pesticides in contaminated feeds or forages or they may eat spilled pesticide. Certain carbamates applied to the skin of animals can cause poisoning by dermal absorption. Generally, carbamates and organophosphates share similar sources with regard to poisoning of animals.

Some common carbamate pesticides are listed under Toxicity. The veterinarian should be acquainted with the names of these compounds to be able to recognize the kinds of pesticides used on the premises or those involved in toxicosis and to treat the toxicosis accordingly.

PROPERTIES OF TOXICOLOGIC IMPORTANCE

These are about the same as for organophosphates, that is, the compounds are not very stable in the environment and not very soluble in water. Organic solvents and oils can carry the compounds across cell barriers. The phenomena of storage activation apparently do not occur with carbamates.

TOXICITY

Buck et al. (1973) have listed LD50 values for five carbamates in several species. Toxicity data are incomplete for domestic animals. Lethal dosages seem to vary up to several hundred mg/kg of body weight according to factors discussed under Organophosphates. The list of LD50 values in rats is given in Table 58.3 and may serve to indicate (roughly) which of the carbamates are potentially most hazardous for domestic animals. Ranges of values are due to differences in source of information and sex of animal.

Carbaryl, probably the least toxic carbamate insecticide, may be applied topically in 1%–4% aqueous suspension in cattle, 1%–2% in sheep, and 1% in goats. Dairy cows can eat 50–200 ppm carbaryl in the diet for a month, or 450 ppm for 2 weeks, without ill effect. In swine, it takes an oral dose of 750 mg carbaryl/kg of body weight to cause acute toxicosis. Smaller dosages (150–300 mg/kg) fed over a period of 8–12 weeks may cause myopathy and muscular dystrophic changes combined with cerebral edema. In dogs, carbaryl may be teratogenic (Radeleff 1970).

Carbofuran, a more hazardous carbamate pesticide, should not be sprayed or

TABLE 58.3. Acute oral LD50 values in rats

Common Name	Trade Name	Acute Oral LD50 *(mg/kg)*
carbofuran	Furadan	5–11
aldicarb	Temik	7
mexacarbate	Zectran	19–37
aminocarb	Matacil	38–40
methiocarb	Mesurol	60–130
propoxur	Unden	83–104
metalkamate	Bux	87–170
landrin	Landrin	178–208
carbaryl	Sevin	307–800

Sources: Clarke and Clarke 1967; Gaines 1969; Buck et al. 1973; Berg 1974.

sprinkled freely on or around animals. Palmer and Schlinke (1973a) produced typical signs of acute toxicosis in dairy calves given oral doses of 0.25 mg/kg of body weight, or more, or topical applications of 0.05% concentration, or more. Tick-infested yearling cattle were poisoned by topical application of a 0.1% concentration of carbofuran. Mild toxicosis resulted when yearling cattle were given an oral dose of 1 mg/kg, but not when the dosage was 0.5 mg/kg. In sheep, oral administration of 2.5 mg carbofuran/kg of body weight caused toxicosis but 1 mg/kg did not. Illness in all these animals was of rapid onset and short (6 hours) duration. A significant conclusion was that the minimal rate of application of carbofuran to a pasture (0.28 kg/ha) could be hazardous for livestock that graze the pasture soon after application of the pesticide.

Some carbamate pesticides may cause leg weakness in chickens, a possible neurotoxic effect. This weakness is produced by a dose of 1600 mg of carbaryl/kg of body weight, or more, and with smaller dosages of two experimental compounds. The leg weakness disappears in 1–24 days. Leg weakness is not produced by aldicarb, mexacarbate, aminocarb, methiocarb, or propoxur (Gaines 1969). This is interesting in view of the fact that the latter compounds are more toxic in rats than carbaryl.

Compounds containing a carbamate moiety are used as fungicidal dressing on seed grains. These are metallic (ferric, zinc, manganese) dithiocarbamates, e.g., ziram (Ziride, rat acute oral LD50 > 5200 mg/kg), maneb (Manzate, rat acute oral LD50, 6750 mg/kg), and ferbam (Fermate, rat acute LD50 > 17,000 mg/kg) (Berg 1974). These particular compounds are relatively nontoxic compared with carbamate insecticides, do not cause toxicosis by the same mechanism as carbamate insecticides, would not cause the same clinical signs as carbamate insecticides, and should *not* be suspected of causing toxicosis in animals manifesting signs of cholinesterase-inhibition. See Buck et al. (1973) for detail on these compounds. Also, some carbamate (dichlormate) and thiocarbamate (diallate, triallate, EPTC, vernolate) herbicides do not cause typical signs of insecticide toxicosis. Toxicity of these compounds in cattle and sheep is only moderate.

Factors that affect toxicity of carbamate pesticides are likely very similar to those affecting toxicity of organophosphates.

TOXICODYNAMIC CONSIDERATIONS

Carbamate pesticides are absorbed from the skin, lungs, and GI tract and distributed throughout the body. They do not accumulate in any particular tissue. Blood esterases would tend to inactivate a portion of the circulating carbamates. Liver microsomal enzymes break the compounds down within hours of exposure. Carbamates do not require activation by liver enzymes and therefore may be more hazardous for very young animals, in which hepatic degradative enzymes are deficient.

MECHANISM OF ACTION

Acute toxicosis is due to inhibition of ACh-E, just as with the organophosphates. The carbamate insecticides occupy both the anionic and esteratic sites of ACh-E, the esteratic site being *carbamylated* rather than phosphorylated as with the organophosphates. Acetylcholinesterase *is* able to hydrolyze carbamate insecticides, although the rate of hydrolysis is not as fast as for the natural substrate ACh. Thus carbamate insecticides are "reversible" inhibitors of ACh-E. Toxicosis develops when the amount of pesticide in the body is so large that the rate of carbamylation of ACh-E exceeds the rate of hydrolysis of pesticide by the enzyme. Acetylcholine then accumulates in neuroeffector and synaptic regions, resulting in clinical signs similar to those of organophosphates.

The leg paralysis (chickens) and muscular degeneration/necrosis and cerebral edema (swine) caused by large dosages of carbaryl may not be due to inhibition of ACh-E; these effects have not been reported for carbamate insecticides that are even more toxic (better ACh-E inhibitors) than carbaryl.

CLINICAL SIGNS

Clinical signs reflect muscarinic and nicotinic cholinergic overstimulation, as already described for organophosphates. The signs are likely to be less severe and/or much shorter in duration than those of the organophosphates.

Signs of muscle weakness/damage or central nervous damage are unlikely under field conditions because the dosage of carbamate compound is not likely to be large enough.

LESIONS

See Organophosphates.

DIFFERENTIAL DIAGNOSIS

See Organophosphates.

TREATMENT

Acute toxicosis responds well to atropine sulfate, 0.2–0.5 mg/kg of body weight, one-fourth given intravenously and the rest subcutaneously or intramuscularly. Atropinization should be maintained for 1 or 2 days. Administration of 2-PAM chloride is not effective and may worsen the animal's condition. Other measures discussed under treatment of organophosphate toxicosis may be taken to ensure rapid recovery. The prognosis is generally good if treatment is instituted soon after onset of clinical signs. Animals may even survive without treatment if clinical signs are not severe because the carbamates are metabolized very quickly.

ANALYSIS

The pesticide may not be detectable in tissues, secretions, or blood because it is rapidly destroyed in the body. Blood ACh-E activity may be depressed, but this effect may be missed because of the reversibility of inhibition of ACh-E by carbamates. Diagnosis is made from the history, clinical signs, lesions (or absence of lesions), response to atropine treatment, and knowledge of exposure to a product containing a carbamate pesticide.

Strychnine

USE

Strychnine is used as a mammalicide, a vertebrate poison, for the control of squirrels, gophers, rabbits, and wild carnivora that become pests about the premises or predators on livestock. Strychnine or its crude source, nux vomica, may be an ingredient in GI medications in which the substance may be touted as a tonic and a bitter stomachic. It is doubtful that the compound accomplishes any "toning up" in any sense of the term in the concentrations used in these medications. Moreover, the efficacy of bitters in animal medicine has not been established. Strychnine seems to be the poison of choice in the malicious destruction of pets.

SOURCE

Strychnine sulfate is readily available wherever pesticides are sold. The compound may be present at 0.5%–1% concentration in colored grain or pelleted baits or it may be sold as a powder to be mixed with other forms of bait. Dogs become poisoned when they eat baits intended for other vertebrate pests or predators. Alternately, strychnine sulfate may be concealed in food and deliberately placed in a dog's yard.

PROPERTIES OF TOXICOLOGIC IMPORTANCE

Strychnine is an alkaloid obtained from the seeds of the tree *Strychnos nux vomica,* which grows in India, Southeast Asia, and northern Australia. The alkaloid is also found in seeds of the climbing shrub *Strychnos ignatii,* which grows in Southeast Asia and the Philippines. Powdered *Strychnos* seeds (nux vomica) also contain brucine, strychnicine, loganin, caffeotannic acid, and proteins. Strychnine is bitter, thus necessitating concealment of the alkaloid in baits intended for carnivora. The alkaloid base forms sulfate, hydrochloride, nitrate, and other salts, which are more water-soluble than the free base. The sulfate is the most commonly used salt of strychnine. It is a white crystalline powder that is insoluble in ether but more or less soluble in alcohol, chloroform, or glycerol. Strychnine is precipitated by alkali, carbonates, bicarbonates, benzoates, dichromates, bromides, iodides, tannic acid, picric acid, salicylates, borax, and proteins. The alkaloid binds to cell membranes, filter papers, and cotton, thus presenting some difficulties in analysis.

TOXICITY

The approximate acute oral lethal dose of strychnine salts in various species is (in mg/kg of body weight): horse and cow, 0.5; swine, 0.5–1; dog, 0.75; cat, 2; rat, 3; and fowl, 5. These dosages can be reduced from 2 to 10 times for the parenteral routes of administration (Buck et al. 1973). In human beings the lethal dose is about 1 mg/kg of body weight (Slater 1971).

Bitter and irritant properties of strychnine can cause emesis in species that can vomit. Thus the presence of food in the stomach may prevent emesis and enhance toxicity. An empty stomach does not necessarily guarantee survival of a dog, cat, or pig that ingests a large amount of strychnine because the alkaloid is absorbed quickly from the gut. Toxicity may be influenced by the rate of ingestion. Small amounts ingested over a period of time may have no ill effect because strychnine is eliminated rapidly from the body.

Individual response to strychnine varies greatly. In 44 dogs that died of acute strychnine poisoning, strychnine concentration ranged from zero to 52 ppm in the liver and from zero to 12,800 ppm in stomach contents (Hatch and Funnell 1968). If all dogs were equally susceptible to strychnine, one would expect the liver concentrations to be about the same in all at death, assuming the alkaloid is distributed the same way in each dog. Time of onset of death is not related to concentration of strychnine in liver or stomach contents. Other species also manifest individual variation in response to strychnine (Clarke and Clarke 1967).

TOXICODYNAMIC CONSIDERATIONS

Strychnine is rapidly absorbed from

the intestinal tract and distributed throughout the body. It does not accumulate in any given tissue, but significant concentrations occur in the liver and kidney. The alkaloid is metabolized in the liver and also excreted unchanged in the urine. Excretion is very rapid; most of a lethal dosage is eliminated within 24 hours. This fact forms one of the bases of therapy: if the animal can be made to survive the first day or so, chances are that no further treatment is needed (see Treatment).

MECHANISM OF ACTION

In the mammalian CNS there is a constant efferent flow of motor impulses from various regions of the brain, down the spinal cord and out to the postural, respiratory, and locomotor muscles. These impulses require *modulation* so that skeletal muscles are not overstimulated; muscle tonus is appropriate for requirements imposed by gravity and by postural changes; and muscle contractions are smooth, properly coordinated, and consistent with requirements of locomotion and respiration.

Modulation of efferent motor impulses is by means of various inhibitory neurons in the brain and spinal cord. A major portion of these neurons are interneurons, which function to inhibit the postsynaptic regions of the motor neuron chain. Postsynaptic inhibition *in the brain* is thought to be mediated by γ-aminobutyric acid (GABA) or other depressant (hyperpolarizing) type amino acids whose inhibitory actions can be blocked in a stereoselective and competitive fashion by convulsant drugs, e.g., picrotoxin and bicuculline, and perhaps by cicutoxin and penicillin (Roberts and Kuriyama 1968; Curtis et al. 1970; Krnjević 1970; Curtis et al. 1971a; Curtis et al. 1971b; Okada et al. 1971; Davidoff 1972; Hill et al. 1972; Huffman and McFadin 1972; Smythies 1974).

Postsynaptic inhibition *in the spinal cord* is analagous to the mechanism outlined for the brain, but with an important difference: the motor inhibitory neurotransmitter in the spinal cord is thought to be glycine (Werman et al. 1967a,b; Curtis et al. 1968). The spinal depressant (hyperpolarizing) effects of glycine (and some other potential inhibitory transmitters) are blocked competitively and stereoselectively by spinal convulsants such as strychnine and thebaine. Thus it is postulated (and becoming generally accepted) that strychnine causes tonic (tetanic) convulsions by competing with spinal glycine for the glycine receptor on motor neurons, thus "demodulating" spinal motor impulses (Curtis et al. 1968; Smythies 1974).

Glycine does occur in some regions of the brain, particularly the medulla (Aprison et al. 1968; Tebēcis and DiMaria 1972; Boehme et al. 1973). Moreover, a large concentration of strychnine can apparently inhibit GABA receptors (Davidoff et al. 1969). Thus supraspinal signs observed in animals (see Clinical Signs) poisoned by strychnine may be due to strychnine inhibition of supraspinal glycine and GABA receptors. It is believed, however, that strychnine toxicosis results mainly from blockade of glycine receptors in the spinal cord.

The nature of the glycine receptor has not been elucidated. On the basis of structure-activity relationships and molecular models, Smythies (1974) has postulated a chemical configuration of the glycine receptor protein. Presumably, when glycine bonds to the receptor protein, conformational changes occur in the receptor. These changes may open adjacent pores in the receptor membrane, thus altering membrane permeability to potassium and chloride ions, with resulting hyperpolarization of the neuronal membrane (Curtis et al. 1968). Recent work (Snyder 1975) seems to establish a cooperative link between the chloride-potassium ion–gating phenomenon and the glycine-recognition area of the glycine receptor. In fact, *the two phenomena, recognition of glycine and subsequent gating of ion flux, are considered two parts of the glycine receptor.* The recognition part binds glycine and the gating mechanism binds strychnine. Thus strychnine is thought to prevent the gating mechanism from operating in response to glycine recognition by the receptor. In this way the motor inhibitory effects of glycine are prevented. An analogous situation exists with the GABA receptor.

Strychnine, bicuculline, and picrotoxin do have some direct depolarizing and firing threshold-lowering effects on neuronal membranes (Freeman 1973), but the relevance of these observations to clinical cases of poisoning is not known.

CLINICAL SIGNS

Having considered the mechanism of action of strychnine, it is not difficult to anticipate that the clinical signs of poisoning are manifestations of too many nerve impulses reaching the skeletal muscles.

In the dog (the species most often presented for treatment), early signs are apparent apprehension, unrest, panting, and possible nausea and vomiting. Then the facial muscles begin to tighten up; the corners of the mouth are drawn back in a "grin"; the eyelids may twitch; and the ears tend to draw together, forming a wrinkled pate. Simultaneously, the dog may be hyperresponsive to auditory or tactile stimuli. Muscles of the neck, chest, and abdomen begin to stiffen, and the stance becomes rigid. If the table is struck or the animal's back is tapped, hyperreflexia is seen. The gait is stiff and the dog may defecate and urinate. As more strychnine is absorbed from the gut, the dog becomes extremely stiff and hyperreflexic. Generalized trembling and twitching of muscles may occur. Then some small stimulus initiates a typical spinal seizure characterized by sudden stiffening of all muscles, collapse, tonic extension of the limbs, opisthotonos, vocalization, and difficult respiration. Extensor muscles are affected most because they are stronger than the flexors. Consciousness is not lost during the initial part of the seizure because strychnine does not depress neural mechanisms of consciousness. Vocalization may be due in part to the severe pain of muscle fatigue.

The initial seizure may terminate in 2 or 3 minutes and the dog lies panting and apparently resting. However, strychnine continues to be absorbed from the gut and soon another tonic seizure occurs, evoked by some stimulus or by the animal's own movements. This time the seizure may be more severe and last longer. The respiratory muscles may be unable to function because they are tonically rigid. Apnea causes cerebral anoxia and loss of consciousness. Anoxic cells in the brain drastically reduce efferent motor activity, with the result that the skeletal muscles relax.

If respiration resumes, the brain becomes oxygenated again. Reoxygenation of the brain allows consciousness to return. Efferent motor activity also returns. By this time the dog may have absorbed enough strychnine so that the next tonic seizure stops respiratory function too long. The dog then dies of cerebral anoxia. Rigor mortis occurs quickly.

The number of convulsions and the total time required for death vary according to dosage of strychnine. Often the dog is simply found dead one morning. A large oral dosage of strychnine may be lethal in 20–30 minutes and produce only 1 convulsion. Smaller dosages may produce 3 or 4 seizures over a period of an hour or more.

Cats manifest about the same signs as dogs, but domestic cats do not gulp down large chunks of poisoned bait as dogs do. Moreover, cats are more likely to reject a bad tasting bait. Thus, cats are only occasionally presented for treatment of strychnine poisoning.

Large species of domestic animals are rarely poisoned by strychnine. Occasionally, swine may be poisoned if they eat rats that died of strychnine poisoning. Meek and Keatts (1971) report that in one horse, ingestion of strychnine-treated oats (used for gopher control) caused sweating, incoordination, shivering, prostration, struggling to rise, tonic-clonic convulsions, and death in about 2 hours.

LESIONS

Significant lesions may not be manifested. If convulsions are prolonged, agonal hemorrhages may occur on the heart or lungs. The haircoat may be muddy or soiled during convulsions. Foreign matter may be aspirated into the bronchi. Early rigor may be seen. Organ congestion, cyanosis, and other evidence of asphyxia may be apparent. The stomach may be empty or it may contain remnants of the last meal. Special attention should be devoted to materials in the stomach because the poisoned bait may be identified as some component that was not fed to the animal in the normal diet.

DIFFERENTIAL DIAGNOSIS

This usually presents little difficulty because the history, clinical signs, necropsy findings, species, and rapid recovery (in animals treated in time) are characteristic of strychnine poisoning. Laboratory analysis of the liver, kidney, stomach contents, and suspect bait may confirm the diagnosis. If the diagnosis is in doubt, the veterinarian must consider other convulsive disorders. There are not many of these for which onset is so rapid, death so quick to follow, and necropsy findings are so inconclusive. In this regard, the organophosphate, carbamate, and chlorinated hydrocarbon pesticides; fluoroacetate; nicotine; fluoride; and 2,4-D weed killer might be considered. Less likely candidates are tetanus toxin, cocaine, carbon monoxide, insulin, metaldehyde, and phenothiazine tranquilizers. Tonic seizures are seen as a component of a variety of seizure disorders. It is important to remember that strychnine does not normally cause very much clonic (epileptiform) activity. Careful questioning of the client may establish the nature of convulsions manifested by the animal.

TREATMENT

The overall objectives are to prevent convulsions so that the animal can breathe and to keep the animal breathing long enough to allow strychnine to be eliminated from the body.

Typically, the animal is presented in a preconvulsive state, having already manifested 1 or 2 seizures. The thing *not* to do is administer an emetic such as apomorphine "to empty the stomach." Chances are that the muscular activity of vomition will precipitate a seizure. Instead, the animal should be given a drug that decreases efferent motor activity in the brain or spinal cord and at the same time restrains the animal so that the trachea can be intubated (to provide a free airway and facilitate artificial respiration if needed). The stomach may be washed out (repeated washing with 2% aqueous tannic acid or sodium bicarbonate or a 1:250 dilution of tincture of iodine, followed by a final wash of plain water) and an intravenous drip initiated (isotonic glucose or saline to accelerate urine formation and elimination of strychnine from the bloodstream). The animal should be provided adequate nursing care and protected from auditory and tactile stimuli.

Traditionally, the drug of choice for dogs has been pentobarbital sodium, 30 mg/kg of body weight, given intravenously. The intraperitoneal or intrathoracic route can be used if the dog is extremely hyperreflexic or in convulsions. Cats are anesthetized with a thiobarbiturate, e.g., thiopental sodium or thiamylal sodium, given intravenously to effect. Cats given pentobarbital or other short-acting barbiturates sleep too long. Cats anesthetized by thiopental or thiamylal given by the intraperitoneal or intrathoracic route require a large total dosage of thiobarbiturate (60–75 mg/kg of body weight) in order that anesthesia be attained. This dosage may make cats sleep too long. Large domestic species can be anesthetized with chloral hydrate–pentobarbital or just heavily sedated or hypnotized with chloral hydrate.

Other drugs can be tried, as an alternative to general anesthesia, to decrease spinal motor activity. Methocarbamol is mentioned by Szabuniewicz et al. (1971). Diazepam has sedative and muscle-relaxant properties. It also mimics glycine in its ability to displace strychnine from the glycine receptor (Snyder 1975). Xylazine might be effective also.

Opiates depress respiration and also stimulate the spinal cord. Ketamine has motor stimulant effects in the brain. Peripheral neuromuscular blocking agents may paralyze respiratory muscles. None of these agents should be used in treatment of strychnine poisoning. Acetylpromazine was not effective in relieving strychnine convulsions in experimental dogs in student laboratory exercises. Glycine infusion is not recommended until research is done with this agent.

When the animal awakens from anesthesia, it should be carefully observed. If convulsive tendencies remain, additional sedation is indicated. Degree of sedation should be light enough to allow periodic reassessment. If the animal survives 24 hours, prognosis for complete recovery is excellent. Care must be taken, however, not to convert a case of strychnine poisoning into a case of anesthetic overdose!

ANALYSIS

Strychnine is never considered to be a "normal" constituent of the body. Thus any concentration of the alkaloid in biological samples from an animal that manifested typical history, signs, and lesions of strychnine poisoning indicates that strychnine was the likely cause of poisoning. Sometimes a sample may be negative for strychnine even when the animal was poisoned by this alkaloid. Stomach contents or liver may be negative (Hatch and Funnell 1968) but *both* of these are not likely to be negative. The veterinarian should send more than one kind of sample for strychnine analysis. Urine may be negative for strychnine if the sample is obtained more than 24 hours after recovery, because the alkaloid is rapidly excreted. The same is true of blood, which does not usually contain much strychnine anyway, due to the fact that strychnine binds to tissue membranes. Stomach washings may be reported negative for strychnine because of extensive dilution during the lavage procedure. The first wash is the best one to analyze.

Fluoroacetate, Fluoroacetamide

USE

Fluoroacetate and fluoroacetamide are used for rodenticidal purposes and for rabbit control.

SOURCE

Domestic animals may ingest baits intended for other species. The baits are usually carrot chunks, bread, bran, or meats. A black dye is mixed with these compounds in order to prevent baits from being mistaken for edible food. Unfortunately, domestic animals do not care how their food looks. Therefore fluoroacetate (Compound 1080) and congeners are further controlled by being available only from a licensed exterminator. The reason for these precautions is that these particular rodenticides are very dangerous for all species.

PROPERTIES OF TOXICOLOGIC IMPORTANCE

These rodenticides are odorless, tasteless, and water-soluble. Rodents do not develop bait shyness to these compounds. Baits left outdoors will gradually lose potency over a period of weeks as the poison is washed or leached away. This fact, however, is no excuse for not retrieving baits after an extermination effort.

TOXICITY

The acute oral lethal dose of fluoroacetate and congeners in various species is (in mg/kg of body weight): dog, 0.05–0.2; cow, 0.25–0.5; pig, 0.3–0.4; cat, 0.3–0.5; sheep, 0.3–0.7; horse, 0.5–1.75; human being, 2–5; rat and mouse, 5–8; fowl, 10–30; and monkey, 14 (Sollmann 1957; Clarke and Clarke 1967; Buck et al. 1973).

It is not known why there is so much species variation in toxicity of fluoroacetate. The variation is apparently not due to differences in size of animal, type of digestive system, or basal metabolic rate. Perhaps it is related to rate of elimination of the poison or rate of condensation of the poison with oxalacetate (see Mechanism of Action).

Dogs, cats, or pigs that eat fluoroacetate-poisoned rats or mice can be fatally poisoned.

TOXICODYNAMIC CONSIDERATIONS

Fluoroacetate is readily absorbed from the gut, lungs, or open wounds, but not through intact skin. The compound is carried throughout the body in the bloodstream, and does not accumulate in a given type of tissue.

MECHANISM OF ACTION

After entry into tissue cells, fluoroacetate condenses with oxalacetate to form fluorocitrate. Fluorocitrate then competes with citrate for the active site of the Krebs cycle enzyme, aconitase, which is the ultimate receptor in fluoroacetate poisoning. The result is that aconitase becomes inhibited by fluorocitrate, thus slowing the Krebs cycle and decreasing cellular respiration. This action occurs in all cells, but brain and heart functions are affected most severely. Ammonia accumulates in the brain and could cause the convulsions typical of fluoroacetate in some species (Benitez et al. 1954).

It takes time for the above processes to occur. Thus in fluoroacetate or fluoroacetamide poisoning, a latent period of 30 minutes to 2 hours exists between ingestion of poison and appearance of signs of metabolic derangement. Once these signs appear, the toxicosis develops rapidly.

CLINICAL SIGNS

Why should inhibition of aconitase have different effects in different mammalian species? Presumably the enzyme has the same biochemical functions in the Krebs cycle of each species. Perhaps the answer lies in the relative degree of importance or toxicity of Krebs cycle intermediates and products in organs of different species. Or, perhaps organs of different species accumulate different amounts of ammonia. In any event, three kinds of clinical manifestations occur with fluoroacetate or fluoroacetamide poisoning.

In dogs and guinea pigs, signs are referable to central nervous excitation but not to cardiac malfunction. After a period of restlessness, vomiting, diarrhea, urination, and hyperirritability, the dog manifests hypermotility, frenzied running in a straight line, barking and yelping, frothing at the mouth, and intermittent clonic-tonic seizures (extensor rigidity and opisthotonos with paddling of the limbs). The seizures are not elicitable by external stimuli. Also, the seizures become weaker as the animal's cellular energy supplies dwindle. Terminal coma and gasping are manifested, and death comes in 2–12 hours. Rigor mortis occurs quickly (Clarke and Clarke 1967; Radeleff 1970; Buck et al. 1973).

In horses, cattle, sheep, goats, rabbits, and monkeys, clinical signs are referable to heart failure but not to central nervous excitation. These species manifest colic, unrest, trembling, staggering, cardiac arrhythmias and tachycardia, and terminal ventricular fibrillation, which is the cause of death. Terminal convulsions may be seen, but these may be secondary to cerebral anoxia. If *all* species manifested the signs described for herbivores, then fluoroacetate would rightly be classified as an agent that causes predominant signs of respiratory insufficiency, which is discussed in Chapter 57. The poison is mentioned in that chapter but discussed in detail here because it is dogs, cats, or pigs, not herbivores, that are usually poisoned by fluoroacetate.

In cats, pigs, and hamsters the signs of fluoroacetate poisoning are a combination of the nervous and cardiac signs already mentioned. There may not be the intense hypermotility and frenzy seen in dogs, but excitation phenomena and cardiac arrhythmias are present.

LESIONS

The occurrence of lesions depends somewhat on whether death was due to sudden ventricular fibrillation or convulsions with respiratory depression. With ventricular fibrillation, there may be no lesions, with the exception of severe enteritis from the irritant effects of fluoroacetate. Death from convulsions and respiratory depression may cause cyanosis, dark colored blood, organ congestion, agonal hemorrhages on the heart, and pulmonary changes in addition to the enteritis. Microscopically, the brain may manifest edema and perivascular infiltration with lymphocytes, but these lesions are not pathognomonic of fluoroacetate or fluoroacetamide toxicosis.

DIFFERENTIAL DIAGNOSIS

Buck et al. (1973) rightly point out that several conditions might be confused with fluoroacetate poisoning and that diagnosis relies on a detailed history and knowledge of clinical signs and lesions. It also helps to know that no other poisons or diseases are present in the animal and that treatment of the condition was to no avail.

In dogs, fluoroacetate poisoning may mimic any severe encephalitic disease; aspects of poisoning by strychnine, lead, chlorinated hydrocarbon pesticides, or bacterial food toxins; and conditions such as hypocalcemia, hypomagnesemia, pancreatic disease, liver necrosis, and cerebral injury. In herbivores, sudden death is also produced by agents discussed in Chapters 57 and 59.

TREATMENT

No specific treatment exists. Convulsions can be controlled with barbiturates given in subanesthetic doses. Oxygen may be administered by positive pressure. The stomach may be washed out with milk or limewater. Attempts to provide cells with excess acetate have not been very rewarding. In this regard, one may administer glyceryl monoacetate, 0.1–0.5 mg/kg of body weight, intramuscularly every hour for a total of 2–4 mg/kg (Szabuniewicz et al. 1971). Alternately, acetate might be provided by oral administration of 8.8 ml/kg of body weight each of 50% ethanol and 5% acetic acid (Buck et al. 1973). The alcohol would be metabolized to acetate in the body, but it might also cause additional respiratory depression.

It seems logical to administer citrate if the biochemical lesion is competitive inhibition of aconitase by fluorocitrate. Indeed, citrate could be given if it did not chelate blood calcium so well and thereby produce hypocalcemia. Perhaps calcium citrate could be given by slow intravenous injection while monitoring the heart for signs of calcium toxicosis. Such therapy has not been tried as far as this author knows, but it might be worth a try in an otherwise doomed animal.

Cardiac arrhythmias might be treatable, but the appropriate antiarrhythmic agent has not been suggested for fluoroacetate-induced arrhythmias. To try one of the drugs empirically would certainly not harm the animal any more than did the fluoroacetate.

ANALYSIS

Fluoroacetate causes citrate accumulation in cells. Kidney tissue may be tested for excess citrate, but an elevated citrate concentration would not be direct proof of exposure to fluoroacetate or congeners. Citrate is also a normal substance in cells.

Organo-monofluorine compounds are not normal substances in cells. Their presence indicates exposure to fluoroacetate or similar compounds or possibly to fluorinated inhalant anesthetics. The analysis for these compounds is extremely complicated and time-consuming. Use of a specific ion electrode for fluorine may simplify tissue and bait analysis for organofluorine compounds (Peters and Baxter 1974).

Nicotine

Animals may ingest nicotine sulfate (Black Leaf 40) from spills of the solution, contaminated containers, or foliage that has been sprayed with the alkaloid. Ingestion of excessive amounts of tobacco leaves (*Nicotiana* spp.) or cured tobacco in cigarettes or cigars may also cause toxicosis.

Nicotine toxicosis reflects initial stimulation and then depolarizing type blockade of all nicotinic cholinergic receptors, i.e., acetylcholine receptors of skeletal muscle motor endplates, autonomic ganglia, and CNS.

Clinical signs are consistent with overstimulation of cholinergic receptors and are similar to signs of organophosphate poisoning. Convulsions of a clonic-tonic type may be very severe; the animal may then become depressed within a few minutes and die of respiratory failure. This is why nicotine sulfate is not a good agent for capture-immobilization of animals.

Postmortem findings might be negative, with the possible exception of the distinctive pungent odor of nicotine in the stomach contents. Nicotine smells like old cigar butts or spittle from a smoker's pipe.

It is unlikely that treatment can be instituted in time to save the poisoned animal. In the very earliest stages of poisoning, a nondepolarizing type ganglion blocker, one that can also pass the blood-brain barrier (e.g., mecamylamine), might be of benefit. This agent would also have partial neuromuscular blocking activity in higher dosages. Treatment with atropine sulfate (the veterinarian's first impulse when there are signs of cholinergic overstimulation) would be without value because atropine does not protect vital nicotinic receptors in respiratory muscles and the CNS from the potent depolarizing effects of nicotine.

If the animal is already in a depressed state and the muscles are flaccid, no drug can help. Artificial respiration becomes the only means of keeping the animal alive. This usually fails.

Plant Poisons

Some plant poisons that cause signs of nervous stimulation through action on a known receptor include nicotine, atropine-like alkaloids in jimson weed (*Datura* spp.) and henbane (*Hyoscyamus* sp.), and thiaminase in horsetails (*Equisetum* spp.). The atropine type alkaloids block muscarinic cholinergic receptors in the brain and periphery. Clinical signs are those of parasympathetic blockade plus agitation, delirium, compulsive motor activity, vocalization, and terminal convulsions. These signs are more or less reversible by adequate dosages of physostigmine (but not neostigmine, which does not readily cross the blood-brain barrier).

The receptor for thiaminase is thiamine. Actually, thiamine is a substrate for destruction by the enzyme. In ruminants (but not in other species) thiaminase causes behavioral excitation and other signs of central nervous stimulation, accompanied by loss of condition, weakness, and diarrhea. The treatment, of course, is thiamine. See Kingsbury (1964) for detail.

POISONS CAUSING NERVOUS STIMULATION OR DEPRESSION BY UNKNOWN MECHANISMS

Chlorinated Hydrocarbon Pesticides

USE

Chlorinated hydrocarbon pesticides are used primarily as contact insecticides.

SOURCE

Although relatively few in number compared with the organophosphates, certain organochlorine insecticides are widely used for prevention and control of insect infestations about commercial, farm, and home premises and on animals. Thus animals may be poisoned by ingestion of contaminated feeds, sprayed foliage, spilled product, or water from "empty" pesticide containers. These pesticides may also be inhaled by the animal or absorbed through the skin when applied topically. Sometimes the source of poisoning cannot be located, having been consumed entirely or washed away. Sometimes the pesticide source is located but no explanation can be found for its presence. Due to their persistence in the environment and their ability to accumulate in biological food chains, organochlorine pesticide residues may appear "naturally" in animal tissues.

Organochlorine insecticides are divided into three groups based on chemical structure: the DDT group, the cyclodiene group, and a group of heterogeneous compounds that can be called a miscellaneous group. The DDT group consists of DDT, related bis-*p*-chlorophenyl compounds and their isomers (which may or may not be commercial insecticides), and the bis-*p*-methoxyphenyl compound methoxychlor. The use of DDT and the related compound TDE is presently restricted, but these may be allowed wider use in later years. Other members of the group, 1,1-dichloro-2,2-bis(*p*-ethylphenyl)ethane (Perthane) and methoxychlor (Marlate), are in use. The cyclodiene group includes the presently banned aldrin and dieldrin and other agents such as chlordane (Octachlor), endrin, endosulfan (Chlorthiepin, Malix), and heptachlor (Velsicol 104). The miscellaneous organochlorine insecticides include toxaphene (Phenatox, Toxakil), which is a mixture of chlorinated camphenes; gamma-benzenehexachloride or lindane (Gammex, Lindafor), which should not be confused with hexachlorobenzene fungicide or with hexachlorophene antiseptic; and mirex (Dechlorane), a presently restricted compound having a 12-chlorine, 10-carbon cage structure.

As more organochlorine pesticides become restricted in use, the incidence of poisoning of animals by these compounds can be expected to decline. As the rough draft of this text was being sent to the typist, the Environmental Protection Agency (EPA) announced the suspension of chlordane and heptachlor on the basis of carcinogenicity in experimental animals.

PROPERTIES OF TOXICOLOGIC IMPORTANCE

Chlorinated hydrocarbon insecticides are poorly soluble in water but soluble in oils and organic solvents. Thus the compounds are used as dusts, wettable powders, emulsions, or suspensions. An oily vehicle or an organic solvent vehicle facilitates penetration of insecticide through intact skin; poisoning has occurred by this mechanism. Volatility is characteristic of this group of insecticides, slow vaporization being responsible for some loss of pesticide from exposed surfaces, uptake of pesticide by foliage of plants, and exposure of insects (and animals) to the pesticide by the inhalation route.

With some exceptions (e.g., endosulfan and Perthane, which are biodegradable) the organochlorine insecticides are very persistent in the environment because they resist chemical or microbial decomposition, especially when protected by layers of soil. Half-lives (in years) of insecticides that are worked into the soil are: aldrin, 1–4; dieldrin, 1–7; lindane, 2; chlordane, 2–4; DDT, 3–10; endrin, 4–8; heptachlor, 7–12; and toxaphene, 10 (Brooks 1974). These half-lives may be reduced to weeks if the pesticides are fully exposed to the elements. The waxy coating of plant materials can be expected to retain these pesticides, as happens with organophosphates.

TOXICITY

Buck et al. (1973) have tabulated some oral and dermal maximum nontoxic dosages, minimum toxic dosages, and some LD50 values of organochlorine insecticides in several species. St. Omer (1970) tabulated the acute oral minimum lethal dosage and also some LD50 values. Additional information is available in Brooks (1974). Still, the literature is incomplete regarding toxicity of chlorinated hydrocarbon pesticides in domestic animals and fowl. Data for calves and some birds can be compared with data for rats with regard to acute oral toxicity. These data, obtained from the above references, are listed in Table 58.4.

It can be seen in the table that the "sick dose" for calves generally relates to the rat oral LD50 and that the "safest" organochlorine pesticides for calves are methoxychlor, Perthane, DDT, and TDE. Endosulfan is also fairly "safe" in mammals because this particular insecticide does not accumulate in the body and is eliminated rather quickly after exposure.

Adult cattle are 2–10 times more resistant than calves to organochlorine insecticides. Sheep and goats may tolerate as much pesticide as adult cattle, or even more, without becoming ill. For dogs, chlordane seems to be a "safe" compound (acute oral LD50, 200–700 mg/kg of body weight).

It can also be seen in Table 58.4 that endrin, aldrin, dieldrin, and toxaphene are very toxic for various birds (this includes chickens) as well as for mammals.

It is misleading to call a pesticide "safe." No matter what the published toxicity values are, if animals or birds become poisoned by a pesticide under a given set of conditions, then that pesticide is *not* safe regardless of how small the dosage was. Toxicity of organochlorine pesticides is affected by a number of factors; it is these factors, listed below, that require attention rather than the actual dosages.

TABLE 58.4. Acutely toxic oral dosages of some chlorinated hydrocarbon pesticides in calves, birds, and rats

Common Name	Trade Name	Calf Acute Oral Toxic Dose	Birds (Various) Acute Oral LD50	Rat Acute Oral LD50
		(mg/kg)	*(mg/kg)*	*(mg/kg)*
endrin	Endrin	. . .	1–6	3–43
aldrin	Octalene	5	10–15	38–60
dieldrin	Dieldrite	10	20–30	40–64
toxaphene	Phenatox	5–10	10–100	40–90
heptachlor	Velsicol 104	20	2000 (M)	40–162
endosulfan	Malix	. . .	. . .	70–110
lindane	Gammex	5	>2000 (M)	76–177
DDT	Gesarol	250	841–>4000	87–400
mirex	Mirex	. . .	>2400 (M)	235–312
chlordane	Octachlor	25	1200 (M)	283–590
TDE	Rothane	250	. . .	400
methoxychlor	Marlate	500–1000	>2000 (M)	5000–6000
perthane	Perthane	250–500	. . .	6600–9000

Note: M means mallard ducks.

1. Age (young animals are more sensitive than adults).
2. Sex (female rats are more sensitive than males to endosulfan, aldrin, dieldrin, endrin, heptachlor, and toxaphene; males are more sensitive to chlordane).
3. Species (see above).
4. Amount of body fat (emaciated, nonlactating animals are more sensitive to lindane and toxaphene than are fat, lactating animals).
5. Stress or illness (enhances toxicity).
6. Presence of other pesticides, poisons, or drugs (chlordane potentiates aldrin, endrin, and parathion in mice) (Keplinger and Deichmann 1967).
7. Route and duration of exposure (the compounds are less toxic if absorbed slowly, as from skin or gut when small dosages have been ingested over a period of time).
8. Size of particles in emulsions used as dips or sprays (large particles adhere to skin and long hair better than small particles do; thus emulsions must be properly made (Radeleff 1970; Ray et al. 1975).

Factors that alter drug response (see Section 2) can also alter response to pesticides.

TOXICODYNAMIC CONSIDERATIONS

After entry into the bloodstream, organochlorine insecticides may be bound to serum lipoproteins (Ecobichon and Saschenbrecker 1968). One would also expect these lipid-soluble compounds to readily enter erythrocyte and leucocyte membranes, to be reversibly bound to lipophilic regions on serum albumin, and to avidly enter chylomicra. Thus the carrier state of chlorinated hydrocarbon pesticides in blood is probably complexly multicompartmented, the pesticide concentration in the different compartments being in dynamic equilibrium.

This equilibrium is influenced by addition to the blood of extra pesticide absorbed from skin, lungs, or gut and by losses of pesticide from the blood due to distribution to body tissues (primarily fat, but also the brain and fetus); breakdown of pesticide by liver microsomal enzymes (a process that can be accelerated by means of enzyme induction if sufficient pesticide is present); and excretion of pesticide and pesticide metabolites in urine, bile, milk, and feces. Thus the dynamic equilibrium of the carrier state of pesticide in blood is an integral part of a larger dynamic equilibrium between intake, distribution, metabolism, and excretion rate of the pesticide.

Under conditions of constant pesticide intake, the concentration of pesticide in the body reaches a plateau at which a balance is achieved in the equilibria discussed. If pesticide intake stops, pesticide concentrations in tissues decline at a rate dependent on the amount of pesticide present, the chemical nature of the pesticide, the rate of metabolism and excretion of pesticide, and the type of tissue. Fat is the main storage tissue for organochlorine pesticides; such tissue, being relatively poorly supplied with blood, can retain some of these compounds (e.g., dieldrin, DDT, lindane) for an extraordinary length of time. This fact is the basis for several aspects of toxicity of these compounds, for persistence of pesticide residues in milk or tissues after just 1 exposure, and for analysis of body fat in the diagnosis of poisoning by these pesticides.

Slow mobilization of pesticide from fat is also the basis for the second (slow) stage of disappearance of pesticide from blood and milk; the first stage is rapid and may account for 40%–50% elimination of pesticide during the first 3–4 days after exposure. The subsequent slow stage of elimination may require months, so that the half-life of some of these pesticides in the body may be very long. Moreover, even after one-half the dosage of pesticide has been eliminated from the body, the remaining one-half can cause excess residues in meat, milk, or eggs for several more months, possibly years (see Chapter 63).

Severe stress such as starvation, a sudden freeze, or forced activity is known to cause release of epinephrine from the adrenal medulla. One of the metabolic functions of epinephrine is to initiate lipolysis. If body fat contains a burden of organochlorine pesticide, sufficient pesticide may be released into the bloodstream to cause clinical signs of poisoning, or even death.

Additional detail on toxicodynamics of organochlorine pesticides is presented by Ecobichon and Saschenbrecker (1968), Radeleff (1970), St. Omer (1970), Buck et al. (1973), Brooks (1974), and Hayes (1974). Brooks also details metabolism and excretion of individual pesticides.

MECHANISM OF ACTION

Chlorinated hydrocarbon insecticides are nonspecific stimulants to the CNS. They have no stereoselective receptor that has yet been identified and therefore no known competitive antagonists.

The molecular mechanism of acute toxicosis has not been determined. A possible mechanism can be postulated, based on experimental findings and some biologic. These lipid-soluble insecticides can easily enter neural membranes. After entry into the membrane or cell, DDT prolongs the time during which some of the sodium channels in the membrane are open during depolarization. Concomitantly, potassium efflux from the cell is hindered (Hille 1968; Buck et al. 1973). The result of these ion imbalances is a decrease in transmembrane resting potential, thus a decrease in firing threshold and an increase in neuronal excitability. These effects are manifested as an increase in spontaneous arousal type electroencephalogram activity, first in the cerebellum and then in other brain regions, occurring *before* the onset of tremors or convulsions (Woolley and Barron 1968).

Also occurring before the onset of clinical signs is an increase in whole brain free ammonia (NH_3 plus NH_4^+) concentration and brain glutamine (which is synthesized from ammonia and glutamate). These changes are produced by several different organochlorine pesticides (St. Omer 1970, 1971). Brain ammonia concentration is also elevated by noninsecticide convulsants such as *m*-fluorotyrosine (St. Omer 1972), fluoroacetate (Benitez et al. 1954), urease, and methionine sulfoxamine (Gibson et al. 1974). It is not known whether elevation of brain ammonia concentration is a cause or an effect of the sodium-potassium flux defect and electroencephalogram changes mentioned above. However, onset and disappearance of convulsions in organochlorine and *m*-fluorotyrosine-poisoned animals is correlated with increase and decrease of brain ammonia concentration (St. Omer 1971, 1972). Thus convulsions produced by these agents may be due to some interference with the production and/or utilization of brain ammonia. In support of this suggestion is the fact that other poisons (e.g., urea, fluoroacetate, ammonium salts) that cause increased tissue concentrations of ammonia also produce clinical signs similar to those of organochlorine insecticides (see Urea in Chapter 59, Fluoroacetate, and Wilson et al. 1968). Moreover, ammonia decreases postsynaptic inhibition of cortical, spinal, and trochlear motor neurons of cats—a decidedly proconvulsant effect (Raabe and Gumnit 1975).

Depression may be produced by some organochlorine pesticides, and this may result from rapid depolarizing blockade of neurons of the reticular activating system. Overdepolarization of medullary neurons may be responsible for respiratory failure, which is the usual cause of death in organochlorine pesticide toxicosis.

In the dog, monkey, and rabbit, DDT can cause sudden ventricular fibrillation. This is attributed to myocardial sensitization to catecholamines and to sympathetic nervous discharges (St. Omer 1970). Not all organochlorine insecticides cause ventricular fibrillation, but it is interesting to note that fluoroacetate and ammonium salts also cause ventricular fibrillation in some species, possibly because of some effect of ammonia on the heart.

Muscle tremors seen in organochlorine pesticide toxicosis are partly central in origin and partly due to direct depolarizing effects on peripheral motor nerve.

Chronic effects of chlorinated hydrocarbon pesticides such as liver damage and eggshell thinning are discussed by Buck et al. (1973). The mechanisms of these phenomena are not known. Behavioral disorders following chronic exposure to dieldrin may relate to depletion of brain serotonin, norepinephrine, and dopamine (Sharma 1973). *Learning disability* occurs in monkeys chronically exposed to small concentrations of dieldrin (Van Gelder and Cunningham 1975). This is correlated with electroencephalogram changes. Behavioral and biochemical correlates are not given.

CLINICAL SIGNS

The signs of acute toxicosis are about the same in all species, but there are differences in onset, number, severity, and duration of signs in individual animals, depending on the kind and quantity of pesticide involved and the existence of factors that influence toxicity of these compounds (see Toxicity). Radeleff's (1970) descriptions of clinical signs have been capsulized by Clarke and Clarke (1967) and Buck et al. (1973). Interesting case histories are presented by Buck et al. (1973), McParland et al. (1973), and Ray et al. (1975).

Onset of signs may take several minutes to several days. Some combination of the following signs is then observed:

1. *Behavioral aberrations,* beginning with apparent anxiety or apprehension, progressing through belligerence or aggressiveness to abnormal posturing (head between legs or kneeling with rump in the air) or jumping over unseen objects, to climbing the walls and manifesting frenzied or maniacal "mindless" behavior.

2. *Nervous phenomena,* beginning with hypersensitivity and fasciculation and twitching of facial and eyelid muscles; then twitching and spasms of cervical, forequarter, and hindquarter muscles (in that order); and progressing through generalized intermittent or continuous coarse spasms and jaw champing to sudden clonic-tonic convulsions accompanied by very high body temperature (possibly off-scale on the rectal thermometer). If death does not occur during the first convulsion, there is postictal coma or depression. More convulsions may occur later or be precipitated by external stimuli.

3. *Autonomic manifestations* such as emesis (in animals that can vomit), profuse salivation, diarrhea, urination, bradycardia (aldrin, dieldrin), or tachycardia with possible cardiac arrhythmias.

4. *Locomotor disturbances,* beginning with stiff gait and "walking on tiptoes" and progressing through incoordination and ataxia to compulsive hypermotility (circling or other motor-encephalitic movements), which may accompany the jaw champing and frenzied behavior.

5. *Dependent signs* such as hot ears or skin (due to fever), increased rate and depth of respiration (due to fever and physical activity), and fluid sounds in the

lungs (due to bronchial secretions and froth generated by dyspnea or convulsive respiratory efforts). Death may occur within minutes or hours, after several days, or not at all. In surviving animals, abortion is not generally seen.

In chronic toxicosis clinical signs may be similar to those of acute toxicosis, perhaps because of a release of pesticide from storage in body fat. Prior to onset of nervous signs there may be interrupted estrous cycles, decrease in weight gain, decreased appetite, decreased milk or egg production, or reproductive problems, all of which are probably nonspecific effects that could occur with a variety of other toxicants.

LESIONS

The carcass may be bruised, lacerated, and dirty due to convulsions. Rigor may be prominent. Cyanosis can be seen. If body temperature was high enough, the heart and intestines may be blanched. Congestion and edema may be found in several organs. Hemorrhages may be seen on the heart and lungs and blood may be present in the pericardial fluid. The heart is generally stopped in systole. There may be excess cerebrospinal fluid. Intestinal contents may be fluid. Liver damage may occur with DDT or mirex.

Microscopically, little can be seen except hemorrhage and edema in various organs. Cloudy swelling may be seen in parenchymatous organs if body temperature was severely elevated. With DDT and mirex, the liver may manifest lipid accumulation in portal regions, hepatocyte enlargement, and glycogen depletion (Kendall 1974).

In chronic poisoning the carcass may be emaciated and devoid of fat and the liver and kidney may manifest degenerative changes.

None of the lesions are specific for organochlorine pesticides. In some instances, such as when the animal is healthy one day and found dead the next morning, no visible lesions may be apparent.

DIFFERENTIAL DIAGNOSIS

If there is a history of recent exposure to an organochlorine pesticide, and if the clinical signs and lesions are classical as described above, then organochlorine toxicosis can be diagnosed presumptively. Other nervous excitatory conditions do not have the identical spectrum and severity of signs described. Infectious disease or brain lesions can cause encephalitic signs, but these conditions can be ruled out by postmortem examination and by clinical pathological and microbiological tests.

"Salt poisoning" can cause signs similar to those of chlorinated hydrocarbon pesticides, but the history and the absence of high body temperature would exclude this condition. Strychnine causes convulsions, but the convulsions are tonic and not preceded by behavioral aberrations or locomotor compulsions. Fluoroacetate causes signs similar to those of organochlorine pesticides, but the convulsions of fluoroacetate are not elicitable by external stimuli and become weaker with time. Moreover, cardiac irregularities are more conspicuous with fluoroacetate. Nicotine causes nicotinic cholinergic signs, not the syndrome described for organochlorine pesticides. Poisoning by moldy or spoiled feed or garbage can cause signs of central nervous stimulation, but again these toxicants do not cause the spectrum of signs produced by organochlorine insecticides.

In practice, the usual question is whether animals that are manifesting muscle tremors, salivation, and apprehension may have been poisoned by an anticholinesterase pesticide or by lead or urea.

With anticholinesterase pesticides, parasympathetic signs are very abundant and there are no behavioral aberrations such as wall climbing or abnormal posturing. Convulsions are either absent or not very severe and body temperature is not severely elevated. Moreover, atropine may cause marked improvement in animals poisoned by organophosphate or carbamate pesticides; this is not the case with organochlorine pesticides, lead, or urea.

Lead does not cause abnormal posturing. Convulsions are less common and there is usually no fever. Lead often causes blindness and all the attendant clinical signs, but organochlorine pesticides do not. Also, lead causes anemia and basophilic stippling of erythrocytes.

In the case of urea, there is no abnormal posturing or jumping over unseen objects. Head pressing and wall climbing are not seen. Urea convulsions are severe and tonic in nature. Between convulsions, the urea-poisoned animal tends to be rigid rather than depressed. Colic is an outstanding sign in urea toxicosis but not with the organochlorine pesticides. Urea does not cause compulsive hypermotility as do lead and organochlorine compounds. The odor of ammonia may be detected in the rumen of animals poisoned by urea.

TREATMENT

Convulsions are treated with pentobarbital (dogs), a thiobarbiturate (cats), or chloral hydrate or pentobarbital (farm species), given intravenously very carefully "to effect." The reason for such caution is that postconvulsive depression may be additive with depression produced by the anesthetic, and the animal may be overdosed with anesthetic. If an animal is already in a depressed state from the pesticide, then anesthetics are contraindicated. Central nervous stimulants are also contraindicated because the depression caused by organochlorine pesticides is probably due to overstimulation of the brain; additional stimulation would only worsen the condition. Artificial respiration and oxygen therapy are indicated.

Assuming that the veterinarian is consulted soon after animals begin to manifest signs of acute toxicosis, many animals in a group may be in preconvulsive states. These are the animals that require immediate attention; that is, time should not be wasted treating convulsing or severely depressed animals because while this is being done, more animals could begin convulsing or become severely depressed.

Sedative doses of barbiturate or chloral hydrate control most of the behavioral, nervous, and locomotor signs. Atropine sulfate may not be needed after sedation, but the drug can be given in small dosage to control parasympathetic signs.

Sedation also allows body temperature to subside slowly. If rapid cooling is necessary (body temperature above 106°–107° F), the animal may be bathed in cool water. Animals with body temperature of 108° F or higher may suffer irreversible brain damage due to denaturation of cellular enzyme and membrane protein constituents.

Sedation can usually be discontinued after 24–48 hours.

If exposure was by the dermal route, the animals must be bathed with soap and water (2–3 lathers) and rinsed thoroughly. If exposure was by the oral route, a saline purgative or gastric lavage is required.

Clarke and Clarke (1967) suggest that calcium borogluconate may be given intravenously, together with glucose in saline. These treatments are said to avoid liver damage and neutralize the effects of preconvulsive hyperkalemia.

Buck et al. (1973) point out that the biological half-life of certain organochlorine pesticides may be shortened in ruminants fed activated charcoal plus phenobarbital. The activated charcoal (0.9 kg/cow/day) supposedly traps pesticide that is excreted into the intestine in the bile and thereby interrupts the enterohepatic-biliary cycle of the pesticide. Phenobarbital (10 mg/kg/day) induces hepatic microsomal enzymes and thus hastens metabolism of certain pesticides. These treatments are logical but they have not been successful in all experiments.

As with any other poison, the source of organochlorine pesticide must be eliminated. Signs of acute toxicosis usually abate in 1 or 2 days, but complete recovery may take weeks or months.

ANALYSIS

Although organochlorine pesticides are not normal metabolites in the biochemical scheme of the body, the pesticides may be found "normally" in body fat as a result of exposure to small concentrations of pesticide in the environment. Thus a positive laboratory test for most organochlorine pesticides does not necessarily mean the animal was poisoned by these pesticides. Generally speaking, parts per *billion* concentrations of insecticide in body fat can be regarded as being of doubtful significance with regard to acute toxicosis. On the other hand, parts per *million* concentrations may be diagnostically meaningful if the history, clinical signs, and postmortem findings are consistent with poisoning by organochlorine pesticides. Brain concentrations of pesticide are better correlated with toxicosis than are concentrations in body fat (Ecobichon and Saschenbrecker 1968).

It is always a good idea to test liver and kidney (dead animal) or blood and milk (live animal). These samples may contain ppm concentrations of pesticide if exposure was recent and excessive. In addition, declining concentrations of pesticide in blood and milk samples obtained weekly may correlate with disappearance of clinical signs and improvement in production, appetite, and weight gains. This would indicate that the pesticide was the original cause of poisoning.

Suspected sources of pesticide should also be tested, in addition to stomach contents, vomitus, or stomach washings. Bile is an excellent biological fluid to test for chlorinated hydrocarbon pesticides, but data on diagnostic usefulness of bile analyses have not yet been accumulated.

Endosulfan is one organochlorine pesticide that is not stored in body fat. It is also rapidly metabolized. In order not to miss detection of this type of compound, samples should be obtained the same day from animals manifesting signs of organochlorine pesticide toxicosis. It is expected that industry will produce more of these readily metabolized, biodegradable pesticides that are not stored in body fat.

For information on residues of organochlorine pesticides, see Chapter 63.

Lead

USE

Lead compounds are common ingredients in a variety of commercial and household products. Metallic lead, once used as plumbing, continues to be used for storage batteries, solder, buckshot, and other applications.

SOURCE

Lead poisoning can result when curious animals ingest lead-based paints (either old dry paint or paint from "empty" paint cans), glazier's putty or other caulking materials, used crankcase oil, greases, linoleum, leaded gasoline, solid lead, solder, roofing materials, asphalt, or industrial effluents in streams or on forage. Grass near busy highways may contain toxic amounts of lead from auto exhausts. Licking of discarded storage batteries can also result in lead poisoning. Water from lead plumbing or glazed crockery pots may contain toxic amounts of lead. Waterfowl can become poisoned by ingesting 6 or 8 buckshot from frequently hunted shorelines. Natural sources of lead such as galena or soils are not particularly toxic but can add to the total body burden of lead. The milk secreted from lead-poisoned animals can be dangerous for the young animal.

Paint seems to be the usual source of lead in poisoned animals. In addition, cattle and calves are often poisoned by ingesting crankcase oil drained from internal combustion engines. The farm dump is often a "smorgasbord" of poisons for animals that gain access to it. The veterinarian should be able to recognize lead-containing materials in such dumps.

PROPERTIES OF TOXICOLOGIC IMPORTANCE

Only 1% or 2% of ingested lead is absorbed from the GI tract because lead can form rather insoluble compounds, even within the gut. Acid conditions favor the dissolution of lead and its inorganic compounds. In nature, lead is persistent indefinitely.

TOXICITY

The acute oral lethal single dose of lead in various species is: calves, 50–600 mg/kg of body weight as lead or lead salts; cattle, 600–800 mg/kg as lead; horses, 500–750 g total dose as lead; sheep, 30–40 g total dose as lead acetate; swine, 10–25 g total dose as lead; dogs, 10–25 g total dose as lead (less in puppies); fowl, 160–600 mg/kg of body weight as absorbed lead from lead salts.

Chronic toxicosis can arise when lead is ingested over a period of days, weeks, or months. The chronic oral lethal dose of lead in different species is: calves, 1–3 g total/day; cattle, 6–7 mg lead acetate/kg body weight/day for 6–8 weeks; horses, 2–7 mg lead/kg/day; sheep (nonpregnant), 8 mg lead acetate/kg/day; sheep (pregnant), as little as 1 mg lead acetate/kg/day, with resulting abortions prior to death; dogs, as little as 0.32 mg lead/kg/day for 5 months, but some dogs may tolerate 1 mg/kg/day for 6 months; and fowl, 320–640 mg lead acetate/kg/day, or (in waterfowl) 16 mg of lead shot/kg of body weight.

Prolonged ingestion of small amounts of lead can eventually cause mild to severe illness in animals (see Clinical Signs).

Cats are not poisoned by lead very often because cats do not chew on foreign objects, lick painted surfaces, or eat materials that are not foodstuffs. Cats can be poisoned if their food or water is contaminated or if they lick lead-containing matter such as grease or oil from their fur.

Toxicity data were obtained from White and Cotchin (1948), Allcroft and Blaxter (1950), Blaxter (1950a), Clarke and Clarke (1967), Aronson (1971), Buck et al. (1973), and Zook (1973).

A number of factors influence the toxicity of lead. These include:

1. Age—young animals are more susceptible.
2. Species—goats, swine, and chickens are more resistant.
3. Reproductive state—pregnant ewes are more sensitive than nonpregnant ewes.
4. Rate of ingestion of lead—large amounts ingested in 1 or 2 days may cause death but smaller amounts ingested over a period of several weeks or months may not.
5. Form of lead—solid lead is not as toxic as more soluble salts of lead, which are more readily absorbed.
6. Route of entry—only 1% or 2% of ingested lead may be absorbed; inorganic lead cannot readily penetrate the skin but organic forms such as tetraethyl lead and tetramethyl lead are absorbed quickly through intact skin; metallic lead shot or bullets lodged in tissues do not dissolve very much because tissue pH is not low enough.
7. Presence of other toxicants or debilitating diseases—these would enhance toxicity of lead.
8. General state of health—poorly nourished, parasitized, poorly kept animals are more susceptible.
9. Amount of ingesta present and condition of the GI tract—ingesta may dilute lead, but a damaged intestinal mucosa may absorb lead better.
10. Past exposure to lead—previous chronic low-level exposure may impart a degree of tolerance to some of the biochemical effects of lead; previous acute exposure may reduce the subsequent amount of lead required to produce a lethal effect (these phenomena relate to rate of lead intake, item 4 above).
11. Individual variation in susceptibility and rate of excretion of lead.
12. Hormonal influences, particularly any effects on bone formation or dissolution—lead is stored in bone.

Other factors could probably be listed by use of medical common sense. Operation of all of these factors may account for the wide variation found in lead concentrations in tissues from lead-poisoned animals (see Analysis).

TOXICODYNAMIC CONSIDERATION

After absorption from the gut, a large proportion of lead is carried on erythrocyte membranes (85%–90% in sheep, 63%–70% in cow blood). The remainder is bound to serum albumin and only a small proportion (less than 1%) is actually free in the serum water (Blaxter 1950b). Nevertheless, unbound lead is in dynamic equilibrium with the lead bound to erythrocytes and serum albumin. Distribution of lead to various tissues takes place from the unbound fraction; it is likely the unbound fraction that is responsible for the toxic effects of lead, just as it is the unbound fraction of a barbiturate anesthetic or an antibiotic that mediates the distribution and actions of these compounds.

As the portal circulation carries lead through the liver, much of the lead is removed and gradually excreted in the bile. Thus liver tissue tends to contain large amounts of lead. The kidneys excrete lead, and the metal is found in the renal cortex in larger concentrations than in the liver. Some workers believe that the bile is the main pathway of excretion of lead in animals and thus the feces are found to contain not only unabsorbed lead but also lead that has been excreted by the liver or even reexcreted in an enterohepatic-biliary cycle (Allcroft 1951; Clarke and Clarke 1967).

Unbound lead from the blood can also be excreted in milk in dangerous concentrations.

Lead readily passes membrane barriers such as the blood-brain barrier and the placenta. Distribution of lead to tissues other than kidney cortex and liver is otherwise unremarkable except for one very important tissue, i.e., bone.

As blood flows through bone, unbound lead is bound to bone substance and immobilized, particularly in the bone-growth regions. The exact mechanism of this trapping of lead in bone is not known, but bone is considered to be a "sink" for lead. The bone sink may contain 90%–98% of the total body burden of lead. This trapping action of bone does not occur suddenly after an acute dosage of lead. Rather, it is a slower process entailing redistribution of lead from the soft tissues of the body. Thus the bone sink is an important detoxification mechanism under conditions of chronic exposure to small concentrations of lead.

Bone cannot hold an infinite amount of lead. When bone becomes saturated, signs of toxicosis may suddenly appear because of rising blood and soft tissue concentrations of lead during exposure to the metal.

If exposure to lead ceases before animals become too ill, lead is gradually lost from bone. Lead concentrations may be elevated in blood for 1–2 months during the natural deleading of bone.

MECHANISM OF ACTION

Lead is probably the primary toxicologic hazard on the farm, judging by the large number of positive cases diagnosed each year. Even the pesticides do not seem to poison as many animals as lead does. Yet we know less about the mechanism of action of lead than about many of the less frequently encountered poisons.

There is a reason for our ignorance about lead. It is not that researchers have ignored lead in favor of more glamorous poisons, but that lead has so many effects in the body that nobody can decide which are relevant to the primary toxic actions of the metal. Indeed, lead has adverse effects on nearly every tissue and organ in the body, thus giving rise to a plethora of clinical signs, biochemical and hematological changes, and lesions. For this reason, lead seems to defy classification in all but the most simplistic approaches to toxicology; often it is just listed as one of the heavy metals or merely discussed in alphabetical order.

If one studies the literature on lead poisoning, particularly in those species most commonly poisoned by lead (calves, cattle, dogs) the clinical signs of poisoning are found to be very similar to those of chlorinated hydrocarbon pesticide and urea toxicosis. There are even certain similarities in postmortem findings between lead and the organochlorine pesticides. Thus the clinical signs of lead poisoning are mainly those of nervous system stimulation, with GI involvement (see Clinical Signs).

The exact mechanism by which lead causes these nervous and GI disorders is not known, but we can speculate about the mechanism of action by using some observed facts and a little reason.

Lead, like mercury and some other metals, is capable of damaging the blood-brain barrier. Whether such damage is necessary for entry of inorganic lead into the brain substance is questionable, but unquestionably lead causes damage to capillary endothelium with resulting cerebral edema and hemorrhage (Christian and Tryphonas 1971; Goldstein et al. 1974). A major question is: what do various gross and microscopic lesions in the brain or in any other organ have to do with lead poisoning? In other words, might not many of the signs, lesions, and biochemical and hematologic changes seen in lead poisoning be secondary to some basic actions of lead at the subcellular or molecular level? Of course! Also, is it not possible that even though the outstanding clinical manifestations of lead poisoning refer to lesions in the brain, that sickness and death due to lead poisoning might be due more directly to some primary metabolic dysfunctions in other organs? Certainly! Let us pursue these questions, beginning with the brain.

After entry into brain cells (neurons and glia) it is probable that the initial actions of lead are exerted on cellular molecular mechanisms. Using single doses of tetraethyl lead in rabbits, Niklowitz (1974) reported that in several regions of the brain, ultrastructural changes such as (in order of appearance) folding of the nuclear membrane, swelling and disruption of mitochondria, hypertrophy of Golgi complexes, and patchy chromatolysis of the ergastoplasm occurred in brain cells. With progressive hypertrophy of Golgi saccules and vacuolization of the ergastoplasm, the cells developed vacuolar hydropic degeneration. Other cells developed pyknosis and increased ribosome content instead of hydrops. Important to note is that the early ultrastructural changes were not visible with light microscopy and they *preceded* onset of severe signs of lead poisoning. Also, the lesions reflected an initial action of lead (actually triethyl lead, the active metabolite of tetraethyl lead) on membranous constituents of brain cells. Niklowitz cited early work in which inorganic lead salts produced ultrastructural changes in nerve cells of other animals also.

Other organs are not immune to ultrastructural damage by lead, but perhaps other organs require a longer time (or larger amounts of lead) before damage is seen. In rats fed small concentrations of lead acetate, the heart cells manifested myofibrillar fragmentation and separation with edema fluid, dilation of sarcoplasmic reticulum, and swelling and disruption of mitochondria (Asokan 1974). These changes, similar to changes found by Niklowitz (1974) in rabbit brain, *preceded* any changes in myocardial electrolytes. No gross lesions were seen.

Presumably, organs such as the liver, kidney, and intestine could also suffer ultrastructural damage by lead. In geese dosed with lead shot, elevated serum glutamic oxaloacetic acid transaminase (SGOT) and serum glutamic pyruvic transaminase (SGPT) values were observed 3 weeks before death (Sileo et al. 1973). These changes, plus a decrease of serum alkaline phosphatase, all reflective of cell damage, were also reported for ducks (Rozman et al. 1974). In dogs, lead acetate feeding caused (among other things) decreased serum alkaline phosphatase, lactic dehydrogenase-I, and increased SGOT and SGPT (Stowe et al. 1973). Buck et al. (1973) state that lead causes rupture of cellular lysosomes and release of acid phosphatase. Chronic administration of lead chloride to rats causes a number of biochemical-enzymatic adaptive changes in the liver and kidney (Singhal et al. 1973). Lead is known to cause gross and microscopic lesions in the liver, kidney, intestine, and other organs (see Lesions). These lesions do not just suddenly appear, but must have some ultrastructural or molecular basis.

Niklowitz (1974) wanted to find out how tetraethyl lead caused ultrastructural changes in rabbit brain cells. He discovered that the ultrastructural changes were coexistent with decreases in local concentrations of the essential trace metals copper, iron, and zinc. He postulated that lead interferes preferentially with these metals as prosthetic groups of enzymes in mitochondria, thus affecting vital metabolic pathways such as cellular respiration, oxidative phosphorylation, and the ATP synthetase complex. This would cause loss of structural integrity of nerve cells, leading to visible lesions and functional disorders.

If Niklowitz's theory is true, lead would be expected to exert profound metabolic and functional effects in all cells, the brain and heart being especially sensitive, but the liver, kidney, and GI mucosa (where there is much enzyme activity) would also be affected. Such *is* the case with lead. Furthermore, if lead acts by interfering with metallic prosthetic groups rather than with enzyme sulfhydryl groups, as some workers think, then one would not expect the sulfhydryl-containing chelator BAL to be highly effective in treatment of lead poisoning. It *is not.*

Niklowitz (1974) goes on to postulate that neural demyelination seen after prolonged exposure to lead may be due to copper deficiency, thus causing defective function of cytochrome oxidase and thereby inhibiting phospholipid synthesis. Konat and Clausen (1974) attribute triethyl lead–induced myelin deficiency to inhibition of brain cell energy metabolism in developing rats.

Whether interference with essential trace metals is the actual mechanism of action of lead remains to be seen. The mechanism does explain all of the clinical signs, biochemical and hematologic changes, microscopic and gross lesions, and death due to lead poisoning and is certainly worthy of vigorous investigation. The only trouble with the trace metal theory is that it does not exclude inhibition of enzyme sulfhydryl groups as at least part of the basic mechanism of action of lead. Many enzymes have sulfhydryl groups; it is conceivable that lead might even act exclusively by sulfhydryl inhibition and that changes in cellular copper, iron, and zinc concentrations, cell ultrastructure, myelination, and cell and organ function might be a result of sulfhydryl inhibition.

Some of the muscle weakness seen in lead poisoning may be due to a prejunctional effect of lead on neuromuscular transmission (Silbergeld et al. 1974). In addition, peripheral nerve segmental demyelination (a probable result of the metabolic inhibitory effects of lead) may contribute to neuromuscular signs.

Behavioral and locomotor effects of small amounts of lead in young animals (see Clinical Signs) have not been satisfactorily explained, but may relate to an increase in brain norepinephrine concentration (Golter and Michaelson 1975) or to effects of lead on neurotransmitter balance, energy metabolism, or myelination of developing brain (Konat and Clausen 1974).

CLINICAL SIGNS

Onset of clinical signs of lead poisoning may take a few hours, days, or weeks, depending on the amount of lead ingested, species, and other factors mentioned under Toxicity. Chronic poisoning may take weeks or months to develop.

The clinical signs manifested by different species do have some differences, but the overall impression is of an encephalopathy preceded and accompanied by GI malfunction. Clinical signs are not classified in the literature (Fenstermacher et al. 1946; White and Cotchin 1948; Allcroft and Blaxter 1950; Clarke and Clarke 1967; Zook et al. 1969; Christian and Tryphonas 1971; Buck et al. 1973; Knight and Burau 1973; Zook 1973). When the signs are classified, the classification looks very much like that of the chlorinated hydrocarbon insecticides, which also produce encephalopathy and GI signs.

Behavioral aberrations are manifested, beginning with apparent anxiety or apprehension and proceeding to such things as hyperexcitability, bellowing or other vocalization, rolling of the eyes and apparent fear or terror, possible belligerence, pressing of the head against a wall or post, attempts to climb the walls, sudden jumping into the air, and frenzied or maniacal behavior. One fascinating aspect of this category of signs is the effect of small amounts of lead in experimental animals. Lead can disrupt conditioned (learned) behavior in adult rats and rabbits (Bryce-Smith 1972) and sheep (Van Gelder et al.

1973). Lead can also disrupt learning and memory in young and adult rats (Snowdon 1973; Avery and Cross 1974) and in lambs born of lead-treated ewes (Carson et al. 1974).

Nervous phenomena such as depression (particularly in sheep and horses, or in chronic poisoning), muscle fasciculations, twitching of ears or muzzle, excessive blinking, muscle spasms, rhythmic jerking of the head and neck, jaw champing, pharyngeal paralysis, laryngeal hemiplegia (causing roaring in horses), tongue lolling, nystagmus, blindness (causing the animal to stumble and blunder into objects), opisthotonos, torticollis, clonic and tonic convulsions, normal body temperature in most cases but occasionally a temperature of 107°–112° F, coma, and either a quiet or convulsive death are also manifested.

Some *autonomic manifestations* of lead poisoning are salivation (or loss of saliva due to inability to swallow), lacrimation, possible sweating, colic (tucked abdomen, tooth gnashing, groaning), thirst, diarrhea or constipation, rumen atony, urinary incontinence, and possible vomiting (even in cattle).

The *locomotor disturbances* of lead poisoning range from a stiff, stilted gait with ataxia and incoordination, through rigidity of all postural muscles, swaying, and posterior weakness, to compulsive hypermotility (circling, pacing, running). In experimental mice and rats, offspring of animals fed low levels of lead developed hypermotility and stereotyped movements (Silbergeld and Goldberg 1973; Michaelson and Sauerhoff 1974; Golter and Michaelson 1975). This condition has been likened to so-called minimal brain dysfunction (a hypermotile learning disability) in children, and it responds to the same drugs (amphetamines) as does minimal brain dysfunction (Silbergeld and Goldberg 1974). The implication is that minimal brain dysfunction in children might relate to prenatal and postnatal exposure to lead. It is conceivable that prenatal or postnatal exposure to lead could cause behavioral, learning, and hypermotility problems in the training of dogs, horses, or other working or pleasure animals, but no evidence supports this speculation.

Some *dependent signs,* obviously secondary to other effects of lead, include rapid, labored breathing, anorexia, weight loss, decreased milk production, dehydration, emaciation, fetal death with either resorption or abortion of the fetus, and general weakness.

The veterinarian does not necessarily see all of these signs. The typical calf or cow has diarrhea and is anorexic, dull or excited, colicky, possibly trembling or blind or pressing the head, bawling or bellowing, and starting to manifest hypermotility. More severe signs may occur later if the condition is not treated.

Sometimes animals ingest so much lead that no signs are observed. Such animals may be found dead.

In waterfowl, lead shot ingestion causes anorexia, loss of weight, weakness, diarrhea, coma, and quiet death (Clemens et al. 1975). Sileo et al. (1973) observed progressive tachycardia in geese as the birds became more and more ill. Some geese developed electrocardiogram abnormalities.

LESIONS

In acute poisoning of calves, cattle, or sheep (farm species most often poisoned by lead) there may be no lesions. Alternately, there may be a marked gastroenteritis and severe kidney damage (sheep) or only a pale liver and hyperemic kidneys (cattle). The stomach may contain paint, paint flakes, black-colored motor oil, or other foreign materials.

Microscopically, the liver of calves and cattle may manifest centrilobular necrosis and some of the hepatocytes may contain eosinophilic, acid-fast intranuclear inclusions. In the brain, histologic changes ranging from diffuse capillary activation to scattered foci of status spongiosus and necrosis of the cerebral cortex may occur.

In subacute poisoning of calves and cattle, few lesions may be manifested. On the other hand, there may be pale muscles, liver, and kidneys and pronounced rigor if the animal had a high body temperature or convulsions prior to death. Transudational lesions such as fluid in the body cavities or pericardium, excess cerebrospinal fluid, lung edema, and cerebral edema may also be seen. Vascular failure may be further manifested by hemolysis; congestion of kidneys, lungs, brain, and abomasal and intestinal mucosa; and petechial or ecchymotic hemorrhages in the subepicardium (particularly along coronary sulci), subendocardium, thymus, and kidneys. Degenerative lesions such as softening of the kidney cortex or cerebral softening and cavitation might be seen. Microscopically, the lesions would be consistent with gross ones. There may be lead-proteinate (Moore et al. 1973), acid-fast eosinophilic intranuclear inclusions in proximal tubular renal epithelium; necrosis of renal tubules; and cerebral status spongiosus with astrocyte swelling, nerve cell degeneration, and vascular proliferation. The brain histopathology may not be readily differentiated from bovine polioencephalomalacia.

In calves and cattle chronically poisoned over 2 or more weeks, lesions may be quite minimal. The carcass may simply be emaciated and lacking in fat. Otherwise, the lesions of subacute toxicosis may be seen, possibly in a more advanced state; that is, hemolysis and hemorrhagic lesions may be more widespread and include hemorrhagic gastroenteritis (very common in abomasum and small gut) and meningitis. The kidneys may manifest fibrotic changes and the brain may be more obviously softened, yellow, and necrotic—particularly at the tips of cerebral gyri. Microscopically, there may be blood-loss anemia with basophilic stippling of erythrocytes and juvenile forms of erythrocytes. More obvious renal and cerebral degenerative changes of the kind mentioned for subacute toxicosis may occur. There may also be an increased number of inclusions in renal tubular epithelium.

Neither basophilic stippling of erythrocytes nor acid-fast eosinophilic inclusions in kidney or liver cells is pathognomonic of lead poisoning, but these microscopic lesions are highly suggestive of it.

For references on lesions of lead toxicosis in calves, cattle, and sheep, see Fenstermacher et al. (1946), White and Cotchin (1948), Allcroft and Blaxter (1950), Allcroft (1951), and Christian and Tryphonas (1971).

In dogs, acute lead poisoning (e.g., from ingestion of paint) may not cause gross lesions. Paint may be found in the stomach or intestines. If dogs have been manifesting clinical signs of poisoning for several days or weeks, a number of gross and microscopic lesions might be found. These lesions are described by Zook et al. (1969), Zook et al. (1972a), Stowe et al. (1973) and Zook (1973). The gross lesions consist of meningeal congestion, very red bone marrow, radio opacity of long bone metaphyses in young animals ("lead lines"), delayed closure of thoracic vertebral epiphyses, and possibly an enlarged, fatty liver, enlarged spleen, and swollen brain.

Microscopic lesions in dogs may include hematologic changes such as basophilic stippling of erythrocytes, immature erythrocytes, anemia due to hemolysis, bone marrow hyperplasia, leucocytosis with neutrophilia and left-shift in neutrophils, eosinopenia, and monopenia or (in chronic cases) neutropenia. There may be eosinophilic acid-fast intranuclear inclusions in renal tubular and hepatic cells, random necrosis of skeletal muscle fibers, peripheral neuropathy, splenic and hepatic hemosiderosis, hepatic fatty metamorphosis, focal proximal renal tubular necrosis, hydropic degeneration of spermatogonia, and granular casts in the urine.

In the brain of the dog the microscopic lesions may include cerebral vasodilation (congestion) with swelling and necrosis of vascular endothelium, capillary proliferation in cortical gray matter, gliosis, vacuolation, hyalinization and necrosis of some arterioles, thrombi in some capillaries, perivascular edema, fibrin deposition, hemorrhage, and necrosis of cortical neurons. Electroencephalogram abnormalities (Zook et al. 1972a) probably reflect these pathological changes.

It is assumed that in many tissues

cellular ultrastructural lesions precede microscopic and gross lesions (see Mechanism of Action).

In geese chronically poisoned with lead shot, microscopic degenerative lesions appear in the myocardium before any electrocardiogram abnormalities are manifested (Sileo et al. 1973). Lesions in mallard ducks given lead shot include destruction of proventricular epithelium, bone medullary osteocytes, and pectoral muscle cells. Renal proximal tubules contain intranuclear inclusions (Clemens et al. 1975).

BIOCHEMICAL CHANGES

Lead causes changes in a number of biochemical processes. Changes in serum enzymes and in brain, liver, and kidney metabolism were mentioned under Mechanism of Action. Two other effects of lead should be mentioned.

Lead inhibits heme synthesis. It does this primarily by inhibiting aminolevulinic acid dehydratase (ALA-D), although more "distal" enzymes in the biosynthetic pathway are also inhibited (Buck et al. 1973). The result of ALA-D inhibition is a "spillover" of the substrate of ALA-D, aminolevulinic acid (ALA), into plasma and urine. Decreased erythrocyte or blood ALA-D or increased plasma or urine ALA concentrations are correlated with blood lead concentration, and this forms the basis for laboratory tests for possible exposure to excessive amounts of lead (Buck et al. 1973; Hilliard et al. 1973; Tomokuni 1974; Roels et al. 1975). It is doubtful that inhibition of ALA-D plays much of a role in lead toxicosis, because poisoned tissues can soon synthesize more ALA-D (Hapke and Prigge 1973).

Another important effect of lead (also cadmium and mercury) is immunosuppression (Koller 1973; Koller and Kovacic 1974). That is, lead can suppress production of antibodies to certain viral and bacterial agents. The implication of this observation with regard to infectious disease needs no elaboration—only experimental investigation.

DIFFERENTIAL DIAGNOSIS

Lead poisoning should be suspected in animals known to have been exposed to lead and that manifest some of the typical signs (head pressing, anorexia, diarrhea, colic, blindness, tremors, hypermotility, vocalization, normal body temperature) and lesions (inflamed abomasum/stomach and small intestine, petechiae on the heart, soft kidneys, pale muscles). The diagnosis is facilitated if the hematologic findings include anemia, juvenile erythrocytes, and basophilic stippling of erythrocytes. In young dogs, radiograms may have "lead lines" in images of the long bones.

Encephalitic diseases and brain disturbances induced by tumor, trauma, hemorrhage, or abscess can cause signs like those of lead poisoning. These conditions should be ruled out by careful questioning, observation, and clinical pathologic or microbiologic testing.

Organochlorine pesticide toxicosis mimics lead in several ways, but organochlorine pesticides generally cause markedly elevated body temperature, marked neuromuscular signs, abnormal posturing, and severe convulsive activity with postictal depression. There is no blindness.

Urea toxicosis also looks like lead poisoning. However, in urea toxicosis there is no abnormal posturing, blindness, head pressing, jumping into the air, or compulsive hypermotility. Also, colic is very prominent with urea, diarrhea is not prominent, and the convulsions are strychninelike and followed by postictal rigidity instead of depression.

Organophosphate and carbamate insecticides mimic some aspects of lead poisoning, but they produce a spectrum of parasympathetic signs, marked neuromuscular signs, and little or no behavioral aberration or convulsive activity. In addition, atropine may alleviate many signs of organophosphate or carbamate pesticide poisoning but will do little more than dry the mouth of a lead-poisoned animal.

Other things to be excluded in the diagnosis of lead poisoning are salt, strychnine, fluoroacetate, nicotine, moldy feed, arsenic, mercury, hypovitaminosis-A, lupinosis (sheep), and nervous acetonemia. The details of history, clinical signs, hematologic findings, and lesions produced by these do not fit lead poisoning.

TREATMENT

Metal toxicoses are treated with chelating agents, which preferentially bond the metal in a nonionized soluble complex (chelate) that is less toxic than the metal and readily excreted in the urine. For lead, the chelator of choice is disodium calcium ethylenediamine tetraacetate (Ca-EDTA, Ca-versenate). The calcium complex is used rather than EDTA-acid or sodium-EDTA so that blood calcium will not be chelated.

In animals, Ca-EDTA apparently chelates lead that is stored in bone and has little ability to chelate lead in soft tissues (Hammond et al. 1967). Ca-EDTA does not chelate erythrocyte lead either, possibly due to the inability of Ca-EDTA to penetrate cell membranes. Removal of lead from vital soft tissues in Ca-EDTA–treated animals is thought to be due to redistribution of lead to the bone sink by means of the bloodstream.

In calves, Ca-EDTA causes illness if dosage exceeds 220 mg/kg of body weight/day for 3 days (Aronson et al. 1968). In dogs the lethal dose of Ca-EDTA is 12 g/kg of body weight (Clarke and Clarke 1967). These values may be materially reduced in lead-poisoned animals because of mobilization of lead from bone. In fact, lead toxicosis can be worsened if Ca-EDTA is used injudiciously; the kidneys may not be capable of excreting a large amount of chelated lead quickly enough.

The recommended therapeutic regimen for cattle and calves (Buck et al. 1973) (presumably other large species too) for Ca-EDTA is to give intraperitoneally or intramuscularly a 1%–2% w/v solution of Ca-EDTA in 5% glucose at the rate of 110 mg/kg of body weight twice a day for 2 days, skip 2 days to allow redistribution of lead to bone, then repeat the treatment for 2 more days. It may require 10–14 days of this interrupted therapy for animals to recover. The treatment works best if blood lead concentration is less than 1 ppm and when neurological signs are minimal. The chelator does not, of course, heal the lesions produced by lead.

In dogs, Ca-EDTA is given subcutaneously in a 1% w/v solution in 5% glucose at the rate of about 25 mg/kg of body weight 4 times a day for 5 days, not to exceed 2 g/day. The treatment is repeated if signs persist (Buck et al. 1973). Other chelators (BAL, *d*-penicillamine) are used in combination with Ca-EDTA in human beings, but such combined therapy has not found general acceptance in veterinary medicine.

Nonspecific treatment for lead poisoning includes sedation or tranquilization to control nervous and behavioral signs, gastric lavage and enemas (dogs), oral administration of magnesium sulfate to precipitate lead and act as a saline purgative, forced feeding (cattle), fluids and electrolytes (contraindicated if nervous signs are severe because of the danger of enhancing cerebral edema), corticosteroids, and antibiotics to prevent bacterial infections. The animal should be kept quiet and comfortable and should not be handled excessively.

The prognosis is grave in acute toxicosis and whenever nervous and behavioral signs are severe.

ANALYSIS

Forage samples normally contain 3–7 ppm of lead, or less. Lambs have safely eaten forage containing lead at 45–60 ppm, but no studies have been made of possible subtle effects (e.g., immunosuppression or hyperkinetic training problems) of so-called nontoxic concentrations of lead in animal feed. Silage containing 140 ppm of lead has poisoned cattle, and herbage containing lead at 216–914 ppm has killed calves (Buck et al. 1973). Presumably, calves could be killed by feedstuffs that contain insufficient lead to cause illness in adult cattle. Lead is ubiquitous in nature; small amounts are to be expected in groundwater, plant materials, and even animal tissues.

The "diagnostically significant" concentration of lead in tissues of animals is difficult to state because of wide variation in individual susceptibilty to lead. In 175 cattle and calves that died of lead poisoning the mean lead concentration and range of lead concentrations found in ingesta, liver, and whole kidney were (in ppm wet weight) 3427 (0–146,200), 43 (0–1300), and 137 (2–2355) (Hatch and Funnell 1969). These data, taken with a review of the literature, prompted the conclusion that the *mere presence* of lead in kidney or liver and ingesta should lead to a presumptive diagnosis of lead poisoning in cattle that die with signs, lesions, and histories characteristic of lead poisoning.

Osweiler et al. (1973) also found very small concentrations of lead in ingesta, liver, and kidney tissue of some cattle that had lead poisoning. It was pointed out that the diagnosis of lead poisoning cannot be confirmed with liver concentrations of lead that are less than 10 ppm unless other tissues have significant amounts of lead. This author agrees, but would add that erythrocyte basophilic stippling, proved access to or ingestion of lead, decreased erythrocyte ALA-D activity, increased plasma or urine ALA, or increased urinary or blood lead following administration of Ca-EDTA can also be used to confirm the diagnosis of lead poisoning.

In most poisoned animals, blood and tissue concentrations of lead are not so small as to provoke diagnostic confusion. In large animals, lead concentrations of 0.35 ppm or more in blood, 10 ppm or more in liver, 15 ppm or more in kidney cortex, 35 ppm or more in feces (recent exposure) or rumen contents support a diagnosis of lead poisoning if the history, signs, and lesions are consistent with lead poisoning (Buck et al. 1973). In chronic poisoning, tissue lead concentration may be very small, but bone lead may be 100 ppm or more, or there may be a large increase in urine lead 24 hours after the start of Ca-EDTA therapy.

In poisoned dogs, hair may contain 88 ppm or more of lead. The blood contains at least 0.35 ppm of lead (sometimes less), the liver contains an average of 17.4 ppm ± 11.7 (standard deviation), or a range of 3.6–50 ppm, and urine lead increases markedly (to 820 ppm or more) 24 hours after commencement of Ca-EDTA therapy. Additionally, basophilic stippling of erythrocytes, decreased erythrocyte ALA-D or increased plasma or urine ALA, and radio opacity of long bone metaphyses (young dogs) may be manifested (Zook et al. 1972b; Buck et al. 1973; Zook 1973).

In poisoned chickens, blood contains about 13 ppm of lead, liver contains more than 10 ppm, and feces may contain 1–2910 ppm (Clarke and Clarke 1967; Buck et al. 1973). Smaller concentrations than these have occasionally been associated with lead poisoning. In mallard ducks the blood lead concentration may be 10 ppm or more, especially if the diet is high in fiber (Clemens et al. 1975).

Erythrocyte ALA-D activity is perhaps a better index of lead exposure (at least acute and subacute exposure) than is plasma or urine ALA. Normal values of erythrocyte ALA-D are given by Hapke and Prigge (1973). The values are expressed in micromoles of porphobilinogen produced/hour/L of erythrocytes. The values in different species are (mean ± standard deviation): human being, 924 ± 284; cattle, 240 ± 128; mongrel dogs, 405 ± 262; beagle dogs, 255 ± 130; pigs 1040 ± 385; horses, 0–0.1; rabbits, 2152 (no standard deviation given); adult rats, 159 ± 40; and 8-week-old rats, 170 ± 50. If lead exposure takes place over a period of several days or weeks, erythrocyte ALA-D activity will be partly or completely restored due to synthesis of new ALA-D, but the fraction of ALA-D that is inhibited by lead can be disinhibited by glutathione, thus unmasking a depressant action of lead on ALA-D activity (Hapke and Prigge 1973).

Fluoride (Acute Poisoning)

Occasionally animals may ingest a quantity of inorganic fluoride such as sodium fluoride (NaF) (formerly used at 1% concentration in dry food for the treatment of roundworms in swine) or sodium fluorosilicate rodenticide. Animals that can vomit generally expel the poison promptly, for fluoride is a strong caustic. Thus signs may be limited to those of gastroenteritis and abdominal pain.

If sufficient fluoride is absorbed (oral acute lethal dose of NaF is about 0.5 g/kg of body weight) fluoride ion increases capillary permeability and also produces a coagulation defect. These actions lead to hemorrhagic gastroenteritis and to hemorrhages, congestion, and edema in various organs including the brain. Fluoride is very reactive and capable of inhibiting a number of enzymes including glycolytic enzymes, phosphatases, and cholinesterase. The result is inhibition of cellular glycolysis and respiration and increased sensitivity of cholinergic mechanisms to acetylcholine. Clinical manifestations of these actions include excitability, muscle tremors, weakness, urination, defecation, salivation, emesis, sudden collapse, clonic convulsions, coma, and death due to respiratory and cardiac failure. Cyanosis and early rigor mortis are seen (Sollmann, 1957; Buck et al. 1973).

The signs and lesions of acute fatal fluoride toxicosis are a blend of signs and lesions that would be produced by any strong caustic (e.g., inorganic arsenic), plus an anticholinesterase pesticide, plus a metabolic inhibitor (e.g. fluoroacetate), plus an anticoagulant rodenticide (e.g., warfarin).

There is no specific treatment for acute fluoride poisoning. Symptomatic treatment may save some animals that did not ingest too much fluoride, but the prognosis is grave.

Mold Toxins

Some mycotoxins that can cause nervous stimulation by unknown mechanisms include ergot alkaloids, tremortin-A, and satratoxins. These are lumped together here for convenience, not because they are in any way related.

SOURCE

Variable combinations of ergot alkaloids (ergotamine, ergonovine, ergocryptine, ergocornine, ergocristine, ergosine) are found in the mature sclerotia of parasitic fungi of the genus *Claviceps*. *Claviceps purpurea* is the most common ergot mold. It attacks the developing ovary (seed) of rye, oats, wheat barley, wild grasses, and Kentucky bluegrass. Seed heads of affected plants manifest replacement of normal seeds by hard, elongated, brown, purple, or black structures which can be larger than the normal seeds. Another ergot mold, *Claviceps paspali,* infects the seed heads of dallisgrass *(Paspalum dilatatum),* a common pasture grass in the southern United States. Argentine bahiagrass *(Paspalum notatum)* may also be attacked by *C. paspali*. The seed heads of affected grass may be misshapen, and several of the seeds may be replaced by hard, globular (2–4 mm diameter), irregularly roughened, yellow to brown sclerotia. *Claviceps cinerea* is an ergot mold that may parasitize tobosagrass *(Hilaria mutica)* and galletagrass *(Hilaria jamesii)*. Warm, moist, humid growing seasons predispose to infection of grasses and grain heads by *Claviceps* spp.

Tremortin-A is one of a number of tremor-inducing (tremorgenic) metabolites produced by species of *Penicillium*. Corn or other feeds manifesting growth of *Penicillium* spp. may be toxic for livestock. Tremortin-A has not been incriminated as a major cause of illness at this time, but the toxin is suspected of having killed sheep that were fed moldy corn and horses that were fed moldy pelletized feed (Wilson 1971; Cysewski 1973).

Satratoxins C, D, F, G, and H (letters refer to chromatographic mobility) are apparently members of the 12,13-epoxy-delta^9-trichothecene group (Eppley and Bailey 1973), the same group of mycotoxins that contains T-2 toxin and diacetoxyscirpenol (Bamburg and Strong 1971). Although they have not yet been recognized as causes of livestock poisoning in the United States, the satratoxins have killed people, sheep, swine, calves, poultry, and thousands of horses in Europe. The disease condition produced by these toxins is known as *stachybotryotoxicosis,* and is related to ingestion of straw, hay, or grain infested with the mold *Stachybotrys atra,* also known as *S. alternans.*

PROPERTIES OF TOXICOLOGIC IMPORTANCE

Ergot toxins, being alkaloids, have the same chemical and physical properties as alkaloids in general. In this regard, incompatibility with tannic acid, albumin, and certain metal salts could serve as one basis for treatment of ergotism, i.e., precipitation of alkaloid in the gut. Ergot alkaloids are pharmacologically active and their smooth muscle stimulant properties have some medical uses (see ergotamine, ergonovine). Ergot alkaloids contain the lysergic acid nucleus. Lysergic acid contains the indole structure. This may explain the central nervous stimulant effects of these compounds since many indoles are central nervous stimulants.

Tremortin-A is soluble in alcohol but not in water. Its empirical formula is $C_{37}H_{44}O_6NCl$ (Wilson 1971). Its chemical structure is apparently complex and has not been determined exactly.

The most important property of the satratoxins, beside their persistence in feeds, is probably their strong irritant effect on skin and mucous membranes. This causes some of the lesions seen in stachybotryotoxicosis and also serves as the basis for detection of the toxins by skin tests in laboratory animals.

TOXICITY

Ergotism occurs in chronic (gangrenous) and acute (nervous or convulsive) forms. The gangrenous form results when animals ingest ergot alkaloids in small amounts over a period of days or weeks. This form of ergotism is discussed in Chapter 60.

Nervous ergotism occurs most commonly in carnivora, horses, and sheep, but only rarely in cattle (Burfening 1973). The amount of ergot sclerotia required to cause nervous signs varies with climate, location, species, and rate of ingestion of toxic feeds. Total alkaloid content and relative amounts of different alkaloids and other mold metabolites in ergot sclerotia also influence toxicity. Data are lacking on the LD50 of ergot sclerotia in various species. Perhaps this is unimportant. If animals eat ergot-infected grain or grass and then develop nervous signs, the grain or grass is toxic, no matter how much was eaten! In other words, if grain or pasture grass is ergotized, animals should not be allowed to eat it. This is a safety precaution that applies to moldy feeds in general. The safety precaution applies notwithstanding USDA tolerance limits for mold or mold toxin content. For ergot, the USDA Grain Division has set 0.3% (on a crude weight basis) as a tolerance limit in grain (Buck et al. 1973). It is doubtful that one would want to feed a prize bull or a winning racehorse 0.3%, 0.2%, or even 0.1% ergot sclerotia in the grain ration, especially in view of the possibility that other molds might also be present.

Tremortin-A is toxic for calves, mice, rats, chickens, rabbits, guinea pigs, hamsters, and probably sheep and horses. In mice, an intraperitoneal injection of 0.25 mg tremortin-A/kg of body weight induces tremors. Larger doses cause more severe signs including convulsions and death. Other species are about as sensitive as mice, although hamsters are more resistant than other laboratory animals. Nephrotoxicity may result with dosages of 0.5 mg toxin/kg of body weight or more, and this effect leads to diuresis with loss of electrolytes and glucose (Wilson 1971; Cysewski 1973).

Satratoxins are toxic for most mammals and fowl. Acute toxicity and death may occur in horses fed as little as 0.5 lb (0.227 kg) of moldy straw over a period of 10 days (Eppley and Bailey 1973). Smaller quantities of toxin are also lethal, but death is probably due to combined effects of a clotting defect, necrotic lesions, and bacterial infection rather than nervous disorder.

MECHANISM OF ACTION

Indoles and lysergic acid derivatives are thought to cause central nervous stimulation by interfering somehow with brain neurotransmitter function. Serotonin is the transmitter of main interest because of chemical structural similarities to indole type stimulants, but other amines such as dopamine and norepinephrine may also be involved in a central imbalance of transmitters elicited by ergotamine and other indole-containing compounds.

Tremors induced by tremortin-A can be alleviated in mice by nonspecific therapy such as mephenesin or diazepam. In calves, chlorpromazine reduces or eliminates tremor and rigidity. Deep anesthesia with pentobarbital also prevents excitatory signs (Wilson 1971; Cysewski 1973). These treatments do not give a clue about the mechanism of action of tremortin-A. The toxin does not produce histologic changes in the brain or spinal cord of calves (Cysewski 1973). The character of muscle impairment produced by tremortin-A (see Clinical Signs) suggests that the toxin somehow upsets central neurotransmitter functions that control muscle activity, but no studies have been made on the effect of synaptic blocking agents or synaptic stimulants on tremortin-A toxicosis.

Satratoxins, being similar to T-2 toxin and diacetoxyscirpenol, may have a mechanism of action similar to those trichothecenes. Skin and mucosal lesions produced by these compounds probably have a common biochemical basis. Clotting defects produced by lower doses of satratoxins may also arise by the same mechanisms as for other trichothecenes. The only problem is, we do not know how T-2 toxin or diacetoxyscirpenol acts; therefore, we do not know how the satratoxins act either. The problem is confounded by the fact that satratoxins produce nervous disorders but other trichothecenes apparently do not (unless perhaps with doses that have not yet been investigated).

CLINICAL SIGNS

Nervous ergotism, whether due to ingestion of *C. purpurea* or *C. paspali,* is characterized by a 1- to 7-day onset of some combination of the following signs: weakness, recumbency, tremors, spasms, hyperexcitability, belligerency, weaving, incoordination, ataxia or staggering gait, falling, nodding of the head, exacerbation of tremors and incoordination by exercise or excitement, excessive limb flexion when walking or running, tonic convulsions with opisthotonos, postical depression and posterior paralysis, and either death or recovery in 10–14 days. Death may be due to anoxia during convulsions or to thirst or accidents suffered during the illness (Goodwin 1967; Buck et al. 1973; Burfening 1973; Cysewski 1973).

Tremortin-A toxicosis is manifested in calves by fine tremor that gets worse with forced exercise or excitement, progressively severe tremors, a stiff "sawhorse" stance, rhythmic swaying of the body, stiff gait, ataxia, falling, lateral recumbency, paddling of the limbs, intermittent extensor rigidity, opisthotonos, and occasionally nystagmus and hypersalivation. In chickens, dyspnea, ataxia, impairment of righting reflex, hypersensitivity to external stimuli, listlessness, and coarse tremors occur (Cysewski 1973). Convulsive and other excitatory signs are produced in laboratory animals (Wilson 1971).

Satratoxins in large dosages produce convulsions and other nervous disorders terminating in death. References cited by Eppley and Bailey (1973) provide more information on stachybotryotoxicosis.

LESIONS

Large amounts of ergot alkaloids, tremortin-A, or satratoxins may not produce any gross lesions. With convulsive ergotism there may be an increased volume of cerebrospinal fluid (Buck et al. 1973), incomplete rigor and empty arteries (Burfening 1973), and agonal changes attributable to convulsions. Ergot sclerotia may be found in the GI tract.

With tremortin-A toxicosis there may be pronounced rigor and a fatty liver (Cysewski 1973).

Satratoxins can produce necrotic lesions on skin and mucous membranes, hemorrhagic gastroenteritis, and possibly agonal lesions due to convulsions.

DIFFERENTIAL DIAGNOSIS

It is important to rule out infectious disease, trauma, neoplasm, abscess, and hemorrhage as possible causes of central excitatory states. When poisoning is suspected, the premises should be carefully inspected for possible sources. This inspection should include examination of pasture grass heads, hay, straw, grain, silage, and prepared feeds for evidence of mold growth. Sclerotia may be found on grass heads or in the grain or hay, thus implicating *Claviceps* sp. A history of ingestion of moldy or ergotized feed, taken with signs and lesions typical of the mold toxins discussed, is suggestive of poisoning by these toxins.

TREATMENT

There are no specific treatments for mycotoxicoses. The offending feed or forage must be removed or fenced away from animals. Animals may be treated symptomatically. Convulsions, tremors, and behavioral aberrations may respond to treatment with chlorpromazine or diazepam. Deep anesthesia with barbiturates is not recommended in sick animals. Orally administered magnesium sulfate may eliminate some toxic feed from the gut. Recovery can occur in a few days. See Chapter 60 for information on other effects of ergot and satratoxins.

ANALYSIS

Feed samples can be examined for ergot sclerotia. If sclerotia have been ground up, the sample can be extracted and tested for ergot alkaloids. Trichothecenes can be detected by their ability to evoke lesions when applied to the skin of laboratory animals. Trichothecenes and tremortin-A can be identified by thin layer chromatography of feed/forage extracts. Laboratory animals may be fed the moldy feed or injected intraperitoneally or intragastrically with extracts of the feed. Culture of the mold is not a productive procedure because molds *will* be found in feed but their toxigenicity under previous conditions of poisoning and storage cannot be established. Animal tissues cannot easily be tested for most mold toxins.

PLANT TOXINS

Several plant poisons cause nervous stimulation or depression by unknown mechanisms. Coniine, from poison hemlock *(Conium maculatum),* produces signs similar to those of the chemically related alkaloid nicotine. Cicutoxin, a resin from water hemlock *(Cicuta maculata),* causes violent convulsions, tremors, fever, and rapid death. Mixed isoquinoline alkaloids in fitweed (*Corydalis* sp.) cause muscle twitching, clonic convulsions, depression, muscle rigidity that is elicitable by external stimuli, staggering, bawling, and biting behavior. Mixed isoquinoline alkaloids in Dutchman's-breeches and squirrel corn (*Dicentra* spp.) cause vomition, trembling, running with head elevated, pain, dyspnea, and opisthotonic rigidity. Lupinine and other quinolizidine alkaloids in lupines (*Lupinus* spp.) cause dyspnea, nervous stimulation or depression, and (in sheep) behavioral aberrations similar to some of those described for lead poisoning.

Strychninelike alkaloids in Carolina jessamine (*Gelsemium* sp.) cause depression, weakness, staggering, mild convulsions, and coma. Lobeline in Indian tobacco (*Lobelia* spp.) causes depression, diarrhea, oral ulcers, hemorrhages, and coma. Solanine in various nightshades (*Solanum* spp.) causes depression, salivation, dyspnea, trembling, paralysis, colic, diarrhea, and coma. Coumarin glycosides in horse chestnut and Ohio buckeye (*Aesculus* spp.) cause depression, vomiting, trembling, paralysis, and inflamed mucous membranes. Alkaloids and glycosides in milkweeds (*Asclepias* spp.) cause depression, weakness, staggering, dyspnea, fever, tetanic seizures, and coma. In monogastric animals, horsetails (*Equisetum* spp.) and bracken fern (*Pteridium* sp.) can cause incoordination and depression, a braced and crouching stance, tremors, collapse, and convulsions. These signs may be due to the presence of thiaminase in the plants or to some factor present (in bracken) that is counteracted by batyl alcohol. Usnic acid in ground lichen (*Parmelia* spp.) causes incoordination, depression, and paralysis. Unknown factors in bitterweed and pingue (*Hymenoxys* spp.) cause depression, weakness, vomiting, and colic.

Treatment for any of these toxicoses is symptomatic. See Kingsbury (1964) for detail.

Central nervous stimulation or depression is seen with many poisons. In a dying animal, convulsions or coma may accompany respiratory insufficiency near terminus. Such convulsions or coma are due to cerebral anoxia. What has been attempted here is to present those poisons causing nervous stimulation or depression as an obvious and integral part of the clinical toxicosis. Some confusion arises when one poison is known to cause both nervous excitation and nervous depression. This confusion can be abolished when one realizes that criteria other than clinical signs are used for diagnosing and treating toxicoses.

REFERENCES

Aaseth, J. 1973. The effect of mercaptodextran on distribution and toxicity of mercury in mice. Acta Pharmacol Toxicol 32: 430.

Allcroft, R. 1951. Lead poisoning in cattle and sheep. Vet Rec 63:583.

Allcroft, R., and Blaxter, K. L. 1950. Lead as a nutritional hazard to farm livestock. V. The toxicity of lead to cattle and sheep and an evaluation of the lead hazard under farm conditions. J Comp Pathol 60:209.

Aprison, M. K.; Shank, R. P.; Davidoff, R. A.; and Werman, R. 1968. The distribution of glycine, a neurotransmitter suspect in the central nervous system of several vertebrate species. Life Sci 7:583.

Aronson, A. L. 1971. Lead poisoning in cattle and horses following long-term exposure to lead. J Am Vet Med Assoc 158: 1870.

Aronson, A. L.; Hammond, P. B.; and Strafuss, A. C. 1968. Studies with calcium ethylenediaminetetraacetate in calves: Toxicity and use in bovine lead poisoning. Toxicol Appl Pharmacol 12:337.

Asokan, S. K. 1974. Experimental lead cardiomyopathy: Myocardial structural changes in rats given small amounts of lead. J Lab Clin Med 84:20.

Avery, D. D., and Cross, H. A. 1974. The effects of tetraethyl lead on behavior in the rat. Pharmacol Biochem Behav 2:473.

Bamburg, J. R., and Strong, F. M. 1971. 12, 13-Epoxytrichothecenes. In S. Kadis and A. Ciegler, eds. Microbial Toxins, vol. 7. New York: Academic Press.

Barrow, M. V.; Simpson, C. F.; and Miller, E. J. 1974. Lathyrism: A review. Q Rev Biol 49:101.

Benetiz, D.; Pscheidt, G. R.; and Stone, W. E. 1954. Formation of ammonium ion in the cerebrum in fluoroacetate poisoning. Am J Physiol 176:488.

Berg, G. L., ed. 1974. Farm Chemicals Handbook 1974. Willoughby, Ohio: Meister.

Blair, D.; Hoadley, E. C.; and Hutson, D. H. 1975. The distribution of dichlorvos in the tissues of mammals after its inhalation or intravenous administration. Toxicol Appl Pharmacol 31:243.

Blaxter, K. L. 1950a. Lead as a nutritional hazard to farm livestock. II. The absorption and excretion of lead by sheep and rabbits. J Comp Pathol 60:140.

———. 1950b. Lead as a nutritional hazard to farm livestock. III. Factors influencing the distribution of lead in the tissues. J Comp Pathol 60:177.

Boehme, D. H.; Fordice, M. W.; Marks, N.; and Vogel, W. 1973. Distribution of glycine in human spinal cord and selected regions of brain. Brain Res 50:353.

Brooks, G. T. 1974. Chlorinated Insecticides, Vol. 2: Biological and Environmental Aspects. Cleveland: CRC Press.

Brown, H. R., and Sharma, R. P. 1975. Inhibition of neural membrane adenosinetriphosphatases by organophosphates. Abstr 14th Ann Meet Soc Toxicol, Williamsburg, Va., Mar. 9–13, 1975.

Bryce-Smith, D. 1972. Behavioural effects of lead and other heavy metal pollutants. Chem Br 8:240.

Buck, W. B.; Osweiler, G. D.; and Van Gelder, G. A. 1973. Clinical and Diagnostic Veterinary Toxicology. Dubuque, Iowa: Kendall/Hunt.

Burfening, P. J. 1973. Ergotism. J Am Vet Med Assoc 163:1288.

Carson, T. L.; Van Gelder, G. A.; Karas, G. C.; and Buck, W. B. 1974. Slowed learning in lambs prenatally exposed to lead. Arch Environ Health 29:154.

Cavagna, G.; Locati, G.; and Vigliani, E. C. 1969. Clinical effects of exposure to DDVP

(Vapona) insecticide in hospital wards. Arch Environ Health 19:112.

Chang, L. W., and Hartmann, H. A. 1972. Blood-brain barrier dysfunction in experimental mercury intoxication. Acta Neuropathol (Berl) 21:179.

Charbonneau, S. M.; Munro, I. C.; Nera, E. A.; Willes, R. F.; Kuiper-Goodman, T.; Iverson, F.; Moodie, C. A.; Stoltz, D. R.; Armstrong, F. A. J.; Uthe, J. F.; and Grice, H. C. 1974. Subacute toxicity of methylmercury in the adult cat. Toxicol Appl Pharmacol 27:569.

Charlton, K. M. 1974. Experimental alkylmercurial poisoning in swine. Lesions in the peripheral and central nervous systems. Can J Comp Med 38:75.

Christian, R. G., and Tryphonas, L. 1971. Lead poisoning in cattle: Brain lesions and hematologic changes. Am J Vet Res 32:203.

Clarke, E. G. C., and Clarke, M. L., eds. 1967. Garner's Veterinary Toxicology, 3rd ed. Baltimore: Williams & Wilkins.

Clarkson, T. W. 1972. The pharmacology of mercury compounds. Annu Rev Pharmacol 12:375.

Clemens, E. T.; Krook, L.; Aronson, A. L.; and Stevens, C. E. 1975. Pathogenesis of lead shot poisoning in the mallard duck. Cornell Vet 65:248.

Curley, A.; Sedlak, V. A.; Girling, E. F.; Hawk, R. E.; Barthel, W. F.; Pierce, P. E.; and Likosky, W. H. 1971. Organic mercury identified as the cause of poisoning in humans and hogs. Science 172:65.

Curtis, D. R.; Hösli, L.; Johnston, G. A. R.; and Johnston, I. H. 1968. The hyperpolarization of spinal motoneurones by glycine and related amino acids. Exp Brain Res 5:235.

Curtis, D. R.; Duggan, A. W.; Felix, D.; and Johnston, G. A. R. 1970. Gaba, bicuculline and central inhibition. Nature 226: 1222.

———. 1971a. Bicuculline, an antagonist of gaba and synaptic inhibition in the spinal cord of the cat. Brain Res 32:69.

Curtis, D. R.; Duggan, A. W.; Felix, D.; Johnston, G. A. R.; and McLennan, H. 1971b. Antagonism between bicuculline and gaba in the cat brain. Brain Res 33:57.

Cysewski, S. J. 1973. Paspalum staggers and tremorgen intoxication in animals. J Am Vet Med Assoc 163:1291.

Davidoff, R. A. 1972. Penicillin and inhibition in the cat spinal cord. Brain Res 45:638.

Davidoff, R. A.; Aprison, M. H.; and Werman, R. 1969. The effects of strychnine on the inhibition of interneurons by glycine and γ-aminobutyric acid. Int J Neuropharmacol 8:191.

Dieter, M. P., and Ludke, J. L. 1975. Studies on combined effects of organophosphates and heavy metals in bird. I. Plasma and brain cholinesterase in coturnix quail fed methylmercury and orally dosed wth parathion. Bull Environ Contam Toxicol 13: 257.

Ecobichon, D. J., and Saschenbrecker, P. W. 1968. Pharmacodynamic study of DDT in cockerels. Can J Physiol Pharmacol 46:785.

Edds, G. T., and Simpson, C. F. 1974. Hexachlorophene-phisohex toxicity in pups. Am J Vet Res 35:1005.

Eppley, R. M., and Bailey, W. J. 1973. 12,13-Epoxy-Δ^9-trichothecenes as the probable mycotoxins responsible for stachybotryotoxicosis. Science 181:758.

Eto, M. 1974. Organophosphorus Pesticides: Organic and Biological Chemistry. Cleveland: CRC Press.

Fenstermacher, R.; Pomeroy, B. S.; Roepke, M. H.; and Boyd, W. L. 1946. Lead poisoning of cattle. J Am Vet Med Assoc 108:1.

Freeman, A. R. 1973. Electrophysiological analysis of the actions of strychnine, bicuculline and picrotoxin on the axonal membrane. J Neurobiol 4:567.

Gaines, T. B. 1969. Acute toxicity of pesticides. Toxicol Appl Pharmacol 14:515.

Ganote, C. E.; Reimer, K. A.; and Jennings, R. B. 1974. Acute mercuric chloride nephrotoxicity, an electron microscopic and metabolic study. Lab Invest 31:633.

Gibson, G. E.; Zimber, A.; Krook, L.; Richardson, E. P., Jr.; and Visek, W. J. 1974. Brain histology and behavior of mice injected with urease. J Neuropathol Exp Neurol 33:201.

Goldstein, G. W.; Asbury, A. K.; and Diamond, I. 1974. Pathogenesis of lead encephalopathy, uptake of lead and reaction of brain capillaries. Arch Neurol 31:382.

Golter, M., and Michaelson, I. A. 1975. Growth, behavior, and brain catecholamines in lead-exposed neonatal rats: A reappraisal. Science 187:359.

Goodwin, D. E. 1967. Ergot poisoning of cattle grazing dallisgrass. J Am Vet Med Assoc 151:204.

Hall, G. A., and Reid, I. M. 1974. The effects of hexachlorophene on the nervous system of sheep. J Pathol 114:241.

Hammond, P. B. 1965. Other beneficial minerals. In L. M. Jones, ed. Veterinary Pharmacology and Therapeutics, 3rd ed. Ames: Iowa State Univ. Press.

Hammond, P. B.; Aronson, A. L.; and Olson, W. C. 1967. The mechanism of mobilization of lead by ethylenediaminetetraacetate. J Pharmacol Exp Ther 157:196.

Hapke, J.-J., and Prigge, E. 1973. Interactions

of lead and glutathione with delta-aminolevulinic acid dehydratase. Arch Toxicol (Berl) 31:153.

Hatch, R. C., and Funnell, H. S. 1968. Strychnine levels in tissues and stomach contents of poisoned dogs: An eleven-year survey. Can Vet J 9:161.

———. 1969. Lead levels in tissues and stomach contents of poisoned cattle: A fifteen-year survey. Can Vet J 10:258.

Hayes, W. J., Jr. 1974. Distribution of dieldrin following a single oral dose. Toxicol Appl Pharmacol 28:485.

Herigstad, R. R.; Whitehair, C. K.; Beyer, N.; Mickelsen, O.; and Zabik, M. J. 1972. Chronic methylmercury toxicosis in calves. J Am Vet Med Assoc 160:173.

Hill, R. G.; Simmonds, M. A.; and Straughan, D. W. 1972. Antagonism of gaba by picrotoxin in the feline cerebral cortex. Br J Pharmacol 44:807.

Hille, B. 1968. Pharmacological modifications of the sodium channels of frog nerve. J Gen Physiol 51:199.

Hilliard, E. P.; Poole, D. B. R.; and Collins, J. D. 1973. Accidental lead intoxication of cattle: Further evidence of an interference in heme biosynthesis. Br Vet J 129:82.

Hooper, P. T. 1972. Spongy degeneration in the brain in relation to hepatic disease and ammonia toxicity in domestic animals. Vet Rec 90:37.

Huffman, R. D., and McFaddin, L. S. 1972 Effects of bicuculline on central inhibition. Neuropharmacology 11:789.

Hughes, H. C., and Lang, C. M. 1973. Effect of orally administered dichlorvos on demodectic mange in the dog. J Am Vet Med Assoc 163:142.

Johnson, M. K. 1974. The primary biochemical lesions leading to the delayed neurotoxic effects of some organophosphorus esters. J Neurochem 23:785.

Jones, D. C. L.; Davis, W. E., Jr.; Newell, G. W.; Sasmore, D. P.; and Rosen, V. J. 1974. Modification of hexachlorophene toxicity by dieldrin and aroclor 1254. Toxicology 2:309.

Jones, M. M., and Harbison, R. D. 1975. Synthesis and study of some new chelating agents to antagonize methylmercury-induced toxicity. Abstr 14th Ann Meet Soc Toxicol, Williamsburg, Va., Mar. 9–13, 1975.

Kahn, M. A. 1973. Toxicity of systemic insecticides, toxicological considerations in using organophosphorus insecticides. Vet Rec 92:411.

Kahrs, R. F. 1968. Chronic mercurial poisoning in swine. A case report of an outbreak with some epidemiological characteristics of hog cholera. Cornell Vet 58:67.

Kasuya, M. 1975. The effect of vitamin E on the toxicity of alkylmercurials on nervous tissue in culture. Toxicol Appl Pharmacol 32:347.

Kendall, M. W. 1974. Acute hepatotoxic effects of mirex in the rat. Bull Environ Contam Toxicol 12:617.

Keplinger, M. L., and Deichmann, W. B. 1967. Acute toxicity of combinations of pesticides. Toxicol Appl Pharmacol 10:586.

Kibler, W. B. 1973. Skeletal muscle necrosis secondary to parathion. Toxicol Appl Pharmacol 25:117.

Kimbrough, R. D. 1973. Review of the toxicity of hexachlorophene, including its neurotoxicity. J Clin Pharmacol 13:439.

Kingsbury, J. M. 1964. Poisonous Plants of the United States and Canada. Englewood Cliffs, N. J.: Prentice-Hall.

Knight, H. D., and Burau, R. G. 1973. Chronic lead poisoning in horses. J Am Vet Med Assoc 162:781.

Koller, L. D. 1973. Immunosuppression produced by lead, cadmium, and mercury. Am J Vet Res 34:1457.

Koller, L. D., and Kovacic, S. 1974. Decreased antibody formation in mice exposed to lead. Nature 250:148.

Konat, G., and Clausen, J. 1974. The effect of long-term administration of triethyllead on the developing rat brain. Environ Physiol Biochem 4:236.

Krnjević, K. 1970. Glutamate and γ-aminobutyric acid in brain. Nature 228:119.

Kushlan, M. C.; Haddow, J. E.; and Lester, R. 1975. *In vitro* enhancement of erythrocyte mercury uptake by spironolactone. Toxicol Appl Pharmacol 31:527.

Leary, J. S.; Keane, W. T.; Fontenot, C.; Feichtmeir, E. F.; Schultz, D.; Koos, B. A.; Hirsch, L.; Lavor, E. M.; Roan, C. C.; and Hine, C. H. 1974. Safety evaluation in the home of polyvinyl chloride resin strip containing dichlorvos (DDVP). Arch Environ Health 29:308.

Loosmore, R. M.; Harding, J. D. J.; and Lewis, G. 1967. Mercury poisoning in pigs. Vet Rec 18:268.

McParland, P. J.; McCracken, R. M.; O'Hare, M. B.; and Raven, A. M. 1973. Benzene hexachloride poisoning in cattle. Vet Rec 93:369.

Meek, D. G., and Keatts, W. H. 1971. Strychnine poisoning in horses. J Am Vet Med Assoc 158:491.

Michaelson, I. A., and Sauerhoff, M. W. 1974. An improved model of lead-induced brain dysfunction in the suckling rat. Toxicol Appl Pharmacol 28:88.

Miller, T. L., and Buhler, D. R. 1974. Effect of hexachlorophene on monovalent cation transport in human erythrocytes, a mechanism for hexachlorophene induced hemolysis. Biochim Biophys Acta 352:86.

Moore, J. F.; Goyer, R. A.; and Wilson, M. 1973. Lead-induced inclusion bodies: Solubility, amino acid content, and relationship to residual acidic nuclear proteins. Lab Invest 29:488.

Niklowitz, W. J. 1974. Ultrastructural effects of acute tetraethyllead poisoning on nerve cells of the rabbit brain. Environ Res 8:17.

Okada, Y.; Nitsch-Hassler, C.; Kim, J. S.; Bak, I. J.; and Hassler, R. 1971. Role of γ-aminobutyric acid (gaba) in the extrapyramidal motor system. I. Regional distribution of gaba in rabbit, rat, guinea pig and baboon CNS. Exp Brain Res 13:514.

Oliver, W. T., and Platonow, N. 1960. Studies on the pharmacology of *N*-(ethylmercuri)-*p*-toluensulfonanilide. Am J Vet Res 21:906.

Olson, K., and Boush, G. M. 1975. Decreased learning capacity in rats exposed prenatally and postnatally to low doses of mercury. Bull Environ Contam Toxicol 13:73.

Osweiler, G. D., and Hurd, J. W. 1974. Determination of sodium content in serum and cerebrospinal fluid as an adjunct to diagnosis of water deprivation in swine. J Am Vet Med Assoc 164:165.

Osweiler, G. D.; Buck, W. B.; and Lloyd, W. E. 1973. Epidemiology of lead poisoning in cattle—A five-year study in Iowa. Clin Toxicol 6:367.

Palmer, J. S., and Schlinke, J. C. 1973a. Toxic effects of carbofuran in cattle and sheep. J Am Vet Med Assoc 162:561.

———. 1973b. Oral toxicity of tributyl phosphorotrithioite, a cotton defoliant, to cattle and sheep. J Am Vet Med Assoc 163:1172.

Palmer, J. S.; Wright, F. C.; and Haufler, M. 1973. Toxicologic and residual aspects of an alkylmercury fungicide to cattle, sheep, and turkeys. Clin Toxicol 6:425.

Peters, J. A., and Baxter, K. J. 1974. Analytical determination of compound 1080 (sodium fluoroacetate) residues in biological materials. Bull Environ Contam Toxicol 11:177.

Piper, R. C.; Miller, V. L.; and Dickinson, E. O. 1971. Toxicity and distribution of mercury in pigs with acute methylmercurialism. Am J Vet Res 32:263.

Potter, S., and Matrone, G. 1974. Effect of selenite on the toxicity of dietary methylmercury and mercuric chloride in the rat. J Nutr 104:638.

Raabe, W., and Gumnit, R. J. 1975. Disinhibition in cat motor cortex by ammonia. J Neurophysiol 38:347.

Radeleff, R. D. 1970. Veterinary Toxicology, 2nd ed. Philadelphia: Lea & Febiger.

Rapoport, S. I. 1970. Effect of concentrated solutions on blood-brain barrier. Am J Physiol 219:270.

Rapoport, S. I., and Thompson, H. K. 1973. Osmotic opening of the blood-brain barrier in the monkey without associated neurological deficits. Science 180:971.

Rapoport, S. I.; Hori, M.; and Klatzo, I. 1971. Reversible osmotic opening of the blood-brain barrier. Science 173:1026.

Rapoport, S. I.; Bachman, D. S.; and Thompson, H. K. 1972. Chronic effects of osmotic opening of the blood-brain barrier in the monkey. Science 176:1243.

Ray, A. C.; Norris, J. D., Jr.; and Reagor, J. C. 1975. Benzene hexachloride poisoning in cattle. J Am Vet Med Assoc 166:1180.

Richardson, R. J., and Murphy, S. D. 1975. Effect of glutathione depletion on tissue deposition of methylmercury in rats. Toxicol Appl Pharmacol 31:505.

Roberts, E., and Kuriyama, K. 1968. Biochemical-physiological correlations in studies of the γ-aminobutyric acid system. Brain Res 8:1.

Roels, H. A.; Lauwerys, R. R.; Buchet, J. P.; and Vrelust, M.-Th. 1975. Response of free erythrocyte porphyrin and urinary δ-aminolevulinic acid in men and women moderately exposed to lead. Int Arch Arbeitsmed 34:97.

Rozman, R. S.; Locke, L. N.; and McClure, S. F. III. 1974. Enzyme changes in mallard ducks fed iron or lead shot. Avian Dis 18:435.

St. Omer, V. V. 1970. Chronic and acute toxicity of the chlorinated hydrocarbon insecticides in mammals and birds. Can Vet J 11:215.

———. 1971. Investigations into mechanisms responsible for seizures induced by chlorinated hydrocarbon insecticides: The role of brain ammonia and glutamine in convulsions in the rat and cockerel. J Neurochem 18:365.

———. 1972. Temporal effect of *m*-fluorotyrosine on brain (prosencephalon and rhombencephalon) ammonia and glutamine during seizures. Brain Res 37:149.

Scott, D. W.; Bolton, G. R.; and Lorenz, M. D. 1973. Hexachlorophene toxicosis in dogs. J Am Vet Med Assoc 162:947.

Sharma, R. P. 1973. Brain biogenic amines: Depletion by chronic dieldrin exposure. Life Sci 13:1245.

Silbergeld, E. K., and Goldberg, A. M. 1973. A lead-induced behavioral disorder. Life Sci 13:1275.

———. 1974. Lead-induced behavioral dysfunction: An animal model of hyperactivity. Exp Neurol 42:146.

Silbergeld, E. K.; Fales, J. T.; and Goldberg, A. M. 1974. The effects of inorganic lead on the neuromuscular junction. Neuropharmacology 13:795.

Sileo, L.; Jones, R. N.; and Hatch, R. C. 1973. The effect of ingested lead shot on the electrocardiogram of Canada geese. Avian Dis 17:308.

Sim, V. M. 1971. Chemicals used as weapons in war. In J. R. DiPalma, ed. Drill's Pharmacology in Medicine, 4th ed. New York: McGraw-Hill.

Singhal, R. L.; Kacew, S.; Sutherland, D. J. B.; and Telli, A. H. 1973. Plumbism: Adaptive changes in hepatic and renal metabolism. Res Commun Chem Pathol Pharmacol 6:951.

Slater, I. H. 1971. Strychnine, picrotoxin, pentylenetetrazol, and miscellaneous drugs. In J. R. DiPalma, ed. Drill's Pharmacology in Medicine, 4th ed. New York: McGraw-Hill.

Smith, H. A.; Jones, T. C.; and Hunt, R. D. 1972. Veterinary Pathology, 4th ed. Philadelphia: Lea & Febiger.

Smythies, J. R. 1974. Relationships between the chemical structure and biological activity of convulsants. Annu Rev Pharmacol 14:9.

Snow, D. H. 1973. The acute toxicity of dichlorvos in the dog. II. Pathology. Aust Vet J 49:120.

Snow, D. H., and Watson, A. D. J. 1973. The acute toxicity of dichlorvos in the dog. I. Clinical observations and clinical pathology. Aust Vet J 49:113.

Snowdon, C. T. 1973. Learning deficits in lead-injected rats. Pharmacol Biochem Behav 1:599.

Snyder, S. H. 1975. The glycine synaptic receptor in the mammalian central nervous system. Br J Pharmacol 53:473.

Sollmann, T. 1957. A Manual of Pharmacology and Its Application to Therapeutics and Toxicology, 8th ed. Philadelphia: W. B. Saunders.

Steinwall, O., and Olsson, Y. 1969. Impairment of the blood-brain barrier in mercury poisoning. Acta Neurol Scand 45:351.

Stowe, H. D.; Goyer, R. A.; Krigman, M. M.; Wilson, M.; and Cates, M. 1973. Experimental oral lead toxicity in young dogs. Arch Pathol 95:106.

Swinyard, E. A. 1969. Laboratory evaluation of antiepileptic drugs, review of laboratory methods. Epilepsia 10:107.

Szabo, S.; Kourounakis, P.; Kovacs, K.; Tuchweber, B.; and Garg, B. D. 1974. Prevention of organomercurial intoxication by thyroid deficiency in the rat. Toxicol Appl Pharmacol 30:175.

Szabuniewicz, M.; Bailey, E. M.; and Wiersig, D. O. 1971. Treatment of some common poisonings in animals. Vet Med Small Anim Clin 66:1197.

Tebēcis, A. K., and DiMaria, A. 1972. Strychnine-sensitive inhibition in the medullary reticular formation: Evidence for glycine as an inhibitory transmitter. Brain Res 40:373.

Tomokuni, K. 1974. δ-Aminolevulinic acid dehydratase test for lead exposure. Arch Environ Health 29:274.

Towfighi, J., Gonatas, N. K.; and McCree, L. 1974. Hexachlorophene changes in central and peripheral myelinated axons of developing and adult rats. Lab Invest 31:712.

Tucker, R. K., and Haegele, M. A. 1971. Comparative acute oral toxicity of pesticides to six species of birds. Toxicol Appl Pharmacol 20:57.

Ulsamer, A. G.; Yoder, P. D.; Kimbrough, R. D.; and Marzulli, F. N. 1975. Effects of hexachlororophene on developing rats: Toxicity, tissue concentrations and biochemistry. Food Cosmet Toxicol 13:69.

Van Gelder, G. A., and Cunningham, W. L. 1975. The effects of low-level dieldrin exposure on the EEG and learning ability of the squirrel monkey. Abstr 14th Ann Meet Soc Toxicol, Williamsburg, Va., Mar. 9–13, 1975.

Van Gelder, G. A.; Carson, T.; Smith, R. M.; and Buck, W. B. 1973. Behavioral toxicologic assessment of the neurologic effect of lead in sheep. Clin Toxicol 6:405.

Walker, A. I. T., and Stevenson, D. E. 1968. Studies on the safety of plastic dog collars containing dichlorvos. Vet Rec 83:538.

Weiss, L. R., and Orzel, R. A. 1967. Enhancement of toxicity of anticholinesterases by central depressant drugs in rats. Toxicol Appl Pharmacol 10:334.

Werman, R.; Davidoff, R. A.; and Aprison, M. H. 1967a. Inhibition of motoneurones by iontophoresis of glycine. Nature 214:681.

———. 1967b. Evidence for glycine as the principal transmitter mediating postsynaptic inhibition in the spinal cord of the cat. J Gen Physiol 50:1093.

White, E. G., and Cotchin, E. 1948. Natural and experimental cases of poisoning of calves by flaking lead paint. Vet J 104:75.

Willes, R. F.; Truelove, J. F.; Krewski, D.; and Munro, I. C. 1975. Effect of methylmercury on electroencephalograms of cats. Abstr 14th Ann Meeting Soc Toxicol, Williamsburg, Va., Mar. 9–13, 1975.

Wilson, B. J. 1971. Miscellaneous *Penicillium* toxins. In A. Ciegler, S. Kadis, and S. J. Ajl, eds. Microbial Toxins, vol. 6. New York: Academic Press.

Wilson, B. J.; Maronpot, R. R.; and Hildebrandt, P. K. 1973. Equine leukoencephalomalacia. J Am Vet Med Assoc 163:1293.

Wilson, R. P.; Davis, L. E.; Muhrer, M. E.; and Bloomfield, R. A. 1968. Toxicologic effects of ammonium carbamate and related compounds. Am J Vet Res 29:897.

Woolley, D. E., and Barron, B. A. 1968. Effects of DDT on brain electrical activity in awake, unrestrained rats. Toxicol Appl Pharmacol 12:440.

Zenick, H. 1974. Behavioral and biochemical consequences in methylmercury chloride toxicity. Pharmacol Biochem Behav 2:709.

Zook, B. C. 1973. Lead intoxication in urban dogs. Clin Toxicol 6:377.

Zook, B. C.; Carpenter, J. L.; and Leeds, E. B. 1969. Lead poisoning in dogs. J Am Vet Med Assoc 155:1329.

Zook, B. C.; Carpenter, J. L.; and Roberts R. M. 1972a. Lead poisoning in dogs: Occurrence, source, clinical pathology, and electroencephalography. Am J Vet Res 33:891.

Zook, B. C.; Kopito, L.; Carpenter, J. L.; Cramer, D. V.; and Schwachman, H. 1972b. Lead poisoning in dogs: Analysis of blood, urine, hair, and liver for lead. Am J Vet Res 33:903.

CHAPTER 59

POISONS CAUSING ABDOMINAL DISTRESS OR LIVER OR KIDNEY DAMAGE

ROGER C. HATCH

POISONS CAUSING SEVERE COLIC

Direct Corrosives and Irritants

ACIDS AND ALKALIS

Strong acids (HCl, HNO_3, H_2SO_4) and alkalis (NaOH, KOH) are not commonly a cause of poisoning in veterinary practice because of the limited access to such agents and because of the disagreeable odor and taste of these materials. Even the curious dairy cow is not likely to taste fuming nitric, sulfuric, or hydrochloric acid, but she might taste some of the weaker acids or alkalis. An animal could be dosed overzealously with an acid or alkaline solution, or the feed could contain something like acid phosphate or calcium hydroxide.

Materials that ionize to form excess hydrogen or hydroxyl ion can cause pH-dependent damage to the cells lining the mouth, esophagus, stomach, and intestine. The mucous membranes may be severely damaged, may become hemorrhagic, and may slough away. Alkalis are especially dangerous because of their ability to penetrate deeply into tissues.

Clinical signs generally include severe colic and visible damage to oropharyngeal membranes. Hematemesis may also occur.

The treatment for acid-induced caustic poisoning is a dilute base such as 2% sodium bicarbonate; for alkali poisoning, treatment is a dilute acid such as 5% acetic acid (vinegar). These treatments are administered in reasonably large amounts, followed by a soothing protective-demulcent. A sedative or tranquilizer may be given to quiet the animal, or a general analgesic may be given to control the pain of severe colic.

The thing *not* to do is to give emetics, strong cathartics, or parasympathomimetic drugs. These agents can cause an acid- or alkali-weakened stomach wall or intestinal wall to rupture during contracture. The consequences of this may be fatal hemorrhage or peritonitis.

CONCENTRATED CHEMICALS

Nearly any chemical, if concentrated enough, can act as a "protoplasmic poison" simply by lying in contact with living tissue. This type of caustic effect is frequently encountered as part of the toxicosis produced by metals such as inorganic arsenic, lead, copper, mercury, and others and by chlorate, nitrates, fluoride, and other agents discussed in these chapters. Many times, the abdominal distress and gastrointestinal (GI) lesions produced by poisons are nonspecific caustic effects of the chemical.

Treatment of the condition of concentration-dependent GI damage is symptomatic. The gut contents should be diluted. Sedatives or analgesics can be used. Internal protectives and demulcents are given. As stated for acids and alkalis, the use of emetics, strong cathartics, and parasympathomimetic drugs is contraindicated because of the danger of gastric or intestinal rupture.

PLANT POISONS

Many plant poisons cause abdominal distress. Outstanding among these because of their direct irritant effects on the intestinal mucosa are solanine from nightshades (*Solanum* spp.), veratramine and zygacine from death camas (*Zigadenus* sp.), glycosides from oleander (*Nerium* sp.), saponins from coffee weed (*Sesbania* sp.), ricin from castor bean (*Ricinus* sp.), abrin from precatory bean (*Abrus* sp.), robin from black locust (*Robinia* sp.), hydroquinone from cocklebur sprouts (*Xanthium* sp.), and unidentified principles in the tung oil tree (*Aleurites* sp.), sneezeweeds (*Helenium* spp.), and the bitterweeds and pingue (*Hymenoxys* spp.). Plants containing soluble or insoluble oxalates are also very irritating to mucous membranes (Kingsbury 1964).

GI irritation is not necessarily the cause of illness or death produced by these plants. Thus several plants listed above are also listed in other chapters. The plants must be considered in differential diagnosis of conditions that cause acute abdominal distress.

Metabolic Poisons

"INORGANIC" ARSENIC

Use. Arsenicals may be present in insecticides (copper acetoarsenite–Paris green; sodium, potassium, or lead arsenate; arsenic trioxide), defoliants/herbicides (sodium or potassium arsenite; sodium, potassium, calcium, or lead arsenate; arsenic acid; monosodium methanearsonate–MSMA; disodium methanearsonate–DSMA; monoammonium methanearsonate–MAMA), livestock dips (lead arsenate), rodenticides (arsenic trioxide), or in medicines such as Fowler's solution (potassium arsenite) and injectable preparations for the control of blood parasites (sodium thiacetarsamide, sodium arsenamide, disodium acetarsenate). Arsenicals may also be found in ruminatoric preparations and tonics. Wood may be treated with the preservative arsenic pentoxide. Arsenic is also found in diverse materials such as vermiculite, paint pigments, detergents, and building materials.

Obviously, not all these forms of arsenic are inorganic, but they all produce toxicosis that is characteristic of the "classical" or "typical" form of arsenic poisoning produced by inorganic arsenicals in general.

Some kinds of organic arsenicals (e.g., the growth promoters) do not do this. They produce peripheral nerve demyelination and are discussed in Chapter 61.

Arsine gas (AsH_3) is a highly toxic gas liberated by the action of water on pyritic ores or by a reducing agent (Fe, Zn, or Sn) plus water or acid in the presence of an arsenic compound. It has no agricultural or household use, but it is an example of an inorganic arsenical that does not cause typical signs of inorganic arsenic poisoning. It causes hemolysis and pulmonary edema and is mentioned in Chapter 57 under Chlorate.

Source. While many arsenicals have been replaced by less dangerous compounds for a number of applications, animals can still be poisoned by this persistent element. Moreover, arsenicals are still used in spite of the availability of less toxic chemicals. Thus animals may ingest sprayed foliage or spilled product. Pastures near smelters may be contaminated with arsenic. "Empty" containers can be licked by animals. Spray tanks and hoses may be rinsed out so as to contaminate drinking water. Paints, a source of lead, may also contain arsenic. Insecticidal arsenicals are not specific for insects—the chemicals will also kill animals. Percutaneous poisoning can occur if animals are dipped in strong solutions of lead arsenate. This practice is obsolete, but the areas around old dipping vats still contain dangerous amounts of arsenic and lead, and so do the vats themselves. The farm dump is a good source of a variety of arsenicals. Arsenic poisoning can also result from intravenous injection of arsenicals used to control blood parasites, even if the correct dosage is used. Milk from arsenic-poisoned cattle may be toxic for calves. Soils normally contain small amounts of arsenic, but not enough to be of toxicologic concern.

Properties of Toxicologic Importance. Arsenic is in Group V of the Periodic Chart of the Elements. It is a metalloid with some properties similar to phosphorus, antimony, and bismuth. Arsenic exists in three oxidation states: —3 (elemental), +3 (trivalent or arsenite), and +5 (pentavalent or arsenate). Arsenic reacts with sulfhydryl groups. This property is the basis for the mechanism of toxic action of arsenic and for treatment of classical arsenic poisoning. Arsenic vaporizes fairly readily when heated, thus causing some difficulties in quantitative analysis of arsenic in biological samples.

Toxicity. In rats, the acute oral single-dose LD50 of some arsenicals is (in mg/kg of body weight): sodium arsenite, 10–50; copper acetoarsenite, 22; arsenic acid, 48–100; arsenic trioxide, 138; MSMA, 700; MAMA, 750; and DSMA, 1000 (Berg 1974). According to Buck et al. (1973), the oral lethal dose of sodium arsenite in most species is 1–25 mg/kg of body weight (but swine may require 100–200 mg/kg in the drinking water). Arsenic trioxide is 3–10 times less toxic than sodium arsenite.

Clarke and Clarke (1967) give some toxicity data for arsenic trioxide and sodium arsenite in domestic species. They state that the average total oral lethal dose of arsenic trioxide and of sodium arsenite, respectively, is: horse, 10–45 g and 1–3 mg; cow, 15–45 g and 1–4 g; sheep and goat, 3–10 g and 200–500 mg; swine, 500–1000 mg and 50–100 mg; dog, 100–150 mg and 50–150 mg; and fowl, 50–300 mg and 10–100 mg.

Chronic arsenic poisoning is not often seen in domestic animals because the metalloid is rapidly excreted

Several factors influence the toxicity of arsenic. Herbivores are commonly poisoned because they eat contaminated forage. Cats are poisoned because they ingest syrupy baits intended for insects. Dogs are occasionally poisoned either maliciously or after being injected intravenously with heartworm remedies containing arsenic. Swine and fowl are rarely poisoned, probably because of limited exposure of these species to arsenic.

Inorganic arsenic in the trivalent state is more toxic than the inorganic pentavalent form which, in turn, is more toxic than organic arsenicals. Toxicity of the pentavalent arsenicals is largely due to conversion *in vivo* to the trivalent state.

Finely divided, soluble arsenic compounds are more toxic than coarse, poorly soluble ones because the latter are poorly absorbed. Toxicity is influenced in part by the rate of excretion of arsenic. Excretion can be slowed and toxicity enhanced in animals that are dehydrated, ill, and in poor condition.

Constant exposure to arsenic may confer some degree of tolerance to the metalloid, but animals may also learn to seek out arsenic and "overdose themselves."

Toxicodynamic Considerations. After absorption, arsenic is distributed throughout the body but tends to accumulate in the liver and kidneys. Pentavalent arsenic may be metabolized to the trivalent state in the liver, although this does not occur with the organic arsenicals discussed in Chapter 61. In domestic animals, arsenic does not stay in the tissues very long. It is rapidly excreted in the urine, feces, bile, milk, saliva, and sweat. A sublethal dosage is eliminated in several days. Arsenic probably crosses the placental barrier, but the paucity of central nervous signs and lesions in poisoned animals suggests that arsenic does not cross the blood-brain barrier very well. Milk from poisoned cows can be toxic for human beings but the flesh of surviving animals is said to be safe for human consumption (Clarke and Clarke 1967).

Mechanism of Action. At the molecular level of inquiry, trivalent arsenic is thought to act primarily by combining with the two sulfhydryl groups of lipoic (thioctic) acid (Clarke and Clarke 1967; Clarkson and DiStefano 1971). *This occurs before there are any other biochemical or structural changes.* Lipoic acid is an essential cofactor for the enzymatic decarboxylation of keto acids such as pyruvate, ketoglutarate, and ketobutyrate. By inactivating lipoic acid, arsenic inhibits the formation of acetyl, succinyl, and propionyl coenzymes-A. Other oxidative decarboxylations that utilize lipoic acid are probably inhibited too. The major consequences of lipoic acid inhibition would appear to be inhibition or slowing of glycolysis and of the citrate cycle.

Secondary molecular actions of trivalent arsenic may include inactivation of sulfhydryl groups of oxidative enzymes and inactivation of the sulfhydryl group of glutathione or other essential monothiols and dithiols (see Selenium, Chapter 57, for the functions of glutathione) (Sollmann 1957; Harvey 1970; Clarkson and DiStefano 1971).

Pentavalent arsenic can uncouple oxidative phosphorylation by forming unstable arsenate esters instead of phosphate esters that are required to provide high-energy phosphate. The importance of this observation is not known (Harvey 1970).

Part of the effects of arsenic on the gut can be attributed to a local corrosive action but GI damage occurs regardless of route of absorption of arsenic. The metalloid seems to prefer tissues rich in oxidative enzymes such as intestine, liver, and kidney. The most sensitive cells seem to be capillary endothelial cells in these organs, because the primary effect of trivalent arsenic at the cellular level of inquiry is a relaxation of capillaries and an increase in capillary permeability. Blood vessels that have smooth muscle in their walls also dilate (Sollmann 1957). The combined metabolic and vascular effects of arsenic explain the signs and lesions described below.

Clinical Signs. The signs of typical arsenic poisoning are similar in different species. In peracute cases there may be no signs observed—the animal is just "found dead." Alternately there may be sudden and severe colic, staggering, collapse, paralysis, and death.

In acute cases signs include severe colic, staggering, weakness, trembling, salivation, vomiting, thirst, diarrhea, possibly blood in the feces, fast and weak pulse, hind-limb paralysis, prostration, normal or subnormal temperature, and death in 1–3 days.

In subacute cases the animal may live several days. Signs include colic, anorexia, depression, staggering, weakness, diarrhea with blood and/or mucosal shreds in the feces, polyuria and then anuria, dehydration, thirst, partial paralysis of hind limbs, trembling, stupor, cold extremities, subnormal temperature, possible hematuria, and (on occasion) convulsions.

Chronic cases are rare and are characterized by wasting, poor condition, thirst, brick red mucous membranes, normal temperature, and a weak, irregular pulse. See Clarke and Clarke (1967), Radeleff (1970), and Buck et al. (1973) for detail.

Lesions. As stated in the above references, the peracute case may manifest no visible lesions. Generally, however, "inorganic" arsenic poisoning in cattle is characterized by a reddened abomasal or duodenal mucosa and submucosal edema and hemorrhages in the abomasum and duodenum, with resulting sloughing of the duodenal mucosa or perforation of the gut wall. The intestinal contents are fluid, foul smelling, bloody, and may contain shreds of intestinal mucosa. The liver may be soft and yellow. The lungs may be edematous and congested. There may be hemorrhages on the heart, peritoneum, kidneys, and liver.

In swine there may be inflamed and edematous fauces. The edema may extend to the larynx and trachea, causing asphyxial signs and lesions.

In the fowl there may be an intense inflammation of the proventriculus and gizzard, and the horny lining of the gizzard may be sloughing away due to an underlying gelatinous exudate. The duodenal mucosa may be slightly reddened and the liver may manifest degenerative changes.

Microscopically, capillary degeneration is observed in the gut, skin, lungs, and other organs. This occurs regardless of route of entry of arsenic. There may also be degenerative changes ranging from cloudy swelling to necrosis in the gut mucosa, liver, kidney, and heart. The degenerative lesions are secondary to the metabolic and vascular effects of arsenic.

Differential Diagnosis. A sudden onset of severe colic, bloody diarrhea, or watery diarrhea containing mucosal shreds, plus postmortem findings of hemorrhagic gastroenteritis and degenerative changes in the liver and kidney should always be interpreted as possible arsenic poisoning. No other metal or metalloid causes such a speedy onset of severe GI damage. Evidence of exposure to arsenic may allow a presumptive diagnosis of arsenic poisoning.

A large number of poisons cause diarrhea and colic, but only such things as caustics, irritant plants, urea, chlorate, pesticides, and enteric diseases are likely to cause GI signs that approach the severity of those seen in the typical case of arsenic poisoning. Lead poisoning, if severe enough, can mimic aspects of arsenic poisoning, but with lead poisoning (as with most other poisons) the spectrum of clinical signs is different from that with arsenic. For example, nervous and behavioral signs are minimal or absent with arsenic poisoning but prominent with lead and pesticides.

Treatment. Specific therapy is aimed at the known affinity of arsenic for sulfhydryl groups, particularly dithiols. Dimercaprol (BAL) is a dithiol-containing chelating agent that can form a relatively nontoxic and easily excretable complex with arsenic. Theoretically, BAL removes arsenic from inhibited sulfhydryl groups of lipoic acid, vital monothiols and dithiols, and enzymes so that metabolic reactions can again proceed at the proper rate.

In practice, however, the response of poisoned animals to BAL is not so dramatic as the idealized antidotal mechanism leads us to believe. The chelator cannot repair cell damage. Also, chelation is not a 100% "tying-up" of a metal—it is an equilibrium reaction that allows some of the metal to remain uncomplexed. Moreover, some enzymes or other sulfhydryl-containing substances may even have as great an affinity for arsenic as does BAL. Thus BAL cannot be expected to disinhibit all sulfhydryl groups to the same degree.

The chelator may mobilize stored arsenic in tissues and cause an initial exacerbation of clinical signs by allowing more arsenic to circulate to target tissues such as gut and liver endothelium. More BAL is required when this happens.

Enzymes that have been inhibited for a long time are not as easily disinhibited by BAL as are enzymes that are freshly poisoned. This is also true for other chelators. Also, if arsenic is present in large excess, neither BAL nor any other chelator can be expected to work very well to regenerate enzyme activity.

As if all this was not enough, BAL also has toxic effects that limit its dosage and frequency of administration. In animals the signs of BAL overdosage include vomiting, tremors, convulsions, coma, and death. Death is not preventable by the control of convulsions because BAL has profound effects on the cardiovascular system. These effects include initial hypertension, capillary damage, marked loss of fluid and protein from the blood, hemoconcentration and reduction in blood volume, and shock. In addition, BAL can cause metabolic disturbances as evidenced by lactic acidemia, acidosis, and hypoglycemia (Levine 1970).

Dimercaprol in small concentrations can inhibit a number of metal-containing enzymes such as polyphenol oxidase, carbonic anhydrase, catalase, and peroxidase. Some nonmetal enzymes are also inhibited. Dimercaprol can compete with glutathione, preventing it from reactivating glutathione-dependent enzymes (see Selenium, Chapter 57). Dimercaprol can also inhibit thiol groups in the pyruvate oxidase system—the same thing that arsenic itself does, but by a different mechanism (Sollmann 1957).

What allows BAL to be used at all in the treatment of arsenic toxicosis is the fact that the metabolic effects of a therapeutic dose of BAL are not severe and they disappear as BAL is excreted over a period of 3–4 hours.

The point of saying all this about BAL is to stress the fact that BAL is not some miracle antidote for metal toxicoses. If administered too late or in insufficient doses at infrequent intervals, the animal may die of arsenic poisoning. If BAL is administered in excess or at too-frequent intervals, the animal may die of BAL poisoning. There *is* a middle ground where, with a little luck and some medical common sense, the animal just might live! This can also be said for every other chelating agent used in the treatment of metal toxicoses.

The dosage of BAL in large animals is 3 mg/kg of body weight given intramuscularly as a 5% solution in a 10% solution of benzyl benzoate in arachis oil. The injection should be repeated every 4 hours for the first 2 days, every 6 hours the 3rd day, and twice a day for the next 10 days until recovery (Buck et al. 1973).

In small animals, a 10% solution of BAL in oil is used. The dosage is 2.5–5 mg/kg (use the 5 mg/kg dose only for acute cases and only on the first day of therapy). The dosage intervals are the same as for large animals (Szabuniewicz et al. 1971).

If BAL therapy seems to worsen the animal's condition initially, this may be due to mobilization of stored arsenic. A little extra BAL might be given. If BAL therapy seems to make the animal worse over a period of 2 or 3 days, the dosage of BAL may be too large for the individual animal.

Chelation therapy, like antibiotic therapy, must continue around the clock. That is, "every 4 hours" means *every 4 hours,* not an injection after breakfast, sometime around noon, and at quitting time. Blood levels of chelators, like those of other drugs, do not respect our work schedules, mealtimes, fatigued muscles, or sleep cycles!

Other measures may be taken in the treatment of arsenic poisoning. The GI tract should be emptied by giving a saline cathartic and (in small animals) a gastric lavage. (Obviously these measures apply only when exposure was by the oral route.) Emetics, strong cathartics, and parasympathomimetic drugs should not be used because they may cause rupture of weakened gut walls. Demulcents are given to coat and soothe the gut lining.

Sodium thiosulfate has been advocated for the treatment of arsenic poisoning. Horses and cattle are given 20–30 g orally in about 300 ml of water, plus 8–10 g intravenously in 10%–20% solution. Sheep and goats are given about a quarter of these dosages (Clarke and Clarke 1967). Other authors suggest that sodium thiosulfate be administered to large animals at the rate of 30–40 mg/kg of body weight intravenously (or twice this dosage orally) 2–3 times a day until recovery (Szabuniewicz et al. 1971). There does not seem to be any rationale for the use of sodium thiosulfate in arsenic poisoning. Conceivably, the sulfur of thiosulfate might react with arsenic and immobilize the metalloid. Ordinarily, the author does not advocate the use of a drug when we do not know what the drug is doing in the body. However, thiosulfate is a normal constituent of the body and its toxicity is in the g/kg range. Thus thiosulfate can probably be used safely in the treatment of arsenic poisoning, but its efficacy is not known.

Sulfhydryl-containing compounds other than BAL have been shown to protect laboratory animals against arsenic poisoning, presumably by forming complexes with arsenic. Such compounds include lipoic acid and other dithiols, cysteine, and glutathione. When British workers found that BAL had better antidotal properties than some other sulfhydryl-containing compounds against arsenical war gases such as Lewisite (the initials BAL for British Anti-Lewisite), BAL became the chelator of choice for the treatment of arsenic poisoning.

In view of the toxicity of BAL, it seems that other monothiols and dithiols should be reevaluated for possible use in combination with BAL or in combination with each other for the treatment of arsenic poisoning. Lipoic acid is especially interesting in this regard because it can actually reverse acute sodium arsenite toxicosis in mice and dogs (Grunert 1960).

Nursing care and supportive therapy are integral parts of the treatment of arsenic poisoning. Thus the animal should be kept warm and comfortable and given fluids and electrolytes, vitamins, nourishment, antibiotics, analgesics, and other symptomatic care. The prognosis is grave if the animal is not treated promptly or if there has been extensive organ damage and the animal is prostrate.

Analysis. Generally, arsenic analysis is performed on stomach or intestinal contents (or feces or vomitus), liver, and kidney. Suspect sources can be tested as well as biological fluids such as blood, urine, and milk. Traces of arsenic (less than 0.5 ppm) can be found normally in animal tissues because of constant ingestion of small amounts of arsenic from the soil. If animals are dipped regularly in arsenical solutions, liver and kidney tissue may contain as much as 8 ppm of arsenic, but the animals will be healthy.

In cattle poisoned by arsenic and not regularly dipped in arsenicals, urine contains 2–200 ppm of arsenic and it may continue to contain elevated concentrations up to 14 days. Liver and kidney concentrations of arsenic range from 2 to 200 ppm, and these tissue levels are directly related to ingesta levels of arsenic, which range from 2 to 104 ppm. Kidney concentrations of arsenic may be the same as, higher than, or lower than liver concentrations in individual animals, but the overall tendency in a group of poisoned cattle is for the average amount of arsenic in kidney and liver tissue to be the same. Calves and old cattle may succumb with very small concentrations of arsenic in liver and kidney tissue.

It is difficult to state a "diagnostic level" of arsenic in animal tissues. Generally, if the liver or kidney contains more than 7–10 ppm, arsenic poisoning is strongly indicated. The history, signs, and lesions must be used to support the diagnosis. Some animals, such as calves or old cattle, may manifest typical signs and lesions, but analysis will reveal only 2 or 3 ppm of arsenic in the tissues. In such cases the ingesta or feces may contain excess arsenic, but not necessarily. Other animals, such as those that are naturally more resistant to arsenic, may have few signs or lesions (they may even die of causes other than arsenic poisoning) but tissue analysis may reveal rather large concentrations of arsenic. Fortunately, the majority of cases of arsenic poisoning do not present these diagnostic difficulties.

For references on diagnosis see Clarke and Clarke (1967), Hatch and Funnell (1969), and Buck et al. (1973).

ORGANOMERCURIALS IN SHEEP

For some reason, organomercurials (e.g., methylmercury and ethylmercury) cause very different signs and lesions in different species. In dogs, cats, calves, rats, primates, and human beings, the signs are of excitation, and central nervous lesions are prominent. In adult cattle, swine, and to some extent in fowl, the clinical signs are of depression, and both central and peripheral nervous lesions are prominent in swine (see Chapter 58).

In sheep, ingestion of organomercurials causes colic, diarrhea, anorexia, nasal discharge, dyspnea, weight loss, stilted gait, lameness, frequent urination, recumbency that is hastened by exercise, and death. Sometimes the signs may be even more nonspecific (anorexia only).

These signs are produced by total dosages of organomercurial equivalent to 6.24–11.52 mg Hg/kg of body weight accumulated over several days' exposure.

Lesions in organomercury-poisoned sheep may include catarrhal enteritis; ulceration and sloughing of the rumen lining; congestion of the liver, kidneys, lungs, intestinal mucosa, and cranial vessels; and pulmonary edema.

In dead sheep, the liver may contain 27.9–121 ppm of mercury, and the kidney may contain 117.5–212 ppm.

Organomercurial toxicosis is difficult to differentiate from other metal toxicoses in sheep. Lead and arsenic come to mind as metals that are frequently encountered causes of metal toxicoses. Lead is apt to cause behavioral and nervous signs, and arsenic is likely to cause a very rapid and severe onset of colic and bloody diarrhea, but both metals can mimic organomercurials. A laboratory test of liver, kidney, and suspect sources is essential to the final diagnosis.

See Chapter 58 for discussion of mechanism of action and treatment of organomercurial toxicosis. See Palmer (1963) and Palmer et al. (1973) for added detail on organomercurial poisoning in sheep.

THALLIUM

Use. Thallium is used as a rodenticide, and only by government agencies.

Source. Dogs and cats used to be poisoned frequently by eating baits intended for rodents. Poisoning by thallium salts is less frequent now that the substance is no longer available to the general public. However, some thallium rodenticides are undoubtedly still in storage in homes and farms. Dogs and cats may obtain thallium-containing baits as long as the substance is used, regardless of who uses it.

Properties of Toxicologic Importance. Thallium salts are odorless, nearly tasteless, and soluble in water. Thallium exists in the +3 (thallic, trivalent) and the +1 (thallous, monovalent) oxidation states. The trivalent ion is readily chelated by ethylenediamine tetraacetate (EDTA) *in vitro,* but EDTA has little or no therapeutic value in thallium poisoning (see Treatment). This suggests that the trivalent form of thallium may not be the active form *in vivo.* The monovalent ion has *s*-valency electrons that partly shield its *d*-electrons and hinder their participation in back-coordination with other ligands (Burger 1973). This is probably why chelating agents are only partly successful in eliminating thallium from the body.

Toxicity. In rats, the acute single-dose oral

LD50 of thallous sulfate is 16–25 mg/kg of body weight (Stecher 1968; Berg 1974) and in other species the acute oral LD50 of thallium salts varies from 10 to 15 mg/kg (Buck et al. 1973). The minimum oral lethal dose of thallium salts in various species is 10–25 mg/kg of body weight, and thallous salts are more toxic than thallic salts (Hammond 1965; Clarke and Clarke 1967; Radeleff 1970).

The toxic (presumably lethal) oral dose of thallous acetate given for different species in mg/kg of body weight is: horse, 27; adult cow, 16; calf, 12; adult sheep, 9; lamb, 20; dog, 18.5; and cat, 10–15 (Clarke and Clarke 1967; Stecher 1968; Zook et al. 1968). Thallous sulfate is only slightly less toxic than the acetate.

Chronic poisoning with thallium is not common but could occur because of accumulation of thallium in the body. The cumulative lethal dosage of thallium is 10–20 mg/kg of body weight (Radeleff 1970).

With some species (human being, sheep) the adult animal is more susceptible to thallium than the young animal. With other species (cattle) the young are more susceptible.

Thallium nitrate toxicity is enhanced by the chelator sodium diethyldithiocarbamate in rats, presumably because this particular thallium chelate is more lipid soluble than thallium ion and, therefore, enters the brain more easily (Rauws et al. 1969). The chelator diphenylthiocarbazone may enhance thallium toxicosis in cats (Zook et al. 1968).

Toxicodynamic Considerations. Thallium is readily absorbed from the gut or skin and is distributed throughout the body. It may accumulate in the kidneys at 5–15 times the concentrations found in other tissues. The biological half-life of thallium is 3–8 days (Hammond 1965). Thallium is excreted mainly in the feces (from the bile) and also in the urine. The element also appears in milk and it can cross the placenta (Sollmann 1957). There is an enterohepatic-biliary cycle for reabsorption and excretion of thallium, and this mechanism is a therapeutic target. Blood concentration of thallium is maximal in dogs 2–4 hours after ingestion of the metal. Four percent of the dosage is excreted the first day, 37% in 7 days, and 60% in 28 days (Buck et al. 1973).

Mechanism of Action. Thallium does not inhibit sulfur-containing enzymes nor does it block the actions of free sulfhydryl groups in human skin (Sollmann 1957; Stavinoha et al. 1959). Yet thallotoxicosis does seem to be related to an inhibition of the metabolism of sulfur-containing compounds, because a high-cystine diet or dietary supplementation with methionine or betaine can protect rats against chronic thallotoxicosis. Moreover, a number of sulfur-containing compounds given parenterally in single doses can prevent and cure thallotoxicosis in mice given an LD90 dosage of thallium sulfate (Stavinoha et al. 1959). Not all sulfur-containing compounds have this effect. Mercaptopropane and α-monothioglycerol have moderate protective action if given 6 hours after thallium. Diphenylthiocarbazone and two analogs of *S*-γ-aminoisothiuronium have good protective action even when given 24 hours after thallium. Other compounds such as glutathione, methionine, and thioacetamide are ineffective. These observations suggest that thallium may act at a fairly specific place in the scheme of sulfur metabolism, but this site is not known.

Thallium is apparently able to substitute for potassium in processes involving active transport of potassium (Gehring and Hammond 1967; Cavieres and Ellory 1974). It is not known whether thallotoxicosis is partly due to this phenomenon, but the implications of potassium exclusion from participation in membrane function of cells (particularly excitable cells such as muscle and nerve cells) are obvious.

Thallium causes a decrease in basal metabolic rate, an initial increase and then a decrease in blood glucose concentration, a decrease in serum calcium concentration (with bone softening and rachitic signs in chronic cases), elevation of serum enzymes that indicates tissue damage, and nonspecific changes in blood chemistry and cell counts (Sollmann 1957; Zook and Gilmore 1967; Zook et al. 1968). None of these changes gives a clue about the mechanism of action of thallium.

Clinical Signs. In dogs and cats (species usually poisoned by thallium) acute, subacute, and chronic thallotoxicoses occur.

In acute poisoning, there is a 1- to 4-day onset of severe colic, vomiting, bloody diarrhea, salivation, anorexia, depression, motor paralysis, trembling, and dyspnea, and death in 3–5 days. Fever is not seen.

Subacute poisoning is characterized by a 3- to 7-day onset of less severe but longer-lasting GI and paralytic signs, tremors, convulsions, red oral mucous membranes, and reddening and pustule formation in the skin beginning with the ears and nose and progressing to the axilla, abdomen, and the rest of the body. Conjunctivitis, pneumonia or bronchitis, fever, and debility are manifested. At 7–10 days the hair begins to fall out and the skin becomes crusty and cracked. The animal may die of thallium poisoning, malnutrition, thirst, or secondary infection.

In chronic toxicosis, mild GI and nervous signs are observed 7–10 days after exposure, and hair loss and dry, scaly skin at 1–3 weeks.

See Clarke and Clarke (1967), Zook and Gilmore (1967), Zook et al. (1968), Radeleff (1970), and Buck et al. (1973) for detail.

Lesions. In acute poisoning there is ulcerative and hemorrhagic gastroenteritis and possible inflammation of the respiratory mucosa. In subacute poisoning there is less gastritis, but degenerative changes occur in the heart, kidneys, and liver. These changes may range from fatty changes to necrosis. There may also be congestion of various organs, including the brain. In chronic poisoning, the skin lesions predominate. Zook et al. (1968) present vivid color pictures of cats poisoned by thallium.

Microscopically, there may be skin hyperkeratosis, parakeratosis, and hyperemia. Also necrotic lesions may be observed in skeletal muscle, heart, and liver. The kidneys may be congested and the brain may manifest edema, neuronal and glial degeneration, demyelination, and perivascular cuffing with leukocytes. There may be demyelination of peripheral nerves. The intestinal mucosa manifests congestion, ulceration, and hemorrhage (see Sollmann 1957; Radeleff 1970; Buck et al. 1973).

Differential Diagnosis. Thallium poisoning is typified by a delayed onset of GI signs, nervous or paralytic signs, and reddening of the mucous membranes and skin, accompanied by bacterial infections such as pneumonia and conjunctivitis. Nothing else is likely to turn a dog's or cat's skin red and also cause alopecia.

If death occurs before typical lesions appear, laboratory tests of tissues and urine are required. Here the tests would include not only thallium but also arsenic, lead, chlorate, and other agents that cause hemorrhagic gastroenteritis.

Thallium poisoning can look very much like any debilitating disease in which there are secondary bacterial infections. In addition, parasitic, fungal, and bacterial skin infections may be mistaken for thallium toxicosis, although systemic illness is not characteristic of simple dermatitic conditions.

Treatment. Specific therapy is aimed at chelation of thallium systemically, competition for potassium-dependent mechanisms supposedly affected by thallium, and trapping of thallium in the intestine so as to interrupt the enterohepatic cycle of reabsorption-bilary excretion of thallium.

Chelation therapy by itself is not a cure for thallotoxicosis because, for reasons given by Burger (1973), thallous ion does not readily participate in complexation reactions. The most effective chelating agent for use in animals seems to be diphenylthiocarbazone (dithizone), and even this agent cannot be used in cats because of toxicity reactions (Zook et al. 1968). In dogs, however, dithizone will hasten the elimination of thallium in the urine. The dosage is 70 mg/kg of body weight given orally 3 times a day for 6 days (Szabuniewicz et al.

1971). Much smaller doses are used in chronic poisoning to minimize the mobilization of too much thallium at one time (Buck et al. 1973). Naturally, vomition must be controlled first. Also, the chelator may have to be discontinued or the dosage reduced if there are signs of enhanced toxicosis.

For competition for potassium-dependent mechanisms supposedly upset by thallium, potassium chloride is given. This chemical should not be given orally because it can cause gastric and intestinal ulcers if given in concentrated form and will interfere with the ion-exchange treatment suggested below. Instead, 2–6 g of potassium chloride can be given in dilute solution by parenteral routes of administration, in divided dosages each day. Care must be taken that urine flow is adequate so that mobilized thallium can be eliminated rather than the blood thallium concentration being increased to dangerous levels. Also, if the intravenous route of administration is used, the heart must be monitored for signs of potassium toxicosis. Regarding the intravenous route, Gehring and Hammond (1967) used a solution of 0.125 mEq of KCl/ml (9.3 mg/ml) infused at the rate of 1.96 ml/minute for two 1-hour periods (2.19 g of KCl total each period) in renal clearance studies in anesthetized dogs.

Trapping of thallium in the intestine is best achieved by ion exchange. The agent of choice may be potassium ferric cyanoferrate-II (potassium-Prussian blue, PPB). Experimentally, PPB can cut the biological half-life of thallium from 4 days to 2 days in rats (Rauws 1974). PPB is not absorbed from the gut and it acts to immobilize thallous ion by an exchange with the potassium of PPB. Fecal excretion of thallium then rises (providing there is no constipation). Once trapped, the thallium is not readily released from Prussian blue except in a very small amount. The beneficial effect of PPB in thallotoxicosis has been confirmed in human beings (Stevens et al. 1974) *but not in domestic animals.* Nevertheless, the relative safety of PPB and its proven efficacy in rats and human beings are strong arguments for its use in treating thallium poisoning in other species. In rats, the dosage is 50 mg PPB/kg of body weight given orally twice a day as a suspension in 1% aqueous Tween-20. In adults and children, the oral dose of PPB is 250–300 mg/kg of body weight (1–5 g total) administered in 12.5–50 ml of a 15% mannitol solution 4 times a day for 10–15 days. This latter dosage regimen also seems appropriate for domestic animals, although this point requires research. PPB can be used in the presence of other drugs since it remains in the GI tract. However, orally administered potassium interferes with the ion exchange between PPB and thallium.

Nonspecific therapy of thallotoxicosis includes gastric lavage, fluids and electrolytes, analgesics or sedatives, antibiotics, vitamins, orally administered charcoal (0.5 g/kg of body weight twice a day), intestinal demulcents, ophthalmic ointments, blood transfusion, peritoneal dialysis, hematinics, soothing and antiinflamatory preparations for the skin, and general nursing care.

The prognosis is always guarded. If the animal is not treated soon after exposure, or if the animal is manifesting signs of extensive damage to internal organs, the prognosis is grave.

Stevens et al. (1974) provide an excellent review of the various methods and substances that have been used to treat thallotoxicosis in human beings and animals.

Analysis. Thallium is not a normal constituent of the body. Therefore, *any* concentration of thallium in urine, blood, or tissues is indicative of thallium poisoning if the history, clinical signs, and lesions are consistent with thallotoxicosis. A rapid test for urine thallium is given by Buck et al. (1973).

UREA

Use. Urea and other organic and inorganic sources of nitrogen, such as biuret and ammonium phosphate, are added to ruminant rations as a source of nonprotein nitrogen. However, urea is the most widely used. Urea is also used as a fertilizer and as a substitute for salts in the melting of snow and ice in residential areas.

Source. Ruminants generally obtain excess urea in feeds or in urea-molasses mixtures. Sometimes the urea is present in too large a concentration, or the feed may not be mixed properly. At other times, the urea is in the proper concentration, but the animals are not accustomed to ingesting urea or they ingest too much of it. Spilling or improper storage of urea fertilizer may also lead to poisoning of animals.

Properties of Toxicologic Importance. The most important property of urea and other commonly used sources of nonprotein nitrogen is their ability to liberate ammonia. Urea is the worst offender in this regard because its hydrolysis is speeded by the enzyme urease. Urease is present in many plants (especially in soybean products) and is therefore present in the rumen. Urea hydrolysis is also speeded by an alkaline pH. Excess urea can liberate sufficient ammonium ion to make the rumen contents more alkaline and thereby accelerate the liberation of more ammonium ion. This process is a therapeutic target.

Toxicity. The usual concentration of urea in ruminant rations is 3% of the grain ration or 1% of the total ration, but larger concentrations have been used with apparent safety. Sheep, for instance, if accustomed to urea, may consume up to 6% urea in the ration (100 g urea/day) (Clarke and Clarke 1967).

In ruminants unaccustomed to urea, ingestion of 0.3–0.5 g urea/kg of body weight may be toxic (Buck et al. 1973). Clarke and Clarke (1967) state that the toxic dosage of urea in (presumably unaccustomed) cattle is 0.45 g/kg (50 g total dosage) but that animals can ingest more urea than this if the dosage is increased gradually. In ruminant nutrition, urea is always introduced in small concentrations and then increased gradually over several days or weeks so that the animals have time to become accustomed to it (i.e., rumen microorganisms have time to adjust to the plentiful supply of usable nitrogen, and the ammonia-detoxication mechanism in the liver has time to adjust to increases in blood ammonia). Sheep that are not accustomed to urea may be poisoned by as little as 8 g total, given as a drench (McBarron and McInnes 1968), or by 0.5 mg urea/kg of body weight (10–15 g total)/day in the ration (Clarke and Clarke 1967). Kromann et al. (1971) give the acute oral LD50 of urea in unaccustomed sheep as 28.5 g/100 kg of body weight, but they point out that this figure is highly variable.

Cattle accustomed to urea can ingest 1 g urea/kg of body weight/day, but this is considered to be a maximum beyond which lethality can occur. In fact, 1–1.5 g/kg of body weight is given as the lethal dosage of urea in ruminants (Buck et al. 1973).

Monogastric animals are susceptible to poisoning by inorganic ammonium salts (which cause toxicosis at an oral dosage of 1.5 mg/kg of body weight) but they are not susceptible to urea poisoning. This is because neither alkaline hydrolysis nor urease activity occurs in monogastrics.

In horses, in which the cecum may contain some urease and a potentially good alkaline medium, urea is lethal when ingested at a rate of 4 g/kg of body weight. Ammonium salts are lethal in this species at a dosage of 1.5 g/kg. This is about the same toxicity as for ruminants, in which the oral lethal dose of ammonium salts is 1–2 g/kg of body weight (Buck et al. 1973).

It should be pointed out here that the inorganic ammonium salts and urea cause poisoning the same way, but there are a number of qualitative differences in response.

A large number of factors alter the toxicity of urea. Degree of adaptation is very important. Animals that are adapted to ingesting urea can tolerate 1 g urea/kg/day, but if the animals go off feed for a few days and then come back on full feed at the same rate of urea intake, toxicosis can result. This is because urea adaptation can wear off quickly.

Very young ruminants are essentially monogastric animals and can tolerate a large amount of urea. As the rumen flora develop and the diet changes, young ruminants become increasingly susceptible to urea toxicosis. They even get more susceptible than adult ruminants.

Other factors that enhance urea toxicosis include rapid ingestion (as in fasted or starving animals), a diet that is low in energy and protein but high in fiber, ingestion of palatable urea concentrate such as urea-molasses mixtures, high pH in the rumen, high body temperature, water deficiency, and feeds rich in urease (McBarron and McInnes 1968; Kromann et al. 1971; Buck et al. 1973).

Toxicodynamic Considerations. In the normal rumen, ammonia that is liberated from nonprotein nitrogen sources is in the form of ammonium ion. This ion is soluble and its charge prevents it from being absorbed across the membranes lining the rumen. If rumen pH is elevated to 11 or thereabouts, which can result when too much urea is ingested and too much ammonia is liberated, the ammonia can also be in the NH_3 form, which is also soluble. Lacking an ionic charge, it can readily be absorbed through the rumen wall and enter the bloodstream.

In the blood there are buffer systems that attempt to maintain blood pH at about 7.4, a pH at which much of the ammonia (but not all of it) is in the ammonium ion form and, therefore, unable to cross cell membranes. Thus, up to a point, ammonia-induced alkalosis is compensated.

Ammonia, a normal by-product of tissue metabolism, is removed from the blood by the liver. In hepatocytes, NH_3 is normally converted to urea by the urea cycle, or it is incorporated into glutamic acid in the synthesis of glutamine (Roberge and Charbonneau 1968). Both of these detoxication processes are enzymatic and both depend on substrates provided by the citric acid cycle.

Ammonium ion in the bloodstream is in equilibrium with NH_3. The NH_3 can cross the blood-brain barrier at a rate that is dependent on the speed of dissociation of NH_3 from NH_4^+ at the level of the cell membrane (Roberge and Charbonneau 1968). Ammonia also crosses the ovine placenta. The fetus can accumulate (and apparently detoxify) more ammonia than the dam, because fetal tissues have larger concentrations of ammonia than those of the dam when the dam is poisoned by urea. Moreover, the dam dies but the fetus does not (Yelverton et al. 1975).

Mechanism of Action. The toxicity of urea and other nonprotein nitrogen sources is due to ammonia absorbed from the stomach. Clinical signs of toxicosis develop only within a narrow range of blood ammonia concentrations (McBarron and McInnes 1968) or when rate of ammonium salt infusion is carefully controlled (Hooper 1972). Presumably, if the absorption of ammonia is below a certain rate, the animal can detoxify the ammonia fast enough to prevent toxicosis. If absorption is too fast, death may occur suddenly, without many of the typical signs of urea toxicosis.

Within the "critical" blood concentration range of ammonia, it appears that the animal cannot detoxify ammonia fast enough to keep ahead of absorption of ammonia from the stomach. In other words, the hepatic urea and glutamine-synthesizing mechanisms are saturated. Ammonia then builds up in the bloodstream and more and more NH_3 accumulates in tissue cells. (Nobody has actually said it is the NH_3 that is toxic rather than NH_4^+, but let us assume it.)

The primary mechanism of ammonia toxicosis appears to be an inhibition of the citric acid cycle. There is an increase in anaerobic glycolysis, blood glucose, and blood lactate (Buck et al. 1973). Acidosis is manifested. The exact means by which ammonia blocks the citric acid cycle is not known. It is postulated that ammonia saturation of the glutamine-synthesizing system causes a backing-up in the citrate cycle, a decrease in its intermediates, and a decrease in energy production and cellular respiration, which leads to convulsions (Roberge and Charbonneau 1968). The decrease of citrate cycle intermediates is postulated to result from reamination of pyruvic, ketoglutaric, and oxaloacetic acids.

As the citrate cycle fails, cells begin to malfunction. Perhaps the central nervous system (CNS) is first to malfunction because it has a large requirement for energy. Behavioral and nervous signs do seem to appear first.

The urea-synthesizing system, being dependent on the citrate cycle, may also begin to fail. Synthesis of urea continues to some extent, however, and blood urea concentration rises.

Cellular energy and respiration deficits probably cause ultrastructural damage and then degenerative changes. Blood potassium, phosphorus, serum glutamic oxaloacetic acid transaminase (SGOT), and serum glutamic pyruvic transaminase (SGPT), increase and urine output decreases.

In urea toxicosis and poisoning by ammonium compounds, the ultimate cause of death is inconsistent. Some animals may die of cardiac standstill induced by hyperkalemia (Buck et al. 1973). Others may die of ventricular fibrillation due to myocardial effects of ammonia itself (Wilson et al. 1968; see also Fluoroacetate, Chapter 58, which also inhibits the citrate cycle and causes accumulation of ammonia in cells and causes ventricular fibrillation in ruminants). Death may also occur from a form of respiratory paralysis in which respiratory effort is apparent but the respiratory muscles do not respond properly. The heartbeat is not primarily affected (Singer and McCarty 1971a). Convulsions can also cause death. In urea poisoning the convulsions are tonic and are elicitable by external stimuli just as with strychnine. Fatal anoxia could develop during a prolonged tonic seizure—the respiratory muscles being unable to relax. During convulsions an animal may aspirate rumen contents. Thus asphyxiation is a possible cause of death, especially if the animal also has pulmonary edema.

Pulmonary edema, if present, is thought to be due to neurogenic adrenergic factors that increase lung capillary permeability (Clarke and Clarke 1967).

For a toxicosis in which central nervous signs can be so prominent, very little has been published about brain lesions in urea toxicosis. A large number of conditions that elevate blood ammonia concentration cause brain damage (Hooper 1972; Gibson et al. 1974). Maybe overt lesions do not have time to develop in most cases of urea poisoning, even though functional nervous disturbances are present. Or perhaps we have been remiss in searching for brain lesions in cases of urea poisoning.

The convulsions seen in urea toxicosis are not clearly linked to decreased cellular respiration and energy in the proposal of Roberge and Charbonneau (1968). The convulsions occur near terminus and could be due to actual cellular damage in the brain. This does not seem likely because such damage would probably cause clonic rather than tonic convulsions. Recently it has been shown that ammonia decreases postsynaptic inhibition of cortical, spinal, and trochlear motor neurons of cats (Raabe and Gumnit 1975). Such an action is consistent with the production of tonic and elicitable convulsions characteristic of urea poisoning.

Clinical Signs. As with many other poisons, animals differ a great deal in the number and intensity of signs of urea toxicosis. Sometimes an animal is found dead. At other times the onset is slightly delayed, but the animal quickly dies after manifesting weakness, dyspnea, severe colic, and terminal tonic convulsions. There are also instances when onset of signs takes several hours and a spectrum of clinical signs is seen. It is this spectrum of signs that is most interesting and informative, because the signs, when classified, are surprisingly similar to those of other encephalopathic poisons such as lead and chlorinated hydrocarbon pesticides.

In urea toxicosis, *behavioral aberrations* such as initial restlessness or uneasiness and dullness are manifested. Later there may be signs of excitation and even belligerency for a brief period. Head pressing has been reported in sheep given a controlled intravenous infusion of ammonium acetate (Hooper 1972). Abnormal posturing, jumping over unseen objects, and maniacal behavior seen in chlorinated hydrocarbon pesticide poisoning has not been reported in urea poisoning. However, near terminus, violent struggling and bellowing occur. There are also *nervous phenomena* such as initial hyperesthesia, tremors, twitching, and spasms of muscles beginning with the eyelids, lips, and neck and progressing to the trunk, limbs, and tail. At terminus, intermittent tonic opisthotonic seizures that are elicitable and exaggerated by external stimuli are manifested. Between convulsive seizures the animal remains rather rigid. *Autonomic manifestations* include initial salivation, bradycardia, hypertension, and severe colic. *The GI signs may be the outstanding feature of urea toxicosis.* They include rumen atony, bloat, tooth grinding, groaning, kicking at the abdomen, and other evidence of colic. Diarrhea is not typical of urea poisoning as it is with lead, arsenic, and pesticide poisoning. Terminally, animals may vomit and aspirate rumen contents during convulsive seizures. *Locomotor disturbances* occur, such as initial incoordination and later staggering and stumbling prior to collapse, but the compulsive hypermotility typical of lead and chlorinated pesticides is not seen in urea toxicosis. Finally, there are *dependent signs* such as hot ears and skin (due to fever generated by convulsive activity), increased and forced or labored respiration (due to acidosis, lung edema, fever), cardiac arrhythmias (due to blood electrolyte and pH changes, epinephrine release, or direct effects of ammonia), frothing at the mouth, tracheal rales, and terminal cyanosis.

It is emphasized that the onset of urea toxicosis may range from 10 minutes to 4 hours, and death may occur in a few hours to 3 or 4 days. Thus all animals do not manifest all the above signs of urea toxicosis. Rather some combination of the signs is seen. The GI and terminal convulsive signs are generally prominent, which is why urea is classified here as a poison causing outstanding signs of abdominal distress.

For detail on clinical signs see Jones (1965), McBarron and McInnes (1968), Wilson et al. (1968), Radeleff (1970), Hooper (1972), Smith et al. (1972), and Buck et al. (1973).

Lesions. The severity and extent of lesions vary. Although this variability has not been studied per se, various accounts of the pathology of urea and ammonium salt toxicosis leave one with the impression that gross and microscopic lesions are most severe and numerous when animals live long enough for the lesions to develop. In other words, hyperammonemia associated with rapid death is likely to produce fewer and milder gross lesions than hyperammonemia associated with clinical signs that last several days before death. The work of Hooper (1972) is consistent with this reasoning. In addition, if duration of survival is held constant, one would expect the most severe and extensive damage to occur in animals in which blood ammonia concentration is the greatest. This logic has not been tested experimentally either, but the concept is consistent with the principles of dose-response relationships.

In urea poisoning there may be no characteristic lesions (Clarke and Clarke 1967). Some animals may manifest only a mild pulmonary edema with lung congestion and petechiation. There may be an odor of ammonia in the rumen (Buck et al. 1973). In other cases lesions include generalized venous stasis and congestion of the organs; more severe pulmonary edema; hydrothorax and hydropericardium; hemorrhages on the heart, lungs, and gut; fatty degeneration of the liver and kidney; and a strong odor of ammonia in the rumen (Jones 1965; McBarron and McInnes 1968; Wilson et al. 1968). The brain may manifest neuronal degeneration, with congestion and hemorrhages in the pia mater (Smith et al. 1972).

Ammonium salt administration tends to cause the more severe and widespread lesions mentioned above, perhaps because of absorption of controlled amounts of ammonia (Clarke and Clarke 1967; Singer and McCarty 1971b). The brain lesions can be made to progress to spongy degeneration with astrocyte changes in ewes infused at a controlled rate with ammonium acetate (Hooper 1972) or in mice in which blood ammonia concentration is elevated by the parenteral injection of urease (Gibson et al. 1974). Such brain lesions are typical of hyperammonemia associated with liver damage from a variety of causes.

Differential Diagnosis. Nonprotein nitrogen toxicosis should be suspected in cattle or sheep that manifest severe colic (without diarrhea), salivation, rapid forced breathing, terminal strychninelike convulsions, and lesions indicative of vascular damage. The odor of ammonia in the rumen may allow a presumptive diagnosis.

The condition can be confused with other agents that cause severe colic (e.g., arsenic or caustics) but such agents generally cause a diarrhea (often a bloody diarrhea) without behavioral, nervous, or motor signs. Lead and organochlorine pesticides cause many of the same kinds of signs that urea causes, but the *spectrum* of signs and lesions caused by these agents is different. Organophosphate toxicosis may mimic aspects of urea toxicosis, but organophosphates cause a variety of parasympathomimetic signs and few or no lesions. Moreover, atropine sulfate may alleviate signs of organophosphate poisoning but does not benefit animals in hyperammonemic states.

Other conditions that can be differentiated from urea poisoning by postmortem examination or laboratory tests include encephalitic disease, enterotoxemia, grain engorgement, and nitrite and cyanide poisoning.

Treatment. In animals that are not too ill, the cold water–acetic acid treatment may work. The adult cow is given 5–10 gal of cold water and 1 gal of 5% acetic acid (or vinegar) orally. This treatment limits absorption of ammonia from the rumen by diluting the rumen contents and slowing the rate of hydrolysis of urea by decreasing rumen pH and temperature. The treatment also promotes urine flow that, if it can be maintained by fluid therapy, may assure recovery from urea toxicosis (Buck et al. 1973). Gaseous or fluid bloat should be relieved before pumping water into the rumen.

Since we do not know exactly how ammonia acts to inhibit cell functions, there is no specific antidote for it. Glucose infusion is liable to cause hyperglycemic signs. Infusion of calcium solution may aggravate cardiac arrhythmias.

It is theoretically possible to decrease blood ammonia concentration by hastening the conversion of ammonia to urea. According to Roberge and Charbonneau (1968) and Paik et al. (1974), rats are protected against ammonia toxicosis by L-arginine or by a combination of L-arginine and *N*-carbamyl-*l*-glutamate. These compounds stimulate the urea cycle. It remains to be seen whether they can benefit animals already poisoned by ammonia-releasing compounds, i.e., when the citrate cycle is already inhibited and cell damage has already occurred.

In prostrate animals, convulsions can be controlled by careful administration of pentobarbital sodium. Fever can be controlled by cold water rinsing. A free airway can be provided and nursing care instituted. Survival is doubtful.

Analysis. Rumen juice and unclotted blood are analyzed. The samples *must* be fresh because the ammonia concentration can increase in biological samples during the process of decomposition. Rumen juice should be frozen and blood should be refrigerated. Suspect feed or molasses should be frozen.

Nonprotein nitrogen toxicosis is indicated when rumen juice contains 800 ppm or more of ammonia and when blood contains 20 ppm or more (Buck et al. 1973). Ammonia concentration in the rumen alone is not closely related to signs of toxicosis because absorption of ammonia from the rumen depends on rumen pH. The pH should be measured. Initial signs of urea toxicosis may be seen at a blood ammonia concentration of 8.4–13 ppm; ataxia may occur at 20 ppm, and death at 50 ppm (Clarke and Clarke 1967). The "significant" blood concentration is different in different animals. Therefore, the final diagnosis depends on the history, signs, and lesions observed.

POISONS CAUSING ABDOMINAL DISTRESS BY UNKNOWN MECHANISMS

Organic Herbicides

If the various synthetic organic herbicides are used properly, they are not a great hazard for animals. Moreover, many of the compounds are rapidly excreted, thus making diagnosis difficult. In addition, there is no specific treatment for organic herbicide poisoning, except for arsenicals that can be treated with BAL (see "Inorganic" Arsenic). All this being so, it is not appropriate to discuss the toxicology of organic herbicides in detail in this particular text. However, some general comments are warranted.

Organic herbicides are classified according to chemical structure. Most of them cause signs of abdominal distress such as anorexia, diarrhea, and possible colic. The *phenoxyacetic acid derivatives* (2,4-D, and 2,4,5-T) also cause weakness, ataxia, and muscle spasms or rigidity. The *triazines* (atrazine, simazine) cause depression and dyspnea. *Chlorinated aliphatic* compounds (dalapon) cause ataxia. The *amides* (diphenamide, Randox) cause salivation, ataxia, and prostration. *Substituted urea* compounds (monuron, linuron, fenuron) cause vomiting, ataxia, and urticaria. The *carbamates* (dichlormate) cause bloat. *Thiocarbamates* (diallate, triallate, EPTC) cause depression, vomiting, salivation, bloat, muscle spasms, and dyspnea. Carbamate and thiocarbamate herbicides should not be confused with carbamate insecticides. *Arsenicals* (MSMA, DSMA, cacodylic acid) cause signs of inorganic arsenic poisoning. The *dinitroaniline derivatives* (nitralin, trifluralin) cause depression, bloat, and prostration. *Dipyridyl compounds* (diquat, paraquat) cause depression and a progressive fibrosing pneumonitis. *Phthalamic acid* (naptalam) causes bloat, and incoordination. *Polychlorobicyclopentadiene isomers* (Bandane) cause depression, tremors, hyperexcitability, incoordination, and prostration. The *picolinic acid compounds* (picloram) cause weakness and depression (Buck et al. 1973).

Necropsy findings with these chemicals include gastroenteritis, congestion in liver, kidney, or lung, and other lesions, depending on the compound.

Buck et al. (1973) have presented useful tables of toxicity, hazard, signs, and lesions of organic herbicides. This source should be consulted for detail on the toxicology of these diverse substances.

Organic Fungicides

A large number of compounds are applied to seed grain, plants, soil, or wood for the purpose of preventing or treating fungal growth. Most of these compounds are not considered to be much of a toxicologic hazard because their LD50 values are high.

Sulfur (250 mg/kg of body weight) can cause violent purgation and colic in cattle and horses.

Dinitro-*o*-cresol (DNOC) and pentachlorophenol PCP) can cause GI distress. The compounds are discussed in Chapter 57.

Organomercurials can also cause abdominal distress. These compounds are no longer used as seed protectants, but some of them may still be in use for other purposes. Organomercurials, specifically methylmercury and ethylmercury compounds, are discussed in Chapter 58 and in this chapter.

For information on relatively nontoxic compounds such as captan, ferbam, nabam, thiram, zineb, ziram, and organic tin fungicides, see Buck et al. (1973).

Plant Poisons

Signs of colic can be produced by almost any plant if ingested in excess. It seems that plant principles are either directly caustic or irritant, as discussed under Direct Corrosives or Irritants, or they produce a more nonspecific irritation of the gut. In other words, we do not know exactly how they cause enteritis. Such plant principles include delphinine from delphiniums (*Delphinium* spp.); alkaloids from box (*Buxus* spp.); the resinoid andromedotoxin from rhododendron (*Rhododendron* spp.), laurels (*Kalmia* spp., *Ledum* spp., *Leucothoe* spp.), and mock azalea (*Menziesia* spp.); and tannic acid from oaks and acorns (*Quercus* spp.). Most of these principles cause severe toxicosis, the GI signs being relatively unimportant. For detail, see Kingsbury (1964).

POISONS CAUSING SEVERE LIVER DAMAGE

Coal Tar

For some reason, pigs like coal tar. They may chew it from tarred walls or floors or they may eat tarpaper. More often, however, pigs root out shards of clay pigeons that may be scattered over shooting ranges. Clay pigeons contain coal tar pitch. The toxicosis in swine has been called "clay pigeon poisoning" and pitch poisoning.

Coal tar is about 50% pitch and 50% mixed volatiles such as benzene, toluene, naphthalene, anthracene, xylene, and other aromatic hydrocarbons; phenol, cresol, and other phenolics; ammonia, pyridine, and other organic bases; and thiophene. Coal tar is a product of the destructive distillation of coal. It is much more toxic than the wood tars (pine tar, creosote) although the tars share some common ingredients.

The toxic factor in coal tar is not known. It is not phenol. The exact toxicity of coal tar is not known either, but typical poisoning results when pigs are fed 15 g of powdered clay pigeon/pig/day for several days.

Clinical signs of coal tar poisoning include anorexia, depression, weakness, sternal recumbency, jaundice, abdominal tenderness, and increased respiratory rate. Death may occur suddenly, without signs being observed, or it may occur in 1–4 days.

Coal tar causes liver hemorrhage and necrosis that is scattered and centrolobular. The liver looks mottled. Tissues are icteric. The liver is engorged and friable. The kidneys are pale and enlarged. There may be anemia, secondary to liver damage. Excess fluid may be found in the abdominal cavity, and the abdominal lymph nodes may be swollen and hemorrhagic. Pigs that manifest the signs and lesions described above should be suspected of having ingested a coal tar–containing material.

There is no specific treatment. The source should be found and removed or fenced away from pigs.

For detail, see Clarke and Clarke (1967) and Buck et al. (1973).

Aflatoxins

source

Aflatoxins are toxic metabolites elaborated by the molds *Aspergillus flavus* and *A. parasiticus*. These molds are ubiquitous in nature and can be found normally in stored feedstuffs. The molds are not inherently toxigenic but can grow rapidly and become so in grains or feeds stored under aerobic conditions when moisture content of the feedstuff exceeds 15% and when the temperature is 24°–25° C (optimum). Toxin production can occur to some extent at lower and higher temperatures (Lillehoj 1973).

Many feedstuffs can support the growth of aflatoxin-producing mold. Peanuts are commonly affected, as are cottonseed meal and cake. Cottonseed growing in the field can be infected with aflatoxin-producing mold (on the lower third of the plant where moisture and temperature conditions are right). Ears of growing corn, if damaged by corn borers, may become moldy and contain large concentrations of aflatoxin. Other products that can be associated with aflatoxicosis are shelled corn, cornmeal, dogmeals, silage, wheat, barley, oats, rice, and other grains or cereal products.

Four major aflatoxins are B_1 and B_2, which fluoresce blue under long-wave ultraviolet light, and G_1 and G_2, which fluoresce green. The most important of these toxins is aflatoxin B_1 because of its toxicity and concentration in moldy feeds.

PROPERTIES OF TOXICOLOGIC IMPORTANCE

Aflatoxins are polycyclic, unsaturated compounds consisting of a coumarin nucleus flanked by an apparently highly reactive bifuran system on one side and either a pentenone (B toxins) or a 6-membered lactone (G series) on the other. These toxins are relatively heat resistant and not soluble in water. They are extractable from feedstuffs by a number of organic solvents. Research is in progress to discover a reliable and practical way of destroying aflatoxins in feedstuffs. The addition of fungicidal dyes (e.g., gentian violet) may help to prevent the production of aflatoxins in feeds, but it will not destroy the aflatoxins already present.

TOXICITY

The aflatoxins are potent carcinogens, mutagens, teratogens, and liver-damaging agents in a variety of animal species. The carcinogenic property, of major concern in public health aspects of foods, will not be discussed here because it is not particularly important in the production of toxicosis in animals. It is sufficient to say that aflatoxins can cause liver tumors in animals. Likewise, the mutagenic and teratogenic properties will not be discussed. For detail on these topics see Detroy et al. (1971).

Liver damage is a very important aspect of aflatoxicosis in animals. Death of animals is due to the consequences of severe liver damage that results when aflatoxins are ingested either acutely in large amounts or chronically in smaller amounts.

According to several sources (Wogan and Shank 1971; Buck et al. 1973; Edds 1973; Ciegler 1975), the acute oral LD50 of aflatoxin B_1 in several species is (in mg/kg of body weight): sheep, 2; young pig, 0.52; dog, 1; puppy, 0.5–1; cat, 0.3–0.6; chicken, 6.3; chick (1-day-old), 0.3–0.6; duckling, 0.5–1; rat (21-day-old), 5.5–17.9; rat (1-day-old), 1; mouse, 9; guinea pig, 1.4–2; hamster, 10.2; monkey, 2.2–7.8; trout (100 g), 0.5–1; and channel catfish, 10–15.

Dietary concentrations of aflatoxins that cause toxicosis (liver damage and/or death) in different species are (in ppm of the diet): heifers, 2.4 for 28 weeks; weanling calves, 0.22 or more for 16 weeks; steers (6- to 8-month-old), 0.7–1 for 16–26 weeks; steers (2-year-old), 0.22 or more for 20 weeks; growing pigs, 0.41 or more for 12–24 weeks; pregnant sows, 0.3–0.5 for 4 weeks; chicks (1-week-old), 0.84 for 10 weeks; chicks (1-day-old), 0.42 for 7 weeks; turkey poults (1-day-old), 0.25 for 4 weeks; and ducklings, 0.3 for 4–6 weeks (Garrett et al. 1968; Buck et al. 1973). In the author's experience, horses may develop typical signs and lesions of toxic hepatopathy and GI upset if they consume mixed feed containing concentrations of aflatoxin B_1 as small as 2–50 parts per billion. It is possible that other mycotoxins could be present in these cases, however. In young pigs as little as 51 parts per billion aflatoxin in the feed eventually causes hepatic and blood biochemical changes indicative of cell damage (Gumbmann and Williams 1969). Presumably, ingestion of minute amounts of aflatoxins over an extended period can cause biochemical aberrations in other species as well, depending on rate of entry and metabolism of aflatoxin in the hepatocyte.

Aside from age, sex, breed, and strain of animal, other factors affect the toxicity of aflatoxin. Toxicity is enhanced by riboflavin; exposure to light; and a diet low in protein, choline, and vitamin B-12. Vitamins A, E, and K in the diet do not protect rats against aflatoxin. Toxicity is decreased by dietary protein, lipids, and carotene (Edds 1973; Newberne et al. 1974).

TOXICODYNAMIC CONSIDERATIONS

Aflatoxins are absorbed from the intestinal tract and bound to serum albumin (Bassir and Bababunmi 1973). The toxins appear in the milk of lactating cattle (Allcroft and Roberts 1968). Liver cells take up aflatoxins from the blood. The rate of uptake depends on the aflatoxin structure and the species. Within the hepatocyte, aflatoxins may exert direct effects on nuclear DNA and RNA synthesis and on sex steroid binding sites on the endoplasmic reticulum. In the microsomes, aflatoxins are metabolized to various forms. One or more of the forms may be major active forms in some species (see Mechanism of Action). For detail on aflatoxin metabolism see the review by Ciegler (1975). Aflatoxins do not accumulate preferentially in any specific tissue but are excreted by the kidneys as nonfluorescent water-soluble sulfates and glucuronides.

MECHANISM OF ACTION

A number of biochemical changes are probably secondary to the cytotoxic actions of aflatoxins. These changes include increases in SGOT, SGPT, blood alkaline phosphatase, isocitric dehydrogenase, and bilirubin. There are decreases in serum protein, nonprotein nitrogen, and urea (Gumbmann and Williams 1969; John and Miller 1969; Buck et al. 1973; Hayes and Hannan 1973). There is also an immunosuppressive effect of aflatoxin (Pier 1973; Thurston et al. 1974). None of these effects helps us to understand how aflatoxin damages the liver.

In rat hepatocytes the first ultrastructural change elicited by aflatoxin B_1 is a change in nucleolar structure (Detroy et al. 1971). This nucleolar change is also produced by the pyrrolizidine alkaloids, which produce the same kinds of liver lesions as aflatoxins. The nucleolar damage is consistent with observations that aflatoxin binds with nuclear DNA. It is postulated (Buck et al. 1973; Wogan 1974, 1975) that binding to DNA prevents DNA from acting as a template. Therefore, nucleic acid polymerases cannot function and this leads to a decrease in ribosomal protein synthesis.

Subsequent ultrastructural changes include a disaggregation and decrease in number of ribosomes, proliferation of smooth endoplasmic reticulum, loss of glycogen, and mitochondrial degeneration (Detroy et al. 1971). These changes are consistent with an inhibition of protein (enzyme) synthesis and are also predictable consequences of two other observations: aflatoxin B_1 inhibits the electron transport system of mitochondria by acting between cytochromes b and c_1 or c *in vitro* (Doherty and Campbell 1972); and aflatoxin B_{2a} (a major metabolite of B_1) covalently binds to rat liver microsomal protein *in vitro* (Gurtoo and Dahms 1974). Such actions could certainly give rise to cell death.

A number of hepatotoxins (including pyrrolizidines) damage the liver by forming reactive intermediates that bind covalently to liver macromolecules (Reid et al. 1973; Gillette et al. 1974; Jerina and Daly 1974). Aflatoxins are thought to be metabolized to highly reactive epoxides and phenolates (the furan system of aflatoxin is involved here) that can bind and theoretically interfere with nucleic acids and proteins (Ciegler 1975). Thus not only is the parent molecule capable of binding to cellular structures, but so are the epoxides and phenolates.

In the papers by Jerina and Daly (1974) and Gillette et al. (1974) it is shown that the epoxides and phenolates of certain monocyclic and polycyclic compounds are normally conjugated with glutathione and that glutathione serves to protect vital macromolecules from these toxic intermediates (see Selenium, Chapter 57, for functions of glutathione). A similar protective mechanism operates against the hepatotoxic metabolites of carbon tetrachloride and chloroform (Brown et al. 1974). Hepatic necrosis is thought to result when glutathione reserves have been drastically depleted by conjugation with toxic intermediates so that the toxic intermediates are free to bind covalently to vital cellular macromolecules. It is not known whether glutathione has anything to do with aflatoxicosis, but it would be very interesting to find out! After all, there is some reason why a high protein diet protects rats against aflatoxin. Maybe the protection is due to the presence of cysteine, a precursor of glutathione. Cysteine (200 mg/kg of body weight) decreases aflatoxin B_1 hepatotoxicity in rats, while the glutathione-depleting agent diethyl maleate (0.6 ml/kg) enhances the hepatotoxicity (Mgbodile et al. 1975).

The big problem in studying the mechanism of action of aflatoxins is in determining which biochemical interactions are closely related to carcinogenesis, mutagenesis, and teratogenesis on the one hand

and hepatic degeneration and necrosis on the other. It appears that the mechanisms overlap considerably.

CLINICAL SIGNS

Acute toxicosis may be characterized by sudden death or by signs such as anorexia, depression, dyspnea, anemia, epistaxis, bloody feces, possible convulsions, and rapid death. In subacute toxicosis, animals develop jaundice, hypoprothrombinemia, hematomas, and hemorrhagic enteritis—a "warfarinlike" condition. Chronic toxicosis is manifested by a gradual decrease in feed efficiency, productivity, and weight gain and rough haircoat, anemia, enlarged abdomen, mild jaundice, depression, and anorexia. Abortion could also occur. Signs differ somewhat for different species, but the overall impression with acute and subacute cases is one of liver damage and a blood coagulation defect (for detail see Buck et al. 1973; Edds 1973; Newberne 1973).

LESIONS

Generally, lesions may include icterus, widespread petechial and ecchymotic hemorrhages, hemorrhagic gastroenteritis, hepatic necrosis and hemorrhage, enlarged liver (acute cases) or hepatic fibrosis (chronic cases), cirrhosis, ascites, hydrothorax, and edema of the wall of the gallbladder.

Microscopic lesions are consistent with gross findings. Hepatic neoplasms may be seen. Acute necrosis and hemorrhage are not generally seen in the liver of cattle, calves, sheep, or chickens, but this could be a dose phenomenon.

Ultrastructural lesions have been described (see Mechanism of Action).

DIFFERENTIAL DIAGNOSIS

A differential diagnosis may be difficult. If animals eat moldy feed and then develop typical signs and lesions of liver damage and blood coagulation defects, a mold toxin can be suspected. Laboratory tests of the feed can detect small amounts of aflatoxins.

Other mold toxins can cause signs and lesions similar to those of aflatoxin. In fact, other mold toxins (T-2 toxin, rubratoxin, ochratoxin A) could even be present in the same feed with aflatoxins. Extensive laboratory tests may be needed to determine which toxin is present.

Other conditions that may mimic aflatoxicosis include warfarin or dicoumarol poisoning (coagulation defect primarily), coal tar poisoning (variegated mottling of the liver), copper poisoning (hemoglobinuria, hemolysis), and poisoning by other hepatotoxins such as carbon tetrachloride, pyrrolizidine alkaloids from ragwort (*Senecio* spp.) or crotalaria (*Crotalaria* spp.), and hepatotoxins from blue-green algae. Inspection of the premises may help rule out these substances, but laboratory tests for aflatoxins are still required. The author has encountered cases of apparent mold toxicosis on a farm where there was also free access to an algae-laden (and toxic) pond, to spilled creosote, to fence posts freshly treated with pentachlorophenol, and to the farm dump!

Infectious diseases such as leptospirosis and infectious hepatitis must also be ruled out.

Mold culture is of no value in diagnosis.

TREATMENT

Surviving animals should be fed an easily digested, low-fat diet containing adequate protein. Multiple vitamins should be given, along with other supportive therapy. Vitamin K in the diet has not been successful in preventing aflatoxicosis in rats, but parenteral dosage of vitamin K could be tried in an effort to combat any coumarinlike anticoagulant effects of aflatoxin. Blood transfusion may be required.

There is no specific therapy for aflatoxicosis. If glutathione has a role in the condition, parenteral administration of its prescursor cysteine or of other sulfhydryl-containing compounds such as BAL or cysteamine could be of some value. These agents are of benefit if given within 1 hour of acetaminophen poisoning in mice. Acetaminophen is a drug that causes hepatic necrosis when its toxic intermediate has exhausted hepatic stores of glutathione (Mitchell et al. 1974). Cysteine, 300 mg/kg of body weight, prevents liver necrosis due to monocrotaline in rats if the cysteine is given 15 minutes before and 2 hours after monocrotaline (McLean 1970). Monocrotaline is a pyrrolizidine alkaloid that may act like aflatoxins in producing hepatic necrosis.

ANALYSIS

According to Food and Drug Administration (FDA) guidelines, ruminant feed should not contain more than 20 ppb (0.02 ppm) aflatoxin (Wessel and Stoloff 1973). The presence of aflatoxin in feed, milk, and urine is indictative of aflatoxicosis in animals that ate moldly feed and then developed the signs and lesions of aflatoxicosis. "Diagnostic" concentrations of aflatoxin do not exist. Reference to the dosages of aflatoxin that cause acute or chronic toxicosis (see Toxicity) may serve as a rough guide to the significance of aflatoxin concentration in feed, but most of the data are for experimental animals under controlled conditions.

RUBRATOXINS

SOURCE

Rubratoxins A and B are hepatotoxic metabolites produced by the molds *Penicillium rubrum* and *P. purpurogenum*. These molds often grow in feedstuffs along with *Aspergillus* spp. and, in fact, rubratoxins and aflatoxins may coexist in the grain or feed product (Moss 1971; Wilson and Harbison 1973). This means that aflatoxicosis may be complicated by rubratoxins and that the conditions favoring aflatoxin production in stored feeds can also favor rubratoxin production.

PROPERTIES OF TOXICOLOGIC IMPORTANCE

The rubratoxins have an unusual polycyclic structure containing stable anhydride functions. Their empirical formula is $C_{26}H_{30}O_{11}$ (Moss 1971). The toxins are poorly soluble in water, insoluble in oils or chloroform, and soluble in ethanol (especially the A toxin), ethyl acetate (especially the B toxin), or acetone. The toxins are stable indefinitely at room temperature.

TOXICITY

Rubratoxicosis is not presently a separate entity in veterinary toxicology because there are no documented cases of uncomplicated rubratoxicosis. Other mold toxins, particularly aflatoxins, have always been present in cases where rubratoxins were present in the moldy feed. But this is no excuse for ignoring the rubratoxins. They do potentiate aflatoxicosis (Moss 1971; Wogan et al. 1971) and under experimental conditions they are capable of causing severe liver damage and hemorrhagic phenomena.

The acute oral LD50 of rubratoxin B (the major and most toxic rubratoxin) in rats is 400–450 mg/kg of body weight. This is when the vehicle is dimethyl sulfoxide, a solvent known to increase the toxicity of rubratoxins (Wogan et al. 1971). Swine are more susceptible to rubratoxins than are laboratory animals. Dogs, cats, goats, and horses are also susceptible to rubratoxins (Moss 1971). Intraperitoneal LD50 values are available for a number of species (Wogan et al. 1971).

It is important to note that rubratoxins are much less toxic than aflatoxins, on an equal weight basis. Rubratoxins are teratogenic, embryocidal, and growth suppressant in mice, but they are not carcinogenic (Hood et al. 1973).

Chronic ingestion of small amounts of rubratoxin may be without effect. On the other hand, rats may ingest small concentrations of toxin for many weeks and then suddenly become ill and die in 3 days. Thus there seems to be a threshold of tolerance for rubratoxins (Wogan et al. 1971).

TOXICODYNAMIC CONSIDERATIONS

The liver apparently metabolizes rubratoxins (Moss 1971; Hayes and Hannan 1973), but the nature of the metabolites is not known.

MECHANISM OF ACTION

Very little is known about biochemical mechanisms of rubratoxin hepatopathy. Apparently the mitochondria are not the primary site of action (Moss 1971; Hayes and Hannan 1973) although there is a depression of oxidation of citrate, malate, and pyruvate in mice.

Rubratoxin does not primarily affect the protein-synthesizing mechanisms. It does not alter amino acid uptake, polyribosome profile, or inducible enzymes (Wogan et al. 1971) although there is a decrease in liver glycogen and protein content.

In dogs, rubratoxin causes an increase in SGOT, serum alkaline phosphatase, blood cholesterol, inorganic phosphate, urea nitrogen, hemoglobin, packed cell volume, and leucocytes (Hayes et al. 1973). There is a surprising decrease in serum lactic dehydrogenase.

CLINICAL SIGNS

Clinical signs include anorexia, dehydration, depression, diarrhea, jaundice, and weight loss. Swine may manifest head pressing, colic, and ventral erythema. Horses may become incoordinated. Death occurs in as few as 12 hours (Moss 1971; Wogan et al. 1971; Hayes et al. 1973).

LESIONS

The general impression is of a severe hemorrhagic necrotizing hepatitis with hemorrhages in various organs. The spleen also may be necrotic. Renal damage is mild or absent. In cats there is edema of the wall of the gall bladder and a massive ascites. In horses there may be brain hemorrhages (see above references).

DIFFERENTIAL DIAGNOSIS

See Aflatoxins. Laboratory tests are required.

TREATMENT

Animals are given symptomatic treatment and nursing care. Field cases in which rubratoxins have been found have been complicated by the presence of aflatoxins, which are more potent than rubratoxins. If a good treatment for aflatoxicosis is ever developed, it will likely benefit animals that ingest rubratoxins in combination with aflatoxins.

ANALYSIS

Rubratoxins can be detected by a chromatographic procedure (Hayes and McCain 1975). Diagnosis depends on a typical history, signs, lesions, and finding rubratoxin in the urine and feed. Aflatoxins can be missed by selective extraction procedures. Therefore, the veterinarian should request tests for hepatotoxic mycotoxins, not just rubratoxins.

Other Mold Toxins

T-2 TOXIN

This mold toxin is discussed in Chapter 57 because the predominant clinical signs and lesions are probably due to extensive hemorrhage and shock. However, T-2 toxin does cause liver and kidney damage that may look like the lesions of aflatoxin or rubratoxin. T-2 toxin and related trichothecenes often cause mucosal and skin sloughing, which may help differentiate them from aflatoxin or rubratoxin. Laboratory tests will confirm the diagnosis.

SPORIDESMINS

The sporidesmins are epipolythiadioxopiperazine compounds produced by certain soil fungi, notably *Pythomyces chartarum*. This mold is thought to be the cause of facial eczema, cholangiohepatitis, and photosensitivity in sheep and cattle in New Zealand. The mold may possibly infect growing rye grass or it may infest decaying herbage. These toxins are mentioned here only because there is no reason to think they will remain forever in New Zealand. In fact, slow growth or weight loss of lambs in parts of Nova Scotia could be related to ingestion of epipolythiadioxopiperazines elaborated from pasture isolates of *Chaetomium* sp. Also, instances of probable mycotoxin-induced photosensitivity reactions have been observed in cattle in the United States (Richard 1973).

AMANITA TOXINS

Mushrooms of the genus *Amanita* contain several toxic principles. The most important of these are cyclic polypeptides called phallotoxins (7 amino acids) and amatoxins (8 amino acids). Phallotoxins (e.g., phalloidin) cause disruption of intracellular membranes such as those of the endoplasmic reticulum, lysosomes, and the cell membrane itself. This action is reportedly antagonized in experimental animals by the dithiol lipoic (thioctic) acid (Hatfield and Brady 1975). Mushroom poisoning of experimental animals is not reversible by lipoic acid (Alleva et al. 1975), because toxic mushrooms also contain amatoxins (e.g., amanitin). Amatoxins cause liver necrosis by attacking the cell nucleus, inhibiting RNA polymerase-II, altering the nucleolus, and inhibiting ribosomal RNA. Eventually, the synthesis of messenger RNA, DNA, and protein is inhibited (Wieland 1968; Hatfield and Brady 1975).

The reason for saying even this much about mushroom poisoning (a rather unimportant condition in veterinary practice) is that the mechanism of hepatotoxic action of amanitin is similar to (but not the same as) that of aflatoxin. When researchers find a good treatment for mushroom poisoning in human beings (the condition being important in this species), they may provide insights into the treatment of aflatoxicosis in animals.

PLANT POISONS

Pyrrolizidine alkaloids are potent hepatotoxins in most species. The alkaloids include monocrotaline from rattlebox *(Crotalaria* sp.); retrorsine from ragwort (*Senecio* spp.); and similar alkaloids in fiddleneck or tarweed (*Amsinckia* sp.), viper's bugloss *(Echium* sp.), and potato weed *(Heliotropium* sp.). These alkaloids apparently cause hepatotoxicity by mechanisms similar to those of aflatoxins. Moreover, clinical signs may be due to direct organ damage by the alkaloids or possibly to liver damage–induced elevation of blood ammonia concentration. For detail and some species differences in response to pyrrolizidine alkaloids, see McLean (1970), Chesney and Allen (1973), Peckham et al. (1974), and McGrath et al. (1975). In rats, monocrotaline hepatopathy has been prevented by timely administration of the glutathione precursor cysteine (300 mg/kg of body weight given 15 minutes before and 2 hours after monocrotaline) (McLean 1970).

Other hepatotoxic plant poisons include polypeptides in blue-green algae, unidentified principles in coneflower *(Rudbeckia laciniata)* and sartwellia *(Sartwellia flaveriae),* tannic acid in oaks and acorns (*Quercus* spp.) (oaks also cause hemorrhagic gastroenteritis and kidney damage), gossypol in cottonseed products *(Gossypium* spp.) (gossypol also causes organ congestion and edema and cardiac enlargement), hydroquinone in cocklebur sprouts *(Xanthium* spp.), and unidentified principles in drymary *(Drymaria* sp.). In addition, a large number of plants cause photosensitivity reactions resulting from damage to the liver. These plants are listed in Chapter 60 because the photosensitivity phenomenon is a striking clinical entity.

POISONS CAUSING SEVERE KIDNEY DAMAGE

ETHYLENE GLYCOL

Ethylene glycol is discussed in Chapter 57 because it affects primarily the respiratory apparatus. Nevertheless, as pointed out in that discussion, renal failure is a component of ethylene glycol toxicosis, particularly in the later stages of the condition. The renal failure is due to deposition of calcium oxalate crystals in the renal tubules, oxalate being a metabolite of ethylene glycol. The renal tubules are partly or completely blocked by the crystals, the tubules are dilated, and tubular epithelial cells are physically damaged. Clinical signs are those of uremia. The history may disclose that the animal (dog or cat) apparently relapsed to a uremic state 12–24 hours after having recovered or partly recovered from a condition of depression, ataxia, partial paralysis, and prostration. Details are given in Chapter 57.

OCHRATOXINS

SOURCE

Ochratoxins are mold toxins produced by the storage molds *Aspergillus ochraceus*, *A. sulphureus*, *A. melleus*, *Penicillium viridicatum*, and *P. cyclopium*. These molds grow on corn, sorghum grain, peanuts, wheat, oats, barley, rye, white beans, and animal feeds. Optimum growth occurs when moisture content of the grain or feed is greater than 16%, and when the temperature is 20°–25° C (Steyn 1971; Munro et al. 1973). At this writing, confirmed instances of ochratoxicosis have not occurred. However, ochratoxins have been found in moldy grains and feeds, and the toxins can produce toxicosis in experimental animals. It is probably only a matter of time until ochratoxicosis is recognized as a problem in the field.

PROPERTIES OF TOXICOLOGIC IMPORTANCE

There are two major ochratoxins, A and B. Ochratoxin A is more toxic and more prevalent. The empirical formulas of these dihydroisocoumarins are $C_{20}H_{18}Cl$-NO_6 (A) and $C_{20}H_{19}NO_6$ (B). They are poorly soluble in water but soluble in chloroform-methanol (Steyn 1971; Munro et al. 1973).

TOXICITY

The acute oral LD50 of ochratoxin A in rats is 20–22 mg/kg of body weight—about twice the LD50 of aflatoxin B_1 in that species. Tumors are not produced in rats. In ducklings the lethal dose is 0.135–0.17 mg total dose and in day-old cockerels it is 0.1–0.2 mg (Steyn 1971; Munro et al. 1973). These workers also report that an intravenous dose of 1 mg ochratoxin A/kg of body weight kills sheep in 12–24 hours. In chickens, chronic ingestion of 4–8 ppm of ochratoxin A in the diet is lethal in 3 weeks. In rats, ingestion of as little as 2.4 ppm causes nephrotoxicity in 24 hours. Death and resorption of rat fetuses also results. Szczech et al. (1973) report that swine fed 0.2–0.6 mg ochratoxin A/kg/day manifest decreased feed intake in 4 days, but overt illness is not seen until 2 weeks later. The economic implication of this observation is obvious. In rats, as little as 0.2 ppm of ochratoxin A in the diet causes kidney damage in 90 days (Munro et al. 1974).

TOXICODYNAMIC CONSIDERATIONS

According to Steyn (1971) and Munro et al. (1973), ochratoxin A is metabolized in the body and excreted in the urine, bile, and feces. The toxin binds to plasma protein and very little toxin crosses the placenta of sheep. Excretion of toxin is nearly complete at 78 hours in the rat.

MECHANISM OF ACTION

In rat liver cells, the first ultrastructural effect of ochratoxin A is proliferation of smooth endoplasmic reticulum, with appearance of hyaline degeneration. Cell necrosis is thought to be due to the endoplasmic reticulum proliferation. The renal proximal tubule cells also manifest necrosis. The toxin does not interact with nucleic acids or their derivatives. The biochemical mechanism of action is thought to be inhibition of a cellular phosphorylase enzyme system, possibly by competition with cyclic 3′,5′-AMP for phosphorylase *b* kinase. Metabolic activation of the toxin is not required (Steyn 1971; Munro et al. 1973).

In cultured monkey kidney cells, ochratoxin A causes abnormal mitoses and cell death. The mitotic effect may relate to abortions seen in rats (Steyn et al. 1975).

Ochratoxin A causes hepatic glycogen depletion, possibly due to inhibition of active transport of glucose into the cell, suppression of glycogenesis, and acceleration of glycogenolysis (Suzuki et al. 1975).

Changes in blood and urine chemistry and character reflect kidney and liver damage. In rats there is a decrease in urine volume and urine specific gravity and protein are increased. Blood urea nitrogen

(BUN) increases (Munro et al. 1973). In pigs the toxin causes increases in packed cell volume, plasma protein, BUN, leucocyte count, and enzymes such as SGOT, lactic dehydrogenase (LDH), and isocitric dehydrogenase (Szczech et al. 1973).

CLINICAL SIGNS

In swine, clinical signs include a decrease in feed intake, weight loss, diarrhea, polyuria, polydipsia, dehydration, and death in 5–6 days (Szczech et al. 1973).

Chicks manifest dehydration, emaciation, decreased growth, and diarrhea. Chickens demonstrate depressed growth, delayed sexual maturity, and decreased size and production (Steyn 1971; Munro et al. 1973). Other species can be expected to manifest signs of renal failure.

LESIONS

Swine manifest enteritis, pale tan liver, edema and hyperemia of lymph nodes, and severe degenerative changes in the kidneys. Microscopically, the kidney tubules and intestinal mucosa are necrotic and the liver is fatty (Szczech et al. 1975).

In chicks, dryness of the gizzard mucosa, petechiation in the proventriculus, and liver damage ranging from fatty foci to necrotic foci are observed. Acute nephrosis and visceral gout are also seen (Steyn 1971; Munro et al. 1973).

DIFFERENTIAL DIAGNOSIS

Mold nephrosis can be suspected when the predominant signs and lesions are of kidney damage and when there is a history of ingestion of moldy feed. Final diagnosis depends on laboratory tests.

A number of poisons damage the kidneys and liver. A list of such poisons is not appropriate here. It behooves the veterinarian to exclude as many poisons as possible by careful inspection of the premises and questioning of the client. The toxicology testing laboratory can exclude such things as metals, and the microbiology and pathology laboratory can exclude diseases. By the process of elimination, mold toxins may be incriminated.

TREATMENT

There is no specific treatment for ochratoxicosis. Supportive therapy and nursing care may enhance survival.

ANALYSIS

There are chromatographic methods of detecting ochratoxin A. The presence of toxin in feed and urine would indicate ochratoxicosis if the history, signs, and lesions are consistent with poisoning by this toxin. However, other mold toxins may also be detected. The dog kidney is very sensitive to ochratoxin A. Szczech et al. (1974) are elucidating the nephrotoxic changes produced in dogs, with the stated objectives of defining alterations that might be of diagnostic and prognostic value if the dog is to be used as a biological test animal.

Penicillium viridicatum Toxins

The storage mold *Penicillium viridicatum* can grow on corn, barley, wheat, rice oats, and decaying vegetation when the moisture content is 17%–22% and the temperature is 4°–30° C (optimum 23° C). Under these conditions the mold elaborates several toxic factors. One factor, *citrinin,* is thought to be the cause of mold nephrosis in swine in Denmark. Other factors in clude *ochratoxins, oxalic acid,* and an *unidentified factor* present in Indiana isolates of *P. viridicatum.*

So far, *P. viridicatum* has not been incriminated in natural outbreaks of nephrosis in the United States. Nevertheless, Indiana isolates of the mold are toxic when fed to pigs and mice. Sooner or later the natural disease will be recognized in the United States.

Results of experimental feeding of toxic isolates of *P. viridicatum* are presented by Carlton et al. (1973), Carlton et al. (1974), McCracken et al. (1974a–d), and Zwicker et al. (1974). The toxicity and pathology of individual toxins such as citrinin and ochratoxin A are under study (Thacker et al. 1975; Kitchen et al. 1975).

In swine the clinical signs of *P. viridicatum* mold nephrosis are anorexia, depression, posterior paralysis, ventral abdominal distension, and edema. The lesions are of a generalized edema, especially perirenal edema, with variable amounts of blood in the transudate around the kidneys.

The signs and lesions mimic those of pigweed *(Amaranthus retroflexus)* poisoning, which occurs mainly in larger swine in the summer months, and edema disease, which occurs in weanling pigs and is characterized by facial edema, encephalomalacia, and necrotic arteritis not seen in pigs fed *P. viridicatum*. The signs and lesions also mimic those of poisoning by ethylene glycol or oxalate-containing plants, which cause deposition of calcium oxalate crystals in the kidneys.

Diagnosis of *P. viridicatum* mold nephrosis depends on integration of history of moldy feed ingestion, clinical signs, lesions, and results of laboratory testing. There is no specific test for all the *P. viridicatum* toxins at present. When mice are fed the suspect mold, they develop renal and hepatic damage. The hepatic damage is ascribed to the unknown toxin produced by *P. viridicatum* (Carlton et al. 1973).

There is no reason to think that swine are the only species that might be affected by *P. viridicatum* toxins under natural conditions.

Plant Poisons

Some of the hepatotoxic plants already discussed also cause nephrotoxicity. Other nephrotoxic plant poisons are hydroquinone from cocklebur sprouts *(Xanthium* spp.); tannic acid from oaks and acorns (*Quercus* spp.); unidentified principles in drymary (*Drymaria* spp.) and pigweed *(Amaranthus retroflexus);* and soluble oxalates in beet (*Beta* spp.), halogeton (*Halogeton* spp.), sorrell (*Oxalis* spp.), purslane (*Portulaca* sp.), rhubarb (*Rheum* spp.), dock (*Rumex* spp.), Russian thistle *(Salsola* sp.), and greaseweed (*Sarcobatus* sp.).

Although many of the poisons discussed in this text can cause abdominal distresss, this chapter attempts to point out some poisons for which abdominal distress (i.e., colic, diarrhea) is very striking. When one excludes poisonous plants (which are generally not readily eaten by animals) and organic fungicides and herbicides (which are relatively nontoxic), it is obvious that only a few poisons need to be considered in the abdominal distress category.

Unfortunately, there are no rigid separations between poisons causing intense colic and those that damage the liver and kidney. Thus arsenic, thallium, and urea may cause renal and hepatic damage in addition to severe colic, and the hepatotoxic and nephrotoxic poisons may cause abdominal distress. The situation is rendered even more confusing by the fact that poisons such as zinc phosphide, copper, lead, selenium, carbon tetrachloride, and several others may cause a host of signs and lesions including colic, liver malfunction, and renal impairment.

Fortunately, each poison produces its own more or less characteristic "fingerprint"of history, signs, and lesions. Thus we are not limited to clinical signs alone when diagnosing a toxicosis.

REFERENCES

Allcroft, R., and Roberts, B. A. 1968. Toxic groundnut meal: The relationship between aflatoxin B, intake by cows and excretion of aflatoxin M in milk. Vet Rec 82:116.

Alleva, F. R.; Balazs, T.; Sager, A. O.; and Done, A. K. 1975. Failure of thioctic acid to cure mushroom-poisoned mice and dogs. Abstr 14th Ann Meet Soc Toxicol, Williamsburg, Va., Mar. 9–13, 1975.

Bassir, O., and Bababunmi, E. A. 1973. The binding of aflatoxin B with serum albumin. Biochem Pharmacol 22:132.

Berg, G. L., ed. 1974. Farm Chemicals Handbook 1974. Willoughby, Ohio: Meister.

Brown, B. R.; Sipes, I. G.; and Sagalyn, A. M. 1974. Mechanisms of acute hepatic toxicity: Chloroform, halothane, and glutathione. Anesthesiology 41:554.

Buck, W. B.; Osweiler, G. D.; and Van Gelder, G. A. 1973. Clinical and Diagnostic Veterinary Toxicology. Dubuque, Iowa: Kendall/Hunt.

Burger, K. 1973. Organic Reagents in Metal Analysis. Elmsford, N.Y.: Pergamon Press.

Carlton, W. W.; Tuite, J.; and Caldwell, R. 1973. *Penicillium viridicatum* toxins and mold nephrosis. J Am Vet Med Assoc 163: 1295.

Carlton, W. W.; Sansing, G.; Szczech, G. M.; and Tuite, J. 1974. Citrinin mycotoxicosis in beagle dogs. Food Cosmet Toxicol 12:479.

Cavieres, J. D., and Ellory, J. C. 1974. Thallium and the sodium pump in human red cells. J Physiol 243:243.

Chesney, C. F., and Allen, J. R. 1973. Resistance of the guinea pig to pyrrolizidine alkaloid intoxication. Toxicol Appl Pharmacol 26:385.

Ciegler, A. 1975. Mycotoxins: Occurrence, chemistry, biological activity. Lloydia 38: 21.

Clarke, E. G. C., and Clarke, M. L. 1967. Garner's Veterinary Toxicology, 3rd ed. Baltimore: Williams & Wilkins.

Clarkson, T. W., and DiStefano, V. 1971. Lead, mercury, arsenic, and chelating agents. In J. R. DiPalma, ed. Drill's Pharmacology in Medicine, 4th ed. New York: McGraw-Hill.

Detroy, R. W.; Lillehoj, E. B.; and Ciegler, A. 1971. Aflatoxin and related compounds. In A. Ciegler, S. Kadis, and S. J. Ajl, eds. Microbial Toxins, vol. 6. New York: Academic Press.

Doherty, W. P., and Campbell, T. C. 1972. Inhibition of rat liver mitochondria electron transport flow by aflatoxin B_1. Res Commun Chem Pathol Pharmacol 3:601.

Edds, G. T. 1973. Acute aflatoxicosis: A review. J Am Vet Med Assoc 162:304.

Garrett, W. N.; Heitman, H. Jr.; and Booth, A. N. 1968. Aflatoxin toxicity in beef cattle. Proc Soc Exp Biol Med 127:188.

Gehring, P. J., and Hammond, P. B. 1967. The interrelationship between thallium and potassium in animals. J Pharmacol Exp Ther 155:187.

Gibson, G. E.; Zimber, A.; Krook, L.; Richardson, E. P., Jr.; and Visek, W. J. 1974. Brain histology and behavior of mice injected with urease. J Neuropathol Exp Neurol 33:201.

Gillette, J. R.; Mitchell, J. R.; and Brodie, B. B. 1974. Biochemical mechanisms of drug toxicity. Annu Rev Pharmacol 14:271.

Grunert, R. R. 1960. The effect of *dl*-α-lipoic acid on heavy-metal intoxication in mice and dogs. Arch Biochem Biophys 86:190.

Gumbmann, M. R., and Williams, S. N. 1969. Biochemical effects of aflatoxin in pigs. Toxicol Appl Pharmacol 15:393.

Gurtoo, H. L., and Dahms, R. 1974. On the nature of the binding of aflatoxin B_{2a} to rat hepatic microsomes. Res Commun Chem Pathol Pharmacol 9:107.

Hammond, P. B. 1965. Toxic minerals: Arsenic, fluorine, selenium, lead, thallium, nitrates. In L. M. Jones, ed. Veterinary Pharmacology and Therapeutics, 3rd ed. Ames: Iowa State Univ. Press.

Harvey, S. C. 1970. Heavy metals. In L. S. Goodman and A. Gilman, eds. The Pharmacological Basis of Therapeutics, 4th ed. New York: Macmillan.

Hatch, R. C., and Funnell, H. S. 1969. Inorganic arsenic levels in tissues and ingesta of poisoned cattle: An eight-year survey. Can Vet J 10:117.

Hatfield, G. M., and Brady, L. R. 1975. Toxins of higher fungi. Lloydia 38:36.

Hayes, A. W., and Hannan, C. J. 1973. Effect of rubratoxin and aflatoxin on oxygen consumption of krebs cycle intermediates. Toxicol Appl Pharmacol 25:30.

Hayes, A. W., and McCain, H. W. 1975. A procedure for the extraction and estimation of rubratoxin B from corn. Food Cosmet Toxicol 13:221.

Hayes, A. W.; Neville, J. A.; and Hollingsworth, E. B. 1973. Acute toxicity of rubratoxin B in dogs. Toxicol Appl Pharmacol 25:606.

Hood, R. D.; Innes, J. E.; and Hayes, A. W. 1973. Effects of rubratoxin B on prenatal development in mice. Bull Environ Contam Toxicol 10:200.

Hooper, P. T. 1972. Spongy degeneration in the brain in relation to hepatic disease and ammonia toxicity in domestic animals. Vet Rec 90:37.

Jerina, D. M., and Daly, J. W. 1974. Arene oxides: A new aspect of drug metabolism. Science 185:573.

John, D. W., and Miller, L. L. 1969. Effect of aflatoxin B_1 on net synthesis of albumin, fibrinogen, and a_1-acid glycoprotein by the isolated perfused rat liver. Biochem Pharmacol 18:1135.

Jones, L. M., ed. 1965. Veterinary Pharmacology and Therapeutics, 3rd ed. Ames: Iowa State Univ. Press.

Kingsbury, J. M. 1964. Poisonous Plants of the United States and Canada. Englewood Cliffs, N.J.: Prentice-Hall.

Kitchen, D. N.; Carlton, W. W.; and Sansing, G. N. 1975. Ochratoxin A and citrinin-induced nephropathy in beagle dogs. Abstr 14th Ann Meet Soc Toxicol, Williamsburg, Va., Mar. 9–13, 1975.

Kromann, R. P.; Joyner, A. E.; and Sharp, J. E. 1971. Influence of certain nutritional and physiological factors on urea toxicity in sheep. J Anim Sci 32:732.

Levine, W. G. 1970. Heavy-metal antagonists. In L. S. Goodman and A. Gilman, eds. The Pharmacological Basis of Therapeutics, 4th ed. New York: Macmillan.

Lillehoj, E. B. 1973. Feed sources and conditions conducive to production of aflatoxin, ochratoxin, *Fusarium* toxins, and zearalenone. J Am Vet Med Assoc 163:1281.

McBarron, E. J., and McInnes, P. 1968. Observations on urea toxicity in sheep. Aust Vet J 44:90.

McCracken, M. D.; Carlton, W. W.; and Tuite, J. 1974a. *Penicillium viridicatum* mycotoxicosis in the rat. I. Ocular lesions. Food Cosmet Toxicol 12:79.

———. 1974b. *Penicillium veridicatum* mycotoxicosis in the rat. II. Scrotal lesions. Food Cosmet Toxicol 12:89.

———. 1974c. *Pencillium viridicatum* mycotoxicosis in the rat. III. Hepatic and gastric lesions. Food Cosmet Toxicol 12:99.

———. 1974d. *Penicillium viridicatum* mycotoxicosis in the rat. IV. Attempts to modify the tissue responses. Food Cosmet Toxicol 12:331.

McGrath, J. P. M.; Duncan, J. R.; and Munnell, J. F. 1975. *Crotalaria spectabilis* toxicity in swine: Characterization of the renal glomerular lesion. J Comp Pathol 85:185.

McLean, E. K. 1970. The toxic actions of pyrrolizidine (senecio) alkaloids. Pharmacol Rev 22:429.

Mgbodile, M. U. K.; Holscher, M.; and Neal, R. A. 1975. A possible protective role for reduced glutathione in aflatoxin B_1 toxicity: Effect of pretreatment of rats with phenobarbital and 3-methylcholanthrene on aflatoxin toxicity. Toxicol Appl Pharmacol 34:128.

Mitchell, J. R.; Thorgeirsson, S. S.; Potter, W. Z.; Jollow, D. J.; and Keiser, H. 1974. Acetaminophen-induced hepatic injury: Protective role of glutathione in man and rationale for therapy. Clin Pharmacol Ther 16:676.

Moss, M. O. 1971. The rubratoxins, toxic metabolites of *Penicillium rubrum* stoll. In A. Ciegler, S. Kadis, and S. J. Ajl, eds. Microbial Toxins, vol. 6. New York: Academic Press.

Munro, I. C.; Scott, P. M.; Moodie, C. A; and Willes, R. F. 1973. Ochratoxin A—Occurrence and toxicity. J Am Vet Med Assoc 163:1269.

Munro, I. C.; Moodie, C. A.; Kuiper-Goodman, T.; Scott, P. M.; and Grice, H. C. 1974. Toxicologic changes in rats fed graded dietary levels of ochratoxin A. Toxicol Appl Pharmacol 28:180.

Newberne, P. M. 1973. Chronic aflatoxicosis. J Am Vet Med Assoc 163:1262.

Newberne, P. M.; Chan, W.-C.M.; and Rogers, A. E. 1974. Influence of light, riboflavin, and carotene on the response of rats to the acute toxicity of aflatoxin and monocrotaline. Toxicol Appl Pharmacol 28:200.

Paik, W. K.; Lawson, D.; and Kim S. 1974. Effect of endocrine glands on the protection of rat from ammonia intoxication. Life Sci 15:1189.

Palmer, J. S. 1963. Mercurial fungicidal seed protectant toxic for sheep and chickens. J Am Vet Med Assoc 142:1385.

Palmer, J. S.; Wright, F. C.; and Haufler, M. 1973. Toxicologic and residual aspects of an alkyl mercury fungicide to cattle, sheep, and turkeys. Clin Toxicol 6:425.

Peckham, J. C.; Sangster, L. T.; and Jones, O. H. 1974. *Crotalaria spectabilis* poisoning in swine. J Am Vet Med Assoc 165:633.

Pier, A. C. 1973. Effects of aflatoxin on immunity. J Am Vet Med Assoc 163:1268.

Raabe, W., and Gumnit, R. J. 1975. Disinhibition in cat motor cortex by ammonia. J Neurophysiol 38:347.

Radeleff, R. D. 1970. Veterinary Toxicology, 2nd ed. Philadelphia: Lea & Febiger.

Rauws, A. G. 1974. Thallium pharmacokinetics and its modification by Prussian blue. Naunyn Schmiedebergs Arch Pharmacol 284:295.

Rauws, A. G.; Ham, M. T.; and Kamerbeek, H. H. 1969. Influence of the antidote dithiocarb on distribution and toxicity of thallium in the rat. Arch Int Pharmacodyn Ther 182:425.

Reid, W. D.; Krishna, G.; Gillette, J. R.; and Brodie, B. B. 1973. Biochemical mechanism of hepatic necrosis induced by aromatic hydrocarbons. Pharmacology 10:193.

Richard, J. L. 1973. Mycotoxin photosensitivity. J Am Vet Med Assoc 163:1298.

Roberge, A., and Charbonneau, R. 1968. Metabolism of ammonia. I. Biochemical aspect of ammonia intoxication. Rev Can Biol 27:321.

Singer, R. H., and McCarty, R. T. 1971a. Acute ammonium salt poisoning in sheep. Am J Vet Res 32:1229.

———. 1971b. Pathologic changes resulting from acute ammonium salt poisoning in sheep. Am J Vet Res 32:1239.

Smith, H. A.; Jones, T. C.; and Hunt, R. D. 1972. Veterinary Pathology, 4th ed. Philadelphia: Lea & Febiger.

Sollmann, T. 1957. A Manual of Pharmacology and Its Application to Therapeutics and Toxicology, 8th ed. Philadelphia: W. B. Saunders.

Stavinoha, W. B.; Emerson, G. A.; and Nash, J. B. 1959. The effects of some sulfur compounds on thallotoxicosis in mice. Toxicol Appl Pharmacol 1:638.

Stecher, P. G., ed. 1968. The Merck Index, 8th ed. Rahway, N. J.: Merck.

Stevens, W.; van Peteghem, C.; Heyndrickx, A.; and Barbier, F. 1974. Eleven cases of thallium intoxication treated with Prussian blue. Int J Clin Pharmacol 10:1.

Steyn, P. S. 1971. Ochratoxin and other dihydroisocoumarins. In A. Ciegler, S. Kadis, and S. J. Ajl, eds. Microbial Toxins, vol. 6. New York: Academic Press.

Steyn, P. S.; Vleggaar, R.; DuPreez, N. P.; Blyth, A. A.; and Seegers, J. C. 1975. The *in vitro* toxicity of analogs of ochratoxin A in monkey kidney epithelial cells. Toxicol Appl Pharmacol 32:198.

Suzuki, S.; Satoh, T.; and Yamazaki, M. 1975. Effect of ochratoxin A on carbohydrate metabolism in rat liver. Toxicol Appl Pharmacol 32:116.

Szabuniewicz, M.; Bailey, E. M.; and Wiersig, D. O. 1971. Treatment of some common poisonings in animals. Vet Med Small Anim Clin 66: 1197.

Szczech, G. M.; Carlton, W. W.; Tuite, J.; and Caldwell, R. 1973. Ochratoxin A toxicosis in swine. Vet Pathol 10:347.

Szczech, G. M.; Carlton, W. W.; and Hinsman, E. J. 1974. Ochratoxicosis in beagle dogs. III. Terminal renal ultrastructural alterations. Vet Pathol 11:385.

Taylor, A. 1971. The toxicology of sporidesmins and other epipolythiadioxopiperazines. In S. Kadis, A. Ciegler, and S. J. Ajl, eds. Microbial Toxins, vol. 7. New York: Academic Press.

Thacker, H. L.; Carlton, W. W.; and Sansing, G. N. 1975. Toxicity of citrinin and ochratoxin A in guinea pigs. Abstr 14th Ann Meet Soc Toxicol, Williamsburg, Va., Mar. 9–13, 1975.

Thurston, J. R.; Deyoe, B. L.; Baetz, A. L.; Richard, J. L.; and Booth, G. D. 1974. Effect of aflatoxin on serum proteins, complement activity, and the antibody response to *Brucella abortus* in guinea pigs. Am J Vet Res 35:1097.

Wessel, J. R., and Stoloff, L. 1973. Regulatory surveillance for aflatoxin and other mycotoxins in feeds, meat, and milk. J Am Vet Med Assoc 163:1284.

Wieland, T. 1968. Poisonous principles of mushrooms of the genus *Amanita.* Science 159:946.

Wilson, B. J., and Harbison, R. D. 1973. Rubratoxins. J Am Vet Med Assoc 163: 1274.

Wilson, R. P.; Davis, L. E.; Muhrer, M. E.; and Bloomfield, R. A. 1968. Toxicologic effects of ammonium carbamate and related compounds. Am J Vet Res 29:897.

Wogan, G. N. 1974. Biochemical effects of aflatoxins. Isr J Med Sci 10:441.

———. 1975. Mycotoxins. Annu Rev Pharmacol 15:437.

Wogan, G. N., and Shank, R. C. 1971. Toxicity and carcinogenicity of aflatoxins. Adv Environ Sci Technol 2:321.

Wogan, G. N.; Edwards, G. S.; and Newberne, P. M. 1971. Acute and chronic toxicity of rubratoxin B. Toxicol Appl Pharmacol 19:712.

Yelverton, C. C.; Roller, M. H.; and Swanson, R. N. 1975. Ammonium nitrogen in fetuses of urea-treated sheep. Am J Vet Res 36:191.

Zook, B. C., and Gilmore, C. E. 1967. Thallium poisoning in dogs. J Am Vet Med Assoc 151:206.

Zook, B. C.; Holzworth, J.; and Thornton, G. W. 1968. Thallium poisoning in cats. J Am Vet Med Assoc 153:285.

Zwicker, G. M.; Carlton, W. W.; and Tuite, J. 1974. Long-term administration of sterigmatocystin and *Penicillium viridicatum* to mice. Food Cosmet Toxicol 2:491.

CHAPTER 60

POISONS CAUSING LAMENESS OR VISIBLE DISFIGUREMENT

ROGER C. HATCH

POISONS CAUSING BONE, TOOTH, HOOF, AND HAIR ABNORMALITIES

FLUORIDE (CHRONIC POISONING)

USE

Whereas acute poisoning by fluorides is related to the use of inorganic and organic fluoride compounds as anthelmintics or rodenticides (see Fluoride [Acute Poisoning] and Fluoroacetate and Fluoroacetamide in Chapter 58), chronic fluoride poisoning (fluorosis) is simply due to prolonged ingestion of excessive amounts of fluorides in feed or water. Another kind of fluoride toxicosis relates to the use of fluorinated inhalant anesthetics such as methoxyflurane and is discussed in Chapter 12.

SOURCE

Fluoride is a normal constituent of forages (especially legumes) and plants that grow in soils rich in fluoride. Grain seeds do not accumulate excessive amounts of fluoride, but herbaceous parts of plants can do so. Natural sources of fluoride are fluorspar (CaF_2), cryolite (Na_3AlF_6), apatite ($CaF_2 \cdot 3Ca_3[PO_4]_2$), and rock phosphate ($CaHPO_4$) with which fluoride associates. Natural waters may contain dissolved fluoride.

Feed and mineral supplements may contain added fluoride, generally associated with rock phosphate.

Pastures can be contaminated with fluoride fallout from nearby industries.

PROPERTIES OF TOXICOLOGIC IMPORTANCE

Fluoride is a highly reactive halogen. It is the most electronegative of the elements and it forms compounds with a variety of other inorganic and organic materials. Fluoride has a strong affinity for calcium, iron, and aluminum.

TOXICITY

The chronic toxicity of fluoride depends on the type and solubility of the compound (soluble NaF is more toxic than CaF_2), the amount ingested, the duration of exposure, the rate of excretion, the age of the animal (young, developing bones and teeth are more susceptible), the nutritional level, the presence of stress factors such as cold or drought, and individual variation in susceptibility. Moreover, ingestion of natural sources of fluoride can enhance the effects of additional fluoride in the body because the element accumulates in bone and teeth. There are also species differences in susceptibility to fluoride. All these factors make it difficult to state absolute toxicity data for chronic poisoning.

The normal intake of fluoride over the lifetime of various species is (in ppm of the dry ration): dairy cow or heifer, 30; beef cow or steer, 40; sheep, 50; pig, 70; horse, 90; turkey, 100; and chicken, 150 (Buck et al. 1973). Cattle and sheep can tolerate 110 ppm over the short interval of fattening.

Fluorosis can occur in mild form in cattle if the diet contains 40 ppm fluoride as NaF. With sheep, 10 ppm of fluoride in the drinking water can cause fluorosis (decreased wool, dental lesions) within 7 years. Fluoride from rock phosphate can cause mild fluorosis in cattle if ingested at a concentration of 100 ppm in the dry ration over a period of 3–5.5 years. Fluorosis from rock phosphate occurs at a dietary fluoride concentration of 350 ppm in chicks and 530 ppm in laying hens (Clarke and Clarke 1967).

TOXICODYNAMIC CONSIDERATIONS

Soluble fluorides are readily absorbed from the intestinal tract and distributed throughout the body. Bone is a natural "sink" for fluoride, just as for lead. In fact, 95%–96% of the body burden of fluoride is in bones and teeth. Tissue fluoride concentration may be elevated only 2–3 times normal in cases of fluorosis. Fluoride is gradually excreted in the urine. Milk fluoride is not readily absorbed. The fetus gains fluoride but is apparently not affected. Unabsorbed fluoride is eliminated in the feces (Hammond 1965; Clarke and Clarke 1967; Buck et al. 1973).

MECHANISM OF ACTION

Bone and teeth can hold only so much fluoride, and only so much can be excreted in the urine. If fluoride intake is constant, pathologic changes develop in bones and teeth, and there are secondary signs and lesions due to the bone and tooth lesions.

In people that have bone-rarefactive disease, chronic administration of sodium fluoride promotes calcium retention. The bones increase in crystallinity and fluoride content (Welt and Blythe 1970). This observation may not have anything to do with fluorosis in animals, but the implication is that the bone lesions of fluorosis in animals could be due in part to a defect in calcium excretion or osteoclast activity. Fluoride is thought to replace the hydroxyl groups of hydroxyapatite, thus altering the crystal structure and crystal lattice dimensions of bone apatite. Mineralization of preenamel, predentine, precementum, and preskeletal matrices may be delayed due to damage to blast cells (Buck et al. 1973).

Fluoride may also inhibit certain enzymes required for bone and tooth formation. It is known that a number of enzymes are inhibited by fluorides. There is a decrease in production of phosphopyruvate, which is a substrate for bone phosphatase (Sollmann 1957).

Fluorosis may involve ascorbate metabolism. In monkeys, fluoride causes typical bone lesions but the lesions regress and may disappear during 12 weeks of continuous ascorbate therapy. Moreover, guinea pigs fed a diet high in fluoride develop "scurvy" and adrenal enlargement even if the diet contains ascorbate. Fluoride may prevent utilization of ascorbate (Sollmann 1957).

Further research is needed to determine the pathogenesis of fluorosis.

CLINICAL SIGNS

There is a 6-month to 1-year or more onset of periodic lameness; painful, stiff gait or posture; decreased feed intake; anorexia; rough haircoat; emaciation; and decreased milk production. Bony exostoses may be seen or felt on the legs, and the teeth have a characteristic mottling and patchy loss of dentine. The teeth also become stained brown around eroded areas, and they wear unevenly. Spontaneous fractures may occur.

LESIONS

The dental lesions are most severe in developing teeth. The bone lesions begin bilaterally on the medial side of the proximal third of the metatarsals of cattle. The lesions consist of hyperostosis, porosis, enlargement, chalky white appearance, and roughening. The lesions progress to the mandible, metacarpals, ribs, and spine. There is spurring and bridging of joints, but the articular surfaces are not involved.

Microscopically, bone manifests a thick cortex due to periosteal hyperostosis, uneven mineralization, zones of immature bone, reabsorption on the endosteal surfaces, and excess osteoid tissue (Radeleff 1970; Buck et al. 1973).

DIFFERENTIAL DIAGNOSIS

The history, signs, and lesions are not generally confused with other conditions in regions known to be contaminated by fluoride. Vitamin deficiency or parathyroid disease might be considered, but laboratory tests for urinary fluoride will rule out these conditions.

TREATMENT

No specific treatment exists at present. There is no known way to mobilize fluoride from bone. Tolerance to fluoride can be increased by a balanced intake of calcium, phosphate, and vitamin D (Hammond 1965). Aluminum salts, calcium carbonate, and defluorinated phosphate can be administered orally to form insoluble compounds with fluoride in the gut. The feed or water containing excess fluoride can be diluted with feed or roughage that is low in fluoride (Buck et al. 1973).

Supportive therapy might include steroids, antibiotics, analgesics, and fluid therapy. Vitamin C in large dosages could possibly help some animals if the intake of fluoride is stopped, but this is merely speculation.

ANALYSIS

The safe concentration of fluoride in the total ration of several species is (in ppm from NaF and rock phosphate, respectively): dairy cow, 30–50 and 60–100; beef cow, 40–50 and 65–100; sheep, 70–100 and 100–120; pig, 70–100 and 100–120; chicken, 150–300 and 300–400; and turkey, 300–400 (NaF) (Hammond 1965). The same reference lists safe fluoride concentrations in mineral mixtures as: cattle, 0.3%; sheep, 0.35%; pig, 0.45%; and poultry, 0.6%.

Pasture contaminated with 25–50 ppm of fluoride (dry weight basis) is potentially dangerous for grazing animals (Clarke and Clarke 1967).

In 2- to 6-year-old dairy cattle with moderate fluorosis, the urine contains 15–20 ppm of fluoride, and excretion is elevated for several months. The normal fluoride concentration in bovine urine is 2–6 ppm. The fluorotic cattle have 3000 ppm or more of fluoride in affected bone. Normal bone fluoride concentration is 400–1200 (possibly up to 2000) ppm or less. Teeth of fluorotic sheep contain 5000 ppm fluoride or more. Normal fluoride concentration in sheep teeth is about 250 ppm (all bone and teeth values are on a dry weight, fat-free basis) (Hammond 1965; Radeleff 1970; Buck et al. 1973).

Urine fluoride concentration can vary. Thus several animals in a herd should be tested whenever fluorosis is suspected.

SELENIUM (CHRONIC POISONING)

In Chapter 57, selenosis is discussed in detail. It is pointed out that in the chronic form of selenosis ("alkali disease") lameness and hoof and hair abnormalities are evident in addition to partial blindness, paresis, incoordination, emaciation, lethargy, and peripheral circulatory insufficiency.

The lameness seen in chronic selenosis is due to erosion of the articular surfaces of long bones and also to painful separation of the hoof wall just below the coronary band. The hoof begins to shed. Shedding may be incomplete, and the old hoof may fuse with new hoof to form an abnormally long rocker-shaped hoof. The fetus may also develop abnormal joints and hooves. The chick embryo may be deformed.

In chronic selenosis, long hair is lost from the tail and mane, and the haircoat is rough.

Other lesions and the possible biochemical basis of selenosis are presented in Chapter 57.

Diagnosis of chronic selenosis is not difficult. The condition occurs in horses, cattle, sheep, and swine raised in arid and semiarid regions in which forage or feed may contain excess selenium.

For details see Hammond (1965), Clarke and Clarke (1967), Radeleff (1970), Smith et al. (1972), and Buck et al. (1973).

Other Elements

LEAD

In young dogs poisoned by lead over a period of several days or weeks, there may be delayed closure of thoracic vertebral epiphyses and radio-opacity of metaphyses. The bone marrow may be very red. These phenomena are helpful in the diagnosis of lead poisoning in young dogs (Chapter 58).

CADMIUM

Among the lesions of experimentally induced chronic cadmium poisoning in rats is a rapid bleaching of the incisor teeth (Clarke and Clarke 1967).

MOLYBDENUM

This element is discussed elsewhere in this text and also by Clarke and Clarke (1967) and Buck et al. (1973). Excessive intake of molybdenum (or deficiency of copper) causes a rough, dry haircoat; depigmentation of hair; osteoporosis and other osteodystrophic and joint changes; lameness; and stunting in several species. Ruminants are particularly sensitive.

THALLIUM

Alopecia is typical of thallium poisoning and is one of the criteria for diagnosis of the condition in dogs and cats. Reddening and secondary bacterial infection of the skin are also seen. See Chapter 59 for details.

Plant Poisons

In Europe, osteolathyrism is a condition of bone deformity caused by toxic principles in sweet peas (*Lathyrus* spp.). Sorghums (*Sorghum* spp.) may contain lathyrogenic nitriles that affect horses (see Van Kampen 1970; Barrow et al. 1974). In Florida, the day-blooming jessamine (*Cestrum diurnum*) has been incriminated in a condition in horses that is characterized by weight loss; lameness; generalized osteopetrosis; calcification of arteries, tendons, and ligaments; and hypercalcemia (Krook et al. 1975). The plant contains a potent substance similar to vitamin D. The lead tree (*Leucaena glauca*) grows in coastal plains from Florida to Texas and in Hawaii. It contains mimosine, an amino acid that causes loss of hair, poor condition, and a slow rate of weight gain in a number of species (Kingsbury 1964).

POISONS CAUSING LESIONS ON SKIN AND MUCOUS MEMBRANES

Corrosives

It hardly seems necessary to say that skin and mucous membranes can be badly damaged by corrosive effects of strong acids, alkalis, or concentrated chemicals. The same points are made in Chapter 59 where the gastrointestinal (GI) tract is the focus of attention. Corrosive lesions on skin and external mucous membranes are irrigated and then treated with neutralizing agents, protective demulcents, and antibiotics. Care must be taken not to "seal in" the irritant with topical dressings.

Chlorinated Naphthalenes

Polychlorinated naphthalenes such as tri-, penta-, hexa-, and octachloronaphthalene were formerly present in lubrication greases and oils and in wood preservatives. Some of these materials may still be around.

In cattle, chlorinated naphthalenes cause severe hyperkeratosis, similar to that of avitaminosis A. It is believed that the poison interferes with utilization of vitamin A and with metabolism of vitamin C. The lesions are generally on the neck and withers but may affect the entire integument. Other signs include depression, variable appetite, lacrimation, salivation, watery nasal discharge, diarrhea, polyuria, red swollen areas in the mouth and on the muzzle, and weight loss (Clarke and Clarke 1967; Radeleff 1970).

In sheep and swine, hyperkeratosis is not seen. These species manifest nonspecific signs such as anorexia, weakness, loss of weight, and nasal discharge. Liver and kidney damage may occur in all species.

Treatment of hyperkeratosis is purely supportive. Antibiotics can be used to prevent bacterial infection. Vitamins A and C should be administered, along with B-complex vitamins. Corticosteroids may be of some benefit. The skin should be kept as pliable as possible and free from flies and ectoparasites.

Other Chemicals

ORGANOMERCURIALS

These are discussed in Chapters 58 and 59. In adult cattle, organomercury poisoning may cause skin manifestations such as eczema, itchiness, pustules, ulcers, hyperkeratinization, and depilation of the tailhead. In swine, there may be red spots on the skin, hyperkeratinization, and ventral abdominal cyanosis. Petechial hemorrhages may occur in mucous membranes. Cattle and swine manifest a number of other signs and lesions of organomercury poisoning. Thus there is little confusion of the condition with other diseases of the skin and mucous membranes.

THALLIUM

The skin is reddened and the hair is lost in dogs and cats poisoned by thallium.

POLYBROMINATED BIPHENYLS

This flame-retardant mixture was accidentally mixed with feeds in Michigan. Losses due to condemnation amounted to 30,000 livestock, nearly 1.6 million poultry, 5 million eggs, 3000 lb of butter, 34,000 lb of dry milk, 18,000 lb of cheese, and 788 tons of contaminated feed (Dunckel 1975). Poisoning in cattle is characterized by initial anorexia and decreased milk production, lameness, and estrus difficulties. Later, there are hematomas or abscesses on the back, under the vulva, along the abdominal veins, and in the hind limbs. Weight loss is marked. Two months after exposure there is abnormal hoof growth (long, curled hooves), matting of hair on the thorax, and alopecia. Hyperkeratosis develops. Liver and kidney damage is seen. The toxicosis is responsive to vitamin A therapy (Jackson and Halbert 1974).

Mold Toxins

ERGOT ALKALOIDS

The ergot alkaloids discussed in Chapter 58, if ingested over a period of several days or weeks, can cause dry gangrene (so-called gangrenous ergotism). All species are susceptible, and the parasitic fungus involved is usually *Claviceps purpurea.* Early signs of gangrenous ergotism are lameness, painful stance or treading and stamping of the feet, and cool extremities. There is a well-defined, constricted band between normal skin and distal parts of the limbs. The ears, nose, and tail are also affected. Pregnant animals may abort. Sows may deliver some live pigs but may be unable to nurse them because the ergot alkaloids also cause agalactia. The distal extremities, tail, ears, and nose slough away, leaving a clean surface that may ooze serum and become encrusted. Secondary bacterial infection readily occurs.

The mechanism by which ergot alkaloids block the blood supply of the extremities is a combination of arteriolar vasoconstriction, damage to capillary endothelium, vascular thrombosis, and stasis of blood.

Treatment of this form of ergotism consists of early detection of clinical signs and removal of the offending feed. The animals should be kept warm to avoid cold-induced vasoconstriction in the extremities. Necrotic lesions are treated with antibacterial agents. Flies and ectoparasites should be kept away from the lesions. Digits and hooves cannot, of course, be replaced.

SATRATOXINS

These mold toxins are also discussed in Chapter 58. They are apparently trichothecene compounds (as are T-2 toxin and diacetoxyscirpenol) and they share with the latter toxins the ability to irritate the skin and mucous membranes on contact. Foci or large areas of necrosis, stomatitis, and mouth fissures develop. Satratoxins are not yet recognized as toxicologic problems in the United States.

BUTENOLIDE

Fescue foot is a condition that closely mimics the peripheral dry gangrene of chronic ergotism in cattle. It occurs in cattle that graze tall fescue grass. Presumably, cold weather favors peripheral vasoconstriction and also toxicity of tall fescue.

According to Yates (1971), fescue foot may be due to ingestion of patches of grass that are infected or metabolically altered by a mold. One mold of interest is *Fusarium tricinctum,* but other molds, particularly those in the family Clavicipitaceae, may be involved too. Isolates of *F. tricinctum* obtained from toxic pastures produce three toxins. One of these, T-2 toxin, is produced in small amounts only and does not cause dry gangrene in animals. Another as yet unidentified toxin is produced in small amounts only. The third toxin is produced in large amounts under controlled conditions. This toxin, which Yates calls "the butenolide," is 4-acetamido-4-hydroxy-2-butenoic acid γ-lactone.

Intramuscular injection of butenolide for 90 days caused necrosis and sloughing of the tail of a heifer (Yates 1971). Oral administration of extracts of moldy fescue hay did not cause signs of fescue foot but did kill cattle. It is possible that fescue must be alive to cause fescue foot, and that a synergism may exist between the plant's metabolism and butenolide. It is also possible that cold temperatures are required for peripheral vasoconstriction and sloughing of the extremities in some cases of fescue foot.

It has not been stated definitely that butenolide is the cause of fescue foot. Because fescue toxicosis resembles ergotism in many ways, and because molds of the family Clavicipitaceae are known to grow as endophytes within fescue and other grasses, the author believes fescue toxicosis may be due to one or more ergot-type alkaloids or their active metabolites. The mechanisms and factors controlling the development of toxic fescue and fescue foot disease are under investigation.

Details on fescue foot are available (Kingsbury 1964; Clarke and Clarke 1967).

T-2 TOXIN

This trichothecene toxin directly irritates the skin and mucous membranes. Stomatitis, oral ulcers, and necrosis of areas of skin that are contacted by moldy plant materials may be seen in addition to hemorrhagic phenomena (Chapter 57).

DIACETOXYSCIRPENOL

This is another trichothecene toxin produced by *Fusarium tricinctum.* It may cause dermal necrosis and gangrene in addition to nonspecific signs such as diarrhea, milk reduction, and weight loss in cattle fed moldy corn. Other trichothecene toxins, some not mentioned in this text, are also capable of causing skin and mucosal lesions. Information on these toxins is given by Bamburg and Strong (1971).

Photosensitizing Plants and Toxins

A large number of plants can cause skin photosensitivity reactions in herbivores. Light-skinned areas of the nose, face, back, escutcheon, and udder react to sunlight by manifesting reddening, subcutaneous edema due to leakage of serum from damaged capillaries, necrosis, and sloughing. There is intense itching and rubbing, which helps to promote tissue injury and secondary bacterial infection.

The photosensitivity reaction is due to activation by long-wave ultraviolet light of chemical toxins circulating in the skin capillaries. The photodynamic toxins may come directly from the plant (e.g., hypericin from St.-John's-wort—*Hypericum perforatum;* fagopyrin from buckwheat—*Fagopyrum sagittatum;* and furanocoumarins from spring parsley—*Cymopterus watsonii*). More commonly, the photodynamic toxin is a metabolite that is normally excreted in the bile. When the liver is damaged or when bile flow is hindered, these metabolites enter the circulation along with the bile pigments that cause icterus. One of these photodynamic metabolites is the chlorophyll breakdown product phylloerythrin. Perhaps this is the only important photodynamic substance.

It is apparent that nearly any poison that causes icterogenic hepatopathy in chlorophyll-eating animals can cause photosensitivity in light-skinned areas of animals that do not die outright from other metabolic effects of the poison.

Plants capable of causing hepatogenous photosensitivity are listed by Kingsbury (1964). Notable among these plants are ragwort (*Senecio* spp.), which contains pyrrolizidine alkaloids; lantana (*Lantana* spp.), which contains a polycyclic triterpene; horsebrush (*Tetradymia* spp.); lechuguilla *(Agave lecheguilla);* sacahuiste *(Nolina texana);* and blue green algae.

Mold toxins that are icterogenic may cause photosensitivity if animals do not die first (see Sporidesmins in Chapter 59). Drugs and diseases that cause liver damage can also cause photosensitivity.

Treatment of photosensitivity includes removal of the cause, switching to a low-chlorophyll diet (if the condition is hepatogenous), protecting light-skinned areas from sunlight (window glass will not do this), and treating the skin lesions with antibiotics and other supportive therapy. Flies and ectoparasites should be kept away from open lesions. Antipruritic tranquilization may be useful. Healing is slow. Hair or wool may not grow in healed areas.

TERATOGENIC PLANT POISONS

Fetal monsters are not a big problem in veterinary practice, but there are instances when pregnant animals may eat sublethal amounts of toxic plants and then give birth to defective offspring.

According to a recent review (Keeler 1975), plant teratogens include alkaloids in tobacco (*Nicotiana* spp.), mimosine in the lead tree (*Leucaena* sp.), lathyrogens in sweet peas (*Lathyrus* spp.), unknown principles in locoweed (*Astragalus* spp.), alkaloids in lupines (*Lupinus* spp.), coniine in poison hemlock (*Conium maculatum*), and alkaloids in false hellebore (*Veratrum californicum*).

Sorghum grasses (*Sorghum* spp.) are reported to cause lathyritic deformities in foals (Van Kampen 1970), possibly because of their nitrile content. Wild cherry *(Prunus serotina)* may cause deformities in pigs (Selby et al. 1971). Jimsonweed *(Datura stramonium)* can also cause deformities in pigs (Leipold et al. 1973).

Any selenium-accumulating plant may cause hoof abnormalities of the fetus.

It is probable that many other plant poisons are teratogenic. Keeler (1975) reports that fetal malformations can be induced in rats by plant toxins not yet known to cause such problems in domestic animals. This is not surprising when one reflects on the fact that a large number of drugs and chemicals (other than plant poisons) are teratogenic in various species.

Generally speaking, the poisons that cause lameness or visible disfigurement are not an important group of poisons as such, but the group does include some very important poisons (e.g., lead, fluoride, selenium, mold toxins, plants) that cause widespread loss of livestock by mechanisms other than making the animal lame or ugly. Diagnosis of some of these toxicoses is facilitated when one knows the external lesions as well as the internal ones.

REFERENCES

Bamburg, J. R., and Strong, F. M. 1971. 12,13-Epoxytrichothecenes. In S. Kadis, A. Ciegler, and S. J. Ajl, eds. Microbial Toxins, vol. 7. New York: Academic Press.

Barrow, M. V.; Simpson, C. F.; and Miller, E. J. 1974. Lathyrism: A review. Q Rev Biol 49:101.

Buck, W. B.; Osweiler, G. D.; and Van Gelder, G. A. 1973. Clinical and Diagnostic Veterinary Toxicology. Dubuque, Iowa: Kendall/Hunt.

Clarke, E. G. C., and Clarke, M. L. 1967. Garner's Veterinary Toxicology, 3rd ed. Baltimore: Williams & Wilkins.

Dunckel, A. E. 1975. An updating on the polybrominated biphenyl disaster in Michigan. J Am Vet Med Assoc 167:838.

Hammond, P. B. 1965. Toxic minerals: Arsenic, fluorine, selenium, lead, thallium, nitrates. In L. M. Jones, ed. Veterinary Pharmacology and Therapeutics, 3rd ed. Ames: Iowa State Univ. Press.

Jackson, T. F., and Halbert, F. L. 1974. A toxic syndrome associated with the feeding of polybrominated biphenyl-contaminated protein concentrate to diary cattle. J Am Vet Med Assoc 165:437.

Keeler, R. F. 1975. Toxins and teratogens of higher plants. Lloydia 38:56.

Kingsbury, J. M. 1964. Poisonous Plants of the United States and Canada. Englewood Cliffs, N.J.: Prentice-Hall.

Krook, L.; Wasserman, R. H.; Shively, J. N.; Tashjian, A. H., Jr.; Brokken, T. D.; and Morton, J. F. 1975. Hypercalcemia and calcinosis in Florida horses: Implication of the shrub, *Cestrum diurnum,* as the causative agent. Cornell Vet 65:26.

Leipold, H. W.; Oehme, F. W.; and Cook, J. E. 1973. Congenital arthrogryposis associated with ingestion of jimsonweed by pregnant sows. J Am Vet Med Assoc 162:1059.

Radeleff, R. D. 1970. Veterinary Toxicology, 2nd ed. Philadelphia: Lea & Febiger.

Selby, L. A.; Menges, R. W.; Houser, E. C.; Flatt, R. E.; and Case, A. A. 1971. Outbreak of swine malformations associated with the wild black cherry, *Prunus serotina.* Arch Environ Health 22:496.

Smith, H. A.; Jones, T. C.; and Hunt, R. D. 1972. Veterinary Pathology, 4th ed. Philadelphia: Lea & Febiger.

Sollmann, T. 1957. A Manual of Pharmacology and Its Application to Therapeutics and Toxicology, 8th ed. Philadelphia: W. B. Saunders.

Van Kampen, K. R. 1970. Sudan grass and sorghum poisoning of horses: A possible lathyrogenic disease. J Am Vet Med Assoc 156:629.

Welt, L. G., and Blythe, W. B. 1970. Anions: Phosphate, iodide, fluoride, and other anions. In L. S. Goodman and A. Gilman, eds. The Pharmacological Basis of Therapeutics, 4th ed. New York: Macmillan.

Yates, S. G. 1971. Toxin-producing fungi from fescue pasture. In S. Kadis, A. Ciegler, and S. J. Ajl, eds. Microbial Toxins, vol. 7. New York: Academic Press.

CHAPTER 61

POISONS HAVING UNIQUE EFFECTS

ROGER C. HATCH

POISONS CAUSING PERIPHERAL NERVE DEMYELINATION

Organic Arsenicals

USE

Certain organic pentavalent arsenicals are added to swine or poultry feeds to improve weight gain and feed efficiency and to combat enteric infections. Arsanilic acid (*p*-aminobenzenearsonic acid) and its sodium salt are most commonly used, particularly for swine. Roxarsone (3-nitro-4-hydroxyphenylarsonic acid—"3-nitro") and the related compound 4-nitro-phenylarsonic acid ("4-nitro") are used mainly in poultry. Other organic arsenicals are discussed in Chapter 59.

SOURCE

Animals or poultry may be poisoned by the benzenearsonic acid compounds if the feed contains too much of the additive or if antibacterial concentrations are ingested for too long a time. If animals or birds have diarrhea and are debilitated or dehydrated, or if the water supply is restricted, even the recommended concentrations of benzenearsonic acid compounds can cause toxicosis.

PROPERTIES OF TOXICOLOGIC IMPORTANCE

In the benzenearsonic acid compounds, arsenic is in the pentavalent state of oxidation. Bonding of arsenic to a substituted benzene ring, a keto oxygen, and 2 hydroxyl groups seems to confer biological stability and toxic properties not shared by other organic or inorganic arsenicals, benzene, or arsenic itself. This statement requires a qualifier. In calves, large dosages of arsanilic acid can cause signs typical of inorganic arsenic poisoning (Buck et al. 1973). It is possible, therefore, that benzenearsonic acid compounds might be partly broken down by rumen microorganisms.

TOXICITY

According to Buck et al. (1973), the recommended feed concentration of arsanilic acid and its sodium salt, when used to promote growth in swine and poultry, is 50–100 ppm. To control swine dysentery, the recommended concentration is 250–400 ppm, fed 5–6 days. Toxicosis can result in 3–10 days in experimental animals fed 1000 ppm or in 3–6 weeks in pigs fed 250 ppm.

The recommended feed concentration of roxarsone (3-nitro), for growth promotion in chickens and turkeys is 25–50 ppm; in swine it is 25–75 ppm. For the control of swine dysentery, 3-nitro is used at a concentration of 200 ppm for 5–6 days. Toxic signs can develop if pigs are fed 250 ppm of 3-nitro for 3–10 days or 100 ppm for 2 months.

For 4-nitro, the recommended feed concentration to promote weight gains in chickens and turkeys is 188 ppm.

Clarke and Clarke (1967) state that a feed concentration of 2000–4000 ppm of arsanilic acid causes convulsions in lambs. If baby chicks consume 3-nitro at a concentration of 90 ppm, growth is suppressed. If the concentration is 450 ppm, the chicks die. The LD100 of 3-nitro in chicks is about 200 mg/kg of body weight.

The toxicity of benzenearsonic acid compounds is enhanced by dehydration, renal impairment, and insufficient water supply. Thus, under certain conditions of health and husbandry, the therapeutic and toxic concentrations of these compounds can overlap.

TOXICODYNAMIC CONSIDERATIONS

The benzenearsonic acid compounds are poorly absorbed from the normal gastrointestinal (GI) tract. Thus they are excreted mainly in the feces. Some absorption does occur, however. After absorption, the compounds are distributed throughout the body and excreted in the urine without being metabolized to a great extent. Thus adequate urine flow is essential for elimination of benzenearsonic acid compounds from the tissues. Elimination of parenterally injected compound is nearly complete in 24–48 hours, but several days are required for elimination of the compound after absorption from the gut (Buck et al. 1973).

MECHANISM OF ACTION

The polyneuritis that results from overdosage with benzenearsonic acid compounds is very similar to that of vitamin B–complex (B_1, B_6) deficiency. Buck et al. (1973) postulate that benzenearsonic acid compounds may produce such a deficiency, but they stress that this is speculative. Biochemical mechanisms of neural demyelination and axonal damage are not known. A Nobel Prize awaits the person who unravels the mysteries of demyelinating diseases.

CLINICAL SIGNS

In acute poisoning by benzenearsonic acid feed additives, there is a 3- to 5-day onset of incoordination, ataxia, and poor control of body movements. Later, pigs develop partial paralysis but they still eat and drink. Blindness may develop with arsanilic acid and sodium arsanilate. There may also be erythema and sensitivity to sunlight. The pigs may recover if the offending feed is withheld prior to complete paralysis.

In chronic cases, there is a gradual onset of blindness and partial paralysis, but the pigs still eat and drink and remain alert. There are gait disturbances and poor weight gains. Poultry manifest incoordination and ataxia after poisoning by 3-nitro. With arsanilic acid and its salt, they manifest ruffled feathers, anorexia, depression, coma, and death (Buck et al. 1973).

LESIONS

Gross lesions are absent except for erythema in white-skinned pigs and possible muscle atrophy in chronic poisoning.

Microscopically, there is peripheral nerve demyelination, degeneration of axons, and gliosis. These changes are prominent in the optic nerves. Peripheral nerve damage occurs after 6–10 days of ingestion of excessive amounts of benzenearsonic acid compounds, and axonal fragmentation occurs several days later. The microscopic lesions worsen with prolonged exposure to the arsenical.

DIFFERENTIAL DIAGNOSIS

Swine or poultry that manifest incoordination and ataxia, partial paralysis without central nervous signs, good appetite, low mortality, and no lesions at autopsy should be suspected of having been poisoned by a benzenearsonic acid compound. Generally, there is a history of ingestion of such a compound in the feed.

Polyneuritis due to vitamin deficiency, infectious disease, or other chemicals may have to be excluded in the differential diagnosis.

TREATMENT

If the offending feed is withheld, the animals or birds may recover. This is assuming that the toxicosis has not continued too long and that plenty of water is available. Multiple vitamin therapy can be instituted, but there is no evidence that vitamins are a specific treatment for poisoning by benzenearsonic acid compounds. Other supportive therapy might include antibiotics to prevent bacterial infection and fluids to promote excretion of the arsenical in the urine.

In rats given a large dosage of either arsanilic acid or *p*-carbamino-phenylarsonic acid intraperitoneally, lethality can be prevented by prior or simultaneous administration of a benzene compound such as *p*-aminobenzoic acid or its isomers, phenylacetic acid, phenylpropionic acid, or others. These compounds are also partially effective if administered within 3–4 hours after the arsenical. There is no antagonistic activity against organic or inorganic trivalent arsenicals (Sandground 1943, 1944). It remains to be seen whether compounds of benzene that are structurally similar to benzenearsonic acids have any therapeutic value in cases of benzenearsonic acid poisoning in domestic animals and fowl.

ANALYSIS

The tissues may be found to contain arsenic (see "Inorganic" Arsenic in Chapter 59). However, the benzenearsonic acid compounds are rapidly excreted. If the animal has not had a constant intake of the compound, it is possible that there will not be significant concentrations of arsenic in the tissues or urine. According to Buck et al. (1973), the excessive feeding of these arsenicals can result in liver and kidney arsenic concentrations of 3–10 ppm (wet weight basis) and blood concentrations of 1–2 ppm.

The suspect feed should also be tested, either for arsenic or for the specific benzenearsonic acid compound. If the feed contains 250 ppm or more of arsanilic acid or 100 ppm or more of 3-nitro, a presumptive diagnosis can be made if the pigs or poultry manifested diarrhea, dehydration, or debility or if water intake was reduced. The diagnosis is confirmed if there are typical signs and neurologic lesions in addition to positive tissue and feed analyses. The neurologic lesions may not be present unless ingestion of the benzenearsonic acid compound has taken place for at least 10 days (optic tract lesions) or 2 weeks (sciatic and brachial nerve lesions) (Buck et al. 1973).

Other Agents

Polyneuritis, or peripheral nerve demyelination, can be produced by poisons other than organic arsenicals. These poisons have been discussed in previous chapters. They include hexachlorophene, cyanates, organomercurials in swine, certain "neurotoxic" organophosphate insecticides, lead, and thallium.

Peripheral nerve demyelination is not necessarily the most worrisome or important lesion with chemicals. Moreover, they do not all produce the same kind of demyelinating lesion. Some cause primary demyelination that may either ascend from the periphery or descend from the central nervous system (CNS). Others cause ascending or descending demyelination secondary to axonal damage. Detailed histopathologic examination is required to differentiate various demyelinating conditions due to chemicals, vitamin deficiency, infectious disease, or genetic factors.

Fortunately, with the chemical-induced demyelinating conditions, other signs and lesions can be of assistance in diagnosis and treatment.

ETHYLENEDIAMINE DIHYDROIODIDE, AN EXPECTORANT AND ANTIINFLAMMATORY AGENT

Use

The organic iodide, ethylenediamine dihydroiodide (EDDI), is fed to cattle to prevent or treat various ailments such as foot rot, mild respiratory conditions, actinomycosis, mastitis, other chronic infections, and iodine deficiency.

Source

EDDI is mixed with trace mineral salt blocks, mineral supplements, feeds, or molasses. If cattle being fed EDDI develop any kind of bacterial or viral infection, the farmer is apt to increase the amount of EDDI in the total ration in an attempt to control the condition. Iodism can result. More significantly, excess iodine may predispose the animals to infections or make existing infections worse.

Properties of Toxicologic Importance

Cattle can develop a taste for EDDI-treated mineral supplements and overdose themselves by eating one lb or more/animal/day. Unlike the inorganic iodides, EDDI is not irritating to GI linings.

Toxicity

The recommended daily intake of EDDI is 50 mg/animal (continuous feeding) or 400–500 mg/animal for 2–3 weeks. These dosages should be curtailed prior to calving, shipping, vaccination, or other stressful situations because stress is a major factor in the development of EDDI-related infections. Should an infection occur during EDDI administration, the compound should be discontinued. If the chemical is not discontinued, animals may manifest more severe or prolonged infection and may also fail to respond to conventional therapy with other drugs.

Toxicodynamic Considerations

Iodides are readily excreted in the milk. Milk from treated cattle is not fit for human consumption. Whether the milk is safe for nursing calves is a matter of conjecture. Iodides are also secreted by glandular cells in the respiratory tract, thus accounting for their expectorant actions. Salivary and lacrimal glands also secrete iodides.

Mechanism of Action

The coughing, lacrimation, salivation, and nasal discharge seen in cattle overdosed with EDDI are probably reflections of the prosecretory actions of iodide. The apparent susceptibility or predisposition of animals to microbial infections has been attributed to a possible antiinflammatory action of iodide, which could result from the ability of iodide to uncouple oxidative phosphorylation. Low-grade fever in animals given excess EDDI may also be due to the uncoupling of oxidative phosphorylation (McCauley et al. 1972, 1973). Rosiles et al. (1975) found that experimentally induced infectious bovine rhinotracheitis (IBR) was not markedly worsened by EDDI (50 or 500 mg/day), although the expectorant action of EDDI did augment the coughing, lacrimation, and nasal discharge in infected feeder calves. Possibly the calves might have manifested more severe illness or death had the dosage of EDDI been increased or had the animals been subjected to stress during the early weeks of illness. More research is needed to characterize the disease-enhancing actions of EDDI reported by practitioners and cattlemen.

Clinical Signs

Excess EDDI causes cattle to manifest coughing, seromucous nasal discharge, lacrimation, dullness or reluctance to move, heavy breathing, and a slight fever (McCauley et al. 1972). Sheep manifest similar signs (McCauley et al. 1973). These signs abate within a few days if EDDI is removed from the ration.

If there is a disease problem in the herd or if the animals are stressed, the clinical signs are worsened. Animals may go off feed, become depressed, and develop a fever of 105°–108° F. Bronchopneumonia or septicemia can occur and many of the cattle may die of these infections in spite of vigorous antibiotic therapy. This is true even if EDDI is removed from the ration (McCauley et al. 1972).

Lesions

No lesions are visible in EDDI toxicosis. Excess fluid may be found in the bronchial tree. Microscopically, there may be a chronic tracheitis. If animals die of viral or bacterial disease complications, the lesions are characteristic of the disease.

Differential Diagnosis

IBR is the main concern in cattle that manifest coughing, lacrimation, nasal discharge, sluggishness, and fever. EDDI toxicosis can look exactly like IBR. In fact, EDDI overfeeding may even trigger an outbreak of IBR in a herd. Thus the role of EDDI in a particular situation may be masked by disease symptoms and by positive serological tests for pathogens such as IBR virus. If EDDI is a significant factor in the disease entity encountered in the herd, the history will indicate exposure to EDDI and serum iodine concentrations will be elevated in the affected animals. Moreover, the animals may not respond well to antibiotic and corticosteroid therapy, and the mortality rate may be very high.

Treatment

There is no antidote for iodism. The source of iodine must be eliminated. Clinical signs may then abate in a few days. If infection is present, conventional therapy is warranted but the prognosis is guarded.

Analysis

In cattle the normal total serum iodine concentration ranges from 5.6 to 14 μg/100 ml (McCauley et al. 1972; Rosiles et al. 1975). In sheep the normal total serum iodine concentration is about 2.3–4.6 μg/100 ml (McCauley et al. 1973). In cases of EDDI-induced iodism and in cases of infection related to the feeding of EDDI, the above authors report total serum iodine concentrations that are 10–100 or more times normal.

ZEARALENONE, AN ESTROGENIC TOXIN

Source

Zearalone (also called F-2 toxin) is one of several toxic metabolites of the mold *Fusarium roseum (Gibberella zeae)* and possibly other *Fusarium* species. These molds proliferate during cold weather and in stored grain (especially corn or pelleted feed containing corn) that has a high moisture content (23% or more). Barley, oats, and wheat can be infected in the field, the disease being known as "scab." In growing corn, the disease is called "gib."

The moldy grain, if fed to animals or fowl, can produce all the signs and lesions of hyperestrogenism. The molds may also produce a "refusal factor" that causes swine to refuse the grain, an emetic factor that causes pigs to vomit, and other toxins such as the trichothecenes. Storage or growing conditions determine the nature and amount of mycotoxin produced. Of primary concern in this chapter is the estrogenic toxin zearalenone and the condition known as porcine vulvovaginitis.

Properties of Toxicologic Importance

Zearalenone is 6-(10-hydroxy-6-oxo-trans-1-undecenyl)-β-resorcylic acid lactone. The compound is stable in grain indefinitely and is not destroyed by roasting or by a variety of other treatments.

Toxicity

Actual LD50 or ED50 values are not available. Feed containing as little as 0.01 ppm zearalenone can cause infertility and abortion in swine (Mirocha et al. 1974). Dairy cattle have developed lethargy, anemia, and feed refusal when the dairy ration contained 1 ppm zearalenone. Bovine abortion has occurred when sorghum contained 12 ppm (Mirocha et al. 1974). Feed may contain more than one estrogenic agent. Diethylstilbestrol (DES) may be a feed contaminant (Nelson et al. 1973).

Toxicodynamic Considerations

Studies of the absorption, distribution,

metabolism, and excretion of zearalenone have not come to the attention of the author.

MECHANISM OF ACTION

On the basis of similarity of signs and lesions to those produced by natural and synthetic estrogens, the mechanism by which zearalenone causes signs of hyperestrogenism must be very similar to the mechanisms of the estrogens themselves. It is beyond the scope of this presentation to discuss the biochemical basis of hyperestrogenism.

CLINICAL SIGNS AND LESIONS

According to Mirocha et al. (1971) and Nelson et al. (1973), the porcine vulvovaginitis syndrome is characterized by edematous swelling and reddening of the vulva, increased vaginal secretions, vaginal prolapse, uterine bleeding, increase in size and secretions of the uterus, mammary growth, lactation, shrunken ovaries, abortion or fetal resorption, infertility, stunting in males and females, and feminization of males. Microscopic lesions include edema and hyperplasia of the uterus, proliferation of mammary ducts, and squamous metaplasia of the cervix and vagina.

If the feed contains the refusal factor, the animals may not eat it. If the emetic factor is present, pigs may vomit. If trichothecenes are present, there may be signs of liver and kidney damage, oral ulcerations, and internal bleeding.

DIFFERENTIAL DIAGNOSIS

Signs of hyperestrogenism associated with ingestion of moldy feed are suggestive of zearalenone or some other estrogenic toxicant in the feed. Laboratory tests are required to determine if zearalenone is actually present.

TREATMENT

The moldy feed must be eliminated. "Dilution" of the feed is not recommended by this author, although the practice is carried out.

ANALYSIS

Zearalenone can be detected by a number of analytical methods (Mirocha et al. 1974). Presence of the toxin in the feed of animals that have the signs and lesions of hyperestrogenism is strong evidence that zearalenone is at fault. Other estrogens such as DES or congeners of zearalenone may be present if zearalenone is not.

PLANT POISONS CAUSING SLOWNESS, STIFFNESS, AND TREMORS

Tremetol is a higher alcohol found in the rayless goldenrod *(Haplopappus heterophyllus)*, in other species of *Haplopappus*, and in white snakeroot *(Eupatorium rugosum)*. Ruminants affected by tremetol manifest slowness, stiff gait, tremors, and eventual collapse. Nursing calves may obtain toxic amounts of tremetol in the milk prior to onset of clinical signs in the dam. Exercise worsens the signs of this condition, which is called "trembles" in animals.

An unknown principle in jimmy fern *(Notholaena sinuata)* causes "jimmies" in sheep. There is lagging behind, incoordination, standing still with the back arched, violent trembling, increased respiration and heartbeat, and prostration. After 15–30 minutes the sheep gets up, but exercise brings on another attack. Death can occur in severe poisoning. The poisonous principle may affect suckling lambs before it affects the dam.

Kingsbury (1964) presents details on these plants.

PONDEROSA PINE, A PLANT POISON CAUSING PREMATURE PARTURITION

Stevenson et al. (1972) reported that range cattle eating the needles of ponderosa pine *(Pinus ponderosa)* do not really abort their fetuses as was formerly thought. Rather, the fetus may be presented alive, and it may survive. The dam may suffer consequences such as retained placenta and secondary bacterial infection. Nevertheless, the condition induced by the pine needles is termed premature parturition rather than abortion. The toxic factor is unknown.

SLAFRAMINE, A TOXIN CAUSING SALIVATION, LACRIMATION, URINATION, AND DEFECATION

Slaframine is an indole alkaloidal mold toxin elaborated by *Rhizoctonia leguminicola,* a mold that infects red clover. The disease in clover is called "black patch." Animals eating infected red clover hay develop a condition that could be called "slobbers." The clinical signs include reduced feed consumption, excessive salivation (thick, tenacious saliva), frequent urination, diarrhea, bloat, and lacrimation. According to Crump (1973), slaframine causes lacrimation in the guinea pig but not in the rat.

Slaframine is apparently activated in the liver after ingestion (Broquist and Snyder 1971). The active molecule, likely a substituted version of the parent indole, seems to have either direct histaminergic effects or possibly a histamine-releasing effect. The clinical signs and laboratory animal responses are consistent with this suggestion. Moreover, in laboratory animals, the signs respond to antihistamines much better than to atropine (Crump 1973).

Slaframine toxicosis is not a major problem in veterinary practice. Infected red clover or red clover hay should not be fed to livestock.

POTENTIALLY HARMFUL RESIDUES

A large number of industrial and agricultural chemicals can find their way into animal feeds and cause "new" kinds of toxicoses. Tissue residues may require the disposal of all animal products intended for human consumption. The flame-retardant polybrominated biphenyls mentioned in Chapter 60 are only one example of compounds that could not possibly be expected to cause toxicologic problems but somehow did.

By-products of the plastics industry such as polychlorinated biphenyls (PCB) and phthalates are not discussed in this section because, so far, they have not caused many toxicologic problems. Their toxicity and hazard are recognized, and vigorous attempts are being made to keep them out of the human food chain.

Other chemicals, such as the fungicides hexachlorobenzene and *p*-chloronitrobenzene, or the newer carbamate pesticides, fungicides, and herbicides may easily enter the human food chain because the chemicals are used in areas close to food-producing animals. Still, these compounds have not presented many toxicologic problems in animals because their toxicity is very low. Thus these compounds are not discussed in much detail.

Lack of acute toxicosis problems in animals, however, is no excuse to disregard various chemicals that animals may ingest. The human food chain must be protected at all costs. Particular attention must be given to residues of drugs and chemicals in edible products. The veterinarian is intimately concerned with problems of drug and chemical residues from two main viewpoints: as a practitioner concerned about the well-being of this clients and the health of their animals and as one of the acknowledged guardians of public health.

Thus veterinary toxicology must include the study of residue problems. Chapter 63 is intended to assist in this study.

REFERENCES

Broquist, H. P., and Snyder, J. J. 1971. Rhizoctonia toxin. In S. Kadis, A. Ciegler, and S. J. Ajl, eds. Microbial Toxins, vol. 7. New York: Academic Press.

Buck, W. B.,; Osweiler, G. D.; and Van Gelder, G. A. 1973. Clinical and Diagnostic Veterinary Toxicology. Dubuque, Iowa: Kendall/Hunt.

Clarke, E. G. C., and Clarke, M. L. 1967. Garner's Veterinary Toxicology, 3rd ed. Baltimore: Williams & Wilkins.

Crump, M. H. 1973. Slaframine (slobber factor) toxicosis. J Am Vet Med Assoc 163: 1300.

Kingsbury, J. M. 1964. Poisonous Plants of the United States and Canada. Englewood Cliffs, N.J.: Prentice-Hall.

McCauley, E. H.; Johnson, D. W.; and Alhadji, I. 1972. Disease problems in cattle associated with rations containing high levels of iodide. Bovine Pract 7:22.

McCauley, E. H.; Linn, J. G.; and Goodrich, R. D. 1973. Experimentally induced iodide toxicosis in lambs. Am J Vet Res 34:65.

Mirocha, C. J.; Christensen, C. M.; and Nelson, G. H. 1971. F-2 (zearalenone) estrogenic mycotoxin from *Fusarium*. In S. Kadis, A. Ciegler, and S. J. Ajl, eds. Microbial Toxins, vol. 7. New York: Academic Press.

Mirocha, C. J.; Schauerhamer, B.; and Pathre, S. V. 1974. Isolation, detection, and quantitation of zearalenone in maize and barley. J Assoc Off Anal Chem 57:1104.

Nelson, G. H.; Christensen, C. M.; and Mirocha, C. J. 1973. *Fusarium* and estrogenism in swine. J Am Vet Med Assoc 163:1276.

Rosiles, R.; Buck, W. B.; and Brown, L. N. 1975. Clinical infectious bovine rhinotracheitis in cattle fed organic iodine and urea. Am J Vet Res 36:1447.

Sandground, J. H. 1943. Studies on the detoxication of organic arsenical compounds. III. The time-factor influencing *p*-aminobenzoate protection of rats receiving lethal doses of phenyl arsonates. J Pharmacol Exp Ther 78:209.

———. 1944. Studies on the detoxication of organic arsenical compounds. V. Additional detoxicants for pentavalent arsenicals. J Pharmacol Exp Ther 80:393.

Stevenson, A. H.; James, L. F.; and Call, J. W. 1972. Pine-needle *(Pinus ponderosa)*-induced abortion in range cattle. Cornell Vet 62:519.

CHAPTER 62

EUTHANATIZING AGENTS

ROGER C. HATCH

WHAT IS EUTHANASIA?

Euthanasia is the humane killing or mercy killing of animals by specially trained personnel. In veterinary practice, animals are generally euthanatized to prevent suffering from incurable or painful conditions. The veterinarian is often asked to kill animals for other reasons. The client may no longer want or be able to keep a pet. Rather than see the pet adopted by "some stranger," the client may ask that the animal be "put to sleep." Animals that are behavior problems are sometimes presented for euthanasia. Dangerously aggressive animals or animals that have annoying or costly vices fit this category. Litters of puppies or kittens may be brought to the veterinarian to be killed because the owner cannot keep them. Once in a while, a client is simply angry about the performance of an animal. Thus the veterinarian may be asked to euthanatize a hunting dog that is gun-shy, or fails to retrieve, or chases rabbits instead of pointing quail. Or, the client may be upset because his animal is a "loser" on the show or race circuit.

No veterinarian enjoys killing animals. Euthanasia is one of the saddest and most disagreeable aspects of practice. Nevertheless, veterinarians euthanatize animals to alleviate suffering. The veterinarian is not obliged to euthanatize animals that are not suffering and may refuse to do so if the animals could be placed with other people. Many veterinarians can offer some sort of unofficial placement service for the occasional unwanted animal.

The terminology of animal killing requires clarification. *Euthanasia,* as discussed above, is a professional term used in preference to more widely understood lay terms such as *killing, mercy killing,* or *humane killing.* The humane killing of domestic animals or fowl for food or disease eradication purposes is termed *slaughter.* The inhumane killing of large numbers of animals or people is also called slaughter. The term offends the sensibilities when used in the wrong context. Home killing of animals for food is termed *butchering.* Curiously, the killing of wild game, fish, or fowl for the purpose of obtaining food and sportful recreation can at times be quite inhumane, but these activities are simply called hunting and fishing!

The killing of animals for materials other than food (pelts, oils, tusks) is often referred to as a *harvest,* as if the animals were plots of earth that had been sown with a special seed the previous spring! A fish catch, on a large scale, is also called a harvest. Hunters are said to harvest game or seals in the name of conservation of a healthy population. Whether the population of game or seals is in fact ready for, or needful of, a large-scale reduction in numbers is often contested bitterly by environmentalists. In a herd, flock, or other large group or population of animals, the killing of aging, weak, poor-producing, or supernumerary animals may be termed *culling* or *thinning.* The mass killing of animal pests, vermin, or other unwanted life forms is called *extermination.* The client should never be asked if he wants his pet exterminated! It is possible to ask if the animal should be *put to sleep,* but care must be taken to make sure that the client understands what is meant. The term *put to sleep* also means to be anesthetized. On the other hand, the phrases *put out of his misery* or *end his suffering* may be less ambiguous.

Professional jargon such as *put him down* (meaning to anesthetize) or *push the plunger* (meaning to euthanatize) should not be used with people who do not understand the jargon and the totally professional attitude with which such terms may be used.

In scientific writing, experimental animals are seldom "killed." Instead, they are usually referred to as being *sacrificed, terminated,* or at worst, *disposed of.* An animal that is sacrificed is one that is offered up to a god or goddess during some sort of ritualistic ceremony. Scientific experiments do not end this way, although one sometimes wonders if it might have helped obtain better experimental results! Animals are not really terminated. Their lives may be terminated, but not the animals themselves. The phrase *at terminus* means at the time of death. It is possible to say that animals were exposed to a certain concentration of lethal gas and observed until terminus, but it is simpler to say the animals were euthanatized or given a lethal dosage of X drug. To dispose of animals means to put them into the garbage can or disposal unit or to have them hauled away. Moreover, the term has the cold connotation that living animals were simply dispensed with. It is possible to dispose of dead animals, but one should not say he disposed of live ones.

News media, when speaking of the killing of diseased, injured, unwanted, or dangerous animals, usually say the animals were *destroyed.* This term is perfectly acceptable in these contexts, but it sometimes has a disturbing connotation of demolition. Buildings are destroyed. Even whole cities may be destroyed. The police may be reported to have destroyed (shot) a dangerous animal. In this case the term is appropriate because gunshot wounds are undeniably destructive. A client should not be asked if he wants his pet dog or cat destroyed. The term is too harsh in this instance.

The ideal euthanatizing agent should satisfy several criteria:

1. It should not cause undue anxiety, alarm, fear behavior, struggling, vocalization, muscle spasms, or clinical signs of autonomic activation. Moreover, the restraint procedure should not precipitate these reactions.

2. It should be painless, or as nearly so as possible under the circumstances of the moment.

3. It should be fast acting, i.e., cause unconsciousness and death instantaneously or within minutes.

4. It should be reliable, i.e., cause death every time when properly used.

5. It should be safe for the properly trained person to use.

6. It should be easy for the properly trained person to use.

7. It should not be known as a drug of abuse in human beings. If it is a drug of abuse, then it must be kept under strict control according to federal regulations.

8. It should be esthetically acceptable to use. Acceptability in this regard depends on who the observers are.

9. It should be compatible with the overall reason and purpose of euthanatizing the animal or animals; i.e., it should be practical to use.

10. It should be economical.

11. It should not create a problem of sanitation or environmental contamination.

12. It should not cause tissue changes that might complicate the postmortem examination. Tissue residues should not interfere with subsequent laboratory tests for poisons or metabolic products.

It is obvious from the above criteria that *there is no such thing as the ideal euthanatizing agent.* Some of the criteria are highly subjective. For example, people can tolerate the pain of a hypodermic injection into their own bodies, but many people cannot bear to see a pet animal react to that very same minor pain stimulus.

One final point must be made before we consider the individual euthanatizing agents. In the veterinarian-client situation, euthanasia should never be performed without the written permission of the client or his legal agent. Veterinarians have been sued by clients who denied giving verbal permission to kill an animal.

The following information is taken from Clifford (1971), Lumb and Jones (1973), Lumb (1974), and Moreland (1974). The presentation by Lumb and Jones (1973) is in large part the text of the Report of the AVMA Panel on Euthanasia (1972) (herein referred to as the Panel), a copy of which was also consulted. The report of the Panel is the latest official information available about euthanasia. This author will comment on recommendations of the Panel whenever such comments seem appropriate.

AGENTS THAT CAN BE USED IN EUTHANASIA

Barbiturates

These drugs come closer than any other agent to meeting the criteria for acceptable euthanatizing agents. Intravenous injection of pentobarbital sodium causes a smooth and rapid onset of unconsciousness. Overdosage of barbiturates causes death by depression of vital medullary respiratory and vasomotor centers. Clinically, the animal simply relaxes, shuts his eyes, and stops breathing, all in rapid order. The heart continues to beat for a few minutes. There is often some minor twitching of muscles just after respiratory arrest.

Barbiturates can be administered by intraperitoneal, intrathoracic, or intracardiac routes. The latter requires precision and may cause some initial struggling during restraint. The former routes require large dosages of barbiturate, and the onset of anesthesia may be marked by ataxia, falling, and struggling to rise. Suitable premedications such as tranquilizers can minimize such activities.

Barbiturates are suitable for euthanasia of individual small animals but not for mass euthanasia. The drugs require professional supervision and control.

Chloral Hydrate

This hypnotic drug is not recommended by the Panel because of the slow onset of action and because it produces restraint difficulties, gasping, spasms of muscles, and vocalization. This author agrees but suggests that the animal can be properly euthanatized with chloral hydrate following premedication with a tranquilizer. Chloral is used this way in veterinary anesthesia, and there is no reason that it cannot be administered beyond the anesthetic stages to produce death.

Chloral hydrate must be given intravenously because of its slow onset of action and its tissue irritant properties. In combination with tranquilizers or other central nervous depressants, the drug is suited to euthanasia of individual large or small animals.

Barbiturate–Choral Hydrate–Magnesium Sulfate

The intravenous injection of a mixture of pentobarbital sodium, chloral hydrate, and magnesium sulfate is a common practice in large animal anesthesia. The mixture is also given to birds by the intramuscular route. Overdosage of such a mixture produces respiratory arrest, cardiac arrest, and muscle relaxation in rapid succession. The mixture is a good alternative to chloral hydrate alone, because the pentobarbital augments and speeds central nervous depression and smooths the onset of anesthesia. The magnesium sulfate prevents muscle spasms and arrests cardiac activity.

T-61 Euthanasia Solution

This product is a mixture of N-2-(methoxyphenyl)-2-ethylbutyl-1-hydroxybutyramide (20%), 4,4′-methylene bis-cyclohexyl-trimethyl ammonium iodide (5%), and tetracaine hydrochloride (0.5%) in aqueous solution with formamide. The mixture has been used for several years in Germany for euthanasia of dogs and cats and has recently been introduced into the United States. It remains to be seen whether T-61 has any important advantages over pentobarbital sodium for euthanasia of pets.

Inhalant Anesthetics in Small Species

The Panel reports ether, chloroform, halothane, and methoxyflurane acceptable for euthanasia of young cats and dogs, birds, rodents, and other small species. Ether vapor is explosive. Ether and methoxyflurane have a slow onset of depression. Halothane and methoxyflurane are expensive. All except ether cause tissue changes. All must be administered in a closed container, and all are hazardous for personnel. Nevertheless, euthanasia is reasonably smooth, marked only by preanesthetic excitement (due to the irritant nature of the agents, or to Stage I and II activity) and attempts of the animals to escape by climbing over each other. Death is rapid when the anesthetic concentration is large enough. These agents are particularly suited to euthanasia of experimental animals such as mice, rats, hamsters, and guinea pigs. It is too expensive and difficult to euthanatize large animals with inhalant anesthetics, although chloroform or halothane can be used in an emergency, when administered by face mask. Preanesthetic sedation or tranquilization is recommended to avoid excitement and struggling during induction.

Carbon Monoxide

Euthanasia of dogs and cats can be carried out in a carbon monoxide chamber. The only problem is that there are a number of precautions and guidelines for proper use of such chambers. These are presented by the Panel and by Moreland (1974). A rather cumbersome technology seems to have evolved with the use of carbon monoxide. The Panel deems the gas suitable for euthanasia under stated conditions of use.

Carbon Dioxide

This gas has been used for a long time to render swine insensible prior to slaughter. Swine are placed on a conveyor belt that moves through a chamber filled with the gas. Emerging from the chamber, the swine are unconscious and can be painlessly exsanguinated. Sheep and calves can be handled similarly.

Carbon dioxide is an anesthetic gas and can be used at a chamber concentration of 30%–40% to euthanatize small laboratory animals. The Panel does not recommend the use of carbon dioxide to kill dogs or cats, primarily because the agent requires more investigation in these species.

Electricity in Large Species

Electrocution is a rather time-consuming, awkward, and dangerous means of killing large animals. The electricity must flow transcranially, not from nose to anus, to cause immediate unconsciousness. The sudden collapse and convulsions associated with electrocution are not pleasant to watch, although convulsions can be prevented by neuromuscular blocking agents. The Panel is not enchanted with electroshock as a means of euthanasia, although the method is acceptable for stunning turkeys or animals prior to slaughter.

Bullets

Large animals may be shot in the head. Death is instantaneous. The procedure is not pretty to watch, but its humaneness is obvious. Naturally, the bullet has to be aimed properly. This requires that the operator be a good shot and that the animal be approached closely. The method lacks reliability in that the bullet may ricochet from a hard skull and only wound the animal. Bystanders can get shot too. The Panel is not enthusiastic about shooting as a means of euthanasia, and the method is not recommended at all for small animals in veterinary practice.

Shooting, however, may be the only way a rancher can destroy predators, or the only way a police officer can destroy a dangerous dog, or the only way a zoo veterinarian can destroy a dangerous elephant. In such instances, the end justifies the means.

Captive Bolt Weapons

In these instruments, a .22 caliber blank cartridge is used to propel a steel bolt against the skull of a large animal. The bolt moves only about an inch, never leaving the barrel of the instrument. The discharge of the cartridge is triggered when the bolt touches the skull. The Panel does not clearly differentiate the captive bolt from the bullet. Actually, the captive bolt is safer to use than a gun. The animal that is properly struck by the bolt drops to the ground instantly and can then be exsanguinated painlessly. It takes an expert to use the captive bolt properly. If the bolt is not positioned properly at the time of firing, the animal may simply be hurt and alarmed.

Concussion

Small laboratory animals can be killed humanely by a sharp blow to the head, followed by thoracotomy or exsanguination.

Vacuum

The high-altitude chamber is becoming popular in some circles for euthanasia of dogs, cats, and other small species. Animals are placed in the chamber and the air in the chamber is quickly pumped out, forming a partial vacuum equivalent to an altitude of 55,000 feet above sea level (68.8 mm Hg or 1.33 lb/square inch or 0.604 kg/square inch). The vacuum is maintained for at least 10 minutes (adult, healthy animals) to 20 minutes (young, old, or sick animals). The animals collapse in less than a minute due to hypoxia. There is reflex muscle movement during unconsciousness.

Rapid decompression in a vacuum chamber should not be confused with the rapid release of air pressure exemplified by explosive decompression, deep sea divers' "bends," or the bends of caisson disease. These latter phenomena are associated with ruptured blood vessels, bubbling-out of dissolved nitrogen in the blood, and considerable pain. These things do not happen in animals euthanatized properly in the high-altitude chamber. The *potential* for blood vessel rupture, gas release from the blood, and severe pain is present if the high-altitude chamber is not operated or maintained properly.

Guillotine, Cervical Dislocation

Small laboratory animals and birds can be killed humanely by quickly chopping off the head or by quickly breaking or crushing the cervical spinal cord.

AGENTS THAT SHOULD NOT BE USED IN EUTHANASIA

Inhalant Anesthetics in Large Species

Except in emergencies, the large animal should not be euthanatized with inhalant anesthetics because of the difficulty and expense involved. Without appropriate premedication, the animal becomes agitated and dangerous to personnel when exposed to inhalant anesthetics. If proper premedication is carried out, as for anesthesia, the whole operation becomes so involved that one is better off to have simply chosen another way to euthanatize the animal.

Nitrogen and Other Inert Gases

Nitrogen has been used to kill mink during harvesting of pelts. According to the Panel, unconsciousness occurs in about 1.5 minutes and death in 5 minutes. The Panel, however, does not actually recommend the use of nitrogen for euthanasia. Instead, the gas is said to have good possibilities in this regard. More research is required to determine the acceptability of nitrogen for euthanasia.

Magnesium Sulfate

When used alone, magnesium sulfate is not a central nervous depressant. It is a neuromuscular blocking agent and myocardial depressant (Aldrete et al. 1968). Although the magnesium ion is capable of blocking central synapses when administered directly into the brain, the ion does not readily cross the blood-brain barrier (Kato et al. 1968). When given intravenously, magnesium sulfate causes a great deal of excitement, alarm, struggling, and vocalization before the animal collapses. Death is due to myocardial depression and inability of the respiratory muscles to function. The animal remains conscious until the brain succumbs to anoxemic anoxia. Magnesium sulfate should be used only in combination with depressants such as pentobarbital and chloral hydrate.

Curariform Drugs

Drugs such as *d*-tubocurarine, gallamine, decamethonium, and succinylcholine cause rapid collapse due to neuromuscular paralysis. Consciousness is not affected. Death is due to anoxemic anoxia, which results from inability of the respiratory muscles to function. These agents should not be used to kill animals. They may be used in proper dosages to restrain animals prior to intravenous administration of a depressant drug such as pentobarbital. They may also be used to "knock down" an animal immediately before using the captive bolt or gun.

Narcotic Analgesics

Opiate derivatives such as morphine and etorphine are central depressants as well as analgesics. Morphine has been used as the sole general anesthetic in animals and human beings. Overdosage with these agents causes death by depression of the respiratory centers in the medulla. On the surface it appears as if these drugs would be acceptable for euthanasia, even though they are subject to strict federal regulations. In fact, there is insufficient information available about euthanasia with narcotic analgesics. Some species are rendered maniacal by large dosages of these drugs. At present, the drugs by themselves are not recommended for euthanasia. Neither are the various analgesic-tranquilizer (neuroleptanalgesic) combinations.

Tranquilizers and Sedatives

The major tranquilizers cause extrapyramidal side effects when administered in large dosages. Both the tranquilizers and the sedatives are capable of causing hypotension and a degree of central nervous depression, but there is no analgesia. Large dosages are required to kill animals. The drugs are not suitable for euthanasia, but they can be used as premedicants to the accepted means of euthanasia.

Central Muscle Relaxants

This group includes glyceryl guaiacolate, mephenesin, methocarbamol, and others. These drugs have central depressant properties, but the depression is exerted mainly in the spinal cord. Large dosages are required to depress the brain. Before this happens, the animal is paralyzed and may be starting to suffer respiratory difficulty. The drugs have no real place in euthanasia except possibly as premedicants for anesthetics.

Strychnine

There is no question that strychnine is lethal. Dogs and cats are especially susceptible. Many pets are poisoned maliciously and accidentally each year by ingesting strychnine. Strychnine is a convulsant poison (see Chapter 58). It does not depress consciousness. Death is due to anoxemic anoxia that results from inability of the tonically rigid respiratory muscles to function. Strychnine is used to exterminate pests and to kill livestock predators, but the alkaloid is not acceptable for euthanasia.

NICOTINE

Dog wardens sometimes use nicotine sulfate in a projectile syringe to capture dogs. Sometimes the dog is captured and sometimes it is killed. Nicotine is an extremely dangerous alkaloid because it has a low therapeutic ratio and because animals vary greatly in susceptibility to it. The drug kills by causing depolarizing blockade of all central and peripheral nicotinic cholinergic receptors (see Chapter 58). The animal develops anoxemic anoxia prior to loss of consciousness. Nicotine acts very quickly, but it is not a humane drug and it is dangerous for personnel to use. It readily penetrates the intact skin.

CYANIDE GAS OR SOLUTION

One would think that if cyanide gas is good enough for execution of people in prisons it is good enough for euthanasia of animals. This is may be so, but cyanide gas is dangerous for personnel. Moreover, the animal manifests severe respiratory difficulty and violent convulsions before death. The injected solution has the same effects. Cyanide causes rapid death by producing histotoxic anoxia. Cells are rendered incapable of using the oxygen in the bloodstream (see Chapter 57). The brain succumbs within minutes to this effect. Cyanide is not recommended for euthanasia. Hydrogen sulfide gas and sulfide injectables act much like cyanide and share all its disadvantages.

CARDIAC DRUGS

Myocardial stimulants, such as digitalis, calcium, and cobalt, and myocardial depressants, such as potassium and magnesium ion, cause death by stopping the heart. The agents do not depress consciousness and they are not analgesic. Cardiac drugs should not be used for euthanasia.

ELECTRICITY IN SMALL SPECIES

Transcranial electroshock is difficult, awkward, and dangerous to apply to large animals. With small animals these factors make electrocution decidedly unreliable unless the animal is suitably premedicated and restrained. If one is to go to all the trouble of premedication and restraint, one might just as well use a better method of euthanasia.

WATER (DROWNING)

For generations, the drowning of unwanted puppies and kittens has been the idiot's delight. Some disturbed people seem to derive pleasure out of watching animals drown. They may even brag about it, much to the distress of the listener. Drowning is not condoned as a means of euthanasia.

AIR EMBOLISM

The injection of air into the bloodstream may have been overexploited in murder mysteries and hospital dramas. Air emboli can certainly cause death if they reach the appropriate areas of the brain or the myocardial circulation. More often, however, the emboli lodge in other places. Severe excitement, pain, and struggling can result. Air embolism may be effective in small laboratory animals, but it may have no effect in large animals. The Panel has no statement about air embolism. The author is of the opinion that there are more reliable and more humane ways to kill animals than to inject air into their veins.

VOLATILE ANESTHETICS GIVEN INTRAVENOUSLY

This sounds like a fast and humane way to euthanatize animals. However, when ether is injected intravenously, it causes massive hemolysis and severe excitement, struggling, and vocalization in the dog.

EXSANGUINATION

Animals should never be bled-out unless they are rendered insensible by agents such as carbon dioxide, captive bolt, electricity, or other means. On the basis of religious freedom, federal regulations exempt kosher killing from this guideline. (Brandly et al. 1966).

While there are innumerable ways to kill animals, it is difficult to find ways that comply with the criteria for acceptability of euthanatizing agents. Nobody with any sense wants to cause animals to suffer, even for a minute. Nevertheless, animals do have to be euthanatized for a variety of reasons. It behooves us to perform this task as professionally and compassionately as possible, while at the same time recognizing that methods of euthanasia can never be without some disadvantages.

In the context of practicality and esthetics of different methods of euthanasia for different purposes, Dr. Lumb (1974) asks the question, "Who is to say that a method of euthanasia can or cannot be used?" The point is well taken, for we do tend to let emotion, sentiment, and empathy influence our judgment about the humaneness of euthanasia methods. Perhaps, however, we should all hold on to our emotions, sentiment, and empathy for animals, lest we kill them as dispassionately as we sometimes kill each other.

REFERENCES

Aldrete, J. A.; Barnes, D. R.; and Aikawa, J. K. 1968. Does magnesium produce anesthesia? Evaluation of its effects on the cardiovascular and neurologic systems. Anesth Analg Curr Res 47:429.

Brandly, P. J.; Migaki, G.; and Taylor, K. E. 1966. Meat Hygiene, 3rd ed. Philadelphia: Lea & Febiger.

Clifford, D. 1971. Euthanasia. In L. R. Soma, ed. Textbook of Veterinary Anesthesia. Baltimore: Willams & Wilkins.

Kato, G.; Kelly, J. S.; Krnjević, K.; and Somjen, G. 1968. Anaesthetic action of magnesium ions. Can Anaesth Soc J 15:539.

Lumb, W. V. 1974. Euthanasia by noninhalant pharmacologic agents. J Am Vet Med Assoc 165:851.

Lumb, W. V., and Jones, E. W. 1973. Veterinary Anesthesia. Philadelphia: Lea & Febiger.

Moreland, A. F. 1974. Carbon monoxide euthanasia of dogs: Chamber concentrations and comparative effects of automobile engine exhaust and carbon monoxide from a cylinder. J Am Vet Med Assoc 165:853.

Smith, C. R.; Booth, N. H.; Fox, M. W.; Jortner, B. S.; Lumb, W. V.; Moreland, A. F.; and Wass, W. M. 1972. Report of the AVMA panel on euthanasia. J Am Vet Med Assoc 160:761.

SECTION 16

Toxicology of Drug and Chemical Residues

CHAPTER 63

DRUG AND CHEMICAL RESIDUES IN THE EDIBLE TISSUES OF ANIMALS

NICHOLAS H. BOOTH

Heavy responsibility is placed on the veterinarian and livestock producer to observe the period for withdrawal of a drug prior to slaughter to assure that illegal concentrations of drug residues in meat, milk, and eggs do not occur. This is essential from a public health standpoint because levels of residues in excess of those legally permitted in edible tissues may produce injurious effects when consumed over a long time span. With greater use of drugs and chemicals required in the production of food crops and animals, the possibility of human beings being continuously exposed to drug and chemical residues for a lifetime is unequivocally evident. Public health authorities and consumers frequently ask questions about the possible adverse effects from continuous exposure to drug and chemical residues. Some of the questions asked are, What will be the allergic, teratogenic, mutagenic, or carcinogenic consequences of consuming foods containing X or Y residues? What will be the effects from exposure to residues upon the prepubertal or postpubertal individual, especially upon gonadal and other endocrine organ development? What will be the effects of residues in the aged as well as those individuals who generally are in poor health?

Greater attention from a public health aspect has centered on the safety of tissue residues, due both to an increased use of veterinary drugs and the expanding general increase of chemicals in the food supply (Fitzhugh 1964). With intensification in the production of animal protein for human consumption, particularly with potential worldwide food shortages, the use of drugs in the diagnosis, prevention, control, and treatment of animal diseases will become increasingly important. Use of drugs in animal production has expanded to the degree that approximately 78%–80% of all animals produced for food purposes receive medication for part or for most of their lives (Yeary 1966; Van Houweling 1971; Shillam 1974). Within a few more years, it is anticipated that nearly all animals produced in the United States for food will have received a chemotherapeutic or prophylactic agent of some type.

Animal drugs and chemicals used for chemotherapeutic and prophylactic purposes are also used as feed additives to promote growth, improve feed efficiency or utilization, synchronize or control the reproductive cycle and breeding performance, enhance feed acceptability, and enhance acceptability by the consumer of the end product. Sixty-five feed additives, including diethylstilbestrol (DES),[1] are used in the United States in animal production (Shillam 1974). Use of feed additives ranging from the antimicrobial to hormone-type agents may improve feed efficiency as much as 17% in beef cattle, 10% in lambs, 15% in poultry, and 15% in swine (Beeson 1963). Although it is evident that drugs are required in the efficient production of meat, milk, and eggs, their indiscriminate use should never be substituted for good management (Aronson 1975). Drugs should be used only when they are required.

Veterinary drugs may be used either for a relatively short period of 1–7 days in the treatment of acute infectious diseases or for long periods, which may cover most of the lifetime of the animal. Most long-term uses are directed toward the promotion of growth, increased weight gain and feed efficiency, or for prophylactic use against one or more diseases (Fitzhugh 1964; Morrison and Munro 1969). All drugs used in food-producing animals are approved by the FDA on the basis that there will be "zero residue" present in the food or that a level of residue not exceeding an FDA tolerance will be present. Under the Delaney Clause, any residue in food resulting from a substance that is a carcinogen is illegal; the concept of no residue or zero tolerance in food is strictly enforced by the FDA under this congressional amendment.

Constantly improving analytical methods make it possible to detect minute quantities of drug and chemical residues in animal tissues ranging from a fraction of a part per million (ppm) to a few parts per billion (ppb) or trillion (ppt). If a noncarcinogen residue is present, a safety margin of at least a 100-fold magnitude is generally applied by toxicologists before the residue can be accepted in food for human consumption. In the past, a "no residue" or "zero tolerance" level was based on the lower limit of sensitivity of the analytical method (Kennedy 1963). For example, if an analytical method was unable to detect a residue below a certain level that could range from 1.0 to 0.1 ppm, the previously accepted minimum level of detection, any level below the limitation of the detection method was defined as no residue or zero tolerance. With the introduction of gas liquid chromatography and other methods of detection such as radioimmunoassay, the detection of residues in animal tissues was improved by a magnitude of 1000 up to 1 million times. This means that drug or chemical residues can be detected in ppb or ppt and that it is virtually impossible to administer a drug to an animal without detecting a level of residue in meat, milk, or eggs even when the prescribed drug withdrawal time is observed.

Any reference to "no residue" or "zero

1. A ban against the use of DES was made by the Food and Drug Administration (FDA) but was later rescinded by a court order. Legislation is pending (1975) in Congress to ban the use of DES in food-producing animals.

tolerance" is scientifically unsound and cannot be enforced by regulatory agencies (Kaemmerer and Butenkötter 1973; WHO 1973). If the "letter of the law" were explicitly enforced under this concept by the Food, Drug and Cosmetic Act, any residue irrespective of how finite in quantity such as 1 ppb, 1 ppt, or less would be considered illegal. The "illegal" food product would therefore be subject to seizure and condemnation even though the quantity of residue in the product might not be a hazard to health. In the establishment of safety factors, toxicologists must be reasonable and be willing to accept levels of residues in foods for human consumption that are considered to be "toxicologically insignificant"; otherwise, we will not be able to produce abundant high-quality or low-cost foods of either plant or animal origin through the use of drugs or chemicals. The return to organic food production would not be a satisfactory solution and would not provide the quantities of food needed to sustain an expanding population in this nation or the world. The question has been asked, If organic procedures for the production of food as often proposed were instituted in the United States to replace the use of all drugs or chemicals, which 50 million or more people would want to be the ones to face starvation first?

DEFINITIONS AND TERMINOLOGY

For the student to better understand the terminology used throughout this discussion, it is necessary to define and discuss the terms commonly used by pharmacologists, toxicologists, and regulatory officials. Unless it is specified otherwise, the terms defined and discussed below are based on the author's own experience or have originated from a number of reports of joint meetings of the Food Agricultural Organization (FAO) and World Health Organization (WHO) during the last 10 years.

Drug or Chemical Residue

A *residue* of a parent drug or chemical and its metabolites may accumulate and be deposited or stored within the cells, tissues, or organs of an animal following the use of drugs and chemicals in the control and treatment of animal diseases or from use of a feed additive used to promote growth and feed efficiency. A residue may also occur when drugs or chemicals are intentionally or unintentionally added to food products. Residual quantities of a drug or chemical and its derivatives are expressed in parts by weight such as mg/kg or mg/L (i.e., ppm), μg/kg or μg/L (i.e., ppb), or ng/kg or ng/L (i.e., ppt).

Feed Additives

Feed additives are defined as drug, chemical, or biological substances added directly to animal feeds in small quantities, usually in concentrations of a few ppm for the purpose of modifying some aspect of performance or production (Shillam 1974).

Target Animal

Use of *target animal* refers to the determination of safety and efficacy of a drug directly within the species for which therapeutic claims are made by the drug manufacturer. In other words, claims made for a drug in the treatment of bovine ketosis must have been tested and evaluated in cattle and not in rats or any other species. Safety and tissue residue data for drugs approved by the FDA in food-producing animals must have been obtained from the so-called target species to coincide with the therapeutic claims made by the manufacturer.

Negligible or Finite Residue

A *negligible* or *finite residue* is an amount of a drug or chemical residue in or on feed or food commodities that would result in a daily intake regarded as toxicologically insignificant on the basis of scientific judgment of adequate safety data (Bevenue and Kawano 1971). This level of residue in the diet would ordinarily be less than 1/200 of the no-effect level observed in feeding trials or in subacute toxicity studies in the most sensitive species tested. The duration of these studies is generally based on 10% of the test animal's lifetime; for a rat with a 30-month life span, this would be

3 months, and for a human being with a life expectancy of 70 years, this would be 7 years (Friedman 1969).

Unintentional Residue

An *unintentional residue* is one that occurs in a feed or food as a result of circumstances not intended to protect the feed or food against the attack of infectious or parasitic diseases. For example, the residue may be acquired at any phase in the growth, production, processing, or storage of feed or food. An intentional or direct additive, on the other hand, is a drug or chemical substance added to a ration for purposes of disease control or promotion of growth.

The unintentional residue also includes a residue of a drug or chemical that occurs as an environmental contaminant but cannot be differentiated from residues due to the actual use of drugs or chemicals. Residues sometimes described as "action level," "indirect additives," "accidental," "incidental," or "background" are encompassed within this term. Regulatory authorities in the FDA often refer to the "action level" for establishment of limits on the background level of uncontrollable residues originating from environmental sources. For example, the action level of dieldrin, a chlorinated hydrocarbon pesticide, in oils and fats intended for use in animal feed is 0.3 ppm and in complete or finished animal feed rations the level for the chemical is 0.03 ppm. In general, the action level for all the chlorinated hydrocarbons is 0.3 ppm in oils and fats; for the organic phosphates and carbamates it is the sensitivity limits of the analytical method.

Action levels must not be misconstrued to mean the same thing as tolerance levels. The law prohibits the intentional or deliberate addition of contaminants such as dieldrin and other pesticidal chemicals to animal feed in any quantity.

Acceptable Daily Intake

The *acceptable daily intake* (ADI) is the daily dosage of a drug or chemical residue that, during the entire lifetime of a human being, appears to be without appreciable risk to health on the basis of all the facts known at the time. "Without appreciable risk" is interpreted to mean the practical certainty that a lifetime exposure to the residue will not result in a deleterious or injurious effect. For a drug or chemical residue, the ADI is established to provide a guide for the maximum quantity that can be taken daily in food without appreciable risk to the consumer. The calculation for the ADI is derived as nearly as possible from feeding trials in animals and/or in human beings. ADI values are always subject to revision whenever new information becomes available and are expressed in mg of drug or chemical/kg of body weight.

The following illustration shows how the ADI of a residue is determined:

1. The level of X drug or chemical when fed in the diet to the most sensitive species revealed the maximum no-adverse-effect or no-effect level to be 100 ppm. (See the discussion below regarding the toxicological significance of the no-adverse effect level of a drug or chemical.) In chronic toxicity studies involving mammalian species, rodent and nonrodent species are used in determining the no-effect levels. When this evaluation was conducted, it turned out that the rat was the most sensitive species tested. Since the average consumption of the mature rat weighing about 200 g is approximately 15 g of feed/day, a dietary intake of 100 ppm (i.e., 100 mg/kg of feed) would result in a total consumption of 1.5 mg of X drug or chemical/a 200-g rat or 7.5 mg/kg of body weight.

2. The Joint FAO and WHO Expert Committee on Food Additives recognizes that the expression ADI in relation to body weight does not reflect the relative exposure of animals of different size as accurately as would the metabolic mass that is equal to $W_b^{0.75}$ (WHO 1974a). Nevertheless, in practice the method of stating the dose level in terms of mg/kg of body weight has proved satisfactory. Moreover, a safety factor of 100 has been widely accepted in extrapolation from the chronic animal toxicity data to human beings. Therefore, the ADI value for the human

being is derived by taking 1/100 of the no-adverse-effect or no-effect level of the X drug level. In this case, 1/100 of 7.5 mg/kg is equal to 0.075 mg/kg for the ADI level in the human being. For additional information regarding the establishment of a safety level or margin for drug residues, see Tolerance Level and Margin of Safety.

PERMISSIBLE RESIDUE

The *permissible level of a residue,* ordinarily a pesticide residue, in or on a food crop is the quantity of the residue permitted when first offered for consumption. The value is calculated from the ADI, the average fraction of the total diet made up by the food in question (also referred to as the food factor), and the average weight of the consumer. The permissible level is expressed in ppm of the fresh weight of the feed or food. The following illustration shows how the permissible level of a pesticide residue is obtained (WHO 1962):

1. A compound X, used as a chemical on a food crop, left a residual level, but not exceeding 1 ppm as established by best agricultural use when it is first presented in the market for human consumption.

2. The food crop in which the residue might occur and the total quantity of food that would be consumed daily by an average person (i.e., 70 kg) on the basis of national food consumption data would be obtained (known as the food factor). If it was determined that the total average consumption of the food product containing the residue was 500 g out of a total daily consumption of 2000 g for an average person, the food factor would be 500/2000 or 0.25. Since the food product when first presented to the consumer does not contain greater than 1 ppm of chemical X, 1 kg of the food product would contain 1 mg of the X chemical (i.e., 1 ppm). Therefore, 500 g of the food product would contain 0.5 mg of X chemical residue.

3. In an average person weighing 70 kg, the daily intake of X chemical would be 0.5 mg/70 kg or 0.007 mg/kg of body weight.

4. If the ADI as derived from the evaluation of toxicological data (procedure for derivation of ADI was discussed above) for chemical X is 0.075 mg/kg of body weight/day (i.e., 70 kg $\times$ 0.075 mg), the total intake for chemical X is equal to 5.25 mg/person/day.

5. Therefore, the permissible level of chemical X in the treated food product would be 10.5 ppm or 10.5 mg/kg of the treated food product. Consumption of 500 g of the food product would result in an ADI of 5.25 mg/person/day (5.25 mg/0.5 kg = 10.5 mg/kg or 10.5 ppm). However, since 10.5 ppm are not necessary or required under good agricultural use of compound X, the tolerance is set at 1 ppm (WHO 1962). It is set at 1 ppm because under good or best agricultural practice no more than this level of compound X is required to accomplish an effective job of pest control. These same tolerance levels, i.e., ones established from good agricultural use or practice on crops, are often transposed by toxicologists in the establishment of animal tissue residue tolerances. When this is done, a safety factor for compound X in the human being becomes much greater than 100. If 10.5 ppm of chemical X can be consumed without appreciable risk based upon the ADI value, it would appear that the safe tolerance should be set at 10.5 ppm rather than at 1 ppm. Certainly no more pesticide or chemical should be used in the production of food than is necessary to accomplish an effective job of pest control. Yet, it appears unreasonable that food of plant or animal origin should have to be condemned because it is higher than the best agricultural use indicates. When such a practice is followed, a considerable economic loss to the producers often results. Also, the condemned food product containing compound X above the 1 ppm tolerance level is unavailable for human consumption. This causes the food costs to rise because of the application of an unnecessarily conservative tolerance level. Regulatory agencies such as the U.S. Department of Agriculture (USDA), the FDA, and the Environmental Protection Agency (EPA) should review and evaluate those tolerance levels, especially for chemicals where they were

transposed from crop use to animal use. Tolerances that are ultraconservative should be revised so that our food supply is not unduly jeopardized. This will become more important in the future if adequate food supplies are maintained to keep pace with the population growth of this nation and the world.

Tolerance Level

A *tolerance level* is the maximum level or concentration of a drug or chemical that is permitted in or on feed or food at a specified time of slaughter and harvesting, processing, storage, and marketing of the feed or food up to the time of consumption by animal or human being. Tolerance levels are expressed in parts by weight of the drug or chemical residue per million or billion parts by weight of the food and are never greater than the permissible level for the feed or food in question. Refer to the illustration above regarding the derivation of the permissible level, including the author's objection to the practice of transposing the same tolerance levels for chemicals as established under best agricultural use for determining the tolerance levels in animal tissues.

Requirements for the establishment of a tolerance demand the demonstration of an adequate margin of safety in experimental trials with two mammalian species. One of the species must be a nonrodent. Avian species are not used in the assessment of the margin of safety because of the difficulty in extrapolating the information to human beings. The experimental trials involve acute, subacute (90-day study), and chronic toxicity studies. Chronic toxicity studies usually extend for the life of the animal. In the case of rodents it is 2 years or more and for other species a lifetime study may be as long as 5–7 years. Also, a three-generation reproductive study is usually required (Food and Drug Administration 1970). In the event of considerable species variation to a drug response, additional studies may be required by the FDA (Kingma 1969).

The FDA and the EPA have the responsibility of establishing tolerances of drugs, chemicals, or biological substances in animal feeds and human foods. Most of the jurisdiction of the EPA pertains to the pesticides, fungicides, and chemicals contaminating the environment. The USDA must enforce the tolerances established by the FDA and the EPA when they apply to meat and poultry products. For milk, enforcement of tolerances is the responsibility of the FDA.

Temporary Tolerance

A *temporary tolerance* is one that is valid for a restricted period and is subject to revision upon the availability of new information. Regulatory agencies such as the FDA, the USDA, and the EPA often refer to the temporary tolerance as an "administrative" or "interim" tolerance level.

No Residue or Zero Tolerance

A *no-residue* or *zero-tolerance* level of a drug or chemical residue by strict definition indicates that absolutely no residue shall be present in or on feed or food commodities for consumption either by animals or human beings. Zero tolerance is the nomenclature used by the FDA for any residue of a compound too toxic to permit a residue in or on feeds or foods. No residue, on the other hand, is the nomenclature used by the USDA, based upon experimental data, to indicate that no residue shall remain from the use of a particular drug or chemical, regardless of the toxic properties of the compound (Bevenue and Kawano 1971). In actual usage and practice, zero tolerance and no residue are used interchangeably by regulatory authorities and are interpreted by most individuals as meaning the same thing.

All veterinary drugs approved by the FDA for use in food-producing animals are on a zero-tolerance (no-residue) basis or are on a specific finite tolerance basis from 0.5 to 8 ppm (Kingma 1969). As pointed out in the introductory portion of this discussion, improvement in analytical methodology has made it possible to detect extremely minute quantities of drug residues beyond the ppm level. Consequently, the terms "zero tolerance" and "no residue" should no longer be used by regulatory agencies because they are scientifically and administratively untenable and should give way in favor of finite residue or negligible residue.

No Effect or Maximum No Adverse Effect

For most biological responses it is assumed that a *threshold* and a *no-effect level* exist. From all evidence, a threshold for biological activities exists within a cell at 4×10^4 molecules (Dinman 1972). In other words, a cellular response would not be expected when the concentration of a drug or chemical is less than 4×10^4 molecules/cell.

The term "effect" must be clarified to avoid semantic misinterpretation. First of all, it must be emphasized that an effect produced within a biological system is not always harmful. In fact, Dinman (1972) defines "effect" as a neutral word implying neither benefit nor harm. According to Dinman, "to assume that the consequence of a drug or chemical agent is a harmful one is to ignore a biological reality; that is, all chemical constituents of the cell are constantly 'turned over,' they are being replaced and renewed."

When toxicologists use the terms *no effect* and *maximum no adverse effect,* they generally refer to a level of a drug or chemical that produces no harmful effect. The terms are also used to denote no change or effect upon physiological activity, no change in organ weight or body weight as well as in the rate of growth, and no change or effect upon cellular structure or enzymatic activity of cells. In most instances, a drug must show no effect when fed for 2 years to the most sensitive species before it can be permitted in the human diet (Kingma 1969). A no-effect or negative observation in toxicologic studies is always subject to severe criticism by the unloving critics and uncritical lovers. As Barnes and Denz (1954) stated, "It is easy to suggest that some positive effect might have been obtained by using a different species, a different criteria of toxicity, and a longer period of toxicity."

Toxicologic Insignificance

In 1969 the National Academy of Sciences, National Research Council (NAS–NRC), prepared a report entitled *Guidelines for Estimating Toxicologically Insignificant Levels of Chemicals in Food.* The report was submitted to the FDA and pointed out that the ADI of a chemical in the total diet (safe level) for human consumption is established through toxicologic evaluation and is commonly expressed as 1/100 of the experimentally no-adverse–effect level. Guidelines proposed by the NAS–NRC for the definition of *toxicologically insignificant levels* were based on the premise that, except for certain nutrients and hormones, certain heavy metals, and certain organic compounds, such as pesticides, no single organic compound in commercial use has been demonstrated to be toxic to animals at dietary levels less than 40 ppm (Oser 1969). Consequently, if a chemical other than one in the above categories has been in commercial production for at least 5 years "without evidence of toxicological hazard incident to its production or use," it is regarded as toxicologically insignificant at a level of 0.1 ppm or less in the diet. For metabolites of pesticides that are generally less toxic than parent compounds, the 0.1 ppm level is also considered as toxicologically insignificant provided the ADI of the pesticide itself is 1 ppm or greater (National Academy of Sciences 1969).

Where the safe levels of organic chemicals have not been determined through animal studies but are functionally effective at concentrations above 0.1 ppm in the diet, it is believed justifiable to consider the structural similarities to other chemical compounds whose toxic and metabolic characteristics are known. Therefore, any pure chemical is considered to be toxicologically insignificant at a level of 1 ppm or less in the diet if its structure is simple, suggestive of ready metabolic handling, and analogous to a closely related group that, without known exception, is or can be assumed to be characterized by a low order of toxicity (Oser 1969). For new chemicals where the chemical structures are "less closely related," the NAS–NRC guidelines suggest that adequate studies be conducted to establish safe levels of a similar magnitude for at least two comparable or analogous compounds. Furthermore, the acute and subacute toxic effects of the new chemical and the analogous chemicals should be similar. If they are similar, the toxicologically insignificant level is then regarded to be 1/10 of the lowest safe level of the analogous substances; if they are dissimilar, a 1/20 factor is recommended by NAS–NRC (Oser 1969).

Carcinogenic Effect

The term *carcinogenic effect* refers to an effect produced by a substance having carcinogenic or cancer-producing activity. Considerable confusion has existed because a carcinogen applies to substances that are so varied in their qualitative and quantitative characteristics (WHO 1974b). Although a preponderance of evidence exists that exposure to carcinogens results in an irreversible biological effect, more information is suggesting that the concept of irreversibility may be subject to modification (Weisburger and Weisburger 1968). Since all chemical carcinogens pose a hazard, human exposure must be reduced to a practical minimum.

The potency of chemical carcinogens can vary in comparable test systems by an order of magnitude as high as 10^7. It is generally recognized that there is no relationship between the toxicity and carcinogenicity of chemical compounds. Ordinarily, the toxic dose of a carcinogen is higher than the carcinogenic dose (Barnes and Denz 1954). The concept prevalently exists that only one molecule of a carcinogenic agent is required to induce cancer in human beings or animals. However, Dinman (1972) stated, "To believe that a single molecule's presence in a cell implies a definite potential for deleterious effect disregards stochastic considerations."

There is good evidence that a large number of molecules/cell are required for a carcinogen to induce its effect (Claus 1974). For example, it requires 1×10^5 molecules/liver cell/day of aflatoxin in feed for 6 months and about 3×10^9 molecules/cell administered orally in a single dose to produce hepatocarcinoma in the rat. Both of these values are well above the postulated 10^4 molecules/cell.

Since cancer induction in human beings may take several decades, a drug or chemical agent may be extensively used for some time before evidence of carcinogenicity appears (WHO 1969a). For example, use of high dose levels of DES to prevent abortion in pregnant women has been associated with the induction of vaginal or cervical adenocarcinoma in their offspring (Greenwald et al. 1971, 1973; Herbst et al. 1971). It has been calculated that a maximum of 50,000 liveborn females/year, born between 1960 and 1970, were exposed to DES *in utero* (Heinonen 1973). Exposure to levels of DES as high as 15 g over more than 200 days has been reported in the literature in the prevention of abortion. According to Cole (1972), a woman would have to consume the carcass and livers of 460 steers weighing 500 lb each for 180 days to receive the same amount of DES prescribed (up to 16.5 g) for a case of threatened abortion. The amount of DES calculated above is based on the recommended *implant* dose of 36 mg/animal and on the assumption that the 120-day withdrawal time after treatment of the animals had not been observed prior to slaughter.

Some scientists believe that the no-effect level for a carcinogen cannot be determined. Consequently, this is the basis of the Delaney Clause, which does not permit any level of a known carcinogen to be added to the food supply of human beings. In food-producing animals treated with or fed carcinogenic compounds, no residues are permitted in the edible tissues at the time of slaughter under this clause. Despite the belief by some scientists that the no-effect level for a carcinogen cannot be determined, it is frequently possible to demonstrate a positive response that is dose related. As previously pointed out, the dosage of known carcinogens required to elicit a response varies by a high order of magnitude. This variability is quite striking between a dose concentration of aflatoxin and

DES that is required to produce cancer in laboratory animals. For example, aflatoxin is capable of inducing a carcinogenic effect at a daily dose level of only a few μg/kg of body weight whereas the dose level for DES to produce such an effect is about 1000 times greater (WHO 1969a). Yet the consumer's concern about 2 ppb of DES in beef liver appears to be much greater than the accepted FDA interim tolerance level of 20 ppb for aflatoxin in cereal grains or peanuts. Inasmuch as aflatoxin is not added by persons but is a naturally occurring toxin in nature, it appears to be much more acceptable to the consumer than manufactured chemical additives.

It is beyond the scope of this discussion to cover the complex and intricate details associated with the assessment of safety of carcinogenic agents. For the interested reader, other literature sources may be consulted (Barnes and Denz 1954; Mantel and Bryan 1961; WHO 1969a; Food and Drug Administration 1971; WHO 1974b).

Mutagenic Effect

The term *mutagen* is used to describe those chemical agents that damage the genetic components of a cell or organism. Genetic material of all living organisms, with the exception of some viruses, is deoxyribonucleic acid (DNA). Several chemicals, including alkylating agents and analogs of DNA bases, have been shown to elicit mutagenic activity (U.S. Senate Hearing 1971). In recent years there has been increasing concern that drugs as well as environmental chemicals may pose a potential hazard to the human population by the production of gene mutations or chromosome aberrations (WHO 1971). Three principal types of genetic injury have been recognized: (1) point mutation, (2) gene elimination, and (3) chromosome breakage (Fahmy and Fahmy 1964). Either the germinal or somatic cells may be affected. Understandably, injury to either cell group may lead to serious consequences. However, from a public health standpoint mutations in the germinal cells are of more immediate importance because of the hazard to future generations.

Testing procedures for assessing mutagenicity of drugs and chemicals have not been clearly established. Recommendations or suggestions in the evaluation of drug or chemical agents for mutagenic potential have been published (WHO 1971, 1974b).

Teratogenic Effect

The term *teratogen* applies to drug or chemical agents that produce a toxic effect on the embryo or fetus during a critical phase of the gestation period. As a consequence, a congenital malformation that affects the structural and functional integrity of the organism is produced. The well-known thalidomide incident involving a number of children in Europe is direct testimony to the hazards that may occur when such an agent is administered during pregnancy. Approximately 5 years after the introduction of thalidomide into clinical use, this drug was identified as the etiologic agent of phocomelia or "seal limbs."

Methallibure, an anterior pituitary activator or estrus cycling control chemical for swine used in the United Kingdom, has been reported as a teratogen. Leftover feed containing this chemical was fed to swine contrary to label instructions. Exposure *in utero* resulted in a significant number of congenital abnormalities in the newborn piglets (Vente et al. 1972). There are a number of other compounds, including those derived from plant sources, that have teratogenic effect in animals.

Experimental methods used in the detection of teratogenic agents involve the design of a three-generation reproductive study (Food and Drug Administration 1970).

Drug Allergy or Hypersensitivity

An allergic or hypersensitive effect following the administration of a drug, i.e., *drug allergy,* is quite similar to that typified by allergic responses to protein, carbohydrate, and lipid macromolecules. Allergic reactions to drugs or chemicals may include anaphylaxis, serum sickness, cutaneous reactions, and a delayed hypersensitive response. In human beings allergic or hypersensitive responses to drugs appear to be more commonly associated with the antibiotics, especially penicillin (Huber 1970, 1971). About 10% of the human population is considered to be hypersensitive to a number of substances, including penicillin (Kautz 1959). In animals the extent of the hypersensitivity to drugs is not well known. Severe or fatal reactions may occur in some species. For example, penicillin may produce a fatal reaction in the guinea pig and chinchilla. In the parakeet procaine in penicillin may have a lethal effect in small concentrations.

For additional information on hypersensitivity in human beings and animals, the reader is referred to Hypersensitivity Due to Antibiotic Residues later in this chapter.

MARGIN OF SAFETY

Before a drug product can be approved for use in food animals, sufficient scientific evidence must be presented to the FDA to show that the product is both safe and efficacious for use in the target animal for which the various claims are made (Booth 1973). In addition, the metabolism characteristics of the drug product, including the tissue decay profile, must be known so that either no residues persist in edible products or any residues that are present are noninjurious when animal products are consumed by human beings (Fitzhugh 1964). Toxicologists have a key role in the evaluation of safety of drugs used in both human beings and animals.

Frequently, the question is asked, How safe is safe? Some scientists believe that society is willing to accept a risk-to-benefit ratio of 1:100,000 up to no less than 1:100,000,000. This means that adverse effects, including the possibility of death, may occur 1 time in 100,000 or only 1 time in 100,000,000 people. At this latter level, virtual safety has been defined by Mantel and Bryan (1961) as a risk level that society might accept. If the level of virtual safety was only acceptable to the public and was universally adopted, most substances (anesthetics, antibiotics, and many other chemotherapeutic agents) would have to be rigidly restricted if not abandoned entirely.

It is obvious from a practical standpoint that absolute safety of a drug or chemical cannot be assured any more than safety can be assured in driving an automobile. Lave (1972) facetiously suggested that 50,000 highway fatalities each year and many thousands of injuries could be prevented in the United States by imposing a speed limit of no more than 2 miles/hour. In a similar manner, all drug products not absolutely or virtually safe should be greatly curtailed or prohibited. It is evident that our regulatory agencies through the request of the people could unknowingly require high safety standards that do not always lead to public benefit and welfare. Safety, according to Oser (1969), "must balance elements of risk associated with normal or intended use, or even in some circumstances with improper or accidental use, against potential advantages resulting from proper use. Assessments of safety must take into account not only the intrinsic chemical, physical, or mechanical attributes of the product in question but also the intelligence, responsibility, and susceptibility of the user or host. Benefits and risks cannot ordinarily be quantitated in comparable terms, and hence it is not possible to write a balanced equation. It must also be accepted as a basic premise that judgments of safety cannot be rendered with absolute certainty, regardless of whether they are based on animal tests or on actual experience in use."

In the assessment of safety, it is necessary to determine the maximum dose or concentration of a drug that does not produce an adverse response or effect in at least two mammalian species; one of the species must be a nonrodent. (See the discussion above under No Effect or Maximum No Adverse Effect.)

In the extrapolation of this information to human beings, a margin of safety can be determined, i.e., an ADI for drug or chemical residues that may persist in edible products such as meat, milk, and eggs. Experimentally, however, it may be difficult to determine whether or not an effect observed is deleterious (WHO 1967). For instance, diarrhea induced by a drug or chemical may be the result of a toxic effect or it could be a nontoxic effect due to osmotic activity often associated with a high dietary intake of the test material. If it is the latter effect that is responsible for the production of the diarrhea as determined by no histopathological changes, it is reasonably acceptable to apply a lower margin of safety than that required for an unequivocal toxic effect.

Joint Expert Committees of FAO and WHO have generally accepted a margin of safety for residual chemicals as food additives that are noncarcinogenic at the 100-fold level following lifetime or chronic toxicity studies in at least two mammalian species. As previously mentioned in this discussion, carcinogenic chemical residues are not permitted in food for human consumption under the Delaney Clause. In a number of instances, a safety margin of 200 has been applied in determining safety of noncarcinogens following chronic toxicity studies. However, FAO and WHO may recommend the use of higher margins of safety than 100 or 200 when toxicological data are inadequate or unavailable from animal studies. Where the data have been derived directly from valid human experimentation, extrapolation from animals is not necessary and may make it possible to use a lower margin of safety. If an intentional food additive is a beneficial component of the diet or is a normal body constituent, there is a reasonable basis for a lower margin of safety. For example, it is unreasonable to apply a 100-fold safety margin to many common additives such as sodium chloride (WHO 1967).

The same principle as cited above for the human being applies to the use of toxicological data obtained in target animals. Understandably, toxicological data obtained in experimental studies on cattle are more meaningful when the information is to be applied in the field to the overall cattle population, i.e., the target species. Experimental data obtained from the rat (i.e., a nontarget species) or other species would not be as useful in its direct application to cattle. When adequate toxicological data have been collected within a target species, a safety factor of 10 is generally accepted. The variation within a specific species (i.e., intraspecies) usually does not vary greater than by a factor of 10; interspecies variation may vary another 10-fold, requiring a safety factor of no less than 100 (Oser 1969).

In the extrapolation of animal toxicity data to human beings, the 100-fold margin of safety (i.e., 1/100 of the maximum no-adverse–effect level) has been uncritically and arbitrarily accepted by national and international regulatory agencies. Its universal acceptance has achieved somewhat sacrosanct status (Oser 1969). Toxicologists have generally accepted this magnitude of safety based on the empirical premise that the human being is about 10 times more sensitive than the most sensitive test animal (usually the rodent) to the effects of drugs and toxic substances. Toxicity data are primarily obtained from acute oral tests and their applicability to the effects of low chronic dosages is of questionable value. Since it is generally recognized that the human being is 10 times more sensitive than the most sensitive test animal (interspecies variation) and variations within human beings (intraspecies variation) cover about a 10-fold range, a safety factor of $1/10 \times 1/10$, or 1/100, has been considered justifiable.

Without question, the pharmacologic effects and dosage relationships are important for assessment of the margin of safety. Dose levels of all chemical substances can be generally classified from a pharmacological basis as ineffective, effective, toxic, and lethal (Frazer 1953). With most common drugs, the general ratio of ineffective, effective, toxic, and lethal dosage in human beings is not greater than 1:10:100:1000, respectively. A similar scale would also be expected to apply in animals of any given species.

PRINCIPLES FOR ESTABLISHING WITHDRAWAL TIMES

The term *withdrawal time* (also known as the depletion or clearance period) refers to the interval from the time an animal is removed from medication until the permitted time of slaughter. This interval is not intended to safeguard the health of the animal but is required to minimize or prevent violative levels of drug residues in edible tissues for human consumption. Withdrawal time intervals vary with each drug preparation and vary among the different species. Depending on the drug product, dosage form, and route of administration, the withdrawal time may vary from a few hours to several days or weeks. A withdrawal period of 120 days is required following the subcutaneous implantation of DES in cattle before they are slaughtered for human consumption. Only 48 hours is required for withdrawal of melengestrol acetate (MGA), a synthetic hormonal agent used orally to prevent estrus in feedlot heifers prior to slaughter.

With approval of the 1958 Food Additives Amendment by Congress, drug manufacturers are now required to submit tissue residue and depletion rate data on all new animal drug applications, including a method for the detection of residues. This requirement pertains only to the food-producing animals. Depletion rate and residue studies are not only required to obtain an understanding of drug concentrations in edible tissues but are also useful in determining when tissue residues are reduced to acceptable tolerance levels or to the limit of detectability. Upon completion of these studies, residue levels in edible tissues may exceed those acceptable to the FDA and other regulatory agencies, and the establishment of a depletion period or withdrawal interval therefore becomes an important part of the 1958 food additives regulation.

Evaluation of the depletion rate of a drug begins with a metabolism study (Sutherland 1969); metabolism and residue studies are ordinarily conducted side by side. This procedure is generally followed because the method for the detection of residues may require modification to enable the detection of metabolites of the parent drug. For example, the metabolites may be more toxic than the residues of the parent drug or chemical. Paraoxon, a metabolite of parathion, is more toxic following degradation in the liver.

In the identification of metabolic pathways as well as the determination of the distribution patterns and presence of residues in tissues, radiolabeled drugs are used. Animals are primed with the unlabeled or nonradio-tagged ("cold") drug or chemical for several dosages before the radiolabeled ("hot") drug is administered in a single dosage. Although the metabolic pathways can be identified in this manner, use of radio-tagged compounds does not necessarily provide correct information on the excretion rate or fate of the more solid bound cold drug. Despite this and other imperfections, use of radiolabeled compounds in metabolism studies have been valuable in the development of a final metabolic flow diagram.

Initially, most metabolism studies are performed in small laboratory animals. Isolation and the biochemical identification of metabolites are generally conducted from the excreta with concomitant studies performed on blood and tissues. Urine provides a good source of metabolites. Metabolite concentrations in urine are often higher than in tissues, making isolation, concentration, and identification relatively easy compared to the use of other body fluids and tissues.

The FDA generally requires depletion data for urine, blood, and bile and in edible tissues such as liver, kidney, skeletal muscle, heart, and fat. Although urine and other body fluids provide reasonable indices of the depletion rate of a drug, concentrations of drug residues or metabolites are variable and are related to water intake of the animal. Depending on the stability and biodegradability of the drug or metabolite, fecal analyses may be of no value because of microbial alteration. On the other hand, the gut flora is capable of converting an inactive compound to highly active or toxic metabolites and should not be discounted entirely in metabolism studies (Smith 1971).

Many depletion curves follow the first-order decay principle (Fig. 63.1). The depletion curve is necessary in the establishment of biological half-life of a drug or metabolite. Simply expressed, the deple-

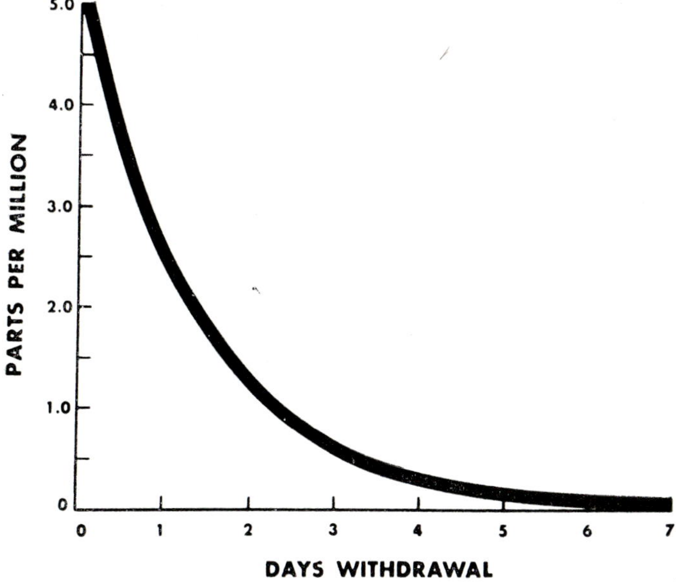

Fig. 63.1. Theoretical depletion of a drug from animal tissue—biological half-life 24 hours. (From Sutherland 1969)

tion curve indicates when one-half of the drug or chemical disappears from the animal in t units of time. The remaining half also requires the same length of time for one-half of it to disappear. In other words, several $t_{1/2}$ times (up to 10 half-lives) may be required before most of the drug is depleted. This knowledge is useful and is the basis for the establishment of a withdrawal interval that will permit tissue residues to decline to or below the acceptable tolerance level.

For many drugs the biological half-life may also indicate the accumulation rate in tissue, including the binding to plasma proteins (Van Rossum 1968). An accumulation to 90% of the plateau may be attained after a time interval of 3.3 times the biological half-life.

The curvilinear form of the depletion curve as shown in Fig. 63.1 is not as easy to use as the semilogarithm form of the curve (see Fig. 63.2). Since the decay curve is an exponential function plotted against time

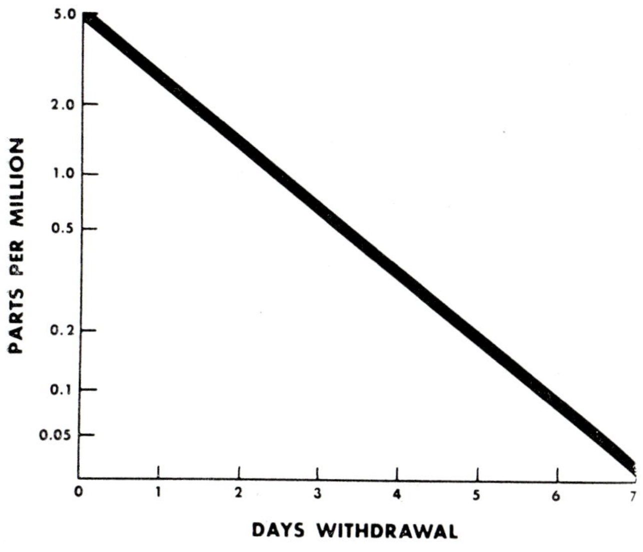

Fig. 63.2. Depletion of a drug from animal tissue—biological half-life 24 hours. (From Sutherland 1969)

(t), the plot on a semilog scale provides a straight line that is much easier to use. Data from depletion studies nearly always can be plotted by a straight or linear line. Biological half-lives usually have a precision within plus or minus 2–3 hours (Sutherland 1969).

It must be made clear that the half-life is related to a given species, a specific tissue of that animal, and a specified route of administration of the drug (Sutherland 1969). Also, it possibly may be related to the duration of administration of the drug. The biological half-lives of a drug given intravenously and in oral dosage are essentially similar. Intramuscular, as well as topical, administration of drugs (e.g., pour-on administration of organophosphate compounds) gives rise to variable half-lives from animal to animal even within the same species. Although the total daily intake of the drug may be the same if administered in water or feed, concentration of the drug in body fluids and tissues may be initially higher following administration in water than in feed. However, a curve or line parallel to the feed line will be observed (Sutherland 1969).

In essence, depletion of a drug from the tissues of an animal never reaches a zero concentration or zero tolerance level. Zero levels of residues following the use of feed additives and veterinary drugs are considered to be something of a scientific impossibility. Sutherland stated that "regulatory changes such as those being effected in pesticide regulations in the United States, in which finite tolerances are substituted for zero, should be considered for meat, milk, and eggs. Present regulations for milk require three successive 'negative' milkings in drug-depletion studies. While this has some merit in the case of mammary infusion products where the possibility of mechanical occlusion of the drug within the udder exists, I can think of no rationale that justifies this requirement in the case of a feed or drinking-water additive. The results of an unadorned, properly conducted depletion study are unequivocal."

It would be misleading if the student were left with the impression that all depletion studies could be plotted by nice straight-line graphs. In Fig. 63.3, the depletion of a drug from fat and skeletal muscle is a linear function whereas it is nonlinear for the kidney and liver. Binding to protein and other biological components accounts for the slower or prolonged disappearance of the drug. Moreover, the analytical method may respond to the metabolites of the parent compound, which will also give a nonlogarithmic depletion

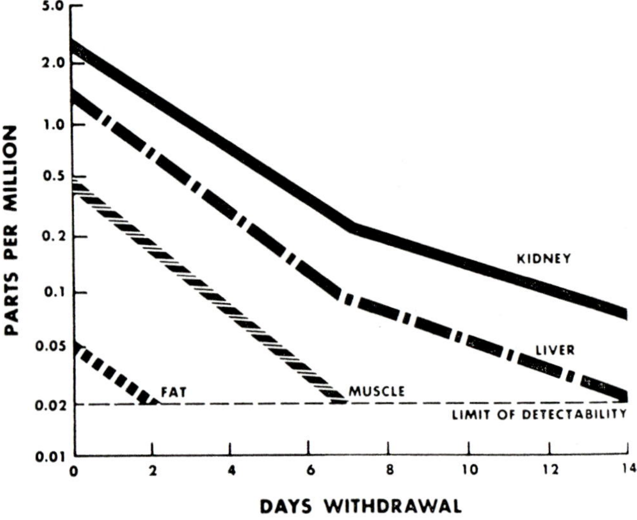

FIG. 63.3. A drug-depletion study, showing drug binding. (From Sutherland 1969)

curve. This complicates the determination of the half-life; the linear and nonlinear portions of the curve are additive and can be used in deriving the half-life by other mathematical treatment.

Figure 63.4 illustrates that the method for detection of tissue residues should be sufficiently sensitive in the measurement of residue concentrations at least as low as the tolerance level set on the basis of toxicologic considerations (Sutherland 1969). In the illustration, Sutherland has modified Fig. 63.3 by assigning it a much higher limit of detectability (0.2 ppm) and has proposed a tolerance level of 0.05 ppm or 50 ppb, which is much lower than this new detectability limit. For liver and kidney, the broken-line portion of the curve is now below the limit or capability of the method to detect the residues. If the lines were "straightened" to extrapolate to the proposed level of tolerance (0.05 ppm), the withdrawal or depletion interval would be about 2 days too short for liver and 5 days too short for the kidney. Analytical methodology must, therefore, be sufficiently sensitive and accurate to detect residues at least down to the proposed tolerance level to avoid the kind of problem illustrated below (Fig. 63.4).

WITHDRAWAL TIMES AND TOLERANCES FOR VETERINARY DRUGS

Drug or chemical feed additives and antimicrobial agents approved by the FDA for use in feed and drinking water of food-producing animals number about 300 or more. Another 100 or more preparations may be administered in single or multiple doses by the oral or parenteral route. Consequently, the veterinary medical practitioner must be familiar with the pharmacodynamic and toxicologic effects of a large number of pharmaceutical preparations that are useful in the diagnosis, prevention, control, and treatment of animal diseases. Also, familiarity with the specified times required for the removal or withdrawal of animals from medication prior to slaughter is imperative. Withdrawal of medication is necessary so violative or illegal levels of drug residues above tolerance are avoided in meat, milk, and eggs marketed for human consumption. The experimental basis for determining the withdrawal interval or depletion rate of drugs and its relation to the tolerance level of residues in tissues has been discussed above.

Whenever drug or chemical preparations are administered to food-producing

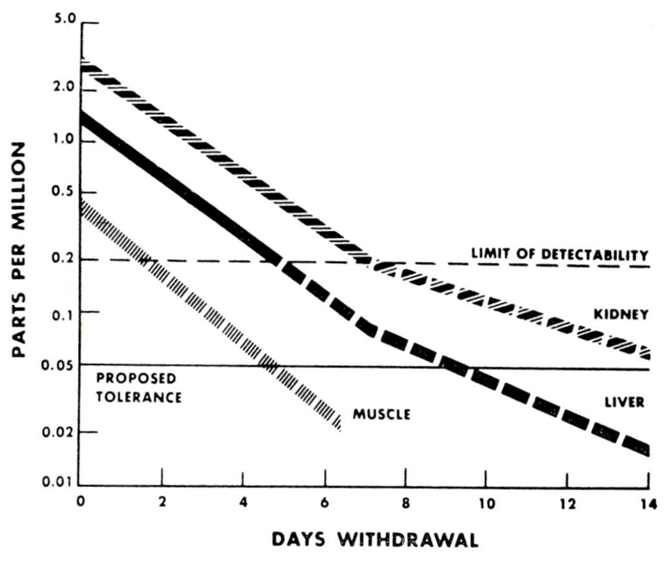

Fig. 63.4. A fictional depletion study, showing inadequate limit of detectability. (From Sutherland 1969)

animals, the veterinarian must alert the livestock owner to the necessity of withholding animals from market or slaughter during and following the treatment period. If the specific withdrawal time for a drug is unobserved, severe penalties can result when residues are detected in edible tissues above the accepted tolerance level. From a regulatory compliance as well as a public health standpoint, every effort must be made to avoid levels of residue in the human food supply that exceed the established tolerance levels.

According to Taylor (1965), most of the violative residues found in food animals are due to the misuse of drug or chemical preparations. This includes (1) slaughtering animals before observing the required period of withholding of drugs or chemicals, (2) using drugs to mask clinical signs at the time of slaughter to avoid condemnation of animals at antemortem inspection and, (3) feeding unapproved or unauthorized medicated feed to animals. Analysis of the probable causes of violative residue levels in edible tissues in 1973 by the FDA revealed that the withdrawal time had not been observed in 76% of the reports. Another 12% of the violations occurred from feed mill or delivery error; 6% were ostensibly due to inadequate cleaning of bins where different medicated feeds had been stored; and 6% were due to the unapproved use of the drug, i.e., the drug was administered to the incorrect species or the incorrect route of administration was employed because of failure to follow the directions on the labeled product.

It is not known what percentage of the violative residues may be due to improper label directions of a drug product. Surveillance studies conducted by the FDA involving antibiotic preparations for intramammary infusion in the treatment of bovine mastitis revealed that approximately 33% of the products tested would not give rise to violative residues in milk when used in accordance with the label directions (Booth 1974). The remaining products tested left residues in the milk from 12 to 140 hours beyond the stated milk-out or milk-discard time; 96 hours is the maximum time allowed by the FDA for the disappearance of drug residues in milk following the use of intramammary infusion products.

The presence of antibiotic residues in meat results primarily from the misuse of drug preparations (Kerr 1972). According to Kerr, of approximately 10,000 samples of red meat and poultry analyzed for drug residues in 1971, 435 samples were reported positive for residues. Of the residues reported in animal tissues, 25 contained DES, 267 contained antibiotics, 47 contained sulfonamides, and 96 contained arsenic. From a monitoring and surveillance aspect, the number of samples analyzed each year for residues is indeed small compared to the number of animals slaughtered each year for food purposes. There is no way that each animal can be tested for all residues; in 1973, well over 114 million livestock and 3 billion poultry were slaughtered (Trabosh 1974). This is a problem area that is recognized by both the USDA and the FDA. Until more practical methods become available for the rapid monitoring and detection of drug residues, this will be a difficult problem to overcome from a regulatory standpoint.

In accordance with the label directions of the drug product, the withdrawal times must be strictly observed so that meat, milk, or egg products will not contain illegal residues when they are sold for human consumption. Also, the drug should be used only for those conditions or circumstances under which approval for use was obtained. For example, the drug should not be administered to lactating dairy cattle when it is specified for use only in nonlactating dairy cattle. Additionally, if the drug product was approved only for intramuscular use, it should not be used by other routes of administration. Use of drug products via an unapproved route of administration, in an unapproved species, or where specified limitations are violated will inevitably lead to the presence of illegal residues in food products intended for human consumption. The proper use of drug prod-

TABLE 63.1. Drug withdrawal times, limitations for use, and tolerance levels of injectable drugs commonly used in cattle

Drug	Preslaughter Withdrawal Time	Discard Time for Milk Prior to Sale	Limitations for Use	Tolerance Level
	(days)	*(hours)*		*(ppm)*
Ampicillin trihydrate	6	48	...	Meat and milk, 0.01
Dihydrostreptomycin sulfate	30	48	...	Meat and milk, zero
Erythromycin	14	72	Do not use in calves	Meat and milk, zero
Hydrochlorothiazine	...	72	...	None published
Levamisole phosphate	7	...	Do not use in dairy animals of breeding age	Meat, 0.1
Oxytetracycline hydrochloride	20	...	Do not use in lactating dairy cattle	Meat, 0.1
Procaine penicillin G	5	72	...	Meat, 0.05; milk, zero
Procaine penicillin G and benzathine penicillin G	30	...	Use only in mature beef animals; do not use in lactating dairy cattle	Meat, 0.05; milk, zero
Procaine penicillin G, dihydrostreptomycin sulfate (DHS), and procaine hydrochloride (Pen-Strep, Combiotic)	30	72	...	Penicillin: meat, 0.05; milk, zero DHS: meat, zero; milk, zero
Sulfachloropyridazine sodium	5	...	Use only in calves; do not use in lactating dairy cows	None published
Sulfaethoxypyridazine	16	72	Do not use for more than 4 days	Meat, 0.1; milk, zero
Sulfamethazine (Sulmet)	10	96	...	Meat and milk, 0.1
Tylosin	8	96	Do not use in calves	Meat, 0.2; milk, 0.05

TABLE 63.2. Drug withdrawal times, limitations for use, and tolerance levels of drugs used orally in cattle

Drug	Preslaughter Withdrawal Time	Discard Time for Milk Prior to Sale	Limitations for Use	Tolerance Level
	(days)	*(hours)*		*(ppm)*
Chlormadinone acetate	28	...	Use only in beef heifers and cows	Zero
Chlorothiazide (Diuril)	...	72	Use only in dairy cattle	None published
Chlortetracycline (5 mg/lb/day)	10	...	Use only in mature beef cattle	Meat, 0.1; fat, zero; milk, zero
Chlortetracycline (Klortet) (350 mg/animal/day)	2	...	...	Meat, 0.1; fat, zero; milk, zero
Chlortetracycline and sulfamethazine	7	...	Use only in mature beef cattle	Meat, 0.1 for both drugs
Chlortetracycline hydrochloride	3	...	Use only in calves	Liver and kidney, 4.0; muscle and fat, 1.0
Chlortetracycline hydrochloride and sulfamethazine	7	...	Use only in mature beef cattle	Meat, 0.1 for both drugs
Dexamethasone and trichlormethiazide	...	72	Use only in dairy cattle	None published
Dihydrostreptomycin (DHS) and vitamin A	10	...	Use only in calves	DHS: meat, zero
Famphur	4	...	Withdraw drug 21 days prior to freshening; use only in nonlactating dairy cattle; do not use in animals exposed to cholinesterase inhibitors	Meat, 0.1
Haloxon	7	...	Do not use in dairy cattle or dairy goats of breeding age	Meat, 0.1
Levamisole hydrochloride	2	...	Use only in mature beef cattle	Meat, 0.1
Melengestrol acetate	2	...	Use only in feedlot heifers	Meat, zero
Ronnel (Trolene)	10	...	Do not use in lactating dairy cattle; withdraw 10 days prior to calving; do not use in animals exposed to cholinesterase inhibitors	Meat, 0.1
Streptomycin (Vetstrep)	2	...	Use only in calves and limit to 5 days of treatment	Meat, zero
Streptomycin, sulfamethazine, and phythalysulfathiazole	10	...	Use only in calves	Streptomycin, zero; sulfas, 0.1 in meat
Sulfabromomethazine	10	96	...	None published
Sulfachloropyridazine	7	...	Use only in calves	None published
Sulfachloropyridazine sodium	7	...	Use only in calves	None published
Sulfadimethoxine	7	60	...	Meat, 0.1; milk, 0.01
Sulfaethoxypyridazine	16	72	...	Meat, 0.1; milk, zero
Sulfamethazine (Spanbolets)	21	...	Do not use in lactating dairy cattle	Meat, 0.1
Sulfamethazine tablets, powder (Sulmet)	10	96	...	Meat and milk, 0.1
Tetracycline hydrochloride (soluble powder)	5	...	Use only in calves and limit to 5 days of treatment	Meat, 0.25
Tetracycline hydrochloride (bolus)	12	...	Use only in calves and limit to 5 days of treatment	Meat, 0.25
Thiabendazole	3	96	...	Meat, 0.1; milk, 0.05

ucts to protect the public health is one of the chief responsibilities of the veterinarian and livestock producer.

The withdrawal times, limitations for use, and tolerance levels for commonly used drugs are given for cattle in Tables 63.1, 63.2, and 63.3; for sheep and goats in Table 63.4; for swine in Tables 63.5 and 63.6; for chickens in Table 63.7; and for turkeys in Table 63.8. The information used in the preparation of these tables was obtained from FDA sources. Many drug products used in animals are not listed in these tables and do have withdrawal times. Also, other formulations may have withdrawal times different from those summarized in Tables 63.1 through 63.8. For these reasons, it is always important to read the label directions of each product carefully to obtain the correct withdrawal time. Inclusion of drugs in the tables should not be interpreted to mean that the author endorses their exclusive use over ones not included.

Withdrawal times are subject to periodic review, change, and revision whenever new information is received by the FDA. To keep up-to-date on actions taken by the FDA, it is necessary to read the *Federal Register.* Any changes published in this document later become a part of Title 21 of the *Code of Federal Regulations.* With the rapid changes occurring in this particular area, it is difficult to compile information on drug withdrawal times that will remain up-to-date. For this reason, the federal documents mentioned above must be continually consulted.

RESIDUES IN EDIBLE TISSUES

Prior to the Food Additives Amendment of 1958, drug manufacturers were not required to provide data on the depletion rate of drug residues, including their metabolites. Consequently, many "old drugs" that did not require this information were approved by the FDA. A number of drugs are in this category such as the sulfonamides, hormonal preparations, antibiotics, and others. Not only is the submittal of residue data now required from the peti-

TABLE 63.3. Drug withdrawal times, limitations for use, and tolerance levels of drugs used by topical, intrauterine, and subcutaneous (implantation) routes of administration in cattle

Drug	Preslaughter Withdrawal Time	Limitations for Use	Tolerance Level
	(days)		*(ppm)*
Topical preparations			
Famphur and xylene (pour-on preparations)	35	Do not use in lactating cattle or in calves	Meat, 0.1
Fenthion (pour-on spray concentrate has a 45-day withdrawal time)	35	Do not use in lactating cattle or in calves	Meat, 0.1
Prolate	21	Use only in mature beef animals; do not use in lactating cattle	None published
Intrauterine preparations			
Tylosin	8	Use only in mature beef cattle; do not use in lactating dairy cattle	Meat, 0.2
Implant preparations			
Diethylstilbestrol*	120	Use only in feedlot cattle	Zero†
Estradiol benzoate and progesterone (Synovex-S)	60	Use only in feedlot steers	Zero†
Estradiol benzoate and testosterone propionate (Synovex-H)	60	Use only in feedlot heifers; not in dairy cattle	Zero†
Zeranol (Ralgro)	65	Use only in feedlot cattle	Zero†

* New animal drug applications for use in feed were withdrawn by the FDA on Jan. 1, 1973, and for implant pellets on Apr. 27, 1973; court action later rescinded the ban pending a hearing. Legislation on banning the use of DES is pending in the U.S. Congress.

† All edible tissues.

TABLE 63.4. Drug withdrawal times and tolerance levels of drugs commonly used in sheep and goats

Drug	Preslaughter Withdrawal Time	Approval Use	Tolerance Level
	(days)	*(species)*	*(ppm)*
Injectable preparations			
Erythromycin	3	Sheep	None published
Procaine penicillin G	5	Sheep	None published
Procaine penicillin G and dihydrostreptomycin sulfate	30	Sheep, lambs, goats	None published
Dihydrostreptomycin sulfate	30	Sheep, lambs	None published
Sulfamethazine (Sulmet)	10	Sheep	None published
Oral preparations			
Chlortetracycline (Klortet)	2	Sheep	None published
Haloxon*	7	Sheep, goats	0.1
Levamisole hydrochloride	3	Sheep	0.1
Ruelene	14	Sheep, goats	None published
Sulfamethazine	10	Sheep	None published
Thiabendazole†	30	Sheep, goats	0.1
Implant preparations			
Flurogestrone acetate (Synchro-Mate)‡	30	Sheep	None published
Zeranol (Ralgro)	40	Lambs	Zero

* Do not use in dairy goats.
† Milk discard time required in dairy goats is 4 hours.
‡ Refers to time of removal of the pessary.

tioner who is applying for approval of a new drug but a practical, specific, reproducible, and sensitive analytical method for the detection of residues is also required.

The amount of work reported in the literature on tissue residues is not extensive. With the exception of analytical procedures published primarily by drug firms, there has been little work at the academic or governmental laboratories involving studies on drug residues in the food-producing animals. Of the studies conducted, most were done on "old veterinary drugs" within the FDA Bureau of Veterinary Medicine during the last few years.

With greater agricultural intensification involving larger production units, cattle feedlot operations in the United States may contain up to 200,000 animals or more on feed with an average turnover rate of greater than 3 times/year. Operations of this magnitude are capable of feeding over 600,000 beef animals each year. In the poultry industry, chicken broilers may be produced in multimillions by a single operational unit each year. Animal production units of this magnitude could expose a significant number of people in the United States to violative levels of residues in their diet if an error in the use of a drug or chemical was made (Kingma 1967). Although the production of food on such a large scale would appear to be a disadvantage, it should be advantageous to regulatory authorities in tracking down the source of the contamination prior to reaching the consumer. Actually, it is less likely that an error of this type would occur

TABLE 63.5. Drug withdrawal times and tolerance levels of injectable drugs commonly used in swine

Drug	Preslaughter Withdrawal Time	Tolerance Level
	(days)	*(ppm)*
Dihydrostreptomycin sulfate	30	Zero
Erythromycin	7	0.1
Lincomycin hydrochloride monohydrate	2	0.1
Oxytetracycline hydrochloride	18	0.1
Procaine penicillin G	5	Zero
Procaine penicillin G and dihydrostreptomycin sulfate (DHS)	30	Penicillin, zero; DHS, unpublished
Tylosin	4	0.2

TABLE 63.6. Drug withdrawal times and tolerance levels of drugs used orally in swine

Drug	Preslaughter Withdrawal Times	Tolerance Level
	(days)	*(ppm)*
Ampicillin trihydrate	1	0.01
Arsanilic acid or sodium arsanilate (in feed or water)	5	Muscle, other byproducts, 0.5; liver, kidney, 2.0
Carbadox	70	Zero
Chlortetracycline (CTC), sulfamethazine, and penicillin (ASP-250)	7	CTC (fat), 0.2; sulfamethazine, 0.1; penicillin, zero
Chlortetracycline hydrochloride	1	Muscle, 1.0; fat, 0.2; kidney, 4.0; liver, 2.0
Dihydrostreptomycin and vitamin A	10	None published
Furazolidone*	5	Zero
Hygromycin B	2	Zero
Levamisole hydrochloride	3	0.1
Pyrantel tartrate	1	Liver, 10; muscle, 1.0
Roxarsone	5	Muscle, 0.5; liver, kidney, 2.0 (calculated as arsenic)
Spectinomycin dihydrochloride pentahydrate	21	None published
Streptomycin, sulfathiazole, and phthalylsulfathiazole	10	Streptomycin, zero; sulfa., 0.1; phthaly., none published
Sulfachloropyridazine sodium	4	0.1
Sulfaethoxypyridazine	10	Zero
Sulfathiazole sodium	10	0.1
Tetracycline hydrochloride	4	0.25
Thiabendazole	30	0.1
Tylosin with vitamins	2	0.2 (for tylosin)
Tylosin phosphate and sulfamethazine	5	Tylosin, 0.2; sulfamethazine, 0.1

* The FDA has proposed withdrawal of furazolidone from the market and has offered its manufacturers an opportunity for a hearing in late 1976.

in the large and more efficiently managed operation.

Drug residue concentrations vary considerably from tissue to tissue and are generally observed to be higher in tissues of storage such as body fat or in organs that actively metabolize and excrete them. For example, residues may be highest in the body fat, in the liver, and/or kidneys. Chlorinated hydrocarbon compounds such as the pesticidal agents have a high affinity for storage in the body fat.

Although some hypersensitive effects reported in human beings have been associated with drinking milk containing antibiotic residues such as penicillin, it is generally recognized that there are no known deleterious effects on human health attributable to drug residues permitted in the food supply. The principal hazards identified occur from occupational exposure and accidents associated with the application of agricultural chemicals. Accidental exposures have been reported in human beings where the food supply had been contaminated with toxic levels of compounds such as the polychlorinated biphenyls (PCB). In Yusho, Japan, a number of individuals were exposed when rice oil was contaminated by a PCB compound; this particular episode has been commonly referred to as the Yusho incident. Also, in Japan, during the 1950s a peculiar fatal disease of unknown origin was reported and later identified as Minimata disease. The disease involved a number of people who had consumed seafood containing heavy concentrations of methylmercuric sulfide. The source of the mercury was from industrial wastes that had been dumped into Minimata Bay. Another well-known incident of mercury toxicity from the consumption of home-slaughtered pork occurred in a family in New Mexico (Storrs et al. 1970a, 1970b). Leftover seed grain that had been treated with a fungicide, an organic mercurial, was fed to fattening pigs. A sufficient level of residue was present in the pork tissues to produce serious toxic effects in some of the members of the family. In Turkey, wheat seed grain treated with hexachlorobenzene, which is used as a substitute for the or-

TABLE 63.7. Drug withdrawal times, limitations for use, and tolerance levels of drugs commonly used in chickens

Drug	Withdrawal Time	Limitations for Use	Tolerance Level
	(days)		*(ppm)*
Aklomide and roxarsone (Aklomix-3)	5	Do not use in egg-laying birds; use as only source of organic arsenic	Aklomide: liver, muscle, 4.5; skin, fat, 3.0 Arsenic: muscle, eggs, 0.5; other byproducts, 2.0
Aklomide, sulfanitran, and roxarsone (Novastat-3)	5	Do not use in egg-laying birds; use as the only source of organic arsenic	Aklomide and arsenic same as above; sulfanitran, zero
Arsanilic acid or sodium arsanilate	5	Use as only source of organic arsenic	Arsenic, same as above
Butynorate, sulfanitran, dinsed and roxarsone (Polystat)	5	Do not use in egg-laying birds; use as only source of organic arsenic	Butynorate and dinsed, none published; arsenic, same as above
Chlortetracycline	1	Do not use in egg-laying birds when used at 500 g/ton of feed	Kidney, 4.0; muscle, liver, fat, skin, 1.0; eggs, zero
Clopidol (Coyden)	0–5	Do not use in chickens over 16 weeks old; withdraw drug 5 days before slaughter when feeding 0.025% or reduce dosage to 0.0125% 5 days before slaughter	Liver and kidney, 15.0; muscle, 5
Erythromycin (Gallimycin)	1–2	Do not use in egg-laying birds when used at a level over 185 g/ton of feed	Eggs, 0.025
Furazolidone (Furox NF-180)*	5	Do not use in egg-laying birds or in replacement birds over 14 weeks	None published
Metoserpate hydrochloride (Pacitron)	3	Do not use in egg-laying birds	0.02
Monesin sodium (Coban)	3	Do not use in egg-laying birds	0.05
Nicarbazin (Nicarb)	4	Do not use in egg-laying birds	None published
Nitarsone (Histostat-50)	5	Use as only source of organic arsenic	None published
Nitrofurazone (NFZ, Amifur)*	5	Do not use for replacement birds over 14 weeks old	None published
Nitromide and sulfanitran (Unistat-2)	5	Do not use in egg-laying birds	Nitromide, none published; sulfanitran, zero
Nitromide, sulfanitran, and roxarsone (Unistat-3)	5	Do not use in egg-laying birds; use as only source of organic arsenic	Nitromide, none published; sulfanitran, zero; arsenic, same as above
Novobiocin (Albamix)	4	Do not use in egg-laying birds	Zero
Robenidine hydrochloride (Robenz)	5	Do not use in egg-laying birds	Skin and fat, 0.2; other edible tissues, 0.1
3-Nitro-4-hydroxyphenylarsonic acid (roxarsone)	5	Use as only source of organic arsenic	Muscle, eggs, 0.5; other byproducts, 2.0
Sulfachloropyrazine, sodium monohydrate	4	Do not use in birds that produce eggs for human food	Zero
Sulfadimethoxine and ormetoprim (Rofenaid)	2	Do not use in birds over 16 weeks old	0.1 for both drugs
Sulfaquinoxaline (SQ 40, Sulquin-40)	10	Do not use in birds producing eggs for human food	None published

* The FDA has proposed withdrawal of furazolidone, nitrofurazone, and other nitrofurans from the market and has offered their manufacturers an opportunity for a hearing in late 1976.

TABLE 63.8. Drug withdrawal times, limitations for use, and tolerance levels of drugs commonly used in the feed of turkeys

Drug	Withdrawal Time	Limitations for Use	Tolerance Level
	(days)		*(ppm)*
Arsanilic acid or sodium arsanilate	5	Do not use in egg-laying birds; use as only source of organic arsenic	Muscle, eggs, 0.5; byproducts, 2.0
Butynorate	7	. . .	None published
Carbarsone (Carb-O-Sep)	5	Use as only source of organic arsenic; high levels of copper may interfere with effectiveness	Arsenic, same as above
Clopidol (Coydon-25)	5	Use only in meat-producing birds and feed as the only ration	Muscle, 5.0; liver, kidney, 15.0
Dimetridazole (Emtrymix)	5	Do not use in birds that produce eggs for human food	Zero
Furazolidone (NF-180, Furox)*	5	Do not use in egg-laying birds	None published
Ipronidazole (Ipropran)	4	Do not use in birds that produce eggs for human food	Zero
Nitarsone (Histostat-50)	5	Use as only source of organic arsenic	Arsenic, same as above
Novobiocin (Albamix)	4	Do not use in egg-laying birds	Zero
3-Nitro-4-hydroxyphenylarsonic acid (roxarsone)	5	Use only as source of organic arsenic	Arsenic, same as above
Sulfadimethoxine and ormetoprim (Rofenaid)	2	Do not use in birds that produce eggs for human food	0.1 for both drugs
Sulfaquinoxaline (SQ)	7	Do not use in birds that produce eggs for human food	None published

* The FDA has proposed withdrawal of furazolidone from the market and has offered its manufacturers an opportunity for a hearing in late 1976.

ganic mercurial fungicide, was converted into flour for human consumption. The flour was consumed by several hundred people and a condition known as porphyria cutanea tarda or "monkey disease" was diagnosed (Cam and Nigogosyan 1963). Conversion of chemically treated seed grains into human food or animal feed is an unwarranted, illegal, and hazardous practice periodically reported (Taylor 1965).

ANTIBIOTIC RESIDUES

Internationally, the levels of antibiotics that may be added to feeds without a veterinary medical prescription vary from country to country. In general, use of antibiotics that might result in deposition of residues in meat, milk, and eggs must not be permitted in food intended for human consumption. However, if the use of antibiotics is necessary as in the treatment of animal diseases, a withholding period must be observed until the residues are negligible or can no longer be detected.

The WHO Expert Committee on the Public Health Aspects of the Use of Antibiotics in Food and Feedstuffs concluded that an antibiotic concentration of 20 ppm used singly or in combination in feeds (on a dry-matter basis) was adequate for promotion of growth and feed-conversion uses (WHO 1963). According to Garrod (1964), antibiotics used in dry feed at less than 20 ppm will not give rise to detectable levels in meat even if administration was continued until the time of slaughter. Under certain circumstances the WHO Expert Committee (1963) acknowledged that it might be necessary to exceed this level. For example, in raising motherless calves and piglets during the suckling period, amounts of 50–80 mg of antibiotic/calf and 30 mg of antibiotic/piglet or lamb were recommended daily in various milk-replacement formulas. These levels exceeded the maximum of 20 ppm recommended by the WHO committee. Under certain other circumstances, use of levels greater than 20 ppm in feed was judged to be justifiable, providing the higher levels were required to prevent or treat infection rather than to promote growth. The WHO committee further recognized that levels of antibiotics exceeding 100 ppm in feed should be administered only upon the recommendation of a veterinarian. In the event the antibiotic exceeds 100 ppm in feed, its use should be discontinued for a sufficient time prior to slaughter to permit depletion or clearance of the drug from the edible tissues. In general, feeding of growth-promotant antibiotics at 20 ppm does not result in violative levels in meat; however, antibiotic levels of 100–200 ppm may be detectable in edible tissues (WHO 1963).

Inasmuch as antibiotics are effective only during the early growth phase of the animal, addition of antibiotics to feed should generally be restricted to the age spans proposed by WHO (see Table 63.9). Feeding antibiotics beyond these age spans not only increases the probability for the accumulation of violative levels of residues in tissues but also is economically unsound.

Concerns have been reflected about the presence of residues in food products and questions have arisen among various public health authorities about the wisdom of using low or subtherapeutic levels of antibiotics in the feed of animals. It is generally accepted that such levels have less than an optimum antimicrobial effect and that the induction of bacterial resistance including transference of R factor can occur (Aronson 1975; Mercer 1975). According to Smith (1974a), antibiotic resistance has become a definite complicating factor in the treatment of animal diseases. There is also concern that resistant organisms shed by animals may transfer R factors to the

TABLE 63.9. Recommendations for the feeding restrictions (i.e., age period) of antibiotics to animals

Species	Age
Poultry, with exception of ducks and geese	8–10 weeks
Swine	4–6 months
Calves	3 months
Beef cattle	18 months
Lambs	2 months
Fur-bearing animals	2–3 months

Source: World Health Organization 1963.

enteric organisms of human beings and could conceivably complicate the treatment of human diseases. Smith (1974b) believes that there is sufficient evidence to indicate that heavily exposed human personnel have a higher incidence of antibiotic-resistant organisms than the general human population and that this higher incidence may be the result of exposure to antibiotics or to antibiotic-fed animals or their food products. However, the degree that animals serve as shedders of antibiotic-resistant pathogens for the general human population remains undetermined.

Hypersensitivity Due to Antibiotic Residues

Of the antibiotics employed as feed additives or in chemotherapy, penicillin and streptomycin and, to a lesser extent, novobiocin and oleandomycin appear from clinical usage in human beings to be more inclined to produce hypersensitivity or allergenicity than others in present use (WHO 1963). Although most of the aminoglycoside antibiotics (streptomycin, dihydrostreptomycin, neomycin, and kanamycin) were once regarded as having little or no allergenic effect, a number of human cases of local hypersensitivity have apparently occurred (WHO 1969b). Residue levels of streptomycin and dihydrostreptomycin, calculated as base, in milk, meat, and eggs as high as 0.2, 1, and 0.5 ppm, respectively, and neomycin base in these respective edible products as high as 0.15, 0.5, and 0.2 ppm are unlikely to produce allergic effects (WHO 1969b).

Allergenic effects of the macrolide antibiotics (erythromycin, oleandomycin, and spiramycin) have not been observed in human beings following their clinical use. Residue levels of erythromycin in milk, meat, and eggs as high as 0.04, 0.3, and 0.3 ppm, respectively; oleandomycin as high as 0.15, 0.3, and 0.1 ppm, respectively; and spiramycin as high as 0.025 ppm (reported only in meat) are not likely to cause allergenic effect (WHO 1969b). The allergenic effect of another macrolide antibiotic, tylosin, in human beings is unknown because it has not been used in human clinical medicine. Allergenic effects from tylosin are not likely to occur at 0.2 ppm in meat (WHO 1969b). However, it is recommended that tylosin not be used for any purpose that would result in detectable residues in human food.

The tolerance level of penicillin G in milk is 0.01 International Unit (IU)/ml (Mercer 1975). However, the evidence is unclear as to what level of penicillin in milk poses an allergenic hazard to human health. It is known that as little as 40 units (0.024 mg) of benzylpenicillin may evoke an allergic response in highly sensitized people (Siegel 1959). A joint FAO/WHO Expert Committee on Food Additives recommended that penicillin should not be permitted to show detectable residues in human food (WHO 1969b). Analytical methods for the detection of penicillin that are sensitive to 0.002–0.005 IU/ml are eventually anticipated (WHO 1970). Through widespread testing and educational programs, the extent of antibiotic residues in milk has decreased to 0.5%–4%. For instance, 7%–30% of the milk examined at one time in the United States, Great Britain, and Australia contained penicillin at concentrations of 0.05 IU/ml and higher.

The principal way that penicillins may enter food for human consumption is the use of intramammary infusion preparations for treatment of bovine mastitis. Penicillins may be ingested in milk that has not been discarded or withheld from sale until free from antibiotic activity.

Novobiocin is used in the treatment of staphylococcal infections in poultry. It has important use in the treatment of staphylococcal infections that are resistant to other antibiotics. Analytical methods in the detection of novobiocin residues make it possible to detect levels in ppm as low as 0.5 in meat, 0.15 in milk, and 0.1 in eggs. Allergic reactions are likely to occur in human beings at levels in food higher than those mentioned above (WHO 1969b). Consequently, use of novobiocin that will result in detectable residues in food for human consumption should not be permitted.

Nystatin is restricted to external use

only and is poorly absorbed; residues in only trace amounts are likely to be present in foods such as meat, milk, and eggs, not exceeding 0–7.1, 0–1.1, and 0–4.3 ppm, respectively (WHO 1969b). Allergic reactions in human beings to nystatin have not been reported.

No reports of allergenicity from the use of the polypeptide antibiotics (bacitracin, polymyxin B) in human beings have appeared. However, if both antibiotics are used, it is recommended that they not be allowed to give rise to detectable residues in food for human consumption (WHO 1969b).

TETRACYCLINE RESIDUES

Although it is rare, allergy to the tetracyclines has been reported in human beings (Weinstein and Welch 1959). Addition of tetracyclines to animal feeds at 5–20 ppm does not seem to produce residues in edible tissues (WHO 1969b). However, detectable levels of tetracycline have been found in the osseous tissues of pigs, calves, and chickens fed 5–80 ppm in the diet. Tetracycline was present in the bones of chickens that were fed only 5 ppm for no longer than 3 days. Tetracycline has also been detected in bones at the level of 5.5 ppm in chickens fed 9.2 ppm for 56 days, 0.52 ppm in swine fed 30 mg/day for 96 days, and 1.79 ppm in calves fed 60 mg/day for 56 days. The tetracyclines are absorbed from the gastrointestinal (GI) tract and may become firmly bound in teeth and skeletal structures. The binding of the tetracyclines to calcium may result in the inhibition of tooth development and skeletal growth. The teeth may become discolored and hypoplasia of the deciduous and permanent teeth has been known to occur. Damage to teeth has been observed from tetracycline usage in human beings between the 4th month of pregnancy and the 7th or 8th year of life (WHO 1969b).

At a residue level of 1 ppm, the tetracyclines are not likely to produce a toxic effect in human beings; a level of 5–7 ppm might be toxic (WHO 1969b). Also photosensitive reactivity following the use of therapeutic or prophylactic dose levels of chlortetracycline has been observed in human beings (WHO 1969b). Use of 5–20 ppm of the tetracyclines in the feed of animals may induce resistance to Enterobacteriaceae.

Tetracycline hydrochloride given intravenously to lactating dairy cattle in an average dosage of 1.8 mg/lb of body weight will result in the excretion of the antibiotic in milk for approximately 36 hours after treatment (Hokanson et al. 1963). In swine, the continuous feeding of chlortetracycline (100 g/ton) in combination with penicillin (50 g/ton) and sulfamethazine (100 g/ton) for 14 weeks resulted in less than 1 ppm for chlortetracycline in all tissues on day 0 of withdrawal (Messersmith et al. 1967). Chlortetracycline residues in muscle and fat were negative (below the level of detectability) 5 days after withdrawal from medication. Oxytetracycline, an antibiotic used in treatment of uterine infections in dairy cattle, is absorbed from the uterus and enters the circulatory system when infused at the dosage level of 4 mg/kg of body weight. The drug is also excreted in milk and can be detected as long as 48 hours after intrauterine infusion (Seguin et al. 1974).

CHLORAMPHENICOL RESIDUES

Chloramphenicol must not be used for any purpose that would result in the presence of residues in food for consumption by human beings. In veterinary medicine, the drug is approved for use only in the nonfood-producing animals. Until recently, there has been no analytical method for the detection of chloramphenicol residues. A gas chromatographic method has been developed with a detection sensitivity of 2 ppb (Mercer 1975).

In human beings chloramphenicol can induce fatal effects such as aplastic anemia and granulocytopenia; other effects include hepatic injury, optic neuritis, and the so-called "grey syndrome" in the newborn infant (WHO 1969b).

PENICILLIN RESIDUES

Probably the most common way milk is contaminated by penicillin is through intramammary infusion of the drug in the treatment of bovine mastitis (Eberhart et al. 1963). However, the administration of penicillin by other routes can also result in the contamination of milk. The allergenic effects in human beings from the consumption of milk containing penicillin and other antibiotic residues was discussed above. The depletion of aqueous penicillin (100,000 units/quarter) in the milk of dairy cattle requires 48 hours and the same dosage in oil requires 72 hours (Peoples and Pier 1960). Low production in cows (less than 9 kg of milk/day) has a delaying effect upon the excretion or depletion rate of antibiotics in milk (Mercer et al. 1970b).

The intrauterine infusion of 600,000 IU of procaine penicillin G and 1 g of dihydrostreptomycin in 5 ml of aqueous suspension given as a single treatment during estrus in dairy cattle did not result in the presence of detectable residues in milk collected at 12, 24, 48, 72, and 96 hours after treatment (Henningson et al. 1963). Use of this preparation following parturition was not reported. The passage of antibiotics from the lumen of the uterus into the systemic circulation following parturition has not been studied extensively. Until more information is available, precautions should be observed similar to the parenteral administration of antibiotic preparations to insure against violative levels of residues from entering milk and other edible products.

In swine the recommended concentration of penicillin (50 g/ton) in combination with recommended concentrations of chlortetracycline (100 g/ton) and sulfamethazine (100 g/ton) was fed continuously for 14 weeks to evaluate the residue concentrations in edible tissues (Messersmith et al. 1967). All edible tissues (liver, muscle, fat, kidneys) were found to be free from penicillin residues after 0, 5, and 7 days of withdrawal. In calves, penicillin residues were present in the injection site and in urine 45 days after treatment with a preparation containing a combination of benzathine penicillin, procaine penicillin, and dihydrostreptomycin (Mercer et al. 1971). This preparation was given as a single intramuscular injection (gluteal region) in an aqueous suspension; the dosage/kg of body weight was 4400 units each of benzathine penicillin G and procaine penicillin G in conjunction with 7.3 mg of dihydrostreptomycin.

DIHYDROSTREPTOMYCIN RESIDUES

When an aqueous suspension of dihydrostreptomycin (0.25 g/ml) in combination with 200,000 units of penicillin was administered intramuscularly to swine at a dosage level of 44 mg/kg (i.e., for dihydrostreptomycin) of body weight/day for 4 days, residues were detected in high concentrations in the liver and kidneys 10 hours after the last injection (Mercer et al. 1970a). The kidney contained 20 times the concentration (235–288 μg of dihydrostreptomycin/g of tissue) of the antibiotic compared to that detected in muscle (1.2–6 μg/g) from the injection site or in the liver (14–21 μg/g). In pigs treated for 3 days with dihydrostreptomycin at a dosage of 26 mg/kg/day in combination with penicillin, dihydrostreptomycin residues were detected for 60 days in the kidneys and muscle-injection sites. Inasmuch as the urine did not contain detectable dihydrostreptomycin at 60 days, an affinity or binding capability of the antibiotic to renal tissue was suspected (Mercer et al. 1970a).

SULFONAMIDE RESIDUES

Many of the sulfonamides were approved prior to the 1958 Food Additives Amendment. Consequently, drug manufacturers were not required to submit data on tissue residues following their use in food-producing animals. In 1973 the FDA ruled that all sulfonamide-containing drugs for oral, injectable, intramammary, and intrauterine use in food-producing animals would be considered new animal drugs.

This meant that a no-effect level in laboratory animals had to be determined and tissue-residue data had to be submitted for the establishment of safe withdrawal periods in the target species. In 1974 the FDA ruled that in addition to this information, studies would be required using thyroid responses as one of the parameters for showing a no-effect level of the drug. Also, it was requested that improved methodology would be required to determine negligible levels of sulfonamide residues in edible tissues in those instances where the sensitivity and specificity of the analytical method were inadequate.

It has been well established that sulfonamides are excreted in milk following their administration (Rasmussen 1958; Sisodia and Stowe 1964). The intrauterine infusion of sulfonamides in cattle is known to give rise to detectable levels in blood and milk for at least 48 hours after administration (Seguin et al. 1974).

Tissue residue studies have been conducted with a number of sulfonamides in poultry, sheep (Righter et al. 1972), and swine (Messersmith et al. 1967; Righter et al. 1971b). In laying hens and cockerels, a withdrawal period greater than 7 days was indicated following the oral administration of sulfaquinoxaline at therapeutic (0.05%) or prophylactic (0.025%) levels (Righter et al. 1970). Residues persisted at a concentration greater than 0.1 ppm 10 days after withdrawal when sulfamerazine was administered to breeder chickens in feed at 0.4% or in water at 0.1% (Righter et al. 1971a). In sheep a 10-day withdrawal period is required for sulfamerazine when given at the recommended therapeutic level of 132 mg/kg for 3 days (Righter et al. 1972). The withdrawal time for sulfamethazine (10 g/100 lb of body weight/day) in fish is 3 weeks (Mercer 1975). According to Mercer, residue data do not exist for several sulfonamides; it is nonexistent for the various routes of administration in several species.

Most of the analytical methodology for the detection of sulfonamide residues in tissues is sensitive to 0.1 ppm (Fellig and Westheimer 1968; Tishler et al. 1968). For blood and serum, sensitivity to 2 ppm has been reported (Righter et al. 1972). In milk a sensitivity of 0.1 ppm has been published (Fechner et al. 1974).

PESTICIDE RESIDUES

In assuring a safe and wholesome food supply through the use of pesticides, the Federal Insecticide and Rodenticide Act (FIRA) of 1947 was passed by the U.S. Congress. In 1954 Public Law 83–518 known as the Miller Amendment to the Food, Drug and Cosmetic Act, was passed assigning to the USDA the responsibility of developing recommendations for the effective uses of pesticides in food production. Under this same amendment, the FDA was assigned the responsibility of establishing safe tolerances for pesticides that might leave residues in or on raw agricultural products at the time of sale for human consumption. Milk and meat were not specifically covered but it was generally accepted that they would be included within the legislative intent of the amendment. Following the establishment of the EPA, most of the responsibilities for regulatory action involving the pesticides and fungicides were transferred to this agency. One of the most significant actions taken by the EPA was the ban of DDT in 1972. This was followed by the ban of other pesticides such as dieldrin and aldrin.

An extensive amount of literature has been published concerning the potential hazards to the health of human beings from the use of pesticidal agents. It is well known that most feed and foodstuffs consumed by animals and human beings contain minute quantities of pesticide residues of one kind or another (Harries et al. 1969). The FDA continually monitors the level of pesticides in the human diet through the conduct of market-basket surveys. Random purchases of foodstuffs at markets and retail stores are made by the FDA throughout the United States to assess the level of residues in the total diet. The food selected and relative amounts taken in the survey are based upon national consumption values of 16-

to 19-year-old males. This age group is selected on the premise that greater amounts of food are consumed by them than by any other segment of the population. The surveys have revealed that the levels of pesticides in foods purchased by American consumers are within the bounds of the established safety allowances even for the segment of the population that consumes the largest amount of food.

Not all safety allowances for residues are based on the 16- to 19-year-old segment of the human population. For example, the diets of infants and invalids are also given consideration in the establishment of safety tolerances for compounds, including the pesticides. Since milk is the predominate item in the diet of these individuals, it should be as free as possible from all residues. In general, no finite or neglible tolerances have been established for pesticide residues in milk and other dairy products.

A large number of pesticides are chlorinated hydrocarbon compounds that have a high affinity for deposition in the body fat of animals (Knipling and Westlake 1966). The amount of storage in the fat of animals appears to be proportional to the concentration of the pesticide in the diet. Feeding trials with a chlorinated hydrocarbon, such as dieldrin, have shown that lambs ingest about twice as much of the pesticide per unit of body weight as steers, while swine ingest only slightly more than steers (Gannon et al. 1959). However, steers store about twice as much dieldrin in fat on a per g weight basis as swine and only one-fifth of the amount in chicken fat (see Table 63.10). Because swine store a higher percentage of fat than steers, it is believed that this may explain the lower concentration (dilution effect) of dieldrin residue in the fat of swine. This, however, cannot explain the differences when sheep are considered because the animals were extremely lean throughout the study. According to Gannon et al., it appears that the propensity of storage of dieldrin in fat may be a characteristic of the species. In lactating cows, less dieldrin is stored in tissues than in steers; losses through excretion in the milk may explain the differences.

TABLE 63.10. Deposition of dieldrin in the body fat of various species

Dieldrin in Feed	Dieldrin in Body Fat			
	Lambs	Swine	Steers	Hens
(ppm)	*(ppm)*			
0.1	0.1	0.4	0.4	4.1
0.25	0.4	0.4	0.8	10.2
0.75	0.6	2.8	3.5	35.7
2.25	1.7	4.3	8.7	. . .
Ratio: ppm in fat/ ppm in feed	0.29	0.83	1.83	9.36

Data used with the permission of Gannon et al. 1959.

The tolerance level for dieldrin in the fat of edible tissues of food-producing animals is 0.3 ppm. As it can readily be seen from the data in Table 63.10, the intake of dieldrin in the diet must be extremely low if the tolerance level of 0.3 ppm is not exceeded. Although dieldrin was banned from use by the EPA on October 1, 1974, it is a good example for showing the degree of storage that occurs in the body fat of the various species. Interestingly, the chicken appears to accumulate dieldrin as well as other chlorinated hydrocarbons in the body fat to a greater extent than other species. For example, the chicken accumulates hexachlorobenzene in the body fat over 30 times the level in the diet (Avrahami and Steele 1972a).

Many more pesticidal agents and other related chlorinated hydrocarbon compounds may concentrate in animal body fat similar to that described above for dieldrin. Only 5 chlorinated hydrocarbon substances have established tolerances under present EPA regulations (see Table 63.11); of these only 2 have established tolerances that apply to all species (Trabosh 1974).

Tolerances for pesticides are established not at the limits of safety but at levels no greater than are necessary to achieve the desired physical or other technical effects (Oser 1971). Whenever the residue levels present exceed the tolerances specified in regulations or in accordance with good agricultural use, the foodstuffs

TABLE 63.11. Environmental Protection Agency tolerance for chlorinated hydrocarbons in fat of food-producing animals (ppm)

Chlorinated Hydrocarbon	Adult Cattle	Calves	Swine	Sheep	Goats	Poultry
Aldrin	*	*	*	*	*	*
BHC	*	*	*	*	*	*
Chlordane	*	*	*	*	*	*
Dieldrin	*	*	*	*	*	*
DDT	7.0	7.0	7.0	7.0	7.0	7.0†
Endrin	*	*	*	*	*	*
HCB	‡	‡	‡	‡	‡	‡
Heptachlor	*	*	*	*	*	*
Lindane	7.0	7.0	4.0	7.0	7.0	4.0†
Methoxychlor	3.0	3.0	3.0	3.0	3.0	3.0
Mirex	0.1	0.1	0.1	0.1	0.1	0.1
PCB	§	§	§	§	§	5.0
Toxaphene	7.0	7.0	7.0	7.0	7.0	7.0†

Source: Permission to use this table was obtained from Trabosh 1974.
* 0.3 ppm, administrative guideline for all species in fat.
† Administrative guidelines for poultry in all tissues; the tolerance level for DDT in red meat animals is now 5 ppm and is administrative at this level for poultry.
‡ 0.5 ppm, administrative guideline for all species in fat.
§ 5.0 ppm, administrative guideline for all species in all tissues.

involved are ruled to be contaminated. This appears unreasonable, particularly with pending food shortages because the residues may not be unsafe.

Those interested in additional information involving tissue residues and established tolerances of other pesticides are referred to the *Code of Federal Regulations* and the journal *Residue Reviews.*

OTHER DRUG AND CHEMICAL RESIDUES

Virginiamycin Residues

The principal use of virginiamycin has been as a feed additive for the promotion of growth in swine and for the prevention and treatment of swine dysentery. Presumably this is an ideal agent since the gram-positive nature of this antibiotic lessens or avoids the problems of resistance transfer through R factor (Di Cuollo et al. 1973). Use of virginiamycin as a feed additive at 155 g/ton (170.5 ppm) for a period of 18 weeks did not result in the detection of tissue residues even in animals not subjected to a withdrawal period.

Tripelennamine (Pyribenzamine) Residues

Tripelennamine is a drug not only used to control allergic manifestations in small and large animals but also used as a stimulant in dairy cows that will not stand up because of various functional disorders (Luders et al. 1970). To assure compliance with FDA regulations, Luders and associates developed an analytical method capable of detecting levels of tripelennamine hydrochloride to less than 10 ppb. Residues in milk were not detected after 48 hours following intramuscular injections of tripelennamine at a dosage of 25 mg/20 kg of body weight administered 3 times at 4-hour intervals.

Metoserpate Residues

A fluorescent method for the detection of metoserpate hydrochloride has been developed by Tishler et al. (1969). To assure compliance with FDA regulations, it was necessary to develop analytical methods suitable for the detection of 20 ppb in certain tissues and 10 ppb in eggs. The method developed by Tishler and co-workers is capable of easily detecting 5 ppb of the drug.

Chlorobutanol Residues

Under the Food Additives Regulation 121.1131, a zero tolerance has been established for residues of chlorobutanol in milk from dairy animals, Wiskerchen and

Weishaar 1972). Chlorobutanol is an ingredient used in intramammary infusion products for the treatment of bovine mastitis. It is permitted as an antibacterial preservative in a concentration of 50 mg anhydrous chlorobutanol in each 10 ml of the product. A gas liquid chromatography method has been developed that is capable of the detection of chlorobutanol in milk to 10 ppb.

Trichlorfon (Neguvon) Residues

Experimental studies have indicated that treatment of dairy cattle with trichlorfon (1 pint of 2% w/v solution applied as a back wash to each animal for warble control) resulted in the presence of residues in milk (Wickham and Flanagan 1962). Residues were detected at 0.1 ppm in the milk taken from the cows more than 6 hours after treatment and contained 0.4 ppm when milk was taken prior to 6 hours after treatment. Insofar as the presence of trichlorfon in meat is concerned, studies have been conducted that show meat eaten raw containing 0.1 ppm or less is not hazardous to human beings.

Aflatoxin Residues

Aflatoxin B_1 is the most potent chemical carcinogen to be discovered. It has been suggested that aflatoxin may be responsible for liver cancer in human beings and animals (Purchase 1972). Ducklings are unusually sensitive to aflatoxin levels in the diet (Armbrecht 1971). Levels of 1.7 ppm were found to be fatal to all Peking white ducks exposed to the chemical in the diet within an 11-day period. Rainbow trout are also very sensitive to the effects of aflatoxin; a no-effect level for the chemical in trout after continuous exposure for 12 months is 1 ppb (Sinnhuber 1967).

Residues appear in meat, milk, and eggs in animals exposed to aflatoxin in the diet at levels much greater than 20 ppb; the temporary tolerance level established by the FDA in food products for aflatoxin is 20 ppb. In swine, feeding of diets containing 233 ppb of aflatoxin did not lead to the presence of residues in the edible tissues (Booth 1969). Feeding of steers at a level of 1 ppm of aflatoxin in the diet for 5 months did not result in the detection of residues in meat or organs. Only traces of residues were found in the blood; they disappeared after a 24-hour withdrawal period (Armbrecht 1971). Aflatoxin residues appear in the milk of lactating animals within 2 days of ingesting a diet containing a total of 8 mg/day (Purchase 1972). Excretion of aflatoxin, i.e., the M_1 metabolite, in milk is proportional to the intake of aflatoxin B_1 (see Fig. 63.5).

Hygromycin B Residues

In a study to determine whether or not residues of hygromycin B were transmitted into the chicken egg, it was learned that no residues could be detected using an analytical method sensitive to 15 ppb (Begue and Kline 1973). The study was conducted for 12 weeks, with the birds receiving the recommended level of hygromycin B in the diet of 12 g/ton of feed. Eggs were analyzed weekly throughout the experiment with no withdrawal of the drug from the diet. The tolerance level (i.e., for each g of tissue) established for hygromycin B in eggs is 0.1 unit; in skeletal muscle and the kidney, the tolerance level is 1 and 1.5 units, respectively (Mercer 1975).

Decoquinate Residues

Decoquinate is used as a broiler chicken coccidiostat in feed. Where twice the recommended use level (0.008%) of decoquinate was fed to chickens, residues reached their maximum levels 3 days after feeding began and remained essentially constant thereafter (Filer et al. 1969). Decoquinate residues were less than 1 ppm in all the tissues analyzed. With the exception of fat and skin, the residues fell rapidly to less than 0.1 ppm in most tissues after 89 hours of withdrawal from medication. At the recommended level of feeding decoquinate (0.004% or 40 g/ton of feed), the drug is excreted quite rapidly (Ferrando et al. 1971). After withdrawal from medication for 2 or 3 days, residues were not detected in many of the tissues examined.

The tolerance established for residues

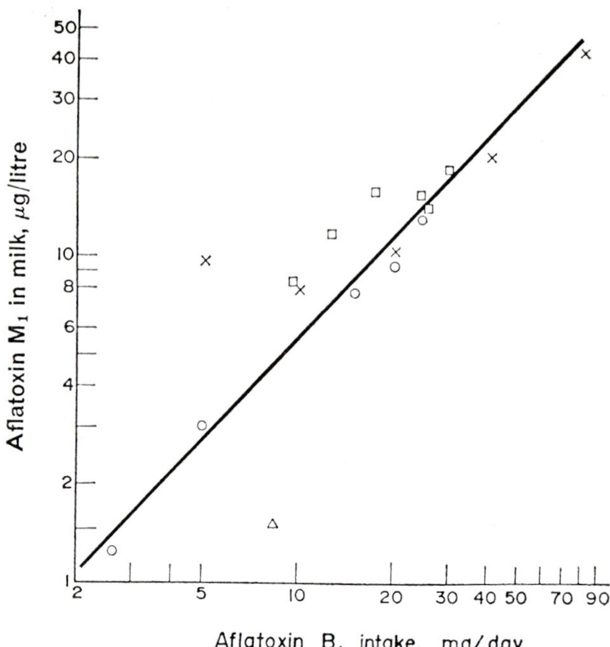

FIG. 63.5. Aflatoxin M_1 levels (converted to µg/L) in milk from cows ingesting various amounts of aflatoxin B_1. These figures were obtained from van der Linde et al. 1964b (Δ), Allcroft and Roberts 1968 (O), Maseri et al. 1969a (×), and Keyl et al. 1968 (□). (Published with the permission of Pergamon Press and I. F. H. Purchase 1972)

of decoquinate in the uncooked edible tissues of chickens is 1 ppm in muscle and 2 ppm in other tissues. A fluorometric method sensitive within 0–2.2 ppm has been developed for the detection of decoquinate residues (Stone 1973). Cooking has little effect on decoquinate.

MERCURY RESIDUES

A dosage of alkylmercury at a level of 0.1 mg/person/day is apparently safe (WHO 1974c). Levels of alkylmercury in fish and shellfish that led to poisoning in Japan were in the range of 5–20 ppm calculated as mercury. In fatal cases, the estimated daily intake of mercury was at the rate of about 1.64 mg/person. In domestic animals fed organomercury compounds, high levels of residues accumulated in the edible tissues (see Table 63.12).

ARSENIC RESIDUES

In 1973 the tolerance level for arsenic in uncooked liver and kidney of swine was increased from 1 to 2 ppm (Food and Drug Administration 1973). For uncooked muscle tissue and by-products of swine, the tolerance level is 0.5 ppm. In edible tissues of chickens and turkeys, the tolerance levels are 0.5 ppm in eggs and uncooked muscle

TABLE 63.12. Examples of residues of mercury in organs and eggs after repeated oral exposure of domestic animals

Compound	Species	Dose	Exposure	Residues in Liver	Kidney	Muscle	Eggs
		(mg/kg)			*(mg/kg)*		
Methylmercury	Pig	5	1 week	80	52	. . .	. . .
	Calf	0.22	10 weeks	80	140	20	. . .
	Chicken	0.15	12 weeks	17	14	6	. . .
		12	8 weeks	16	20	8	. . .
	Hen	0.5	7 weeks	. . .	. . .	. . .	12
Ethylmercury	Cattle	0.48	30 days	50	100	20	. . .
Phenylmercury	Pig	4.6	13 days	72	220	1	. . .
Methoxyethylmercury	Pig	3–5	30–60 days	. . .	50	0.1	. . .

Source: Data used with the permission of World Health Organization 1974c.

tissue; for uncooked by-products of chickens and turkeys it is 1 ppm. The withdrawal times for the various arsenical preparations (arsanilic acid, sodium arsanilate, 3-nitro-4-hydroxy-phenylarsonic acid) in poultry and swine are 5 days (see Tables 63.6, 63.7, 63.8).

Prednisolone and Prednisone Residues

A tolerance of zero has been established by the FDA for residues of prednisolone and prednisone in milk. Milk from cows treated with 3 consecutive intramuscular injections of 9α-fluoroprednisolone acetate (20 mg) at 12-hour intervals showed no residues of this drug or its metabolite, 9α-fluoroprednisolone, when milk samples were collected at —24, —12, and 0 hours and +12 and +24 hours posttreatment (Krzeminski et al. 1974). The analytical method used for the detection of these residues was sensitive within the range of 5–20 ppb. In beef heifer calves injected intramuscularly with 20 mg of 9α-fluoroprednisolone acetate for 3 consecutive days and slaughtered at 0, 1, 3, 5, 7, 10, and 13 days posttreatment, no residues were detected in muscle, liver, fat, and kidney 7 days after the last injection.

CHEMICAL RESIDUES FROM ACCIDENTAL OR ENVIRONMENTAL CONTAMINATION

Polychlorinated Biphenyls

Within the last few years it has become readily apparent that aroclors of PCB compounds are capable of entering the animal and human food chain (Booth 1974). In 1971 fish meal processed in North Carolina for use in poultry feeds became accidentally contaminated with Aroclor 1242, a PCB compound, during its pasteurization in the elimination of *Salmonella* organisms (Pichirallo 1971). Many tons of this contaminated feed were distributed to ten southeastern states and were fed to millions of chickens. As a consequence, poor hatchability of eggs and many death losses of young chicks occurred. In addition, many thousands of broilers and eggs were condemned as unfit for human food purposes because the level of PCB in the edible products exceeded the temporary tolerance level of 5 ppm (on a fat basis) established by the FDA.

Feeding of Aroclor 1254 at levels of 0.1–10 ppm to White Leghorn chickens for 8 or 32 weeks did not produce any toxic signs (Teske et al. 1974). However, 20 ppm of Aroclor 1232, 1242, 1248, and 1254 fed to White Leghorn hens reduced the hatchability of eggs, and teratogenic effects were also observed in the embryos (Cecil et al. 1974). These investigators also reported that PCB residues in fertile eggs were not related to the incidence of embryotoxic and teratogenic effects in unhatched embryos. Interestingly, as the percentage chlorination of the PCB compounds increased, the total PCB residues in eggs also generally increased. The last two digits of the aroclor series represent the percent chlorination of the PCB compounds. For example, 1248 and 1254 contain 48% and 54% chlorine, respectively. Also, the depletion rate of the higher chlorinated compounds from eggs and body fat is generally greater than for the lower chlorinated compounds (Fig. 63.6).

A linear relationship between the concentration of PCBs added to the diet and in the tissues of chickens has been demonstrated (Fig. 63.7). As the level of aroclor in the diet is increased, the accumulation of the chemical in the edible tissues increased (Table 63.13). If the level of Aroclor 1254 in poultry feed exceeds 0.2 ppm, the tissue residue levels will in all probability exceed the interim safe tolerance level of 5 ppm that was set by the FDA.

Most avian and mammalian species appear to be relatively tolerant to the toxic effects of PCBs (Hammond 1972). However, mink seem to be most susceptible to the toxicity of these compounds; levels of 1–5 ppm of Aroclor 1254 in the diet may reduce reproductive performance after only 4 months of exposure. The reproductive performance of swine is affected when 20 ppm of Aroclor 1242 is fed throughout the gestation period (Hansen et al. 1975).

PCB RESIDUES

EGG
FAT

ppm PCB

% DEPLETION:	1221	1232	1242	1248	1254	1268
EGG	0	17	80	67	42	92
FAT	66	48	93	56	26	17

Fig. 63.6. PCB residues after 9 weeks of feeding 20 ppm Aroclors 1221 to 1268 and % depletion of PCB residues after a subsequent 7 weeks of feeding uncontaminated feed. (From Cecil et al. 1974)

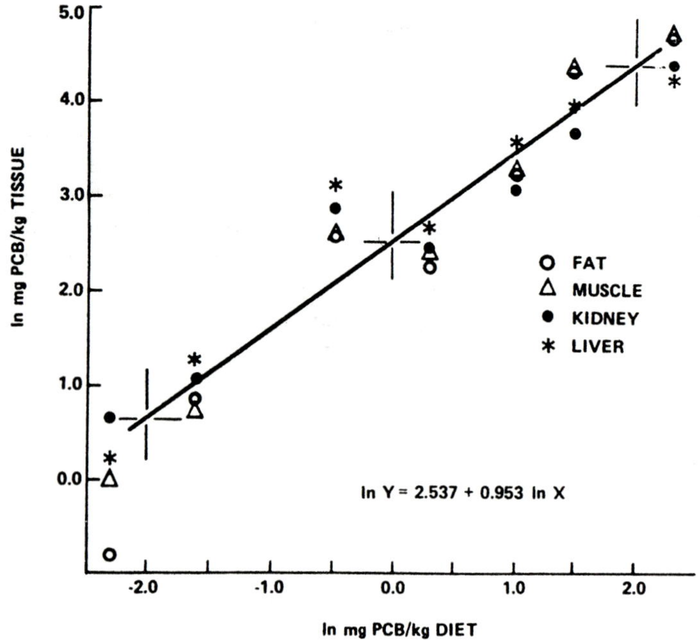

Fig. 63.7. Linear relationship between the concentration of Aroclor 1254 added to the diet and the concentration of PCB in the tissues of 8-week-old White Leghorn chickens. Natural logarithms of the PCB concentrations were used to maintain homogeneity of error variances. (From Teske et al. 1974)

TABLE 63.13. PCB concentrations (ppm) on an extractable fat basis, in dissectable fat, liver, kidney, and muscle of 8-week-old White Leghorn hens given diets containing Aroclor 1254 for 8 weeks*

Group	Dietary Level	Dissectable Fat	Liver	Kidney	Muscle†
	(mg/kg)				
1	0	0.48	1.3	2.09	1.09
2	0.1	1.89	4.2	3.53	2.15
3	0.5	11.3	28.3	18.8	12.8
4	1.0	9.52	18.5	11.5	10.9
5	3.0	25.1	36.8	21.8	30.7
6	5.0	66.4	61.8	49.3	69.8
7	10.0	110.6	98.1	87.4	109.0

Source: Data used with the permission of Teske et al. 1974.
* Values are means of 6 hens.
† Composited from breast and thigh.

There was an increased number of mummified fetuses in animals treated with PCB, and body fat concentrations of the chemical in the sows ranged from 4 to 20 ppm.

Fish are susceptible to the toxic effects of PCB compounds; concentrations of 20 and 50 ppb are lethal to catfish and bluegill when exposed for several weeks. Trout died at about 8 ppb and shrimp were killed by concentrations as low as 1 ppb. Concern has been reported (Harvey et al. 1974) about the buildup of PCB compounds in the Atlantic Ocean, especially in the marine diatoms, since these represent the basic energy source for marine life. Concentrations of PCBs as low as 10–25 ppb will reduce the growth rates of two species of marine diatoms (Mosser et al. 1972).

Hexachlorobenzene

During 1973, the FDA became concerned that hexachlorobenzene (HCB) appeared to be a contaminant of the environment (Booth and McDowell 1975). One of the current agricultural uses of HCB, a fungicidal agent, is in the treatment of seed grains. Inasmuch as HCB is also a byproduct of chlorine gas and chlorinated hydrocarbon production and because it is used in the manufacture of pentachlorophenol, a wood preservative, it also enters the environment from industrial sources. HCB was not detected in the tissues of food-producing animals in the United States until late 1972 or early 1973. The first episode was reported by the USDA in cattle located near Darrow, Louisiana (United States Environmental Protection Agency 1973). Quarantine restrictions were imposed surrounding this region, which involved about 120 square miles and about 20,000 cattle. Biopsy fat samples were obtained from 555 animals in 157 herds. HCB was detected in 34% of the herds above 0.5 ppm in 29% of the cattle tested. After the USDA discovered HCB in the body fat of cattle, the EPA established an interim tolerance of 0.5 ppm in the fat of cattle, sheep, goats, and horses. Edible meat products containing HCB at this concentration are violative and cannot be used as a source of food for human consumption.

Episodes of HCB toxicosis in human beings, associated with the consumption of HCB-treated wheat, have been reported in Turkey (Schmid 1960; Cam and Nigogosyan 1963). Several hundred people, mostly children, were affected by the intoxication, which was diagnosed as porphyria cutanea tarda. Some of the clinical signs consist of blistering and epidermolysis of the skin involving exposed parts of the body (face and hands), causing the skin to be unusually sensitive to sunlight (photosensitization) and to minor trauma.

Experimental studies in sheep have revealed that HCB is stored in body fat to the extent of 7–9 times the concentration in the feed at all gradations of intake from 0.1 to 100 ppm (Avrahami and Steele

1972a). On withdrawal or discontinuance of the HCB for 42 weeks, it was apparent that HCB was released more slowly than it accumulated in adipose tissue. Also, this study revealed that HCB elimination from fat was more rapid in the animals in the higher dosages, suggesting that this process is not a simple first-order reaction. Thus the approximate half-life of HCB in fat varied between 10 and 18 weeks where the maximum concentration in fat associated with these half-lives varied between 650 ppm and 0.9 ppm, respectively.

When 100 ppm of HCB was fed to laying pullets, it was also found in tissues in amounts roughly proportional to the dietary intake (Avrahami and Steele 1972b). After 16 months of feeding, the concentrations of HCB in body fat were 21 to 31 times the concentration in the feed, and the relative HCB concentrations in body fat, egg yolk, liver, and skeletal muscle were 175, 40, 4, and 1, respectively. Concentrations of HCB in the diet as great as 100 ppm had no deleterious effect on the health of the pullets or on fertility or hatchability of eggs. HCB stored in tissues of these pullets at the end of the HCB dosing period was still being eliminated in eggs laid 24 weeks later. Under these conditions, the calculated half-life for HCB in eggs was 11 $\pm$ 3 weeks.

Polybrominated Biphenyl Contamination

A toxic syndrome associated with the feeding of polybrominated biphenyl (PBB)–contaminated feed to dairy cattle was reported in the state of Michigan (Jackson and Halbert 1974). PBB is used as a flame retardant in the textile industry. The manufacturer of this compound also markets magnesium oxide for the supplementation of dairy cattle rations to prevent hypomagnesemic tetany. PBB was inadvertently placed in shipping bags or containers intended for magnesium oxide.

In May 1974, more than 30 Michigan dairy herds had been quarantined, unable to market milk or meat due to contamination by PBB (Jackson and Halbert 1974). By the end of the year, about 30,000 livestock and 1.6 million poultry on 507 premises became contaminated by concentrations of PBB requiring their destruction (Dunckel 1975).

Effective November 1974, the FDA established interim tolerances for PBB; a tolerance of 0.3 ppm was set for milk and meat and 0.05 ppm was set for eggs and finished feeds (Dunckel 1975). Inasmuch as PBB has a marked affinity for fat and does not appear to be biotransformed, elimination or clearance of the chemical from the body below 1 ppm may not occur during a normal lifetime of the animal. Approximately 7 months after the last feeding of PBB-contaminated feed, tissue residues ranged from 43 ppm in milk fat to 310 ppm in liver fat of cattle (Jackson and Halbert 1974).

As pointed out above with PCBs, HCB, and PBB, the accidental contamination of the animal feed supply by chemicals is a potential source of contamination of the food supply for human beings. Fortunately, most of the episodes have first involved animals so corrective action could be instituted by regulatory agencies such as the FDA, the USDA, and the EPA without the involvement of human exposure. For this reason, animals are excellent monitors in the detection of toxic agents that may enter the food chain from accidental or environmental contamination. The field veterinarian is the most likely person trained in the biomedical sciences to first observe the clinical signs of toxicoses in animals exposed to chemicals entering the environment. Furthermore, the veterinarian is the most likely individual to utilize the multidisciplinary principles of ecology in solving field problems. Inasmuch as veterinarians deal with more of the human total environment than most other biomedical professionals, they rank at the top as "practical ecologists."

DRUG AND CHEMICAL RESIDUES FROM THE USE OF RECYCLED ANIMAL WASTES

Due to potential hazards from possible pathogens and drug residues, the FDA does not sanction the use of animal and poultry wastes as feed (Taylor et al. 1974). However, with the development of sufficient scientific information, the FDA believes that animal waste products could be removed from the "do not sanction" category and be placed in the same category as feed ingredients. If feeding of animal wastes is eventually sanctioned, it is anticipated that the pollution problem due to animal excreta could be reduced about 30% (Blair 1974). Not only would feeding of wastes reduce environmental pollution but it would serve as an economic source of energy in the production of food animals. Some sources of animal waste products are already recognized as feed ingredients by the Association of American Feed Control Officials. These are meat meal tankage, blood meal, hydrolyzed poultry feathers, poultry by-product meal, and dehydrated paunch products.

According to Blair (1974), the disease risk from pathogens as a result of recycling dehydrated poultry wastes appears to be low. Feeding of poultry wastes to beef cattle and sheep has not resulted in any disease problems. However, risks from drug or chemical residues appear greater when animal wastes are fed. The primary concern in the feeding of animal wastes will be the evaluation of animal and human safety. Evaluations must consider the source of the raw animal excreta (i.e., the species) and what possible harmful substances it may contain such as antibiotics, sulfonamides, arsenicals and other heavy metals, coccidiostats, trace metals, pesticides, hormones, mycotoxins, and others. Due to the variable sources of wastes, the type and amount of research data needed to establish safety will vary for each product (Taylor et al. 1974). For instance, litter collected and processed from caged laying birds would probably be free from potential harmful substances. Litter from broilers, however, would more likely contain several substances (coccidiostats, arsenicals, antibiotics, and others). Examination of broiler litter obtained from several broiler-producing areas in Virginia revealed the presence of oxytetracycline, chlortetracycline, penicillin, nicarbazin, amprolium, arsenic, and copper residues; neomycin and zinc bacitracin residues were not detected (Webb and Fontenot 1975). When litter containing some of these residues (arsenic and copper) was fed to cattle for 121–198 days, there was no problem with tissue residues following a 5-day withdrawal of litter.

Adverse effects have been reported from feeding poultry litter to livestock. For example, copper toxicity has been observed in ewes fed poultry litter containing high levels of copper (Fontenot and Webb 1974). The high copper levels in the litter occurred from feeding chicks copper sulfate. Inasmuch as sheep are more sensitive to the effects of copper than cattle, this problem would not be as great in cattle. However, the problem of tissue residues and excretion of copper residues in the milk of lactating animals must be considered.

Griel and co-workers (1969) found that abortions in a beef breeding herd were associated with the feeding of chicken litter containing dinestrol diacetate, with an estrogenic activity greater than 10 μg of DES equivalents/100 g of litter.

Before the use of recycled animal wastes as feed ingredients in the production of food animals can be sanctioned, a number of studies are necessary to demonstrate the safety as well as efficacy of such a practice. Where tissue residues are apt to occur, information of various types will be required by the FDA to establish safe residue tolerances compatible with human safety (Taylor et al. 1974). This is especially true where a safety tolerance for a particular compound has not been established. For example, the feeding of broiler litter containing arsenic residues to ruminants is known to produce tissue residues. Although tissue tolerances for arsenic compounds have been established for poultry and swine, none has been established in ruminant tissues. According to Taylor et al., a determination has to be made whether or not the increased arsenic burden in human diets resulting from the extension of the tolerance to beef tissues would pose a health hazard. In the case of clopidol, a poultry coccidiostat, a different problem emerges (Taylor et al. 1974). Tissue tolerances have been established for this drug in milk and in poultry, sheep, cattle, swine, and goats. However, information is unavailable on the quantity of poultry litter containing clopidol residues that can be fed to animals without producing a tissue residue in excess of the established tolerance level. Similar problems such as the ones mentioned above for arsenic and clopidol also exist for a number of other residue substances that are found in animal wastes.

EFFECT OF COOKING AND FREEZING UPON TISSUE RESIDUES

Tolerance for drugs or chemicals is established only in the raw, fresh, or uncooked food product. This practice is followed because a number of people eat rare or semicooked food products.

It is known that cooking degrades the tetracycline antibiotics (chlortetracycline, oxytetracycline) in food products containing as much as 5–10 ppm; levels remaining after heat inactivation are calculated to be less than 1 ppm (WHO 1963). Properties of the inactivated tetracyclines or breakdown products are unknown. Streptomycin is essentially unaffected when heated at 100° C for 2 hours (Mercer 1975). Chloramphenicol is also quite heat stable; levels of the antibiotic were reduced by only about 80% in tissues cooked for 30 minutes at 100° C (Mercer 1975).

Freezing temperatures will degrade penicillin in tissues; however, detectable levels may persist from 8 to 21 days (Mercer 1975). According to Mercer, freezing appears to have little effect upon the degradation of oxytetracycline and dihydrostreptomycin.

Ostensibly, trichlorfon (Neguvon) is destroyed by cooking meat containing 10 ppm for at least 1 hour. Sheep treated orally with this drug at 120 mg/kg of body weight and cattle treated with 100 mg/kg of body weight may have tissue residues up to 10 ppm when slaughtered within 6 hours following treatment. Animals slaughtered 6 hours following treatment had trichlorfon residues at 0.1 ppm or less.

Fat drippings from cooking usually contain concentrated levels of chlorinated hydrocarbons. Draining off the melted fat has been used to lower the residue levels of compounds such as DDT, dieldrin, and others in meat products. Heat does not appear to inactivate the chlorinated hydrocarbon compounds.

Cooking of chicken wrapped in aluminum foil at 220° C appears to have no effect on decoquinate residues (Ferrando et al. 1971). Decoquinate, which is mainly present in body fat, is in the upper layer (fat portion) of the cooking juices.

BENEFITS VERSUS PUBLIC HEALTH RISKS

The benefits of using drug and chemical compounds in the production of food animals must always be evaluated against the public health risks. Also, the benefits versus the risks of not using these compounds are equally if not more important to consider. With the current annual increase in the world human population of 80 or more million people, it is evident that human beings must depend more and more on the use of drugs and chemicals to control infectious and parasitic diseases of plants and animals.

World food production increase, until 1972, exceeded the world increase in population; food production had been increasing at an annual rate of 2.8% compared with a 2.6% increase in the population. Since then, the world grain reserves have steadily declined. Factors such as adverse weather conditions, fuel and resource shortages, and socioeconomic instability have been contributing to the decline of food production.

Future estimates of the world population and food supply suggest a greater deficiency of the raw materials currently used in concentrate feeds in semiintensive and intensive systems of food-animal production (Burt 1973). This deficit is probable because the human population will increase more rapidly than the production of food crops. This will result in an increased demand for foods of animal origin and a concomitant decrease in a surplus of food crops to be used in their production. If a deficit in cereal grains develops as anticipated, because of an increasing world population, greater diversion of cereals directly into the human diet will be necessary. This means that the supply of cereal grains for use in concentrate feeds for animals will decline. Such a decline will adversely affect the pork and poultry industries to a greater extent than the production of ruminants. Utilization of recycled wastes and the by-products of plants and animals in the diet of ruminants needs to be explored to a greater degree because the world supply of concentrate feeds will be in substantial deficit by the end of this century (Burt 1973). Ruminants will play a greater role in the future in the production of animal protein in the human diet when compared to other domestic species. This is because most of the land surface of the world does not lend itself to cereal crop production. The capability of ruminants to survive on land of varying topography and vegetation as well as to convert plant materials such as cellulose and other fibrous substances into high quality protein is well recognized.

With greater deficits in the production of cereal crops, animal production will need to become more efficient than it is now. This can occur by improvement of the nutritional requirements and utilization of feed by animals through the benefits derived from chemical additives and use of drugs to prevent and control animal diseases. In addition, advances in genetic selection of animals that are more efficient in the production of meat, milk, and eggs will be required. Continued genetic improvement of milk production is anticipated, with a yield of 50% more milk/lb of feed (Naber 1974). It is also anticipated that the broiler feed conversion factor will be reduced from 2 lb of feed/lb/broiler to 1.7 lb by the year 2000. Egg production is expected to reach 260 eggs/hen/year by the end of this century compared to the present 220 eggs produced annually. Weaning weights of beef animals are anticipated to increase up to 500 or 600 lb compared to the present 400–450 lb. Feed conversion in beef animals is expected to decline to a ratio of 6:1 from the present levels of 8:1 or 9:1 and daily weight gains in the feedlot will probably attain an average of 3.5 lb compared to the present 2.75 lb (Naber 1974).

In the future, improved feed efficiency of livestock and poultry is necessary or more cereal grains may be directed to the diet of human beings. Improved efficiency will decrease the amount of feed to produce meat as well as decrease the time animals spend in the feedlot or poultry batteries prior to slaughter. This will reduce the amount of animal waste per animal and hence alleviate the problem of environmental pollution. For competitive reasons, the stimulus to improve efficiency in the production of animals will be beneficial to the consumer in the reduction of food costs. The future role of drugs and chemicals in this endeavor will be more important than in the past in providing a wholesome and ample food supply.

REFERENCES

Armbrecht, B. H. 1971. Aflatoxin residues in food and feed derived from plant and animal sources. Residue Rev 41:13.

Aronson, A. L. 1975. Potential impact of the use of antimicrobial drugs in farm animals on public health. Presented at the meeting on Pharmacology in the Animal Health Sector, Sept. 23–24, 1975. Colorado State Univ., Fort Collins.

Avrahami, M., and Steele, R. T. 1972a. Hexachlorobenzene. I. Accumulation and elimination in sheep after oral dosing. NZ J Agric Res 15:476.

———. 1972b. Hexachlorobenzene. II. Residues in laying pullets fed HCB in their diet and the effects on egg production, egg hatchability, and on chickens. NZ J Agric Res 15:482.

Barnes, J. M., and Denz, G. A. 1954. Experimental methods used in determining chronic toxicity. Pharmacol Rev 6:191.

Beeson, W. M. 1963. The influence of feed additives on the production of food. J Agric Food Chem 11:374.

Begue, W. J., and Kline, R. M. 1973. Semiquantitative microbiological residue method for hygromycin B in chicken eggs. J Assoc Off Anal Chem.

Bevenue, A., and Kawano, Y. 1971. Pesticides, pesticide residues, tolerances and the law (U.S.A.). Residue Rev 35:103.

Blair, R. 1974. Evaluation of dehydrated poultry waste as a feed ingredient for poultry. Fed Proc 33:1934.

Booth, A. N. 1969. Review of the biological effects of aflatoxins on swine, cattle, and poultry. J Am Oil Chem Soc (Abstr) 46: 154.

Booth, N. H. 1973. Development of a regulatory and research program in veterinary medical toxicology. Vet Toxicol 15:100.

———. 1974. The relationship of research regulatory programs of the Bureau of Veterinary Medicine. Food Drug Cosmet Law J 29:44.

Booth, N. H., and McDowell, J. R. 1975. Toxicity of hexachlorobenzene and associated residues in edible animal tissues. J Am Vet Med Assoc 166:591.

Burt, A. W. A. 1973. Requirements and opportunities for upgrading raw materials for use in animal feeds. J Sci Food Agric 24:493.

Cam, C., and Nigogosyan, G. 1963. Acquired toxic porphyria cutanea tarda due to hexachlorobenzene. J Am Med Assoc 183:88.

Cecil, H. C.; Bitman, J.; Lillie, R. J.; Fries, G. F.; and Verrett, J. 1974. Embryotoxic and teratogenic effects in unhatched fertile eggs from hens fed polychlorinated biphenyls (PCB's). Bull Environ Contam Toxicol 11:489.

Claus, G. 1974. Environmental carcinogens: Is there a threshold of exposure? Clin Toxicol 7:497.

Cole, H. H. 1972. A strong case for DES implants. Calf News 10:52.

Di Cuollo, C. J.; Miller, J. A.; and Miller, C. R. 1973. Tissue residue studies in swine treated with virginiamycin. J Agric Food Chem 21:818.

Dinman, B. D. 1972. "Non-concept" of "no-threshold": Chemicals in the environment. Science 175:495.

Dunckel, A. E. 1975. An updating on the polybrominated biphenyl disaster in Michigan. J Am Vet Med Assoc 167:838.

Eberhart, R. J.; Watrous, G. H.; Hokanson, J. F.; and Burch, G. E. 1963. Persistence of antibacterial agents in milk after intramammary treatment of clinical mastitis. J Am Vet Med Assoc 143:390.

Fahmy, O. G., and Fahmy, M. J. 1964. Mutagenesis in relation to genetic hazards in man. Proc R Soc Med 57:646.

Fechner, G.; Topfer, H.; and Pannwitz, E. 1974. Beitrag zur Ruckstands-analytik und -dynamik von Sulfonamiden in Milch. Arch Exp Veterinaermed 28:261.

Fellig, J., and Westheimer, J. 1968. Determination of sulfadimethoxine in animal tissues. J Agric Food Chem 16:738.

Ferrando, R.; Laurent, M. R.; Terlain, B. L.; and Caude, M. C. 1971. Decoquinate: Estimation of residues in chicken tissues before and after cooking. J Agric Food Chem 19:52.

Filer, W. W.; Hiscock, D. R.; and Parnell, E. W. 1969. Decoquinate. I. An absorption and elimination study in broiler chickens using 14C-labelled decoquinate. J Sci Food Agric 20:65.

Fitzhugh, O. G. 1964. Appraisal of the safety of residues of veterinary drugs and their metabolites in edible animal tissues. Ann NY Acad Sci 111:665.

Fontenot, J. P., and Webb, K. E., Jr. 1974. Poultry wastes as feedstuffs for ruminants. Fed Proc 33:1936.

Food and Drug Administration. 1970. On protocols for safety evaluations: Panel on reproduction studies in the safety evaluation of food additives and pesticide residues. Toxicol Appl Pharmacol 16:264.

———. 1971. Advisory committee on protocols for safety evaluation: Panel on carcinogenesis report on cancer testing in the safety evaluation of food additives and pesticides. Toxicol Appl Pharmacol 20:419.

———. 1973. Title 21, Food and Drugs, Section 135. g. 33. Code of Federal Regulations, p. 305. Washington, D.C.: U.S. Government Printing Office.

Frazer, A. C. 1953. Pharmacological aspects of chemicals in food. Endeavour 12:43.

Friedman, L. 1969. Symposium on the evaluation of the safety of food additives and chemical residues. II. The role of the laboratory animal study of intermediate duration for evaluation of safety. Toxicol Appl Pharmacol 16:498.

Gannon, N.; Link, R. P.; and Decker, G. C. 1959. Storage of dieldrin in tissues of steers, hogs, lambs and poultry fed dieldrin in their diets. J Agric Food Chem 7:826.

Garrod, L. P. 1964. Sources and hazards to man of antibiotics in foods. Proc R Soc Med 57:1087.

Greenwald, P.; Barlow, J. J.; Nasca, P. C.; and Burnett, W. S. 1971. Vaginal cancer after maternal treatment with synthetic estrogens. N Engl J Med 285:390.

Greenwald, P.; Nasca, P. C.; Burnett, W. S.; and Polan, A. 1973. Prenatal stilbestrol experience of mothers of young cancer patients. Cancer 31:568.

Griel, L. C., Jr.; Kradel, D. C.; and Wickersham, E. W. 1969. Abortion in cattle associated with the feeding of poultry litter. Cornell Vet 59:226.

Hammond, A. L. 1972. Chemical pollution: Polychlorinated biphenyls. Science 175:155.

Hansen, L. G.; Byerly, C. S.; Metcalf, R. L.; and Bevill, R. F. 1975. Effect of a polychlorinated biphenyl mixture on swine reproduction and tissue residues. Am J Vet Res 36:23.

Harries, J. M.; Jones, C. M.; and Tatton, J. O'G. 1969. Pesticide residues in the total diet in England and Wales, 1966–67. I. Organisation of a total diet study. J Sci Feed Agric 20:242.

Harvey, G. R.; Miklas, H. P.; Bowen, V. T.; and Steinhauer, W. G. 1974. Observations on the distribution of chlorinated hydrocarbons in Atlantic Ocean organisms. J Marine Res 32:103.

Heinonen, O. P. 1973. Diethylstilbestrol in pregnancy. Cancer 31:573.

Henningson, R. W.; Hurst, V.; Moore, S. L.; and Kelly, J. W. 1963. Effect of intrauterine infusion of penicillin-streptomycin and furacin and vaginal deposition of furacin on chemical residue levels in milk. J Dairy Sci 46:195.

Herbst, A. L.; Ulfelder, H.; and Poskanzer, D. C. 1971. Adenocarcinoma of the vagina. N Engl J Med 284:878.

Hokanson, J. F.; Watrous, G. H.; Burch, G.; and Eberhart, R. J. 1963. Persistence of antibacterial agents in milk after intravenous treatment of acute bovine mastitis. J Am Vet Med Assoc 143:395.

Huber, W. G. 1970. The public health hazards associated with the non-medical and animal health usage of antimicrobial drugs. Pure Appl Chem 21:377.

———. 1971. The impact of antibiotic drugs and their residues. Adv Vet Sc Comp Med 15:101.

Jackson, T. F., and Halbert, F. L. 1974. A toxic syndrome associated with the feeding of polybrominated biphenyl-contaminated protein concentrate to dairy cattle. J Am Vet Med Assoc 165:437.

Kaemmerer, K., and Butenkötter, S. 1973. The problem of residues in meat of edible domestic animals after application or intake of organophosphate esters. Residue Rev 46:1.

Kautz, H. D. 1959. Penicillin and other antibiotics in milk. J Am Med Assoc 171:49.

Kennedy, E. E. 1963. The impact on the analytical chemist of government regulations pertaining to tissue residues. J Agric Food Chem 11:392.

Kerr, E. E. 1972. Residues—Facts or fallacies. Bull Assoc Food Drug Off 36:186.

Kingma, F. J. 1967. Residue problems compounded by big feedlots. J Am Vet Med Assoc 151:741.

———. 1969. Criteria for establishing and monitoring permissible drug residue levels. In Proceedings of a Symposium on the Use of Drugs in Animal Feeds. No. 1679, p. 270. Washington, D. C.: National Academy of Sciences.

Knipling, E. F., and Westlake, W. E. 1966. Insecticide use in livestock production. Residue Rev 13:1.

Krzeminski, L. F.; Cox, B. L.; and Hogg, D. D. 1974. Residue determination of 9α-fluoroprednisolone acetate and its metabolite 9α-fluoroprednisolone in bovine tissues. J Agric Food Chem 22:882.

Lave, L. B. 1972. Risk, safety and the role of government. In Perspectives on Benefit-Risk Decision Making, p. 96. Washington, D.C.: National Academy of Engineering.

Luders, R. C.; Williams, J.; Fried, K.; Rehm, C. R.; and Tishler, F. 1970. Determination of Pyribenzamine (tripelennamine) residues in bovine milk. J Agric Food Chem 18:1153.

Mantel, N., and Bryan, W. R. 1961. "Safety" testing of carcinogenic agents. J Natl Cancer Inst 27:455.

Mercer, H. D. 1975. Antimicrobial drugs in food-producing animals. Vet Clin North Am 5:3.

Mercer, H. D.; Geleta, J. N.; Carter, G. G.; and Kramer, J. 1970a. Dihydrostreptomycin: Tissue residues and certain physicopharmacologic properties in swine. Am J Vet Res 31:1589.

Mercer, H. D.; Geleta, J. N.; Schultz, E. J.; and Wright, W. W. 1970b. Milk-out rates for antibiotics in intrammary infusion products used in the treatment of bovine mastitis: Relationships of somatic cell counts, milk production level and drug vehicle. Am J Vet Res 31:1549.

Mercer, H. D.; Rollins, L. D.; Garth, M. A.; and Carter, G. G. 1971. A residue study and comparison of penicillin and dihydrostreptomycin concentrations after intramuscular and subcutaneous administration in cattle. J Am Vet Med Assoc 158:776.

Messersmith, R. E.; Sass, B.; Berger, H.; and Gale, G. O. 1967. Safety and tissue residue evaluations in swine fed rations containing chlortetracycline, sulfamethazine and penicillin. J Am Vet Med Assoc 151:719.

Morrison, A. B., and Munro, I. C. 1969. Appraisal of the significance to man of drug residues in edible animal tissues. In Proceedings of a Symposium on the Use of Drugs in Animal Feeds. No 1679, p. 255. Washington, D.C.: National Academy of Sciences.

Mosser, J. L.; Fisher, N. S.; Teng, T-C.; and Wurster, C. F. 1972. Polychlorinated biphenyls: Toxicity to certain phytoplankters. Science 175:191.

Naber, E. C. 1974. Food and the year 2000. Poult Meat 25:62.

National Research Council. 1969. Guidelines for estimating toxicologically insignificant levels of chemicals in food. Washington, D.C.: National Academy of Sciences.

Oser, B. L. 1969. Much ado about safety. Food Cosmet Toxicol 7:415.

———. 1971. Contaminants from food processing—hazard or not. Food Cosmet Toxicol 9:245.

Peoples, S. A., and Pier, A. C. 1960. Drug levels in milk. Mod Vet Pract 41:26.

Pichiarallo, J. 1971. PCB's: Leaks of toxic substances raises issue of effects, regulation. Science 173:899.

Purchase, I. F. H. 1972. Aflatoxin residues in food of animal origin. Food Cosmet Toxicol 10:531.

Rasmussen, F. 1958. Mammary excretion of sulphonamides. Acta Pharmacol Toxicol 15:139.

Righter, H. F.; Worthington, J. M.; and Mercer, H. D. 1971a. Tissue residue depletion of sulfamethazine in calves and chickens. Am J Vet Res 32:1003.

———. 1971b. Tissue-residue depletion of sulfathiazole in swine. J Anim Sci 33:797.

———. 1972. Tissue residue depletion of sulfamerazine in sheep. J Agric Food Chem 20:876.

Righter, H. F.; Worthington, J. M.; Zimmerman, H. E., Jr.; and Mercer, H. D. 1970. Tissue-residue depletion of sulfaquinoxaline in poultry. Am J Vet Res 31:1051.

Schmid, R. 1960. Cutaneous porphyria in Turkey. N Engl J Med 263:397.

Seguin, B. E.; Morrow, D. A.; and Oxender, W. D. 1974. Intrauterine therapy in the cow. J Am Vet Med Assoc 164:609.

Shillam, K. W. G. 1974. The use of feed additives in the production of food. J Sci Food Agric 25:227.

Siegel, B. B. 1959. Hidden contacts with penicillin. WHO 21:703.

Sinnhuber, R. O. 1967. Aflatoxin in cottonseed meal and liver cancer in rainbow trout. Trout Hepatoma Res Conf Res Rep 70:48.

Sisodia, C. S., and Stowe, C. M. 1964. The mechanism of drug secretion into bovine milk. Ann NY Acad Sci 111:650.

Smith, H. W. 1974a. Veterinary and food aspects of drug resistance. J Sci Food Agric 25:227.

———. 1974b. Antibiotic-resistant bacteria in animals: The dangers to human health. Br Vet J 130:110.

Smith, R. L. 1971. The role of the gut flora in the conversion of inactive compounds to active metabolites. In W. N. Aldridge, ed. Mechanisms of Toxicity, p. 229. New York: St. Martin.

Stone, L. R. 1973. Fluorometric determination of decoquinate in chicken tissues. J Assoc Off Anal Chem 56:71.

Storrs, B.; Thompson, J.; Fair, G.; Dickerson, M. S.; Nickey, L.; Barthel, W.; and Spaulding, J. E. 1970a. Organic mercury poisoning. Morb Mortal 19:25.

Storrs, B.; Thompson, J.; Nickey, L.; Barthel, W.; and Spaulding, J. C. 1970b. Follow-up organic mercury poisoning. Morb Mortal 19:169.

Sutherland, G. L. 1969. Principles for establishing withdrawal periods for feeds containing drugs. In Proceedings of a Symposium on the Use of Drugs in Animal Feeds. No. 1679, p. 244. Washington, D.C.: National Academy of Sciences.

Taylor, J. C.; Gable, D. A.; Graber, G.; and Lucas, E. W. 1974. Health criteria for processed wastes. Fed Proc 33:1945.

Taylor, K. E. 1965. Toxic residues in meat products. Proc 69th Ann Meet Livest Sanit Assoc, Oct. 25–29, p. 294.

Teske, R. H.; Armbrecht, B. H.; Condon, R. J.; and Paulin, H. J. 1974. Residues of polychlorinated biphenyl in products from poultry fed Aroclor 1254. J Agric Food Chem 22:900.

Tishler, F.; Hagman, G. E.; Birecki, J.; and Bathish, J. N. 1969. Spectrophotofluorometric determinations of metoserpate in biological systems. J Agric Food Chem 17:1403.

Tishler, F.; Sutter, J. L.; Bathish, J. N.; and Hagman, H. E. 1968. Improved method for determination of sulfonamides in milk and tissues. J Agric Food Chem 16:50.

Trabosh, H. M. 1974. Testing and enforcement of food safety standards by meat and poultry inspection personnel. J Am Vet Med Assoc 165:1006.

United States Environmental Protection Agency. 1973. Open public hearing of the Hazardous Materials Advisory Committee chaired by E. Mrak, August 6–7, Washington, D.C.

United States Senate Hearing. 1971. Chemicals and the future of man. 92nd Congr, 1st Ses, April 6, 7.

Van Houweling, C. D. 1971. The Food, Drug and Cosmetic Act, animal drugs, and the consumer. Ann NY Acad Sci 182:411.

Van Rossum, J. M. 1968. Pharmacokinetics of accumulation. J Pharm Sci 57:2162.

Vente, J. Ph.; Wrathall, A. E.; and Hebert, N. 1972. Quantitative anatomical study of methallibure-induced malformations in piglets. Res Vet Sci 13:169.

Webb, K. E., Jr., and Fontenot, J. P. 1975. Medicinal drug residues in broiler litter and tissues from cattle fed litter. J Anim Sci 41:1212.

Weinstein, H. I., and Welch, H. 1959. Sensitivity to the tetracyclines. Antibiotic Annals, p. 643. New York: Medical Encyclopedia.

Weisburger, J. H., and Weisburger, E. K. 1968. Food additives and chemical carcinogens: On the concept of zero tolerance. Food Cosmet Toxicol 6:235.

Wickham, J. C., and Flanagan, P. 1962. Residues of trichlorphon (Neguvon) in milk after dermal application to cattle. J Sci Food Agric 13:449.

Wiskerchen, J. E., and Weishaar, J. 1972. Quantitative determination of chlorbutanol in milk by gas-liquid chromatography. J Assoc Off Anal Chem 55:948.

World Health Organization. 1962. Principles governing consumer safety in relation to pesticide residues. WHO Tech Rep Ser 240.

———. 1963. The public health aspects of the use of antibiotics in food and feedstuffs. WHO Tech Rep Ser 260.

———. 1967. Procedures for investigating intentional and unintentional food additives. WHO Tech Rep Ser 348.

———. 1969a. Principles for the testing and evaluation of drugs for carcinogenicity. WHO Tech Rep Ser 426.

———. 1969b. Specifications for the identity and purity of food additives and their toxicological evaluation: Some antibiotics. WHO Tech Rep Ser 430.

———. 1970. Joint FAO/WHO Expert Committee on Milk Hygiene. Third report. WHO Tech Rep Ser 453.

———. 1971. Evaluation and testing of drugs for mutagenicity: Principles and problems. WHO Tech Rep Ser 482.

———. 1973. Pesticide residues in food. Report of the 1972 joint FAO/WHO meeting. WHO Tech Rep Ser 525.

———. 1974a. Toxicological evaluation of certain food additives with a review of general principles and specifications. WHO Tech Rep Ser 539.

———. 1974b. Assessment of the carcinogenicity and mutagenicity of chemicals. WHO Tech Rep Ser 546.

———. 1974c. The use of mercury and alternative compounds as seed dressings. WHO Tech Rep Ser 555.

Yeary, R. A. 1966. Public health significance of chemical residues in foods. J Am Vet Med Assoc 149:145.

Index